ASE's Comprehensive Echocardiography

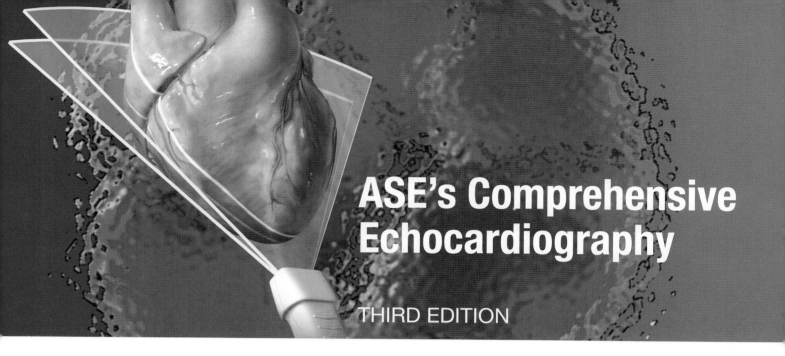

ASE's Comprehensive Echocardiography

THIRD EDITION

ROBERTO M. LANG, MD, FASE, FACC, FESC

Professor of Medicine
Director, Noninvasive Cardiac Imaging Laboratories
Section of Cardiology
University of Chicago Heart and Vascular Center
Chicago, Illinois

STEVEN A. GOLDSTEIN, MD, FASE, FACC

Professor of Medicine
Georgetown University Medical School
MedStar Heart and Vascular Institute
Washington Hospital Center
Washington, DC

ITZHAK KRONZON, MD, FASE, FACC, FAHA, FESC, FACP

Professor of Medicine
Department of Cardiology
Donald and Barbara Zucker School of Medicine at
    Hofstra/Northwell
Northwell Health-Lenox Hill Hospital
New York, New York

BIJOY K. KHANDHERIA, MD, FASE, FACC, FESC, FACP

Director, Echocardiography Center for Research and
    Innovation – Aurora Research Institute
Aurora Cardiovascular and Thoracic Services
Aurora Sinai/Aurora St. Luke's Medical Centers
University of Wisconsin School of Medicine and Public Health
Milwaukee, Wisconsin

MUHAMED SARIC, MD, PhD, FASE, FACC

Professor of Medicine
Director, Non-invasive Cardiology
Leon H Charney Division of Cardiology
New York University Langone Health
New York, New York

VICTOR MOR-AVI, PhD, FASE

Research Professor
Director of Cardiac Imaging Research
Director of Cardiovascular Research Training and Mentorship
Department of Medicine/Section of Cardiology
University of Chicago Medical Center
Chicago, Illinois

ELSEVIER

Elsevier
1600 John F. Kennedy Blvd.
Ste 1800
Philadelphia, PA 19103-2899

ASE's COMPREHENSIVE ECHOCARDIOGRAPHY, THIRD EDITION

ISBN: 9780323698306

Notice

Practitioners and researchers must always rely on their own experience and knowledge in evaluating and using any information, methods, compounds or experiments described herein. Because of rapid advances in the medical sciences, in particular, independent verification of diagnoses and drug dosages should be made. To the fullest extent of the law, no responsibility is assumed by Elsevier, authors, editors or contributors for any injury and/or damage to persons or property as a matter of products liability, negligence or otherwise, or from any use or operation of any methods, products, instructions, or ideas contained in the material herein.

Previous editions copyrighted 2016, 2011.

Library of Congress Control Number: 2020945518

Content Strategist: Robin Carter
Content Development Specialist: Anne Snyder
Content Development Manager: Rebecca Gruliow
Publishing Services Manager: Shereen Jameel
Senior Project Manager: Karthikeyan Murthy
Design Direction: Brian Salisbury

Printed in Canada

Last digit is the print number: 9   8   7   6   5   4   3   2   1

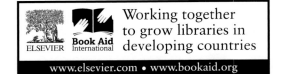

Contributors

Amr E. Abbas, MD, FASE
Professor of Medicine
Director of Cardiovascular Research
Department of Cardiovascular Medicine
Oakland University William Beaumont
  School of Medicine and Beaumont
  Hospital
Royal Oak, Michigan

Karima Addetia, MD, FASE
Assistant Professor of Medicine
Section of Cardiology
University of Chicago Heart and Vascular
  Center
Chicago, Illinois

Jonathan Afilalo, MD, MSc
Associate Professor of Medicine
McGill University
Azrieli Heart Center, Department of
  Medicine
Jewish General Hospital
Montreal, Quebec, Canada

Hanna N. Ahmed, MD, MPH
Assistant Professor
Cardiovascular Medicine
University of Massachusetts Medical
  School
Worcester, Massachusetts

Mohamed Ahmed, MD
Genesis Heart and Vascular Center
Zanesville, Ohio

Ahmadreza Alizadeh, MD
Chief, GI Radiology
Department of Radiology
Lenox Hill Hospital
New York, New York

Talal S. Alnabelsi, MD
Gill Heart and Vascular institute
University of Kentucky
Lexington, Kentucky

Carlos L. Alviar, MD
Assistant Professor of Cardiovascular
  Medicine
Division of Cardiology
University of Florida
Gainesville, Florida

Bonita Anderson, DMU (Cardiac),
M Appl Sc (Med Ultrasound), ACS, FASE
School of Clinical Sciences
Queensland University of Technology
Advanced Cardiac Scientist
Cardiac Sciences Unit
The Prince Charles Hospital
Brisbane, Queensland, Australia

Mohamed-Salah Annabi, MD, MSc
Institut Universitaire de Cardiologie et de
  Pneumologie de Québec
Université Laval
Quebec, Canada

Reza Arsanjani, MD
Cardiovascular Medicine
Mayo Clinic
Scottsdale, Arizona

Federico M. Asch, MD, FACC, FASE
Director, Cardiovascular Core
  Laboratories
MedStar Health Research Institute at
  Washington Hospital Center
Associate Professor of Medicine
Department of Cardiology
Georgetown University
Washington, DC

Gerard P. Aurigemma, MD, FASE
Professor of Medicine and Radiology
Cardiovascular Medicine
University of Massachusetts Medical
  School
UMassMemorial Healthcare
Worcester, Massachusetts

Kelly Axsom, MD
Assistant Professor
Division of Cardiology
Columbia University Irving Medical Center
New York, New York

Luigi P. Badano, MD, PhD, FESC,
FACC, Honorary FASE
Professor
School of Medicine and Surgery
University of Milano-Bicocca
Department of Cardiac, Neural and
  Metabolic Sciences
Istituto Auxologico Italiano, IRCCS
Milan, Italy

Revathi Balakrishnan, MD
Director, Bellevue Cardiology Clinic
Leon H Charney Division of Cardiology
New York University School of Medicine
New York, New York

Daniel Bamira, MD
Clinical Instructor of Medicine
Leon H Charney Division of Cardiology
New York University Langone Health
New York, New York

Manish Bansal, MD, DNB Cardiology,
FACC, FASE
Director, Clinical and Preventive
  Cardiology
Heart Institute
Medanta, The Medicity
Gurgaon, Haryana, India

Jeroen J. Bax, MD, PhD
Professor of Cardiology
Director, Cardiac Imaging Unit
Leiden University Medical Center
Leiden, The Netherlands

Roy Beigel, MD
Director
Department of Cardiology
Sheba Medical Center
Sackler School of Medicine, Tel Aviv
  University
Tel Hashomer, Israel

Eric Berkowitz, MD, FACC
Clinical Affiliate Assistant Professor
Department of Cardiovascular Disease
FAU Charles E. Schmidt College of
  Medicine
Boca Raton Regional Hospital
Boca Raton, Florida

Samuel Bernard, MD
Cardiac Ultrasound Laboratory
Massachusetts General Hospital
Boston, Massachusetts

Philippe B. Bertrand, MD, PhD
Cardiac Ultrasound Laboratory
Massachusetts General Hospital
Boston, Massachusetts

Daniel G. Blanchard, MD, FASE
Professor of Medicine
Department of Cardiology
University of California
San Diego, California

Matthew Bruce, MD
Northwestern University Feinberg School
    of Medicine
Chicago, Illinois

Jonathan Buggey, MD
Harrington Heart & Vascular Institute
University Hospital Cleveland Medical
    Center
Cleveland, Ohio

**Darryl J. Burstow, MBBS, FRACP,
FASE**
Associate Professor
Department of Cardiology
University of Queensland
The Prince Charles Hospital
Brisbane, Queensland, Australia

Benjamin Byrd III, MD, FASE, FACC
Professor
Department of Medicine
Vanderbilt University School of Medicine
Nashville, Tennessee

Ludovica Carerj, MD
Department of Clinical and Experimental
    Medicine
Section of Radiology
Azienda Ospedaliera Universitaria
    "Policlinico G. Martino" and Universita'
    Degli Studi di Messina
Messina, Italy

Scipione Carerj, MD
Professor
Department of Clinical and Experimental
    Medicine
Section of Cardiology
Azienda Ospedaliera Universitaria
    "Policlinico G. Martino" and Universita'
    Degli Studi di Messina
Messina, Italy

John D. Carroll, MD
Professor of Medicine
Division of Cardiology
University of Colorado
Director of Interventional Cardiology,
    University of Colorado Hospital
Aurora, Colorado

Hari P. Chaliki, MD
Associate Professor of Medicine
Mayo Clinic College of Medicine
Division of Cardiovascular Medicine
Mayo Clinic
Scottsdale, Arizona

**Mohammed A. Chamsi-Pasha, MD,
FASE**
Assistant Professor
Cardiovascular Imaging Section
Department of Cardiology
Houston Methodist DeBakey
    Heart & Vascular Center
Houston, Texas

**Jonathan Chan, MBBS(Hons), PhD,
FRACP, FRCP, FCSANZ, FSCCT, FACC**
Professor of Cardiology
Griffith University School of Medicine
Department of Cardiology
The Prince Charles Hospital
Brisbane, Queensland, Australia

Kwan-Leung Chan, MD
Professor of Medicine
Division of Cardiology
University of Ottawa Heart Institute
Ottawa, Ontario, Canada

Michael Chetrit, MD
Cardiovascular Imaging
Cleveland Clinic
Cleveland, Ohio

Alexandra Maria Chitroceanu, MD
University of Liège Hospital
GIGA Cardiovascular Sciences
Department of Cardiology
Liège, Belgium
Carol Davila University of Medicine and
    Pharmacy
Department of Cardiology
University Emergency Hospital
Bucharest, Romania

Geoff Chidsey, MD
Assistant Professor
Department of Cardiology
Vanderbilt University Medical Center
Nashville, Tennessee

Quirino Ciampi, MD, PhD
Director, Echocardiography Laboratory
Division of Cardiology
Fatebenefratelli Hospital
Benevento, Italy

Marie-Annick Clavel, DVM, PhD
Associate Professor of Medicine
Institut Universitaire de Cardiologie et de
    Pneumologie de Québec
Université Laval
Quebec, Canada

Jennifer Conroy, MD
Assistant Professor
Zucker School of Medicine at Hofstra/
    Northwell
Department of Cardiology
Lenox Hill Hospital, Northwell Health
New York, New York

Vivian W. Cui, MD, MSc, RDCS
Research/Education Echocardiographer
Pediatric Cardiology
Advocate Children's Hospital
Heart Institute
Oak Lawn, Illinois

Maurizio Cusmà-Piccione, MD
Department of Clinical and Experimental
    Medicine
Section of Cardiology
Azienda Ospedaliera Universitaria
    "Policlinico G. Martino" and Universita'
    Degli Studi di Messina
Messina, Italy

Daniel A. Daneshvar, MD
Department of Cardiology
Kaiser-Permanente
Woodland Hills, California

Jacqueline S. Danik, MD, DrPH
Clinical Director of Echocardiography
Cardiology Division
Massachusetts General Hospital
Assistant Professor of Medicine
Harvard Medical School
Boston, Massachusetts

Ravin Davidoff, MBBCh, FASE
Chief Medical Officer
Section of Cardiovascular Medicine
Boston Medical Center
Professor of Medicine
Boston University School of Medicine
Boston, Massachusetts

Brian P. Davidson, MD, FASE
Associate Professor
Knight Cardiovascular Institute
Oregon Health & Science University
VA Portland Health Care System
Portland, Oregon

Jeanne M. DeCara, MD
Professor of Medicine
Section of Cardiology
University of Chicago Medicine
Chicago, Illinois

Victoria Delgado, MD, PhD
Associate Professor
Department of Cardiology
Leiden University Medical Center
Leiden, Netherlands

Anthony N. DeMaria, MD, FASE
Professor of Medicine
Department of Cardiology
University of California
San Diego, California

Ankit A. Desai, MD
Assistant Professor of Medicine
Division of Cardiology
Sarver Heart Center
University of Arizona
Tucson, Arizona

Neda Dianati-Maleki, MD, MSc, FACC
Division of Cardiovascular Medicine
Stony Brook University Medical Center
Stony Brook, New York

John B. Dickey, MD, FASE
Assistant Professor of Medicine
Division of Cardiovascular Diseases
University of Massachusetts Medical
School
Worcester, Massachusetts

Bryan Doherty, MD, FACC
Non-Invasive Cardiology
Dickson Medical Associates
Dickson, Tennessee

Robert Donnino, MD
Assistant Professor
Departments of Medicine and Radiology
New York University Langone Medical
Center
Veterans Affairs New York Harbor
Healthcare System
New York, New York

Pamela S. Douglas, MD, FASE
Ursula Geller Professor of Research in
Cardiovascular Disease
Department of Medicine (Cardiology)
Duke University School of Medicine
Durham, North Carolina

Adam M. Dryden, MD, FRCPC
Cardiac Anesthesiologist
Department of Anesthesiology and Pain
Medicine
University of Ottawa Heart Institute
Ottawa, Ontario, Canada

Raluca Elena Dulgheru, MD, PhD
University of Liège Hospital
GIGA Cardiovascular Sciences
Department of Cardiology
University Hospital Sart Tilman
Liège, Belgium

Jean G. Dumesnil, MD, FASE (Hon)
Professor of Medicine
Institut Universitaire de Cardiologie et de
Pneumologie de Québec
Université Laval
Quebec, Canada

**Natalie F.A. Edwards, MCardiac
Ultrasound, BExSci, ACS, AMS, FASE,
FASA**
Senior Cardiac Scientist
Echocardiography Laboratory
The Prince Charles Hospital
Brisbane, Queensland, Australia

Benjamin W. Eidem, MD, FASE
Professor of Pediatrics and Medicine
Divisions of Pediatric Cardiology &
Cardiovascular Disease
Mayo Clinic
Rochester, Minnesota

Nadia El Hangouche, MD
Division of Cardiology
Northwestern University Feinberg School
of Medicine
Chicago, Illinois

Uri Elkayam, MD
Professor of Medicine
Division of Cardiology
University of Southern California
Los Angeles, California

Francine Erenberg, MD
Assistant Professor
Pediatric Cardiology
Cleveland Clinic Lerner College of
Medicine of Case Western Reserve
University
Cleveland, Ohio

Arturo Evangelista, MD, PhD
Cardiac Imaging Department
Vall d´Hebron Research Institute (VHIR)
Hospital Universitari Vall d´Hebron
Barcelona, Spain

Nadeen N. Faza, MD
Assistant Professor
Cardiovascular Imaging Section
Department of Cardiology
Houston Methodist DeBakey Heart and
Vascular Center
Houston, Texas

Afsoon Fazlinezhad, MD, RDCS, FASE
Echocardiography Laboratory
Department of Cardiovascular Diseases
Mayo Clinic
Scottsdale, Arizona

Beatriz Ferreira, MD, PhD
Director
Maputo Heart Institute
Maputo, Mozambique

Nowell M. Fine, MD, SM, FASE
Libin Cardiovascular Institute
Assistant Professor
Cardiac Sciences
University of Calgary
Calgary, Alberta, Canada

Laura Flink, MD
Cardiologist
The Permanente Medical Group
San Leandro Medical Center
San Leandro, California

Nir Flint, MD
Cardiology Division
Tel Aviv Sourasky Medical Center
Sackler School of Medicine, Tel Aviv
University
Tel Aviv, Israel

**Christopher B. Fordyce, MD, MHS,
MSc**
Clinical Assistant Professor
Division of Cardiology
University of British Columbia
Vancouver, British Columbia, Canada

Benjamin H. Freed, MD, FASE, FACC
Associate Professor of Medicine
Division of Cardiology
Northwestern University Feinberg School
of Medicine
Chicago, Illinois

Christos Galatas, MD, CM
Division of Cardiology
Hôpital Cité-de-la-Santé
Laval, Quebec, Canada

Julius M. Gardin, MD, MBA, FASE
Professor of Medicine
Division of Cardiology
Rutgers New Jersey Medical School
Newark, New Jersey

Edward A. Gill, MD, FASE
Professor of Medicine
University of Colorado School of
Medicine, Division of Cardiology
Aurora, Colorado

Kudrat Gill, MD
Department of Radiology
Lenox Hill Hospital
New York, New York

Linda D. Gillam, MD, MPH, FASE
Dorothy and Lloyd Huck Chair of
Cardiovascular Medicine
Morristown Medical Center/Atlantic
Health System
Morristown, New Jersey
Professor of Medicine
Thomas Jefferson University
Philadelphia, Pennsylvania

Steven Giovannone, MD
Cardiology Associates
Schenectady, New York

Mina Girgis, MD, FRCPC
Division of Cardiology
Toronto General Hospital, University
Health Network
University of Toronto
Toronto, Ontario, Canada

Mark Goldberger, MD
Assistant Clinical Professor of Medicine
Division of Cardiology
Columbia University Medical Center
New York, New York

Steven A. Goldstein, MD, FASE, FACC
Professor of Medicine
Georgetown University Medical School
MedStar Heart and Vascular Institute
Washington Hospital Center
Washington, DC

Fei Fei Gong, MBBS, BMedSc
Division of Cardiology
Northwestern University Feinberg School
    of Medicine
Chicago, Illinois

John Gorcsan III, MD, FASE
Professor of Medicine
Director of Clinical Research
Division of Cardiology
Washington University in St. Louis
St. Louis, Missouri

Julia Grapsa, MD, PhD, FASE
Cardiology Department
Guys and St Thomas
Barts Health Trust
London, United Kingdom

Erin S. Grawe, MD
Assistant Professor of Anesthesia
University of Cincinnati
Cincinnati, Ohio

Pooja Gupta, MD, FASE
Associate Professor
Pediatric Cardiology
Central Michigan University
Children's Hospital of Michigan
Detroit, Michigan

Vedant A. Gupta, MD
Assistant Professor
Internal Medicine–Cardiology
Gill Heart and Vascular Institute
University of Kentucky
Lexington, Kentucky

Swaminatha V. Gurudevan, MD, MS
Invasive Cardiology
Arch Health Medical Group
Escondido, California

Ezequiel Guzzetti, MD
Institut Universitaire de Cardiologie et de
    Pneumologie de Québec
Cardiology
Université Laval
Quebec, Canada

Rebecca T. Hahn, MD, FASE
Professor of Medicine
Division of Cardiology
Columbia University Irving Medical
    Center
The New York Presbyterian Hospital
New York, New York

Jennifer Hellawell, MD
Medical Director
Early Development, Cardiometabolic
    Division
Amgen
Thousand Oaks, California

Brian D. Hoit, MD, FASE
Professor of Medicine, Physiology and
    Biophysics
Case Western Reserve University
Director of Echocardiography
University Hospital Cleveland Medical
    Center
Cleveland, Ohio

Sara Hoss, MD
Division of Cardiology
Toronto General Hospital
University of Toronto
Toronto, Ontario, Canada

Grace Hsieh, MD
Section of Cardiovascular Medicine
Boston Medical Center
Boston, Massachusetts

Richard Humes, MD
Professor
Pediatric Cardiology
Central Michigan University
Children's Hospital of Michigan
Detroit, Michigan

Judy Hung, MD, FASE
Director of Echocardiography
Cardiology Division
Massachusetts General Hospital
Professor of Medicine
Harvard Medical School
Boston, Massachusetts

Sabrina Islam, MD, MPH, FASE
Assistant Professor of Medicine
Temple Heart and Vascular Institute
Lewis Katz School of Medicine
Temple University
Philadelphia, Pennsylvania

Eric M. Isselbacher, MD
Co-director
Thoracic Aortic Center
Massachusetts General Hospital
Associate Professor of Medicine
Harvard Medical School
Boston, Massachusetts

Kamari C. Jackson, MD
Northwestern University Feinberg School
    of Medicine
Chicago, Illinois

Renuka Jain, MD, FACC, FASE
Clinical Adjunct Associate Professor of
    Medicine
University of Wisconsin
Aurora St. Luke's Medical Center
Milwaukee, Wisconsin

Bernard Kadosh, MD
Leon H. Charney Division of Cardiology
New York University School of Medicine
New York, New York

Peter A. Kahn, MD, MPH, ThM
Department of Internal Medicine
Yale University School of Medicine
New Haven, Connecticut

Minako Katayama, MD
Assistant Professor of Medicine
Mayo Clinic College of Medicine
Mayo Clinic
Scottsdale, Arizona

Martin G. Keane, MD, FASE
Professor of Medicine
Temple Heart and Vascular Institute
Lewis Katz School of Medicine
Temple University
Philadelphia, Pennsylvania

Benjamin B. Kenigsberg, MD
Departments of Cardiology and Critical
    Care
MedStar Washington Hospital Center
Washington, DC

**Bijoy K. Khandheria, MD, FASE,
FACC, FESC, FACP**
Director, Echocardiography Center for
    Research and Innovation
Aurora Sinai/Aurora St. Luke's Medical
    Centers
University of Wisconsin School of
    Medicine and Public Health
Milwaukee, Wisconsin

Benjamin Khazan, MD
Temple Heart and Vascular Institute
Lewis Katz School of Medicine
Temple University
Philadelphia, Pennsylvania

Bruce J. Kimura, MD
Medical Director
Scripps Mercy Cardiovascular
    Ultrasound
Department of Cardiology
University of California
San Diego, California

James N. Kirkpatrick, MD, FASE
Professor of Medicine
Section of Cardiology
University of Washington Medical Center
Seattle, Washington

Allan L. Klein, MD, FRCP(C), FACC, FAHA, FASE, FESC
Professor of Medicine
Cleveland Clinic Lerner College of
 Medicine of Case Western Reserve
 University
Department of Cardiovascular Medicine
Heart, Vascular and Thoracic Institute
Cleveland Clinic
Cleveland, Ohio

Arber Kodra, MD
Department of Cardiology
Northwell Health–Lenox Hill Hospital
New York, New York

Payal Kohli, MD
Cardiologist
Cherry Creek Heart
Denver, Colorado

Smadar Kort, MD, FACC, FASE, FAHA
Director, Noninvasive Cardiovascular
 Imaging
Professor of Medicine
Division of Cardiovascular Disease
Stony Brook University Medical Center
Stony Brook, New York

Wojciech Kosmala, MD, PhD
Professor
Department of Cardiology
Wroclaw Medical University
Wroclaw, Poland

Frederick W. Kremkau, PhD
Professor of Radiologic Sciences
Center for Experiential and Applied
 Learning
Wake Forest University School of
 Medicine
Winston Salem, North Carolina

Eric V. Krieger, MD
Associate Professor
Departments of Medicine and
 Cardiology
University of Washington
Seattle, Washington

Itzhak Kronzon, MD, FASE, FACC, FAHA, FESC, FACP
Professor of Medicine
Department of Cardiology
Donald and Barbara Zucker School of
 Medicine at Hofstra/Northwell
Northwell Health–Lenox Hill Hospital
New York, New York

Preetham Kumar, MD
Department of Cardiology
MedStar Washington Hospital Center
Washington, DC

Agatha Kwon, BSc (Hons), GradDipCardiacUltrasound
Senior Clinical Measurement Scientist
Cardiac Investigations Unit
Royal Brisbane Women's Hospital
Brisbane, Queensland, Australia

Wyman W. Lai, MD, MPH, MBA
Clinical Professor
Department of Pediatrics
UCI School of Medicine
Irvine, California
Director of Echocardiography
CHOC Children's
Orange, California

A. Stephane Lambert, MD, MBA, FRCPC
Professor of Anesthesiology
Department of Anesthesiology and Pain
 Medicine
University of Ottawa Heart Institute
Ottawa, Ontario, Canada

Patrizio Lancellotti, MD, PhD, FESC, FACC
Professor
University of Liège Hospital
GIGA Cardiovascular Sciences
Department of Cardiology
University Hospital Sart Tilman
Liège, Belgium

Roberto M. Lang, MD, FASE, FACC, FESC
Professor of Medicine
Director, Noninvasive Cardiac Imaging
 Laboratories
University of Chicago Heart and Vascular
 Center
Chicago, Illinois

Katherine Lau, MBBS, FRACP
Lecturer, School of Clinical Medicine
Staff Specialist, Department of
 Echocardiography
The Prince Charles Hospital
The University of Queensland
Brisbane, Queensland, Australia

Florent Le Ven, MD, PhD
Hopital de La Cavale Blanche
Cardiology
University Hospital
Brest, France

Hanna Lee, MD, FRCPC
Division of Cardiology
Peter Munk Cardiac Centre
Toronto General Hospital, University
 Health Network
University of Toronto
Toronto, Ontario, Canada

Kyle R. Lehenbauer, MD
Saint Luke's Mid America Heart Institute
Kansas City, Missouri

Steven J. Lester, MD, FASE
Cardiovascular Medicine
Mayo Clinic
Scottsdale, Arizona

Steve W. Leung, MD, FASE
Associate Professor
Departments of Cardiovascular Medicine
 and Radiology
Gill Heart and Vascular Institute
University of Kentucky
Lexington, Kentucky

Aaron C.W. Lin, MBChB, FRACP
Department of Cardiology
The Prince Charles Hospital
Brisbane, Queensland, Australia

Jonathan R. Lindner, MD, FASE
M. Lowell Edwards Professor of
 Cardiology
Knight Cardiovascular Institute
Oregon National Primate Research
 Center
Oregon Health and Science University
Portland, Oregon

Stephen H. Little, MD, FASE
Associate Professor
Cardiovascular Imaging Section
Department of Cardiology
Houston Methodist DeBakey
 Heart & Vascular Center
Houston, Texas

Shiying Liu, MD
Cardiac Ultrasound Laboratory
Massachusetts General Hospital
Boston, Massachusetts

Luca Longobardo, MD
Department of Clinical and Experimental
 Medicine
Section of Cardiology
Azienda Ospedaliera Universitaria
 "Policlinico G. Martino" and Universita'
 Degli Studi di Messina
Messina, Italy

Leo Lopez, MD, FASE
Clinical Professor of Pediatrics
Stanford University
Medical Director of Echocardiography
Lucile Packard Children's Hospital
Palo Alto, California

Ángela López Sainz, MD, PhD
Cardiac Imaging Department
Hospital Universitario Vall Hebrón
Barcelona, Spain
Vall Hebron Research Institut
Universitat Autónoma de Barcelona
CiBERCV
Spain

Sushil Allen Luis, MBBS, FRACP, FACC, FASE
Associate Professor of Medicine
Department of Cardiovascular Medicine
Mayo Clinic
Rochester, Minnesota

Michael L. Main, MD, FASE
Co-Executive Medical Director
Saint Luke's Mid America Heart
    Institute
Kansas City, Missouri

Judy R. Mangion, MD, FASE
Associate Director of Echocardiography
Division of Cardiovascular Medicine
Brigham and Women's Hospital
Boston, Massachusetts

Sunil V. Mankad, MD, FACC, FASE
Professor of Medicine
Department of Cardiovascular Medicine
Mayo Clinic
Rochester, Minnesota

Dimitrios Maragiannis, MD, FESC, FASE, FACC, FAHA
Department of Cardiology
General Military Hospital of Athens
Athens, Greece

Rachel Marcus, MD, FASE
Medstar Union Memorial Hospital
Baltimore, Maryland

Thomas H. Marwick, MD, PhD, MPH
Professor
Director, Baker Heart and Diabetes
    Institute
Melbourne, Victoria, Australia

S. Carolina Masri, MD
Assistant Professor
Section of Cardiology
University of Wisconsin
Madison, Wisconsin

Priti Mehla, MD
Assistant Professor
Zucker School of Medicine at Hofstra/
    Northwell
Department of Cardiology
Lenox Hill Hospital, Northwell Health
New York, New York

Sudhir Ken Mehta, MD, MBA
Clinical Associate Professor of Pediatrics
Cleveland Clinic Lerner College of
    Medicine of Case Western Reserve
    University
Cleveland, Ohio

Todd Mendelson, MD, MBE
Assistant Professor of Clinical Medicine
University of Pennsylvania
Philadelphia, Pennsylvania

Hassan Mir, MD, FRCPC
Division of Cardiology
Peter Munk Cardiac Centre
Toronto General Hospital, University
    Health Network
University of Toronto
Toronto, Ontario, Canada

Carol Mitchell, PhD, ACS, RDMS, RDCS, RVT, RT(R), FASE
Associate Professor
University of Wisconsin School of
    Medicine and Public Health
Madison, Wisconsin

Farouk Mookadam, MD
Department of Cardiovascular Medicine
Mayo Clinic
Scottsdale, Arizona

Tyler B. Moran, MD, PhD
Assistant Professor
Section of Cardiology, Department of
    Medicine
Baylor College of Medicine
Houston, Texas

Michael Morcos, MD
Department of Cardiology
University of Washington Medical Center
Seattle, Washington

Denisa Muraru, MD, PhD, FESC, FACC, FASE
Department of Medicine and Surgery
University of Milano-Bicocca
Department of Cardiovascular, Neural and
    Metabolic Sciences
Istituto Auxologico Italiano, IRCCS
Milan, Italy

Sherif F. Nagueh, MD, FACC, FAHA, FASE
Professor of Medicine
Division of Cardiology
Weill Cornell Medical College
Medical Director of Echocardiography
    Laboratory
Methodist DeBakey Heart and Vascular
    Center
Houston, Texas

Mayooran Namasivayam, MBBS, PhD
Division of Cardiology
Massachusetts General Hospital, Harvard
    Medical School
Boston, Massachusetts

Tasneem Z. Naqvi, MD, FRCP(UK), MMM, FASE
Professor of Medicine, Consultant
Department of Cardiovascular Diseases
Mayo Clinic
Scottsdale, Arizona

Akhil Narang, MD, FASE
Assistant Professor of Medicine
Division of Cardiology
Northwestern University
Chicago, Illinois

Kazuaki Negishi, MD, PhD, FASE
Professor of Medicine
Nepean Clinical School
University of Sydney
Kingswood, New South Wales, Australia

Talha Niaz, MBBS
Assistant Professor
Division of Pediatric Cardiology
Mayo Clinic
Rochester, Minnesota

Arvind Nishtala, MD
Division of Cardiology
Northwestern University
Chicago, Illinois

Vuyisile T. Nkomo, MD, MPH, FASE
Associate Professor of Medicine
Mayo Clinic College of Medicine
Division of Cardiovascular Medicine
Mayo Clinic
Rochester, Minnesota

Thomas F. O'Connell, MD
Department of Cardiovascular Medicine
Beaumont Hospital
Royal Oak, Michigan

Erwin Oechslin, MD
The Bitove Family Professor of Adult
    Congenital Heart Disease
Professor of Medicine
University of Toronto
Peter Munk Cardiac Centre, University
    Health Network
Toronto, Ontario, Canada

Joan Olson, RDCS, RVT, FASE
Echocardiography Laboratory
University of Nebraska
Omaha, Nebraska

Julio A. Panza, MD, FACC, FAHA
Chief of Cardiology
Westchester Medical Center
Professor of Medicine
New York Medical College
Valhalla, New York

Alexander I. Papolos, MD
Assistant Professor of Medicine
Department of Cardiology
MedStar Washington Hospital Center
Washington, DC

Roosha K. Parikh, MD
Houston Methodist DeBakey Heart &
    Vascular Center
Houston Methodist Hospital
Houston, Texas

Matthew W. Parker, MD, FASE
Director of Echocardiography
UMassMemorial Healthcare
Associate Professor of Medicine
Division of Cardiovascular Medicine
University of Massachusetts Medical
    School
Worcester, Massachusetts

Amit R. Patel, MD
Associate Professor
Medicine and Radiology
University of Chicago
Chicago, Illinois

Aneet Patel, MD
Cardiology Department
Kaiser Permanente
Seattle, Washington

Hena N. Patel, MD
Section of Cardiology
University of Chicago
Chicago, Illinois

Yash Patel, MD, MPH
Department of Cardiovascular Medicine
Morristown Medical Center/Atlantic
    Health System
Morristown, New Jersey

Gila Perk, MD, FASE
Associate Professor of Medicine
Director, Interventional Echocardiography
Icahn School of Medicine at Mount Sinai
New York, New York

Andrew C. Peters, MD
Division of Cardiology
Northwestern University Feinberg School
    of Medicine
Chicago, Illinois

**Ferande Peters, MBBCH, FCP, FESC,
FACC, FRCP(London)**
Associate Professor
Cardiovascular Pathophysiology and
    Genomic Unit
University of the Witwatersrand Medical
    School
Johannesburg, South Africa

Duc Thinh Pham, MD
Associate Professor of Surgery
Division of Cardiac Surgery
Northwestern University Feinberg School
    of Medicine
Chicago, Illinois

**Philippe Pibarot, DVM, PhD, FACC,
FAHA, FASE**
Professor of Medicine
Institut Universitaire de Cardiologie et de
    Pneumologie de Québec
Université Laval
Quebec, Canada

Eugenio Picano, MD, PhD
Professor
Biomedicine Department
Institute Clinical Physiology
National Council Research
Pisa, Italy

**Michael H. Picard, MD, FASE, FACC,
FAHA**
Professor of Medicine
Harvard Medical School
Massachusetts General Hospital
Boston, Massachusetts

Juan Carlos Plana, MD, FASE
Don W. Chapman, M.D. Endowed Chair of
    Cardiology
Section of Cardiology
Department of Medicine
Baylor College of Medicine
Houston, Texas

Zoran B. Popović, MD, PhD
Department of Cardiovascular Medicine
Heart and Vascular Institute
Cleveland Clinic
Cleveland, Ohio

Thomas R. Porter, MD, FASE
Professor of Medicine
Division of Cardiovascular Medicine
University of Nebraska
Omaha, Nebraska

Adriana Postolache, MD
University of Liège Hospital
GIGA Cardiovascular Sciences
Department of Cardiology
University Hospital Sart Tilman
Liège, Belgium

Shawn C. Pun, MD, FRCPC
Division of Cardiology
Royal Inland Hospital
Kamloops, British Columbia, Canada

Robert A. Quaife, MD
Professor of Medicine
Division of Cardiology
University of Colorado, Anshutz Medical
    Campus
Director of Advanced Cardiac Imaging,
    University of Colorado Hospital
Aurora, Colorado

Peter S. Rahko, MD, FACC, FASE
Professor of Medicine
University of Wisconsin School of
    Medicine and Public Health
Director, Adult Echocardiography
    Laboratory
University of Wisconsin Hospital
Madison, Wisconsin

**Harry Rakowski, MD, FRCPC, FACC,
FASE**
Professor of Medicine
University of Toronto
Douglas Wigle Chair in HCM Research
Division of Cardiology
Peter Munk Cardiac Centre
Toronto General Hospital
Toronto, Ontario, Canada

**Jay Ramchand, MBBS BMedSci
FRACP**
Cardiovascular Imaging, Heart and
    Vascular Institute
Cleveland Clinic
Cleveland, Ohio

Kate Rankin, MBBS (Hons.), FRACP
University Hospital Geelong
Geelong, Victoria, Australia
Peter Munk Cardiac Centre
Toronto General Hospital, University
    Health Network
Toronto, Ontario, Canada

Rajeev V. Rao, MD, FRCPC, FACC
Medical Director of Echocardiography
    Laboratory
Division of Cardiology
Royal Victoria Regional Health Centre
Barrie, Ontario, Canada

Nina Rashedi, MD, FASE
Cardiovascular Imaging
University of Chicago
Chicago, Illinois

Corey Rearick, MD
Department of Medicine
University of Chicago
Chicago, Illinois

Vera H. Rigolin, MD, FASE
Professor of Medicine
Northwestern University Feinberg School
   of Medicine
Medical Director
Echocardiography Laboratory
Northwestern Memorial Hospital
Chicago, Illinois

David A. Roberson, MD, FASE
Director of Echocardiography
Advocate Children's Heart Institute
Hope Children's Hospital
Chicago, Illinois

**José F. Rodríguez Palomares, MD,
PhD**
Director
Cardiac Imaging Department
Hospital Universitari Vall d´Hebron
   CIBER-CV
Barcelona, Spain

Sarah M. Roemer, RDCS, FASE
Echocardiography Laboratory
Advocate Aurora Health
Milwaukee, Wisconsin

Eleanor Ross, MD
Pediatric Cardiology
Advocate Children's Hospital
Heart Institute for Children
Oak Lawn, Illinois

Frederick L. Ruberg, MD
Associate Chief, Cardiovascular Medicine
Associate Professor of Medicine
Boston Medical Center
Boston University School of Medicine
Boston, Massachusetts

**Lawrence G. Rudski, MD, FRCPC,
FASE, FACC**
Professor of Medicine
McGill University
Director, Azrieli Heart Center
Department of Medicine
Jewish General Hospital
Montreal, Quebec, Canada

Carlos E. Ruiz, MD, PhD
Professor of Cardiology in Pediatrics and
   Medicine
Hackensack Meridian Health–Seton Hall
   University
Hackensack, New Jersey

Erwan Salaun, MD, PhD
Institut de Cardiologie et Pneumologie de
   Québec
Quebec Heart and Lung Institute
Quebec, Canada

Ernesto E. Salcedo, MD, FASE
Professor of Medicine
Division of Cardiology
University of Colorado
Director of Echocardiography, University
   of Colorado Hospital
Aurora, Colorado

**Danita M. Yoerger Sanborn, MD,
MMSc, FASE**
Echocardiography Laboratory, Cardiology
   Division
Massachusetts General Hospital
Assistant Professor of Medicine
Harvard Medical School
Boston, Massachusetts

Yamuna Sanil, MD, FASE
Associate Professor
Pediatric Cardiology
Central Michigan University
Children's Hospital of Michigan
Detroit, Michigan

**Muhamed Saric, MD, PhD, FASE,
FACC**
Professor of Medicine
Director, Non-invasive Cardiology
Division of Cardiology
New York University Langone Health
New York, New York

**Gregory M. Scalia, MBBS, MMedSc,
FRACP, FCSANZ, FACC, FASE**
Professor of Cardiology
University of Queensland
Brisbane, Australia
Director of Echocardiography
The Prince Charles Hospital
Brisbane, Queensland, Australia

Nelson B. Schiller, MD
Professor
Division of Cardiology
San Francisco Veterans Affairs Medical
   Center
Cardiovascular Research Institute
University of San Francisco
San Francisco, California

**Partho P. Sengupta, MD, DM, FACC,
FASE**
Professor of Cardiology
Chief of Cardiology
West Virginia University Heart and
   Vascular Institute
Morgantown, West Virginia

Atman P. Shah, MD
Associate Professor of Medicine
Clinical Director, Section of Cardiology
The University of Chicago
Chicago, Illinois

Jack S. Shanewise, MD, FASE
Professor of Anesthesiology
Columbia University Vagelos College of
   Physicians & Surgeons
New York, New York

Miriam Shanks, MD, PhD
Associate Professor
Mazankowski Alberta Heart Institute
University of Alberta
Edmonton, Alberta, Canada

Stanton K. Shernan, MD, FAHA, FASE
Professor of Anaesthesia
Department of Anesthesiology,
   Perioperative and Pain Medicine
Brigham & Women's Hospital
Harvard Medical School
Boston, Massachusetts

Rosa Sicari, MD, PhD
Research Director
Institute of Clinical Physiology, National
   Council of Research
Pisa, Italy

Omar K. Siddiqi, MD
Assistant Professor
Boston Medical Center
Boston University School of Medicine
Boston, Massachusetts

Robert J. Siegel, MD, FASE
Director Cardiac Non-Invasive Laboratory
Smidt Heart Institute
Cedars-Sinai Medical Center
Los Angeles, California

Amita Singh, MD
Assistant Professor of Medicine
Section of Cardiology
University of Chicago Hospitals
Chicago, Illinois

Gregory J. Sinner, MD, MPT
Division of Cardiovascular Medicine
Gill Heart and Vascular Institute
University of Kentucky
Lexington, Kentucky

Samuel Siu, MD, SM, MBA, FASE
Professor of Medicine
Western University
London, Ontario, Canada

Vincent L. Sorrell, MD, FASE
The Anthony N. DeMaria Professor of
   Medicine
Gill Heart and Vascular Institute
University of Kentucky
Lexington, Kentucky

Simona Sperlongano, MD
University of Liège Hospital
Department of Cardiology
University Hospital Sart Tilman
Liège, Belgium
University of Campania "Luigi Vanvitelli"
Department of Translational Medical
    Sciences
Monaldi Hospital
Naples, Italy

Raymond F. Stainback, MD, FASE
Chief, Noninvasive Cardiology
Department of Cardiology
Baylor St Luke's Medical Center Hospital
Texas Heart Institute
Associate Professor of Medicine
Baylor College of Medicine
Houston, Texas

Masaaki Takeuchi, MD, PhD
Professor
Department of Laboratory and Transfusion
    Medicine
University of Occupational and
    Environmental Health Hospital
Kitakyushu, Japan

Balaji K. Tamarappoo, MD, PhD
Smidt Heart Institute
Cedars Sinai Medical Center
Los Angeles, California

Astha Tejpal, MD
Department of Cardiology
Lenox Hill Hospital
New York, New York

**Paaladinesh Thavendiranathan, MD,
MSc, FRCPC, FASE**
Associate Professor of Medicine
Peter Munk Cardiac Centre
Toronto General Hospital
University of Toronto
Toronto, Ontario, Canada

James D. Thomas, MD, FASE
Division of Cardiology
Feinberg School of Medicine
Northwestern University
Chicago Illinois

Biana Trost, MD
Assistant Professor of Cardiology
Director of Echocardiography
Zucker School of Medicine at Hofstra/
    Northwell
Lenox Hill Hospital, Northwell Health
New York, New York

Michael Y.C. Tsang, MD
Clinical Assistant Professor
Division of Cardiology
University of British Columbia
Vancouver, Canada

Wendy Tsang, MD, SM
Assistant Professor of Medicine,
    University of Toronto
Division of Cardiology
Toronto General Hospital, University
    Health Network
Toronto, Ontario, Canada

Matt M. Umland, ACS, RDCS, FASE
Echocardiography Quality Director
Advocate Aurora Health
Milwaukee, Wisconsin

Alan F. Vainrib, MD
Assistant Professor
Leon H Charney Division of Cardiology
New York University Langone Health
New York, New York

Joseph M. Venturini, MD
Attending Cardiologist
Advocate Heart Institute
Downers Grove, Illinois

Philippe Vignon, MD, PhD
Medical-Surgical Intensive Care Unit
Limoges Teaching Hospital
Faculty of Medicine
University of Limoges
Limoges, France

Rachel Wald, MD, FRCPC
Associate Professor
University of Toronto
Peter Munk Cardiac Centre, University
    Health Network
Toronto, Ontario, Canada

**Nozomi Watanabe, MD, PhD, FJCC,
FACC**
Director, Department of Clinical
    Laboratory
Chief, Noninvasive Cardiovascular
    Imaging
Miyazaki Medical Association Hospital
    Cardiovascular Center
Miyazaki, Japan

Kevin Wei, MD, FASE
Professor of Medicine
Knight Cardiovascular Institute
Oregon Health and Science University
Portland, Oregon

Neil J. Weissman, MD, FASE
Chief Scientific Officer
MedStar Health Research Institute
Georgetown University
Washington, DC

Mariko Welch, MD
Virginia Mason Medical Center
Seattle, Washington

Brent White, MD
Division of Cardiology
Northwestern University Feinberg School
    of Medicine
Chicago, Illinois

Lynne Williams, MBBCh, MRCP, PhD
Department of Cardiology
Royal Papworth Hospital NHS Foundation
    Trust
Cambridge, United Kingdom

Anna Woo, MD, SM, FRCPC, FACC
Director, Echocardiography
Peter Munk Cardiac Centre
Toronto General Hospital, University
    Health Network
University of Toronto
Toronto, Ontario, Canada

Feng Xie, MD
Professor of Medicine
Division of Cardiovascular Medicine
University of Nebraska
Omaha, Nebraska

Concetta Zito, MD, PhD
Department of Clinical and Experimental
    Medicine
Section of Cardiology
Azienda Ospedaliera Universitaria
    "Policlinico G. Martino" and Universita'
    Degli Studi di Messina
Messina, Italy

William A. Zoghbi, MD, FASE
Professor and Chair
Department of Cardiology
Houston Methodist DeBakey Heart &
    Vascular Center
Houston, Texas

Preface

For more than a half a century, Doppler echocardiography has made unparalleled contributions to clinical cardiology as a tool for real-time imaging of cardiac anatomy and physiology. Echocardiography is currently used daily in hospitals and clinics around the world for assessing cardiac structure and function while simultaneously providing invaluable noninvasive information required for the diagnosis and prognosis of multiple disease states. The American Society of Echocardiography (ASE) is an organization of more than 17,000 professionals committed to advancing cardiovascular ultrasonography and improving lives through excellence in education, research, innovation, advocacy, and service to the profession and the public. ASE's goal is to be the primary resource for education, knowledge exchange, and professional development in echocardiography. The previous editions of this book, *ASE's Comprehensive Echocardiography*, constituted a major step toward the achievement of this goal while at the same time becoming a highly popular educational and clinical resource for echocardiographers worldwide.

This new edition of the book is the result of a large-scale collaborative effort of more than 100 ASE members, who have contributed chapters on their topics of expertise. In contrast to previously published textbooks on echocardiography, this book covers a full range of topics in a succinct format that is well illustrated by multiple figures, tables, and an extensive collection of online videos.

Since the preparation of the second edition of this textbook and its publication in 2016, ASE has developed and updated professional guidelines pertaining to multiple aspects of echocardiographic practice. These guidelines were mostly driven by the need to incorporate novel quantitative techniques in our practice, as well as the incorporation of myocardial strain and three-dimensional imaging technology that not only has "pushed the envelope of echocardiography" but, in fact, significantly expanded this modality into new, previously uncharted territories.

The publication of many of these guidelines, as well as the expansion of clinical knowledge in many areas, were the principal motivations for the need to revise *ASE's Comprehensive Echocardiography* and thus provide up-to-date information that includes the most recent developments. Accordingly, the material in this book, including text, figures, and references, has been extensively revised to achieve this goal.

As with the previous editions, we encourage the readers to also review the accompanying online video clips of cardiac diseases, which provide additional insights to the hundreds of images included in the print version. We believe that this combined approach is the most effective way of learning clinical echocardiography. Our hope is that physicians and cardiac sonographers will continue to use this new text and the companion material as a reference and educational aide for echocardiography laboratories around the world.

The ASE and the editors thank the authors for selflessly contributing their time, effort, and expertise for the completion and success of this project. We also wish to thank the sonographers, who with their expert hands have generated and provided us with the spectacular images that illustrate this text, without which this educational endeavor would not have been possible. Importantly, we wish to thank those who contributed to the previous editions of the book but could not participate in this most recent update. The editors also want to thank our ASE colleagues, who have tirelessly worked with us on this project from conception to fruition, including Robin Wiegerink, Alyssa Lawrentz, and Christina LaFuria, as well as the expert help from the Elsevier staff.

Roberto M. Lang, MD, FASE

Steven A. Goldstein, MD, FASE

Itzhak Kronzon, MD, FASE

Bijoy K. Khandheria, MD, FASE

Muhamed Saric, MD, FASE

Victor Mor-Avi, PhD, FASE

Acknowledgments

We wish to thank our families for their continuous support while we worked on this project: our spouses Lili, Simoy, Ziva, Priti, Amy, and Andy; our children Daniella, Gabriel, Lindsey, Lauren, Derek, Iris, Rafi, Shira, Vishal, Trishala, Malik, Elias, Eden, and Yarden; and our grandchildren Ella, Adam, Lucy, Eli, Jacob, and Levi. Dr. Kronzon also thanks Dr. Arbor Kodra for his valuable help with editing and proofreading.

Contents

Video Contents

The following chapters include videos of case presentations online that correspond to select images in the chapters:

1 General Principles of Echocardiography

Frederick W. Kremkau

Echocardiography is diagnostic imaging with ultrasound (sonography) of the heart. *Sonography* comes from the Latin *sonus* (sound) and the Greek *graphein* (to write). Diagnostic sonography is medical, real-time, two-dimensional (2D) and three-dimensional (3D) anatomic, motion, and flow imaging using ultrasound.

ULTRASOUND

Ultrasound is sound, a traveling pressure wave, of frequency higher than what humans can hear. Frequencies used in echocardiography range from about 2 MHz for adult transthoracic studies to about 10 MHz for higher-frequency applications such as harmonic imaging and pediatric and transesophageal studies. Higher frequencies produce images with improved detail resolution but with less penetration because the weakening of the ultrasound as it travels (attenuation) increases with increasing frequency. Ultrasound provides a live, noninvasive view of the heart. Echocardiography is accomplished with a pulse-echo technique.[1] Pulses of ultrasound, two to three cycles long, are generated by a transducer (Fig. 1.1) and directed into the patient, where they produce echoes at organ boundaries and within tissues. These echoes then return to the transducer, where they are detected and presented on the display of the sonographic instrument (Fig. 1.2). The ultrasound instrument processes the echoes and presents them as visible dots, which form the anatomic image on the display. The brightness of each dot represents the echo strength (amplitude), producing what is known as a *grayscale image*. The location of each dot corresponds to the anatomic location of the echo-generating object. Positional information is determined by knowing the path of the pulse as it travels and measuring the time it takes for each echo to return to the transducer. From a starting point at the top of the display, the proper location for presenting each echo is determined. Because the speed of the sound wave is known, the echo arrival time can be used to determine the depth of the object that produced the echo.

When a pulse of ultrasound is sent into tissue, a series of dots (one scan line, data line, or echo line) is displayed. Not all of the ultrasound pulse is reflected from any single interface. Rather, most of the original pulse continues into the tissue and is reflected from deeper interfaces. The echoes from one pulse appear as one scan line. Subsequent pulses go out in slightly different directions from the same origin. The result is a sector scan (sector image), which is shaped like a slice of pie (Fig. 1.3A). The resulting cross-sectional image is composed of many (typically 96 to 256) of these scan lines. For decades, sonography was limited to 2D cross-sectional scans (or slices) through anatomy such as that in Fig. 1.3A. 2D imaging has been extended into 3D scanning and imaging, also called *volume imaging,* as described in Chapter 2. This requires scanning the ultrasound through many adjacent 2D tissue cross sections to build up a 3D volume of echo information (see Fig. 1.3B), like a loaf of sliced bread in which each slice represents a 2D image and the loaf represents the 3D volume.

TRANSDUCER

The transducer used in echocardiography is a phased array that electronically steers the ultrasound beam in the sector format. It is energized by an electrical voltage from the instrument that produces each outgoing ultrasound pulse. The returning echo stream is received by the transducer and converted to an echo voltage stream that is sent into the instrument, ultimately appearing on the display as a scan line. This process occurs a few thousand times per second (called the *pulse repetition frequency* [PRF]). A coupling gel is used between the transducer and the skin to eliminate the air that would block the passage of ultrasound across that boundary. Transducers (see Fig. 1.1) are designed for transthoracic (see Section II) and for transesophageal (see Section III) imaging. The latter provides a shorter acoustic path (with less attenuation, allowing higher frequencies and improved resolution) to the heart that avoids intervening lung and ribs.

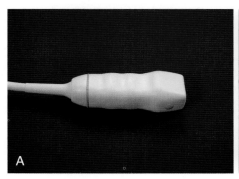
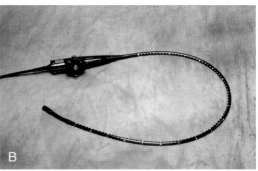

Figure 1.1. A, Transthoracic transducer. **B,** Transesophageal transducer.

INSTRUMENT

The echocardiographic instrument has a functional block diagram as shown in Fig. 1.2B. The beam former drives the transducer and receives the returning echo streams, amplifying (this is called *gain*) and digitizing them. Attenuation compensation occurs in the reception side of the beam former. This is an amplification process that equalizes echo strengths (amplitudes) by increasing gain with depth. This compensates for the weakening of echo amplitude with depth caused by attenuation. The signal processor, among other functions, detects the amplitude of each echo voltage. Echo amplitudes are stored digitally in the image memory, which is part of the image processor. Upon completion of a single scan (one frame of a real-time presentation), the stored image is sent to the flat-panel display. The echo information enters the image memory in ultrasound scan-line sector format but is read out to the display in horizontal-line display format, with each horizontal line on the display corresponding to a row of echo data in the image memory.

ARTIFACTS

In imaging, an artifact is any presentation that does not correctly display the structure or function (tissue motion and blood flow) imaged. Artifacts are caused by problematic aspects of the imaging process. They can hinder correct interpretation and diagnosis. These artifacts must be avoided or managed properly when encountered to avoid the errors they can cause. Some artifacts are produced by improper equipment operation or settings (e.g., incorrect gain and compensation settings). Other artifacts are inherent in the sonographic methods and can occur even with proper equipment and technique. The assumptions inherent in the sonographic process include the following:

- Sound travels in straight lines.
- Echoes originate only from objects located on the beam axis.
- The amplitude of returning echoes is related directly to the reflecting or scattering properties of the objects that produces them.
- The distance to reflecting or scattering objects is proportional to the round-trip travel time at a speed of 1.54 mm/µs.

If any of these assumptions are violated, artifacts occur. Fig. 1.4 and Video 1.4 provide examples of artifacts in echocardiography.

VIRTUAL BEAMFORMING

Two alternative fundamental principles of operation are now present in the array of commercially available echocardiographic equipment. The first, termed *conventional echocardiography*, has been the operating principle for more than 50 years and is described earlier in this chapter. Recently, a second principle has appeared, termed *virtual-beam echocardiography*.[1,2] These two operating principles are fundamentally different, and there are implications for the resulting anatomic images and motion information presented. Virtual-beam sonography improves nearly every aspect of echocardiographic, anatomic imaging, motion, and flow presentation. Rather than a one-to-one relationship of pulse to scan line, characteristic of conventional echocardiography, virtual-beam echocardiography acquires each image with a few broad, unfocused beams and then through massive, high-speed, retrospective computation accomplished with graphics processing units determines the amplitude (and Doppler shift if needed) of the echo at each pixel location (Fig. 1.5). This computational, retrospective beamforming capitalizes on the fact that an echo arrives at the elements of the transducer in a sequence uniquely characteristic of the location from which it originated. The challenge is to sort out each echo from the mixed-up combination in

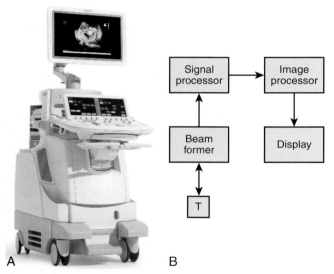

Figure 1.2. A, Echocardiographic instrument. **B,** Block diagram of an echocardiographic instrument. *T,* transducer.

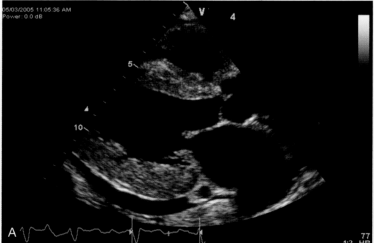
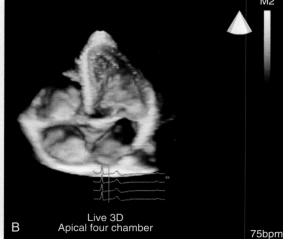

Figure 1.3. A, Two-dimensional cardiac sector image. **B,** Three-dimensional cardiac image.

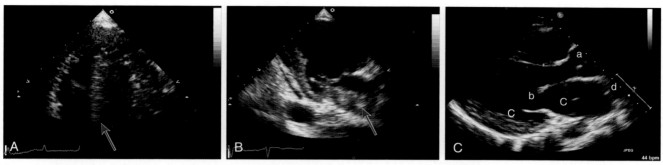

Figure 1.4. A, Comet-tail artifact *(arrow)*. **B,** Grating-lobe artifact *(arrow)* mimicking a mass in the atrium. **C,** Aortic valve (a), mitral valve (b), grating lobe (c) duplication of (b), and mirror-image (d) duplication of (a). See also Video 1.4.

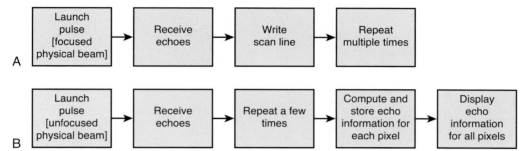

Figure 1.5. A, Sequence of operations for conventional, pulse-echo echocardiography. **B,** Sequence of operations for virtual-beam echocardiography.

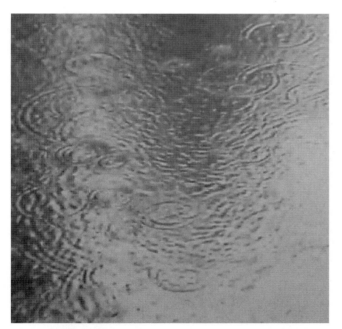

Figure 1.6. Raindrops falling on a puddle are an example of the computational challenge with virtual beamforming. Note that the wave emanating from each drop travels away to be combined with all the others. If they can be sorted out as they arrive at any edge of the photo, the location of their origins and strengths can be individually determined based on their arrival characteristics. This is analogous to what the retrospective computational process accomplishes virtual beamforming. See also Video 1.6.

which they arrive at the transducer, similar to waves from raindrops combining as they travel (Fig. 1.6 and Video 1.6). When the computational process for a frame is complete, the results are sent to the display to show that frame. Virtual beamforming produces images that are in focus throughout, with higher frame rates, increased sensitivity and penetration, and improved contrast resolution compared with conventional echocardiography (Fig. 1.7 and Video 1.7).

Artificial intelligence, machine learning, and deep learning are invading echocardiography, taking on some optimization functions that formerly were the responsibility of the echocardiographer, and automating some functions. This transition to instrument optimization and automation will continue, will alter the role of echocardiographers, and will improve the accuracy and efficiency of diagnostic echocardiography.

Advanced features and techniques, including 3D echocardiography, Doppler principles, tissue Doppler imaging, speckle tracking, and strain, are covered in the following chapters in this section. Expansion of all the topics covered in this chapter can be found in Kremkau.[1,2]

Please access ExpertConsult to view the corresponding videos for this chapter.

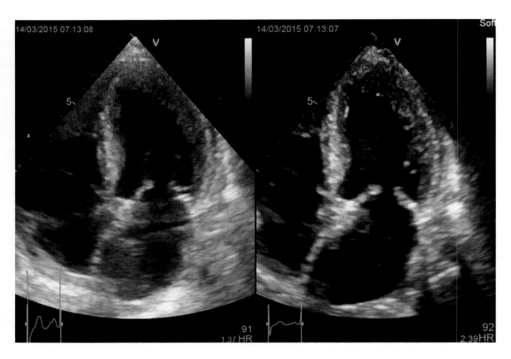

Figure 1.7. Comparison of conventional pulse-echo imaging *(left)* with virtual beamforming *(right)*. See also Video 1.7.

REFERENCES

1. Kremkau FW. *Sonography: Principles and Instruments*. 10th ed. Philadelphia: Elsevier/Saunders; 2020.

2. Kremkau FW. Your new paradigm for understanding and applying sonographic principles. *J Diag Med Sonography*. 2019;35(5):439–446.

2   Three-Dimensional Echocardiography

Luigi P. Badano, Denisa Muraru

The milestone in the history of three-dimensional echocardiography (3DE) has been the development of fully sampled matrix-array transthoracic transducers based on advanced digital processing and improved image formation algorithms that allowed the operators to obtain on-cart transthoracic real-time volumetric imaging with short acquisition times and high spatial and temporal resolution. Further technological developments (i.e., advances in miniaturization of the electronics and in element interconnection technology) made it possible to insert a full matrix array into the tip of a transesophageal probe for real-time volumetric imaging. In addition to transducer engineering, improved computer processing power and the availability of dedicated software packages for both on- and offline postprocessing have allowed 3DE to become a practical clinical tool.

COMPARISON BETWEEN TWO- AND THREE-DIMENSIONAL ECHOCARDIOGRAPHY ULTRASOUND TRANSDUCERS

The backbone of the 3DE technology is the transducer. A conventional two-dimensional (2D) phased array transducer is composed of 128 piezoelectric elements, electrically isolated from each other, arranged in a single row (Fig. 2.1). Ultrasound wave fronts are generated by firing individual elements in a specific sequence with a delay in phase with respect to the transmit initiation time. Each element adds and subtracts pulses to generate a single ultrasound wave with a specific direction that constitutes a radially propagating scan line (Fig. 2.2). Because the piezoelectric elements are arranged in a single row, the ultrasound beam can be steered in two dimensions—vertical (axial) and lateral (azimuthal)—while resolution in the z-axis (elevation) is fixed by the thickness of the tomographic slice, which in turn is related to the vertical dimension of the piezoelectric elements.

Currently, 3DE matrix-array transducers are composed of approximately 3000 individually connected and simultaneously active (fully sampled) piezoelectric elements with operating frequencies ranging from 2 to 4 MHz and 5 to 7 MHz for transthoracic and transesophageal transducers, respectively. To steer the ultrasound beam in 3D space, a 3D array of piezoelectric elements needs to be used in the probe; therefore, piezoelectric elements are arranged in rows and columns to form a rectangular grid (matrix configuration) within the transducer (see Fig. 2.1, *right*). The electronically controlled phasic firing of the elements generates a scan line that propagates radially (y or axial direction) and can be steered both laterally (x or azimuthal direction) and in the elevation plane (z direction) to acquire a volumetric pyramid of data (see Fig. 2.1, *right*). Matrix-array probes can also provide real-time multiple simultaneous 2D views at high frame rates in predefined or user-selected plane orientations (Fig. 2.3). The main technological breakthrough that allowed manufacturers to develop fully sampled matrix

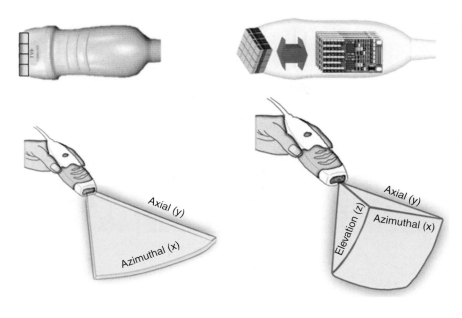

Figure 2.1. Two- (2D) and three-dimensional (3D) transducers. Schematic drawing showing the differences between a 2D *(left)* and a 3D *(right)* transducer.

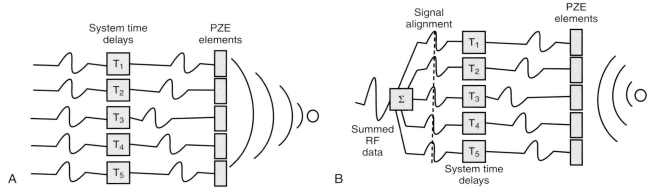

Figure 2.2. Two-dimensional (2D) beamforming. Schematic drawing of beamforming using a conventional 2D phased array transducer. During transmission *(left)*, focused beams of ultrasound are produced by pulsing each piezoelectric (PZE) element with precalculated time delays (i.e., phasing). During reception *(right)*, focusing is achieved by applying selective delays at echo signals received by the different piezoelectric elements to create isophase signals that are summed in a coherent way. RF, Radio frequency.

transducers has been the miniaturization of electronics that drove the development of individual electrical interconnections for every piezoelectric element, which could be independently controlled, both in transmission and reception.

Beamforming is a technique used to process signals to produce directionally or spatially selected signals sent or received from arrays of sensors. In 2D echocardiography (2DE), all the electronic components for the beamforming (high-voltage transmitters, low-noise receivers, analog-to-digital converter, digital controllers, digital delay lines) are in the system and consume a lot of power (~100W and 1.500 cm² of personal computer electronics board area). If the same beamforming approach would have been used for matrix-array transducers used in 3DE, it would require around 4 kW of power consumption and a huge PC board area to accommodate the needed electronics. To reduce both power consumption and the size of the connecting cable, several miniaturized circuit boards have been incorporated into the transducer, allowing partial beamforming to be performed in the probe (Fig. 2.4). This unique circuit design results in an active probe, which allows micro-beamforming of the signal with low power consumption (<1 W) and avoids the need to connect every piezoelectric element to the ultrasound machine. The 3000-channel circuit boards within the transducer

control the fine steering by delaying and summing signals within subsections of the matrix, known as patches (see Fig. 2.4). This micro-beamforming allows reduction of the number of the digital channels to be put into the cable that connects the probe to the ultrasound system from 3000 (which would make the cabling too heavy for practical use) to the conventional 128 to 256, allowing the same size of the 2D cable to be used with 3D probes. Coarse steering is controlled by the ultrasound system in which the analog-to-digital conversion occurs using digital delay lines (see Fig. 2.4). However, the electronic circuitry inside the probe produces heat, the level of which is directly proportional to the mechanical index used during imaging; therefore, the engineering of active 3DE transducer should include thermal management.

Finally, new and advanced crystal manufacturing processes allow production of single crystal materials with homogeneous solid-state technology and unique piezoelectric properties. These new transducers result in reduced heating production by increasing the efficiency of the transduction process, which improves the conversion of transmit power into ultrasound energy and of received ultrasound energy into electrical power. Increased efficiency of the transduction process together with a wider bandwidth results in increased ultrasound penetration and

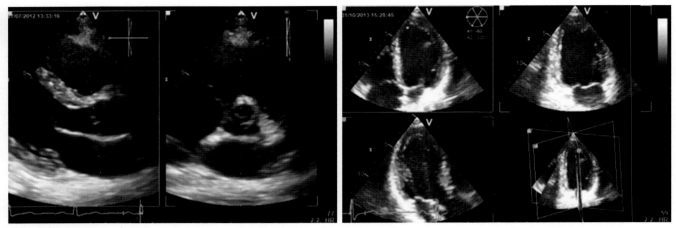

Figure 2.3. Multiplane acquisition using the matrix-array transducer. Bi- and triplane acquisitions with matrix-array transducers. *CW,* Continuous wave.

Figure 2.4. Three-dimensional (3D) beamforming. Beamforming with 3D matrix-array transducers has been split into two: the transducer and the ultrasound (US) machine levels. At the transducer level, interconnection technology and integrated analog circuits control transmit and receive signals using different subsection of the matrix (patches) to perform analog pre-beamforming and fine steering. Signals from each patch are summed to reduce the number of digital lines in the coaxial cable that connects the transducer to the ultrasound system from 3000 to the conventional 128 or 256 channels. At the ultrasound machine level, analog-to-digital (A/D) convertors amplify, filter, and digitize the elements signals, which are then focused (coarse steering) using digital delay (DELAY) circuitry and summed together (Ξ) to form the received signal from a desired object.

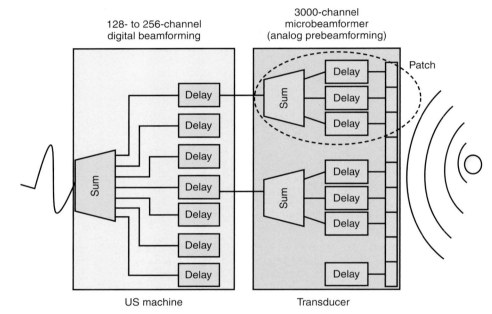

resolution, which improves image quality with the additional benefits of reducing artifacts, lowering power consumption, and increasing Doppler sensitivity.

Further developments in transducer technology have resulted in a reduced transducer footprint, improved side-lobe suppression, increased sensitivity and penetration, and the implementation of harmonic capabilities that can be used for both grayscale and contrast imaging. The latest generation of matrix transducers are significantly smaller than the previous ones, and the quality of 2D and 3D imaging has improved significantly, allowing a single transducer to acquire both 2D and 3DE studies, as well as having the ability of acquiring the entire left and right ventricular cavity in a single beat.

Three-Dimensional Echocardiography Physics

3DE is an ultrasound technique, and the physical limitation of the constant speed of sound in human body tissues (~1540 m/s) cannot be overcome. The speed of sound in human tissues divided by the distance a single pulse has to travel forth and back (determined by the image depth) results in the maximum number of pulses that can be fired each second without interference. Based on the acquired pyramidal angular width and the desired beam spacing in each dimension

(spatial resolution), this number is related to the volumes per second that can be imaged (temporal resolution). Therefore, similar to 2DE imaging, in 3DE imaging, there is an inverse relationship between volume rate (temporal resolution), acquisition volume size, and the number of scan lines (spatial resolution). Any increase in one of these factors results in a decrease in the other two.

The relationship between volume rate, number of parallel receive beams, sector width, depth, and line density can be described by the following equation:

$$\text{Volume rate} = \frac{1540 \times \text{No. of parallel received beams}}{2 \times (\text{Volume width/Lateral resolution})^2 \times \text{Volume depth}}$$

Accordingly, the volume rate can be adjusted to the specific needs by changing either the volume width or depth. The 3D system allows the user to control the lateral resolution by changing the density of the scan lines in the pyramidal sector. However, a decrease in spatial resolution also affects the contrast of the image. Volume rate can also be increased by increasing the number of parallel receive beams, but in this way, the signal-to-noise ratio and the image quality are affected.

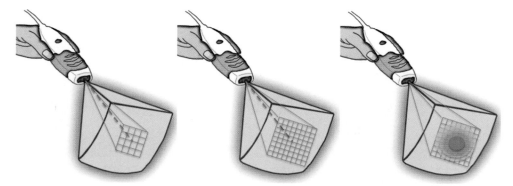

Figure 2.5. Parallel receive beamforming. Schematic representation of the parallel receive or multiline beamforming technique receiving 16 *(left)* or 64 *(center)* beams for each transmit pulse *(dashed red line)*. The *right panel* shows the degradation of the power and resolution of the signal (from red maximal to bright yellow minimal) from the parallel receiving beams steered farther away from the center of the transmit beam.

To put all this in perspective, let us assume that we want to image up to 16 cm depth in the body and acquire a 60- × 60-degree pyramidal volume. With the speed of sound of 1540 m/s and each pulse propagating 16 cm × 2 (from to the transducer and back), 1540/0.32 = 4812 pulses may be fired per second without getting interference between the pulses. Assuming that 1-degree beam spacing in both X and Z dimensions is sufficient, one would need 3600 beams (60 × 60) to spatially resolve the 60- × 60-degree pyramidal volume. As a result, the temporal resolution (volume rate) would be 4812/3600 = 1.3 Hz, which is practically useless in clinical echocardiography.

This example shows that the fixed speed of sound in body tissues is a major challenge to the development of 3DE imaging. Manufacturers have developed several techniques, such as parallel receive beamforming, multibeat imaging, and real-time zoom acquisition, to cope with this challenge, but in practice, this is usually achieved by selecting the appropriate acquisition mode for different purposes (see the "Image Acquisition" and "Image Display" sections later).

Parallel receive beamforming or multiline acquisition is a technique in which the system transmits one wide beam and receives multiple narrow beams in parallel. In this way, the volume rate is increased by a factor equal to the number of the received beams. Each beamformer focuses along a slightly different direction that was insonated by the broad transmit pulse. As an example, to obtain a 90- × 90-degree, 16-cm depth pyramidal volume at 25 vps, the system needs to receive 200,000 lines/s. Because the emission rate is around 5000 pulsed/s, the system should receive 42 beams in parallel for each emitted pulse. However, increasing the number of parallel beams to increase temporal resolution leads to an increase in size, costs, and power consumption of the beamforming electronics and deterioration in the signal-to-noise ratio and contrast resolution. With this technique of processing the received data, multiple scan lines can be sampled in the amount of time a conventional scanner would take for a single line, at the expense of reduced signal strength and resolution, because the received beams are steered farther and farther away from the center of the transmit beam (Fig. 2.5).

Another technique to increase the size of the pyramidal volume and maintain the volume rate (or the opposite, namely maintaining the volume rate and increasing the pyramidal volume) is the multibeat acquisition. With this technique, a number of electrocardiography (ECG)-gated subvolumes acquired from consecutive cardiac cycles are stitched together to build up the final pyramidal volume (Fig. 2.6). Multibeat acquisition is effective only if the different subvolumes are fixed in position and size; therefore, any transducer movement, cardiac translation caused by respiration, or change in cardiac

cycle length results in subvolume malalignment and stitching artifacts (Fig. 2.7).

Finally, the quality of the 3DE images of the cardiac structures is affected by the point-spread function of the system. The point-spread function describes the imaging system's response to a point input. A point input, represented as a single pixel in the "ideal" image, is represented by something other than a single pixel in the actual image (Fig. 2.8). The degree of spreading (blurring) of any point object varies according to the dimension used. In current 3DE systems, it is around 0.5 mm in the axial (y) dimension, around 2.5 mm in the lateral (x) dimension, and around 3 mm in the elevation (z) dimension. As a result, the best images (less degree of blurring, i.e., distortion) are obtained when using the axial dimension and the worst (greatest degree of spreading) when using the elevation dimension.

These concepts have an immediate practical application in the choice of the best approach to image a cardiac structure. According to the point-spread function of 3DE, the best results for imaging the aortic valve using transesophageal 3DE is expected to be obtained by using the short-axis view as the reference plane because the aortic valve is mostly imaged in the axial and lateral dimensions. Conversely, the worst result is expected when using the long-axis view as the reference plane, which mostly uses the lateral and elevation dimensions (Fig. 2.9).

Image Acquisition

Currently, 3D acquisition can be easily incorporated into standard echocardiographic examination by either switching between 2D and 3D probes or with the newest all-in-one probes by switching between 2D and 3D modes available in the same probe. The latter probes are also capable of providing single-beat full-volume data-sets, as well as real-time 3D color Doppler imaging. At present, three different methods for 3D dataset acquisition are available[1]: multiplane imaging, "real-time" (or "live") 3D imaging, and multibeat ECG-gated imaging.

In the multiplane mode, multiple simultaneous 2D views can be acquired at a high frame rate using predefined or user-selected plane orientations and displayed using the split-screen option (see Fig. 2.3). The first view on the left is usually the reference plane that is orientated by adjusting the probe position, while the other views represents views obtained from the reference view by simply tilting or rotating the imaging planes. Multiplane imaging is a real-time acquisition, and secondary imaging planes can only be selected during acquisition. Doppler color flow can be superimposed on 2D images, and in some systems, both tissue Doppler and speckle tracking analysis can be performed. Although strictly not a 3D acquisition, this imaging mode is useful in situations when assessment of multiple views from the

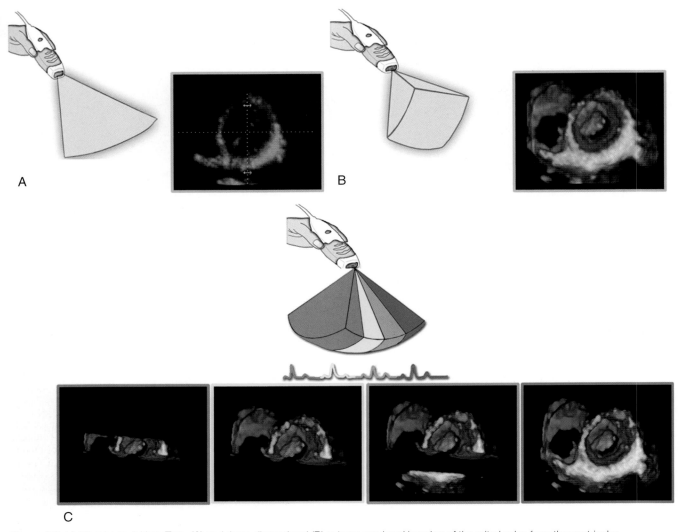

Figure 2.6. Multibeat acquisition. Two- (**A**) and three-dimensional (**B**) volume-rendered imaging of the mitral valve from the ventricular perspective. The latter has been obtained from a four-beat full-volume acquisition (**C**). The four pyramidal subvolumes. The colors show the relationships between the pyramidal subvolumes, the electrocardiographic beats, and the way the 3D dataset has been built up in the lower part of the figure.

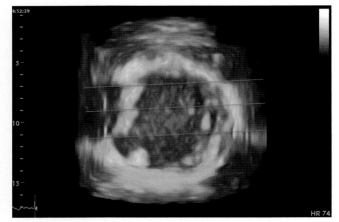

Figure 2.7. Stitching artifacts. Volume-rendered image displayed with respiratory gating artifacts. The *blue lines* highlight the misalignment of the pyramidal subvolumes.

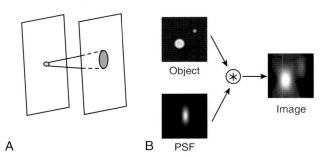

Figure 2.8. Point-spread function (PSF). **A,** Graphical representation of the extent of degradation (blur) of a point passing through an optical system. **B,** Effect of the PSF on the final image of a circular object.

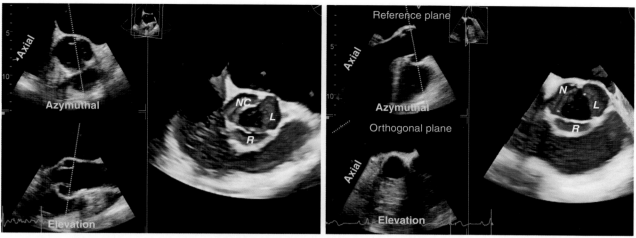

Figure 2.9. Orientation of the acquisition views and three-dimensional echocardiography dataset quality. Transesophageal zoom-mode acquisition of the aortic valve. Using the short-axis view as the reference plane *(left)*, the thin valve leaflets are imaged using the axial and lateral dimensions of the probe. Conversely, using the long-axis view as the reference plane *(right)*, the thin valve leaflets are imaged using the axial and elevation dimensions with worse spatial resolution of the dataset.

same cardiac cycle is useful (e.g., atrial fibrillation or other irregular arrhythmias, stress echo, evaluation of interventricular dyssynchrony).

In the real-time mode, a pyramidal 3D volumetric dataset is obtained from each cardiac cycle and visualized live, beat after beat, as during 2D scanning. As the dataset is updated in real time, the image orientation and plane can be changed by rotating or tilting the probe. Analysis can be done with limited postprocessing, and the dataset can be rotated (independent of the transducer position) to view the heart from different orientations. Heart dynamics are visualized in a realistic way, with instantaneous online volume-rendered reconstruction. It allows fast acquisition of dynamic pyramidal structures from a single acoustic view that can encompass the entire heart without the need of a reference system, ECG, and respiratory gating. Although this acquisition mode overcomes rhythm disturbances or respiratory motion limitations, it still suffers from relatively poor temporal and spatial resolution. Real-time imaging can be used in the following modes:

Live 3D: After the desired cardiac structure has been imaged in two dimensions, it can be converted to a 3D image by pressing a specific button on the control panel. The 3D system automatically switches to a narrow sector acquisition (~30- × 60-degree pyramidal volume) to preserve spatial and temporal resolution. The size of the pyramidal volume can be increased to visualize larger structures, but both scan line density (spatial resolution) and volume rate (temporal resolution) will be reduced. 3D live imaging mode is used to (1) guide full-volume acquisition, (2) visualize small structures (e.g., aortic valve, masses), (3) record short-lived events (i.e., bubble passage), (4) image patients with irregular rhythm or dyspnea that prevent full-volume acquisition, and (5) monitor interventional procedures.

Live 3D color: Color flow can be superimposed on a live 3D dataset to visualize blood flow in real time. Temporal resolution is usually very low.

3D zoom: This imaging mode is an extension of the live 3D mode and allows a focused real-time view of a structure of interest. A crop box is placed on a 2D single- or multiplane image (see Fig. 2.9) to allow the operator to adjust the lateral and elevation width to include the structure of interest in the dataset; then the system automatically crops the adjacent structures to provide a real-time display of the structure of interest with high spatial and temporal resolution. The drawback of the 3D zoom mode is that the spatial relationships of the structure of interest

with surrounding structures is lost. This is mainly used during transesophageal studies for detailed anatomical analysis of a specific structure of interest.

Full volume: The full-volume mode has the largest acquisition volume possible (up to 90 × 90 degrees). Real-time (or "single-beat") full-volume acquisition is affected by low spatial and temporal resolution and is used for the quantification of cardiac chambers when multibeat ECG-gated acquisition is not possible (e.g., irregular cardiac rhythm, patient unable to cooperate for breath-holding). In contrast to real-time or live 3D imaging, multibeat acquisition is realized through sequential acquisitions of narrow, smaller volumes obtained from several ECG-gated consecutive heart cycles (from 2 to 6) that are subsequently stitched together to create a single volumetric dataset (see Fig. 2.6). After acquisition, the dataset cannot be changed by manipulating the probe as in live 3D imaging, and analysis requires offline slicing, rotation, and cropping of the acquired dataset. It provides large datasets with high temporal and spatial resolution that can be used for quantifying cardiac chamber size and function or assessing spatial relationships among cardiac structures. However, this 3D imaging mode has the disadvantage of the ECG gating because the images are acquired over several cardiac cycles, and the final dataset is available to be visualized by the operator only after the last cardiac cycle has been acquired. In essence, it is "near real-time" imaging, which is prone to artifacts caused by patient or respiratory motion or irregular cardiac rhythms. Multibeat imaging can be performed with or without color-flow mapping, and usually more cardiac cycles are required for 3D color datasets.

Image Display and Analysis

3D datasets can be sectioned in several planes and rotated to visualize the cardiac structure of interest from any desired perspective, irrespective of its orientation and position within the heart. This allows the operator to easily obtain unique views that may be difficult or impossible to achieve using conventional 2DE (e.g., en-face views of the tricuspid valve or cardiac defects). Three main actions are undertaken by the operator to obtain the desired view from a 3D volumetric dataset: cropping, slicing, and rotating. Similar to what anatomists or the surgeons do to expose an anatomic structure, the operator needs to remove the surrounding structures within a 3DE dataset to visualize the structure of interest. This process of virtually removing the irrelevant neighboring tissue is referred to as "cropping" (Fig. 2.10) and can be

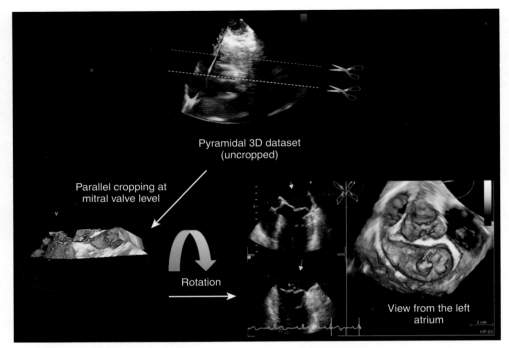

Figure 2.10. Dataset cropping and rotation. To display the mitral valve from the left atrial perspective (surgical view), a full-volume pyramidal dataset has been cropped to remove part of the left ventricle from above and part of the left atrium from below. Then the remaining dataset has been rotated to the desired perspective and to put the cardiac structures in an anatomical sound position.

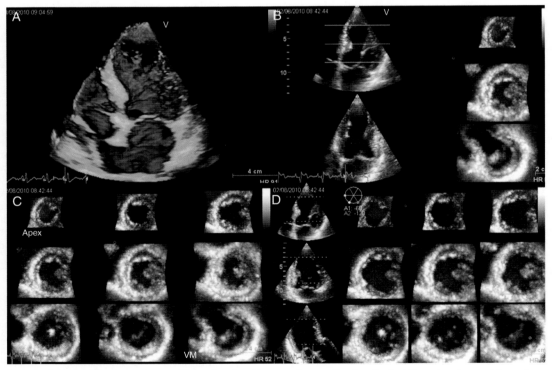

Figure 2.11. Dataset slicing. A full-volume dataset (**A**) can be sliced in several ways. Two longitudinal (four-chamber and the orthogonal view) plus three transversal slices at different levels of the left ventricle *(yellow lines)* (**B**). Nine transversal slices of the left ventricle from the mitral valve (MV) to the apical (apex) level (**C**). Three longitudinal slices (four- and two-chamber plus the long-axis apical views) and nine transversal views (**D**). The position of the lowest and the highest transversal planes are adjustable by the operator, and the slices in between are automatically repositioned to be equidistant. The positions of the longitudinal planes are adjustable as well both during acquisition and postprocessing.

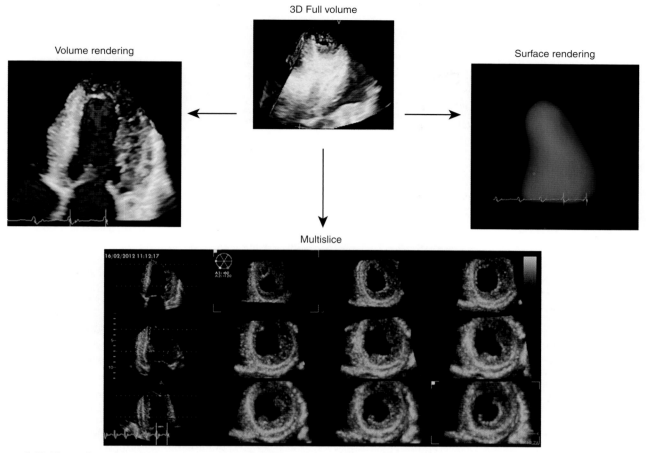

Figure 2.12. Three-dimensional (3D) dataset display. From the same pyramidal 3D dataset, the left ventricle can be visualized using different display modalities: volume rendering to visualize morphology and spatial relationships among adjacent structures, surface rendering for quantitative purposes, and multislice (multiple two-dimensional tomographic views extracted automatically from a single 3D dataset) for morphologic and functional analysis at different regional levels.

performed either during or after acquisition. In contrast with 2D images, displaying a cropped image also requires dataset rotation (see Fig. 2.10) and the definition of the viewing perspective because the same 3D structure can be visualized en face either from above or below, as well as from any desired view angle.[1] Slicing refers to a virtual "cutting" of the 3D dataset into one or more (≤12) 2D grey-scale images (Fig. 2.11). Finally, irrespective of its acquisition window, a cropped or sliced image should be displayed according to the anatomical orientation of the heart within the human body, and this is usually obtained by rotating the selected images.

Acquisition of volumetric images leads to the challenge of rendering depth perception on a flat 2D monitor. Three-dimensional images can be visualized using three display modalities (Fig. 2.12), including volume rendering, surface rendering, and tomographic slices. In the volume-rendering mode, various color maps are applied to create depth perception. Generally, lighter shades (e.g., bronze; see Fig. 2.6) are used for

structures closer to the observer, and darker shades (e.g., blue hues; see Fig. 2.6) are used for deeper structures. Surface-rendering mode displays the 3D surface of cardiac structures, identified either by manual tracing or by using automated border detection algorithms on multiple 2D cross-sectional images of the structure or cavity of interest. This stereoscopic approach is useful for the assessment of shape and better appreciation of the geometry and function during the cardiac cycle. Finally, the pyramidal dataset can be automatically sliced in several tomographic views that can be displayed simultaneously (see Fig. 2.11). Cut planes can be orthogonal, parallel, or freely oriented, selected as desired by the echocardiographer for optimized cross-sections of the heart, to answer specific clinical questions and to perform accurate and reproducible measurements.

REFERENCE

1. Duffin JM. The cardiology of R.T.H. Laennec. *Med Hist.* 1989;33:42–71.

3 Doppler Principles

Frederick W. Kremkau

Echocardiography provides noninvasive, real-time, diagnostic cardiac anatomic imaging (see Chapter 1) and motion and flow information. In the present context, the motion and flow are myocardial motion of contraction and relaxation and the resulting flow of blood, respectively. Motion and flow information are provided by implementing the Doppler effect.

DOPPLER EFFECT

The *Doppler effect* is a change in frequency caused by motion of a sound source, receiver or observer, or reflector. If a reflector is moving toward the source and receiver (the ultrasound transducer in our context), the received echo has a higher frequency than would be experienced without the motion. Conversely, if the motion is away (receding), the received echo has a lower frequency. The amount of increase or decrease in the frequency depends on the speed of the reflector motion, the angle between the sound propagation direction and the motion direction, and the frequency of the wave emitted by the source. The change in frequency (difference between emitted and received frequencies) caused by the reflector motion is called the Doppler-shift frequency or, more commonly, the *Doppler shift* (f_D). The Doppler shift is equal to the received frequency (f_R) minus the source frequency (f_T). For approaching reflectors (e.g., blood cells in circulation), the Doppler shift is positive; that is, the received frequency is greater than the source frequency. For a receding reflector, the Doppler shift is negative; that is, the received frequency is less than the source frequency. The proportional relationship between the Doppler shift and the reflector speed (v) is given by the Doppler equation:

$$f_D = f_R - f_T = \frac{2f_T\, v \cos\theta}{c}$$

in which c is the sound speed in tissue and θ is the Doppler angle, the angle between the sound beam direction and the motion direction. Take, for example, a source frequency of 5 MHz, an approaching flow speed of 50 cm/s, a propagation (sound) speed of 1.54 mm/µs in tissue, and a zero Doppler angle (cos = 1). The blood is approaching the source, so the received frequency is greater than the source frequency, with a positive Doppler shift of 0.0032 MHz or 3.2 kHz. For flow away from the transducer, the Doppler shift is −3.2 kHz. The Doppler shift is what the instruments described in this chapter detect and measure. The fact that the Doppler shift is proportional to the blood flow speed explains why the Doppler effect is so useful in medical diagnosis. Doppler operation measures the Doppler shift. The myocardial motion and blood flow are what interest us. The measured shifts are proportional to tissue or flow speed, which is the information we seek. Doppler shift is measured by the instrument and the Doppler equation is solved to yield calculated flow-speed information.[1] Tissue Doppler is described in Chapter 4.

If the direction of sound propagation is parallel to the flow direction, the maximum Doppler shift is obtained. If the angle between these two directions (Fig. 3.1) is nonzero (nonparallel), lesser Doppler shifts will occur. Half the original Doppler shift occurs at an angle of 60 degrees. No Doppler shift occurs at 90 degrees. The Doppler shift depends on the cosine of the Doppler angle as shown in the Doppler equation. Estimation of the angle is done by orienting an indicator line on the anatomic display so that it is parallel to the presumed direction of flow. This is a

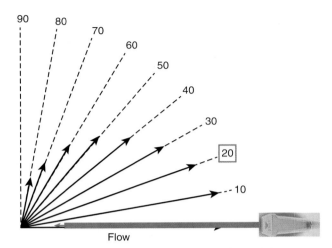

Flow

Figure 3.1. Doppler shift decreases as Doppler angle increases.

subjective operation performed by the instrument operator. In much echocardiographic work (e.g., apical view with flow from atrium to ventricle), the Doppler angle is 20 degrees or less, and angle incorporation can be ignored. In that case, the instrument assumes an angle of zero, and the error in calculated flow speed is a 6% or less underestimation of the flow speed.

COLOR DOPPLER DISPLAYS

Doppler operation presents information on the presence, direction, speed, and character of blood flow and on the presence, direction, and speed of tissue motion. This information is presented in audible, color Doppler, and spectral Doppler forms. Color Doppler imaging presents two-dimensional (2D), cross-sectional, real-time blood flow or tissue motion information along with 2D, cross-sectional, grayscale anatomic imaging. 2D real-time presentations of flow information allow the observer readily to locate regions of abnormal flow for further evaluation using spectral analysis. The direction of flow is appreciated readily, and disturbed or turbulent flow is presented dramatically in 2D form. Color Doppler operation presents anatomic information in the conventional grayscale form but also rapidly detects Doppler-shift frequencies at several locations along each scan line, presenting them in color at appropriate locations in the cross-sectional image. The color map decodes the arbitrary color assignments. In Fig. 3.2, the map in the upper right-hand corner shows red and yellow colors for increasing positive Doppler shifts above the black (zero Doppler shift) baseline and blue and cyan colors for increasing negative Doppler shifts below the baseline.

SPECTRAL-DOPPLER DISPLAYS

The term "spectral" relates to a spectrum, an array of the frequency components of a wave, separated and arranged in order of increasing frequency. The term *analysis* comes from a Greek word meaning to break up or to take apart. Thus, spectral analysis is the breaking up of the frequency components of a complex wave or signal and spreading them out in order of increasing frequency.

A mathematical process called the fast Fourier transform (FFT) is used to analyze the frequency spectrum of the Doppler signal. The spectral display presents a display of the Doppler shift spectrum (converted to flow speed by solving the Doppler equation) on the vertical axis and time on the horizontal axis (Fig. 3.3). Whereas a broad spectrum is associated with turbulent flow, a narrow spectrum is associated with laminar flow.

Two types of spectral Doppler operation are used for detection of flow in the heart: continuous wave (CW) and pulsed wave (PW). CW operation detects Doppler-shifted echoes in the relatively large region of overlap between the beams of the transmitting and receiving elements of a transducer. PW operation emits ultrasound pulses and receives echoes using a single element transducer or an array. Through range gating on reception, PW Doppler selects information from a particular depth along the beam based on echo arrival time, thus forming a small sample volume. If the electronic gate opens later, the sample volume moves deeper. To use PW Doppler effectively, it is combined with grayscale sonography, so the anatomic location of the sample volume is known. Spectral Doppler operation provides continuous or pulsed voltages to the transducer and converts echo voltages received from the transducer to audible and visual information corresponding to blood flow. CW

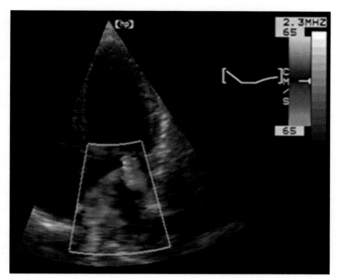

Figure 3.2. Apical view in color-Doppler form. The *red region* shows upward flow toward the apex and the transducer. The *blue region* shows regurgitant flow into the atrium.

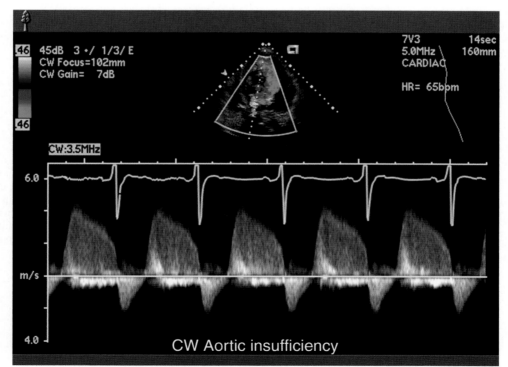

Figure 3.3. Color Doppler *(upper)* and spectral Doppler *(lower)* presentations.

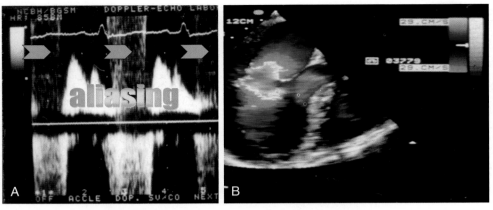

Figure 3.4. A, Spectral Doppler display with aliasing. The peak systolic portions of the signal are chopped off at the lower boundary and reappear at the upper boundary. The peak value is buried and unrecoverable with baseline shifting. Uncovering the correct presentation requires a scale increase in this case. **B,** Transesophageal echocardiography color Doppler display with aliasing (*red-orange-yellow* area in the region of the mitral valve). The flow is downward from the atrium the to ventricle and should be blue (negative Doppler shifts) according to the map. However, the blood accelerates as it passes through the mitral valve, and the Doppler shifts exceed the negative Nyquist limit. The color then jumps to the upper Nyquist limit, turning to yellow and progressing down the map through orange to red. Then the reverse sequence occurs as the blood decelerates into the ventricle. The upward flow in the outflow tract correctly shows as positive shifts (red).

operation detects flow that occurs anywhere within the intersection of the transmitting and receiving beams of the dual-transducer assembly. The sample volume is the region from which Doppler-shifted echoes return and are presented audibly or visually. In this case, the sample volume is the overlapping region of the transmitting and receiving beams. Because the sample volume is large, CW Doppler systems can give complicated and confusing presentations if two or more different motions or flows are included in the sample volume. PW systems solve this problem by detecting motion or flow at a selected depth with a relatively small sample volume. However, the large sample volume of a CW system is helpful when searching for a Doppler maximum (e.g., to calculate pressure drop across a valvular stenosis).

When observing blood flow, to eliminate the high-intensity, low-frequency Doppler-shifted echoes *called* clutter caused by heart wall or cardiac valve motion with pulsatile flow, a wall filter that rejects frequencies below an adjustable value is used. Sometimes called a *wall-thump filter*, the filter rejects these strong echoes that otherwise would overwhelm the weaker echoes from the blood. These strong echoes have low Doppler-shift frequencies because the tissue structures do not move as fast as the blood does. The upper limit of the filter is adjustable.

ALIASING

Pulsed-Doppler operation (color-Doppler and pulsed-spectral Doppler) does not detect the entire Doppler shift frequency as CW operation does but rather obtains samples of it because pulsed operation is a sampling process, with each pulse yielding a sample of the Doppler-shift signal. The samples are connected and smoothed (filtered) to yield the sampled waveform. If the pulsing (sampling) rate is not sufficient, aliasing occurs. Aliasing is the most common artifact encountered in Doppler ultrasound. Contemporary meanings for *alias* include (as an adverb) "otherwise called" or "otherwise known as" and (as a noun) "an assumed or additional name." Aliasing in its technical use indicates improper representation of information that has been sampled insufficiently. An optical form of temporal aliasing occurs in motion pictures when wagon wheels appear to rotate at various speeds and in reverse direction. Similar behavior is observed when a fan is illuminated with a strobe light. Depending

---

BOX 3.1 Doppler Operation Improvements With Virtual Beamforming

1. Simultaneous grayscale, color Doppler, and spectral Doppler (no time sharing)
2. Color flash reduced or eliminated (Fig. 3.5)
3. Retrospective sample volume (Fig. 3.6)
4. Flow velocity vector mapping (Fig. 3.7)
5. Automation of some functions (e.g., sample-volume positioning and aliasing correction)

---

on the flashing rate of the strobe light, the fan may appear stationary or rotating clockwise or counterclockwise at various speeds (Video 3.1). Fig. 3.4 illustrates aliasing in spectral and color displays. The Nyquist limit describes the minimum number of samples required to avoid aliasing. At least two samples per cycle of the measured Doppler shift must be acquired for the image to present correctly. For a complicated signal, such as a Doppler signal containing many frequencies, the sampling rate must be such that at least two samples occur for each cycle of the highest frequency encountered. To restate this rule, if the highest Doppler-shift frequency present in a signal exceeds half of the sampling frequency (which is the pulse repetition frequency transmitted), aliasing will occur. There are two common methods for correcting aliasing. Baseline shifting is a cut-and-paste method that moves the misplaced portions of the spectral displays to their correct locations (where they would be if there were no aliasing). Increasing the spectral display vertical scale increases the sampling rate to achieve the necessary Nyquist limit to avoid aliasing. In extreme cases, both methods are used.

VIRTUAL-BEAMFORMING

The fact that there are two fundamental operating principles involved in commercially available echocardiography systems today is discussed in Chapter 1. The advantages of virtual-beamforming[2] in cardiac Doppler are listed in Box 3.1.

Please access ExpertConsult to view the corresponding videos for this chapter.

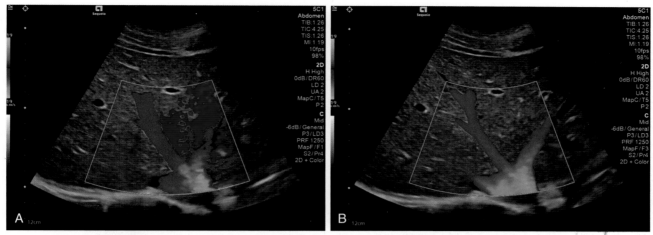

Figure 3.5. Abdominal image with color Doppler. **A,** Red is the flash artifact. **B,** The flash artifact eliminated.

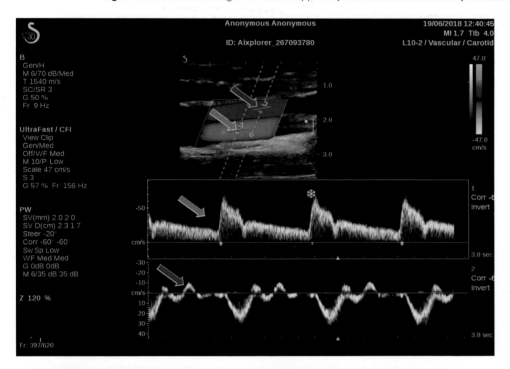

Figure 3.6. Retrospective sample volumes from saved color Doppler image. Sample volume 1 (upper spectral display) shows flow in the artery. Sample volume 2 (lower spectral display) shows flow in the vein. Note that the color Doppler frame rate is 156 Hz (frames/sec).

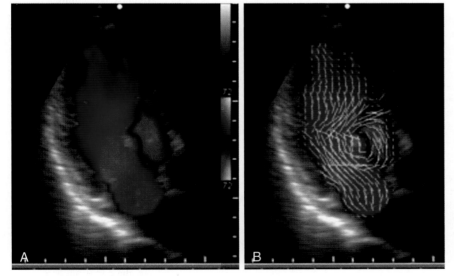

Figure 3.7. A, Conventional cardiac color-flow image. **B,** Cardiac vector-flow image. The *arrows* indicate flow speed and direction at each location in the flow. The color scale is calibrated in centimeters per second.

REFERENCES

1. Kremkau FW. *Sonography: Principles and Instruments*. 10th ed. Philadelphia: Elsevier/Saunders; 2020.

2. Kremkau FW. The new paradigm for understanding, teaching and testing sonographic principles. *J Vasc Ultrasound*. 2018;42(4):198–202.

4 Tissue Doppler, Myocardial Work: Physics and Techniques

Jonathan Chan, Gregory M. Scalia, Natalie F.A. Edwards

TISSUE DOPPLER IMAGING

Doppler shifts within the heart return either from moving red blood cells or moving myocardial tissue. Blood flow is high velocity; therefore, pulsed-wave Doppler assessment requires backscatter of high velocities and low amplitudes.[1] In comparison, tissue Doppler imaging (TDI) focuses on myocardial velocities at specific locations within the heart that are much slower and amplitudes that are much higher.[1] Distinction between Doppler signals originating from the myocardium and blood flow requires adjustment of gain, wall filters (high-pass filter for blood flow and lower-pass filter for tissue velocity), and velocity scale of the Doppler spectral or color display.[2] TDI velocities may by displayed as a spectral Doppler trace with the signal recorded from a specific sample volume site as a color-encoded M-mode or color-encoded two-dimensional (2D) trace.[1]

Limitations of Tissue Doppler Imaging

TDI interrogates the motion of the myocardium at a single point with reference to the ultrasound transducer. Therefore, it is limited by myocardial tethering and translational motion.[1,2] Using TDI for the assessment of systolic ventricular function suffers from an inability to differentiate actively contracting myocardium from passive myocardial motion caused by tethering. As a result, normal velocities may be detected in a hypokinetic or akinetic segment when it is being pulled on by normally contracting adjacent myocardial segment.[3] TDI is also dependent on achieving parallel orientation between the ultrasound beam and the direction of myocardial motion.[2–4] Ideally, the incident beam angle should not exceed 15 degrees to maintain underestimation of velocity to 4% or less.[2]

Tissue Doppler Imaging–Derived Strain and Strain Rate

Strain and strain rate imaging overcomes the limitation of passive myocardial motion caused by tethering because measurement of myocardial deformation is independent of adjacent segments.[5] TDI-based strain was the initial echocardiographic approach to measure myocardial deformation and measures strain in the direction of the ultrasound beam. Natural strain and strain rate are derived from tissue Doppler myocardial velocities from the velocity gradient calculated as the difference of two instantaneous velocities (V_a and V_b) normalized for the distance (d) between them (measured in units of s^{-1} or 1/s) (Fig. 4.1):

$$SR = (V_b - V_a) \div d$$

Whereas shortening rate of a myocardial segment in relation to its original length is represented by a negative value, lengthening rate is represented by a positive value. Strain (measured as a percentage) is derived from the time integral of strain rate:

$$S = \int_{to}^{t} SRn \, dt$$

Speckle-Tracking Echocardiography

Speckle-tracking echocardiography (STE) is based on tracking natural acoustic markers that appear as bright and dark spots

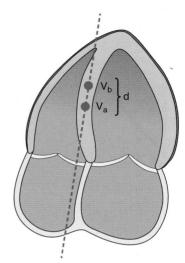

Figure 4.1. From the apical four-chamber view, strain rate from the interventricular septum is measured from two neighboring velocity points (V_a and V_b) located with a known distance (d) apart along the ultrasound beam.

on the grayscale image within the myocardium over subsequent frames.[2,5] The speckles are the result of constructive and destructive interference patterns caused by backscattered signals from structures smaller than the ultrasound wavelength.[2,3] A cluster of speckles (a kernel) are tracked from frame to frame with respect to their original position to allow for assessment of strain in two dimensions (Fig. 4.2). From apical images, speckles can be tracked in the longitudinal direction, and from parasternal short-axis images, speckles can be tracked in the radial and circumferential direction.

Compared with TDI, STE is a largely angle-independent technique and provides a direct measurement of strain.[2] Image quality must be of a high enough quality to track a region of interest accurately, and it is important to minimize foreshortening.[4] Frame rate is an important consideration in STE with an optimal frame rate considered to be in the range of 40 to 80 frames/sec. A frame rate that is too high may not provide enable speckle displacement for the tracking algorithm, but a frame rate that is too low leads to the loss of speckles because they may move out of the plane of the subsequent frame.[2]

Speckle-Tracking Echocardiography–Derived Strain and Strain Rate

STE-derived strain is based on Lagrangian strain because the analysis is based on the original length (l_o). Strain or deformation of a myocardial segment is defined as the difference between the final (*l*) and original length (l_o) divided by the original length:

$$Strain = [(1 - 1_0) / 1_0] \times 100\%$$

STE-derived strain tracks the speckles and determines the distance between two markers in a defined myocardial region and

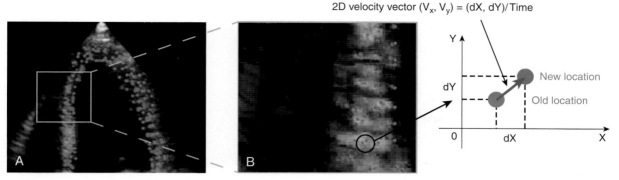

Figure 4.2. Principle of speckle-tracking echocardiography. The strain software identifies natural acoustic makers within the myocardial wall segments (**A**), which is also shown in a zoom image (**B**). The *green dot* in the graphical representation displays the old location, and the *red dot* represents the new location of the same natural acoustic marker during two consecutive frames. *2D,* Two dimensional. (Modified with permission from Leitman M, et al.: Two-dimensional strain—a novel software for real time quantitative echocardiographic assessment of myocardial function, *J Am Soc Echocardiogr* 17:1021–1029, 2004.)

plots this distance over the cardiac cycle. Strain rate is then derived as the first derivative, or the slope of the graph of strain over the cardiac cycle.

GLOBAL LONGITUDINAL STRAIN

Global longitudinal strain (GLS) is the most frequently used parameter for left ventricular (LV) systolic deformation. Peak GLS is the relative length change of the LV myocardium between end-diastole and end-systole as an average of all segments:

$$GLS\,(\%) = (MLs - MLd)\,/MLd$$

in which ML is the myocardial length at end-systole (MLs) and end-diastole (MLd).[6] Because the systolic length is smaller than the diastolic length (because of shortening of the myocardium), peak GLS is a negative number, which has caused confusion. The American Society of Echocardiography cardiac chamber guidelines recommend the use of an absolute value of strain (%) with reference to an increase or decrease in strain.[6]

GLS has been shown to be more reproducible for quantification of LV function than circumferential and radial strains.[7] Whereas GLS values as low as 18% to 20% are now acceptable as within normal range, a severe reduction in GLS being less than 12%.[8] LV ejection fraction (EF) has traditionally been used to assess LV systolic function, but there are limitations of volumetric measurements compared with the more sensitive myocardial deformation by strain imaging. This means that EF can remain normal despite reduced GLS in early subclinical myocardial dysfunction.[7,8]

MYOCARDIAL WORK

More recently, myocardial strain, especially GLS, has been shown to be more sensitive than traditional EF to detect early subclinical myocardial dysfunction and has important prognostic implications. However, both EF and longitudinal strain are sensitive to changes in preload and afterload.[9–11] This load-dependent limitation may affect accurate assessment of LV systolic function.

Afterload is commonly defined as the stress that the ventricle must work against to eject blood during ventricular contraction in systole. Afterload is related to ventricular wall stress and can be expressed by Laplace's law:

$$LV\ wall\ stress\,\left(dynes\,/\,cm^2\right) =$$

$$(LV\ pressure \times Radius)\,/2 \times LV\ wall\ thickness$$

Therefore, LV afterload is directly proportional to LV pressure and geometric changes in LV chamber dimensions but inversely related to LV wall thickness. An increase in afterload reduces the ability of the ventricle to eject blood. Studies have shown that an increase in afterload results in decreased longitudinal strain in patients with preserved systolic function, resulting in misinterpretation of true myocardial contractile function.[10,12–14] A true representation of myocardial function cannot be determined solely by myocardial strain deformation parameters, particularly when LV wall stress is substantially increased.

The concept of myocardial work was developed to enable more accurate assessment of LV systolic function by taking into account changes in afterload. By incorporating instantaneous LV pressure recordings with LV volumetric changes, Suga[15] demonstrated a linear correlation between myocardial oxygen consumption and the area of the LV pressure–volume loop measured using invasive hemodynamic techniques. Similarly, another technique measuring the area of the myocardial force-segment length loops also reflected myocardial oxygen consumption under variable loading conditions.[16] However, because of the invasive nature of these techniques, they have not been widely adopted in clinical practice.

Recently, Russell and coworkers[17,18] developed a new noninvasive method for calculating myocardial work that allows incorporation of afterload through noninvasive LV pressure–strain loops. The area of the non-invasive pressure–strain loop is a new index of myocardial work and metabolism and has been shown to provide similar physiological information to that obtained from invasive force-segment length and pressure–volume loops.[17,18] The LV pressure–strain loop is constructed from data obtained by strain analysis during 2D STE and combining them with noninvasive LV pressure data estimated from brachial artery blood pressure (BP). Noninvasive pressure–strain loops have been validated against invasively measured LV pressures and demonstrated a strong correlation with oxygen consumption as well as regional glucose cardiac metabolism assessed by 18-flurodeoxyglucose positron emission tomography.[17,18] The noninvasive nature of this new technique makes it more attractive and feasible for potential clinical use.

Physics of Myocardial Work

Work is defined as the magnitude of force multiplied by the magnitude of displacement and is expressed in joules:

$$Work = Force \times Displacement$$

The physical principle of work can also be applied to the LV, where myocardial contraction or longitudinal strain is substituted for displacement. Calculation of myocardial force is difficult, so

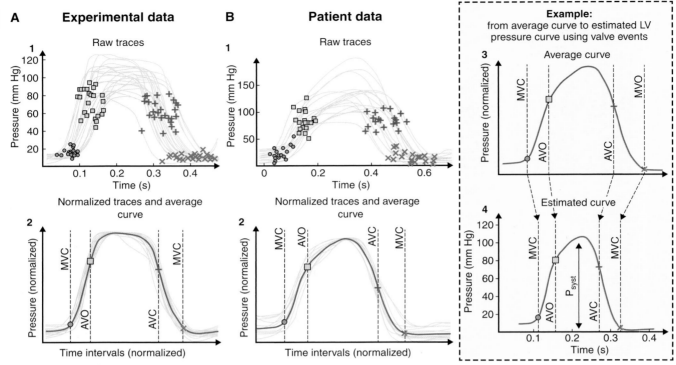

Figure 4.3. A1, Pressure recordings obtained were obtained using a dog model under a wide range of hemodynamic conditions with the valvular timing events for both the mitral and aortic valves indicated on each individual trace. **A2,** The pressure traces initially obtained *(light grey curves)* were stretched or compressed along the time axis (*x*-axis) to enable valvular timing events to coincide for each recording. The traces were then scaled vertically to have the same peak value. An average *(black curve)* pressure trace was subsequently used for predicting pressures. **B1** and **B2,** This was then performed using patients under a wide range of hemodynamic conditions. *3,* An averaged pressure waveform obtained from *B2* is displayed with arbitrary time intervals. *4,* Using the reference pressure waveform (*3*), estimation of the noninvasive left ventricular pressure is obtained by adjusting the valvular timing events along the *x*-axis according to the visualization of these events on two-dimensional echocardiography, and the amplitude of the signal (*y*-axis) was scaled according to the systolic arterial cuff pressure. (Modified with permission from Russell K, et al: A novel clinical method for quantification of regional left ventricular pressure-strain loop area: a non-invasive index of myocardial work, *Eur Heart J* 33:724–733, 2012.)

LV pressure is used as a substitute. Although this estimation is not a perfect calculation of true myocardial work, the area of the LV pressure–strain loop represents a good index of myocardial work because both longitudinal strain and LV pressure are dynamic throughout the cardiac cycle. Whereas noninvasive LV pressure–strain loops are derived from estimation of LV pressure from brachial artery cuff BP, strain is measured by STE.

Russell and coworkers[17] devised a method to estimate noninvasive LV pressure by first developing a general normalized reference LV pressure curve by pooling data from invasive hemodynamic measurements (intracardiac micromanometry) of many participants with different cardiac pathologies under a wide range of loading conditions. This normalized reference LV pressure curve was then individualized by incorporating noninvasive data from individual brachial artery BP and valvular timing of events obtained by echocardiography (Fig. 4.3). The reference LV pressure curve was synchronized with valvular timing events (isovolumic contraction, ejection period, isovolumic relaxation) of the individual participant. The peak amplitude of the LV pressure curve was adjusted to be equivalent to be the individual's brachial artery systolic BP. Myocardial work calculated from this method of noninvasive LV pressure estimation has been shown to be accurate and equivalent to invasive LV pressure measurements.[9]

Segmental work is calculated by combining longitudinal strain values with data from LV pressure curve as illustrated in Fig. 4.4. The first step requires the differentiation of strain to strain rate. The strain rate is then multiplied by the instantaneous LV pressure to obtain instantaneous power. In the final step, power is further integrated over time to derive myocardial work. Myocardial work is measured throughout the cardiac cycle from mitral valve closure (MVC) to mitral valve opening (MVO). The calculated work is approximately equivalent to the area represented within the LV pressure–strain loop. Work is measured in units of mm Hg%.

Noninvasive Left Ventricular Pressure–Strain Loop

An example of a normal LV pressure–strain loop is presented in Fig. 4.5. Instantaneous LV pressure is plotted on the vertical *y*-axis, and LV longitudinal strain is plotted on the horizontal *x*-axis. The resultant LV pressure–strain curve relationship forms an almost rectangular shaped closed loop and can be divided temporally into different phases of the cardiac cycle.

Isovolumic contraction: From MVC to aortic valve opening (AVO), there is an initial rapid rise in LV pressure with minimal change in strain.
Ejection period: From AVO to aortic valve closure (AVC). After the aortic valve opens, ventricular ejection leads to an increase in strain magnitude because of myocardial shortening, with myocardial deformation reaching its peak at AVC.
Isovolumic relaxation: AVC to MVO. LV pressure then falls rapidly with little change in myocardial strain.
Diastasis: MVO to MVC. LV pressure falls below left atrial pressure in early diastole corresponding to MVO; then the LV relaxes during diastasis with a decrease in strain magnitude and a gradual rise in LV filling pressure.[19,20]

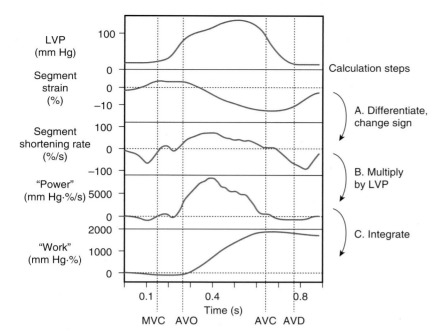

Figure 4.4. Step-by-step algorithm for calculation of myocardial work that is performed on all myocardial segments. Segment strain (%) is differentiated to obtain segmental shortening rate (%/s) or the strain rate. Segmental shortening rate is then multiplied by the estimated instantaneous left ventricular pressure to obtain power (mm Hg %/s). Power is then integrated over time to provide an estimate of work as a function of time. *AVC,* Aortic valve closure; *AVO,* aortic valve opening; *MVC,* mitral valve closure; *MVO,* mitral valve opening. (Modified with permission from Russell K, et al.: Assessment of wasted myocardial work: a novel method to quantify energy loss due to uncoordinated left ventricular contractions, *Am J Physiol Heart Circ Physiol* 305:H996–H1003, 2013.)

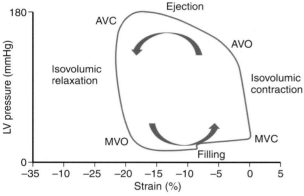

Figure 4.5. Left ventricular (LV) pressure–strain loop showing the relationship between timing of the cardiac events to changes in LV pressure and global longitudinal strain. The LV pressure–strain loop rotates in an anticlockwise direction. *AVC,* Aortic valve closure; *AVO,* aortic valve opening; *MVC,* mitral valve closure; *MVO,* mitral valve opening. (Modified with permission from Chan J, et al.: A new approach to assess myocardial work by non-invasive left ventricular pressure–strain relations in hypertension and dilated cardiomyopathy, *Eur Heart J Cardiovasc Imag* 20:31–39, 2019.)

Myocardial Work Indices

The global myocardial work index (GWI) is the measure of the total amount of work performed by the LV and is the average work performed by the sum of all the LV segments. GWI can be represented by the area within the LV pressure–strain loop. There are also additional components of work that can be derived from noninvasive measurements showing contraction patterns of individual segments (see Fig. 4.5).

Constructive work (CW) represents work contributing to effective ventricular contraction. This is the sum of work performed by myocardial fiber shortening during systole plus lengthening during isovolumic relaxation.

Wasted work (WW) represents negative work not contributing to LV ejection. This is the sum of work performed by myocardial fiber lengthening during systole plus shortening during isovolumic relaxation.

Myocardial work efficiency (WE) is the ratio of constructed work divided by the sum of constructive and wasted work (WW) and is expressed as a percentage: WE (%) = CW/(CW + WW).

Normal ventricles with all segments contracting and relaxing synchronously throughout the cardiac cycle will have a myocardial WE approaching 100%. Edwards and colleagues[20] reported a group of healthy control patients to have a global myocardial WE of 96% ± 2%. In contrast, Chan and coworkers[19] have recently shown that patients with ischemic and nonischemic cardiomyopathy have significantly lower global myocardial WE of 83% ± 9%.

From the EACVI NORRE study, normal reference values for GWI and related indices were estimated in 226 healthy individuals (Table 4.1) with subtle differences noted for global WW and global myocardial WE for gender and age (women only).[21] Similarly, a study by El Mahdiui and colleagues[22] showed a global myocardial WE of 96.0% (interquartile range [IQR], 95.0%–96.3%) in healthy individuals, which did not differ from patients with cardiovascular risk factors (96.0%; IQR, 95.0%–97.0%).

Potential Clinical Applications of Myocardial Work

Indices of myocardial work provide more advanced assessment of LV systolic function, beyond left ventricular ejection fraction (LVEF) and GLS, by incorporating changes in loading condition. Myocardial work can now be measured noninvasively using brachial artery pressure and strain imaging by echocardiography. At the time of publishing this book, there is only one commercially available vendor-specific software that calculates work. The automated functional imaging module is relatively simple to use and is merely an extension to the existing GLS protocol with additional steps of entering the BP and valvular timing events (Fig. 4.6). The results are displayed typically as bull's eye plots, LV pressure–strain loops, and tabulated numerical data (Fig. 4.7). The results have been proven to be highly reproducible among independent blinded observers.[19–21] The simplicity and ease of offline analysis coupled with highly reproducible measurements makes it more attractive for clinical use. To date, there are a few published studies in the literature

TABLE 4.1 Global Myocardial Work Values Obtained in a Group of 226 Healthy Individuals[a]

	Total (*n* = 226)	Male (*n* = 85)	Female (*n* = 141)	*P* Value (between genders)
GWI (mm Hg %)	1896 ± 308	1849 ± 295	1924 ± 313	0.07
GCW (mm Hg %)	2232 ± 331	2228 ± 295	2234 ± 352	0.9
GWW (mm Hg %)	78.5 (53–122.2)	94 (61.5–130.5)	74 (49.5–111)	0.013
GWE (%)	96 (94–97)	95 (94–97)	96 (94–97)	0.026

GWE, Global myocardial work efficiency; *GWI,* global myocardial work index; *GCW,* global constructive work; *GWW, global* wasted work.

Modified with permission from Manganaro R, et al: Echocardiographic reference ranges for normal non-invasive myocardial work indices: results from the EACVI NORRE study. *Eur Heart J Cardiovasc Imag* 20:582–590, 2019.

[a]Data in the table are mean ± standard deviation or median (interquartile range).

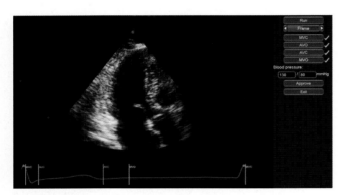

Figure 4.6. After derivation of global longitudinal strain using the automated functional imaging module, myocardial work is estimated after selection of valvular timing events on the two-dimensional apical long-axis view, and the blood pressure is also entered. *AVC,* Aortic valve closure; *AVO,* aortic valve opening; *MVC,* mitral valve closure; *MVO,* mitral valve opening.

that have demonstrated its potential, and the outlook is promising for inclusion in the following areas of clinical practice.

Cardiac Resynchronization Therapy

One of the best examples to highlight the relevance of different myocardial work parameters is in the dyssynchronous LV with left bundle branch block conduction delay. There is often early septal activation and contraction before AVO when the LV pressure is low followed by septal lengthening during systole. There is also delayed contraction of the lateral segments. The septal segments contribute minimally to LV ejection, resulting in elevated WW and reduced myocardial WE. Myocardial work can improve after successful cardiac resynchronization therapy (CRT).

Early studies assessing the clinical utility of myocardial work have found global CW to be a strong predictor of LV remodeling and response to CRT.[23,24] Recently, Galli and coworkers[25] demonstrated that global CW of 888 mm Hg % or less was the best predictor of cardiac mortality (area under the curve, 0.71; *P* = .007) after CRT in a group of 166 patients. Patients had a very poor prognosis if they were nonresponders to CRT with CW less than 888 mm Hg %.[25] There is a potential for myocardial work indices to help in the better selection of patients who may benefit from CRT.

Ischemic Heart Disease

Myocardial work has been shown to be superior to LVEF and longitudinal strain in identifying acute coronary occlusion in patients with non–ST-segment elevation myocardial infarction acute coronary syndromes.[26] El Mahdiui and colleagues[22] also recorded a lower global myocardial WE in patients with residual myocardial

ischemia despite percutaneous intervention, which could be attributed to an element of LV dyssynchrony after acute coronary syndrome. Ischemic myocardium can sometimes exhibit the phenomena of early systolic lengthening as well as postsystolic shortening after AVC. Myocardial work may have the potential to improve selection of suitable post-infarct patients for revascularization.

More recently, Edwards and coworkers[20] have shown that global myocardial work is more sensitive than GLS in the detection of early subclinical myocardial dysfunction in significant coronary artery disease (single and multivessel lesions ≥70%) with no resting regional wall motion abnormalities and normal EF.[20] Because of a reduction in global CW, patients with significant coronary artery disease also had reduced global WE (94.0% ± 3.0%) compared with control participants. This study suggests that there is potential for myocardial work indices to improve the diagnosis and early detection of stable coronary artery disease.

Hypertensive Heart Disease

Chan and coworkers[19] compared myocardial work in a group of control participants and those with uncontrolled hypertension. Increased systolic BP resulted in significantly elevated global myocardial work, indicating that the LV is working at a higher energy level, compensating for increased afterload. There was no difference in myocardial WE compared with control participants because of a proportional increase in global CW and global WW.[19] There were no changes in longitudinal strain and EF, which confirms the inability of traditional methods to detect increased load imposed on the LV. Myocardial work may be useful for the serial assessment of myocardial function assessment compensating for variable loading conditions (e.g., patients undergoing cardiotoxic chemotherapy) or monitoring response to hypertensive treatment.

Dilated Cardiomyopathy

Patients with LV dysfunction from ischemic and nonischemic dilated cardiomyopathy with reduced EF and GLS have significant increases in global WW and impaired global work index and global WE.[19] Myocardial work indices are good indicators for evaluating impaired myocardial performance at least equivalent to EF and GLS. It would be interesting to use myocardial work to evaluate dilated ventricles with only mildly reduced or preserved LVEF in the early stages of cardiomyopathy. A recent study demonstrated that the presence of LV contractile reserve by myocardial work during exercise correlates with clinical response to spironolactone treatment in heart failure with preserved EF.[27]

FUTURE DIRECTIONS

According to the principles of Laplace's law, patients with dilated ventricles demonstrate higher wall stress at any given pressure compared with smaller ventricles; therefore, work performed by the myocardium can be underestimated in the dilated LV.[19,28] This

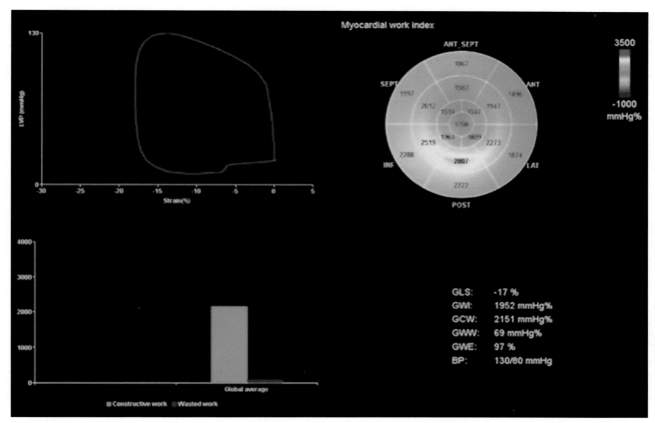

Figure 4.7. Display format of myocardial work results using the automated functional imaging module from EchoPAC software (version 203, GE, Horton, Norway). The *top left panel* displays the left ventricular (LV) pressure–strain loop, which provides a graphical representation of the relationship between estimated LV pressure and strain through the cardiac cycle. The *top right panel* displays the 17-segment bull's eye model of myocardial work. *Green shading* indicates normal ranges of myocardial work, *red shading* indicates elevated myocardial work, and *blue shading* indicates reduced myocardial work. The *bottom left panel* is a graphical representation of the proportion of constructive work *(green)* and wasted work *(blue)*. The *bottom right panel* displays the tabulated results. *BP,* Blood pressure; *GWE,* global myocardial work efficiency; *GWI,* global myocardial work index; *GLS,* global longitudinal strain; *GCW,* global constructive work; *GWW,* global wasted work.

is a limitation of myocardial work estimated from LV pressure–strain loops because it does not take into account LV geometry for variable LV chamber sizes. A fair comparison of work between ventricles of different sizes requires incorporation of myocardial wall stress.[19,29] Future directions in measuring myocardial work should include LV geometry and wall thickness for calculation of wall stress and there may be a role for three-dimensional echocardiography.

Noninvasive assessment of myocardial work through LV pressure–strain loop offers a new and promising technique that allows incorporation of afterload in the assessment of LV systolic function. This may add incremental value to echocardiographic parameters of EF and GLS, which are load dependent. Different myocardial work indices offer new insight in quantifying intrinsic myocardial contractility under different LV loading conditions. These indices have great potential for further research, but more large-scale studies and data are needed to determine their utility in clinical decision-making processes.

REFERENCES

1. Abraham TP, Dimaano VL, Liang H-Y. Role of tissue Doppler and strain echocardiography in current clinical practice. *Circulation.* 2007;116:2597–2609.
2. Mor-Avi V, Lang RM, Badano LP, et al. Current and evolving echocardiographic techniques for the quantitative evaluation of cardiac mechanics: ASE/EAE consensus statement on methodology and indications. *J Am Soc Echocardiogr.* 2011;24:277–313.
3. Blessberger H, Binder T. Two dimensional speckle tracking echocardiography: basic principles. *Heart.* 2010;96:716–722.
4. Geyer H, Caracciolo G, Abe H, et al. Assessment of myocardial mechanics using speckle tracking echocardiography: fundamentals and clinical applications. *J Am Soc Echocardiogr.* 2010;23:351–369.
5. Anderson B. *The Normal Examination and Echocardiographic Measurements.* ed 3. Brisbane, Australia: Echotext Pty Ltd; 2017.
6. Lang RM, Badano LP, Mor-Avi V, et al. Recommendations for cardiac chamber quantification by echocardiography in adults. *J Am Soc Echocardiogr.* 2015;28:1–39.
7. Chan J, Shiino K, Obonyo NG, et al. Left ventricular global strain analysis by two-dimensional speckle-tracking echocardiography: the learning curve. *J Am Soc Echocardiogr.* 2017;30:1081–1090.
8. Potter E, Marwick TH. Assessment of left ventricular function by echocardiography: the case for routinely adding global longitudinal strain to ejection fraction. *JACC Cardiovasc Imag.* 2018;11(2 pt 1):260–274.
9. Hubert A, Le Rolle V, Leclercq C, et al. Estimation of myocardial work from pressure–strain loops analysis: an experimental evaluation. *Eur Heart J Cardiovasc Imag.* 2018;19:1372–1379.
10. Murai D, Yamada S, Hayashi T, et al. Relationships of left ventricular strain and strain rate to wall stress and their afterload dependency. *Heart Ves.* 2017;32:574–583.
11. Burns AT, La Gerche A, D'Hooge J, et al. Left ventricular strain and strain rate: characterization of the effect of load in human subjects. *Eur J Echocardiogr.* 2010;11:283–289.
12. Donal E, Bergerot C, Thibault H, et al. Influence of afterload on left ventricular radial and longitudinal systolic functions: a two-dimensional strain imaging study. *Eur J Echocardiogr.* 2009;10:914–921.
13. Rösner A, Bijnens B, Hansen M, et al. Left ventricular size determines tissue Doppler-derived longitudinal strain and strain rate. *Eur J Echocardiogr.* 2009;10:271–277.
14. Fredholm M, Jörgensen K, Houltz E, et al. Load-dependence of myocardial deformation variables—a clinical strain–echocardiographic study. *Acta Anaesthesiol Scand.* 2017;61:1155–1165.

15. Suga H. Total mechanical energy of a ventricle model and cardiac oxygen consumption. *An J Physiol*. 1979;236:H498–H505.
16. Hisano R, Cooper G. Correlation of force-length area with oxygen consumption in ferret papillary muscle. *Circ Res*. 1987;61:318–328.
17. Russell K, Eriksen M, Aaberge L, et al. A novel clinical method for quantification of regional left ventricular pressure-strain loop area: a non-invasive index of myocardial work. *Eur Heart J*. 2012;33:724–733.
18. Russell K, Eriksen M, Aaberge L, et al. Assessment of wasted myocardial work: a novel method to quantify energy loss due to uncoordinated left ventricular contractions. *Am J Physiol Heart Circ Physiol*. 2013;305:H996–H1003.
19. Chan J, Edwards NFA, Khandheria BK, et al. A new approach to assess myocardial work by non-invasive left ventricular pressure–strain relations in hypertension and dilated cardiomyopathy. *Eur Heart J Cardiovasc Imag*. 2019;20:31–39.
20. Edwards NFA, Scalia GM, Shiino K, et al. Global myocardial work is superior to global longitudinal strain to predict significant coronary artery disease in patients with normal left ventricular function and wall motion. *J Am Soc Echocardiogr*. 2019;32:947–957.
21. Manganaro R, Marchetta S, Dulgheru R, et al. Echocardiographic reference ranges for normal non-invasive myocardial work indices: results from the EACVI NORRE study. *Eur Heart J Cardiovasc Imag*. 2019;20:582–590.
22. El Mahdiui M, van der Bijl P, Abou R, et al. Global left ventricular myocardial work efficiency in healthy individuals and patients with cardiovascular disease. *J Am Soc Echocardiogr*. 2019;32:1120–1127.
23. Galli E, Leclercq C, Hubert A, et al. Role of myocardial constructive work in the identification of responders to CRT. *Eur Heart J Cardiovasc Imag*. 2018;19:1010–1018.
24. Vecera J, Penicka M, Eriksen M, et al. Wasted septal work in left ventricular dyssynchrony: a novel principle to predict response to cardiac resynchronization therapy. *Eur Heart J Cardiovasc Imag*. 2016;17:624–632.
25. Galli E, Hubert A, Le Rolle V, et al. Myocardial constructive work and cardiac mortality in resynchronization therapy candidates. *Am Heart J*. 2019;212:53–63.
26. Boe E, Russell K, Eek C, et al. Non-invasive myocardial work index identifies acute coronary occlusion in patients with non-ST-segment elevation-acute coronary syndrome. *Eur Heart J Cardiovasc Imag*. 2015;16:1247–1255.
27. Przewlocka-Kosmala M, Marwick TH, Mysiak A, et al. Usefulness of myocardial work measurement in the assessment of left ventricular systolic reserve response to spironolactone in heart failure with preserved ejection fraction. *Eur Heart J Cardiovasc Imag*. 2019;20(10):1138–1146.
28. Alter P, Rupp H, Rominger MB, et al. A new methodological approach to assess cardiac work by pressure–volume and stress–length relations in patients with aortic valve stenosis and dilated cardiomyopathy. *Pflügers Arch*. 2008;455:627–636.
29. Boe E, Skulstad H, Smiseth OA. Myocardial work by echocardiography: a novel method ready for clinical testing. *Eur Heart J Cardiovasc Imag*. 2019;20:18–20.
30. Leitman M, Lysyansky P, Sidenko S, et al. Two-dimensional strain—a novel software for real time quantitative echocardiographic assessment of myocardial function. *J Am Soc Echocardiogr*. 2004;17:1021–1029.

5

Speckle-Tracking and Strain Measurements: Principles, Techniques, and Limitations

Luca Longobardo, Concetta Zito, Scipione Carerj, Bijoy K. Khandheria

GENERAL CONCEPTS

The word "strain," which in everyday language means "stretching," in echocardiography indicates a measure of tissue deformation; the "strain rate" is the rate at which the deformation occurs. Considering a given one-dimensional object under either lengthening or shortening deformation, the initial length could be indicated as L_0 and its length at a given time as $L(t)$. The normalized deformation, strain ε, can be mathematically represented by the following equation:

$$\varepsilon(t) = \frac{L(t) - L_0}{L_0}$$

This is called Lagrangian strain, which occurs when the initial length is known. However, whenever the original length is unknown, strain can be assessed considering its small temporal variations $d\varepsilon_N(t)$ during an infinitesimal time increment dt, as mathematically translated by the equation:

$$d\varepsilon_N(t) = \frac{L(t + dt) - L(t)}{L(t)}$$

This is the natural strain and represents variations during the total process of shortening or lengthening. Regarding small changes, Lagrangian and natural strain share almost the same values. Nevertheless, considering the large cardiac deformations that occur during systole and diastole, natural strain seems to be more appropriate to use.

Left ventricular (LV) muscular wall has been commonly considered to be shaped by three different layers, called the endocardium, myocardium, and epicardium. In the past years, several studies have explored the three-dimensional (3D) deformation of the ventricular tissue, describing myocyte arrangements as a continuum of two helical fiber geometries and not as three separated layers. These studies, performed using cardiac magnetic resonance imaging (MRI),[1] demonstrated that the subendocardial region shows a right-handed helical myofiber geometry, which changes gradually into a left-handed helical geometry in the subepicardium. This position of fibers allows a better pump function of the ventricle. Sallin in 1969 reported that the degree of shortening of the left ventricle would be 15% if fibers were disposed only longitudinally, 30% with circumferential fibers, and 60% or more with fibers oriented in an oblique spiral direction, as really occurs.[2] This myocardial structure broadly determines the components of myocardial deformation. We can also distinguish longitudinal, radial, and circumferential strains. Longitudinal and circumferential strains are shown as negative curves because they are the expression of myocardial shortening, whereas the radial strain produces a positive curve because it is the representation of myocardial lengthening. In addition, the helical nature of the heart muscle determines a wringing motion during the cardiac cycle, with counterclockwise rotation of the apex and clockwise rotation of the base around the LV long axis, when observed from the apical perspective. This deformation is called *twisting*. The subsequent recoil of twisting is defined *untwisting* and is associated with the release of restoring forces that contribute to diastolic suction and facilitate early LV filling.[3] In general, longitudinal LV strain is the most sensitive to the presence of myocardial disease, and it explains why longitudinal strain is considered the most sensitive parameter for the assessment of subtle systolic dysfunction and why it can already be reduced in the early phases of cardiac diseases when LV ejection fraction (EF), the most robust parameter for the evaluation of systolic dysfunction, is still normal. Indeed, when endocardial function is impaired but midmyocardial and epicardial function are unaffected, it may result in normal or nearly normal circumferential and twist mechanics with relatively preserved LV pump function and EF. On the other hand, an acute transmural insult or progression of disease results in simultaneous midmyocardial and subepicardial dysfunction, leading to a reduction in LV circumferential and twist mechanics and a reduction in EF.

A GLANCE AT THE HISTORY: TISSUE DOPPLER–DERIVED STRAIN

The first echocardiographic technique available for the assessment of strain was the tissue Doppler imaging (TDI)–derived strain. Tissue Doppler allowed assessment of the velocity of movement of myocardium relative to the transducer displayed as a parametric color image. However, because this approach is particularly susceptible to tethering of adjacent tissue, myocardial motion may be measured relative to the adjacent myocardium within the sample volume.[4] Dedicated software processes the instantaneous gradient of velocity along a sample length and generates a strain rate curve; the integration of this curve provides instantaneous data on deformation, that is, strain.[4,5] Although TDI strain showed to be a sensitive and accurate tool for quantitative assessment of cardiac function, it is affected by several technical limitations. The most evident TDI strain limitation is angle dependency, an intrinsic limitation of all Doppler techniques, particularly influential in the evaluation of myocardial segments such as the apex where the vectors of contraction change frequently along the scan line.[6] The high sensitivity to signal noise and the limited spatial resolution represent the other most important limitations of TDI strain and strain rate.

FROM THE PRESENT TO THE FUTURE: TWO- AND THREE-DIMENSIONAL SPECKLE-TRACKING ECHOCARDIOGRAPHY

In the past two decades, TDI strain has been completely replaced by speckle-tracking echocardiography (STE)–derived strain. STE allows a frame-by-frame tracking of natural acoustic markers, called "speckles," within the myocardium with standard echocardiographic images and is not based on Doppler velocities. Speckles result from interactions (e.g., reflections, scattering, or interference) of an ultrasound beam with myocardial tissue[7] and appear as bright and dark spots within the LV wall in a typical B-mode image. Tracked frame to frame over the cardiac cycle, distances between speckles or their spatiotemporal displacement (regional strain velocity vectors) provide non-Doppler information about global and segmental myocardial deformation.[8] For these reasons, STE measurements are angle independent, not influenced by translational movement caused by respiration and tethering from adjacent myocardium and less sensitive to signal noise, significantly overcoming the intrinsic limitations of TDI strain.[9–11]

The reliability of this technique has been widely demonstrated; comparing STE with sonomicrometry and cardiac magnetic resonance, authors found an excellent correlation between STE measurements and these gold-standard techniques.[12,13] STE allows an accurate evaluation of all the three components of the myocardial contraction (longitudinal, radial, and circumferential) and provides information on global and regional function. However, among STE parameters, the most robust one, widely used in literature and recommended by the current 2015 American Society of Echocardiography guidelines[14] for the assessment of LV systolic function, is global longitudinal strain (GLS). Indeed, circumferential and radial strain, as well as strain rate measurements, suffer from high variability to be routinely used in clinical practice.[8] Moreover, the global strain value is obtained from mean values over the entire length of the myocardial wall, overcoming the variability that affects measures of the regional strain. The current guidelines[14] suggest −20% ±2% as cutoff values of the LV GLS. More recently, a multicenter study reported the cutoff values for all strain parameters in a healthy population[15] (Table 5.1). The authors found that the lowest expected values of LV strains and twist calculated as ± 1.96 standard deviations from the mean in healthy participants were −16.7% in men and −17.8% in women for longitudinal strain, −22.3% and −23.6% for circumferential strain, 20.6% and 21.5% for radial strain, and 2.2 degrees and 1.9 degrees for twist, respectively. Moreover, longitudinal strain decreased with age, whereas the opposite occurred with circumferential and radial strain. Male gender was associated with lower strain for longitudinal, circumferential, and radial strain.

The calculation of GLS requires the identification of the so-called "regions of interest" (ROIs), through the automated or manual selection of fiducial landmarks in the apical three-, four-, and two-chamber views (Fig. 5.1A). The software provides the tracing of endocardial borders and the definition of the ROIs (Fig. 5.1B). This process must be particularly accurate because a wrong placement of the landmarks or inappropriately narrow or wide ROIs can cause an unreliable measurement. The placement of landmarks, for example, on the atrial side of the mitral annulus or into the LV outflow tract should be avoided, and often manual adjustment of segmental contours is essential to obtain accurate measurements. Increasing or decreasing the ROI width, it is possible to select endocardial, midwall, and epicardial GLS or, with the most recent software, the multilayer GLS (Fig. 5.2). There is a natural gradient from the endocardium, where GLS is highest, to the epicardium.[16] Although there is no evidence that favors one over another,[8] the endocardial GLS is the only one that is provided by all vendors.[17] After adjusting aortic valve closure, and repeating the same process for each apical view, the software provides the strain curves for each segment in each view, the median value, and the bull's eye polar map (Fig. 5.1C and D).

Image quality is particularly important for an accurate estimation of GLS as well, and a proper frame rate plays a pivotal role because a frame rate that is too low can cause the loss of speckles because they may move out of the plane on subsequent frames; however, a frame rate that is too high may not yield enough speckle displacement for the tracking algorithm to operate reliably. Thus, a frame rate between 40 and 80 frames/s seems to be the most appropriate.

The role of 2D STE GLS in the assessment of not only the systolic function of the left ventricle[18] but also of right ventricle,[19] left atrium,[20] and so on has been widely demonstrated and is discussed elsewhere in this book. However, 2D STE strain is affected by significant limitations that should be kept in mind.

TABLE 5.1 Two-Dimensional Speckle-Tracking Echocardiographic Parameters Cutoff Values from the EACVI NORRE Study

	Male (mean ± SD)	Male (95% CI)	Female (mean ±SD)	Female (95% CI)
Longitudinal strain (%)	−21.7 ± 2.5	−16.7 to −26.7	−23 ± 2.7	−17.8 to −28.2
Circumferential strain (%)	−31.4 ± 4.6	−22.3 to −40.5	−32.2 ± 4.4	−23.6 to −40.7
Radial strain (%)	36.3 ± 8	20.6 to 52.1	38.2 ± 8.5	21.5 to 54.8
Twist, degrees	7.4 ± 2.6	2.2 to 12.6	8.3 ± 3.3	1.9 to 14.8

CI, Confidence interval; *EACVI, NORRE,* European Association of Cardiovascular Imaging Normal Reference Ranges for Echocardiography; *SD,* standard deviation.

Reproduced with permission from Sugimoto T, et al: Echocardiographic reference ranges for normal left ventricular 2D strain: results from the EACVI NORRE study, *Eur Heart J Cardiovasc Imaging* 18:833–840, 2017.

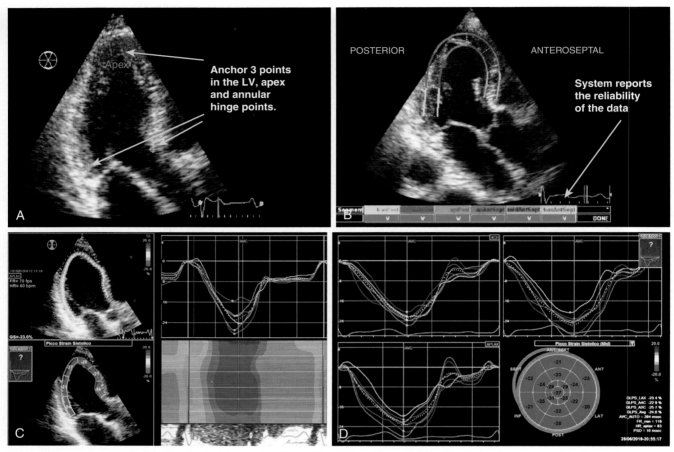

Figure 5.1. How to perform global longitudinal strain using General Electric's software. Starting from the three-chamber view, three fiducial landmarks are anchored in the left ventricular (LV) apex and annular hinge points (**A**). The software automatically traces the regions of interest (ROIs) and reports the reliability of the data (**B**). ROIs can be manually adjusted if incorrect. Then after adjusting aortic valve closure, the software provides the strain curves from the three-chamber view (**C**). Repeating these steps for the four- and two-chamber views, the software provides the strain curves from each view, the median value, and the bull's eye polar map (**D**).

Reproducibility is the most important point. As already discussed, it can be affected by technical issues, including poor image quality that reduces endocardial border and speckle detection, a too low or high frame rate, wrong placement of fiducial landmarks, the foreshortening of the LV apex, and so on. Accordingly, it would be reasonable that strain analysis should be performed by expert echocardiographers with specific training to avoid technical mistakes that affect the accuracy of the measurement.

Another important cause of low reproducibility, in past years considered one of the most significant technical limitations of strain analysis, is intervendor variability. However, important efforts have been made to reduce differences among vendors,[17,21] and a multicenter study recently found that no significant intervendor differences were noted in longitudinal strain, but intervendor differences were observed for circumferential and radial strain despite the use of vendor-independent software.[15]

Reproducibility can be affected by clinical issues as well. As already discussed, it is well known that strain range values change with age and sex. Moreover, hemodynamic factors and the volume status of the patient play important roles in this context. In particular, load dependency should be carefully considered, especially when serial evaluations of GLS are performed in patients who could experience significant change of preload, such as patients treated by chemotherapy, who often are affected by vomiting and diarrhea, and patients with severe renal failure treated with dialysis.[18]

In more recent years, 3D strain was developed to overcome the well-known intrinsic limitations of 2D echocardiography.

3D acquisition obtains a simultaneous computation of all three orthogonal strain values (radial, longitudinal, and circumferential) in the entire LV myocardium, as well as other more complex parameters such as area strain, a new measurement that includes both longitudinal and circumferential strain. In addition, more accurate LV torsion values can be calculated through the simultaneous measurement of rotations in each short-axis plane and the distance between the planes.[22] Excellent correlation with sonomicrometry and cardiac magnetic resonance imaging has been reported for 3D strain and area strain.[23,24] However, currently, the routine use of this technique is hindered by the limited availability of 3D echocardiography and the low spatial and temporal resolution of 3D echocardiography imaging.

Interestingly, 2D speckle tracking–derived parameters, so far used only as research tools with promising results, are myocardial mechanical dispersion and myocardial work (MW). Myocardial mechanical dispersion can be described as inhomogeneous contraction of LV segments caused by the dispersion of ventricular repolarization. This parameter can be accurately assessed by 2D STE longitudinal strain as the standard deviation of time to peak longitudinal strain of each segment of the LV, and it is related to the risk of malignant arrhythmias in patients with nonischemic dilated cardiomyopathy, myocardial infarction, and hypertrophic cardiomyopathy.[25–27]

MW was created to overcome the load dependency that affects strain measurements. Indeed, this new parameter incorporates both deformation and load into its analysis and investigates LV

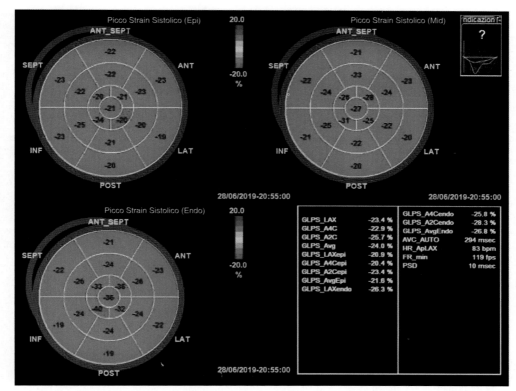

Figure 5.2. Example of multilayer assessment of two-dimensional speckle tracking left ventricular global longitudinal strain (GLS). As reported in the figure, the bull's eye map on the top left reported epicardial strain, on the top right midwall strain, and on the bottom left endocardial strain. The table shows each layer of GLS values for three-, four-, and two-chamber views, respectively, and the average values *(circled)*. *ANT,* Anterior; *INF,* inferior; *LAT,* lateral; *POST,* posterior; *SEPT,* septal.

performance in cases of changes in afterload that could lead to misleading conclusions if relying only on strain analysis. The calculation of MW requires blood pressure, from which the estimation of LV pressure curves is obtained, and the identification of valvular event times. A bull's eye with the segmental MW values and global values is provided from the software, and work is evaluated from mitral valve closure to mitral valve opening (in other words, the mechanical systole including isovolumetric relaxation). Along with segmental and global values for MW, a set of additional indices is also provided, including the "constructive work" (i.e., the work performed by a segment during shortening in systole), the "wasted work" (i.e., the contraction performed after aortic valve closure during lengthening in systole), and the "myocardial work efficiency" (i.e., the constructive work divided by the sum of constructive and wasted work). To date, this technique has been applied in myocardial ischemia and in identification of cardiac resynchronization therapy responders with good results.[28,29] Moreover, a recent multicenter study identified the cutoff values for these new parameters.[30]

REFERENCES

1. Rohmer D, Sitek A, Gullberg GT. Reconstruction and visualization of fiber and laminar structure in the normal human heart from ex vivo diffusion tensor magnetic resonance imaging (DTMRI) data. *Invest Radiol.* 2007;42:777–789.
2. Sallin EA. Fiber orientation and ejection fraction in the human left ventricle. *Biophys J.* 1969;9:954–964.
3. Sengupta PP, Tajik AJ, Chandrasekaran K, et al. Twist mechanics of the left ventricle: principles and application. *JACC Cardiovasc Imag.* 2008;1:366–376.
4. Marwick TH. Measurement of strain and strain rate by echocardiography: ready for prime time? *J Am Coll Cardiol.* 2006;47:1313–1327.
5. D'hooge J, Heimdal A, Jamal F, et al. Regional strain and strain rate measurements by cardiac ultrasound: principles, implementation and limitations. *Eur J Echocardiogr.* 2000;1:154–170. Erratum in: Eur J Echocardiogr 1:295–299, 2000.
6. Urheim S, Edvardsen T, Torp H, et al. Myocardial strain by Doppler echocardiography. Validation of a new method to quantify regional myocardial function. *Circulation.* 2000;102:1158–1164.
7. Helle-Valle T, Crosby J, Edvardsen T, et al. New noninvasive method for assessment of left ventricular rotation: speckle tracking echocardiography. *Circulation.* 2005;112:3149–3156.
8. Collier P, Phelan D, Klein A. A Test in context: myocardial strain measured by speckle-tracking echocardiography. *J Am Coll Cardiol.* 2017;69:1043–1056.
9. Leung DY, Ng AC. Emerging clinical role of strain imaging in echocardiography. *Heart Lung Circ.* 2010;19:161–174.
10. Leitman M, Lysyansky P, Sidenko S, et al. Two-dimensional strain—a novel software for real-time quantitative echocardiographic assessment of myocardial function. *J Am Soc Echocardiogr.* 2004;17:1021–1029.
11. Artis NJ, Oxborough DL, Williams G, et al. Two-dimensional strain imaging: a new echocardiographic advance with research and clinical applications. *Int J Cardiol.* 2008;123:240–248.
12. Geyer H, Caracciolo G, Abe H, et al. Assessment of myocardial mechanics using speckle tracking echocardiography: fundamentals and clinical applications. *J Am Soc Echocardiogr.* 2010;23:351–369. quiz 453–455. Erratum in: J Am Soc Echocardiogr 23:734, 2010.
13. Amundsen BH, Helle-Valle T, Edvardsen T, et al. *Noninvasive Myocardial Strain Measurement by Speckle Tracking Echocardiography: Validation against Sonomicrometry and Tagged Magnetic Resonance Imaging.* 2006;47:789–793.
14. Lang RM, Badano LP, Mor-Avi V, et al. Recommendations for cardiac chamber quantification by echocardiography in adults. *J Am Soc Echocardiogr.* 2015;28:1–39.e14.
15. Sugimoto T, Dulgheru R, Bernard A, et al. Echocardiographic reference ranges for normal left ventricular 2D strain: results from the EACVI NORRE study. *Eur Heart J Cardiovasc Imaging.* 2017;18:833–840.
16. Leitman M, Lysiansky M, Lysyansky P, et al. Circumferential and longitudinal strain in 3 myocardial layers in normal subjects and in patients with regional left ventricular dysfunction. *J Am Soc Echocardiogr.* 2010;23:64–70.
17. Farsalinos KE, Daraban AM, Ünlü S, et al. Head-to-head comparison of global longitudinal strain measurements among nine different vendors: the EACVI/ASE inter-vendor comparison study. *J Am Soc Echocardiogr.* 2015;28:1171–1181.
18. Zito C, Longobardo L, Citro R, et al. Ten years of 2D Longitudinal strain for early myocardial dysfunction detection: a clinical overview. *BioMed Res Int.* 2018:8979407. 2018.
19. Longobardo L, Suma V, Jain R, et al. Role of two-dimensional speckle-tracking echocardiography strain in the assessment of right ventricular systolic function and comparison with conventional parameters. *J Am Soc Echocardiogr.* 2017;30:937–946. e6.

20. Longobardo L, Todaro MC, Zito C, et al. Role of imaging in assessment of atrial fibrosis in patients with atrial fibrillation: state-of-the-art review. *Eur Heart J Cardiovasc Imag.* 2014;15:1–5.
21. Yang H, Marwick TH, Fukuda N, et al. Improvement in strain concordance between two major vendors after the strain standardization initiative. *J Am Soc Echocardiogr.* 2015;28:642–648.
22. Seo Y, Ishizu T, Atsumi A, et al. Three-dimensional speckle tracking echocardiography. *Circ J.* 2014;78:1290–1301.
23. Seo Y, Ishizu T, Enomoto Y, et al. Validation of 3D speckle tracking imaging to quantify regional myocardial deformation. *Circ Cardiovasc Imag.* 2009;2:451–459.
24. Seo Y, Ishizu T, Enomoto Y, et al. Endocardial surface area tracking for assessment of regional LV wall deformation with 3D speckle tracking imaging. *JACC Cardiovasc Imag.* 2011;4:358–365.
25. Haugaa KH, Goebel B, Dahlslett T, et al. Risk assessment of ventricular arrhythmias in patients with nonischemic dilated cardiomyopathy by strain echocardiography. *J Am Soc Echocardiogr.* 2012;25:667–673.
26. Ersbøll M, Valeur N, Andersen MJ, et al. Early echocardiographic deformation analysis for the prediction of sudden cardiac death and life-threatening arrhythmias after myocardial infarction. *JACC Cardiovasc Imag.* 2013;6:851–860.
27. Haland TF, Almaas VM, Hasselberg NE, et al. Strain echocardiography is related to fibrosis and ventricular arrhythmias in hypertrophic cardiomyopathy. *Eur Heart J Cardiovasc Imag.* 2016;17:613–621.
28. Boe E, Russell K, Eek C, et al. Non-invasive myocardial work index identifies acute coronary occlusion in patients with non-ST-segment elevation-acute coronary syndrome. *Eur Heart J Cardiovasc Imag.* 2015;16:1247–1255.
29. Galli E, Leclercq C, Fournet M, et al. Value of myocardial work estimation in the prediction of response to cardiac resynchronization therapy. *J Am Soc Echocardiogr.* 2018;31:220–230.
30. Manganaro R, Marchetta S, Dulgheru R, et al. Echocardiographic reference ranges for normal non-invasive myocardial work indices: results from the EACVI NORRE study. *Eur Heart J Cardiovasc Imag.* 2019;20:582–590.

6 Clinical Utility of Global Longitudinal Strain

Luca Longobardo, Concetta Zito, Scipione Carerj, Bijoy K. Khandheria

In the past two decades, two-dimensional speckle-tracking global longitudinal strain (GLS) has become one of the most important new echocardiographic parameters for the assessment of cardiac diseases. Indeed, it has been widely demonstrated that GLS provides reliable and early information regarding the diagnosis and prognosis in several clinical settings, and it is more practical than conventional parameters such as left ventricular ejection fraction (LVEF) because it detects early alterations that other parameters do not. Indeed, compared with LVEF, GLS was superior in predicting major adverse cardiac events in patients with heart failure, acute myocardial infarction, valvular heart disease, and miscellaneous cardiac diseases.[1] Moreover, it can provide an estimation not only of global but also of regional function through its polar projection, the so-called bull's eye map, that identifies typical patterns of myocardial damage that can help obtain the correct diagnosis[2,3] (Fig. 6.1).

GLS was developed as a parameter for the assessment of LV systolic function, and its effectiveness is well recognized in the current American Society of Echocardiography recommendations.[4] However, more recently, the use of GLS has been extended to different cardiac structures, including the right ventricle and atria, providing interesting results that require further study. Technical issues concerning how to perform GLS, and the limitations of this measurement have been widely discussed in other chapters of this book. This chapter discusses the diagnostic and prognostic role of GLS for the assessment of LV systolic function in the main clinical settings; moreover, data about the effectiveness of this measurement in the evaluation of right ventricle (RV) and left atrium (LA) are provided.

EVALUATION OF LEFT VENTRICULAR SYSTOLIC FUNCTION

Left Ventricular Hypertrophy

LV hypertrophy (LVH) is a very common finding, but often it is quite difficult to distinguish between physiologic and pathological hypertrophy, and, within the latter group, to identify the underlying disease. In this context, GLS and regional longitudinal strain (LS) have had a significant role in detecting myocardial dysfunction correlated to fibrosis or storage or infiltrative cardiac disease. Indeed, it has been widely demonstrated that GLS is normal in athletes (see Fig. 6.1A), who show benign LVH caused by systematic training.[5] On the contrary, GLS is reduced in patients with asymptomatic hypertension (see Fig. 6.1B) even when LVH has not occurred yet.[6] GLS is also markedly reduced in all cardiomyopathies that cause LVH, including hypertrophic cardiomyopathy (HCM) (see Fig. 6.1C), cardiac amyloidosis (CA) (see Fig. 6.1D), and Anderson-Fabry disease. HCM is the most noticeable example of severe pathological LVH. In this context, a pronounced impairment of GLS with a significant gradient of decreasing LS from the apex to the base,[7] although EF is often normal or supernormal. The regional alterations of strain in the polar maps identify the most damaged myocardial segments with increased fibrosis, with a very high correspondence with cardiac magnetic resonance. Moreover, the impairment of GLS can be an independent predictor of cardiac death or defibrillator discharge in this population of patients.[8] Similarly, GLS and regional LS plays an important role in the diagnosis of CA. Indeed, even if EF can be normal in the first stage of the disease, GLS is always reduced. In addition, the bull's eye polar map shows a very typical pattern, characterized by a regional and progressive variations in LS from the base to the apex with a relative LV "apical-sparing" pattern.[2] The evidence of this pattern, even not exclusive of CA, is quite accurate in the diagnosis of the disease, providing a significant support in the differential diagnosis. On the other hand, in Anderson-Fabry cardiomyopathy, a decrease of LS at the basal posterolateral wall has been reported.[2] However, this finding needs to be further confirmed.

Coronary Artery Disease

LS has an important diagnostic and prognostic role in patients with coronary artery disease (CAD). Indeed, as discussed in Chapter 5, LS evaluates the systolic function of endocardial fibers, the most sensitive to ischemia. Thus, it is easily understandable that LS is particularly accurate in the detection of subtle ischemia in patients with acute coronary occlusion and non–ST-segment elevation acute coronary syndrome that cannot be assessed by wall motion score index.[9] Moreover, regional LS allows a reliable estimation of coronary involvement because the regional alterations of LS identified in the bull's eye maps typically recall the coronary artery distribution (see Fig. 6.1E). In this context, the regional pattern of LS impairment provides the differential diagnosis with

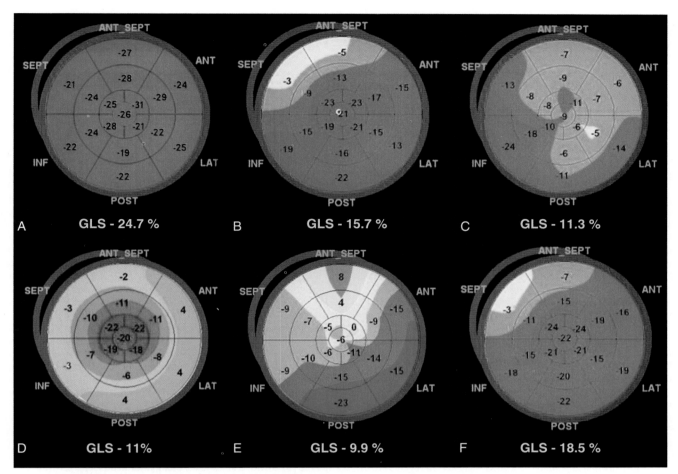

Figure 6.1. Bull's eye maps of global longitudinal strain (GLS) depicting different patterns of left ventricular hypertrophy: a normal subject (**A**), hypertension (**B**), hypertrophic cardiomyopathy (**C**), amyloidosis with the classical "apical-sparing" pattern (**D**), anterior myocardial infarction (**E**), and aortic stenosis with hypertrophy of basal segments (**F**). *ANT,* anterior; *ANT SEPT,* anteroseptal; *INF,* inferior; *LAT,* lateral; *POST,* posterior; *SEPT,* septal. (Modified from Zito C, et al: Ten years of 2D longitudinal strain for early myocardial dysfunction detection: a clinical overview, *Biomed Res Int* 8979407, 2018.)

Takotsubo syndrome, characterized by a reduction of LS in the apical segments with increased contractility of basal segments, and with myocarditis, characterized by an impairment of myocardial contractility without the typical distribution of coronary arteries.[2] As a prognostic parameter, reduced GLS has been shown to predict negative LV remodeling and poor outcomes, including death, heart failure, and reinfarction in patients with acute myocardial infarction.[10] These findings suggest a significant prognostic role of GLS not only in patients with acute CAD but also in patients with chronic CAD, who should undergo GLS assessment during follow-up.

Heart Valve Disease

The role of GLS in patients with heart valve disease has been reevaluated over the past years. The most solid data have been reported on aortic stenosis (AS). Indeed, it has been demonstrated that GLS gradually decreases while AS severity increases without any simultaneous change in LVEF[2,11] and that in asymptomatic patients with severe AS and normal EF, reduced GLS is associated with an abnormal exercise response.[12] Maybe more interesting is the prognostic role of GLS in this population. Indeed, it has been reported that GLS was associated with an increased risk of cardiac events over EF[13] and AS gradient even in asymptomatic patients and that a cutoff value of −14.7% was associated with increased mortality rate in patients with severe AS and normal LVEF.[14] These findings explain why in the recent recommendations for the

multimodality imaging strategies for the assessment of AS, GLS was included as a parameter for the risk stratification of patients with asymptomatic severe AS for the evaluation of an early surgical treatment (class IIb).[15]

The regional distribution of myocardial contractility impairment in patients with severe AS is similar to that reported in CA, with a significant decrease of LS in the basal segments and relative apical sparing (see Fig. 6.1F).[2,3] This evidence again underlines the difficulty of the differential diagnosis in patients with LVH, the most common finding also in patients with AS, and the role of regional LS that, together with other parameters, can help narrow down the field of diagnostic hypotheses.

Less robust but growing evidence is available about the prognostic role of GLS in patients with aortic (AR) and mitral regurgitation (MR). It has been reported that a reduced GLS is associated with AR progression over time. Indeed, Di Salvo and coworkers[16] studied a population of young patients with congenital isolated moderate to severe AR and found that LV LS was significantly reduced in patients with progressive AR compared with those with stable AR and that the only significant risk factor for progressive AR was average LV LS. Moreover, Alashi and colleagues[17] evaluated a cohort of asymptomatic patients with severe chronic AR and preserved LVEF and found that reduced GLS correlated with a reduced survival rate at 5-year follow-up. In addition, in patients with moderate to severe AR reduced GLS was associated with disease progression during conservative management and with impaired outcome after surgery.[18] These data seem to suggest a role for GLS in the risk stratification of these patients, but so far, there are no recommendations for the use of this measurement in the assessment of patient with AR. Similarly, GLS was shown to be reduced in patients with severe MR,[19] and in asymptomatic patients with degenerative MR, GLS was able to identify subtle LV systolic dysfunction.[20] Moreover, Witkowski and coworkers[21] analyzed a large series of patients treated with mitral valve replacement and found that reduced GLS was a major independent predictor of long-term LV dysfunction after adjustment for EF and LV end-diastolic diameter. Despite these data, GLS has not been included in the guidelines for the management of patients with MR.

Cancer Therapeutics–Related Cardiac Dysfunction

According to current guidelines, cancer therapeutics–related cardiac dysfunction (CTRCD) can be diagnosed when a decrease in LVEF of more than 10% to a value less than 53% occurred in patients treated with chemotherapy.[22] However, EF decreases late during chemotherapy, and Thavendiranathan and colleagues reported that the interoperator variability of EF was about 10% in the assessment of LV systolic function in their cohort of patients treated with chemotherapy.[23] On the contrary, GLS showed to be a sensible parameter for the early assessment of subtle LV systolic dysfunction, for example, in women with breast cancer treated with anthracycline, taxanes and trastuzumab.[24] Moreover, it has been reported that GLS was able to detect preclinical changes in LV systolic function, before conventional changes in LVEF, in human epidermal growth factor receptor 2–positive patients with breast cancer treated with trastuzumab.[25] Accordingly, the use of GLS for the evaluation of patients treated with chemotherapy has been recently recommended by the expert consensus for multimodality imaging evaluation of adult patients during and after cancer therapy.[22] In this document, authors stated that a relative percentage reduction in GLS of more than 15% from baseline should be considered abnormal and a marker of early LV subclinical dysfunction in patients treated with chemotherapy and that this parameter should be used together with LVEF for the surveillance of these patients. In addition, it has been reported that anthracycline causes more myocardial damage of the septal and apical segments of the left ventricle;[2] however, these data need further study.

EVALUATION OF THE RIGHT VENTRICLE

The fundamental role that the right side of the heart plays in many diseases has been only recently considered. RV function influences the prognosis of patients with heart failure, heart valve disease, myocardial infarction, cardiomyopathies, and so on. The echocardiographic assessment of RV systolic function relies on the so-called conventional parameters, including tricuspid annular plane systolic excursion (TAPSE), right-sided index of myocardial performance, Doppler tissue imaging S′ wave, and fractional area change. However, in the past decade, the application of GLS to the study of the right ventricle demonstrated that LS is able to detect subtle RV systolic dysfunction earlier and with greater accuracy than conventional parameters in several clinical settings.[26] RV GLS is commonly assessed in the apical four-chamber view only and could include both the RV free wall and septal segments or the RV free wall alone. There is not unanimous agreement about which method should be preferred; currently, the use of the RV free wall alone seems to have the largest body of evidence and is suggested by the current guidelines.[4] The same guidelines indicated a RV free wall longitudinal strain cutoff value of −20% to −21% to define normal RV systolic function.[4] Of course, the use of GLS for the study of RV is affected by the same limitations already described for the LV and by peculiar limitations. Indeed, RV chamber shape is more complex than LV one, with the inflow and outflow portions in different planes and a thin RV wall that makes it difficult to limit the width of the region of interest to the

myocardium; moreover, software originally designed for analysis of LV strain must be "tricked" to calculate RV strain because the images are inverted compared with LV assessment; therefore, the bull's eye figures cannot be considered.[26]

The role of GLS for the assessment of RV systolic function has been studied in several clinical settings, but the most robust data have been obtained in patients with pulmonary hypertension (PH) and thromboembolic disease, heart failure, and arrhythmogenic RV dysplasia. In patients with PH[27] or acute and chronic thromboembolism,[28] RV GLS showed a better correlation with invasive hemodynamic parameters of RV performance than conventional measurements. Indeed, Fukuda and colleagues[27] found that RV LS was significantly lower in patients with PH than in normal control participants (Fig. 6.2) and that RV LS was an independent echocardiographic predictor not only of hemodynamic RV performance, including mean pulmonary artery pressure and pulmonary vascular resistance, but also of RV EF and RV end-systolic volume measured by cardiac magnetic resonance imaging and with 6-min walking distance. Moreover, it showed to be a powerful predictor of cardiovascular events and death with high sensitivity and good specificity in these patients.[29] A similar efficacy as a prognostic parameter has been reported in the setting of heart failure with reduced LV EF, in which a reduced RV GLS was associated with death, need for emergency transplantation, and acute HF admissions on short-term follow-up[30] even with an incremental prognostic value to LV EF.[31] Moreover, RV GLS is an important tool in risk stratification for RV failure in patients eligible for LV assist device implantation; a significantly reduced RV strain value obtained before or immediately after implantation can identify patients who are at higher risk of death.[32] Finally, RV GLS seems to be superior to conventional parameters in the assessment of subtle RV systolic dysfunction in patients with initial stages of arrhythmogenic RV dysplasia[33] and in the detection of subclinical RV functional abnormalities in asymptomatic carriers of pathogenic mutations.[34]

EVALUATION OF LEFT ATRIAL FUNCTION

The pathophysiological role of LA in several disease states has been widely elucidated, demonstrating that LA plays a relevant role in several conditions directly or indirectly affecting the heart. LA strain provides additional information compared with the conventional parameters for the assessment of atrial function.[35] Three different LA functions can be recognized during the cardiac cycle: (1) the reservoir phase, when during LV systole, the LA receives blood from the pulmonary veins, characterized by a positive strain deformation (this seems to be the most effective LA strain parameter for the assessment of LA function); (2) the conduit phase, when during early diastole, LA serves as a conduit, passively filling LV cavity according to pressure gradient; and (3) the pump function, when during late diastole it contributes to ventricular filling with an atrial contraction, characterized by a negative strain deformation. LA reservoir LS has been tested in several clinical settings, but the most robust data have been reported so far in the context of atrial fibrillation (AF)[36] and in the assessment of diastolic function in patients with heart failure and preserved ejection function (HFpEF). In particular, LA strain is an effective tool for the indirect assessment of early atrial remodeling and fibrosis, the main pathophysiological background of the onset and persistence of AF.[12] Accordingly, LA strain is reduced in patients with AF even before atrial dilatation has occurred,[37] and a normal LA strain shows to be an independent predictor of sinus rhythm maintenance in patients with lone AF undergoing AF ablation or external electrical cardioversion.[38] In the context of the assessment of diastolic function in patients with HFpEF, it has been reported that LA strain was able to improve the evaluation of diastolic function even when distinction between grades was difficult with conventional echocardiographic parameters (Fig. 6.3).[39]

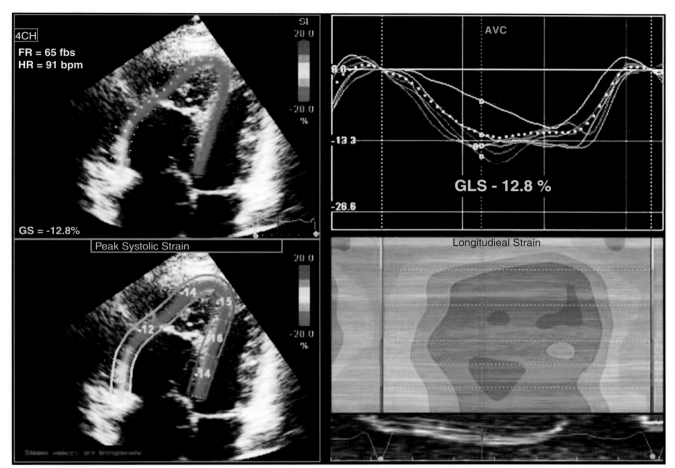

Figure 6.2. Example of reduced global longitudinal strain (GLS) of the right ventricle in a patient with pulmonary hypertension. *AVC,* aortic valve closure; *FR,* frame rate; *HR,* heart rate.

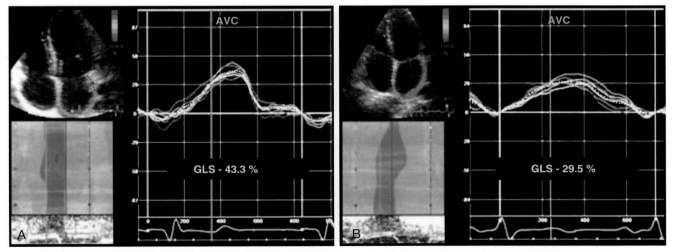

Figure 6.3. Example of left atrial reservoir longitudinal strain (GLS) in a normal participant (**A**) and in a patient with heart failure and preserved ejection function and grade 3 diastolic dysfunction (restrictive pattern) (**B**). *AVC,* aortic valve closure.

REFERENCES

1. Kalam K, Otahal P, Marwick TH. Prognostic implications of global LV dysfunction: a systematic review and meta-analysis of global longitudinal strain and ejection fraction. *Heart*. 2014;100:1673–1680.
2. Zito C, Longobardo L, Citro R, et al. Ten years of 2D longitudinal strain for early myocardial dysfunction detection: a clinical overview. *BioMed Res Int*. 2018:8979407.
3. Singh A, Voss WB, Lentz RW, et al. The diagnostic and prognostic value of echocardiographic strain. *JAMA Cardiol*. 2019;4:580–588.
4. Lang RM, Badano LP, Mor-Avi V, et al. Recommendations for cardiac chamber quantification by echocardiography in adults. *J Am Soc Echocardiogr*. 2015;28:1–39.e14.
5. Caselli S, Montesanti D, Autore C, et al. Patterns of left ventricular longitudinal strain and strain rate in Olympic athletes. *J Am Soc Echocardiogr*. 2015;28:245–253.
6. Imbalzano E, Zito C, Carerj S, et al. Left ventricular function in hypertension: new insight by speckle tracking echocardiography. *Echocardiography*. 2011;28(6):649–657.
7. Popović ZB, Kwon DH, Mishra M, et al. Association between regional ventricular function and myocardial fibrosis in hypertrophic cardiomyopathy assessed by speckle tracking echocardiography and delayed hyperenhancement magnetic resonance imaging. *J Am Soc Echocardiogr*. 2008;21:1299–1305.
8. Tower-Rader A, Betancor J, Popovic ZB, et al. Incremental prognostic utility of left ventricular global longitudinal strain in hypertrophic obstructive cardiomyopathy patients and preserved left ventricular ejection fraction. *J Am Heart Assoc*. 2017;6.
9. Eek C, Grenne B, Brunvand H, et al. Strain echocardiography predicts acute coronary occlusion in patients with non-ST-segment elevation acute coronary syndrome. *Eur J Echocardiogr*. 2010;11:501–508.
10. Antoni ML, Mollema SA, Delgado V, et al. Prognostic importance of strain and strain rate after acute myocardial infarction. *Eur Heart J*. 2010;31:1640–1647.
11. Miyazaki S, Daimon M, Miyazaki T, et al. Global longitudinal strain in relation to the severity of aortic stenosis: a two-dimensional speckle-tracking study. *Echocardiography*. 2011;28:703–708.
12. Lafitte S, Perlant M, Reant P, et al. Impact of impaired myocardial deformations on exercise tolerance and prognosis in patients with asymptomatic aortic stenosis. *Eur J Echocardiogr*. 2009;10:414–419.
13. Kearney LG, Lu K, Ord M, et al. Global longitudinal strain is a strong independent predictor of all-cause mortality in patients with aortic stenosis. *Eur Heart J Cardiovasc Imag*. 2012;13:827–833.
14. Magne J, Cosyns B, Popescu BA, et al. Distribution and prognostic significance of left ventricular global longitudinal strain in asymptomatic significant aortic stenosis: an individual participant data meta-analysis. *JACC Cardiovasc Imag*. 2019;12:84–92.
15. Dulgheru R, Pibarot P, Sengupta PP, et al. Multimodality imaging strategies for the assessment of aortic stenosis: viewpoint of the heart valve clinic International Database (HAVEC) group. *Circ Cardiovasc Imag*. 2016;9:e004352.
16. Di Salvo G, Rea A, Mormile A, et al. Usefulness of bidimensional strain imaging for predicting outcome in asymptomatic patients aged ≤ 16 years with isolated moderate to severe aortic regurgitation. *Am J Cardiol*. 2012;110:1051–1055.
17. Alashi A, Mentias A, Abdallah A, et al. Incremental prognostic utility of left ventricular global longitudinal strain in asymptomatic patients with significant chronic aortic regurgitation and preserved left ventricular ejection fraction. *JACC Cardiovasc Imag*. 2018;11:673–682.
18. Olsen NT, Sogaard P, Larsson HB, et al. Speckle-tracking echocardiography for predicting outcome in chronic aortic regurgitation during conservative management and after surgery. *JACC Cardiovasc Imag*. 2011;4:223–230.
19. Marciniak A, Claus P, Sutherland GR, et al. Changes in systolic left ventricular function in isolated mitral regurgitation. A strain rate imaging study. *Eur Heart J*. 2007;28:2627–2636.
20. Lancellotti P, Cosyns B, Zacharakis D, et al. Importance of left ventricular longitudinal function and functional reserve in patients with degenerative mitral regurgitation: assessment by two-dimensional speckle tracking. *J Am Soc Echocardiogr*. 2008;21:1331–1336.
21. Witkowski TG, Thomas JD, Debonnaire PJ, et al. Global longitudinal strain predicts left ventricular dysfunction after mitral valve repair. *Eur Heart J Cardiovasc Imag*. 2013;14:69–76.
22. Plana JC, Galderisi M, Barac A, et al. Expert consensus for multimodality imaging evaluation of adult patients during and after cancer therapy. *J Am Soc Echocardiogr*. 2014;27:911–939.
23. Thavendiranathan P, Grant AD, Negishi T, et al. Reproducibility of echocardiographic techniques for sequential assessment of left ventricular ejection fraction and volumes: application to patients undergoing cancer chemotherapy. *J Am Coll Cardiol*. 2013;61:77–84.
24. Sawaya H, Sebag IA, Plana JC, et al. Assessment of echocardiography and biomarkers for the extended prediction of cardiotoxicity in patients treated with anthracyclines, taxanes, and trastuzumab. *Circ Cardiovasc Imag*. 2012;5:596–603.
25. Fallah-Rad N, Walker JR, Wassef A, et al. The utility of cardiac biomarkers, tissue velocity and strain imaging, and cardiac magnetic resonance imaging in predicting early left ventricular dysfunction in patients with human epidermal growth factor receptor II-positive breast cancer treated with adjuvant trastuzumab therapy. *J Am Coll Cardiol*. 2011;57:2263–2270.
26. Longobardo L, Suma V, Jain R, et al. Role of two-dimensional speckle-tracking echocardiography strain in the assessment of right ventricular systolic function and comparison with conventional parameters. *J Am Soc Echocardiogr*. 2017;30:937–946.e6.
27. Fukuda Y, Tanaka H, Sugiyama D, et al. Utility of right ventricular free wall speckle-tracking strain for evaluation of right ventricular performance in patients with pulmonary hypertension. *J Am Soc Echocardiogr*. 2011;24:1101–1108.
28. Lee JH, Park JH, Park KI, et al. A comparison of different techniques of two-dimensional speckle-tracking strain measurements of right ventricular systolic function in patients with acute pulmonary embolism. *J Cardiovasc Ultrasound*. 2014;22:65–71.
29. Motoji Y, Tanaka H, Fukuda Y, et al. Efficacy of right ventricular free-wall longitudinal speckle-tracking strain for predicting long-term outcome in patients with pulmonary hypertension. *Circ J*. 2013;77:756–763.
30. Cameli M, Lisi M, Righini FM, et al. Right ventricular longitudinal strain correlates well with right ventricular stroke work index in patients with advanced heart failure referred for heart transplantation. *J Card Fail*. 2012;18:208–215.
31. Motoki H, Borowski AG, Shrestha K, et al. Right ventricular global longitudinal strain provides prognostic value incremental to left ventricular ejection fraction in patients with heart failure. *J Am Soc Echocardiogr*. 2014;27:726–732.
32. Grant AD, Smedira NG, Starling RC, et al. Independent and incremental role of quantitative right ventricular evaluation for the prediction of right ventricular failure after left ventricular assist device implantation. *J Am Coll Cardiol*. 2012;60:521–528.
33. Aneq MÅ, Engvall J, Brudin L, et al. Evaluation of right and left ventricular function using speckle tracking echocardiography in patients with arrhythmogenic right ventricular cardiomyopathy and their first degree relatives. *Cardiovasc Ultrasound*. 2012;10:37.
34. Teske AJ, Cox MG, Te Riele AS, et al. Early detection of regional functional abnormalities in asymptomatic ARVD/C gene carriers. *J Am Soc Echocardiogr*. 2012;25:997–1006.
35. Longobardo L, Zito C, Khandheria BK. Left atrial function index: did we end up waiting for Godot? *Eur Heart J Cardiovasc Imag*. 2017;18:128–129.
36. Longobardo L, Todaro MC, Zito C, et al. Role of imaging in assessment of atrial fibrosis in patients with atrial fibrillation: state-of-the-art review. *Eur Heart J Cardiovasc Imag*. 2014;15:1–5.
37. Todaro MC, Choudhuri I, Belohlavek M, et al. New echocardiographic techniques for evaluation of left atrial mechanics. *Eur Heart J Cardiovasc Imag*. 2012;13:973–984.
38. Hammerstingl C, Schwekendiek M, Momcilovic D, et al. Left atrial deformation imaging with ultrasound based two-dimensional speckle-tracking predicts the rate of recurrence of paroxysmal and persistent atrial fibrillation after successful ablation procedures. *J Cardiovasc Electrophysiol*. 2012;23:247–255.
39. Singh A, Addetia K, Maffessanti F, et al. LA strain for categorization of LV diastolic dysfunction. *JACC Cardiovasc Imaging*. 2017;10:735–743.

7 Transthoracic Echocardiography: Nomenclature and Standard Views

Carol Mitchell, Peter S. Rahko

IMAGING PLANES

The imaging planes are the long-axis (images acquired in the parasternal long-axis [PLAX] views), short-axis (images acquired in the parasternal short-axis [PSAX] views), and apical (images acquired in the apical views) planes (Fig. 7.1).[1]

IMAGE ACQUISITION WINDOWS

The following windows are used to acquire transthoracic echocardiography (TTE) images. The windows are the parasternal, apical, subcostal, and suprasternal notch (SSN). The parasternal window is located adjacent to the sternum and at the level of the third or fourth intercostal space. Images are acquired from the anterior surface of the body and can be acquired from the left or right window. The location of the window is described in relationship to the sternum. A *left parasternal window* refers to a window on the left side of the sternum. A *right parasternal window* refers to a window to the right of the sternum. The apical window is located over the area where the maximal apical impulse is felt. With normal cardiac situs (levocardia), the apical impulse is felt on the patient's left side usually in alignment with the midaxillary line in the fifth intercostal space. This location is typically where the transducer is placed for starting the acquisition of the apical window views; however, it should be noted that multiple apical windows may be used to acquire all apical images of the heart. The subcostal window is located just below the xiphoid process. The SSN window is located just superior to the manubrium of the sternum (Fig. 7.2).[1]

SCANNING MANEUVERS: TRANSDUCER MOVEMENT DESCRIPTIONS

Transducer movements are described using the terms *tilt, sweep, rotate, slide, rock,* and *angle* (Figs. 7.3 to 7.7). The term *tilt* is used to describe movements in which the transducer remains in a stationary position and the face of the transducer is manipulated to demonstrate additional image planes in the same axis.[1]

The term *sweep* refers to the intentional action of capturing a long video clip demonstrating anatomical relationships. For example, using tilt, capturing a long video clip from the apical window imaging from the coronary sinus (CS; posterior heart) to the apical five-chamber view (anterior heart) is an example of a sweep. The term *rotate* refers to a movement in which the transducer stays in the same position but the orientation index marker is moved from one location to another in a clockwise or counterclockwise fashion (see Fig. 7.4).[1,2] Moving the transducer orientation index marker from pointing toward the right shoulder to pointing toward the left shoulder (i.e., moving from the long-axis plane to the parasternal short-axis plane) is an example of the rotation maneuver. The term *slide* refers to a movement in which the transducer is physically moved from one location to another. Moving up or down a rib space is an example of the slide maneuver

(see Fig. 7.5).[1,2] *Rock* and *angle* refer to smaller movements used to optimize an image. The term *rock* is used to describe a small movement of the transducer toward or away from the orientation marker while staying in the same imaging plane (see Fig. 7.6).[1] This movement is often used to center a structure. *Angle* refers to a movement in which the transducer remains in the same position, but the sound beam is directed toward an anatomic structure of interest.[1] An example of the angle movement is directing the sound beam toward the tricuspid valve (TV) and then toward the pulmonic valve (PV) while imaging in the parasternal window, short-axis view at the level of the great vessels (see Fig. 7.7).

TRANSDUCER ORIENTATION

All ultrasound imaging transducers have an orientation index marker. For each view described in the two-dimensional (2D) imaging section of this chapter, information is provided regarding the placement of the orientation index marker.

STANDARD VIEWS: TWO-DIMENSIONAL IMAGING

The TTE examination begins with the patient in the left lateral decubitus position and with acquisition of the parasternal window long-axis (PLAX) view images.[1] The transducer is placed in the third to fourth intercostals space in the left parasternal window with the orientation index marker directed toward the patient's right shoulder at approximately the 9 to 10 o'clock position.[1] Images acquired in the PLAX views are depicted in Table 7.1.

The first image acquired in the PLAX view is a view of the left ventricle (LV) with an increased imaging depth. The image should display the long axis of the interventricular septum perpendicular to the ultrasound beam and positioned with the leaflet tips of the mitral valve (MV) in the center of the image, and the ventricle should be elongated. If the ventricle appears tipped, the transducer can be moved closer to the sternum and up a rib space to bring the LV more perpendicular (horizontal) to the ultrasound beam. Alternative maneuvers to "level off" the tipped-up ventricle include (1) sitting the patient more upright and (2) having the patient exhale strongly and hold the exhalation. If the ventricle appears rounded or foreshortened, the transducer should be adjusted by rotating, tilting, or angling to maximize the LV cavity length within the field of view. This image is taken to assess for pericardial and pleural effusions. This image should be taken as a clip.

The next image clip acquired is the PLAX LV view. For this view, the depth should be adjusted to leave about 1.0 cm of depth beyond the pericardium. This view should be optimized to demonstrate movement of the aortic valve (AV) and MV leaflets. From this view, 2D linear measurements of the right ventricle (RV) diameter, interventricular septum thickness, LV diameter, and LV posterior wall thickness can be made in

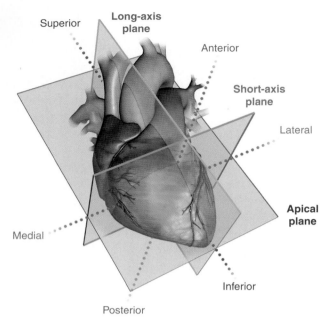

Figure 7.1. Imaging planes of the heart. Long-axis *(blue)*, short-axis *(green)*, and apical *(purple)* views. (From Mitchell C, et al: Guidelines for performing a comprehensive transthoracic echocardiographic examination in adults: recommendations from the American Society of Echocardiography. *J Am Soc Echocardiogr* 32:1–64, 2019.)

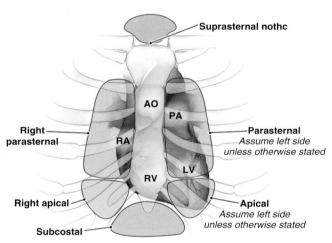

Figure 7.2. Image acquisition windows. *AO,* Aorta; *LV,* left ventricle; *PA,* pulmonary artery; *RA,* right atrium; *RV,* right ventricle. (From Mitchell C, et al: Guidelines for performing a comprehensive transthoracic echocardiographic examination in adults: recommendations from the American Society of Echocardiography, *J Am Soc Echocardiogr* 32:1–64, 2019.)

end-diastole. After performing these measurements, one can scroll to the end-systole frame and measure the LV diameter in systole. The next measurement to be made from this view is the proximal right ventricular outflow tract (RVOT) diameter at end-diastole followed by measurement of the left atrium (LA) diameter in end-systole. After acquiring this clip, zoom on the AV and left ventricular outflow tract (LVOT). After assessing the zoomed AV, the transducer should be slid slightly toward the sinotubular junction and ascending aorta, and another video clip should be acquired. Measurements of the LVOT and aortic

annulus should be made inner edge to inner edge at midsystole where the diameter is the largest. Next, the diameter of the aortic sinus of Valsalva, sinotubular junction, and ascending aorta should be measured. These structures are measured leading edge to leading edge in end-diastole. An alternative view for imaging the ascending aorta is the right parasternal view of the aorta. To acquire this image, place the patient in the right lateral decubitus position with the right arm moved above the head. The transducer should be placed in the second or third intercostal space with the orientation index marker directed to the patient's right shoulder.[1] The next image clip to acquire is the zoomed view of the MV. The region of interest should be positioned over the MV and should include the LA and inflow portion of the LV.[1,3]

The next PLAX view to acquire is the RVOT. This view demonstrates the RVOT, pulmonary valve (PV), and proximal pulmonary artery (PA). From the PLAX LV view, tilt the transducer anteriorly and rotate the orientation index marker clockwise.[1] This image should be recorded as a clip.

After interrogation of the RVOT, the RVOT should be imaged and a clip recorded. From the RVOT view, return to the PLAX LV view and then tilt the transducer inferiorly toward the right hip.[1] The transducer may also need to be rotated counterclockwise to best image the TV. When the image is optimized, the TV should be visualized in the center of the sector, and the right atrium (RA) and RV should be visible. Color Doppler images should be acquired after each grayscale clip.

Typically, after acquiring the PLAX images, the transducer is rotated clockwise to have the orientation index marker pointing toward the patient's left shoulder.[1] The patient remains in the left lateral decubitus position, and the parasternal short-axis (PSAX) views are acquired. Images to acquire from the PSAX views are provided in Table 7.2.[1]

The first PSAX view to acquire is at the level of the great vessels (aorta and pulmonary artery). In this view, the image is acquired superior to the level of the AV, and the image demonstrates the pulmonary valve, pulmonary artery, and in some cases the left and right branch pulmonary arteries.[1] This image should be recorded as a clip. After this view, the transducer should be tilted inferiorly to demonstrate the AV, TV, and PV. A clip should be recorded. After imaging with the wide sector, the sector should be narrowed and the transducer angled to focus on the TV and then the PV. After acquiring these structures, zoom on the AV to evaluate leaflet excursion and the number of leaflets.[1] Although not part of the routine examination, at this level, small movements of the transducer can be performed to demonstrate the origins of the coronary arteries.[1,4]

After examining the anatomic structures at the great vessel level, the transducer is tilted inferiorly and slightly leftward to image the MV. At this level, the motion of the MV leaflets should be examined; the RV is seen anterior to the LV as a crescent-shaped structure, and the anterior, lateral, and inferior walls of the LV are seen.[1] A video clip should be acquired at this level.

Next, the transducer is tilted inferiorly to acquire a clip at the level of the papillary muscles. At this level, the ventricle should appear circular, and both papillary muscles should be visualized. This image represents the mid-LV cavity and is particularly important in evaluating global and regional function of the LV. The RV is also seen at this level. Two clips should be acquired at this level with images optimized to evaluate myocardial thickening and LV function. The final PSAX image acquired as a clip is an image of the LV apex. Often the transducer needs to be tilted inferiorly and may need to also be slid down an intercostal space to best visualize the apex.[1] Color Doppler images should be acquired after each grayscale clip.

The next set of images to acquire are from the apical window. To locate the apical window, feel for the maximal apical impulse below the breast tissue. This is typically at

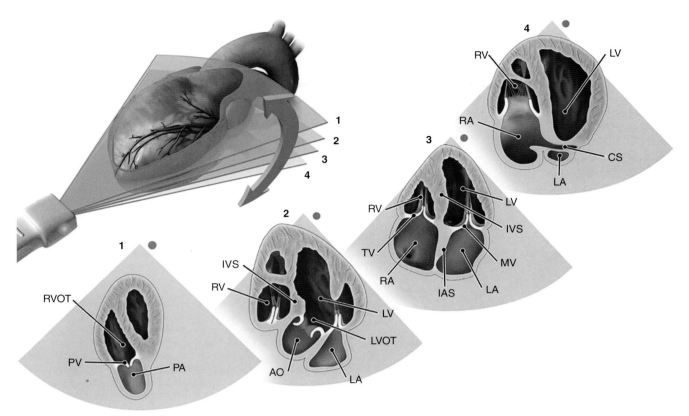

Figure 7.3. Tilting transducer movement. The *blue dot* represents the orientation index marker. *AO,* Aorta; *CS,* coronary sinus; *IAS,* interatrial septum; *IVS,* interventricular septum; *LA,* left atrium; *LV,* left ventricle; *LVOT,* left ventricular outflow tract; *MV,* mitral valve; *PA,* pulmonary artery; *PV,* pulmonary valve; *RA,* right atrium; *RV,* right ventricle; *RVOT,* right ventricular outflow tract; *TV,* tricuspid valve. (From Mitchell C, et al: Guidelines for performing a comprehensive transthoracic echocardiographic examination in adults: recommendations from the American Society of Echocardiography, *J Am Soc Echocardiogr* 32:1–64, 2019.)

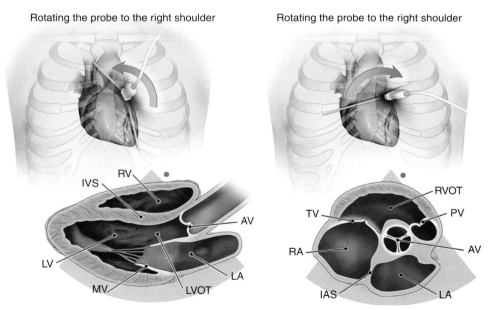

Figure 7.4. Rotation scanning maneuver. The *blue dot* represents the index orientation marker as it is related to the image. In the parasternal long-axis image, the *blue dot* represents the orientation index marker located on the superior aspect of the image. In the parasternal short-axis image, the *blue dot* represents the position of the orientation index marker and the lateral aspect of the image. *IAS,* interatrial septum; *AV,* aortic valve; *IVS,* interventricular septum; *LA,* left atrium; *LV,* left ventricle; *LVOT,* left ventricular outflow tract; *MV,* mitral valve; *PV,* pulmonary valve; *RA,* right atrium; *RV,* right ventricle; *RVOT,* right ventricular outflow tract; *TV,* tricuspid valve. (From Mitchell C, et al: Guidelines for performing a comprehensive transthoracic echocardiographic examination in adults: recommendations from the American Society of Echocardiography, *J Am Soc Echocardiogr* 32:1–64, 2019.)

the level of the fifth intercostal space and aligned near the midaxillary line.[1] Images to acquire from the apical window are listed in Table 7.3.

The first view acquired in the apical window is the apical four-chamber (A4C) view. To acquire this view, place the transducer over the apical impulse with the orientation index marker in the 4 to 5 o'clock position toward the bed. The image should be optimized so that all four chambers are seen. Left-sided structures are displayed on the right side of the display monitor. The heart should be aligned so that the apex of the LV is in the center of the sector, and maximal length of the LV should be demonstrated. As a guide, typically the LV should make up to two-thirds of the length and the LA one-third of the length from the deepest portion of the LA wall to the LV apex. The LV should also taper to an ellipsoid shape at the apex. If the LV appears short in length or the LV apex appears rounded, the image may be foreshortened, and the transducer should be further manipulated to demonstrate the LV at its maximum length. The RV is displayed on the left side of the monitor, and the moderator band should be identified in the apical portion of the RV. Motion of the atrioventricular valves (MV and TV) should be evaluated in this view along with assessment of size of all four chambers. Instrumentation settings should be optimized to assess performance and demonstrate good visualization of the walls and septa of all chambers. The first clip should demonstrate all four chambers to assist with evaluation of chamber size. After this initial view, the sector size and depth should be adjusted to focus on the LV for further assessment of the regional wall motion and global function. The sector should be narrowed to focus on the LV and the depth adjusted to see the LV, MV, and a portion of the LA. A ventricular focus clip should be acquired in the A4C view.[1,2]

The next image to acquire is the apical two-chamber (A2C) view. From the A4C view, the transducer orientation index marker is rotated 60 degrees counterclockwise. The A2C view demonstrates the LA, MV, LV, and CS in cross section in the atrioventricular groove. Two clips should be acquired from the A2C view, one with depth adjusted to demonstrate the entire LA, MV, and LV and a second with sector width and depth adjusted to focus on the LV. For this second clip the entire LV and MV and a portion of the LA should be demonstrated.[1]

After the A2C views, the apical long-axis views should be acquired. To acquire this view, rotate the transducer orientation index marker 60 degrees counterclockwise from the A2C view. Adjust the depth and sector width to demonstrate the entire LA,

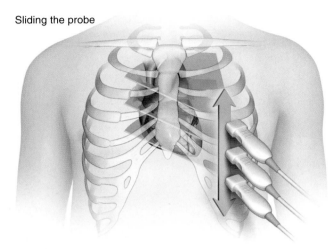

Sliding the probe

Figure 7.5. Sliding scanning maneuver. (From Mitchell C, et al: Guidelines for performing a comprehensive transthoracic echocardiographic examination in adults: recommendations from the American Society of Echocardiography, *J Am Soc Echocardiogr* 32:1–64, 2019.)

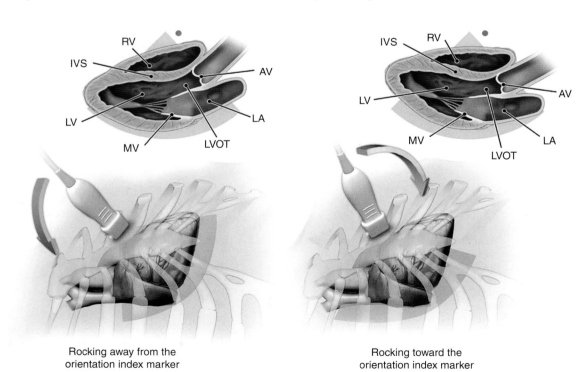

Rocking away from the orientation index marker

Rocking toward the orientation index marker

Figure 7.6. Rocking scanning maneuver. The blue dot represents the index orientation marker. *AV,* Aortic valve; *IVS,* interventricular septum; *LA,* left atrium; *LV,* left ventricle; *LVOT,* left ventricular outflow tract; *MV,* mitral valve; *RV,* right ventricle. (From Mitchell C, et al: Guidelines for performing a comprehensive transthoracic echocardiographic examination in adults: recommendations from the American Society of Echocardiography, *J Am Soc Echocardiogr* 32:1–64, 2019.)

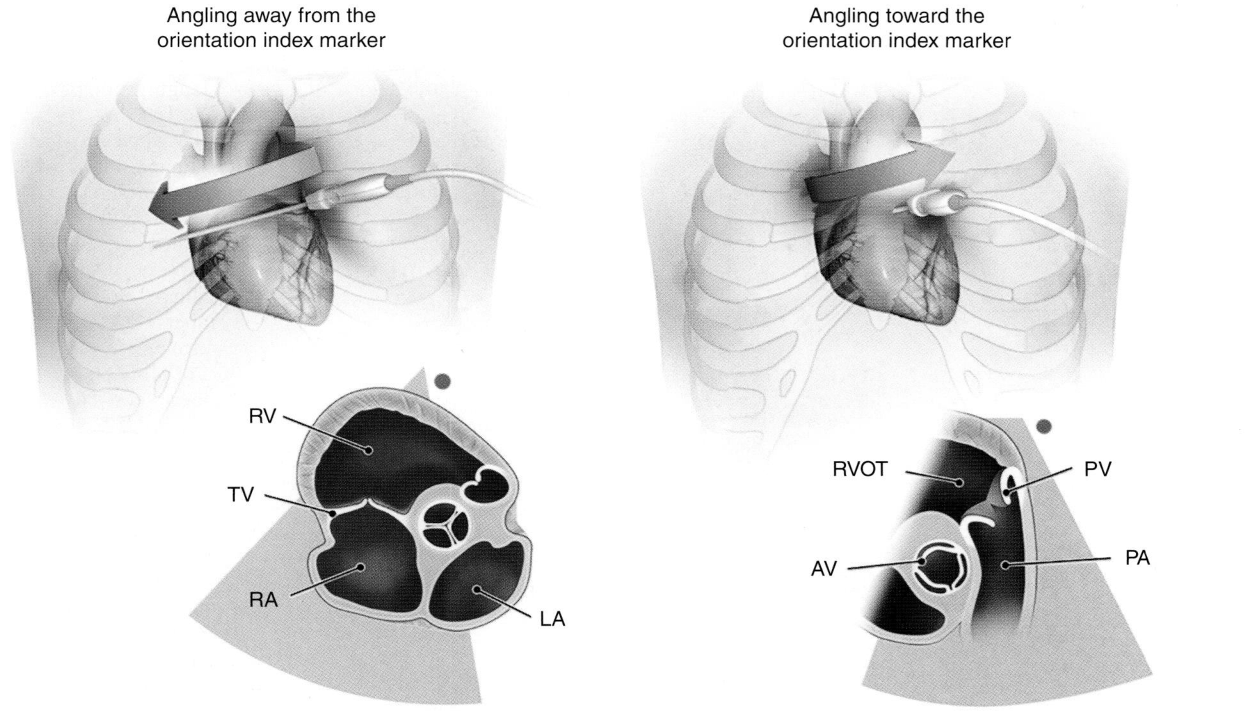

Angling away from the
orientation index marker

Angling toward the
orientation index marker

Figure 7.7. Angle scanning maneuver. The blue dot represents the index orientation marker. *AV,* Aortic valve; *LA,* left atrium; *PA,* pulmonary artery; *PV,* pulmonary valve; *RA,* right atrium; *RV,* right ventricle; *RVOT,* right ventricular outflow tract; *TV,* tricuspid valve. (From Mitchell C, et al: Guidelines for performing a comprehensive transthoracic echocardiographic examination in adults: recommendations from the American Society of Echocardiography, *J Am Soc Echocardiogr* 32:1–64, 2019.)

MV, LV, LVOT, AV, and ascending aorta. Next, adjust the depth and sector width to focus on the LV and acquire a second clip demonstrating the entire LV and MV and a portion of the LA. 2D measurement of LV volumes should be done with the biplane summation-of-disks methods. Using the focused LV A4C and A2C views, the LV cavity should traced along the interface of the compacted and noncompacted myocardium. Measurements are made at end-diastole and then using the same cardiac cycle advanced to the end-systolic frame to be traced with the same method.[1,3] Tracings are made at the interface of the noncompacted and compacted myocardium (Fig. 7.8).[1] If three-dimensional (3D) imaging is available, an ejection fraction should be calculated from the 3D data set.[5]

Focused views demonstrating the pulmonary veins draining into the LA should be acquired in the A2C and A4C views. For these views, the depth needs to be optimized to demonstrate the pulmonary veins entering the atria. Adjustment of the focal zone (if available) to the level of the pulmonary veins may help with visualization of these structures.[1] A clip should be acquired. After acquiring this image, focus on optimizing the LA image. Often, the optimized LV view is not the best view for imaging the LA. Adjust the transducer to clearly demonstrate the maximum width of the base and length of the LA. This image should be used for measuring LA volumes. LA volumes are measured in 2D by tracing the endocardial border in end-systole in the A4C and A2C views. After measuring the LA volume, the RA image should be optimized, and the endocardial border should be traced at the maximum width and length of the RA.[1–3]

The next image series to acquire is a sweep starting with the A4C view and tilting posterior to image the CS and then tilting anterior through the apical five-chamber (A5C) view and RVOT-to-PA view.

Next image the A5C view. From the A4C view, tilt the transducer anteriorly until the LVOT, AV, and ascending aorta are seen. The

A5C view demonstrates the LV, LVOT, AV, ascending aorta, and MV. Record a clip of this view.[1,2]

The final image series to acquire from the apical window is the RV-focused view and measurements of the RV. The RV-focused view is obtained by rotating slightly counterclockwise from the A4C view and maximizing the length of the ventricle. The plane is still maintained in the center of the LV, but small transducer movements allow for optimizing visualization of the RV and maximizing area. This is the view that the RV should be measured in. Tricuspid annular-plane systolic excursion, an M-mode measurement, can be made from either the A4C or the focused RV view, whichever aligns the vector of the TV annulus the best. RV linear measurements to be made are basal diameter, midcavity diameter, and length. RV area can also be measured at end-diastole.[1,6]

After apical images are acquired, the subcostal window images should be acquired. For these images, the patient is positioned in the supine position, and the transducer is placed just inferior to the xiphoid process with the orientation index marker directed toward the patient's left side in the 3 o'clock position.[1] Images to be acquired from the subcostal view are listed in Table 7.4.

The first image acquired in the subcostal window, is the subcostal four-chamber (4C) view. This view demonstrates the RA, TV, RV, LV, IVS, MV, LA, and interatrial septum (IAS). This view is particularly helpful for evaluating the atrial and ventricular septa because these structures are imaged perpendicular to the sound beam in this view. An additional alternative view that can be acquired in this same image plane is a zoomed focused view of the IAS. This view assists with focusing on the septum for evaluation of patent foramen ovale and atrial septal defects.[1] RV free wall thickness can also be evaluated from this view.[1,3] Record a clip of this view.

Next the inferior vena cava (IVC) and hepatic veins should also be imaged from this window.[1] To acquire the image of the IVC, the transducer orientation index marker should be rotated from the 3 o'clock position 90 degrees to demonstrate the heart

Text continues on p. 47

TABLE 7.1 Parasternal Window Long-Axis Plane Views Acquired With Protocol[a]

View	Anatomic Drawing	Ultrasound Image
Increased depth left ventricle	A	B Depth: 210 mm Video 7.1
Left ventricle normal depth	A	B Video 7.2
Measurement at end-diastole; IVS thickness (1), LV internal diameter (2), LV posterior wall (3), RV diameter (4)		
Measurement: LV systole (1)		

View	Anatomic Drawing	Ultrasound Image
Measurement: RVOT end-diastole (1)		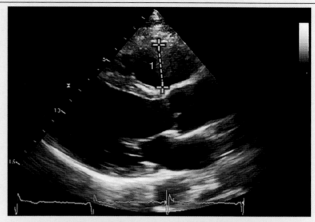
Measurement: LA diameter (1)		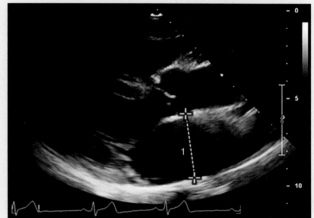
Zoomed AV	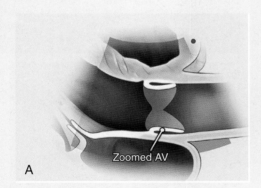	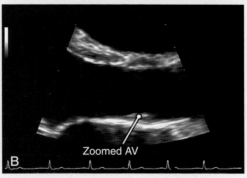 Video 7.3
Measurement: LVOT diameter (1) and AV annulus (2) at midsystole		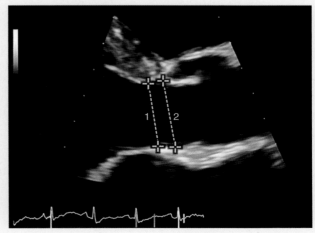

TABLE 7.1 Parasternal Window Long-Axis Plane Views Acquired With Protocol[a]—cont'd

View	Anatomic Drawing	Ultrasound Image
Measurement: diameter sinus of Valsalva (1) and sinotubular junction (2) at end-diastole		
Measurement: diameter of the Asc Ao at end-diastole		
Right parasternal Asc Ao (alternative view for imaging Asc Ao)		
Zoomed MV		

Video 7.4

TABLE 7.1 Parasternal Window Long-Axis Plane Views Acquired With Protocol[a]—cont'd

View	Anatomic Drawing	Ultrasound Image
RVOT		
RVIT		

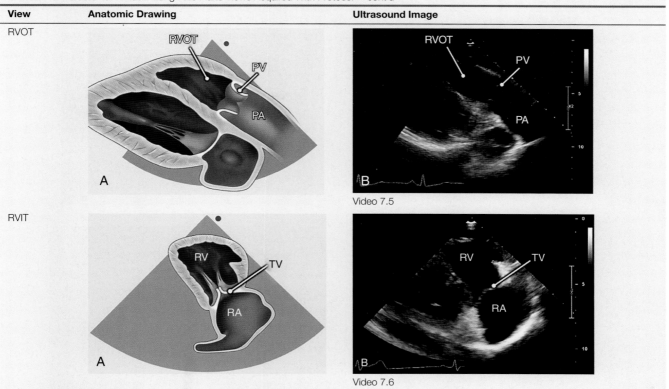

Video 7.5

Video 7.6

[a]All images should be acquired as a clip except for two-dimensional measurement images.

Ao, Aorta; *Asc Ao,* ascending aorta; *AV,* aortic valve; *IVS,* interventricular septum; *LA,* left atrium; *LVOT,* left ventricular outflow tract; *LV,* left ventricle; *MV,* mitral valve; *PA,* pulmonary artery; *PLAX,* parasternal long axis; *PV,* pulmonic valve; *RV,* right ventricle; *RA,* right atrium; *RVIT,* right ventricular inflow tract; *RVOT,* right ventricular outflow tract; *TV,* tricuspid valve.

Modified from Mitchell C, et al: Guidelines for performing a comprehensive transthoracic echocardiographic examination in adults: recommendations from the American Society of Echocardiography, *J Am Soc Echocardiogr* 2019; 32:1–64, 2019.

TABLE 7.2 Parasternal Window Short-Axis Plane Views Acquired With Protocol[a]

View	Anatomic Drawing	Ultrasound Image
Level great vessels		
Level RV, AV, and PV		

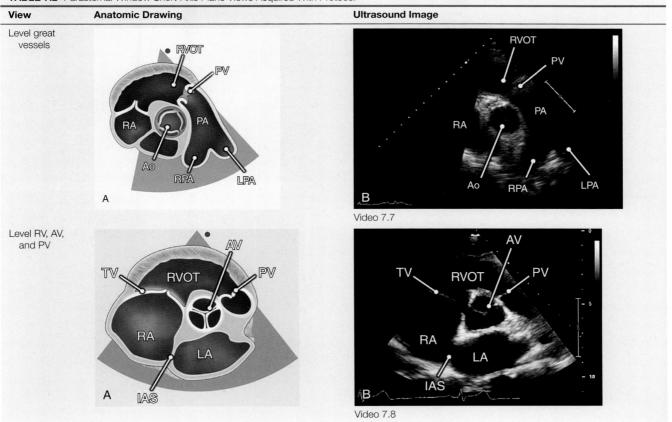

Video 7.7

Video 7.8

Continued

View	Anatomic Drawing	Ultrasound Image
Zoomed AV	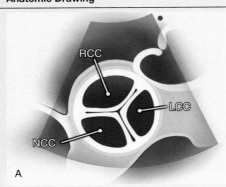	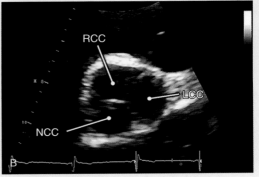 Video 7.9
Coronary artery origins (alternative view)	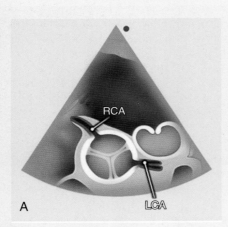	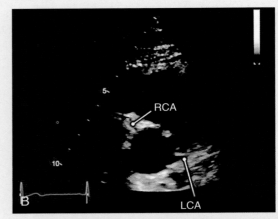

Measurement: proximal (1) and distal (2) RVOT at end-diastole

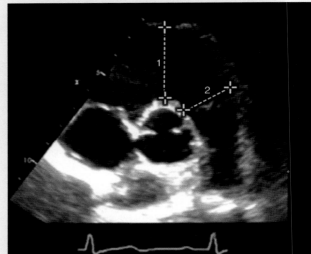

Measurement: main PA diameter (1) at end-diastole

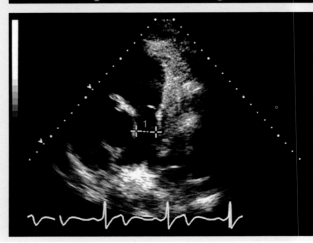

TABLE 7.2 Parasternal Window Short-Axis Plane Views Acquired With Protocol[a]—cont'd

View	Anatomic Drawing	Ultrasound Image
Focused TV	A	B Video 7.10
Focused PV	A	B Video 7.11
Level MV	A	B Video 7.12
Level papillary muscles	A	B Video 7.13

Continued

TABLE 7.2 Parasternal Window Short-Axis Plane Views Acquired With Protocol[a]—cont'd

View	Anatomic Drawing	Ultrasound Image
Level LV apex		

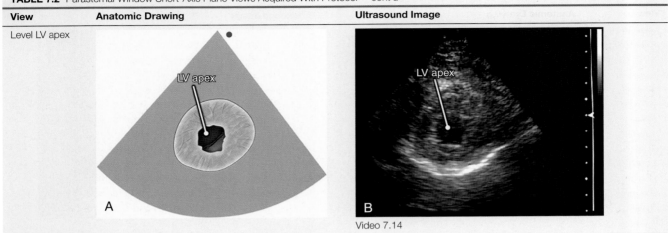

Video 7.14

[a]All images should be acquired as a clip except for two-dimensional measurement images.

ALPap, Anterior lateral papillary muscle; *AMVL,* anterior mitral valve leaflet; *Ao,* aorta; *AV,* aortic valve; *IVS,* interventricular septum; *LA,* left atrium; *LPA,* left pulmonary artery; *LV,* left ventricle; *LVOT,* left ventricular outflow tract; *MV,* mitral valve; *PMPap,* posterior medial papillary muscle; *PMVL,* posterior mitral valve leaflet; *PSAX,* parasternal short axis; *RA,* right atrium; *RPA,* right pulmonary artery; *RV,* right ventricle; *RVOT,* right ventricular outflow tract; *PA,* pulmonary artery; *PV,* pulmonic valve; *TV,* tricuspid valve.

Modified from Mitchell C, et al: Guidelines for performing a comprehensive transthoracic echocardiographic examination in adults: recommendations from the American Society of Echocardiography, *J Am Soc Echocardiogr* 32:1–64, 2019.

TABLE 7.3 Apical Window, Apical Plane Views Acquired With Protocol[a]

View	Anatomic Drawing	Ultrasound Image
A4C	IVS, RV, TV, LV, RA, LA, MV, IAS	IVS, RV, TV, LV, RA, LA, MV, IAS
		Video 7.15
A4C ventricular focus	LV	LV
		Video 7.16

TABLE 7.3 Apical Window, Apical Plane Views Acquired With Protocol[a]—cont'd

View	Anatomic Drawing	Ultrasound Image
A2C		
A2C ventricular focus		
Apical long axis		
Apical long-axis ventricular focus		

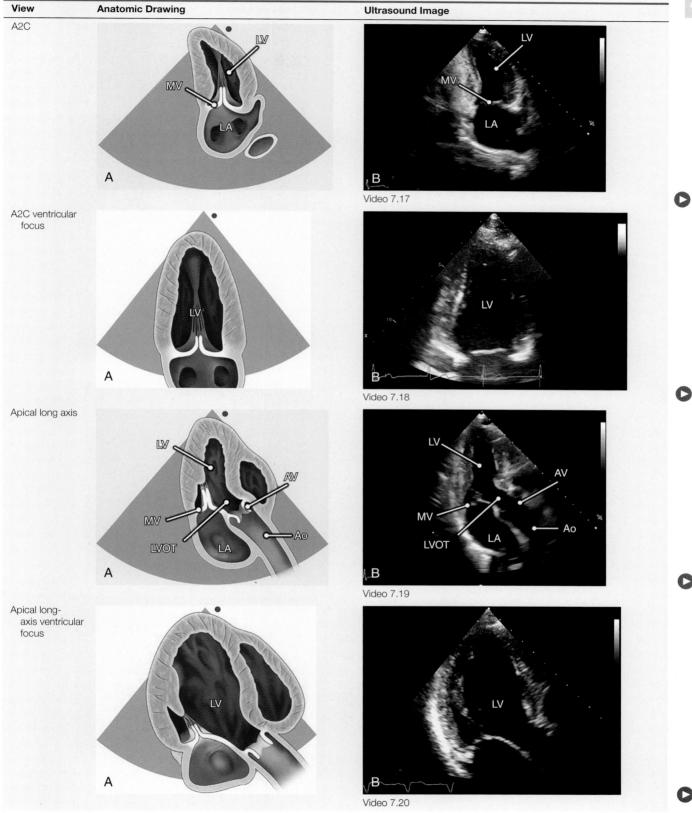

Video 7.17

Video 7.18

Video 7.19

Video 7.20

Continued

TABLE 7.3 Apical Window, Apical Plane Views Acquired With Protocol[a]—cont'd

View	Anatomic Drawing	Ultrasound Image
A4C pulmonary veins and focused view of pulmonary veins	

Videos 7.21 and 7.22 |
| A5C | |

Video 7.23 |
| Apical RVOT and PV | |

Video 7.24 |

View	Anatomic Drawing	Ultrasound Image

Measurement: LV volumes (A4C and A2C views end-diastole [1] and A4C and A2C views end-systole [2])

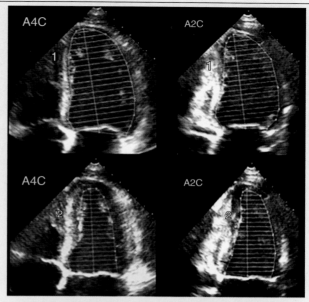

Measurement: 3D LV ejection fraction (should be performed if available)

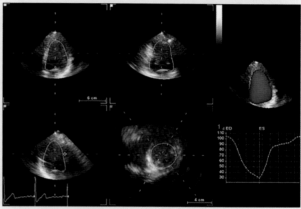

Measurement: LA volume A4C and A2C. *1*, LA length; *2*, LA area.

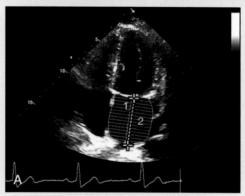

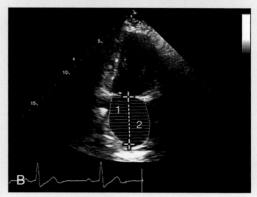

Continued

TABLE 7.3 Apical Window, Apical Plane Views Acquired With Protocol[a]—cont'd

View	Anatomic Drawing	Ultrasound Image
Measurement: RA volume four chamber. *1,* RA length; *2,* RA area.		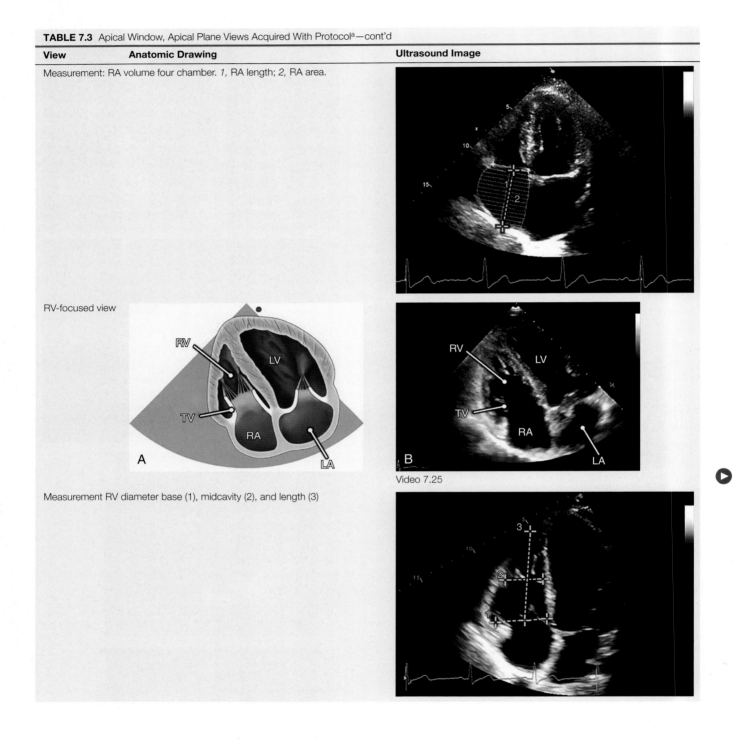
RV-focused view		
Measurement RV diameter base (1), midcavity (2), and length (3)		

Video 7.25

TABLE 7.3 Apical Window, Apical Plane Views Acquired With Protocol^a—cont'd

View	Anatomic Drawing	Ultrasound Image
Measurement RV area (1)		

^{a}All images should be acquired as a clip except for two-dimensional measurement images.

A2C, Apical two-chamber view; *A4C,* apical four-chamber view; *A5C,* apical five-chamber view; *ALPap,* anterior lateral papillary muscle; *AMVL,* anterior mitral valve leaflet; *Ao,* aorta; *AV,* aortic valve; *IVS,* interventricular septum; *LA,* left atrium; *LPA,* left pulmonary artery; *LV,* left ventricle; *LVOT,* left ventricular outflow tract; *MV,* mitral valve; *PA,* pulmonary artery; *PMPap,* posterior medial papillary muscle; *PMVL,* posterior mitral valve leaflet; *PSAX,* parasternal short axis; *Pulvns,* pulmonary veins; *PV,* pulmonic valve; *RA,* right atrium; *RV,* right ventricle; *RPA,* right pulmonary artery; *RVOT,* right ventricular outflow tract; *TV,* tricuspid valve.

Modified from Mitchell C, et al: Guidelines for performing a comprehensive transthoracic echocardiographic examination in adults: recommendations from the American Society of Echocardiography, *J Am Soc Echocardiogr* 32:1–64, 2019.

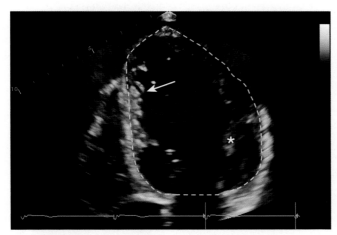

Figure 7.8. Tracing the interface of the compacted and noncompacted myocardium in a patient with dilated cardiomyopathy. Structures of the noncompacted myocardium (trabeculae [*arrow*] and papillary muscles [*asterisk*]) are considered part of the left ventricular cavity. (From Mitchell C, et al: Guidelines for performing a comprehensive transthoracic echocardiographic examination in adults: recommendations from the American Society of Echocardiography, *J Am Soc Echocardiogr* 32:1–64, 2019.)

in short axis and the IVC in long axis. From this view, the IVC diameter can be measured, and the IVC diameter changes with respiration can monitored.[3,6] A clip should be recorded of this image. After the IVC has been imaged, small manipulations of the transducer are performed to demonstrate the hepatic veins draining into the IVC. A clip should be recorded of the hepatic veins. A color Doppler image should be recorded after each grayscale image.

The final image acquired is the longitudinal view of the aortic arch from the SSN window. For this view, the transducer is moved to the SSN window, located superior to the manubrium. Images are acquired with the patient in the supine position and a pillow behind the shoulders so that the head may be tilted back. Also, position the patient's head slightly leftward. The transducer orientation index marker is positioned toward the patient's left shoulder.[1] The images to acquire from the SSN view are demonstrated in Table 7.5.

The longitudinal plane of the aortic arch can be acquired from this window. Position the transducer orientation index marker at the 12 to 1 o'clock position. Slowly rotate the orientation index marker until it cuts through a plane from the tip of the left scapula to the right nipple. In this plane, the ascending aorta, transverse arch and its branches (innominate artery, left common carotid artery, and left subclavian artery), and the descending aorta are visualized. The right pulmonary artery is seen in cross section behind the ascending aorta.[1] In some instances, a structure may be seen anterior to the aortic arch, which is the innominate vein. To fully evaluate this structure, imaging in the SSN short-axis plane can provide an alternative view that can be used to evaluate the innominate vein and superior vena cava. This view is acquired by rotating the transducer orientation index marker clockwise until the aorta is demonstrated in cross section. Then tilt the transducer inferior until the innominate vein and superior vena cava are seen.[1]

A color Doppler clip should be acquired after the grayscale image acquisition. Color Doppler is helpful to differentiate arterial and venous structures.

The images discussed in this chapter represent the standard 2D images to acquire for the comprehensive transthoracic imaging protocol. A full listing of the protocol images can be found in Tables e7.1 to Table e7.3. Spectral Doppler measurements that also should be included in the comprehensive protocol are described in Chapters 11 and 35 and Table e7.2.

Please access ExpertConsult to view the corresponding videos for this chapter.

TABLE 7.4 Subcostal Window Image Views Acquired With Protocol[a]

View	Anatomic Drawing	Ultrasound Image
Subcostal four-chamber view		Video 7.26
Focused IAS (alternative view for imaging the IAS)		
IVC		Video 7.27
Measurement of IVC diameter		

TABLE 7.4 Subcostal Window Image Views Acquired With Protocol[a]—cont'd

View	Anatomic Drawing	Ultrasound Image
Hepatic veins	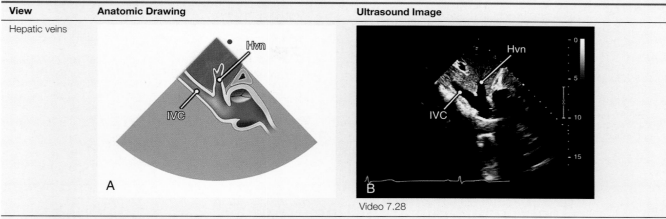	

Video 7.28

[a]All images should be acquired as a clip except for two-dimensional measurement images.

Ao, Aorta; *AV,* aortic valve; *Hvn,* hepatic vein; *IVC,* inferior vena cava; *IAS,* interatrial septum; *IVS,* interventricular septum; *LA,* left atrium; *LV,* left ventricle; *LVOT,* left ventricular outflow tract; *MV,* mitral valve; *PSAX,* parasternal short axis; *PA,* pulmonary artery; *PV,* pulmonic valve; *RA,* right atrium; *RV,* right ventricle; *RVOT,* right ventricular outflow tract; *TV,* tricuspid valve.

Modified from Mitchell C, et al: Guidelines for performing a comprehensive transthoracic echocardiographic examination in adults: recommendations from the American Society of Echocardiography, *J Am Soc Echocardiogr* 32:1–64, 2019.

TABLE 7.5 Suprasternal Notch Window Views Acquired With Protocol[a]

View	Anatomic Drawing	Ultrasound Image
Apical four chamber		

Video 7.29

View	Anatomic Drawing	Ultrasound Image
Left innominate vein, SVC, RAP (alternative view to evaluate the innominate vein, SVC, and PA)		

[a]All images should be acquired as a clip.

AscAo, Ascending aorta; *Desc Ao,* descending aorta; *Innom a,* innominate artery; *LCCA,* left common carotid artery; *LSA,* left subclavian artery; *PA,* pulmonary artery; *RPA,* right pulmonary artery; *SVC,* superior vena cava.

Modified from Mitchell C, et al: Guidelines for Performing a Comprehensive Transthoracic Echocardiographic Examination in Adults: recommendations from the American Society of Echocardiography, *J Am Soc Echocardiogr* 32:1–64, 2019.

REFERENCES

1. Mitchell C, Rahko PS, Blauwet LA, et al. Guidelines for performing a comprehensive transthoracic echocardiographic examination in adults: recommendations from the American Society of Echocardiography. *J Am Soc Echocardiogr.* 2019;32:1–64.
2. Anderson B. The two-dimensional echocardiographic examination. In: Anderson B, ed. *Echocardiography: The Normal Examination and Echocardiographic Measurements.* 3rd ed. Australia: Echotext Pty Ltd; 2017.
3. Lang RM, Badano LP, Mor-Avi V, et al. Recommendations for cardiac chamber quantification by echocardiography in adults: an update from the American Society Echocardiography and the European Association of Cardiovascular Imaging. *J Am Soc Echocardiogr.* 2015;28:1–39.
4. Brown LM, Duffy CE, Mitchell C, Young L. A practical guide to pediatric coronary artery imaging with echocardiography. *J Am Soc Echocardiogr.* 2015;28:379–391.
5. Lang RM, Badano LP, Tsang W, et al. EAE/ASE recommendations for image acquisition and display using three-dimensional echocardiography. *J Am Soc Echocardiogr.* 2012;25(3–46).
6. Rudski LG, Lai WW, Afilalo J, et al. Guidelines for the echocardiographic assessment of the right heart in adults: a report from the American Society of Echocardiography endorsed by the European Association of Echocardiography, a registered branch of the European Society of Cardiology, and the Canadian Society of Echocardiography. *J Am Soc Echocardiogr.* 2010;23(7):685–713; quiz 786–788.

8 Technical Quality and Tips

Bonita Anderson, Agatha Kwon

OPTIMIZING TWO-DIMENSIONAL IMAGES

The most commonly used controls for optimizing two-dimensional (2D) images are summarized in Table 8.1. These controls can be used to improve spatial, contrast, and temporal resolution. *Spatial resolution* refers to the ability of the ultrasound machine to detect structures that are anatomically separate and to display them as being separate. The best spatial resolution occurs at higher transducer frequencies, where the spatial pulse length (and wavelength) is smallest, and at the focal zone, where the ultrasound beam is narrowest.[1] Therefore, the operator should use the highest possible transducer frequency that allows adequate depth penetration, and the focus should be positioned at the center of the region of interest. Because higher frequency transducers improve spatial resolution, the measurement of small structures is more accurate, and the distinction between closely related anatomic structures is more apparent (Fig. 8.1 and Video 8.1).

Contrast resolution refers to the ability of the ultrasound machine to differentiate subtle differences in echogenicity between anatomic structures and to then display these as visually distinguishable structures. Controls that can be manipulated to improve contrast resolution include the overall gain, time-gain compensation (TGC), and dynamic range (DR) and the use of harmonic imaging. The overall gain increases the amplitude (or gain) of returning ultrasound signals. As echoes returning from deeper structures become progressively weaker as the ultrasound beam is attenuated, compensation for this effect is required. This is achieved via the adjustment of TGC whereby deeper echo signals are amplified more than shallower echo signals. The general aim of gain and TGC is to ensure that signals arising from tissues of similar acoustic properties are displayed at the same echo amplitude.

Dynamic range refers to the ratio of the maximum to minimum signal level; that is, the DR is the ratio of the strongest to the weakest echo. The aim of adjusting the DR is to provide the optimal amount of grayscale information so that the image is not too grainy, the contrast is not too high, and the image is not too hazy or soft. Essentially, the DR is increased when images are of a high quality (softens the images and increases the gray scale),

TABLE 8.1 Common Two-Dimensional Image Optimization Controls

2D Control	Desired Adjustment	Aim of Adjustment
Transducer frequency	Highest possible for given image depth (use harmonic imaging as a default)	Improves spatial and contrast resolution
Field of view (FOV)	Smallest FOV to display region of interest	Maximizes frame rate (improves temporal resolution)
Focus	To center of region of interest	Improves lateral resolution
Gain and TGC	Ensure blood pool is echo free and that structures of similar acoustic properties along imaging depth are displayed at similar amplitudes	Amplify received echo signals
Zoom (write-zoom)	Magnifies region of interest	Increases frame rate (improves temporal resolution), improves spatial resolution and measurement accuracy
Dynamic range	Increased for high-quality images	Softens images and increases grayscale
	Decreased for poor-quality images	Enhances strongest echoes, eliminates weaker echoes and reduces noise
Edge enhancement	Increased	Sharpens borders and edges of structures
Reject	Set to reject low-level echoes	Reduces noise by eliminating weak echoes; improves spatial and contrast resolution
B-color maps	Various maps	Improves contrast resolution; enhances subtle tissue differences
Postprocessing curves	Various maps	Modifies grayscale intensities on the display; improves contrast resolution

TGC, Time-gain compensation

Adapted from Anderson B. Chapter 1 *Basic Principles of Two-Dimensional Ultrasound Imaging in Echocardiography: The Normal Examination and Echocardiographic Measurements* (3rd Edition): Echotext Pty Ltd; 2017, with permission.

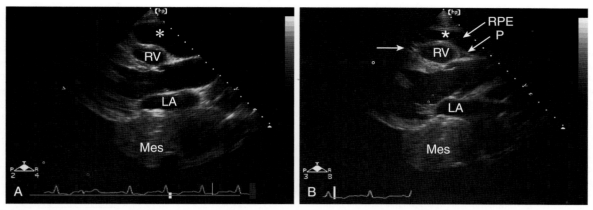

Figure 8.1. Systolic frames acquired from the parasternal long-axis view of the left ventricle in the same patient. An echo-free space *(asterisk)* is seen anterior to the right ventricle (RV), and a mesothelioma (Mes) is seen posterior to the left atrium (LA). **A,** In an image acquired using a transducer frequency of 3 MHz, the echo-free space anterior to the RV appears to be a pericardial effusion. **B,** In an image acquired using a transducer frequency of 5 MHz, the distinction between the pericardium (P) and pleural space can be appreciated, thus identifying the echo-free space as a right pleural effusion (RPE) rather than as a pericardial effusion. Also see accompanying Video 8.1.

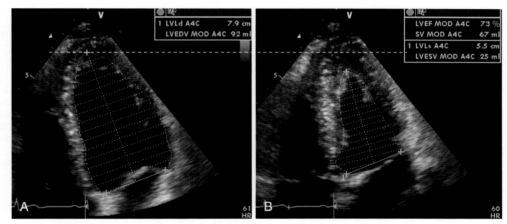

Figure 8.2. Apical four-chamber end-diastolic (**A**) and end-systolic (**B**) frames. Note that the position of the apex in the end-systolic frame is approximately 1 cm lower than in the end-diastolic frame, which indicates apical foreshortening.

and DR is decreased when image quality is poor (enhances the strongest echoes, eliminates the weaker signals, and reduces background noise). Harmonic imaging, which typically uses the second harmonic frequencies that arise from native tissue, has revolutionized 2D imaging by significantly reducing background noise and near-field artifacts and by improving endocardial border delineation.[2,3] Harmonic imaging should be used to improve bubble visualization in agitated-saline contrast studies, and harmonic imaging at a low or very low mechanical index should be used when performing studies using ultrasound enhancement agents.[4–6]

Temporal resolution refers to the ability of the ultrasound machine to accurately show the position of moving structures at a particular instant in time. Temporal resolution is discussed in terms of the frame rate so that the higher the frame rate, the better the temporal resolution. High frame rates are desirable in echocardiography because of the dynamic nature of cardiac motion; in addition, high frame rates are required for advanced imaging modalities such as 2D speckle-tracking echocardiography.[7,8] The frame rate can be increased by decreasing the image depth (decreases the pulse travel time) and by narrowing sector width (decreases the number of scan lines).

AVOIDING APICAL FORESHORTENING

Apical foreshortening results from the ultrasound imaging plane improperly transecting the left ventricular (LV) major axis. This limitation is important to recognize because it can lead to measurement error in the estimation of the LV ejection fraction and measurement variability in global longitudinal strain measurements.[8,9] Apical foreshortening can also mask the presence of apical regional abnormalities and apical thrombus. Foreshortening of the apical views can be easily recognized by scrutinizing the LV shape and its apical motion. In a foreshortened apical view, the ventricle appears wider and shorter, and the LV apex appears thickened and squeezes downward during systole. Another clue to foreshortening is the location of the apex. As the heart shortens from the base during systole, the LV apex between end-diastolic and end-systolic frames should be at the same horizontal point on the image display. When there is foreshortening, the LV apex in the end-systolic frame is farther from the transducer than is the LV apex in the end-diastolic frame (Fig. 8.2). The most common cause of apical foreshortening is having the transducer too high on the chest wall. Therefore, foreshortening is often rectified by moving the transducer one or two intercostal spaces lower (see Video 8.2) or by repositioning the patient into a steeper left lateral position to maximize the length of the left ventricle.

OPTIMIZING SPECTRAL DOPPLER TRACES

The most important technical factor affecting the optimal display of spectral Doppler traces and thus the accuracy of measurements is the alignment between blood flow and the ultrasound beam. When blood flow is parallel to the ultrasound beam, the maximum Doppler shift, and thus the maximum velocity is accurately detected. However, when blood flow is not parallel to the ultrasound beam, the Doppler shift is reduced, and the derived velocity is underestimated. Furthermore, because pressure gradients are derived from the Doppler velocity, the accuracy of pressure gradient estimation is also influenced by the alignment between blood flow and the ultrasound beam. For these reasons, blood flow must be interrogated from echocardiographic views in which flow is aligned as parallel to the ultrasound beam as possible; this often requires multiple acoustic views, including off-axis imaging. This is especially important in the assessment of aortic stenosis because the direction of the aortic jet is unpredictable and usually cannot be visualized.[10]

Controls that can be adjusted to improve spectral Doppler traces are summarized in Table 8.2. In particular, the velocity scale and baseline should be adjusted to ensure that the signal of interest fills the spectral display. For example, in the evaluation of valvular regurgitation, both forward and regurgitant flow should be displayed simultaneously on the same Doppler display because the velocity of forward flow and the intensity of the regurgitant jet compared with forward flow can also be used as qualitative measures of regurgitation severity.[11,12]

Wall filters, which allow the elimination of low-velocity signals, should be set sufficiently high to eliminate low-velocity signals but not so high that the beginning and end of flow are obscured or ambiguous. The sweep speed, which is the horizontal display rate of the spectral Doppler trace, can affect the accuracy of time-related measurements. Therefore, a minimum sweep speed of 100 mm/s is recommended for time-related measurements such as flow durations, velocity-time integrals, and time-velocity slopes. Slower sweep speeds are useful for averaging velocities that vary with respiration and for observing respirophasic variation related to pathologies such as cardiac tamponade and constrictive pericarditis.[13]

Optimization of spectral Doppler traces is especially important in the measurement of the peak tricuspid regurgitant velocity, which is used for the estimation of the right ventricular systolic pressure (RVSP). When there are very strong spectral Doppler signals, the signal may display a stronger intensity, lower velocity "chin" and a less intense, higher velocity "beard." "Bearding" may occur as a result of intrinsic spectral broadening or nonlaminar flow. It has been shown that the accuracy of the RVSP is increased using the peak velocity measured at the "chin" rather than the "beard."[14] To avoid erroneous measurements, the "beard" of the signal can be removed by decreasing the DR or compression, or by increasing the reject (Fig. 8.3). The control that best achieves this effect is dependent on the available controls on the ultrasound instrument being used.

Sample volume size is also important for pulsed-wave Doppler assessment. The appropriate sample volume size changes depending on which structure is being interrogated.[6] Generally, smaller sample

TABLE 8.2 Common Spectral Doppler Optimization Controls

Spectral Doppler Control	Desired Adjustment
Incident angle	Aligned parallel with blood flow (off-axis imaging may be required)
Doppler gain	Amplifies received Doppler signals without excessive background noise
Velocity scale and baseline	The signal of interest or the signal being measured fills the display
Wall filters	Eliminate or reduce unwanted signals from vessel walls or tissue movement
	Set to the lowest practical level (without eliminating genuine signals from low-velocity blood flow)
Sweep speed	Display two cardiac cycles per trace
	Increased to 100 mm/s for time-related measurements (e.g., time intervals, integrals, and velocity slopes)
	Decreased for observing respiratory variation
Sample volume position	Placed along the cursor line to the desired site of interrogation
Sample volume length	Conventional PWD: as small as possible to minimize spectral broadening and to provide a crisp, clean signal
	TDI: 5–10 mm to cover a larger sample area
Dynamic range (compression)	Decreased to enhance strongest signals, eliminate weaker signals, and reduce noise
Reject	Increased to eliminate weaker signals and reduce noise
Color-scale maps	Enhance spectral Doppler signals

PWD, Pulsed-wave Doppler; *TDI*, tissue Doppler imaging.
Adapted from Anderson B: Basic principles of spectral Doppler in echocardiography. In: B. Anderson, ed. *Echocardiography: The Normal Examination and Echocardiographic Measurements*. 3rd ed. Brisbane, Australia: Echotext Pty Ltd; 2017, with permission.

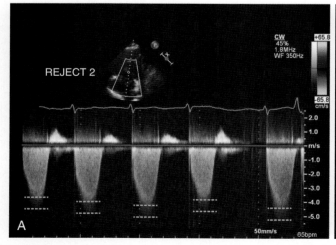
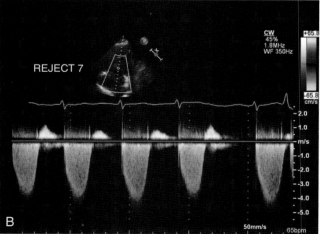

Figure 8.3. Two spectral Doppler traces acquired from a patient with significant tricuspid regurgitation (TR). **A,** The continuous-wave Doppler trace shows a "chin" *(pink line)* and a "beard" *(blue line)*. **B,** This trace was acquired after the reject was increased; observe that there is less background noise and that the "beard" on the TR has been eliminated.

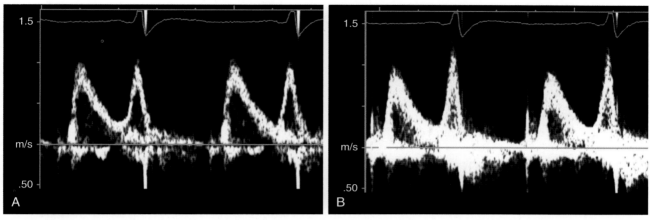

Figure 8.4. The effect of sample volume size is illustrated in these two transmitral inflow traces acquired with a pulsed-wave Doppler sample volume of 1.5 mm (**A**) and 5 mm (**B**). The trace recorded with a 1.5-mm sample volume displays minimal spectral broadening (narrow spectral width), an obvious spectral window (*dark area* under the spectral Doppler curve), and a crisper profile. The trace recorded with the larger sample volume displays significant spectral broadening (filling-in of the spectral window), which occurs because a greater volume of blood is being sampled from around the mitral valve leaflet tips. Measurements from the trace with the smaller sample volume will be more accurate.

TABLE 8.3 Common Color Doppler Optimization Controls

Color Doppler Control	Desired Adjustment or Usage
Color box size	As narrow and as short as possible while ensuring the region of interest (including surrounding structures) are adequately interrogated
Velocity scale	Set to 50–70 cm/s allowing adequate filling of color box
	Decrease to enhance detection of low velocity flow or when there is underfilling of the color box
Color gain	Increased to the point of random colored pixels (speckling) and then decreased to just below speckling
Wall filter	Increased to eliminate low velocity signals and "noise"
	May be decreased when investigating low-velocity flow
Color baseline	Remains at the default position in the center of color bar; May be moved to decrease color Nyquist limit in one direction
Color maps	Select color map (including variance maps) based on the sonographer's or institution's preference
2D–color image comparison	Useful when trying to determine the cause of regurgitation or other abnormal flow

2D, Two-dimensional.
Adapted from Anderson B: Basic principles of two-dimensional ultrasound imaging in echocardiography. In: B. Anderson, ed. *Echocardiography: The Normal Examination and Echocardiographic Measurements*. 3rd ed. Brisbane, Australia: Echotext Pty Ltd; 2017, with permission.

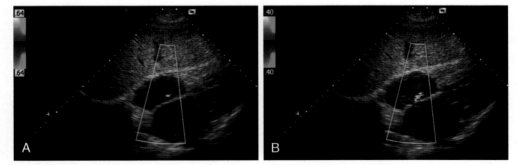

Figure 8.5. The effect of color velocity scale is illustrated in these two subcostal four-chamber images acquired with the color velocity scale set at maximum (**A**) and at 40 cm/s (**B**). Observe that at the maximum color velocity scale of 64 cm/s, there is significant underfilling of the color box. By decreasing the color velocity scale to 40 cm/s, there is enhanced detection of low-velocity flow, and a small patent foramen ovale is apparent. Also see accompanying Video 8.5.

volumes produce "cleaner" spectral waveforms, and larger sample volumes lead to increased spectral broadening (Fig. 8.4). Increased spectral broadening may falsely display laminar flow as turbulent flow and may lead to erroneous measurements.

OPTIMIZING COLOR DOPPLER IMAGES

Key controls that are adjusted to optimize color Doppler images are summarized in Table 8.3. Importantly, to ensure maximum frame rates and an acceptable color velocity scale (Nyquist limit), the color box should be adjusted to visualize the structure in question. Because widening the color box width increases the processing time and therefore lowers the frame rate, the color box should be as narrow as possible. Likewise, a color box deeper into the image may decrease the pulse repetition frequency and therefore lower the color velocity scale; therefore, the color box should be as shallow as possible. The recommended default color velocity scale for all routine color Doppler interrogation is between 50 and 70 cm/s.[12] In situations when the color box is underfilled, despite adequate color gain or when flow velocity is low, the color scale should be reduced until there is adequate filling of the color box (Fig. 8.5 and Video 8.5).

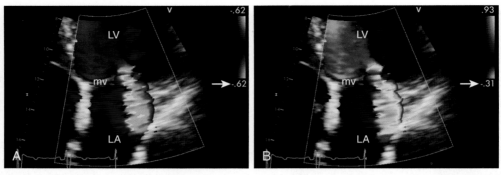

Figure 8.6. Two images acquired from a zoomed apical four-chamber view of the mitral valve (mv) in the same patient. Mitral regurgitation (MR) into the left atrium (LA) is evident. In **A,** The color baseline is set to the center of the color bar, and the color Nyquist limit is 0.62 m/s. **B,** The color baseline has been shifted downward in the direction of the MR jet, so now the color Nyquist limit at the bottom of the color bar is at 0.31 m/s *(arrow)*; observe that this baseline shift has enhanced the flow convergence radius on the left ventricular (LV) side of the mitral valve. (Reproduced with permission from Anderson B: Basic principles of two-dimensional ultrasound imaging in echocardiography. In: B. Anderson, ed. *Echocardiography: The Normal Examination and Echocardiographic Measurements.* 3rd ed. Brisbane, Australia: Echotext Pty Ltd; 2017.)

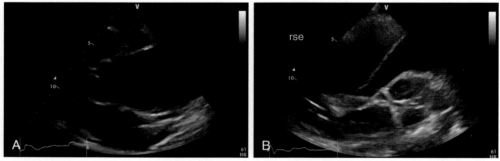

Figure 8.7. Two images acquired from the same patient. **A,** Image acquired from a high left parasternal window; the ascending aorta appears dilated, measuring at 6.3 cm. **B,** Image acquired from the right sternal edge (rse); a linear structure is noted within the aortic lumen consistent with a dissection flap. Importantly, the dissection flap was not apparent from the high left parasternal window, and this highlights the importance of imaging a dilated aorta from the right sternal border. Also see accompanying Video 8.7.

Color Doppler gain, which adjusts the degree of amplification of received Doppler signals, should be set just below the threshold for background speckling or noise, and it should be optimized for every view.

By default, the color baseline is set in the middle of the color bar. Color baseline shift for the evaluation of regurgitant valves is recommended for measuring the flow convergence radius and for estimation of the effective regurgitant orifice area via the proximal isovelocity surface area (PISA) method.[12] Baseline shift is performed in the direction of the regurgitant jet with the aim of increasing the hemispherical flow convergence zone profile and highlighting the aliasing contour (Fig. 8.6).

Author Tip

Although many controls on ultrasound machines are similar regardless of the manufacturer, it is important to also be aware of the different image optimization methods for different ultrasound systems. Therefore, operators should be familiar with the various technicalities of the machines that they operate. Details regarding the effective manipulation of these image optimization controls can usually be found in the user manual or may be explained by an applications specialist.

ALTERNATE WINDOWS

In cases when images from conventional transthoracic acoustic windows are suboptimal or provide incomplete clinical information,

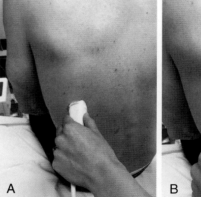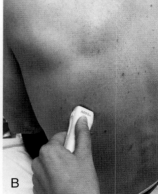

Figure 8.8. Two photos demonstrating the patient and probe positions for obtaining long-axis (**A**) and short-axis views of the left ventricle (**B**) from the posterior imaging window through a left pleural effusion. See text for details.

the operator should consider extending from the normal imaging protocol to explore imaging from other nonstandard imaging windows or nonstandard patient positioning. When imaging from nonstandard windows, the operator needs to apply anatomical knowledge to interpret the heart's orientation within the thoracic cavity and to apply knowledge of imaging planes to acquire interpretable views of the heart.

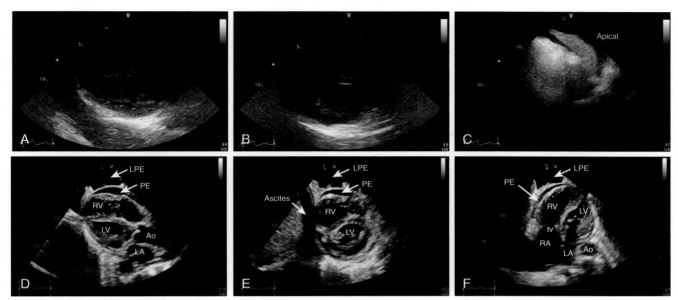

Figure 8.9. These images were acquired from a patient with carcinoid heart disease. The top images are attempted parasternal long-axis (**A**), parasternal short-axis (**B**) and apical four-chamber (**C**) views. Image quality is poor, but the apical view shows a left pleural effusion (LPE) with a banana-shaped collapsed lung. The bottom images were acquired from the posterior imaging window through an LPE: long-axis (**D**), short-axis (**E**), and four-chamber views (**F**). These images show a dilated right ventricle (RV) and thickened and retracted tricuspid valve leaflets (tv) and a small pericardial effusion (PE). Also see accompanying Video 8.9. *Ao,* Aorta; *LA,* left atrium; *LV,* left ventricle; *RA,* right atrium.

The right sternal border can be very useful in imaging the ascending aorta in patients with a dilated aorta. As the ascending aorta dilates, it tends to take a more anterior and rightward course; therefore, the middle and distal segments of the ascending aorta can be imaged better by moving the transducer to the right third or fourth intercostal spaces (Fig. 8.7 and Video 8.7). This window may also be used to image the interatrial septum and the openings of the superior and inferior vena cava into the right atrium.

When there is a left pleural effusion, the posterior imaging window provides an alternate acoustic window to image the heart.[15,16] The patient can be scanned either lying in a right lateral decubitus position or sitting upright with the transducer placed in the left subscapular space roughly in the fifth intercostal space (Fig. 8.8). A long-axis view of the left heart can be obtained with the index marker directed toward the patient's right shoulder, and short-axis views of the left heart can be obtained with the index marker directed toward the patient's left shoulder. A four-chamber view can also be obtained with more lateral placement of the transducer with anterior tilt. A case example of posterior imaging compared with transthoracic imaging is illustrated in Fig. 8.9 and Video 8.9.

SUMMARY

Transthoracic echocardiography remains an important imaging tool for the assessment of cardiac disease. To obtain the most diagnostically accurate information from this examination, it is imperative that the operator has a comprehensive understanding of how various imaging controls can be adjusted to improve image quality and to be aware of limiting factors that may reduce measurement accuracy. Operators should also be familiar with imaging from alternative windows that may provide additional diagnostic information.

Please access ExpertConsult to view the corresponding videos for this chapter.

ACKNOWLEDGMENT

The authors acknowledge the valuable input and suggestions offered by Dr. Andy Pellett, PhD, RDCS, who reviewed this chapter.

REFERENCES

1. Anderson B. Basic principles of two-dimensional ultrasound imaging in echocardiography. In: Anderson B, ed. *Echocardiography: The Normal Examination and Echocardiographic Measurements.* 3rd ed. Brisbane, Australia: Echotext Pty Ltd; 2017.
2. Becher H, Tiemann K, Schlosser T, et al. Improvement in endocardial border delineation using tissue harmonic imaging. *Echocardiography.* 1998;15(5):511–518.
3. Kasprzak JD, Paelinck B, Ten Cate FJ, et al. Comparison of native and contrast-enhanced harmonic echocardiography for visualization of left ventricular endocardial border. *Am J Cardiol.* 1999;83(2):211–217.
4. Ha JW, Shin MS, Kang S, et al. Enhanced detection of right-to-left shunt through patent foramen ovale by transthoracic contrast echocardiography using harmonic imaging. *Am J Cardiol.* 2001;87(5):669–671. A11.
5. Porter TR, Mulvagh SL, Abdelmoneim SS, et al. Clinical applications of ultrasonic enhancing agents in echocardiography: 2018 American Society of Echocardiography Guidelines Update. *J Am Soc Echocardiogr.* 2018;31(3):241–274.
6. Mitchell C, Rahko PS, Blauwet LA, et al. Guidelines for performing a comprehensive transthoracic echocardiographic examination in adults: recommendations from the American Society of Echocardiography. *J Am Soc Echocardiogr.* 2019;32(1):1–64.
7. Mor-Avi V, Lang RM, Badano LP, et al. Current and evolving echocardiographic techniques for the quantitative evaluation of cardiac mechanics. *J Am Soc Echocardiogr.* 2011;24(3):277–313.
8. Collier P, Phelan D, Klein A. A test in context: myocardial strain measured by speckle-tracking echocardiography. *J Am Coll Cardiol 28.* 2017;69(8):1043–1056.
9. Lang RM, Badano LP, Mor-Avi V, et al. Recommendations for cardiac chamber quantification by echocardiography in adults: an update from the American Society of Echocardiography and the European Association of Cardiovascular Imaging. *J Am Soc Echocardiogr.* 2015;28(1):1–39.
10. Baumgartner H, Hung J, Bermejo J, et al. Recommendations on the echocardiographic assessment of aortic valve stenosis: a focused update from the European Association of Cardiovascular Imaging and the American Society of Echocardiography. *J Am Soc Echocardiogr.* 2017;30(4):372–392.
11. Anderson B. Doppler quantification of regurgitant lesions in echocardiography. In: Anderson B, ed. *Echocardiography: The Normal Examination and Echocardiographic Measurements.* 3rd ed. Brisbane, Australia: Echotext Pty Ltd; 2017.
12. Zoghbi WA, Adams D, Bonow RO, et al. Recommendations for noninvasive evaluation of native valvular regurgitation: a report from the American Society of Echocardiography developed in collaboration with the Society for Cardiovascular Magnetic Resonance. *J Am Soc Echocardiogr.* 2017;30(4):303–371.
13. Klein AL, Abbara S, Agler DA, et al. American Society of Echocardiography clinical recommendations for multimodality cardiovascular imaging of patients with pericardial disease. *J Am Soc Echocardiogr.* 2013;26(9):965–1012.
14. Kyranis SJ, Latona J, Platts D, et al. Improving the echocardiographic assessment of pulmonary pressure using the tricuspid regurgitant signal—the "chin" vs the "beard". *Echocardiography.* 2018;35(8):1085–1096.
15. Naqvi TZ, Huynh HK. A new window of opportunity in echocardiography. *J Am Soc Echocardiogr.* 2006;19(5):569–577.
16. Waggoner AD, Baumann CM, Stark PA. "Views from the back" by subscapular retrocardiac imaging: technique and clinical application. *J Am Soc Echocardiogr.* 1995;8(3):257–262.

9 Transthoracic Echocardiography Tomographic Views

Wendy Tsang, Roberto M. Lang, Itzhak Kronzon

This chapter describes the main set of echocardiographic images that should be obtained for standardization and facilitation of image interpretation. Standard examination images are acquired from several transducer positions on the chest wall. Each window, angulation, and rotation of the transducer about its axis enables acquisition of several tomographic echocardiographic views. The sonographer acquiring the images may sit on either the left side of the patient, scanning with the left hand, or on the right side of the patient, scanning with the right hand. Nomenclature of the transthoracic views is primarily based on the position of the transducer (i.e., parasternal, apical, subxiphoid, suprasternal). In addition, nomenclature of the transthoracic views is based on three orthogonal planes: long-axis, short-axis, and apical views. The views not encompassed by this nomenclature are named by the anatomic structures they visualize. Two-dimensional (2D) grayscale images are typically acquired first, and then, while maintaining the image plane, color Doppler images are superimposed.

PARASTERNAL WINDOW

The parasternal window provides the parasternal long-axis, right ventricular (RV) inflow and outflow, and short-axis views. The parasternal long-axis (PLAX) view is typically the first image acquired in a transthoracic study (Fig. 9.1). A high-depth image should be obtained to exclude pleural and pericardial effusion (see Fig. 9.1C) and other pathology posterior to the heart. A low-depth image should be subsequently obtained to assess the cardiac anatomy (see

Fig. 9.1D and Video 9.1). From this view, the left atrium (LA), left ventricle (LV), right ventricular outflow tract (RVOT), and aortic root are visualized. The right and either noncoronary cusps or left coronary cusp, depending on the cut-plane, of the aortic valve are seen, as well as the anterior and posterior mitral valve leaflets. Occasionally, the right coronary artery can be seen (Fig. 9.2). If the image is obtained from a high rib space, the LV will point apically resulting in a "booted" heart. This can be corrected by moving the transducer down a rib space. In some patients, visualization of the LV and the aorta in the same plane is not possible, so an image of the LV should be obtained at a lower rib space and then the transducer moved up a rib space to image the aortic root and proximal ascending aorta. In the PLAX view, the mitral valve and aortic valve should be inspected and interrogated with color Doppler to identify the presence of regurgitation or stenosis.

Although no longer recommended, the linear left atrial anteroposterior dimension can be measured in this view.[1] It is measured from the trailing edge of the aortic root to the leading edge of the LA at end-systole, when the LA is largest. Also, from this view, M-mode measurements of the aortic root and LV are obtained, although measurements directly from the 2D images are preferred. If M-mode LV measurements are being obtained, the 2D targeted M-mode cursor should be placed at the level of the papillary muscle tips, oriented perpendicular to the LV walls. Left ventricular internal dimensions should be measured at end-diastole (LVIDd) and end-systole (LVIDs). The leading edge–to–leading edge convention should be

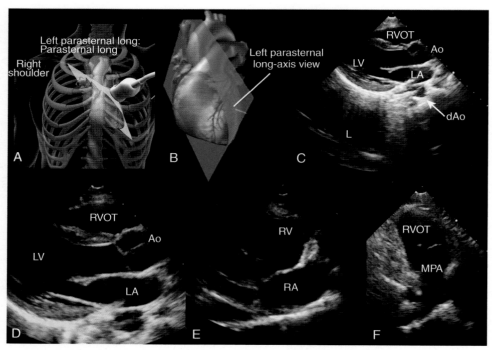

Figure 9.1. The parasternal long-axis view is acquired from the second left intercostal space (**A**). Schematic demonstrating the parasternal long-axis view cut plane through the heart (**B**). Parasternal long-axis view in low depth (**C**) and high depth (**D**). Parasternal right ventricular inflow (**E**) and right ventricular outflow view (**F**). *Ao,* Aortic root; *dAo,* descending aorta; *L,* lung; *LA,* left atrium; *LV,* left ventricle; *MPA,* main pulmonary artery; *RA,* right atrium; *RV,* right ventricle; *RVOT,* right ventricular outflow tract.

used.[2,3] From these measurements, the fractional shortening can be computed as:

$$FS = (LVIDd - LVIDs) / (LVIDd)$$

Intraventricular septal (IVS) and posterior wall thicknesses (PWT) (see Fig. 9.1D) are measured at end-diastole. LV mass can be estimated using the formula:

$$LVmass = 0.8 \times (1.04 \left[(LVIDd + PWTd + IVSd)^3 - (LVIDd)^3 \right] + 0.6 \text{ g}$$

in which PWTd is posterior wall thickness at end-diastole and IVSd is interventricular septal wall thickness at end-diastole.[4]

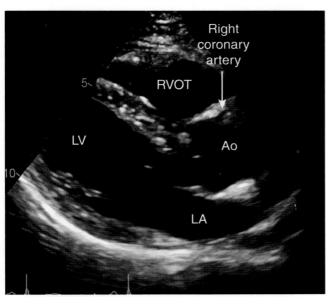

Figure 9.2. A parasternal long-axis view in which the right coronary artery can be seen at the aortic root *(arrow)*. *Ao,* Aortic root; *LA,* left atrium; *LV,* left ventricle; *RVOT,* right ventricular outflow tract.

From the parasternal long-axis window, the RV inflow view is obtained by tilting the end of the transducer toward the patient's head (see Fig. 9.1E). This allows imaging of the RA, RV, and tricuspid valve. This view is primarily used for visualizing the anterior and either the posterior (if no coronary sinus or septum is seen) or septal tricuspid valve leaflets if the coronary sinus or septum is seen. This view also allows assessment for the presence of tricuspid valve regurgitation with color Doppler. In contrast, by tilting the transducer toward the patient's feet, the RVOT comes into view (see Fig. 9.1F). From this perspective, the pulmonic valve and the bifurcation of the pulmonary artery are visualized. A patent ductus arteriosus may be seen in this view using color Doppler. By rotating the transducer 90 degrees from the parasternal long-axis view, the parasternal short-axis (PSAX) views are obtained. With angulation of the transducer superiorly, structures at the aortic valve level are imaged (Fig. 9.3). These structures include cusps of the aortic valve, pulmonary artery, pulmonic valve, RVOT, septal and anterior leaflets of the tricuspid valve, RA, LA, and interatrial septum. The left main coronary artery and bifurcation can be seen in this window (Fig. 9.4). The left upper pulmonary vein is closest to the left atrial appendage in this view with flow away from the transducer. The left lower pulmonary vein will be closer to the descending aorta with flow toward the transducer. By tilting the transducer anteriorly, the RVOT can be seen (see Fig. 9.2B). The mitral valve can be inspected by returning to the short-axis view of the aortic valve and then directing the transducer inferiorly (see Fig. 9.2C). Continued inferior angulation of the transducer allows acquisition of multiple short-axis cuts of the LV from the base to the apex, allowing assessment of overall LV performance, wall motion, and papillary muscle position (see Fig. 9.2D and E; Videos 9.2 to 9.4). For patients with increased LV septal wall thickness on the PLAX images, LV wall thickness may be measured in the short-axis images for confirmation.[5] It is also in the short-axis images that identification of an increased ratio of noncompacted to compacted myocardium should be assessed.[6]

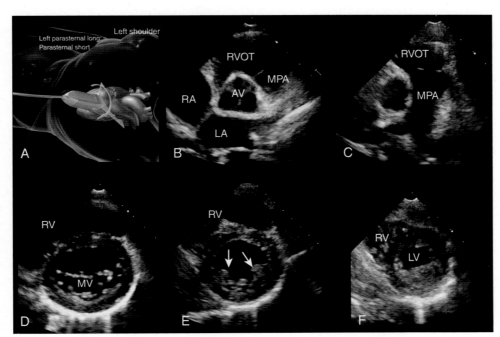

Figure 9.3. Rotation of the probe 90 degrees clockwise from the parasternal long-axis window brings the parasternal short-axis view into the imaging plane (**A**). Parasternal short-axis view of the aortic valve (**B**). Parasternal right ventricular outflow view (**C**). Parasternal short-axis view of the mitral valve at the basal LV (**D**), the mid–left ventricle (**E**) at the papillary muscles *(arrows)* and left ventricular apex (**F**). *AV,* Aortic valve; *LA,* left atrium; *LV,* left ventricle; *MPA,* main pulmonary artery; *MV,* mitral valve; *RA,* right atrium; *RV,* right ventricle; *RVOT,* right ventricular outflow tract.

TRANSTHORACIC APICAL WINDOW

The apical window is typically best obtained with the patient in a shallow left lateral decubitus position with the transducer placed at the apical cardiac impulse and then adjusted to obtain an optimal image (Fig. 9.5A). Care should be taken to prevent foreshortening of the LV.

Clues to recognizing foreshortening of the LV are listed in Box 9.1. Three-dimensional echocardiography is instrumental in avoiding this potential problem. From the apical transducer position, all four cardiac chambers should be well visualized (see Fig. 9.5B and Video 9.5). This view allows excellent Doppler interrogation of the mitral and tricuspid valves as well as the pulmonary veins. Typically, the right lower pulmonary vein is seen in the apical four-chamber view with flow parallel to the interatrial septum (Videos 9.6 and 9.7). Anterior angulation of the transducer, while in the four-chamber view, allows the aortic valve to come into plane (see Fig. 9.5C). With this angulation, the right upper pulmonary vein can be seen (Fig. 9.6).

After the apical four-chamber view has been acquired, the transducer is rotated counterclockwise approximately 60 degrees to obtain the apical two-chamber view and then an additional 60 degrees to obtain the apical three-chamber view (see Fig. 9.5D and E; Video 9.8). The two-chamber view allows evaluation of the anterior and inferior walls of the LV as well as color Doppler evaluation of the mitral valve. In some patients, the left atrial appendage and left

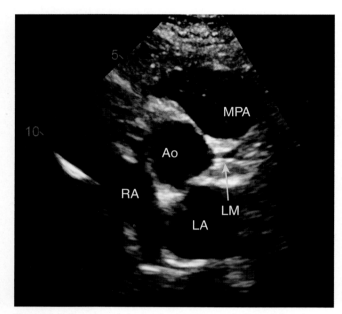

Figure 9.4. Parasternal short-axis view demonstrating a left main coronary artery and its bifurcation *(arrow)*. *Ao,* Aortic root; *LA,* left atrium; *LM, l*eft main; *MPA,* main pulmonary artery; *RA,* right atrium.

BOX 9.1 Clues to Recognize Foreshortening of the Left Ventricle

LV has a globular appearance that is wider and shorter with a rounded apex (normally >8 cm long and tapers toward the apex)
LV apex appears thickened
LV apex "squeezes" or moves downward systole (normally the LV apex should remain at the same horizontal level between end-diastole and end-systole)
LV in apical four- and two-chamber views should have similar lengths

LV, Left ventricle.

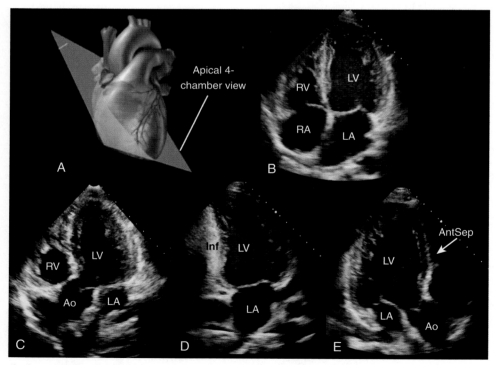

Figure 9.5. Schematic demonstrating the apical four-chamber cut plane through the heart (**A**). Apical four-chamber (**B**), five-chamber (**C**), two-chamber (**D**) and three-chamber (**E**) views. *AntSep,* Anteroseptal wall; *Ao,* aortic root; *Inf,* inferior wall; *LA,* left atrium; *LV,* left ventricle; *RA,* right atrium; *RV,* right ventricle.

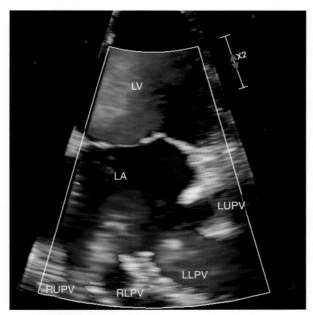

Figure 9.6. Focus apical four-chamber view demonstrating the four pulmonary veins. *LLPV,* Left lower pulmonary vein; *LUPV,* left upper pulmonary vein; *RLPV,* right lower pulmonary vein; *RUPV,* right upper pulmonary vein.

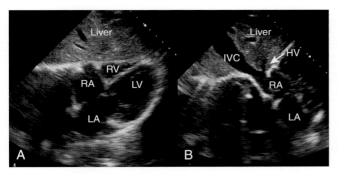

Figure 9.7. Subcostal four-chamber view (**A**) and inferior vena cava view (**B**). *HV,* Hepatic vein; *IVC,* inferior vena cava; *LA,* left atrium; *LV,* left ventricle; *RA,* right atrium; *RV,* right ventricle.

upper pulmonary vein are well seen in this view. The apical three-chamber view is similar to the PLAX view, wherein the anteroseptal and inferolateral walls can be assessed (Video 9.9). Color Doppler evaluation of the mitral and aortic valves should be repeated in the apical three-chamber view.

SUBCOSTAL WINDOW

Subcostal images are obtained with the patient supine, often with the knees bent to relax the abdomen. From this window, visualization of all four cardiac chambers is possible (Fig. 9.7). This view is particularly helpful for evaluating the pericardium, RV free wall thickness, and the interatrial septum. A short-axis image of the LV obtained from the subcostal view can provide images comparable with those obtained from the PSAX views. Because the subcostal short-axis images are acquired at greater depth, they are typically only recorded if the parasternal images are inadequate. Finally, from this view, the inferior vena cava and hepatic veins should be visualized (Fig. 9.7). In patients with good subcostal windows, the superior vena cava (SVC) could be visualized entering the RA. If this view can be obtained, assessment for the presence of a superior sinus venosus defect can be performed. One additional structure that should be scanned routinely from the subcostal view is the abdominal aorta. Pulsed-wave Doppler images obtained in this view are also helpful for examining flow patterns of the abdominal aorta.

TRANSTHORACIC SUPRASTERNAL WINDOW

With the patient supine and the neck hyperextended, the transducer is placed in the suprasternal notch. This allows visualization of the ascending aorta, aortic arch, and proximal descending aorta in the long axis and the right pulmonary artery in the short axis (Fig. 9.8). Continuous-wave Doppler recordings from this transducer position can be used to measure the maximum velocity across a coarctation site. Rotation of the probe 90 degrees in this view allow visualization of the aorta in cross section and the right pulmonary artery in a long view with the LA below it. In patients with good image quality, the pulmonary veins entering the LA can be seen in this view. Also, pulsed-wave Doppler can be used to document the flow patterns of the proximal thoracic descending aorta. The pediatric blind probe can be used in this position to obtain the highest gradient across a stenotic aortic valve. If the

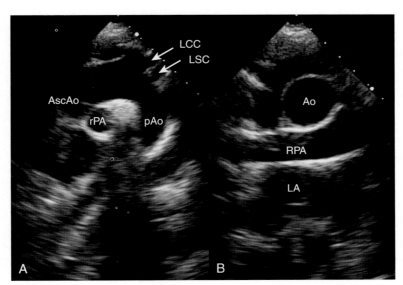

Figure 9.8. Suprasternal notch long-axis view (**A**) and short-axis (**B**) view of the aorta. *AscAo,* Ascending aorta; *Ao,* aorta; *LA,* left atrium; *LCC,* left common carotid; *LSC,* left subclavian; *pAo,* proximal thoracic descending aorta; *rPA,* right pulmonary artery.

transducer is placed on the right side, then the SVC can be visualized, and flow to the RA can be imaged.

OFF-AXIS VIEWS

The views described previously can be acquired in the majority of patients. Causes for suboptimal images include the patient's body habitus, inability of the patient to be positioned properly, congenital heart disease, patients' postsurgical status, and variability in patients' anatomy. One approach to these patients is to use nontraditional imaging windows such as the right parasternal position or off-axis views. Labeling the site from where images were obtained is important, especially in patients who require serial studies. In addition, off-axis views play a role in demonstrating findings such as pleural or pericardial effusions.

Please access ExpertConsult to view the corresponding videos for this chapter.

REFERENCES

1. Lang RM, Badano LP, Mor-Avi V, et al. Recommendations for cardiac chamber quantification by echocardiography in adults. *J Am Soc Echocardiog*. 2015;28:1–39.
2. Schiller NB, Shah PM, Crawford M, et al. Recommendations for quantitation of the left ventricle by two-dimensional echocardiography. *J Am Soc Echocardiogr*. 1989;2:358–367.
3. Lang RM, Badano LP, Tsang W, et al. EAE/ASE recommendations for image acquisition and display using three-dimensional echocardiography. *J Am Soc Echocardiogr*. 2012;25:3–46.
4. Devereux RB, Alonso DR, Lutas EM, et al. Echocardiographic assessment of left ventricular hypertrophy: comparison to necropsy findings. *Am J Cardiol*. 1986;57:450–458.
5. Elliott PM, Anastasakis A, Borger MA, et al. ESC Guidelines on diagnosis and management of hypertrophic cardiomyopathy. *Eur Heart J*. 2014;35(39):2733–2779. 2014.
6. Gati S, Rajani R, Carr-White GS, Chambers JB. Adult left ventricular noncompaction: reappraisal of current diagnostic imaging modalities. *JACC Cardiovasc Imag*. 2014;7:1266–1275.

10 M-Mode Echocardiography

Itzhak Kronzon, Gerard P. Aurigemma

Historically, M-mode (motion mode) echocardiography was the first effective modality for the ultrasonic evaluation of the heart. M-mode echocardiography provides an ice pick, one-dimensional (1D; depth only) view of the heart.[1,2] The ultrasound echoes reflected from the various cardiac interfaces are represented as dots and their intensities by brightness (B-mode). With the sweep of the screen (or the recording paper), the location of each interface is represented by a line, which provides information about its temporal location (Fig. 10.1). The two-dimensional (2D) appearance of the tracing is the result of presenting depth (expressed as the up–down dimension of the tracing) and width (left-to-right dimension, which expresses time).

An important attribute of M-mode echocardiography, compared with 2D imaging, is its superior temporal resolution. In the current 2D-directed M-mode echocardiography, data are acquired at a rate up to 1000 frames per second, compared with 15 to 100 frames per second for 2D echocardiography, depending on sector width and heart rate.[1,2] Thus M-mode echocardiography remains important in daily clinical use for its ability to time events during the cardiac cycle and assess fast-moving structures (e.g., valves) (see Fig. 10.1).

The limitations of M-mode echocardiography are related to its 1D nature. Although the interrogating ultrasound beam can be tilted to visualize different structures and their anatomic relations, it may miss other structures. Also, it may produce erroneous information about chamber and vessel dimensions by scanning them obliquely. Therefore, M-mode tracings should always be obtained with the guidance of the 2D images.

Some echocardiographers consider M-mode echocardiography to be an historical relic. Many of its initial uses during the earliest decade of echocardiography have been supplanted by the newer, more anatomically correct 2D, three-dimensional (3D), and Doppler modalities. We and others believe that, like history itself, older experience is still worth studying.[1] Furthermore, in selected situations, M-mode echocardiography remains a fundamental part of the routine echocardiographic examination and provides an important supplement to the newer echocardiographic modalities. Accordingly, this chapter demonstrates classic M-mode images, with emphasis on its continued value in the era of 2D and 3D Doppler echocardiography.

LEFT VENTRICLE

The most common use for echocardiography, in any of its forms, is to assess size and function of the left ventricle (LV).[3] At present, 2D-directed M-mode echocardiography is still used to establish cardiac chamber size and wall thickness (Fig. 10.2). Given its superior temporal resolution, M-mode echocardiography is perfectly suited to diagnosing abnormal LV contraction patterns, such as those seen with left bundle branch block (see Fig. 10.2B).[4,5]

It has long been appreciated that normal systolic function includes the descent of the mitral and tricuspid annulus toward the apex, which remains relatively stationary.[5] The extent of the descent of the base, measured in millimeters, is reflective of global systolic function. Acronyms for this descent of the base are TAPSE[6] (tricuspid annular plane systolic excursion) and MAPSE (mitral annular plane systolic excursion) (see Fig. 10.2E).[6]

MITRAL VALVE
Normal Motion

During the rapid ventricular filling in early diastole, the anterior mitral leaflet moves from its end-systolic closed position (D point) toward the opening position, that is, anteriorly toward the interventricular septum (E point); there is a reciprocal motion of the posterior leaflet (se Fig. 10.1A and C). The nadir of this backward motion is called the *F point*. Atrial contraction reopens the leaflets (the A point). Near the onset of systole, the leaflets move to the closed position (at the C point), where they remain throughout systole.

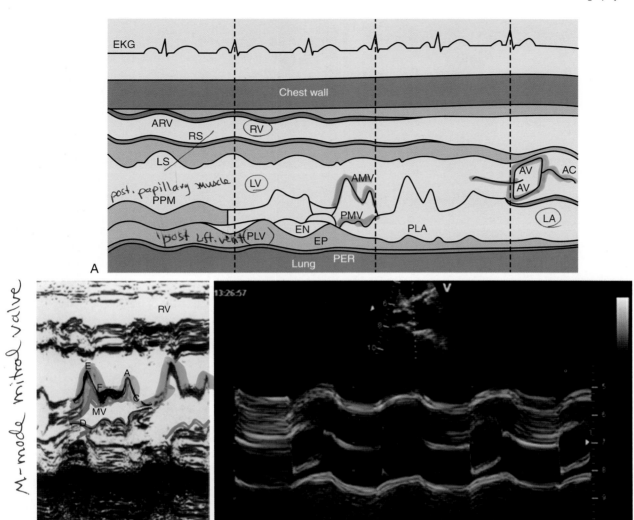

Figure 10.1. Left ventricle. **A,** Schematic shows the four principal M-mode views of the heart. *AMV,* Anterior mitral valve; *ARV,* anterior right ventricle; *EKG,* electrocardiograph; *EN,* endocardial edge; *EP,* epicardial surface; *LA,* left atrial; *LS,* left ventricular septum; *LV,* left ventricle; *PLA,* plasminogen activator; *PLV,* posterior left ventricle; *PMV,* posterior mitral valve; *PPM,* posterior papillary muscle; *RS,* right ventricular septum; *RV,* right ventricle. **B,** M-mode view of the mitral valve. **C,** M-mode transducer is directed through the RV, proximal aorta, and LA. Aortic valve leaflets and AC aortic closure line, which, in normal individuals, is in the midportion of the aorta. A, Anteriormost excursion of the anterior leaflet with atrial systole; C, closure of the mitral valve and end-diastole; D, posteriormost excursions of the mitral leaflets in early diastole; E, anteriormost excursions of the mitral leaflets in early diastole; F, closure point of the mitral valve in early diastasis; *MV,* mitral valve; *RV,* right ventricle. (Part A adapted with permission from Feigenbaum H: *Echocardiography,* ed 5. Philadelphia: Lea & Febiger; 1993.)

Mitral Stenosis

The mitral leaflets open at early diastole. The leaflets are thickened with commissural fusion. The larger anterior leaflet moves anteriorly, which also pulls the smaller posterior leaflet anteriorly. Because of the pressure gradient across the valve throughout diastole and the lack of rapid ventricular filling phase, the leaflets do not return toward the closure position as in normal valves.[1,2] The E-F slope (see Fig. 10.1B) is flatter than normal. The M-mode combination of leaflet thickening, anterior motion of the posterior mitral leaflet, and flat E-F slope is diagnostic of mitral stenosis (Fig. 10.3A).

Mitral Valve Prolapse

Unlike mitral stenosis, the valve diastolic motion is normal, and the leaflets remain closed in systole. In mitral valve prolapse, the closed mitral leaflets sag backward. This motion may occur in mid to late systole (see Fig. 10.3B) and may be associated with mid-systolic click or pansystolic (and be associated with a pansystolic mitral regurgitation murmur).[7–9]

Systolic Anterior Motion of the Anterior Mitral Leaflet

An anterior mitral leaflet that demonstrates systolic anterior motion (SAM) is seen mainly in patients with hypertrophic cardiomyopathy; high velocity in the left ventricular outflow tract results in SAM of the anterior mitral leaflet[10,11] because of the Venturi effect. In these patients, the diastolic mitral valve motion is normal. During systole, however, the anterior leaflet moves toward the interventricular septum and may coapt with the ventricular surface. The duration and degree of coaptation are related to the pressure gradient (see Fig. 10.3C).[10,11]

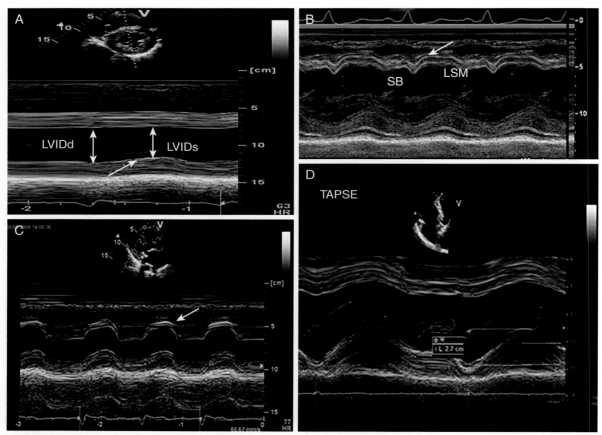

Figure 10.2. Left ventricle (LV). **A,** LV of a patient with infiltrative cardiomyopathy caused by amyloidosis. The walls are thick, and the fractional shortening is low. **B,** Left bundle branch block. Compared with the normal LV echocardiogram (**A**), the initial downward motion of the septum (ESM) is absent, and there is a prominent downward motion of the septum in early ventricular systole (the septal :beak: [*SB*]), which represents unopposed right ventricular (RV) contraction caused by delayed activation of the posterior and lateral LV. Also, during ventricular systole, the septum moves anteriorly *(arrow)*. Finally, there is a posterior septal motion (PSM), which occurs after the peak upward excursion of the posterior wall (LSM) and coincides with RV filling. **C,** Septal motion in severe tricuspid regurgitation (TR). Notice the abrupt rightward motion *(arrow)* of the interventricular septum as the RV unloads into the right atrium (RA) during isovolumic systole. **D,** Example of normal tricuspid annular plane systolic excursion (TAPSE), defined as 16 mm or greater.[6] *LVIDd,* Diastolic left ventricular dimensions; *LVIDs,* systolic left ventricular dimensions.

The Mitral Valve in Aortic Insufficiency

In acute aortic regurgitation, the diastolic pressure in the ventricle rises rapidly during diastole as a result of aortic runoff. In fact, in some instances, the LV pressure may rise above the left atrial (LA) pressure, leading to premature closure of the mitral valve (see Fig. 10.3D and E).[12,13] When the aortic regurgitation jet strikes the anterior mitral leaflet, a fine, fluttering motion can be seen. This finding suggests the presence of aortic insufficiency but is not a marker of its severity (see Fig. 10.3F). None of these findings in aortic regurgitation are reliably demonstrated by 2D echocardiography because of its inferior temporal resolution. Therefore, M-mode data complement the assessment of valve regurgitation severity in contemporary practice.

The Mitral Valve in Left Ventricular Dysfunction

Normally, the mitral E point is close to the interventricular septum (E point septal separation). In patients with left ventricular dilatation and reduced stroke volume, the E point of the anterior leaflet is separated from the septum by a distance of at least 8 mm. Interestingly, this expression of unfavorable LV remodeling was the first echocardiographic finding that appeared directly related to

prognosis (see Fig. 10.3G).[14–16] A second M-mode sign of LV dysfunction is a disturbance in the A-C line, which is usually rapid and straight. In patients with noncompliant LVs, atrial systole results in a significant elevation in LV diastolic pressures. The M-mode reflection of this phenomenon is an interruption in the normal A-C closure line, which is known as the *A-C shoulder* or *B bump* (see Fig. 10.3H).[17,18]

Color M-Mode Echocardiography

This multiparametric display features flow events superimposed on the M-mode display and is perhaps the best method available to time regurgitant events. As is shown in Figure 10.3I, color M-mode echocardiography graphically demonstrates both systolic and diastolic mitral regurgitation in the same patient. Doppler color M-mode echocardiography can be used for the measurement of the hemisphere maximum radius in the calculation of the proximal isovelocity area (PISA)[19] (Fig. 10.3J). This technique can be used when the MV leaflets are not well visualized, making it difficult to decide where to place the measurement of the PISA radius. We have also found this technique useful in cases of atrial fibrillation in which the average of several PISA radii must be determined.

10

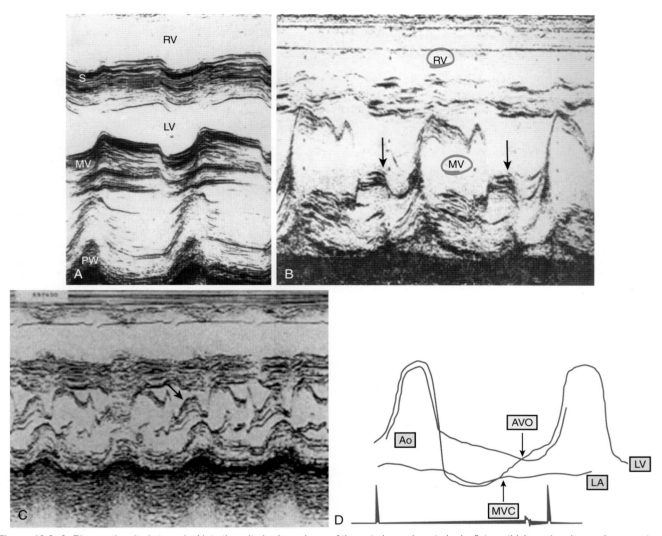

Figure 10.3. A, Rheumatic mitral stenosis. Note the mitral valve echoes of the anterior and posterior leaflet are thickened and move in concert because of inflammatory valvulitis. The E-F slope is diminished. **B,** Severe mitral valve prolapse; *arrows* indicate late systolic sagging or "hammocking" of the mitral valve. **C,** Anterior motion of the mitral valve in a patient with hypertrophic obstructive cardiomyopathy *(arrow)*. **D,** Hemodynamic tracing illustrating the principle behind the early opening of the aortic valve in a patient with acute severe aortic regurgitation. Notice that there is pressure equilibration between the aorta and left ventricle (LV), which occurs at end-diastole. See text for details. *Ao,* Aorta; *AVO,* atrial valve opening; *LA,* left atrium; *MV,* mitral valve; *MVC,* mitral valve closing; *PW,* posterior wall; *RV,* right ventricle; *S,* septum.

AORTIC VALVE
Normal Motion

The aortic valve can be seen in the middle of the aortic root. The right and the noncoronary cusps move in systole to the opened position, and they move in diastole toward the closed position, creating the impression of rectangles connected by strings (see Fig. 10.1A and C). The ejection time, a descriptor of forward stroke volume, can be timed from the aortic valve opening to its closure. Fine fluttering of the opened leaflets is not uncommon and actually suggests that the leaflets are thin and relatively normal. In patients with aortic stenosis, the leaflets appear thickened and calcified and have diminished excursion. A bicuspid aortic valve may have eccentric closure line (Fig. 10.4A).

The Aortic Valve in Hypertrophic Obstructive Cardiomyopathy

In hypertrophic obstructive cardiomyopathy the SAM may result in left ventricular outflow obstruction, and therefore flow across the aortic valve will be decreased in mid-systole. M-mode echocardiography will show a midsystolic closure of the aortic valve (see Fig. 10.4B). In discrete subaortic stenosis caused by a subaortic membrane, by contrast, the valve opens well in early systole and then suddenly returns to near closure position, where it stays for the rest of systole (Fig. 10.4C). Midsystolic closure of the aortic valve is also seen in other causes of dynamic outflow tract obstruction and has been observed in some instances of stress cardiomyopathy (see Fig. 10.4D) when hyperdynamic function of the base of the left ventricle, coupled with suitable LV geometry, creates a Venturi effect in the LV outflow tract.

Premature Aortic Valve Opening

With severe aortic regurgitation, there are a rapid rise of LV diastolic pressure and a rapid decline in the aortic diastolic pressure. With LA contraction, the LA (and LV) diastolic pressure may rise above the aortic diastolic pressure, resulting in premature (end-diastolic) aortic valve opening (see Fig. 10.4E).

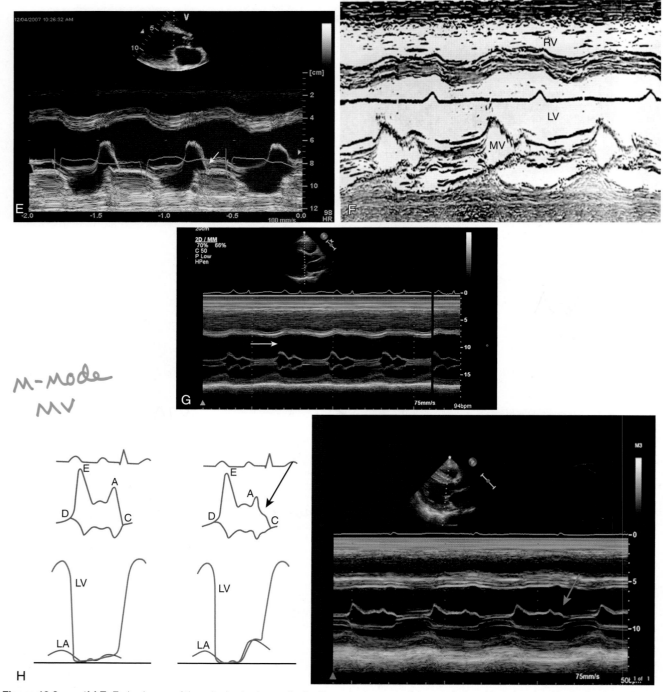

M-Mode
MV

Figure 10.3, cont'd E, Early closure of the mitral valve in a patient with acute severe aortic regurgitation. Note that the mitral valve *(arrow)* closes well before the QRS complex, indicative of pressure equilibration between the LV and left atrium in this patient. **F,** Fine fluttering of the mitral valve at end diastole in a patient with aortic regurgitation. **G,** E point septal separation *(arrow)* in a patient with idiopathic dilated cardiomyopathy. *LV,* Left ventricle; *MV,* mitral valve; *RV,* right ventricle. **H,** Schematic diagram *(left panel)* and M-mode recording in a patient with elevated left ventricular diastolic pressure showing the so-called B-bump *(black arrow, right panel* of schematic; *blue arrow* in patient M-mode image).

Continued

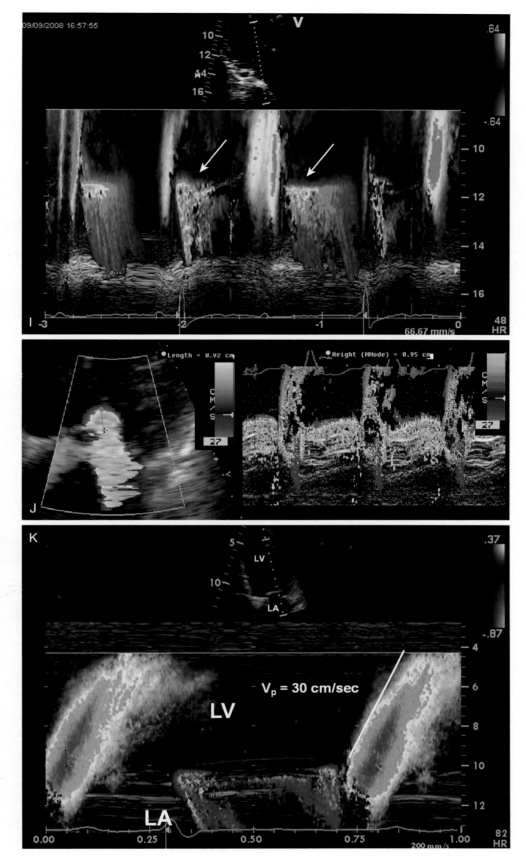

Figure 10.3, cont'd I, Color M-mode in a patient with complete heart block. The *left arrow* points to superimposed mitral regurgitation jet, which occurs in isovolumic systole. The *right arrow* points to diastolic mitral regurgitation seen in the left atrium after nonconducted atrial depolarization. **J,** Use of M-mode echocardiography to estimate size of a proximal isovelocity systolic area (PISA). This adaptation of color M-mode allows for easy recognition of the extent of the PISA. A, Anteriormost excursion of the anterior leaflet with atrial systole; C, closure of the mitral valve and end-diastole; D, posteriormost excursions of the mitral leaflets in early diastole; E, anteriormost excursions of the mitral leaflets in early diastole; *LA,* left atrial pressure; *LV,* left ventricular pressure. **K,** Color M-mode (see Fig. 10.5A) Vp (or flow propagation velocity) in a normal individual. Ao, Aortic pressure; *AVO,* aortic valve opening; *LA,* left atrial pressure; *LV,* left ventricular pressure; *MVC,* mitral valve closure. (Part H adapted with permission from Feigenbaum H: *Echocardiography*, ed 5. Philadelphia: Lea & Febiger; 1993. Part J schematic adapted with permission from Feigenbaum H: *Echocardiography*, ed 5. Philadelphia: Lea & Febiger; 1993. Part J figure courtesy of Dr. Roberto Lang.)

M-Mode
Ao

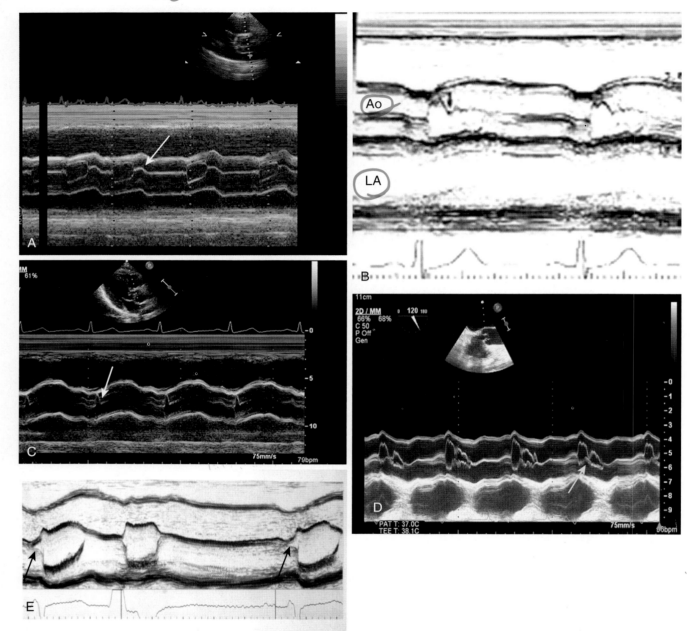

Figure 10.4. Aortic valve. **A,** M-mode echocardiogram in a patient with a bicuspid aortic valve. *Arrow* indicates eccentric closure line. **B,** In hypertrophic cardiomyopathy (HCM), there is midsystolic closure *(arrows)* indicating left ventricular (LV) outflow tract obstruction with diminution in forward flow. As the LV pressure rises and then overcomes the dynamic obstruction, the aortic valve opens a second time. Opening of the aortic valve is associated with reduced forward stroke volume. **C,** In the subaortic membrane, the aortic valve envelope shows a rapid upward swing followed by restoration to a midaortic position without secondary opening *(white arrow)*. This is in contrast to the M-shaped envelope in patients with hypertrophic obstructive cardiomyopathy. **D,** Midsystolic closure of the aortic valve seen in a patient with stress cardiomyopathy, Takotsubo phenotype, complicated by dynamic LV outflow tract obstruction. This patient had refractory hypotension and was being treated with positive inotropic agents. Recognition of dynamic LV outflow tract obstruction by two-dimensional echocardiography and supported by this M-mode finding led to a different strategy: volume resuscitation, withdrawal of beta-agonist agents, and administration of alpha agonists. **E,** Early aortic valve opening *(black arrow)* in a patient with acute severe aortic regurgitation. In the first and third beats after a longer cycle, there is more opportunity for pressure equilibration between the LV and the aorta because the filling of the left ventricle is augmented. This leads to premature opening of the aortic valve. *Ao,* Aorta; *LA,* left atrium. (Image courtesy of Dr. Theo E. Meyer.)

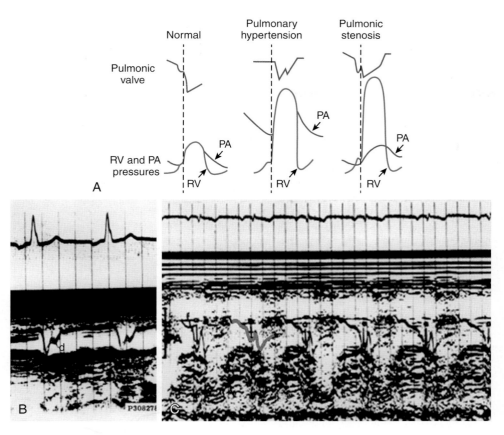

Figure 10.5. Pulmonary valve. **A,** Schematic of the pulmonary valve in a normal individual, a patient with pulmonary hypertension, and a patient with pulmonic stenosis. The *lower part* of the diagram demonstrates right ventricular (RV) and pulmonary artery (PA) pressures in the three scenarios. **B,** The "flying W" sign in a patient with severe pulmonary hypertension. **C,** Taken from a study of a patient with severe valvular pulmonic stenosis; note the exaggerated atrial contraction motion, as shown in the schematic. *Red overlay* has been placed to simulate schematic shown in *A*. (Part A reproduced with permission from Feigenbaum H: *Echocardiography*, ed 5. Philadelphia: Lea & Febiger;1993.)

PULMONIC VALVE
Normal Motion

In most cases in which motion is normal, only the anterior leaflet of the pulmonic valve can be depicted on M-mode echocardiography. This leaflet moves posteriorly and remains opened during systole. At end-diastole, with right atrial (RA) contraction, the right ventricular (RV) pressure approaches the pulmonary arterial end-diastolic pressure, resulting in posterior motion of the pulmonic valve (A-wave) (Fig. 10.5A).[2,20,21]

Severe Pulmonary Hypertension

In severe pulmonary hypertension, the pulmonary artery diastolic pressure is much higher than the RV diastolic pressure. In this hypertension situation, the RA contraction has no effect on the pulmonic valve end-diastolic position. Reduced or no A-wave is seen despite normal sinus rhythm (see Fig. 10.5B). Another finding seen in pulmonary hypertension is the "flying W" sign seen during pulmonic valve systolic opening. This unusual motion, with midsystolic closure and late systolic opening, may be the result of increased pulmonary vascular resistance.[20,21] The abnormal absence of the pulmonic valve A wave, together with the presence of flying W sign, is highly suggestive of severe pulmonary hypertension. They can be used when Doppler estimation of pulmonary artery pressure is not possible because of the lack of tricuspid or pulmonic regurgitation.

PERICARDIAL DISEASE

Pericardial effusion is better demonstrated by 2D echocardiography than by M-mode echocardiography. However, the timing of the abnormalities seen in cardiac tamponade and constrictive pericarditis can contribute to the understanding of the pathophysiology of these conditions; this issue is reviewed in Fig. 10.6.

CARDIAC TAMPONADE

M-mode echocardiography can demonstrate pericardial effusion as well as the respiratory variations in ventricular size and valve excursion. Because of ventricular interdependence, inspiration results in less pulmonary venous return and transmitral flow, which leads to a phasic decline in left ventricular volume. This process is reversed during inspiration. The M-mode echocardiogram (recorded simultaneously with respiratory tracing) shows the septal inspiratory shift toward the LV. This is the echocardiographic equivalent of the paradoxical pulse.[22–24]

The exact timing of diastolic RV collapse can also be demonstrated by M-mode echocardiography (see Fig. 10.6A and B). In some cases of pulmonary hypertension or chronic right-sided pressure overload with RV hypertrophy, LA or even LV collapse may occur before RV or RA collapse is seen. This may also be seen in instances of low filling pressure. The elevation of RA pressure seen in most cases of tamponade can be confirmed by M-mode tracing of the inferior vena cava (IVC) near its communication with the RA. An IVC diameter of more than 20 mm with a reduced (<50%) decrease during inspiration or "sniff" indicates elevated RA pressure, usually greater than 15 mm Hg (IVC plethora) (see Fig. 10.6C).

CONSTRICTIVE PERICARDITIS

This difficult clinical diagnosis can still be supported by an array of M-mode echocardiographic findings.[25,26] These findings include (1) pericardial thickening; (2) IVC plethora (see earlier discussion); (3) inspiratory septal shift toward the LV (the RV cavity dimension

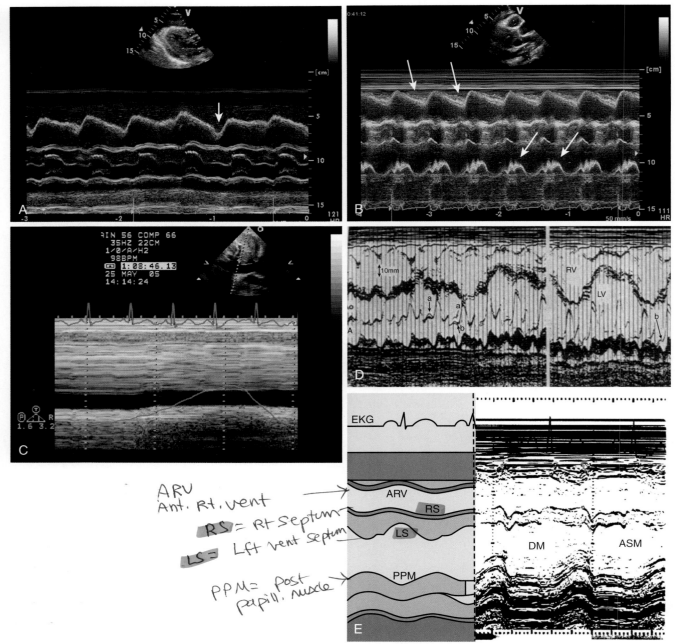

Figure 10.6. Pericardial disease. **A,** Cardiac tamponade: large pericardial effusion and diastolic collapse of the right ventricular free wall, indicated by the *arrow*. **B,** Large circumferential pericardial effusion *(upper pair of downward arrows)* and left atrial collapse *(lower pair of downward arrows)*, indicating increased intrapericardial pressure leading to ventricular diastolic and left atrial systolic collapse. When filling pressures are low, this constellation of findings is called *low-pressure cardiac tamponade.* **C,** In a patient with tamponade, the vena cava is dilated and does not collapse. **D,** Constrictive pericarditis. **E,** Schematic of normal septal motion *(left)* and recording from a patient with constrictive pericarditis. Note the diastolic posterior motion of the septum (DM) and the second reverberation in the septum (ASM), which corresponds to atrial systole. *ARV,* Anterior right ventricle; *EKG,* electrocardiograph; *LS,* left ventricular septum; *RS,* right ventricular septum; *PPM,* posterior papillary muscle.

increases during inspiration and decreases during expiration, and there are reciprocal changes in the LV; during expiration, the mitral valve opening duration is longer than that during inspiration; see Fig. 10.6D); (4) diastolic septal "bounce" (characteristic early diastolic notch) as well as a late diastolic reverberation in the septum, around the time of atrial contraction (Fig. 10.6, *D, E*); and (5) premature opening of the pulmonic valve caused by elevation of the RV end-diastolic pressure without pulmonary hypertension and relatively low pulmonary artery diastolic pressure.

REFERENCES

1. Feigenbaum H. Role of M-mode technique in today's echocardiography. *J Am Soc Echocardiogr.* 2010;23:240–257.
2. Feigenbaum H. *Echocardiography.* ed 5. Malvern, PA: Lea & Febiger; 1993.
3. Lang RM, Bierig M, Devereux RB, et al. Recommendations for chamber quantification. *J Am Soc Echocardiogr.* 2005;18:1440–1463.
4. Grines CL, Bashore TM, Boudoulas H, et al. Functional abnormalities in isolated left bundle branch block. The effect of interventricular asynchrony. *Circulation.* 1989;79:845–853.
5. Jones CJ, Raposo L, Gibson DG. Functional importance of the long axis dynamics of the human left ventricle. *Br Heart J.* 1990;634:215–220.

6. Rudski LG, Lai WW, Afilalo J, et al. Guidelines for the echocardiographic assessment of the right heart in adults. *J Am Soc Echocardiogr.* 2010;23:685–713. quiz 786–688.
7. Dillon JC, Haisse CL, Chang S, et al. Use of echocardiography in patients with prolapsed mitral valve. *Circulation.* 1971;43:503–507.
8. Kerber RE, Isaeff DM, Hancock EW. Echocardiographic patterns in patients with the syndrome of systolic click and late systolic murmur. *N Engl J Med.* 1971;284:691–693.
9. Popp RE, Brown OR, Silverman JF, et al. Echocardiographic abnormalities in the mitral valve prolapsed syndrome. *Circulation.* 1974;49:428–433.
10. Henry WL, Clark CE, Griffith JM, et al. Mechanism of left ventricular outflow obstruction in patients with obstructive asymmetric septal hypertrophy (idiopathic hypertrophic subaortic stenosis). *Am J Cardiol.* 1975;35:337–345.
11. Pollick C, Rakowski H, Wigle ED. Muscular subaortic stenosis: the quantitative relationship between systolic anterior motion and the pressure gradient. *Circulation.* 1984;69:43–49.
12. Botvinick EH, Schiller NB, Wickramasekaran R, et al. Echocardiographic demonstration of early mitral valve closure in severe aortic insufficiency. Its clinical implications. *Circulation.* 1975;51:836–847.
13. Perez JE, Cordova F, Cintron G. Diastolic opening of the aortic valve (AV) in a case of aortic insufficiency due to AV fenestration. *Cardiovasc Dis.* 1978;5:254–257.
14. Ahmadpour H, Shah AA, Allen JW, et al. Mitral E point septal separation: a reliable index of left ventricular performance in coronary artery disease. *Am Heart J.* 1983;106:21–28.
15. Child JS, Krivokapick J, Perloff JK. Effect of left ventricular size on mitral E point to ventricular septal separation in assessment of cardiac performance. *Am Heart J.* 1981;101:797–805.
16. Massie BM, Schiller NB, Ratshin RA, et al. Mitral-septal separation: new echocardiographic index of left ventricular function. *Am J Cardiol.* 1977;39:1008–1016.
17. Konecke LL, Feigenbaum H, Chang S, et al. Abnormal mitral valve motion in patients with elevated left ventricular diastolic pressures. *Circulation.* 1973;47:989–996.
18. Ambrose JA, Teichholz LE, Meller J, et al. The influence of left ventricular late diastolic filling on the A wave of the left ventricular pressure trace, *Circulation.* 1979;60:510–519.
19. Zoghbi WA, Enriquez-Sarano M, Foster E, et al. Recommendations for evaluation of the severity of native valvular regurgitation with two-dimensional and Doppler echocardiography. *J Am Soc Echocardiogr.* 2003;16:777–802.
20. Weyman AE, Dillon JC, Feigenbaum H, et al. Echocardiographic patterns of pulmonic valve motion with pulmonary hypertension. *Circulation.* 1974;50:905–910.
21. Nanda NC, Gramiak R, Robinson TI, et al. Echocardiographic evaluation of pulmonary hypertension. *Circulation.* 1974;50:575–581.
22. Armstrong WF, Schilt BF, Helper DJ, et al. Diastolic collapse of the right ventricle with cardiac tamponade: an echocardiographic study. *Circulation.* 1982;65:1491–1496.
23. Feigenbaum H, Zaky A, Grabhorn LL. Cardiac motion in patients with pericardial effusion. A study using reflected ultrasound. *Circulation.* 1966;34:611–619.
24. Leimgruber PP, Klopfenstein HS, Wann LS, et al. The hemodynamic derangement associated with right ventricular diastolic collapse in cardiac tamponade: an experimental echocardiographic study. *Circulation.* 1983;68:612–620.
25. Pool P, Seagren C, Abbasi A, et al. Echocardiographic manifestations of constrictive pericarditis: abnormal septal motion. *Chest.* 1975;68:684–688.
26. Candell-Rivera J, Garcia del Castillo H, Permanyer-Miralda G, et al. Echocardiographic features of the interventricular septum in chronic constrictive pericarditis. *Circulation.* 1978;57:1154–1158.

11

11 Doppler Echocardiography: Normal Antegrade Flow Patterns

Matthew W. Parker, Mohamed Ahmed, Gerard P. Aurigemma

BASIC CONCEPTS

Four modalities of Doppler echocardiography are currently available for use with a wide variety of applications: pulsed-wave (PW) Doppler, continuous-wave (CW) Doppler, color-flow imaging, and tissue Doppler imaging. The various Doppler modalities each complement M-mode and two-dimensional (2D) or three-dimensional (3D) B-mode structural data with hemodynamic (CW and PW Doppler and color-flow Doppler) and functional (tissue Doppler imaging) data. Doppler echocardiography is the modality on which noninvasive assessment of cardiac hemodynamics depends. The purpose of this chapter is to review the normal antegrade intracardiac flow using PW and CW Doppler.

Christian Johann Doppler (b. 1803) first observed that when a sound source and observer are moving closer together, the observed frequency of the sound is higher than when the source and observer are both not moving, and when the sound source and observer are moving away from each other, the observed frequency is lower than when not moving. The Doppler shift or frequency is proportionate to the velocity of movement between the source and observer. This principle applies equally to ultrasound backscattered by moving blood cells in the beating heart:

$$\Delta F = \frac{V \times 2F_0 \times \cos\theta}{C}$$

In this equation, ΔF represents the Doppler shift, V is the velocity of tissue, F_0 is the transducer frequency, $\cos\theta$ is the cosine of the angle of incidence between the direction of flow and the long axis of the ultrasound beam, and C is the speed of sound in tissue. All commercially available ultrasound machines calculate the velocity of blood flow by assuming that the average speed of sound in the body is 1540 m/s and that the ultrasound beam is parallel to flow so that $\cos\theta=1$:

$$V = \frac{\Delta F \times 1540 \, m/s}{2F_0}$$

Quantification of flow velocity is obtained with either PW or CW Doppler. PW Doppler records velocity at one specific location, whereas CW Doppler records flow velocity along the entire pathway of the ultrasound beam (Fig. 11.1).

CW Doppler permits accurate measurement of any flow velocity but cannot determine the location of the peak velocity it measures because all velocity signals along the length of the ultrasound beam are merged into one reflected signal. The reflected Doppler signal is converted to a velocity and displayed as a spectrum with velocity on the *y*-axis and time on the *x*-axis. By convention, flow toward the transducer is displayed, spectrally, above the zero baseline and flow away, below the zero baseline. CW Doppler is used to measure high velocities across stenotic or regurgitant valves.

PW Doppler can measure flow at a precisely defined location but with a more limited range of measurable velocities. PW Doppler is used to assess velocities across normal valves or vessels to calculate flow and assess cardiac function. PW Doppler velocity spectra can be displayed and measured similar to CW Doppler. Because PW Doppler allows measurement of velocity at a specific anatomic site, the 2D echocardiographic measurements of a valve or orifice can be combined with PW flow data to calculate stroke volume (SV), cardiac output (CO), and measurement of diastolic filling parameters. PW Doppler of multiple sample regions can also be displayed as a color map integrated into a 2D or 3D echocardiogram to screen for flow acceleration (stenosis) or regurgitation.

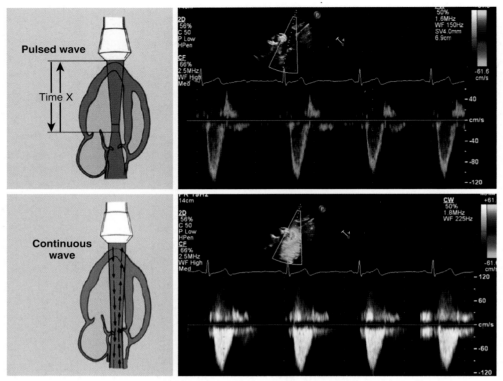

Figure 11.1. Pulsed-wave (PW) and continuous wave (CW) Doppler imaging. The PW signal *(upper panel)* is optimized to show the modal velocity without spectral broadening. Note the high density of the CW velocity jet as it records flow velocity along the pathway of the ultrasound beam *(lower panel)*. The flow away from the transducer is displayed below the zero line.

Daniel Bernoulli (b. 1700) described the phenomenon by which the increase in velocity of a fluid occurs simultaneously with a decrease in pressure (potential energy). Doppler frequencies therefore correspond to pressure gradients in the heart that can be calculated using the simplified Bernoulli equation:

$$\Delta P = 4V^2$$

in which ΔP represents the pressure gradient and V represents the blood flow velocity. Common clinical applications include estimation of pressure gradients across valves and estimation of pulmonary artery pressure from the velocity of tricuspid regurgitation.

TECHNICAL CONSIDERATIONS FOR OPTIMAL DOPPLER RECORDINGS
Maintain Parallel Orientation Between the Ultrasound Beam and the Direction of Blood Flow

Ultrasound machines calculate velocity from the Doppler shift with the assumption that flow (or motion) is parallel to the ultrasound beam. Incident angles smaller than 20 degrees produce errors smaller than 6% based on this assumption but more oblique angles produce significant errors as the (unmeasured) $\cos\theta$ increases rapidly above 30 degrees. Color Doppler and anatomic landmarks may be helpful to identify the likely direction of flow for alignment. Angle-correction tools available on some ultrasound systems for vascular imaging are generally not recommended for cardiac use because the true direction of flow is unknown and often dynamic in 3D space. Any clinically significant flow should be interrogated in at least two windows with different incident angles and the higher observed Doppler shift (velocity) taken as the more accurate measurement.[1,2]

Flow of Fluids Can Be Laminar or Turbulent

Normal flow through the cardiac chambers and great vessels is laminar, with essentially all blood cells traveling in the same direction and within a narrow range of velocities. Near the walls of vessels or when crossing a stenotic orifice, flow becomes turbulent, with blood cells moving in many directions across a wide range of velocities. Doppler sampling should be performed as near the center of the stream of flow as is feasible with adjustment of the PW sample size to capture a dense modal flow velocity with minimal spectral broadening.[1]

Use Optimal Gain Settings and Wall Filters

Gain should be adjusted to display a smooth flow signal with a clear modal velocity. Generally, the background should show slight speckling to ensure adequate sensitivity. High gain settings may emphasize weak signals outside of the modal velocity and reduce reproducibility of measurements. The width of the PW sample volume must be adjusted to avoid spectral broadening. The wall filter removes high-intensity, low-velocity signals from Doppler spectra but can obscure the exact onset and end of the flow signal of interest when set too high (Fig. 11.2).

Use Appropriate Velocity Scale to Display the Entire Velocity Spectrum of the Flow of Interest

Larger signals are more easily measured than small ones. The velocity scale should allow the Doppler tracing to be displayed as large as possible without aliasing. This generally means adjusting the baseline up or down the screen, depending on the direction of the flow signal, in addition to adjusting the scale to accommodate the observed velocity in the available height

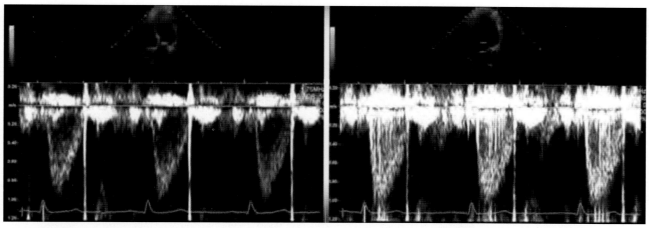

Figure 11.2. Pulsed-wave Doppler signals from the left ventricular outflow tract (LVOT). The *left panel* clearly shows the modal velocity in the LVOT. The *right panel* was acquired with a wider sample volume and higher gain, causing spectral broadening so that the modal velocity is obscured.[1] (Reproduced with permission from Mitchell C, et al. Guidelines for performing a comprehensive transthoracic echocardiographic examination in adults: recommendations from the American Society of Echocardiography, *J Am Soc Echocardiogr* 32(1):1–64, 2019.)

of the display. Automated tools are available on many ultrasound platforms and can quickly position the baseline, gain, and wall filter as a "starting point" for further refinement by the echocardiographer.

Signal Aliasing Is the Phenomenon That Occurs When the Nyquist Limit Is Exceeded

The key limitation of PW Doppler is that aliasing occurs when a Doppler shift exceeds one-half the pulse repetition frequency being transmitted, referred to as the Nyquist limit. The pulse repetition frequency determines the depth of the PW sample, and the velocity of the signal of interest produces the Doppler shift observed, so that some flows cannot be observed without aliasing. High-pulse repetition frequency offers a partial solution by introducing additional sample volumes along the length of the ultrasound beam, trading some range ambiguity for a higher Nyquist limit. CW Doppler has no Nyquist limit but at the cost of complete range ambiguity.

Measure Cross-Sectional Area at the Same Location That Is Used for Doppler Sampling

SV calculations assume the modal velocity and the cross-sectional area of an orifice or annulus are measured at the same plane, but the optimal view for cross-sectional area (CSA) measurement is perpendicular to the walls of a structure, and the optimal view for Doppler measurement is parallel to blood flow. For many applications, the CSA of an outflow tract or annulus is calculated from the diameter; the largest observed diameter avoids underestimation of CSA. Use of landmarks during acquisition and attention to localizing features such as end-ejection valve clicks to verify position of the PW Doppler sample can minimize errors when combining anatomic and Doppler measurements.

Average Velocity and Cross-Sectional Area Measurements Over at Least Three Beats

Ectopic beats may produce different loading conditions and flow states and so Doppler signals should be preferably obtained at least three beats after an ectopic beat. More than three beats may be required when the rhythm is irregular, such as in atrial fibrillation.

INDIVIDUAL FLOW PROFILES
Left Ventricular Outflow

For left ventricular (LV) outflow recordings, a 5-mm PW Doppler sample is positioned in the LV outflow tract (LVOT) just proximal to the aortic valve. Apical five-chamber (anterior angulation of the four-chamber view) or apical long-axis views are usually used. The typical shape of the spectral envelope is a smooth curve with a well-defined steep acceleration slope that peaks at maximal velocity; the slope of this curve represents dP/dt of the LV and normally exceeds 1200 mm Hg/sec. This peak is followed by a deceleration slope (Fig. 11.3). The normal LVOT velocity is 0.6 to 1.3 m/s.[2] In the normal heart, the maximum recorded velocities by CW or PW Doppler at the LV outflow are similar, with the exception that there may be a modestly higher velocity measured by CW caused by some degree of acceleration across the aortic valve, up to 1.7 m/s.

Measuring SV is one of many important applications of Doppler echocardiography. The area of the spectral profile of a Doppler signal, referred to as the velocity time integral (VTI), is equal to the distance travelled by the blood cells in the PW sample volume in one cardiac cycle. The flow (SV) across an orifice such as the LVOT can be calculated as the product of the PW VTI at the level of the orifice and the CSA of that orifice:

$$SV\left(cm^2\right) = CSA\left(cm^2\right) \times VTI\,(cm)$$

CSA can be calculated for a circular orifice such as the LVOT using the formula $CSA = \pi r^2$ or measured from a 3D multiplanar reconstruction. Because the LVOT diameter is readily measured from the parasternal long-axis view, the formula may be rearranged to:

$$SV_{LVOT} = LVOT\ diameter^2 \times 0.785 \times LVOT\ VTI$$

The normal LVOT VTI is 17 to 23 cm, and the average LVOT diameter 2.1 to 2.3 cm, yielding an approximate SV of 68 to 84 cm³ in a normal adult heart.[6,7] The per-beat stroke volume can be multiplied by the heart rate to calculate the minute CO. SV and CO can be quantified across all valves and great vessels in similar fashion but are typically measured at the LVOT because it is technically straightforward to image with both 2D and Doppler, increasing reproducibility. Special attention is needed in measuring the LV outflow diameter because any error is magnified when the diameter is raised to the second power in the formula given earlier. PW Doppler sampling and diameter measurements should be recorded as close as possible to the same level.

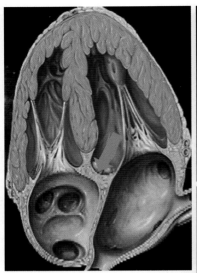

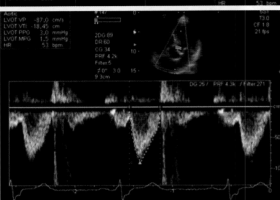

Figure 11.3. The typical shape of a left ventricular outflow tract (LVOT) Doppler recording. The velocity envelope is a smooth curve with a well-defined steep acceleration slope. After peaking at the maximal LVOT velocity, there is a gradual deceleration slow. Note the aortic valve closing click at the end of envelope, confirming the Doppler signal was acquired at the plane of the aortic annulus. Stroke volume can be calculated by multiplying the cross-sectional area (CSA) of the LVOT at the annulus by the velocity time integral (VTI) of the spectral Doppler velocities.

Forward stroke volume
= CSA x VTI

$$\pi D^2/4 \times VTI = 0.785\ D^2 \times VTI$$

SV and CO provide noninvasive estimates of LV function and allow monitoring of hemodynamic changes after therapeutic interventions. Other uses include calculation of regurgitant volume in valvular insufficiency and determining the pulmonary-to-systemic flow ratio (Qp:Qs) in the quantification of shunts; these applications are reviewed in other chapters.

Right Ventricular Outflow

In a manner similar to the LV outflow recordings, blood flow can be quantified at the right ventricular (RV) outflow by placing the PW Doppler sample volume just proximal to the pulmonary valve. The RV outflow view, obtained from either the parasternal short-axis or the subcostal views at the aortic valve level, is used to align the Doppler beam with the long axis of the RVOT (Fig. 11.4). Compared with the spectral profile obtained in the LVOT, the RVOT flow is characterized by a slower acceleration slope followed by a mid- to late-peaking systolic velocity. The RVOT spectral profile thus has a more rounded contour than the LVOT, reflecting the lower downstream pulmonary vascular resistance compared with the systemic vascular resistance faced by the LV. The maximum velocity in the RVOT is typically 0.8 to 1.0 m/s.[2]

The PW Doppler recording across the pulmonary valve allows measurement of the pulmonary artery acceleration time, which is normally greater than 130 ms and shortens in proportion to elevations in pulmonary artery pressure. For measuring the pulmonary artery acceleration time (PAAT), a 5-mm PW Doppler sample volume should be placed in the center of the RVOT just proximal to the pulmonic valve; the opening valve click serves as a highly reproducible signal for the onset of flow and the time from valve opening to the peak systolic velocity is measured. The PAAT can also be used to estimate the mean pulmonary artery pressure using validated regression equations.

In a normal heart, the RVOT and LVOT stroke volumes are equal. Any difference represents either shunt or regurgitation of one of the semilunar valves and can therefore be used to quantify those lesions.

Left Ventricular Inflow

PW Doppler recordings of diastolic transmitral flow are the cornerstone of the echocardiographic assessment of diastolic function and LV filling pressure. A 1- to 3- mm PW Doppler sample is placed at the level of the mitral leaflet tips in the apical four-chamber or apical long-axis view.[1] The normal LV inflow starts after the opening of the mitral valve, with rapid acceleration of flow from the left atrium (LA) to the LV caused by the LA–LV pressure gradient. The maximum early diastolic flow velocity (E velocity) is reached and followed by a flow deceleration (deceleration time). In most individuals, depending on heart rate, loading conditions, and the PR interval, there is a period of diastasis with minimal flow. Near the end of diastole, a second peak velocity (A velocity) is produced when the LA pressure again exceeds LV pressure because of atrial contraction (Fig. 11.5).

The normal E velocity varies significantly with age. Average peak E velocity is 0.8 m/s for individuals younger than 40 years and decreases with advancing age. Conversely, the A velocity increases with normal aging. Accordingly, the normal E/A ratio decreases with age. Moreover, increase in age is associated with prolongation of the E wave deceleration time.[8] Both the E and A velocities tend to be slightly higher in women than in men across all age groups (Table 11.1).[6,7]

Comprehensive evaluation of diastolic filling is reviewed in other chapters. It is worth mentioning that in addition to age, parameters such as heart rate can confound the evaluation of diastolic function. Faster heart rates shorten the diastolic filling time producing a higher A velocity and at the extreme, fusing the E and A waves. Similarly, a prolonged PR interval can cause fusion of the E and A waves.

Velocity recorded with PW Doppler at the mitral annulus can be used to calculate the stroke volume:

$$SV_{Mitral\ Valve} = Mitral\ annulus\ CSA \times Mitral\ annulus\ VTI$$

The mitral annulus diameter measured in the parasternal long-axis view can be used to calculate the mitral annular area, assuming a circular shape, or the area of the mitral annulus can be measured

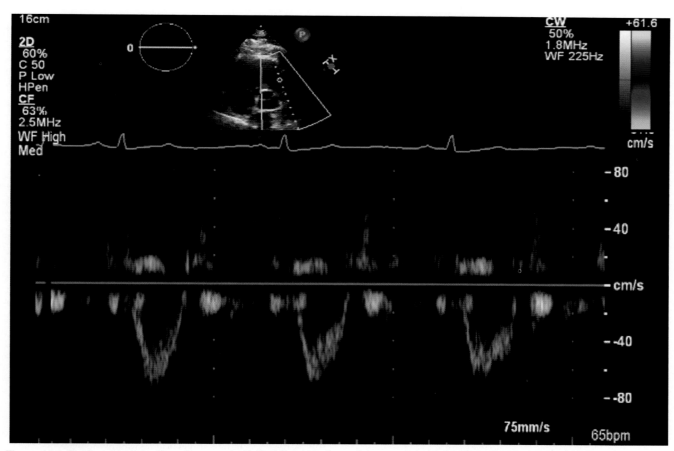

Figure 11.4. Right ventricular outflow. Compared with the left ventricular outflow recordings, the velocity at the right ventricular outflow is characterized by a slower acceleration slow followed by a late peaking systolic velocity and an overall more rounded contour.

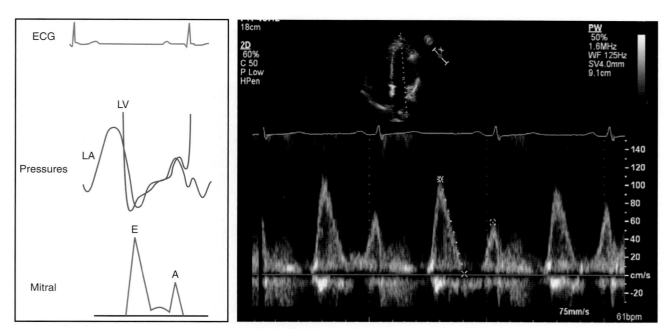

Figure 11.5. The normal left ventricular (LV) inflow starts after the mitral valve opens; flow from the left atrium (LA) to the LV rapidly accelerates. The maximum early diastolic flow velocity (E velocity) is produced by the early diastolic pressure gradient and a flow deceleration (deceleration time) follows as the LA empties to the point that pressure there falls. Note the period of minimal flow (diastasis) following the deceleration time. A second peak velocity (A velocity) is produced when LA pressure exceeds LV pressure because of atrial contraction. *ECG,* Electrocardiogram.

from a 3D multiplanar reconstruction. In distinction to the diastolic filling velocities, which are recorded at the level of the mitral leaflet tips, the flow for mitral stroke volume must be recorded at the level of the mitral annulus. The tubular shape of the LVOT provides a more reproducible stroke volume measurement in most cases, but comparison of the mitral valve (MV) and LVOT stroke volumes can be useful for estimation of aortic or mitral regurgitant volumes.

Right Ventricular Inflow

The Doppler pattern and quantification are essentially the same for the RV (tricuspid) inflow as for the LV inflow but with a PW sample volume placed at the tricuspid leaflet tips. The apical four-chamber view or a parasternal RV inflow view may be used. The peak E velocity of the RV inflow is lower than the mitral E velocity of the LV inflow, usually only 0.3 to 0.7 m/s, because of the larger tricuspid annulus.

Pulmonary Vein Flow

PW Doppler evaluation of the pulmonary venous flow can provide important insights into the diastolic filling of the LA and LV. From the transthoracic window, starting with a standard four-chamber view, slight anterior angulation of the probe allows visualization of the right superior pulmonary vein. From the midesophageal window, clockwise rotation of the transesophageal probe allows visualization of the right-sided pulmonary veins, and counterclockwise rotation displays the left-sided pulmonary veins. Color-flow imaging can facilitate detection of blood entering the atrium from the vein(s) to aid in localizing them. A 2- to 3-mm PW Doppler sample placed at least 5 mm into the vein produces optimal recordings.

The typical pulmonary venous flow pattern is triphasic (Fig. 11.6). Atrial filling from the pulmonary veins occurs most prominently during ventricular systole (S) with a second phase during ventricular diastole (D); a brief systolic atrial reversal (Ar) follows atrial contraction late in diastole because there is no valve between the LA and the pulmonary circuit. Depending on the relative contributions of the transmitted right ventricular pressure wave and the AV valve descent on LA filling in an individual, the S wave may have two components, S1 and S2. The maximum velocities and durations of each of these waves can be measured and allow the calculation of the S/D ratio; the systolic filling fraction [SVTI/(SVTI + DVTI)]; duration of Ar; the difference in the duration of the Ar and the mitral (forward) A-wave (Ar − A); and the D velocity deceleration time.[4]

In normal subjects, the S/D ration is greater than 1. As with other diastolic parameters, the pulmonary venous inflow velocities are influenced by age, with the S/D ratio increasing with age. The Ar velocity also increases with age but rarely exceeds 35 cm/s in normal individuals.[5]

TABLE 11.1 Normal Flow Velocities in the Left Heart

	Younger than 40 Years	40–60 Years	>60 Years
LV Ejection			
Women			
LVOT peak velocity, m/s	1.01 ± 0.17	1.02 ± 0.16	1.01 ± 0.17
LVOT VTI, cm	20.8 ± 3.5	21.6 ± 3.4	21.7 ± 3.7
Men			
LVOT peak velocity, m/s	0.99 ± 0.17	0.99 ± 0.18	0.96 ± 0.18
LVOT VTI, cm	20 ± 3.3	20.4 ± 3.6	20.3 ± 3.7
Mitral Inflow			
Women			
E velocity, m/s	0.80 ± 0.16	0.74 ± 0.15	0.69 ± 0.16
A velocity, m/s	0.48 ± 0.15	0.59 ± 0.15	0.75 ± 0.18
E/A ratio	1.85 ± 0.76	1.32 ± 0.40	0.96 ± 0.32
E wave deceleration, ms	212 ± 55	220 ± 66	244 ± 79
Men			
E velocity, m/s	0.75 ± 0.15	0.64 ± 0.15	0.61 ± 0.14
A velocity, m/s	0.44 ± 0.14	0.52 ± 0.14	0.65 ± 0.18
E/A ratio	1.86 ± 0.64	1.30 ± 0.42	0.99 ± 0.34
E wave deceleration, ms	212 ± 65	232 ± 81	269 ± 97
Pulmonary Vein Flows			
Women			
PV S velocity, m/s	0.58 ± 0.12	0.59 ± 0.12	0.62 ± 0.12
PV D velocity, m/s	0.55 ± 0.11	0.48 ± 0.12	0.43 ± 0.11
Men			
PV S velocity, m/s	0.52 ± 0.11	0.55 ± 0.11	0.62 ± 0.13
PV D velocity, m/s	0.55 ± 0.12	0.47 ± 0.11	0.43 ± 0.11

A, Active diastolic filling; *D,* diastolic; *E,* early diastolic; *LV,* left ventricle; *LVOT,* left ventricular outflow tract; *PV,* pulmonary vein; *S,* systolic; *VTI,* velocity time integral.

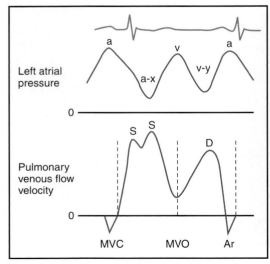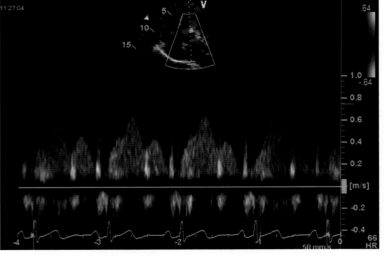

Figure 11.6. The typical pulmonary venous flow pattern consists of a triphasic waveform: prominent atrial filling during ventricular systole (S velocity), a second atrial filling phase during ventricular diastole (D velocity), and a brief systolic reversal with backflow of blood into the pulmonary veins (Ar velocity) when the atrium contrasts during late diastole. *AR,* Atrial reversal; *MVC,* mitral valve closure; *MVO,* mitral valve opening.

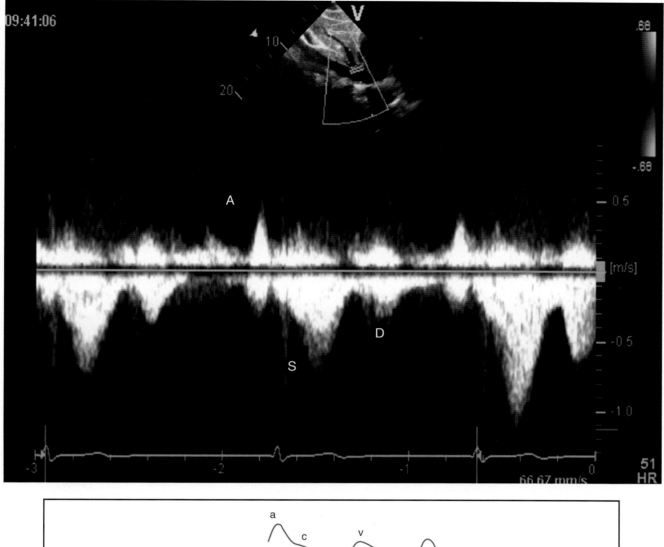

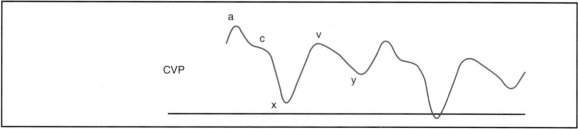

Figure 11.7. Normal hepatic vein flow consists of a small reversal of flow (A wave caused by RA contraction) that is followed by a large systolic (S) wave as the blood flows from hepatic vein into the right atrium (RA). A brief end-systolic flow reversal of flow is observed and followed by a diastolic (D) filling phase when the RA serves as a conduction for blood from the hepatic vein to the right ventricle. Note the correlation between the hepatic vein flow and the central venous pressure. *CVP,* Central venous pressure.

Physiologically, the S velocity is dependent on LA pressure, and the D velocity is determined by the balance between LV compliance and filling pressure. An increase in LA pressures decreases the S/D ratio to less than 1 by decreasing the S velocity and increasing the D velocity. Ar velocity and duration are influenced by LA contractility, atrial preload, and LV end-diastolic pressure. With an increase in LV end diastolic pressure, Ar velocity and duration increase.

Hepatic Vein Flow

Both hepatic venous flow from the subcostal view and superior vena caval flow from the suprasternal view can be used to evaluate the right atrial (RA) filling. The hepatic vein is a useful surrogate for the inferior vena cava (IVC) because it is parallel to the insonifying beam in the subcoastal window.

To record hepatic venous flow, the IVC is first visualized entering the RA; then a hepatic vein is identified converging into the inferior caval flow, usually 2 to 3 cm from the IVC–RA junction. Color-flow imaging can help in localizing this confluence and identifying the course of the hepatic vein. The Doppler cursor is then aligned with the hepatic vein.

The typical hepatic vein flow consists of a small reversal of flow after RA contraction (A wave) that is followed by a systolic (S) phase during which blood flows from the hepatic vein into the proximal vena cava and RA. A brief end-systolic reversal of flow may be observed corresponding to the RA V wave and is followed by a diastolic (D) phase when the RA serves as a conduit of blood from the caval veins into the RV (Fig. 11.7). Typically, the S wave is slightly larger than the D wave. An increase in RA pressure results in a decrease of

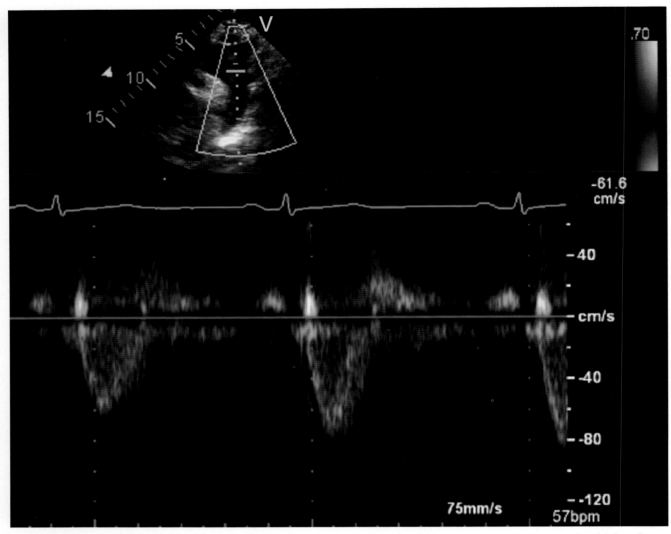

Figure 11.8. Flow in the descending aorta consists of a systolic antegrade flow, early diastolic flow reversal, and a low-velocity mid-diastolic antegrade flow. Note the beam is directed along the middle of the aorta.

the systolic component of the hepatic vein flow. Disorders in which the hepatic vein flow assessment are most useful include tricuspid regurgitation, pulmonary hypertension, restrictive cardiomyopathy, and constrictive pericarditis.[3]

Descending Thoracic Aortic Flow

PW and CW Doppler recordings of the descending thoracic aorta can be obtained from the suprasternal notch. Two-dimensional echocardiographic images of the aortic arch and descending aorta are highly variable because of the surrounding bony structures and aerated lung tissue, but Doppler flow signals are usually high quality, given the parallel angle of intercept with flow along the aorta. The smaller footprint of the nonimaging (PEDOF) Doppler probe may facilitate obtaining flow in the descending thoracic aorta because it fits more comfortably in the suprasternal notch than larger imaging probes.

The typical flow consists of systolic antegrade flow, usually at a velocity approximately 1 m/s followed by a brief diastolic flow reversal (i.e., lasting less than one-third of diastole) and a low-velocity antegrade flow for the remainder of diastole (Fig. 11.8). Care should be taken to place the Doppler sample volume near the center of the aorta because retrograde diastolic flows may be normal

along the walls of the aorta. Coarctation of the aorta (persistent forward flow throughout diastole), patent ductus arteriosus (high antegrade flow velocity and diastolic flow reversal beyond the level of the ductus), and severe aortic regurgitation (holodiastolic flow reversal) all produce characteristic alterations in the thoracic aortic flow signal.

EMERGING APPLICATIONS OF DOPPLER: INTRACARDIAC FLOW ANALYSIS

Three-dimensional phase contrast magnetic resonance imaging has demonstrated that LV filling and ejection relies on the interaction of circular, swirling motions that store the kinetic energy of blood while changing directions. These vortices cannot be measured with Doppler alone because a portion of the circular vortex is always perpendicular to the ultrasound beam. Recent computational advances allow real-time calculation of the lateral velocity of blood based on speckle tracking of the myocardium to augment color-flow Doppler measurement of the longitudinal velocity, producing flow velocity vector maps of intracardiac flow and pressure gradients. The normal LV filling involves a clockwise-spinning vortex anterior to the mitral valve and a smaller, counterclockwise-spinning vortex posteriorly (Fig. 11.9). During early diastole, the

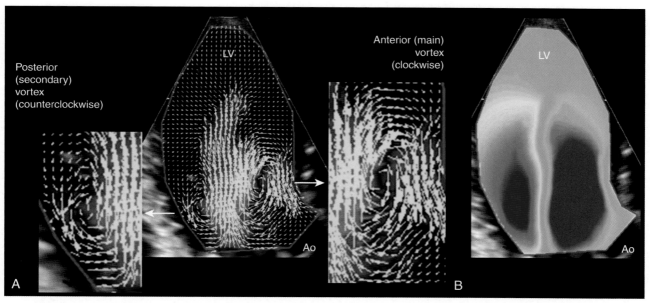

Figure 11.9. A, Flow velocity vector map showing mitral inflow with a pair of counterrotating vortices, one anterior (main clockwise vortex at *right*) and one posterior (secondary counterclockwise vortex at *left*). Velocity vectors forming the two vortices are magnified in the *insets*. **B,** Circulation parametric map. Vortices are the compact readers show in *blue (clockwise vortex)* and red *(counterclockwise vortex)*. Both images refer to an apical long-axis view obtained in a normal subject without contrast.[9] *Ao,* Aorta; *LV,* left ventricle. (Reproduced with permission from Mele D, et al. Intracardiac flow analysis: techniques and potential clinical applications, *J Am Soc Echocardiogr* 32:319–332, 2019.)

spinning vortices promote suction by avoiding the inertial effects of static blood, and later, during the pre-ejection period, the energy of the vortex redirects blood toward the outflow tract without losing kinetic energy (i.e., without stopping and redirecting blood in the LV). Vortex imaging with color-flow Doppler mapping is not currently in clinical use but may provide future insights into hemodynamic function and dysfunction.

REFERENCES

1. Mitchell C, Rahko PS, Blauwet LA, et al. Guidelines for performing a comprehensive transthoracic echocardiographic examination in adults: recommendations from the American Society of Echocardiography. *J Am Soc Echocardiogr.* 2019;32(1):1–64.
2. Hatle L, Angelsen B. *Doppler Ultrasound in Cardiology: Physical Principles and Clinical Applications.* ed 2. Philadelphia: Lea & Febiger; 1985.
3. Reynolds T, Appleton CP. Doppler flow velocity patterns of the superior vena cava, inferior vena cava, hepatic vein, coronary sinus, and atrial septal defect: a guide for the echocardiographer. *J Am Soc Echocardiogr.* 1991;4(5):503–512.
4. Smiseth O. Pulmonary veins: an important side window into ventricular function. *Eur Heart J Cardiovasc Imag.* 2015;16(11):1189–1190.
5. Klein AL, Tajik AJ. Doppler assessment of pulmonary venous flow in healthy subjects and in patients with heart disease. *J Am Soc Echocardiogr.* 1991;4:379–392.
6. Caballero L, Koy S, Dulgheru R, et al. Echocardiographic reference ranges for normal cardiac Doppler data: results from the NORRE Study. *Eur Heart J Cardiovasc Imag.* 2015;16(9):1031–1041.
7. Dalen H, Thorstensen A, Vatten LJ, et al. References values and distribution of conventional echocardiographic Doppler measures and longitudinal tissue Doppler velocities in a population free from cardiovascular disease. *Circ Cardiovasc Imag.* 2010;3:614–622.
8. Tighe DA, Vinch CS, Hill JC, et al. Influence of age on assessment of diastolic function by Doppler tissue imaging. *Am J Cardiol.* 2003;91(2):254–257.
9. Mele D, Smarrazzo V, Pedrizzetti G, et al. Intracardiac flow analysis: techniques and potential clinical applications. *J Am Soc Echocardiogr.* 2019;32:319–332.

12 Introduction to Transesophageal Echocardiography: Indications, Risks, Complications, and Protocol

Renuka Jain

The field of transesophageal echocardiography (TEE) has evolved significantly since its initial development.[1] The esophageal transducer was developed to obtain ultrasound images from the esophagus, an ideal location because of its direct location behind the heart and associated structures. This allowed for the improvement of image resolution and avoidance of the standard artifacts of transthoracic imaging. The contemporary TEE transducer is a flexible transducer, housing a phased matrix array at the distal end, controlled by proximal knobs and manual movements.

PREPROCEDURAL ASSESSMENT

Before performance of TEE, a detailed review of indications and contraindications to procedure is required. The indications for TEE are listed in Table 12.1 and are classified into four general categories.[2] The contraindications for TEE are listed in Table 12.2 and are divided into absolute and relative contraindications.[2] Caution should be given to patients on chronic steroid therapy; those with a history of prior radiation to the oropharynx, scleroderma, or achalasia; or when the procedure time is expected to be prolonged.[2] Recent data suggest that TEE can be safely performed in appropriately selected patients with esophageal varices and thrombocytopenia.[3,4] Consultation with gastroenterology may be helpful in evaluating specific contraindications.

The risk of TEE derives from two sources: (1) the risk of sedation and (2) injury to the gastrointestinal (GI) tract from probe insertion and manipulation. Sedation used for TEE can lead to respiratory depression, altered mental status, and hypotension; consultation with anesthesiology may be helpful when assessing the preprocedure risk.[5] Mallampati airway score and American Society of Anesthesiologist Physical Status (ASA) classification are useful guides in determining patients at higher risk for complications.[2] Injuries to the gastric tract can be minor or major; the most serious complication is esophageal perforation, which does not always present with the classic Meckel's triad of vomiting, pain, and subcutaneous emphysema.[6] Pharyngeal or cervical perforations occur more typically in patients under moderate sedation, usually as a complication of TEE insertion[6]; in operative settings, perforations occur more frequently in the thoracic or abdominal esophagus.[7] The risks and complications of TEE are listed in Table 12.3 along with their overall incidence.[2] Detailed assessment of the risk-to-benefit ratio should be reviewed with patients as part of the informed consent.

ANESTHESIA AND SEDATION

After the decision is made to proceed with TEE, the choice of anesthesia and sedation must be determined. Localized anesthesia is commonly used to improve ease of probe insertion by diminishing gag reflex. Multiple techniques can be used to numb the oropharynx using oral formulations of benzocaine or lidocaine in aerosolized spray or gargling. A rare but significant complication from the agents used for topical anesthesia (primarily benzocaine products) is methemoglobinemia, characterized by cyanosis, tachycardia, and abnormally low blood oxygen level. Methylene blue should be readily administered if this condition is suspected; it is given as 1.5 to 2 mg/kg intravenous infusion over 5 to 10 minutes. Methylene blue should not be administered to patients also receiving selective serotonin reuptake inhibitors, given the risk of serotonin syndrome.[2]

Moderate sedation is typically used for awake and stable patients who present for TEE performed in the nonoperative setting. A combination of an opioid and benzodiazepine is preferred as they are short-acting agents and have synergistic amnestic and analgesic effects. Midazolam (given in 1- or 2-mg increments) and fentanyl (given in 25- or 50-mcg increments) are administered at regular intervals with close monitoring of vital signs and patient's level of consciousness. If respiratory depression complicates the procedure, initial maneuvers are performed, such as increasing oxygen, and verbal or physical stimuli should be used to awaken the patient. Respiratory depression that does not respond to initial maneuvers may require reversal agents—flumazenil for benzodiazepines (0.2-mg starting dose) and naloxone for opiates (0.04- to 0.1-mg starting dose with escalating doses every 2–3 minutes until respirations improve).[2] For intensive care unit patients with mechanical ventilation who are already receiving sedation, critical care or anesthesiology teams can aid in determining further sedation strategies. An anesthesiologist is typically present for all TEE procedures performed in the operating room using propofol or general anesthesia.[5]

TABLE 12.1 General Indications for Transesophageal Echocardiography

Evaluation of cardiac structures when TTE is nondiagnostic or would be inadequate	Detailed evaluation of left atrial appendage, aorta, prosthetic valves, paravalvular spaces for abscess or leaks; chest wall injuries; poor imaging windows on TTE
Intraoperative guidance	All open-heart procedures involving valves and thoracic aorta; some coronary artery bypass surgeries; noncardiac surgery if knowledge of cardiovascular structures is needed
Transcatheter procedure guidance	Transcatheter valve procedures, left atrial appendage occlusion, atrial or ventricular septal defect closures
Critically ill patients	Ventilated patients with possible cardiovascular pathology that will impact ICU management

ICU, Intensive care unit; *TTE,* transthoracic echocardiography.
Adapted with permission from Hahn RT, et al: Guidelines for performing a comprehensive transesophageal echocardiographic examination, *J Am Soc Echocardiogr* 26:921–964, 2013.

TABLE 12.2 Contraindications to Transesophageal Echocardiography

Absolute Contraindications	Relative Contraindications
Esophageal related: esophageal tumor, stricture, fistula, or perforation	Barrett esophagus
	History of dysphagia (may require gastroenterology consultation)
Active upper GI bleed	Active esophagitis
Perforated bowel or bowel obstruction	High-grade esophageal varices
	Active peptic ulcer disease
Unstable cervical spine	Neck immobility (severe cervical arthritis, atlantoaxial joint disease)
Uncooperative patient	Severe hiatal hernia
	Severe coagulopathy or thrombocytopenia
	Prior neck or chest radiation
	Prior GI surgery
	Esophageal diverticulum
	Loose teeth (may require dental consultation)

GI, Gastrointestinal.
Adapted with permission from Hahn RT, et al: Guidelines for performing a comprehensive transesophageal echocardiographic examination, *J Am Soc Echocardiogr* 26:921–964, 2013.

MOVEMENTS OF TEE TRANSDUCER

There are several ways to maneuver the TEE transducer, as shown in Fig. 12.1:

- *Anteflexion* and *retroflexion* are usually accomplished by turning the largest wheel on the probe. A neutral position is always denoted on the wheel notch (Fig. 12.1A).
- *Insertion* and *withdrawal* are performed manually, and all probes are designed with depth markers to ascertain distance in the GI tract. These maneuvers are frequently used to improve image quality by improving contact with the esophagus (Fig. 12.1B). During insertion and withdrawal, the probe should be in a neutral position to prevent esophageal injury.
- *Rotation* occurs by turning the probe to the patient's right (clockwise) or to the left (counterclockwise) (Fig. 12.1C).
- *Omniplane angulation* changes the angle of the ultrasound beam, from 0 to 180 degrees. Contemporary TEE transducers have biplane and triplane imaging so that orthogonal views can be obtained simultaneously (Fig. 12.1D).
- *Lateral steering* of the probe is accomplished by turning the smaller wheel on probe (Fig. 12.1E).

TRANSDUCER INSERTION AND MANIPULATION

Several factors improve success of TEE insertion. The left lateral decubitus position is preferred for nonintubated patients under moderate sedation. The probe should be coated with a small quantity of ultrasound gel to improve patient comfort but not cause the patient to aspirate significant quantities. If possible, removal of any oral or nasogastric tubing can help prevent interference with probe insertion and imaging windows. A disposable bite block device prevents injury to the patient, probe, and operator. For ventilated patients who are also sedated, a lateral position for the bite block can be used; in patients under general anesthesia, the bite block can be placed over the probe initially for insertion and then placed into the mouth. For patients with tracheostomy, deflation of tracheostomy cuff can aid in TEE insertion.[8]

A small amount of anteflexion is placed on the transducer, and it is inserted into the posterior oropharynx. If the individual is awake, asking the patient to swallow or waiting for the patient to naturally swallow may be sufficient for passing the probe into the esophagus. A

TABLE 12.3 Risks and Complications of Transesophageal Echocardiography

Complications	Incidence for Diagnostic TEE (%)
Mortality	<0.01–0.02
Major bleeding	<0.01
Major morbidity	0.2
Esophageal perforation	<0.01
Dysphagia	1.8
Hoarseness	12
Bronchospasm	0.06–0.07
Laryngospasm	0.14
Minor pharyngeal bleeding	0.01–0.2
Dental injury	0.1
Lip injury	13
Heart failure	0.05
Arrhythmia	0.06–0.3

TEE, Transesophageal echocardiography.
Adapted with permission from Hahn RT, et al: Guidelines for performing a comprehensive transesophageal echocardiographic examination, *J Am Soc Echocardiogr* 26:921–964, 2013.

one-handed approach (one hand near the tip of transducer and the other hand on the controls) can be used. A two-handed approach can also be used, with one hand near the transducer tip and one finger placed into the mouth to guide probe when placed by the opposite hand. For most standard TEE probes, the control wheels should be facing downward when the transducer is inserted, so that anteflexion is in the correct direction (following the curvature of the tongue) during insertion.

For cases in which TEE insertion is difficult, alternative strategies are needed. Placement under direct visualization can be performed using a laryngoscope. Alternatively, another individual may tilt head and chin downward to open up the posterior oropharynx and facilitate probe insertion. In an intubated and sedated patient, as in those under general anesthesia, the operator may stand at the head of the bed of a supine patient; one hand can insert the probe while the other holds the lower jaw and lifts it out and upward. Force should never be used when inserting the probe because this can injure the oropharynx. This is especially true in intubated and heavily sedated patients, who are not be able to provide feedback to noxious stimuli. To prevent injury, the probe should also never be in a locked position or forcefully inserted or withdrawn.[8]

After the TEE transducer has been placed, the probe should ideally be controlled with two hands at all times. Otherwise, the probe may move or come out if the patient becomes agitated. Only the hand near the mouth should control probe insertion and withdrawal to keep the probe in place. This hand should not be used to rotate the probe because this can put unnecessary tension on the TEE probe and make proper manipulation less predictable.

The probe should not be heavily anteflexed for prolonged periods; this position is more likely to lead to esophageal damage with prolonged contact.[6] When moving between imaging planes, the probe should be moved to a neutral position and then inserted or withdrawn. Anteflexion or retroflexion can then be reapplied. In addition, in prolonged procedures, the transducer should be paused when not in use, reducing thermal injury. These maneuvers reduce the possibility of esophageal and gastric injury from TEE.

SAMPLE PROTOCOL

The following is a general protocol that describes sequence for performing TEE:

1. *Preprocedural planning:* After acquiring patient history and performing a physical examination, assess whether TEE is indicated and ensure that no contraindications are present. Decide on a method of sedation. Obtain informed consent for procedure and sedation.

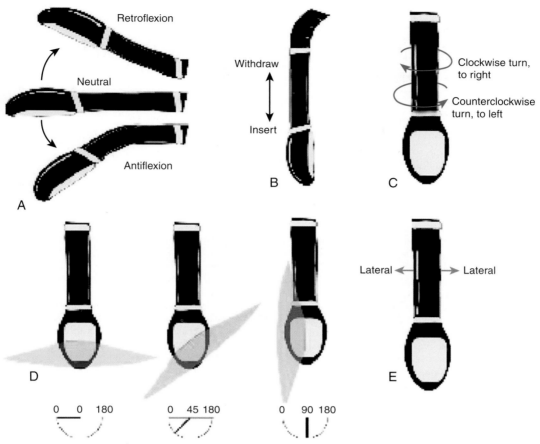

Figure 12.1. The transesophageal echocardiography transducer has five categories of motion: anteflexion and retroflexion (**A**), insertion and withdrawal (**B**), rotation (**C**), omniplane angulation (**D**), and lateral steering (**E**).

2. *Prepare the room for TEE:* Ensure appropriate equipment and patient monitoring for sedation. This includes noninvasive blood pressure measurements every 2 to 3 minutes, continuous oxygen saturation monitoring, suctioning catheter, and adequate intravenous access. Capnography should be used because it has been noted to reduce respiratory complications in cases using moderate sedation.[5] If determined that patient is ASA classification 3 or higher, telemetry should be used.[5] Adequate doses of sedation agents and sedation reversal agents should be acquired. A code cart and advanced airway equipment should be readily available.

3. *Prepare the patient for TEE:* To minimize risk of aspiration, ensure that NPO (nothing by mouth) status is maintained as per local guidelines (typically at least 6 hours for solids and at least 4 hours for liquids), including tube feedings. Dentures should be removed. Ideally, nasogastric or orogastric tubes should be removed. Endotracheal tubes may need to be moved to one side of mouth. Topical anesthesia should be administered. A disposable "bite block" should be placed in mouth to protect the teeth and TEE probe.

4. *Procedure:* Ensure the ultrasound machine and TEE transducer are working properly. Administer sedation, and after the patient is appropriately sedated, insert the TEE transducer using the techniques described. Perform all TEE views that will answer the clinical question and then complete a comprehensive examination as indicated.

5. *Postprocedural monitoring:* After the TEE probe has been removed, the patient should be examined for signs of complications, including visual inspection of the oropharynx. The transducer should also be inspected for blood and damage. The patient should be allowed to recover from sedation and

monitored closely. The patient should remain NPO for at least 1 hour after the procedure to allow topical anesthesia to wane and should not drive the rest of that day. Results should be communicated to the patient and ordering provider.

Acknowledgment

The author would like to acknowledge the contributions of Drs. Elyse Foster and Atif Qasim, who were the authors of this chapter in previous edition.

REFERENCES

1. Frazin L, Talano JV, Stephanides L, et al. Esophageal echocardiography. *Circulation.* 1976;54:102–108.
2. Hahn RT, Abraham T, Adams MS, et al. Guidelines for performing a comprehensive transesophageal echocardiographic examination. *J Am Soc Echocardiogr.* 2013;26:921–964.
3. Liu E, Guha A, Dunleavy M, Obarski T. Safety of transesophageal echocardiography in patients with esophageal varices. *J Am Soc Echocardiogr.* 2019;32:676–677.
4. Kithungvan D, Kalluru D, Lunagariya A, et al. Safety of transesophageal echocardiography in patients with thrombocytopenia. *J Am Soc Echocardiogr.* 2019;32:1010–1015.
5. Practice guidelines for moderate procedural sedation and analgesia 2018. *Anesthesiology.* 2018;128:437–479.
6. Hilberath JN, Oakes DA, Shernan SK, et al. Safety of transesophageal echocardiography. *J Am Soc Echocardiogr.* 2010;23:1115–1127.
7. Sainathan S, Andaz S. A systematic review of transesophageal echocardiography-induced esophageal perforation. *Echocardiography.* 2013;30:977–983.
8. Hauser ND, Swanevedler J. Transoesophageal echocardiography: contraindications, complications, and safety of perioperative TEE. *Echo Res Practice.* 2018;5:101–113.

13 Transesophageal Echocardiography Tomographic Views

Rebecca T. Hahn

Transesophageal echocardiography (TEE) has proven utility in a number of clinical scenarios, including the operating room, intensive care unit, and outpatient setting.[1-5] The rapid growth of structural heart disease interventions has led to a greater appreciation of the role of TEE in both disease diagnosis as well as procedural guidance.[6-8] Thus, TEE has become an essential interdisciplinary imaging tool for cardiac surgeons, anesthesiologists, cardiac interventionalists, and clinical cardiologists. The "Guidelines for Performing a Comprehensive Transesophageal Echocardiography Examination: Recommendations from the American Society of Echocardiography and the Society of Cardiovascular Anesthesiologists"[9] reviews all aspects of TEE training and image acquisition, provides a current definition of a "Comprehensive TEE Examination" and names a set of 28 TEE views (see Figures 13.1–13.4), utilizing four levels of imaging (see Figure 13.5) intended to facilitate and provide consistency in training, reporting, archiving, and quality assurance in the multiplane TEE examination. Eight additional views have been added to the prior "ASE/SCA Guidelines for Performing a Comprehensive Intraoperative Multiplane Transesophageal Echocardiography Examination"[10] and include:

1. Midesophageal (ME) five-chamber view
2. ME modified bicaval tricuspid valve (TV) view
3. Upper esophageal (UE) right and left pulmonary veins view
4. ME left atrial appendage (LAA) view
5. Transgastric (TG) apical short-axis (SAX) view
6. TG long-axis (LAX) view
7. TG right ventricular basal view
8. TG right ventricular inflow–outflow view

With these additional views, complete imaging of right and left heart structures can be performed for either a diagnostic or intraprocedural TEE.

The new guidelines present a suggested imaging protocol to facilitate a description of probe manipulation for image acquisition. However, the number and order of image acquisition may vary based on the indication for study and the patient's clinical status. In addition, the comprehensive imaging views in the protocol are not intended to represent all the imaging planes that can be obtained when imaging specific structures. The following is a summary of the 28 recommended views with discussion of additional views that may be obtained by small adjustments in position of the probe or transducer angle, which may allow a more comprehensive evaluation of specific structures (Videos 13.1 to 13.28). A discussion of the specific indications for TEE (i.e., endocarditis or cardiac source of embolus) is beyond the scope of this chapter.

Three-dimensional (3D) imaging includes both the use of simultaneous biplane imaging and acquisition of 3D volumes and may be acquired at any point in the routine protocol but should be guided by the intended structure to be imaged. Because of the way the 3D volume is generated (typically sweeping from front to back of the acquired volume) and depending on the acquisition protocol (i.e., single-beat vs multibeat acquisitions or narrow sector vs user-defined sector) resolution of structures imaged may be determined by primary imaging planes. Some of these considerations are discussed within the individual imaging views and covered more extensively in other chapters.

Key Points From the Imaging Protocol

- The comprehensive transesophageal echocardiographic (TEE) examinations should include the 28 views outlined with addition of a Doppler examination for functional assessment when appropriate (Figs. 13.1 to 13.4). The performance of a comprehensive or complete TEE examination should be performed whenever possible.
- Use of all five manipulations of the TEE probe is typically required during image acquisition (Fig. 13.5): advancing or withdrawing the transducer, manual rotation (clockwise [toward the right] and counterclockwise [toward the left] rotation), right and left lateral flexion, anterior and posterior flexion, and mechanical rotation.
- To avoid injury to the esophagus, a neutral probe position is used to rotate or advance or withdraw the probe before adjusting flexion.
- Three-dimensional imaging (which includes simultaneous multiplane imaging) is an essential tool to describe the morphology of complex structures.

MIDESOPHAGEAL FIVE-CHAMBER VIEW

After initially passing the probe into the esophagus, it is slowly advanced until the aortic valve (AV) and left ventricular (LV) outflow tract (LVOT) come into view at a probe depth of about 30 cm. Slight transducer angle manipulation (10-degree rotation) allows image optimization of the AV and LVOT. In this plane, the LA, right atrium (RA), LV, right ventricle (RV), mitral valve (MV), and TV are also imaged, hence the name "ME five-chamber view" (see Fig. 13.1). This view allows visualization of the A_2A_1 and P_1P_2 scallops (from left to right on the imaging plane) of the MV and two of the three AV cusps. Color-flow Doppler can be applied to aid in identifying aortic, mitral, and tricuspid regurgitation. In the neutral probe position, the true apex of the ventricles may not be imaged; simultaneous multiplane imaging can confirm that the apex is not centered in the orthogonal plane. To image the apex and acquire the longest axis of the LV, retroflexion is typically required.

Key Points

- The midesophageal five-chamber view is usually the initial image obtained when inserting the probe in the neutral position.
- Retroflexion of the probe is typically required to image the apex of the heart.

MIDESOPHAGEAL FOUR-CHAMBER VIEW

From the ME five-chamber view, if the apex of the LV has been imaged using retroflexion, then mechanical rotation of approximately 10 to 20 degrees to eliminate the AV or LVOT from the image display results in the ME four-chamber view (see Fig. 13.1). If the

Imaging Plane	3D Model	2D TEE Image	Acquisition Protocol	Structures Imaged

Midesophageal Views

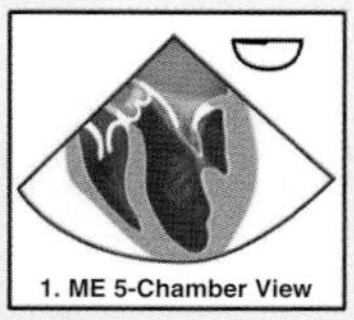	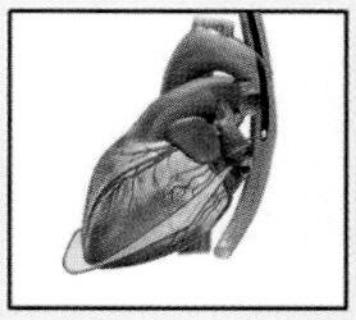	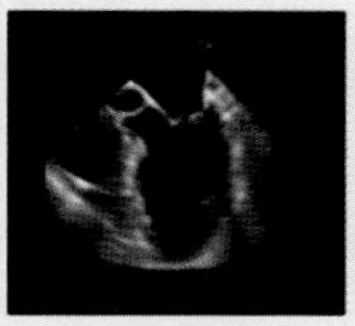	Transducer angle: ~0–10° Level: Midesophageal Maneuver (from prior image): NA	Aartic valve LVOT LA/RA LV/RV/IVS MV (A_2A_1–P_1) TV
1. ME 5-Chamber View				
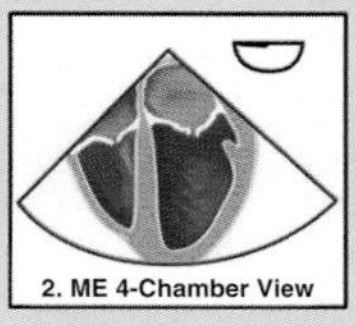 2. ME 4-Chamber View	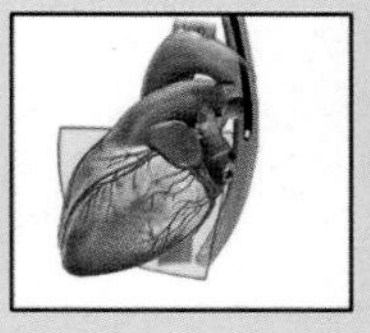	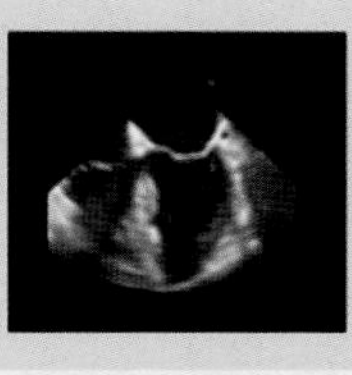	Transducer angle: ~0–10° Level: Midesophageal Maneuver (from prior image): Advance ± retroflex	LA/RA IAs LV/RV/IVS MV (A_3A_2–P_2P_1) TV
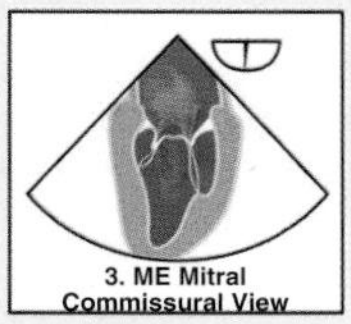 3. ME Mitral Commissural View	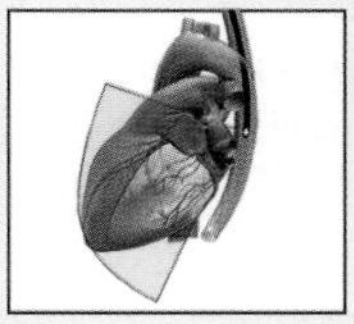	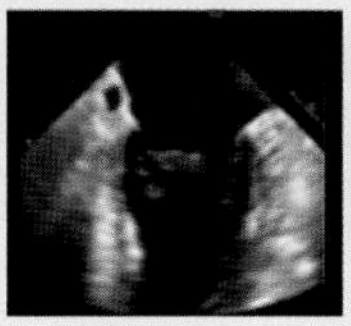	Transducer angle: ~50–70° Level: Midesophageal Maneuver (from prior image): NA	LA Coronary sinus LV MV (P_3–$A_3A_2A_1$–P_1) Papillary muscles chordae tendinae
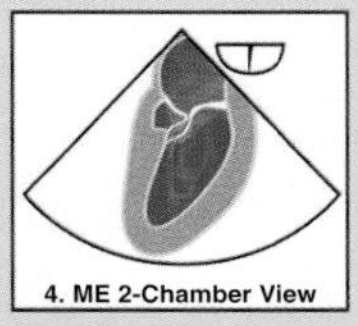 4. ME 2-Chamber View	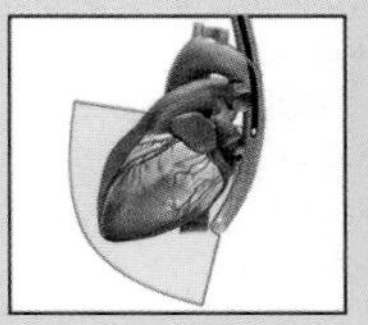	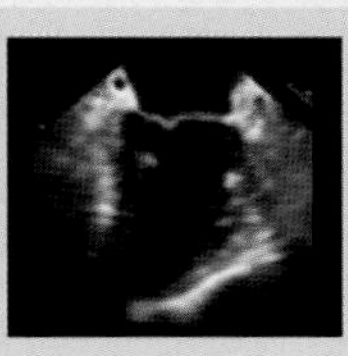	Transducer angle: ~80–100° Level: Midesophageal Maneuver (from prior image): NA	LA Coronary sinus LAA LV MV (P_3–$A_3A_2A_1$)
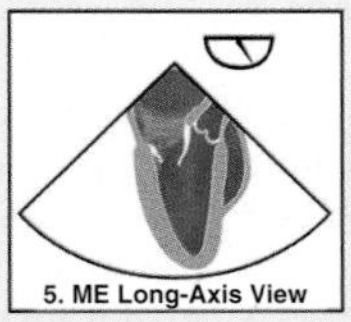 5. ME Long-Axis View	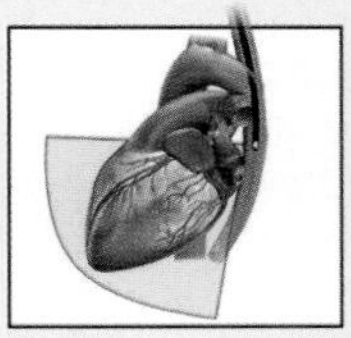	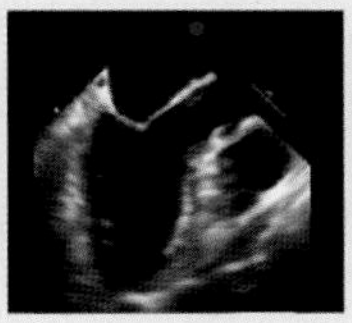	Transducer angle: ~120–140° Level: Midesophageal Maneuver (from prior image): NA	LA LV LVOT RVOT MV (P_2–A_2) Aortic valve Proximal ascending aorta
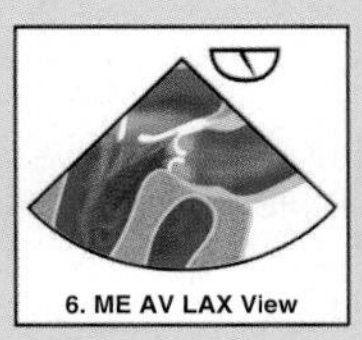 6. ME AV LAX View	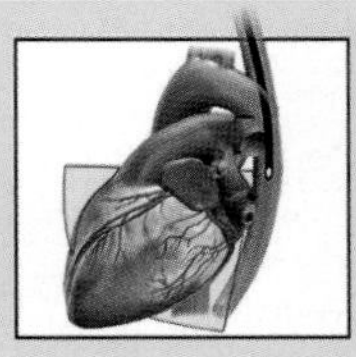	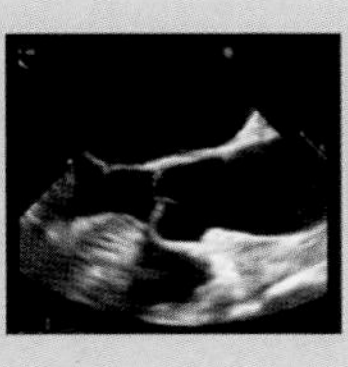	Transducer angle: ~120–140° Level: Midesophageal Maneuver (from prior image): Withdrawl ± anteflex	LA LVOT RVOT MV (A_2–P_2) Aortic valve Proximal ascending aorta
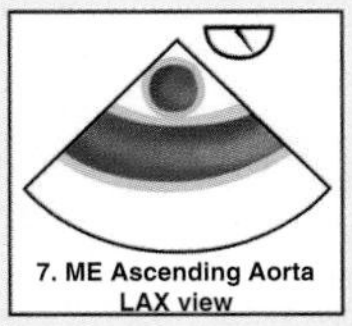 7. ME Ascending Aorta LAX view	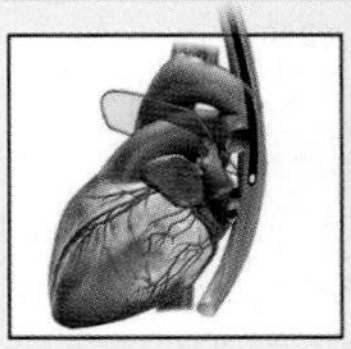	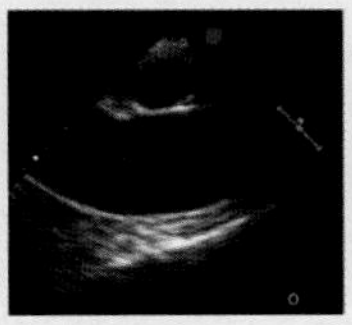	Transducer angle: ~90–110° Level: UE Maneuver (from prior image): Withdrawl	Mid-ascending aorta Right pulmonary artery
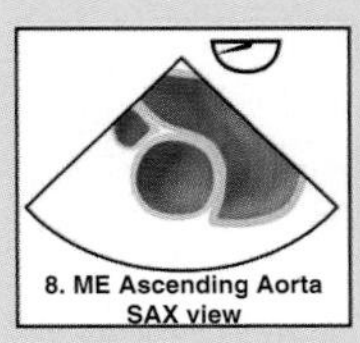 8. ME Ascending Aorta SAX view	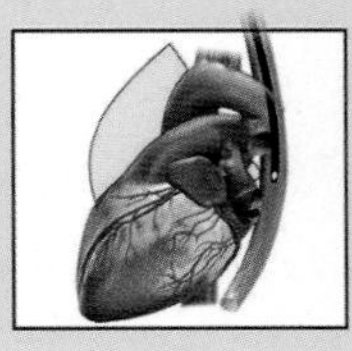	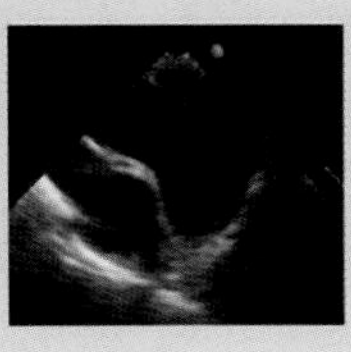	Transducer angle: ~0–30° Level: UE Maneuver (from prior image): CW	Mid-ascending aorta (SAX) Main/bifurcation Pulmonary artery SVC

Figure 13.1. Imaging views 1 through 8 (midesophageal level) of the comprehensive transesophageal echocardiographic examination. The first column shows the tomographic view of the image. The second column shows the position of the transesophageal probe. The third column shows the two-dimensional image of the view. Column 4 describes the acquisition protocol with each successive view working from the prior view. Column 5 lists the structures imaged in each view. See text for abbreviations.

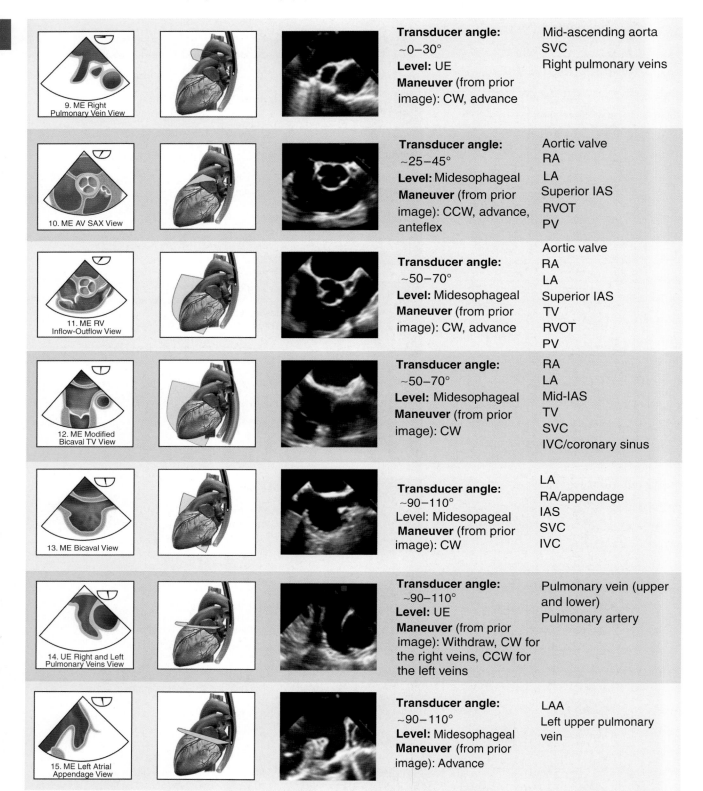

			Transducer angle: ~0–30° **Level:** UE **Maneuver** (from prior image): CW, advance	Mid-ascending aorta SVC Right pulmonary veins
9. ME Right Pulmonary Vein View				
10. ME AV SAX View			**Transducer angle:** ~25–45° **Level:** Midesophageal **Maneuver** (from prior image): CCW, advance, anteflex	Aortic valve RA LA Superior IAS RVOT PV
11. ME RV Inflow-Outflow View			**Transducer angle:** ~50–70° **Level:** Midesophageal **Maneuver** (from prior image): CW, advance	Aortic valve RA LA Superior IAS TV RVOT PV
12. ME Modified Bicaval TV View			**Transducer angle:** ~50–70° **Level:** Midesophageal **Maneuver** (from prior image): CW	RA LA Mid-IAS TV SVC IVC/coronary sinus
13. ME Bicaval View			**Transducer angle:** ~90–110° Level: Midesopageal **Maneuver** (from prior image): CW	LA RA/appendage IAS SVC IVC
14. UE Right and Left Pulmonary Veins View			**Transducer angle:** ~90–110° **Level:** UE **Maneuver** (from prior image): Withdraw, CW for the right veins, CCW for the left veins	Pulmonary vein (upper and lower) Pulmonary artery
15. ME Left Atrial Appendage View			**Transducer angle:** ~90–110° **Level:** Midesophageal **Maneuver** (from prior image): Advance	LAA Left upper pulmonary vein

Figure 13.2. Imaging views 9 through 15 (midesophageal level) of the comprehensive transesophageal echocardiographic examination. See Fig. 13.1 for further description. See text for abbreviations.

Transgastric Views

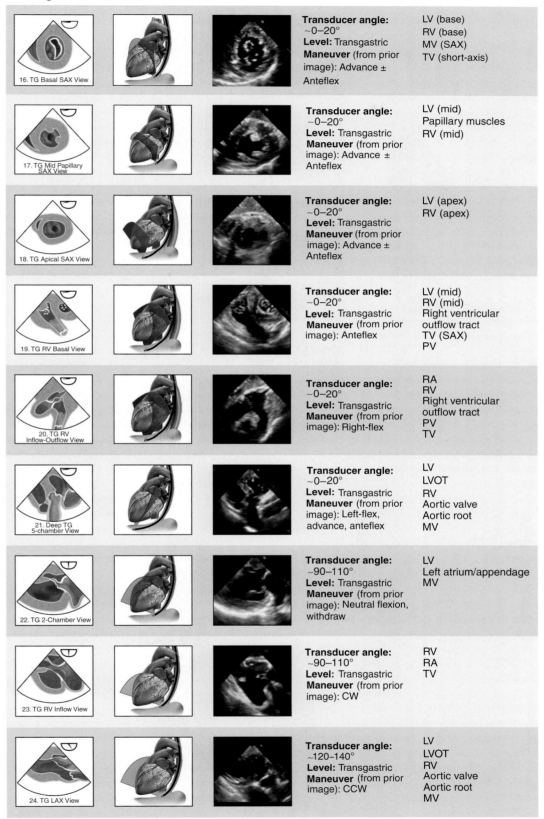

			Transducer angle / Level / Maneuver	Structures
16. TG Basal SAX View			**Transducer angle:** ~0–20° **Level:** Transgastric **Maneuver** (from prior image): Advance ± Anteflex	LV (base) RV (base) MV (SAX) TV (short-axis)
17. TG Mid Papillary SAX View			**Transducer angle:** ~0–20° **Level:** Transgastric **Maneuver** (from prior image): Advance ± Anteflex	LV (mid) Papillary muscles RV (mid)
18. TG Apical SAX View			**Transducer angle:** ~0–20° **Level:** Transgastric **Maneuver** (from prior image): Advance ± Anteflex	LV (apex) RV (apex)
19. TG RV Basal View			**Transducer angle:** ~0–20° **Level:** Transgastric **Maneuver** (from prior image): Anteflex	LV (mid) RV (mid) Right ventricular outflow tract TV (SAX) PV
20. TG RV Inflow-Outflow View			**Transducer angle:** ~0–20° **Level:** Transgastric **Maneuver** (from prior image): Right-flex	RA RV Right ventricular outflow tract PV TV
21. Deep TG 5-chamber View			**Transducer angle:** ~0–20° **Level:** Transgastric **Maneuver** (from prior image): Left-flex, advance, anteflex	LV LVOT RV Aortic valve Aortic root MV
22. TG 2-Chamber View			**Transducer angle:** ~90–110° **Level:** Transgastric **Maneuver** (from prior image): Neutral flexion, withdraw	LV Left atrium/appendage MV
23. TG RV Inflow View			**Transducer angle:** ~90–110° **Level:** Transgastric **Maneuver** (from prior image): CW	RV RA TV
24. TG LAX View			**Transducer angle:** ~120–140° **Level:** Transgastric **Maneuver** (from prior image): CCW	LV LVOT RV Aortic valve Aortic root MV

Figure 13.3. Imaging views 16 through 24 (transgastric level) of the comprehensive transesophageal echocardiographic examination. See Fig. 13.1 for further description. See text for abbreviations.

Aortic Views

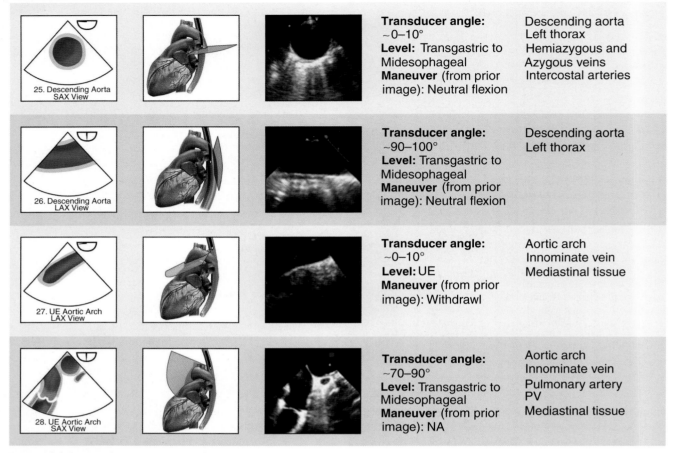

Figure 13.4. Imaging views 25 through 28 (aortic views) of the comprehensive transesophageal echocardiographic examination. See Fig. 13.1 for further description. See text for abbreviations.

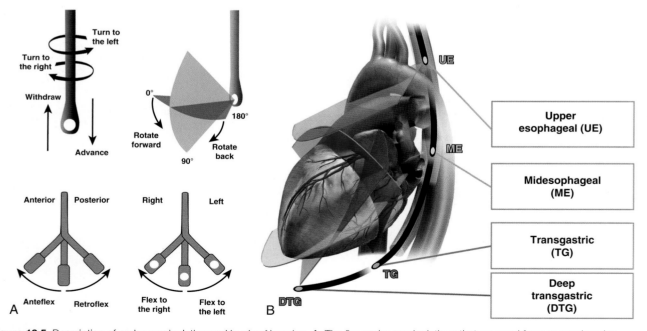

Figure 13.5. Description of probe manipulation and levels of imaging. A, The five probe manipulations that are used for a comprehensive transesophageal echocardiographic examination. B, The four standard levels of probe position.

AV is still imaged, the probe may need to be advanced. The image depth is then adjusted to ensure viewing of the LV apex. Note that this view is typically deeper than the ME five-chamber view, and the AV and LV outflow tract will not be visualized. Furthermore, the transducer angle may need to be rotated to maximize the tricuspid annular dimension. To better align the MV and LV apex, slight probe retroflexion may be necessary. With an appropriately aligned four-chamber view, a single-plane measurement of the mitral annulus can be made for the assessment of diastolic transmitral stroke volume; a pulsed Doppler sample volume should be placed at the annulus to acquire a spectral Doppler profile for velocity time integral measurement. Diastolic function assessment by TEE has been validated using the lateral mitral annular e′ velocity (abnormal <10 cm/s) and transmitral E to e° ratio (normal ≤8) as indicative of diastolic dysfunction.[11] Structures seen include the LA, RA, interatrial septum, LV, RV, interventricular septum, MV (A_3A_2 and P_2P_1 scallops), and TV. The TV septal leaflet adjacent to the interventricular septum is to the right of the sector display, and the TV posterior leaflet is adjacent to the RV free wall, to the left of the display.

The ME four-chamber view is one of the most comprehensive views available for evaluating cardiac anatomy and function. Turning the probe to the left (counterclockwise) allows imaging of primarily left heart structures. Turning the probe to the right (clockwise) allows imaging of primarily right heart structures. Diagnostic information obtained from this view include MV and TV function, assessment of global LV and RV systolic function and of regional left (inferoseptal and anterolateral), and right (lateral) wall function. Color-flow Doppler can be applied to aid in identifying aortic, mitral, and tricuspid regurgitation. After slight probe advancement, the coronary sinus is imaged in the long axis immediately above the attachment of the TV septal leaflet to the interventricular septum.

Simultaneous multiplane imaging is unique to the matrix array transducer and permits the use of a dual screen to simultaneously display two real-time two-dimensional (2D) images (Fig. 13.6).[12] The primary image is the reference view, and the second view can be generated with typically two modifiable manipulations. First, the angle of the secondary view in reference to the primary view can be modified (typical default angle of 90 degrees). Second, the lateral location of the secondary view in reference to the primary view but can be manipulated (typical default position in the midline of the sector). The 90-degree orthogonal image is oriented as if forward rotated from the primary view. Thus, when the primary imaging plane reaches 90 degrees, the orthogonal multiplane image may appear "reversed" compared with standard single-plane imaging. The orthogonal view obtained during simultaneous biplane imaging of the ME four-chamber view is the ME two-chamber view (see Fig. 13.2). 3D full-volume acquisitions of the ventricle can be performed for assessment of ejection fraction.

Key Points

- The midesophageal four-chamber view is one of the most comprehensive views available for evaluating cardiac anatomy and function. Measurement of the mitral annulus from this (or the two-chamber view) can be used to quantify diastolic stroke volume.
- To obtain the four-chamber view, the transducer angle may need to be rotated to approximately 10 to 20 degrees to eliminate the aortic valve or left ventricular (LV) outflow tract from the image display and to maximize the tricuspid annular dimension, with slight probe retroflexion to image the true LV apex.

MIDESOPHAGEAL MITRAL COMMISSURAL VIEW

From the ME four-chamber view, rotating the transducer angle to between 50 and 70 degrees generates the ME mitral commissural view (see Fig. 13.1). The MV scallops on the image display (from left to right) are P_3, A_2, and P_1, although frequently, adjacent A_3 and A_1 segments can also be imaged (P_3–$A_3A_2A_1$–P_1). From this neutral probe orientation, rotating the probe leftward (counterclockwise) may allow imaging of the length of the posterior leaflet ($P_3P_2P_1$), and continued counterclockwise rotation will image the posterior mitral annulus, coronary sinus, or circumflex artery. Turning the probe rightward (clockwise from the neutral position) may allow imaging of the length of the anterior leaflet ($A_3A_2A_1$).[13] In addition, the anterolateral and posteromedial papillary muscles with their corresponding chordae are prominent structures in the ME commissural view. Diagnostic information obtained from this view includes global and regional LV function (anterior/anterolateral and inferior/inferolateral walls) and MV function. Color-flow Doppler can be applied to aid in identifying commissural mitral regurgitation jets.

The orthogonal view obtained during simultaneous biplane imaging is the ME LAX view (see Fig. 13.6). Sweeping across the commissural plane with simultaneous biplane imaging allows for evaluation of the entire line of mitral leaflet coaptation: medial P_1/A_1, mid P_2/A_2, and lateral P_3/A_3. 3D narrow sector acquisition (with or without color) to assess the MV orifice can be performed from this view; the entire mitral coaptation length is imaged in the lateral plane with the coaptation of the two leaflets in the elevational plane.

Key Points

- The midesophageal mitral commissural view images the medial (to the left of the screen) and lateral (to the right of the screen) commissures of the mitral valve and usually the largest annular dimension.
- Using simultaneous multiplane imaging (i.e., biplane imaging) to scan through the commissures, the orthogonal view allows for evaluation of the entire line of mitral leaflet coaptation: medial P_1/A_1, mid P_2/A_2, and lateral P_3/A_3.

MIDESOPHAGEAL TWO-CHAMBER VIEW

From the ME mitral commissural view, rotating the transducer angle to between 80 and 100 degrees generates the ME two-chamber view (see Fig. 13.1). Structures seen include the LA, LA appendage, LV, and MV (P_3-$A_3A_2A_1$). Diagnostic information obtained from this view includes global and regional LV function (anterior and inferior walls) and MV function. Color-flow Doppler applied over the MV to aid in identification of valvular pathology (regurgitation, stenosis, or both). The coronary sinus is seen in short axis immediately above the basal inferior LV segment. The orthogonal view obtained during simultaneous biplane imaging is the ME four-chamber view (see Fig. 13.6); however, the left heart is now to the left of the display (mirror image of 0-degree view). Rotating to the right (clockwise) at this transducer angle results in the ME bicaval view (see view #13, Fig. 13.2). Rotating to the left (counterclockwise) at this transducer angle results in the ME LAA view (see view #15, Fig. 13.2).

Key Point

- The simultaneous multiplane image default is 90 degrees forward rotated from the primary image (Fig. 13.6). Thus, the orthogonal view obtained using the midesophageal two-chamber view would be 180 degrees forward rotated, resulting in an left-right inverted four-chamber view: the left heart is now to the left of the display (mirror image of 0-degree view).

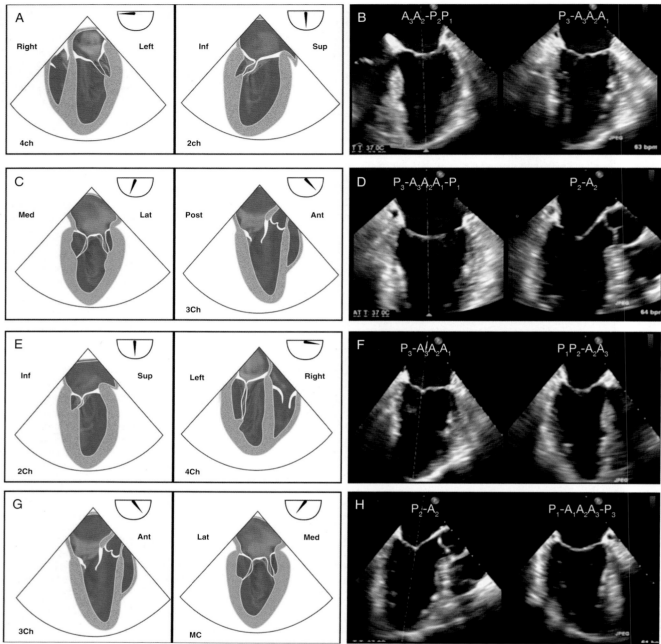

Figure 13.6. Simultaneous multiplane transesophageal echocardiographic image display. Simultaneous multiplane imaging permits the use of a dual screen to simultaneously display two real-time 2D images. In these examples, the primary image (on the left in each panel) is the reference view, with the second view (on the right in each panel) orthogonally rotated 90° to the primary view, but any tilt angle can be used for the secondary view. The typical 90° orthogonal second image is oriented as if the rotation has occurred in a clockwise manner and, for some views, appears "left-right reversed" compared with single-plane imaging. A, B, The primary view is the mid-esophageal (ME) four-chamber (4Ch) view. C, D, The primary view is the ME mitral commissural (MC) view. E, F, The primary view is the ME two-chamber (2Ch) view. G, H, The primary view is the ME LAX view. *A,* anterior; *Ant,* anterior; *Inf,* inferior; *Lat,* lateral; *MC,* mitral commissural; *Med,* medial; *P,* posterior; *Sup,* superior.

MIDESOPHAGEAL LONG-AXIS VIEW

From the ME two-chamber view, the transducer angle is rotated to approximately 120 to 140 degrees to image the ME LAX view, which is the same as the transthoracic three-chamber view. Structures seen include the LA, LV, LVOT, AV, proximal ascending aorta, coronary sinus, and MV (P_2–A_2). Diagnostic information obtained from this view includes global and regional LV function (inferolateral and anterior septal walls), MV, and AV function. The membranous interventricular septum as well as the RV wall that subtends the RV outflow tract (RVOT) can also be imaged. The orthogonal view obtained during simultaneous biplane imaging is the ME mitral commissural view (see Fig. 13.6); however, the anterior/anterolateral LV wall is now to the left of the display (mirror image of 60-degree view). Color-flow Doppler can be applied to identify aortic regurgitation.

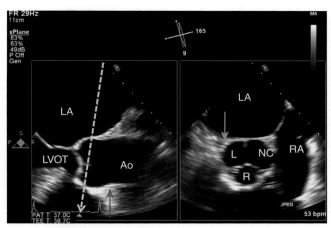

Figure 13.7. Simultaneous multiplane imaging of the aortic valve. From the midesophageal long-axis view of the aorta (view #6), the simultaneous orthogonal view is the short-axis view of the aorta. However, this view appears inverted from the single-plane midesophageal short-axis view (view #10). From these views, the right coronary artery (*red arrow*) and left coronary artery (*green arrow*) can be imaged. See text for abbreviations.

Key Points

- The midesophageal long-axis view is a key view to image the relationship between the mitral valve, the aortic valve, and the left ventricular outflow tract and ascending aorta. The mitral-aortic angle can be measured from this view.
- Measurements of mitral leaflet lengths to inform surgical or transcatheter devices may be performed from this view.

MIDESOPHAGEAL AORTIC VALVE LONG-AXIS VIEW

From the ME LAX view, anteflexion of the probe while maintaining a transducer angle of 120 to 140 degrees results in the ME AV LAX view (see Fig. 13.1). Optimizing the image to bisect the largest aortic root diameter can be accomplished with slight insertion and right or left rotation. Reducing the depth of field allows concentrated imaging of the LVOT, AV, and proximal aorta, including the sinus of Valsalva and sinotubular junction. This view is useful in evaluating the AV function and obtaining the dimensions of the annulus and sinotubular junction. The anterior (far-field) AV cusp is the right coronary cusp; frequently, the right coronary ostium is imaged from this view. The posterior (near-field) cusp can be the noncoronary cusp or the left coronary cusp, depending on the window; when perfectly centered on the aorta, however, the plane of imaging may be at the commissure between these two cusps. The orthogonal view obtained during simultaneous biplane imaging is a SAX view of the AV (see Fig. 13.7); however, the right heart is now to the right of the display (mirror image of the single 2D AV SAX imaging view #10). Color-flow Doppler can be applied to identifying aortic regurgitation as well as flow within the right coronary ostium.

The ME AV LAX view is one of the main views used for transcatheter AV procedures.[14,15] The sagittal plane measurement of the annulus and LVOT is performed from this view. The use of simultaneous biplane imaging may assist acquisition of the largest annular diameter. A user-defined (zoomed) 3D volume of the AV can be obtained from this view (or the AV SAX view) to measure annular area and perimeter,[16,17] as well as the location of the coronary ostia.[15] Color Doppler 3D acquisition can be useful for assessing the severity of aortic regurgitation.[18]

MIDESOPHAGEAL ASCENDING AORTA LAX VIEW

Key Points

- The midesophageal (ME) aortic valve (AV) long-axis view is useful in evaluating AV function and obtaining the dimensions of the annulus and sinotubular junction.
- The simultaneous multiplane orthogonal view is the ME AV short-axis view (see later); however, the left heart is now to the left of the display (mirror image of 0-degree view).

From the ME AV LAX view, withdrawal of the probe, typically with backward rotation to approximately 90 degrees, results in the ME ascending aorta LAX view (see Fig. 13.1). This view allows for evaluation of the proximal ascending aorta. The right pulmonary artery (PA) lies posterior to the ascending aorta in this view. Although aortic flow is typically perpendicular to the insonation beam from this view, color-flow Doppler may still be useful in some pathologies. By centering the image plane on the SAX image of the right PA (in the near field), turning the probe to the left (counterclockwise) with possible retroflexion results in LAX imaging of the main PA and the PV. This view aligns the insonation beam with PA flow and optimizes the imaging plane for pulsed-wave (PW), continuous-wave (CW), and color Doppler of the RVOT, PV, or main PA. The orthogonal view obtained during simultaneous biplane imaging is mirror image of the ME ascending aortic SAX view (view #8) with the PA to the left of the aorta.

MIDESOPHAGEAL ASCENDING AORTA SHORT-AXIS VIEW

From the ME AV and ascending aorta view, backward transducer rotation to approximately 0 to 40 degrees results in the ME ascending aorta SAX view (see Fig. 13.1). In addition to the ascending aorta in SAX and superior vena cava (SVC), the main PA and right lobar PA can be seen. From this neutral probe orientation, turning the probe to the left (counterclockwise) allows imaging of the PA bifurcation. Turning the probe to the right from the neutral position allows imaging of a greater extent of the right lobar PA. The left lobar PA is difficult to image because of the left main stem bronchus. The pulmonary valve (PV) can also be imaged from this plane in some patients. The orthogonal view obtained during simultaneous biplane imaging is the 90-degree view of the right pulmonary veins. PW, CW, and color Doppler of the PA may be useful. Careful insertion of the probe should allow imaging of the proximal left coronary artery, as well as the bifurcation to the left anterior descending and circumflex coronary arteries.

MIDESOPHAGEAL RIGHT PULMONARY VEIN VIEW

From the ME ascending aorta SAX view (and typically at 0 degrees), advancing the probe in addition to turning to the right (clockwise) results in the ME right pulmonary vein view (see Fig. 13.2). The inflow of the inferior pulmonary vein is typically perpendicular to the insonation beam; however, superior pulmonary vein inflow is typically parallel to the beam, and Doppler from this view can be performed. In addition to the right pulmonary veins, the SVC (SAX) and ascending aorta (SAX) are also imaged. The orthogonal view obtained during simultaneous biplane imaging is the ME ascending aorta LAX view (view #7). The right pulmonary veins can also be imaged from the 90- to 110-degree view by first obtaining a ME bicaval view (view #13) and rotating the probe to the right (clockwise). Note that the left pulmonary veins may be imaged by turning the probe to the left (counterclockwise).

MIDESOPHAGEAL AORTIC VALVE SHORT-AXIS VIEW

From the ME right pulmonary vein view, reposition the probe (turning to the left, counterclockwise) to center the aorta in the display (as in the ME ascending aorta SAX view) and advance and rotate the transducer angle to between 25 and 40 degrees to obtain the ME AV SAX view (see Fig. 13.2). Slight anteflexion may be required. For a trileaflet valve, the left coronary cusp will be posterior and to the right on the display, the noncoronary cusp will be adjacent to the interatrial septum, and the right coronary cusp will be anterior and adjacent to the RVOT. AV morphology and function can be evaluated from this view. In addition, with a subtle degree of withdrawal, the left coronary artery (arising from the left coronary cusp) and the right coronary artery (arising from the right coronary cusp) can be imaged. In addition to the AV, a portion of the superior LA, interatrial septum, and RA are imaged. This superior portion of the interatrial septum is important because frequently, shunting from a patent foramen ovale may be imaged. In addition, the RVOT and PV may be seen in the far field. Color-flow Doppler (and, when appropriate, PW and CW Doppler) should be used to assess all imaged structures. The orthogonal view obtained during simultaneous biplane imaging is the ME AV LAX view. 3D imaging of the AV from this view should be considered, particularly for the assessment of coronary ostia position.

MIDESOPHAGEAL RIGHT VENTRICLE INFLOW–OUTFLOW VIEW

> ### Key Point
>
> - The midesophageal aortic valve short-axis view images the left coronary cusp posterior. To the right on the display, the noncoronary cusp is adjacent to the interatrial septum, and the right coronary cusp is anterior and adjacent to the right ventricular outflow tract. Evaluating both the left and right coronary arteries is also possible (Fig. 13.7).

From the ME AV SAX view, slight advancement of the probe and rotating the transducer angle to 50 to 70 degrees until the RVOT and PV appear in the display results in the ME RV inflow–outflow view (see Fig. 13.2). Structures seen in the view include the LA, RA, interatrial septum, TV, RV (on left of display), RVOT (on right of display), PV, and proximal (main) PA. From this view, one can evaluate RV size and function (with RVOT diameter), TV morphology and function, and PV morphology and function.

The ME RV inflow–outflow view is one of the most important views for imaging the TV. The anterior TV leaflet is near the aorta and posterior leaflet near the lateral RV wall; the septal leaflet is out of plane. Similar to the mitral "commissural" view, a simultaneous multiplane imaging sweep across the commissural plane allows for evaluation of the entire line of tricuspid septal leaflet coaptation: anteroseptal from the aorta to midvalve and posteroseptal from the midvalve to the lateral wall. Because most tricuspid regurgitant jets arise between the septal leaflet and one of the other two leaflets, 3D narrow-sector acquisition (with or without color) to assess the TV orifice can be performed from this view. The entire tricuspid septal leaflet coaptation length is imaged in the lateral plane and the coaptation with the anterior or posterior leaflets in the elevational plane.

Visualization of two of the PV leaflets (typically the left or right and anterior) is frequently limited by acoustic noise from the AV or periaortic fibrous tissue. Advancing the probe and placing the RVOT perpendicular to the insonation beam enhances imaging for measurement of RVOT diameter. Color-flow Doppler as well as spectral Doppler of both valves should be performed. This view and the subsequent view can be particularly useful for imaging tricuspid regurgitant jets directed toward the interatrial septum.

MIDESOPHAGEAL MODIFIED BICAVAL TRICUSPID VALVE VIEW

> ### Key Points
>
> - The midesophageal (ME) right ventricular (RV) inflow–outflow view is a key view for assessing the tricuspid valve. Simultaneous multiplane imaging sweep across the tricuspid commissural plane allows for evaluation of the entire line of tricuspid septal leaflet coaptation: anteroseptal from the aorta to the midvalve and posteroseptal from the midvalve to the lateral wall.
> - The ME RV inflow–outflow view is a key view for imaging the pulmonic valve measurement of right ventricular outflow tract (RVOT) diameter. Advancing the probe and counterclockwise rotation places the RVOT perpendicular to the insonation beam.

From the ME RV inflow–outflow view, maintaining a transducer angle of 50 to 70 degrees, the probe is turned to the right (clockwise) until primarily the TV is centered in the view, resulting in the ME modified bicaval TV view (see Fig. 13.2). The LA, RA, interatrial septum, inferior vena cava (IVC), and TV are well imaged. Occasionally, the right atrial appendage as well as the SVC will be seen. Because of the radially short septal TV leaflet, many tricuspid regurgitant jets are eccentric and directed toward the interatrial septum; from this view, the septal TV leaflet is imaged en face, and jets directed toward the interatrial septum are parallel to the insonation beam. Color-flow Doppler and spectral Doppler (particularly CW Doppler) should be performed in this view.

MIDESOPHAGEAL BICAVAL VIEW

From the ME modified bicaval TV view, the transducer angle is rotated forward to 90 to 110 degrees, and the probe is turned to the right (clockwise) to obtain the ME bicaval view (see Fig. 13.2). Imaged in this view are the LA, RA, IVC, SVC RA appendage, and interatrial septum. Motion of the interatrial septum should be observed because atrial septal aneurysms are associated with interatrial shunts. From this view, interatrial septum morphology and function should be assessed. In addition, IVC and SVC inflow are well imaged. The orthogonal view obtained during simultaneous biplane imaging is a ME four-chamber view focused on the interatrial septum. Further right (clockwise) rotation with slight withdrawal of the probe allows imaging of the right pulmonary veins (orthogonal to view #9). With 3D imaging using the bicaval image as the near-field image, the TV and MV can be seen in the far field. This 3D imaging plane can be useful when guiding devices toward the atrioventricular valves.

MIDESOPHAGEAL RIGHT AND LEFT PULMONARY VEINS VIEW

At a transducer angle of 90 to 110 degrees, imaging of either the right or left pulmonary veins can be performed. From the ME bicaval view, turning the probe farther to the right (clockwise) results in imaging of the right pulmonary veins with the superior vein to the right of the display. Turning the probe to the left (counterclockwise) takes the imaging through the entire heart (past the LA) to the ME left pulmonary veins view (see Fig. 13.2). The left superior vein is to the right of the display, and typically inflow is parallel to the insonation beam, allowing for accurate spectral Doppler assessment.

MIDESOPHAGEAL LEFT ATRIAL APPENDAGE VIEW

From the ME left pulmonary veins view (at a transducer angle of 90–110 degrees), rotating the probe to right (clockwise) with possible advancement and/or anteflexion of the probe opens the LAA for the ME LAA view (see Fig. 13.2). Often the left superior pulmonary vein is also imaged.

Given the complex and highly variable anatomy of the LA appendage, a complete assessment of morphology typically requires imaging the LA appendage from 0 to 150 degrees of mechanical rotation or using simultaneous biplane imaging to achieve the equivalent complete assessment. Typically, the LA appendage is an ellipse with the widest orifice diameter between 135 and 150 degrees. Color-flow Doppler and PW Doppler may be useful particularly for assessment of contractile function. The assessment of the LAA by 3D echocardiography has been well described.[19–22] Using the simultaneous imaging modality may be helpful in excluding thrombus as well as positioning catheters during percutaneous procedures. Real-time 3D TEE is useful to define the variable anatomy of the orifice and the relationship to the pulmonary veins both pre- and intraprocedurally.

TRANSGASTRIC BASAL SHORT-AXIS VIEW

> **Key Point**
>
> - To obtain the ideal midesophageal left atrial appendage (LAA) view (long axis of the LAA aligned parallel to the insonation beam), advancement (deeper probe position) with anteflexion of the probe may be useful.

From the ME views and at a transducer angle of 0 degrees, the probe is placed in a neutral position and advanced into the stomach, frequently imaging the coronary sinus inflow as well as the IVC and hepatic vein in the distal esophageal (DE) position before reaching the TG level. The DE view of the TV as well as the coronary sinus are frequently possible without intervening left heart structures. When the probe is in the gastric cavity, anteflexion typically results in the TG basal SAX view (see Fig. 13.3). This view demonstrates the typical SAX view or "fish mouth" appearance of the MV in the TG imaging plane with the anterior leaflet on the left of the display and the posterior leaflet on the right. The medial commissure is in the near field with the lateral commissure in the far field. An assessment of MV morphology and function as well as LV size and function can be performed from this view. The orthogonal view obtained during simultaneous biplane imaging is a two-chamber view of the base of the LV (including the MV), which may be useful for assessing MV morphology and function. Color-flow Doppler of the MV in this view may help characterize regurgitant orifice morphology.

TRANSGASTRIC MIDPAPILLARY SHORT-AXIS VIEW

While maintaining contact with the gastric wall, the anteflexed probe for the TG basal SAX view can be relaxed to a more neutral position, or the probe may be advanced farther into the stomach to obtain the TG midpapillary SAX view (see Fig. 13.3). Proper positioning may require multiple probe manipulations using varying probe depths and degrees of anteflexion. The transducer angle should typically remain at 0 degrees. The TG midpapillary SAX view provides significant diagnostic information and can be extremely helpful in assessing LV size and volume status and global and regional function. This is the primary TG view for intraoperative monitoring because myocardium supplied by the left anterior descending, circumflex, and right coronary arteries can be seen. The orthogonal image during simultaneous multiplane imaging is the TG two-chamber view, which may be useful to ensure an on-axis SAX view. This orthogonal view should be perpendicular to the insonation beam. If the MV (seen on the right of the secondary image) is higher (closer to the apex of the sector) than the apex, the probe should be advanced. If the MV is deeper than the apex, the probe should be withdrawn. Ensuring on-axis imaging of these views permits more accurate assessment of wall motion.

TRANSGASTRIC APICAL SHORT-AXIS VIEW

From the TG midpapillary SAX view, the probe is slightly advanced and/or retroflexed while maintaining contact with the gastric wall to obtain the TG apical SAX view (see Fig. 13.3). The RV apex is imaged from this view by turning to the right (clockwise). This view allows for evaluation of the apical segments of the LV and RV. This image may be difficult to obtain because retroflexion within the stomach may prevent adequate probe contact with the gastric wall. Advancing the probe to the level of the LV apex with slight flexion can also image the apical segments of ventricles.

TRANSGASTRIC RIGHT VENTRICULAR BASAL VIEW

Returning to the TG basal SAX view (anteflexed, at a transducer angle of approximately 0–30 degrees) by turning the probe toward the patient's right (clockwise), the TG basal RV view (see Fig. 13.3) can be seen. The TV is imaged in SAX view while the RVOT is imaged in LAX view. The orthogonal view obtained during simultaneous biplane imaging of the TV is with the TG RV Inflow view (view #23, described later). The orthogonal view obtained during simultaneous biplane imaging of the RVOT is with the TG RV inflow–outflow view (mirror image of view #20 described later). Color-flow Doppler of the TV in this view may help characterize regurgitant orifice morphology.

TRANSGASTRIC RIGHT VENTRICULAR INFLOW–OUTFLOW VIEW

> **Key Points**
>
> - The transgastric basal right ventricular (RV) view produces a short-axis view of the tricuspid valve and is essential for assessing leaflet coaptation and the shape of the regurgitant orifice (with or without color Doppler). It is important to image the tips of all three leaflets.
> - Doppler of the RV outflow tract for calculation of RV stroke volume can be performed from this view.

From the TG basal RV view (transducer angle of 0 degrees), maximal right flexion with or without anterior flexion results in the TG RV inflow–outflow view (see Fig. 13.3). In this view, typically the anterior and posterior leaflets of the TV are imaged as well as the left and right cusps of the PV. Advancing the probe may be necessary to align RVOT flow with the insonation beam. The mirror image of this view can be also be obtained from a neutral probe position (no flexion) with the probe turned to the right (clockwise) so that the right ventricle is in view and then forward-rotating to 90 to 120 degrees. TG views of the PV can be used to align transpulmonic flow with the Doppler beam.

DEEP TRANSGASTRIC FIVE-CHAMBER VIEW

> **Key Points**
>
> - Imaging the right heart typically requires using right flexion of the probe, as well as clockwise rotation.
> - Maximal right flexion with or without anterior flexion from the transgastric position should result in the transgastric right ventricular inflow–outflow view.

From the TG RV inflow–outflow view (transducer angle of 0 degrees), advancing the probe to the deep TG level, maximum left flexion with gradual anteflexion results in the deep TG five-chamber view (see Fig. 13.3). Because of parallel Doppler beam alignment with the LVOT, AV, and proximal aortic root, spectral Doppler interrogation of the LVOT and AV is possible. The MV is also imaged, and complete Doppler interrogation of this valve may also be attempted.

TRANSGASTRIC TWO-CHAMBER VIEW

The probe is returned to the TG midpapillary SAX view, and the transducer angle is rotated to approximately 90 to 110 degrees to obtain the TG two-chamber view (see Fig. 13.3). The anterior and inferior walls of the LV are imaged in addition to the papillary muscles, chordae, and MV. Although the LA and LAA are often seen, far-field imaging may not allow accurate assessment of LA appendage pathology.

TRANSGASTRIC RIGHT VENTRICLE INFLOW VIEW

From the TG two-chamber view (transducer angle of 90–110 degrees), rotating to the right (clockwise) results in the TG RV inflow (or RV two-chamber) view (see Fig. 13.3). The anterior and inferior walls of the RV are imaged in addition to the papillary muscles, chordae, and TV. The proximal RVOT is also frequently seen, and slight advancement of the probe may allow imaging of the PV.

TRANSGASTRIC LONG-AXIS VIEW

From the TG RV inflow view, rotating to the left to return to the TG two-chamber view, rotate the transducer angle to 120 to 150 degrees to obtain the TG LAX view (see Fig. 13.3). Sometimes turning the probe slightly to the right is necessary to bring the LVOT and AV into view. Portions of the inferolateral and anterior septum are imaged, as well as the LVOT, AV, and proximal aorta. With parallel Doppler beam alignment of the LVOT, AV, and proximal aortic root, spectral Doppler interrogation of the LVOT and AV is possible. This view is most equivalent to a right parasternal view of the AV and can often yield the highest transvalvular velocities.

DESCENDING AORTA SHORT-AXIS AND DESCENDING LONG-AXIS VIEWS

Imaging of the descending aorta with TEE is easily performed because the aorta is immediately adjacent to the stomach and esophagus. From the TG LAX view, the transducer angle is returned to 0 degrees· and the probe is turned to the left (counterclockwise). Although one can begin imaging the descending aorta below the diaphragm (typically beginning at the celiac artery), abdominal gas and variable aortic position may prevent adequate imaging, and withdrawing the probe to just above the diaphragm allows imaging of the descending thoracic aorta (see Fig. 13.4). The short axis of the aorta is obtained at a transducer angle of 0 degrees, while the long axis is obtained at a transducer angle of approximately 90 degrees; slight retroflexion may be needed if Doppler of the aorta is needed (i.e., to assess for holodiastolic flow reversal in the setting of aortic regurgitation). Image depth should be decreased to enlarge the size of the aorta and the focus set to be in the near field. Finally, gain should be increased in the near field to optimize imaging. While keeping the aorta in the center of the image, the probe can be advanced or withdrawn to image the entire descending aorta. Because there are no internal anatomic landmarks in the descending aorta, describing the location of pathology is difficult. One approach to this problem is to identify the location in terms of distance from the incisors. The descending thoracic aorta is located posterior and to the left of the esophagus, and when imaging this structure, the TEE probe faces the left thoracic cavity. Thus, intercostal arteries are typically seen arising from the aorta toward the right side of the screen. When imaging the descending thoracic aorta, the hemiazygous vein (which drains the left posterior thorax) may be seen in the far field of imaging. In the mid to upper thorax,

this vein joins the azygous vein (which drains the right posterior thorax). This venous structure is typically parallel to the aorta and aortic arch, eventually draining into the SVC. Because their walls are contiguous, the two structures could be mistaken for a dissection flap within the aorta; color-flow Doppler or pulsed Doppler easily distinguishes venous from arterial flow within each lumen.

UPPER ESOPHAGEAL AORTIC ARCH LONG-AXIS VIEW

As one is evaluating the descending aorta SAX view (transducer angle of 0 degrees) and withdrawing the probe, the aorta eventually becomes elongated, and the left subclavian artery may be imaged, indicating the beginning of the distal aortic arch. At this location, the aorta is positioned anterior to the esophagus, and thus the UE aortic arch LAX view (see Fig. 13.4) is best imaged by then turning to the right (clockwise) so the probe faces anterior. This allows imaging of the midaortic arch. In addition to the aorta, the left innominate vein is frequently imaged with venous flow by color-flow Doppler. Because the left main stem bronchus typically crosses between the esophagus and the aorta, a portion of the proximal aortic arch and distal ascending aorta may not be visualized.

UPPER ESOPHAGEAL AORTIC ARCH SHORT-AXIS VIEW

From the UE aortic arch LAX view, the transducer angle is advanced toward 70 to 90 degrees to obtain the UE aortic arch SAX view (see Fig. 13.4). The main PA and PV can frequently be seen in long axis in the far field but may require adjustment of imaging depth, probe frequency, and focal zone. Because of parallel Doppler beam alignment of the PV and main PA, spectral Doppler interrogation of the PV may be performed. Because of the curvature of the aorta, between the LAX and SAX view of the aortic arch, the right brachiocephalic and left common carotid arteries may be seen arising from the aorta, typically in the near field and to the right of the screen.

Please access ExpertConsult to view the corresponding videos for this chapter.

> **Key Point**
>
> - The deep transgastric five-chamber view is essential for Doppler assessment of aortic valve function. To obtain this view, the probe should be inserted into the fundus of the stomach near the left ventricular (LV) apex. With maximum left flexion with gradual anteflexion, the LV outflow tract and aortic valve should be imaged.

> **Key Point**
>
> - The transgastric long-axis view is most equivalent to a right parasternal view of the aortic valve and can often yield the highest transvalvular velocities.

REFERENCES

1. Kallmeyer IJ, Collard CD, Fox JA, Body SC, Shernan SK. The safety of intraoperative transesophageal echocardiography: a case series of 7200 cardiac surgical patients. *Anesth Analg.* 2001;92:1126–1130.
2. Peterson GE, Brickner ME, Reimold SC. Transesophageal echocardiography: clinical indications and applications. *Circulation.* 2003;107:2398–2402.
3. Maffessanti F, Marsan NA, Tamborini G, et al. Quantitative analysis of mitral valve apparatus in mitral valve prolapse before and after annuloplasty: a three-dimensional intraoperative transesophageal study. *J Am Soc Echocardiogr.* 2011;24:405–413.

4. Heidenreich PA, Stainback RF, Redberg RF, et al. Transesophageal echocardiography predicts mortality in critically ill patients with unexplained hypotension. *J Am Coll Cardiol.* 1995;26:152–158.
5. Meier B, Frank B, Wahl A, Diener HC. Secondary stroke prevention: patent foramen ovale, aortic plaque, and carotid stenosis. *Eur Heart J.* 2012;33:705–713.
6. Hahn RT, Nicoara A, Kapadia S, et al. Echocardiographic imaging for transcatheter aortic valve replacement. *J Am Soc Echocardiogr.* 2018;31:405–433.
7. Nyman CB, Mackensen GB, Jelacic S, et al. Transcatheter mitral valve repair using the edge-to-edge clip. *J Am Soc Echocardiogr.* 2018;31:434–453.
8. Hahn RT, Nabauer M, Zuber M, et al. Intraprocedural imaging of transcatheter tricuspid valve interventions. *JACC Cardiovasc Imag.* 2019;12:532–553.
9. Hahn RT, Abraham T, Adams MS, et al. Guidelines for performing a comprehensive transesophageal echocardiographic examination. *J Am Soc Echocardiogr.* 2013;26:921–964.
10. Shanewise JS, Cheung AT, Aronson S, et al. ASE/SCA guidelines for performing a comprehensive intraoperative multiplane transesophageal echocardiography examination. *Anesth Analg.* 1999;89:870–884.
11. Swaminathan M, Nicoara A, Phillips-Bute BG, et al. Utility of a simple algorithm to grade diastolic dysfunction and predict outcome after coronary artery bypass graft surgery. *Ann Thorac Surg.* 2011;91:1844–1850.
12. Lang RM, Badano LP, Tsang W, et al. EAE/ASE recommendations for image acquisition and display using three-dimensional echocardiography. *J Am Soc Echocardiogr.* 2012;25(3–46).
13. Foster GP, Isselbacher EM, Rose GA, et al. Accurate localization of mitral regurgitant defects using multiplane transesophageal echocardiography. *Ann Thorac Surg.* 1998;65:1025–1031.
14. Zamorano JL, Badano LP, Bruce C, et al. EAE/ASE recommendations for the use of echocardiography in new transcatheter interventions for valvular heart disease. *Eur J Echocardiogr.* 2011;12:557–584.
15. Bloomfield GS, Gillam LD, Hahn RT, et al. A practical guide to multimodality imaging of transcatheter aortic valve replacement. *JACC Cardiovasc Imag.* 2012;5:441–455.
16. Santos N, de Agustin JA, Almeria C, et al. Prosthesis/annulus discongruence assessed by three-dimensional transoesophageal echocardiography: a predictor of significant paravalvular aortic regurgitation after transcatheter aortic valve implantation. *Eur Heart J Cardiovasc Imag.* 2012;13:931–937.
17. Hahn RT, Khalique O, Williams MR, et al. Predicting paravalvular regurgitation following transcatheter valve replacement: utility of a novel method for three-dimensional echocardiographic measurements of the aortic annulus. *J Am Soc Echocardiogr.* 2013;26:1043–1052.
18. Pirat B, Little SH, Igo SR, et al. Direct measurement of proximal isovelocity surface area by real-time three-dimensional color Doppler for quantitation of aortic regurgitant volume: an in vitro validation. *J Am Soc Echocardiogr.* 2009;22:306–313.
19. Nucifora G, Faletra FF, Regoli F, et al. Evaluation of the left atrial appendage with real-time 3-dimensional transesophageal echocardiography: implications for catheter-based left atrial appendage closure. *Circ Cardiovasc Imag.* 2011;4:514–523.
20. Nakajima H, Seo Y, Ishizu T, et al. Analysis of the left atrial appendage by three-dimensional transesophageal echocardiography. *Am J Cardiol.* 2010:106885–106892.
21. Latcu DG, Rinaldi JP, Saoudi N. Real-time three-dimensional transoesophageal echocardiography for diagnosis of left atrial appendage thrombus. *Eur J Echocardiogr.* 2009;10:711–712.
22. Shah SJ, Bardo DM, Sugeng L, et al. Real-time three-dimensional transesophageal echocardiography of the left atrial appendage: initial experience in the clinical setting. *J Am Soc Echocardiogr.* 2008;21:1362–1368.

14   Applications of Transesophageal Echocardiography

Amita Singh

Transesophageal echocardiography (TEE) is a widely available imaging modality with an extensive spectrum of indications for diagnostic and intraprocedural imaging. Owing to the proximity of the TEE probe to cardiac structures and thus the improved spatial resolution, TEE offers invaluable clinical information for commonly encountered cardiac diseases, with guideline-based recommendations for its use spanning from: assessment of mechanism and severity of native and prosthetic valvular disease, evaluation of structural and congenital anomalies, detection of intracardiac thrombus, characterization of cardiac masses, and assessment of aortic pathologies, among others. TEE has long been used for diagnostic imaging in echocardiographic laboratories and operating rooms and has rapidly expanding applications with the concurrent rise in performance of structural heart interventions.

DIAGNOSTIC APPLICATIONS
Mitral Valve Disease

Mitral valve (MV) pathology is readily identified by TEE because of systematic visualization of the complex saddle-shaped annulus, leaflets and sub-valvular apparatus. This can be achieved using both conventional two- (2D) and three-dimensional (3D) imaging techniques, the latter of which often provides incrementally valuable information.

In cases of mitral regurgitation (MR), TEE permits a thorough assessment for the underlying morphologic cause and quantification of severity by visualizing constituent elements of the regurgitant jet with color flow and spectral doppler. Delineation of primary versus secondary etiologies of MR is paramount because ensuing options for management are directed by this categorization. Although

mechanisms of MR can be appropriately classified by transthoracic echocardiography (TTE), TEE has been shown to better localize pathology in cases of mitral regurgitation undergoing surgical or percutaneous repair, particularly with 3D renderings of the valve.[1] TEE can also offer objective but nuanced data regarding dynamic changes in annular geometry throughout the cardiac cycle, the details of which lie beyond the scope of this chapter. The use of TEE in cases of unexplained MR can yield observations of novel pathology, as evidenced by the relatively recent description of posterior leaflet indentations as a form of congenital valvular disease and atrial functional mitral regurgitation in patients with atrial fibrillation[2,3] (Fig. 14.1). The multitude of these insights inform the basis that 3D TEE should be used routinely to evaluate patients with significant MR.

Although the diagnosis of mitral stenosis is not predicated on performance of TEE, therapeutic options may be better informed if TEE is performed. Rheumatic mitral disease, historically the most common etiology of mitral stenosis, can be adequately evaluated by TTE, but TEE can also assess suitability of anatomy for valvuloplasty. An entity of degenerative mitral stenosis causing a growing clinical dilemma stems from severe annular calcification, in which the exuberant calcification of the fibrous mitral annulus poses limitations for TTE because of acoustic shadowing. TEE may be useful in such patients for more accurate assessment of severity of mitral disease by clarification of valve area and detection of underappreciated regurgitation, allowing for accurate assessment of valve dysfunction.[4]

Aortic Valve Disease

TEE is an important adjunctive method in the assessment of aortic valvular pathology when TTE is limited by image quality,

Anterior mitral valve clefts

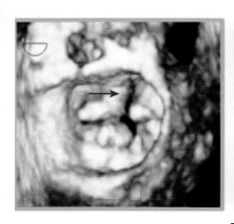
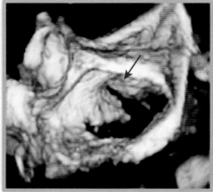
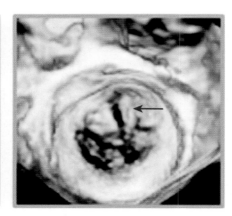

Posterior mitral valve indentations

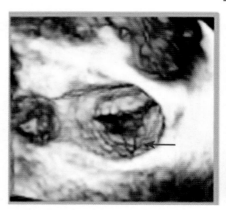
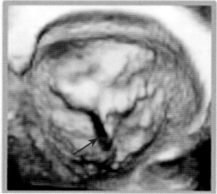
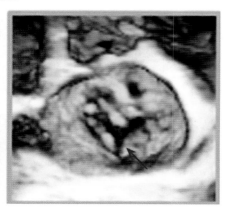

Figure 14.1. Representative cases of anterior cleft morphologies *(top row)* and posterior mitral cleft indentations *(bottom row)* as visualized by three-dimensional imaging of the mitral valve en face using surgeon's view.

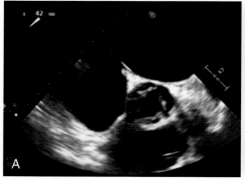
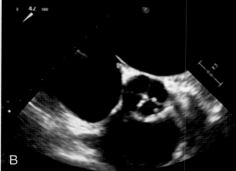

Figure 14.2. Quadricuspid aortic valve morphology in systole (**A**) and diastole (**B**). See accompanying Video 14.2.

calcification burden, or discrepant findings. TEE can also assist in the identification of congenital causes of aortic valvulopathy with excellent reliability and precision[5] (Fig. 14.2 and Video 14.2).

In cases of aortic stenosis, there can be challenges in the assessment of aortic valve area by TTE because of acoustic shadowing from calcification or suboptimal image quality. TEE can precisely measure left ventricular outflow tract diameter, which is an integral component in the calculation of effective aortic valve area. TEE further improves estimation of valve area with 2D and 3D planimetry, demonstrating good agreement with invasively determined and multidetector computed tomography (CT)–derived valve areas.[6] Additionally, 3D TEE may also be more accurate in the estimation of aortic valve area in patients with bicuspid aortic valves, for whom the domed leaflets may lead to overestimation with conventional 2D methods.[7] The widespread adoption of 3D TEE imaging in the evaluation of aortic stenosis has yielded important insights regarding the dynamic, ellipsoid morphology of the aortic annulus, with more eccentric variations noted in bicuspid valves.[8] These observations have important implications for transcatheter aortic valve replacement planning and outcomes.

TEE provides a similarly complimentary role in the clarification of aortic regurgitation etiology and severity, with a role primarily reserved for when TTE is insufficient. With recent guidelines emphasizing the importance of identifying the mechanism of aortic regurgitation, TEE can offer important and accurate classification in patients planned for aortic surgery[9] (Fig. 14.3). TEE evaluation may also help to highlight patients at risk of adverse events, including failure of surgical repair.[10]

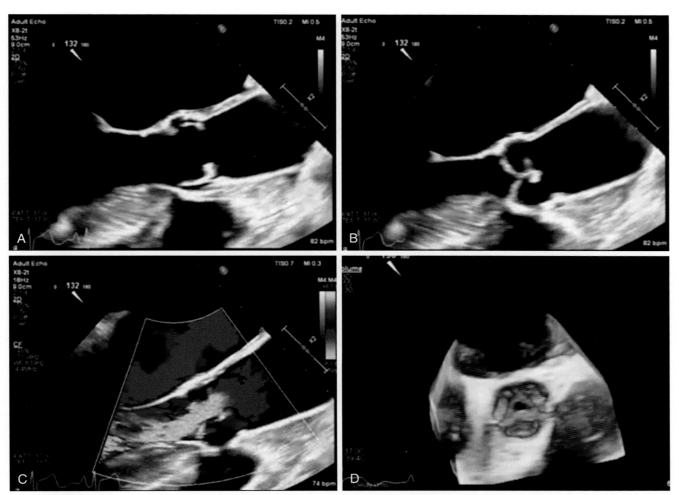

Figure 14.3. Case of moderate aortic regurgitation with unclear etiology. Two-dimensional imaging with systolic doming (**A**) and thickening in diastole (**B**). Central moderate to severe regurgitant jet (**C**) with three-dimensional demonstrating central malcoaptation (**D**).

Tricuspid and Pulmonic Valves

The anterior location of the tricuspid and pulmonic valves and their associated apparatus can pose challenges to visualization by TEE, but it remains an option in patients when TTE is suboptimal. In such cases, use of multiple views from the mid- and lower esophageal as well as transgastric positions can help to fully elucidate right-sided valve pathology. The tricuspid valve is composed of three nonuniformly sized leaflets (with occasional accessory leaflets described), an ellipsoid, vertically oriented annulus, and subvalvular apparatus (Fig. 14.4 and Video 14.4). The annulus itself can exhibit dynamic changes in size and contour according to loading conditions and right heart geometry. Tricuspid annular dimensions are well elucidated using 3D applications, though some data suggest that 3D TTE is probably equivalent to TEE.[11] Pulmonic valve pathology prompting TEE evaluations is most commonly related to preexisting congenital disease, concern for endocarditis, or evaluation of pulmonic valve prostheses.

Prosthetic Valves

TEE is frequently used for the investigation of suspected or confirmed prosthetic valve dysfunction. Image quality of bioprosthetic and mechanical prosthesis is invariably enhanced by the use of TEE because of less acoustic shadowing and less obscuration of far-field structures. TEE is standardly performed for concern of prosthetic valve endocarditis because of its superior sensitivity and ability to

evaluate for vegetation, abscess, or fistulous complications. With 2D and 3D TEE, careful delineation of prosthetic leaflet motion, degenerative changes, and the presence of pathologic thrombus, vegetations, or pannus can be performed, with consequential implications for clinical management (Fig. 14.5 and Video 14.5). The introduction of 3D color imaging with adequate temporal resolution can also help to coregister abnormal regurgitant jets to the valvular or perivalvular space, as well as define the associated lesion severity (Fig. 14.6 and Video 14.6). Real-time TEE guidance is now standardly used for percutaneous valve interventions, including perivalvular leak closure.

INTRACARDIAC THROMBUS AND MASS EVALUATION

Left Atrium and Appendage

Evaluation of the left atrium (LA) and appendage (LAA) is a common step in the management of patients with atrial fibrillation or flutter. Because of the posterior location of the L, and the complex morphologies of the LAA, TEE provides excellent resolution for the detection of thrombus, which poses an absolute contraindication to chemical and electrical cardioversion. The administration of microbubble contrast during TEE may improve the ability to correctly discern the presence of LAA thrombus.[12] TEE also permits the assessment of spontaneous echo contrast or "smoke" and

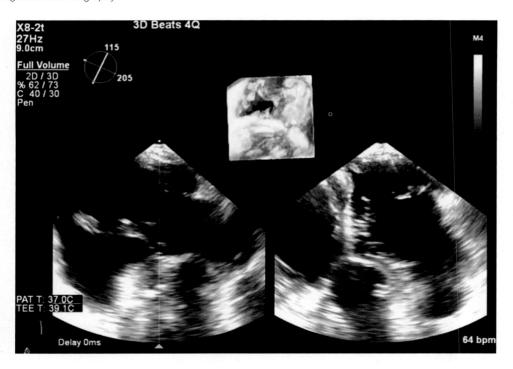

Figure 14.4. Representative three-dimensional acquisition of tricuspid valve from transgastric view. See accompanying Video 14.4.

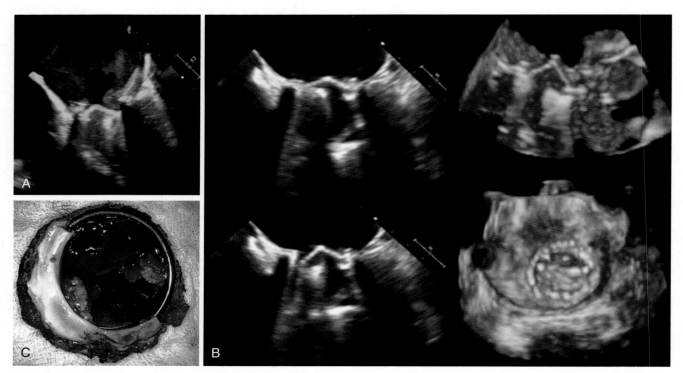

Figure 14.5. A, Mechanical mitral prosthesis thrombosis with left atrial and valve-associated thrombus and dense spontaneous echo contrast in the left atrium. **B,** Mechanical mitral prosthesis dysfunction with immobile posterior mechanical leaflet on two- and three-dimensional imaging with pathology demonstrating amalgam of acute and chronic thrombus, with pannus formation (**C**). See accompanying Videos 14.5A and B.

detection of reduced appendage emptying velocities, both of which are predictors of increased thromboembolic risk in patients with atrial arrhythmias (Fig. 14.7). Evaluation for occult LA or LAA thrombus is routinely performed before invasive pulmonary vein isolation or cryoablation. Applications of 3D TEE have underscored the complex and dynamic geometries of the LAA, with increasing relevance given the availability of implantable LAA closure devices. Use of TEE for the evaluation of patients presenting with cryptogenic stroke is common, but recent studies have suggested the yield of TEE in terms of findings of LAA thrombus or spontaneous echo contrast leading to initiation of anticoagulation occur in only 3% to 4% of cases.[13]

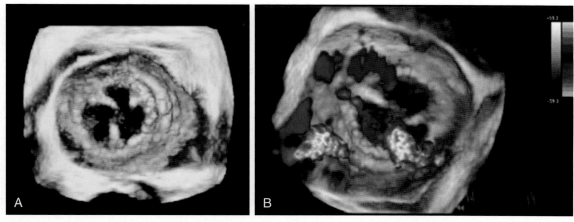

Figure 14.6. Three-dimensional (3D) imaging of bioprosthetic MV (**A**) with 3D color imaging (**B**) revealing two distinct perivalvular leaks at the 6 and 9 o'clock positions. See accompanying Video 14.6.

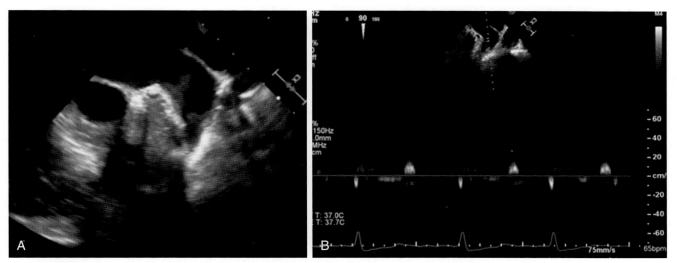

Figure 14.7. Left atrial appendage with thrombus and spontaneous echo contrast in the appendage (**A**) with evidence of reduced left atrial emptying velocities (**B**).

Intracardiac Masses

Although the overall incidence of cardiac masses is extremely low, assessment by TEE has utility in their evaluation by offering comprehensive visualization of size, attachment point, mobility, and typical morphologic appearance, particularly for smaller or valvular-associated masses (Figs. 14.8 and 14.9 and Video 14.8). The use of contrast agents can help in the determination of perfusion within cardiac masses, which is suggestive of malignant etiologies. Calcified, hemorrhagic, and mobile components can also be delineated by TEE. 3D TEE correlates well with ex vivo mass size and extent, based on small case series.[14] TEE may also aid in planning of surgical resection, particularly when valvular masses are involved.

PATENT FORAMEN OVALE AND SEPTAL DEFECTS

TEE has a significant role in the diagnosis and monitoring of patent foramen ovale (PFO) closure, when applicable. Because of the dynamic nature of transient shunting across a PFO, TTE can miss small PFO, particularly if provocative maneuvers are not well performed.[15] TEE is used in cases when TTE is equivocal, a high clinical index of suspicion exists, or TTE is positive for interatrial shunt. Although a PFO does not constitute a true atrial septal defect, TEE proves valuable in its ability to delineate the specific location and

size with 3D en-face visualization, detection of multiple defects, and demarcation of adequate tissue rims.

The detection of atrial septal defects (ASDs) is much improved by the use of TEE, which is able to acquire comprehensive views of the interatrial septum, vena cava, coronary sinus, and pulmonary veins, all of which can be variably involved. Location of the defect, directionality of shunting, and morphology are all enhanced by 3D TEE applications and is now considered standard in the diagnosis of ASD as well as in preprocedural planning.[16]

Ventricular septal defects (VSDs) can be caused by congenital abnormalities or iatrogenic after trauma, surgery, or myocardial infarction. 3D TEE provides detailed information regarding the morphology of these defects, quantification of abnormal shunting, and guidance during percutaneous closure.[17]

ENDOCARDITIS

In patients for whom endocarditis is suspected and principally in patients with preexisting prosthetic valves, TEE is considered the diagnostic test of choice. This relates to the improved spatial resolution and ability to detect even small vegetations. Vegetation location and size, along with any associated valvular dysfunction, are critical to identifying patients at increased risk for adverse events, including systemic embolism, when early surgical intervention

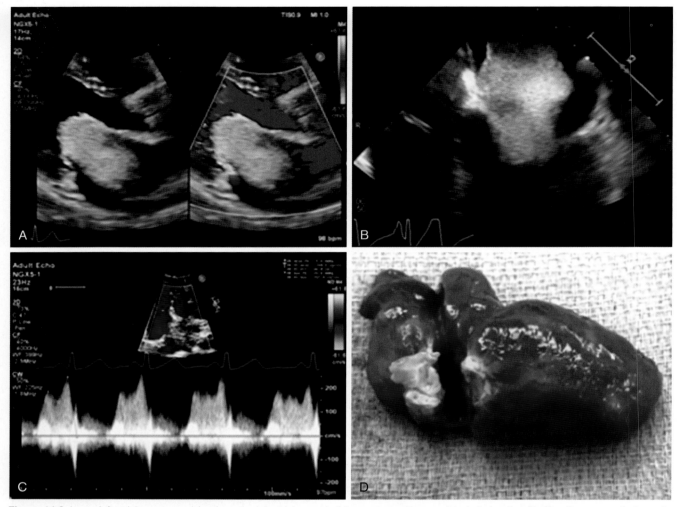

Figure 14.8. Large left atrial myxoma arising from the left atrial aspect of the septum with associated obstruction (**A–C**), with gross pathology at resection (**D**). See accompanying Video 14.8.

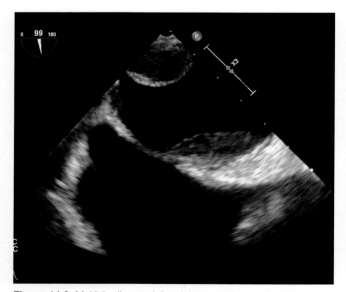

Figure 14.9. Multiple discrete left atrial masses in a patient 6 months after transplant, later identified as thrombus.

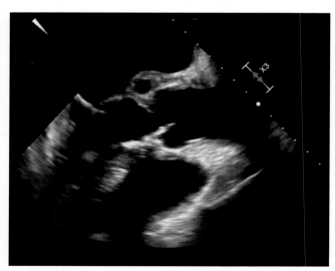

Figure 14.10. Intervalvular fibrosa and aortic root abscess and valvular vegetation in a patient with aortic homograft. See accompanying Video 14.10.

may be favored. Direct visualization of vegetations, if present, may also point to noninfectious causes, including Liebman-Sacks disease. Complications such as abscess, fistulous rupture, or contact lesions are better appreciated with TEE, though cardiac CT may offer a complementary role in such cases[18] (Fig. 14.10 and Video 14.10). TEE has a growing role in the assessment of cardiovascular implantable electronic device infections, in which left sided-valvular involvement or lead-associated vegetations may be present.[19]

AORTIC DISEASE

TEE is able to systemically evaluate for the presence and extent of atheromatous disease, which is a common finding in older patients after presenting with unexplained transient ischemic attacks or stroke.[20,21] In cases of suspected or confirmed aortic dissection, TEE has the ability to concomitantly characterize dissection type, identify the true and false lumen, define the entry site and involvement of coronary and branch vessels, and evaluate the severity of aortic valvular disease, all of which have significant implications for surgical repair. With improvements in CT angiography and MR angiography, TEE is not routinely used for the diagnosis of aortic dissection but remains a reliable adjunctive tool given its ability to visualize the majority of the thoracic aorta.

CRITICAL CARE APPLICATIONS OF TRANSESOPHAGEAL ECHOCARDIOGRAPHY

In the care of critically ill or hemodynamically unstable patients, TEE appears safe and effective when performed by experienced intensivist operators and is facilitated by the use of a miniaturized probe (mTEE). The incremental information regarding cardiac function and estimation of filling pressures aids in the assessment of hemodynamic status. Although more recent data would support equipoise in the routine use of mTEE in this population, there may be a particular benefit noted in patients with mechanical circulatory support devices.[22,23]

INTRAOPERATIVE APPLICATIONS OF TRANSESOPHAGEAL ECHOCARDIOGRAPHY

Pre- and postcardiopulmonary bypass TEE is recommended in patients undergoing cardiac surgery, with some studies estimating findings alter clinical management in up to 11% of cases with patients undergoing valvular surgery. The postcardiopulmonary bypass TEE has prognostic importance in patients undergoing MV repair and can help inform the need for additional pump runs as a result of findings.[24]

INTRAPROCEDURAL AND STRUCTURAL APPLICATIONS OF TRANSESOPHAGEAL ECHOCARDIOGRAPHY

TEE has been historically used in the cardiac catheterization laboratory in performance of mitral balloon valvuloplasty, percutaneous closure of atrial and VSDs, and closure of perivalvular leaks. Rapid growth in the introduction and implantation of percutaneous valve interventions have bolstered the role of TEE in the arena of structural interventions, with TEE playing an integral role in appropriate patient selection, intraprocedural monitoring, and postprocedural assessment for complications. Detailed discussion of structural intervention imaging is provided in further chapters.

Mitral Valvuloplasty

Percutaneous balloon valvuloplasty is a validated and effective treatment for mitral stenosis resulting from commissural fusion, with limited case reports detailing performance in bioprosthetic MVs TEE offers important periprocedural insights, including baseline presence of regurgitation, detection of LAA thrombus, and precise MV area estimation with 3D TEE, and intraprocedural assessment of MV area and any incurred MR after percutaneous mitral balloon valvuloplasty (PMBV) (Figs. 14.11 to 14.13).[25]

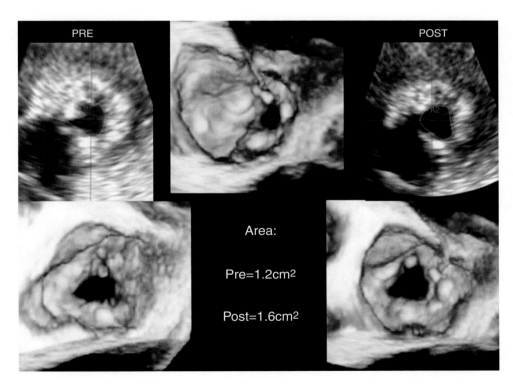

Figure 14.11. Valvuloplasty of the mitral valve with demonstration of three-dimensional planimetry for valve area with pre- and postvalvuloplasty measurements.

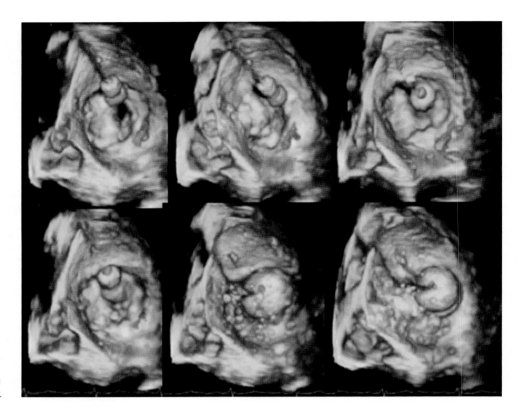

Figure 14.12. Real-time three-dimensional imaging of balloon position and deployment in stenotic mitral valve from the surgeon's view.

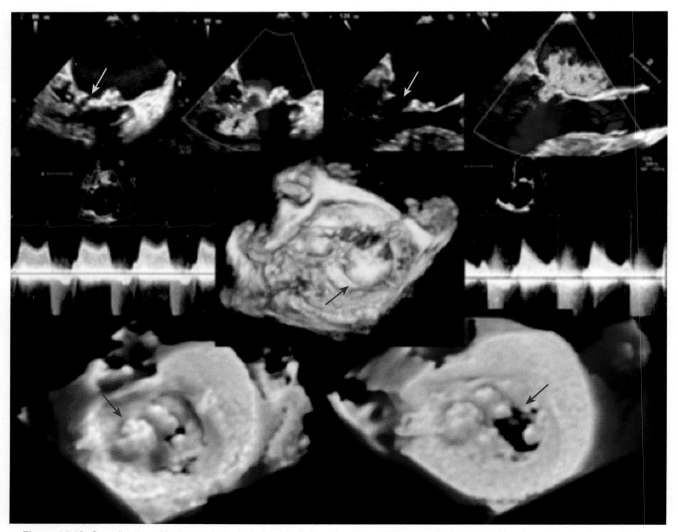

Figure 14.13. Complication of balloon valvuloplasty for mitral stenosis of tear of the posterior leaflet resulting in severe mitral regurgitation.

Transaortic Valve Replacement

Early experience with transaortic valve replacement (TAVR) involved routine use of TEE in the preprocedural planning stage for annular sizing, assessment of risk for coronary obstruction, periprocedural monitoring of valve deployment for appropriate positioning, and postprocedural assessment of perivalvular regurgitation. The use of TEE for annular sizing remains well validated and comparable to multidetector CT but relies on experience with 3D acquisition and careful reconstruction of the inherently ellipsoid annular topography.[26]

Perivalvular Leak Closure

Identification of perivalvular leak and its associated severity constitutes an important clinical finding and mandates assessment of suitability of the defect for closure. 3D TEE with and without color-flow Doppler plays a fundamental role in defining the shape, size, and circumferential involvement of perivalvular abnormalities. Real-time guidance with simultaneous 2D and 3D imaging during perivalvular leak (PVL) closure can facilitate several of the important procedural steps while monitoring for immediate complications.[27]

Percutaneous Mitral Repair and Replacement

As outlined previously, 2D and 3D TEE has immense utility in the identification of mechanisms of MR. TEE holds an important role in preprocedural assessment of patients being considered for MitraClip therapy. Real-time 3D TEE imaging allows for understanding of clip alignment and positioning in proximity to the causative pathology, monitoring of device steering in the LA and LV, and immediate assessment of MR reduction.[28] Transcatheter MV replacement in failed surgical valve replacement is another area of growth, which relies on real-time TEE for intraprocedural guidance of transseptal and transapical access, valve positioning, and assessment for complications.

Left Atrial Appendage Closure and Isolation

TEE is well suited to LAA visualization and is performed in patients undergoing LAA closure with occluder devices. TEE is typically obtained in advance of the procedure to rule out thrombus, as well as size the LAA. Intraprocedural TEE guides transseptal puncture and confirms adequacy of the "seal" around the occlude device, after it is deployed. Postprocedurally, TEE is performed to assess for peridevice flow and thrombus.

Atrial Septal Defect and Ventricular Septal Defect Closure

Multiple series have supported improved procedural outcomes when 3D TEE is used to guide ASD and VSD closure in the pediatric and adult populations. This is primarily because of improved accuracy of sizing and geometry, which has been shown to have good correlation compared to intraoperative evaluation.[29,30]

CONCLUSIONS

TEE continues to be an essential tool in imaging of numerous common cardiac conditions with an expanding domain of indications. 3D TEE has allowed for improved ability to categorize cardiac pathology and tailor accurate diagnoses, and real-time TEE guidance has emerged as a pivotal tool in the practice of percutaneous structural interventions.

Please access ExpertConsult to view the corresponding videos for this chapter.

REFERENCES

1. Ben Zekry S, Nagueh SF, Little SH, et al. Comparative accuracy of two- and three-dimensional transthoracic and transesophageal echocardiography in identifying mitral valve pathology in patients undergoing mitral valve repair: initial observations. *J Am Soc Echocardiogr.* 2011;24:1079–1085.
2. Narang A, Addetia K, Weinert L, et al. Diagnosis of isolated cleft mitral valve using three-dimensional echocardiography. *J Am Soc Echocardiogr.* 2018;31:1161–1167.
3. Kagiyama N, Hayashida A, Toki M, et al. Insufficient leaflet remodeling in patients with atrial fibrillation: association with the severity of mitral regurgitation. *Circ Cardiovasc Imag.* 2017;10.
4. Eleid MF, Foley TA, Said SM, et al. Severe mitral annular calcification: multimodality imaging for therapeutic strategies and interventions. *JACC Cardiovasc Imag.* 2016;9:1318–1337.
5. Espinola-Zavaleta N, Munoz-Castellanos L, Attie F, et al. Anatomic three-dimensional echocardiographic correlation of bicuspid aortic valve. *J Am Soc Echocardiogr.* 2003;16:46–53.
6. Klass O, Walker MJ, Olszewski ME, et al. Quantification of aortic valve area at 256-slice computed tomography: comparison with transesophageal echocardiography and cardiac catheterization in subjects with high-grade aortic valve stenosis prior to percutaneous valve replacement. *Eur J Radiol.* 2011;80:151–157.
7. Machida T, Izumo M, Suzuki K, et al. Value of anatomical aortic valve area using real-time three-dimensional transoesophageal echocardiography in patients with aortic stenosis: a comparison between tricuspid and bicuspid aortic valves. *Eur Heart J Cardiovasc Imag.* 2015;16:1120–1128.
8. Chamberland CR, Sugeng L, Abraham S, et al. Three-dimensional evaluation of aortic valve annular shape in children with bicuspid aortic valves and/or aortic coarctation compared with controls. *Am J Cardiol.* 2015;116:1411–1417.
9. le Polain de Waroux JB, Pouleur AC, Goffinet C, et al. Functional anatomy of aortic regurgitation: accuracy, prediction of surgical repairability, and outcome implications of transesophageal echocardiography. *Circulation.* 2007;116:I264–I1269.
10. le Polain de Waroux JB, Pouleur AC, Robert A, et al. Mechanisms of recurrent aortic regurgitation after aortic valve repair: predictive value of intraoperative transesophageal echocardiography. *JACC Cardiovasc Imag.* 2009;2:931–939.
11. Volpato V, Lang RM, Yamat M, et al. Echocardiographic assessment of the tricuspid annulus: the effects of the third dimension and measurement methodology. *J Am Soc Echocardiogr.* 2019;32:238–247.
12. von der Recke G, Schmidt H, Illien S, et al. Use of transesophageal contrast echocardiography for excluding left atrial appendage thrombi in patients with atrial fibrillation before cardioversion. *J Am Soc Echocardiogr.* 2002;15:1256–1261.
13. Katsanos AH, Giannopoulos S, Frogoudaki A, et al. The diagnostic yield of transesophageal echocardiography in patients with cryptogenic cerebral ischaemia: a meta-analysis. *Eur J Neurol.* 2016;23:569–579.
14. Asch FM, Bieganski SP, Panza JA, Weissman NJ. Real-time 3-dimensional echocardiography evaluation of intracardiac masses. *Echocardiography.* 2006;23:218–224.
15. Rodrigues AC, Picard MH, Carbone A, et al. Importance of adequately performed Valsalva maneuver to detect patent foramen ovale during transesophageal echocardiography. *J Am Soc Echocardiogr.* 2013;26:1337–1343.
16. Martin-Reyes R, Lopez-Fernandez T, Moreno-Yanguela M, et al. Role of real-time three-dimensional transoesophageal echocardiography for guiding transcatheter patent foramen ovale closure. *Eur J Echocardiogr.* 2009;10:148–150.
17. Mercer-Rosa L, Seliem MA, Fedec A, et al. Illustration of the additional value of real-time 3-dimensional echocardiography to conventional transthoracic and transesophageal 2-dimensional echocardiography in imaging muscular ventricular septal defects: does this have any impact on individual patient treatment? *J Am Soc Echocardiogr.* 2006;19:1511–1519.
18. Kim IC, Chang S, Hong GR, et al. Comparison of cardiac computed tomography with transesophageal echocardiography for identifying vegetation and intracardiac complications in patients with infective endocarditis in the era of 3-dimensional images. *Circ Cardiovasc Imag.* 2018;11:e006986.
19. Baddour LM, Epstein AE, Erickson CC, et al. Update on cardiovascular implantable electronic device infections and their management. *Circulation.* 2010;121:458–477.
20. Van Woerkom RC, Lester SJ, Demaerschalk BM, et al. Comparison of the utility of transesophageal echocardiography in patients with acute ischemic stroke and transient ischemic attack stratified by age group. *Am J Cardiol.* 2018;122:2142–2146.
21. Guidoux C, Mazighi M, Lavallee P, et al. Aortic arch atheroma in transient ischemic attack patients. *Atherosclerosis.* 2013;231:124–128.
22. Merz TM, Cioccari L, Frey PM, et al. Continual hemodynamic monitoring with a single-use transesophageal echocardiography probe in critically ill patients with shock: a randomized controlled clinical trial. *Intensive Care Med.* 2019;45:1093–1102.
23. Lau V, Priestap F, Landry Y, et al. Diagnostic accuracy of critical care transesophageal echocardiography vs cardiology-led echocardiography in ICU patients. *Chest.* 2019;155:491–501.
24. Practice guidelines for perioperative transesophageal echocardiography: an updated report by the American Society of Anesthesiologists and the Society of Cardiovascular Anesthesiologists Task Force on transesophageal echocardiography. *Anesthesiology.* 2010;112:1084–1096.
25. Wunderlich NC, Beigel R, Siegel RJ. Management of mitral stenosis using 2D and 3D echo-Doppler imaging. *JACC Cardiovasc Imag.* 2013;6:1191–1205.

26. Rong LQ, Hameed I, Salemi A, et al. Three-dimensional echocardiography for transcatheter aortic valve replacement sizing: a systematic review and meta-analysis. *J Am Heart Assoc.* 2019;8:e013463.
27. Eleid MF, Cabalka AK, Malouf JF, et al. Techniques and outcomes for the treatment of paravalvular leak. *Circ Cardiovasc Interv.* 2015;8:e001945.
28. Altiok E, Hamada S, Brehmer K, et al. Analysis of procedural effects of percutaneous edge-to-edge mitral valve repair by 2D and 3D echocardiography. *Circ Cardiovasc Imag.* 2012;5:748–755.
29. Cheng TO, Xie MX, Wang XF, et al. Real-time 3-dimensional echocardiography in assessing atrial and ventricular septal defects: an echocardiographic-surgical correlative study. *Am Heart J.* 2004;148:1091–1095.
30. Charakida M, Pushparajah K, Anderson D, Simpson JM. Insights gained from three-dimensional imaging modalities for closure of ventricular septal defects. *Circ Cardiovasc Imag.* 2014;7:954–961.

15 Pitfalls and Artifacts in Transesophageal Echocardiography

Arvind Nishtala, Akhil Narang

Transesophageal echocardiography (TEE) is an invaluable tool for diagnosing and evaluating cardiac pathophysiology, and a well-performed TEE provides critical information to aid medical decision making. Therefore, it is of utmost importance that physicians recognize pitfalls and artifacts in TEE imaging that could lead to misdiagnosis and unnecessary invasive procedures. *Pitfalls* generally refers to misinterpretation of properly represented structures or variants of normal anatomy as pathology. *Artifacts* refers to phenomena that do not properly represent the structures that are being imaged, thus creating the potential for erroneous interpretation.

PITFALLS OF TRANSESOPHAGEAL ECHOCARDIOGRAPHY

The most common pitfalls seen with TEE during clinical practice are the result of variant anatomic structures that are misdiagnosed as abnormal findings but do not necessarily denote pathology.

Crista Terminalis

The crista terminalis is a well-defined fibromuscular ridge formed by the junction of the sinus venosus and primitive right atrium; it extends along the posterolateral aspect of the right atrial wall. The crista terminalis originates from regression of the septum spurium as the sinus venosus is incorporated into the right atrial wall. The regression of the crista terminalis shows wide variations, and thus the appearance of the crista terminalis exhibits variability on TEE. Occasionally, this structure can be prominent and can mimic a mass-like tumor, thrombus, or vegetation in the right atrium.[1–5] The crista terminalis is best visualized in the midesophageal (ME) bicaval view on TEE as a protuberance into the right atrial cavity at the junction of the superior vena cava and right atrium (Fig. 15.1). An understanding of its variable anatomy can prevent misdiagnosis and unnecessary additional tests.

Eustachian Valve and Chiari Network

The eustachian valve and the Chiari network may often be misdiagnosed as right atrial intracardiac lesions. The eustachian valve is an embryologic remnant of the right valve of the sinus venosus and can occasionally persist into adulthood, with variable size on echocardiographic imaging. It commonly appears as a flap of tissue originating from the anterior rim of the inferior vena cava of variable length and motion. The Chiari network is

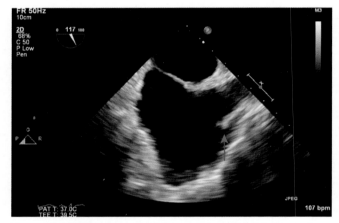

Figure 15.1. Midesophageal 117-degree view of a crista terminalis *(red arrow)* mimicking a right atrial mass. (Also see Video 15.1.)

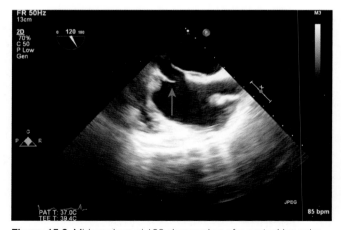

Figure 15.2. Midesophageal 122-degree view of a eustachian valve *(red arrow)* misdiagnosed as an atrial intracardiac lesion. (Also see Video 15.2.)

also a remnant of incomplete resorption of the right sinus venosus valve and appears as a reticulated network of fibers originating from the eustachian valve and connecting to different parts of the right atrium[6] (Fig. 15.2). On TEE, the Chiari network is seen as a long, thin, highly mobile structure with variable insertion sites.

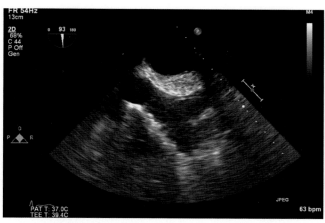

Figure 15.3. Midesophageal 93-degree view of lipomatous hypertrophy of the atrial septum. (Also see Video 15.3.)

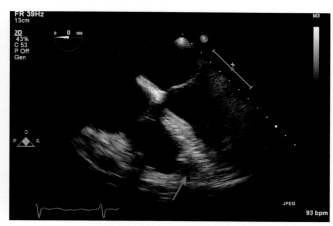

Figure 15.5. Midesophageal 0-degree view of a moderator band *(red arrow)* located in the right ventricular apex. (Also see Video 15.5.)

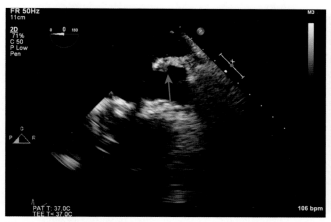

Figure 15.4. Midesophageal 0-degree view of a Coumadin ridge *(red arrow)* mimicking an intracardiac lesion. (Also see Video 15.4.)

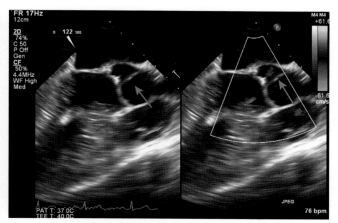

Figure 15.6. Midesophageal 122-degree view of Lambl excrescences *(red arrow)* misinterpreted as an aortic valve vegetation. (Also see Video 15.6.)

Both of these structures are best visualized in the ME bicaval view on TEE. Neither are of pathologic importance, although, when prominent, they can appear to be pathological structures, such as tumor, thrombus, or vegetation.[7–9] In rare cases, these structures can be implicated with endocarditis, intracardiac thrombus, and catheter entrapment.

Lipomatous Hypertrophy of the Atrial Septum

Lipomatous hypertrophy of the atrial septum (LHAS) is a benign condition caused by the excessive deposition of adipose tissue in the atrial septum and that is most often detected as an incidental finding on echocardiography.[10] The classic echocardiographic finding is a homogeneous, bilobed configuration of the atrial septum with sparing of the fossa ovalis in the ME four-chamber or bicaval views[11] (Fig. 15.3). LAHS is benign and most commonly detected as an incidental finding.

Coumadin Ridge and Pectinate Muscles

A prominent muscle ridge covered by endocardium is formed between the left atrial appendage and the atrial insertion of the left upper pulmonary vein. This prominence, best seen in the ME two-chamber view and referred to as a coumadin ridge, has the appearance of a "Q-Tip," and vigilance is needed to prevent its misdiagnosis as an atrial tumor or thrombus[12,13] (Fig. 15.4). The right and left atrial appendages also have pectinate muscles that appear

as a number of parallel ridges that protrude into the lumen of the appendage and can be mistaken for thrombus.

Moderator Band

The moderator band is in the right ventricular apex and connects the ventricular septum to the anterior papillary muscle, serving as a primary conduction pathway for electrical activation of the free wall of the right ventricle. It appears as a prominent trabecula, which does not seem to be attached to a single side but crosses the lower portion of the right ventricular chamber. This prominence is best seen in the ME four-chamber view and can be misconstrued as an intracardiac mass[14] (Fig. 15.5).

Lambl Excrescences

Lambl excrescences are thin, mobile, filiform structures, often referred to as valvular strands in the echocardiography literature.[15] These strands may occur singly, in rows, or in clusters, often originating from the aortic or the mitral valve in older adult patients. The differential diagnosis for these strands includes papillary fibroelastoma, valvular vegetation or thrombus, and cardiac neoplasms or metastases. Lambl excrescences have been associated with stroke, but the definitive guidelines for their management are controversial. They are best seen in the ME three-chamber view of the long axis of the aortic valve (Fig. 15.6).

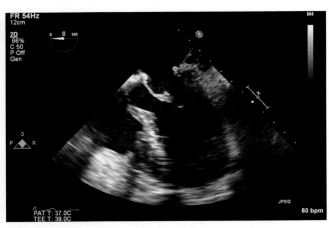

Figure 15.7. Midesophageal 0-degree view of a mitral valve ring misinterpreted as valve calcification. (Also see Video 15.7.)

Prosthetic Valve Structures

Prosthetic valve strands are thin, mildly echogenic, filamentous structures that are several millimeters long and move independently from the valve. Strands are found in 6% to 69% of patients with prosthetic valves, usually located at the inflow site of the prosthetic valve.[16] Prosthetic valve sutures appear as linear, thick, bright, multiple structures at the periphery of the sewing ring of a prosthetic valve and can be susceptible to blurring artifact on three-dimensional TEE imaging. Both prosthetic valve strands and sutures can be misdiagnosed as valvular lesions[17] (Fig. 15.7).

Pericardial Fat

Pericardial fat often appears as a gelatinous structure within the pericardial space adjacent to the visceral pericardium and can be misinterpreted to be a pericardial effusion or mass.[18,19] Pericardial fat can be differentiated from intrapericardial hematomas because the latter are often free-floating within the pericardial space and not attached to the visceral pericardium.

Pleural Effusion

Hypoechogenic areas of the lung can sometimes be misidentified as pleural effusions. Normal pulmonary parenchyma can mimic pleural effusion in TEE.[9]

Hiatal Hernia

Hiatal hernias often raise suspicions of extracardiac masses in echocardiography and usually present as a mass compressing the left atrium, best seen in the ME four-chamber view.[20,21] Tomographic imaging is usually necessary to make the diagnosis.

TRANSESOPHAGEAL ECHOCARDIOGRAPHY ARTIFACTS

Artifacts are generated when the basic assumptions of ultrasound imaging and physics are violated and with the interference of external devices, equipment, or internal cardiac structures. When artifacts occur, they fail to convey anatomic information or accurately represent the structures that are being imaged, and structures can appear to be there when they are in fact not; structures may not appear when they are in fact present, or structures can also look different from reality or appear in the wrong location. The basic assumptions made by ultrasound systems are as follows:

1. Ultrasound echoes travel in a straight line.
2. Echoes return to the transducer after one reflection.
3. Echoes originate only from the main transducer beam and reflectors located within it.
4. The ultrasound beam travels at a constant speed of 1540 m/s in human tissue, and the position of the reflected structure is directly proportional to the travel time of the ultrasound beam.

Artifacts that arise from violation of these assumptions can be classified into those that arise from multiple reflections, misplaced reflections, and missed reflections.[22]

Reverberation Artifact

Reverberation artifact occurs when the primary ultrasound beam is reflected off a strong second reflector as it returns to the transducer, thus violating the assumption that echoes return to the transducer after one reflection. Because the ultrasound beam takes twice as long to return to the transducer, the artifactual image appears at twice the distance between the structure and the transducer. The second reflector is commonly the ultrasound transducer itself but can also be the thoracic aorta, other calcified structures, and intracardiac devices. In TEE imaging, reverberation artifacts are common within the thoracic aorta[23] and the left atrial appendage.[24,25] Decreasing gain, using M-mode echocardiography, seeking multiple imaging planes, and identifying parallel motion at the depth of the suspected artifact are ways to identify and mitigate reverberation artifact.[26,27]

Comet-Tail Artifact

When two strong reflectors are closely spaced with one another, the multiple reverberations that arise create a "comet-tail" artifact. The signal intensity decreases with the number of reflections taken (and thus distance traveled) by the ultrasound beam, thereby creating the appearance of a comet tail. Comet-tail artifacts are commonly seen during TEE imaging of prosthetic valves or aortic plaques.

Mirror and Refraction Artifacts

Mirror image artifact occurs beneath a strongly reflective surface when the ultrasound beam is reflected off this surface toward structures closer to the transducer, which then reflect the beam back onto the reflector surface and back to the transducer. The ultrasound scanner interprets these artifactual structures to be below the reflector surface at an equal distance to that between the reflector surface and the real structures. The pleural surface is a strong reflector and can commonly cause mirror artifacts, especially in the ME view of the descending thoracic aorta on TEE.[26] Similarly, a refraction artifact can occur when an intracardiac structure refracts the ultrasound beam onto a reflective surface, which then refracts the beam back to its original angle of projection, creating a duplicate image of the structure adjacent to its true location. Structures such as the pleura, pericardium, or rib cartilage may induce refraction of the ultrasound beam resulting in refraction artifacts.[28]

Acoustic Shadowing and Enhancement Artifacts

Acoustic shadowing occurs when the ultrasound beam meets an interface of two structures with marked differences in acoustic impedance, resulting in reflection and scattering of the ultrasound beam and minimal distal transmission. Because of the lack of echoes distally, acoustic shadowing appears as hypoechoic or anechoic areas in otherwise uniform tissue. Common examples include structures with a high level of acoustic impedance, such as calcific or prosthetic valves, other calcified structures, and intracardiac devices. In TEE imaging, the acoustic shadowing of prosthetic mitral valves make ultrasound evaluation of aortic regurgitation

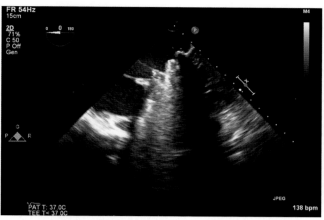

Figure 15.8. Midesophageal 0-degree view of mechanical mitral valve shadowing causing lack of signal in the sector beyond the mechanical valve. (Also see Video 15.8.)

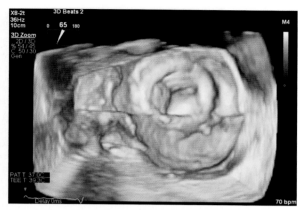

Figure 15.9. Stitch artifact generated from two-beat acquisition.

challenging[29] (Fig. 15.8). Seeking an alternate imaging plane is the best way to mitigate acoustic shadowing.

Enhancement artifacts are the opposite of acoustic shadowing and occur when the ultrasound beam is differentially weakly attenuated by a structure it encounters, resulting in greater distal transmission of echoes with the reflected waves being of higher amplitude than other structures at an identical depth. The ultrasound system depicts these returning waves as areas of relative increased echogenicity. Manipulation of time-gain compensation can serve to mitigate the appearance of enhancement artifacts.

Side-Lobe and Beam-Width Artifacts

The main ultrasound beam is concentrated in the center, but there exist smaller "side lobes" of energy directed to either side of the central beam. These side lobes usually dissipate in tissue without any prominent reflections, but side lobe artifacts can arise when strong reflectors reflect these echoes back to the transducer, with the ultrasound system incorrectly misplacing the image because of the assumption that it was generated by a structure in the path of the central beam.[30] Side-lobe artifacts may appear as narrow, curvilinear densities at a radial distance from the transducer smeared over the beam's entire width.[22] Beam-width artifacts occur because ultrasound waves are three-dimensional conical structures, not just two-dimensional planar structures, and the ultrasound beam widens beyond the focal zone. Structures adjacent to the imaging plane but still within the cone of the ultrasound beam can be displayed in the imaging plane. They can appear as structures, leads, or thrombi.[31,32]

Medical Devices

Intracardiac devices such as pacemakers or implantable cardioverter-defibrillator leads, central venous catheters, prosthetic valves, septal occluders, and mechanical support devices present strong reflective surfaces for the generation of multiple types of artifacts (including reverberations, comet-tail, and mirroring artifacts; acoustic shadowing and enhancement; and beam-width and side-lobe artifacts). Careful attention has to be paid to the interpretation of echocardiographic images in the presence of such medical devices to achieve an accurate evaluation.

Artifacts in Three-Dimensional Transesophageal Echocardiography

Three-dimensional (3D) TEE allows the study of cardiac structures in a 3D format and projection that replicates anatomic specimens. 3D TEE is prone to the same types of artifacts as standard

two-dimensional (2D) TEE; however, some additional types of artifacts are unique to 3D image acquisition and processing.[33,34]

Stitching Artifacts

Stitching artifacts are unique to 3D multibeat acquisitions of volumetric data obtained from several sequential electrocardiography-gated cardiac cycles.[35] Although this imaging mode is associated with high 3D spatial and temporal resolution, the 3D image that is acquired is not viewed in real time and is prone to stitch artifacts caused by patient or respiratory motion and irregular heart rhythms.[33] Stitch artifacts can be seen as a displacement of sequential subvolumes in the postprocessed 3D image (Fig. 15.9). The key to eliminating stitch artifacts is to minimize patient and probe motion during the multibeat acquisition and to ideally use this modality of imaging in patients with regular heart rhythms.

Dropout Artifacts

Dropout artifact appears on 3D acquisitions as a loss of tissue and arise because of poor ultrasound signal strength combined with structures parallel to the ultrasound beam and can potentially eliminate anatomic structures that otherwise exist.[35] It is important to manipulate the probe position and adjust the gain setting to confirm the presence of and eliminate these artifacts.

Blurring Artifacts

Blurring artifacts create the appearance that structures are thicker in 3D images than they may be in reality or in 2D images because of the creation of an image from nonisotropic voxels.[33] During image processing, the type of resolution predominantly being used to generate the 3D image may create the appearances of thin structures appearing thicker than they are. For example, the stitches around an annuloplasty ring may appear exaggeratedly thickened, and the ruptured chordae from a degenerative mitral valve may appear thicker or as a single thick chord on 3D images.

Catheter- and Device-Related Artifacts

3D TEE is used for imaging guidance of percutaneous interventions because of its enhanced visualization of intracardiac catheters and devices. Intracardiac catheters and devices are strong reflectors of ultrasound echoes and are sources of reverberation and shadowing artifacts. Reverberation artifacts may appear to lengthen a catheter and may be misinterpreted for being the catheter tip. Shadowing can create dropout artifacts just distal to the catheter or device; the area of dropout has the same footprint as the catheter or device and follows its motion. Blooming artifacts arise from metallic guidewires being intersected by the ultrasound beam and make metallic structures appear to have thick, irregular edges. Catheters with wide lumens can appear as two linear structures, known as railroad-shaped artifacts, caused by the ultrasound image being generated from the two surfaces that are perpendicular to the transducer generating the most reflective echoes while the tangential surfaces produce weak echoes.[33]

CONCLUSIONS

Image artifacts and diagnostic pitfalls are commonly encountered in TEE and arise from improper scanning technique, intracardiac devices, violations of the assumptions of ultrasound physics, and image postprocessing. TEE pitfalls can be understood and prevented with comprehensive knowledge of the anatomic, structural, and functional properties of the heart. A keen awareness of the different types of artifacts, the mechanisms that lead to them, the impact on acquired images, and methods to mitigate them is of utmost importance to prevent misdiagnoses and medical errors.

Please access ExpertConsult to view the corresponding videos for this chapter.

Acknowledgments

The authors thank Drs. Stamatios Lerakis, John Palios, and Randolph P. Martin for their contributions to the previous edition of this chapter.

REFERENCES

1. Akcay M, Bilen ES, Bilge M, et al. Prominent crista terminalis: as an anatomic structure leading to atrial arrhythmias and mimicking right atrial mass. *J Am Soc Echocardiogr.* 2007;20(197):e9–e10.
2. Salustri A, Bakir S, Sana A, et al. Prominent crista terminalis mimicking a right atrial mass: case report. *Cardiovasc Ultrasound.* 2010;8:47.
3. D'Amato N, Pierfelice O, D'Agostino C. Crista terminalis bridge: a rare variant mimicking right atrial mass. *Eur J Echocardiogr.* 2009;10:444–445.
4. Salim H, Palit A, Maher A. When is a mass not a mass? An unusual presentation of prominent crista terminalis. *BMJ Case Rep.* 2016. bcr2015211532 2016.
5. Pharr JR, West MB, Kusumoto FM, Figueredo VM. Prominent crista terminalis appearing as a right atrial mass on transthoracic echocardiogram. *J Am Soc Echocardiogr.* 2002;15:753–755.
6. Pothineni KR, Nanda NC, Burri MV, et al. Live/real time three-dimensional transthoracic echocardiographic visualization of Chiari network. *Echocardiography.* 2007;24:995–997.
7. Carson W, Chiu SS. Eustachian valve mimicking intracardiac mass. *Circulation.* 1998;97:2188.
8. Malaterre HR, Kallee K, Périer Y. Eustachian valve mimicking a right atrial cystic tumor. *Int J Card Imag.* 2000;16:305–307.
9. Schneider B, Hofmann T, Justen MH, Meinertz T. Chiari's network: normal anatomic variant or risk factor for arterial embolic events? *J Am Coll Cardiol.* 1995;26:203–210.
10. O'Connor S, Recavarren R, Nichols LC, Parwani AV. Lipomatous hypertrophy of the interatrial septum: an overview. *Arch Pathol Lab Med.* 2006;130:397–399.
11. Fyke FE, Tajik AJ, Edwards WD, Seward JB. Diagnosis of lipomatous hypertrophy of the atrial septum by two-dimensional echocardiography. *J Am Coll Cardiol.* 1983;1:1352–1357.
12. Strachinaru M, Gazagnes MD, Mabiglia C, Costescu I. Coumadin ridge mass assessed on three-dimensional transoesophageal echocardiography. *Acta Cardiol.* 2013;68:193–196.
13. Sanchez DR, Bryg RJ. Normal variants in echocardiography. *Curr Cardiol Rep.* 2016;18:104.
14. Mittal SR. Moderator band wrongly interpreted as RV mass. *J Assoc Physicians India.* 2012;60:42.
15. Jaffe W, Figueredo VM. An example of Lambl's excrescences by transesophageal echocardiogram: a commonly misinterpreted lesion. *Echocardiography.* 2007;24:1086–1089.
16. Rozich JD, Edwards WD, Hanna RD, et al. Mechanical prosthetic valve-associated strands: pathologic correlates to transesophageal echocardiography. *J Am Soc Echocardiogr.* 2003;16:97–100.
17. Van Den Brink RBA. Evaluation of prosthetic heart valves by transesophageal echocardiography: problems, pitfalls, and timing of echocardiography. *Semin CardioThorac Vasc Anesth.* 2006;10:89–100.
18. Najib MQ, Ganji JL, Raizada A, et al. Epicardial fat can mimic pericardial effusion on transoesophageal echocardiogram. *Eur J Echocardiogr.* 2011;12:804.
19. Ansari A, Rholl AO. Pseudopericardial effusion: echocardiographic and computed tomographic correlations. *Clin Cardiol.* 1986;9:551–555.
20. Yang SS, Wagner P, Dennis C. Hiatal hernia masquerading as left atrial mass. *Circulation.* 1996;93:836.
21. Gupta R, Chamoun A, Ahmad M, Birnbaum Y. Hiatal hernia masquerading as an extracardiac mass on transesophageal echocardiogram. *Clin Cardiol.* 2003;26:353.
22. Pamnani A, Skubas NJ. Imaging artifacts during transesophageal echocardiography. *Anesth Analg.* 2014;118:516–520.
23. Evangelista A, Garcia-Del-Castillo H, Gonzalez-Alujas T, et al. Diagnosis of ascending aortic dissection by transesophageal echocardiography: utility of M-mode in recognizing artifacts. *J Am Coll Cardiol.* 1996;27:102–107.
24. Schneider B, Stöllberger C, Schneider B. Diagnosis of left atrial appendage thrombi by multiplane transesophageal echocardiography: interlaboratory comparative study. *Circ J.* 2007;71:122–125.
25. Maltagliati A, Pepi M, Tamborini G, et al. Usefulness of multiplane transesophageal echocardiography in the recognition of artifacts and normal anatomical variants that may mimic left atrial thrombi in patients with atrial fibrillation. *Ital Hear J.* 2003;4:797–802.
26. Bertrand PB, Levine RA, Isselbacher EM, Vandervoort PM. Fact or artifact in two-dimensional echocardiography: avoiding misdiagnosis and missed diagnosis. *J Am Soc Echocardiogr.* 2016;29:381–391.
27. Quien MM, Saric M. Ultrasound imaging artifacts: how to recognize them and how to avoid them. *Echocardiography.* 2018;35:1388–1401.
28. Spieker LE, Hufschmid U, Oechslin E, Jenni R. Double aortic and pulmonary valves: an artifact generated by ultrasound refraction. *J Am Soc Echocardiogr.* 2004;17:786–787.
29. Zabalgoitia M, Garcia M. Pitfalls in the echo–Doppler diagnosis of prosthetic valve disorders. *Echocardiography.* 1993;10:203–212.
30. Laing FC, Kurtz AB. The importance of ultrasonic side-lobe artifacts. *Radiology.* 1982;145:763–768.
31. Kyavar M, Sadeghpour A, Alizadehasl A, Salehi N. Thrombosis on implanted device for atrial septal defect closure or echocardiographic beam width artifact? A diagnostic enigma! *Int J Cardiovasc Imag.* 2012;28:1851–1852.
32. Skubas N, Brown NI, Mishra R. Diagnostic dilemma: a pacemaker lead inside the left atrium or an echocardiographic beam width artifact? *Anesth Analg.* 2006;102:1043–1044.
33. Faletra FF, Ramamurthi A, Dequarti MC, et al. Artifacts in three-dimensional transesophageal echocardiography. *J Am Soc Echocardiogr.* 2014;27:453–462.
34. Lang RM, Badano LP, Mor-Avi V, et al. Recommendations for cardiac chamber quantification by echocardiography in adults. *J Am Soc Echocardiogr.* 2015;28:1–39.
35. Lang RM, Badano LP, Tsang W, et al. EAE/ASE recommendations for image acquisition and display using three-dimensional echocardiography. *Eur Heart J Cardiovasc Imag.* 2012;13:1–46.

16 Cardiac Point-of-Care Ultrasound: Background, Instrumentation, and Technique

Bruce J. Kimura, Daniel G. Blanchard, Anthony N. DeMaria

WHEN A STAT ECHO IS NOT FAST ENOUGH

Developed for military triage, POCUS techniques easily translated to use by trauma surgeons and emergency room physicians, exemplified by the development of the Focused Abdominal Sonography for Trauma (FAST) exam in the early 1990s to diagnose traumatic intraperitoneal bleeding.[1] Point-of-care ultrasound (POCUS) capitalizes on the immediacy and utility of ultrasound at the bedside, especially when initial triage and clinical urgency demand action or when findings are intermittent and fleeting.

The immediate clinical value of limited cardiac ultrasound data obtained from POCUS disrupts the standard conventions of the detailed-oriented philosophy and comprehensive format of standard echocardiography. The advent of portable devices (Fig. 16.1) opened new markets for development in emergency, critical care, internal medicine, and family medicine and has created novel terminology distinct from the practice of echocardiography, using descriptors such as "hand-carried" or "handheld" ultrasound, "quick-look" studies, "focused cardiac ultrasound," and more recently "point-of-care ultrasound."[2] No term has yet sufficiently distinguished POCUS practice from that of echocardiography because a "stat echo" also can be performed at the "point of care" using the smaller echocardiographs and recording equivalent data.

POCUS: INTENTS AND PURPOSES

Defining characteristics of current POCUS practice include the imaging of only a few ultrasound findings, performance by the treating physician, and indications to assist in the *immediate* diagnosis, treatment, triage, or risk stratification of the patient (Table 16.1). With on-the-spot imaging and diagnosis, POCUS will change current standards of imaging and interpretation in ultrasonography. Despite common features in individual specialty use, cardiac POCUS practice is evolving but appears bounded by two distinct imaging philosophies:

1. A generalized practice, in which POCUS is used routinely whenever a stethoscope is used in ultrasound-augmented physical examination (UAPE) or,
2. A subspecialized practice, as a formal limited echocardiogram directed to answer specific clinical questions that may arise after initial clinical evaluation.

Although real-world POCUS practice often consists of both philosophies to some degree, these two polar boundaries of POCUS have differential impact on medical education, competency requirements, and the approach to medical testing and reimbursement.

POCUS, when practiced to augment the physical examination, is best done by the physician taking care of the patient as a directed search for a simplified ultrasound *signs*, each a clue to formation of a preliminary diagnosis. The POCUS equivalents of cardiac physical findings improve their detection while allowing the continued use of the same time-honored cardiac physiologic concepts taught in medical school (Table 16.2)[3]. Potential applications are similar to the use of the stethoscope and include initial and frequent reapplications at initial presentation, during subsequent hospital rounds, or in clinic visits. An evidence-based POCUS technique named cardiovascular-limited ultrasound examination (CLUE) has been validated and is a compilation of six easily learned, quick-look ultrasound signs performed within a 2-minute examination (Fig. 16.2).[4] Notably, the CLUE has shown both diagnostic and prognostic value in outpatients[5] and inpatients referred for echocardiography,[6,7] as well as in patients admitted by hospitalists.[8] The CLUE represents a proof-of-concept POCUS exam—one that improves traditional bedside physical examination techniques for prognostic findings and has been successfully incorporated into the curriculum of an internal medicine residency program[9] in which residents have proven its effectiveness.[5] Any significant abnormality found on bedside examination—whether by ultrasound or auscultation and palpation—can be documented as a part of the physical examination and is taken into consideration for confirmation by formal echocardiographic study or consultation, time permitting. Because clinically relevant ultrasound techniques can be successfully taught in medical school[10,11] or internal medical residency,[9,12] ultrasound-augmented physical examination may be a gateway for all physicians to learn POCUS. Ultimately, physicians' use of UAPE to improve their evaluation and management is an individual assessment of its incremental value in clinical context.

POCUS, when practiced as a form of limited echocardiography, can be differentiated from UAPE in an expert consensus document of the American Society of Echocardiography.[13] In UAPE, the number of views and interpretation are limited to only ultrasound signs suggesting cardiac disease, in contrast to a limited echocardiogram, in which the user is responsible for all diagnoses, primary and incidental, manifest in the limited number of views in the imaging protocol (Table 16.3). Under these terms, the term "limited" refers to the number of views and not the number of diagnoses. Limited echocardiography is a formal medical imaging test requiring imaging standards, study archival, and an all-inclusive interpretation and report. The evolving practice of POCUS is clearly different from the current practice of limited echocardiography because no formal diagnostic medical imaging test has the potential of being applied with such repetition and frequency by multiple physicians on the same patient.

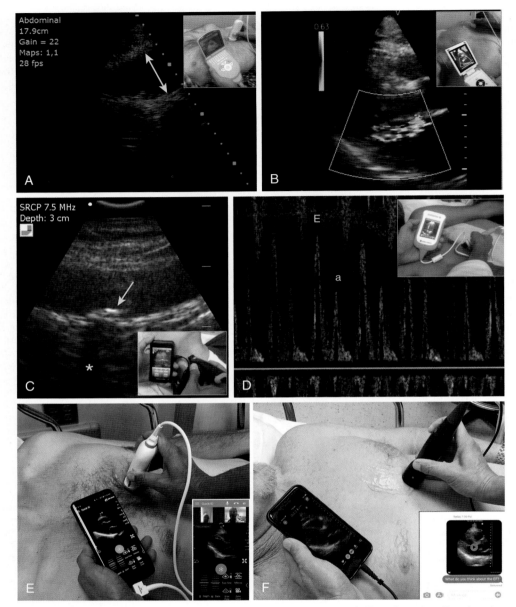

Figure 16.1. Point-of-care ultrasound instrumentation and technique, pocket-sized devices. **A,** Two-dimensional imaging shows midline longitudinal view of a nonpalpable 4.0-cm abdominal aortic aneurysm (Acuson P10, 2- to 4-MHz phased array transducer, Siemens Medical Solutions USA, approved 2007). **B,** Color Doppler can localize murmurs as specific valvular lesions such as severe mitral regurgitation causing left atrial enlargement (Vscan, 1.7- to 3.8-MHz phased array transducer, GE Healthcare, approved 2009). **C,** High-frequency probe detects subclinical atherosclerosis as carotid plaque *(arrow)* (MobiUS SP1, 7.5- to 12-MHz mechanical interchangeable transducer, smartphone connected, Mobisante, approved 2011). **D,** Spectral pulsed-wave Doppler can assess left ventricular diastolic filling patterns (Sonimage P3, 3- to 5-MHz mechanical interchangeable transducer, Konica Minolta Healthcare Americas, approved 2013). **E,** Device connectivity to smartphone allows app-based remote imaging guidance *(inset)* (Lumify, S4-1 MHz phased array transducer, Philips Healthcare, approved 2015). **F,** Multifrequency imaging probe with connection to smartphone allows cloud-based image texting *(inset)* (Butterfly iQ, approved 2017).

INSTRUMENTATION: FORM FITS FUNCTION

The form of developing POCUS equipment follows its intended function by maximizing portability and simplicity but also for documentation, limited quantitation, and connectivity. By far the most controversial development has been in pocket-sized ultrasound devices, bringing to the forefront issues of device ownership and use in the hospital—as either a personally owned ultrasound stethoscope or a hospital-purchased device with compatibility to archive studies into hospital-based systems. Currently, additional features vary by manufacturer and include color or Spectral Doppler, interchangeable or multifrequency transducers, and varying forms of image storage and transmission. Image setting presets are available to allow quick "boot-ups" for cardiac, abdominal, or obstetrics and gynecology imaging. Color or spectral Doppler gives the user the capability to differentiate an anechoic region such as a cyst as opposed to a vessel and allows a gross visual assessment of flow patterns as arterial or venous. For more advanced users, the presence of color Doppler can also be used to estimate valvular regurgitation and severity.[14] Pulsed-wave spectral Doppler also provides the potential to assess diastolic filling patterns. Battery-life generally provides 1 to 2 hours of continuous imaging, further promoting brief quick-look application and recharging every 1 to 2 days. Remote real-time imaging with "telementoring" has already been reported as a feasible and inexpensive method for health care delivery and training.[15]

Today, portable ultrasound devices have a wide range of cost, from $2000 for a pocket-sized device to $25,000 for a bedside tablet or laptop ultrasound device. No specific payor reimbursement exists for use of any device when used to augment bedside physical examination. However, cost savings to a health care system will be significant by improving diagnostic efficiency in outpatient echo

referral,[5] timeliness of triage, and appropriateness of consultation. For inpatients, assuming billing is performed for limited echocardiography and fully overread by a cardiologist, a preliminary reimbursement model (with application on approximately 30%–40% of medical admissions) predicted remuneration capable of funding POCUS equipment purchase and training.[16,17] Presently, partnerships, call groups, hospital departments, and clinics often share a POCUS device given the limited number of trained users.

POCUS: DIVERSITY IN PRACTICE AND OUTCOMES

POCUS was created to fulfill an unmet imaging need in cardiac ultrasound. Diversity in patient populations and POCUS goals has resulted in diversity in practice and expectations of POCUS. POCUS is the test of choice in the emergency department (ED) for emergency triage and cardiac arrest because echocardiography laboratories are unable to provide such stat coverage around the clock. In intensive care units (ICUs), POCUS can be applied multiple times per day for decision making and monitoring in critically ill patients, whereas it would be difficult for a hospital echo lab to cover for every on-the-spot clinical change. When applied to the heart during routine outpatient evaluation, POCUS has the advantage of providing a more accurate screening exam to determine referral for a standard echo and risk stratification. Currently, many different sets of diagnosis-based, symptom-based, or "focused" imaging protocols for specific clinical indications have been created. Each has its own specific accuracies and limitations, for each physician's own particular practice and patient mix. For example,

TABLE 16.1 Characteristics of Point-Of-Care Ultrasound Examinations

1. Performed by the physician at the bedside during clinical evaluation
2. Limited number of findings sought, usually brief (<5 minutes)
3. Can encompass more than one organ system
4. Has indication and value to immediately affect diagnosis, management, or triage
5. Uses small, inexpensive portable devices with limited data entry and measurement packages
6. Limited reporting, often semiquantitative
7. Often repeated by subsequent physicians and used for monitoring or follow-up
8. Often lacks characterization of incidental findings
9. Variable imaging and training for each physician

TABLE 16.2 Physical Exam and Point-Of-Care Ultrasound Findings

Entity	Physical Finding (SN, SP)	POCUS Finding (SN, SP)	Notes
LV systolic dysfunction	S3 (11%–51%, 85%–98%), (13%, 98%) in ED	Subjective estimation of contraction and/or EPSS >1 cm (69%–94%, 88%–94%)[5]	US criteria vary between studies; both are easily learned and are reproducible by noncardiologists Prevalence of physical findings in LVSD is <20%, and even lower in asymptomatic LVSD
	Displaced apical impulse (5%–66%, 93%–99%) 15% incidence in symptomatic HFrEF cohort		
Elevated LA filling pressures	S4 (35%–71%, 50%–70%)	LAE (53%–75%, 72%–94%)	LAE is prognostic and not found by physical examination US is learned after brief training
Pulmonary edema or interstitial disease	Rales (19%–64%, 82%–94%), (62%, 68%) in ED	B lines (85%–98%, 83%–93%)	B lines are US artifacts and potentially vary between devices US is easily learned by novices Prevalence of 13% in HFrEF cohort
Pleural effusion	Dullness to percussion (73%–89%, 81%–91%)	Fluid in thorax (64%–90%, 72%–95%)	Studies of physical findings used CXR as gold standard, whereas US used CT Significant increases in SN with US, especially for small effusions
RV enlargement or pulmonary hypertension	Sustained left parasternal lift (71%, 80%)	RV/LV > 1 (55%, 69%)	Nonspecific finding of RVE is seen RVMI, submassive PE, and chronic or pulmonale Expert US practice needed to use spectral Doppler
Elevated central venous pressures	JVP (47%–92%, 93%–96%) (37%, 87%) in ED, 22% incidence in HFrEF cohort	IVC plethora (73%, 85%)	POCUS advantages in supine ICU patients POCUS data include nonexperts JVP by US correlates with physical estimates but underestimates catheter-confirmed pressure
Valve regurgitation	Murmur for mild or worse: MR (56%–75%, 89%–93%) or AI (54%–87%, 75%–98%)	Color Doppler (82%, 93%) for mild severity	Color Doppler jet area limitations apply Expert practice likely necessary to quantify severity
Severe AS	Late-peaking murmur (83%–90%, 72%–88%)	Restricted cusp mobility (85%, 89%)	Expert auscultation coupled with POCUS may be the best screening method

AI, Aortic insufficiency; *CXR,* chest radiography; *AS,* aortic stenosis; *ED,* emergency department; *EPSS,* E-point septal separation: *HFrEF,* heart failure with reduced ejection fraction; *ICU,* intensive care unit; *IVC,* inferior vena cava; *JVP,* jugular venous pulsations; *LA,* left atrium; *LAE,* left atrial enlargement; *LV,* left ventricle; *LVSD,* left ventricular systolic dysfunction; *MR,* mitral regurgitation; *PE,* pulmonary embolism; *POCUS,* point-of-care ultrasound; *RV,* right ventricular; *RVE,* right ventricular enlargement; *RVMI,* right ventricular myocardial infarction; *SN,* sensitivity; *SP,* specificity; *US,* ultrasound.
From Kimura BJ: *Point-of-care cardiac ultrasound techniques in the physical exam: better at the bedside.* Heart 103:987–994, 2017.

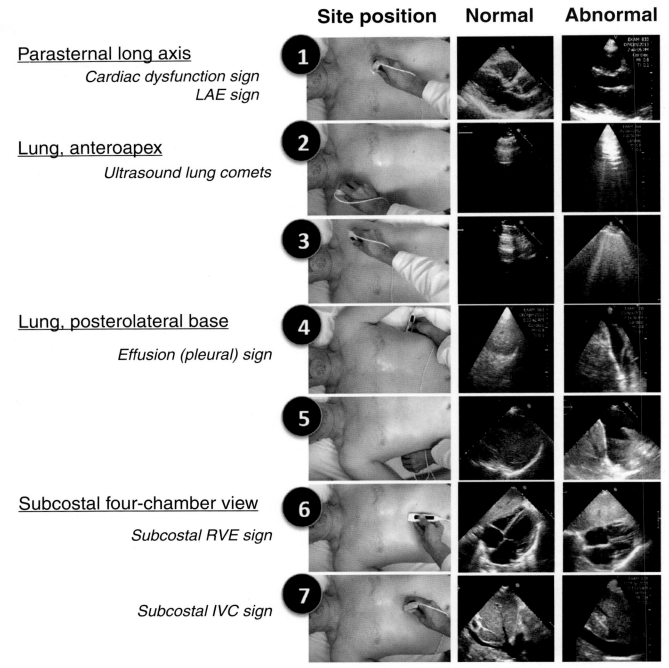

Figure 16.2. Cardiovascular-limited ultrasound examination (CLUE) protocol, hand position, and normal versus abnormal findings. The six CLUE signs and seven hand positions are probe sited shown with resultant views, when the sign is absent *(normal)* or present *(abnormal)*. Longitudinal images are oriented with cranial to the right. *IVC,* Inferior vena cava; *LAE,* left atrial enlargement; *RVE,* right ventricular enlargement. (Reproduced with permission from Kimura BJ, et al: Cardiac limited ultrasound exam techniques to augment the bedside cardiac physical, *J Ultrasound Med* 34:1683–1690, 2015.)

in the emergency and critical care literature, more than 15 separate acronyms and imaging protocols are used for the single indication of unexplained hypotension.[18] If such heterogeneity continues, user training will be variable, and a standardized curriculum would be difficult to develop for undergraduate medical education.

The outcome value of POCUS is intimately linked to the value of comprehensive echocardiography itself and the nature of the indication for imaging. In comprehensive echocardiography, imaging standards routinely measure chamber dimensions, valve function, and parameters of systolic and diastolic performance. These metrics can serve as a valuable baseline with which to track disease progression or treatment effects by comparison to future studies, regardless of the indication for the current echocardiogram. Although the outcome value of time spent in such endeavors is uncertain, no one argues against the immediate benefit of a quick-look diagnosis afforded by POCUS in emergencies, such as pericardial tamponade. At this point in time, similar to many diagnostic techniques, outcome data from treatments specifically changed by POCUS are primarily limited to case reports and series. Mortality data from randomized trials are difficult to reconcile without uniformly

TABLE 16.3 Point-of-Care Ultrasound as a Physical Examination Technique Versus Limited Ultrasound Examination

	POCUS as Ultrasound-Augmented Physical Exam	POCUS as Limited Echocardiogram
Clinical use	• Applied during any physical examination • Simplified, brief imaging protocol for "signs" of disease • Frequent, repeated, daily use • Abnormalities should prompt echo referral or consultation, time allowing	• Applied as a diagnostic test for a single entity • Applied once initially but can be repeated as follow-up exam (e.g., pericardial effusion)
Indication	• Obtaining structural data to help form clinical diagnosis • Screening • Risk stratification	• Documentation of medical necessity • For diagnosis or exclusion of an entity after initial considerations
Equipment	• Simplified, 2D imaging, limited Doppler • Ideally pocket sized, portable • Inexpensive • Battery powered • Individually owned • Short boot times	• Standard echocardiograph, fully featured • Expensive with shared ownership or hospital ownership • Often connected to PACS
Accuracy	• Moderate sensitivity and high specificity for signs related to disease • Early, subclinical disease often detected	• High sensitivity and specificity for diagnosis sought by imaging protocol. • Can be gold standard exam
Potential liability	• Only for signs sought	• For all findings manifest, primary and incidental
Medicare CPT	• As a part of Evaluation and Management codes	• 93308
Documentation	• As a part of physical exam in the history and physical • Image archival optional	• Images archived to PACS • Separate formal report
Education	• Medical school, residency	• Subspecialty (cardiology, anesthesiology, critical care and emergency medicine)
Competency	• User discretion, depending on personal accuracy	• Evolving standards (ASCeXAM) within specialty • ASE examination

ASE, American Society of Echocardiography; *CPT,* Current Procedural Terminology; *PACS,* Picture Archiving and Communication System; *2D,* two-dimensional.

controlling the treatment strategies to the various POCUS findings. In one randomized study of low-risk echo referrals,[19] no benefit of POCUS on length of stay was found even though it changed some form of management in 37%. Despite having prognostic value for triage and medical decision making, cardiac POCUS, much like echocardiography, has yet to show a mortality benefit when applied to a diverse clinical population for which it was determined to be indicated. When ultrasound is applied to specific patient populations, such as septic patients in the ICU, a recent database analysis demonstrated a significant reduction in 28-day mortality rate when comparing the use of transthoracic echocardiography (TTE) versus no TTE (odds ratio, 0.78; 95% confidence interval, 0.68–0.90; $p < .001$), suggesting some beneficial association with the presence of the test.[20] In addition, the subtle value in patient and physician reassurance may have clinical impact that is difficult to measure but still worth the application of noninvasive ultrasound imaging. Ultimately, future POCUS investigation may finally define and validate specific echocardiographic techniques and imaging protocols for outcomes when applied in clinical context.

POCUS CAN AFFECT REFERRAL FOR ECHOCARDIOGRAPHY

The overall effect of POCUS on echocardiographic referral is unknown, but both a reduction of unnecessary referrals for low-risk indications is anticipated along with an increase of referrals for confirmation of abnormal POCUS findings. For example, a recent outcome study projected a 30% savings at minimal risk in outpatient echo costs if a physician's echo referral was guided by simplified detection of left atrial enlargement, patient's age, and the presence of diabetes.[5] An evidence-based bedside physical that incorporates POCUS, when normal, provides reassurance to both the patient and physician, can reduce unnecessary imaging referrals in low-risk patients, and should be further investigated as a cost-conscious, value-driven health care method.

The practice of POCUS will likely improve triage for inpatient echocardiography when used to clarify nonspecific presentations of dyspnea or hypotension. However, until the archiving, reporting, and display of images become standardized, confusion may exist

over the specific pathology any particular POCUS application was meant to identify and which specialist made the interpretation. The coexistence of echo practices in the EDs, ICUs, and hospital echo labs will necessitate the delineation and coordination of services and development of a unified plan of image archival and reports to specifically communicate the result of each POCUS examination to the referring clinician. When limited imaging protocols are applied as an initial test, the referring physician must be made aware of the clinical entities excluded, considered unlikely, or not imaged, to continue the patient's evaluation.

The conundrum of whether to also order an additional standard comprehensive echocardiogram in the setting of POCUS clearly depends on the findings and the decision-making process of the physician. Knowledge of the POCUS indication, the clinical context, and presence of more definitive data are unique data points understood by the imaging physician at the point of care and not by the echocardiographer at a remote echo reading station. The cancellation of a request for a standard echo for a minor POCUS abnormality would be driven by responsible cost utilization.

INCIDENTAL FINDINGS: THE ACHILLES HEEL OF POCUS?

One of the advantages of POCUS is the ability to efficiently evaluate the issue of primary concern. However, the performance of a limited imaging protocol risks either incomplete or absent characterization of all findings and measurements that would have been obtained during standard echocardiography. One risk of POCUS practice therefore lies in either the inadvertent missed finding or a pertinent coexisting finding that is an alternate explanation for the indication used to perform POCUS. For instance, in hypotension and suspected cardiomegaly on chest radiograph, a limited subcostal POCUS view may be sufficient to exclude pericardial tamponade and yet poorly characterize or miss ruptured mitral chordae that is causing cardiogenic shock. Similarly, aortic stenosis, intracardiac thrombosis, or pulmonary hypertension could be easily missed in limited studies unless specifically interrogated in addition to the prespecified limited imaging protocol. Significant incidental findings are common, with up to a 45% prevalence, in hospitalized populations referred for echocardiography and increase with age.[21] In particular, subtle wall motion abnormalities, small vegetations in infective endocarditis, and potential sources of cardioembolism can be easily missed by small portable POCUS devices. Thus, the use of limited ultrasound views may help to exclude a primary diagnosis but may inadvertently fail to record a significant finding that was partly displayed. The reassurance to the POCUS practitioner, the patient, or referring physician of a normal cardiac POCUS may be unfounded in high-risk cases, and therefore referral for standard echocardiography should remain under consideration. Conversely, the automatic echo referral of any irrelevant, suspected incidental finding discovered by POCUS has uncertain patient benefit and will increase immediate costs.

The goal of POCUS to determine the simple presence or absence of a diagnosis in the shortest time possible separates this field from the traditional expectations of diagnostic medical imaging and comprehensive interpretations. In other bedside tests, such as formal chest radiographs and electrocardiograms, readings have always met the standard of complete interpretation of all recorded findings manifest to an expert. Conversely, the urgency of POCUS may permit limiting its diagnostic obligations to only findings sought immediately. The FAST exam may serve as a precedent for an examination that searches for only for fluid collections consistent with traumatic hemorrhage despite the imaging of multiple organs, including the heart.[1] Similarly, for critical care applications, the omnipresent mortality risk of an unstable ICU patient could justify the focus on only specific cardiopulmonary findings that directly relate to hypotension or respiratory failure. In both situations, the delay in treatment caused by acquiring and performing a standard exam could be considered deleterious to patient care. For nonacute POCUS applied in primary care, arguments can be made based on the fact that the incidental detection of common noncardiac findings (e.g., thyroid nodules, renal cysts) in asymptomatic individuals have not been shown to improve survival in screening outcome studies.

Defining the extent of diagnostic responsibility of the POCUS user for the primary diagnosis and incidental findings is critical to the role of the technique, has implications regarding the magnitude of training and competency, and relates to the utility of standard comprehensive studies. In the future, only organ systems or entities in which the user was formally trained or sought hospital privileges for could be considered user responsibility, which would help define teaching and competency protocols at appropriate levels for each specialty. At this point, the diagnostic burden of cardiac POCUS remains unclear, and professional societies may benefit from collaboration to formulate appropriate practice guidelines based on their philosophy and roles of their constituents. Protecting the Achilles heel of POCUS may ultimately require societal input to set a new standard of care in imaging, one that multiple specialists can each have separate, limited diagnostic responsibility for data contained within the same single image based on their contextual involvement in the case.[22]

THE VALUE OF LUNG POCUS DATA IN ECHOCARDIOGRAPHY

Lung ultrasonography is a rapidly developing field pertinent to cardiac presentations of dyspnea, pulmonary edema, and congestive heart failure (CHF) and provides complementary data of a more advanced clinical stage to the echocardiogram's estimation of elevated LA pressures.[23] One of the main findings in lung ultrasound is not a real finding at all but an artifact, the B-line. Although there have been no ex vivo validation studies, this "ring-down" or reverberation artifact (see Fig. 16.1, sites 2–5, and Figs. 16.3 and 16.4)[4,7] has been attributed to the ultrasound beam becoming trapped within interstitial regions near the pleural surface, which have been thickened by edema, infiltration, or fibrosis. More sensitive than rales, the B-line artifact appears to have a 85% to 90% accuracy for CHF when it occurs bilaterally in the lungs in the appropriate populations.[24,25] Despite the fact that B lines vary with transducer frequencies and signal processing and are evanescent, this artifact has consistently been shown to relate to prognosis when obtained using different devices on various clinical populations. Pleural effusions are readily detected at the lung bases by ultrasound, even in the supine position, and can show septation or particulates in inflammatory disease. The presence of bilateral echolucent pleural effusions strongly argues for CHF, with 90% accuracy,[26] and portends a poorer inpatient and 1-year prognosis.[7] Persistent lung findings at discharge may portend readmission,[27] and dedicated POCUS views are critical to detect smaller effusions. Echocardiography can often estimate left atrial pressures using advanced Doppler techniques[28]; however, the presence of lung B lines and pleural effusions denotes a decompensated state with a worse New York Heart Association class and prognosis.[27,29] B lines and effusions have been related to mortality in outpatients and inpatients with CHF, even more than

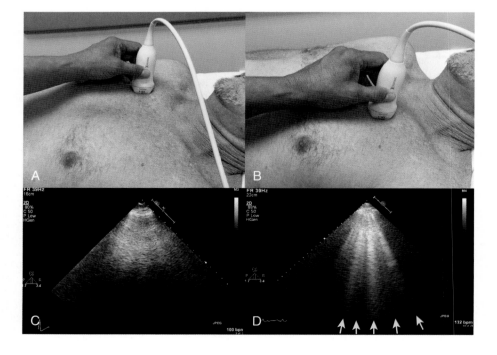

Figure 16.3. Lung B lines. **A,** Hand position used to direct ultrasound into the right lung apex with the transducer oriented sagittally. **B,** Same, for left lung apex. **C,** Normal lung. **D,** Abnormal B lines *(arrows)* or a comet-tail artifact, defined as three or more vertical lines. (Reproduced with permission from Garibyan VN, et al: The prognostic value of lung ultrasound findings in hospitalized patients undergoing echocardiography, *J Ultrasound Med* 37:1641–1648, 2018.)

left ventricular ejection fraction.[7] POCUS assessment for B lines and effusions is easily learned and performed and is endorsed by expert panels[30] and professional societies in emergency and critical care medicine.

DISCREPANCIES BETWEEN POCUS AND ECHOCARDIOGRAPHIC RESULTS

Discrepant data between POCUS and echocardiography often occur when POCUS has been performed first and was temporally followed by echocardiography, often hours later. The bias of such error analysis ignores the immediate value that fleeting POCUS data may have provided to the care of the patient before echocardiography was performed.

Errors in POCUS imaging can often be the result of the inability to move or position the patient optimally, by limited access to imaging windows, or by hurried imaging by the physician. Aside from such errors of inconvenience, data discrepancies between initial POCUS and subsequent echocardiography can also be related to (1) interpretative biases caused by clinical factors not known to the echo lab, such as the presence of cardiac ischemia, hypoxia, sepsis, pressor or inotrope use, and the dynamics of ventilation; (2) insensitivity of a POCUS limited imaging technique in determination of severity of a lesion; (3) the detection of incidental findings that either support or refute the primary diagnosis or are significant by themselves; or (4) the transient nature of the finding resulting in POCUS detection but resolve by the time of echocardiography. Echocardiographers should become familiarized with the favored ultrasound techniques often used by emergency and critical care medicine to diagnose volume status or cardiac failure as to help reconcile differences between POCUS and subsequent echocardiography (Table 16.4).

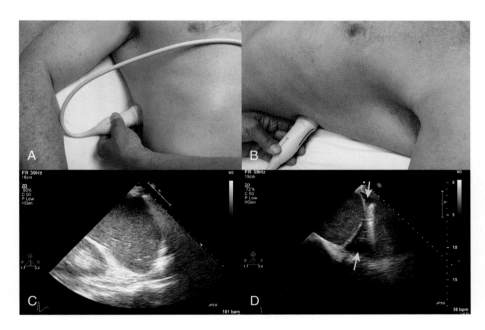

Figure 16.4. Pleural effusions. **A,** Hand position used to direct ultrasound into the right lung base with the transducer directed on a coronal posterior plane. **B,** Same, for the left lung base. **C,** Normal lung without effusion (cranial to the right). **D,** Abnormal pleural fluid (*arrows,* cranial to the right). (Reproduced with permission from Garibyan VN, et al: The prognostic value of lung ultrasound findings in hospitalized patients undergoing echocardiography, *J Ultrasound Med* 37:1641–1648, 2018.)

TABLE 16.4 Reasons for Discrepant Point-of-Care Ultrasound Findings From Echocardiography

Finding Sought	POCUS Method	Limitations	Pertinent Notes for Echocardiographer
LVEF	Subjective estimation, EPSS, MAPSE	1. Compensatory hyperkinesis of normal, nonischemic walls confounds overall EF 2. Poor endocardial definition often biases to a lower EF 3. Rapid ventricular response in atrial fibrillation "lowers" apparent EF 4. Transient stunning, changes in sepsis, resuscitation, and with catecholamines (Takotsubo) 5. Effect of septal dyskinesis, LBBB 6. EPSS estimates of LVEF can be confounded by eccentric AI, wall motion asymmetry, or acute ischemia 7. MAPSE confounded by lateral hypokinesis	1. Contrast-enhanced border delineation can be useful 2. HR, BP, CVP measurements and ventilator status should be displayed at time of estimation 3. Recent clinical events, inotropic or pressor infusions, or hypothermia should be noted 4. EF often "better" when stable in echo lab
CVP: IVC distensibility SVC collapsibility	IVCCI: a <50% diameter reduction; SVCCI: >36% variability = fluid responsive	1. IVC excursion may be related to diaphragmatic motion 2. Size of IVC can vary because of body size, liver weight, or intraabdominal pressure 3. Right ventricular cardiac output, central shifting of volume, or vasoparesis of sepsis can change size, without a change in "intravascular volume" 4. Difficult to interpret with positive-pressure ventilation 5. Differential SVC >IVC flow in the critically ill	1. CVP often misequated to volume status 2. CO often a determinant "fluid responsiveness." 3. HR, BP, CVP measurements and ventilator status should be known

Continued

TABLE 16.4 Reasons for Discrepant Point-of-Care Ultrasound Findings From Echocardiography—cont'd

Finding Sought	POCUS Method	Limitations	Pertinent Notes for Echocardiographer
Cardiac output	Passive leg raise	1. Difficult estimation caused by noncircular LVOT 2. Standardization of maneuvers unclear and may not be reproducible 3. Volume responsiveness more representative of RV output; unclear effects in TR	1. Presence of LVOT obstruction could confound estimates of CO 2. Presence of pressors or inotropes
Regurgitant valvular lesions	Color Doppler jet area	1. Underestimation of volume of eccentric jets; overestimation of functional, central jets 2. Unable to detect small vegetations 3. Acute AR or MR may be underestimated because of tachycardia	1. HR parameters critical 2. Acuity of lesions correlate to symptoms
AS	Calcification and immobility of aortic valve	1. Severity can only be an estimate by 2D imaging 2. Low-gradient AS requires careful Doppler assessment	POCUS is overly sensitive for aortic valve calcification, often resulting in echo referral
PA pressure	Doppler-based Bernoulli estimation using TR jet peak velocity	1. Not angle corrected 2. Coupled often with unreliable CVP estimate 3. PA systolic pressure dependent on CO 4. Gradient represents highest instantaneous value, not mean	1. Tendency to underestimate TR jet velocity, particularly with poor envelope 2. Can use agitated blood–saline mixture 3. Use invasive CVP value at time of study
RV function	RV-to-LV ratio TAPSE 60/60 sign McConnell sign	1. Difficult to obtain true long-axis because foreshortening of the LV is common in supine patients 2. Differentiate acute vs chronic cor pulmonale or with RV MI still problematic 3. Acceleration time often short in tachycardic states; difficult to obtain in intubated patients	Despite echocardiographic data of RV function, POCUS remains an insensitive technique to diagnose PE, particularly in the setting of prior pulmonary HTN
Diastolic dysfunction	Doppler of MV inflow	1. Confounded by tachycardia in acute setting	Knowledge of hemodynamics and inotropic or pressor therapies needed between studies
Pericardial effusion	IVC dilation, RV or RA collapse	1. Effusion size not always prognostic or diagnostic 2. M-mode to time collapse in tachycardia often difficult	Tamponade physiology dependent upon central venous pressure. Confounded in constrictive-effusive states
Wall motion analysis	2D subjective	1. Not all segments are visualized 2. Endocardial definition is critical 3. Acute vs chronic often difficult 4. Ischemia can be transient	1. Septum often nonspecific 2. Use of contrast agents may be helpful
Pleural effusions	2D	1. Small effusions can be missed if transducers are not posterior enough. 2. Confusion with ascites or gastric contents 3. Dedicated views much more accurate than echocardiography	Echo is insensitive for pleural effusions; left pleural fluid is seen from PLAX, right pleural fluid occasionally from subcostal view
Ultrasound B lines for pulmonary edema		Difficult to differentiate CHF, ARDs, and interstitial lung disease	LA pressure data critical to determine cardiogenic vs noncardiogenic pulmonary edema

ARDS, Acute Respiratory Distress Syndrome; *AS,* Aortic stenosis; *AR,* aortic regurgitation; *BP,* blood pressure; *CHF,* congestive heart failure; *CO,* cardiac output; *CVP,* central venous pressure; *EF,* ejection fraction; *EPSS,* E-Point Septal Separation; *HR,* heart rate; *HTN,* hypertension; *IVC,* inferior vena cava; *IVCCI,* inferior vena cava collapsibility index; *LA,* left atrium; *LBBB,* left bundle branch block; *LV,* left ventricle; *LVEF,* left ventricular ejection fraction; *LVOT,* left ventricular outflow tract; *MAPSE,* mitral annular plane systolic excursion; *MI,* myocardial infarction; *MR,* mitral regurgitation; *PA,* pulmonary artery; *PLAX,* parasternal long-axis; *POCUS,* point-of-care ultrasound; *RA,* right atrium; *RV,* right ventricle; *SVC,* superior vena cava; *SVCCI,* superior vena cava collapsibility index; *TAPSE,* tricuspid annular plane systolic excursion; *TR,* tricuspid regurgitation; *2D,* two-dimensional.

CONCLUSION

As a health care technique, cardiac POCUS, as a derivative of echocardiography, may ultimately prioritize the value of specific echocardiographic findings based on clinical context, ease of acquisition, or general outcome data. The optimal pathways for cardiac POCUS will involve a collaborative effort among echocardiographers, bedside clinicians, and medical educators.

REFERENCES

1. Rozycki GS, Ochsner MG, Jaffin JH, et al. Prospective evaluation of surgeons' use of ultrasound in the evaluation of trauma patients. *J Trauma.* 1993;34(4):516–527.
2. Via G, Hussain A, Wells M, et al: International evidence-based recommendations for focused cardiac ultrasound, *J Am Soc Echocardiogr.* 27:683
3. Kimura BJ. Point-of-care cardiac ultrasound techniques in the physical exam: Better at the bedside. *Heart.* 2017;103:987–994.
4. Kimura BJ, Shaw DJ, Amundson SA, et al. Cardiac limited ultrasound exam techniques to augment the bedside cardiac physical. *J Ultrasound Med.* 2015;34(9):1683–1690.
5. Han PJ, Tsai BT, Martin JW, et al. Evidence basis for a point-of-care ultrasound exam to refine referral for outpatient echocardiography. *Am J Med.* 2019;132(2):227–233.
6. Kimura BJ, Yogo N, O'Connell C, et al. Cardiopulmonary limited ultrasound examination for "quick-look" bedside application. *Am J Cardiol.* 2011;108(4):586–590.
7. Garibyan VN, Amundson SA, Shaw DJ, et al. Lung ultrasound findings detected during inpatient echocardiography are common and associated with short- and long-term mortality. *J Ultrasound Med.* 2018;37(7):1641–1648.
8. Kimura BJ, Lou MM, Dahms EB, et al. Prognostic implications of a point-of-care ultrasound examination on hospital ward admission. *J Ultrasound Med.* 2020;39(2):289–297.

9. Kimura BJ, Amundson SA, Phan JN, et al. Observations during development of an internal medicine residency training program in cardiovascular limited ultrasound examination. *J Hosp Med*. 2012;7(7):537–542.

10. Hoppmann RA, Rao VV, Bell F, et al. The evolution of an integrated ultrasound curriculum (iUSC) for medical students: 9-year experience. *Crit Ultrasound J*. 2015;7(18).

11. Tarique U, Tang B, Singh M, Kulasegaram KM, et al. Ultrasound curricula in undergraduate medical education: a scoping review. *J Ultrasound Med*. 2018;37(1):69–82.

12. LoPresti CM, Jensen TP, Dversdal RK, et al. Point-of-care ultrasound for internal medicine residency training: a position statement from the Alliance of Academic Internal Medicine. *Am J Med*. 2019;132(11):1356–1360.

13. Spencer KT, Kimura BJ, Korcarz CE, et al. Focused cardiac ultrasound: recommendations from the American Society of Echocardiography. *J Am Soc Echocardiogr*. 2013;26(6):567–581.

14. Testuz A, Müller H, Keller PF, et al. Diagnostic accuracy of pocket-size handheld echocardiographs used by cardiologists in the acute care setting. *Eur Heart J Cardiovasc Imaging*. 2013;14:38–42.

15. Mai TV, Ahn DT, Phillips C, et al. Feasibility of remote real-time guidance of a cardiac examination performed by novices using a pocket-sized ultrasound device. *Emerg Med Int*. 2013;2013:627230.

16. Tsai BT, Dahms EB, Waalen J, et al. Actual use of pocket-sized ultrasound devices for cardiovascular examination by trained physicians during a hospitalist rotation. *J Community Hosp Intern Med Perspect*. 2016;6(6):33358.

17. Nguyen DT, Espinosa RF, Phan JN, Shaw DJ, Kimura BJ. Would hospitalist use of point-of-care ultrasound pay for itself? A return-on-investment prediction model using unincentivized, ultrasound-trained residents. *J Hosp Med*. 2017;12(suppl 2).

18. Seif D, Perera P, Mailhot T, et al. Bedside ultrasound in resuscitation and the rapid ultrasound in shock protocol. *Crit Care Res Pract*. 2012;2012:503254.

19. Lucas BP, Candotti C, Margeta B, et al. Hand-carried echocardiography by hospitalists: a randomized trial. *Am J Med*. 2011;124:766–774.

20. Feng M, McSparron JI, Kien DT, et al. Transthoracic echocardiography and mortality in sepsis: analysis of the MIMIC-III database. *Intensive Care Med*. 2018;44:884–892.

21. Kimura BJ, Pezeshki B, Frack SA, et al. Feasibility of "limited" echo imaging: characterization of incidental findings. *J Am Soc Echocardiogr*. 1998;11(7):746–750.

22. Kimura BJ, DeMaria AN. Contextual imaging: a requisite concept for the emergence of point-of-care ultrasound. *Circulation* 2020;142:1025–1027.

23. Miglioranza MH, Gargani L, Sant'Anna RT, et al. Lung ultrasound for the evaluation of pulmonary congestion in outpatients: a comparison with clinical assessment, natriuretic peptides, and echocardiography. *JACC Cardiovasc Imaging*. 2013;6:1141–1151.

24. Liteplo AS, Marill KA, Villen T, et al. Emergency thoracic ultrasound in the differentiation of the etiology of shortness of breath (ETUDES): sonographic B-lines and N-terminal pro-brain-type natriuretic peptide in diagnosing congestive heart failure. *Acad Emerg Med*. 2009;16:201–210.

25. Price S, Platz E, Cullen L, et al. Expert consensus document: echocardiography and lung ultrasonography for the assessment of acute heart failure. *Nat Rev Cardiol*. 2017;14:427–440.

26. Kataoka H, Takada S. The role of thoracic ultrasonography for evaluation of patients with decompensated chronic heart failure. *J Am Coll Cardiol*. 2000;35:1638–1646.

27. Coiro S, Rossignol P, Ambrosio G, et al. Prognostic value of residual pulmonary congestion at discharge assessed by lung ultrasound imaging in heart failure. *Eur J Heart Fail*. 2015;17:1172–1181.

28. Mitter SS, Shah SJ, Thomas JD. A test in context: E/A and E/e' to assess diastolic dysfunction and LV filling pressure. *J Am Coll Cardiol*. 2017;69:1451–1464.

29. Frassi F, Gargani L, Tesorio P, et al. Prognostic value of extravascular lung water assessed with ultrasound lung comets by chest sonography in patients with dyspnea and/or chest pain. *J Card Fail*. 2007;13(10):830–835.

30. Volpicelli G, Elbarbary M, Blaivas M, et al. International evidence-based recommendations for point-of-care lung ultrasound. *Intensive Care Med*. 2012;38:577–591.

17 Focused Cardiac Ultrasound in Emergency Clinical Settings

Brian P. Davidson, Jonathan R. Lindner

Focused cardiac ultrasound (FoCUS) refers to a point-of-care ultrasound examination that is goal oriented in a specific clinical setting.[1,2] These "focused" bedside echocardiographic examinations differ from diagnostic echocardiography in that they are performed to answer specific clinical questions that are based on a clinically derived differential diagnosis, and they are increasingly performed by clinicians who have not necessarily achieved competency in comprehensive cardiovascular ultrasound.[3] These brief echocardiographic studies are increasingly being performed with small handheld devices and are playing a growing role in the evaluation and management of patients in emergency situations.

In many ways, echocardiography is ideally suited for use in urgent clinical settings. It is the only modality that can be performed portably at the bedside, allowing examination of patients who are too unstable for transport. The acquisition time is short (usually <10 minutes) and provides immediate information regarding life-threatening conditions. The technology does not expose patients to iodinating contrast or ionizing radiation and can be performed safely and serially on virtually any patient. Echocardiography technology, particularly portable devices, is relatively inexpensive to purchase and easy to maintain and store. Finally, echocardiography is well suited to imaging many of the cardiovascular conditions that can threaten life. This chapter reviews the major applications of FoCUS in patients presenting with medical emergencies. These applications are broadly discussed as both common clinical scenarios in which

FoCUS is useful and in the evaluation of specific life-threatening conditions.

CHEST PAIN

Diagnostic Algorithms for Acute Coronary Syndrome

More than 8 million patients in the United States present annually to emergency departments (EDs) with symptoms concerning for acute coronary syndrome (ACS).[4] A minority of these patients (10%–30%) are ultimately diagnosed with either acute myocardial infarction (MI) or other forms of ACS. In those with ACS, the correct diagnosis is often delayed or even missed in up to 5% of cases because of limitations in the accuracy and time required for standard diagnostic algorithms that include patient history, physical examination, 12-lead electrocardiogram (ECG), and circulating biomarkers.[5] Noninvasive echocardiography is now routinely used in many centers to rapidly diagnose ACS, to identify those who have high-risk features of their ACS, and to reduce health care costs by confidently excluding ischemia in those whose symptoms are not from ACS. The use of comprehensive echocardiography in patients with chest pain (CP) caused by suspected acute myocardial ischemia is a recommended when the baseline ECG is nondiagnostic.[6] Many patients presenting with ACS are hemodynamically stable, and urgent bedside echocardiography is not indicated. Conversely, unstable patients can benefit from FoCUS to evaluate CP caused by life-threatening conditions (Fig. 17.1), including complications of acute myocardial infarction, pulmonary embolus, and aortic dissection (discussed later).

Evaluation for Wall Motion Abnormalities

Transthoracic echocardiography (TTE) has a high sensitivity but moderate specificity for the diagnosis of acute MI.[7] When patients are evaluated during symptoms or within a short period of resolution, the sensitivity of echocardiography for detecting regional wall motion abnormalities is as high as 90% in those with non-diagnostic findings on ECG. Echocardiographic evidence of wall motion has also been shown to provide earlier diagnosis of ACS than conventional (non–high-sensitivity) troponin assays.[8,9] In particular, echocardiography can be useful for rapid diagnosis of ACS caused by left circumflex disease, which is often "silent" on the standard 12-lead ECG.[8] Assessment of regional wall motion by echocardiography in the acute setting can also provide useful prognostic information in patients with CP. The presence of a definitive wall motion abnormality in those with ACS increases likelihood for related late adverse events by approximately fourfold.[7]

Perhaps more important is the high negative predictive value of echocardiography. The presence of completely normal wall motion is able to exclude ischemia with a greater than 95% negative predictive value provided that imaging is performed during symptoms or soon after its resolution.[9] It should be cautioned that echocardiography may be falsely negative in situations when imaging is performed late after resolution of symptoms or if there is incomplete or inadequate visualization of all myocardial segments. Given that segmental wall motion

and wall thickening analysis are some of the most technically demanding aspects of echocardiographic interpretation, FoCUS should be used to exclude ACS only in clinical settings when the value of a negative diagnostic test is high and by those who are competent in the interpretation of wall motion and use of ultrasound contrast agents when necessary.

Contrast-Enhanced Echocardiography

Encapsulated microbubble ultrasound contrast agents that are stable after intravenous injection improve endocardial border delineation of the left ventricle (LV) in otherwise technically suboptimal studies.[10] This issue is of particular importance in the evaluation of patients in whom ACS is suspected because (1) every segment needs to be visualized, (2) a high level of reader confidence is needed, and (3) the imaging environment in the ED is often suboptimal. Clinical studies have demonstrated that ultrasound contrast agents substantially increase the number of interpretable segments, decrease interobserver variability, and increase reader confidence. The evaluation of regional wall motion with contrast echocardiography specifically for ED patients with chest pain has been demonstrated to provide incremental value to clinical information, the ECG, and initial troponin.[9] LV opacification with contrast echocardiography in those with already recognized ACS can also reveal the presence of ventricular pseudoaneurysms or ventricular thrombus. The use of ultrasound-enhancing agents (UAEs) with handheld ultrasound devices, however, is constrained by limited contrast-specific imaging technologies on the current generations of these devices. Although UEAs can be visualized using two-dimensional harmonic imaging available on handheld devices, administration of the agents is best matched to ultrasound systems that optimize contrast signal to noise via adjustable acoustic output controls and contrast-specific imaging sequences.

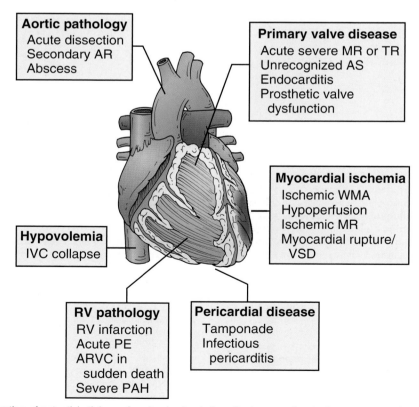

Figure 17.1. Graphic illustration of potential etiology of acute chest pain in patients presenting to the emergency department. *AR,* Aortic regurgitation; *ARVC,* arrhythmogenic right ventricular cardiomyopathy; *AS,* aortic stenosis; *IVC,* inferior vena cava; *MR,* mitral regurgitation; *PAH,* pulmonary arterial hypertension; *PE,* pulmonary embolism; *RV,* right ventricular; *TR,* tricuspid regurgitation; *VSD,* ventricular septal defect; *WMA,* wall motion abnormality.

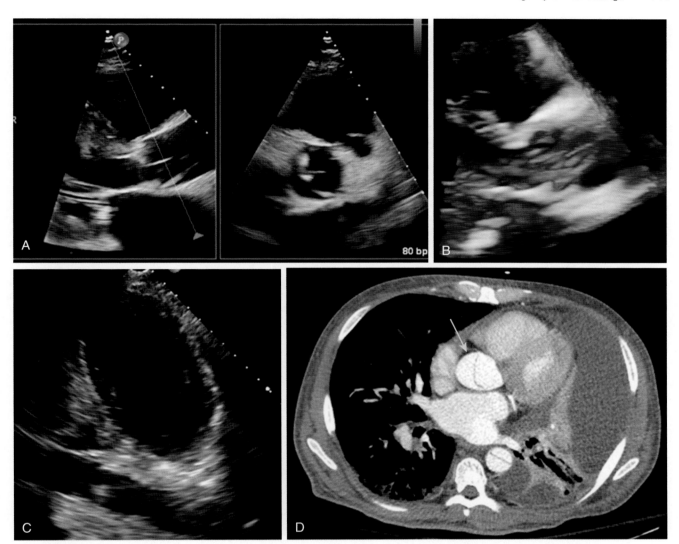

Figure 17.2. Images of a Stanford type A aortic dissection on transthoracic echocardiography using parasternal biplane imaging of the aortic root (**A**), live three-dimensional parasternal imaging of the aortic root (**B**), and modified apical view of the descending thoracic aorta (**C**). **D**, Contrast-enhanced computed tomography image of the chest demonstrating the presence of a true and false lumen in the aortic root *(arrow)*. See corresponding Video 17.2.

Aortic Dissection

The symptoms that herald an acute aortic syndrome (AAS), including chest pain, are often nonspecific. Accordingly, delay in the diagnosis is common because a broad differential diagnosis is considered. Aortic dissection is the most common form of AAS found in approximately 80% to 90% of cases; acute intramural hematoma and penetrating atherosclerotic ulcer make up the remaining causes.[11] A high index of suspicion and rapid imaging is required in these potentially life-threatening conditions given that the morbidity and mortality are time dependent.

TTE has limitations in its ability to visualize the entire thoracic aorta. In those with suspected AAS, right parasternal imaging can be added to the left parasternal long-axis view to extend visualization of the ascending thoracic aorta. For the detection of dissection, the aortic arch can be interrogated in the suprasternal view, and the descending aorta is often visualized behind the left atrium in the parasternal long-axis view and on subcostal imaging (Fig. 17.2 and Video 17.2). Although the image quality of the aorta is often poor (particularly for the distal ascending aorta and the proximal thoracic descending aorta),

FoCUS is vital in the emergency setting for the rapid assessment of complications of dissection, such as aortic valve dysfunction, pericardial tamponade, or wall motion abnormalities that occur from ostial coronary involvement.

Typical features on transthoracic imaging in patients with acute aortic dissection are a dilated aorta, thickened aortic walls, and the presence of an intimal flap that separates the true and false lumens. The overall sensitivity of TTE in diagnosing all forms of aortic dissection is only 59% to 83%, and specificity is 63% to 93% compared with other modalities.[11] Although the findings of a visible flap in the thoracic aorta or new aortic insufficiency on echo are supportive of the diagnosis, the absence of such findings is often inadequate to exclude the diagnosis. Yet in patients in whom poor windows preclude accurate assessment for an aortic intimal flap, other associated findings can be useful for elevating the likelihood of AAS, such as aortic enlargement, a bicuspid aortic valve, new or acute aortic insufficiency, or nonaortic findings of connective tissue diseases. If there is a high index of suspicion for aortic dissection, definitive imaging approaches such as computed tomography should not be delayed by the performance of FoCUS imaging.

HYPOTENSION

Acute Complications of Myocardial Infarction

Although heart failure from LV systolic dysfunction and arrhythmias are common complications of MI, there are several specific acute mechanical complications in which urgent echocardiography plays an important role. These complications include ventricular free wall rupture, ventricular septal defect (VSD), acute mitral regurgitation (MR) from papillary muscle rupture, and right ventricular (RV) infarction, which can produce life-threatening hypotension. Ventricular free wall rupture is thought to account for more than 15% of deaths occurring early in acute MI. Although the true incidence is not clearly established, risk factors for rupture have been identified and include ST-segment elevation myocardial infarction, hypertension in the early phase, fibrinolytic therapy, age, and female sex.[12] These ruptures may present on echocardiography as circumferential or focal pericardial effusion with tamponade, an overt pericardial hematoma (Fig. 17.3 and Video 17.3), or contained rupture from a pseudoaneurysm. Ventricular septal rupture (Fig. 17.4) has many of the same risk factors as free wall rupture and are more common in large and anterior MI. On echocardiography, there is often RV dysfunction when shunt flow is high. When evaluating for ischemic VSD, scrutiny of the entire interventricular septum with color-flow Doppler and nonstandard views is necessary.

Acute severe MR from papillary muscle rupture complicating MI should be suspected in patients post MI who present with acute severe pulmonary edema, shock, and a murmur. Because the anterolateral papillary muscle often possesses dual coronary supply, rupture of the posterior medial papillary muscle is more

frequent.[13] It should be noted that the murmur and corresponding color Doppler pattern of MR on echocardiography can be very brief, occupying only the first portion of systole, because of the large amount of acute regurgitant volume. Because these patients also are often tachycardic, approaches for maximizing temporal resolution are often helpful including narrow sector imaging and even color M-mode. The appearance of a mobile mass attached to the mitral leaflets, indirect evidence of very poor forward stroke volume despite hyperdynamic LV systolic function in noninfarcted segments, and pulmonary venous systolic flow reversal are all ancillary findings. It should also be recognized that acute severe MR from myocardial infarction can also occur, especially after inferior or posterior MI, from asymmetric leaflet tethering, which occurs from dyskinesis or sudden loss of systolic inward excursion.

RV infarction occurs in 30% to 50% of cases of inferior wall MI and is usually caused by a very proximal right coronary artery occlusion. This importance of detecting RV infarction is underscored by the hypotension that frequently occurs when these patients are treated with nitrates or have low intravascular volume status. Echocardiography can be very useful in detecting RV infarction through visual detection of global or segmental RV dysfunction, reduced quantitative measures of RV function (tricuspid annular plane excursion, tricuspid annular tissue Doppler, RV strain), RV enlargement, inferior vena cava (IVC) plethora, and acute secondary tricuspid regurgitation.

Tamponade

Echocardiography is the primary imaging modality used in the diagnosis and evaluation of a pericardial effusion. FoCUS has shown a

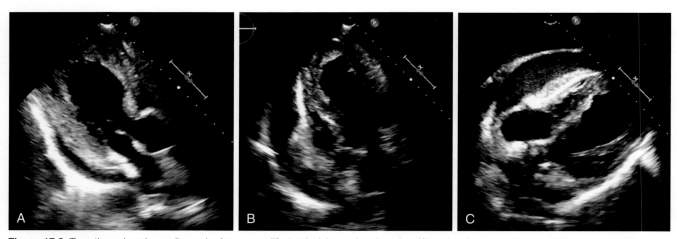

Figure 17.3. Transthoracic echocardiography from a modified apical three-chamber view (**A**), apical four-chamber view (**B**), and subcostal view (**C**) demonstrating the presence of mixed pericardial effusion and hematoma in a patient with recent acute myocardial infarction. Corresponding Video 17.3 shows a tissue defect at the apical-anterior portion of the infarcted left ventricle.

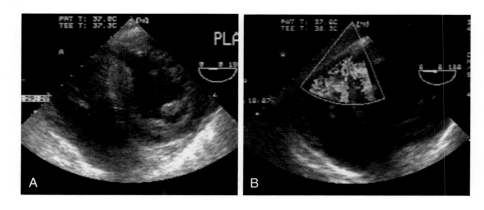

Figure 17.4. Transesophageal echocardiography demonstrating the presence of discontinuity of ventricular septal tissue on two-dimensional imaging (**A**) and the presence of high-velocity left-to-right flow with spectral broadening on color Doppler (**B**).

high degree of sensitivity and specificity in the detection of effusions in emergency settings or at the bedside.[14] Echocardiographic findings for both the diagnosis of pericardial effusion and the assessment of tamponade physiology are provided in a separate chapter. However, there are some concepts of using echocardiography to guide urgent treatment in the emergent setting that deserve highlighting. In an unstable patient, FoCUS can be helpful for identifying low volume status, assessing changes in positive end-expiratory pressure (PEEP) in ventilated patients, early identification of effusive-constrictive physiology, and identifying the site, accessibility, and even drainage potential of fluid or thrombus collection. Because critically ill patients are tachycardic, techniques to aid in tamponade assessment include using simultaneous ECG display during the echo or using M-mode imaging to mitral valve opening and the RV free wall motion.

In hypotensive patients who recently have undergone cardiac surgery, bedside FoCUS is often challenging because of poor imaging quality associated with surgical dressings, mechanical ventilation, and postoperative changes including mediastinal air or indwelling drains.[15] Care must be used in evaluating for tamponade because fluid collections or hematoma can be localized, and clot may be difficult to discriminate from surrounding mediastinal tissues. Additionally, Doppler-based findings of tamponade can sometimes be found from other conditions that create the appearance of ventricular interdependence such as acute postoperative RV dysfunction, lung hyper-expansion (PEEP), and loculated pleural effusions.

Undifferentiated Hypotension and Shock

The bedside FoCUS examination can provide clinically impactful real-time information in patients presenting with undifferentiated hypotension.[1] The FoCUS examination is often part of regimented multisystem imaging protocols including the Focused Assessment with Sonography for Trauma (FAST) and Rapid Ultrasonography for Shock and Hypotension (RUSH) algorithms.[16] Cardiovascular causes of systemic hypotension include, but are not limited to, left- and right-sided systolic dysfunction, acute severe valvular regurgitation, outflow obstructions (severe aortic stenosis, hypertrophic cardiomyopathy), pericardial tamponade, and acute aortic dissection. Negative findings with FoCUS are also helpful for raising awareness for noncardiac causes of hypotension. In nontrauma patients, a hyperdynamic LV with low end-systolic dimensions is particularly helpful for predicting the presence of sepsis.[17] In addition, cardiac ultrasound examination can often be helpful for identifying signs of severe hypovolemia, including a completely collapsed IVC or end-systolic LV cavity obliteration in spontaneously breathing adults.

The contribution of ultrasound to medical decision making has been shown in randomized controlled trials.[18] In hypotensive patients in the ED, the FoCUS examination has been shown to lead clinicians to significantly narrow their differential diagnoses and increased overall diagnostic accuracy.[19] Studies of hypotensive patients in EDs have demonstrated that bedside FoCUS leads to a change in management in 41% to 66% of all patients, with a particularly high impact (96% of patients) in those older than the age of 65 years.[18,20] In intensive care units (ICU), FoCUS can assist in the decision to use volume resuscitation, vasoactive drugs, diuretics, or vasodilators. Finally, in ICUs, focused ultrasound has been demonstrated to improve outcomes. In a prospective study of patients referred to medical intensive care, patients were randomized to receive point-of-care ultrasound performed by intensivists trained in level II echocardiography within 24 hours of admission to the ICU versus standard management. The 28-day survival rate was improved in patients randomized to bedside ultrasound (66% vs 56%; $P = .04$) compared with standard care.[21]

DYSPNEA

Dyspnea is a common feature of many of the cardiovascular conditions that can acutely threaten life. Causes of dyspnea that involve the heart, lungs, or deep veins of the legs can be visualized with ultrasound. Some common assessment approaches include the assessment of LV systolic function, pericardial effusion, RV size and function, and estimated central venous pressure through imaging of the IVC. FoCUS is now often also combined with lung ultrasonography, which can provide evidence in the lungs for pulmonary edema, pneumothorax, pneumonia, and pleural effusion.[22]

The impact of focused ultrasound on the evaluation of undifferentiated dyspnea has been demonstrated in the ED setting. In a prospective trial, patients undergoing ultrasound compared with a standard care were more likely to have a primary diagnosis for dyspnea at 4 hours (88% vs 64%; $P < .0001$).[23] In another study, ED ultrasound reduced the average time needed to formulate a diagnosis for dyspnea by two-thirds.[24] Finally in addition to accelerating the diagnosis, focused ultrasound in one study identified 14% of patients presenting with respiratory symptoms with an acute life-threatening condition missed at the primary assessment.[25]

Acute Decompensated Heart Failure

Decompensated heart failure is one of the most common causes of acute dyspnea. Current guidelines provide a class I indication for comprehensive echocardiography in all patients with acute decompensated heart failure.[26] FoCUS, however, can be useful as a supplement to the initial clinical examination but should not replace the comprehensive echocardiography examination. The addition of FoCUS to the clinical examination has been shown to increase sensitivity, but not specificity, for identifying left-sided ventricular dysfunction or valve disease.[27] Recognition of the presence of major valve disease on the basis of simple morphologic findings is now feasible with pocket-sized devices used by a diverse group of examiners. The benefit of FoCUS while awaiting comprehensive echocardiography is to distinguish those with reduced or preserved LV systolic function and identify significant valvular heart disease, allowing more targeted immediate therapy.[28]

Pulmonary Embolism

Performing FoCUS as part of the bedside evaluation for acute pulmonary embolism (PE) is becoming common but requires an understanding of the diagnostic performance of this imaging. Most studies of FoCUS for this application have used identification of RV enlargement and RV dysfunction as the surrogate evidence for PE. Although evidence of RV "strain" with FoCUS is most commonly defined as an RV-to-LV diameter ratio greater than 0.6 in the apical four-chamber view, this criteria has low sensitivity (55%) and specificity (69%) for diagnosing submassive PE (Fig. 17.5 and Video 17.5).[29] The challenge of using FoCUS to rule out RV strain was demonstrated in an ED study comparing focused echocardiography with conventional echocardiography within 72 hours for patients presenting with shortness of breath, hypotension, or chest pain. The specificity of RV dilation on FoCUS for RV strain was 98%, but sensitivity was only 26% compared with comprehensive echocardiography.[30] Some of the reasons for the discrepancy between FoCUS and conventional echocardiography has been thought to be falsely increased RV relative to LV caused by foreshortening of the LV during imaging and underestimation of RV enlargement in the setting of LV enlargement. The specificity of RV enlargement for PE in unselected populations is limited by recognition that other conditions result in RV dilation, including chronic pulmonary hypertension, RV infarction, chronic severe tricuspid regurgitation, atrial septal defect, acute ventricular septal rupture, and RV dysplastic syndromes. Based on the challenges and limitations, FoCUS as a diagnostic test for PE is best applied in the appropriate emergency clinical context (tachycardia, hypotension, chest pain, hypoxia). In this setting, findings such as RV enlargement, new tricuspid regurgitation, or a hyperdynamic or underfilled

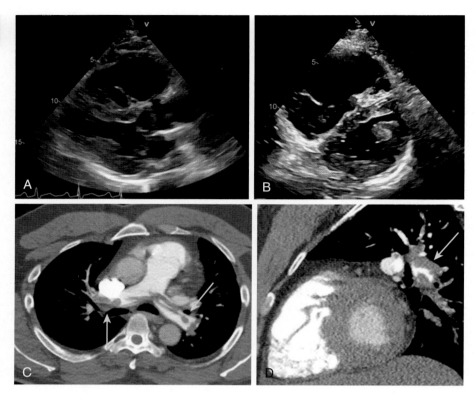

Figure 17.5. Transthoracic echocardiography from the parasternal long-axis (**A**) and short-axis (**B**) planes demonstrating marked increase in right ventricular (RV) end-systolic dimensions in a patient with acute pulmonary embolus. Corresponding Video 17.5 illustrates RV enlargement and segmental RV dysfunction. The corresponding contrast-enhanced computed tomography images in the transaxial (**C**) and sagittal (**D**) planes illustrate the presence of bilateral pulmonary emboli (arrows).

LV occur in 27% to 55% of cases of PE and are specific; however, the absence of such findings is insufficient to rule out PE entirely.

Chest Trauma

Focus bedside cardiac ultrasound is a recognized critical component to the rapid assessment of patients who have experienced chest trauma. Ultrasound can be used to detect intraperitoneal hemorrhage, pericardial tamponade, and hemothorax or pneumothorax in a triage environment. Direct injury to the myocardium can result from either blunt or penetrating trauma. The contused myocardium is dysfunctional (Video 17.6) and can show increased echogenicity and thickness from tissue edema. The spectrum of injury can range from myocardial contusions to myocardial rupture that invariably causes fatal consequences. Blunt cardiac injury can also result in valvular trauma. Tricuspid valve trauma is the most frequent valvular blunt trauma. Finally, traumatic brain injury can cause a systemic massive catecholamine release, leading to an abrupt surge in the sympathetic nervous system outflow. Stress cardiomyopathy or Takotsubo is the most common form of myocardial injury in this presentation with its characteristic regional LV dysfunction caused by the distribution of sympathetic innervation throughout the heart.[31]

CARDIAC ARREST (ADVANCED CARDIAC LIFE SUPPORT)

In patients experiencing sudden cardiac arrest, the application of FoCUS to the evaluation surrounding Advanced Cardiac Life Support (ACLS) interventions has both diagnostic and prognostic value. Imaging from the subcostal window is recommended to minimize interruption of compressions that would occur with parasternal and apical imaging. The primary aims are to identify treatable causes of cardiac arrest and to determine whether return of spontaneous circulation has occurred. For the latter, FoCUS can identify cardiac motion and contractile function. There is also increasing evidence that FoCUS is particularly helpful in pulseless

electrical activity arrest in that it can differentiate between those with electromechanical dissociation and those with organized myocardial activity.[1] Cardiac motion on ultrasound has a high sensitivity (95%) and specificity (80%) to predict return of spontaneous circulation during cardiac arrest.[32] FoCUS has also been used to guide vasopressor therapy based on the presence of organized cardiac activity.

Please access ExpertConsult to view the corresponding videos for this chapter.

REFERENCES

1. Via G, Hussain A, Wells M, et al. International evidence-based recommendations for focused cardiac ultrasound. *J Am Soc Echocardiogr.* 2014;27:683.e1–683.e33.
2. Labovitz AJ, Noble VE, Bierig M, et al. Focused cardiac ultrasound in the emergent setting: a consensus statement of the American Society of Echocardiography and American College of Emergency Physicians. *J Am Soc Echocardiogr.* 2010;23:1225–1230.
3. Ryan T, Berlacher K, Lindner JR, et al. COCATS 4 Task Force 5: training in echocardiography. *J Am Coll Cardiol.* 2015;65:1786–1799.
4. Nawar EW, Niska RW, Xu J. National Hospital Ambulatory medical care Survey: 2005 emergency department summary. *Advance Data 1–32.* 2007.
5. Pope JH, Aufderheide TP, Ruthazer R, et al. Missed diagnoses of acute cardiac ischemia in the emergency department. *N Engl J Med.* 2000;342:1163–1170.
6. Rybicki FJ, Udelson JE, Peacock WF, et al. 2015 ACR/ACC/AHA/AATS/ACEP/ASNC/NASCI/SAEM/SCCT/SCMR/SCPC/SNMMI/STR/STS appropriate utilization of cardiovascular imaging in emergency department patients with chest pain. *J Am Coll Cardiol.* 67:853–879. 2016.
7. Sabia P, Abbott RD, Afrookteh A, et al. Importance of two-dimensional echocardiographic assessment of left ventricular systolic function in patients presenting to the emergency room with cardiac-related symptoms. *Circulation.* 1991;84:1615–1624.
8. Parato VM, Mehta A, Delfino D, et al. Resting echocardiography for the early detection of acute coronary syndromes in chest pain unit patients. *Echocardiography.* 2010;27:597–602.
9. Rinkevich D, Kaul S, Wang XQ, et al. Regional left ventricular perfusion and function in patients presenting to the emergency department with chest pain and no ST-segment elevation. *Eur Heart J.* 2005;26:1606–1611.
10. Porter TR, Mulvagh SL, Abdelmoneim SS, et al. Clinical applications of ultrasonic enhancing agents in echocardiography. *J Am Soc Echocardiogr.* 2018;31:241–274.
11. Baliga RR, Nienaber CA, Bossone E, et al. The role of imaging in aortic dissection and related syndromes. *JACC Cardiovasc Imag.* 2014;7:406–424.

12. Becker RC, Gore JM, Lambrew C, et al. A composite view of cardiac rupture in the United States National Registry of Myocardial Infarction. *J Am Coll Cardiol.* 1996;27:1321–1326.

13. Voci P, Bilotta F, Caretta Q, et al. Papillary muscle perfusion pattern. *Circulation.* 1995;91:1714–1718.

14. Alerhand S, Carter JM. What echocardiographic findings suggest a pericardial effusion is causing tamponade? *Am J Emerg Med.* 2019;37:321–326.

15. Price S, Prout J, Jaggar SI, et al. "Tamponade" following cardiac surgery: terminology and echocardiography may both mislead. *Eur J Cardio Thorac Surg.* 2004;26:1156–1160.

16. Ultrasound Guidelines: emergency, point-of-care and clinical ultrasound guidelines in medicine. *Ann Emerg Med.* 2017;69:e27–e54.

17. Jones AE, Craddock PA, Tayal VS, Kline JA. Diagnostic accuracy of left ventricular function for identifying sepsis among emergency department patients with non-traumatic symptomatic undifferentiated hypotension. *Shock.* 2005;24:513–517.

18. Breitkreutz R, Price S, Steiger HV, et al. Focused echocardiographic evaluation in life support and peri-resuscitation of emergency patients: a prospective trial. *Resuscitation.* 2010;81:1527–1533.

19. Jones AE, Tayal VS, Sullivan DM, Kline JA. Randomized, controlled trial of immediate versus delayed goal-directed ultrasound to identify the cause of nontraumatic hypotension in emergency department patients. *Crit Care Med.* 2004;32:1703–1708.

20. Ferrada P, Evans D, Wolfe L, et al. Findings of a randomized controlled trial using limited transthoracic echocardiogram (LTTE) as a hemodynamic monitoring tool in the trauma bay. *J Trauma Acute Care Surg.* 2014;76:31–37.

21. Kanji HD, McCallum J, Sirounis D, et al. Limited echocardiography-guided therapy in subacute shock is associated with change in management and improved outcomes. *J Crit Care.* 2014;29:700–705.

22. Bekgoz B, Kilicaslan I, Bildik F, et al. BLUE protocol ultrasonography in Emergency Department patients presenting with acute dyspnea. *Am J Emerg Med.* 2019;37(11):2020–2027.

23. Laursen CB, Sloth E, Lassen AT, et al. Point-of-care ultrasonography in patients admitted with respiratory symptoms: a single-blind, randomised controlled trial. *Lancet Respir Med.* 2014;2:638–646.

24. Zanobetti M, Scorpiniti M, Gigli C, et al. Point-of-care ultrasonography for evaluation of acute dyspnea in the. In: *Chest.* Vol. 151. 2017:1295–1301.

25. Laursen CB, Sloth E, Lambrechtsen J, et al. Focused sonography of the heart, lungs, and deep veins identifies missed life-threatening conditions in admitted patients with acute respiratory symptoms. *Chest.* 2013;144:1868–1875.

26. Yancy CW, Jessup M, Bozkurt B, et al. 2013 ACCF/AHA guideline for the management of heart failure: a report of the American College of Cardiology Foundation/American Heart Association Task Force on practice guidelines. *Circulation.* 2013;128:e240–327.

27. Marbach JA, Almufleh A, Di Santo P, et al. Comparative accuracy of focused cardiac ultrasonography and clinical examination for left ventricular dysfunction and valvular heart disease: a systematic review and meta-analysis. *Ann Intern Med.* 2019;171:264–272.

28. Price S, Platz E, Cullen L, et al. Expert consensus document: echocardiography and lung ultrasonography for the assessment and management of acute heart failure. *Nat Rev Cardiol.* 2017;14:427–440.

29. Fields JM, Davis J, Girson L, et al. Transthoracic echocardiography for diagnosing pulmonary embolism: a systematic review and meta-analysis. *J Am Soc Echocardiogr.* 2017;30:714–723. e4.

30. Taylor RA, Moore CL. Accuracy of emergency physician-performed limited echocardiography for right ventricular strain. *Am J Emerg Med.* 2014;32:371–374.

31. Medina de Chazal H, Del Buono MG, Keyser-Marcus L, et al. Stress cardiomyopathy diagnosis and treatment. *J Am Coll Cardiol.* 2018;72:1955–1971.

32. Tsou PY, Kurbedin J, Chen YS, et al. Accuracy of point-of-care focused echocardiography in predicting outcome of resuscitation in cardiac arrest patients: a systematic review and meta-analysis. *Resuscitation.* 2017;114:92–99.

18   Ultrasound-Enhancing Agents

Joan Olson, Feng Xie, Thomas R. Porter

CURRENTLY AVAILABLE SECOND-GENERATION ULTRASOUND CONTRAST AGENTS

The 2018 American Society of Echocardiography Guidelines recommended changing the terminology of ultrasound contrast agents to ultrasound-enhancing agents (UEAs) for the purpose of distinguishing UEAs from traditional iodinated or magnetic resonance agents.[1] The currently available UEAs in the United States are Optison (General Electric Healthcare), Lumason (Bracco Healthcare), and Definity (Lantheus Imaging). Lumason is the same as what is marketed as Sonovue in 44 other countries, including all of Europe, Brazil, India, and China. Sonozoid (General Electric Healthcare) is approved in Japan and Norway for liver tumor imaging but not for cardiac applications (Table 18.1). Lumason, Optison, and Definity are currently approved only for left ventricular opacification (LVO), but Lumason is also approved for adult and pediatric liver and vesicular imaging. In Europe, SonoVue is approved for improving the detection of coronary artery disease and Doppler enhancement. However, all of these agents have been used to examine myocardial blood flow with perfusion imaging techniques available for almost 20 years on commercially available ultrasound systems.[1,2]

ULTRASOUND CONTRAST AGENT COMPOSITION

The improvement in LVO achieved with UCAs after venous injection or infusion has been related to the incorporation of high-molecular-weight gases inside the microbubble shell (see Table 18.1). High-molecular-weight gases (sulfur hexafluoride or perfluorocarbons like perfluoropropane) have both lower diffusivity and lower blood solubility, which prolongs their gas phase in blood. Imaging techniques have been modified to image microbubbles at very low mechanical indices (<0.2) using fundamental nonlinear imaging.[2]

TECHNICAL CONSIDERATIONS TO OPTIMIZE CONTRAST ENHANCEMENT

The success of contrast imaging depends on optimizing the gain, time gain compensation, and mechanical index (MI) for imaging,

as well as controlling the contrast infusion rate or bolus size so as to obtain myocardial contrast enhancement without shadowing in the left ventricular cavity. Current guidelines recommend very low MI imaging with fundamental nonlinear imaging for optimal LVO and endocardial border resolution (Table 18.2). The advantage of fundamental nonlinear imaging is that enhanced contrast signal is achieved at MIs that are below what would produce adequate contrast from harmonic imaging. This very low MI has the added advantage of eliciting virtually no nonlinear signal from tissue, resulting in inherent background subtraction. Moreover, because the received frequency is the fundamental frequency, there is minimal attenuation in the far field (Fig. 18.1 and Video 18.1).

ROLE OF HEALTH CARE PROFESSIONALS IN MAINTAINING ULTRASOUND-ENHANCING AGENT QUALITY

The physician is responsible for the overall quality control of the procedure, which begins by ensuring all personnel (cardiology fellows, nurses, and sonographers) are adequately educated in the concepts of LVO optimization that is necessary for both bolus injections and continuous infusions of microbubble contrast. Physicians should work with their ultrasound vendors to ensure that a good portion of their system fleet have fundamental nonlinear imaging software for both rest and stress echocardiography. The physician needs to work with the lead sonographer and nursing team to develop a standard operating procedure to be followed whenever UEAs are used. The physician assigned to the laboratory that uses UEAs needs to be Level II or III trained in echocardiography and be trained in the performance and interpretation of contrast-enhanced examinations before operating independently. This includes knowing the vendor-specific ultrasound imaging equipment for accessing fundamental nonlinear imaging techniques and optimizing time gain compensation, focus, MI, and flash high MI impulses for each technique (Table 18.3).

TABLE 18.1 Commercially Available Second-Generation Ultrasound Contrast Agents

Agent	Manufacturer	Shell	Gas	Approved
Optison	GE Healthcare	Albumin A-type protein	Perfluoropropane	LVO: United States, Europe
Definity	Lantheus Medical Imaging	Phospholipid	Perfluoropropane	LVO: United States, Europe
SonoVue/Lumason	Bracco Diagnostics	A-type lipid	Sulfur hexafluoride	LVO and Doppler: United States, Europe, Brazil, India, China[a]
Sonozoid[a]	Ge Healthcare	Lipid	Perfluorobutane	Noncardiac liver tumor imaging: Japan and Norway

LVO, Left ventricular opacification.

[a]Highest population countries and continents listed. SonoVue is approved in a total of 44 countries.

TABLE 18.2 Current Imaging Techniques Recommended for Left Ventricular Opacification With Ultrasound-Enhancing Agents

Imaging Technique	Pulse Sequence Scheme	Recommended MI	Advantages	Disadvantage
Amplitude modulation	Alternating amplitude/receives fundamental nonlinear responses	<0.2	High contrast sensitivity and minimal attenuation	Less resolution
Amplitude or phase modulation	Alternating amplitude and phase/receives fundamental and harmonic nonlinear responses	<0.2	High contrast sensitivity and minimal attenuation of far field	Less resolution
Phase inversion (pulse inversion)	Alternating phase only; receives even order harmonics	<0.2	High resolution	Attenuation far field
Tissue harmonic imaging	Transmit one frequency/receive at the second harmonic	0.2–0.4	High resolution	Attenuation far field

MI, Mechanical index.

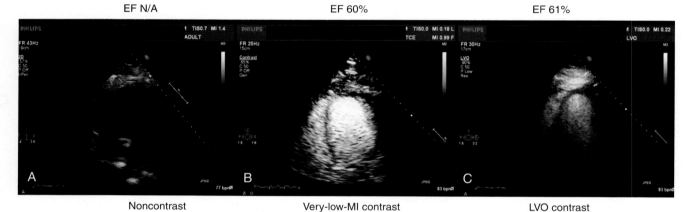

EF N/A   EF 60%   EF 61%

Noncontrast   Very-low-MI contrast   LVO contrast

Figure 18.1. Improved delineation of distal segments and apex with the use of a small bolus injection and slow "infusion-like flush" of saline in an intensive care unit patient. **A,** Noncontrast. **B,** With imaging with a very low mechanical index (MI), there is improved delineation of basal, mid, and distal segments (transmit and receive frequencies were 1.8 MHz using fundamental nonlinear imaging). **C,** With low-MI harmonic imaging, there was attenuation of the basal segments because only the high-frequency harmonic signals were being analyzed. See accompanying Video 18.1. *EF,* Ejection fraction; *LVO,* left ventricular opacification; *N/A,* not applicable.

ROLE OF SONOGRAPHER/NURSE

UEAs are used to enhance images, improve border detection, and provide information on myocardial perfusion at rest and during functional stress echocardiographic studies. The agent is administered by a registered nurse or other qualified medical personnel, including sonographers, when hospital policies permit. One of the most important things to avoid is excessive contrast in the LV cavity causing acoustic shadowing (Fig. 18.2). This is typically from too large a bolus injection or flush rate, resulting in both the inability to see the basal and midsegments of the LV cavity and the loss of a large proportion of the contrast you prepared being rendered useless as it passes through the LV cavity. Therefore, a continuous infusion or small bolus injection of any agent should be used, with 5-mL saline flushes that are given over a 10-second period or longer. The recommended infusion is an approximate 3% infusion for Definity (1.5-cc vial in 50 mL of saline) and 15% Optison infusion (3 mL in 20 mL of saline). These can be subdivided into two separate aliquots for rest and stress imaging if needed. For Lumason, it is recommended that small (0.5- to 1.0-mL) boluses be used followed by slow 5- to 10-mL saline flushes over 10 to 20 seconds as discussed later.

The nurse or sonographer prepares the contrast solution before acquiring images. Definity is activated by agitating the vial for 45 seconds in an activation device called a Vialmix. Optison and Lumason (SonoVue) are distributed in glass vials that are ready for use. For bolus injections, it is recommended that initial doses be low (0.1 mL for Definity, 0.2–0.3 mL for Optison, and 0.5–1.0 mL for Lumason) and that the flush be 5 to 10 mL of saline over 10 to 20 seconds (a slow saline infusion flush). This prevents excessive opacification and shadowing in the far field (see Fig. 18.2). For any continuous infusion of diluted contrast, the recommended initial infusion rate of the dilutions described is approximately 4 cc per minute by hand, watching the clock. The solution should be mixed back and forth by hand periodically so that the enhancing agent does not settle in the bottom of the syringe.

SAFETY OF ULTRASOUND CONTRAST AGENTS

The safety of UEAs has now been well established. Despite early concerns by the Food and Drug Administration, there has been no increased risk compared with an equivalent patient population not receiving contrast. This now includes data from well over 250,000 patients,[1] including patients in intensive care settings, patients with potential acute coronary syndromes undergoing resting or stress echocardiography, and patients after acute myocardial infarction.[3–15] Data obtained from the large Premier Database has demonstrated the potential lifesaving impact of using a UEA with echocardiography. Critically ill patients undergoing contrast-enhanced echocardiography within the first 24 hours after admission had significantly lower 48-hour and hospital mortality rates than propensity-matched patients undergoing unenhanced echocardiography.[12] These critical data imply that the

TABLE 18.3 Concepts that Optimize Ultrasound-Enhancing Agent Use for Left Ventricular Opacification and Myocardial Perfusion When Using Fundamental Versus Harmonic Nonlinear Imaging

System Setting	Amplitude Modulation	Amplitude and Phase Modulation	Low-MI Harmonic
Gain and time gain compensation (TGC)	Higher TGC in the near field and occasionally far field (in large patients); gain then adjusted so that myocardial signal is void after high-MI impulse	Higher TGC in the near field and occasionally far field (in large patients); gain then adjusted so that myocardial signal is void after high-MI impulse	Higher TGC in the near field and far field
Focus	Far field behind the mitral valve	Far field behind the mitral valve	Near field to decrease scan line density and prevent swirling artifact while at 0.2–0.3 MI
MI	0.12–0.20	0.12–0.20	0.2–0.3 to balance cavity contrast enhancement and reduce swirling artifact in apex 0.4 to improve delineation of noncompaction
# "Flash high MI impulses"	2–4 frames under resting conditions 5–15 frames during peak stress conditions during stress echocardiography[a]	2–4 frames under resting conditions 5–15 frames during peak stress conditions during stress echocardiography[a]	No high-MI option for this application

[a]This range of high mechanical index (MI) impulses is what has been required to get myocardial clearance without cavity clearance.

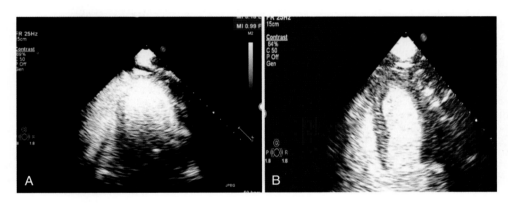

Figure 18.2. Acoustic shadowing (**A**), which typically occurs with a bolus injection and too rapid a flush. With a slower "infusion saline flush" after a small bolus injection or continuous infusion of a diluted contrast agent, there is less attenuation (**B**) and better delineation of basal, mid, and apical segments with fundamental nonlinear imaging.

increased diagnostic accuracy afforded by the use of contrast may lead to earlier correct diagnoses and subsequent reduced mortality.

A rare anaphylactoid reaction may occur in response to Definity; this is estimated to have a frequency of 0.006%.[1] Because of this, it is recommended that all nurses and sonographers using Definity have hospital policies in place that ensure recognition of this rare reaction and how to treat (epinephrine, Advanced Cardiac Life Support measures for maintenance of airway, volume resuscitation, and antihistamines). The safety and efficacy of ultrasound contrast agents in patients with pulmonary hypertension and right-to-left shunts have also been demonstrated,[1–3,6,16,17] and UEAs are no longer contraindicated in these patients.

Please access ExpertConsult to view the corresponding videos for this chapter.

REFERENCES

1. Porter TR, Mulvagh SL, Abdelmoneim SS, et al. Clinical applications of ultrasonic enhancing agents in echocardiography. *J Am Soc Echocardiogr.* 2018;31:241–274.
2. Porter TR, Abdelmoneim S, Belcik JT, et al. Guidelines for the cardiac sonographer in the performance of contrast echocardiography. *J Am Soc Echocardiogr.* 2014;27:797–810.
3. Wei K, Main ML, Lang RM, et al. The effect of Definity on systemic and pulmonary hemodynamics in patients. *J Am Soc Echocardiogr.* 2012;25:584–588.
4. Wever-Pinzon O, Suma V, Ahuja A, et al. Safety of echocardiographic contrast in hospitalized patients with pulmonary hypertension: a multi-center study. *Eur Heart J Cardiovasc Imag.* 2012;13:857–862.
5. Exuzides A, Main ML, Colby C, et al. A Retrospective comparison of mortality in critically ill hospitalized patients undergoing echocardiography with and without an ultrasound contrast. *J Am Coll Cardiol Imag.* 2010;3:578–585.
6. Abdelmoneim SS, Bernier M, Scott CG, et al. Safety of contrast agent use during stress echocardiography in patients with elevated right ventricular systolic pressure a cohort study. *Circ Cardiovasc Imag.* 2010;3:240–248.
7. Abdelmoneim SS, Bernier M, Scott CG, et al. Safety of contrast agent use during stress echocardiography; a 4-year experience form a single-center cohort study of 26,774 patients. *J Am Coll Cardiol Imag.* 2009;2:1048–1056.
8. Dolan MS, Gala S, Dodla S, et al. Safety and efficacy of commercially available ultrasound contrast agents for rest and stress echocardiography: a multicenter experience. *J Am Coll Cardiol.* 2009;53:32–38.
9. Gaibazzi N, Squeri A, Ardissino D, et al. Safety of contrast flash-replenishment stress echocardiography in 500 patients with a chest pain episode of undetermined origin within the last 5 days. *Eur J Echocardiogr.* 2009;10:726–732.
10. Anantharam B, Chahal N, Chelliah R, et al. Safety of contrast in stress echocardiography in stable patients and in patients with suspected acute coronary syndrome but negative 12-hour troponin. *Am J Cardiol.* 2009;104:14–18.
11. Main ML, Ryan AC, Davis TE, et al. Acute mortality in hospitalized patients undergoing echocardiography with and without an ultrasound contrast agent. *Am J Cardiol.* 2008;102:1742–1746.
12. Main ML, Hibberd MG, Ryan A, et al. Acute mortality in critically ill patients undergoing echocardiography with or without an ultrasound contrast agent. *J Am Coll Cardiol Imag.* 2014;7:408.
13. Wei K, Mulvagh SL, Carson L, et al. The safety of Definity and Optison for ultrasound image enhancement: a retrospective analysis of 78,383 administered contrast doses. *J Am Soc Echocardiogr.* 2008;11:1202–1206.
14. Kusnetzky LL, Khalid A, Khumri TM, et al: Acute mortality in hospitalized patients undergoing echocardiography with and without an ultrasound contrast agent: results in 18,671 consecutive patients, *J Am Coll Cardiol.* 51:1704–1706.
15. Shaikh K, Chang SM, Peterson L, et al. Safety of contrast administration for endocardial enhancement during stress echocardiography compared with non-contrast stress. *Am J Cardiol.* 2008;102:1444–1450.
16. Herzog C. Incidence of adverse events associated with use of perflutren contrast agents for echocardiography. *J Am Med Assoc.* 2008;99:2023–2025.
17. Parker JM, Weller MW, Feinstein LM, et al. Safety of ultrasound contrast agents in patients with known or suspected cardiac shunts. *Am J Cardiol.* 2013;112:1039–1045.

19 Physical Properties of Microbubble Ultrasound Contrast Agents

Jonathan R. Lindner

MICROBUBBLE CONTRAST AGENTS

A wide variety of ultrasound-enhancing agents (UEAs), or contrast agents, have been developed for use in diagnostic imaging. Agents that have been approved by regulatory agencies for routine diagnostic use in humans are composed of encapsulated microbubbles.[1] Key considerations that have guided the design of these agents are that they must be safe, able to transit the pulmonary and systemic microcirculation unimpeded, and sufficiently stable after intravenous injection to reach the left ventricular cavity and the myocardium and to produce strong acoustic signals. To satisfy these requirements, microbubbles must be smaller than the effective diameter of the pulmonary and systemic capillary beds (<6–7 μm) and yet contain enough gas volume to undergo cavitation that can be readily detected by ultrasound. The in vivo stability of microbubbles has been achieved by two strategies. Encapsulation of the microbubbles using lipid surfactant (arranged in a monolayer) or albumin "shells" has been used to reduce outward diffusion of the gas core and to reduce microbubble surface tension, which allows for the production of stable yet small microbubbles. Microbubble stability has been enhanced further by using biocompatible high-molecular-weight gases such as perfluorocarbons (octafluoropropane [C_3F_8], decafluorobutane [C_4F_{10}]) or sulfur hexafluoride (SF_6). These gases have both low solubility (low Ostwald coefficient) and low diffusion coefficients, which, according to Epstein-Plesset modeling of the stability of free bubbles, markedly increase their life span.[2] A partial list of microbubble agents approved for use in humans is provided in Fig. 19.1.

The behavior of commercially produced microbubbles in the microcirculation, or their rheology, has been well characterized. This issue is of importance when considering their safety, their ability to transit to the peripheral circulation after intravenous injection, and their application as flow tracers when performing perfusion imaging. Rheology studies have relied on either (1) comparing microbubble transit rates on imaging with those of labeled erythrocytes or (2) intravital microscopy where microbubble transit can be directly visualized (Fig. 19.2). These techniques have definitively demonstrated that microbubble behavior is similar to that of erythrocytes, and they transit the microcirculation of normal tissues unimpeded, with the exception of reticuloendothelial organs (e.g., the liver) where uptake occurs for many microbubbles as part of their normal clearance pathway.[3,4]

The acoustic detection of gas-filled microbubbles within the vascular compartment is based on their compressibility (Fig. 19.3). The gases that have been used in microbubble contrast agents are several orders of magnitude more compressible than water or tissue. Because they are smaller than ultrasound wavelengths, they undergo volumetric oscillation, whereby they compress and expand during the pressure peaks and troughs of the ultrasound pulse.[5] When imaging at low acoustic power, the degree of signal enhancement is governed by the magnitude of oscillation, also called *stable cavitation*. The mechanical index (MI), defined as the peak negative acoustic pressure divided by the square root of the transmit frequency, at which stable cavitation occurs, is less than 0.25 for most agents. At higher acoustic pressures (MI generally >0.5), exaggerated microbubble oscillation produces microbubble destruction, which is termed *inertial cavitation*. This activity produces very strong broadband ultrasound signals by a variety of mechanisms, the most important of which is the abrupt release of free gas microbubbles from the confines of their shell, which than can undergo nondamped exaggerated oscillation.[6] The inertial cavitation phenomenon is also important for nullifying contrast signal when performing quantitative perfusion imaging, which is discussed elsewhere.

The schemes used clinically to augment microbubble signal relative to tissue rely on the detection of specific acoustic signatures produced by nonlinear oscillation. Nonlinear oscillation is defined by a variety of microbubble vibration behaviors in which the changes in microbubble volume are eccentric and not linearly related to the applied ultrasound pressure. The magnitude of oscillation and nonlinear behavior in turn depends on the compressibility and density of the gas, the viscosity and density of the surrounding medium, the frequency and power of ultrasound, and equilibrium radius of the microbubbles.[7] Viscoelastic damping from the shell is a particularly important issue. Ideally, microbubbles should have "flexible" shells. With regard to frequency, there is an ideal resonant frequency at which all forms of radial oscillation become efficient and exaggerated. This "resonant frequency" is inversely related to the square of the microbubble's radius and is also influenced by the viscoelastic and compressive properties of the shell and gas.[7] When performing contrast echocardiography in patients, selection of the ideal frequency for microbubble resonance is generally not a major consideration because the range of frequencies used in clinical practice are generally close to the ideal resonant frequency for

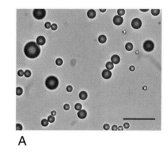

Figure 19.1. Illustration of lipid microbubbles on microscopy (**A**) and a table listing some of the commercially available microbubble agents (**B**). *Asterisk* indicates agents currently approved for use by the US Food and Drug Administration.

Shell	Gas	Size	Proprietary Name
Lipid	C_3F_8	1-3 μm	Definity*
	C_4F_{10}	2 μm	Sonazoid
	SF_6	2-3 μm	Sonovue/Lumason*
	Air	2-3 μm	Levovist
Albumin	C_3F_8	2-4 μm	Optison*

A   B

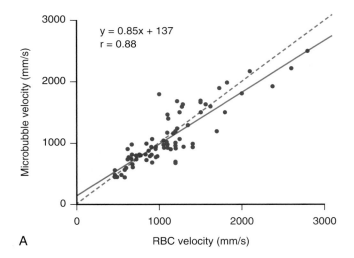

$$y = 0.85x + 137$$
$$r = 0.88$$

A

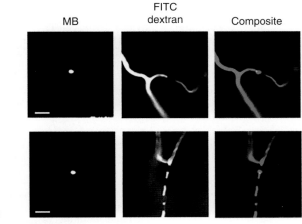

MB | FITC dextran | Composite

B

Figure 19.2. A, Relationship between capillary and noncapillary microvascular velocities for a lipid-shelled perflutren microbubble agent and that for red blood cells (RBC) determined by intravital microscopy of the cremaster muscle. **B,** Examples from intravital microscopy showing two separate fluorescently labeled microbubbles in the *left panels,* the microcirculation imaged by injection of fluorescein isothiocyanate (FITC)–labeled dextran in the *middle panel* (*dark intravascular shadows* representing RBCs), and a pseudocolorized composite image (*red* = microbubble, *green* = intravascular dextran) in the *right panels* illustrating microbubbles in the microvascular compartment. Adapted from Ref. (4).

contrast agents approved for use in humans. This is not necessarily the case for high- and ultrahigh frequency probes that are used for intravascular and preclinical imaging in small animals.

CONTRAST-SPECIFIC IMAGING TECHNIQUES

The general principle underlying two-dimensional ultrasound imaging is to receive and filter ultrasound signals that are reflected from tissues to generate an image that defines anatomic boundaries and texture. Contrast echocardiography, whether for left ventricular opacification or for myocardial perfusion, is based on different principles. The aim is to minimize tissue signal and amplify microbubble signal to better define endocardial borders or measure the concentration of microbubbles in the myocardial microcirculation. To accomplish this, several pulse schemes have been developed and incorporated into contrast-specific features on most echocardiography imaging systems.

Perfusion imaging and certain research applications (molecular imaging, cavitation-related gene therapy, sonothrombolysis) have been performed with high-power ultrasound imaging to generate robust signals. When imaging microbubble agents at high power, inertial cavitation produces very strong but transient broadband signals that contain somewhat higher peaks at the harmonic frequencies occurring at multiples of the transmission frequency (see Fig. 19.3).[8] The main limitation, other than the transient nature of the microbubble contrast effect, is that the tissue signal is strong, so it becomes difficult to discern microbubble from tissue signal. Although filtering to receive signals at twice the fundamental (transmission) frequency, called *second harmonic imaging,* improves microbubble signal-to-tissue ratio, tissue still continues to produce backscatter at the second harmonic frequency, primarily because the ultrasound beam is distorted as it travels through tissue. Tissue signal is more concentrated at the fundamental and harmonic peaks, whereas microbubble inertial cavitation produces a signal response with a much broader band, so off-harmonic imaging either between the fundamental and harmonic frequencies or just beyond the second harmonic (ultraharmonic imaging) are approaches that have been used to increase high-power contrast signal relative to tissue.

A second approach to augmenting microbubble signal-to-noise ratio during high-power imaging is to use signal processing that further reduces tissue clutter by decorrelation imaging. This approach relies on either radiofrequency decorrelation or Doppler processing to measure the degree to which a packet of sequential ultrasound pulses along a single line differ from each other (Fig. 19.4). Provided there is little tissue motion during the pulse sequences, signals from tissue alone are similar. Therefore, the degree of noncorrelation, which determines pixel intensity, is low for tissue and below the wall filter settings. In contrast, microbubbles resident within tissue are destroyed rapidly so that the sequential returning signals are dissimilar, and the degree of decorrelation is high, denoted by high pixel intensity.

When performing contrast imaging at low power, tissue does not produce much of a nonlinear signal. However, the amplitude of the nonlinear signal produced by microbubbles at low MI is rather small. Compensation by increasing the gain solves little because it also increases the existing tissue noise. Hence it is important again to eliminate tissue signal to maximize the microbubble signal-to-noise ratio. One approach, termed *pulse inversion* or *phase inversion,* relies on successive pulses of ultrasound that have inverted phases (are mirror images of each other) (Fig. 19.5A). At these low transmission powers, tissue produces mostly linear backscatter, so ultrasound is reflected at the fundamental frequency. By summing the two returning signals, tissue signal can be eliminated. However, microbubbles produce nonlinear signals that do not cancel and are displayed according to the amplitude. Tissue signal during low-power imaging may also be suppressed online by alternating acoustic power rather than phase, often called *amplitude modulation* or *power modulation* (Fig. 19.5B).[6] Several successive pulses are transmitted for each line alternating between low power and *very* low power (half-amplitude of the low-power pulse). Linear signals that return from tissue are similar in phase and frequency. Accordingly, this signal can be eliminated by doubling the half-amplitude (very low power) signal and subtracting from the low-power signal. Because microbubbles produce a nonlinear signal at low but not very low power, doubling the low-power linear signal does not completely cancel the signal. Signals that are not cancelled are again displayed according to amplitude. Because noncancellation occurs even at the fundamental frequency, the received bandwidth can be broadened to include even the relatively stronger fundamental frequencies. A final approach has to use a "chirp" technique, in which frequency is gradually

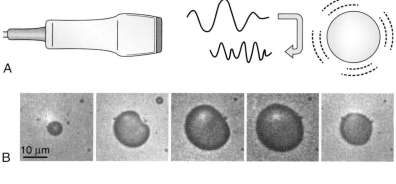

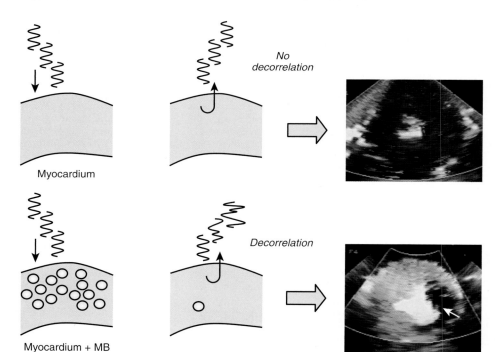

Figure 19.3. A, Schematic illustrating stable cavitation of a microbubble in the oscillating pressures of the ultrasound field with resultant microbubble cavitation and return of broadband signals. **B,** High-speed microscopy illustrating expansion and compression of a lipid microbubble in the pressure fluctuations of an ultrasound field. **C,** Acoustic signal of microbubbles measured from a passive cavitation detector. f_0, Fundamental frequency; Arrows show harmonic frequency range. (*Part B courtesy Nico De Jong, PhD.*)

Figure 19.4. Illustration of high-power multipulse decorrelation techniques for detecting microbubbles (MB) in the myocardium. After transmission of several ultrasound pulses, in the absence of microbubbles, tissue returns signals at a similar frequency (fundamental) to transmitted signals. In the presence of microbubbles, broadband nonlinear signal generation is produced by inertial cavitation in the first several pulses which then become linear (fundamental) after microbubbles are destroyed. Pixel intensity is then displayed according to the degree of pulse decorrelation (difference). The contrast echocardiography images show microbubbles signal in the myocardium except in the inferolateral wall during left circumflex artery occlusion.

increased during a long power pulse, which permits detection of a wider range of the microbubble size distribution.

CLINICAL PERSPECTIVE

The physical properties of microbubbles with regard to rheology and behavior in an acoustic field are important for safety considerations and understanding and optimizing contrast-enhanced ultrasound. Although imaging systems have incorporated many of the microbubble signal detection schemes discussed in this chapter, there are many more user adjustments (power, dynamic range, acoustic focus, line density, and so on) that require knowledge of the interactions between ultrasound and microbubble contrast agents.

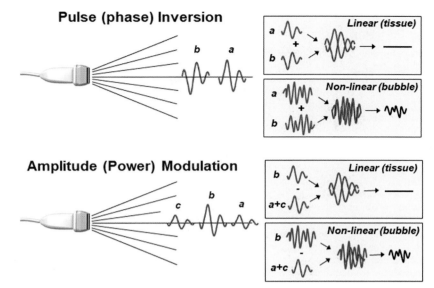

Figure 19.5. Contrast-specific multipulse ultrasound imaging protocols used to increase microbubble signal relative to background or tissue. **A,** During pulse-inversion or phase-inversion imaging, each focused transmit line contains at least two pulses that are phase-inverted by 180 degrees. Returning signals are then summed. Tissue produces linear backscatter at low mechanical index resulting in signal cancellation. Nonlinear signals produced by microbubbles are encoded with many frequencies and do not cancel on summation. **B,** During amplitude modulation imaging, alternating in-phase pulses are transmitted at full and half amplitude. Two received half-amplitude pulses are summed and then subtracted from the full amplitude pulse. Tissue produces linear backscatter at the full and half-amplitude, resulting in signal cancellation. For microbubbles, nonlinear signal generation is much greater for the full-amplitude pulse, resulting in incomplete cancellation by subtraction of the summed half-amplitude signals.

REFERENCES

1. Kaufmann BA, Wei K, Lindner JR. Contrast echocardiography. *Curr Probl Cardiol.* 2007;32:51–96.
2. Kabalnov A, Klein D, Pelura T, et al. Dissolution of multicomponent microbubbles in the bloodstream: 1. *Theory Ultrasound Med Biol.* 1998;24:739–749.
3. Jayaweera AR, Edwards N, Glasheen WP, et al. In vivo myocardial kinetics of air-filled albumin microbubbles during myocardial contrast echocardiography. Comparison with radiolabeled red blood cells. *Circ Res.* 1994;74:1157–1165.
4. Lindner JR, Song J, Jayaweera AR, et al. Microvascular rheology of Definity microbubbles after intra-arterial and intravenous administration. *J Am Soc Echocardiogr.* 2002;15:396–403.
5. Dayton PA, Morgan KE, Klibanov AL, et al. Optical and acoustical observations of the effects of ultrasound on contrast agents. *IEEE Trans Ultrason Ferroelectr Freq Control.* 1999;46:220–232.
6. Chomas JE, Dayton P, Allen J, et al. Mechanisms of contrast agent destruction. *IEEE Trans Ultrason Ferroelectr Freq Control.* 2001;48:232–248.
7. de Jong N, Hoff L, Skotland T, Bom N. Absorption and scatter of encapsulated gas filled microspheres: theoretical considerations and some measurements. *Ultrasonics.* 1992;30:95–103.
8. Burns PN. Harmonic imaging with ultrasound contrast agents. *Clin Radiol.* 1996;51(suppl 1):50–55.

20 | Applications of Ultrasound Contrast Agents

Jonathan R. Lindner, Kevin Wei

Echocardiography plays a critical role in the management of patients, especially in its ability to evaluate left ventricular (LV) global and regional function. Its clinical utility, however, may be affected by image quality. In approximately 10% to 15% of routine echocardiograms and up to 25% to 30% of studies performed in intensive care units, the endocardial border is not clearly defined.[1] Ultrasound contrast agents have been shown in numerous studies to enhance delineation of the endocardial border, which improves both the qualitative and quantitative assessment of LV function and decreases interobserver and intraobserver variability.[2–6]

Several ultrasound-enhancing agents (UEAs) are currently available for clinical use, which are listed in previous chapters. They are approved by regulatory agencies in multiple countries for left ventricular opacification (LVO), which enhances definition of LV endocardial borders in patients with "technically suboptimal" echocardiograms at rest.[7] Some of the agents are also approved for enhancement of Doppler signals.[7] Apart from helping to improve assessment of LV systolic function, ultrasound contrast agents have been shown to enhance the detection and evaluation of other structural abnormalities. This chapter provides examples of common scenarios in which ultrasound contrast agents can provide better delineation of not only cardiac function but also pathology. Not all current clinical applications can be reviewed within the scope of this chapter, and for more details, readers are referred to the most recent consensus statement about contrast agents released by the American Society of Echocardiography.[7]

CLINICAL APPLICATIONS
Assessment of Cardiac Function

The evaluation of right ventricular and LV systolic function is a cornerstone for echocardiography, and it is one of the most common indications for requesting an echocardiographic study. For LV function, inadequate visualization of two or more endocardial borders has been used to define a study as "technically difficult" or "suboptimal." However, ultrasound contrast agents could be used even in studies that are technically adequate. Clinical scenarios in which UEAs for left LVO are thought to be most impactful include (1) when echocardiography is otherwise unable to fully examine LV dimensions or volume in patients in whom all myocardial segments cannot be fully seen; (2) to guide management in critically ill patients who, because of positive-pressure ventilation or an inability to cooperate with the ultrasound examination, have technically difficult windows; and (3) when echocardiography is integrated in critical decision making based on accurate quantification of systolic function or LV dimension at rest or during stress or whether there is a segmental wall motion abnormality in patients with chest pain where every myocardial region needs to be well seen with a high degree of confidence (i.e., during active chest pain).

Studies have consistently demonstrated that UEAs improve feasibility, accuracy, and reproducibility of echocardiography for qualitative and quantitative assessment of LV structure and function at rest and during exercise or pharmacologic stress.[8–12] In one large study evaluating 632 inpatients and outpatients who were considered to have technically difficult or uninterpretable resting echocardiograms, the use of contrast markedly decreased the number of uninterpretable studies from 11.7% to 0.3% and increased the number of technically adequate from 1.6% to 89.9%.[13] The use of ultrasound contrast agents significantly improved patient management as well; additional diagnostic procedures were rendered unnecessary in 32.8% of patients, and drug management was changed in 10.4%.[13]

Accurate determination of LV ejection fraction (EF) provides important prognostic information for patients who have had myocardial infarction and in those with congestive heart failure.[14] Echocardiography can be used serially to assess cardiac function because it uses no ionizing radiation and is easily accessible, portable, and relatively inexpensive compared with other imaging techniques. It is therefore often used to monitor patients receiving cardiotoxic drugs and to determine which patients qualify for device implantation. The use of ultrasound contrast agents improves the accuracy of EF quantification compared with harmonic imaging,[15,16] and measurements of LV volumes and EF have been shown to correlate more closely with those obtained from radionuclide, magnetic resonance, and computed tomographic methods.[17–19]

When using echocardiography to evaluate for wall motion abnormalities at rest, the use of LVO has consistently been shown to increase not only the number of interpretable studies but also the number of interpretable segments. In multicenter studies, the administration of UAEs during echocardiography improved the identification of wall motion abnormalities when using magnetic resonance imaging (MRI) as a gold standard and had the lowest interobserver variability for regional wall motion assessment compared with MRI or echocardiography without contrast.[20,21]

Both pharmacologic and exercise stress echocardiography have been shown to have high sensitivity and specificity for the diagnosis of coronary artery disease, but they mainly rely on the subjective assessment of wall thickening. As such, their accuracy is highly dependent on image quality. Complete visualization of every LV endocardial border is required to confidently document or exclude abnormalities of regional myocardial wall thickening. Studies may be nondiagnostic in up to 30% of patients because of challenges with image acquisition from tachycardia, tachypnea, body habitus, and other causes.[22] With

state-of-the-art LVO, adequate endocardial border resolution can be obtained in up to 95% of patients at peak stress.[8] LVO during stress echocardiography improves reader confidence and the accuracy of this technique for detecting coronary artery disease,[11,12,23,24] resulting in less downstream resource use and greater cost-effectiveness.[23] The use of UEAs in particular helps with the delineation of myocardial segments that often have poor endocardial discrimination, such as the basal portions of the inferior or lateral walls, and the LV apex, which is subject to foreshortening and near-field clutter artifact.

The evaluation of regional cardiac function by echocardiography can be used to triage patients with acute chest pain. The presence of a new resting regional wall motion abnormality (RWMA) has a high sensitivity for detecting cardiac ischemia.[25–28] Those with RWMA were 6.1 times more likely to have cardiac death, acute myocardial infarction, unstable angina, congestive heart failure, or revascularization within 48 hours of presentation ($P < .0001$), and an abnormal echocardiogram was an independent and more useful prognostic indicator than clinical evaluation and electrocardiogram (ECG) findings.[27] Conversely, patients with normal wall motion have a primary event (nonfatal acute myocardial infarction or total mortality) rate of only 0.4%.[28] It should be mentioned that 2.3% of patients discharged from the emergency department after a routine evaluation may have an acute myocardial infarction.[29]

Delineation of Intracardiac Pathology

Ultrasound contrast agents are particularly helpful for defining pathologic findings in the near field, such as at the LV apex. Apical abnormalities may be difficult to delineate clearly because of near-field clutter, lack of harmonic generation, power heterogeneity, and the predisposition towards foreshortening. Contrast can facilitate the identification and assessment of intracardiac masses such as tumors and apical thrombi, apical hypertrophy, isolated LV noncompaction, and apical aneurysms or pseudoaneurysms, among others.

Fig. 20.1 shows an example of a pedunculated thrombus at the apex, which appears as a "filling defect" protruding into the LV cavity. The typical clinical context is a patient with a cardiomyopathy or an associated apical wall thickening abnormality. Occasionally, a sessile or laminated thrombus may be difficult to differentiate from a mass or tumor. In these situations, changing imaging settings to evaluate myocardial perfusion could help differentiate a thrombus from a benign or malignant neoplasm.[30] Thrombi are completely avascular and demonstrate no contrast enhancement. Masses that are brighter than the surrounding myocardium (or hyperenhanced) suggest a highly vascular or malignant tumor, and stromal tumors (e.g., myxomas, lipomas, or fibromas) have a poor blood supply and appear hypoenhanced. Fig. 20.2 shows images from a patient with hypereosinophilia and endomyocardial fibroelastosis who has an unusually "thick" apex delineated on an LVO image (Fig. 20.2A). In Fig. 20.2B, the myocardium and LV cavity are both enhanced with contrast, revealing an obliterative apical thrombus, which appears as a stark filling defect juxtaposed against the contrast-enhanced myocardium and LV cavity.

Fig. 20.3 shows images from a patient with a nonischemic cardiomyopathy who was diagnosed with an apical thrombus (Fig. 20.3A, *arrows*) and treated with anticoagulants; but subsequent contrast-enhanced images revealed that the correct diagnosis (as well as the cause of the patient's LV dysfunction) was isolated LV noncompaction (Fig. 20.3B). The prominent trabeculations and deep intertrabecular recesses are clearly demarcated by the ultrasound contrast agent.

Fig. 20.4 shows images from a patient who had an abnormal ECG and was referred for echocardiography; the patient had suboptimal apical windows and was found to have apical hypertrophic cardiomyopathy. Ultrasound contrast agents may also be used to improve visualization of the right ventricle[31] and great vessels[32] and to enhance systemic Doppler signals[33] (e.g., pulmonary venous inflows or aortic outflow). Fig. 20.5 shows images from a patient

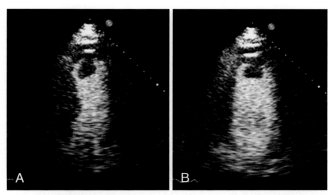

Figure 20.1. Contrast-enhanced systolic (**A**) and diastolic (**B**) frames illustrating a pedunculated apical thrombus. See text for details.

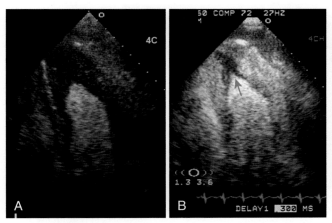

Figure 20.2. Contrast left ventricular opacification image (**A**) from a patient with endomyocardial fibroelastosis, with improved delineation of the apical thrombus using myocardial perfusion imaging settings (**B**, *arrow*). See text for details.

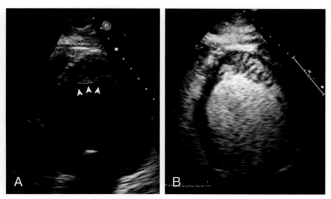

Figure 20.3. Apical four-chamber images before (**A**) and after contrast administration (**B**) illustrating non-compacted myocardium. See text for details.

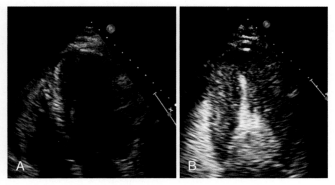

Figure 20.4. Apical 4-chamber view images from a patient with Apical hypertrophic cardiomyopathy before (**A**) and after contrast administration (**B**). See text for details.

with an extensive aortic dissection, but the dissection flap is poorly seen from the subcostal window (Fig. 20.5A). After administration of contrast, the true lumen (Fig. 20.5B) shows much denser contrast enhancement than the false lumen.

Perfusion Imaging With Myocardial Contrast Echocardiography

The commercially available UEAs act as pure intravascular tracers.[34] Accordingly, the degree of signal enhancement in any tissue is proportional to the relative blood volume within that tissue. Hence, signal enhancement during myocardial contrast echocardiography (MCE) is dominated by signal from the capillary compartment. Myocardial perfusion can be assessed by destroying microbubbles within the microcirculation and then examining the rate at which microbubble signal replenishes (microvascular flux rate) and the extent of replenishment (microvascular blood volume). The product of the flux rate and blood volume is an index of perfusion.[35]

When echocardiography is performed to assess segmental wall motion abnormalities at rest, the addition of MCE perfusion imaging can provide incremental information even when a wall motion abnormality is identified. In this situation, perfusion information allows one to determine that the wall motion abnormality is from (1) complete lack of perfusion, (2) hypoperfusion with some antegrade or collateral flow, or (3) stunning when perfusion has normalized but a wall motion abnormality persists (Fig. 20.6).

Perfusion imaging may also be helpful for discerning patterns typical for other conditions, such as stress cardiomyopathy. The use of MCE as a point-of-care technique in patients with acute chest pain has been shown to increase the predictive accuracy for the diagnosis of ischemia beyond clinical information, ECG, and early cardiac enzymes, as well as to provide valuable prognostic information.[27,28] Myocardial perfusion imaging has also been used to improve the performance of exercise or pharmacologic (inotropic or vasodilator) stress testing for the diagnosis of coronary artery disease in stable symptomatic patients. Clinical studies have demonstrated that MCE used together with a variety of different stressors is at least comparable, and possibly superior, to radionuclide single-photon emission computed tomography imaging for the detection of ischemia.[36,37] When compared with wall motion assessment during stress, MCE perfusion imaging results in higher sensitivity for the detection of stenosis, particularly for moderate rather than severe stenosis, or when target work level is not achieved, as well as for detecting multivessel coronary artery disease.[38,39] MCE assessment of myocardial perfusion has also been used for a variety of other applications. These include the assessment of myocardial viability in those with acute and chronic coronary artery disease, differentiating intracardiac mass as thrombus versus tumor, and assessment of microvascular dysfunction (Fig. 20.7).[28,40,41]

SUMMARY

Ultrasound contrast agents can significantly improve the ability of echocardiography to define cardiac function and to more clearly delineate the presence of intracardiac pathologic findings. The use

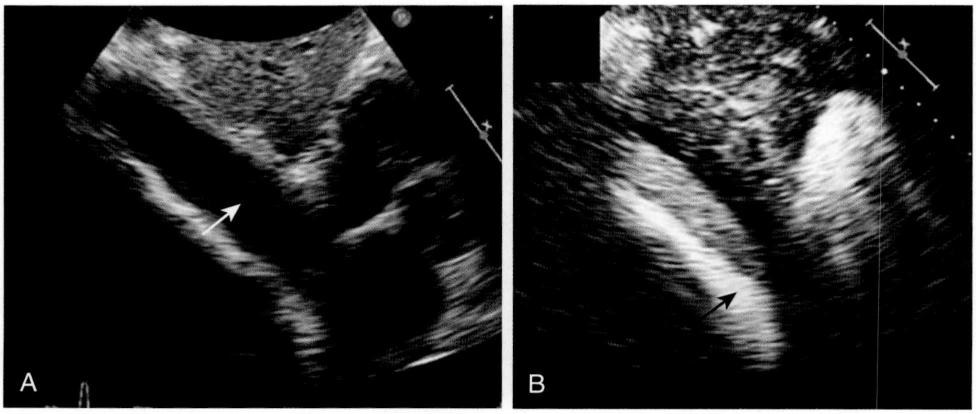

Figure 20.5. Abdominal aorta with dissection before (**A,** *arrow*) and after contrast administration (**B**). The true lumen demonstrates denser signal enhancement (**B,** *black arrow*) compared with the false lumen. See text for details.

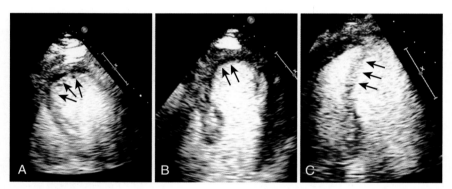

Figure 20.6. Three separate patients presenting with acute coronary syndromes and wall motion abnormality in the left anterior descending (LAD) territory with different myocardial contrast echocardiography perfusion patterns on apical four-chamber view imaging. **A,** Images after destruction-replenishment illustrating transmural lack of perfusion *(arrows)* caused by LAD occlusion. **B,** Images early after microbubble destruction showing subendocardial hypoperfusion of the distal septum and apex. **C,** Images obtained early after a high-power pulse illustrating hyperemic flow in the distal septum *(arrows)*, which was akinetic in a patient who in whom thrombolytic therapy resulted in epicardial artery recanalization.

Figure 20.7. Myocardial contrast echocardiography perfusion imaging in two patients with intracardiac masses *(arrows)* demonstrating partial perfusion at the base of a cardiac metastasis from soft tissue sarcoma (**A**) and widespread spatial extent of tumor perfusion in a metastatic melanoma lesion (**B**). See corresponding Video 20.7.

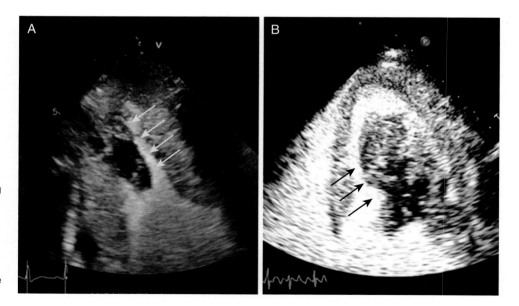

of an ultrasound contrast agent is currently approved for technically suboptimal studies. This definition is intentionally vague. If the presence of pathologic findings is suspected in any cardiac chamber or vascular structure that is not well defined by unenhanced two-dimensional or Doppler images, or accurate and reproducible assessment of chamber volumes or ejection fraction are required, then the study could be considered suboptimal, and use of ultrasound contrast agent is required.

Please access ExpertConsult to view the corresponding videos for this chapter.

REFERENCES

1. Senior R, Dwivedi G, Hayat S, Lim TK. Clinical benefits of contrast-enhanced echocardiography during rest and stress examinations. *Eur J Echocardiogr.* 2006;6(suppl 2):S6–S13.
2. Cohen JL, Cheirif J, Segar DS, et al. Improved left ventricular endocardial border delineation and opacification with OPTISON (FS069), a new echocardiographic contrast agent: results of a phase III multicenter trial. *J Am Coll Cardiol.* 1998;32(3):746–752.
3. Hundley WG, Kizilbash AM, Afridi I, et al. Effect of contrast enhancement of transthoracic echocardiographic assessment of left ventricular regional wall motion. *Am J Cardiol.* 1999;84:1365–1369.
4. Kitzman DW, Goldman ME, Gillam LD, et al. Efficacy and safety of the novel ultrasound contrast agent perflutren (Definity) in patients with suboptimal baseline left ventricular echocardiographic images. *Am J Cardiol.* 2000;86(6):669–674.
5. Lang RM, Mor-Avi V, Zoghbi WA, et al. The role of contrast enhancement in echocardiographic assessment of left ventricular function. *Am J Cardiol.* 2002;90:28J–34J.
6. Nanda NC, Kitzman DW, Dittrich HC, Hall G. Imagent improves endocardial delineation, inter-reader agreement, and the accuracy of segmental wall motion assessment. *Echocardiography.* 2003;20:151–161.
7. Porter TR, Mulvagh SL, Abdelmoneim SS, et al. Clinical applications of Ultrasonic enhancing agents in echocardiography: 2018 American Society of echocardiography Guidelines Update. *J Am Soc Echocardiogr.* 2018;31:241–274.
8. Porter TR, Xie F, Kricsfeld A, et al. Improved endocardial border resolution during dobutamine stress echocardiography with intravenous sonicated dextrose albumin. *J Am Coll Cardiol.* 1994;23:1440–1443.
9. Yokoyama N, Schwarz KQ, Steinmetz SD, et al. Prognostic value of contrast stress echocardiography in patients with image quality too limited for traditional noncontrast harmonic echocardiography. *J Am Soc Echocardiogr.* 2004;17:15–20.
10. Dolan MS, Riad K, El-Shafei A, et al. Effect of intravenous contrast for left ventricular opacification and border definition on sensitivity and specificity of dobutamine stress echocardiography compared with coronary angiography in technically difficult patients. *Am Heart J.* 2001;142:908–915.
11. Rainbird AJ, Mulvagh SL, Oh JK, et al. Contrast dobutamine stress echocardiography: clinical practice assessment in 300 consecutive patients. *J Am Soc Echocardiogr.* 2001;14:378–385.
12. Vlassak I, Rubin DN, Odabashian JA, et al. Contrast and harmonic imaging improves accuracy and efficiency of novice readers for dobutamine stress echocardiography. *Echocardiography.* 2002;19:483–488.
13. Kurt M, Shaikh KA, Peterson L, et al. Impact of contrast echocardiography on evaluation of ventricular function and clinical management in a large prospective cohort. *J Am Coll Cardiol.* 2009;53:802–810.
14. Aronow WS. Epidemiology, pathophysiology, prognosis, and treatment of systolic and diastolic heart failure. *Cardiol Rev.* 2006;14:108–124.
15. Yu EHC, Sloggett CE, Iwanochko RM, et al. Feasibility and accuracy of left ventricular volumes and ejection fraction determination by fundamental, tissue harmonic, and intravenous contrast imaging in difficult-to-image patients. *J Am Soc Echocardiogr.* 2000;13:216–224.
16. Dias BF, Yu EHC, Sloggett CE, et al. Contrast-enhanced quantitation of left ventricular ejection fraction: what is the best method? *J Am Soc Echocardiogr.* 2001;14:1183–1190.
17. Hundley WG, Kizilbash AM, Afridi I, et al. Administration of an intravenous perfluorocarbon contrast agent improves echocardiographic determination of left ventricular volumes and ejection fraction: comparison with cine magnetic resonance imaging. *J Am Coll Cardiol.* 1998;32:1426–1432.
18. Hoffmann R, von Bardeleben S, ten Cate F. Assessment of systolic left ventricular function: a multi-centre comparison of cineventriculography, cardiac magnetic resonance imaging, unenhanced and contrast-enhanced echocardiography. *ACC Curr J Rev.* 2005;14:33–34.
19. Malm S, Frigstad S, Sagberg E, et al. Accurate and reproducible measurement of left ventricular volume and ejection fraction by contrast echocardiography: a comparison with magnetic resonance imaging. *J Am Coll Cardiol.* 2004;44:1030–1035.
20. Hoffmann R, Barletta G, von Bardeleben S, et al. Analysis of left ventricular volumes and function: a multicenter comparison of cardiac magnetic resonance imaging, cine ventriculography, and unenhanced and contrast-enhanced two-dimensional and three-dimensional echocardiography. *J Am Soc Echocardiogr.* 2014;27:292–301.
21. Hoffmann R, von Bardeleben S, Kasprzak JD, et al. Analysis of regional left ventricular function by cineventriculography, cardiac magnetic resonance imaging, and unenhanced and contrast-enhanced echocardiography: a multicenter comparison of methods. *J Am Coll Cardiol.* 2006;47:121–128.
22. Marwick TH, Nemec JJ, Pashkow FJ, et al. Accuracy and limitations of exercise echocardiography in a routine clinical setting. *J Am Coll Cardiol.* 1992;19:74–81.
23. Thanigaraj S, Nease RF, Schechtman KB, et al. Use of contrast for image enhancement during stress echocardiography is cost-effective and reduces additional diagnostic testing. *Am J Cardiol.* 2001;87:1430–1432.
24. Plana JC, Mikati IA, Dokainish H, et al. A randomized cross-over study for evaluation of the effect of image optimization with contrast on the diagnostic accuracy of dobutamine echocardiography in coronary artery disease: the OPTIMIZE trial. *JACC Cardiovasc Imag.* 2008;1:145–152.
25. Sabia P, Afrookteh A, Touchstone DA, et al. Value of regional wall motion abnormality in the emergency room diagnosis of acute myocardial infarction: a prospective study using two-dimensional echocardiography. *Circulation.* 1991;84(Suppl I). I-85–I-92.
26. Kontos MC, Arrowood JA, Paulsen WH, Nixon J. Early echocardiography can predict cardiac events in emergency department patients with chest pain. *Ann Emerg Med.* 1998;31(5):550–557.
27. Rinkevich D, Kaul S, Wang X-Q, et al. Regional left ventricular perfusion and function in patients presenting to the emergency department with chest pain and no ST-segment elevation. *Eur Heart J.* 2005;26(16):1606–1611.
28. Tong KL, Kaul S, Wang X-Q, et al. Myocardial contrast echocardiography versus thrombolysis in myocardial infarction score in patients presenting to the emergency department with chest pain and a nondiagnostic electrocardiogram. *J Am Coll Cardiol.* 2005;46(5):920–927.
29. Lee TH, Rouan GW, Weisberg MC, et al. Clinical characteristics and natural history of patients with acute myocardial infarction sent home from the emergency room. *Am J Cardiol.* 1987;60:219–224.
30. Kirkpatrick JN, Wong T, Bednarz JE, et al. Differential diagnosis of cardiac masses using contrast echocardiographic perfusion imaging. *J Am Coll Cardiol.* 2004;43:1412–1419.
31. Masugata H, Cotter B, Ohmori K, et al. Feasibility of right ventricular myocardial opacification by contrast echocardiography and comparison with left ventricular intensity. *Am J Cardiol.* 1999;84:1137–1140.
32. Kimura BJ, Phan JN, Housman LB. Utility of contrast echocardiography in the diagnosis of aortic dissection. *J Am Soc Echocardiogr.* 1999;12:155–159.
33. Terasawa A, Miyatake K, Nakatani S, et al. Enhancement of Doppler flow signals in the left heart chambers by intravenous injection of sonicated albumin. *J Am Coll Cardiol.* 1993;21(3):737–742.
34. Lindner JR, Song J, Jayaweera AR, et al. Microvascular rheology of Definity microbubbles after intra-arterial and intravenous administration. *J Am Soc Echocardiogr.* 2002;15:396–403.
35. Wei K, Jayaweera AR, Firoozan S, et al. Quantification of myocardial blood flow with ultrasound-induced destruction of microbubbles administered as a constant venous infusion. *Circulation.* 2002;97:473–483.
36. Jeetley P, Hickman M, Kamp O, et al. Myocardial contrast echocardiography for the detection of coronary artery stenosis: a prospective multicenter study in comparison with single-photon emission computed tomography. *J Am Coll Cardiol.* 2006;47:141–145.
37. Senior R, Moreo A, Gaibazzi N, et al. Comparison of sulfur hexafluoride microbubble (SonoVue)-enhanced myocardial contrast echocardiography with gated single-photon emission computed tomography for detection of significant coronary artery disease: a large European multicenter study. *J Am Coll Cardiol.* 2013;62:1353–1361.
38. Shah BN, Chahal NS, Bhattacharyya S, et al. The feasibility and clinical utility of myocardial contrast echocardiography in clinical practice: results from the incorporation of myocardial perfusion assessment into clinical testing with stress echocardiography study. *J Am Soc Echocardiogr.* 2014;27:520–530.
39. Elhendy A, O'Leary EL, Xie F, et al. Comparative accuracy of real-time myocardial contrast perfusion imaging and wall motion analysis during dobutamine stress echocardiography for the diagnosis of coronary artery disease. *J Am Coll Cardiol.* 2004;44:2185–2191.
40. Kaufmann BA, Wei K, Lindner JR. Contrast echocardiography. *Curr Probl Cardiol.* 2007;32:51–96.
41. Taqui S, Ferencik M, Davidson BP, et al. Coronary microvascular dysfunction by myocardial contrast echocardiography in nonelderly patients referred for computed tomographic coronary angiography. *J Am Soc Echocardiogr.* 2019;32:817–825.

21 Use of Contrast in the Intensive Care Unit and Emergency Department

Kyle R. Lehenbauer, Michael L. Main

CONTRAST USE IN THE INTENSIVE CARE UNIT

Patients in the intensive care unit (ICU) setting have a variety of illnesses, and echocardiography can offer real-time information on cardiac function, hemodynamics, and, in certain patients, potential causes of their illnesses. Furthermore, because echocardiography is noninvasive, portable, and free of ionizing radiation, it is an ideal tool for ICU patient care. However, the ICU is an often hostile environment for acquisition of transthoracic echocardiography (TTE) images. ICU patient rooms are often crowded with less than ideal lighting, and patient- and disease-state related factors, including endotracheal intubation and mechanical ventilation; obscuration of optimal imaging windows because of surgical dressings, chest tubes, and other support devices; and inability to properly position the patient because of a lack of a drop section, presence of restraints, and inability of the patient to cooperate (among many others), all increase the degree of imaging difficulty and worsen the odds for completion of a technically adequate examination, which completely answers the attending physician's clinical questions.

Following approval of the first transpulmonary ultrasound-enhancing agent (UEA) (Optison, GE Healthcare, 1995), several early studies described the efficacy of UEAs in improving image quality and diagnostic accuracy in the ICU. UEAs improve image quality, wall motion scoring, and left ventricular ejection fraction (LVEF) calculation in both unselected ICU patients[1] and in patients who are mechanically ventilated.[2] Additionally, in ICU patients with baseline very technically difficult echocardiograms (>50% of the myocardial segments not visualized from any view), UEA use improved the ability to estimate ejection fraction from 31% of studies to 97% and improved agreement with transesophageal echocardiography (TEE) for regional wall motion assessment from 48% at baseline to 70% with UEAs. Furthermore, contrast echocardiography was cost-effective in comparison with TEE.[3]

In 2007, the United States Food and Drug Administration (FDA) issued a Black Box warning, contraindicating the use of UEA in most ICU patients, including patients with the following diagnoses: "acute myocardial infarction or acute coronary syndromes, worsening or decompensated heart failure, serious ventricular arrhythmias or patients at high risk for arrhythmias based on QT interval prolongation, as well as respiratory failure, severe emphysema, pulmonary emboli or other conditions which may cause pulmonary hypertension."[4]

These warnings followed spontaneous healthcare provider reports of four patient deaths, which occurred in close temporal relationship to UEA administration. Critics of the FDA action noted the lack of a documented causal relationship between UEA administration and these outcomes, the previously described excellent safety and efficacy profile of UEAs, the potential risks of alternative procedures such as TEE and nuclear scintigraphy, and the likely contribution of "pseudo complications" to these serious adverse events (complications caused by progression of the underlying disease state rather than a contemporaneous procedure or diagnostic examination).[4,5]

In early 2008, Kusnetzky and colleagues described acute mortality rates in a large cohort of 18,671 hospitalized patients who underwent echocardiography. A total of 12,475 patients underwent unenhanced echocardiography, and 6196 patients underwent echocardiography with the UEA Definity (Lantheus Medical Imaging). At 24 hours after the transthoracic echocardiogram, 0.37% of patients in the unenhanced echocardiography arm and 0.42% of patients in the UEA arm had died (not significant). The authors concluded that there was no demonstrable increased mortality risk with UEA administration, even in sick patients (and in fact in this study, there were no deaths in the contrast arm within 1 hour of UEA administration).[6]

Over the next several years, multiple studies were conducted in the inpatient and ICU settings (several of which were mandated by the FDA) that have better informed us regarding both the safety and efficacy of UEAs.[6–14] These studies are summarized in Table 21.1. Based on this evidence and other considerations, the FDA modified the Black Box warning, and there is now widespread agreement that these agents are not only safe but also indicated in the ICU setting, including patients with clinical diagnoses previously on the FDA contraindication list.

One risk of UEA has been identified in several series, serious allergic (anaphylactoid) reactions, occurred in ~1:10,000 patients.[7,9] These reactions are categorized as CARPA reactions (complement activation–related pseudoallergy), a recently described variant of the classic type 1 hypersensitivity reaction.[15] Unlike common food and drug type 1 hypersensitivity reactions, CAPRA reactions are not immunoglobulin E mediated, do not require prior exposure, tend to me milder or absent on repeat exposure, and usually resolve spontaneously. Additionally, there is a higher reaction rate among the general population, particularly in women and individuals with preexisting food and drug allergies, so-called "atopic" individuals. CARPA reactions may occasionally be life threatening and manifest similar to any other anaphylactic reaction. Although there is no evidence that these reactions occur more frequently in the critically ill patient population, patients with serious illness may be more likely to succumb given lack of clinical reserve. Rapid point-of-care administration of intramuscular epinephrine may be lifesaving in very serious CARPA reactions, and this medication (and other drugs used in the treatment of serious allergic reactions such as inhaled beta-agonists) should be readily available at the point of care (and particularly in ICUs) outside of the usual "crash cart" provision.

Several studies have also confirmed the association between UEA use in ICUs and improved patient outcomes. Main and colleagues used the Premier database (Premier Inc., the largest US hospital–based service-level comparative database) to compare 48-hour mortality and hospital stay mortality in a cohort of critically ill, propensity-matched patients undergoing echocardiography either with (16,217 patients) or without (16,217 patients) a UEA.[13] At 48 hours, mortality in the UEA group was lower than the unenhanced echocardiography group (1.7% vs 2.5%; 95% confidence interval [CI], 0.54–0.80) (Fig. 21.1). This difference between the two groups persisted until hospital discharge. Although the underlying etiologic explanation for lower mortality rate in the UEA group was beyond the scope of this study, potential mechanisms include earlier and more accurate diagnosis leading to better patient management and the avoidance of inherent

TABLE 21.1 Large Studies (>1000 patients) That Have Evaluated Contrast Use in the Inpatient or Intensive Care Unit Setting

Author, Publication Date	Study Design	ECA	Total Patients	UEA Patients	Control Patients	Inpatient or Outpatient	Rest or Stress	Outcomes
Herzog et al.,[7] 2008	Retrospective	Definity or Optison	16,025	16,025	NA	Both	Both	No short-term deaths; serious adverse events in 0.031%
Kusnetzky et al.,[6] 2008	Retrospective	Definity	18,671	6196	12,475	Inpatients	Rest	No increased mortality rate in UEA patients
Main et[8] al., 2008	Retrospective	Definity	4,300,966	58,254	4,242,712	Inpatients	Rest	No increased mortality rate in UEA patients
Wei et al.,[9] 2008	Retrospective	Definity or Optison	78,383	78,383	NA	Both	Both	Severe allergic reactions in 0.01% and anaphylactoid reactions in 0.006%
Exuzides et al.,[10] 2019	Retrospective	Optison	14,500	2900	11,600	Inpatients	Rest	No increased mortality rate in UEA patients
Goldberg et al.,[11] 2012	Retrospective	Definity	96,705	2518	94,187	Both	Both	No increase mortality rate in UEA patients
Wever-Pinzon et al.,[12] 2012	Retrospective	Definity	1513	1513	NA	Inpatients	Both	No deaths or SAE attributed to UEA in patients with pulmonary hypertension
Main et al.,[13] 2014	Retrospective	Definity	32,434	16,217	16,217	Inpatients	Rest	UEA use associated with a 28% lower mortality rate

SAE, serious adverse event; *UEA,* ultrasound-enhancing agent.

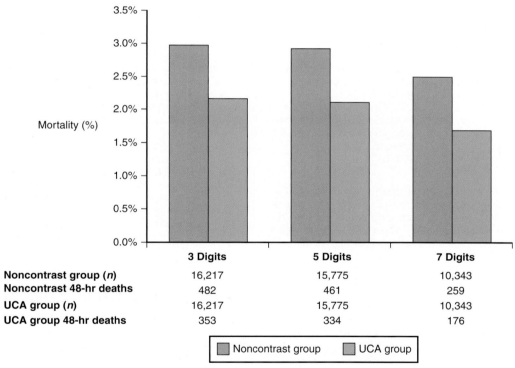

Figure 21.1. Mortality at 48 h in the UEA and Noncontrast Echocardiography Groups. At 3-, 5-, and 7-decimal-place matching, patients undergoing echocardiography with an ultrasound contrast agent (UCA) had lower 48-h mortality than patients undergoing unenhanced echocardiography. (Reproduced with permission from Main et al: Acute mortality in critically ill patients undergoing echocardiography with or without an ultrasound contrast agent, JACC Cardiovasc Imaging 7:40-48, 2014.)

risks associated with downstream testing. In fact, limited data have documented clinical utility and safety even in patients with left ventricular assist devices[16] and patients undergoing extracorporeal membrane oxygenation[17] (although a perfusionist or critical care physician should be present during the UEA examination given propensity of these systems to automatically shut down if bubbles are detected by the sensing mechanism).[18]

In a pivotal outcomes study by Kurt and colleagues,[19] 632 consecutive patients with baseline technically difficult or uninterpretable studies underwent both an unenhanced and a UEA

study. After UEA, the percent of uninterpretable studies decreased from 11.7% to 0.3%, and the technically difficult rate decreased from 86.7% to 9.8%. This dramatic improvement in study quality was associated with important management changes: overall, 35.6% of patients had a downstream procedure avoided, a change in medication, or both a medication and procedure change because of the UEA examination. This effect was even more dramatic in the surgical ICU, where approximately two-thirds of patients had an important management change attributable to the UEA study (Fig. 21.2).

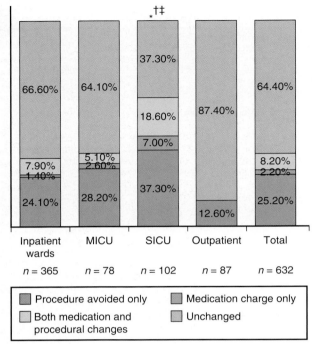

Figure 21.2. "Frequency of total impact of contrast use on patient management. The highest impact was observed for inpatients, particularly in the SICU." *Asterisk* indicates p < 0.0001 comparing SICU with inpatient ward, *dagger* indicates p < 0.0001 comparing SICU with outpatients, and *double dagger* indicates p = 0.0004 comparing SICU and MICU. *MICU,* Medical intensive care unit; *SICU,* surgical intensive care unit. (Reproduced with permission from Kurt M, et al. Impact of contrast echocardiography on evaluation of ventricular function and clinical management in a large prospective cohort. *J Am Coll Cardiol* 53:802–810, 2009)

Confirmation of these findings was recently presented in a follow-up study using the Premier database.[14] A total of 1,538,864 ICU patients from 773 hospitals underwent transthoracic echocardiography either with (n = 51,141) or without (n = 1,487,723) a UEA. After adjusting for patient, clinical, and hospital characteristics, patients in the UEA cohort were less likely to undergo a subsequent TTE or TEE (odds ratio [OR], 0.704 for TTE; OR, 0.841 for TEE; P < .001 for both). Additionally, the mean ICU length of stay was shorter in the UEA cohort (4.15 days vs 4.59 days, P <0.001), and UEA patients were more likely to experience either an initiation or discontinuation of a parenteral inotrope, anticoagulant, or vasopressor on the day of or the day after the echocardiographic study, consistent with results of the study by Kurt and colleagues.

Pulmonary hypertension is frequently encountered in ICUs and was identified in 2007 as a disease state contraindication by the FDA. In conjunction with the FDA, two invasive cardiac catheterization studies were conducted to evaluate the effect of UEAs on pulmonary hemodynamics in patients with normal and elevated baseline pulmonary artery systolic pressure. No significant changes in pulmonary artery systolic pressure or pulmonary vascular resistance were noted after intravenous injection of clinically relevant does of Optison[20] or Definity.[21] More recently, Wever-Pinzon and colleagues[12] evaluated the potential effects of the UEA Definity in 1513 hospitalized patients with pulmonary hypertension (60% mild pulmonary hypertension, 34% moderate pulmonary hypertension, and 6% severe pulmonary hypertension). The incidence of adverse events was extremely low (0.002%), and no events were attributable to the UEA. Based on these three studies, UEA use in patients with pulmonary hypertension is considered safe and is no longer contraindicated by the FDA.

UEA use may be particularly helpful in cardiac ICUs in the treatment of patients with acute myocardial infarction. With drug and device therapy increasingly dependent on LVEF partition values, accurate and reproducible LVEF data are critical. UEA use improves LVEF agreement with cardiac magnetic resonance imaging (the standard reference technique) in unselected patients[22] and improves interobserver agreement in assessment of left ventricular (LV) systolic function even in patients with good baseline endocardial border resolution.[23] Additionally, contrast markedly improves our ability to diagnose or exclude LV thrombus. In the Kurt study of 632 patients with technically difficult echocardiograms,[19] an LV thrombus was suspected in 35 patients and thought to be definitely present in 3 patients at baseline; with addition of an UEA, only 1 patient had a suspected thrombus, and 5 additional patients with thrombus were identified (P < 0.0001). Finally, myocardial contrast echocardiography can differentiate myocardial stunning from necrosis immediately after percutaneous intervention in acute myocardial infarction, and aids in risk stratification.[24]

In light of this data, the 2018 American Society of Echocardiography (ASE) Guidelines Update for Clinical Applications of Ultrasonic Enhancing Agents lists the following recommendations for UEA use in the ICU setting[25]:

1. "Given a demonstrated impact on patient management and an association with mortality reduction, UEAs are recommended in all technically difficult ICU and ED patients to more quickly and accurately diagnose potentially life-threatening conditions and to reduce the need for downstream diagnostic testing. Contrast echocardiography should not be withheld on the basis of any particular diagnosis or co-morbidity." (Class I recommendation, Level of Evidence B-NR [moderate-quality evidence from one or more well-designed nonrandomized trials, observational studies, or registry studies of meta-analysis of such studies.])
2. "Myocardial contrast echocardiography with very low mechanical index imaging may be used in post-STEMI patients to evaluate for LV-systolic function, intracavitary thrombi, and microvascular flow within the infarct territory at institutions with sonographer and physician expertise in performance and interpretation of myocardial perfusion echocardiography." (Class IIa recommendation, Level of Evidence B-NR [moderate-quality evidence from one or more well-designed nonrandomized trials, observational studies, or registry studies of meta-analysis of such studies.])

CONTRAST USE IN THE EMERGENCY DEPARTMENT

Patients presenting to the emergency department (ED) with chest pain pose a significant diagnostic challenge. Typically, decision making is based on the clinical history, physical examination, cardiac enzyme analysis, and electrocardiogram (ECG), which are then incorporated into overall clinical risk calculators to aid in patient triage.

In most patients presenting to the ED with chest pain, there is no clear ST-segment elevation on the presenting ECG, and these patients often wait several hours in the ED (for repeat cardiac enzyme analysis) before disposition. Point-of-care echocardiographic assessment of regional and global LV systolic function and myocardial perfusion (MP) may be a powerful adjunct to existing diagnostic strategies.

In an early study by Kaul and colleagues in the ED setting,[26] contrast echocardiographic assessment of regional wall motion and MP was comparable to single-photon computed tomography; contrast echocardiography provided 17% incremental information over demographic, clinical, and ECG parameters for the prediction of cardiac events.

Rinkevich et al.[27] studied 1017 patients who presented to the ED with chest pain, all of whom underwent contrast echocardiography

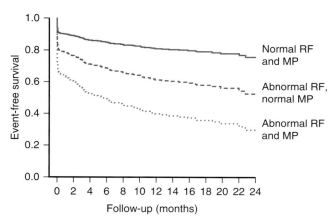

Figure 21.3. Event-free survival in patients with an intermediate-risk modified Thrombolysis in Myocardial Infarction score (3 or 4). *MP,* Myocardial perfusion; *RF,* regional function. (Reproduced with permission from Tong KL, et al: Myocardial contrast echocardiography versus Thrombolysis In Myocardial Infarction score in patients presenting to the emergency department with chest pain and a nondiagnostic electrocardiogram, *J Am Coll Cardiol* 46:920–927, 2005.)

for assessment of regional function (RF) and MP. Early assessment of these echocardiographic variables added significantly to risk stratification for subsequent cardiac-related death, acute myocardial infarction, unstable angina, heart failure, and revascularization. Patients with abnormal RF were 6.1 times (CI, 3.5–10.6) more likely to experience an early event compared with patients with normal RF, and patients with abnormal MP were 2.4 times (CI, 1.5–3.7) more likely to experience an early event compared with patients with normal MP. When both RF and MP were abnormal, the odds ratio for an early cardiac event was 14.2 times (CI, 8.3–24.8) higher than in patients with normal echocardiographic findings.

Tong and colleagues[28] extended these findings in a study of 957 patients with chest pain and a nondiagnostic ECG who underwent RF and MP assessment in the ED. In this study, the modified Thrombolysis In Myocardial Infarction score was unable to differentiate between intermediate- and high-risk patients at early, intermediate, or late follow-up, whereas RF provided incremental prognostic data for predicting intermediate and late events. In patients with abnormal RF, MP offered additional refinement of risk for classification into intermediate- and high-risk groups (Fig. 21.3).

Although abnormal findings of RF and MP are predictors of adverse cardiac events, it is important to note that an overwhelming number of patients presenting to the ED with chest pain do not have an underlying acute coronary syndrome or even obstructive coronary artery disease. Therefore, the negative predictive value of contrast echocardiography in the ED also makes it a powerful triaging tool. Patients with normal contrast echocardiography findings (both wall motion analysis and perfusion analysis) have an acute myocardial infarction rate estimated at 0.6% within 24 hours of ED presentation. Furthermore, it is estimated that up to 55% of patients in the ED could avoid hospital admission and downstream resource utilization if they are found to have normal RF and MP. Finally, Wyrick and colleagues[29] have estimated an average savings of at least $900 per patient using a contrast echocardiography strategy in the ED setting.

Based on these studies, the 2018 ASE Guidelines Update for Clinical Applications of Ultrasonic Enhancing Agents lists the following recommendations for UEA use in the ED setting:[25]

1. "In patients presenting to the ED with suspected myocardial ischemia (and non-diagnostic ECG), regional function assessment with UEAs adds incremental diagnostic and prognostic value over traditional clinical and electrocardiographic evaluation and may reduce healthcare costs." (Class I recommendation, Level of Evidence B-NR [moderate-quality evidence from one or more well-designed nonrandomized trials, observational studies, or registry studies of meta-analysis of such studies.])

2. "In patients presenting to the ED with suspected myocardial ischemia (and non-diagnostic ECG), myocardial perfusion assessment with UEAs adds incremental diagnostic and prognostic value (over traditional clinical, electrocardiographic, and regional function assessment) and may reduce costs. This technique should be considered at centers with sonographer and physician expertise in performance and interpretation of myocardial perfusion echocardiography." (Class IIa recommendation, Level of Evidence B-NR [moderate-quality evidence from one or more well-designed nonrandomized trials, observational studies, or registry studies of meta-analysis of such studies])

SUMMARY

Contrast echocardiography is safe and effective in the ICU and ED settings. In the ICU, contrast echocardiography directly influences patient management, resulting in a reduction in downstream testing and important changes in therapeutic intervention. Large studies in the ICU population have shown an association between contrast echocardiography and reduced mortality rates. In the ER, contrast echocardiography affords assessment of both RF and MP, which in turn improves patient triage; predicts early, intermediate, and late cardiac events; and has the potential to reduce health care costs.

REFERENCES

1. Reilly JP, Tunick PA, Timmermans RJ, et al. Contrast echocardiography clarifies uninterpretable wall motion in intensive care unit patients. *J Am Coll Cardiol.* 2000;35:485–490.
2. Kornbluth M, Liang DH, Brown P, et al. Contrast echocardiography is superior to tissue harmonics for assessment of left ventricular function in mechanically ventilated patients. *Am Heart J.* 2000;140:291–296.
3. Yong Y, Wu D, Fernandes V, et al. Diagnostic accuracy and cost-effectiveness of contrast echocardiography on evaluation of cardiac function in technically very difficult patients in the intensive care unit. *Am J Cardiol.* 2002;89:711–718.
4. Muskula PR, Main ML. Safety with echocardiographic contrast agents. *Circ Cardiovasc Imaging.* 2017;10. e005459.
5. Main ML, Goldman JH, Grayburn PA. Thinking outside the "box"—the ultrasound contrast controversy. *J Am Coll Cardiol.* 2007;50:2434–2437.
6. Kusnetzky LL, Khalid A, Khumri TM, et al. Acute mortality in hospitalized patients undergoing echocardiography with and without an ultrasound contrast agent: results in 18,671 consecutive studies. *J Am Coll Cardiol.* 2008;51(17):1704–1706.
7. Herzog CA: Incidence of adverse events associated with use of perflutren contrast agents for echocardiography, *JAMA* 2008;299:2023–2025..
8. Main ML, Ryan AC, Davis TE, et al. Acute mortality in hospitalized patients undergoing echocardiography with and without an ultrasound contrast agent (multicenter registry results in 4,300,966 consecutive patients). *Am J Cardiol.* 2008;102:1742–1746.
9. Wei K, Mulvagh SL, Carson L, et al. The safety of Definity and Optison for ultrasound image enhancement: a retrospective analysis of 78,383 administered contrast doses. *J Am Soc Echocardiogr.* 2008;21:1202–1206.
10. Exuzides A, Main ML, Colby C, et al. A retrospective comparison of mortality in critically ill hospitalized patients undergoing echocardiography with and without an ultrasound contrast agent. *JACC Cardiovasc Imaging.* 2010;3:578–585.
11. Goldberg YH, Ginelli P, Siegel R, et al. Administration of perflutren contrast agents during transthoracic echocardiography is not associated with a significant increase in acute mortality risk. *Cardiology.* 2012;122:119–125.
12. Wever-Pinzon O, Suma V, Ahuja A, et al. Safety of echocardiographic contrast in hospitalized patients with pulmonary hypertension: a multi-center study. *Eur Heart J Cardiovasc Imaging.* 2012;13:857–862.
13. Main ML, Hibberd MG, Ryan A, et al. Acute mortality in critically ill patients undergoing echocardiography with or without an ultrasound contrast agent. *JACC Cardiovasc Imaging.* 2014;7:40–48.
14. Main ML, Weleski Fu J, Gundrum J, et al. Impact of contrast echocardiography on clinical outcomes in critically ill patients. *Am J Cardiol.* 2020 (under review).
15. Szebeni J. Complement activation-related pseudoallergy: a new class of drug-induced acute immune toxicity. *Toxicology.* 2005;216:106–121.

16. Fine NM, Abdelmoneim SS, Dichak A, et al. Safety and feasibility of contrast echocardiography for LVAD evaluation. *JACC Cardiovasc Imaging*. 2014;7:429–430.

17. Bennett CE, Tweet MS, Michelena HI, et al. Safety and feasibility of contrast echocardiography for ECMO evaluation. *JACC Cardiovasc Imaging*. 2017;10:603–604.

18. Grecu L, Fishman MA. Beware of life threatening activation of air bubble detector during contrast echocardiography in patients on venoarterial extracorporeal membrane oxygenator support. *J Am Soc Echocardiogr*. 2014;27:1130–1131.

19. Kurt M, Shaikh KA, Peterson L, et al. Impact of contrast echocardiography on evaluation of ventricular function and clinical management in a large prospective cohort. *J Am Coll Cardiol*. 2009;53:802–810.

20. Main ML, Grayburn PA, Lang RM, et al. Effect of Optison on pulmonary artery systolic pressure and pulmonary vascular resistance. *Am J Cardiol*. 2013;112:1657–1661.

21. Wei K, Main ML, Lang RM, et al. The effect of Definity on systemic and pulmonary hemodynamics in patients. *J Am Soc Echocardiogr*. 2012;25:584–588.

22. Malm S, Frigstad S, Sagberg E, et al. Accurate and reproducible measurement of left ventricular volume and ejection fraction by contrast echocardiography: a comparison with magnetic resonance imaging. *J Am Coll Cardiol*. 2004;44:1030–1035.

23. Nayyar S, Magalski A, Khumri TM, et al. Contrast administration reduces interobserver variability in determination of left ventricular ejection fraction in patients with left ventricular dysfunction and good baseline endocardial border delineation. *Am J Cardiol*. 2006;98:1110–1114.

24. Main ML, Magalski A, Chee NK, et al. Full-motion pulse inversion power Doppler contrast echocardiography differentiates stunning from necrosis and predicts recovery of left ventricular function after acute myocardial infarction. *J Am Coll Cardiol*. 2001;38:1390–1394.

25. Porter TR, Mulvagh SL, Abdelmoneim SS, et al. Clinical applications of ultrasonic enhancing agents in echocardiography: 2018 American Society of Echocardiography guidelines update. *J Am Soc Echocardiogr*. 2018;31:241–274.

26. Kaul S, Senior R, Firschke C, et al. Incremental value of cardiac imaging in patients presenting to the emergency department with chest pain and without ST-segment elevation: a multicenter study. *Am Heart J*. 2004;148:129–136.

27. Rinkevich D, Kaul S, Wang XQ, et al. Regional left ventricular perfusion and function in patients presenting to the emergency department with chest pain and no ST-segment elevation. *Eur Heart J*. 2005;26:1606–1611.

28. Tong KL, Kaul S, Wang XQ, et al. Myocardial contrast echocardiography versus Thrombolysis in Myocardial Infarction score in patients presenting to the emergency department with chest pain and a nondiagnostic electrocardiogram. *J Am Coll Cardiol*. 2005;46:920–927.

29. Wyrick JJ, Kalvaitis S, McConnell KJ, et al. Cost-efficiency of myocardial contrast echocardiography in patients presenting to the emergency department with chest pain of suspected cardiac origin and a nondiagnostic electrocardiogram. *Am J Cardiol*. 2008;102(6):649–652.

22 Technical Aspects of Contrast Echocardiography

Matt M. Umland, Sarah M. Roemer

In 2001, the American Society of Echocardiography (ASE) published a position paper that provided guidelines for sonographers performing contrast-enhanced echocardiographic studies. This chapter focuses on the sonographer's role in four specific areas: (1) understanding of microbubble physics and ultrasound instrumentation, (2) recognition of indications for the use of contrast media, (3) need for establishment of intravenous (IV) access privileges, and (4) development of written policies for contrast agent infusion or injection.[1] The purpose of this chapter is to discuss the technical aspects and provide tips for the use of contrast enhancement to optimize the visualization of endocardial borders and cardiac structures.

INDICATIONS

The 2008 ASE guidelines suggested that ultrasound-enhancing agents (UEAs) should be used when two or more left ventricular (LV) segments cannot be adequately visualized for the assessment of LV function, including ejection fraction and regional wall motion (RWM).[2,3] The use of UEAs for LV opacification improves the feasibility, accuracy, and reproducibility of echocardiography for the qualitative and quantitative assessment of LV structure and function at rest and during exercise or pharmacologic stress testing. Contrast enhancement facilitates the identification and assessment of intracardiac masses, such as tumors and thrombi; improves the visualization of the right ventricle and great vessels; and enhances Doppler signals used for evaluating valvular function.[4] UEAs should be considered to document or exclude the following structural abnormalities: apical hypertrophy, noncompaction, thrombus, endomyocardial fibrosis, LV apical ballooning, LV aneurysm, LV pseudoaneurysm, and myocardial rupture. UEAs may also be considered to identify and characterize intracardiac masses and to differentiate cardiac structural variants.[4]

AVAILABLE TYPES OF CONTRAST AGENTS

Software and presets for LV opacification using low mechanical index (MI) harmonic imaging have been available on nearly all commercial systems for more than a decade. Three UEAs (Optison, Definity, and Lumason) are approved by the US Food and Drug Administration for the indication of LV opacification; all other applications in cardiovascular imaging constitute off-label uses.

STEP-BY-STEP PROTOCOL

The first step after recognition of the need for UEA and assuring exclusion of any potential allergic reaction is to gain IV access. IV access remains one of the biggest obstacles to administering UEAs in clinical echocardiography laboratories. It is critical that echocardiography laboratories work with administrators to adopt a user-friendly IV insertion program that will promote the use of UEAs in technically difficult studies in both the outpatient and inpatient settings. The 2001 statement released by ASE supports IV training for sonographers in hospital and clinic settings. This training requires knowledge of aseptic technique, venous anatomy, appropriate sites of access, risks to patients, and hospital approval to perform the procedure. In addition, individual echocardiographic laboratories should work together with their institutional review board committees to decide on the appropriate manner to obtain consent from the patients.

The second step includes proper setup of the ultrasound systems and administration of the contrast agent. In general, low-MI harmonic imaging requires lowering the MI to less than 0.3 while using the harmonic imaging mode and the administration of small contrast boluses followed by slow saline flushes (3–5 mL over 5–10 sec).[1] If the MI setting is too high, it may cause a destruction of the microbubbles and swirling of contrast, resulting in nonuniform LV opacification. Fig. 22.1 and Video 22.1 demonstrate imaging with a low MI setting of 0.19, which is then increased to 0.50 in the same video clip, transitioning from full opacification to a swirling presentation. After IV injection, the microbubbles transit rapidly through the lungs, cardiac chambers, and myocardium without affecting LV function, coronary or systemic hemodynamics, ischemic markers, or pulmonary gas exchange.[4] Adequate opacification can be seen from the apex to the mitral annular plane in the apical view (Fig. 22.2 and Video 22.2). In addition to proper

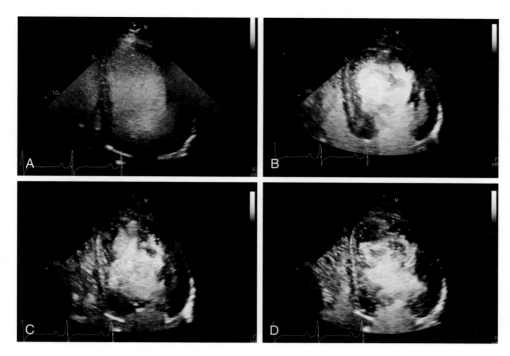

Figure 22.1. Example of contrast administration at different mechanical index settings: 0.09 (**A**), 0.30 (**B**), 0.40 (**C**), and 0.50 (**D**). See accompanying Video 22.1.

administration techniques, system settings, including gain and compression, should be properly adjusted to reduce background noise.[1] Compression settings allow for adjustment of the black-and-white interface of the structures.

UEA opacification can be challenging because of various artifacts (Table 22.1). UEA-related artifacts are most commonly caused by suboptimal administration techniques. A high-bolus dosage is likely to cause an attenuation artifact in the LV apex, resulting in acoustic shadowing of the LV base and midsegments. This artifact will spontaneously resolve over time but can be actively avoided with proper administration. On the other hand, a lower-bolus dosage is to likely cause a swirling artifact in the LV apex due to insufficient amount of contrast being administered (see Fig. 22.1 and Video 22.1). If available, a high-MI "flash" technique can be used to enhance endocardial definition. This high-power impulse delivers a quick burst of power lasting three to five frames and clearing contrast from the myocardium to improve image quality.[1]

Additional system adjustments are recommended to also improve image quality (see Table 22.1). After injection of UEA, the opacified blood in the left ventricle fills the intertrabecular spaces up to the compacted myocardium, allowing more accurate and reproducible tracing of the endocardial boundaries. According to the recent ASE/European Association of Cardiovascular Imaging recommendations for LV chamber quantification, volumetric measurements should be based on tracings at the interface between the compacted and noncompacted myocardium.[4,5] Care should be taken to avoid foreshortening of apical images, which is likely to result in an underestimation of ventricular volumes and an overestimation of LV ejection fraction. Standard imaging planes should include the apical four-chamber, two-chamber, long-axis, and parasternal long- and short-axis views. Additional aliquots of UEAs may be necessary for opacification of all views.

COMPLICATIONS OF ULTRASOUND-ENHANCING AGENTS

Although anaphylactoid reactions to UEAs are rare, it is advised that sonographers follow a preestablished policy for early

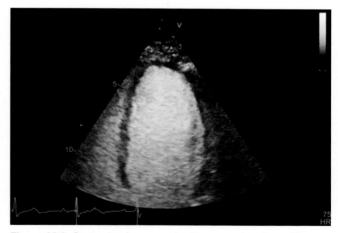

Figure 22.2. Contrast enhancement using proper imaging settings, resulting in optimal left ventricular opacification. See accompanying Video 22.2.

recognition and effective management of these rare acute life-threatening reactions. This policy needs to outline the process required for activation and implementation of the roles of team members involved in the treatment of acute allergic reactions to UEAs. Cardiopulmonary resuscitation personnel and equipment should be readily available before UEA administration, and all patients should be monitored for acute reactions. Allergy kits should be readily available in all echocardiography laboratories that administer UEAs. The kits should be placed in areas where contrast materials are frequently administered. The nurses or designated medical personnel should be responsible for maintaining the kits and performing monthly checks for expiration dates. When an allergic reaction is identified, the nurse should assess the patient, initiate treatment on the basis of the symptoms, and immediately notify the supervising physician. Depending on the severity of the anaphylactic reaction, assistance of the rapid-response team or code team may be required. Although

TABLE 22.1 Image Artifacts Associated With Suboptimal Administration of Contrast Media

Artifact Location	Artifact or Problem	Correction Strategy	Key Points
LV cavity contrast	Swirling	Decrease MI, increase dosage, adjust focal zone to near field	Lower frame rate prevents apical bubble destruction
LV cavity contrast	Shadowing of basal or midsegments	Reduce dosage (bolus or infusion rate)	Infusion compared with bolus reduces shadowing issues
LV apex contrast	Insufficient contrast	Increase near-field TGC, move focus position to near field, increase dosage	Reduced contrast concentration may assist trabeculation or thrombus visualization in some cases

LV, Left ventricular; *MI,* mechanical index; *TGC,* time-gain compensation.

respiratory distress caused by bronchospasm is the most serious concern, other reactions include shock; urticarial, facial, or laryngeal edema; seizures; and convulsions.[2]

Please access ExpertConsult to view the corresponding videos for this chapter.

REFERENCES

1. Porter T, Abdelmoneim S, Belcik JT, et al. Guidelines for the cardiac sonographer in the performance of contrast echocardiography. *J Am Soc Echocardiogr.* 2014;27:797–810.
2. Porter T, Mulvagh S, Abdelmoneim S, et al. Clinical applications of ultrasonic enhancing agents in echocardiography: 2018 American Society of Echocardiography guidelines update. *J Am Soc Echocardiogr.* 2018;31:241–274.
3. Intersocietal Accreditation Commission. IAC Standards and Guidelines for Adult Echocardiography Accreditation. https://www.intersocietal.org/echo/standards/IACAdultEchocardiographyStandards2017.pdf.
4. Mulvagh SL, Rakowski H, Vannan MA, et al. American Society of Echocardiography Consensus Statement on the Clinical Applications of Ultrasonic Contrast Agents in Echocardiography. *J Am Soc Echocardiogr.* 2008;21:1179–1201.
5. Herzog CA. Incidence of adverse events associated with use of perflutren contrast agents for echocardiography. *J Am Med Assoc.* 2008;299:2023–2025.

23 | Left Ventricular Systolic Function: Basic Principles

Zoran B. Popović, James D. Thomas

FUNCTIONAL ANATOMY OF THE LEFT VENTRICLE

The left ventricle is a hollow muscular shell that is capable of ejecting more than 100 mL of blood at over 200 mm Hg of pressure and then filling with the same quantity of blood at less than 10 mm Hg and in less than 100 ms during exercise. This action becomes all the more remarkable when one realizes that the fundamental contractile unit of the cardiac myocyte, the sarcomere, is only capable of shortening by about 13%, whereas the ventricle shortens in length and circumference by about 20% with more than 40% radial thickening, leading to the ejection of more than 60% of the end-diastolic volume. The transduction of this small degree of sarcomere shortening into a 60+% ejection fraction (EF) is only possible because of a very specific counterwoven double helix arrangement of muscle fibers.

Before a discussion of the actual anatomy, consider an alternative, simpler arrangement consisting only of fibers coursing circumferentially around the cavity. The sarcomeres generate force most efficiently in a narrow range around 13%, but as shown in Fig. 23.1, to reduce the cross-sectional area by 60% with an incompressible material such as myocardium requires fiber shortening of about 15% at the midwall (near optimal for the sarcomere), but at the epicardium, there is only 7% shortening, too little for optimal force generation. Furthermore, at the endocardium, conservation of mass requires the fibers to shorten by 26%, well beyond what a sarcomere can do, requiring inefficient crumpling of the fibers. To generate ejection with pressure requires an arrangement of myofibrils that allows each sarcomere to contribute optimally to contraction.

In reality, as Fig. 23.2 demonstrates, the left ventricular (LV) myofibrils are arranged roughly in a left-handed helix in the epicardium and a right-handed helix in the endocardium, with a circumferential arrangement in the midwall. These are not discrete layers but rather show a continuous gradation from roughly +60 degrees to −60 degrees (relative to the circumferential midwall fibers) as one goes from endocardium to epicardium.[1] Although this helps to normalize sarcomeric shortening, a further feature is required, with the fibers arranged in discrete sheets defined by perimysial collagen so that during systole, they can tilt inward, allowing for much greater regional deformation while keeping sarcomere shortening in the optimal zone (Fig. 23.3).[2]

The counterwoven helical architecture contributes to ventricular torsion, the wringing motion that helps to eject blood while also storing energy in the interstitium and the sarcomeric molecular spring, titin, to be released during diastole to assist in the low pressure filling of the heart.[3,4] The left-handed fibers in the epicardium, being farther from the ventricular centroid, have a mechanical advantage over the right-handed endocardial fibers and thus can rotate the apex counterclockwise (as viewed in the typical short-axis echo plane) while pulling the base in a clockwise direction, generating about 13 to 15 degrees of twist at rest.

LEFT VENTRICULAR VOLUME AND ITS DYNAMIC GEOMETRY

The resulting left ventricle is a complex ellipsoid structure that is characterized by one major and two minor axes. The two minor axes, although similar in length, are not identical because the axis lying in the septolateral (horizontal) plane is shorter than the one lying in the intercommissural (vertical) plane because of lower curvature of the interventricular septum. During cardiac contraction, after initially becoming more spherical, the left ventricle becomes more elliptical at end-systole. Hearts with systolic failure characteristically become more spherical. LV geometry is also influenced by right ventricular (RV) pathology—characteristically, septolateral dimensions decrease in the setting of RV pressure overload. These changes are relevant because flattening of the septum elicits profound changes in regional LV contractility caused by interference with Starling mechanism.[5,6]

GENERATING LEFT VENTRICULAR EJECTION FROM CONTRACTION OF MYOFIBRILLS

Myofibrillar contraction leads to shortening of the left ventricle along the long axis and around its circumference, which then results in radial thickening. The parameter that quantifies this deformation in the longitudinal, circumferential, and radial directions is called *strain*. How much each of these strain components contributes to LV ejection varies and depends on LV geometry. A recent study has shown that thicker ventricles need lower strains to generate the same amount of EF (Fig. 23.4A).[7] The same study also showed that, in general, ejection is affected less by longitudinal than by circumferential strain (Fig. 23.4B). Thus, a decrease in longitudinal (long-axis) strain, often seen as an early marker of LV dysfunction, can be offset by a lesser increase in circumferential strain to result in a falsely reassuring normal EF (see Fig. 23.4).

CARDIAC CYCLE

The cardiac cycle itself is one of the most complex physiologic phenomena in existence. It refers to the interplay between electrical and mechanical events in the heart that lead to sequential filling and emptying of various cardiac chambers. This interplay can be viewed as a sequence in time (time domain) or in a framework of pressure-volume loops of the individual cardiac chambers. We limit discussion here to the LV cardiac cycle (Fig. 23.5).

The contraction of the left ventricle is initiated by the arrival of electrical impulse, which in a normal heart starts a depolarization wave from the base of the septum and when reaching the "superhighway" of the Purkinje conduction system moves rapidly toward the LV apex, engulfing the entire heart, reaching the posterior base of the left ventricle within the next 35 ms. Depolarization of the muscle does not immediately start mechanical contraction: another 10 to 15 ms is needed for the actual fiber shortening to start. Thus, the usual definition of end-diastole is nadir of the Q wave (beginning of the R wave) because it is assumed that at this time, most of the cardiac tissue, even if electrically activated, has not yet started to contract. This time point precedes the closure of the mitral valve (assessed by Doppler, M-mode echocardiography, or phonocardiography), although, when viewed with high temporal resolution echocardiography, closure of the mitral valve appears more of a process than a discrete phenomenon. The time interval between the Q wave and mitral valve closure is called *electromechanical delay*. In the presence of wide QRS complex, it is much more difficult to define the point of end-diastole because in that setting, the peak Q wave or the beginning of the R wave can precede the actual beginning of contraction by more than 100 ms; a typical way of overcoming this is to assume the time point just before mitral valve closure as end-diastole. Yet another way to define end-diastolic pressure (more relevant to the catheterization laboratory but that can be applied in the echocardiography) is the time when LV dP/dt (first derivative of pressure) reaches 10% of maximum LV dP/dt. Regardless of its definition, the end-diastolic point closely corresponds to the lower right-hand corner of the LV pressure-volume loop diagram (Fig. 23.6).

Although discussion of how to define end-diastole may seem academic, it is of crucial importance whenever we assess LV systolic function, whether by using familiar LV volumes but especially novel parameters such as strain. With the closure of mitral valve LV pressure starts to rise, the left ventricle becomes more spherical, finally resulting in the aortic valve opening and the beginning of ejection. The period between MV closure and aortic valve opening is the isovolumic contraction time (IVCT), and the period between the beginning of depolarization and aortic valve opening is the pre-ejection period (PEP). Several phenomena occur with aortic valve opening: the LV starts decreasing its dimensions and becomes less spherical, while pressure stops its rapid rise. This is reflected by the first derivative of LV pressure (LV dP/dt) reaching its maximum (LV dP/dtmax) almost coincidental with the aortic valve opening (see more later). The LV ejection period (defined as the time between aortic valve opening and closure) is classically characterized by two parts: rapid (early) and slow (late) ejection, although the differentiation between these two periods is obscured in the setting of high afterload or low contractility. Interestingly, most of the ejection of blood volume ejected occurs while LV pressure is relatively constant (see pressure-volume [PV] loop diagram). As we near the end of ejection, a relatively rapid pressure drop occurs. In the PV loop diagram, this is marked as the left upper point on the diagram and defines physiologic end systole (in mathematical terms, maximum of the pressure–volume ratio). This time point usually precedes aortic valve closure by 15 to 30 ms except in some pathologic states (e.g., mitral regurgitation) and marks the beginning of relaxation. With aortic valve closure, the rate of pressure drop increases rapidly (as the pressure vent of the aortic valve gets closed), leading to the occurrence of peak negative dP/dt (dP/dtmin), a marker of relaxation (see next section). LV pressure continues to drop, albeit more slowly, until the mitral valve opens ending this isovolumic relaxation time (IVRT) period. This pressure drop during IVRT follows an approximately exponential decay curve characterized by the time constant of isovolumic pressure decay (again see next section). With mitral valve opening, there is an interplay with continued relaxation and early filling of the left ventricle, which leads first to short period of pressure drop up to minimum LV diastolic pressure (with an increase in volume and thus, instantaneously, "negative" compliance). There follows a relatively long period of continuous pressure increase, augmented by atrial contraction and culminating with mitral valve closure and end of this LV filling period.

DETERMINANTS OF LEFT VENTRICULAR PERFORMANCE

The basis of LV performance is summed up by Harvey's principle of continuous (closed-loop) circulation of the blood and the Starling mechanism of cardiac output regulated by its preload (i.e., input), enabling it to work as a servo motor. Determinants of LV performance are usually identified as preload, afterload,

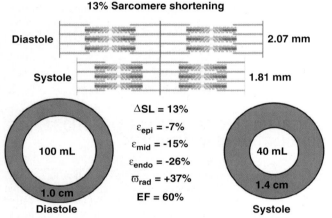

13% Sarcomere shortening

Diastole — 2.07 mm
Systole — 1.81 mm

$\Delta SL = 13\%$
$\varepsilon_{epi} = -7\%$
$\varepsilon_{mid} = -15\%$
$\varepsilon_{endo} = -26\%$
$\varpi_{rad} = +37\%$
EF = 60%

100 mL   40 mL
1.0 cm   1.4 cm
Diastole   Systole

Figure 23.1. Schematic representation of sarcomere shortening (optimally near 13%) and the circumferential and radial deformation necessary to ejection 60% of the cavity volume. A simple circumferential wrapping of fibers would lead to incomplete sarcomeric shortening in the epicardium and a crumpling of myofibrils in the subendocardium. *ΔSL,* Change in sarcomere length; *ε,* regional strain, with the subscripts *epi, mid,* and *endo* referring to circumferential shortening at these respective myocardial levels and *rad* referring to radial thickening; *EF,* ejection fraction.

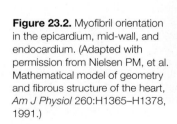

Figure 23.2. Myofibril orientation in the epicardium, mid-wall, and endocardium. (Adapted with permission from Nielsen PM, et al. Mathematical model of geometry and fibrous structure of the heart, *Am J Physiol* 260:H1365–H1378, 1991.)

Epicardium   Midwall   Endocardium

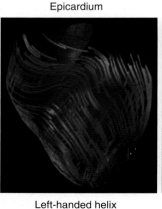 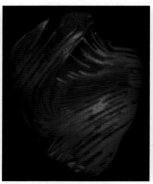 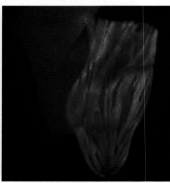

Left-handed helix   Circumferential   Right-handed helix

contractility (inotropy), and diastolic function (lusitropy and chamber compliance; see later); however not all of them are completely independent.

LV preload refers to initial sarcomere length and is linked to cardiac performance through the Starling mechanism. In sum, an increase in preload (i.e., the amount of blood coming into the heart) leads to an increase in force generation of sarcomeres, which in turn leads to increased LV pressure, power, and work. The amount of work generated in each heart stroke is quantified by the area of the pressure volume loop: one can easily see that the two ways one can increase the stroke work is by increasing the difference between diastolic and systolic pressures, by increasing the difference between diastolic and systolic volumes, or both. Because we cannot measure sarcomere length, preload is quantified by end-diastolic volume. As a surrogate, one can use pulmonary capillary wedge pressure, mean left atrial pressure, LV end-diastolic pressure, or LV mean diastolic pressure, all of them strongly correlated but with somewhat different physiologic determinants.

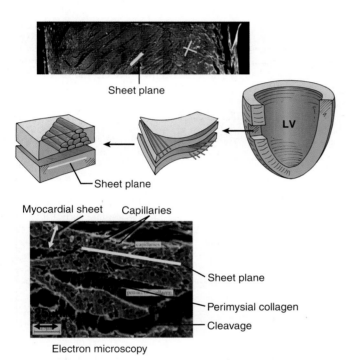

Sheet plane

LV

Sheet plane

Myocardial sheet   Capillaries

Sheet plane

Perimysial collagen

Cleavage

Electron microscopy

Figure 23.3. Further subdivision of myofibrils into discrete sheets, which can tilt relative to the circumferential plane during systole to maintain optimal sarcomere shortening.

LV afterload is the amount of resistance that the heart encounters as it ejects. It is very important to understand that afterload under normal condition is "good": most of the vital organs need some level of blood pressure so they can operate their autoregulatory blood supply systems. If blood pressures were in the 50–mm Hg range, no matter how many liters of blood pumped through the circulatory system, the brain, kidneys and heart would not be able to extract sufficient oxygen for proper function. In this regard, septic shock can be considered a situation of inadequate afterload. On the other hand, however, too much of the afterload leads obviously to a decrease in stroke volume because pressure and flow are linked together within the pressure-volume loop. Afterload is usually separated in two components, oscillatory and static. The static component represents capillary resistance and can be quantified simply by a systemic vascular resistance equation as cardiac output divided by the difference between mean systolic and central venous pressure. The oscillatory component reflects elasticity of the aorta and big vessels and is defined by the interplay between arterial pressure and flow that can only be quantified using complex computational methods. Yet another measure that theoretically represents sum of both components is arterial elastance, the ratio between end systolic pressure and stroke volume.

We have already mentioned that LV force, power, and work are determined by preload, increasing with increased preload. So how do we then define LV contractility? Although there are several possible ways, potentially the easiest one is that LV contractility represents the amount of force, power, or work increase per unit increase in preload (i.e., end-diastolic volume). Experimental work has shown that the relationship between cardiac performance parameters and end-diastolic volume is nearly linear, with the slope of this relationship representing contractility (Fig. 23.7). When dP/dtmax is used as the parameter of interest, the name of the slope is the *elastance derivative* (dE/dt).[8] When stroke work is used, the name is *preload-recruitable stroke work*.[9] Finally, when LV power is used, the name of relationship is *preload-adjusted maximal power*.[10]

Yet another way, and more complicated, way to understand is through assessment of end-systolic pressure–-volume relationships. In brief, if a sudden decrease of preload occurs, blood pressure drops precipitously because the end-systolic volume becomes simultaneously smaller and smaller, and the afterload is suddenly reduced by the blood pressure drop. The relationship between blood pressure and end-systolic volume decrease is again linear, with the slope of relationship representing end-systolic elastance. Of note, there are several other closely related but not identical concepts such as time-varying maximum elastance, which we will not cover because of their complexity and paucity of actual use even in physiology community. Elastance is difficult to understand in the context of Starling law. One way to gain an insight to what

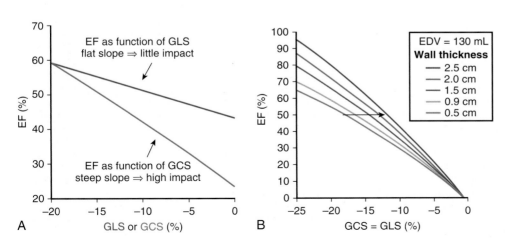

A   EF (%) vs GLS or GCS (%)

EF as function of GLS
flat slope ⇒ little impact

EF as function of GCS
steep slope ⇒ high impact

B   EF (%) vs GCS = GLS (%)

EDV = 130 mL
Wall thickness
— 2.5 cm
— 2.0 cm
— 1.5 cm
— 0.9 cm
— 0.5 cm

Figure 23.4. Ejection fraction is approximately two times more sensitive to increase in circumferential, than to increase in longitudinal, strain (**A**). In ventricles with thicker walls, less longitudinal and circumferential strain is required to maintain normal ejection fraction. *EDV,* End-diastolic volume; *EF,* ejection fraction; *GCS,* global circumferential strain; *GLS,* global longitudinal strain. (Adapted with permission from Stokke TM, et al: Geometry as a confounder when assessing ventricular systolic function: Comparison between ejection fraction and strain, *J Am Coll Cardiol* 70:942–954, 2017.)

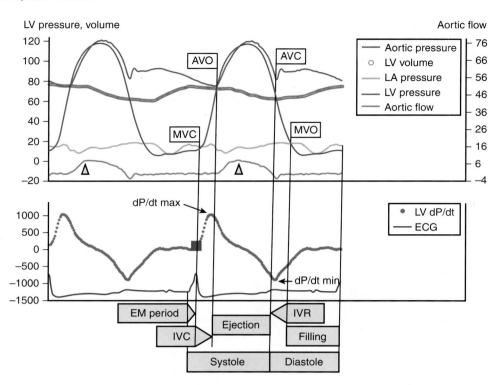

Figure 23.5. Cardiac cycle. Hemodynamic data obtained from an experiment in a dog with tachycardia induced cardiomyopathy. See text for details. The *red cross* marks a point when dP/dt (first derivative of pressure) reaches 10% of its maximum value. *Blue arrows* point to the peak of the aortic flow that separates rapid (early) from slow (late) aortic ejection. *AVC(O),* Aortic valve closure (opening); *ECG,* electrocardiogram; *EM,* electromechanical; *IVC,* isovolumic contraction; *IVR,* isovolumic relaxation; *LA,* left atrial; *LV, left ventricular; MVC(O),* mitral valve closure (opening).

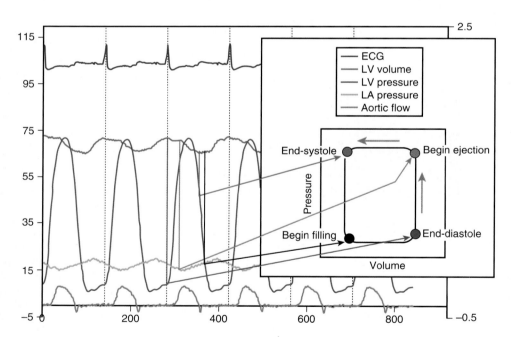

Figure 23.6. A schematic diagram of how the pressure-volume loop is constructed from left ventricular (LV) tracings of pressure and volume. *ECG,* Electrocardiogram; *LA,* left atrial.

it actually means is to interpret it as a measure of resistance of the left ventricle to increase its size with increasing systolic blood pressure: one might imagine what would happen if the aorta were constricted. A heart with high elastance will maintain initial end-systolic volume, but one with low elastance will increase its end-systolic volume.

And that leads to a final method for assessing contractility, that is, the wall stress versus EF (or fractional shortening) relationship. Wall stress is a force acting in a given direction per unit area and is represents a measure of a force that opposes myocardial fiber contraction or, in other words, afterload. Besides intracavitary pressure, two additional factors influence stress: LV cavity size and wall thickness. For a same pressure, force (stress)

will be larger in a larger ventricle as the ventricular surface over which intracavitary pressure is acting is larger. Inversely, larger wall thickness decreases stress as it distributes force over a larger linear dimension. The final concept is similar to the concept of elastance: hearts with high contractility are able to have high EF despite high stress, but the opposite is true for a failing heart. Plotting wall stress on the *x*-axis and EF on the *y*-axis in Cartesian coordinates enables comparison with previously ascertained normal stress–EF values without the need of further preload manipulation (Fig. 23.8).[11]

Of note, in clinical cardiology, parameters that require preload manipulation in their calculation are seldom used. A key reason for that is one needs to know the minimum LV volume that elicits

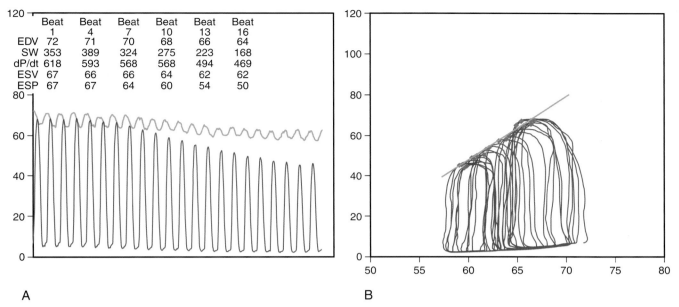

	Beat 1	Beat 4	Beat 7	Beat 10	Beat 13	Beat 16
EDV	72	71	70	68	66	64
SW	353	389	324	275	223	168
dP/dt	618	593	568	568	494	469
ESV	67	66	66	64	62	62
ESP	67	67	64	60	54	50

A　　　　　　　　　B

Figure 23.7. A, Left ventricular (LV) pressure *(dotted line)* and volume *(full line)* during sudden vena cava occlusion performed during the evaluation of a dog with tachycardia-induced cardiomyopathy. *Numbers on the top table* represent parameters of LV function measured on every third beat. Notice continuous and parallel decrease of LV end-diastolic (EDV) and end-systolic (ESV) volumes, stroke work (SW), maximum LV dP/dt (first derivative of pressure), and end-systolic pressures during vena cava occlusion. By pairing end-diastolic volume measured at every beat with corresponding stroke work, maximum LV dP/dt (or ventricular power, one calculate parameters of contractility (see text for details). **B,** The same data shown as LV pressure-volume loops. The *diamond-shaped dots* represent end-systolic pressure-volume points of individual beats. The *straight line* is a regression line passed through individual end-systolic pressure volume points, whose slope represents end-systolic elastance (see text for details).

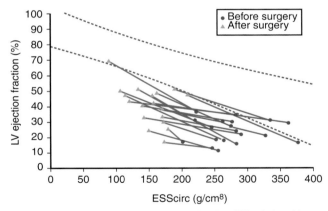

Figure 23.8. End systolic stress–ejection fraction (EF) relationship in patients with nonischemic dilated cardiomyopathy before and after partial left ventriculectomy. This, now abandoned, procedure increased EF by reducing left ventricular end-systolic stress. The figure shows that this increase in EF was caused by decreased afterload (stress). *ESScirc,* circumferential end-systolic stress. (Adapted with permission from Popovic Z, et al: Effects of partial left ventriculectomy on left ventricular performance in patients with nonischemic dilated cardiomyopathy, *J Am Coll Cardiol* 32:1801–1808, 1998.)

a cardiac response-the so called V0. Although there are several methods to estimate V0, these are usually taken as rough estimates and not as actual measures. EF–wall stress relationships are also almost never explicitly used in modern adult cardiology because they often exhibit low sensitivity to depressed contractility.[12] However, one point is critical: any echocardiography examination is diminished in value unless one records the blood pressure during the examination.

RESPONSE TO EXERCISE

Exercise elicits a complex and powerful response of the cardiovascular system brought about sympathetic activation and multiple autoregulatory cardiac mechanisms. Muscle mobilization leads to decreased venous capacitance and increased preload; in other words, contraction of muscles pumps out the blood out of the limb vasculature into the central circulation.[13] This in turn leads to reflex tachycardia (Bainbridge reflex) and increased contractility through the Bowditch (force-frequency)[14] phenomenon. There is a decrease of peripheral resistance caused by muscle arteriolar vasodilation, leading to decreased afterload and increased cardiac output. At the same time, sympathetic activation leads further to increased contractility, heart rate, and relaxation rate. All of these phenomena lead to the heart delivering more cardiac output in a hemodynamically optimized (less afterload) environment. These phenomena lead to moderately increased blood pressure, a decrease in end-systolic volume that is larger than the decrease in the end-diastolic volume, a mild increase in stroke volume, and am overall increase in the cardiac output mostly because of increased heart rate. Heart rate increase is not a necessary mechanism because cardiac output occurs even in the setting of a fixed heart rate; however, the total increase in cardiac output is compromised if an increase does not occur. Cardiac exercise also leads to a mild increase in LV filling pressures.[15] Of interest is to note that although changes in EF and strain are minimal, there is a dramatic increase in strain rate, both positive and negative.

REFERENCES

1. Nielsen PM, Le Grice IJ, Smaill BH, Hunter PJ. Mathematical model of geometry and fibrous structure of the heart. *Am J Physiol.* 1991;260:H1365–H1378.
2. Young AA, Legrice IJ, Young MA, Smaill BH. Extended confocal microscopy of myocardial laminae and collagen network. *J Microsc.* 1998;192:139–150.
3. Notomi Y, Popovic ZB, Yamada H, et al. Ventricular untwisting: a temporal link between left ventricular relaxation and suction. *Am J Physiol Heart Circ Physiol.* 2008;294:H505–H513.

4. Notomi Y, Martin-Miklovic MG, Oryszak SJ, et al. Enhanced ventricular untwisting during exercise: a mechanistic manifestation of elastic recoil described by doppler tissue imaging. *Circulation*. 2006;113:2524–2533.

5. Moon MR, Bolger AF, DeAnda A, et al. Septal function during left ventricular unloading. *Circulation*. 1997;95:1320–1327.

6. Puwanant S, Park M, Popovic ZB, et al. Ventricular geometry, strain, and rotational mechanics in pulmonary hypertension. *Circulation*. 2010;121:259–266.

7. Stokke TM, Hasselberg NE, Smedsrud MK, et al. Geometry as a confounder when assessing ventricular systolic function: comparison between ejection fraction and strain. *J Am Coll Cardiol*. 2017;70:942–954.

8. Little WC. The left ventricular dp/dtmax-end-diastolic volume relation in closed-chest dogs. *Circ Res*. 1985;56:808–815.

9. Glower DD, Spratt JA, Snow ND, et al. Linearity of the Frank-Starling relationship in the intact heart: the concept of preload recruitable stroke work. *Circulation*. 1985;71:994–1009.

10. Sharir T, Feldman MD, Haber H, et al. Ventricular systolic assessment in patients with dilated cardiomyopathy by preload-adjusted maximal power. Validation and noninvasive application. *Circulation*. 1994;89:2045–2053.

11. Popovic Z, Miric M, Gradinac S, et al. Effects of partial left ventriculectomy on left ventricular performance in patients with nonischemic dilated cardiomyopathy. *J Am Coll Cardiol*. 1998;32:1801–1808.

12. Starling MR, Kirsh MM, Montgomery DG, Gross MD. Impaired left ventricular contractile function in patients with long-term mitral regurgitation and normal ejection fraction. *J Am Coll Cardiol*. 1993;22:239–250.

13. Shepherd JT. Changes in tone of limb veins during supine exercise. *J Appl Physiol*. 1965;20:1–8.

14. Mulieri LA, Hasenfuss G, Leavitt B, et al. Altered myocardial force-frequency relation in human heart failure. *Circulation*. 1992;85:1743–1750.

15. Higginbotham MB, Morris KG, Williams RS, et al. Regulation of stroke volume during submaximal and maximal upright exercise in normal man. *Circ Res*. 1986;58:281–291.

24 Global Left Ventricular Systolic Function: Ejection Fraction Versus Strain

Thomas H. Marwick, Kazuaki Negishi

The assessment of global left ventricular (LV) systolic function is a cornerstone of risk evaluation and management in most cardiac diseases. The simplest and most widely used parameter for this purpose has been ejection fraction (EF) and regional wall motion analysis, but over the past decade, new parameters such as global longitudinal strain (GLS) have become available.

INDICATIONS FOR SYSTOLIC FUNCTION EVALUATION

Echocardiography is appropriately indicated when cardiac related symptoms or conditions are suspected, most commonly in the setting of suspected heart failure (HF).[1] Despite the value of LV dysfunction as an important component of risk evaluation for decision making, the methodologies and cut-offs used in studies that have defined these EF criteria for the guidance of management are highly variable, with few studies using core laboratories (Table 24.1).[2] The EF criteria for implantable defibrillators or cardiac resynchronization therapy (CRT)[3,4] or for intervention in regurgitant valve lesions[5] have not been gathered with a high degree of accuracy, and it seems irrational to use them as exact thresholds.

In asymptomatic subjects at risk for HF, the use of echocardiography to detect reduced EF or subtle structural heart disease reclassifies the patient from stage A to stage B of HF, with resulting management implications.[6] These patients with a subclinical phase to their cardiomyopathy include those treated with cardiotoxic chemotherapy and those with gene-positive cardiomyopathies, amyloidosis, or other infiltrative conditions. The detection of subclinical disease not only includes global but also regional dysfunction (in ischemic heart disease, sarcoidosis, and myocarditis).

Finally, although the temporal analysis of LV contraction carries prognostic information, the clinical application of this remains uncertain. There are very strong prognostic reasons to undertake CRT in patients with HF symptoms, systolic dysfunction, and left bundle branch block, irrespective of the measurement of mechanical synchrony, and there are reasonable grounds to doubt the reliability of some of the literature on prediction of response.[7] Paradoxically, measurement of synchrony may come into clinical use in the selection of patients for implantable defibrillators rather than CRT because measurements of dispersion of mechanical activation may be of value in understanding the risk of arrhythmia.[8]

LIMITATIONS OF EJECTION FRACTION

EF has become an indispensable component of cardiac evaluation. Its presence pervades the guidelines, and it is instrumental in the multitude of decisions, ranging from medical management of HF, medical devices, and surgical timing in asymptomatic patients.[9]

Despite the breadth of its use, EF has a number of important limitations (Table 24.2):

1. The most common EF limitations that are specific to echocardiography are technical issues related to image quality and assumptions about LV geometry, which are avoidable with the use of contrast LV opacification and three-dimensional (3D) echocardiography, respectively.

2. EF is load dependent, meaning that it cannot be interpreted as a reflection of contractility in the absence of knowledge about afterload and preload. Although properties of an ideal index of contractility might include sensitivity to changes in inotropy, independence of load, heart size and mass, ease and safety of application, and proof in the clinical setting,[10] no perfect index currently exists. Perhaps the best way to integrate the role of loading in the evaluation of LV function is to ensure that the measurement of blood pressure (as an analog of central pressure) and, to a lesser extent, inferior vena cava characteristics should be included in imaging studies that could be used clinically to estimate contractility.[9]

3. EF is also influenced by heart rate. The increased stroke volume associated with bradycardia may lead to overestimation of the true EF, and conversely in tachycardia the reduced stroke volume may lead to underestimation of the actual function. There is no technique that corrects for this, so heart rate needs to be kept in mind in the application of EF data.

4. EF is a function of LV size. In LV hypertrophy, EF may not correspond well to the real interest of the clinician, which is function in the midmyocardium.[11]

5. Although EF is a good marker of gross LV dysfunction, it may be insufficiently sensitive to identify mild degrees of systolic dysfunction, perhaps evidenced by the inability to identify

TABLE 24.1 Multicenter Studies That Have Defined Ejection Fraction Criteria for the Guidance of Management in Heart Failure

Study, Year	Intervention	Patients (n)	Technique	Core Lab	Entry Criteria
SOLVD, 1991	Enalapril	2569	Echo, RNV, LVgram	Yes	EF ≤35%
Hydralazine–nitrate, 1991	Enalapril vs hydralazine–nitrate	804	Echo, RNV	Yes	EF <45%, LVEDD >27 mm/m² BSA
CIBIS, 1994	Bisoprolol	641	RNV, LVgram	No	EF <40%
US Carvedilol, 1996	Carvedilol	1094	Echo	Yes	EF ≤35%
MERIT-HF, 1999, 2000	Metoprolol XL	3991	Unspecified	No	EF ≤40%
CIBIS II, 1999	Bisoprolol	2647	Echo, RNV, LVgram	No	EF ≤35%
Capricorn, 2001	Carvedilol	1959	Echo, RNV, LVgram	No	EF ≤40%, WMSI ≤1.3
Carvedilol, 2001	Carvedilol	2289	Unspecified	No	EF <25%
BEST, 2001	Bucindolol	2708	RNV	No	EF <35%
MIRACLE-ICD, 2003	CRT/ICD	369	Echo	Yes	EF ≤35%
COMET, 2003	Carvedilol vs metoprolol	1511	Echo, RNV	No	EF <35%
CHARM, 2003	Candesartan	2548	Unspecified	No	EF ≤40%
SCD-HeFT, 2005	ICD	3521	Unspecified	No	EF<35%
CARE-HF, 2005	CRT	813	Echo	Yes	EF ≤35%, LVEDD >30 mm/m height

BSA, Body surface area; *CRT,* cardiac resynchronization therapy; *echo,* echocardiography; *EF,* ejection fraction; *ICD,* implantable cardioverter-defibrillator; *LVEDD,* left ventricular end-diastolic dimension; *LVgram,* contrast ventriculography; *RNV,* radionuclide ventriculography; *WMSI,* wall motion score index. Studies, in order of appearance: SOLVD, Studies of Left Ventricular Dysfunction; CIBIS, The Cardiac Insufficiency Bisoprolol Study; MERIT-HF, Metoprolol CR/XL Randomized Intervention Trial in Chronic Heart Failure; BEST, Beta-Blocker Evaluation in Survival Trial; MIRACLE-ICD - Multicenter InSync ICD Randomized Clinical Evaluation; COMET, Carvedilol Or Metoprolol European Trial; CHARM, Candesartan in Heart failure—Assessment of moRtality and Morbidity; SCDHeFT, Sudden Cardiac Death in Heart Failure Trial; CARE-HF, Cardiac Resynchronization—Heart Failure.

TABLE 24.2 Limitations of Ejection Fraction

Problem	Circumstances of Inaccuracy	Potential Solution
Geometry dependence	LBBB, extensive wall motion abnormality, off-axis imaging	3D imaging, geometry-independent techniques
Load dependence	Extremes of afterload, mitral regurgitation	Pressure-volume loops, pre-ejection markers
High and low HR	Heart block, tachycardias (especially atrial fibrillation)	None
Marker of endocardial shortening	LV hypertrophy	Midmyocardial shortening
Insensitivity to minor change	Prognostic value close to EF 50%	Non-EF techniques for assessing subclinical dysfunction
Expertise	Wide use of EF	Quantitation

3D, Three-dimensional; *EF,* ejection fraction; *HR,* heart rate; *LBBB,* left bundle branch block; *LV,* left ventricular.

a gradation of risk in patients with EF greater than 45%.[12] In contrast, the use of global longitudinal strain offers the greatest increment in predictive power in patients with EF greater than 35% and without motion abnormality.[13] Finally, the wide use of EF suggests that not all assessment is performed at the same level of expertise, indicating that more formal quality control, automation, and quantitation may be desirable.[14]

THE ROLE OF GLOBAL LONGITUDINAL STRAIN

We need to recognize that EF was defined in the 1960s, when the practice of cardiology was significantly different from now. The evaluation of five significant current challenges in cardiology is facilitated by GLS but not by EF:

1. HF with preserved EF has become the dominant manifestation of HF and is likely to become even more important as the population ages and the consequences of obesity diabetes and hypertension impact the aging heart. Although EF is not useful in the recognition of this entity, GLS is consistently impaired in these patients. GLS falls as EF worsens, but the two are not necessarily closely linked. In particular, a small ventricle with LV hypertrophy will have preserved EF despite compromised myocardial function and GLS. Moreover, GLS is related to prognosis when EF is not (e.g., in patients with EF >40%).[9]

2. Stage B HF is a precursor to the development of clinical HF and is recognized on the basis of normal LV structure and function in the absence of symptoms. The conventional criteria for the definition of stage B HF are prior myocardial infarction, LV remodeling, including LV hypertrophy, and low EF. Mounting evidence suggests that GLS, together with LV hypertrophy and diastolic dysfunction, should be used as markers of nonischemic stage B HF.[15] Moreover, GLS is also helpful in asymptomatic valvular disease, especially aortic stenosis, mitral regurgitation, and aortic regurgitation.[16]

3. A number of situations require the surveillance of LV function over time, the most frequent topic being the assessment of chemotherapy patients treated with potentially cardiotoxic drugs. Currently, two-dimensional (2D) EF is the most widely performed echocardiographic measure of LV function, but its wide confidence intervals (~12%) make it difficult to discern minor changes of function from random noise. Although 3D EF is preferred,[17] its confidence intervals are still greater than 6%. This means that many alterations of EF are difficult to distinguish from background noise. GLS is not only a sensitive marker of LV impairment but also a very robust and reproducible one. The use of GLS in patients at risk of cardiotoxicity has shown its ability to identify LV dysfunction at an earlier stage than EF, and this is potentially useful as a guide to initiating cardioprotective therapy.

4. Patients with impaired LV function at risk of sudden cardiac death, and current criteria for defibrillator implantation are based on EF less than 35%. Nonetheless, there are more people (and therefore more absolute numbers of sudden death) with mildly than severely impaired LV function, so the current EF threshold neglects many patients at risk of sudden cardiac death. This is particularly problematic in patients with nonischemic HF because trials have provided a confusing signal about who best to treat. LV contractile dispersion can be measured from segmental strain, and a number of studies have documented that LV dispersion provides incremental information to EF and other clinical predictors of cardiac death.[18] Although timing parameters are more variable than magnitude parameters with strain measurement, this is an application that is likely to attract ongoing attention.

5. The assessment of diastolic dysfunction is frustratingly complex, with LV untwist, relaxation, compliance, and filling pressure exerting different influences on LV filling at different stages of the disease. The most recent diastolic function guidelines[19] have improved sensitivity and specificity from the previous guidelines but at the cost of more patients designated as nondiagnostic. Left atrial strain may be a solution to this problem because it appears to deteriorate in a linear fashion as LV function worsens.[20]

CHOICE FOR ASSESSMENT TOOL OF LEFT VENTRICULAR SYSTOLIC FUNCTION IN MULTIMODALITY ERA

LV systolic function is currently assessed with various modalities. The right tool can be selected by fundamental characteristics of each modality (Table 24.3). These include spatial, temporal, and contrast resolution; 3D acquisition and display; repeatability; and intra- and interobserver variation.[21]

Echocardiography, cardiac magnetic resonance imaging (CMR) and computed tomography (CT) have a spatial resolution of a millimeter or a few millimeters.[22] In contrast, nuclear cardiology techniques have a lower spatial resolution of up to 1.0 cm. Techniques with lower spatial resolution are inherently less suited to the generation of exact information regarding regional wall motion disturbances, wall thickness, and dimension.

The highest temporal resolution is available using echocardiographic techniques. Generally, this component of imaging is considered important when assessing the rate of contraction or the presence and degree of LV dyssynchrony. This underlies the assessment of LV synchrony with techniques of low temporal resolution such as 3D echocardiography and single-photon emission computed tomography (SPECT). Another aspect of temporal resolution that is often neglected is the importance of measuring and averaging a large number of cardiac cycles in patients with stable cardiac rhythm. Failure to do so is one of the weaknesses of echocardiography, which then exposes measurements to the risk of sampling error based on individual cardiac cycles.

Contrast resolution is the ability to accurately segment the LV wall from the blood pool. The best contrast resolution is obtainable using magnetic resonance imaging (MRI). Contrast techniques such as contrast echocardiography and ventriculography improve the contrast resolution of the underlying technique. These considerations are vital in the accurate measurement of LV dimensions and volumes. From the standpoint of contrast resolution, as well as tissue characterization, MRI is the optimal tool.

3D imaging is available with echocardiography, CMR, and CT. The main attraction of 3D imaging is to avoid geometric assumptions in calculations of LV volumes and to avoid errors created by cutting a 3D structure in two dimensions. In a generic sense,[23] 3D imaging using any technique is superior to 2D imaging for the purpose of calculating volumes and to a lesser extent EF. The latter is true because the errors in volume calculations tend to cancel out when expressed in a ratio to obtain EF.

Repeatability, precision, or test–retest variation relates to the ability to obtain the same measurement on multiple tests when there has been no interval change of function.[24] This parameter is often neglected but is extremely important in patient follow-up; clearly, a technique with a high degree of test–retest variation is unfavorable for follow-up applications. This is particularly a problem with 2D imaging because of the previously mentioned variations in cut-planes from episode to episode of imaging. 3D techniques are generally more repeatable, as are techniques that are independent of volumetric considerations such as global strain. Intra- and interobserver variability is often related to image quality. Although techniques with limited intra- and interobserver variability may still be used with appropriate training, less variable methods have the potential attraction of operating at a high level of quality in less expert hands.

Combining these fundamental aspects of imaging technologies with situations when LV imaging is required can provide some clues as to the most appropriate imaging choices. First, situations when accurate sequential follow-up is needed are most favored using 3D imaging, for example, MRI, with 3D echocardiography being a good alternative. Although nuclear ventriculography has been used for this purpose, it may be less sensitive to minor change.[25] Subtle disturbances of systolic function may not be apparent on EF. In these situations, such as the follow-up of patients on cytotoxic chemotherapy, strain techniques could become the test of choice. Decisions requiring an accurate calculation of LV volumes or EF should be performed using an inherently 3D technique such as MRI or 3D echocardiography. Such circumstances might include decisions for device therapy in HF[26] or when quantitative methods are used to facilitate surgical decision making in patients with valvular heart disease.[27] Assessment of regional wall motion is best performed using a high-resolution technique, such as echocardiography or MRI. Contrast should be used with echocardiography whenever indicated by the failure to visualize more than two segments[28]; the benefit of contrast in the absence of suboptimal imaging is unproven and may be detrimental.

CONCLUSIONS

Despite its limitations, EF is accepted by the cardiology community. The evidence base for modern cardiology is so heavily based on this simple measurement that it is unlikely to disappear. However, this information is readily supplemented by

TABLE 24.3 Selecting the Right Tool for the Job: Imaging Characteristics of Various Tests

	Technique	Application
High spatial resolution	CMR	LV hypertrophy, infiltration
High temporal resolution	Tissue Doppler, strain	LV synchrony
High contrast resolution	CMR, contrast echocardiography	LV volumes
High repeatability	CMR, 3D echocardiography	Sequential follow-up
Sensitivity to minor change	Strain	Subclinical cardiomyopathy

3D, Three-dimensional; *CMR,* cardiac magnetic resonance imaging; *LV,* left ventricular.

GLS. The ubiquitous presence of cardiovascular diseases in current aging societies mandates an inexpensive, widely available test that is able to provide hemodynamic assessment, so echocardiography is likely to remain as the workhorse of LV functional assessment.

REFERENCES

1. Douglas PS, Garcia MJ, Haines DE, et al. ACCF/ASE/AHA/ASNC/HFSA/HRS/SCAI/SCCM/SCCT/SCMR 2011 appropriate use criteria for echocardiography. *J Am Soc Echocardiogr*. 2011;24:229–267.
2. Marwick TH. Methods used for the assessment of LV systolic function: common currency or tower of Babel? *Heart*. 2013;99:1078–1086.
3. Gregoratos G, Abrams J, Epstein AE, et al. ACC/AHA/NASPE 2002 Guideline Update for Implantation of Cardiac Pacemakers and Antiarrhythmia Devices—summary article. *J Am Coll Cardiol*. 2002;40:1703–1719.
4. Vardas PE, Auricchio A, Blanc JJ, et al. Guidelines for cardiac pacing and cardiac resynchronization therapy. *Eur Heart J*. 2007;28:2256–2295.
5. Bonow RO, Carabello BA, Chatterjee K, et al. Focused update incorporated into the ACC/AHA 2006 guidelines for the management of patients with valvular heart disease. *J Am Coll Cardiol*. 2008;52:e1–e142. 2008.
6. Hunt SA, Abraham WT, Chin MH, et al. Focused update incorporated into the ACC/AHA 2005 Guidelines for the Diagnosis and Management of Heart Failure in Adults. *J Am Coll Cardiol*. 2009;53:e1–e90. 2009.
7. Francis DP. How easily can omission of patients, or selection amongst poorly-reproducible measurements, create artificial correlations? Methods for detection and implications for observational research design in cardiology. *Int J Cardiol*. 2013;167:102–113.
8. Haugaa KH, Goebel B, Dahlslett T, et al. Risk assessment of ventricular arrhythmias in patients with nonischemic dilated cardiomyopathy by strain echocardiography. *J Am Soc Echocardiogr*. 2012;25:667–673.
9. Potter E, Marwick TH. Assessment of left ventricular function by echocardiography: the case for routinely adding global longitudinal strain to ejection fraction. *JACC Cardiovasc Imag*. 2018;11:260–274.
10. Carabello BA. Evolution of the study of left ventricular function: everything old is new again. *Circulation*. 2002;105. 2701–273.
11. Wachtell K, Gerdts E, Palmieri V, et al. In-treatment midwall and endocardial fractional shortening predict cardiovascular outcome in hypertensive patients with preserved baseline systolic ventricular function: the Losartan Intervention for Endpoint reduction study. *J Hypertens*. 2010;28:1541–1546.
12. Curtis JP, Sokol SI, Wang Y, et al. The association of left ventricular ejection fraction, mortality, and cause of death in stable outpatients with heart failure. *J Am Coll Cardiol*. 2003;42:736–7342.
13. Stanton T, Leano R, Marwick TH. Prediction of all-cause mortality from global longitudinal speckle strain: comparison with ejection fraction and wall motion scoring. *Circ Cardiovasc Imag*. 2009;2:356–364.
14. Johri AM, Picard MH, Newell J, et al. Can a teaching intervention reduce interobserver variability in LVEF assessment: a quality control exercise in the echocardiography lab. *JACC Cardiovasc Imag*. 2011;4:821–829.
15. Marwick TH, Shah SJ, Thomas JD. Myocardial strain in the assessment of patients with heart failure. *JAMA Cardiol*. 2019;4:287–294.
16. Magne J, Cosyns B, Popescu BA, et al. Distribution and prognostic significance of left ventricular global longitudinal strain in asymptomatic significant aortic stenosis: an individual participant data meta-analysis. *JACC Cardiovasc Imag*. 2019;12:84–92.
17. Plana JC, Galderisi M, Barac A, et al. Expert consensus for multimodality imaging evaluation of adult patients during and after cancer therapy. *J Am Soc Echocardiogr*. 2014;27:911–939.
18. Kawakami H, Nerlekar N, Haugaa KH, et al. Prediction of ventricular arrhythmias with left ventricular mechanical dispersion: a systematic review and meta-analysis. *JACC Cardiovasc Imag*. 2020;13:562–5672.
19. Nagueh SF, Smiseth OA, Appleton CP, et al. Recommendations for the evaluation of left ventricular diastolic function by echocardiography. *J Am Soc Echocardiogr*. 2016;29:277–314.
20. Singh A, Medvedofsky D, Mediratta A, et al. Peak left atrial strain as a single measure for the non-invasive assessment of left ventricular filling pressures. *Int J Cardiovasc Imag*. 2019;35:23–32.
21. Lin E, Alessio A. What are the basic concepts of temporal, contrast, and spatial resolution in cardiac CT? *J Cardiovasc Comput Tomogr*. 2009;3:403–408.
22. Lang RM, Bierig M, Devereux RB, et al. Recommendations for chamber quantification. *J Am Soc Echocardiogr*. 2005;18:1440–1463.
23. Hibberd MG, Chuang ML, Beaudin RA, et al. Accuracy of three-dimensional echocardiography with unrestricted selection of imaging planes for measurement of left ventricular volumes and ejection fraction. *Am Heart J*. 2000;140:469–475.
24. Streiner DL, Norman GR. "Precision" and "accuracy": two terms that are neither. *J Clin Epidemiol*. 2006;59:327–330.
25. Streeter RP, Nichols K, Bergmann SR. Stability of right and left ventricular ejection fractions and volumes after heart transplantation. *J Heart Lung Transplant*. 2005;24:815–818.
26. Goldenberg I, Moss AJ, Hall WJ, et al. Predictors of response to cardiac resynchronization therapy in the Multicenter Automatic Defibrillator Implantation Trial with Cardiac Resynchronization Therapy (MADIT-CRT). *Circulation*. 2011;124:1527–1536.
27. Thavendiranathan P, Liu S, Datta S, et al. Automated quantification of mitral inflow and aortic outflow stroke volumes by three-dimensional real-time volume color-flow Doppler transthoracic echocardiography: comparison with pulsed-wave Doppler and cardiac magnetic resonance imaging. *J Am Soc Echocardiogr*. 2012;25:56–65.
28. Mulvagh SL, Rakowski H, Vannan MA, et al. American Society of Echocardiography consensus statement on the clinical applications of ultrasonic contrast agents in echocardiography. *J Am Soc Echocardiogr*. 2008;21:1179–1201.

25 Regional Left Ventricular Systolic Function

Manish Bansal, Partho P. Sengupta

Given its considerable diagnostic, prognostic, and therapeutic implications, the assessment of left ventricular (LV) regional systolic function forms an important part of any echocardiographic examination. Because coronary artery disease (CAD) is by far the commonest cause resulting in regional LV systolic dysfunction, the mere presence of regional wall motion abnormality (RWMA) usually confirms the presence of underlying CAD. Additionally, the distribution of RWMA helps in predicting the location of stenosis in the coronary arterial tree, whereas the extent of RWMA and its potential reversibility help in guiding several therapeutic decisions in these patients.

ASSESSMENT OF REGIONAL LV SYSTOLIC DYSFUNCTION

Numerous qualitative, semiquantitative, and quantitative methods have been developed over the years to evaluate LV regional systolic function (Table 25.1).[1] All of these techniques rely on a segmental approach that divides LV myocardium into a number of segments and the contractile function of each segment is then assessed individually.

Left Ventricular Myocardial Segmentation

For the purpose of standardization, the American Society of Echocardiography had recommended a 16-segment model in 1989,[2] but a 17th segment, the apical cap, was added later to allow comparison with other imaging modalities, such as nuclear imaging (Fig. 25.1).[3,4] Although either model can be used for assessment of LV systolic function by echocardiography, the 16-segment model remains clinically applicable because the apical cap normally does not exhibit any apparent contractile function. However, when the WMA is localized to the true apex, the 16-segment model may lead to overestimation of systolic dysfunction during scoring. In comparison, strain imaging software typically divide the left ventricle into 18 segments.

Methods for Assessment of Regional Left Ventricular Systolic Function

Visual Wall Motion Analysis

Visual analysis of segmental wall motion is the most commonly used method for the assessment of LV regional systolic function. Each myocardial segment is carefully assessed for the extent of wall thickening and motion and is graded as normal, hypokinetic, akinetic, or dyskinetic or aneurysmal. These different grades of wall motion can also be assigned a score, as outlined in Table 25.2. The score for each segment is added, and the total score is divided by the number of segments analyzed to obtain a wall motion score index, which provides a semiquantitative estimate of overall LV systolic function. A higher wall motion score index signifies worse LV systolic function. The use of ultrasound contrast is recommended to improve endocardial border delineation when two or more LV myocardial segments cannot be visualized adequately for assessment of regional wall motion.[5]

TABLE 25.1 Methods for Assessment of Regional Left Ventricular Systolic Function

Modality	Method
M-mode	• Regional thickening
2D echocardiography	• Visual assessment of wall motion
	• Percent radian shrinkage
	• Percent segmental area reduction or fractional area change
	• Center-line chordal shortening
	• Acoustic quantification with color kinesis
3D echocardiography	• Regional volume change
Tissue Doppler imaging	• Segmental velocity
	• Segmental displacement
	• Segmental strain and strain rate
Speckle-tracking echocardiography (can be 2D or 3D)	• Segmental longitudinal, radial, and circumferential strain and strain rate
	• Layer-specific strain and strain rate

2D, Two-dimensional; *3D,* three-dimensional.

Although the visual assessment has been extensively used and validated in clinical and research settings, its subjective and qualitative nature remains a major challenge. This subjective interpretation renders regional wall motion assessment highly operator dependent and susceptible to interobserver variability. Considerable expertise is required to ensure adequate accuracy and reproducibility of the interpretation.[6,7] Additionally, because of its qualitative nature, visual inspection is unable to detect subtle changes in regional systolic function, which is particularly relevant when interpreting stress echocardiograms.

Quantitative Techniques for Assessment of Left Ventricular Regional Systolic Function

To overcome the challenges inherent in visual wall motion analysis, several quantitative methods for the assessment of regional LV function have been developed over the years. These include percent radial shortening, fractional area change, centerline approach, and acoustic quantification with color kinesis.[1] These techniques depend on detection of the endocardial border during different phases of cardiac cycle, either manually or through acoustic quantification. The computerized algorithms then analyze the extent of endocardial displacement to derive information about segmental systolic function. Although seemingly promising, none of these techniques gained wide acceptance in clinical practice because (1) they are dependent on grayscale image quality, (2) it is not possible to differentiate between true myocardial contraction and translational movement, and (3) the incremental information obtained is relatively limited when compared with conventional wall motion analysis. More recently, a similar approach based on automated border recognition during three-dimensional echocardiography has been developed. It estimates regional LV systolic function by calculating fractional change in the LV cavity subvolumes subtended by the individual myocardial segments. However, it is even more dependent on grayscale image quality than two-dimensional echocardiography.

Doppler-based tissue velocity imaging offers an alternative approach to assessment of regional myocardial function. The technique has been used quite frequently in the past but has now been largely superseded by strain imaging. The major problem with tissue velocity imaging is that it only measures myocardial motion

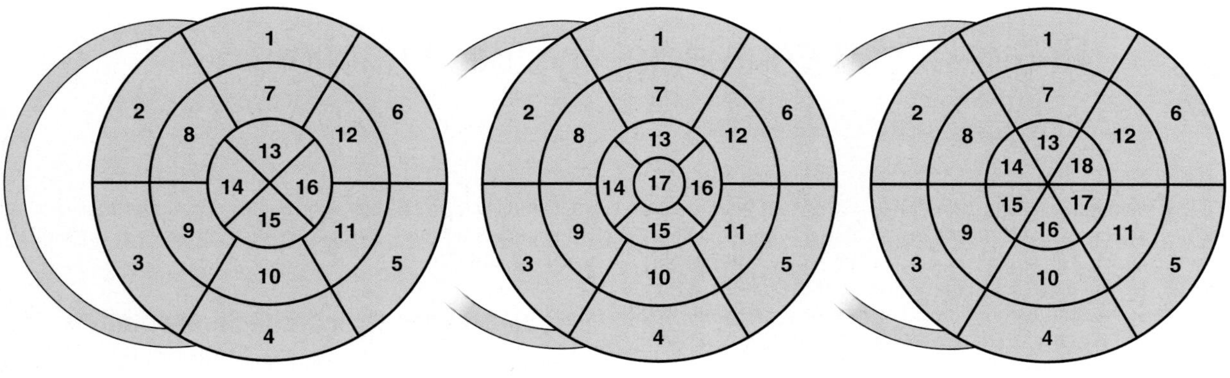

All models

1. basal anterior
2. basal anteroseptal
3. basal inferoseptal
4. basal inferior
5. basal inferolateral
6. basal anterolateral

7. mid anterior
8. mid anteroseptal
9. mid inferoseptal
10. mid inferior
11. mid inferolateral
12. mid anterolateral

16 and 17 segment model

13. apical anterior
14. apical septal
15. apical inferior
16. apical lateral

17 segment model only

17. apex

18 segment model only

13. apical anterior
14. apical anteroseptal
15. apical inferoseptal
16. apical inferior
17. apical inferolateral
18. apical anterolateral

Figure 25.1. Schematic diagram of the different left ventricular segmentation models: 16-segment model *(left)*, 17-segment model *(center)*, and 18-segment model *(right)*. (Reproduced with permission from Lang RM et al: Recommendations for cardiac chamber quantification by echocardiography in adults, *J Am Soc Echocardiogr* 28:1–39, 2015.)

relative to the transducer and not true myocardial deformation. Additionally, being a Doppler-based technique, its dependence on the angle of insonation is another major limitation.

Strain imaging, which measures myocardial deformation, is currently the preferred quantitative technique for assessment of regional LV systolic function. There are two main forms of myocardial strain imaging: tissue Doppler based and grayscale based. Doppler-based strain imaging offers higher temporal resolution and is more suited for imaging at fast heart rates. However, its angle dependence is a major limitation that seriously compromises its accuracy in dilated and distorted ventricles. Moreover, because of the angle dependence, tissue Doppler imaging cannot be used for measuring radial and circumferential strain and LV rotation and torsion. For these reasons, grayscale-based strain imaging or speckle-tracking echocardiography (STE) is currently the most commonly used technique for this purpose.[8] It relies on tracking the spatial movement of acoustic speckles in a grayscale image, generated by tissue–ultrasound interactions. The STE software recognizes these speckles and automatically tracks them frame by frame through the cardiac cycle to derive velocity, displacement, strain, and strain rate data. The apical four-chamber, two-chamber, and long-axis views are used for measuring longitudinal strain, whereas the short-axis views are used for quantification of radial strain, circumferential strain, rotation, and twist.

Although STE has become a very useful modality for assessment of global LV systolic function, several challenges remain, particularly for regional function assessment. First, it is highly dependent on grayscale image quality. Second, significant intervendor variability still exists, especially for segmental strain.[9] And third, and the most relevant to regional function assessment, the reproducibility of strain measurements at segmental level is currently poor.[10] As a result, the technique is not yet suitable for routine clinical application for assessment of LV regional systolic function.

CLINICAL APPLICATIONS
Recognition of Underlying Coronary Artery Disease and Culprit Coronary Artery

CAD typically affects the left ventricle in a regional manner. This, combined with the high prevalence of CAD, makes it the commonest cause of regional LV systolic dysfunction. Accordingly, the mere presence of regional involvement in a patient with LV systolic dysfunction is considered indicative of underlying CAD. Furthermore, because the distribution of RWMA corresponds to the coronary vascular supply, it helps in identifying the site of stenosis in the coronary arterial tree. Although variations in coronary vascular distribution exist, Fig. 25.2 depicts the most commonly found pattern. Atypical distribution may be seen in patients with previous coronary bypass graft surgery because of varying contributions of native and grafted vessels to the myocardial blood supply.

In patients presenting with acute coronary syndrome, the wall motion abnormalities may be quite subtle initially and difficult to recognize. In such situations, strain imaging may help recognize

TABLE 25.2 Visual, Semiquantitative Assessment of Left Ventricular Segmental Myocardial Systolic Function as Recommended by the American Society of Echocardiography

Wall Motion Type	Description	Wall-Motion Score
Normal or hyperkinetic	Normal thickening (usually >30% thickening from end-diastole)	1
Hypokinetic	Reduced thickening (usually 10%–30% thickening from end-diastole)	2[a]
Akinetic	Markedly reduced or no thickening (<10% thickening from end-diastole)	3
Dyskinetic or aneurysmal	Dyskinesia: paradoxical thinning and/or outward motion during systole	4
	Aneurysm: diastolic deformation of the shape with dyskinetic movement	

[a]Some schemes assign scores of 1.5 and 2.5 to denote mild hypokinesis and severe hypokenesis, respectively.
Reproduced with permission from Lang RM et al: Recommendations for cardiac chamber quantification by echocardiography in adults, *J Am Soc Echocardiogr* 28:1–39, 2015.

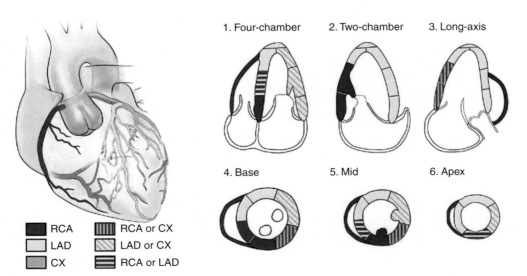

Figure 25.2. The typical distribution of coronary vascular supply. *CX,* Circumflex; *LAD,* left anterior descending; *RCA,* right coronary artery. (Reproduced with permission from Lang RM et al: Recommendations for cardiac chamber quantification by echocardiography in adults, *J Am Soc Echocardiogr* 28:1–39, 2015.)

early myocardial dysfunction. In a study involving patients with non–ST-elevation myocardial infarction, reduced endocardial territorial longitudinal strain (<−16%) was found to have 89% sensitivity and 81% specificity for diagnosing significant CAD.[11] Similarly, endocardial global circumferential strain below −21% identified significant CAD with 85% sensitivity and specificity. However, it must be reiterated that the reproducibility of segmental strain analysis is currently not good enough to justify its routine clinical application.

Nonischemic Causes of Regional Left Ventricular Systolic Dysfunction

Apart from CAD, several nonischemic cardiac conditions can result in regional LV systolic dysfunction (Box 25.1). Although these conditions are much less common than CAD, it is important to be aware of them to avoid misdiagnosis.

Left bundle branch block (LBBB) and other conduction abnormalities that interfere with the normal electrical activation of the left ventricle represent the commonest nonischemic cause of regional LV systolic dysfunction. LBBB results in a typical septal contraction pattern characterized by brief, early, inward motion followed by a later outward motion (Fig. 25.3). The pattern of RWMA in other conduction abnormalities varies depending on the sequence of LV myocardial depolarization. Abnormal septal motion is also seen in some other conditions, such as postpericardiotomy state, constrictive pericarditis, and right ventricular pressure and volume overload.

Many systemic illnesses such as sarcoidosis and hemochromatosis can also result in RWMA, although global involvement is more common. RWMA affecting the basal posterolateral and septal regions is common in people with sarcoidosis and can mimic CAD. Similarly, nonischemic dilated cardiomyopathy can also present with regional LV systolic dysfunction, usually characterized by marked impairment of septum and inferior wall and relative preservation of anterior and lateral walls. Finally, some normal variants can also produce RWMA. These include physiologic heterogeneity in LV contraction and early relaxation patterns.

Several important clues can help differentiate true ischemic RWMA from regional dysfunction resulting from the nonischemic causes mentioned. Atypical distribution of RWMA not conforming to any particular vascular territory, abnormal myocardial motion with preserved myocardial thickening, and wall motion abnormalities confined only to a brief period of the cardiac cycle generally favor a nonischemic cause. However, stress cardiomyopathy, also known as apical ballooning syndrome or Takotsubo cardiomyopathy, is a distinct form of regional LV systolic dysfunction that is almost indistinguishable from CAD. The underlying clinical setting, relatively less impressive electrocardiographic changes or rise in cardiac enzymes, and spontaneous, complete recovery of LV systolic function are helpful in diagnosing this condition. However, the confirmation of diagnosis requires demonstration of normal coronary arteries during coronary angiography.

Assessment of Inducible Myocardium Ischemia

Stress echocardiography is one of the commonest modalities used for diagnosing inducible myocardial ischemia. Induction of an RWMA in response to some form of stressor (exercise, pharmacologic, or pacing) is the fundamental concept underlying stress echocardiography. Visual wall motion analysis is the most common method used for recognition of inducible myocardial ischemia during stress echocardiography. Although inherent subjectivity of visual wall motion analysis remains a challenge, it has been demonstrated to have good accuracy with expert interpreters. In a large meta-analysis, the average sensitivity and specificity of exercise echocardiography were found to be 83% and 84%, respectively.[12] The sensitivity and specificity of dobutamine echocardiography were 80% and 85%, respectively, and were 71% and 92% for dipyridamole echocardiography and 68% and 81%, respectively, for adenosine stress echocardiography.[12] Addition of strain imaging to visual wall motion analysis has been shown to enhance the accuracy of stress echocardiography.[13,14] Tissue Doppler strain appears more suitable for this purpose owing to its better temporal resolution at faster heart rates. However, STE has also been used, with reasonable accuracy, at least in the anterior circulation.[15]

Assessment of Myocardial Viability and Transmural Extent of Infarct

In patients with significant, ischemic LV systolic dysfunction, the presence of myocardial viability is an important prognostic marker and is associated with greater likelihood of functional recovery after revascularization and better clinical outcomes.[16–20] Accordingly, myocardial viability assessment is often performed in these patients to determine the need for and the mode of revascularization.

The simple measurement of end-diastolic wall thickness may itself be helpful in predicting myocardial viability. A thinned-out (<6 mm) myocardial segment, especially with increased echogenicity, is highly suggestive of scar tissue, and this finding has 93% negative predictive value for the lack of viability.[21] However, the converse is not true because a dysfunctional segment with diastolic wall thickness larger than 6 mm may not necessarily recover after revascularization.

Dobutamine echocardiography is the standard echocardiographic modality used for assessment of myocardial viability. In a dysfunctional myocardium, improvement in contractile function with low-dose dobutamine indicates the presence of viability. However, a biphasic response, which refers to initial improvement at low-dose followed by worsening at peak dose, is the most specific for functional recovery after revascularization.[22] In a meta-analysis comparing different modalities for myocardial viability assessment, dobutamine echocardiography was reported to have a sensitivity of 84% and specificity of 81% for predicting functional recovery after revascularization.[23] The specificity of dobutamine

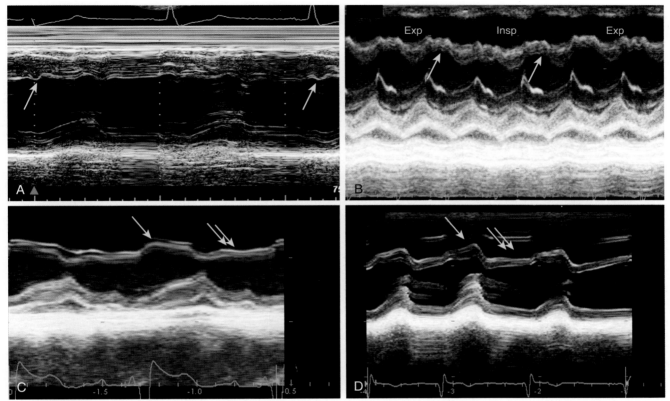

Figure 25.3. Examples of nonischemic left ventricular regional wall motion abnormality. **A,** Left bundle branch block with the characteristic early systolic beak *(arrows)*. **B,** Constrictive pericarditis, characterized by oscillatory movements of ventricular septum. Please also note respirophasic changes in right ventricular size with smaller size during expiration (Exp) and larger size during inspiration (Insp). **C,** Right ventricular pressure overload. There is septal compression toward the left ventricle during both systole *(single arrow)* and diastole *(double arrows)*. **D,** Right ventricular volume overload. The interventricular septum assumes normal position during systole *(single arrow)* but gets compressed toward the left ventricle during diastole *(double arrows)*.

echocardiography was highest among all the modalities included in this analysis. Quantitative techniques, such as strain imaging, have been explored to enhance the diagnostic accuracy of dobutamine echocardiography for myocardial viability assessment. The studies have shown that a combination of visual wall motion analysis and strain imaging may yield greater accuracy compared with either modality alone.[24,25]

Yet another approach to assess myocardial viability is to evaluate the transmural extent of myocardial infarction. With increasing transmural extent, the infarcted segment becomes less likely to recover functionally and is more likely to undergo scarring, thinning, and adverse remodeling with consequent reduction in LV ejection fraction.[26]

Experimental models have previously established that coronary occlusion beyond 20 minutes results in a wave front of necrosis that extends from the subendocardium to the subepicardium.[27] With only 20% of myocardial involvement, segments start showing systolic thinning, and no further increase is seen in the severity of systolic thinning with an increasing extent of transmural infarction.[28] Thus systolic thinning of a myocardial segment as seen on conventional M-mode and two-dimensional echocardiography suggests the presence of an infarct greater than 20% but cannot be used to differentiate more profound degrees of transmural infarction.

However, STE may be helpful in this regard.[29,30] The muscle fibers in LV myocardium are arranged in the form of helically oriented layers. The fibers in the subendocardial layer are responsible mainly for the long-axis contraction of the left ventricle, whereas those in the midmyocardial and subepicardial layers mainly determine

radial thickening and circumferential shortening.[8,30] Coronary ischemia causes subendocardial dysfunction, resulting in reduced longitudinal strain, with relative preservation of circumferential and radial strain. Subendocardial infarction similarly causes reduction in longitudinal strain, whereas transmural infarction is associated with loss of all the strain components (Fig. 25.4). Thus, nontransmural disease is characterized by disparity among principal myocardial strains. STE, by demonstrating this disparity, can help differentiate a subendocardial from a transmural infarction.[29,30]

Other Applications

Echocardiography has also been used for assessment of mechanical dyssynchrony in patients with LV systolic dysfunction undergoing cardiac resynchronization therapy (CRT).[31] Dispersion in time to peak contraction of different myocardial segments assessed using tissue velocity imaging has been the most commonly used parameter. Initial single-center studies showed it to have incremental value in predicting response to CRT.[32,33] However, these findings were not supported by a multicenter study performed subsequently.[34] Several other indices based on longitudinal strain, radial strain, and so on have also been tried, but none of these approaches are currently in routine clinical use because of significant interobserver variability, lack of clear incremental benefit over conventional modalities, and various technical challenges.[31] More recently, segmental radial strain has been shown to be helpful in identifying the optimum site for LV lead placement by allowing simultaneous assessment of activation delay as well as the scar extent.[35,36] The best outcomes can be achieved when LV lead is placed adjacent to

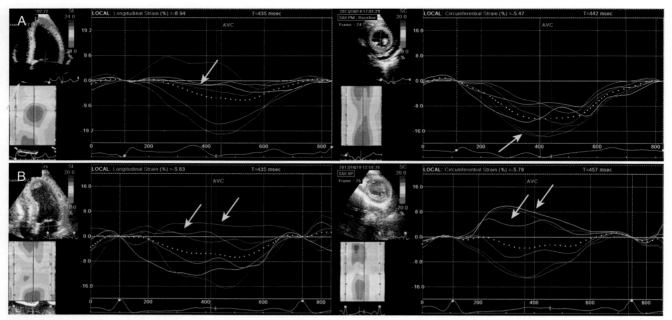

Figure 25.4. Speckle-tracking echocardiography–derived measurements of segmental longitudinal (**A**) and circumferential (**B**) strain from the apical four-chamber and apical short-axis views, respectively. Note the relatively preserved strains in the basal segments *(single arrow)* but the significantly impaired strain values in the apical segments *(double arrows)*, particularly the apical lateral segment.

the latest activated myocardial segment that is not scarred. However, technical challenges preclude its wider clinical application.

In patients with depressed LV ejection fraction, dispersion in time to peak segmental contraction has also been used as a predictor of the risk for serious ventricular arrhythmias.[37–39] Such disparity reflects nonuniform electrical activation of the left ventricle, which is a substrate for arrhythmogenesis. However, the clinical utility of this finding remains unclear at present.

REFERENCES

1. Echocardiography and coronary artery disease. In: Armstrong WF, Ryan T, eds. *Feigenbaum's Echocardiography*. Philadelphia: Wolters Kluwer; 2019:427–459.
2. Schiller NB, Shah PM, Crawford M, et al. Recommendations for quantitation of the left ventricle by two-dimensional echocardiography. *J Am Soc Echocardiogr.* 1989;2:358–367.
3. Cerqueira MD, Weissman NJ, Dilsizian V, et al. Standardized myocardial segmentation and nomenclature for tomographic imaging of the heart. *Circulation.* 2002;105:539–542.
4. Lang RM, Badano LP, Mor-Avi V, et al. Recommendations for cardiac chamber quantification by echocardiography in adults. *J Am Soc Echocardiogr.* 2015;28:1–39.
5. Mulvagh SL, Rakowski H, Vannan MA, et al. American Society of Echocardiography consensus statement on the clinical applications of ultrasonic contrast agents in echocardiography. *J Am Soc Echocardiogr.* 2008;21:1179–1201.
6. Hoffmann R, Lethen H, Marwick T, et al. Analysis of interinstitutional observer agreement in interpretation of dobutamine stress echocardiograms. *J Am Coll Cardiol.* 1996;27:330–336.
7. Hoffmann R, Lethen H, Marwick T, et al. Standardized guidelines for the interpretation of dobutamine echocardiography reduce interinstitutional variance in interpretation. *Am J Cardiol.* 1998;82:1520–1524.
8. Geyer H, Caracciolo G, Abe H, et al. Assessment of myocardial mechanics using speckle tracking echocardiography: fundamentals and clinical applications. *J Am Soc Echocardiogr.* 2010;23:351–369.
9. Mirea O, Pagourelias ED, Duchenne J, et al. Intervendor differences in the accuracy of detecting regional functional abnormalities. *JACC Cardiovasc Imag.* 2017;11:25–34.
10. Mirea O, Pagourelias ED, Duchenne J, et al. Variability and reproducibility of segmental longitudinal strain measurement. *JACC Cardiovasc Imag.* 2017;11:15–24.
11. Sarvari SI, Haugaa KH, Zahid W, et al. Layer-specific quantification of myocardial deformation by strain echocardiography may reveal significant CAD in patients with non-ST-segment elevation acute coronary syndrome. *JACC Cardiovasc Imag.* 2013;6:535–544.
12. Noguchi Y, Nagata-Kobayashi S, Stahl JE, Wong JB. A meta-analytic comparison of echocardiographic stressors. *Int J Cardiovasc Imag.* 2005;21:189–207.

13. Voigt JU, Exner B, Schmiedehausen K, et al. Strain-rate imaging during dobutamine stress echocardiography provides objective evidence of inducible ischemia. *Circulation.* 2003;107:2120–2126.
14. Ng AC, Sitges M, Pham PN, et al. Incremental value of 2D speckle tracking strain imaging to wall motion analysis for detection of coronary artery disease in patients undergoing dobutamine stress echocardiography. *Am Heart J.* 2009;158:836–844.
15. Hanekom L, Cho GY, Leano R, et al. Comparison of two-dimensional speckle and tissue Doppler strain measurement during dobutamine stress echocardiography: an angiographic correlation. *Eur Heart J.* 2007;28:1765–1772.
16. Senior R, Kaul S, Lahiri A. Myocardial viability on echocardiography predicts long-term survival after revascularization in patients with ischemic congestive heart failure. *J Am Coll Cardiol.* 1999;33:1848–1854.
17. Allman KC, Shaw LJ, Hachamovitch R, Udelson JE. Myocardial viability testing and impact of revascularization on prognosis in patients with coronary artery disease and left ventricular dysfunction: a meta-analysis. *J Am Coll Cardiol.* 2002;39:1151–1158.
18. Afridi I, Grayburn PA, Panza JA, et al. Myocardial viability during dobutamine echocardiography predicts survival in patients with coronary artery disease and severe left ventricular systolic dysfunction. *J Am Coll Cardiol.* 1998;32:921–926.
19. Bax JJ, Poldermans D, Elhendy A, et al. Improvement of left ventricular ejection fraction, heart failure symptoms and prognosis after revascularization in patients with chronic coronary artery disease and viable myocardium detected by dobutamine stress echocardiography. *J Am Coll Cardiol.* 1999;34:163–169.
20. Meluzin J, Cerny J, Frelich M, et al. Prognostic value of the amount of dysfunctional but viable myocardium in revascularized patients with coronary artery disease and left ventricular dysfunction. *J Am Coll Cardiol.* 1998;32:912–920.
21. Cwajg JM, Cwajg E, Nagueh SF, et al. End-diastolic wall thickness as a predictor of recovery of function in myocardial hibernation: relation to rest-redistribution T1-201 tomography and dobutamine stress echocardiography. *J Am Coll Cardiol.* 2000;35:1152–1161.
22. Afridi I, Kleiman NS, Raizner AE, Zoghbi WA. Dobutamine echocardiography in myocardial hibernation. Optimal dose and accuracy in predicting recovery of ventricular function after coronary angioplasty. *Circulation.* 1995;91:663–670.
23. Bax JJ, Wijns W, Cornel JH, et al. Accuracy of currently available techniques for prediction of functional recovery after revascularization in patients with left ventricular dysfunction due to chronic coronary artery disease: comparison of pooled data. *J Am Coll Cardiol.* 1997;30:1451–1460.
24. Hanekom L, Jenkins C, Jeffries L, et al. Incremental value of strain rate analysis as an adjunct to wall-motion scoring for assessment of myocardial viability by dobutamine echocardiography: a follow-up study after revascularization. *Circulation.* 2005;112:3892–3900.
25. Bansal M, Jeffriess L, Leano R, et al. Assessment of myocardial viability at dobutamine echocardiography by deformation analysis using tissue velocity and speckle-tracking. *JACC Cardiovasc Imag.* 2010;3:121–131.
26. Thanavaro S, Krone RJ, Kleiger RE, et al. In-hospital prognosis of patients with first nontransmural and transmural infarctions. *Circulation.* 1980;61:29–33.

27. Kloner RA, Jennings RB. Consequences of brief ischemia: stunning, preconditioning, and their clinical implications: part 1. *Circulation*. 2001;104:2981–2989.
28. Lieberman AN, Weiss JL, Jugdutt BI, et al. Two-dimensional echocardiography and infarct size: relationship of regional wall motion and thickening to the extent of myocardial infarction in the dog. *Circulation*. 1981;63:739–746.
29. Chan J, Hanekom L, Wong C, et al. Differentiation of subendocardial and transmural infarction using two-dimensional strain rate imaging to assess short-axis and long-axis myocardial function. *J Am Coll Cardiol*. 2006;48:2026–2033.
30. Bansal M, Sengupta PP. Longitudinal and circumferential strain in patients with regional LV dysfunction. *Curr Cardiol Rep*. 2013;15:339.
31. Gorcsan 3rd J, Abraham T, Agler DA, et al. Echocardiography for cardiac resynchronization therapy: recommendations for performance and reporting. *J Am Soc Echocardiogr*. 2008;21:191–213.
32. Yu C-M, Fung W-H, Lin H, et al. Predictors of left ventricular reverse remodeling after cardiac resynchronization therapy for heart failure secondary to idiopathic dilated or ischemic cardiomyopathy. *Am J Cardiol*. 2003;91:684–688.
33. Yu C-M, Fung JW-H, Zhang Q, et al. Tissue Doppler imaging is superior to strain rate imaging and postsystolic shortening on the prediction of reverse remodeling

in both ischemic and nonischemic heart failure after cardiac resynchronization therapy. *Circulation*. 2004;110:66–73.
34. Chung ES, Leon AR, Tavazzi L, et al. Results of the Predictors of Response to CRT (PROSPECT) trial. *Circulation*. 2008;117:2608–2616.
35. Khan FZ, Virdee MS, Palmer CR, et al. Targeted left ventricular lead placement to guide cardiac resynchronization therapy. *J Am Coll Cardiol*. 2012;59:1509–1518.
36. Saba S, Marek J, Schwartzman D, et al. Echocardiography-guided left ventricular lead placement for cardiac resynchronization therapy. *Circ Heart Fail*. 2013;6:427–434.
37. Haugaa KH, Smedsrud MK, Steen T, et al. Mechanical dispersion assessed by myocardial strain in patients after myocardial infarction for risk prediction of ventricular arrhythmia. *JACC Cardiovasc Imag*. 2010;3:247–256.
38. Haugaa KH, Grenne BL, Eek CH, et al. Strain echocardiography improves risk prediction of ventricular arrhythmias after myocardial infarction. *JACC Cardiovasc Imag*. 2013;6:841–850.
39. Ersboll M, Valeur N, Andersen MJ, et al. Early echocardiographic deformation analysis for the prediction of sudden cardiac death and life-threatening arrhythmias after myocardial infarction. *JACC Cardiovasc Imag*. 2013;6:851–860.

26 Myocardial Strain in Valvular Heart Disease

John Gorcsan III

Myocardial strain measurement using speckle-tracking echocardiography (STE) has made major contributions to the care of patients with cardiac diseases. This chapter focuses on emerging applications specific to patients with valvular heart disease. Most of the recent studies on myocardial strain and valvular disease have been retrospective or registry data but have made important exciting observations that have potential to make a major impact on patient management. This chapter is limited to topics of the use of myocardial strain with the most common valve diseases, including mitral regurgitation (MR), aortic stenosis (AS), and aortic regurgitation (AR). Important new data demonstrating the prognostic value of global longitudinal strain (GLS) are discussed in patients with: asymptomatic severe MR, severe AS undergoing surgical valve replacement, asymptomatic severe AS, and asymptomatic severe AR. Combined, these data demonstrate that GLS is a powerful new diagnostic measure that can contribute to the care of patients with valvular heart disease.

STRAIN AS AN ADDITIVE TO EJECTION FRACTION IN VALVULAR HEART DISEASE

The unique features that speckle tracking strain contributes to the evaluation of patients with valvular heart disease relates to valve effects on left ventricular (LV) mechanical function. Myocardial strain occurs in three dimensions, including vectors of longitudinal strain, circumferential strain, radial strain, and torsion.[1] The measure most commonly represented currently to quantify LV function is the index of GLS.[2] The standard approach of obtaining GLS is from the apical four-chamber, apical two-chamber, and apical long-axis views, combining the longitudinal shortening data from these three views into a single index (Fig. 26.1). Other vectors of myocardial strain may have important clinical utility, but the focus of this chapter remains on GLS because of its widespread clinical adoption and relative simplicity. In this review, GLS is often reported in absolute values with higher GLS representing better LV function for ease of understanding.

LV volumes and ejection fraction (EF) are the well-established means to quantify LV function in patients with MR, AS, and AR. GLS has been shown to be additive to LVEF, in particular with associations with prognosis, and the implication that GLS may influence future clinical decision-making processes for surgical or percutaneous valve interventions. EF describes the

blood displacement within the LV, whereas strain measures the deformation of the wall of the chamber.[3] It is clear that measures of wall deformation of the chamber must relate to the blood displacement within the chamber; however, GLS and LVEF are not precisely correlated.[4] It is believed that GLS is additive to LVEF because it includes wall properties that cannot be measured by LV volumes, including fibrosis, hypertrophy, and infiltration.

Myocardial fibrosis, including macroscopic fibrosis from ischemic disease and myocardial infarction and microscopic interstitial fibrosis,[5] has been shown to have the potential to influence greatly values of strain. Myocyte hypertrophy, in which cells increase in width, resulting in LV hypertrophy, is another principal mechanism of disease that can affect GLS in a manner different than LVEF. The additive value of strain to LVEF has been shown with elegant computer simulations and in patients with heart failure and preserved ejection fraction.[6,7] Furthermore, infiltrative diseases, most commonly cardiac amyloidosis, have profound effects on LV wall properties, which can be measured by strain imaging in a manner different than LVEF.[7]

Valvular heart disease may have important effects on ventricular function. For example, in patients with significant MR associated with LV unloading to the lower pressure left atrium (LA), the measure of LVEF may be misleadingly elevated. In other words, patients with MR and LVEF in the lower range of normal may actually have LV dysfunction that is masked by the effects of unloading.[8] It should be stressed that GLS and other measures of strain are also load dependent and are subject to the same influences of load as LVEF. However, GLS appears additive to LVEF in valvular heart disease by likely including wall properties of fibrosis, hypertrophy, and infiltration (discussed earlier), which are not captured by LVEF. Accordingly, GLS may be less load dependent than LVEF in certain clinical scenarios, but GLS is not load independent.

STRAIN IN MITRAL REGURGITATION
Strain in Asymptomatic Mitral Regurgitation With Preserved Left Ventricular Ejection Fraction

Factors influencing the important decision for patients with MR as to when to intervene with surgical mitral valve repair, replacement, or percutaneous intervention, such as mitral clip, continue

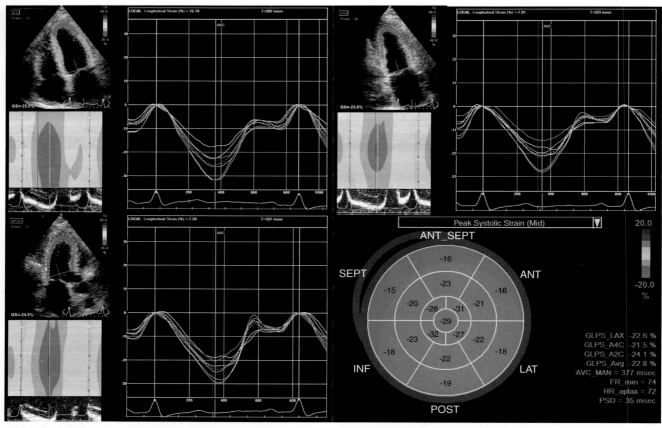

Figure 26.1. An example of longitudinal strain used to determine global longitudinal strain (GLS). The apical four-chamber view *(upper left)*, apical two-chamber view *(upper right)*, apical long-axis view *(lower left)*, and bull's-eye polar plot *(bottom right)*. The GLS in this example is 22.8% (in absolute values).

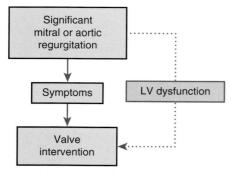

Figure 26.2. Flow diagram of relationships of significant mitral or aortic regurgitation to symptoms and surgical or percutaneous valve intervention, with the onset of symptoms as an indication for intervention. A clinical goal is to identify patients who may develop subclinical left ventricular (LV) dysfunction and are at high risk before they present with symptoms.

to evolve.[9,10] One of the most difficult clinical decisions remains when to intervene with mitral intervention with the goal to prevent irreversible LV dysfunction in patients with severe MR who are apparently asymptomatic (Fig. 26.2). Clinical practice has included exercise tolerance testing with or without imaging, or deciding to intervene based on the morphology of the mitral valve, such as P2 prolapse or flail with a high likelihood of success with an experienced surgical team for mitral valve repair.[11] Although evidence has emerged supporting early mitral valve intervention based on the above characteristics, controversy remains, and many patients who are asymptomatic choose not to have an intervention and wait for the development of symptoms. Accordingly, there is an opportunity for strain imaging to identify patients with severe MR and subclinical LV dysfunction who are more likely to benefit from early surgical intervention despite being asymptomatic.

The potential clinical utility of strain imaging in asymptomatic patients with severe MR was first reported by Mentias and colleagues in a retrospective analysis of 737 patients referred for evaluation for mitral valve surgery.[12] They examined incremental prognostic utility of GLS and exercise testing in asymptomatic patients with primary MR and preserved LVEF. They used vendor neutral strain imaging software applied to archived Digital Imaging and Communications in Medicine (DICOM) data to assess GLS and documented patient outcomes with mortality as the primary endpoint. Patients with MR were selected with preserved LV function documented by routine measures of LVEF, end-systolic dimension (ESD), and end-diastolic dimension (EDD): (1) moderate to severe or severe (3+ or 4+) MR, (2) LVEF greater than 60%, and (3) nondilated left ventricle (EDD <3.3 cm/m^2 and ESD <4 cm).

They found that age, gender-adjusted exercise metabolic equivalents, resting right ventricular systolic pressure, Society of Thoracic Surgeons score, and mitral valve surgery were significantly associated with patient survival, as has been observed previously. Their new observation was that baseline lower GLS magnitude was associated with a worse long-term survival (hazard ratio [HR], 1.60; 95% confidence interval, 1.47–1.73; P < .001) (Fig. 26.3). Using the median GLS of 21.7% (in absolute values), better baseline GLS was highly associated with long-term survival. When risk of death at 5 years was estimated by GLS, risk began to increase with strain worse than 21%,

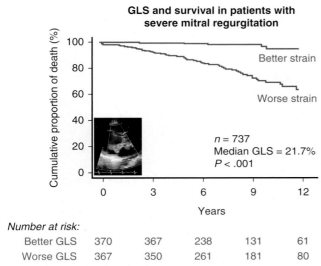

Figure 26.3. Kaplan-Meier time to event analysis of asymptomatic patients with severe mitral regurgitation grouped by medial global longitudinal strain (GLS). Patients with worse GLS (<21.7% in absolute values) were at higher risk of death than patients with better strain higher than the median. The *lower left inset* is a parasternal long-axis view example of a patient with posterior leaflet prolapse and severe mitral regurgitation. (Modified with permission from Mentias A et al: Strain echocardiography and functional capacity in asymptomatic primary mitral regurgitation with preserved ejection fraction, *J Am Coll Cardiol* 68:1974–1986, 2016.)

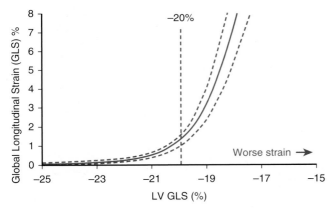

Figure 26.4. A plot of estimated risk of death over 5 years by global longitudinal strain (GLS) in asymptomatic patients with severe mitral regurgitation (MR). Risk of death increases with strain worse than 21% (in absolute values) and significantly increases with GLS worse than 20%. (Modified with permission from Mentias A et al: Strain echocardiography and functional capacity in asymptomatic primary mitral regurgitation with preserved ejection fraction, *J Am Coll Cardiol* 68:1974–1986, 2016.)

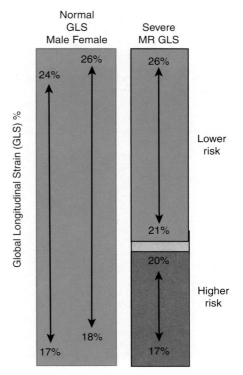

Figure 26.5. Comparisons of the normal range of global longitudinal strain (GLS) values using the same software in normal individuals and asymptomatic patients with severe mitral regurgitation (MR) and preserved left ventricular ejection (LV) fraction. Note that MR patients with GLS usually considered within the lower range of normal are at higher risk for death with values worse than 21%, in absolute values. This is because of the LV unloading that occurs with severe MR and can mask subclinical LV dysfunction.

dramatically increasing with strain worse than 20% (Fig. 26.4). This is remarkable because all of these patients had preserved LV function by routine measures such as LVEF and LV dimensions. Furthermore, GLS using similar strain analysis software was reported as normal between 17% to 24% for men and 18% to 26% for women in a large international series.[13] By comparison, in patients with significant MR, risk increased with GLS values usually considered in the normal range (Fig. 26.5). These data suggest that GLS, like LVEF, is load dependent and that with the unloading of severe MR, GLS with truly preserved LV function should be higher than 21%. In other words, GLS less than 21% (in absolute values) may represent subclinical LV dysfunction and is a marker of increased risk in these patients.

The prognostic value of GLS in patients with primary severe MR who underwent mitral surgery was supported by another study by Hiemstra and coworkers They studied 593 patients with severe MR and preserved LVEF (60% ± 8%) in which 99% underwent mitral valve repair.[14] GLS was determined at preoperative baseline, and patients were followed for on the average 6 years with all-cause mortality as the primary endpoint. The GLS cut-off of 20.6% was significantly associated with survival with higher strain magnitude having a better prognosis (Fig. 26.6). Furthermore, GLS was similarly predictive of patient outcomes regardless of mitral valve pathology as the cause of severe MR. These two complementary studies combine to support the concept that GLS is an important prognostic marker in asymptomatic patients with severe MR and may be a marker of subclinical LV dysfunction. The message is also consistent that GLS values in association with significant LV unloading that occurs with severe MR should be in the high-normal range with truly preserved LV function. Patients with GLS in the low-normal range may have LV dysfunction masked by the LV unloading of MR. The cut-off value of GLS at approximately 21% (in absolute values) was chosen because it was the median in these investigators' retrospective series.[14] Although it may be clinically useful as a guide, GLS may likely need to be tested prospectively to gain scientific validity in patients with severe MR to determine patient treatment.

Strain in Secondary Mitral Regurgitation With Depressed Left Ventricular Ejection Fraction

Interest has increased in patients with reduced LVEF and severe secondary MR because of the success of percutaneous mitral clip interventions.[10] Namazi and colleagues studied a large series of 650 patients with severe secondary MR by GLS and followed outcome.[15] In contrast to patients with preserved LV function in the aforementioned studies, the group mean LVEF was 29% ± 10% in these patients, and the group mean baseline GLS was markedly reduced at 7.2%. Of interest, GLS with a median cut-off of 7.0% was highly associated with survival (*P* < .001) (Fig. 26.7A). When adjusting for confounding baseline variables, impaired LV GLS (<7.0%) remained independently associated with all-cause mortality (HR, 1.337; 95% CI, 1.038–1.722; *P* < .024), whereas LVEF 30% or below was not associated with clinical outcome. A statistical model showed that the probability of death in patients with severe secondary MR progressively increased with worsening GLS, in particular with GLS values below 10% (Fig. 26.7B). A minor limitation of this study was that 70% of patients had cardiac resynchronization therapy, which is higher than most patient series with heart failure, but the prognostic utility of GLS was strongly supported in patients with severe secondary MR.

STRAIN IN AORTIC STENOSIS
Strain Before Surgical Aortic Valve Replacement for Severe Aortic Stenosis

Severe AS is a significant valve pathology with devastating clinical outcomes without surgical or percutaneous intervention. The prognostic role of GLS was demonstrated in patients undergoing surgical aortic valve replacement (AVR) for symptomatic severe AS[16] (Fig. 26.8). A total of 125 patients with aortic valve area smaller than 1.0 cm^2 had baseline preoperative GLS recorded as a substudy of a prospective single-center randomized study to evaluate the effect of candesartan compared with conventional treatment on reverse remodeling. The composite primary endpoint was a major adverse cardiac event (MACE), defined as cardiovascular mortality and cardiac hospitalization due to worsening of heart failure. Although baseline LVEF was similar in both groups of patients with or without MACE at 54% ± 8%, GLS had significant prognostic significance. When divided into quartiles, GLS was 20.0% ± 1.6% in the first quartile, 16.9% ± 0.7% and 14.3% ± 0.9% in the two middle quartiles, respectively, and 10.3% ± 1.4% in the fourth quartile. GLS in the top two quartiles was associated with a favorable postoperative prognosis, whereas GLS in the third and fourth quartiles was associated with significantly higher incidence of MACE.[16] These data suggest that GLS is measuring LV dysfunction not detected by LVEF, such as wall properties of degree of fibrosis or hypertrophy. Of interest, Medvedofsky and colleagues studied the prognostic value of GLS in a final cohort of 213 patients with severe symptomatic AS who underwent transcatheter aortic valve replacement (TAVR).[17] They observed baseline GLS not to be predictive of 1-year mortality as an endpoint.

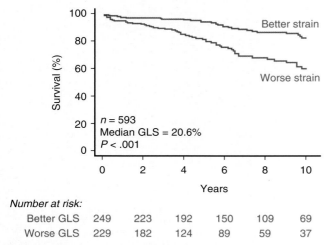

Figure 26.6. Kaplan-Meier plots of asymptomatic patients with severe primary mitral regurgitation (MR) and preserved left ventricular ejection fraction grouped by median global longitudinal strain (GLS) above and below 20.5% (absolute values). Patients with better strain had better survival and patients with worse strain had worse survival, indicating GLS is a marker of risk for these patients. (Modified with permission from Hiemstra YL et al: Prognostic value of global longitudinal strain and etiology after surgery for primary mitral regurgitation, *JACC Cardiovasc Imag* 13:577–585, 2020.)

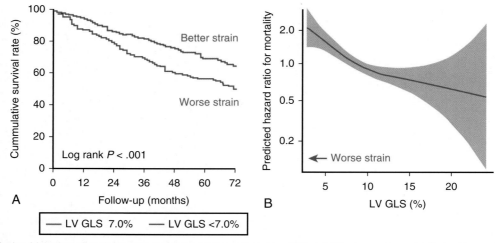

Figure 26.7. A, Kaplan-Meir plots of patients with severe secondary mitral regurgitation (MR) who underwent mitral valve repair surgery grouped by median global longitudinal strain above and below 7% (absolute values). In these patients with depressed left ventricular ejection fraction (LVEF), GLS had additive prognostic value to LVEF. **B,** A plot of the predicted hazard ratio for mortality in patients with severe secondary MR with risk significantly increasing when GLS is worse than 10%. (Modified with permission from Namazi F et al: Prognostic value of left ventricular global longitudinal strain in patients with secondary mitral regurgitation, *J Am Coll Cardiol* 75:750–758, 2020.)

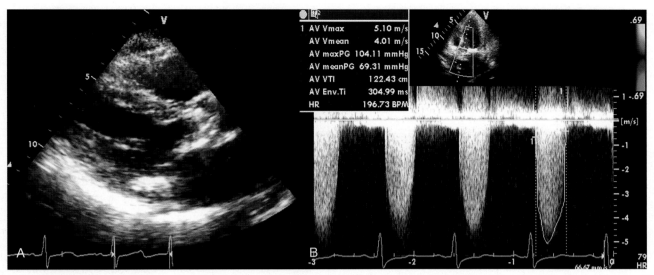

Figure 26.8. An example of an older woman with severe aortic stenosis. **A,** Parasternal long-axis view showing severely calcified aortic valve. **B,** Continuous wave Doppler velocity across aortic valve demonstrating severely elevated velocities and gradients.

The reason for these observed differences in prognostic value in surgical AVR patients versus those treated with TAVR are not clear, and further study of TAVR patients is warranted.

Strain in Asymptomatic Aortic Stenosis

The management of patients with severe AS discovered in patients who are apparently asymptomatic remains a difficult clinical problem. It is known that echocardiographic Doppler measures of AS severity have powerful prognostic significance.[18] A common clinical scenario is that progression of AS severity occurs gradually, and patients gradually modify their activities as to not be aware of symptoms. This may occur in patients with congenital bicuspid valve disease and AS who have altered their physical activities over years. AS may also gradually progress to a severe disease in older adult patients who have cut down on their physical exertion by attributing their feelings as part of the normal aging process. Alternatively, patients may tolerate a severe degree of AS for unclear reasons. Several approaches to determine timing of aortic valve replacement, most commonly with TAVR, commonly have been used. Exercise testing is an option, but there is also a risk associated with exercising patients with severe AS, and this approach is not universally adopted.[11] Accordingly, the hypothesis has been investigated that GLS can be a marker of subclinical LV dysfunction and a predictor of outcomes in asymptomatic patients with severe AS.

A three-center international study[19] was conducted including 220 asymptomatic patients with preserved LVEF greater than 50% and severe AS by the following criteria: (1) aortic valve area smaller than 0.6 cm^2/m^2 and/or (2) mean aortic gradient 40 mm Hg or greater and/or (3) peak aortic velocity 4 m/s or greater. After baseline GLS was recorded, the timing for AVR was left at the discretion of the treating physicians at each of the three centers. The time to symptom development and AVR and the date of all-cause mortality were recorded as clinical endpoints. A total of 118 (54%) developed symptoms during an average follow-up period of 1 year. GLS values lower than the median of 18.2% were significantly associated with development of symptoms ($P = 0.02$), showing the prognostic value of GLS. Similarly, the intervention by surgical AVR in 80% or TAVR in 27% (3% with balloon valvuloplasty) was associated with lower absolute GLS less than 18.2%.

The impression that GLS is a marker of risk in patients with asymptomatic AS was supported by a meta-analysis of 10 studies, including 1067 asymptomatic patients with significant AS and LVEF greater than 50%.[20] Using receiver operator curve analysis, the best cut-off value predictive of mortality was a GLS of 14.7% (in absolute values). The hazard ratio for mortality for GLS worse than 14.7% was strikingly increased by 2.69 (95% CI, 1.53–4.47; $P < .001$). Interestingly, the relationship between GLS and mortality remained significant in patients with clearly preserved LVEF of 60% or greater (Fig. 26.9). Although a clear cut-off value has not been established to identify patients with asymptomatic severe AS by these retrospective data, they represent compelling information for risk prediction by GLS in these patients. It is thought that declining GLS may be an early marker of LV dysfunction and potentially an indicator of patients who are most likely to benefit from earlier TAVR or surgical AVR interventions. It is unknown if this additional information readily obtained from an echocardiogram at the same time that AS severity is assessed will influence clinical decision making for AVR; this remains of interest for future investigation.

STRAIN IN AORTIC REGURGITATION

The decision for surgical intervention with AVR in patients with AR who are symptomatic is straightforward. A subset of patients with chronic severe AR, from a congenital bicuspid valve, for example, can develop compensatory adaptive mechanisms, including lowering peripheral vascular resistance and LV remodeling in which they are able to tolerate even severe chronic AR without symptoms. Since the classic work of Bonow and coworkers in 1983 describing the natural history of asymptomatic patients with AR and normal LV function, clinical decisions for AVR have been made based on routine measures of LV EF and LV dimensions.[21] Specifically, an asymptomatic patient with significant AR and LVEF less than 50% is considered a candidate for AVR as are patients with LVEF 50% or greater and LVESD greater than 50 mm or LVEDD 65 mm.[11] A variation has been to index dimensions to body surface area in asymptomatic patients with severe AR, and risk significantly increases when indexed LVESD has become greater than 2.0 cm/m^2.[22] Because the follow-up by echocardiography for LVEF and dimensions has been so well established, it has been difficult to prove that additional measures can impact on surgical decision making because they have

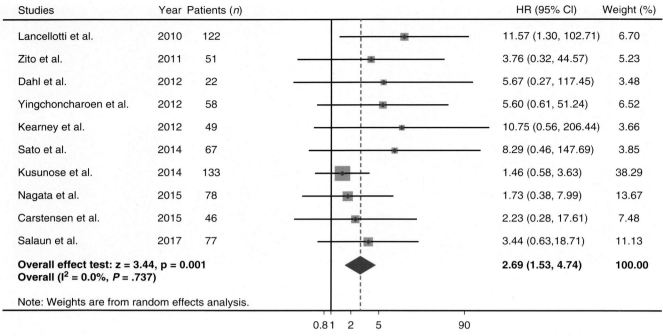

Studies	Year	Patients (n)		HR (95% CI)	Weight (%)
Lancellotti et al.	2010	122		11.57 (1.30, 102.71)	6.70
Zito et al.	2011	51		3.76 (0.32, 44.57)	5.23
Dahl et al.	2012	22		5.67 (0.27, 117.45)	3.48
Yingchoncharoen et al.	2012	58		5.60 (0.61, 51.24)	6.52
Kearney et al.	2012	49		10.75 (0.56, 206.44)	3.66
Sato et al.	2014	67		8.29 (0.46, 147.69)	3.85
Kusunose et al.	2014	133		1.46 (0.58, 3.63)	38.29
Nagata et al.	2015	78		1.73 (0.38, 7.99)	13.67
Carstensen et al.	2015	46		2.23 (0.28, 17.61)	7.48
Salaun et al.	2017	77		3.44 (0.63,18.71)	11.13
Overall effect test: z = 3.44, p = 0.001 **Overall (I^2 = 0.0%, *P* = .737)**				**2.69 (1.53, 4.74)**	**100.00**
Note: Weights are from random effects analysis.					

0.8 1   2   5   90

Figure 26.9. Results of a meta-analysis of 10 studies of global longitudinal strain (GLS) in asymptomatic patients with severe aortic stenosis (AS) and preserved left ventricular (LV) function shown as a forest plot. The pooled average increase in risk of death was 2.69 using a GLS value of worse than 14.7% (in absolute values). (Modified with permission from Magne J et al: Distribution and prognostic significance of left ventricular global longitudinal strain in asymptomatic significant aortic stenosis: an individual participant data meta-analysis, *JACC Cardiovasc Imag* 12:84–92, 2019.)

been shown to be strongly associated with mortality in patients with asymptomatic severe AR.

Alashi and colleagues reported the potential incremental prognostic utility of GLS in asymptomatic patients with significant AR (either 3+ or 4+ AR) in a large series of 1063 patients in a retrospective analysis.[23] Patients were selected with preserved LV function defined by routine measures LV EF 50% or greater and indexed LVESD less than 2.5 cm/m² for GLS determination (Fig. 26.10). Interestingly, only 63% of these patients eventually underwent AVR. In this series, the median absolute GLS was 19.5%, which was not quite as high as the 21% median GLS in their severe MR population. GLS of 19.5% was found to be significantly associated with survival over 12 years with 11% dying with better GLS versus 17% dying with worse GLS (*P* = 0.005). However, AVR had the greatest impact on patient survival with 9% dying with AVR versus 23% dying without AVR. When the associated impact of GLS and AVR were compared together, the prognostic value was most apparent in patients who did not undergo AVR with risk of dying with absolute GLS worse than 19% (Fig. 26.11). When interpreting these retrospective data, the decision for AVR was made at the discretion of the clinicians caring for these patients, and not all factors influencing the decision for AVR can be accounted for. Furthermore, patients with normal LVEF and nondilated LVs were not randomly assigned to AVR based on GLS in this retrospective analysis. It would be of future interest to demonstrate the potential

utility of GLS to identify the value of earlier AVR in asymptomatic patients with severe AR and preserved LVEF whose LVs and not yet severely dilated. Before definitive data emerge, the use of GLS remains an intriguing possibility for identifying subclinical LV dysfunction in symptomatic patients at risk with 3+ or 4+ AR with LVEF greater than 50% and LVESD greater than 50 mm (indexed LVESD <2.5 cm/m²) or LVEDD 65 mm. Whether GLS will gain enough support to influence the clinical medical and surgical standards for AVR in these patients remains to be seen.

In summary, the technique of speckle tracking echocardiography to measure GLS has become widely adopted and has been successfully applied to patients with valvular heart disease. The role of GLS for identifying subclinical LV dysfunction in patients with asymptomatic significant MR, AS, or AR and preserved LV function by routine means, such as LVEF, appears to be most promising. At this point, these compelling and exciting data were derived from retrospective analysis of GLS from stored digital echocardiograms and patient registries. One may conclude that there is currently enough evidence for GLS to become a standard component of the echocardiographic examination to follow patients with valvular heart disease. The impact of GLS to directly influence surgical or percutaneous valve intervention in asymptomatic patients with preserved LVEF will be an exciting advance but may likely require future prospective studies.

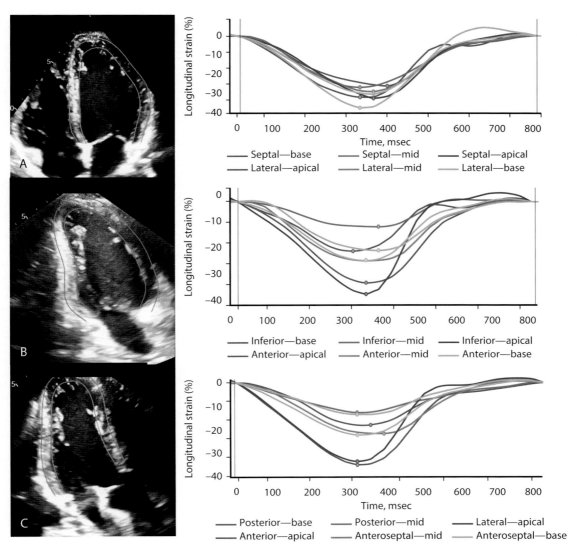

Figure 26.10. An example of global longitudinal strain using vendor-neutral software to determine global longitudinal strain. Apical four-chamber view (**A**), apical two-chamber view (**B**), and the apical long-axis view (**C**) with corresponding longitudinal strain curves to the *right*.

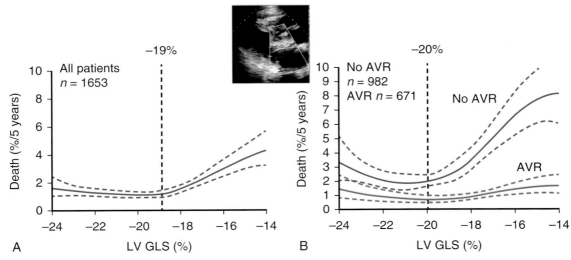

Figure 26.11. Plot of estimated risk of death by global longitudinal strain (GLS) in asymptomatic patients with severe aortic regurgitation (AR). **A,** All patients showing risk of death increases with GLS worse than 19% (in absolute values). **B,** Patients grouped by those with surgical aortic valve replacement (AVR) versus no AVR. Risk of death increases with GLS worse than 20% (in absolute values) in patients who did not undergo AVR. In contrast, GLS does not confer prognostic value in the patients who underwent AVR. *Top center inset* is example of parasternal long-axis view from a patient with severe AR. (Modified with permission from Alashi A et al: Incremental prognostic utility of left ventricular global longitudinal strain in asymptomatic patients with significant chronic aortic regurgitation and preserved left ventricular ejection fraction, *JACC Cardiovasc Imag* 11:673–682, 2018.)

Acknowledgments

Dr. Gorcsan was supported, in part, by research grants from Medtronic, EBR Systems, GE Medical Systems, and V-Wave Ltd.

REFERENCES

1. Gorcsan 3rd J, Tanaka H. Echocardiographic assessment of myocardial strain. *J Am Coll Cardiol*. 2011;58:1401–1413.
2. Marwick TH, Shah SJ, Thomas JD. Myocardial strain in the assessment of patients with heart failure: a review. *JAMA Cardiol*. 2019;4:287–294.
3. Onishi T, Saha SK, Delgado-Montero A, et al. Global longitudinal strain and global circumferential strain by speckle-tracking echocardiography and feature-tracking cardiac magnetic resonance imaging: comparison with left ventricular ejection fraction. *J Am Soc Echocardiogr*. 2015;28:587–596.
4. Park JH, Park JJ, Park JB, Cho GY. Prognostic value of biventricular strain in risk stratifying in patients with acute heart failure. *J Am Heart Assoc*. 2018;7:e009331.
5. Schelbert EB, Piehler KM, Zareba KM, et al. Myocardial fibrosis quantified by extracellular volume is associated with subsequent hospitalization for heart failure, death, or both across the spectrum of ejection fraction and heart failure stage. *J Am Heart Assoc*. 2015;4.
6. Lumens J, Prinzen FW, Delhaas T. Longitudinal strain: "Think globally, track locally. *JACC Cardiovasc Imag*. 2015;8:1360–1363.
7. Kraigher-Krainer E, Shah AM, Gupta DK, et al. Impaired systolic function by strain imaging in heart failure with preserved ejection fraction. *J Am Coll Cardiol*. 2014;63:447–456.
8. Enriquez-Sarano M, Akins CW, Vahanian A. Mitral regurgitation. *Lancet*. 2009;373:1382–1394.
9. Nishimura RA, Otto C. ACC/AHA valve guidelines: earlier intervention for chronic mitral regurgitation. *Heart*. 2014;100:905–907. 2014.
10. Stone GW, Lindenfeld J, Abraham WT, et al. Transcatheter mitral-valve repair in patients with heart failure. *N Engl J Med*. 2018;379:2307–2318.
11. Nishimura RA, Otto CM, Bonow RO, et al. AHA/ACC focused update of the 2014 AHA/ACC guideline for the management of patients with valvular heart disease. *J Am Coll Cardiol*. 2017;70:252–289. 2017.
12. Mentias A, Naji P, Gillinov AM, et al. Strain echocardiography and functional capacity in asymptomatic primary mitral regurgitation with preserved ejection fraction. *J Am Coll Cardiol*. 2016;68:1974–1986.
13. Asch FM, Miyoshi T, Addetia K, et al. Similarities and differences in left ventricular size and function among races and nationalities: results of the World Alliance Societies of Echocardiography normal values study. *J Am Soc Echocardiogr*. 2019;32:1396–1406 e2.
14. Hiemstra YL, Tomsic A, van Wijngaarden SE, et al. Prognostic value of global longitudinal strain and etiology after surgery for primary mitral regurgitation. *JACC Cardiovasc Imag*. 2020;13:577–585.
15. Namazi F, van der Bijl P, Hirasawa K, et al. Prognostic value of left ventricular global longitudinal strain in patients with secondary mitral regurgitation. *J Am Coll Cardiol*. 2020;75:750–758.
16. Dahl JS, Videbaek L, Poulsen MK, et al. Global strain in severe aortic valve stenosis: relation to clinical outcome after aortic valve replacement. *Circ Cardiovasc Imag*. 2012;5:613–620.
17. Medvedofsky D, Koifman E, Miyoshi T, et al. Usefulness of longitudinal strain to assess remodeling of right and left cardiac chambers following transcatheter aortic valve implantation. *Am J Cardiol*. 2019;124:253–261.
18. Harris AW, Pibarot P, Otto CM. Aortic stenosis: guidelines and evidence gaps. *Cardiol Clin*. 2020;38:55–63.
19. Vollema EM, Sugimoto T, Shen M, et al. Association of left ventricular global longitudinal strain with asymptomatic severe aortic stenosis: natural course and prognostic value. *JAMA Cardiol*. 2018;3:839–847.
20. Magne J, Cosyns B, Popescu BA, et al. Distribution and prognostic significance of left ventricular global longitudinal strain in asymptomatic severe aortic stenosis: an individual participant data meta-analysis. *JACC Cardiovasc Imag*. 2019;12:84–92.
21. Bonow RO, Rosing DR, McIntosh CL, et al. The natural history of asymptomatic patients with aortic regurgitation and normal left ventricular function. *Circulation*. 1983;68:509–517.
22. Popovic ZB, Desai MY, Griffin BP. Decision making with imaging in asymptomatic aortic regurgitation. *JACC Cardiovasc Imag*. 2018;11:1499–1513.
23. Alashi A, Mentias A, Abdallah A, et al. Incremental prognostic utility of left ventricular global longitudinal strain in asymptomatic patients with significant chronic aortic regurgitation and preserved left ventricular ejection fraction. *JACC Cardiovasc Imag*. 2018;11:673–682.

27 Right Ventricular Anatomy

Judy R. Mangion

Historically, the echocardiographic assessment of diseases affecting the right ventricle (RV) has lagged behind that of the left ventricle (LV), despite knowledge demonstrating that diseases affecting the right side of the heart have been shown to have important clinical consequences.[1] The geometry of the RV is very complex in normal subjects and even more complex in diseased states, which makes it especially difficult to assess with two-dimensional (2D) techniques (Video 27.1). The RV has a thin wall and has a circumferential arrangement of myofibers in the subepicardium and longitudinal fibers in the endocardium (Fig. 27.1).[2,3] The RV assumes a flattened, pear-shaped appearance folded over the LV. It consists of three components: (1) an inlet portion consisting of the tricuspid valve, chordae tendineae, and papillary muscles; (2) a trabecular apical myocardium; and (3) an infundibulum or conus, which encompasses the smooth-walled RV outflow tract, beneath the pulmonic valve (Fig. 27.2).[4]

CORONARY FLOW TO THE RIGHT VENTRICLE

It is important to think about RV anatomy in the context of coronary flow to the RV (Fig. 27.3).[5] Coronary flow to the RV is unique in that it occurs during both systole and diastole. The right coronary artery (RCA) provides predominant flow, supplying the lateral wall through acute marginal branches, and supplies the posterior wall and posterior interventricular septum through the posterior descending artery. The anterior wall of the RV is supplied by the conus artery branch of the RCA and by branches of the left anterior descending artery.[6,7]

ECHOCARDIOGRAPHIC ASSESSMENT OF RIGHT VENTRICULAR ANATOMY

It is also useful to think about RV anatomy in segmental terms, similar to the LV. The segments of the RV include an anterior RV, inferior

RV, lateral RV, and RV outflow tract (RVOT) (Fig. 27.4).[5] A segmental approach to the evaluation of right ventricular systolic function begins with each of the standard 2D transthoracic views. In the parasternal long-axis view (Fig. 27.5A and Video 27.5A), the RVOT is visualized. In the parasternal short-axis view (Fig. 27.5 B and Video 27.5B), the anterior free wall, lateral free wall, and inferior free wall of the RV are visualized. In the RV inflow tract view (Fig. 27.5C and Video 27.5C), the anterior free wall and inferior free wall of the RV are visualized. In the standard apical four-chamber view (Fig. 27.5D and Video 27.5D), the lateral free wall and right ventricular apex are visualized. In the subcostal four-chamber view (Fig. 27.5E and Video 27.5E), the inferior free wall of the RV or diaphragmatic surface of the RV is visualized.[5] It should be emphasized that the standard apical four-chamber view optimizes the visualization of the left ventricle (Fig. 27.6A and Video 27.6A). To optimize the visualization of the RV, the transducer needs to be moved slightly laterally (Fig. 27.6B and Video 27.6B). This prevents dropout of the lateral free wall of the RV and right ventricular apex.

The extent of right ventricular regional wall motion abnormalities has been shown to correlate with the site of coronary occlusion. Gemayel and coworkers[8] studied 25 patients with clinical evidence of right ventricular infarction who underwent echocardiography and coronary angiography. Video 27.7 illustrates significant hypokinesis of the RVOT, anterior free wall, inferior free wall, and lateral free wall of the RV in a 72-year-old man with presenting symptoms of an acute inferior wall myocardial infarction. Fig. 27.7 shows the coronary angiogram obtained in the same patient demonstrating a proximal occlusion of the RCA. This case illustrates that the more proximal the right coronary occlusion, the more extensive the RV infarction. Contrast this clinical scenario with that of another patient who also presented with symptoms of an acute inferior myocardial infarction (Video 27.8). In this patient, on the apical four-chamber

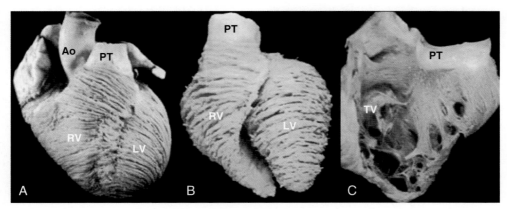

Figure 27.1. Gross anatomic specimens of the right ventricle (RV) demonstrating circumferential arrangement of subepicardial myofibers (**A** and **B**) and longitudinal arrangement of myofibers in the subendocardium (**C**). *Ao,* Aorta; *LV,* left ventricle; *PT,* pulmonary trunk; *TV,* tricuspid valve. (Reproduced with permission from Ho SY, et al: Anatomy, echocardiography and normal right ventricular dimensions, *Heart* 92(Suppl 1): i2–i13, 2006.)

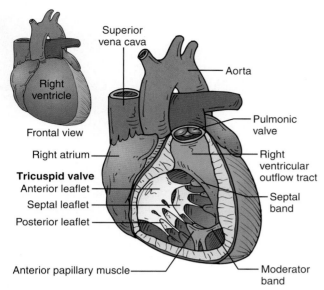

Figure 27.2. Anatomy of the right ventricle (RV). The RV has three distinct parts: an inlet component, which includes the tricuspid valve, chordae tendineae, and papillary muscles; an apical trabecular component, which includes the apical myocardium; and an infundibular or outlet component, which includes the smooth RV outflow tract up to the pulmonic valve. (Reproduced with permission from Bulwer BE, et al: Echocardiographic assessment of ventricular systolic function. In Solomon SD, editor: *Essential Echocardiography*, Totowa, NJ: Humana Press; 2007.)

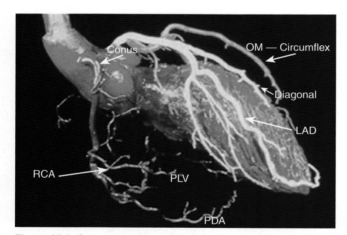

Figure 27.3. Coronary artery supply to the right ventricle (RV). The right coronary artery (RCA) supplies the predominant flow to the right ventricle. The conus branch of the RCA and branches of the left anterior descending coronary artery (LAD) supply the anterior wall of the RV, and the marginal branches of the RCA supply the lateral wall of the RV. The posterior descending artery (PDA) supplies the posterior wall of the RV and the posterior interventricular septum. *OM,* posterior left ventricular branch; *PLV,* posterior left ventricular branch. (Reproduced with permission from Mangion JR: Right ventricular imaging by two-dimensional and three-dimensional echocardiography, *Curr Opin Cardiol* 22:423–429, 2010.)

view, the lateral free wall of the RV contracts normally, whereas the inferior free wall of the RV on the subcostal view is akinetic. The site of RCA occlusion in this patient is distal (Fig. 27.8). This case highlights the importance of subcostal 2D echocardiographic views in the evaluation of patients with suspected RV infarction.

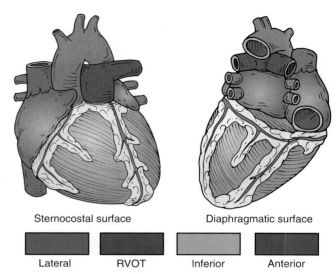

Figure 27.4. The right ventricle (RV) consists of a sternocostal surface and a diaphragmatic surface. It is subdivided into an anterior wall *(purple)*, inferior wall *(yellow)*, lateral wall *(green)*, and right ventricular outflow tract (RVOT; *blue*; see Fig. 27.5). (Reproduced with permission from Mangion JR: Right ventricular imaging by two-dimensional and three-dimensional echocardiography, *Curr Opin Cardiol* 22:423–429, 2010.)

If the subcostal view is not routinely obtained, RV infarction may be missed when the RCA occlusion is distal.[8]

Intravenously injected echocardiographic contrast agents that are capable of opacifying the LV and improving definition of the endocardial border are valuable but underused tools in 2D transthoracic echocardiography.[9] Despite their ability to improve the accuracy and reproducibility of echocardiographic structure and function, they are less often used to define the right ventricular endocardial border. Intravenous saline contrast is a less expensive tool that could also be used to facilitate visualization of the RV, although its effects last only seconds, whereas the echocardiographic contrast agents last several minutes. Imaging the RV with echocardiographic contrast agents requires slow injection of contrast media to prevent attenuation artifacts. Imaging with contrast agents also requires optimizing transducer position for visualizing the RV (Fig. 27.9 and Video 27.9). These agents are administered using the same preprogrammed settings on the ultrasound machine that are used for visualizing the LV.

REFERENCE VALUES FOR RIGHT VENTRICULAR STRUCTURE

The American Society of Echocardiography published in 2010 guidelines for the echocardiographic assessment of the right side of the heart in adults, including reference values for right ventricular structure (eFig. 27.1).[10] The American Society of Echocardiography also published updates to right ventricular chamber quantification in the 2015 Cardiac Chamber Quantification Guidelines, which were also endorsed by the European Association of Cardiovascular Imaging.[11] It is important to note that current values are based on large populations or pooled values from several studies and they are not based on body surface area or gender. Reference data have not yet been classified into mild, moderate, or severe categories. More recent publications have indicated that both gender and body surface area (BSA) play an important part in determining normal RV reference ranges. In general, the RV is 10% to 15% larger in volume than the LV with a thinner free wall (3–5 mm in adults) and one-third to one-sixth smaller mass. It is likely that future published RV

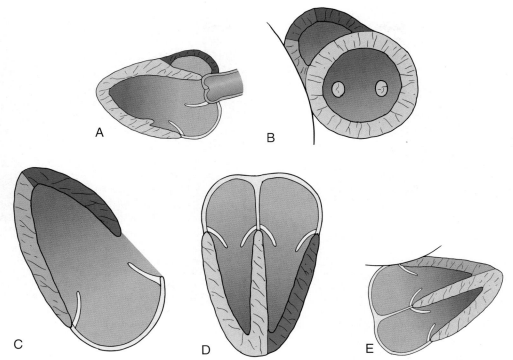

Figure 27.5. With two-dimensional (2D) transthoracic echocardiography in the parasternal long-axis view (**A**), the right ventricular outflow tract (RVOT) is visualized. **B,** In the parasternal short-axis view, the anterior wall, lateral wall, and *inferior* wall of the right ventricle (RV) are visualized. From the RV inflow tract view (**C**), the anterior free wall and inferior free wall of the RV are visualized. In the apical four-chamber view (**D**), the lateral free wall is visualized. In the subcostal four-chamber view (**E**), the inferior free wall of the RV or diaphragmatic surface of the RV is visualized. (Reproduced with permission from Mangion JR: Right ventricular imaging by two-dimensional and three-dimensional echocardiography, *Curr Opin Cardiol* 22:423–429, 2010.)

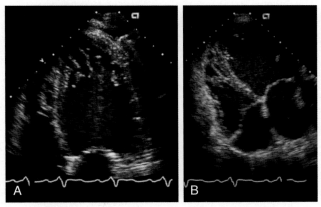

Figure 27.6. The standard apical four-chamber view (**A**) optimizes visualization of the left ventricle (RV). To optimize visualization of the RV, the transducer should be moved more laterally, as this case illustrates (**B**).

guidelines will include upper and lower reference ranges corrected for both BSA and gender as well as ethnicity.[12–14]
Please access ExpertConsult to view the corresponding videos for this chapter.

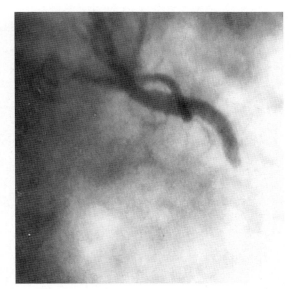

Figure 27.7. Note the proximal occlusion of the right coronary artery in this patient. The more proximal the RCA occlusion, the more extensive the RV infarction.

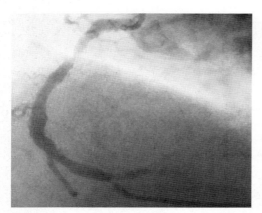

Figure 27.8. In contrast to Figure 27.7, the site of RCA occlusion in this patient is distal. This illustrates the importance of subcostal views in diagnosing right ventricle infarction when the RCA occlusion is distal.

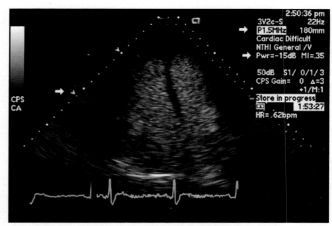

Figure 27.9. Apical four-chamber view demonstrating ultrasound contrast enhancement of the right ventricle and left ventricle. The contrast agent should be delivered slowly to prevent attenuation artifact. (Reproduced with permission from Mangion JR: Right ventricular imaging by two-dimensional and three-dimensional echocardiography, *Curr Opin Cardiol* 22:423–429, 2010.)

Acknowledgment

The author thanks Dr. Scott D. Solomon for his contribution to the previous edition of this chapter.

REFERENCES

1. Zornoff LA, Skali H, Pfeffer MA, et al. SAVE Investigators: right ventricular dysfunction and risk of heart failure and mortality after myocardial infarction. *J Am Coll Cardiol.* 2002;39:1450–1455.
2. Ho SY, Nihoyannoupoulos P. Anatomy, echocardiography and normal right ventricular dimensions. *Heart.* 2006;92(suppl 1):i2–i13.
3. Shiota T. Two-dimensional and three-dimensional echocardiographic evaluation of the right ventricle. In: Gillam LD, Otto CM, eds. *Advanced Approaches in Echocardiography.* Philadelphia: Saunders; 2012.
4. Bulwer BE, Solomon SD, Janardhanan R. Echocardiographic assessment of ventricular systolic function. In: Solomon SD, ed. *Essential Echocardiography.* Totowa, NJ: Humana Press; 2007.
5. Mangion JR. Right ventricular imaging by two-dimensional and three-dimensional echocardiography. *Curr Opin Cardiol.* 2010;22:423–429.
6. Cross CE. Right ventricular pressure and coronary flow. *Am J Physiol.* 1962;202:12–16.
7. Kinch JW, Ryan TJ. Right ventricular infarction. *N Engl J Med.* 1994;330:1211–1217.
8. Gemayel CY, Fram DB, Gillam LD, et al. In vivo correlation of the site of right coronary artery occlusion and echocardiographically defined right ventricular infarction. *Circulation.* 2000;102:II–542.
9. Mulvagh S, Rakowski H, Vannan MA, et al. American Society of Echocardiography consensus statement on the clinical applications of ultrasonic contrast agents in echocardiography. *J Am Soc Echocardiogr.* 2008;21:1179–1201.
10. Rudski LG, Lai WW, Afilalo J, et al. Guidelines for the echocardiographic assessment of the right heart in adults. *J Am Soc Echocardiogr.* 2010;23:685–713.
11. Lang RM, Badano LP, Mor-Avi V, et al. Recommendations for cardiac chamber quantification by echocardiography in adults. *J Am Soc Echocardiogr.* 2015;28:1–39.
12. Willis J, Augustine D, Shah R, et al. Right ventricular normal measurements: time to index? *J Am Soc Echocardiogr.* 2012;25:1259–1267.
13. D'Oronzio U, Senn O, Biaggi P, et al. Right heart assessment by echocardiography: gender and body size matters. *J Am Soc Echocardiogr.* 2012;25:1251–1258.
14. Sanz J, Sanchez-Quintana D, Bossone E, et al. Anatomy, function, and dysfunction of the right ventricle. *J Am Coll Cardiol.* 2019;73:1463–1482.

28 The Physiologic Basis of Right Ventricular Echocardiography

Laura Flink, Payal Kohli, Nelson B. Schiller

The right ventricle (RV), which had been deemed the *forgotten ventricle,* is now recognized as a central player in cardiovascular function. Its physiology, shape, function, and coronary blood flow are complex and impose impediments to noninvasive imaging. This chapter reviews the physiology of the RV and describes echocardiographic, functional, and structural correlates.

The RV was first described as more than a passive conduit in 1616 by Sir William Harveyin, who recognized that the "right ventricle may be said to be made for the sake of transmitting blood through the lungs, not for nourishing them." In the following centuries, studies focused on the left ventricle (LV) overshadowed studies of the RV. It was not until the 1970s when the RV became fully recognized as a key player in cardiovascular disease states, such as heart failure and pulmonary hypertension. In the final decades of the 20th century, standard two-dimensional (2D) transthoracic echocardiographic (TTE) imaging of the RV became a mainstay for its evaluation. Recently, advances in imaging modalities such as three-dimensional (3D) TTE[1] have improved detection and characterization of RV pathophysiologic states.

Evaluation of the RV by echocardiography relies on knowledge of its anatomy and physiology and involves characterization of wall thickness, shape, ventricular cavity size, and regional and global contractile function. A complete RV examination includes both qualitative and quantitative parameters, including RV size, right atrial (RA) size, RV systolic function, and pulmonary hemodynamics.[2]

STRUCTURE AND ANATOMY OF THE RIGHT VENTRICLE

The location of the right ventricle in the thorax as the most anterior cardiac structure places it retrosternally and in the near field of the ultrasound beam, thus limiting optimal echocardiographic imaging windows and resolution (Fig. 28.1, *top right*). Several anatomic features distinguish the RV from the LV (Table 28.1). These include (1) relative apical displacement of the tricuspid valve (TV) compared with the mitral valve (MV), (2) the presence of bands and coarse apical trabeculations, (3) the presence of more than three papillary muscles, and (4) a trileaflet TV with septal papillary muscle attachments.

Anatomically, the RV may be separated into three unique components: (1) the RV inlet, which consists of the TV, chordae tendineae, and papillary muscles (PMs); (2) the RV body, which is made up of the highly trabeculated apical myocardium; and (3) the smooth outlet conus (also known as the infundibulum). The positioning of the RV places its body as the most rightward cardiac structure and the end of the outflow tract as the most leftward. Therefore, a single 2D sector does not encompass the entire ventricle. The anterior location and thin walls of the RV mandate the use of the transducer with the highest available carrier frequency that permits adequate penetration. Most often, the use of higher frequencies, which are optimal for RV imaging, are less successful in imaging the left ventricle. Therefore, the RV tends to be imaged at suboptimal resolution (see Fig. 28.1, *top right*).

The RV inlet can be best imaged in the RV inflow (RVI) view (see Fig. 28.1 *left, third from top*), which allows for visualization of the tricuspid annular plane and can be useful in identifying congenital lesions involving the annulus and the TV; these include prolapse, vegetations, and Ebstein anomaly.[3] In most 2D TTE tomographic planes, only two of three of the TV leaflets are visualized,[4] and multiple views are needed to adequately image all leaflets. In the RVI view, the anterior and either septal or posterior leaflets are best visualized, whereas the apical four-chamber (A4C) view (see Fig. 28.1 *right, second from top*) allows observation and characterization of the anterior and septal leaflets.

The RV body can be fully imaged on 2D TTE. From a segmental point of view, it is also useful to divide the chamber into its respective anatomic walls (anterior, lateral, inferior, basal mid, and apical). This anatomic classification allows for localization of RV pathologic states, such as occlusion of the right coronary artery, which can result in localized right ventricular infarction (Fig. 28.2). The thin but variable thickness of the walls is an additional factor in segmental susceptibility to ischemia and infarction. In the standard A4C view of the body of the RV, the basal wall, lateral wall (also known as the free wall), and apical segments are readily visualized, whereas the RVI view (see Fig. 28.1 *left, third from top*) allows for visualization of the inferior wall of the RV and the anterior and posterior leaflets of the TV. The parasternal short-axis (PSAX) view at the base of the heart allows visualization of the right ventricular outflow tract (RVOT), along with the anterior and lateral cusps of the pulmonic valve (PV) (see Fig. 28.1, *left, third from bottom*).

Similar to the division of its walls, the trabeculations of the ventricle are subdivided into three anatomically distinct bands: parietal, septomarginal, and moderator. The crista supraventricularis (CSV) consists of the parietal band and the infundibular septum, and the septomarginal band is continuous with the moderator band (Fig. 28.3). The CSV is an important anatomic marker of RV dimensions that also serves multiple other functions, including narrowing of the TV annulus during systole.[5]

Unlike the LV, where the MV and aortic valve (AV) are in fibrous continuity, the TV and PV are anatomically separated by the ventriculoinfundibular fold, which creates a spatial boundary that may have physiologic significance. For example, endovascular infections can spread directly from the mitral to aortic valves (or vice versa), but this is much less common on the right side because of the presence of ventriculoinfundibular fold. The moderator band, when particularly complex, may also connote RV dysplasia.[6]

The geometry of the right ventricle is also complex. Unlike the ellipsoid LV, the RV is triangular when viewed from the side and crescentic when viewed in cross section (see Fig. 28.1, *top right*, and Table 28.1).[7] This complex three-dimensional shape complicates the echocardiographic quantitation of RV size and ejection fraction (EF). Importantly, only the compact muscle layers of the ventricle should be included in this measurement, and the trabecular layer should be systematically excluded. Because the infundibulum can account for 25% to 30% of RV volume, awareness of its absence should attend the analysis of measurements of the RV body.[8] Owing to the complex geometry of the RV when qualitatively evaluating RV size by 2D TTE, multiple complementary views should be considered before suggesting RV enlargement (Fig. 28.4). Note that the image of the body of the RV in the four-chamber view often includes an outpouching that is a normal anatomic structure known as the *acute margin of the heart*. The American Society of Echocardiography (ASE) reference limits for normal RV linear dimensions in the A4C view are basal RV diameter, 2.5 to 4.1 cm; mid-RV diameter, 1.9 to 3.5 cm; and base-to-apex length, 5.9 to 8.3 cm. The normal RVOT proximal diameter is 2.1 to 3.5 cm, and the distal diameter is 1.7 to 2.7 cm. The normal end-diastolic areas indexed to body surface area for men and women are 5 cm/m^2 to 12.6 cm/m^2 and 4.5 to 11.5 cm/m^2, respectively. The normal end-systolic areas indexed to body surface area for men and women are 2 to 7.4 cm/m^2 and 1.6 to 6.4 cm/m^2, respectively. The normal end-diastolic volumes indexed to body surface area for men and women are 35 to 87 mL/m^2 and 32 to 74 mL/m^2, respectively. The normal end-systolic volumes indexed to body surface area for men and women are 10 to 44 mL/m^2 and 8 to 36 mL/m^2, respectively.[9,10]

Echocardiographic measures of RV size are significantly different in men and women, as demonstrated in a study using 2D and 3D. In one study, the authors found that RV end-diastolic volume using 3D echocardiography was larger in men than women (129 ± 25 mL vs 102 ± 33 mL P < .01).[9,10] In our lab, we performed 3D measurements of the RV on 29 normal participants without known cardiovascular disease and found these to be more rational volumes as they are more similar to the LV volumes. Fig. 28.5 demonstrates how we measured RV volumes in our cohort. Given the irregular shape of the RV, 3D volume measurements may become the method of choice. We found the normal RV volume in a healthy cohort of adults was 100 ± 22 mL (52 ± 10 mL/m^2). In women, the volume was 79 ± 13 mL (45 ± 7 mL/m^2), and in men, the volume was 107 ± 20 mL (54 ± 10 mL/m^2) (Table 28.2).

In addition to RV function and dimensions, measurement of RV mass also poses a clinical challenge. The RV mass is one-sixth that of the LV, but its volume is larger, and the mass is asymmetrically distributed. RV wall thickness can be measured in diastole, from the subcostal view (using either M-mode or 2D TTE) or in the left parasternal view. Agitated saline or microbubble contrast may be helpful in measuring wall thickness by distinguishing the compact from the trabecular muscle. Standard practice calls for using RV free-wall thickness greater than 5 mm to define RV hypertrophy, but quantification of total RV mass has not been satisfactorily performed with 2D TTE.[2] During normal loading conditions, the RV retains its crescentic shape. However, in the setting of pressure or volume overload because of ventricular interdependence, the RV may hypertrophy and become more circular or spheroid, whereas the LV may assume a crescentic shape. Such geometric transformations may alter the mathematical assumptions that are used in normally shaped hearts to extrapolate EF from linear dimensions to become particularly inaccurate once ventricular remodeling has occurred. 2D biplane measurements from apical views continue to provide accurate information about volume and function in this setting. A summary of some of the aforementioned challenges to assessing the right ventricle by transthoracic echocardiography are listed in Box 28.1.

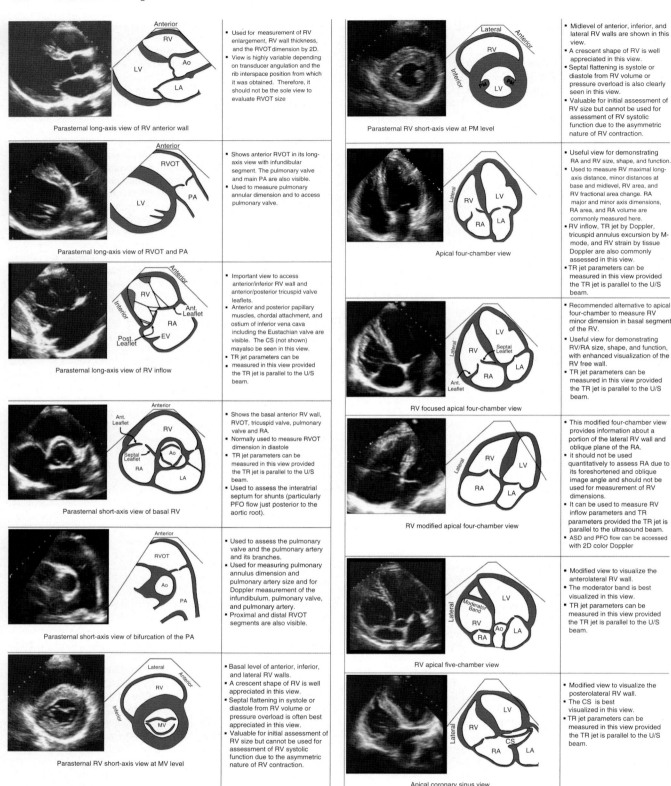

Figure 28.1. Views used to perform comprehensive evaluation of the right heart. Each view is accompanied by uses, advantages, and limitations of that particular view. *2D,* Two dimensional; *Ao,* aorta; *ASD,* atrial septal defect; *CS,* coronary sinus; *EF,* ejection fraction; *EV,* Eustachian valve; *LA,* left atrium; *LV,* left ventricle; *MV,* mitral valve; *PA,* pulmonary artery; *PFO,* patent foramen ovale; *PM,* papillary muscle; *RA,* right atrium; *RV,* right ventricle; *RVOT,* right ventricular outflow tract; *TR,* tricuspid regurgitation. *U/S,* ultrasound. (Reproduced with permission from Rudski LG, et al: Guidelines for the echocardiographic assessment of the right heart in adults: a report from the American Society of Echocardiography, *J Am Soc Echocardiogr* 23:685–713, 2010.)

TABLE 28.1 Comparison of Normal Right Ventricular and Left Ventricular Parameters

	Right Ventricle[a]	Left Ventricle[a]
Structure	Thin compacta, heavily trabeculated cavity	Thicker compacta
Shape	Crescentic with triangular base	Truncated ellipse[39]
End-diastolic volume	75 ± 13 (49–101)	66 ± 12 (44–89)[40]
Mass, g/m²	26 ± 5 (17–34)[40]	87 ± 12 (64–109)[40]
Wall thickness, mm	2–5	7–11
Ventricular pressures, mm Hg		
Systolic	25 (15–30)	130 (90–140)
Diastolic	4 (1–7)	8 (5–12)
RVEF, %	> 40–45[40]	> 50[40]
Ventricular elastance (Emax), mm Hg	1.30 ± 0.84[41]	5.48 ± 1.23[15]
Afterload resistance, WU	0.88 (0.25–1.63)	13.75 (8.75–20)
Stroke work index, g/m² per beat	8 ± 2	50 ± 20
Major vector of contraction	Longitudinal	Circumferential and longitudinal

[a]Parentheses indicate range of values.
RVEF, Right ventricular ejection fraction.
Adapted from Haddad F, et al: Right ventricular function in cardiovascular disease, part I: anatomy, physiology, aging, and functional assessment of the right ventricle, *Circulation* 117:1436–1448, 2008.

RIGHT VENTRICULAR HEMODYNAMICS

As with the LV, RV function is based on preload, contractility, and afterload, and each of these will be sequentially discussed in the following sections.

Right Ventricular Preload

The RV has a thin wall and operates at low filling pressure, making it very sensitive to changes in preload. Physiologically, this sensitivity becomes apparent during exaggerated respiration or when pericardial restraint is increased. For this reason, the free wall of the RV, in the absence of pulmonary hypertension, collapses during states of cardiac tamponade. This collapse is in proportion to the elevation in intrapericardial pressure and is respirophasic, reflecting increased sensitivity to the waxing and waning of caval filling. This is in turn dictated by the respiratory cycling of the thoracic pump as it overcomes or succumbs to inflow obstruction imposed by elevated intrapericardial pressures. The LV has a thick wall and higher filling pressure, so it resists collapse from elevated intrapericardial pressures during early tamponade. As tamponade worsens, however, transmural pressure rises, and the LA may also phasically collapse.

Right Ventricular Contractility

A discussion of the contraction of the RV and its hemodynamic correlates is informed by considering the myocyte configuration unique to this thin-walled ventricle. There are two layers of muscle

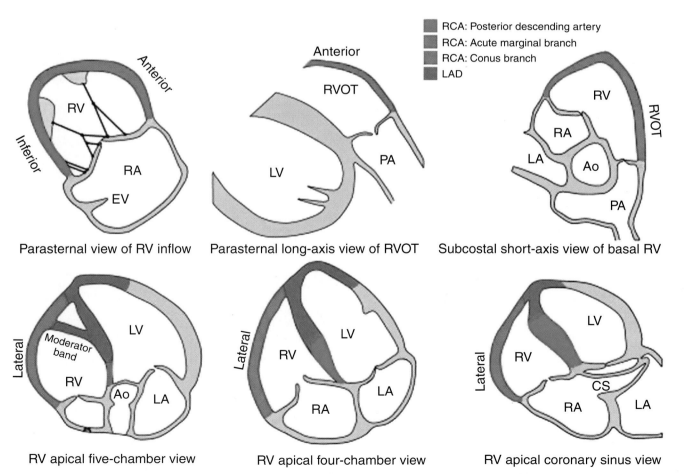

Figure 28.2. Segmental nomenclature of the right ventricular walls, along with their coronary supply. *Ao,* Aorta; *CS,* coronary sinus; *EV,* Eustachian vein; *LA,* left atrium; *LAD,* left anterior descending artery; *LV,* left ventricle; *PA,* pulmonary artery; *RA,* right atrium; *RCA,* right coronary artery; *RV,* right ventricle; *RVOT,* right ventricular outflow tract.

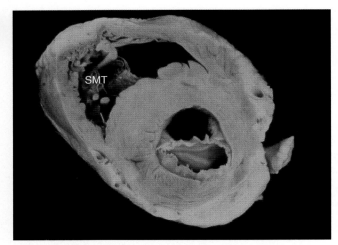

Figure 28.3. Cross section of the heart at the level of the mitral valve demonstrates the crescentic shape of the right ventricle, the ellipsoid shape of the left ventricle, and the relative thickness of the walls (see Table 28.1). Note that the septomarginal trabeculation (SMT), which in this area of the ventricle is termed the *moderator band*, extends into the right ventricular outflow tract, where it is termed the *crista supraventricularis*. (Courtesy of Nelson B. Schiller.)

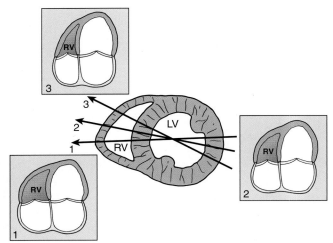

Figure 28.4. Diagram showing the recommended apical four-chamber (A4C) view with focus on the right ventricle (RV) (*1*) and the sensitivity of right ventricular size with angular change (*2, 3*) despite similar size and appearance of the left ventricle (LV). The lines of intersection of the A4C planes (*1, 2, 3*) with a mid–left ventricular short-axis view are shown on top and corresponding A4C views at the bottom. (Reproduced with permission from Rudski LG, et al: Guidelines for the echocardiographic assessment of the right heart in adults: a report from the American Society of Echocardiography, *J Am Soc Echocardiogr* 23:685–713, quiz 786–688, 2010.)

fibers in the RV wall (superficial and deep) with a complex over-lapping pattern that forms a 3D network.[11] The superficial muscle layer is parallel to the atrioventricular groove and the right coronary artery, whereas the deep fibers are longitudinally aligned from the base to the apex.[11–13] The superficial RV fibers are continuous with those of the LV, resulting in continuity between the ventricles. The functional consequences of this continuous layer include coordination of the RV and LV, ventricular interdependence, and traction on the RV free wall caused by LV contraction.

Although the normal RV operates at lower pressure than the LV, the ventricles are connected in series, and their effective stroke volume must be equal. Many factors maintain this equality, including the pericardium (so-called fifth chamber), the interatrial and interventricular septa, and great veins and pulmonary veins (Dr. John Tyberg, personal communication). For echocardiographers, the motion and position of the interatrial septa during respiration is one among many examples of how small pressure and volume changes in the atria during the respiratory cycle are constantly modulating interventricular output.

The contraction of the RV occurs in a sequential fashion, beginning with the trabeculations and ending with the contraction of the conus, about 25 to 50 milliseconds apart.[12,13] During RV systole, the free wall moves inward, then the long axis shortens, and the base descends toward the apex. Because of the deeper longitudinal fibers, the RV shortens longitudinally more than it shortens horizontally,[12,14] which is different from the LV. A higher surface area–to-volume ratio of the RV allows for less inward motion than the LV for same volume ejected. In addition, bulging of the ventricular septum into the right ventricular cavity contributes to ejection.

The fiber orientation of the RV musculature makes the longitudinal vector of its contraction the most important; this is appreciated in real-time imaging by the highly visible descent of the RV base (also known as the movement of the tricuspid annulus toward the apex) that occurs during systole. This motion is best appreciated in the apical and subcostal views of the RV.

A first step in evaluating right ventricular contractile function is visual inspection of the real-time 2D echocardiogram. Because the wall of the RV is thin, careful adjustments of instrument gain and settings and judicious selection of transducers may be needed to accurately detect RV inward systolic motion or wall thickening. In addition, the RV is extremely sensitive to loading conditions. For example, a high pulmonary vascular resistance (afterload) may affect contractility and EF of the RV much more than it would

impact the LV. Given that the RV and LV stroke volumes are identical in the absence of a shunt, a decrease in RV stroke volume may significantly decrease the preload of the LV (Table 28.3), thus diminishing its volume and obscuring preexisting pathology as well as diminishing cardiac output. Therefore, it is important to note comprehensive RV hemodynamics in any complete echocardiographic assessment.

Pressure–volume loops are particularly helpful for understanding the complex interplay of RV hemodynamics as they contribute to RV function.[1] The slope of the end-systolic pressure–volume relationship is defined as the elastance. Elastance is a measure that is relatively independent of load and therefore a reliable index of contractility.[15] The end-systolic volume index of the LV, an expression of elastance, is a relatively load-independent indicator of LV function and offers independent prognostic information about adverse cardiovascular outcomes such as mortality and heart failure in patients with coronary artery disease.[16,17] However, because of geometric constraints, RV end-systolic volume is difficult to measure accurately by 2D TTE, and a noninvasive expression of its elastance is not readily available. Hopefully, future research in this area, particularly with 3D volumes of the RV, will provide this potentially valuable clinical information (Fig. 28.6).

Right ventricular stroke work index (SWI), a combined expression of the pressure and volume work done by the right ventricle, is another useful parameter. It can be calculated by subtracting right atrial pressure from mean pulmonary artery pressure and multiplying this difference by stroke volume index. Because of the difference in structure and contractile properties of the LV and RV, their relative stroke work indices are quite different, whereby the RV SWI is only approximately 15% of LV SWI.

Right Ventricular Afterload

The RV has heightened sensitivity to increased afterload for several reasons: (1) coronary flow is more vulnerable, and increases in pressure can readily lead to RV ischemia (see the discussion of RV perfusion later); and (2) the RV has a thin wall, so wall stress, which is estimated by Laplace law (and is inversely proportional to twice wall thickness), increases more rapidly with pressure increase than

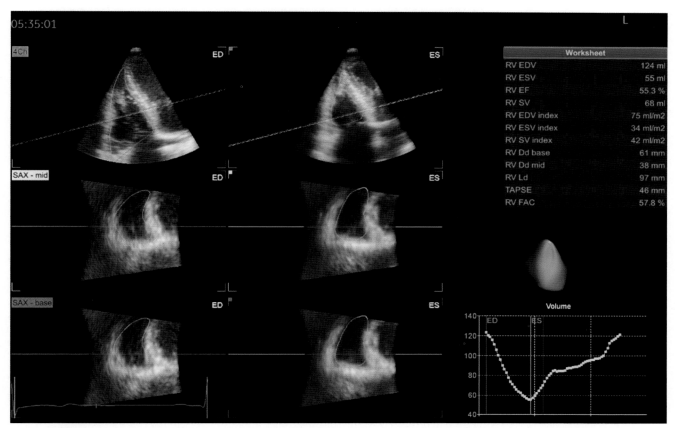

Figure 28.5. Three-dimensional measurement of right ventricular volumes. (Courtesy of Dwight Bibby at Research Cardiology Physiology Laboratory of the Health eHeart Study, Cardiovascular Research Institute, University of California-San Francisco.)

TABLE 28.2 Right Ventricular Three-Dimensional Volume and Strain (Two- and Three-Dimensional) in Our Normal Cohort

	All (*n* = 29)	Women (*n* = 7)	Men (*n* = 22)
3D RV end-diastolic volume	100 ± 22	79 ± 13	107 ± 20
3D RV end-systolic volume	50 ± 18	45 ± 13	52 ± 19
3D RV end-diastolic volume index	52 ± 10	45 ± 7	54 ± 10
3D RV end-systolic volume index	26 ± 10	25 ± 6	27 ± 11
3D RV septal wall strain	20 ± 7	20 ± 5	20 ± 8
3D RV free-wall strain	28 ± 9	26 ± 6	28 ± 10
2D RV septal wall strain	16 ± 3	16 ± 3	15 ± 3
2D RV free-wall strain	28 ± 4	29 ± 3	28 ± 4

RV, Right ventricular.
Data from the Research Cardiology Physiology Laboratory of the Health eHeart Study, Cardiovascular Research Institute, University of California-San Francisco, CA.

BOX 28.1 Limitations of Two-Dimensional Echocardiographic Assessment of the Right Ventricle

- Anterior retrosternal position
- Complex asymmetric shape
- Poor demarcation of the RV endocardial border because of a heavily trabeculated inner contour
- Difficult to image all portions of the RV in perpendicular views; separate inflow and outflow portions require visualization from separate views
- Asymmetric distribution of RV mass
- Load dependency

RV, Right ventricular.

TABLE 28.3 Echocardiographic Measurements in Normal Control Participants and Patients With Cor Pulmonale Demonstrate the Reversal in Right and Left Heart Ratios With Chronic Pressure Overload

	Control Participants	Cor Pulmonale
Right ventricle/left ventricle	0.6 ± 7	1.1 ± 0.6
Right atrium/left atrium	0.8 ± 0.3	1.3 ± 0.7

Modified with permission from Himelman RB, et al: Improved recognition of cor pulmonale in patients with severe chronic obstructive pulmonary disease, *Am J Med* 84:891–898, 1988.

in the LV. Normally, the resting peak systolic pulmonary pressure achieved by the RV is less than 30 mm Hg, but this value varies by age and cardiac output. With exercise, the pulmonary pressure may rise as high as 40 mm Hg in unconditioned normal individuals and as high as 55 mm Hg in athletes or persons older than age 65 years. Characteristically, normal systolic pulmonary pressure rises slowly through grades of cardiac output that attend increasing exercise levels. Rapid increases in pressure are more characteristic of a pathologic response. Thus, the healthy RV has considerable reserve as long as the pressure load increases slowly and is not

accompanied by elevated pulmonary vascular resistance.[18] Abrupt increases in pulmonary pressures are poorly tolerated by the thin-walled RV because the wall stress increases rapidly. Examples of situations in which this intolerance is manifest are acute pulmonary embolism and the abrupt dilation of a transplanted heart

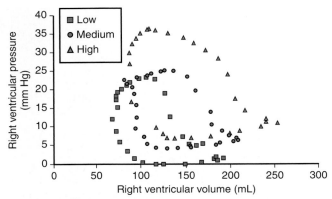

Figure 28.6. Right ventricular (RV) pressure–volume (PV) loops demonstrating a parallel vertical shift from low-loading (nitroprusside), to medium-loading, to high-loading (phenylephrine) conditions. The PV loops of the normal RV response to phenylephrine shows good response (elastance) of end-systolic volume (ESV). As pressure rises, the ESV stays nearly the same, and thus contractility behaves in a nearly load-independent manner. However, at the highest pressure, the loop suggests that the RV dilates. This dilation seems to mirror what often occurs after a pulmonary embolism. (Reproduced with permission from Starling MR, et al: Value of the tricuspid valve echogram for estimating right ventricular end-diastolic pressure during vasodilator therapy, *Am J Cardiol* 45:966–972, 1980.)

when the recipient has underlying elevated pulmonary vascular resistance. Deterioration of RV function in these circumstances is accompanied by rapid dilatation of the chamber and by a sudden drop in contractile function. One feature of pulmonary embolism that affords insight into the vulnerability of normal RV function is the segmental loss of RV midwall function that is said to be a diagnostic feature of major pulmonary embolism.[19] We theorize that an abrupt rise in pulmonary pressure and subsequent oxygen demand of the RV myocardium is likely to cause midwall ischemia because the timing of right coronary flow is, contrary to left coronary flow, systolic dominant. An acute elevation of RV wall stress may markedly impair right coronary blood flow, especially at the midwall. The rise in troponin and the location of the wall motion in acute pulmonary embolism appear to support this pathophysiologic explanation.[20]

The use of Doppler to determine pulmonary artery pressure is a mainstay of current echocardiography practice. The first step is the demonstration of tricuspid regurgitation by color-flow Doppler in the A4C view (Fig. 28.7). Then the continuous wave beam is placed across the jet, and the peak velocity is used to calculate the peak gradient between the right atrium and right ventricle with the Bernoulli equation: peak gradient (mm Hg) = 4 × peak velocity.[2] Provided that there is no pulmonary stenosis, this gradient added to the RA pressure is equal to peak systolic pulmonary artery pressure. RA pressure is determined by the respiratory behavior of the inferior vena cava (IVC).[21] An alternative method of estimating RA pressure has been published by the ASE and is as follows. For an IVC diameter of 2.1 cm or less that collapses more than 50% with a sniff, a normal RA pressure of 3 mm Hg is assigned. For an IVC diameter of at least 2.1 cm that collapses less than 50% with a sniff, an elevated RA pressure of 15 mm Hg is assigned. In cases in which the IVC diameter and collapse do not fit this paradigm, an intermediate value of 8 mm Hg is assigned.[2] Additional information to validate RA pressure may be obtained from Doppler imaging of the hepatic vein. Normal RA pressure (<5 mm Hg) is assumed if the hepatic vein is systolic dominant, and low RA pressure (2 mm Hg or negative) is assumed if flow is continuous.[22] If the IVC is not visualized, skilled sonographers may image the superior vena cava (SVC) and obtain the flow profile of pulsed-wave Doppler

(PWD), seeking the same flow patterns seen in the hepatic vein. Another method of judging RA pressure is to observe the curvature and respiratory responses of the interatrial septum. The chamber with the higher pressure will dictate the curvature. Usually, when the septum is bidirectional, the pressure in both chambers is low.[23]

In addition to peak systolic pressure, it is useful to measure end-diastolic pulmonary regurgitation (EDPR) gradient and then add it to RA pressure, which provides a direct correlate of PA diastolic pressure (an indirect correlate of left ventricular end-diastolic pressure [LVEDP]). The gradient, as a standalone measurement without RA pressure, suggests abnormal hemodynamics when it is greater than 5 mm Hg.[24] Mean PA pressure may be calculated by three methods. First, mean pressure can be calculated from the peak (opening) PR gradient + RA when this measurement is available. Second, planimetry of the TR signal + RA provides a validated estimate of mean pulmonary pressure. Third, the formula used for calculating mean arterial systolic pressure {mean pressure = [systole + (2 × diastole)]/3} may be applied if diastolic pressure from EDPR is available. Resistance may also be estimated from the simple ratio of peak TR velocity to PA velocity time integral.[18] Use of noninvasive pulmonary vascular resistance (PVR) prevents mistaking elevated pulmonary pressure that is caused by increased flow for pressure that is mediated by elevated resistance. Central to understanding hemodynamics of the right side of the heart is PA velocity time integral, or stroke distance, as an indicator of cardiac output. In individuals with high blood flow, such as patients with sickle cell disease or end-stage liver disease, a high stroke distance with borderline elevated PA pressure indicates normal PVR. Conversely, a very low stroke distance (velocity time integral well below 17 cm) may be a sign of markedly increased PVR even when pulmonary artery systolic pressure (PASP) is only mildly elevated.[25]

Overall, despite the hemodynamic sensitivity of the RV to acute changes in preload, contractility, and afterload, the RV is highly adaptable and can even take on the role of the systemic ventricle if needed.[26,27] We care for a patient in his eighth decade with L-transposition and a systemically functioning subaortic right ventricle with normal resting hemodynamics and above average formally measured exercise tolerance.

QUANTITATIVE ASSESSMENT OF RIGHT VENTRICULAR FUNCTION

Despite the complexity of the RV anatomy and assessing the RV size, there are options for global quantitation of RV function. These include RVEF and fractional area shortening from the four-chamber view of RV body, tricuspid annular plane systolic excursion (TAPSE) (Fig. 28.8A), and RV dP/dt from the acceleration of the tricuspid regurgitation signal, RV index of myocardial performance (RIMP, the Tei) index and Doppler tissue imaging (DTI) (Fig. 28.8B) may also describe the systolic velocity of the tricuspid annulus (S′), and RV strain.[10]

Right Ventricular Ejection Fraction

Whereas the difference between mathematical volume of an ellipsoid in systole and diastole can be used to estimate the LVEF, the estimation of the RV systolic function is more challenging. The systolic and diastolic right ventricular volumes (minus the RVOT volume) is computed by the area length algorithm using values obtained by tracing the outline of the cavity in the four-chamber view in systole and diastole. The RVEF is calculated as follows: RVEF = (RV end-diastolic volume − RV end-systolic volume)/RV end-diastolic volume. The area length method correlates reasonably well with the EF obtained by radionuclide blood pool imaging. One study was able to replicate quantitative angiography of the RV volume in children by adding the area length volume of the apical view to the volume from the subcostal view.[28] 3D TTE has been validated against cardiac MRI, and an RVEF below 45%

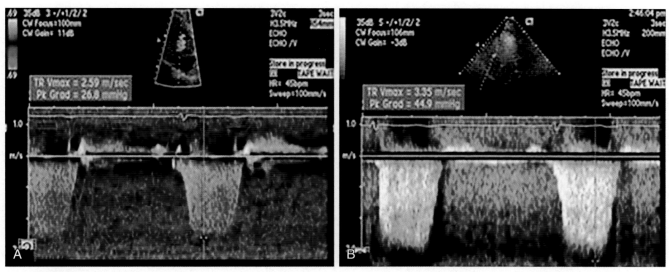

Figure 28.7. A, Tricuspid regurgitation signal that is not contrast enhanced and correctly measured at the peak velocity. **B,** After contrast enhancement, the clear envelope has been obscured by noise, and the reader erroneously estimated a gradient several points higher. As this example shows, it is critical that only well-defined borders be used for velocity measurement because slight errors are magnified by the second-order relationship between velocity and derived pressure. (Reproduced with permission from Rudski LG, et al: Guidelines for the echocardiographic assessment of the right heart in adults: a report from the American Society of Echocardiography, *J Am Soc Echocardiogr* 23:685–713, quiz 786–688, 2010.)

is likely abnormal. RV using the disk summation method to calculate RVEF.[29] Compared with the LV, the base-to-apex shortening contributes more to RV emptying (see Table 28.1). The body of RV volume and hence EF can be estimated by measuring the body of the RV (i.e., the RV in the four-chamber view) during systole and diastole and applying either the fractional area change or area–length volume estimation to calculate RVEF.[12]

Fractional Area Change

An alternative method of measuring RV contractile function is the RV fractional area change as measured in the A4C view looking at the change in RV end-diastolic area to RV end-systolic area. Normal RV fractional area change is 32% to 60%, mildly reduced is 25% to 31%, moderately reduced is 18% to 24%, and severely reduced is 17% or less.[9] A fractional area change of less than 35% indicates RV systolic dysfunction.

TAPSE

Basal descent may be measured as a surrogate for RV systolic function and is also known as TAPSE. TAPSE is quantitated as a linear M-mode measurement through the lateral annulus of the TV; TAPSE greater than 16 mm is consistent with normal RV systolic function. A failing RV, such as in end-stage cor pulmonale or severe pulmonary hypertension, rarely has a TAPSE that measures above 1 cm. Although TAPSE measures only longitudinal function and is a focal measurement that is angle dependent, it has shown good correlation with techniques estimating RV global systolic function, such as radionuclide-derived RVEF,[2] TAPSE less than 17 mm is suggestive of RV dysfunction.

Right Ventricular dP/dt

The ratio of change in pressure to change in time is a measurement of RV systolic function as it describes the pressure produced by the RV during systole. For convenience, this is measured as the change in pressure in the tricuspid regurgitation jet from 1 to 2 m/s. Using the modified Bernoulli equation, the change in pressure is equal to

$4v^2$ (12 mm Hg) over the time this takes. Values less than 400 mm Hg/s indicate reduced RV function. This has been shown to correlate well with RVEF on cardiac MRI.[30]

S' Velocity

RV dysfunction has also been defined by using tissue Doppler S' velocity, which is the myocardial systolic excursion velocity. This measurement is performed using tissue Doppler imaging at the level of the lateral tricuspid annulus in the A4C view. It is highly reproducible and correlates well with RVEF. An S' velocity less than 9.5 cm/s indicates RV dysfunction.[10]

Right Ventricular Index of Myocardial Performance, the Tei Index

This measure looks at the ratio of nonejection time to ejection time. This can be done using pulsed-wave Doppler or tissue Doppler of the lateral annulus measuring these two times. An RIMP greater than 0.43 by pulse wave Doppler and greater than 0.54 by tissue Doppler indicates RV dysfunction.[10] Note that the Tei index measures a combination of both systolic and diastolic function.

Right Ventricular Strain

Last, RV strain and strain rate have become important parameters for estimating global RV function and recognizing subtle and early RV dysfunction. Strain imaging is an echocardiographic method of measuring the cyclic deformity of cardiac chambers during the cardiac cycle. Analysis of digitized images (grayscale or 3D) may be applied to any of the chambers. Speckle tracking or DTI may yield similar strain results. Strain data (dimensional or rate) may be segmental or global and conducted in radial, longitudinal, or z-axes. Although initially developed as a parameter for assessing subtle LV dysfunction, it has also been adapted to assess RV function. RV global longitudinal strain (GLS) is the measurement most used and has been adapted from LV strain measurement software. RV GLS initially described an RV free wall and septum; however, currently,

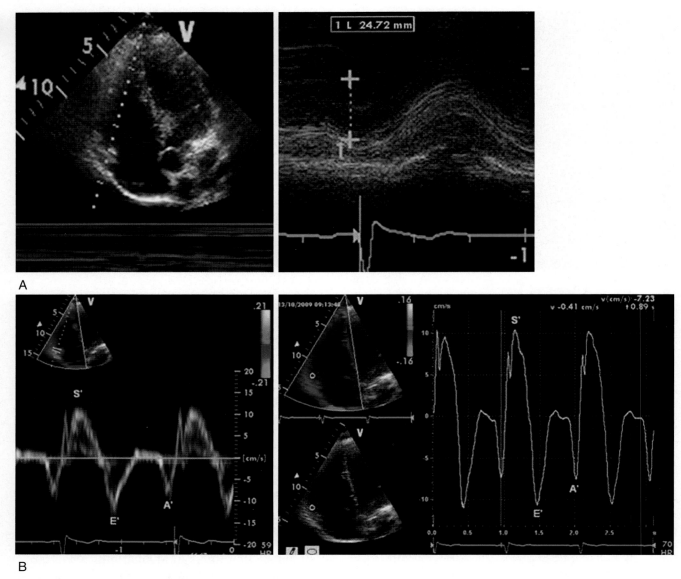

A

B

Figure 28.8. A, Measurement of tricuspid annular plane systolic excursion (TAPSE). **B,** Tissue Doppler imaging of the tricuspid annulus in a patient with normal right ventricular systolic function: pulsed (*left*) and color-coded offline analysis (*right*). (Reproduced with permission from Rudski LG, et al: Guidelines for the echocardiographic assessment of the right heart in adults: a report from the American Society of Echocardiography, *J Am Soc Echocardiogr* 23:685–713, quiz 786–688, 2010.)

it is recommended to measure and report only RV free-wall strain. Peak strain (strain of the RV free wall alone) has been shown to have prognostic meaning in various disease states such as congenital heart disease, coronary artery disease, pulmonary hypertension, amyloidosis, heart failure, and myocardial infarction and after mechanical LV support implantation.[10,31] Pooled data have generated reference values for free-wall strain, and the accepted normal value for RV free-wall strain is −29% ± 4.5% with the abnormality threshold therefore being greater than −20% (values closer to 0 are abnormal), which are similar to the normal values for LV strain. RV free-wall strain measurements are now thought to be reproducible and feasible for clinical use.[10] We measured 2D and 3D strain in our lab of 29 normal participants without known cardiovascular disease (Fig. 28.9). We found normal free-wall strain measured in 2D to be −29% ± 4.5% in all participants, −29% ± 3% in women, and −28% ± 4% in men. Using 3D strain imaging, we found similar normal values: −28% ± 9% in all participants, −26% ± 6% in women, and −28% ± 10% in men. In our cohort, we also measured

RV septal strain in 2D and in 3D. In 2D, normal values were −6% ± 3% in all participants, −16% ± 3% in women, and −15% ± 4% in men. Using 3D strain imaging, we found normal values −20% ± 7% in all participants, −20% ± 5%, in women, and −20% ±8 % in men(see Table 28.2).

CORONARY BLOOD FLOW OF THE RIGHT VENTRICLE

In the majority of individuals (~80%), the coronary arterial tree is right dominant (defined as a posterior descending artery [PDA] from the right coronary artery [RCA]), and the RCA supplies most of the RV. The lateral wall is supplied by marginal branches of the RCA, and the posterior wall is supplied by the PDA. The anterior wall and anteroseptal region, including the RV apex, receives its blood flow from the left anterior descending artery (LAD). For this reason, the RV apex is often spared during RV infarction or in acute massive pulmonary embolism with RV strain (so-called McConnell sign[20]), as discussed earlier. Conversely, a LAD infarction or

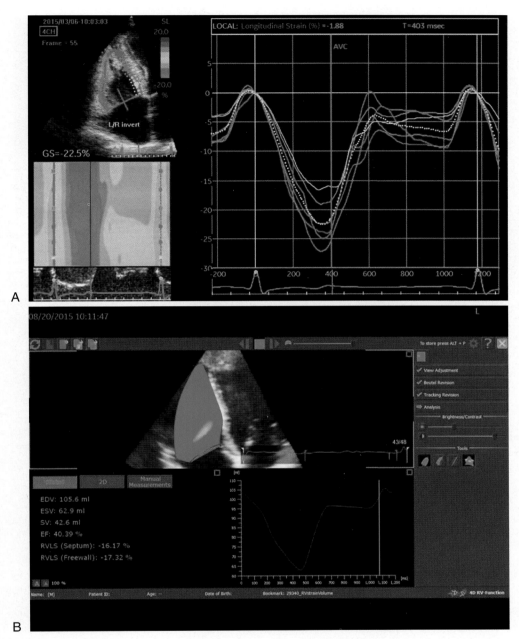

Figure 28.9. A, Two-dimensional right ventricular strain measurement. **B,** Three-dimensional right ventricular strain measurement. (Courtesy of Dwight Bibby at Research Cardiology Physiology Laboratory of the Health e Heart Study, Cardiovascular Research Institute, University of California–San Francisco.)

anterior infarction often spills over to involve the RV apex. The perfusion of the RVOT originates from a conus branch with a separate origin in 30% of individuals.[2]

Because of the thin-walled structure and low intraventricular filling pressures of the RV, baseline coronary blood flow to the RV is primarily systolic. However, blood flow to the LV is likely more diastolic or equally diastolic and systolic because of high filling pressures. The proximal RCA has blood flow that is both systolic and diastolic, but beyond marginal branches, diastolic flow predominates. This becomes highly relevant because this right ventricle is especially vulnerable to changes in loading conditions, and certain areas, which are thinner, are more susceptible to developing wall motion abnormalities or becoming ischemic during periods of increased wall stress.[32] For example, during acute

massive pulmonary embolism or after orthotopic heart transplant in a patient with a history of pulmonary hypertension, there is a sudden increase in RV afterload (and RV systolic filling pressures), which results in a decreased coronary perfusion pressure to the branches of the RCA that are perfused during systole. Therefore, relative hypokinesia develops in the midventricular wall, which is the thinnest part of the RV free wall.

The ramus limbi dextri is an interesting feature of the right coronary anatomy. This coronary branch runs from the midwall of the RV through the moderator band (or septal marginal trabeculation) and collaterizes the LAD. Because of this branch, patients with unoccluded proximal RCA who have LAD occlusion beyond the ramus are noted to have a small region of preserved midseptal wall motion.

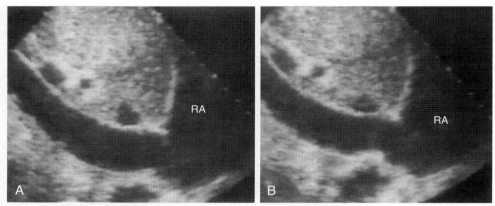

Figure 28.10. Long-axis two-dimensional subxiphoid image of the inferior vena cava and right atrium (RA) showing end-expiratory (**A**) and end-inspiratory (**B**) phases. The inferior vena cava is plethoric and shows minimal response to respiration. (Reproduced with permission from Bleeker GB, et al: Assessing right ventricular function: the role of echocardiography and complementary technologies, *Heart* 92(Suppl 1): i19–i26, 2006.)

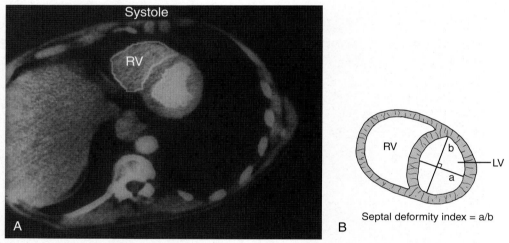

Figure 28.11. A, Computed tomography imaging showing right ventricular septal flattening and interventricular dependence that occurs as the right ventricle enlarged. **B,** Septal deformity index (a/b) to quantitate the degree of septal flattening in setting of right ventricular enlargement. *LV,* Left ventricle; *RV,* right ventricle.

The most important and common cause of RV segmental abnormalities is RV infarction. Most clinically important RV infarctions are seen in the setting of inferior wall myocardial infarction, although clinically unapparent involvement of the RV apex may be seen in anteroapical infarction.[33] The M-mode echocardiogram in RV infarction shows an enlarged ventricle.[34] On 2D TTE, the RV is dilated, and portions of the anterior midwall and inferior RV wall may appear akinetic or even aneurysmal; a hinge point may demonstrate infarcted segments, and the descent of the RV base is impaired.[33] The first clue to the presence of RV infarction may come from the short-axis view, where the distinctive akinesis is noted in the contiguous walls of the RV, inferior septum, and inferoposterior left ventricular walls. Inspection of the RV in the A4C view will reveal dilatation and may also show segmental midwall dyskinesis and remodeling.

An indication of the hemodynamic severity of the infarction is provided by the degree of RV dilation as well as the degree of IVC plethora (Fig. 28.10).[33,35] When RV infarction is clinically suspected, an echocardiogram is the method of choice for making the diagnosis and is the best means of establishing its hemodynamic severity.

INTERVENTRICULAR DEPENDENCE

The ventricles interact, so changes in size, systolic pressure of one chamber, and diastolic pressure of one chamber affect the size, shape, and function of the other. The ventricles may interact through the shape and direction of curvature of the interventricular septum (IVS); indirectly through the pericardium, where high pressure in one ventricle is transmitted to the other; or through the atria, where the interatrial septum may shift to reflect transmitted pressures (Figs. 28.11 and 28.12). Examples of this physiology include hemodynamically significant pericardial tamponade and any situation involving pericardial restraint, such as pericardial constriction. Physiologically, the Valsalva maneuver can alter the relationship of the ventricles; pathologically, pericardial diseases, pulmonary hypertension, acute pulmonary embolism, or RV infarction alter the geometry of the LV through interventricular dependence and decrease in preload (Table 28.3).

Changes in loading conditions can also affect the ventricular curvature and cause flattening of the IVS (see Fig. 28.12). Acute volume overload can lead to the flattening of the IVS during diastole, whereas severe pressure overload can result in flattening of the IVS during systole.[36,37]

RIGHT VENTRICULAR DIASTOLIC FUNCTION

Similar to the systolic function of the RV, the diastolic function of the RV is also difficult to capture comprehensively with any given standard 2D TTE parameter. A number of physiologic and pathophysiologic conditions can lead to RV diastolic dysfunction. Just as its left-sided counterpart, the aging RV can develop variable

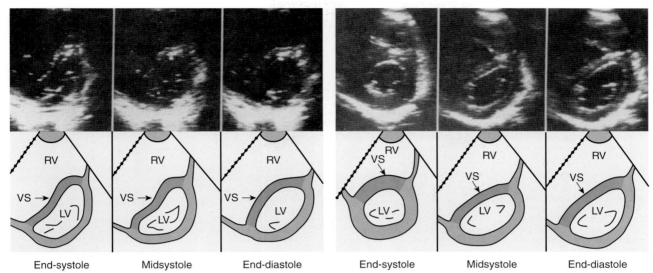

| End-systole | Midsystole | End-diastole | | End-systole | Midsystole | End-diastole |

Figure 28.12. Serial stop-frame short-axis two-dimensional echocardiographic images of the left ventricle at the mitral chordal level with diagrams from a patient with isolated right ventricular (RV) pressure overload caused by primary pulmonary hypertension (*left*). Images and diagrams on the *right* are from a patient with isolated RV volume overload caused by tricuspid valve resection. Although the left ventricular (LV) cavity maintains a circular profile throughout the cardiac cycle in normal participants, in RV pressure overload, leftward ventricular septal (VS) shift and reversal of septal curvature are present throughout the cardiac cycle, with most marked distortion of the left ventricle at end-systole. In a patient with RV volume overload, the septal shift and flattening of VS curvature occur predominantly in mid to late diastole, with relative sparing of LV deformation at end-systole. (Reproduced with permission from Louie EK, et al: Doppler echocardiographic demonstration of the differential effects of right ventricular pressure and volume overload on left ventricular geometry and filling, *J Am Coll Cardiol* 19:84–90, 1992.)

> **BOX 28.2** Clues to Right Ventricular Diastolic Dysfunction
>
> - Dilated inferior vena cava
> - Dilated right atrium
> - RV free-wall thickness >5 mm
> - Reduced transtricuspid E/A ratio (<0.8)
> - Elevated end-diastolic velocity of PR Doppler signal
> - Diastolic flow predominance in the hepatic veins

degrees of diastolic dysfunction, especially in the setting of pulmonary hypertension or other chronically increased RV afterload. On 2D TTE, the same pulsed wave Doppler measurements made across the mitral valve and tissue Doppler imaging of the septum and lateral wall can be roughly applied to the RV with its corresponding right-sided structures (see Fig. 28.8B).[2] Similarly, the isovolumetric relaxation time and deceleration time (DT) can be measured.[2] Some clues to right ventricular diastolic dysfunction are listed in Box 28.2.

RHYTHM DISTURBANCES ORIGINATING FROM THE RIGHT VENTRICLE

Arrhythmogenic right ventricular dysplasia is a genetically mediated disorder characterized by increased fat content of the RV myocardium and a propensity for fatal arrhythmia. Several attempts to develop echocardiography criteria for this disorder have been made, and criteria include depressed TAPSE, DTI abnormalities, and chamber enlargement. Recently, strain imaging has shown promise in increasing the yield of echocardiography in this condition.[38]

CONCLUSION

The unique anatomy and physiology of the RV is effectively evaluated by echocardiography, which is most often the only modality needed to characterize this ventricle. Now that we have enhanced

methods of evaluating RV size and function with 3D volume measurements and RV strain, respectively, the RV can now move into a more central place of systematic evaluation alongside the left-sided chambers.

REFERENCES

1. Bleeker GB, Steendijk P, Holman ER, et al. Assessing right ventricular function: the role of echocardiography and complementary technologies. *Heart*. 2006;92(suppl 1):i19–i26.
2. Rudski LG, Lai WW, Afilalo J, et al. Guidelines for the echocardiographic assessment of the right heart in adults: a report from the American Society of Echocardiography. *J Am Soc Echocardiogr*. 2010;23:685–713. quiz 786–688.
3. Lundstrom NR. Echocardiography in the diagnosis of Ebstein's anomaly of the tricuspid valve. *Circulation*. 1973;47:597–605.
4. Badano LP, Agricola E, Perez de Isla L, et al. Evaluation of the tricuspid valve morphology and function by transthoracic three-dimensional echocardiography. *Eur J Echocardiogr*. 2009;10:477–484.
5. James TN. Anatomy of the crista supraventricularis: its importance for understanding right ventricular function, right ventricular infarction and related conditions. *J Am Coll Cardiol*. 1985;6:1083–1095.
6. Gallucci V, Scalia D, Thiene G, et al. Double-chambered right ventricle: Surgical experience and anatomical considerations. *Thorac Cardiovasc Surg*. 1980;28(13–17).
7. Jiang L. *Principle and Practice of Echocardiography*. Baltimore: Lippincott Williams & Wilkins; 1994.
8. Nesser HJ, Tkalec W, Patel AR, et al. Quantitation of right ventricular volumes and ejection fraction by three-dimensional echocardiography in patients: comparison with magnetic resonance imaging and radionuclide ventriculography. *Echocardiography*. 2006;23:666–680.
9. Lang RM, Bierig M, Devereux RB, et al. Recommendations for chamber quantification: a report from the American Society of Echocardiography's Guidelines and standards Committee and the chamber quantification Writing Group. *J Am Soc Echocardiogr*. 2005;18:1440–1463.
10. Lang RM, Badano LP, Mor-Avi V, et al. Recommendations for chamber quantification by echocardiography in adults: an update from the American Society of Echocardiography and the European Association of Cardiovascular Imaging. *J Am Soc Echocardiogr*. 2015;28:1–39.
11. Ho SY, Nihoyannopoulos P. Anatomy, echocardiography, and normal right ventricular dimensions. *Heart*. 2006;92(suppl 1):i2–i13.
12. Haddad F, Hunt SA, Rosenthal DN, Murphy DJ. Right ventricular function in cardiovascular disease, part I: anatomy, physiology, aging, and functional assessment of the right ventricle. *Circulation*. 2008;117:1436–1448.
13. Dell'Italia LJ. The right ventricle: anatomy, physiology, and clinical importance. *Curr Probl Cardiol*. 1991;16:653–720.

14. Petitjean C, Rougon N, Cluzel P. Assessment of myocardial function: a review of quantification methods and results using tagged MRI. *J Cardiovasc Magn Reson.* 2005;7:501–516.

15. Starling MRWR, Dell'Italia LJ, Mancini GB, et al. The relationship of various measures of end-systole to left ventricular maximum time-varying elastance in man. *Circulation.* 1987;76:32–43.

16. McManus DD, Shah SJ, Fabi MR, et al. Prognostic value of left ventricular end-systolic volume index as a predictor of heart failure hospitalization in stable coronary artery disease: data from the Heart and Soul Study. *J Am Soc Echocardiogr.* 2009;22:190–197.

17. Turakhia MP, McManus DD, Whooley MA, Schiller NB. Increase in end-systolic volume after exercise independently predicts mortality in patients with coronary heart disease: data from the Heart and Soul Study. *Eur Heart J.* 2009;30:2478–2484.

18. Abbas AE, Franey LM, Marwick T, et al. Noninvasive assessment of pulmonary vascular resistance by Doppler echocardiography. *J Am Soc Echocardiogr.* 2013;26:1170–1177.

19. McConnell MV, Solomon SD, Rayan ME, et al. Regional right ventricular dysfunction detected by echocardiography in acute pulmonary embolism. *Am J Cardiol.* 1996;78:469–473.

20. Sosland RP, Gupta K. Images in cardiovascular medicine: McConnell's sign. *Circulation.* 2008;118:e517–e518.

21. Simonson JS, Schiller NB. Sonospirometry: a new method for noninvasive estimation of mean right atrial pressure based on two-dimensional echographic measurements of the inferior vena cava during measured inspiration. *J Am Coll Cardiol.* 1988;11:557–564.

22. Nagueh MF, Kopelen HA, Zoghbi WA, et al. Estimation of mean right atrial pressure using tissue Doppler imaging. *Am J Cardiol.* 1999;84:1448–1451. A1448.

23. Kusumoto FM, Muhiudeen IA, Kuecherer HF, et al. Response of the interatrial septum to transatrial pressure gradients and its potential for predicting pulmonary capillary wedge pressure: an intraoperative study using transesophageal echocardiography in patients during mechanical ventilation. *J Am Coll Cardiol.* 1993;21:721–728.

24. Ristow B, Ahmed S, Wang L, et al. Pulmonary regurgitation end-diastolic gradient is a Doppler marker of cardiac status: data from the Heart and Soul Study. *J Am Soc Echocardiogr.* 2005;18:885–891.

25. Schiller NB, Ristow B. Doppler under pressure: it's time to cease the folly of chasing the peak right ventricular systolic pressure. *J Am Soc Echocardiogr.* 2013;26:479–482.

26. Dobson R, Danton M, Nicola W, Hamish W. The natural and unnatural history of the systemic right ventricle in adult survivors. *J Thorac Cardiovasc Surg.* 2013;145:1493–1501. discussion 1501–1493.

27. Sim MM. Adaptation of the systemic right ventricle in a congenitally corrected transposition of the great arteries. *Circulation.* 2013;127:e448–e450.

28. Silverman NH, Hudson S. Evaluation of right ventricular volume and ejection fraction in children by two-dimensional echocardiography. *Pediatr Cardiol.* 1983;4:197–203.

29. Horton KD, Meece RW, Hill JC. Assessment of the right ventricle by echocardiography: a primer for cardiac sonographers. *J Am Soc Echocardiogr.* 2009;22:776–792. quiz 861–772.

30. Singbal Y, Vollbon W, Huynh L, et al. Exploring noninvasive tricuspid dP/dt as a marker of right ventricular function. *Echocardiography.* 2015;32(9):1347–1351.

31. Chang WT, Tsai WC, Liu YW, et al. Changes in right ventricular free wall strain in patients with coronary artery disease involving the right coronary artery. *J Am Soc Echocardiogr.* 2013.

32. Kinch JW, Ryan TJ. Right ventricular infarction. *N Engl J Med.* 1994;330:1211–1217.

33. Goldberger JJ, Himelman RB, Wolfe CL, Schiller NB. Right ventricular infarction: recognition and assessment of its hemodynamic significance by two-dimensional echocardiography. *J Am Soc Echocardiogr.* 1991;4:140–146.

34. Sharpe DN, Botvinick EH, Shames DM, et al. The noninvasive diagnosis of right ventricular infarction. *Circulation.* 1978;57:483–490.

35. Kircher BJ, Himelman RB, Schiller NB. Noninvasive estimation of right atrial pressure from the inspiratory collapse of the inferior vena cava. *Am J Cardiol.* 1990;66:493–496.

36. Ryan T, Petrovic O, Dillon JC, et al. An echocardiographic index for separation of right ventricular volume and pressure overload. *J Am Coll Cardiol.* 1985;5:918–927.

37. Kingma I, Tyberg JV, Smith ER. Effects of diastolic transseptal pressure gradient on ventricular septal position and motion. *Circulation.* 1983;68:1304–1314.

38. Marcus FI, McKenna WJ, Sherrill D, et al. Diagnosis of arrhythmogenic right ventricular cardiomyopathy/dysplasia: proposed modification of the Task Force Criteria. *Eur Heart J.* 2010;31:806–814.

39. Starling MR, Crawford MH, Walsh RA, O'Rourke RA. Value of the tricuspid valve echogram for estimating right ventricular end-diastolic pressure during vasodilator therapy. *Am J Cardiol.* 1980;45:966–972.

40. Louie EK, Rich S, Levitsky S, Brundage BH. Doppler echocardiographic demonstration of the differential effects of right ventricular pressure and volume overload on left ventricular geometry and filling. *J Am Coll Cardiol.* 1992;19:84–90.

41. Himelman RB, Struve SN, Brown JK, et al. Improved recognition of cor pulmonale in patients with severe chronic obstructive pulmonary disease. *Am J Med.* 1988;84:891–898.

29 Imaging the Right Heart: Limitations and Technical Considerations

Sabrina Islam, Benjamin Khazan, Martin G. Keane

The anatomy of the right ventricle (RV) creates significant technical challenges to an accurate echocardiographic assessment. Proper image acquisition is highly dependent on precise movements and angulations of the transducer as well as the volume and pressure states of the ventricle. Numerous measurements such as estimation of RV function, calculation of RV hemodynamics, and assessment of the right atrium (RA) rely on meticulous image procurement and are thus prone to error. Attention to core imaging guidelines and machine adjustments, reviewed here, optimizes echocardiographic right heart imaging and reduces miscalculations. Advanced imaging techniques, including three-dimensional echocardiography (3DE), use of commercial contrast, computed tomography, and magnetic resonance imaging (MRI), can overcome some of the pitfalls of two-dimensional echocardiography (2DE), though they remain largely supplemental and have limitations of their own.

which is acoustically challenging to capture and places portions of the RV and right ventricular outflow tract (RVOT) in the near field of the ultrasound beam, which is detrimental to imaging. Second, the RV has an exquisite but highly complex architecture that includes three anatomically distinct segments—RV inflow, RV body, and RV outflow (see Chapter 27). This complexity precludes imaging of the entire RV in any single 2DE view. Third, the thin-walled and highly trabeculated nature of the RV chamber require careful technical considerations for precise delineation of wall thickness, thickening, and motion. Finally, in addition to all of the technical considerations already mentioned, a complete functional assessment of the RV is compounded by the ability to quantify the complex contractile function of the ventricle. Right heart imaging therefore requires careful attention to all technical aspects of transthoracic echocardiography (TTE) 2D and Doppler imaging.

CORE LIMITATIONS OF IMAGING

The right heart presents numerous technical challenges to echocardiographic assessment of size, structure and function. First, the right heart is largely positioned retrosternal and anterior,

CHALLENGES IN EVALUATING RV SIZE AND STRUCTURE

The RV body itself has a complex pyramidal structure, which appears crescentic in short-axis views and roughly triangular

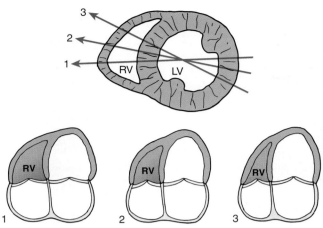

Figure 29.1. Diagram of the "right ventricular (RV)–focused" apical four-chamber (A4C) view (plane *1*). The upper short-axis diagram demonstrates the counterclockwise rotation from the "standard" A4C orientation *(2)* that is necessary to display the maximal diameter of the RV chamber. The corresponding A4C views below demonstrate the appearance of the RV-focused view *(1)* compared with the other imaging planes *(2, 3)*, which could lead to underestimation of RV longitudinal diameter and area. (Adapted from Lang RM, et al: Recommendations for cardiac chamber quantification by echocardiography in adults, *J Am Soc Echocardiogr* 28:1–39, 2015.)

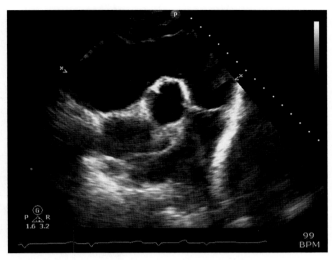

Figure 29.2. Proper orientation of the parasternal short-axis view for displaying the full right ventricular outflow tract (RVOT) to allow accurate measurement of RVOT diameter.

in long-axis views. Complete volumetric assessment of the RV based on 2D TTE linear or area measurements is impossible, given the fact that no simple geometric assumptions exist for the more asymmetrical RV. Nonetheless, there is value in assessment of RV size by linear and area measurement in clinical echocardiography. Given the paucity of fixed reference points, however, the perceived morphology and dimensions of the RV depend significantly on the plane of imaging and small rotations in the transducer.[1,2]

The Right Ventricle–Focused View

The standard apical four-chamber (A4C) view focuses predominantly on the left ventricle (LV), and consequently portions of the RV may not be visible.[3] To overcome these limitations, the "RV-focused view" should be obtained in all studies interrogating the right heart (Fig. 29.1). This view provides enhanced visualization of the RV free wall and reveals the maximal diameter of the ventricle without foreshortening, thus improving estimation of RV dimensions and reducing interobserver variability of structure. Therefore, the RV-focused view is essential for measuring fractional area change and is recommended for accurate assessment of longitudinal strain.[4] Additionally, its unique angle may allow for better capture of a TR jet or establishment of ASDs or PFOs.[1,5-9]

To generate the RV-focused view, the standard A4C view should first be obtained. With the LV apex remaining at the center of the scanning sector, the transducer should be slightly rotated counterclockwise to focus on the RV until the maximal transverse plane is displayed (typically the basal RV diameter); this avoids foreshortening.[1,2,9,10] Often, the transducer will require medial or lateral movements to produce this image.[4,6,9] To improve image quality, the frame rate can be increased by reducing sector size.[4] A high-frequency transducer may be of benefit given that the RV is a near-field structure.[9] The RV may also be preferentially viewed with small adjustments in transducer angle and position from the apical two- and three-chamber views, yielding a modified three-chamber view (RA, RV, and RVOT), and a modified two-chamber view (RA and RV), respectively.[1]

Technical Considerations for Other Standard Transthoracic Echocardiography Views

In addition to the RV-focused A4C view, a comprehensive multiplane examination of the right heart also includes the parasternal long-axis (PLAX), RV inflow, and short-axis (PSAX) views; the standard A4C view; and subcostal views.[1,2] All of these views are essential given the complex geometry of the RV, its poor anatomic reference points, and the inability to image the three anatomical components (inlet, body, and outlet) simultaneously in any single 2D plane.[2,6] These obstacles create pitfalls in imaging of the RV in "standard views."

The PLAX view produces views of the proximal RVOT, which may vary based on the rib interspace used for imaging as well as the angulation of the transducer. Excessively oblique positioning may lead to underestimation or overestimation of RVOT size.[1,2] Furthermore, careful adjustments in the gain may be necessary for ideal visualization.[2] The PSAX view reveals the proximal and distal RVOT (RV outflow) as well as the RA and tricuspid valve (RV inflow). The aortic valve or root should be seen in short axis in the center of the picture, often necessitating movement of the transducer superiorly along the chest wall (Fig. 29.2). Image quality and accuracy in this view are again dependent on transducer angle and position. RVOT dimensions may be inaccurate in patients with chest or spine deformities, and even without these confounders, 2D PSAX views do not typically achieve an accurate morphologic assessment.[2] Moreover, measurements may vary with patient position (RV dimension will be smaller if the patient is supine compared to sitting up at a 30- or 45-degree angle). RV functional assessment is limited in this view as well given the asymmetric nature of RV contraction; contraction by the RV inflow and RV outflow are longitudinal and circumferential, respectively, and are thus perpendicular to one another.[1,9]

Linear and area measurements of the RV and concurrent functional assessment of the RV in the standard A4C and RV-focused apical four views depend on suitable endocardial definition of the RV free wall (Fig. 29.3). The free wall, however, is usually retrosternal and is thus difficult to visualize. Other confounders of RV size and area include the presence of trabeculations and foreshortening caused by improper transducer positioning. Furthermore, the RV's crescentic shape, combined with the LV's twisting contractile motion, frequently results in end-diastolic images and end-systolic images of the RV residing in different planes.[2] Finally, even when using the RV-focused A4C view, if the center of the sector is located over the RV (instead of the LV, as recommended), the RV may appear falsely dilated.[10]

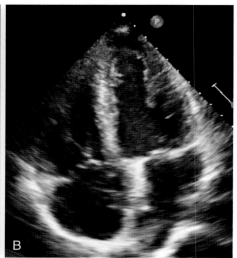

Figure 29.3. Images obtained from the same study demonstrate how careful transducer placement and medial-lateral positioning can result in complete visualization of the right ventricular (RV) free wall (**A**) versus incomplete definition of RV free-wall endocardium (**B**).

The subcostal view allows for assessment of inferior vena cava (IVC) size and collapsibility and thus right atrial pressures. While the IVC is typically viewed in long axis, changes in its diameter may simply be reflective of movement/translation of the vessel into another plane, and thus a cross-section evaluation may be more appropriate. Filling pressures may be overestimated if the patient is not in the left lateral decubitus position or if the patient is intubated, because IVC collapse in this instance is confounded by positive pressure ventilation. Last, although the subcostal view allows accurate assessment of RV wall thickness caused by perpendicular beam trajectory, caution with measurement is recommended in the presence of epicardial fat (Fig. 29.4).

Overload States

The shape of the RV can vary dramatically with volume loading, with the overall shape becoming more globular and with varying degrees of diastolic flattening of the interventricular septum. Adequate semiquantitative evaluation of the dilated RV size still depends on linear measurements of basal and midcavity RV diameters, as well as RV longitudinal dimension in the RV-focused four-chamber view.[9] However, because the volume-loaded RV becomes apex forming, careful adjustments in the RV-focused view planes are essential to avoid foreshortening. Even with such adjustments, TTE assessment of volume-loaded RV size is significantly less accurate/reproducible than that of normal RVs compared with cardiac magnetic resonance imaging (CMR).[11]

Pressure overload of the RV may manifest with some degree of RV dilatation but predominantly with significant hypertrophy of the ventricular walls. Assessment of RV wall thickness is preferably performed in the subcostal view in the vicinity of the tip of the anterior tricuspid leaflet, with the ultrasound beam directed perpendicular to wall. Hypertrophied trabeculae in the pressure-overloaded RV introduce increased scatter, however, leading to overestimation of the thickness of the nontrabeculated free wall.[12] Use of fundamental imaging with higher-frequency beam focused on the near field is essential in these situations to maximize detail and accuracy (Fig. 29.5).

PITFALLS IN ASSESSMENT OF RV FUNCTION

All echocardiographic studies of the RV must include assessment of systolic function. There are several ways in which to accomplish this, though it is essential to measure at least one of the following: fractional area change (FAC), tricuspid annular plane systolic excursion (TAPSE), systolic excursion velocity (S′), or RV index of myocardial performance (RIMP).

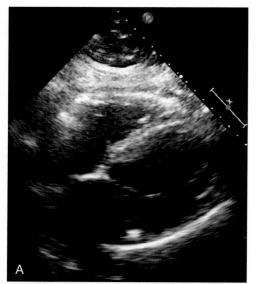

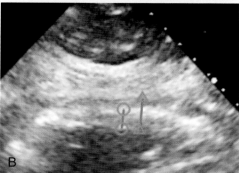

Figure 29.4. Even with appropriate perpendicular beam orientation and clear definition of right ventricular wall thickness in the subcostal view (**A**), the presence of overlying epicardial fat may lead to inaccurate wall thickness measurement. Careful measurement of the free wall itself is essential. Inclusion of epicardial fat pad must be avoided (**B**).

Fractional Area Change

Measurements of RV ejection fraction using FAC correlate well with results from CMR[1] because FAC is not angle dependent and accounts for both the longitudinal and radial components of RV contraction.[3] To adequately assess FAC, the entire ventricle must be

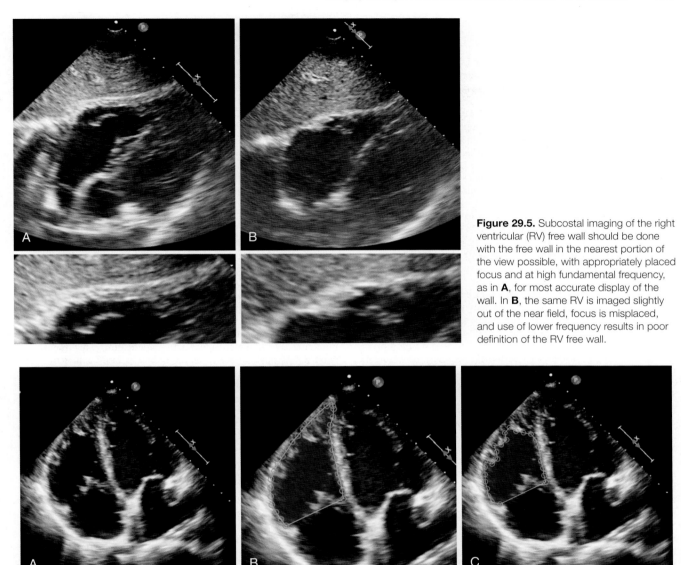

Figure 29.5. Subcostal imaging of the right ventricular (RV) free wall should be done with the free wall in the nearest portion of the view possible, with appropriately placed focus and at high fundamental frequency, as in **A**, for most accurate display of the wall. In **B**, the same RV is imaged slightly out of the near field, focus is misplaced, and use of lower frequency results in poor definition of the RV free wall.

Figure 29.6. Measurement of right ventricular (RV) area for fractional area change calculations requires orientation in an appropriate RV-focused apical four-chamber view (**A**). When tracing the RV area, all major trabeculations and the moderator band must be included as part of the RV ventricular area (**B**). Excluding major trabeculations (**C**) leads to significant underestimation of RV area, both in systole and diastole.

in view (apex and lateral free wall) in both systole and diastole.[1,13] Excellent endocardial border definition is essential, and thus the RV-focused view may be required.[4,7,8] While measuring cavity size, operators must take care to include trabeculations and the moderator band within the traced volume of the RV (Fig. 29.6). The propensity to undertrace the cavity has resulted in limited reproducibility of FAC.[1,6,10] It is important to remember that evaluation of true RV cavity size by FAC is limited by the ventricle's complex geometry.[14] Importantly, FAC neglects the RVOT's contribution to the ejection fraction, which contains up to 25% to 30% of total RV volume.[5,9–13]

TAPSE and S′

TAPSE and S′ represent other elementary evaluation techniques for RV systolic function—from the viewpoint of longitudinal shortening—and are both performed from the A4C window. These measurements correlate with radionuclide angiography, with TAPSE also correlated to assessment of ejection fraction via the Simpson biplane method and FAC.[1] Both techniques examine single segments of the RV (TAPSE at the lateral tricuspid annulus and S′

at the annulus or RV free wall) and are highly angle dependent because the sampled segment must be parallel to the direction of annular motion.[1,4,6,13] Given their small region of interest at the basal lateral aspect, TAPSE and S′ rely on the assumption that the displacement of these segments are representative of the function of the entire RV. In instances of chamber remodeling that differentially affects contractile function of other segments, both may be inaccurate. TAPSE does not accurately describe global RV function in patients with tetralogy of Fallot or prior cardiac surgery and is also load dependent, because increased values in the setting of severe tricuspid regurgitation can result in overestimation of true RV function.[4] Measurements of S′ may also be inaccurate after a thoracotomy, pulmonary thromboendarterectomy, or heart transplant and have not been validated in nonsinus rhythm.[6,8,13]

Right Ventricular Index of Myocardial Performance

The RIMP, also known as the myocardial performance index (MPI) or Tei index, is an adjunctive measure of RV systolic function that should not be used alone for quantitation of RV function.[1,13] RIMP addresses a composite of RV systolic and diastolic function by measuring work done during ejection and non-ejection and is useful in that it can be used in the presence of tricuspid regurgitation and avoids geometric assumptions.[1] There are two methods to achieve a RIMP measurement, each with its own pitfalls. The pulsed Doppler technique requires measurement from the end of an A wave to the beginning of an E wave. Because this necessitates at least two heartbeats, variations in the R-R interval (e.g., atrial fibrillation) can make pulsed Doppler RIMP measurements unreliable.[1,3] Alternatively, use of the tissue Doppler technique yields an accurate assessment of isovolumic contraction time and isovolumic relaxation time within a single heartbeat and thus overcomes this limitation. However, both pulsed and tissue Doppler methodologies are load dependent, and quantification can vary with pressure and volume status.[1,3,10] In conditions that increase RA pressure, such as RV infarction or pulmonary hypertension, the IVRT will decrease because of a rapid equilibration of RA and RV pressures and can thus falsely lower RIMP calculations.

Right Ventricular Hemodynamics: Doppler Assessment

In addition to estimation of RV function by way of morphologic and 2D area or volume changes, hemodynamic features of systolic performance such as RV stroke volume (SV) and RV cardiac output can be derived from combined 2D and Doppler measurements. Measurement of RV SV can be calculated by multiplying the RVOT cross-sectional area to the RV velocity time integral (VTI). The echocardiographer must be vigilant to pitfalls in these measurements because the structural complexities of imaging the RVOT present unique challenges.[15] Imaging of the RVOT region (infundibulum or conus) is typically best performed in the left PSAX view, which demonstrates the RVOT at the level of the pulmonic valve and the proximal portion of the main pulmonary artery. Although the RVOT can also be visualized in the left PLAX view, this view shows only the most proximal portion of the RVOT, frequently off-axis and not suitable for cross-sectional area measurements.[1] Measurements should be made in diastole and are complicated by noncylindrical geometry, retrosternal position, and inaccuracies introduced by chest and spine deformities.[2]

In the PSAX view, the RVOT falls into the nearfield of the beam, a location often not optimally visualized, particularly with limited resolution of the anterior free-wall endocardium. For improved visualization and accuracy, focus depth should be set at a shallow level, and a higher-frequency beam may be helpful to distinguish the thin-walled, trabeculated structure (seef Fig. 29.2). A transducer producing a higher-frequency beam, however, may

be unavailable or may be too large to be used within a standard intercostal space to adequately optimize RVOT visualization.[16] Because of the oblique view, neither the RVOT diameter nor the RVOT VTI can be confidently measured. Additionally, in the setting of these limitations and less attention traditionally focused on the RV, there are limited data available for normative values.

Echocardiographic evaluation of RV SV assumes that the cross-sectional area of the RVOT is circular in morphology and calculates the area based on the radius of the RVOT. However, 3DE, cardiac computed tomography (CT), and MRI have demonstrated that for the majority of the population the RV is noncircular in morphology. It has been found to be elliptical[17-19] (Fig. 29.7). Hence, when using a circular cross-sectional area (πr^2) for RVOT, error is inherently introduced. Additionally, oblique imaging of the RVOT diameter/radius can lead to significant over- or underestimation of its size,[1] an error only magnified because of squaring of the radius. Nonetheless, when performed with care, estimation of RV SV (and by default RV cardiac output) can provide important supplementary information for assessment of overall RV performance.

Oblique imaging of the RVOT is also an important consideration with Doppler VTI measurement. To start measuring RVOT VTI, pulsed-wave Doppler should be placed in the center of the RVOT, 5 to 10 mm proximal to the pulmonic valve.[20] The RVOT peak velocity and VTI should be measured here. Optimal Doppler imaging requires a parallel angle to blood flow. With oblique imaging, the Doppler signal will underestimate the RVOT VTI and RVOT peak velocity, thus introducing significant error in RV SV and cardiac output evaluations. Often, the Doppler signal from the PSAX is insufficient, and alternate imaging planes should be attempted, such as use of the subcostal view, in which the Doppler cursor can frequently be oriented parallel to blood flow.

OVERCOMING TECHNICAL CHALLENGES OF TWO-DIMENSIONAL TRANSTHORACIC ECHOCARDIOGRAPHY WITH ADVANCED IMAGING

Advanced imaging techniques can be used to further evaluate right ventricular structure and function. They can be adjunct imaging modalities to confirm and supplement data obtained by TTE; however, each technique comes with its own limitation.

Three-Dimensional Echocardiography

Evaluation of the RV with 3D TTE techniques has become a reasonable alternative method of evaluation of RV size, structure,

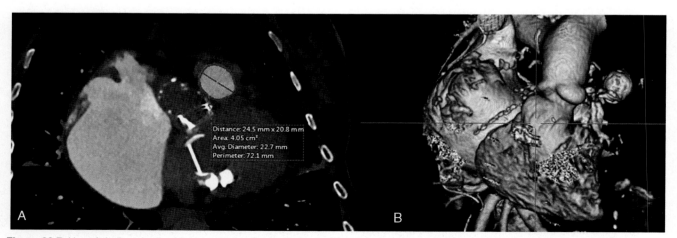

Figure 29.7. Use of shallow depth of field and higher-frequency beam (**A**) for measurements of right ventricular outflow tract (RVOT) diameter are preferred over excessively deep depth of field and lower-frequency imaging (**B**). Significant differences in RVOT diameter measurement may result.

and function. Typically, an A4C RV-focused view of reasonable technical quality is required for data acquisition over four to six beats. Three-dimensional echo technique does not rely on geometric assumptions, which are typically inaccurate when applied to the RV. Given the previously described challenges for adequate imaging of the RV with 2DE, visualization can be suboptimal when attempting to acquire a 3D dataset.[5] RV volumes obtained from 3D datasets are often underestimated when compared with MRI-obtained values. This is often a result of poor endocardial definition of the RV because of limited visualization. Additionally, the heavily trabeculated RV apex can result in blurring of 3D image borders, leading to inaccurate endocardial tracings. Difficulties with defining the RV anterior wall in the region of the RVOT on 2D imaging typically translates into poor 3D RVOT assessment, which is a necessary component for accurate volume assessments. Finally, there is significant overall 3D quality variability between novice and experienced operators, thus introducing significant potential error when applied by inexperienced operators.

Transesophageal Echocardiography

Transesophageal echocardiography (TEE) can be a useful modality for interrogating the RV for size and function, particularly in instances of limited visualization with 2DE. The TEE probe is manipulated to obtain views in the midesophagus and in superficial and deep transgastric views.[19] The TEE probe is limited in the locations and views that can be obtained. Often this makes it difficult to obtain supplemental or optimized views of right-sided structures. In the available imaging planes, the RV is often foreshortened. The RV is an anterior structure and therefore located in the far field during TEE. This can result in limited endocardial definition and accuracy when evaluating endocardial structures such as when attempting to evaluate RV wall thickness. Additionally, there is limited information outlining the correct orientation of the RV when attempting to evaluate its size and function, which can lead to significant variability in the accuracy of size estimates based on TEE. Volumetric assessment with transesophageal 3DE, however, have been noted to be similar to those obtained with 3D TTE and may be able to overcome the variability of transesophageal 2DE. Because of these issues, TEE imaging has limited use in supplementing traditional 2D transthoracic techniques.

Speckle Tracking and Strain

RV global longitudinal peak systolic strain (RVGLS) and RV free-wall strain (RV FWLS) have been shown to provide valuable information regarding RV systolic function, supplemental to traditional 2DE techniques. Doppler tissue imaging (DTI) and 2D and 3D speckle-tracking echocardiography (STE) techniques are available. RVGLS is typically evaluated from a single RV-focused A4C view (Fig. 29.8). Although Fig. 29.8 illustrates RVGLS that includes the ventricular septum, newer software is becoming available that measures only RV free-wall strain, which is preferable. 2D STE is the accepted modality for evaluation of RVGLS and RV FWLS and has been validated when compared with RVEF by CMR as well as invasive hemodynamic assessment of RV function.[3] This relationship was particularly apparent in populations at risk for RV dysfunction such as in heart failure, pulmonary hypertension, pulmonary embolism, valvular disease, and myocardial infarction. In a structurally normal RV, the majority of systolic function is due to longitudinal shortening as detected by TAPSE and S′. In the setting of significant RV impairment and alteration of the RV structure or with the introduction of regional wall motion abnormalities, the basal motion of the RV may be distorted. STE is angle independent and often independent of the translational motion of respiration or tethering to adjacent myocardium, allowing it to overcome the challenges of evaluating a dysfunctional or distorted RV. However, technical challenges caused by the thin walls of the RV, the complex anatomy of the RV, and significant translational and rotational motion of portions of the RV throughout the cardiac cycle introduce significant errors of RV visualization. Alternate modes of evaluating global RVLS have been proposed to use multiple views similar to GLS evaluation of the LV; however, these have not yet been validated or adopted as standard practice.

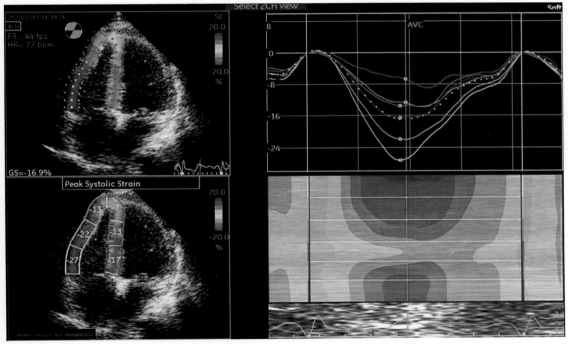

Figure 29.8. Right ventricular global longitudinal strain measured from the right ventricle–focused apical four-chamber view, as demonstrated here.

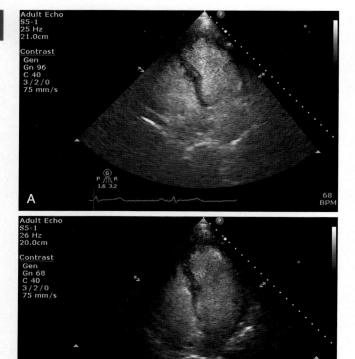

Figure 29.9. Although use of contrast is highly effective for evaluation of right ventricular size and function in technically difficult studies, the amount of contrast used, mechanical index, and positioning of the image must be optimized to ensure adequate endocardial border enhancement (**A**). Inadequate contrast optimization (**B**) results in poor free-wall border definition and inaccuracy of assessment of size and function.

Contrast Echocardiography

The challenges of inadequate endocardial visualization limiting the ability to adequately delineate the RV wall morphology and motion often leads to suboptimal 2D and 3D image acquisition. In these situations, it is important to recognize that commercial contrast enhancement can provide enhanced visualization of the RV in both 2DE and 3DE.[21] Contrast echocardiography is also promising as an adjunct tool for refining RV volume and functional assessment in complex or difficult cases. With contrast echocardiography, 3DE images can be obtained that provide reproducible RV systolic measurements that are comparable to those obtained on CMR.[21] Contrast echocardiography itself, however, is subject to temporal technical limitations because there is often rapid clearance of contrast from the RV. Additionally, images are typically optimized for LV visualization, leading to inadequate RV assessments (Fig. 29.9).

Computed Tomography

Gated cardiac CT imaging is an excellent supplemental imaging modality for visualization of the right heart. This is particularly true when potential normal variants are noted on TTE but concerns for possible pathologic abnormalities exist.[22] CT imaging can often clarify and confirm normal structures that are aberrant from typical appearances and can be misidentified as abnormal structures, such as a prominent RV moderator band that may mimic an RV mass. CT imaging is also noted to be superior in determining the RV structure, volume, and function compared with TTE, with greater reproducibility. The drawbacks of CT include limited availability of advanced or high-resolution

scanners in some institutions, as well as limited access to image interpreters with expertise in RV reconstruction. Additionally, CT imaging entails exposure to IV contrast and radiation, which may make the modality prohibitive in many cases. In cases of excessive arrhythmia burden including tachycardia, appropriate gating may not be feasible. Valvular and hemodynamic evaluations—easily obtained by 2DE and CMR—cannot be assessed by CT.

Cardiac Magnetic Resonance Imaging

In cases of severe technical limitations to TTE visualization, CMR is an additional complementary imaging modality for improved structural and functional assessment of the RV. Although 2DE has superior spatial and temporal resolution, CMR imaging has become the established gold standard for RV structure, volume, and global and regional function assessment.[23] The traditional CMR method of volume assessment approximates a method of discs approach for reconstruction of the RV. This method has been noted to have variability and often overestimates end-systolic volumes because of difficulty in identification of the base of trabeculations. This can potentially be corrected through manual retracing methods by experienced operators. Newer CMR techniques have also been proposed for more accurate estimation of RV size and function using a knowledge-based reconstruction database. These databases of known baseline RV healthy and diseased shapes are used as the models for the geometric assumptions applied in reconstruction algorithms. Such algorithms can also improve the accuracy of volumes acquired by 2DE and 3DE as well. Limitations of this modality include the constraints placed on CMR, particularly in those with other implantable devices, which may be incompatible. Additionally, exposure to contrast agents may be prohibitive in those individuals with intolerance or renal impairment. In cases of significant arrhythmia burden, gated imaging may not be feasible, diminishing the data available for interpretation from the modality.

Machine Learning

Despite improvements in acquisition of 3D imaging, there remains limited utilization of this imaging modality. Because of variability in image quality based on operator skill and experience as well as time necessary to obtain accurate and reproducible images, 3D imaging is not as widely or readily available. With the development and application of machine learning–based algorithms, however, 3D imaging of the RV may eventually be obtained and interpreted with increasing accuracy and reproducibility.[24] RV volumes and ejection fractions can be obtained with minimal image manipulation in a reasonable time frame to allow the modality to be implemented more readily. However, this technology is not widely available, limiting the utility of the modality at present.

RIGHT ATRIUM

TTE provides limited potential for accurate evaluation of the RA. Primary evaluation of the chamber is typically performed in the A4C view, where size can be assessed at end-systole by linear dimensions, area–length volume, or via method of disks.[1,2] 3D TTE provides a more accurate assessment of volume[25] but may underestimate RV volume in comparison with CT and CMR techniques.[26] TEE allows a more comprehensive assessment of all sections of the RA, including the RA appendage, insertion of venae cavae, and interatrial septum. TEE may also be required for clarification of RA anatomic variants (Chiari network, eustachian valve, and so on) from possible pathologic states in cases of technically limited TTE evaluation. In any assessment of RA size, attention must be paid to the easy extrinsic compressibility of the RA by pericardial and pleural effusions or masses of the liver or mediastinum. Function of the RA is poorly assessed by standard 2DE techniques and may be best supplemented by strain imaging.[27]

REFERENCES

1. Rudski LG, Lai WW, Afilalo J, et al. Guidelines for the echocardiographic assessment of the right heart in adults. *J Am Soc Echocardiogr.* 2010;23:685–713.
2. Lang RM, Badano LP, Mor-Avi V, et al. Recommendations for cardiac chamber quantification by echocardiography in adults. *J Am Soc Echocardiogr.* 2015;28:1–39.
3. Longobardo L, Suma V, Jain R, et al. Role of two-dimensional speckle-tracking echocardiography strain in the assessment of right ventricular systolic function and comparison with conventional parameters. *J Am Soc Echocardiogr.* 2017;30:937–946.
4. Wu VC, Takeuchi M. Echocardiographic assessment of right ventricular systolic function. *Cardiovasc Diagn Ther.* 2018;8:70–79.
5. Partington SL, Kilner PJ. How to image the dilated right ventricle. *Circ Cardiovasc Imag.* 2017;10:e004688.
6. Abouzeid CM, Shah T, Johri A, Weinsaft JW, Kim J. Multimodality imaging of the right ventricle. *Curr Treat Options Cardiovasc Med.* 2017;19:1–11.
7. Sokalskis V, Peluso D, Jagodzinski A, Sinning C. Added clinical value of applying myocardial deformation imaging to assess right ventricular function. *Echocardiography.* 2017;34:919–927.
8. Schneider M, Binder T. Echocardiographic evaluation of the right heart. *Wien Klin Wochenschr.* 2018;130:413–420.
9. Venkatachalam S, Wu G, Ahmad M. Echocardiographic assessment of the right ventricle in the current era: application in clinical practice. *Echocardiography.* 2017;34:1930–1947.
10. Portnoy SG, Rudski LG. Echocardiographic evaluation of the right ventricle: a 2014 perspective. *Curr Cardiol Rep.* 2015;17:1–8. article 21.
11. Lu KJ, Chen JX, Profitis K, et al. Right ventricular global longitudinal strain is an independent predictor of right ventricular function: a multimodality study of cardiac magnetic resonance imaging, real time three-dimensional echocardiography and speckle tracking echocardiography. *Echocardiography.* 2015;32:966–974.
12. Harrison A, Hatton N, Ryan JJ. The right ventricle under pressure: evaluating the adaptive and maladaptive changes in the right ventricle in pulmonary arterial hypertension using echocardiography. *Pulm Circ.* 2015;5:29–47.
13. Alsoos F, Khaddam A. Echocardiographic evaluation methods for right ventricular function. *J Echocardiogr.* 2015;13:43–51.
14. Rajagopal S, Forsha DE, Risum N, et al. Comprehensive assessment of right ventricular function in patients with pulmonary hypertension with global longitudinal peak systolic strain derived from multiple right ventricular views. *J Am Soc Echocardiogr.* 2014;27:657–665.
15. Vitarelli A, Terzano C. Do we have two hearts? New insights in right ventricular function supported by myocardial imaging echocardiography. *Heart Fail Rev.* 2010;15:39–61.
16. Armstrong WF, Ryan T, Feigenbaum H. 7th ed. *Feigenbaum's Echocardiography.* Philadelphia: Wolters Kluwer Health/Lippincott Williams & Wilkins; 2010:13–14. 106–107.
17. Izumo M, Shiota M, Saitoh T, et al. Non-circular shape of right ventricular outflow tract: a real-time 3-dimensional transesophageal echocardiography study. *Circ Cardiovasc Imag.* 2012;5:621–627.
18. Saremi F, Ho SY, Cabrera JA, Sanchez-Quintana D. Right ventricular outflow tract imaging with CT and MRI: part 1, morphology. *AJR Am J Roentgenol.* 2013;200:W39–W50.
19. Tadic M. Multimodality evaluation of the right ventricle: an updated review. *Clin Cardiol.* 2015;38:770–776.
20. Mitchell C, Rahko PS, Blauwet LA, et al. Guidelines for performing a comprehensive transthoracic echocardiographic examination in adults. *J Am Soc Echocardiogr.* 2019;32:1–64.
21. Medvedofsky D, Mor-Avi V, Kruse E, et al. Quantification of right ventricular size and function from contrast-enhanced three-dimensional echocardiographic images. *J Am Soc Echocardiogr.* 2017;30:1193–1202.
22. Malik SB, Chen N, Parker 3rd RA, Hsu JY. Transthoracic echocardiography: pitfalls and limitations as delineated at cardiac CT and MR imaging. *Radiographics.* 2017;37:383–406.
23. Laser KT, Horst JP, Barth P, et al. Knowledge-based reconstruction of right ventricular volumes using real-time three-dimensional echocardiographic as well as cardiac magnetic resonance images: comparison with a cardiac magnetic resonance standard. *J Am Soc Echocardiogr.* 2014;27:1087–1097.
24. Genovese D, Rashedi N, Weinert L, et al. Machine learning-based three-dimensional echocardiographic quantification of right ventricular size and function: validation against cardiac magnetic resonance. *J Am Soc Echocardiogr.* 2019;32:969–977.
25. Peluso D, Badano LP, Muraru D, et al. Right atrial size and function assessed with three-dimensional and speckle tracking echocardiography in 200 healthy volunteers. *Eur Heart J Cardiovasc Imag.* 2013;14:1106–1114.
26. Khalique OK, Cavalcante JL, Shah D, et al. Multimodality imaging of the tricuspid valve and right heart anatomy. *JACC Cardiovasc Imag.* 2019;12:516–531.
27. Rai A, Lima E, Munir F, et al. Speckle tracking echocardiography of the right atrium: the neglected chamber. *Clin Cardiol.* 2015;38:692–697.

30 Assessment of Right Ventricular Systolic and Diastolic Function

Lawrence G. Rudski, Denisa Muraru, Jonathan Afilalo

The right ventricle (RV) plays a key role in the outcome of many disease states. RV dysfunction is associated with excess morbidity and mortality in patients with chronic left-sided heart failure (HF), acute myocardial infarction (MI), pulmonary embolism (PE), pulmonary arterial hypertension (PAH), and congenital heart disease. Despite this knowledge, a standardized approach toward the echocardiographic assessment of the RV was only developed and applied a decade ago, with revised recommendations in 2015.[1,2] This chapter focuses on how to assess RV function, with an emphasis on newer techniques.

ANATOMY AND PHYSIOLOGY

The right side of the heart receives the systemic venous return from the superior and inferior venae cavae. The right atrium serves as a conduit and a pump, filling the right ventricle via the tricuspid valve. The right ventricle then ejects its stroke volume (SV) through the pulmonary veins (PVs) and into the pulmonary artery (PA). In the absence of a shunt, right-sided SV should be equal to that of the left side. The right side of the heart differs from the left in terms of anatomy and physiology in several important ways. Although the left ventricle (LV) can be modeled as a prolate ellipse, the RV loosely resembles a pyramid that wraps around the LV and is composed of three portions: the inlet, the body, and the outflow tract. Contraction is generated by a deep subendocardial layer of longitudinal fibers that cause a base-to-apex motion and a superficial layer of circumferential fibers that cause inward contraction.[3] Recent data from three-dimensional (3D) imaging suggest that this inward motion is more important than previously thought. The RV lacks the third layer of spiral fibers that are present in the LV. The RV end-diastolic volume (EDV) is slightly greater than that of the LV, and as a result, the RV has a slightly lower ejection fraction (EF). This is accomplished with a mass that is approximately one-fifth that of the LV. Accordingly, the RV is well suited as a volume pump, but is prone to failure when faced with an acute pressure challenge.[4,5] In chronic volume overload states, such as in the setting of severe tricuspid regurgitation (TR) or pulmonic regurgitation (PR), or in the presence of a shunt, the RV responds by enlarging in an attempt to restore forward SV. With chronic pressure overload, such as with pulmonary

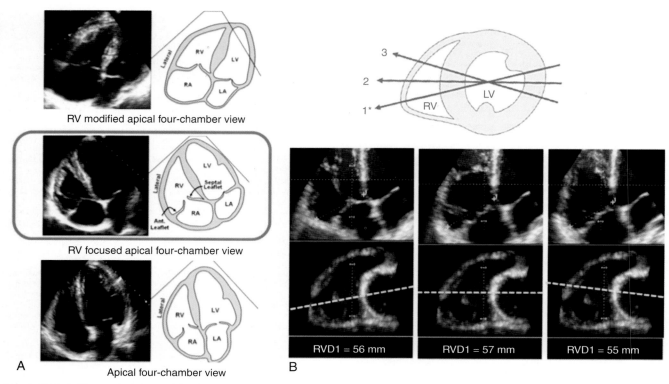

Figure 30.1. A, Three apical views of the right ventricle (RV): the RV-modified, RV-focused, and standard apical four-chamber views. B, The rationale for using the RV-focused view in ensuring the maximal dimension by demonstrating the relationship between rotation of the transducer and the RV measurement. *LA,* Left atrium; *LV,* left ventricle, *RA,* right atrium; *RVD1,* basal RV dimension. (Reproduced with permission from Lang RM, et al: Recommendations for cardiac chamber quantification by echocardiography in adults, *J Am Soc Echocardiogr* 28:1–39.e14, 2015.)

hypertension (PH) or pulmonic stenosis, the RV initially responds with hypertrophy of the wall in an attempt to normalize wall tension. Eventually, when compensatory mechanisms fail in the setting of severe PH and increased transmural pressure, myocardial blood flow decreases because of the loss of coronary flow during systole.

The complex anatomic and physiologic differences just described present many challenges in the noninvasive echocardiographic evaluation of the dimensions and function of the right side of the heart. A wide variety of methods to describe RV size and function have been developed, none of which provide a complete picture, but recent advances in 3D echocardiography (3DE) and new understanding of the assessment of myocardial contractility have yielded new insights and methods of standardization.[6]

QUANTITATIVE EVALUATION BY ECHOCARDIOGRAPHY

Right Ventricular Size

Two-Dimensional Measurements

Quantitation of RV dimensions is critical and improves inter-rater variability when compared with visual assessment alone.[7] Measurements by two-dimensional echocardiography (2DE) are challenging because the geometry of the RV is complex and it lacks specific right-sided anatomic landmarks to be used as reference points. The conventional apical four-chamber (A4C) view (i.e., focused on the left ventricle) results in too much variability on how the right side of the heart is projected, and consequently, RV linear dimensions and areas may vary widely in the same patient with relatively minor rotations in transducer position (Fig. 30.1). RV dimensions are best estimated from a RV-focused A4C view with

an upper reference limit of 42 mm (Fig 30.2). The RV-focused view consistently results in larger values than the traditional A4Cview and has less inter- and intraobserver variability and reduced test–retest variability.[8] Care should be taken to obtain the image with the LV apex at the center of the scanning sector while simultaneously displaying the largest basal RV diameter that prevents foreshortening. Other dimensions that can be measured are the midchamber (35-mm limit), longitudinal diameter (83 mm but of little clinical utility), and RV outflow tract (RVOT). The proximal RVOT diameter is used to diagnose arrhythmogenic right ventricular cardiomyopathy (ARVC), whereas the distal RVOT diameter can be used to help calculate the ratio of pulmonic to systemic flow (Qp:Qs) in the presence of a shunt.

Recent data have suggested that indexing RV size to body surface area (BSA) may be relevant in some circumstances; however, the measurements used in these studies lacked the reference points of the RV-focused view and frequently use RV areas rather than linear dimensions.[9,10] As such, indexing should be considered only at the extremes of BSA but may be used in assessing RV volumes (see later).

Three-Dimensional Volumes

Because of the complex asymmetric shape of the RV, only a volumetric method such as 3DE can provide a truly reliable measure of its size. Unlike 2DE, accuracy of 3DE does not depend on the imaging view or unverified geometric assumptions regarding RV shape. If image quality is accurate and heart rhythm is fairly regular, RV volumes measured by 3DE have excellent reproducibility and are in close agreement with those obtained using cardiac magnetic resonance (CMR).[11,12] Measurement of RV volumes is recommended for the clinical evaluation of RV size in laboratories with experience in 3DE.[2] Age, gender, and body size are important determinants of RV volumes measured either by 3DE or by CMR (Fig. 30.3).[13] Preliminary results from the World Alliance Societies of Echocardiography (WASE)

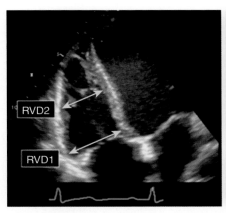
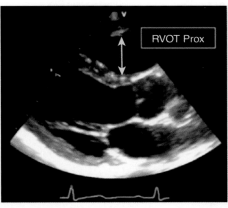
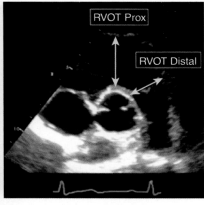

Figure 30.2. Right ventricular dimensions demonstrated from the right ventricle–focused view, the proximal right ventricular outflow tract (RVOT) from the parasternal long-axis view, and the proximal (Prox) and distal RVOT in the parasternal short-axis view. *RVD1,* basal RV dimension; *RVD2,* mid RV dimension. (Reproduced with permission from Lang RM, et al: Recommendations for cardiac chamber quantification by echocardiography in adults, *J Am Soc Echocardiogr* 28:1–39.e14, 2015.)

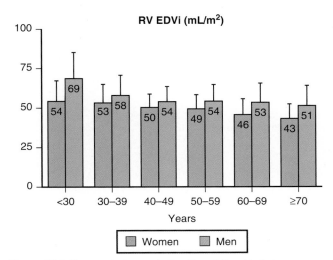

Figure 30.3. Bar graph demonstrating the relationship between right ventricular (RV) volumes and age, gender, and body size. *EDVi,* indexed end-diastolic volume.

study suggest that RV volumes also depend on ethnicity.[14] An RV EDV of 87 mL/m[2] in men and 74 mL/m[2] for women and an RV ESV of 44 mL/m[2] for men and 36 mL/m[2] for women have been recommended by American Society of Echocardiography (ASE)/European Association of Cardiovascular Imaging (EACVI) guidelines as the upper limits of the corresponding normal ranges.[2] Patient-specific normative ranges from allometric equations may be applied when confirming RV enlargement using 3DE.[13]

Right Ventricular Systolic Function

Fractional Area Change

Fractional area change (FAC) is a measure of global RV systolic function that has been shown to correlate with RV EF by cardiac MRI.[15,16] To calculate FAC, end-diastolic and end-systolic RV area are obtained by planimetry of the endocardial border in the RV focused A4C view (when the cavity is largest and smallest, respectively), in which FAC = [(end-diastolic area − end-systolic area)/end-diastolic area] × 100 (abnormal is <35%). A common pitfall of this measure is undertracing the cavity inside trabeculations, moderator band, or both (Fig. 30.4).

Tricuspid Annular Plane Systolic Excursion and Velocity

Tricuspid annular plane systolic excursion (TAPSE) and velocity (S′) are measures of longitudinal function, reflecting the contraction of the RV's dominant deep fibers and correlating with RV EF.[17,18] After aligning the cursor parallel to the RV annular plane systolic excursion, M-mode is activated to measure the displacement of the annular plane (TAPSE; abnormal <1.7 cm), whereas tissue Doppler is activated to measure the velocity (S′; abnormal <9.5 cm/sec). A pitfall of the S′, like any Doppler-based measure, is the risk of underestimating the annular velocity if interrogation is not parallel to the plane of motion (Fig. 30.5). Slightly higher values and greater reproducibility are seen when these parameters are measured from the RV-focused view but there are insufficient data to provided reference limits using this view.[8]

Unlike the gold standard measure of 3D RV EF, these 2D measures do not capture the contraction of the entire RV. FAC neglects the contribution of the RVOT, whereas TAPSE and S′ also neglect the contribution of the free wall and septum. Two scenarios warrant mention in this regard. In patients after cardiac surgery, TAPSE and S′ are markedly reduced, whereas compensatory inward bellows motion of the septum causes FAC to be normal or near normal.[19,20] Conversely, in patients with PAH, TAPSE and S′ are often preserved, but FAC may be frankly abnormal.[21]

Right Ventricular Index of Myocardial Performance

Right ventricular index of myocardial performance (RIMP) is a nonvolumetric measure of global ventricular function. RIMP is defined as the ratio of the isovolumic time (isovolumic contraction and relaxation time) to the ventricular ejection time:

$$RIMP = (IVCT + IVRT)/ET$$

in which IVCT is the isovolumic contraction time, IVRT is the isovolumic relation time, and ET is the ejection time.

Because RIMP is a ratio of time intervals, its determination is independent of the geometric shape of the ventricle, which is important given the complex geometry of the right ventricle.

RIMP can be obtained with standard Doppler echocardiographic techniques (Fig. 30.6). Note that when measuring RIMP using spectral blood pool Doppler signals, measures from two separate heartbeats is required, and thus it is important to ensure that heartbeats with similar R-R intervals are used. In a strict sense, when there is TR, the IVCT) and IVRT do not exist. Perhaps more appropriate terms are the duration of cessation of tricuspid

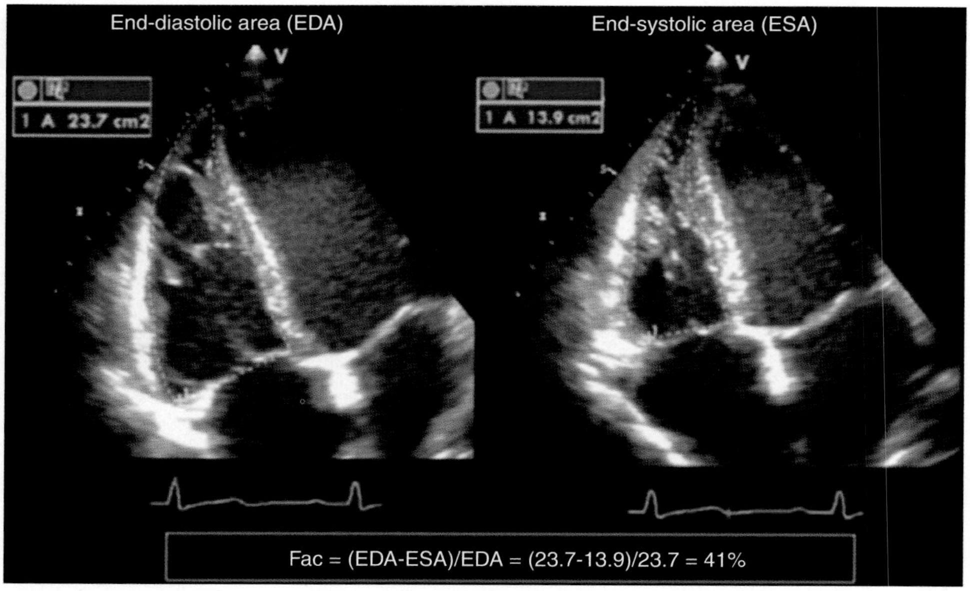

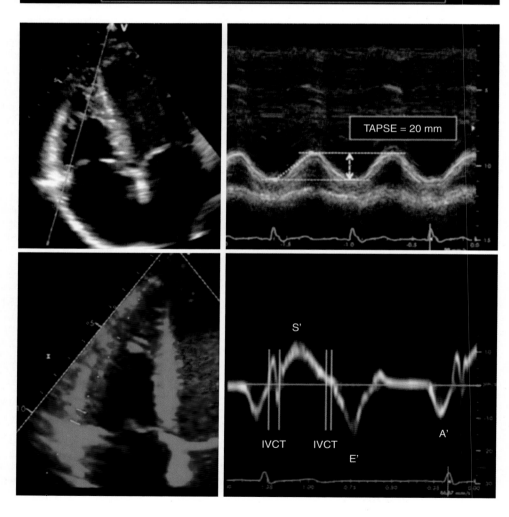

Figure 30.4. Measurement of fractional area change (Fac) is calculated as end-diastolic area minus end-systolic area divided by end-diastolic area. In this normal participant, the calculated Fac is 41%. (Reproduced with permission from Lang RM, et al: Recommendations for cardiac chamber quantification by echocardiography in adults, *J Am Soc Echocardiogr* 28:1–39.e14, 2015.)

Figure 30.5. Measurement of longitudinal velocity and motion. The *upper panel* demonstrates the tricuspid annular plane systolic excursion (TAPSE) wherein an M-mode cursor is placed through the annulus and the excursion distance is measured off the M-mode trace. The *lower panel* shows the systolic excursion velocity of the tricuspid annulus (S′), performed with a sample volume placed at the level of the annulus and tissue Doppler activated. The S′ must be distinguished by the isovolumic contraction spike; the latter is seen prior to the end of the QRS complex on the electrocardiogram. *IVCT,* Isovolumic contraction time. (Reproduced with permission from Lang RM, et al: Recommendations for cardiac chamber quantification by echocardiography in adults, *J Am Soc Echocardiogr* 28:1–39.e14, 2015.)

inflow to the onset of pulmonary ejection flow and the cessation of pulmonary ejection flow to the onset of tricuspid inflow. The upper reference limits are 0.43 when RIMP is calculated from spectral blood pool Doppler signals and 0.54 when calculated by tissue Doppler imaging.

It is important to understand that RIMP varies with pressure and volume status and may not be a true measure of the intrinsic properties of right ventricular myocardial function. An understanding of the impact of changes in arterial and atrial pressure on the value of RIMP is crucial in the clinical interpretation of the values obtained.

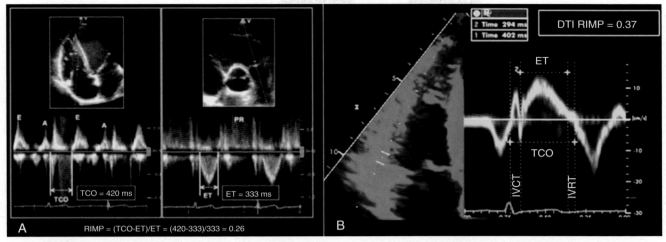

Figure 30.6. Calculation of the right ventricular (RV) index of myocardial performance using spectral Doppler of blood flow velocity profiles (**A**) and spectral tissue Doppler imaging (**B**). In **A**, the time between the end of the transtricuspid A wave to the onset of the transtricuspid E wave of the following beat or the duration of the tricuspid regurgitation velocity is measured. The ejection time (ET) is measured as the duration of the pulsed-wave Doppler signal from the right ventricular outflow tract. In **B**, a pulsed wave sample volume is placed in the right ventricular free wall annulus, and the time intervals in milliseconds are measured. The right ventricular index of myocardial performance (RIMP) is derived from pulsed-wave tissue Doppler of the RV annulus (image displayed with RV on right side of sector). *DTI,* Doppler tissue imaging; *IVCT,* isovolumic contraction time; *IVRT,* isovolumic relation time; *TCO,* time from closure to opening of tricuspid valve. (Reproduced with permission from Lang RM, et al: Recommendations for cardiac chamber quantification by echocardiography in adults, *J Am Soc Echocardiogr* 28:1–39.e14, 2015.)

Three-Dimensional Ejection Fraction

3D RVEF is a truly global measure of RV systolic function because it integrates both radial and longitudinal components of RV contraction (Fig. 30.7) and the relative contribution of all the regions (inflow, outflow, and apex) to overall RV performance.[22] It has particular clinical value in patients after cardiac surgery or heart transplant, when longitudinal RV function indices (i.e., TAPSE, S wave) are generally reduced and may no longer be representative of global RV systolic function.[19] 3D RVEF has been rigorously validated against CMR measurements in various cardiac conditions[23] and is the recommended method for quantifying RV systolic function if appropriate experience is available.[2] In patients with various cardiovascular diseases, 3D RVEF has been reported to have incremental prognostic value with respect conventional 2DE RV function parameters and independent of 3D left ventricular EF.[11,24,25]

Although currently available 3DE scanners may allow RV quantitation using single-beat, full-volume acquisitions, 3D RVEF is routinely obtained by acquiring a four- or six-beat full-volume dataset of the RV to achieve an optimal spatial and temporal resolution (at least 20 vps for heart rates <80/min; at least 30 vps for heart rates >80/min).[14] Most patients with relatively normal or moderately enlarged RVs are optimally imaged from the RV-focused view because RV imaging through the apex-forming LV helps improve penetration and increases RV free-wall definition. Conversely, with apex-forming RVs, the apicomedial approach (closer to the sternum) may be more useful because the dilated RV is anteriorly positioned. The RV dataset is subsequently analyzed onboard or offline with dedicated fully automated or semiautomated software to derive RV volumes and RVEF (Fig. 30.8). Visualizing the RV dataset in a multislice display during 3D acquisition is necessary to verify that the whole RV is included within the dataset and to rule out stitching artifacts before storing; it can also be used to assess RV regional wall motion (Fig. 30.9). RV fully automated analysis is faster yet leads to larger underestimation of RVEF and RV volumes in comparison with semiautomated analysis (i.e., with manual correction of endocardial borders).[12]

3D RVEF is influenced by age and gender, with slightly higher RVEFs reported in older adult patients than in young patients and RVEFs are higher in women than in men.[13] An RVEF of 45% has been recommended as the lower limit of normality,[2] and RVEF of 41% to 45%, 31% to 40%, and less than 30% were recently identified as partition values to stratify mild, moderate, and severe RV dysfunction, respectively, based on the risk of cardiac death and MACE.[26] Because RVEF reflects the interaction between RV contractility and load, RVEF may overestimate RV systolic function in conditions evolving with markedly increased preload (e.g., severe TR, large atrial septal defects) or underestimate true RV performance in settings with high afterload (e.g., pulmonary thromboembolism, PH).

Feasibility of 3DE acquisition of RV depends on patient acoustic window and operator expertise, being generally lower than for the LV. Transthoracic 3DE is challenging in patients with marked obesity, obstructive pulmonary disease, highly irregular arrhythmias, very enlarged and deformed RVs, or mechanical support devices or in postoperative setting with mechanical ventilation. When the transthoracic acoustic window is poor and RVEF is clinically relevant, contrast-enhanced transthoracic 3DE or transesophageal 3DE can be occasionally used.[27,28]

Strain

There is a growing body of evidence showing that assessing RV longitudinal strain (RVLS) provides incremental information in several pathologic conditions.[29] RVLS is considered a clinically useful noninvasive index of RV contractility because it is less confounded by heart motion and geometric changes and less dependent on load than conventional RV functional indices or 3D RVEF. RVLS is routinely assessed in the RV-focused four-chamber view (Fig. 30.10) because this view allows a better definition of RV free wall and provides more reproducible measurements of RVLS than the standard four-chamber view centered on the LV.[8] Speckle-tracking echocardiography (STE) is currently recommended to analyze RVLS for clinical use[2] as a sensitive and reproducible index of RV performance. It is less dependent on angle and more practical and reproducible than tissue Doppler strain. For several conditions (e.g., HF, PH, significant functional TR, acute MI, chronic obstructive pulmonary disease [COPD]), RVLS has prognostic value.[30–35] In HF with reduced EF, RVLS by STE

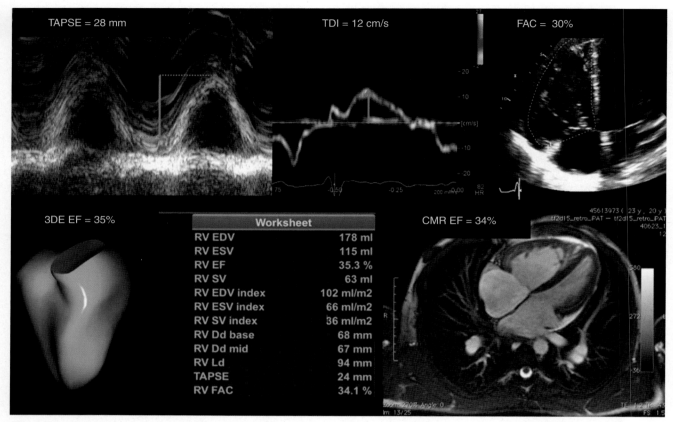

Figure 30.7. The *upper panels* demonstrate tricuspid annular plane systolic excursion (TAPSE) and systolic velocity by tissue Doppler imaging (TDI S'), which both measure longitudinal function of the base. The *upper right panel* shows fractional area change, a more "global" parameter that incorporated some radial motion. Three-dimensional right ventricular ejection fraction (3D RVEF) by MRI or echocardiography, by contrast, is a truly global measure of right ventricular (RV) systolic function because it integrates both radial and longitudinal components of RV contraction. *CMR,* Cardiac magnetic resonance; *Dd,* diastolic dimension; *EDV,* end-diastolic volume; *ESV,* end-systolic volume; *FAC,* fractional area change; *Ld,* length in diastole; *SV,* stroke volume.

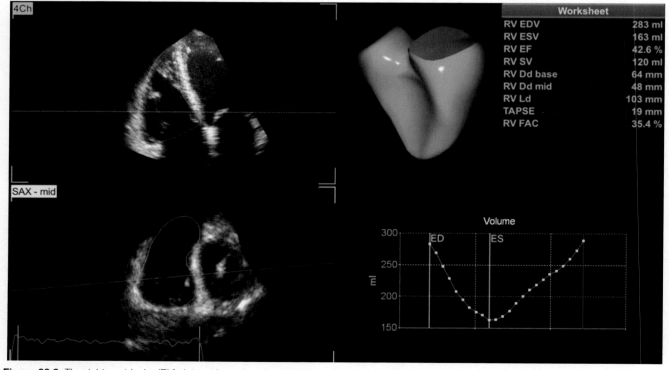

Figure 30.8. The right ventricular (RV) dataset is analyzed onboard or offline with dedicated fully automated or semiautomated software to derive RV volumes and RV ejection fraction (EF). *Dd,* diastolic dimension; *EDV,* end-diastolic volume; *ESV,* end-systolic volume; *FAC,* fractional area change; *Ld,* length in diastole; *SAX,* short axis; *SV,* stroke volume; *TAPSE,* tricuspid annular plane systolic excursion.

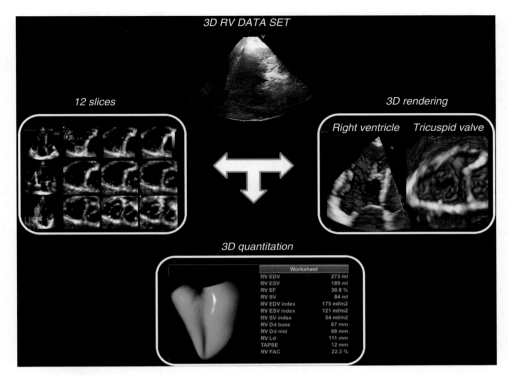

Figure 30.9. Three-dimensional (3D) echocardiography enables a comprehensive assessment of the right ventricular (RV) morphology and function from a single pyramidal full-volume dataset *(top)*: multiple longitudinal and transversal slices displayed simultaneously for a fast check of 3D dataset quality and for regional motion assessment of the RV *(left)*; RV and tricuspid valve anatomy *(right)*; and RV endocardial surface reconstruction for quantitation of RV volumes and ejection fraction *(bottom)*. *Dd,* dimension in diastole; *EDV,* end-diastolic volume; *EF,* ejection fraction; *ESV,* end-systolic volume; *FAC,* fractional area change; *Ld,* length in diastole; *SV,* stroke volume; *TAPSE,* tricuspid annular plane systolic excursion.

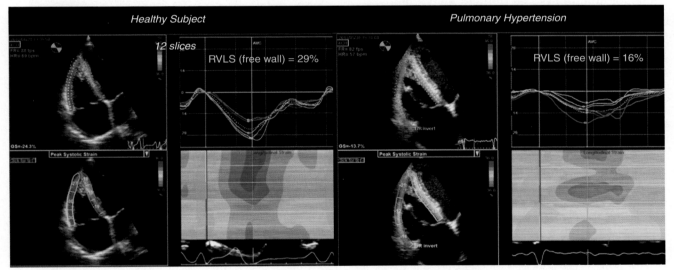

Figure 30.10. Right ventricular (RV) longitudinal strain is routinely assessed in the RV-focused four-chamber view because this view allows a better definition of the RV free wall and provides more reproducible measurements of RV longitudinal strain (RVLS) than the standard four-chamber view centered on the left ventricle. The *left panel* shows normal free-wall strain (average of three free-wall segments), and the *right panel* shows reduced free-wall strain in a patient with increased afterload in pulmonary hypertension.

seems to provide stronger prognostic value than CMR-derived RVEF or RVLS, TAPSE, or FAC.[36] However, STE strain is highly dependent on a good image quality with adequate temporal resolution (40–80 frames/sec) and no artifacts.

Various STE software tools incorporate diverse algorithms in calculating strain and analyze different myocardial layers (subendocardial, midwall, or full wall strain). As a result, different equipment might not yield equivalent strain values in the same subject. In 2018, the EACVI/ASE/Industry Task Force published recommendations for the standardization of RV strain image acquisition and analysis for both clinical and scientific purposes.[37] Also, more robust sex-specific normative values have become available,[38,39] showing that women have larger RVLS magnitude

than men. RVLS analysis is usually limited to the RV inlet free wall (see Fig. 30.5). The inclusion of the RV interventricular septal component in the computation of global RV strain is controversial but could be useful for quantifying RV dyssynchrony. Uncoordinated longitudinal RV contraction may serve as an early sign of RV dysfunction and may decrease RV systolic function to a greater extent than what might be expected from the impairment of contractility alone.[40]

Because RV function is sensitive to increased afterload, the ratio of RVLS to pulmonary arterial systolic pressure (RVLS/PASP) has been suggested as a surrogate of RV–pulmonary arterial coupling. The RVLS/PASP and TAPSE/PASP appear to predict prognosis in patients with HF and TAVR.[41-43]

RIGHT VENTRICULAR DIASTOLIC FUNCTION

The most common cause of right-sided diastolic dysfunction is PH from primary or secondary causes such as connective tissue disease, lung disease, thromboembolic disease, mitral valve disease, or left-sided HF. Other causes include RV ischemia and congenital heart disease. RV diastolic dysfunction has been associated with worse functional class and clinical outcomes in patients with HF and reduced EF,[44] HF and preserved EF,[45] hypertrophic cardiomyopathy,[46] mitral stenosis,[47] PAH,[48] COPD,[49] chronic thromboembolic PH,[50] Ebstein anomaly,[51] and tetralogy of Fallot.[52] In conditions such as systemic sclerosis, RV diastolic dysfunction has been proposed as an early marker of RV involvement[53] and end-organ damage.[54] The echocardiographic parameters used to evaluate right-sided diastolic function are reviewed in this section.

Tricuspid Inflow Doppler Velocities

Early passive filling velocities (E), deceleration time (DT), and late active filling velocities (A) can be measured using pulsed wave Doppler interrogation at the tips of the tricuspid leaflets during held end-expiration. Similar to the assessment of left-sided diastolic function, a reduced E/A ratio suggests impaired relaxation, whereas an elevated E/A ratio suggests restrictive filling. The practical utility of transtricuspid Doppler has been limited by its sensitivity to respiration.[55] The E/A ratio decreases modestly by 0.1 per decade of advancing age.[56]

Tricuspid Annulus Tissue Doppler Velocities

Early passive myocardial velocities (e′) and late active myocardial velocities (a′) can be measured using tissue Doppler interrogation at the lateral tricuspid annulus, with the beam parallel to the RV annulus systolic excursion. Tissue Doppler parameters have been shown to approximate invasive hemodynamic measures; the e′ is negatively correlated with the isovolumetric active relaxation time constant tau, and the E/e′ ratio is positively correlated with the RA mean pressure. The E/e′ ratio does not change significantly with advancing age, although it is on average 0.5 higher in men than women,[56] and it is less reliable in patients with congestive HF or recent cardiac surgery.[57] Speckle-tracking strain parameters have emerged in recent studies; the RV longitudinal early-diastolic strain rate (SRe) and the E/SRe ratio appear to be even more closely correlated with tau and RA mean pressure, respectively.[50,58] Larger studies are needed to determine the prognostic implications and normal reference values of diastolic strain parameters.

Supportive Signs

A number of indirect signs are suggestive of RV diastolic dysfunction, including RV hypertrophy, RA enlargement, and other signs of RA hypertension[59] such as greater than 21-mm dilatation and less than 50% inspiratory collapse of the inferior vena cava, leftward bulge of the interatrial septum, or diastolic dominance in the hepatic vein flow tracing (diastolic wave velocity > systolic wave velocity on pulsed-wave Doppler interrogation). End-diastolic forward flow in the pulmonary artery flow tracing, initially thought to reflect pathological transmission of flow from atrial contraction through the noncompliant "restrictive" RV, was recently debunked and shown to be affected by factors other than diastolic compliance.[60] Prolonged postsystolic isovolumetric time—alone or as part of the Tei index—was thought to reflect impaired diastolic relaxation but subsequently shown to be affected mostly by pathological postsystolic contraction.[61]

Grading Diastolic Function

Gradation of right-sided diastolic filling may be divided into normal filling, impaired relaxation (mild diastolic dysfunction), pseudonormal filling (moderate diastolic dysfunction), and restrictive filling (severe diastolic dysfunction).[1] E/A ratio less than 0.8 or e′/a′ ratio less than 0.5 is consistent with impaired relaxation. E/A ratio of 0.8 to 2.1 or e′/a′ ratio of 0.5 to 1.9, combined with evidence of elevated RA pressure (particularly a dilated or noncollapsing inferior vena cava or an increased E/e′ ratio greater than 6) is consistent with pseudonormal filling. E/A ratio greater than 2.1 or e′/a′ ratio greater than 1.9, with DT less than 120 msec and evidence of elevated RA pressure, is consistent with restrictive filling.

CLINICAL IMPACT OF RIGHT VENTRICULAR SIZE AND FUNCTION: PROGNOSIS

As stated previously, the RV contributes just as much to cardiac output as the LV does. With a closed circulation, these two chambers are inexorably linked. RV failure is often associated with both elevated jugular venous pressure (JVP) and peripheral edema. More severe dysfunction may result in hepatic congestion and dysfunction and hepatorenal syndrome. RV failure, however, may provoke symptoms typically associated with LV failure; the most notable is dyspnea, the result of reduced cardiac output. Although echocardiographic parameters have not been related to most of the previously mentioned findings, there is a significant association between parameters of RV function and prognosis. In patients with left-sided HF, right-sided myocardial performance index (MPI),[62] S′,[63] TAPSE,[64] and RV percent FAC (FAC%)[65] all have proven value in prognostication. In patients who have had surgery to repair tetralogy of Fallot, a variety of echocardiographic measures of RV function correlate with prognosis and quality of life.[66,67] The presence of RV enlargement in patients with acute PE is associated with poor prognosis, and it is included in a decision algorithm for patient care that leads to treatment with thrombolytic agents. In patients with PAH, a number of measures of RV systolic function, most recently strain detected with 2D STE, assist in prognostication.[68] 3D echocardiography studies have demonstrated that RVEF provides incremental value when combined with LVEF in predicting outcomes in a variety of conditions, including coronary artery disease, valvular heart disease, and cardiomyopathies. It also was superior to TAPSE and %FAC.[11] Remaining challenges relate to identifying which parameter is best to use in a given disease condition, given the diverse effects of pressure overload, volume overload, or intrinsic myocardial diseases. In addition, feasibility and expertise with 3DE continue to limit its broad applicability. Initial experience with machine learning algorithms that automatically identify endocardial borders and calculate RV volumes and RVEF have demonstrated accuracy in a minority of studies, but it is anticipated that this technology will evolve and increase uptake of 3DE assessment of the RV.[69]

SUMMARY AND RECOMMENDATIONS

Assessment of the right side of the heart is a critical part of every echocardiographic study. Evaluation of RV size and systolic function present challenges to the interpreter because the RV has complex geometry, and the many methods of assessment may provide discordant findings. Nevertheless, a quantitative assessment of RV size and function provide important diagnostic and prognostic information to guide short- and long-term care. Measurement of chamber dimensions and volumes, when feasible; evaluation of RV systolic function by one of the several methods endorsed by current guidelines; and estimation of systolic pulmonary artery pressure are required in all reports when the study permits. Guidelines and recommendations for the echocardiographic assessment of the right side of the heart should be used as a template.[1,2]

REFERENCES

1. Rudski LG, Lai WW, Afilalo J, et al. Guidelines for the echocardiographic assessment of the right heart in adults. *J Am Soc Echocardiogr*. 2010;23:685–713.
2. Lang RM, Badano LP, Mor-Avi V, et al. Recommendations for cardiac chamber quantification by echocardiography in adults. *J Am Soc Echocardiogr*. 2015;28:1–39. e14.
3. Ho SY, Nihoyannopoulos P. Anatomy, echocardiography, and normal right ventricular dimensions. *Heart*. 2006;92(suppl 1):i2–13.
4. Haddad F, Hunt SA, Rosenthal DN, Murphy DJ. Right ventricular function in cardiovascular disease, part I: anatomy, physiology, aging, and functional assessment of the right ventricle. *Circulation*. 2008;117:1436–1448.
5. Haddad F, Doyle R, Murphy DJ, Hunt SA. Right ventricular function in cardiovascular disease, part II: pathophysiology, clinical importance, and management of right ventricular failure. *Circulation*. 2008;117:1717–1731.
6. Rudski LG, Afilalo J. The blind men of Indostan and the elephant in the echo lab. *J Am Soc Echocardiogr*. 2012;25:714–717.
7. Ling LF, Obuchowski NA, Rodriguez L, et al. Accuracy and interobserver concordance of echocardiographic assessment of right ventricular size and systolic function: a quality control exercise. *J Am Soc Echocardiogr*. 2012;25:709–713.
8. Genovese D, Mor-Avi V, Palermo C, et al. Comparison between four-chamber and right ventricular-focused views for the quantitative evaluation of right ventricular size and function. *J Am Soc Echocardiogr*. 2019;32:484–494.
9. D'Oronzio U, Senn O, Biaggi P, et al. Right heart assessment by echocardiography: gender and body size matters. *J Am Soc Echocardiogr*. 2012;25:1251–1258.
10. Willis J, Augustine D, Shah R, et al. Right ventricular normal measurements: time to index? *J Am Soc Echocardiogr*. 2012;25:1259–1267.
11. Surkova E, Muraru D, Genovese D, et al. Relative prognostic importance of left and right ventricular ejection fraction in patients with cardiac diseases. *J Am Soc Echocardiogr*. 2019;32(e3):1407–1415.
12. Muraru D, Spadotto V, Cecchetto A, et al. New speckle-tracking algorithm for right ventricular volume analysis from three-dimensional echocardiographic data sets: validation with cardiac magnetic resonance and comparison with the previous analysis tool. *Eur Heart J Cardiovasc Imag*. 2016;17:1279–1289.
13. Maffessanti F, Muraru D, Esposito R, et al. Age- and body size- and gender-specific reference values for right ventricular volumes and ejection fraction by three-dimensional echocardiography: a multicenter echocardiographic study in 507 healthy volunteers. *Circ Cardiovasc Imag*. 2013;6:700–710.
14. Asch FM, Miyoshi T, Addetia K, et al. Similarities and differences in left ventricular size and function among races and nationalities: results of the World Alliance Societies of Echocardiography Normal Values study. *J Am Soc Echocardiogr*. 2019;32(e2):1396–1406.
15. Lai WW, Gauvreau K, Rivera ES, et al. Accuracy of guideline recommendations for two-dimensional quantification of the right ventricle by echocardiography. *Int J Cardiovasc Imag*. 2008;24:691–698.
16. Anavekar NS, Gerson D, Skali H, et al. Two-dimensional assessment of right ventricular function: an echocardiographic-MRI correlative study. *Echocardiography*. 2007;24:452–456.
17. Lopez-Candales A, Dohi K, Rajagopalan N, et al. Defining normal variables of right ventricular size and function in pulmonary hypertension: an echocardiographic study. *Postgrad Med J*. 2008;84:40–45.
18. Miller D, Farah MG, Liner A, et al. The relation between quantitative right ventricular ejection fraction and indices of tricuspid annular motion and myocardial performance. *J Am Soc Echocardiogr*. 2004;17:443–447.
19. Maffessanti F, Gripari P, Tamborini G, et al. Evaluation of right ventricular systolic function after mitral valve repair: a 2D Doppler, speckle-tracking, and 3D echocardiographic study. *J Am Soc Echocardiogr*. 2012;25:701–708.
20. Tamborini G, Muratori M, Brusoni D, et al. Is right ventricular systolic function reduced after cardiac surgery? A two- and three-dimensional echocardiographic study. *Eur J Echocardiogr*. 2009;10:630–634.
21. Brown SB, Raina A, Katz D, et al. Longitudinal shortening accounts for the majority of right ventricular contraction and improves after pulmonary vasodilator therapy in normal subjects and patients with pulmonary arterial hypertension. *Chest*. 2011;140:27–33.
22. Addetia K, Muraru D, Badano LP, Lang RM. New directions in right ventricular assessment using 3D echocardiography. *J Am Coll Cardiol*. 2019;4:936–944.
23. Shimada YJ, Shiota M, Siegel RJ, Shiota T. Accuracy of right ventricular volumes and function determined by three-dimensional echocardiography in comparison with magnetic resonance imaging: a meta-analysis study. *J Am Soc Echocardiogr*. 2010;23:943–953.
24. Nagata Y, Wu VC-C, Kado Y, et al. Prognostic value of right ventricular ejection fraction assessed by transthoracic 3D echocardiography. *Circ Cardiovasc Imag*. 2017;10.
25. Vitarelli A, Barillà F, Capotosto L, et al. Right ventricular function in acute pulmonary embolism: a combined assessment by three-dimensional and speckle-tracking echocardiography. *J Am Soc Echocardiogr*. 2014;27:329–338.
26. Muraru D, Badano LP, Nagata Y, et al. Development and prognostic validation of partition values to grade right ventricular dysfunction severity using 3D echocardiography. *Eur Heart J Cardiovasc Imaging*. 2020;21:10–21.
27. Fusini L, Tamborini G, Gripari P, et al. Feasibility of intraoperative three-dimensional transesophageal echocardiography in the evaluation of right ventricular volumes and function in patients undergoing cardiac surgery. *J Am Soc Echocardiogr*. 2011;24:868–877.
28. Medvedofsky D, Mor-Avi V, Kruse E, et al. Quantification of right ventricular size and function from contrast-enhanced three-dimensional echocardiographic images. *J Am Soc Echocardiogr*. 2017;30:1193–1202.
29. Mor-Avi V, Lang RM, Badano LP, et al. Current and evolving echocardiographic techniques for the quantitative evaluation of cardiac mechanics. *J Am Soc Echocardiogr*. 2011;24:277–313.
30. Goedemans L, Abou R, Hoogslag GE, et al. Comparison of left ventricular function and myocardial infarct size determined by 2-dimensional speckle tracking echocardiography in patients with and without chronic obstructive pulmonary disease after st-segment elevation myocardial infarction. *Am J Cardiol*. 2017;120:734–739.
31. Hamada-Harimura Y, Seo Y, Ishizu T, et al. Incremental prognostic value of right ventricular strain in patients with acute decompensated heart failure. *Circ Cardiovasc Imag*. 2018;11:e007249.
32. Park SJ, Park J-H, Lee HS, et al. Impaired RV global longitudinal strain is associated with poor long-term clinical outcomes in patients with acute inferior STEMI. *JACC Cardiovasc Imag*. 2015;8:161–169.
33. Prihadi EA, van der Bijl P, Dietz M, et al. Prognostic implications of right ventricular free wall longitudinal strain in patients with significant functional tricuspid regurgitation. *Circ Cardiovasc Imag*. 2019;12:e008666.
34. Schuh A, Karayusuf V, Altiok E, et al. Intra-procedural determination of viability by myocardial deformation imaging: a randomized prospective study in the cardiac catheter laboratory. *Clin Res Cardiol*. 2017;106:629–644.
35. Shukla M, Park J-H, Thomas JD, et al. Prognostic value of right ventricular strain using speckle-tracking echocardiography in pulmonary hypertension. *Can J Cardiol*. 2018;34:1069–1078.
36. Houard L, Benaets M-B, de Meester de Ravenstein C, et al. Additional prognostic value of 2d right ventricular speckle-tracking strain for prediction of survival in heart failure and reduced ejection fraction: a comparative study with cardiac magnetic resonance. *JACC Cardiovasc Imag*. 2019;12:2373–2385.
37. Badano LP, Kolias TJ, Muraru D, et al. Standardization of left atrial, right ventricular, and right atrial deformation imaging using two-dimensional speckle tracking echocardiography. *Eur Heart J Cardiovasc Imag*. 2018;19:591–600.
38. Muraru D, Onciul S, Peluso D, et al. Sex- and method-specific reference values for right ventricular strain by 2D speckle-tracking echocardiography. *Circ Cardiovasc Imag*. 2016;9:e003866.
39. Park J-H, Choi J-O, Park SW, et al. Normal references of right ventricular strain values by two-dimensional strain echocardiography according to the age and gender. *Int J Cardiovasc Imag*. 2018;34:177–183.
40. Kalogeropoulos AP, Georgiopoulou VV, Howell S, et al. Evaluation of right intraventricular dyssynchrony by two-dimensional strain echocardiography in patients with pulmonary arterial hypertension. *J Am Soc Echocardiogr*. 2008;21:1028–1034.
41. Bosch L, Lam CSP, Gong L, et al. Right ventricular dysfunction in left-sided heart failure with preserved versus reduced ejection fraction. *Eur J Heart Fail*. 2017;19:1664–1671.
42. Guazzi M, Dixon D, Labate V, et al. RV Contractile function and its coupling to pulmonary circulation in heart failure with preserved ejection fraction: stratification of clinical phenotypes and outcomes. *JACC Cardiovasc Imag*. 2017;10:1211–1221.
43. Sultan I, Cardounel A, Abdelkarim I, et al. Right ventricle to pulmonary artery coupling in patients undergoing transcatheter aortic valve implantation. *Heart*. 2019;105:117–121.
44. Bistola V, Parissis JT, Paraskevaidis I, et al. Prognostic value of tissue Doppler right ventricular systolic and diastolic function indexes combined with plasma B-type natriuretic peptide in patients with advanced heart failure secondary to ischemic or idiopathic dilated cardiomyopathy. *Am J Cardiol*. 2010;105:249–254.
45. Morris DA, Gailani M, Vaz Pérez A, et al. Right ventricular myocardial systolic and diastolic dysfunction in heart failure with normal left ventricular ejection fraction. *J Am Soc Echocardiogr*. 2011;24:886–897.
46. Pagourelias ED, Efthimiadis GK, Parcharidou DG, et al. Prognostic value of right ventricular diastolic function indices in hypertrophic cardiomyopathy. *Eur J Echocardiogr*. 2011;12:809–817.
47. Saricam E, Ozbakir C, Yildirim N, et al. Evaluation of the relationship between functional capacity and right ventricular diastolic function in patients with isolated mitral stenosis and sinus rhythm: a tissue Doppler study. *Echocardiography*. 2007;24:134–139.
48. Utsunomiya H, Nakatani S, Nishihira M, et al. Value of estimated right ventricular filling pressure in predicting cardiac events in chronic pulmonary arterial hypertension. *J Am Soc Echocardiogr*. 2009;22:1368–1374.
49. Fenster BE, Holm KE, Weinberger HD, et al. Right ventricular diastolic function and exercise capacity in COPD. *Respir Med*. 2015;109:1287–1292.
50. Moriyama H, Murata M, Tsugu T, et al. The clinical value of assessing right ventricular diastolic function after balloon pulmonary angioplasty in patients with chronic thromboembolic pulmonary hypertension. *Int J Cardiovasc Imag*. 2018;34:875–882.
51. Akazawa Y, Fujioka T, Kühn A, et al. Right ventricular diastolic function and right atrial function and their relation with exercise capacity in Ebstein anomaly. *Can J Cardiol*. 2019;35:1824–1833.
52. Aboulhosn JA, Lluri G, Gurvitz MZ, et al. Left and right ventricular diastolic function in adults with surgically repaired tetralogy of Fallot: a multi-institutional study. *Can J Cardiol*. 2013;29:866–872.
53. Lindqvist P, Caidahl K, Neuman-Andersen G, et al. Disturbed right ventricular diastolic function in patients with systemic sclerosis: a Doppler tissue imaging study. *Chest*. 2005;128:755–763.
54. Meune C, Khanna D, Aboulhosn J, et al. A right ventricular diastolic impairment is common in systemic sclerosis and is associated with other target-organ damage. *Semin Arthritis Rheum*. 2016;45:439–445.

55. Berman GO, Reichek N, Brownson D, Douglas PS. Effects of sample volume location, imaging view, heart rate and age on tricuspid velocimetry in normal subjects. *Am J Cardiol*. 1990;65:1026–1030.
56. D'Andrea A, Vriz O, Carbone A, et al. The impact of age and gender on right ventricular diastolic function among healthy adults. *J Cardiol*. 2017;70:387–395.
57. Sade LE, Gulmez O, Eroglu S, et al. Noninvasive estimation of right ventricular filling pressure by ratio of early tricuspid inflow to annular diastolic velocity in patients with and without recent cardiac surgery. *J Am Soc Echocardiogr*. 2007;20:982–988.
58. Chowdhury SM, Goudar SP, Baker GH, et al. Speckle-tracking echocardiographic measures of right ventricular diastolic function correlate with reference standard measures before and after preload alteration in children. *Pediatr Cardiol*. 2016;38:27–35.
59. Deschamps J, Lipes J, Weinstock A, et al: Ultrasound assessment of central venous pressure: a systematic review and meta-analysis, *Cardiovasc Ultrasound*.
60. Kutty S, Valente AM, White MT, et al. Usefulness of pulmonary arterial end-diastolic forward flow late after tetralogy of Fallot repair to predict a "restrictive" right ventricle. *Am J Cardiol*. 2018;121:1380–1386.
61. Mauritz GJ, Marcus JT, Westerhof N, et al. Prolonged right ventricular post-systolic isovolumic period in pulmonary arterial hypertension is not a reflection of diastolic dysfunction. *Heart*. 2011;97:473–478.
62. Field ME, Solomon SD, Lewis EF, et al. Right ventricular dysfunction and adverse outcome in patients with advanced heart failure. *J Card Fail*. 2006;12:616–620.
63. Meluzín J, Spinarová L, Dusek L, et al. Prognostic importance of the right ventricular function assessed by Doppler tissue imaging. *Eur J Echocardiogr*. 2003;4:262–271.
64. Kjaergaard J, Akkan D, Iversen KK, et al. Right ventricular dysfunction as an independent predictor of short- and long-term mortality in patients with heart failure. *Eur J Heart Fail*. 2007;9:610–616.
65. Anavekar NS, Skali H, Bourgoun M, et al. Usefulness of right ventricular fractional area change to predict death, heart failure, and stroke following myocardial infarction. *Am J Cardiol*. 2008;101:607–612.
66. Lu JC, Ghadimi Mahani M, Agarwal PP, et al. Usefulness of right ventricular free wall strain to predict quality of life in "repaired" tetralogy of Fallot. *Am J Cardiol*. 2013;111:1644–1649.
67. Cetin I, Tokel K, Varan B, et al. Evaluation of right ventricular function by using tissue Doppler imaging in patients after repair of tetralogy of Fallot. *Echocardiography*. 2009;26:950–957.
68. Fine NM, Chen L, Bastiansen PM, et al. Outcome prediction by quantitative right ventricular function assessment in 575 subjects evaluated for pulmonary hypertension. *Circ Cardiovasc Imag*. 2013;6:711–721.
69. Genovese D, Rashedi N, Weinert L, et al. Machine learning-based three-dimensional echocardiographic quantification of right ventricular size and function: validation against cardiac magnetic resonance. *J Am Soc Echocardiogr*. 2019;32:969–977.

31   Right Ventricular Hemodynamics

Reza Arsanjani, Steven J. Lester

Echocardiography is the primary clinical method for the noninvasive measurement of right heart hemodynamic parameters and is an indispensable tool for the initial assessment, diagnosis, longitudinal follow-up, and prognostication of patients with abnormal right heart function. Ohm's law describes the relationship between flow, pressure, and resistance in an electric circuit, where the electrical potential between two points (pressure gradient) is equivalent to the product of current (flow) and resistance; $\Delta P = Q \times R$. Ohm's law principles applied to the circulation are the foundation for a complete hemodynamic evaluation of the right heart with the need to resolve for parameters of flow, pressure, and resistance.

FLOW

Doppler echocardiography is able to quantify blood flow through its ability to resolve for blood flow velocities. Christian Andreas Doppler described the mathematic relationship between the magnitude of the frequency shift, which is the difference in the reflected frequency from the emitted frequency and the velocity of the target (red blood cell) relative to the source (the transducer). Doppler echocardiography is able to then record instantaneous velocities throughout the cardiac cycle. Flow (cm^3/sec) can be derived as the product of blood flow velocity (cm/sec) multiplied by the cross-sectional area (cm^2) of the structure through which the blood is flowing; flow = area × velocity. Because flow in the cardiovascular system is pulsatile, individual velocities during the ejection phase must be sampled and integrated to measure flow volume. The sum of these individual velocities is called the time velocity integral (TVI) and is equal to the area enclosed by the Doppler velocity profile. The TVI then represents a linear distance, the average distance a red blood cell travels per beat, and stroke volume (cm^3) is calculated as the product of the TVI (cm) and cross-sectional area (cm^2) of the structure through which the blood is flowing (Fig. 31.1).

PRESSURE

Doppler provides the ability to resolve for blood flow velocities. Daniel Bernoulli described the relationship between blood flow

velocities and pressure gradient. The Bernoulli equation is founded on the principle of conservation of energy: although energy may change its position or form, the total amount of energy within a closed system must remain constant:

$$\Delta P = 1/2\rho \left(V_2^2 - V_1^2 \right) (\text{Convective acceleration})$$
$$+ \rho \int^2 (dv/dt)^* ds \, (\text{Flow acceleration})$$
$$+ R(\mu) (\text{Viscous friction})$$

in which ΔP is the pressure gradient; ρ is the mass density of blood; V_1 and V_2 are the velocity proximal and distal to obstruction, respectively; R is the viscous resistance; and μ is viscosity.

Under most physiologic conditions, the latter two terms (flow acceleration and viscous friction) are negligible and can be ignored, and $V_2 >>> V_1$; thus, V_1 can be ignored. Therefore, under most physiologic conditions, a simplified Bernoulli equation can be applied to the peak velocity obtained to derive the peak instantaneous gradient:

$$\Delta P = 4(V_2)^2$$

It is crucial that one pays close attention to the technical aspects of Doppler interrogation, ensuring as parallel as possible an intercept angle with the axis blood flow, so as not to underestimate the velocity and subsequently the derived pressure gradient. Therefore, imaging from multiple windows and the use of color Doppler to help guide the position of spectral Doppler interrogation are critical to ensure capture of the true (highest) velocity signal. When measuring either the peak velocity or tracing the spectral Doppler profile to determine the TVI, the Doppler gain must not be set too high, and one must avoid tracing the "fuzz," but rather the modal velocities (Fig. 31.2). Suboptimal spectral Doppler signals can be enhanced with the use of either agitated saline (air, blood, saline) contrast or manufactured ultrasound-enhancing agents.

RESISTANCE

Vascular resistance is the static resistance that must be overcome to permit the flow of blood through the circulatory system. Vascular

31

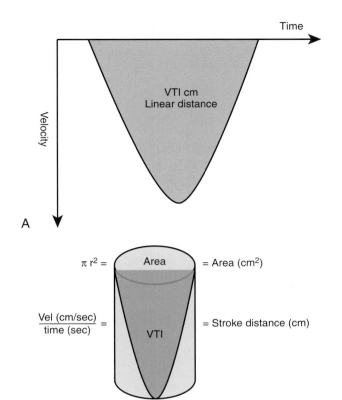

Figure 31.1. A, Schematic of a Doppler velocity profile with the integration of instantaneous velocities measured throughout the ejection period to derive the time velocity integral (TVI). **B,** Schematic of the stroke volume calculation. The volume of a cylinder is the product of its cross-sectional area and its length, in which length is the TVI (a linear distance).

resistance is calculated as the ratio of the driving pressure (pressure gradient) to flow across the vascular circuit:

$$\text{Resistance} = \frac{\Delta P}{Q}$$

in which ΔP is the pressure difference and Q is the flow across the circuit.

RIGHT HEART HEMODYNAMIC MEASURES

With its ability to resolve for the fundamental components of a complete hemodynamic evaluation, echocardiography can been seen as a "PA catheter in a box."

Right Atrial Pressure

Vessels such as the inferior and superior vena cavae and hepatic veins, which carry flow that empties into the right atrium (RA), have features that correlate with RA pressure. The size of the inferior vena cava (IVC) and its response to inspiration is most commonly used for the evaluation of RA pressure. Imaging of the IVC is most commonly obtained from the long-axis, subcostal view, performed in the supine position, taking note that IVC size is significantly influenced by patient position, being largest in the right lateral position, intermediate in the supine position, and smallest in the left lateral position. Measurement of the IVC diameter should be made at end-expiration just proximal to the hepatic veins.[1] IVC diameter varies with respiration, with minimal size observed at end-inspiration. A caval respiratory index (% decrease in diameter of the IVC with inspiration or a sniff) is then obtained. An IVC diameter less than 2.1 cm that collapses greater than 50% with a sniff suggests a normal RA pressure of 3 mm Hg (range, 0–5 mm Hg), whereas an IVC diameter greater than 2.1 cm that collapses less than 50% with a sniff suggests a high RA pressure of 15 mm Hg (range, 10–20 mm Hg) (Table 31.1). There are clinical scenarios, such as with severe tricuspid regurgitation (TR), whereby the RA pressure may exceed 20 mm Hg, and this constitutes one of the limitations of the caval respiratory approach.

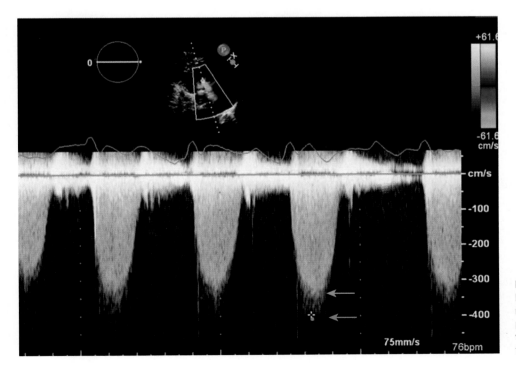

Figure 31.2. Continuous-wave Doppler tracing of a tricuspid regurgitant jet illustrating the preference of using the modal velocities *(blue arrow)* and avoiding the "fuzz" *(green arrow)*.

TABLE 31.1 Echocardiographic Estimation of Right Atrial Pressure Based on the Size of the Inferior Vena Cava and the Percent of Collapse During Sniffing[9]

IVC Size (mm)	Sniffing (% Collapse)	RA Pressure (mm Hg)
≤21>	50	3 (0–5)
	<50	8 (5–10)
>21	50	
	<50	15 (10–20)

IVC, Inferior vena cava.

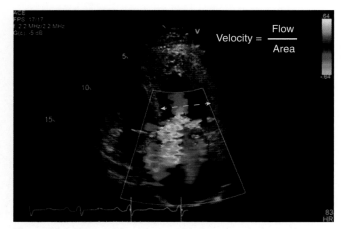

$$\text{Velocity} = \frac{\text{Flow}}{\text{Area}}$$

Figure 31.3. Image of the right ventricle from an apical transducer position demonstrating tricuspid annular dilatation with severe tricuspid regurgitation (TR). The TR velocity is inversely related to the area through which the blood flows; therefore, as the area increases, the velocity decreases for any given flow volume. The peak velocity could be underestimated in the setting of tricuspid annular dilatation and severe TR.

IVC size and response to inspiration are confounded by varying force of inspiratory effort and patient cooperation. In addition, the presence of a dilated IVC may be a normal variant in younger patients and athletes. The presence of a prominent Eustachian valve may also buttress open the IVC in some individuals, resulting in IVC dilatation despite normal systemic venous pressures. As such, there are clinical scenarios whereby there is discordance between estimate of RA pressure based on the size of the IVC and the caval respiratory index. In these indeterminate cases, it has been suggested that an intermediate value of 8 mm Hg (range, 5–10 mm Hg) be used for RA pressure. Also in these cases, one should evaluate other secondary indices of RA pressure to help further stratify the RA pressure estimate such that if these secondary indices suggest a normal RA pressure then the value reported may be reduced to 3 mm Hg.

SECONDARY INDICES OF RIGHT ATRIAL PRESSURE

1. *Hepatic vein flow velocity profile*: The hepatic venous systolic filling fraction (calculated as the ratio between the TVI of the hepatic venous systolic wave and sum of the TVI of the systolic and diastolic hepatic venous waves [excluding atrial reversal]) has been shown to be a predictor of RA pressure with dichotomous separation of RA pressure greater than 8 mm Hg by a hepatic vein systolic filling fraction less than 55%.[2] Note that the systolic filling fraction used to estimate RA pressure has reduced specificity in those with a normal LV ejection fraction or in atrial fibrillation.
2. *Right-sided E/e′ ratio*: As RA pressure increases, the early diastolic tricuspid inflow velocity (E) increases, and the right

ventricular free-wall early diastolic annular velocity (e′) decreases. Therefore, for the most part, as RA pressure increases, so too does the E/e′ ratio. An E/e′ ratio greater than 6 has modest test characteristics with which to predict a mean RA pressure of 10 mm Hg or greater.[3]

3. *RA size:* RA enlargement and an intraatrial septum that bows leftward (toward the left atrium) throughout the cardiac cycle are qualitative and supportive signs of increased RA pressure.

Right Ventricular Systolic Pressure

Right ventricular systolic pressure (RVSP) can be derived by applying the simplified Bernoulli equation to the peak TR velocity and adding to this value an estimate of right atrial pressure. Note that an assumption made during the assessment of right ventricular systolic pressure using echocardiography is that velocity is only dependent on pressure. Blood flow velocity, however, is directly related to flow and inversely related to the cross-sectional area through which the blood flows. Therefore, for any given flow volume, as the cross-sectional area through which the blood flows increases, the blood flow velocity decreases. When there is dilatation of the tricuspid annulus (increased effective regurgitant orifice), simply applying the simplified Bernoulli equation to the peak TR velocity may result in an underestimation of RVSP. In addition, when there is severe TR and rapid equalization of RV and RA pressure (large RA V waves), our methods to estimate RA pressure (see earlier) may woefully underestimate the RA pressure. Finally, with severe TR and more laminar flow between the RV and RA, the assumption in the convective acceleration component of the Bernoulli equation that the proximal velocity is much less than distal velocity, and as such can be ignored, is no longer valid (Fig. 31.3).

Pulmonary Artery Pressure (Fig. 31.4)

1. *Pulmonary artery systolic pressure (PASP)*: The PASP is equal to the RVSP in the absence of flow obstruction between the RV and pulmonary artery. When there is such flow obstruction, the PASP is estimated as the RVSP minus the pressure gradient across the RVOT and/or pulmonic valve.
2. *Pulmonary artery diastolic pressure (PADP):* Applying the simplified Bernoulli equation to the end-diastolic pulmonary regurgitation velocity and adding an estimate of RA pressure provides an estimate of PADP.
3. *Pulmonary artery mean pressure (mPAP):* There are a number of echocardiographic methods with which to derive mPAP:
   a. Apply the simplified Bernoulli equation to the peak pulmonary regurgitation velocity and add to this value an estimate of RA pressure.
   b. Calculate mPAP as (PASP + 2PADP)/3.
   c. Obtain the mean RV–RA gradient by tracing the TR velocity profile to obtain the TVI and subsequent mean gradient and adding to the mean gradient an estimate of RA pressure: (mPAP = $\text{TR}_{\text{mean gradient}}$ + RA pressure).
   d. Measure the pulmonary artery acceleration time (AT) and calculate mPAP as 79 – (0.45 × AT). If the AT is 120 ms or less, the equation 90 – (0.62 × AT) should be used.[4–6]

Pulmonary Vascular Resistance

Pulmonary vascular resistance (PVR) is calculated by dividing the pressure difference across the pulmonary circuit by the transpulmonary flow. By using the peak tricuspid regurgitation velocity (TRV) as a surrogate for pressure and the right ventricular outflow tract TVI (RVOT_{TVI}) as a surrogate for flow, PVR can be estimated by the ratio of TRV to RVOT_{TVI}.[7] If the $\text{TRV/RVOT}_{\text{TVI}}$ ratio is greater than 0.175, this suggests that the PVR is elevated beyond 2 Wood units. If the $\text{TRV/RVOT}_{\text{TVI}}$ ratio is greater than 0.175 and 0.275

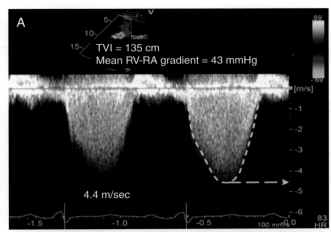

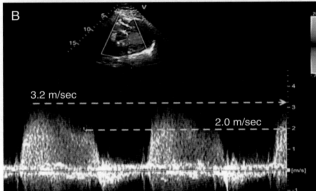

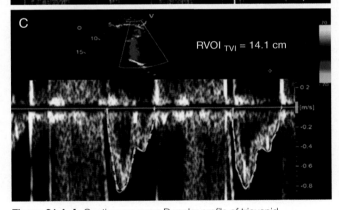

Figure 31.4. A, Continuous-wave Doppler profile of tricuspid regurgitation (TR). The peak TR velocity is 4.4 m/sec. The right ventricular (RV) systolic pressure = $4*(4.4)^2$ + right atrial (RA) pressure or 77 mm Hg + RA pressure. The mean pulmonary artery pressure can be estimated as the mean gradient between the RV and RA (43 mm Hg) + RA pressure. **B,** Continuous-wave Doppler profile of pulmonary regurgitation. The peak pulmonary regurgitation velocity is 3.2 m/sec. The mean pulmonary artery pressure can be estimated as $4 \times (3.2)^2$ + RA pressure or 41 mm Hg + RA pressure. The pulmonary artery diastolic pressure = $4 \times (2.0)^2$ + RA pressure. **C,** RV outflow tract time velocity integral ($RVOT_{TVI}$): TRV/ $RVOT_{TVI}$ = 4.4/14.1 = 0.31. Because this ratio is greater than 0.275, the equation to calculate pulmonary vascular resistance is $TRV^2/ RVOT_{TVI} \times 5 = [(4.4)^2/14.1] \times 5 = 6.9$ Wood units.

or less, then the equation $TRV/RVOT_{TVI} \times 10$ provides a good estimate of PVR. However, because of the quadratic relationship between velocity and the pressure gradient, in patients with a $TRV/ RVOT_{TVI}$ ratio greater than 0.275 indicative of marked elevation in PVR, the equation $TRV^2/RVOT_{TVI} \times 5$ should be used to estimate PVR (Fig. 31.4, C).[8]

SUMMARY

With its ability to resolve for flow, pressure, and resistance coupled with its configurability and harmless energy source, echocardiography has become the principal tool used for the evaluation of right heart hemodynamics. The clinical integration of multiple parameters and avoidance of overreliance on any single measure help to circumvent potential pitfalls in any one calculation and ensure the most accurate interpretation of right heart hemodynamics.

Acknowledgments

The authors would like to thank Drs. Laurence G. Rudsky and Amr E. Abbas for their contributions to this chapter in the previous edition.

REFERENCES

1. Moreno FL, Hagan AD, Holmen JR, et al. Evaluation of size and dynamics of the inferior vena cava as an index of right-sided cardiac function. *Am J Cardiol*. 1984;53:579–585.
2. Nagueh SF, Kopelen HA, Zoghbi WA. Relation of mean right atrial pressure to echocardiographic and doppler parameters of right atrial and right ventricular function. *Circulation*. 1996;93:1160–1169.
3. Nageh MF, Kopelen HA, Zoghbi WA, et al. Estimation of mean right atrial pressure using tissue Doppler imaging. *Am J Cardiol*. 1999;84:1448–1451. A1448.
4. Abbas AE, Fortuin FD, Schiller NB, et al. Echocardiographic determination of mean pulmonary artery pressure. *Am J Cardiol*. 2003;92:1373–1376.
5. Dabestani A, Mahan G, Gardin JM, et al. Evaluation of pulmonary artery pressure and resistance by pulsed doppler echocardiography. *Am J Cardiol*. 1987;59:662–668.
6. Aduen JF, Castello R, Daniels JT, et al. Accuracy and precision of three echocardiographic methods for estimating mean pulmonary artery pressure. *Chest*. 2011;139:347–352.
7. Abbas AE, Fortuin FD, Schiller NB, et al. A simple method for noninvasive estimation of pulmonary vascular resistance. *J Am Coll Cardiol*. 2003;41:1021–1027.
8. Abbas AE, Franey LM, Marwick T, et al: Noninvasive assessment of pulmonary vascular resistance by Doppler echocardiography, J Am Soc Echocardiogr 26:1170–1177.
9. Lang RM, Badano LP, Mor-Avi V, et al. Recommendations for cardiac chamber quantification by echocardiography in adults. *J Am Soc Echocardiogr*. 2015;28:1–39.

32 The Right Atrium

Christos Galatas, Julia Grapsa, Lawrence G. Rudski

The right atrium (RA) is an important but often overlooked cardiac chamber. It is situated in the most anterolateral region of the heart, and it normally receives deoxygenated blood from the superior vena cava (SVC), inferior vena cava (IVC), and coronary sinus. The RA is not simply a blood reservoir. When the tricuspid valve opens during ventricular diastole, the RA serves as conduit and subsequently pumps blood into the right ventricle (RV) during atrial contraction. Various anatomical, physiological, electrophysiological, and pathological features of the RA are recognized as unique, and echocardiographic parameters of RA dysfunction have been shown to correlate with severity and prognosis in several disease states.

ANATOMY

The RA is divided into two parts: the thin-walled *sinus venosus* posteriorly and the *auricle* or *RA appendage* anteriorly. The sinus venosus is attached medially to the left atrium (LA) and posterolaterally to the crista terminalis. It includes the venous portion (insertion of the IVC and SVC), the vestibulum, and the atrial septum. The pectinated RA appendage merges posterolaterally from the crista terminalis and overlies the aortic root.

Anatomic Landmarks

The orifice of the SVC lies on the upper posterolateral wall, and the orifice of the IVC lies on the inferior posterolateral wall. The *crista terminalis*, a crescent-shaped, smooth, muscular ridge, extends from the SVC to the IVC. The *tricuspid valve* (TV) separates the RA from the RV. Just posterior to the TV at its most superior edge is the orifice of the *coronary sinus* (CS). A membranous structure, the *thebesian valve*, is often seen at the opening of the CS.

The *fossa ovalis*, a thin membrane between the right and left atria, lies at the middle of the posterior wall of the RA, at the lower part of the septum, above and to the left of the orifice of the IVC. The *limbus fossa ovalis* is a prominent oval margin of the fossa ovalis.

The *Eustachian valve* (valve of the IVC) is a crescentic tissue fold arising from the anterior rim of the IVC, with variable length and shape. In the fetus, this valve serves to direct blood from the IVC through the foramen ovale and into the LA. The *Chiari network* is a congenital remnant of the right valve of the sinus venosus. It is generally more extensive than a prominent Eustachian valve (from which is should be differentiated) and attaches to two or more regions of the RA (Fig. 32.1).

PHYSIOLOGY

The RA acts a reservoir for systemic venous return through the SVC, the IVC, and the small-caliber CS that drains blood from the coronary system. The filling pattern is divided into three phases: a dominant systolic phase, a diastolic phase, and a third short atrial contraction phase with small reversal (upstream) flow from the RA into the system veins. During diastole, the TV opens, and blood from the RA is drained into the RV in two phases, early and late diastolic filling. The first phase is passive, with a pressure gradient driving the flow, and the second phase is active atrial contraction. The RA pressure varies significantly with the respiratory cycle and is usually between 3 and 8 mm Hg.

The RA increases in size and volume in response to prolonged increases in pressure or volume loads (e.g., pulmonary hypertension and significant TV regurgitation, respectively) or both. The RA also enlarges in response to chronic atrial fibrillation. The increase of RA size and volume has prognostic value in assessing right-sided (and left-sided) heart diseases.[1,2]

ECHOCARDIOGRAPHIC VIEWS

Multiple views are used to assess the RA, including the RV inflow view of the parasternal long-axis, the parasternal short-axis, the apical four-chamber (A4C), and the subcostal views (Fig. 32.2). Of these, the A4C view is most important and is commonly used to determine RA volume. Transesophageal echocardiography (TEE) affords a more complete visualization of the interatrial septum, the entrance of both venae cavae, the RA appendage, and the ostium of the coronary sinus. TEE visualization is particularly important when excluding RA compression by clot after cardiac surgery.

ANATOMIC VARIANTS

The *Eustachian valve* is a remnant of the fetal stage. In an adult heart, the Eustachian valve is quite variable in length and shape, extending sticklike from the inferior vena cava. It is best seen by transthoracic echocardiography (TTE) from the RV inflow view but can usually be visualized in other views as well (Fig. 32.3).

Rarely (1% of congenital heart disease), the Eustachian valve divides the right atrium into two components, a state known as *cor triatriatum dexter*. This finding should not be confused with the crista terminalis, which is seen in many routine TTE studies in the A4C view (see Fig. 32.3) or with the interatrial septum on TEE.

The *crista terminalis*, or terminal ridge, is a crescent-shaped muscular ridge that extends from the SVC to the IVC. When prominent, this muscular ridge can protrude into the right atrial cavity and resemble a mass, such as a neoplasm or thrombus. Thus, awareness of this structure is important to prevent the misdiagnosis of a "tumor."

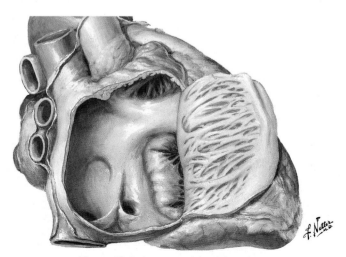

Figure 32.1. Anatomy of the right atrium.

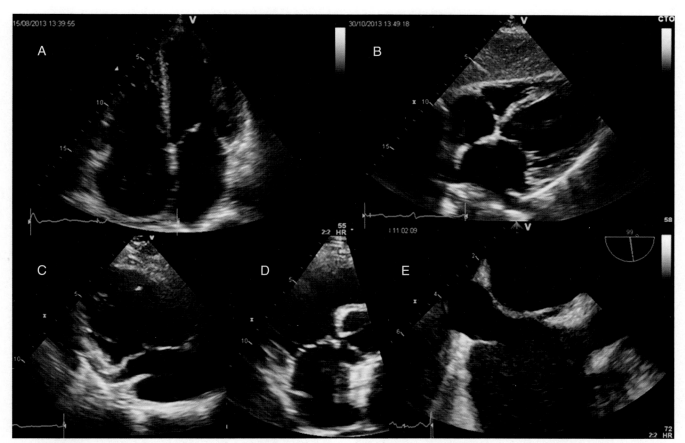

Figure 32.2. Standard two-dimensional views of the right atrium. **A,** Apical four-chamber view. **B,** Subcostal view. **C,** Parasternal short-axis view. **D,** Right ventricular inflow view. **E,** Transesophageal bicaval view.

The *Chiari* network (see Fig. 32.3) is a congenital remnant of the right valve of the sinus venosus, which is resorbed to varying degrees in utero. It has been found in 1.3% to 4% of autopsy studies and is believed to be of little clinical consequence by itself. When seen, there is a greater prevalence of both a patent foramen ovale (PFO) and a greater degree of shunting across the PFO with agitated saline contrast.[3] The network appears as a fine filamentous floating mass or "tangle" in the RA is several views, and it usually has more than one attachment. This highly mobile structure tends to move into and out of the scan plane. Because of its fenestrations, it does not cause obstruction to flow—unlike *cor triatriatum dexter*, with which it can be confused.

Box 32.1 lists a number of structures (anatomic variants and foreign objects) that should be recognized on a two-dimensional (2D) echocardiogram. A more detailed description of these variants is present in Chapter 129.

RIGHT ATRIAL SIZE AND FUNCTION
Right Atrial Volume Measurement by Two-Dimensional Echocardiography

Quantification of the RA size is most commonly performed using the A4C view. The maximal long-axis distance of the RA is measured from the center of the tricuspid annular plane to the center of the superior RA wall, parallel to the interatrial septum. The minor axis is measured from a plane perpendicular to the long axis of the right atrium, extending from the lateral border of the right atrium to the interatrial septum. The RA volume can be calculated from the A4C view using a single plane diameter–length measurement, a single plane area–length measurement, or a disc calculation based on Simpson's rule (Fig. 32.4).

There are inherent limitations in determining the volume of a three-dimensional (3D) structure using a single plane. However, the American Society of Echocardiography and the European Association of Cardiovascular Imaging currently recommend assessing RA size using the single plane area-length method or disk summation technique.[4] Normative values have been established from two studies enrolling more than 900 healthy patients: 25 ± 7 mL/m^2 in men and 21 ± 6 mL/m^2 in women.[5,6] In contrast to the LA, normal RA volume appears to vary based on gender, and indexing to body size does not eliminate this discrepancy.[7] Moreover, the RA volumes appear to be smaller than LA volumes when calculated using this 2D method.

In a small study comparing magnetic resonance imaging (MRI)–calculated RA volume as a gold standard, single-plane derived volumes by echocardiography were highly sensitive for detecting RA enlargement and demonstrated a high interobserver reliability. In addition, the volumes obtained by echocardiography were highly correlated with the MRI-derived values.[8]

Right Atrial Volume Measurement by Three-Dimensional Echocardiography

Several publications have examined three-dimensional echocardiography (3DE) as a more accurate and reproducible method to assess RA volume. The geometric assumptions made with single plane, 2D echocardiography (2DE) are not required using 3DE, and RA volume may be calculated using the summation of discs method (Fig. 32.5). One study that included 166 healthy patients found that the indexed RA volume ranged from 20 to 47 mL/m^2 with significant gender-based differences.[9] Subsequent studies confirmed that 3DE-derived RA volumes are higher in men and

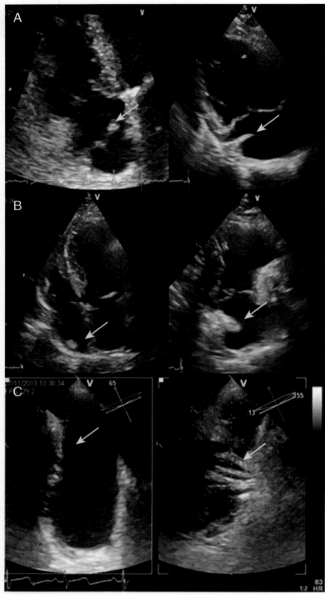

Figure 32.3. A, *Left,* A large Chiari network in the right atrium (RA). *Right,* A prominent Eustachian ridge in the inflow view. **B,** A prominent Crista Terminalis in the apical four-chamber and inflow views. **C,** Prominent ridges of the RA wall using biplane imaging on a transesophageal echocardiogram.

BOX 32.1 Important-to-Recognize Right Atrial Findings

NORMAL VARIANTS
- Eustachian valve
- Chiari network
- Eustachian ridge
- Crista terminalis
- Lipomatous hypertrophy of the septum
- Fatty infiltration of tricuspid annulus

ABNORMAL FINDINGS
- Thrombus on pacemaker wire
- Vegetation or endocarditis
- Myxoma
- Extrinsic compression of the right atrium by thrombus
- Foreign bodies
- Pacemaker or defibrillator wires
- Central venous catheters, including dialysis catheters
- Extracorporeal membrane oxygenation catheters
- Atrial septal defect occluder devices

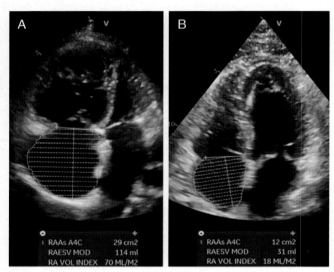

Figure 32.4. Method to trace the right atria (RA) area and volume using single plane by single plane area–length method. **A,** A severely dilated RA in a patient with pulmonary arterial hypertension. **B,** A normal RA volume.

showed that RA volume determined by 3DE tends to be higher than by 2DE.[6] Therefore, RA volumes obtained with 3DE cannot be used interchangeably with 2DE-derived volumes. Both 2DE and 3DE demonstrated very good intra- and interobserver reproducibility; however, interobserver reproducibility was superior with 3DE-derived volumes. Despite the limitations of 2DE, it is currently more widely used in clinical practice.

Right Atrial Strain

Assessment of myocardial strain as a marker of subclinical or early dysfunction has been used in other cardiac chambers, and several studies have examined right atrial strain. Negative strain (LSneg) can be measured during RA contraction, positive RA strain (LSpos) can be measured during RA filling, and total strain (LStot) can be

measured using both the positive and negative strain phases. Unlike RA volume reference values, which are gender specific, parameters of RA function such as strain may be age specific. Data from a single study involving 200 healthy volunteers suggested normative strain values: LSpos, 27 ± 9; LSneg, −17 ± 4; and LStot, 44 ± 10.[6] Further study to confirm normal strain values is required.

CLINICAL IMPLICATIONS OF RIGHT ATRIAL ENLARGEMENT AND DYSFUNCTION

RA enlargement and RA dysfunction are correlated with severity and prognosis in several disease states. In patients with heart failure (HF) and a left ventricular ejection fraction of 35% or less, increasing RA volume was predictive of death, need for transplant, or HF hospitalization and remained an independent factor after adjusting for several clinical, biochemical, and echocardiographic parameters.[2] In a separate, prospective study of patients with dilated cardiomyopathy, elevated RA volume was independently predictive of adverse cardiovascular outcomes and provided incremental value

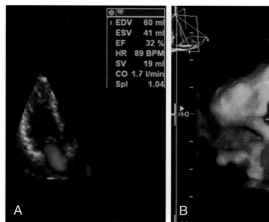 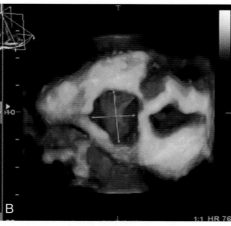

Figure 32.5. A, Measurement of right atrial (RA) volume using the three-dimensional volumetric approach. **B,** Technique to measure the RA eccentricity index.

to well-validated cardiomyopathy risk scores.[10] Higher-indexed RA volumes are also associated with lower functional capacity in patients with HF.[11] RA strain is significantly correlated with hemodynamically assessed pulmonary artery pressure greater than 50 mm Hg in patients with HF and in left ventricular assist device recipients and predicts the need for right-sided assist device and mortality.[12,13]

Increased RA size has consistently been associated with poor prognosis in pulmonary arterial hypertension (PAH).[14,15] Several of the original studies demonstrated that RA area correlates with adverse outcomes. Consequently, current international guidelines recommend including RA size in the risk assessment of patients with PAH.[16] RA enlargement is also associated with increasing severity of tricuspid regurgitation in these patients.[17] The 1-year follow-up of patients with PAH demonstrated that RA sphericity index measured by 3DE had a sensitivity of 96% and a specificity of 90% (area under the curve [AUC], 0.97) in predicting clinical deterioration, with a cutoff value of 0.24.[1] Furthermore, right atrial isthmus ablation in patients with severe pulmonary hypertension and atrial flutter improves functional capacity and clinical outcomes.[18,19]

More recently, several studies have demonstrated the prognostic value of RA strain in pulmonary hypertension patients.[20–22] Strain has been associated with increased hospitalization or death, adverse clinical outcomes, and higher invasively determined right atrial pressure and end-diastolic RV pressure. However, the absence of universally accepted reference values and lack of familiarity with this technique limit its widespread use at this time.

In patients with paroxysmal atrial fibrillation (AF), RA enlargement is associated with increased AF reoccurrence.[23] The same study suggested that indexed RA volume may be superior to indexed LA volume in predicting AF reoccurrence (AUC, 0.77 vs 0.64, respectively). Both RA indexed volume and RA strain are independent predictors of AF development in the postoperative period of patients undergoing coronary artery bypass grafting.[24]

RIGHT ATRIUM PRESSURE AND PERFORMANCE
Assessment of Right Atrial Pressure by Two-Dimensional Echocardiography

Using 2DE in the subcostal view, RA pressure is most frequently estimated by the IVC diameter and the degree of inspiratory collapse with either spontaneous respiration or sniffing. Guidelines from the American Society of Echocardiography suggest that the measurement of the IVC diameter should be made at end-expiration, 0.5 to 3.0 cm proximal to the entrance to the RA.[25] An IVC diameter less than 2.1 cm that collapses more than 50% suggests a normal RA pressure of 3 mm Hg (range, 0–5 mm Hg), whereas an IVC diameter

greater than 2.1 cm that collapses less than 50% suggests a high RA pressure of 15 mm Hg (range, 10–20 mm Hg). In indeterminate cases in which the IVC diameter and IVC collapse are discordant, an intermediate value of 8 mm Hg (range, 5–10 mm Hg) may be used. The cutoffs of 2.1 cm and 50% may not be optimal in all patient populations, and indexed values (11 mm/m²) may correlate better with RA pressure.[26,27]

Unfortunately, this technique may significantly underestimate RA pressure when it is markedly elevated. Moreover, the sonographer must also ensure that the apparent collapse of the IVC does not simply represent a transition out of the imaging plane. Use of short-axis imaging of the IVC may alleviate this problem.

In patients whose lungs are being ventilated using positive pressure, the degree of IVC collapse cannot be used to reliably estimate RA pressure. RA pressure measured by transduction of a central line should be used in these cases if available. However, an IVC diameter of 12 mm or less appears to identify patient with RA pressures less than 10 mm Hg. In this same patient group, a small and collapsed IVC suggests the presence of hypovolemia. The IVC may also be dilated in normal young athletes, and a dilated IVC in this population may not reflect an elevated RA pressure. Repeat imaging with the patient in the left lateral decubitus position often restores IVC pliability.

CONCLUSIONS

Assessment of the RA is an essential component of the routine 2DE. Although sometimes underappreciated, the RA has an important role in both normal and pathologically altered hearts. RA volume as determined by 2DE should be performed in all patients, and the difference between normal indexed values in men and women should be recognized. 3DE overcomes the geometric assumptions made with 2DE and may eventually supplant 2DE in the assessment of RA volume; however, more studies and familiarity with this technique are required before becoming widely adopted. RA volume and strain yield important prognostic information in several conditions such as PAH, HF, and AF. Therefore, the RA should be carefully examined in these diseases. The RA is clearly more important than a simple blood reservoir.

Acknowledgment

The authors acknowledge the contributions of Dr. Nimrod Blank, who was a coauthor of this chapter in the previous edition.

REFERENCES

1. Grapsa J, Gibbs JS, Cabrita IZ, et al. The association of clinical outcome with right atrial and ventricular remodeling in patients with pulmonary arterial hypertension. *Eur Heart J Cardiovasc Imaging.* 2012;13:666–672.
2. Sallach JA, Tang WH, Borowski AG, et al. Right atrial volume index in chronic systolic heart failure and prognosis. *JACC Cardiovasc Imag.* 2009;2:527–534.

3. Schneider B, Hofmann T, Justen MH, et al. Chiari's network: normal anatomic variant or risk factor for arterial embolic events? *J Am Coll Cardiol.* 1995;26:203–210.
4. Lang RM, Badano LP, Mor-Avi V, et al. Recommendations for cardiac chamber quantification by echocardiography in adults. *J Am Soc Echocardiogr.* 2015;28:1–39.
5. Kou S, Caballero L, Dulgheru, et al. Echocardiographic reference ranges for normal cardiac chamber size: results from the NORRE study. *Eur Heart J Cardiovasc Imaging.* 2014;15:680–690.
6. Peluso D, Badano LP, Muraru D, et al. Right atrial size and function assessed with three-dimensional and speckle-tracking echocardiography in 200 healthy volunteers. *Eur Heart J Cardiovasc Imaging.* 2013;14:1106–1114.
7. D'Oronzio U, Seen O, Biaggi P, et al. Right heart assessment by echocardiography: gender and body size matters. *J Am Soc Echocardiogr.* 2012;25:1251–1258.
8. Ebtia M, Murohy D, Gin K, et al. Best method for right atrial volume assessment by 2D echocardiography: validation with magnetic resonance imaging. *Echocardiography.* 2015;32:734–739.
9. Aune E, Baekkevar M, Roislien J, et al. Normal reference ranges for left and right atrial volume indexes and ejection fractions obtained with real-time three-dimensional echocardiography. *Eur J Echocardiogr.* 2009;10:738–744.
10. Moneghetti K, Giraldeau G, Wheeler MT, et al. Incremental value of right heart metrics and exercise performance to well-validated risk scores in dilated cardiomyopathy. *Eur Heart J Cardiovasc Imag.* 2018;19:916–925.
11. Mantziari L, Kamperidis V, Ventoulis I, et al. Increased right atrial volume index predicts low duke activity status index in patients with chronic heart failure. *Hellenic J Cardiol.* 2013;54:32–38.
12. Padeletti M, Cameli M, Lisi M, et al. Right atrial speckle tracking analysis as a novel noninvasive method for pulmonary hemodynamics assessment in patients with chronic systolic heart failure. *Echocardiogr.* 2011;28:658–664.
13. Charisopoulou D, Banner N, Demetrescu C. Right atrial and ventricular echocardiographic strain analysis predicts requirement for right ventricular support after left ventricular assist device implantation. *Eur Heart J Cardiovasc Imag.* 2019;20:199–208.
14. Raymond RJ, Hinderliter AL, Willis PW, et al. Echocardiographic predictors of adverse outcomes in primary pulmonary hypertension. *J Am Coll Cardiol.* 2002;39:1214–1219.
15. Bustamante-Labarta M, Perrone S, De La Fuente RL, et al. Right atrial size and tricuspid regurgitation severity predict mortality or transplantation in primary pulmonary hypertension. *J Am Soc Echocardiogr.* 2002;15:1160–1164.
16. Galiè N, Humbert M, Vachiery JL, et al. ESC/ERS Guidelines for the diagnosis and treatment of pulmonary hypertension. *Eur Heart J.* 2015;37:67–119. 2016.
17. Mutlak D, Aronson D, Lessick J, et al. Functional tricuspid regurgitation in patient with pulmonary arterial hypertension: is pulmonary artery pressure the only determinant of severity? *Chest.* 2009;135:115–121.
18. Showkathali R, Tayebjee MH, Grapsa J, et al. Right atrial flutter isthmus ablation is feasible and results in acute clinical improvement in patients with persistent atrial flutter and severe pulmonary arterial hypertension. *Int J Cardiol.* 2011;149:279–280.
19. Garlitski AC, Mark Estes NA. Ablation of atrial flutter in severe pulmonary hypertension: pushing the outside of the envelope. *J Cardiovasc Electrophysiol.* 2012;23:1191–1192.
20. Alenezi F, Mandawat A, Il'Giovine ZJ, et al. Clinical utility and prognostic value of right atrial function in pulmonary hypertension. *Circ Cardiovasc Imaging.* 2018;11.
21. Liu W, Wang Y, Zhou J, et al. The association of functional capacity with right atrial deformation in patients with pulmonary arterial hypertension: a study with two-dimensional speckle tracking. *Heart Lung Circ.* 2018;27:350–358.
22. Fukuda Y, Tanaka H, Ryo-Koriyama K, et al. Comprehensive functional assessment of right-sided heart using speckle tracking strain for patients with pulmonary hypertension. *Echocardiography.* 2016;33:1001–1008.
23. Luong C, Thompson DJ, Bennett M, et al. Right atrial volume is superior to left atrial volume for prediction of atrial fibrillation recurrence after direct current cardioversion. *Can J Cardiol.* 2015;31:29–35.
24. Aksu U, Kalkan K, Gulcu O, et al. The role of the right atrium in development of postoperative atrial fibrillation: a speckle tracking echocardiography study. *J Clin Ultrasound.* 2019;47:470–476.
25. Rudski L, Wyman WL, Afilalo J, et al. Guidelines for the echocardiographic assessment of the right heart in adults. *J Am Soc Echocardiogr.* 2010;23:685–713.
26. Kawata T, Daimon M, Lee SL, et al. Reconsideration of inferior vena cava parameters for estimating right atrial pressure in an east Asian population: comparative simultaneous ultrasound-catheterization study. *Circ J.* 2017;81:346–352.
27. Taniguchi T, Ohtani T, Nakatani S, et al. Impact of body size on inferior vena cava parameters for estimating right atrial pressure: a need for standardization? *J Am Soc Echocardiography.* 2015;28:1420–1427.

33 Pulmonary Embolism

Hanna N. Ahmed, Gerard P. Aurigemma

Pulmonary embolism (PE) is a common and often fatal disease. In the United States, more than 250,000 people are diagnosed with PE annually, and more than 60,000 die from the disease each year.[1–3] However, PE is one of the most underdiagnosed serious acute diseases. Although the overall 3-month mortality rate for all patients who develop PE is 15%,[4,5] if it is not recognized, it carries a higher mortality rate of approximately 30%. Because treatment can reduce this high mortality rate, prompt and accurate diagnosis is essential. Unfortunately, the clinical signs and symptoms (e.g., dyspnea, chest pain, tachypnea, and hypotension) are nonspecific and may be mistaken for acute coronary syndrome. Moreover, many critically ill patients have coexisting cardiopulmonary disorders that may divert attention from the diagnosis.

DIAGNOSIS

Chest radiography and electrocardiograms (ECGs) have limited diagnostic value because they often are normal in patients with PE. The classic Westermark sign on chest radiograph (focal oligemia on a pulmonary segment) is seldom seen;[6] other signs such as the Hampton hump (wedged-shaped density above the diaphragm) are also uncommon. ECGs are abnormal in 80% to 90% of patients, but the changes are usually nonspecific and nondiagnostic.[7,8]

Computed tomography pulmonary angiography (CTPA) is usually the noninvasive diagnostic test of choice when acute PE is suspected. It can also be used to detect other intrathoracic pathologic changes that may explain the patient's clinical presentation. Compared with pulmonary angiography, CTPA is minimally invasive, more readily available, rapid, and cost effective. It is highly accurate for detection of emboli in main lobar and segmental pulmonary arteries, more accurate than conventional angiography (Fig. 33.1). The sensitivity of CTPA varies from 45% to 100%, and the specificity varies from 78% to 100%.[9–13] A multidetector CT scanner can be used to evaluate pulmonary vessels down to sixth-order branches, and it significantly increases the detection rate of PE in the segmental and subsegmental levels.[14] There is some evidence that the more sensitive multidetector CT scanners allow the diagnosis of smaller pulmonary emboli that are less likely to cause significant sequelae.[15,16]

In the Prospective Investigation On Pulmonary Embolism Diagnosis (PIOPED) II study, CTPA had a sensitivity of 83% and a specificity of 96% for PE diagnosis. In PIOPED II, the pretest clinical probability as determined by the Wells' criteria also influenced the predictive value of CTPA. A negative CTPA had a high negative predictive value for PE for those with a low or intermediate clinical probability of PE (96% and 89%, respectively). If, however, the pretest probability was high, the negative predictive value was only 60%. The positive predictive value of a positive CTPA in those with an intermediate- or high-risk clinical probability was high (92% and 96%, respectively). The

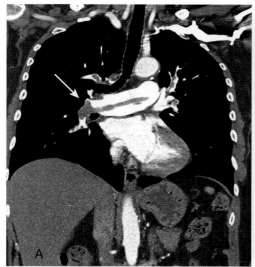
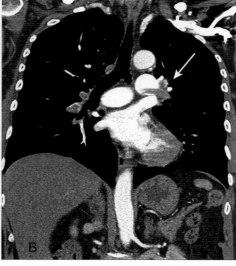

Figure 33.1. A and B, Computed tomography angiogram of the chest shows an extensive pulmonary embolism involving both pulmonary arteries *(arrows)*.

positive predictive value of a positive CTPA in those with a low pretest likelihood was only 58%.[17] The radiation exposure from a CT scan can be significant, particularly in institutions without a major focus on reducing radiation dose. The lifetime risk of cancer must be included in the risk-to-benefit calculation.

The ventilation-perfusion lung scan (V/Q scan), once a first-line diagnostic test for PE, is generally reserved for situations when contrast allergy or renal dysfunction limit the use of CTPA. Unfortunately, about 35% to 40% of nuclear lung scans are considered nondiagnostic,[9,10] and further testing is usually required.

TRANSTHORACIC ECHOCARDIOGRAPHY

The potential roles for echocardiography in the diagnosis and evaluation of patients with PE are listed in Box 33.1. Echocardiography can be of critical help in hemodynamically unstable patients, in which the absence of any signs of right ventricular (RV) overload or dysfunction may lead to consideration of a different cause of the instability, such as tamponade, severe left ventricular (LV) dysfunction, aortic dissection, hypovolemia, or acute valvular dysfunction. Another role for echocardiography in the hemodynamically unstable patient would be in those whom immediate CTPA is not available or feasible. In such cases, if the pretest clinical probability is high and there are otherwise unexplained echocardiographic signs of RV pressure overload and dysfunction, more aggressive therapeutic measures may be entertained (eg, thrombolytic therapy or catheter-directed thrombolysis).[18]

PE is associated with variable degrees of pulmonary arterial obstruction. With large emboli, the degree of pulmonary vascular obstruction typically leads to increased pulmonary artery pressure. Unlike the left ventricle, the normal right ventricle can only tolerate a narrow range of acute increase in afterload. This sudden increase in RV afterload can be accompanied by RV dilatation, because the diastolic compliance of the right ventricle is high. RV end-diastolic pressure (RVEDP) may remain relatively low until dilatation is limited by pericardial restraint. If the increase in RV afterload is significant, as is the case with significant PE, it should be expected that RV systolic function would decline. With the increase in RV end-diastolic volume (RVEDV) and RVEDP, the interventricular septum starts to bulge to the left, leading to underfilling of the left ventricle with a resultant decrease in stroke volume.[19,20]

Unfortunately, although RV dilatation and dysfunction (Figs. 33.2 and 33.3) may suggest PE, these findings are nonspecific and may result from other cardiopulmonary conditions that are commonly found in patients with suspected PE (e.g., chronic obstructive pulmonary disease [COPD], acute respiratory distress

BOX 33.1 Potential Roles of Echocardiography for Evaluation of Known or Suspected Pulmonary Emboli

1. Contribute to the diagnosis.
2. Evaluate the hemodynamic consequences.
3. Assess the cardiopulmonary responses to therapeutic interventions.
4. Determine management.
5. Exclude other entities that may present like pulmonary emboli.

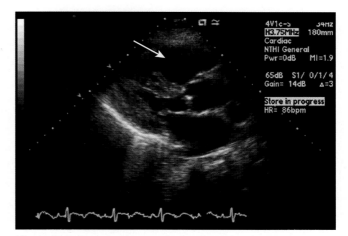

Figure 33.2. Parasternal long-axis view illustrating right ventricular dilatation *(arrow)*.

syndrome). Other causes of RV dilatation and dysfunction that should be considered include congestive heart failure, RV infarction, chronic tricuspid regurgitation, pulmonic stenosis, and atrial septal defect.

In contrast to signs of RV dysfunction, LV ejection fraction (LVEF) may be normal or even hyperdynamic in PE. Pulmonary vascular obstruction and reduced stroke volume may reduce LV preload, producing an echocardiographic appearance of an underfilled left ventricle (Fig. 33.4). In addition, increased sympathetic tone and neurohormonal changes may produce both tachycardia and hypercontractility of the left ventricle.

Visualization of emboli in the right-sided chambers or pulmonary arteries is an uncommon but extremely valuable finding. Nevertheless,

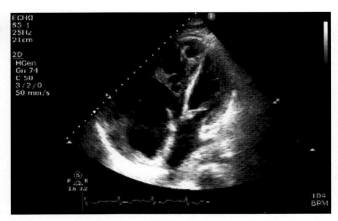

Figure 33.3. Apical four-chamber view showing a dilated right ventricle.

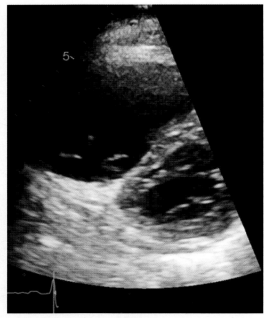

Figure 33.4. Flattening of the interventricular septum. (Image courtesy of Gerard P. Aurigemma, MD.)

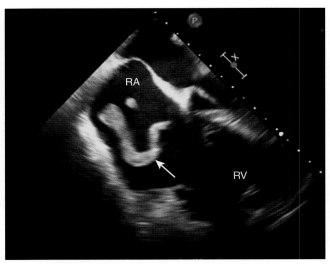

Figure 33.5. Transesophageal echocardiogram four-chamber view (centered over the right side of the heart) illustrating a mobile, somersaulting, unattached tubular mass *(arrow)* in the right atrium (RA) that is pathognomonic for a pulmonary embolus-in-transit. *RV,* Right ventricle. See corresponding Video 33.5.

BOX 33.2 Echocardiographic Findings in Acute Pulmonary Embolism

1. Direct visualization of thromboemboli in the right side of the heart or pulmonary artery
2. Right ventricular dilatation
3. Right ventricular dysfunction
   a. Global
   b. Regional
4. Normal or hyperdynamic left ventricular function
5. Ventricular septal "flattening" and paradoxical septal motion
6. Pulmonary artery dilatation
7. Unusual degree of tricuspid or pulmonary regurgitation
8. Increased pulmonary artery pressure

---

this is a dramatic finding in the small subset of patients who are discovered to have thrombi trapped in chambers of the right side of the heart. These thrombi, on their way from the systemic veins to the pulmonary circulation, appear on two-dimensional echocardiography as mobile, long, snakelike masses that are often unattached and appear to somersault (Fig. 33.5 and Video 33.5). The prevalence of echocardiographically detected thrombi in the right side of the heart was generally considered low (in the range of 1%–2%). However, in the International Cooperative Pulmonary Embolism Registry, intracardiac thrombi were visualized in 45 of 1135 patients (4%).[21]

The true sensitivity and specificity of transthoracic echocardiography (TTE) in the diagnosis of acute PE is difficult to assess. Reported sensitivities range from 20% to 60%, and specificities range from 80% to 95%.[22–26] Most of the reported studies only included patients with proven pulmonary emboli, so that the specificity of the various echocardiographic abnormalities could not be assessed. Some echocardiographic signs found in PE are listed in Box 33.2. At present, computed tomographic pulmonary angiography (CTPA) remains the diagnostic method of choice for patients with suspected PE. TTE should be considered

as a supportive test. Its value as a diagnostic test is based primarily on its wide availability and low risk. However, its sensitivity is insufficient to exclude PE.

Some echocardiographic signs that have been reported in association with PE are the McConnell sign (McCS) and the 60/60 sign. McCS is defined as normo- or hyperkinesis of the apical segment of the RV free wall despite hypo- or akinesis of the remaining parts of the RV free wall (Fig. 33.6 and Video 33.6).[27] Of additional value is the "60/60" sign, defined as an RV ejection (or pulmonary ejection) acceleration time (AT) of 60 msec or less in the presence of a tricuspid insufficiency pressure gradient that is 60 mm Hg or less (Figs. 33.7 and 33.8).[28]

Kurzyna and coworkers[28] prospectively examined 100 consecutive patients with suspected acute PE and demonstrated that the sensitivity and specificity were 19% and 100% for McCS and 25% and 94% for the 60/60 sign, respectively. An advantage of the McCS and the 60/60 sign is that in patients with previous cardiorespiratory diseases, the specificities of these two signs are not significantly altered. In contrast, the classic RV overload criteria (RV dilatation, systolic flattening of the interventricular septum, and increased tricuspid regurgitation pressure gradient in the absence of RV hypertrophy) are not useful in the group of patients with known cardiorespiratory diseases such as COPD, with the specificity dropping to as low as 21%.[28]

There is no one single reliable diagnostic echocardiographic parameter that is found in patients with acute PE. Various studies

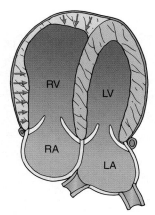

Figure 33.6. Diagram illustrating a dilated right ventricle (RV) with hypokinesis of a portion of the RV and preservation of contractility at the RV apex *(three arrows)*, the so-called McConnell sign. *LA,* Left atrium; *LV,* left ventricle.

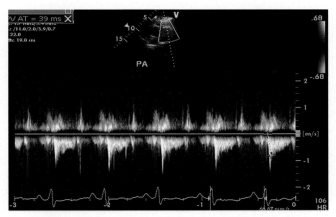

Figure 33.7. Spectral Doppler across the pulmonic valve shows that the acceleration time of the flow is significantly decreased (<60 msec). Combined with a tricuspid regurgitant peak gradient less than 60 mm Hg, these findings are consistent with a positive 60/60 sign.

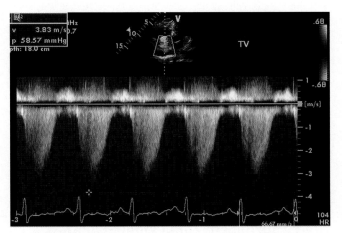

Figure 33.8. The tricuspid regurgitant peak gradient is calculated to be 59 mm Hg. Right ventricular systolic pressure is estimated to be 65 to 70 mm Hg, which is consistent with severe pulmonary hypertension.

have evaluated many different echocardiographic signs. Fields and colleagues conducted a systematic review and meta-analysis of 22 articles to summarize the test characteristics of various echo signs in the diagnosis of PE using CTPA, V/Q scan, surgery, or autopsy as gold standard in adults who presented with signs or symptoms suggestive of PE.[29] The prevalence of disease was 40.8%. Their conclusion was that TTE has high specificity but low sensitivity for TTE in the diagnosis of PE. They looked at 12 echocardiographic signs (listed in Table 33.1). Evidence of undefined "right heart strain" in 16 of the 22 articles had a sensitivity of 53% and specificity of 83%. Other signs included the 60/60 sign, RV hypokinesis, McCS, pulmonary arterial hypertension (PAH), right heart (RH) thrombus, RV:LV ratio, right ventricular end-diastolic diameter (RVEDd), abnormal or paradoxical septal motion, tricuspid regurgitation (TR), tricuspid annular plane systolic excursion (TAPSE), and right ventricular systolic pressure (RVSP). In general, there was high specificity for echocardiography. However, sensitivity for echocardiography was low. Also of note is that there is variability in PE presentation, clot burden, and physiologic reserve that contributes to pulmonary vascular resistance (PVR) and acute RH strain. Not studied was whether multiple signs together improve diagnostic accuracy.

Several recent studies were not included in Fields and coworkers' meta-analysis.[29] Kurnicka and colleagues conducted a study in 511 patients at a single center in Poland whose aim was to study the frequency of RV dysfunction, echocardiography signs of PE (McCS, 60/60 sign, right heart thrombus), and any incidental abnormalities (defined as LVEF ≤35%, moderate or severe aortic stenosis or insufficiency, moderate or severe mitral regurgitation) in patients who had confirmed at least segmental acute PE diagnosed by CTPA.[30] Most of these patients were hemodynamically stable on admission; 3.1% were considered high risk. RV dysfunction (RVD) in this study was defined as RV free-wall hypokinesis plus RVEDd:LVedd ratio greater than 0.9 in the apical four-chamber (A4C) view. This combined finding of RVD was present in only 20% of patients. Of the hemodynamically stable patients, only 18% had RVD on TTE. Of the unstable patients only 3 (18.8%) did not have signs of RV dysfunction as defined in this study, though all had some measure of RV overload present. Interestingly, normal RV morphology and preserved function were found in 33.4% of patients in this study, all of whom were hemodynamically stable. As for particular echocardiographic signs, the authors made the following observations. For RV overload signs, RV enlargement (>42 mm at the base) in the A4C view was present in 27.4% of patients, moderate RV free-wall hypokinesis in 26.6%, interventricular septum flattening in 18.4%, Tricuspid regurgitation peak systolic gradient (TRPG) greater than 30 mm Hg in 46.6%, pulmonary AT less than 80 msec in 37.2%, distended inferior vena cava with decreased collapsibility in 12.9%. For typical echocardiographic signs of PE in high-risk PE, McCS was present in 75% of patients, the 60/60 sign in 31.3%, and RH thrombus in 18.8%. For typical echocardiographic signs of PE in non–high-risk PE, McCS was present in 18% of patients, the 60/60 sign in 12.3%, and RH thrombus in 1.2%. Incidental abnormalities were found in 9% of the whole group. There is no generally accepted echocardiography definition of RVD used for PE diagnosis or risk stratification in hemodynamically unstable patients. The authors suggest that a combination of a dilated, hypokinetic RV together with McCS and the 60/60 sign might be most useful, but this needs to be further evaluated.

Mediratta and coworkers studied a group of 81 patients at a single center with McCS on echocardiogram.[31] They underwent CT or V/Q scan for suspected PE. In this group, 55 of 81 (68%) had PE, and 26 of 81 (32%) did not have PE; of those that did not have PE, 69% had pulmonary hypertension (PH). There were also 40 normal control participants in the study. Compared with normal control participants, McCS-positive patients had lower fractional area change (FAC), early tricuspid annular velocity S' by tissue Doppler (TDI S'), TAPSE, RV free wall global longitudinal strain (GLS), and RV regional free wall strain (RFWS) in all segments. In McCS-positive patients, the authors looked at several variables and found the following:

TABLE 33.1 Sensitivity and Specificity of Echocardiographic signs in Pulmonary Embolism

Echocardiographic Sign	Sensitivity (95% CI)	Specificity (95% CI)
Undefined "right heart strain"	0.53 (0.45, 0.61)	0.83 (0.74, 0.90)
60/60 sign	0.24 (0.16, 0.33)	0.84 (0.45, 0.97)
RV hypokinesis	0.38 (0.31, 0.44)	0.91 (0.88, 0.94)
McConnell's sign	0.22 (0.16, 0.29)	0.97 (0.95, 0.99)
PAH	0.44 (0.19, 0.72)	0.84 (0.70, 0.92)
RH thrombus	0.05 (0.02, 0.09)	0.99 (0.96, 1.00)
RV:LV ratio	0.55 (0.49, 0.60)	0.86 (0.83, 0.89)
RVEDd	0.80 (0.61, 0.92)	0.80 (0.67, 0.89)
Abnormal or paradoxical septal motion	0.26 (0.22, 0.31)	0.95 (0.93, 0.97)
TR	0.40 (0.35, 0.46)	0.83 (0.79, 0.86)
TAPSE	0.64 (0.54, 0.73)	0.61 (0.56, 0.67)
RVSP	0.47 (0.34, 0.61)	0.73 (0.65, 0.80)

CI, Confidence interval; *LV,* left ventricle; *PAH,* pulmonary arterial hypertension; *RH,* right heart; *RV,* right ventricle; *RVEDd,* right ventricular end-diastolic diameter; *RVSP,* right ventricular systolic pressure; *TAPSE,* tricuspid annular plane systolic excursion; *TR,* tricuspid regurgitation.
Modified from Fields JM, et al: Transthoracic echocardiography for diagnosing pulmonary embolism: A systematic review and meta-analysis, J Am Soc Echocardiogr 30:714–723, 2017.

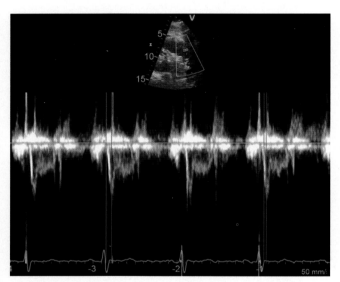

Figure 33.9. Early systolic notching. (Image courtesy of Gerard P. Aurigemma, MD.)

pulmonary arterial systolic pressure (PASP), TR by vena contracta (VC) width, and fractional area change (FAC) were all lower in PE-positive, McCS-positive patients than PE-negative, McCS-positive patients. There was no significant difference in TAPSE or TDI S′ between the two groups with McCS. The authors also looked at speckle tracking echo (STE) RV global longitudinal and regional free wall strain (four segments: apex, midapical, midbasal, basal). They found that global, basal, and apical segmental RV strain values were lower in PE-positive, McCS-positive patients compared with PE-negative, McCS-positive patients. The highest area under the curve (AUC) values were for TR severity, PASP, RV FAC, and GLS. Their conclusion was that McCS was not synonymous with acute PE. Any cause of acute increase in PVR could result in McCS. RV free wall strain might be useful in patients with McCS being evaluated for acute PE because PE-positive, McCS-positive patients had lower global LGS and lower apical and basal segmental strain values than PE-negative, McCS-positive patients.

Afonso and colleagues studied early systolic notching (ESN) of the RV outflow tract (RVOT) Doppler profile in 277 participants (187 with PE and 90 control participants).[32] ESN was defined visually as a narrow peaked initial wave (spike) with early deceleration of the RVOT envelope making a sharp notch in the first half of systole followed by a second Doppler wave (dome) that was more curvilinear (Fig. 33.9). ESN is a highly specific sign of elevated PVR and can be found in PE, pulmonary artery compression, or pulmonary arterial hypertension. ESN reflects the proximity of increased afterload to the RVOT and the markedly elevated PVR. Midsystolic notching (MSN) is defined as a distinct notch falling in the middle of the second half of the systolic ejection period. MSN or late systolic notching is commonly observed in patients with less severe grades of chronic precapillary pulmonary hypertension. Systolic notching is not characteristically observed in patients with postcapillary or left-sided pulmonary venous hypertension who by definition have normal PVR. Notching is strongly suggestive of elevated PVR but may be dissociated from pulmonary artery pressure in patients with acute PE. In this study, the authors found that 92% of patients who had massive PE (MPE) and submassive PE (SMPE) had ESN. In contrast, none of the control participants had ESN. They reported that for MPE or SMPE, ESN had a sensitivity of 92%, specificity of 99%, positive predictive value (PPV) of 98%, negative predictive value (NPV) of 96%, and AUC of 0.96. They also looked at McCS and the 60/60 sign in their study and found McCS in this study had a sensitivity of 52%, specificity 97%, PPV of 90%, NPV of 82%, and AUC of 0.75, and the 60/60 sign in this study had a sensitivity of 51%, specificity of 96%, PPV of 93%, NPV of 70%, and AUC of 0.74. One important limitation of their study is that they excluded patients with known pulmonary hypertension or prior PE, so this sign may not be applicable in those patients. This finding would need to be validated in other studies with less stringent inclusion criteria.

TTE can also be useful when examining patients with suspected pulmonary emboli by helping to exclude other causes of hemodynamic compromise or clinical syndromes that present in a similar fashion. For example, LV failure, acute myocardial infarction, cardiac tamponade, and aortic dissection may often be excluded. Notably, in patients with shock, an echocardiogram that shows no signs of RV pressure overload or dilatation effectively excludes major PE as a cause of shock. In these cases, alternative diagnoses should be pursued (Figs. 33.10 and 33.11). In summary, as per the most recent European Society of Cardiology (ESC) guidelines, in suspected high-risk PE, as indicated by the presence of hemodynamic instability, bedside echocardiography or emergency CTPA (depending on availability and clinical circumstances) is recommended for diagnosis (class I; level of evidence: C).[18]

TRANSESOPHAGEAL ECHOCARDIOGRAPHY

A major advantage of transesophageal echocardiography (TEE) over TTE is improved visualization of the proximal pulmonary arteries. The main pulmonary artery may be visualized in its long axis by

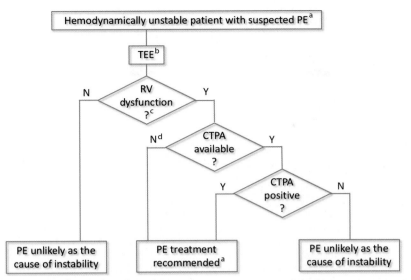

Figure 33.10. Diagnostic algorithm for patients with suspected high-risk pulmonary embolism (PE) presenting with hemodynamic instability. *CTPA,* Computed tomography pulmonary angiography; *RV,* right ventricular; *TTE,* transthoracic echocardiography. (Based on Konstantinides SV, et al: 2019 ESC Guidelines for the diagnosis and management of acute pulmonary embolism, *Eur Heart J* 41:543–603, 2020.)
[a]See Table 4 for definition of haemodynamic instability and high-risk PE.
[b]Ancillary bedside imaging tests may include TOE, which may detect emboli in the pulmonary artery and its main branches; and bilateral venous CUS, which may confirm DVT and thus VTE.
[c]In the emergency situation of suspected high-risk PE, this refers mainly to a RV/LV diameter ratio >1.0; the echocardiographic findings of RV dysfunction, and the corresponding cut-off levels, are graphically presented in Figure 3, and their prognostic value summarized in Supplementary Data Table 3.
[d]Includes the cases in which the patient's condition is so critical that it only allows bedside diagnostic tests. In such cases, echocardiographic findings of RV dysfunction confirm high-risk PE and emergency reperfusion therapy is recommended

withdrawing the TEE probe from the four-chamber view (midesophagus) to the upper esophagus, with maximal anteflexion of the probe. With the probe still at 0 degrees, the right pulmonary artery can also be imaged in its long axis. Usually a long portion of the right pulmonary artery can be imaged, at least to the point where it branches into lobar arteries. The left pulmonary artery is less well imaged because the proximal left pulmonary artery falls in a relatively blind spot for TEE because the left main stem bronchus runs between the esophagus and the left pulmonary artery. By slowly rotating the probe toward 90 degrees, a distal portion of the left pulmonary artery can sometimes be identified by its position relative to the thoracic aorta. Injection of agitated saline may be used to identify either the right or the left pulmonary artery.

The echocardiographic features of a thrombus include distinct borders, different echodensity than blood and the vascular wall, protrusion into the arterial lumen, alteration of blood flow by Doppler, and visualization in more than one imaging plane. These features help differentiate a true thrombus from artifacts and minimize false-positive diagnoses. In addition to imaging the pulmonary arteries, the atrial septum should also be evaluated for the presence of a patent foramen ovale and possible lodged thrombi. Both the inferior and superior venae cavae should also be imaged. Examination of the venae cavae is especially important when an intracardiac catheter is present because thrombi may be attached to catheters within the right side of the heart.

Early studies suggest that TEE is highly sensitive for detecting emboli in the main and right pulmonary arteries, but as mentioned earlier, TEE is quite limited in detecting distal or left pulmonary artery emboli. The visualization of an embolus, as shown in Fig. 33.5, can be considered diagnostic, but negative results must be confirmed with alternative tests such as helical CT scan, pulmonary magnetic resonance angiography, or pulmonary angiography.

Even though TEE may permit a diagnosis in some instances, it should not be implemented as a first-line test in patients suspected of having PE. The diagnostic accuracy of TEE remains to be established

in a population of patients with a wide range in severity of PE, from minor to massive. TEE can be considered as an alternative diagnostic tool for detecting central pulmonary arterial pulmonary thromboemboli in patients with suspected PE, especially in patients in intensive care units and receiving mechanical ventilation. In these patients, other diagnostic tests are logistically difficult.

PROGNOSIS

Several studies have suggested that the degree of RV dysfunction on echocardiogram can serve as a predictor of mortality. A correlation has been reported between echocardiographic RV dysfunction and clinical outcome in patients with confirmed PE. Patients with echocardiographic RV dysfunction have been shown to be at increased risk for subsequent clinical worsening and death related to PE. Some authors have extrapolated that such patients may benefit from more aggressive therapeutic strategies, including thrombolytic treatment.[21,26] However, this approach has not yet been validated in appropriate prospective studies. Moreover, the majority of these patients had hypotension. Therefore, the prognostic value of RV dysfunction in patients with PE and normal blood pressure has not been determined. Because normotensive patients with RV dysfunction represent a large proportion of patients with PE, the benefits of extending thrombolytic therapy to this subgroup must be weighed against the potential risk for bleeding. In addition, there are limited data on the relevance of echocardiographic screening for the identification of low-risk patients.

SUMMARY

PE is a serious condition that affects a large number of patients. Several diagnostic tools are available to aid in the diagnosis of this condition. Although echocardiography is not the gold standard test to detect PE, it can be used as an adjunct tool for evaluating patients with high-risk PE. In addition to providing direct visualization of

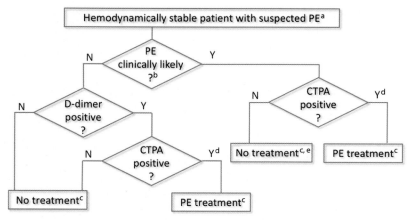

Figure 33.11. Diagnostic algorithm for patients with suspected pulmonary embolism (PE) without hemodynamic instability. *CTPA,* Computed tomography pulmonary angiography. (Based on Konstantinides SV, et al: 2019 ESC Guidelines for the diagnosis and management of acute pulmonary embolism, *Eur Heart J* 41:543–603, 2020.)

[a]The proposed diagnostic strategy for pregnant women with suspected acute PE is discussed in section 9.

[b]Two alternative classification schemes may be used for clinical probability assessment, i.e. a three-level scheme (clinical probability defined as low, intermediate, or high) or a two-level scheme (PE unlikely or PE likely).When using a moderately sensitive assay, D-dimer measurement should be restricted to patients with low clinical probability or a PE-unlikely classification, while highly sensitive assays may also be used in patients with intermediate clinical probability of PE due to a higher sensitivity and negative predictive value. Note that plasma D-dimer measurement is of limited use in suspected PE occurring in hospitalized patients.

[c]Treatment refers to anticoagulation treatment for PE.

[d]CTPA is considered diagnostic of PE if it shows PE at the segmental ormore proximal level.

[e]In case of a negative CTPA in patients with high clinical probability, investigation by further imaging testsmay be considered before withholding PE-specific treatment.

thrombus within the right-sided chambers and pulmonary arteries, echocardiography provides important information about RV function. RV regional or global dysfunction is often present and can be identified by TTE. However, in a population of unselected patients with suspected PE, TTE is of limited diagnostic value because it fails to identify approximately half of the patients with angiographically proven PE. Because of its poor sensitivity, TTE should not be used for routine screening for suspected PE.

Nevertheless, echocardiography can provide both supportive diagnostic and prognostic information. Patients with echocardiographic evidence of RV dilatation, RV dysfunction, or both have a higher incidence of death and recurrent PE. Thus, echocardiography might prove useful in identifying patients at high risk after PE who would benefit from aggressive therapies, including thrombolysis and open or suction embolectomy.

More recently, the improved imaging quality of TEE has provided greater sensitivity for the visualization of pulmonary emboli. Unfortunately, although the incidence of visualized thrombi in patients with suspected PE is unknown, it is probably under 20% to 30%. Nevertheless, despite a limited accuracy for detecting overall pulmonary emboli, TEE, when positive, can clarify the diagnosis at the bedside within a few minutes. Thus, TEE can reduce the need for further diagnostic procedures. TEE can also exclude other causes simulating PE and is of special value in patients receiving mechanical ventilation.

Acknowledgments

The authors would like to acknowledge the contributions of Drs. Zhao, Rigolin, and Goldstein, who were the authors of this chapter in a previous edition.

REFERENCES

1. Yusuf H, Tsai J, Atrash H, et al. Venous thromboembolism in adult hospitalizations in the United States 2007–2009. *MMWR Morb Mortal Wkly Rep.* 2012;61:401–404.
2. Beckman MG, Hooper WC, Critchley SE, et al. Venous thromboembolism: a public health concern. *Am J Prev Med.* 2010;38(4 Suppl):S495–S501.
3. Stein PD, Kayali F, Olson RE. Regional differences in rates of diagnosis and mortality of pulmonary thromboembolism. *Am J Cardiol.* 2004;93:1194–1197.
4. Kearon C. Natural history of venous thromboembolism. *Circulation.* 2003;107:I 22–I 30.
5. Stein PD, Beemath A, Olsen RE. Trends in the incidence of pulmonary embolism and deep venous thrombosis in hospitalized patients. *Am J Cardiol.* 2005;95:1525.
6. Westermark N. On the roentgen diagnosis of lung embolism. *Acta Radiol.* 1938;19:357–372.
7. Murin S, Romano PS, White RH. Comparison of outcomes after hospitalization for deep venous thrombosis or pulmonary embolism. *Thromb Haemost.* 2002;88:407–414.
8. Stein PD, Dalen JE, McIntyre KM, et al. The electrocardiogram in acute pulmonary embolism. *Prog Cardiovasc Dis.* 1975;17:247–257.
9. Garg K, Welsh CH, Feyerabend AJ, et al. Pulmonary embolism: diagnosis with spiral CT and ventilation-perfusion scanning—correlation with pulmonary angiographic results or clinical outcome. *Radiology.* 1998;208:201–208.
10. Mayo JR, Remy-Jardin M, Muller NL, et al. Pulmonary embolism: prospective comparison of spiral CT with ventilation- perfusion scintigraphy. *Radiology.* 1997;205:447–452.
11. Drucker EA, Rivitz SM, Shepard JA, et al. Acute pulmonary embolism: Assessment of helical CT for diagnosis. *Radiology.* 1998;209:235–241.
12. Goodman LR, Curtin JJ, Mewissen MW, et al. Detection of pulmonary embolism in patients with unresolved clinical and scintigraphic diagnosis: helical CT versus angiography. *AJR Am J Roentgenol.* 1995;164:1369–1374.
13. Eng J, Krishnan JA, Segal JB, et al. Accuracy of CT in the diagnosis of pulmonary embolism: a systematic literature review. *AJR Am J Roentgenol.* 2004;183:1819–1827.
14. Ghaye B, Szapiro D, Mastora I, et al. Peripheral pulmonary arteries: How far in the lung does multi-detector row spiral CT allow analysis? *Radiology.* 2001;219:629–636.
15. Araoz P, Haramati L, Mayo J, et al. Panel discussion: pulmonary embolism and outcomes. *AJR Am J Roentgenol.* 2012;198:1313–1319.
16. Patel S, Kazerooni EA, Cascade PN. Pulmonary embolism: Optimization of small pulmonary artery visualization at multi-detector row CT. *Radiology.* 2003;227:455–460.
17. Stein PD, Fowler SE, Goodman LR, et al. Multidetector computed tomography for acute pulmonary embolism. *N Engl J Med.* 2006;354:2317–2327.
18. Konstantinides SV, Meyer G, Becattini C, et al. ESC Scientific Document Group, 2019 ESC Guidelines for the diagnosis and management of acute pulmonary embolism. *Eur Heart J.* 2020;41:543–603.

19. Matthews JC, McLaughlin V. Acute right ventricular failure in the setting of acute pulmonary embolism or chronic pulmonary hypertension: a detailed review of the pathophysiology, diagnosis, and management. *Curr Cardiol Rev.* 2008;4:49–59.

20. Bryce YC, Perez-Johnston R, Bryce EB, et al. Pathophysiology of right ventricular failure in acute pulmonary embolism and chronic thromboembolic pulmonary hypertension: a pictorial essay for the interventional radiologist. *Insights Imag.* 2019;10(18).

21. Goldhaber SZ, Visani L, De Rosa M. Acute pulmonary embolism: clinical outcomes in the International Cooperative pulmonary embolism Registry (ICOPER). *Lancet.* 1999;353:1386–1389.

22. Roy PM, Colombet I, Durieux P, et al. Systematic review and meta-analysis of strategies for the diagnosis of suspected pulmonary embolism. *Br Med J.* 2005;331:259.

23. Ribeiro A, Lindmarker P, Juhlin-Dannfelt A, et al. Echocardiography Doppler in pulmonary embolism: right ventricular dysfunction as a predictor of mortality rate. *Am Heart J.* 1997;134:479–487.

24. Miniati M, Monti S, Pratali L, et al. Value of transthoracic echocardiography in the diagnosis of pulmonary embolism: results of a prospective study in unselected patients. *Am J Med.* 2001;110:528–535.

25. Kasper W, Konstantinides G, Geibel A, et al. Prognostic significance of right ventricular afterload stress detected by echocardiography in patients with clinically suspected pulmonary embolism. *Heart.* 1997;77:346–349.

26. Torbicki A, Perrier A, Konstantinides S, et al. The Task Force for the diagnosis and management of acute pulmonary embolism of the European Society of Cardiology (ESC). Guidelines on the diagnosis and management of acute pulmonary embolism. *Eur Heart J.* 2008;29:2276–2315.

27. McConnell MV, Solomon SD, Rayan ME, et al. Regional right ventricular dysfunction detected by echocardiography in acute pulmonary embolism. *Am J Cardiol.* 1996;78:469–473.

28. Kurzyna M, Torbicki A, Pruszczyk P, et al. Disturbed right ventricular ejection pattern as a new Doppler echocardiographic sign of acute pulmonary embolism. *Am J Cardiol.* 2002;90:507–511.

29. Fields JM, Davis J, Girson L, et al. Transthoracic echocardiography for diagnosing pulmonary embolism: a systematic review and meta-analysis. *J Am Soc Echocardiogr.* 2017;30:714–723.

30. Kurnicka K, Lichodzieiewska B, Goliszek S, et al. Echocardiographic pattern of acute pulmonary embolism: analysis of 511 consecutive patients. *J Am Soc Echocardiogr.* 2016;29:907–913.

31. Mediratta A, Addetia K, Medvedofsky D, et al. Echocardiographic diagnosis of acute pulmonary embolism in patients with McConnell's sign. *Echocardiography.* 2016;33:696–702.

32. Afonso L, Sood A, Akintoye E, et al. A Doppler echocardiographic pulmonary flow marker of massive or submassive acute pulmonary embolus. *J Am Soc Echocardiogr.* 2019;32:799–806.

33

34 Physiology of Diastole

Sherif F. Nagueh

Normal diastole consists of four time intervals: isovolumic relaxation time (IVRT), early diastolic filling (rapid filling or E phase), diastasis, and late diastolic filling (atrial kick or A phase). Left ventricular (LV) diastole conventionally begins with the closure of the aortic valve (AV), which ushers the drop in LV pressure. The time interval between AV closure and mitral valve (MV) opening is the isovolumic relaxation time (IVRT). During IVRT, LV pressure is decreasing while its volume is unchanged, assuming no significant mitral and aortic regurgitation. This period ends with the opening of the MV. MV opening follows the drop in LV pressure below left atrial (LA) pressure. LV filling during the early diastolic filling period (rapid filling or E phase) occurs as LV relaxation leads to lower LV early diastolic pressures and a positive transmitral pressure gradient. With ongoing LV filling, LA pressure drops, and LV pressure rises, leading to a decreased transmitral pressure gradient and reduced rate of LV filling in mid diastole. The rate of decline in early diastolic filling is related to LV stiffness such that higher LV stiffness leads to faster deceleration of LV filling. In late diastole, the LA contracts and leads to another positive transmitral pressure gradient and another peak of LV filling (atrial kick or A phase) in late diastole (Fig. 34.1). The time period between the end of the E phase and the beginning of the A phase is referred to as *diastasis*.

LEFT VENTRICULAR RELAXATION

LV relaxation is affected by load, inactivation, and dyssynchrony.[1–3] In general, increased LV afterload (LV end-systolic wall stress) leads to delayed and slow relaxation.[2] The effects of dyssynchrony have been examined in animal models as well as human disease, including patients with aortic stenosis, hypertension, and hypertrophic obstructive cardiomyopathy. There are data showing an improvement in LV relaxation with a reduction in LV dyssynchrony. It is also worth noting that increased load can affect LV relaxation both directly and indirectly because it can contribute to dyssynchrony.[3] *Inactivation* refers to the mechanisms leading to actin–myosin detachment and reducing calcium level in the sarcoplasm.

In ventricles with normal relaxation, LV minimal pressure is low, but with impaired relaxation, this pressure is increased. Both the rate and the extent of LV relaxation affect LV diastolic pressures.[4] The effect of impaired LV relaxation on LV filling pressures is more notable at fast heart rates.[4] In this situation, LV filling is reduced (which can be detected by imaging) along with increased LV diastolic pressures.[5] LV systolic duration is another important factor that affects filling pressures. For any given degree of LV relaxation, LV filling pressures increase as systolic duration increases.[4]

LV relaxation is measured invasively by the time constant, tau (τ). The relation between LV pressure and time can be mathematically represented by several models. These include monoexponential decay to a zero asymptote, monoexponential decay to a nonzero asymptote, linear fit between LV pressure and its first differential (dP/dt), and a hybrid logistic regression model. Another approach to assess LV relaxation includes the time for dP/dt to decline to 50% of its initial value (t½). Of these methods, the monoexponential decay of LV pressure to a zero asymptote has been more frequently used, and LV relaxation would be considered complete after 3.5 τ. The equation is given by:

$$P(t) = P_o\, e^{-t/\tau}$$

in which Po is LV pressure at time of dP/dt min.

Taking the natural logarithm of both sides:

$$\mathrm{Ln}\, P(t) = \mathrm{Ln}\, P_o - t/\tau,\ \text{or}$$

$$t/\tau = \mathrm{Ln}\, P_o - \mathrm{Ln}\, P_t.$$

Therefore, τ can be derived as:

$$\tau = t/(\mathrm{Ln}\, P_o - \mathrm{Ln}\, P_t).$$

At the time of mitral valve opening, t = IVRT, and τ can be given as:

$$\tau = \mathrm{IVRT}/(\mathrm{Ln}\, P_o - \mathrm{Ln}\, P_{LAP}).$$

It is possible to use noninvasive estimates of LAP and LV end systolic pressure and thus obtain τ using entirely noninvasive measurements. This approach has been validated against invasive standards, though it has its limitations.[6]

On the cellular level, several factors affect relaxation.[7] These include calcium transport into the sarcoplasmic reticulum (SERCA 2a), outside the cell (sodium calcium exchanger and calcium pump in the sarcolemma) and into the mitochondria, energy levels (ADP/ATP ratio and inorganic phosphate), the phosphorylation status of troponin I (desensitizes the contractile proteins to calcium), and myosin heavy chain mutations. These factors are affected by the sympathetic nervous system and circulating catecholamines, atrial natriuretic peptide and brain natriuretic peptide levels, the renin–angiotensin–aldosterone system, and inducible nitric oxide. In particular, active reuptake of calcium into the sarcoplasmic reticulum by SERCA 2a is reduced in patients with heart failure. The activity of SERCA 2a is under control by phospholamban, the phosphorylation of which releases the inhibitory effect of the protein on SERCA 2a activity.

LEFT VENTRICULAR STIFFNESS

LV stiffness determines the diastolic pressure–volume (PV) relationship (Fig. 34.2). It is possible to derive LV chamber stiffness using conductance catheters that simultaneously measure LV volume and pressure. Several factors affect chamber stiffness, including LV geometry, myocardial stiffness, and factors extrinsic to the LV as pericardial, RV, and LV interactions. Of note, incomplete relaxation can contribute to elevated LV diastolic pressures

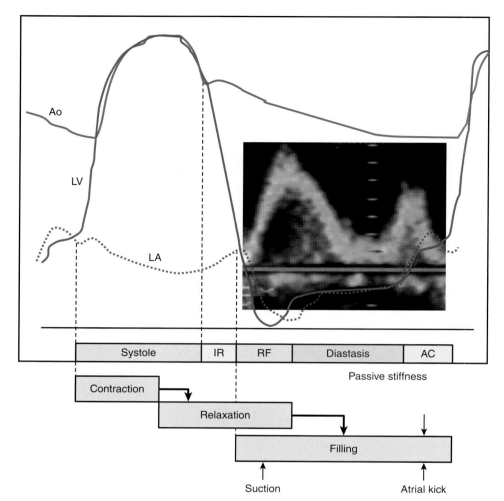

Figure 34.1. The relationship between aortic (Ao), left ventricular (LV), and left atrial (LA) pressure and mitral inflow. *AK,* Atrial kick; *IR,* isovolumic relaxation period; *RF,* rapid filling.

| Systole | IR | RF | Diastasis | AC |

Passive stiffness

Contraction

Relaxation

Filling

Suction   Atrial kick

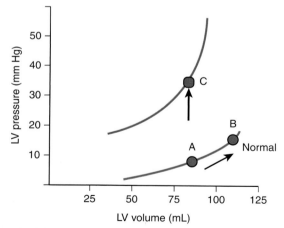

Figure 34.2. The left ventricular (LV) diastolic pressure–volume relationship from a normal heart (*A*) and one with increased LV chamber stiffness (*C*). Notice that the normal ventricle can still develop elevated diastolic pressures as its volume increase (*A* to *B*) even though the LV stiffness constant has not increased.

for any given volume. Myocardial stiffness is determined by the sarcomeric proteins, microtubules, and extracellular matrix composition.[7]

The diastolic pressure–volume relationship has been represented by several mathematical models, including exponential, cubic, and power models. The exponential models have been more frequently used as for example:

$$P = b\ e^{kV}.$$

Differentiating this equation:

$$dP/dV = k\ \left(b\ e^{kV}\right)\ \text{or}\ dP/dV = kP$$

in which *k* is the chamber stiffness constant.

For any given volume, LV diastolic pressure is higher for stiffer ventricles. There are two general approaches to derive k: either rely on LV pressure and volume measurements without altering load or use preload alterations by varying venous return through inflating a balloon in the inferior vena cava. The limitations of deriving k without preload alteration include not accounting for the effects of relaxation as early diastolic data points are represented and failing to detect dynamic changes in stiffness as stiffness can be load dependent in a number of cardiac diseases.[8]

Notwithstanding these methods that are used to compare stiffness between different ventricles,[9] it is important to note that for any given ventricle, as LV volume increases, LV diastolic pressure rises steeply. This is because of the curvilinear relation between LV volumes and pressures. Therefore, for any given segment of a unique pressure–volume curve, one can expresses the PV relation by the operating chamber stiffness, which is lower in the flat portion of the curve and is higher in the steep segment at larger LV volumes.

On a cellular level, myocardial tension is primarily determined by titin (TTN). TTN has isoforms, the ratio of which, determines passive tension and passive stiffness. Of note, TTN phosphorylation can modulate myocardial stiffness, and this has been shown in animal models as well as in patients with heart failure.[7] In a normal heart, collagen does not affect tension at the normal sarcomere length. However, higher levels of collagen isoform I and increased collagen cross-linking contribute to increased stiffness in patients with heart failure. Recent studies have reported abnormalities as well in matrix metalloproteinases with respect to their synthesis and degradation.

VENTRICULAR–ARTERIAL COUPLING

Increased arterial elastance (Ea) can contribute to the development of heart failure with preserved ejection fraction (HFpEF). Ea is derived as the ratio between end-systolic pressure and LV stroke volume. In turn, end-systolic pressure can be reliably estimated as 0.9 × systolic blood pressure. Furthermore, the ratio of Ea to LV end-systolic stiffness (Ees) can be derived and used to assess ventricular arterial coupling. With aging, both Ea and Ees increase. Some reports have noted abnormal Ea/Ees ratio in patients with HFpEF, but others did not.

DIAGNOSIS OF HEART FAILURE WITH PRESERVED EJECTION FRACTION

This diagnosis is established in the presence of symptoms and signs of heart failure usually with a LV end-diastolic volume index below 97 mL/m^2 and LV ejection fraction greater than 50%. Evidence of abnormal LV diastolic function is needed and can be established by invasive and noninvasive criteria. Invasive measurements include mean wedge pressure greater than 15 mm

Hg, LV end-diastolic pressure greater than 16 mm Hg, τ greater than 48 ms, or LV chamber stiffness constant greater than 0.27.[10] It is important to carefully establish this diagnosis because it is common to have several other reasons of dyspnea in the older adult population, and HFpEF diagnosis carries high morbidity and mortality.

REFERENCES

1. Brutsaert DL, Sys SU, Gillebert TC. Diastolic failure: pathophysiology and therapeutic implications. *J Am Coll Cardiol.* 1993;22:318–325.
2. Leite-Moreira AF, Correia-Pinto J, Gillebert TC. Afterload induced changes in myocardial relaxation: a mechanism for diastolic dysfunction. *Cardiovasc Res.* 1999;43:344–353.
3. Gillebert TC, Lew WY. Nonuniformity and volume loading independently influence isovolumic relaxation rates. *Am J Physiol.* 1989;257:H1927–H1935.
4. Hay I, Rich J, Ferber P, et al. Role of impaired myocardial relaxation in the production of elevated left ventricular filling pressure. *Am J Physiol Heart Circ Physiol.* 2005;288:H1203–H1208.
5. Nagueh SF, Appleton CP, Gillebert TC, et al. Recommendations for the evaluation of left ventricular diastolic function by echocardiography. *J Am Soc Echocardiogr.* 2009;22:107–133.
6. Scalia GM, Greenberg NL, McCarthy PM, et al. Noninvasive assessment of the ventricular relaxation time constant (tau) in humans by Doppler echocardiography. *Circulation.* 1997;95:151–155.
7. Kass DA, Bronzwaer JG, Paulus WJ. What mechanisms underlie diastolic dysfunction in heart failure? *Circ Res.* 2004;94:1533–1542.
8. Pak PH, Maughan L, Baughman KL, Kass DA. Marked discordance between dynamic and passive diastolic pressure-volume relations in idiopathic hypertrophic cardiomyopathy. *Circulation.* 1996;94:52–60.
9. Zile MR, Baicu CF, Gaasch WH. Diastolic heart failure—abnormalities in active relaxation and passive stiffness of the left ventricle. *N Engl J Med.* 2004;350:1953–1959.
10. Paulus WJ, Tschope C, Sanderson JE, et al. How to diagnose diastolic heart failure. *Eur Heart J.* 2007;28:2539–2550.

---

35 Echo Doppler Parameters of Diastolic Function

Michael Chetrit, Allan L. Klein

Diastolic heart failure, or heart failure with preserved ejection fraction (HFpEF), is not only a commonly encountered syndrome that accounts for approximately 50% of all heart failure but also a well-recognized contributor to clinical heart failure with increased morbidity and mortality similar to systolic heart failure.[1] Diastole is a complex and dynamic phenomenon that is influenced by age, loading condition, heart rate, and peripheral vascular tone. Routine assessment of diastolic function as part of the comprehensive echocardiography was recommended by the American Society of Echocardiography (ASE) and the European Association of Cardiovascular Imaging (EACVI) guidelines.[2] The purpose of this chapter is to describe the Doppler parameters of diastolic function used in clinical practice and their prognostic implications.

DOPPLER MITRAL FLOW VELOCITY PATTERNS

Doppler measurement of the mitral flow velocity provides unique information about the velocity of blood flow across the mitral valve into the ventricle during diastole. This velocity is a complex function of the pressure gradient across the mitral valve, defined by the law of conservation of energy equation. Hence, flow velocity represents the intermediate link between hemodynamic conditions indicated by instantaneous left atrial and left ventricular pressures and the filling characteristics of the ventricle.

Mitral flow velocity variables are recorded from the apical four-chamber (A4C) view with pulsed-wave (PW) Doppler by placing a 1- to 2-mm sample volume between the mitral leaflet tips at their narrowest point, which is visualized with two-dimensional echocardiography (2DE) at end-expiration during normal breathing. The Doppler gain and filter settings should be as low as possible, with sweep speed at 50 to 100 mm/s and the spectral Doppler baseline one-third to halfway up on the monitor display. Variables that can be measured include peak mitral flow velocity in early diastole (E wave) and during atrial contraction (A wave), mitral E wave deceleration time (DT), the E wave velocity just before atrial contraction (E at A), the duration of mitral A wave velocity (Adur) (sample volume at the mitral annulus level), and isovolumic relaxation time (IVRT). In young, healthy individuals, there is a rapid acceleration of blood flow from the left atrium (LA) to the left ventricle (LV) after mitral valve opening.

E wave: Early peak filling velocity of 0.6 to 0.8 m/s occurs 90 to 110 ms after the onset of mitral valve opening. This E wave occurs simultaneously with the maximum pressure gradient between the LA and LV that in turn depends on the pressure difference along the flow stream, LV relaxation, and the relative compliance of the two chambers. The normal E wave pattern shows rapid acceleration and deceleration; normal deceleration slope is 4.3 to 6.7 m/s.[3] Mitral DT, as defined by the time interval from the peak

E wave to its extrapolation to baseline, typically ranges from 150 to 240 ms (normal values range from 160–200 ms).[4]

E wave deceleration time (DT): DT is prolonged in patients with LV relaxation abnormalities because it takes longer for LA and LV pressure to equilibrate. A low normal DT, on the other hand, can be seen in normal young subjects, in whom there is vigorous LV relaxation and elastic recoil, and a short DT if there is a decrease in LV compliance or marked increase in LA pressure as in advanced diastolic dysfunction (DT <150 ms).

Diastasis: Early diastolic filling is then followed by a variable period of minimal flow (diastasis). The duration of diastasis is dependent on heart rate; it is longer with slow heart rates and entirely absent with faster rates.

A wave: Last, the A wave, which is the result of an atrial contraction ("atrial kick") pushing the remaining blood from the LA to the LV, follows the diastasis and is influenced by LV compliance and LA contractility (Fig. 35.1).[3] The normal A wave velocity typically ranges from 0.19 to 0.35 m/s and is significantly smaller than the E wave.

E/A ratio: In young, healthy individuals, the E/A ratio is greater than 1. Sinus tachycardia, premature atrial contraction, and first-degree atrioventricular block may result in fusion of the E and A waves. The peak A wave velocity in fused E and A velocity, with an E-at-A wave velocity greater than 20 cm/s is larger than it would have been at a slower heart rate, when mitral flow velocity has time to decrease before atrial contraction.[5] In these cases, the E/A wave ratio may be reduced compared with values obtained at a slower heart rate, so that more reliance on other Doppler variables is needed when interpreting the fused LV filling pattern.

With aging, the LV relaxation takes longer, primarily because there is a gradual increase in systolic blood pressure and LV mass, resulting in reduced LV filling in early diastole and increased filling at atrial contraction. The peak E and A wave velocities become approximately equal during the sixth and seventh decade of life. DT and IVRT become longer with age, and atrial contraction contributes up to 35% to 40% (as opposed to 10%–15% in adolescents) of LV diastolic stroke volume.[6] With progressively worsening diastolic function, transmitral flow evolves in a recognizable pattern.

Grade 1 diastolic dysfunction (abnormal relaxation): There is a low E wave (<50 cm/s) and a high A wave, resulting in an E/A ratio less than 1. DT is prolonged and is usually longer than 240 ms, and IVRT, the earliest Doppler manifestation of diastolic dysfunction (measured by PW or continuous-wave [CW] Doppler), is longer than 110 ms. Often considered the transition from grade 1a to grade 1b, abnormal relaxation is followed by a decrease in late LV compliance, resulting in a rise in LV end-diastolic pressure (LVEDP). This rise in end-diastolic pressures truncates atrial systole causing a shortened duration of the mitral A wave with a more rapid (i.e., shorter) A wave deceleration time.[4] In fact, an A-wave deceleration time 60 ms or less predicts an LVEDP greater than 18 mm Hg.[4]

Grade 2 diastolic dysfunction (pseudonormalization): This occurs when there is a rise in mean left atrial pressure and a decrease in early and late compliance of the left ventricle (LV). It is associated with a normal appearance of the transmitral inflow ("pseudonormal" pattern) with an E/A ratio between 0.8 and 2.0 and a DT between 150 and 200 ms.

Grade 3 diastolic dysfunction (restrictive filling): With disease progression, grade 3 diastolic dysfunction or restrictive filling develops. There are a very high E wave, a low A wave, and a significantly decreased DT. The E/A ratio is typically greater than 2, and the DT is less than 150 ms. In previous iterations, restrictive filling pressures were subcategorized to either reversible grade 3 or fixed restrictive pattern (grade 4) depending on the response to the Valsalva maneuver or other preload reducing maneuvers. This categorization has since been removed from the current

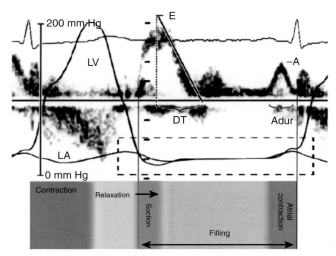

Figure 35.1. Mitral inflow represents pressure difference between the left ventricle and left atrium: simultaneous invasive pressure curves and Doppler echocardiography during the phases of left ventricular filling (relaxation, suction, filling, and atrial contraction). *A,* Mitral filling at atrial contraction; *Adur,* duration of mitral A wave; *DT,* mitral deceleration time; *E,* mitral early filling wave; *LA,* left atrial pressure curve; *LV,* left ventricular pressure curve.

2016 ASE/EACVI joint recommendations for the assessment of LC diastolic function.[2] Doppler criteria used to define grades of diastolic dysfunction are summarized in Table 35.1.

Mid-diastolic (L) wave: The Doppler imaging of mitral inflow may have additional forward flow during mid-diastole. The prominent mid-diastolic filling "hump" has been described as a mitral L-wave. The L-wave is often seen in patients with a markedly prolonged LV relaxation or with elevated LV filling pressures, though it can be seen in healthy individuals with bradycardia.[7]

VALSALVA MANEUVER

Because diastolic function is affected by preload change, the Valsalva maneuver is a test used to modify cardiac loading condition, which is helpful in the measurement of mitral inflow parameters. The Valsalva maneuver is performed by forceful attempted expiration (~40 mm Hg) against a closed glottis, resulting in a complex hemodynamic process involving four phases. During the strain phase of the maneuver, preload (mean LA pressure) is reduced, and peak mitral E wave velocity decreases by at least 20%. There is also a simultaneous, albeit smaller, decrease in peak A wave velocity during the strain phase as well.[8] With pseudonormal mitral flow patterns, the Valsalva strain lowers the elevated LA pressure and reveals the underlying impaired LV relaxation, resulting in a measured E/A ratio below 1.[9] Patients with restrictive filling patterns or individuals who have a sensitivity to preload revert to a pseudonormal or even impaired relaxation pattern. Patients who have restrictive filling patterns and exhibit no change with Valsalva have severe irreversible or fixed diastolic function. The primary limitation of the routine use of the Valsalva maneuver is that it is difficult to obtain adequate tracings.[10,11] Occasionally, the position of the sample volume may move during the maneuver. In addition, the inherent difficulties in performing an adequate Valsalva maneuver may limit its use in routine practice. In current guidelines, the Valsalva maneuver can be considered an ancillary technique to assess for elevated filling pressures.

PULMONARY VENOUS FLOW

Accurate pulmonary vein (PV) flow velocity can be obtained from the A4C view with PW Doppler in 85% to 90% of patients. The right upper PV is the most frequently visualized and accessible

TABLE 35.1 Doppler Parameters in Normal Population and Various Grades of Diastolic Dysfunction.

Criteria	Normal Young	Normal Adult	Impaired Relaxation (Grade 1)	Pseudonormal (Grade 2)	Restrictive (Grade 3)
E/A ratio	≥0.8	≥0.8	≤0.8 + E <50 ms	0.8–2.0 (reverses with Valsalva maneuver)	>2.0

Deceleration time (ms)	<240	150–240	≥240	150–200	<150

IVRT (ms)	70–90	70–90	>90	<90	<70
PV S/D ratio	<1	≥1	≥1	<1	<1

PV AR-MV A wave duration (ms)	≥30	≤0	≤0 or ≥30	≥30	≥30

AR velocity (cm/s)	<35	<35	<35	≥35	≥35

Continued

TABLE 35.1 Doppler Parameters in Normal Population and Various Grades of Diastolic Dysfunction.

Criteria	Normal Young	Normal Adult	Impaired Relaxation (Grade 1)	Pseudonormal (Grade 2)	Restrictive (Grade 3)
Propagation velocity (cm/s)	>55	>55	>45	<45	<45

Mitral e′ velocity (cm/s)	>10	>8	<8	<8	<8

Mitral E/e′	<10	<10	>10	>10	>10

TR velocity (m/s)	<2.8	<2.8	>2.8	>2.8	>2.8s

PASP (mm Hg)	<25	<36	>36	>36	>36

AR, Atrial regurgitation; *E/A,* Doppler ratio of early to late transmitral flow velocity; *IVRT,* isovolumetric relaxation time; *MV,* mitral valve; *PASP,* pulmonary artery systolic pressure; *PV,* pressure volume; *S/D,* systolic velocity/diastolic velocity; *TR,* tricuspid regurgitation.

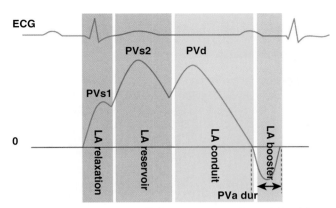

ECG

PVs2   PVd

PVs1

0

LA relaxation

LA reservoir

LA conduit

LA booster

PVa dur

Figure 35.2. Pulmonary vein (PV) flow, corresponding to left atrial (LA) function. *ECG*, electrocardiogram; *PVs1,* early systolic pulmonary vein flow; *PVs2,* late systolic pulmonary vein flow; *PVd,* diastolic pulmonary vein flow; *PVa dur,* duration of peak reverse flow velocity at atrial contraction. (Image courtesy of Luke J. Burchill, MBBS, PhD.)

from the transthoracic echocardiographic examination.[12] To properly obtain the PV flow with Doppler, the sample volume should be placed approximately 1 to 2 cm into the pulmonary vein, with the box size adjusted to 3 to 4 mm, Doppler filter set to 200 Hz, and sweep speed adjusted to 50 to 100 mm/s. The flow from the PV to the RA occurs in three phases: antegrade systolic, antegrade diastolic, and retrograde after atrial contraction. The normal pulmonary venous waveforms are quadriphasic, though they area often seen as triphasic. In 70% of patients, it is difficult to discriminate between the two systolic components of the PV flow. However, in patients with low filling pressures, systolic forward flow becomes biphasic, and the PV flow pattern is quadriphasic. The first phase is early systolic (PVs1). It occurs in early systole and represents the increase in pulmonary venous flow secondary to atrial relaxation. The second phase, late systolic (PVs2), occurs in mid to late systole. It is caused by the increase in pulmonary venous pressure propagated through the pulmonary arterial tree from the right side of the heart. The apical systolic annular motion of the mitral annulus is also believed to contribute to this finding. This phase reflects the reservoir function of the LA. The next phase is early diastole (PVd), which occurs during ventricular relaxation and is influenced by LV filling. It corresponds to transmitral E velocity and represents LA conduit function. The last phase is peak reversed flow velocity at atrial contraction (PVa or PV Ar), which occurs in late diastole; is influenced by late diastolic pressures in the LV, atrial preload, and LA contractility[13]; and reflects the LA booster function (Fig. 35.2). The PVa velocity and duration depend on atrial preload and contractility. Similar to the Valsalva maneuver, PV sampling has consistently ranked among the least feasible parameters but can be used as ancillary information when assessing LV filling pressures.

Pulmonary Veins Systolic/Diastolic Ratio

Under normal conditions, the PVs2 (S) wave should be greater than the PVd (D) wave, resulting in an S/D ratio is greater than 1. The PV flow pattern, however, is affected by several factors worth considering whenever interrogated. In young adults (age younger than 40 years), the diastolic wave typically predominates, reflecting rapid diastolic suction and filling during myocardial relaxation. With increasing age, the S/D ratio increases. As LA pressure increases, particularly with elevated LV filling pressures, the S wave velocity decreases, and the S/D ratio falls to less than 1. This comes as no surprise given systolic flow is governed by the pressure gradient between the pulmonary veins and the LA. The PV systolic fraction, which is the ratio of the velocity time integral (VTI) of the S wave to the sum of the S and D waves (PV systolic fraction = $S_{VTI}/[S_{VTI} + D_{VTI}]$), was shown predict LA pressure.[14] A PV systolic fraction

of less than 55% predicted a pulmonary capillary wedge pressure (PCWP) of 15 mm Hg or less, with a sensitivity of 91% and specificity of 87%.[14] A reduced PV systolic fraction (<40%) is related to decreased LA compliance and increased mean LA pressure in patients with poor LV systolic function. There is limited accuracy in patients with preserved LV systolic function (velocity >50%), atrial fibrillation, significant mitral regurgitation, and hypertrophic cardiomyopathy.

Reversed Pulmonary Venous Flow at Atrial Contraction

Atrial contraction results in flow within the LV as well as retrograde within the PVs. In normal subjects, reversed flow during the atrial contraction (Ar) velocities increase with age but rarely exceeds 35 cm/s. Consequently, increased Ar velocities (>35 cm/s) suggest elevated LVEDP.[15] In the presence of a noncompliant ventricle, the A wave duration is shortened (see earlier), and the Ar is prolonged. The prolonged time difference between Ar and mitral A wave duration (Ar-A) also indicates elevated LVEDP and can separate patients with abnormal LV relaxation from those with normal filling pressures and those with elevated LVEDPs but normal LA pressures. An Ar-A duration longer than 30 ms is predictive of an LVEDP greater than 20 mm Hg with high sensitivity (82%) and specificity (92%).[16] Additionally, Ar-A duration is the only indication of increased LV A wave pressure that is independent of age[15] and reliable in patients with depressed and preserved LV ejection (LVEF) fraction.[17] Atrial fibrillation results in a blunted S wave and the absence of Ar velocity. The primary limitation in interpreting PV flow is the difficulty in obtaining adequate Doppler signal, especially when assessing the Ar wave, which is often obscured by low-velocity LA wall motion.[18]

COLOR M-MODE FLOW PROPAGATION VELOCITY

During isovolumetric relaxation, the LV pressure drops without LV filling. The time constant of LV pressure decline known as tau (τ) is an index of LV relaxation that is relatively independent of heart rate and preload. It is well recognized that in early diastole, small but significant intraventricular mitral-to-apex pressure gradients are generated; these gradients are proposed to exert a ventricular suction effect.[19] Color M-mode velocity propagation (Vp) index, a noninvasive index of fluid acceleration, can mirror these intraventricular pressure gradients (IVPGs). It is also inversely related to the ventricular relaxation time constant τ: a faster rate of ventricle relaxation leads to a more rapid propagation of flow into the ventricle.[20] Color M-mode Doppler is a Doppler technique in which mean velocities are color coded and exhibited in time (on the horizontal axis) and depth (on the vertical axis), providing a spatiotemporal map of flow velocity along the scan line. Acquisition is made at end expiration in the A4C view using color flow imaging with a narrow color sector and the depth is adjusted to include the entire LV from the mitral leaflets to the apex. The M-mode scan line is located through the midline of the LV inflow blood column from the mitral valve to the apex. Then the color flow baseline is adapted to lower the Nyquist limit to plus or minus 75% of the spectral E velocity to obtain overflow ("aliasing") so that the central highest velocity jet is blue. The sweep speed of M-mode is typically set to 100 mm/s. Vp should be measured as the slope of the first aliasing velocity (red to blue) during early filling, from the mitral valve plane to 4 cm distally into the LV cavity.[21] A Vp less than 50 cm/s is consistent with diastolic dysfunction.

The most widely used index is E/Vp, which has been validated in a healthy population and in patients with hypertrophic cardiomyopathy,[22] dilated cardiomyopathy, and ischemic heart disease.[21] An E/Vp ratio greater than 1.5 can predict LVEDP greater than 12 mm Hg with high accuracy (sensitivity, 79%; specificity, 89%; positive predictive value, 93%; negative predictive value, 70%).[23] In addition, the E/Vp ratio has also been applied in patients with atrial fibrillation, and it is reasonably accurate for assessing

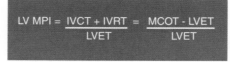

$$LV\ MPI = \frac{IVCT + IVRT}{LVET} = \frac{MCOT - LVET}{LVET}$$

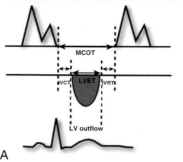

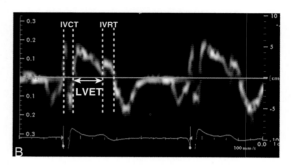

Figure 35.3. Myocardial performance (Tei) index obtained by (A) continuous wave/pulse wave Doppler and (B) tissue Doppler measured as the sum of isovolumetric contraction time *(IVCT)* and isovolumetric relaxation time *(IVRT)*, divided by the LV ejection time *(LVET)*. *MCOT,* Mitral valve closure to opening time (ms).

LVEDP. The measurement should be averaged for more than three heartbeats, and an E/Vp ratio of at least 1.4 yields a 100% specificity and 72% sensitivity in predicting a PCWP greater than 15 mm Hg.[24]

There are several potential limitations of the use of Vp as a measure of LV diastolic function. First, in many situations, the isovelocity contour may not be accurately described by a straight line, and Vp varies with the method used to determine the isovelocity contour. Also, E/Vp should be interpreted with caution in patients with preserved LVEF, especially in patients with normal LV volumes, because abnormal filling pressures can have a misleading normal Vp. Additionally, there are reports showing a positive influence of preload on Vp in patients with normal LVEF as well as those with depressed LVEF.[6] Overall, color M-mode for the evaluation of diastolic function is less used in most echocardiography laboratories but can be used as an ancillary measurement in assessing diastolic function.

TISSUE DOPPLER ANNULAR VELOCITY

The velocity of the mitral annulus represents velocity of changes in the LV long-axis dimension. In systole, the mitral annulus moves toward the LV apex. In diastole, it returns to its initial position in two phases generating two waveforms: (1) a rapid filling waveform (e′) dependent on active LV relaxation, elastic recoil, and the lengthening ventricle and (2) an atrial contraction waveform (a′) dependent on the contracting atrial fibers that pull the mitral annulus away from the apex.[4] This manifests on the tissue Doppler signal of mitral annulus as s′ (systolic velocity), e′ (early diastolic velocity), and a′ (late diastolic velocity).

The measurement of mitral annular velocities is an important component in interpreting the diastolic filling pattern, estimating LV filling pressures, and differentiating constrictive pericarditis from restrictive cardiomyopathies. These velocities are recorded from the A4C view by placing a 5- to 6-mm sample volume over the lateral or medial portion of the mitral annulus to cover the longitudinal excursion of the mitral annulus in both systole and diastole. The velocity scale should be set at about 20 cm/s above and below the zero-velocity baseline, and the angulation between the ultrasound beam and the plane of cardiac motion should be minimized. The recommendation for spectral recordings is a sweep speed of 50 to 100 mm/s at end-expiration, and measurements should be averaged for at least three consecutive cardiac cycles.[2]

The velocity of mitral annulus movement during early filling (e′) correlates modestly with the invasively measured time constant τ, but it is not solely determined by myocardial relaxation.[25] The e′ velocity is a measure of myocardial relaxation that is relatively independent of preload in patients with cardiac disease, whereas it appears load dependent in patients with normal systolic function.[8] In healthy and young persons, lateral e′ is 10 cm/s or greater, and

septal e′ is 7 cm/s or greater. These velocities increase with exercise and underlie diastolic LV suction. The e′ velocities fall with corresponding elevated E/e′ ratio because myocardial relaxation worsens with aging.[3] In patients with diastolic dysfunction, e′ is even more reduced than with age and remains reduced in all grades of diastolic dysfunction. Typically, the septal e′ is lower than the lateral e′ velocity. Early studies suggested septal E/e′ ratio of 8 or less is associated with normal PCWP, and an E/e′ ratio of 15 or higher suggests elevated PCWP.[11] When the value is between 8 and 15, other echocardiographic indices should be used. In the recent past, if E/e′ ratio is used, E/e′ ratio of at least 12 is a marker of elevated LV filling pressures in patients with preserved LVEF.[26] Based on the Normal Reference Ranges for Echocardiography Study (NORRE) study,[27] the current ASE guidelines for assessment of diastolic function recommends using an average of the septal and lateral annular velocities, in which an average E/e′ ratio of 14 or greater supports the presence of diastolic dysfunction and can also support the presence of elevated filling pressures, though this is not absolutely required.[2] However, there are certain situations when E/e′ may not provide an accurate assessment of PCWP, such as in normal hearts, in which e′ behaves as a load-dependent variable; in constrictive pericarditis, in which E/e′ does not increase despite elevated PCWP (annulus paradoxus)[28]; in mitral valve disease (mitral annular calcification, mitral stenosis, significant mitral regurgitation); and after mitral valve surgery (mitral valve annuloplasty or mitral valve replacement).[29] Additionally, several studies with conflicting results have questioned the robustness of the E/e′ ratio in estimating filling pressures in the setting of acutely decompensated advanced systolic heart failure, especially in patients with dilated LV, severely impaired cardiac output, cardiac resynchronization therapy,[30] and symptomatic hypertrophic cardiomyopathy.[31]

Several studies have assessed the time interval between the onset of the mitral E velocity and annular e′ velocity as an alternative for assessing LV filling pressure.[32,33] The ratio of isovolumic relaxation time to the time interval between E and e′ velocities has also been used to estimate filling pressures in patients with primary mitral valve disease.[29] Throughout the years, E/e′ has consistently demonstrated important prognostic information when elevated. In a recent meta-analysis of 18 manuscripts providing information on the prognostic implications of the studied echocardiographic parameters, E/e′ was associated with the highest risk of all-cause mortality and cardiovascular hospitalization.[34]

MYOCARDIAL PERFORMANCE INDEX

The myocardial performance index, or the Tei index, is based on Doppler-derived time intervals that combines both systolic and diastolic cardiac performance. Tei and colleagues[35] have shown that the Tei index is simply derived using conventional

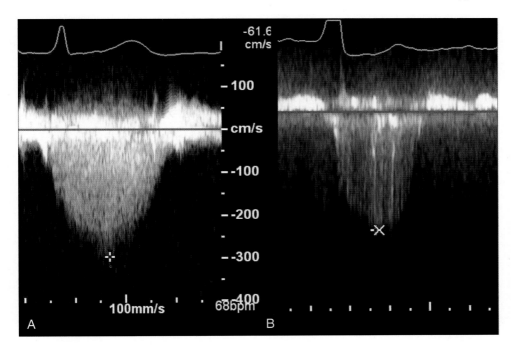

Figure 35.4. A, Continuous-wave (CW) Doppler of the tricuspid regurgitant jet demonstrating a peak velocity of 3 m/s (pulmonary artery systolic pressure, 36 mm Hg). **B,** Bubble contrast–enhanced CW Doppler of the insufficient regurgitant jet demonstrating a peak velocity of 2.4 m/s (23 mm Hg).

PW Doppler or tissue Doppler echocardiography, as shown in Fig. 35.3 A–B. An interval *a* between cessation and re-onset of mitral filling flow includes isovolumetric contraction time (IVCT), ejection time (ET), and IVRT. Interval *b* between onset and cessation of aortic ejection flow equals ET.[35] The mean normal value of the LV Tei index is 0.39 ± 0.05.[35] In adults, values of the LV Tei index below 0.40 are considered normal. Higher index values are correlated with more pathologic states of overall cardiac dysfunction. In systolic dysfunction, prolonged IVCT, prolonged IVRT, and a shortened ET were observed. In diastolic dysfunction, IVRT is the main feature.

The advantages of the Tei index are that it is noninvasive, easy to obtain, and reproducible. Moreover, a number of studies have proven that the Tei index is independent of arterial pressure, heart rate, atrioventricular valve regurgitation, ventricular geometry, afterload, and preload in patients who are supine. The Tei index has been shown to have robust prognostic value in several cardiac diseases, including dilated cardiomyopathy, pulmonary hypertension, cardiac amyloidosis, and myocardial infarction.[36] Similar to other methods, the limitations of this technique include (1) the impracticality of assessing the Tei index in patients with atrial fibrillation, frequent supraventricular and ventricular extra systoles and intraventricular conduction disturbances, ventricular pacing, and significant atrial tachycardia with mixing of the two transmitral flow waves; (2) its partial dependence on preload, although it is believed to be less dependent than other diastolic Doppler parameters; and (3) pseudonormalization of the index in patients who have restrictive physiology with preserved LV systolic function. In consequence, it has been removed from the recent recommendations for the assessment of LV diastolic function.

PULMONARY ARTERY SYSTOLIC PRESSURES

The association between heart disease and pulmonary hypertension is well described. Although pulmonary hypertension can complicate valvular heart disease or congenital heart defects, HFpEF remains the most studied population.[37] Pulmonary hypertension develops in response to a backward transmission of elevated filling pressure. These increased filling pressures can occur in the presence of diastolic dysfunction, mitral regurgitation, or a noncompliant LA. Bouchard and coworkers, in a cohort of 69 patients with preserved systolic function and in the setting or normal pulmonary vascular resistance, demonstrated a close correlation between pulmonary artery systolic pressure and PCWP.[38] In a community-based study of 1049 residents from Olmsted county, there was a significant association between pulmonary pressures and left atrial volume index, diastolic function grade, and left ventricular filling pressures (E/e').[38] Furthermore, long-standing backward transmission of pressures results in pulmonary arteriolar remodeling, medial hyperplasia, and intimal fibrosis, resulting in an increase in pulmonary pressures and eventually adding a precapillary component to a postcapillary problem.

Echocardiography remains a reliable tool to estimate pulmonary artery systolic pressures[39] by using the tricuspid regurgitation (TR) jet in the absence of pulmonary valve stenosis. Specifically, sampling the tricuspid regurgitant jet using CW Doppler determines the maximum velocity across the valve. Multiple angles and acoustic windows are often needed to sample this very direction dependent jet. It is recommended that the Doppler sweep speed be 100 mm/s for all tracings and that the baseline be shifted so as to have the tip of the dense envelope represent two-thirds of the frame. If the signal is weak or unreliable, contrast agents, including agitated saline (Fig. 35.4), are an excellent alternatives with caution to trace only the dense well-defined envelope and avoid overestimating.[6]

In patients with very severe TR, there is rapid equalization of the RV and RA pressures, resulting in a characteristic triangular-shaped Doppler profile, which is known to underestimate the maximum velocities. After a reliable sample of the maximum TR jet velocity is acquired, the simplified Bernoulli equation is applied in combination with the estimated right atrial pressures (Fig. 35.5) to give the estimated right ventricular systolic pressure and pulmonary artery systolic pressure (PASP) (in the absence of pulmonic valve stenosis). The literature is rather unclear on what is a normal estimated PASP. Normal invasive cutoffs, currently endorsed by the World Health Organization and the European Society of Cardiology,[37] is a PASP of 25 mm Hg. Moreover, PASP increases with age.[38] Consequently, normal cutoffs suggested in most echocardiography laboratories and endorsed by the ASE are pressures of 35 to 36 mm Hg, representing a Vmax of 2.8 m/s to 2.9 m/s.[40]

PASP is the latest addition to the arsenal of Doppler-based parameters for both the assessment of diastolic dysfunction as well as the grade of dysfunction[2] in the 2016 diastolic guidelines. This comes as no surprise given the link to elevated filling pressure, diastolic dysfunction, and its overall feasibility in most community and hospital-based studies.[38] Furthermore, PASP is an excellent tool to differentiate HFpEF from patients with hypertensive heart disease demonstrating incremental value to Doppler indices of

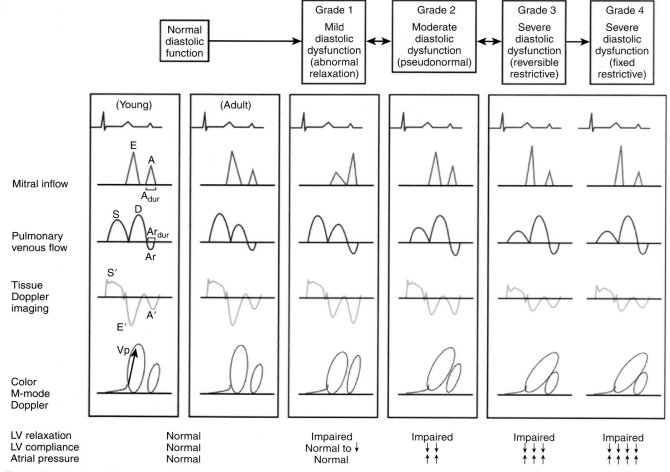

Figure 35.5. Grades of diastolic dysfunction. *A,* Mitral filling wave at atrial contraction; *a',* tissue Doppler mitral annular late diastolic velocity; *Adur,* mitral filling wave at atrial contraction duration; *Ar,* pulmonary venous reverse flow velocity at atrial contraction; *D,* pulmonary venous diastolic flow; *Diast,* diastole; *E,* mitral early filling wave; *e',* tissue Doppler mitral annular early diastolic tissue velocity; *LV,* left ventricular; *S,* pulmonary venous systolic flow; *s',* tissue Doppler mitral annular systolic velocity; *Syst,* systolic; *Vp,* color M-mode velocity propagation.

diastolic dysfunction such as (E/e').[41] PASP has very important prognostic value. In the two largest community-based studies investigating the role of PASP and heart disease, PASP has consistently demonstrated a strong association with mortality, whether it is in the presence of HFpEF (log rank $P = .003$) or in a community-based setting (hazard ratio, 2.07; 95% confidence interval, 1.62–2.64).[38]

INTEGRATION OF DOPPLER ECHOCARDIOGRAPHY PARAMETERS

The diastolic filling pattern is separated into distinct categories and simplified into LV diastolic function grades (see Fig. 35.5.) One should also take into consideration the effects of loading conditions on the diastolic filling pattern.

CONCLUSION

Integration of multiple Doppler echocardiography variables allows a comprehensive assessment of diastolic function in a wide variety of patients. It enables the diagnosis of underlying cardiac dysfunction, gives an estimate of LV filling pressures, guides heart failure therapy, and provides important prognostic information. The development of novel echocardiography techniques allows more advanced assessment of diastolic function; however, standard Doppler echocardiography remains the keystone of diastolic function assessment.

REFERENCES

1. Redfield MM, Jacobsen SJ, Burnett Jr JC, et al. Burden of systolic and diastolic ventricular dysfunction in the community. *J Am Med Assoc.* 2003;289:194.
2. Nagueh SF, Smiseth OA, Appleton CP, et al. Recommendations for the evaluation of left ventricular diastolic function by echocardiography. *J Am Soc Echocardiogr.* 2016;29:277–314.
3. Ommen SR, Nishimura RA. A clinical approach to the assessment of left ventricular diastolic function by Doppler echocardiography. *Heart.* 2003;89(suppl 3):iii18–23.
4. Silbiger JJ. Pathophysiology and echocardiographic diagnosis of left ventricular diastolic dysfunction. *J Am Soc Echocardiogr.* 2019;32:216–232.
5. Appleton CP. Influence of incremental changes in heart rate on mitral flow velocity: assessment in lightly sedated, conscious dogs. *J Am Coll Cardiol.* 1991;17:227–236.
6. Nagueh S, Appleton C, Gillebert T, et al. Recommendations for the evaluation of left ventricular diastolic function by echocardiography. *J Am Soc Echocardiog.* 2009;22:107–133.
7. Ha J-W, Oh JK, Redfield MM, et al. Triphasic mitral inflow velocity with mid-diastolic filling: clinical implications and associated echocardiographic findings. *J Am Soc Echocardiogr.* 2004;17:428–431.
8. Nagueh SF, Middleton KJ, Kopelen HA, et al. Doppler tissue imaging: a noninvasive technique for evaluation of left ventricular relaxation and estimation of filling pressures. *J Am Coll Cardiol.* 1997;30:1527–1533.
9. Dumesnil JG, Gaudreault G, Honos GN, Kingma JGJ. Use of Valsalva maneuver to unmask left ventricular diastolic function abnormalities by Doppler echocardiography in patients with coronary artery disease or systemic hypertension. *Am J Cardiol.* 1991;68:515–519.
10. Khan S, Bess RL, Rosman HS, et al. Which echocardiographic Doppler left ventricular diastolic function measurements are most feasible in the clinical echocardiographic laboratory? *Am J Cardiol.* 2004;94:1099–1101.
11. Ommen SR, Nishimura RA, Appleton CP, et al. Clinical utility of Doppler echocardiography and tissue Doppler imaging in the estimation of left ventricular filling pressures: a comparative simultaneous Doppler-catheterization study. *Circulation.* 2000;102:1788–1794.

12. Quinones MA, Otto CM, Stoddard M, et al. Recommendations for quantification of Doppler echocardiography. *J Am Soc Echocardiogr.* 2002;15:167–184.
13. Cameli M, Sparla S, Losito M, et al. Correlation of left atrial strain and Doppler measurements with invasive measurement of left ventricular end-diastolic pressure in patients stratified for different values of ejection fraction. *Echocardiography.* 2016;33:398–405.
14. Kuecherer HF, Muhiudeen IA, Kusumoto FM, et al. Estimation of mean left atrial pressure from transesophageal pulsed Doppler echocardiography of pulmonary venous flow. *Circulation.* 1990;82:1127–1139.
15. Klein AL, Tajik AJ. Doppler assessment of pulmonary venous flow in healthy subjects and in patients with heart disease. *J Am Soc Echocardiogr.* 1991;4:379–392.
16. Dini FL, Michelassi C, Micheli G, Rovai D. Prognostic value of pulmonary venous flow Doppler signal in left ventricular dysfunction: contribution of the difference in duration of pulmonary venous and mitral flow at atrial contraction. *J Am Coll Cardiol.* 2000;36:1295–1302.
17. Yamamoto K, Nishimura RA, Burnett JCJ, Redfield MM. Assessment of left ventricular end-diastolic pressure by Doppler echocardiography: contribution of duration of pulmonary venous versus mitral flow velocity curves at atrial contraction. *J Am Soc Echocardiogr.* 1997;10:52. –59.
18. Bess RL, Khan S, Rosman HS, et al. Technical aspects of diastology: why mitral inflow and tissue Doppler imaging are the preferred parameters. *Echocardiography.* 2006;23:332–339.
19. Courtois M, Kovacs SJJ, Ludbrook PA. Transmitral pressure-flow velocity relation. Importance of regional pressure gradients in the left ventricle during diastole. *Circulation.* 1988;78:661–671.
20. Brun P, Tribouilloy C, Duval AM, et al. Left ventricular flow propagation during early filling is related to wall relaxation: a color M-mode Doppler analysis. *J Am Coll Cardiol.* 1992;20:420–432.
21. Garcia MJ, Ares MA, Asher C, et al. An index of early left ventricular filling that combined with pulsed Doppler peak E velocity may estimate capillary wedge pressure. *J Am Coll Cardiol.* 1997;29:448–454.
22. Nagueh SF, Lakkis NM, Middleton KJ, et al. Doppler estimation of left ventricular filling pressures in patients with hypertrophic cardiomyopathy. *Circulation.* 1999;99:254–261.
23. Firstenberg MS, Levine BD, Garcia MJ, et al. Relationship of echocardiographic indices to pulmonary capillary wedge pressures in healthy volunteers. *J Am Coll Cardiol.* 2000;36:1664–1669.
24. Nagueh SF, Kopelen HA, Quinones MA. Assessment of left ventricular filling pressures by Doppler in the presence of atrial fibrillation. *Circulation.* 1996;94(9):2138–2145.
25. Opdahl A, Remme EW, Helle-Valle T, et al. Determinants of left ventricular early-diastolic lengthening velocity: independent contributions from left ventricular relaxation, restoring forces, and lengthening load. *Circulation.* 2009;119:2578–2586.
26. Gabriel RS, Klein AL. Modern evaluation of left ventricular diastolic function using Doppler echocardiography. *Curr Cardiol Rep.* 2009;11:231–238.
27. Caballero L, Kou S, Dulgheru R, et al. Echocardiographic reference ranges for normal cardiac Doppler data: results from the NORRE Study. *Eur Heart J Cardiovasc Imag.* 2015;16:1031–1041.
28. Oh JK, Hatle L, Tajik AJ, Little WC. Diastolic heart failure can be diagnosed by comprehensive two-dimensional and Doppler echocardiography. *J Am Coll Cardiol.* 2006;47:500–506.
29. Diwan A, McCulloch M, Lawrie GM, et al. Doppler estimation of left ventricular filling pressures in patients with mitral valve disease. *Circulation.* 2005;111:3281–3289.
30. Mullens W, Borowski AG, Curtin RJ, et al. Tissue Doppler imaging in the estimation of intracardiac filling pressure in decompensated patients with advanced systolic heart failure. *Circulation.* 2009;119:62–70.
31. Geske JB, Sorajja P, Nishimura RA, Ommen SR. Evaluation of left ventricular filling pressures by Doppler echocardiography in patients with hypertrophic cardiomyopathy: correlation with direct left atrial pressure measurement at cardiac catheterization. *Circulation.* 2007;116:2702–2708.
32. Rivas-Gotz C, Khoury DS, Manolios M, et al. Time interval between onset of mitral inflow and onset of early diastolic velocity by tissue Doppler: a novel index of left ventricular relaxation: experimental studies and clinical application. *J Am Coll Cardiol.* 2003;42:1463–1470.
33. Sohn D-W, Kim Y-J, Park Y-B, Choi Y-S. Clinical validity of measuring time difference between onset of mitral inflow and onset of early diastolic mitral annulus velocity in the evaluation of left ventricular diastolic function. *J Am Coll Cardiol.* 2004;43:2097–2101.
34. Nauta JF, Hummel YM, van der Meer P, et al. Correlation with invasive left ventricular filling pressures and prognostic relevance of the echocardiographic diastolic parameters used in the 2016 ESC heart failure guidelines and in the 2016 ASE/EACVI recommendations. *Eur J Heart Fail.* 2018;20:1303–1311.
35. Tei C, Ling LH, Hodge DO, et al. New index of combined systolic and diastolic myocardial performance: a simple and reproducible measure of cardiac function-a study in normals and dilated cardiomyopathy. *J Cardiol.* 1995;26:357–366.
36. Karatzis EN, Giannakopoulou AT, Papadakis JE, et al. Myocardial performance index (Tei index): evaluating its application to myocardial infarction. *Hellenic J Cardiol.* 2009;50:60–65.
37. Galie N, Humbert M, Vachiery J-L, et al. 2015 ESC/ERS Guidelines for the diagnosis and treatment of pulmonary hypertension. *Eur Heart J.* 2016;37:67–119.
38. Bursi F, McNallan SM, Redfield MM, et al. Pulmonary pressures and death in heart failure: a community study. *J Am Coll Cardiol.* 2012;59:222–231.
39. Yock PG, Popp RL. Noninvasive estimation of right ventricular systolic pressure by Doppler ultrasound in patients with tricuspid regurgitation. *Circulation.* 1984;70:657–662.
40. Badesch DB, Champion HC, Sanchez MAG, et al. Diagnosis and assessment of pulmonary arterial hypertension. *J Am Coll Cardiol.* 2009;54(1 Suppl):S55–S66.
41. Lam CSP, Roger VL, Rodeheffer RJ, et al. Pulmonary hypertension in heart failure with preserved ejection fraction: a community-based study. *J Am Coll Cardiol.* 2009;53(13):1119–1126.

36 Clinical Recommendations for Echocardiography Laboratories for Assessment of Left Ventricular Diastolic Function and Filling Pressures

Sherif F. Nagueh

Many patients are referred to the echocardiography laboratory with complaints of dyspnea. These include patients with normal and depressed left ventricular (LV) ejection fraction (EF). It is important to determine whether symptoms in these patients have a cardiac cause or not because this can have therapeutic implications for decisions that include the use and titration of diuretics. Of note, many patients with LV systolic dysfunction have normal LV filling pressure and have dyspnea from noncardiac causes. Therefore, one should not rely solely on LVEF to draw inferences about LV filling pressures.

A comprehensive echocardiographic examination is essential for reaching the correct diagnosis. This includes acquisition of satisfactory two-dimensional (2D) and Doppler signals, including mitral inflow, pulmonary venous flow, pulmonary regurgitation (PR) and tricuspid regurgitation (TR) peak velocities by continuous-wave (CW) Doppler from multiple windows, and mitral annulus velocities by tissue Doppler (TD). For patients who can perform a Valsalva maneuver, the change in mitral inflow pattern may be helpful in identifying patients with increased LV filling pressures. The inflow pattern in these cases changes from pseudo-normal filling to an impaired relaxation pattern.[1] In addition, in some cases, flow propagation velocity (Vp) and untwisting measurements can provide useful insights into the mechanisms behind diastolic dysfunction, though they are usually not needed in day-to-day clinical applications.[1,2] On the other hand, there is growing interest in the clinical applications of LV diastolic strain rate during the isovolumic relaxation period and during early diastole, as well as left atrial (LA) reservoir strain.[2] Echocardiographic Doppler parameters of diastolic function are discussed in detail in Chapter 35.

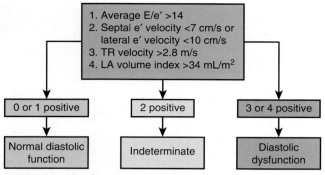

Figure 36.1. Algorithm for assessment of left ventricular diastolic function in patients without apparent myocardial disease. *LA*, Left atrium; *TR*, tricuspid regurgitation.

ESTIMATION OF LEFT VENTRICULAR FILLING PRESSURE AND LEFT VENTRICULAR DIASTOLIC FUNCTION GRADING

In 2016, the American Society of Echocardiography (ASE) and the European Association of Cardiovascular Imaging (EACVI) published an updated diastolic function assessment guidelines document with the objectives of simplifying the approach and decreasing the interobserver variability in determining LV filling pressure and grading LV diastolic function.[2] Emphasis was placed on fewer variables, namely (1) mitral inflow velocities, (2) biplane LA maximum volume, (3) peak tricuspid regurgitation (TR) velocity, and (4) mitral annulus early diastolic velocity (e′) at the septal and lateral sides of the mitral annulus.

The guidelines emphasized the importance of taking the clinical context into account, as well as other 2D and Doppler findings. The writing group recognized the coexistence of LV systolic and diastolic dysfunction in most patients with cardiac disease. This relation highlights the importance of identifying LV systolic dysfunction, whether it is with LVEF or global longitudinal strain (GLS). Other indicators of myocardial disease and diastolic dysfunction include pathologic LV hypertrophy and LA enlargement in patients with hypertension or aortic stenosis in the absence of atrial fibrillation and mitral valve disease. Likewise, segmental dysfunction in patients with coronary artery disease (CAD) is often associated with diastolic dysfunction. Specific Doppler signals that by themselves are indicative of abnormal elevated LV filling pressure include the change in mitral inflow pattern with Valsalva as described earlier, the presence of pathologic middiastolic L wave in mitral inflow (≥50 cm/s), increased amplitude or duration of pulmonary vein atrial wave (Ar), and discordant mitral inflow and tricuspid inflow. In patients with normal intravascular volume and filling pressure, right ventricular (RV) inflow and LV inflow are concordant in that predominant early diastolic filling of RV and LV occurs. However, when there are LV diastolic dysfunction and elevated LA pressure but still normal mean right atrial (RA) pressure, the tricuspid E/A ratio is less than 1, whereas the mitral E/A ratio is greater than 1.

The ASE/EACVI guidelines provide two algorithms for assessment of LV diastolic function and filling pressures. Algorithm A is for patients with normal LVEF and no myocardial disease (Fig. 36.1), and algorithm B for patients with depressed LVEF and patients with myocardial disease and normal LVEF (Fig. 36.2).

Algorithm A

This algorithm applies to subjects with normal LVEF and no myocardial disease (see Fig. 36.1). In the absence of myocardial disease and in situations when it is not possible to determine if myocardial disease is present, the 2016 guidelines update recommends relying on four signals: septal and lateral e′ velocities, average E/e′ ratio (based on average of septal and lateral e′ velocities), peak TR jet,

and biplane LA maximum volume index. Based on the number of available variables indicative of diastolic dysfunction (variables with values that met or exceeded the cutoff values), one of three conclusions is reached: normal, abnormal, or indeterminate diastolic function. The proportion of cases with indeterminate diastolic function is lower in laboratories that acquire more complete datasets and that take into account all clinical, 2D, and Doppler findings.

Algorithm B

This algorithm applies to patients in sinus rhythm who have either depressed LVEF or have myocardial disease and normal LVEF (see Fig. 36.2). This algorithm allows for simultaneous estimation of LV filling pressures and grading of LV diastolic dysfunction. The guidelines explicitly state that the recommendations are geared for estimating early diastolic pressures, namely mean LA pressure, mean wedge pressure, mean LV diastolic pressure, and mean LV pre-A diastolic pressure. All of these previously mentioned pressures have strong correlations with one another in the absence of mitral valve disease and have similar Doppler correlates. This algorithm, which applies to patients in sinus rhythm, starts with mitral E/A ratio and peak E velocity. Patients are classified into one of three groups:

- Grade I diastolic dysfunction with impaired relaxation and normal LV filling pressures (E/A ratio ≤0.8 and E ≤50 cm/s)
- Grade II diastolic dysfunction (E/A ratio >0.8 but <2 or E/A ratio ≤0.8 but E>50 cm/s)
- Grade III diastolic dysfunction (E/A ratio ≥2)

For patients to be assigned to group II diastolic dysfunction, additional variables should be evaluated, including average E/e′ ratio, biplane LA maximum volume index, and peak TR velocity. The majority of the available variables (two of two, two of three, or three of three) should be in the abnormally elevated range to support assigning a given patient grade II diastolic dysfunction (average E/e′ >14, biplane LA maximum volume index >34 mL/m², peak TR velocity >2.8 m/s).

This approach does not apply to patients with hypertrophic cardiomyopathy, mitral stenosis or mitral regurgitation (MR), severe aortic regurgitation, moderate or severe mitral annulus calcification, atrial fibrillation, or left bundle branch block or ventricular paced rhythm; patients with group I or groups III, IV, or V pulmonary hypertension; patients with advanced heart block; heart transplant recipients; and patients with LV assist devices.

STRESS TESTING FOR ASSESSMENT OF DIASTOLIC FUNCTION

When patients have symptoms of exertional dyspnea but normal LV filling pressure at rest, one should proceed to diastolic stress testing to determine if the patient develops increased LV filling pressure with exercise (average E/e′ ratio >14) along with increased peak TR velocity (>2.8 m/s) with exercise (thus increased pulmonary artery [PA] systolic pressure). If confirmed, the latter findings support the diagnosis of cardiac cause of dyspnea and heart failure with preserved LVEF. The guidelines were validated in a large multicenter study that included 450 patients. In the study, echocardiographic assessment of LV filling pressure was superior to clinical evaluation and had good accuracy in patients with normal LV EF, obesity, or pulmonary disease.[3] Furthermore, the guidelines update has excellent interobserver reproducibility.[4]

ESTIMATION OF LEFT VENTRICULAR FILLING PRESSURES IN PATIENTS WITH ATRIAL FIBRILLATION

Frequently, patients with atrial fibrillation are referred for the assessment of LV function, including filling pressures. Similar

Clinical Recommendations for Echocardiography Laboratories for Assessment of Left Ventricular Diastolic Function and Filling Pressures **223**

36

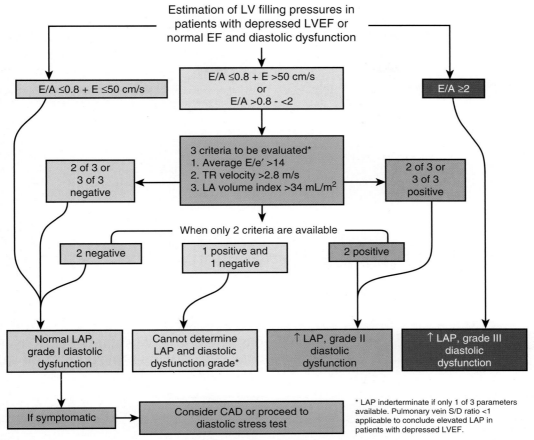

Figure 36.2. Algorithm for assessment of left ventricular (LV) filling pressures and grading diastolic function in patients with myocardial disease, including patients with normal or depressed LV ejection fraction (LVEF). *CAD,* Coronary artery disease; *LAP,* left atrial pressure.

to patients in sinus rhythm, mitral inflow relates well to filling pressures in patients with depressed LVEF and a short E-wave deceleration time (DT) (≤150 ms) has good accuracy in identifying these patients. When LVEF is normal, other parameters can be applied. LV filling pressures are elevated with a septal E/e′ ratio greater than 11, an IVRT 65 ms or less, a peak acceleration rate of mitral E velocity 1900 cm/s^2 or greater, an E/Vp ratio ≥1.4, a DT of pulmonary vein diastolic velocity 220 ms or less, and PA systolic pressure greater than 35 mm Hg. Furthermore, examining the beat-to-beat variability in mitral inflow in patients with atrial fibrillation can be of value in predicting filling pressures. When LA pressure is elevated, there is usually little variation in Doppler measurements (peak and mean E velocity, peak acceleration rate and DT) when cycle length varies. However, with a normal or reduced LA pressure, the coefficient of variation in Doppler measurements is large and is related to the RR interval.[5] These findings need not be quantified but could be used as a screening tool in Doppler recordings at slower sweep speeds of 25 to 50 mm/s.

ESTIMATION OF LEFT VENTRICULAR FILLING PRESSURES IN PATIENTS WITH MITRAL REGURGITATION

Moderately severe and severe MR affect LV filling independent of diastolic function. Therefore, it is often challenging to estimate filling pressures in these patients. Similar to the approach outlined earlier, evaluation of LV diastolic function depends on whether LVEF is normal or depressed. With depressed EF,

a short DT and increased E/e′ ratio usually predict elevated LV filling pressures as well as clinical outcomes.[1,2] With normal EF, other measurements are needed including pulmonary vein Ar (atrial reversal velocity) duration and the time delay between mitral E velocity and annular e′ velocity because patients with impaired LV relaxation have a reduced and a delayed e′ velocity.[6] Furthermore, an elevated PA systolic pressure in this population when it occurs is usually caused by increased LA pressure. However, elevated LA pressure can occur because of severe MR in the absence of LV diastolic dysfunction; therefore, pulmonary vein Ar velocity and annular e′ delay are unique markers identifying the presence of increased LV end-diastolic pressure and impaired LV relaxation and thus diastolic dysfunction.

PROGNOSTIC POWER OF AMERICAN SOCIETY OF ECHOCARDIOGRAPHY/EUROPEAN ASSOCIATION OF CARDIOVASCULAR IMAGING DIASTOLIC FUNCTION GRADE

Grading of LV diastolic function is an important predictor of outcomes. This has been shown in several studies including community-based studies.[7,8] More recently, the 2016 guidelines update was shown to successfully predict outcome in several patient populations, including patients presenting with acute myocardial infarction and patients referred for evaluation of heart failure.[9–11] Therefore, it is important to include comments on LV filling pressures and diastolic function grade in echocardiography reports.

REFERENCES

1. Nagueh SF, Appleton CP, Gillebert TC, et al. Recommendations for the evaluation of left ventricular diastolic function by echocardiography. *J Am Soc Echocardiogr.* 2009;22:107–133.
2. Nagueh SF, Smiseth OA, Appleton CP, et al. Recommendations for the evaluation of left ventricular diastolic function by echocardiography. *J Am Soc Echocardiogr.* 2016;29:277–314.
3. Andersen OS, Smiseth OA, Dokainish H, et al. Estimating left ventricular filling pressure by echocardiography. *J Am Coll Cardiol.* 2017;69:1937–1948.
4. Nagueh SF, Abraham TP, Aurigemma GP, et al. Interobserver variability in applying American Society of Echocardiography/European Association of Cardiovascular Imaging 2016 guidelines for estimation of left ventricular filling pressure. *Circ Cardiovasc Imag.* 2019;12:e008122.
5. Nagueh SF, Kopelen HA, Quiñones MA. Assessment of left ventricular filling pressure by Doppler in the presence of atrial fibrillation. *Circulation.* 1996;94:2138–2145.
6. Diwan A, McCulloch M, Lawrie G, et al. Doppler estimation of left ventricular filling pressures in patients with mitral valve disease. *Circulation.* 2005;111:3281–3289.
7. Kane GC, Karon BL, Mahoney DW, et al. Progression of left ventricular diastolic dysfunction and the risk of heart failure. *J Am Med Assoc.* 2011;306:856–863.
8. Aljaroudi W, Alraies MC, Halley C, et al. Impact of progression of diastolic dysfunction on mortality in patients with normal ejection fraction. *Circulation.* 2012;125:782–788.
9. Prasad SB, Lin AK, Guppy-Coles KB, et al. Diastolic dysfunction assessed using contemporary guidelines and prognosis following myocardial infarction. *J Am Soc Echocardiogr.* 2018;31:1127–1136.
10. Sanchis L, Andrea R, Falces C, et al. Differential clinical implications of current recommendations for the evaluation of left ventricular diastolic function by echocardiography. *J Am Soc Echocardiogr.* 2018;31:1203–1208.
11. Tennøe AH, Murbræch K, Andreassen JC, et al. Left ventricular diastolic dysfunction predicts mortality in patients with systemic sclerosis. *J Am Coll Cardiol.* 2018;72:1804–1813.

37 Causes of Diastolic Dysfunction

John B. Dickey, Gerard P. Aurigemma

DEFINITIONS

Diastolic dysfunction can be defined as an abnormality in the ability of the left ventricle to fill at normal pressure. Diastolic dysfunction, unlike heart failure with preserved ejection fraction (HFpEF) or diastolic heart failure, is not a clinical diagnosis but rather refers to a pathophysiologic abnormality that can be the basis of the clinical syndrome HFpEF.

Two principal mechanisms are responsible for diastolic dysfunction: impaired active ventricular relaxation and increased passive myocardial stiffness (or decreased compliance). Relaxation comprises a series of energy-consuming steps starting with the release of calcium from troponin C and ending with extension of the sarcomeres to their resting length. This process encompasses two distinct phases: isovolumetric relaxation (drop in left ventricular [LV] pressure at a constant volume) and auxotonic relaxation (contraction to accommodate an increasing volume load during LV filling). The relationship between LV diastolic pressure and volume characterizes ventricular stiffness ($\Delta P/\Delta V$) and ventricular compliance ($\Delta V/\Delta P$). Both intracellular and extracellular structures affect stiffness, including LV mass and LV mass-to-volume ratio, in addition to the intrinsic stiffness of the myocardium.[1,2] Echocardiographic assessment of diastolic dysfunction is performed using two-dimensional (2D) imaging, transmitral and pulmonary vein Doppler, tissue Doppler of the mitral annulus, and strain imaging. These are each addressed in their respective chapters.

DIASTOLIC HEART FAILURE VERSUS HEART FAILURE WITH PRESERVED EJECTION FRACTION

Diastolic heart failure and HFpEF refer to a clinical syndrome of heart failure; the terms are overlapping but not synonymous. As we use the terms, HFpEF is a broader clinical syndrome wherein LV diastolic dysfunction may or may not be the primary pathophysiologic derangement. In this usage, HFpEF can be caused by valvular (e.g., acute, severe mitral regurgitation), pericardial disease (e.g., constrictive pericarditis), or myocardial (diastolic heart failure) disease. The term *diastolic heart failure* implies myocardial disease and is the most common cause of HFpEF. In this chapter, myocardial causes of diastolic dysfunction are discussed; pericardial and valvular etiologies are discussed elsewhere.

COMORBIDITIES ASSOCIATED WITH HEART FAILURE WITH PRESERVED EJECTION FRACTION

Diastolic dysfunction is highly prevalent.[3–8] Using predefined echocardiographic criteria, some degree of diastolic dysfunction was found in nearly 30% of the total population, whereas systolic dysfunction was found in only 6.0%. Redfield and colleagues established that nearly 6% of patients had moderate to severe diastolic dysfunction.[4] The incidence increases with age, and at any given age, it is more common among women by a factor of 2 to 1. It is associated with multiple comorbidities, such as hypertension, diabetes mellitus, obesity, coronary heart disease (CHD), and infiltrative cardiomyopathies (Fig. 37.1). The prevalence of these comorbidities in diastolic dysfunction has been established through multiple large-scale, cross-sectional studies (Table 37.1).[9–13] Multiple population-based studies showing that 40% to 50% of all patients with congestive heart failure (CHF) can have a normal EF.[4–6] As noted earlier, the term *HFpEF* is increasingly applied to this syndrome. The prevalences of preclinical (i.e., no diagnosis of CHF before participation in the study) diastolic dysfunction were 20.6% for mild diastolic dysfunction and 6.8% for moderate to severe diastolic dysfunction. In a high-risk population (age at least 65 years of age plus presence of hypertension or coronary artery disease [CHD]), the prevalence of preclinical diastolic dysfunction increased significantly to 47.6% in mild diastolic dysfunction and 16.5% in moderate to severe diastolic dysfunction. Table 37.2 lists the conditions resulting in diastolic dysfunction as well as their predominant mechanisms.

Hypertension

Hypertension is the most common reason for development of diastolic dysfunction and occurs in 55% to 86% of patients with HFpEF.[14] Often, echocardiographic evidence of diastolic dysfunction is present in hypertensive patients far in advance of any heart failure symptoms.[4,15] Chronic pressure overload causes progressive cardiomyocyte hypertrophy, enhanced collagen deposition, and microvascular rarefaction with subclinical myocardial ischemia. Over time, this results in LV hypertrophy (LVH) with higher myocardial oxygen demand, eventually leading to increased myocardial stiffness during both systole and diastole and impaired relaxation.[1,2]

The kidneys are also intricately entwined in this process. Glomerular filtration declines as arterial stiffness and pulse pressure increase, causing renal dysfunction, which in turn worsens hypertension.[15] As vascular stiffness increases with age, so too does the prevalence of diastolic dysfunction, although studies have demonstrated that systolic and diastolic myocardial stiffness also both increase with age, independent of arterial load.[16]

Coronary Heart Disease

It has long been established that acute ischemia can cause diastolic dysfunction. Recurrent transient ischemia in patients with CHD and stable angina, however, has been shown to lead to patchy fibrosis in predominantly subendocardial tissue of

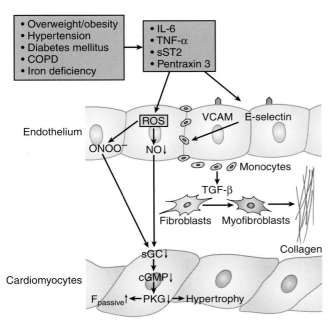

Figure 37.1. Myocardial remodeling in heart failure with preserved ejection fraction: importance of comorbidities. *COPD,* Chronic obstructive pulmonary disease; $F_{passive}$, resting tension; *cGMP,* cyclic guanosine monophosphate; *IL-6,* interleukin-6; *NO,* nitric oxide; *ONOO–,* peroxynitrite; *PKG,* cGMP-dependent protein kinase; *ROS,* reactive oxygen species; *sGC,* soluble guanylyl cyclase; *sST2,* somatostatin receptor 2; *TGF-β,* transforming growth factor-β; *TNF-α,* tumor necrosis factor-α; *VCAM,* vascular cell adhesion protein.

patients with exercise-induced ischemia.[17] The exercise-induced dysfunction of the ischemic segments places a chronic stress overload on the nonischemic segments, however, and structural changes in the nonischemic segments (cardiomyocyte hypertrophy and fibrosis) can be seen here as well. The structural changes in chronic ischemia can be similar to those seen in chronic pressure overload.[17,18] Diastolic dysfunction is detectable at rest in ischemic segments in chronic CHD, and the extent of these changes correlates with the degree of ischemia as determined by coronary angiography.[19]

Diabetes Mellitus

Distinctly separate from diabetes-related CHD is the entity of diabetic cardiomyopathy, a common and, in the opinion of some, underdiagnosed cause of cardiovascular morbidity in patients with diabetes. First described by Rubler and coworkers,[20] diabetic cardiomyopathy is defined as abnormal myocardial function in the absence of hypertension, valvular disease, or CHD. Because these conditions frequently coexist, an isolated diagnosis of its prevalence is thought to range from 30% to 60%.[4,21–24] The mechanisms of diabetic cardiomyopathy remain under investigation and are believed to include chronic hyperglycemia, insulin resistance, altered lipid metabolism with cardiac steatosis, microvascular disease, cardiac autonomic dysfunction, and changes in the renin–angiotensin system.[25]

Hyperglycemia exerts its detrimental effects on ventricular function via multiple direct and indirect pathways. Increased glucose metabolism escalates the mitochondrial production of reactive oxygen species (ROS), which damage DNA and accelerate cardiomyocyte apoptosis and myocardial fibrosis.[26] Advanced glycation end products (AGEs), which are present at higher levels in people with diabetes, further contribute by cross-linking collagen and elastin both within and outside the cell. The presence of AGEs leads to increased myocardial stiffness and impaired relaxation.[26–28] By upregulating certain receptors, AGEs activate transcription factors (e.g., nuclear factor κB [NF-κB]) and proinflammatory cytokines (including tumor necrosis factor-α [TNF-α]).[29]

Chevali and associates[30] hypothesized that cardiac remodeling in diabetic cardiomyopathy progresses through three stages. An early, usually asymptomatic stage with myocardial damage primarily at the molecular level can manifest as LVH with abnormal diastolic function. These structural changes are subtle and can only be ascertained using very sensitive techniques such as strain imaging, strain rate, and tissue velocity. During the middle stage, cardiomyocyte hypertrophy and fibrosis progress with worsening of diastolic function, which can be assessed using conventional echocardiographic techniques. These

TABLE 37.1 Characteristics of Patients With Heart Failure With Preserved Ejection Fraction in Epidemiologic Studies

	Tribouilloy et al.,[9] 2008	Buris et al.,[74] 2006	Owan et al.,[10] 2006	Bhatia et al.,[11] 2006	Masoudi et al.,[12] 2003	Lenzen et al.,[13] 2004
Country	France	United States	United States	Canada	United States	Europe
HFpEF Definition						
Patients, *n*	368	308	2167	880	6754	3148
Age, yr	76	77	74	75	80	71
Male sex, %	47	43	44	34	29	45
LVEF, %	63	—	61	62	—	56
Comorbidities, %						
Hypertension	74	86	63	55	69	59
Diabetes	26	36	33	32	37	26
Myocardial infarction	9	36	—	17	21	—
CHD or ischemia	28	—	53	36	46	59
Stroke or TIA	5	—	—	15	17	16
Atrial fibrillation	36	31	41	32	36	25

CHD, Coronary heart disease; *HFpEF,* heart failure with preserved ejection fraction; *LVEF,* left ventricular ejection fraction; *TIA,* transient ischemic attack.
Adapted with permission from Zile MR, Brutsaert DL: New concepts in diastolic dysfunction and diastolic heart failure: part II: causal mechanisms and treatment, *Circulation* 105:1503–1508, 2002.

TABLE 37.2 Conditions Resulting in Diastolic Dysfunction and Their Predominant Mechanisms

Condition	Predominant Mechanism	Diastolic Dysfunction Present
Hypertension	Increased afterload Myocardial fibrosis	+ − +++
Coronary artery disease	Ischemia Myocardial fibrosis	+ − +++
Diabetes mellitus	Hyperglycemia Coexistent CHD and HTN	+ − +++
Hypertrophic cardiomyopathy	Myocardial disarray Fibrosis Afterload	++ − +++++
Restrictive cardiomyopathy	Fibrosis Direct cellular injury Infiltration	+++ − +++++

CHD, Coronary heart disease; *DM*, diabetes mellitus; *HCM*, hypertrophic cardiomyopathy; *HTN*, hypertension; *RCM*, restrictive cardiomyopathy.

processes continue, and eventually systolic dysfunction occurs. The late stage is often accompanied by overt heart failure, microvascular and macrovascular CHD, hypertension, and cardiac autonomic neuropathy.

Obesity

Obesity is much more common in patients with diastolic dysfunction than those with systolic dysfunction. It contributes directly to development of diastolic dysfunction by increasing the hemodynamic load on the heart. Obesity also has indirect effects; as a state of chronic inflammation, obesity is associated with elevated levels of proinflammatory cytokines, which can cause diastolic dysfunction, as described earlier. Obese patients frequently also have hypertension, CHD, and diabetes, all of which are independent risk factors for development of diastolic dysfunction. Finally, both obstructive and central sleep apnea are common in obese individuals, and these have been implicated in the progression of diastolic dysfunction to clinically apparent heart failure.[31]

Hypertrophic Cardiomyopathy

Hypertrophic cardiomyopathy (HCM) is another frequently encountered condition (1 in 500 among the general population worldwide[32]) in which diastolic dysfunction is prevalent. HCM is the most common of the inherited cardiac disorders,[32] and it is discussed in detail in other chapters. HCM results from 1 or more of 1400 mutations in 11 genes coding for sarcomere proteins. The age of manifestation as well as disease progression can vary considerably between individuals. Diastolic dysfunction is one of the defining characteristics of HCM and can be caused by several mechanisms, including increased afterload, myocardial fibrosis, and myocardial hypertrophy. Olivotto and associates[33] have proposed a classification of this phenotypically heterogeneous disease into four clinical grades, which differ in mechanism: (1) nonhypertrophic (grade I), (2) "classic" phenotype (grade II), (3) adverse remodeling (grade III), and (4) overt dysfunction (grade IV). Even in patients with genotype-positive nonhypertrophic disease, sarcomere function is altered to the extent that intracellular calcium and energy homeostasis are disrupted, and subtle echocardiographic evidence of diastolic dysfunction, such as impaired relaxation and left atrial (LA) dilatation, may already be evident.[34] These become more pronounced as HCM progresses and are generally accompanied by a gradual decline in LVEF.[33] In grade II, LVH is believed to result from both disrupted energy balance within the sarcomere (increased adenosine triphosphate requirement) and impaired relaxation caused by malfunction of mechanisms by which contraction normally ceases at low cytosolic calcium concentrations.[35,36]

These processes culminate in grades III and IV, when cardiomyocyte energy depletion results in apoptosis with myocyte loss and fibrotic transformation of the myocardium. These are compounded by microvascular ischemia inherent in the progression of LVH.[35,36] More recent research by Coppini and coworkers[37] suggests that enhanced late sodium currents in cardiomyocytes of patients with HCM also interfere with intracellular calcium handling, independent of sarcomeric mutations. This late sodium current may offer a target for therapeutic intervention. The resultant prolongation of the cardiomyocyte action potential with increased intracellular calcium concentrations during diastole was shown to be reversible. Ranolazine, an inhibitor of the late sodium current, was able to accelerate the contraction–relaxation cycle and thereby improve diastolic function.

DIASTOLIC DYSFUNCTION IN RESTRICTIVE CARDIOMYOPATHY

Restrictive cardiomyopathy (RCM) can be thought of as a phenotype in which diastolic dysfunction is the dominant pathophysiologic derangement. RCM can result from a number of different diseases, all with distinct histological changes but all featuring diastolic dysfunction as a hallmark. To varying degrees, this is caused by myocardial fibrosis.

Amyloidosis

The most commonly encountered RCM is cardiac amyloidosis. In this disorder, deposition of abnormal extracellular protein begins in the subendocardium, gradually extending into the myocardium between the myocytes.[38] The muscle fibers themselves are not infiltrated and do not hypertrophy. Both the LV and the right ventricle (RV) can be affected with significant increases in wall thickness and stiffness. Of the several forms of amyloidosis, primary or light chain amyloidosis most commonly affects the heart (in 90% of cases).

Hemosiderosis

Iron overload can result either from hereditary hemochromatosis, in which the iron transport capacity of transferrin is overwhelmed by abnormally high plasma iron levels, or from increased erythrocyte catabolism as seen in frequent transfusions. In both conditions, iron is taken up by reticuloendothelial macrophages, which, when saturated, spill excess iron into parenchymal cells of various organs, causing tissue damage and fibrosis. Myocardial fibrosis in this setting can present as either restrictive diastolic dysfunction or a dilated cardiomyopathy.[38,39]

Cardiac Sarcoidosis

Another systemic disease with both environmental and genetic risk factors, sarcoidosis involves the CD4 + T cell–mediated formation of granulomas (macrophages, epithelioid cells, giant cells, T cells), which may either resolve or persist with or without fibrosis. Only about 5% of patients with clinically diagnosed sarcoidosis have cardiac involvement; however, cardiac granulomas are found in nearly 25% of all autopsies. The granulomas are usually along the LV free wall and basal ventricular septum. The resultant fibrosis is best visualized on cardiac magnetic resonance imaging, whereas echocardiographic findings are nonspecific.[38,40]

Hypereosinophilic Syndrome

Hypereosinophilic syndrome is a systemic disease affecting multiple organs. It can occur as a result of certain malignancies, vasculitides, and parasitic infections, or it may be idiopathic (Loeffler endocarditis). Injury results from the progressive dissolution of toxic granules, which cause endomyocardial fibrosis. This is often accompanied by thrombus formation along the damaged endocardium.[38,41]

Systemic Sclerosis

Extensive fibrosis is the hallmark of scleroderma, an autoimmune disease that can cause severe dysfunction of any organ, including the vasculature. Fibrosis is mediated by autoantibodies against various cellular antigens and is preceded by vascular injury of small vessels, especially arterioles. Coexistent hypertension, which is prevalent in this condition, likely contributes to diastolic dysfunction.[38]

PHYSIOLOGIC CHANGES ASSOCIATED WITH HEART FAILURE WITH PRESERVED EJECTION FRACTION

Several physiologic states are associated with diastolic dysfunction and HFpEF. Chronic elevation in LV filling pressure cause an elevation in LA pressure, leading to changes in LA geometry and function. Beyond absolute increase in LA volume, patients with HFpEF have increased LA stiffness as well reduced LA function by strain analysis.[42,43] Increased hydrostatic pressure also increases pulmonary venous pressure, leading to pulmonary hypertension, a physiologic state present in at least 70% of patients with diastolic dysfunction.[44] Although much of this elevation in pulmonary pressure is caused by "passive" pulmonary venous hypertension, some patients develop pulmonary vascular remodeling in response to elevated pressure, evidenced by elevated transpulmonary gradients. Although data are lacking on the exact pathophysiologic mechanism of this remodeling, histopathologic studies have suggested increase in global vascular intimal thickness, most prominently in the venous system.[45] Pulmonary vascular dysfunction can be worsened or triggered by exercise, leading to exercise intolerance.[46,47] As pulmonary hypertension persists, right ventricular dilation and dysfunction also occur and can result in progressive tricuspid regurgitation from annular dilation.

Physiologic changes in HFpEF are also seen on the systemic side. Increased arterial stiffness and decreased aortic compliance, increase afterload, and lead to an increase in reflected arterial pressure waves.[48–50] Beyond the contribution of increased afterload to alterations in diastolic relaxation patterns and systolic contractility, changes in peripheral vascular compliance lead to increased lability in central blood pressure, making patients more susceptible to the effects of vasoactive agents and changes in plasma volume with diuretics.[51] Microvascular changes in skeletal[52] and cardiac muscle[53] have also been described. Paulus and associates have proposed a paradigm for the development of HFpEF in which multiple comorbidities predispose to systemic inflammation, leading to inflammation of the microvascular endothelium, producing inflammatory cytokines such as interleukin-6 and TNF-α. This reduces levels of nitric oxide, cyclic guanosine monophosphate (cGMP), and protein kinase G (PKG) in neighboring cardiomyocytes.[54] In the periphery, the ability of tissues to augment oxygen extraction is impaired,[55] and in older persons, overall capillary density is decreased.[52] Furthermore, chronotropic incompetence occurs frequently in HFpEF and further limits cardiac output in response to physical activity.[56,57]

PHENOTYPING HEART FAILURE WITH PRESERVED EJECTION FRACTION

The contributions of multiple comorbid conditions to the development of diastolic dysfunction and the syndrome of HFpEF combined with the failure of multiple randomized clinical trials to demonstrate efficacy of neurohormonal inhibition in this population[58–62] has led to the proposal of a new paradigm: HFpEF is not a simply a manifestation of abnormalities in diastolic function but a syndrome with several phenotypes. However, even after moving away from a "one size fits all" model of HFpEF, it is clear that classifying patients into different "phenotypes" is complicated because

of the heterogeneity in patient signs and symptoms, comorbidities, and response to therapies. (It is worth noting that such heterogeneity also exists in HFrEF.) Highlighting this difficulty, in a study by Prasad and colleagues, who tried to identify the underlying pathophysiologic abnormalities in LV diastolic function in patients with "diastolic heart failure," nearly 2100 patients needed to be screened to find 23 without other comorbid conditions.[63] Use of cluster analysis to identify groups of patients with phenotypes more similar to each other than to others[64] has allowed the development of schema for classifying HFpEF.[65–67]

Classification by Clinical Features

In this system, patients are classified by patterns shared between patient populations,[68] which include HFpEF in obesity,[31,69] hypertension,[15,70,71] metabolic syndrome,[54] diabetes,[21–23,25,30] or chronic kidney disease (so-called "garden variety" HFpEF); HFpEF in CHD; atrial fibrillation predominant; HCM; pulmonary vascular disease and right heart failure predominant; valvular heart disease; "high-output" HFpEF caused by arteriovenous fistulae, anemia, or thyroid disease; and restrictive cardiomyopathies (e.g., cardiac amyloidosis). Advantages to this system are that these categories are relatively simple for clinicians to identify. However, there tends to be significant overlap between these classifications. Additionally, patients can move between classifications, making long-term treatment challenging

Classification by Risk Factor Phenotype and Clinical Presentation

To attempt to address the variability in patient symptoms at presentation and underlying pathophysiology, Shah and colleagues proposed a classification scheme based on a matrix of "predisposition phenotypes" (e.g., metabolic syndrome, hypertension, chronic kidney disease, CHD) and "clinical presentation phenotypes" (e.g., pulmonary congestion, atrial fibrillation, pulmonary hypertension)[66] (Fig. 37.2 and Table 37.3). Then specific therapeutic options based on the features present in that individual are suggested, changing based on the clinical findings. This "roadmap" retains the advantage of easily identifiable clinical risk factors and clinical findings while adding in nuance necessary in managing patients with complex and often shifting physiology across multiple organ systems.

IMPACT ON SURVIVAL

Longitudinal studies have shown an increased rate of all-cause mortality in patients with diastolic dysfunction (hazard ratio [HR], 8.31, for mild diastolic dysfunction compared with normal diastolic function; HR, 10.17, for moderate to severe diastolic dysfunction compared with normal diastolic function) when controlled for age, sex, and EF.[4] Several large longitudinal studies, including the Organized Program To Initiate Lifesaving Treatment In Hospitalized Patients With Heart Failure (OPTIMIZE-HF) Registry, have shown equivalent rates of survival and readmission for patients with heart failure; populations compared were patients with HFpEF and patients with heart failure with reduced EF (HFrEF) at various intervals of follow-up.[3,11,72] However, because patients with diastolic dysfunction tend to be older and have more comorbid conditions, they are more likely to die of noncardiovascular causes than patients with HFrEF, as seen in The Effect of Digoxin on Mortality and Morbidity in Patients with Heart Failure (DIG) and Irbesartan in Patients with Heart Failure and Preserved Ejection Fraction (I-PRESERVE) trials.[60,62] A community-based study showed that the decrease in cardiovascular deaths among patients with diastolic dysfunction was primarily attributable relatively fewer deaths from coronary disease, with similar rates of deaths related to heart failure (Table 37.4).[73]

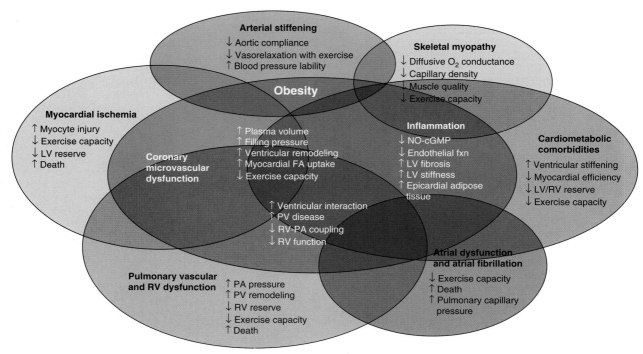

Figure 37.2. There are key clinical phenotypes that demonstrate distinct pathophysiologic features compared with the "garden variety" of heart failure with preserved ejection fraction (HFpEF). *FA,* Fatty acid; *fxn,* function; *HR,* heart rate; *LA,* left atrial; *LV,* left ventricular; *NO-cGMP,* nitric oxide–cyclic guanosine monophosphate signaling; *O₂,* oxygen; *PA,* pulmonary artery; *PH,* pulmonary hypertension; *PV,* pulmonary vascular; *RV,* right ventricular. (Reproduced with permission from Obokata M, et al: Diastolic dysfunction and heart failure with preserved ejection fraction: understanding mechanisms by using noninvasive methods, *JACC Cardiovasc Imag* 13:245–257, 2020.)

TABLE 37.3 "Roadmap" of Phenotype-Specific Heart Failure With Preserved Ejection Fraction Treatment Strategy Using a Matrix of Predisposition Phenotypes and Clinical Presentation Phenotypes[a]

		HFpEF Clinical Presentation Phenotypes				
HFpEF Predisposition Phenotype		Lung congestion	+ Chronotropic incompetence	+ Pulmonary hypertension (CpcPH)	+ Skeletal muscle weakness	+ Atrial fibrillation
	Overweight, obesity, metabolic syndrome, type 2 DM	• **Diuretics (loop diuretics in DM)** • Caloric restriction • Statins • Inorganic nitrite or nitrate • Sacubitril • Spironolactone	+ Rate-adaptive atrial pacing	+ Pulmonary vasodilators (e.g., PED5i)	**+ Exercise training program**	+ Cardioversion or rate control **+ anticoagulation**
+ Arterial hypertension		+ ACEi or ARB	+ ACEi or ARB + rate-adaptive atrial pacing	+ ACEi or ARB + pulmonary vasodilators (e.g., PED5i)	**+ Exercise training program**	+ ACEi or ARB + cardioversion or rate control **+ anticoagulation**
+ Renal dysfunction		+ Ultrafiltration (if needed)	+ Ultrafiltration (if needed) + rate-adaptive atrial pacing	+ Ultrafiltration (if needed) + pulmonary vasodilators (e.g., PED5i)	+ Ultrafiltration (if needed) **+ exercise training program**	+ Ultrafiltration (if needed) + cardioversion or rate control **+ anticoagulation**
+ CAD		+ ACEi + revascularization	+ ACEi + revascularization + rate-adaptive atrial pacing	+ ACEi + revascularization + pulmonary vasodilators (e.g., PED5i)	+ ACEi + revascularization **+ exercise training program**	+ ACEi + revascularization + cardioversion or rate control **+ anticoagulation**

[a]Phenotype-specific heart failure with preserved ejection fraction (HFpEF) treatment strategy using a matrix of predisposition phenotypes and clinical presentation phenotypes. A stepwise approach is proposed that begins in the left-hand upper corner of the matrix with general treatment recommendations, presumed to be beneficial to the vast majority of HFpEF patients as they address the presentation phenotype of lung congestion and the predisposition phenotype of overweight or obesity present in >80% of patients with HFpEF. Subsequently, supplementary (+) recommendations are suggested for additional predisposition-related phenotypic features when moving downward in the matrix and for additional presentation-related phenotypic features when moving rightward in the matrix. Only therapeutic measures indicated in bold are currently established. All other therapeutic measures require further testing in specific phenotypes.

ACEi, Angiotensin-converting enzyme inhibitor; *ARB,* angiotensin II receptor blockers; *CAD,* coronary artery disease; *CpcPH,* combined pre- and postcapillary Pulmonary Hypertension; *DM,* diabetes mellitus; *PDE5I,* phosphodiesterase 5 inhibitor.

Adapted with permission from Shah SJ, et al: Phenotype-specific treatment of heart failure with preserved ejection fraction: a multiorgan roadmap, *Circulation* 134:73–90, 2016.

TABLE 37.4 Diastolic Heart Failure: Effects of Age on Prevalence and Prognosis

	Age <50 Years	Age 50–70 Years	Age >70 Years
Prevalence (%)	15	33	50
Mortality (%)	15	33	50
Morbidity (%)	25	50	50

Adapted with permission from Volpe M, et al: Hypertension as an underlying factor in heart failure with preserved ejection fraction, *J Clin Hypertens* 12:277–283, 2010.

Acknowledgment

The authors acknowledge the contributions of Dr. Rebecca Lynn Baumann, who was the author of this chapter in the previous edition.

REFERENCES

1. Zile MR, Brutsaert DL. New concepts in diastolic dysfunction and diastolic heart failure: Part II: causal mechanisms and treatment. *Circulation*. 2002;105:1503–1508.
2. Zile MR, Brutsaert DL. New concepts in diastolic dysfunction and diastolic heart failure: part I: diagnosis, prognosis, and measurements of diastolic function. *Circulation*. 2002;105:1387–1393.
3. Tsutsui H, Tsuchihashi-Makaya M, Kinugawa S. Clinical characteristics and outcomes of heart failure with preserved ejection fraction: lessons from epidemiological studies. *J Cardiol*. 2010;55:13–22.
4. Redfield MM, Jacobsen SJ, Burnett JC, et al. Burden of systolic and diastolic ventricular dysfunction in the community: appreciating the scope of the heart failure epidemic. *J Am Med Assoc*. 2003;289:194–202.
5. Devereux RB, Roman MJ, Liu JE, et al. Congestive heart failure despite normal left ventricular systolic function in a population-based sample: the Strong Heart Study. *Am J Cardiol*. 2000;86:1090–1096.
6. Kitzman DW, Gardin JM, Gottdiener JS, et al. Importance of heart failure with preserved systolic function in patients > or = 65 years of age. CHS Research Group. Cardiovascular Health Study. *Am J Cardiol*. 2001;87:413–419.
7. Vasan RS, Larson MG, Benjamin EJ, et al. Congestive heart failure in subjects with normal versus reduced ventricular ejection fraction: prevalence and mortality in a population-based cohort. *J Am Coll Cardiol*. 1999;33:1948–1955.
8. Aurigemma GP, Gaasch WH. Clinical practice. Diastolic heart failure. *N Engl J Med*. 2004;351:1097–1105.
9. Tribouilloy C, Rusinaru D, Mahjoub H, et al. Prognosis of heart failure with preserved ejection fraction: a 5 year prospective population-based study. *Eur Heart J*. 2008;29:339–347.
10. Owan TE, Hodge DO, Herges RM, et al. Trends in prevalence and outcome of heart failure with preserved ejection fraction. *N Engl J Med*. 2006;355:251–259.
11. Bhatia RS, Tu JV, Lee DS, et al. Outcome of heart failure with preserved ejection fraction in a population-based study. *N Engl J Med*. 2006;355:260–269.
12. Masoudi FA, Havranek EP, Smith G, et al. Gender, age, and heart failure with preserved left ventricular systolic function. *J Am Coll Cardiol*. 2003;41:217–223.
13. Lenzen MJ, Scholte op Reimer WJ, Boersma E, et al. Differences between patients with a preserved and a depressed left ventricular function. *Eur Heart J*. 2004;25:1214–1220.
14. Glezeva N, Baugh JA. Role of inflammation in the pathogenesis of heart failure with preserved ejection fraction and its potential as a therapeutic target. *Heart Fail Rev*. 2014;19:681–694.
15. Volpe M, McKelvie R, Drexler H. Hypertension as an underlying factor in heart failure with preserved ejection fraction. *J Clin Hypertens*. 2010;12:277–283.
16. Borlaug BA, Redfield MM, Melenovsky V, et al. Longitudinal changes in left ventricular stiffness: a community-based study. *Circ Heart Fail*. 2013;6:944–952.
17. Hess OM, Schneider J, Nonogi H, et al. Myocardial structure in patients with exercise-induced ischemia. *Circulation*. 1988;77:967–977.
18. Hess OM, Ritter M, Schneider J, et al. Diastolic stiffness and myocardial structure in aortic valve disease before and after valve replacement. *Circulation*. 1984;69:855–865.
19. Hoffmann S, Mogelvang R, Olsen NT, et al. Tissue Doppler echocardiography reveals distinct patterns of impaired myocardial velocities in different degrees of coronary artery disease. *Eur J Echocardiogr*. 2010;11:544–549.
20. Rubler S, Dlugash J, Yuceoglu YZ, et al. New type of cardiomyopathy associated with diabetic glomerulosclerosis. *Am J Cardiol*. 1972;30:595–602.
21. Nicolino A, Longobardi G, Furgi G, et al. Left ventricular diastolic filling in diabetes mellitus with and without hypertension. *Am J Hypertens*. 1995;8:382–389.
22. Di Bonito P, Cuomo S, Moio N, et al. Diastolic dysfunction in patients with non-insulin-dependent diabetes mellitus of short duration. *Diabet Med*. 1996;13:321–324.
23. Di Bonito P, Moio N, Cavuto L, et al. Early detection of diabetic cardiomyopathy: usefulness of tissue Doppler imaging. *Diabet Med*. 2005;22:1720–1725.
24. Poirier P, Bogaty P, Garneau C, et al. Diastolic dysfunction in normotensive men with well-controlled type 2 diabetes: importance of maneuvers in echocardiographic screening for preclinical diabetic cardiomyopathy. *Diabetes Care*. 2001;24:5–10.
25. Fang ZY, Prins JB, Marwick TH. Diabetic cardiomyopathy: evidence, mechanisms, and therapeutic implications. *Endocr Rev*. 2004;25:543–567.
26. Aragno M, Mastrocola R, Medana C, et al. Oxidative stress-dependent impairment of cardiac-specific transcription factors in experimental diabetes. *Endocrinology*. 2006;147:5967–5974.
27. Petrova R, Yamamoto Y, Muraki K, et al. Advanced glycation endproduct-induced calcium handling impairment in mouse cardiac myocytes. *J Mol Cell Cardiol*. 2002;34:1425–1431.
28. Gawlowski T, Stratmann B, Stork I, et al. Heat shock protein 27 modification is increased in the human diabetic failing heart. *Horm Metab Res*. 2009;41:594–549.
29. Burgess ML, McCrea JC, Hedrick HL. Age-associated changes in cardiac matrix and integrins. *Mech Ageing Dev*. 2001;122:1739–1756.
30. Chavali V, Tyagi SC, Mishra PK. Predictors and prevention of diabetic cardiomyopathy. *Diabetes Metab Syndr Obes*. 2013;6:151–160.
31. Powell BD, Redfield MM, Bybee KA, et al. Association of obesity with left ventricular remodeling and diastolic dysfunction in patients without coronary artery disease. *Am J Cardiol*. 2006;98:116–120.
32. Maron BJ, Maron MS. Hypertrophic cardiomyopathy. *Lancet*. 2013;381:242–255.
33. Olivotto I, Cecchi F, Poggesi C, Yacoub MH. Patterns of disease progression in hypertrophic cardiomyopathy: an individualized approach to clinical staging. *Circ Heart Fail*. 2012;5:535–546.
34. Ho CY, Lopez B, Coelho-Filho OR, et al. Myocardial fibrosis as an early manifestation of hypertrophic cardiomyopathy. *N Engl J Med*. 2010;363:552–563.
35. Ashrafian H, McKenna WJ, Watkins H. Disease pathways and novel therapeutic targets in hypertrophic cardiomyopathy. *Circ Res*. 2011;109:86–96.
36. Marston SB. How do mutations in contractile proteins cause the primary familial cardiomyopathies? *J Cardiovasc Transl Res*. 2011;4:245–255.
37. Coppini R, Ferrantini C, Yao L, et al. Late sodium current inhibition reverses electromechanical dysfunction in human hypertrophic cardiomyopathy. *Circulation*. 2013;127:575–584.
38. Nihoyannopoulos P, Dawson D. Restrictive cardiomyopathies. *Eur J Echocardiogr*. 2009;10(iii):23–33.
39. Pietrangelo A. Hereditary hemochromatosis—a new look at an old disease. *N Engl J Med*. 2004;350:2383–2397.
40. Iannuzzi MC, Rybicki BA, Teirstein AS. Sarcoidosis. *N Engl J Med*. 2007;357:2153–2165.
41. Chew CY, Ziady GM, Raphael MJ, et al. Primary restrictive cardiomyopathy. Non-tropical endomyocardial fibrosis and hypereosinophilic heart disease. *Br Heart J*. 1977;39:399–413.
42. Santos AB, Roca GQ, Claggett B, et al. Prognostic relevance of left atrial dysfunction in heart failure with preserved ejection fraction. *Circ Heart Fail*. 2016;9:e002763.
43. Melenovsky V, Hwang SJ, Redfield MM, et al. Left atrial remodeling and function in advanced heart failure with preserved or reduced ejection fraction. *Circ Heart Fail*. 2015;8:295–303.
44. Gorter TM, Hoendermis ES, van Veldhuisen DJ, et al. Right ventricular dysfunction in heart failure with preserved ejection fraction: a systematic review and meta-analysis. *Eur J Heart Fail*. 2016;18:1472–1487.
45. Fayyaz AU, Edwards WD, Maleszewski JJ, et al. Global pulmonary vascular remodeling in pulmonary hypertension associated with heart failure and preserved or reduced ejection fraction. *Circulation*. 2018;137:1796–1810.
46. Singh I, Rahaghi FN, Naeije R, et al. Right ventricular-arterial uncoupling during exercise in heart failure with preserved ejection fraction: role of pulmonary vascular dysfunction. *Chest*. 2019;156:933–943.
47. Borlaug BA, Kane GC, Melenovsky V, Olson TP. Abnormal right ventricular-pulmonary artery coupling with exercise in heart failure with preserved ejection fraction. *Eur Heart J*. 2016;37:3293–3302.
48. Chirinos JA, Kips JG, Jacobs Jr DR, et al. Arterial wave reflections and incident cardiovascular events and heart failure: MESA (Multiethnic Study of Atherosclerosis). *J Am Coll Cardiol*. 2012;60:2170–2177.
49. Zamani P, Bluemke DA, Jacobs Jr DR, et al. Resistive and pulsatile arterial load as predictors of left ventricular mass and geometry: the multi-ethnic study of atherosclerosis. *Hypertension*. 2015;65:85–92.
50. Weber T, Wassertheurer S, O'Rourke MF, et al. Pulsatile hemodynamics in patients with exertional dyspnea: potentially of value in the diagnostic evaluation of suspected heart failure with preserved ejection fraction. *J Am Coll Cardiol*. 2013;61:1874–1883.
51. Borlaug BA, Kass DA. Ventricular-vascular interaction in heart failure. *Cardiol Clin*. 2011;29:447–459.
52. Kitzman DW, Nicklas B, Kraus WE, et al. Skeletal muscle abnormalities and exercise intolerance in older patients with heart failure and preserved ejection fraction. *Am J Physiol Heart Circ Physiol*. 2014;306:H1364–H1370.
53. Shah SJ, Lam CSP, Svedlund S, et al. Prevalence and correlates of coronary microvascular dysfunction in heart failure with preserved ejection fraction: PROMIS-HFpEF. *Eur Heart J*. 2018;39:3439–3450.
54. Paulus WJ, Tschope C. A novel paradigm for heart failure with preserved ejection fraction: comorbidities drive myocardial dysfunction and remodeling through coronary microvascular endothelial inflammation. *J Am Coll Cardiol*. 2013;62:263–271.

55. Dhakal BP, Malhotra R, Murphy RM, et al. Mechanisms of exercise intolerance in heart failure with preserved ejection fraction: the role of abnormal peripheral oxygen extraction. *Circ Heart Fail*. 2015;8:286–294.

56. Borlaug BA, Melenovsky V, Russell SD, et al. Impaired chronotropic and vasodilator reserves limit exercise capacity in patients with heart failure and a preserved ejection fraction. *Circulation*. 2006;114:2138–2147.

57. Brubaker PH, Joo KC, Stewart KP, et al. Chronotropic incompetence and its contribution to exercise intolerance in older heart failure patients. *J Cardiopulm Rehabil*. 2006;26:86–89.

58. Yusuf S, Pfeffer MA, Swedberg K, et al. Effects of candesartan in patients with chronic heart failure and preserved left-ventricular ejection fraction: the CHARM-Preserved Trial. *Lancet*. 2003;362:777–781.

59. Pitt B, Pfeffer MA, Assmann SF, et al. Spironolactone for heart failure with preserved ejection fraction. *N Engl J Med*. 2014;370:1383–1392.

60. Massie BM, Carson PE, McMurray JJ, et al. Irbesartan in patients with heart failure and preserved ejection fraction. *N Engl J Med*. 2008;359:2456–2467.

61. Redfield MM, Chen HH, Borlaug BA, et al. Effect of phosphodiesterase-5 inhibition on exercise capacity and clinical status in heart failure with preserved ejection fraction: a randomized clinical trial. *J Am Med Assoc*. 2013;309:1268–1277.

62. Digitalis Investigation G. The effect of digoxin on mortality and morbidity in patients with heart failure. *N Engl J Med*. 1997;336:525–533.

63. Prasad A, Hastings JL, Shibata S, et al. Characterization of static and dynamic left ventricular diastolic function in patients with heart failure with a preserved ejection fraction. *Circ Heart Fail*. 2010;3:617–626.

64. Ahmad T, Pencina MJ, Schulte PJ, et al. Clinical implications of chronic heart failure phenotypes defined by cluster analysis. *J Am Coll Cardiol*. 2014;64:1765–1774.

65. Shah SJ, Katz DH, Deo RC. Phenotypic spectrum of heart failure with preserved ejection fraction. *Heart Fail Clin*. 2014;10:407–418.

66. Shah SJ, Kitzman DW, Borlaug BA, et al. Phenotype-specific treatment of heart failure with preserved ejection fraction: a multiorgan roadmap. *Circulation*. 2016;134:73–90.

67. Obokata M, Reddy YNV, Borlaug BA. Diastolic dysfunction and heart failure with preserved ejection fraction: understanding mechanisms by using noninvasive methods. *JACC Cardiovasc Imag*. 2020;13:245–257.

68. Kao DP, Lewsey JD, Anand IS, et al. Characterization of subgroups of heart failure patients with preserved ejection fraction with possible implications for prognosis and treatment response. *Eur J Heart Fail*. 2015;17:925–935.

69. Obokata M, Reddy YNV, Pislaru SV, et al. Evidence supporting the existence of a distinct obese phenotype of heart failure with preserved ejection fraction. *Circulation*. 2017;136:6–19.

70. Bogaty P, Mure P, Dumesnil JG. New insights into diastolic dysfunction as the cause of acute left-sided heart failure associated with systemic hypertension and/or coronary artery disease. *Am J Cardiol*. 2002;89:341–345.

71. Yamamoto K, Wilson DJ, Canzanello VJ, Redfield MM. Left ventricular diastolic dysfunction in patients with hypertension and preserved systolic function. *Mayo Clin Proc*. 2000;75:148–155.

72. Fonarow GC, Stough WG, Abraham WT, et al. Characteristics, treatments, and outcomes of patients with preserved systolic function hospitalized for heart failure: a report from the OPTIMIZE-HF Registry. *J Am Coll Cardiol*. 2007;50:768–777.

73. Henkel DM, Redfield MM, Weston SA, Gerber Y, Roger VL. Death in heart failure: a community perspective. *Circ Heart Fail*. 2008;1:91–97.

74. Bursi F, Weston SA, Redfield MM, et al. Systolic and diastolic heart failure in the community. *JAMA*. 2006;296(18):2209–2216.

38   Assessment of Left Atrial Size

Denisa Muraru

A wealth of imaging and hemodynamic data have documented that the left atrium (LA) is not only a simple conduit for left ventricular filling; it also represents a critical structure for overall cardiac performance. It not only acts as a contractile pump that delivers 15% to 30% of the entire left ventricular filling volume but also acts as a reservoir that collects pulmonary venous return during ventricular systole allowing passage of the atrial stored blood into the left ventricle (LV) during early ventricular diastole. Given its important physiological role, changes to normal LA size or function have been associated with adverse cardiovascular outcomes. Previously, only LA maximal size was considered to be a clinically relevant prognostic marker.[1] Recently, both LA minimum volume[2] and phasic function parameters[3] have been reported to be powerful predictors of outcome in various cardiac conditions. LA volume is a surrogate marker of the severity and chronicity of diastolic dysfunction.[4] Additionally, maximal LA volume (LAV$_{max}$) is a biomarker for adverse cardiac events in healthy individuals and in various cardiovascular conditions,[5] including myocardial infarction,[6] heart failure,[7] stroke,[8] degenerative mitral regurgitation,[9] and atrial fibrillation (AF).[10] Echocardiography, traditionally two-dimensional echocardiography (2DE), and more recently three-dimensional echocardiography (3DE), is the most commonly used noninvasive imaging modality to evaluate LA size.[3,4] Measurement of LA size is best accomplished with transthoracic echocardiography, which allows complete visualization of the LA.[11] With transesophageal echocardiography, the LA cannot be fit in the image sector thereby precluding the ability to measure its actual size.

Historically, the anteroposterior (AP) LA diameter by M-mode or 2D images from the parasternal long-axis view was used to estimate LA size (Fig. 38.1). From this approach, the AP dimension of the LA can be measured. Because this measurement is easy to perform and highly reproducible, it has become the most frequently used metrics of LA size by echocardiography laboratories worldwide. However, LA AP diameter underestimates LA size.[12] LA enlargement is asymmetrical, occurring in the mediolateral and superoinferior axes, with relatively limited enlargement in the AP dimension because of the constraints of the spine and the sternum (Fig. 38.2). LA AP dimension identified only 49% of patients with an enlarged LA versus 76% identified by evaluating LA volume.[13] Accordingly, the use of the LA AP diameter to estimate LA size is currently discouraged by the guidelines[11] except in patients with hypertrophic cardiomyopathy in whom this parameter is included in the score to stratify the risk of sudden cardiac death.[14]

Biplane LA volume by 2DE is the currently recommended measurement to evaluate LA size[11] because it is a stronger predictor of outcomes than linear dimensions.[1] However, accurate measurement of LA volume by 2DE requires dedicated acquisitions of apical views optimized for the LA with proper endocardial border tracing.[11] The long axis of the LV is not parallel to the long axis of the LA, and this has been more clearly demonstrated with the adoption of 3DE for LA assessment[11,15] (Fig. 38.3). Accordingly, measurements should be obtained from dedicated apical four- and two-chamber views. In the correct imaging plane and time of the cardiac cycle, the base of

the LA should be at its largest size, indicating that the imaging plane passes through the maximal short-axis dimension. The LA length should also be maximized to ensure alignment along the true long axis of the LA and the length of the LA long-axes measured in the two- and four-chamber views should be similar.

Measurements should be taken at the end of left ventricular systole because this is when the LA chamber is at its greatest dimension. When tracing the endocardial border, the LA appendage, the confluence of the pulmonary veins and the space between the mitral valve leaflets and annulus should be excluded from LA volume measurements (Fig. 38.4). Phasic LA volumes can be calculated by measuring LA volumes at various times of the cardiac cycle: maximal LA volume is measured just before mitral valve opening, LA pre A volume at the onset of the P wave on the electrocardiographic tracing, and minimal LA volume at end-diastole (before mitral valve closure) (Fig. 38.5). Parameters of phasic LA function (active and passive emptying volume and fraction and conduit volumes) are calculated from these volumes (Table 38.1).

Using 2DE, biplane LA volume can be measured using two algorithms: the modified Simpson's method of disk summation and the area–length method.[13] With the Simpson's method, the LA endocardial border is traced and volume computed by adding the volume of a stack of 20 cylinders of height equal to L/20 (in which L is the length of the LA) and bases calculated by orthogonal minor and major transverse axes (a$_i$ and b$_i$) assuming an oval shape

$$\text{LA volume} = \left(\frac{\pi}{4}\right) \sum_{i=1}^{20} a_i \times b_i \times \frac{L}{20}$$

Alternatively, a biplane calculation could also be performed using the area–length algorithm with LA areas and lengths obtained from both the apical four- (A1) and two-chamber (B1) views. LA volume is calculated as:

$$\text{LA volume} = \frac{\left(\frac{8}{3\pi}\right) \times A1 \times B1}{L} = \frac{0.85 \times A1 \times B1}{L}$$

The length (L) of the LA is the shortest distance between the midline of the plane of the mitral annulus to the opposite superior side (roof) of the LA measured in either the four- or two-chamber views. To avoid significant miscalculations caused by foreshortening of one of these two views, the difference between L measured in the two- and four-chambers views should be less than 1 cm. Although the area–length method still assumes an ellipsoidal LA shape, it has the advantage of reducing linear dimensions to a single measurement.[16] Both methods have been reported to be accurate compared with measurements obtained using computed tomography.[17] The biplane area–length method systematically yields larger LA volumes than the disk summation method.[18,19] However, both methods have comparable prognostic power.[19]

Body size is a major determinant of LA size, with absolute LA volumes being larger in men than in women.[15] However, indexation

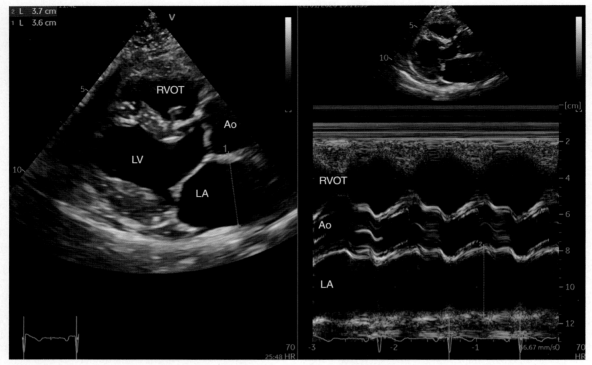

Figure 38.1. Leading edge-to-leading edge linear measurement *(dotted blue line)* of left atrial anteroposterior diameter using two-dimensional (left) and M-mode (right) echocardiography. *Ao,* Aorta; *LA,* left atrium; *LV,* left ventricle; *RVOT,* right ventricular outflow tract.

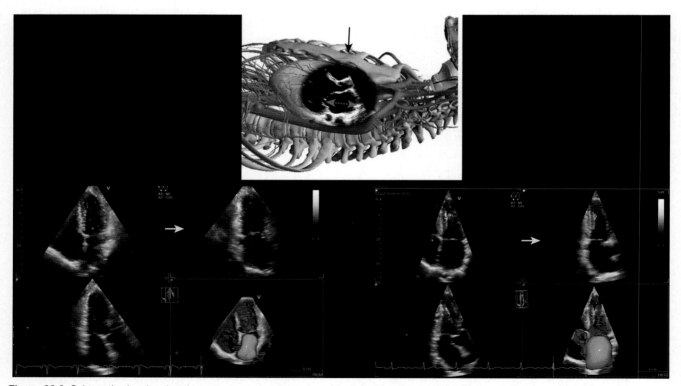

Figure 38.2. Schematic showing that the anteroposterior dimension of the left atrium is constrained between the sternum and the spine and therefore the largest expansion may only occur in the superoinferior dimension *(red dashed double arrow)*. Normal left atrium with three-dimensional reconstruction of actual volume size *(bottom left)* and a dilated left atrium in the same patient *(bottom right)* showing the change in left atrial size and shape.

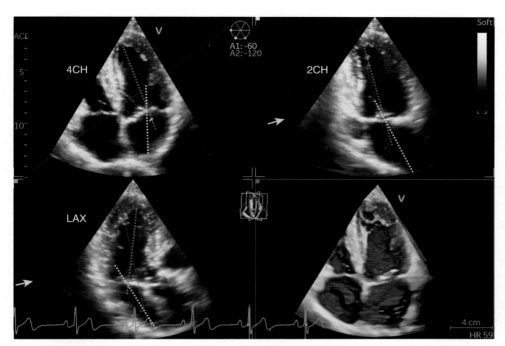

Figure 38.3. Apical views of the heart obtained from a three-dimensional echocardiography dataset to illustrate the fact that the long axis of the left ventricle *(red pointed line)* and left atrium *(yellow pointed line)* do not lie in the same plane. Left atrial (LA) size displayed in the four-chamber view optimized for the left ventricle (4CH) is significantly shorter than the LA size displayed in the two-chamber (2CH) and apical longa-axis (LAX) views.

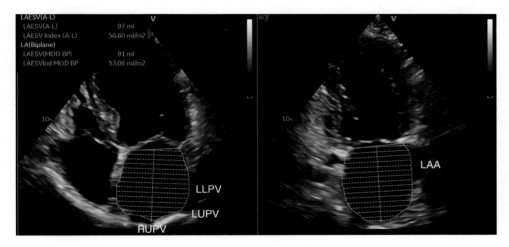

Figure 38.4. Two-dimensional measurements to obtain the left atrial volume using the apical four- *(left)* and two-chamber *(right)* views (see text for details). Using the same endocardial border tracings, the left atrial volume obtained with the area–length method (LAESV A-L) was larger than the one obtained with the Simpson's (MOD BP) algorithm. *LAA,* Left atrial appendage; *LLPV,* left lower pulmonary vein; *LUPV,* left upper pulmonary vein; *RUPV,* right upper pulmonary vein.

of LA volumes to body surface area (LAVI) leads to similar values between men and women and corrects for the effect of gender.[11,18] Reference values for LA volumes derived from 2DE have been similar in population-based studies[20] and in normative studies of healthy volunteers.[21] The effects of healthy aging on LA volume have been controversial, with some studies reporting an increase in LA volumes only at extremes of age[20] and others demonstrating a progressive age-related increase in LA volumes.[22] Differences in LA size according to ethnicity suggested larger LA size for Europeans compared with South and East Asians.[23]

The threshold value to diagnose LA enlargement by 2DE has recently been revised in the 2015 European Association of Cardiovascular Imaging/American Society of Echocardiography guidelines for chamber quantification.[11] Thus, the previous cut-off of maximal LA volume (LAV_{max}) greater than 28 mL/m^2 has been raised to 34 mL/m^2 based on pooled data coming from larger cohorts of healthy participants.[11] This revision aligns the "enlarged LA" cut-off value with the one recommended in the algorithm to diagnose LV diastolic function.[24] Moreover, the revised value of greater than 34 mL/m^2 used to define LA enlargement, is perhaps more clinically relevant because a LAV_{max} greater than 32 mL/m^2 was associated to adverse outcomes in ischemic stroke, diabetes,

and heart failure.[1,25–27] Finally, the revised threshold value to define an enlarged LA allowed a reclassification into normal LA size for 21% of patients previously reported as having an enlarged LA, without any loss of the prognostic power associated with an enlarged LA.[19]

The problem with currently recommended partition values (mild LA enlargement – LAV_{max} = 35–41 mL/m^2, moderate LA enlargement LAV_{max} = 42 to 48 mL/m^2, and severe LA enlargement – LAV_{max} >48 mL/m^2) is the narrow range of the varying grades of LA volume enlargement. Thus, even small measurement errors can result in misclassification of the grade of LA enlargement. The recent multicenter Normal Reference Ranges for Echocardiography (NORRE) study, which included 734 healthy individuals, suggested upper normal limits for LAV_{max} to be even larger than the current 34-mL/min cut-off (42 mL/m^2 using the area–length method and 37 mL/m^2 using the Simpson's method).[18]

2DE LA volume correlates with LA volumes obtained using 3DE,[28] CT,[29] and cardiac magnetic resonance (CMR),[30] with 2DE demonstrating a systematic underestimation of LA volumes.[31,32] This is likely caused by some foreshortening of the LA in the absence of dedicated acquisitions which maximize the LA long axis. Moreover, 2DE is associated with more difficult endocardial

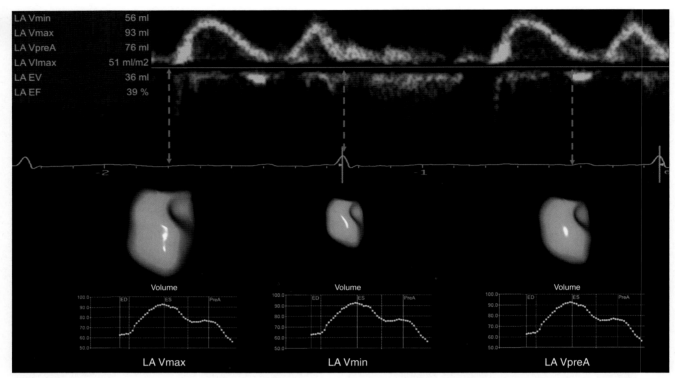

Figure 38.5. Phasic left atrial volumes. *From the top:* spectral Doppler of left ventricular filling, electrocardiography tracing, three-dimensional left atrial surface and volume–time curves to show the time *(red lines)*, and volumes of the left atrium at left ventricular end-systole (LA Vmax), at end-diastole (LA Vmin), and before the P-wave on the EKG (LA VpreA).

TABLE 38.1 Reference Values for Two- and Three-Dimensional Echocardiographic Measurements of the Left Atrium

	Left Atrial Size				
	3DE	**2DE**	**P Value**	**NL 3DE**	**NL 2DE**
Maximal volume (mL/m²)	32 ±4	24 ± 6	< .001	<46	<34
Minimal volume (mL/m²)	11 ± 3	8 ± 3	< .001	<17	<14
PreA volume (mL/m²)	18 ± 5	15 ± 5	< .001	<28	<25
Total emptying volume (mL)	38 ± 10	29 ± 7	< .001	—	—
Passive emptying volume (mL)	25 ± 7	17 ± 6	< .001	—	—
Active emptying volume (mL)	14 ± 6	12 ± 4	< .001	—	—

2DE, Two-dimensional echocardiography; *3DE,* three-dimensional echocardiography; *NL,* normal limit.

border definition, particularly in the two-chamber view,[28] with consequent suboptimal accuracy of 2DE method.[32] Despite these limitations, the ease of use and wide availability of 2DE makes it a clinically powerful tool, and it boasts the largest body of evidence on the alterations in LA volumes, as well as on its prognostic value (discussed in detail later).

3DE is fast becoming the modality of choice to measure cardiac chamber volumes. Its lower interobserver variability and higher test–retest reproducibility compared with 2DE make 3DE particularly important and the preferred method for serial measurements.[33] With the most recent technological advances, 3DE datasets of the LA are easily obtained with acceptable frame rate using single-beat acquisition. Regarding 3DE work flow, both semiautomated and fully automated contour detection of 3DE datasets have shown good correlation with manual tracing methods, with significant reduction in analysis times and increase in measurement reproducibility.[34] In a multicenter study, the agreement for classification of an enlarged LA using a cut-off of 34 mL/m² had a κ coefficient of interrater agreement of 0.88 (4 false negatives and 7 false positives) between 3DE LA volume and CMR compared with a κ coefficient of 0.71 (25 false negatives and 2 false positives) for 2DE.[31] Although Simpson's method of disks was previously applied,[35] more recently, the 3DE speckle-tracking and pattern recognition methods have been developed to achieve a fully automated identification of endocardial border to measure LA volumes,[36] though these newer algorithms require further clinical validation (see Fig. 38.5).

3DE LA volumes correlate better than 2DE with the volumes obtained by either CT[35] or CMR[30,31] because 3DE includes no geometrical assumptions regarding LA chamber shape. Moreover, 3DE-derived LA volumes have demonstrated better reproducibility than those derived from 2DE. Two studies sought to define reference values of 3D LA volumes by adapting 3DE software algorithms developed for the LV to measure the LA.[34,37] A recent study of 276 of healthy participants used a 3D software package specific for the LA, showing that 3DE LA phasic volumes were significantly larger than those obtained by 2DE[15] (Table 38.1). Similar to 2DE LA volume, indexation to body surface area of 3DE LA volumes eliminated gender differences,

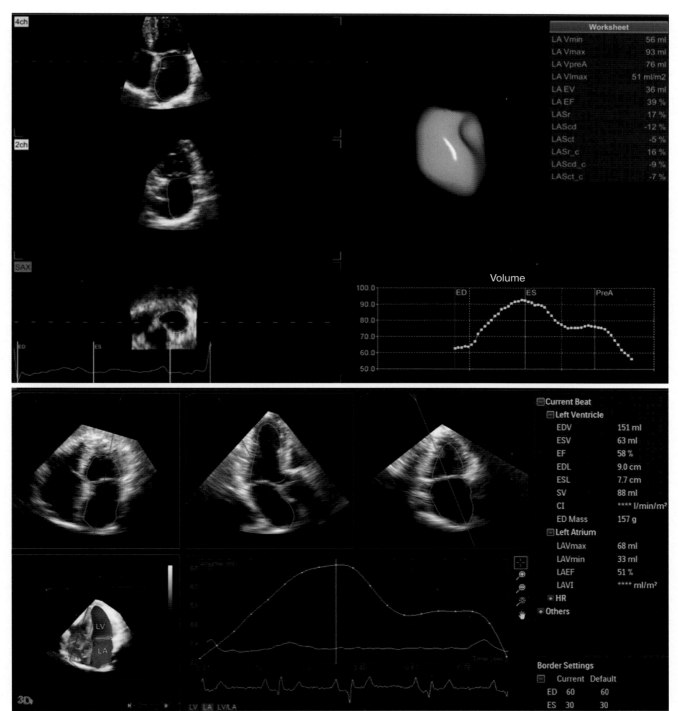

Figure 38.6. Automated measurements of the LA volumes using three-dimensional echocardiography. *Top,* Auto LA Q (GE Vingmed) that provides also automated measurements of longitudinal and circumferential strain, in addition to volumes. *Bottom,* HeartModel (Philips Medical Systems). *EF,* Emptying fraction; *EV,* emptying volume; *LA,* left atrial; *LASr,* left atrial longitudinal strain reservoir; *LAScd,* left atrial longitudinal strain conduit; *LASct,* left atrial longitudinal strain contraction; *LASr_c,* left atrial circumferential strain reservoir; *LAScd_c,* left atrial circumferential strain conduit; *LASct_c,* left atrial circumferential strain contraction; *LV,* left ventricular; *Vmax,* maximal volume; *Vmin,* minimal volume; *VpreA,* volume before atrial contraction.

and a small yet significant increase in 3DE LA volume was observed with aging.

3DE may be the way to measure LA volume in the future because novel fully automated, dedicated software packages are available on high-end ultrasound systems (Fig. 38.6), which will allow more robust test–retest reproducibility for serial measurements. The availability of fully automated quantitation algorithms using single-beat volume datasets allows a reliable LA 3DE quantification even in patients with AF. The major limitations at present are the limited spatial resolution of 3DE datasets and the relative paucity of data for both normative values, as well as prognostic value of 3DE LA volumes and phasic function indices.

PROGNOSTIC VALUE OF LEFT ATRIAL SIZE

Current recommendations encourage the reporting of the LAV_{max}.[11] There is a large body of evidence supporting LAV_{max} to stratify cardiovascular risk,[38] so LAV_{max} is routinely included in most echocardiogram reports. However, there is recent evidence suggesting that LAV_{min} may be a more important prognostic indicator using either 2DE or 3DE.[2,39] The correlation with LV filling pressures has also been reported to be stronger for LAV_{min} than for LAV_{max}.[40]

In patients with AF, the addition of LA strain during the reservoir phase and LAV_{max} to statistical models has been consistently reported as incremental to the $CHADS_2$ score in predicting hospitalization or death.[41] Moreover, abnormal reservoir function, obtained from 3D LA volumes, was associated with an increased recurrence of AF after catheter ablation procedure.[41] Therefore, LA reservoir function might be used for best predicting the success rate of the procedure and to individualize treatment and follow-up.

LAV_{max} is a predictor of the development of HF, irrespective of LV systolic function. In patients with dilated cardiomyopathy, and when HF is present, LA enlargement and dysfunction are important predictors of clinical outcomes.[42,43] Similar predictive value for adverse events has been reported in patients with HF of ischemic etiology.[44] In patients with heart failure with preserved ejection fraction (HFpEF), the relevance of LA volume is perhaps even greater, LAV_{max} having both diagnostic and prognostic value.[46,47]

The role of LA function assessment to optimize timing of surgery in asymptomatic patients with moderate mitral regurgitation has not been demonstrated yet, but LAV_{max} greater than 60 mL/m² has been acknowledged as an important prognostic marker[11] and an indication for surgery in asymptomatic patients with severe degenerative mitral regurgitation by current guidelines.[48] In patients with aortic valve stenosis, guidelines do not recommend the assessment of the LA to address their management.[48] Nevertheless, LA dilation is associated with LV remodeling and provides prognostic information in severe asymptomatic aortic valve stenosis.[49,50]

CONCLUSIONS

Measurements of the LA have hitherto been limited to evaluation of maximal LA volume. However, there are emerging data to support the prognostic role of minimal and phasic LA volumes as well as LA phasic function. The particular clinical areas of relevance are evaluation of diastolic dysfunction, HFpEF, and AF, all of which are common and growing problems. Although normative data and prognostic utility of 3DE are warranted, it is likely that evaluation of LA parameters will be included in guidelines for evaluation of patients.

Acknowledgment

The author thanks Dr. Theresa S.M. Tsang for her contribution to the previous edition of this chapter.

REFERENCES

1. Tsang TSM, Abhayaratna WP, Barnes ME, et al. Prediction of cardiovascular outcomes with left atrial size: is volume superior to area or diameter? *J Am Coll Cardiol*. 2006;47:1018–1023.
2. Russo C, Jin Z, Homma S, et al. Left atrial minimum volume and reservoir function as correlates of left ventricular diastolic function: impact of left ventricular systolic function. *Heart*. 2012;98:813–820.
3. Vieira MJ, Teixeira R, Goncalves L, Gersh BJ. Left atrial mechanics: echocardiographic assessment and clinical implications. *J Am Soc Echocardiogr*. 2014;27:463–478.
4. Thomas L, Marwick TH, Popescu BA, et al. Left atrial structure and function, and left ventricular diastolic dysfunction: JACC state-of-the-art review. *J Am Coll Cardiol*. 2019;73:1961–1977.
5. Kizer JR, Bella JN, Palmieri V, et al. Left atrial diameter as an independent predictor of first clinical cardiovascular events in middle-aged and elderly adults: the Strong Heart Study (SHS). *Am Heart J*. 2006;151:412–418.
6. Moller JE, Hillis GS, Oh JK, et al. Left atrial volume: a powerful predictor of survival after acute myocardial infarction. *Circulation*. 2003;107:2207–2212.
7. Ristow B, Ali S, Whooley MA, Schiller NB. Usefulness of left atrial volume index to predict heart failure hospitalization and mortality in ambulatory patients with coronary heart disease and comparison to left ventricular ejection fraction. *Am J Cardiol*. 2008;102:70–76.
8. Benjamin EJ, D'Agostino RB, Belanger AJ, et al. Left atrial size and the risk of stroke and death. *The Framingham Heart Study, Circulation*. 1995;92:835–8341.
9. Essayagh B, Antoine C, Benfari G, et al. Prognostic implications of left atrial enlargement in degenerative mitral regurgitation. *J Am Coll Cardiol*. 2019;74:858–870.
10. Vaziri SM, Larson MG, Benjamin EJ, Levy D. Echocardiographic predictors of nonrheumatic atrial fibrillation. The Framingham Heart Study. *Circulation*. 1994;89:724–730.
11. Lang RM, Badano LP, Mor-Avi V, et al. Recommendations for cardiac chamber quantification by echocardiography in adults. *J Am Soc Echocardiogr*. 2015;28:1–39.
12. Badano LP, Pezzutto N, Marinigh R, et al. How many patients would be misclassified using M-mode and two-dimensional estimates of left atrial size instead of left atrial volume? A three-dimensional echocardiographic study. *J Cardiovasc Med*. 2008;9:476–484.
13. Barbieri A, Bursi F, Zanasi V, et al. Left atrium reclassified: application of the American Society of Echocardiography/European Society of Cardiology cutoffs to unselected outpatients referred to the echocardiography laboratory. *J Am Soc Echocardiogr*. 2008;21:433–438.
14. Elliott PM, Anastasakis A, Borger MA, et al. 2014 ESC guidelines on diagnosis and management of hypertrophic cardiomyopathy. *Eur Heart J*. 2014;35:2733–2779.
15. Badano LP, Miglioranza MH, Mihaila S, et al. Left atrial volumes and function by three-dimensional echocardiography: reference values, accuracy, reproducibility, and comparison with two-dimensional echocardiographic measurements. *Circ Cardiovasc Imag*. 2016;9. e004229.
16. Nistri S, Galderisi M, Ballo P, et al. Determinants of echocardiographic left atrial volume implications for normalcy. *Eur J Echocardiogr*. 2011;12:826–833.
17. Al-Mohaissen MA, Kazmi MH, Chan KL, Chow BJ. Validation of two-dimensional methods for left atrial volume measurement: a comparison of echocardiography with cardiac computed tomography. *Echocardiography*. 2013;30:1135–1142.
18. Kou S, Caballero L, Dulgheru R, et al. Echocardiographic reference ranges for normal cardiac chamber size: results from the NORRE study. *Eur Heart J Cardiovasc Imag*. 2014;15:680–690.
19. Surkova E, Badano LP, Genovese D, et al. Clinical and prognostic implications of methods and partition values used to assess left atrial volume by two-dimensional echocardiography. *J Am Soc Echocardiogr*. 2017;30:1119–11129.
20. Boyd AC, Schiller NB, Leung D, et al. Atrial dilation and altered function are mediated by age and diastolic function but not before the eighth decade. *JACC Cardiovasc Imag*. 2011;4:234–242.
21. Pritchett AM, Jacobsen SJ, Mahoney DW, et al. Left atrial volume as an index of left atrial size: a population-based study. *J Am Coll Cardiol*. 2003;41:1036–1043.
22. Nikitin NP, Witte KK, Thackray SD, et al. Effect of age and sex on left atrial morphology and function. *Eur J Echocardiogr*. 2003;4:36–42.
23. Ethnic-specific normative reference values for echocardiographic LA and LV size, LV Mass, and systolic function: the EchoNoRMAL study. *JACC Cardiovasc Imag*. 2015;8:656–665.
24. Nagueh SF, Smiseth OA, Appleton CP, et al. Recommendations for the evaluation of left ventricular diastolic function by echocardiography. *J Am Soc Echocardiogr*. 2016;29:277–314.
25. Barnes ME, Miyasaka Y, Seward JB, et al. Left atrial volume in the prediction of first ischemic stroke in an elderly cohort without atrial fibrillation. *Mayo Clin Proc*. 2004;79:1008–1014.
26. Poulsen MK, Dahl JS, Henriksen JE, et al. Left atrial volume index: relation to long-term clinical outcome in type 2 diabetes. *J Am Coll Cardiol*. 2013;62:2416–2421.
27. Takemoto Y, Barnes ME, Seward JB, et al. Usefulness of left atrial volume in predicting first congestive heart failure in patients > or = 65 years of age with well-preserved left ventricular systolic function. *Am J Cardiol*. 2005;96:832–836.
28. Russo C, Hahn RT, Jin Z, et al. Comparison of echocardiographic single-plane versus biplane method in the assessment of left atrial volume and validation by real time three-dimensional echocardiography. *J Am Soc Echocardiogr*. 2010;23:954–960.
29. Kircher B, Abbott JA, Pau S, et al. Left atrial volume determination by biplane two-dimensional echocardiography: validation by cine computed tomography. *Am Heart J*. 1991;121(3 Pt 1):864–871.
30. Buechel RR, Stephan FP, Sommer G, et al. Head-to-head comparison of two-dimensional and three-dimensional echocardiographic methods for left atrial chamber quantification with magnetic resonance imaging. *J Am Soc Echocardiogr*. 2013;26:428–435.
31. Mor-Avi V, Yodwut C, Jenkins C, et al. Real-time 3D echocardiographic quantification of left atrial volume: multicenter study for validation with CMR. *JACC Cardiovasc Imag*. 2012;5:769–777.
32. Agner BF, Kuhl JT, Linde JJ, et al. Assessment of left atrial volume and function in patients with permanent atrial fibrillation: comparison of cardiac magnetic resonance imaging, 320-slice multi-detector computed tomography, and transthoracic echocardiography. *Eur Heart J Cardiovasc Imag*. 2014;15:532–540.
33. Jenkins C, Bricknell K, Marwick TH. Use of real-time three-dimensional echocardiography to measure left atrial volume: comparison with other echocardiographic techniques. *J Am Soc Echocardiogr*. 2005;18:991–997.

34. Wu VC, Takeuchi M, Kuwaki H, et al. Prognostic value of LA volumes assessed by transthoracic 3D echocardiography: comparison with 2D echocardiography. *JACC Cardiovasc Imag*. 2013;6:1025–1035.

35. Iwataki M, Takeuchi M, Otani K, et al. Measurement of left atrial volume from transthoracic three-dimensional echocardiographic datasets using the biplane Simpson's technique. *J Am Soc Echocardiogr*. 2012;25:1319–1326.

36. Perez de Isla L, Feltes G, Moreno J, et al. Quantification of left atrial volumes using three-dimensional wall motion tracking echocardiographic technology: comparison with cardiac magnetic resonance. *Eur Heart J Cardiovasc Imag*. 2014;15:793–799.

37. Aune E, Baekkevar M, Roislien J, et al. Normal reference ranges for left and right atrial volume indexes and ejection fractions with real-time three-dimensional echocardiography. *Eur J Echocardiogr*. 2009;10:738–744.

38. Hoit BD. Left atrial size and function: role in prognosis. *J Am Coll Cardiol*. 2014;63:493–505.

39. Caselli S, Canali E, Foschi ML, et al. Long-term prognostic significance of three-dimensional echocardiographic parameters of the left ventricle and left atrium. *Eur J Echocardiogr*. 2010;11:250–256.

40. Appleton CP, Galloway JM, Gonzalez MS, et al. Estimation of left ventricular filling pressures using two-dimensional and Doppler echocardiography in adult patients with cardiac disease. *J Am Coll Cardiol*. 1993;22:1972–1982.

41. Montserrat S, Gabrielli L, Borras R, et al. Left atrial size and function by three-dimensional echocardiography to predict arrhythmia recurrence after first and repeated ablation of atrial fibrillation. *Eur Heart J Cardiovasc Imag*. 2014;15:515–522.

42. Gottdiener JS, Kitzman DW, Aurigemma GP, et al. Left atrial volume, geometry, and function in systolic and diastolic heart failure of persons > or =65 years of age. *Am J Cardiol*. 2006;97:83–89.

43. Quinones MA, Greenberg BH, Kopelen HA, et al. Echocardiographic predictors of clinical outcome in patients with left ventricular dysfunction enrolled in the SOLVD registry and trials: significance of left ventricular hypertrophy. *J Am Coll Cardiol*. 2000;35:1237–1244.

44. Tamura H, Watanabe T, Nishiyama S, et al. Increased left atrial volume index predicts a poor prognosis in patients with heart failure. *J Card Fail*. 2011;17:210–216.

45. Meris A, Amigoni M, Uno H, et al. Left atrial remodeling in patients with myocardial infarction complicated by heart failure, left ventricular dysfunction, or both: the VALIANT Echo study. *Eur Heart J*. 2009;30:56–65.

46. Pedersen F, Raymond I, Madsen LH, et al. Echocardiographic indices of left ventricular diastolic dysfunction in 647 individuals with preserved left ventricular systolic function. *Eur J Heart Fail*. 2004;6:439–447.

47. Otterstad JE, St John Sutton MG, Froeland GS, et al. Prognostic value of two-dimensional echocardiography and N-terminal proatrial natriuretic peptide following an acute myocardial infarction. *Eur Heart J*. 2002;23:1011–1020.

48. Nishimura RA, Otto CM, Bonow RO, et al. 2014 AHA/ACC Guideline for the management of patients with valvular heart disease. *Circulation*. 2014;129:e521–e643.

49. Rusinaru D, Bohbot Y, Salaun E, et al. Determinants of left atrial volume index in patients with aortic stenosis. *Arch Cardiovasc Dis*. 2017;110:525–533.

50. Christensen NL, Dahl JS, Carter-Storch R, et al. Relation of left atrial size, cardiac morphology, and clinical outcome in asymptomatic aortic stenosis. *Am J Cardiol*. 2017;120:1877–1883.

39 Assessment of Left Atrial Function

Brian D. Hoit, Wendy Tsang

The recent interest in left atrial (LA) function has enhanced our understanding of the atrial contributions to cardiovascular performance in both health and disease. The development of sophisticated, noninvasive indices of LA function has been critical to this resurgence. Although echocardiography is most often used because of its availability, safety, versatility, and ability to image in real time with high temporal and spatial resolution, cardiac computed tomography (CCT) and cardiac magnetic resonance imaging (CMRI) are useful in specific clinical instances.[1] For example, CMRI quantifies scar and predicts the risk of recurrence of atrial fibrillation after LA ablation,[2] and CCT plays an important role before, during, and after LA ablation. Despite increasing interest, quantifying LA function is difficult in part because of its complex geometry and intricate fiber orientation.[3] Further increasing complexity and confounding functional analysis are interactions between atrial and ventricular performance.

LEFT ATRIAL FUNCTION

The principal role of the LA is to modulate left ventricular (LV) filling and cardiovascular performance. This is accomplished by its roles as a *reservoir* for pulmonary venous return during ventricular systole, a *conduit* for pulmonary venous return during early ventricular diastole, and a *booster pump* for ventricular filling during late ventricular diastole. In normal patients, the atrial contribution to ventricular stroke volume by the reservoir, conduit, and booster phases are 40%, 35%, and 25%, respectively. The interplay between these atrial functions and ventricular performance throughout the cardiac cycle is fundamental to understanding changes in the LA functional indices. For example, although reservoir function is governed by atrial compliance during ventricular systole, reservoir capacity is influenced by atrial contractility and relaxation, systolic descent of the LV base, and the LV end-systolic volume. Conduit function is influenced by atrial compliance and is reciprocally related to reservoir function, but because the mitral valve is opened, it is closely related to LV relaxation and compliance. Finally, atrial booster pump function reflects the magnitude and timing of atrial contractility but is dependent on the degree of venous return (atrial preload), left ventricular end-diastolic pressures (atrial afterload), and LV systolic reserve.

LA function is most often assessed by echocardiography using LA volumetric analysis; spectral Doppler of transmitral, pulmonary venous, and left atrial appendage (LAA) flow; and tissue Doppler and deformation analysis (strain and strain rate imaging) of the LA body (Table 39.1 and Fig. 39.1). LA volumetric and Doppler methods were the earliest methods used to assess LA function but have been overtaken by speckle-tracking deformation analysis as the primary method used. It must be noted that results obtained from deformation and volumetric analysis are not directly comparable.[4] Although atrial pressure–volume loops can be generated in humans using invasive and semi-invasive means,[5] these methods are cumbersome, time consuming, and difficult to apply.

Generally, LA volumetric and speckle-tracking deformation analyses are obtained from two-dimensional (2D) echocardiograms

TABLE 39.1 Volumetric Indices of Left Atrial Function

LA Function	LA Volume Fraction	Calculation
Global function; reservoir	LAEF (or total EF)	$(LA_{max} - LA_{min})/LA_{max}$
Reservoir function	Expansion index	$[(LA_{max} - LA_{min})/LA_{min}]$
Conduit	Passive EF	$[(LA_{max} - LApre\text{-}A)/LA_{max}]$
Booster pump	Active EF	$[(LApre\text{-}A - LA_{min})/LApre\text{-}A]$

EF, Ejection (or emptying) fraction; *LA*, left atrial; *LA_max*, maximal LA volume; *LA_min*, minimal LA volume; *LApre-A*, LA volume immediately before atrial systole.

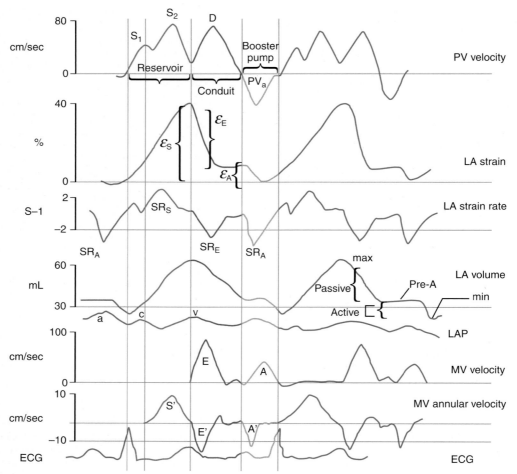

Figure 39.1. Functions of the left atrium and their color-coded relation to the cardiac cycle (*red*, reservoir; *blue*, conduit; *yellow*, booster pump). Displayed are pulmonary venous (PV) velocity, left atrial (LA) strain, LA strain rate, LA volume and pressure, and mitral spectral and tissue Doppler imaging. *a* and *A*, Late diastole; *A'*, atrial contraction; *D*, ventricular diastole; *E* and *E'*, early diastole; *ECG*, electrocardiogram; ε, strain; *LAP*, left atrial pressure; *MV*, mitral valve; PV_a, pulmonary venous reversal velocity; *S'*, ventricular systole; SR_A, strain rate in late diastole; SR_E, strain rate in early diastole; SR_S, strain rate in ventricular diastole. (Reproduced with permission from Hoit BD: Left atrial size and function: role in prognosis, *J Am Coll Cardiol* 63:493–505, 2014.)

using two- and four-chamber focused views of the LA when the LA is not foreshortened.[6] However, obtaining LA functional data from three-dimensional (3D) echocardiography is preferred because it is more accurate because of visualization of all the LA walls in a dataset (Fig. 39.2).[7] Although there have been concerns in the past regarding the time and expertise required to analyze 3D LA datasets, advancements in semi- or fully automated analysis programs are resolving this issue.[8] CCT and CMRI have also been used to assess volumetric LA functions but are not as popular because of radiation exposure and accessibility issues.[9]

VOLUMETRIC METHODS

Volumetric assessment of LA reservoir, conduit, and booster pump function can be obtained from LA volumes at their maximum (at end-systole, just before mitral valve opening), minimum (at end-diastole, when the mitral valve closes), and immediately before atrial systole (before the electrocardiographic P wave). From these volumes, total, passive, and active ejection or emptying fractions, representative of reservoir, conduit, and booster pump function, respectively, can be calculated (see Fig. 39.1 and Table 39.1). The expansion index, which normalizes total LA emptying volume to minimum LA volume is an index that may be more closely related to reservoir function than LA total ejection fraction (LAEF). The

LA functional index (LAFI) is a novel measure that incorporates the LAEF, the LV outflow tract velocity time integral (LVOTvti), and the maximum LA volume indexed to body surface area (LAVi): [LAFI = (LAEF × LVOTvti)/LAVi].[10] Although the passive ejection fraction is used as a surrogate of conduit function, conduit volume is actually the volume of blood that passes through the LA that cannot be accounted for by reservoir or booster pump functions. This volume of blood requires simultaneous measurement of LV and LA volumes: [LV stroke volume – (LA_{max} – LA_{min})].

SPECTRAL DOPPLER

Doppler waveforms of pulmonary venous flow (LA filling) and transmitral flow (LA emptying) can be used to estimate relative atrial functions (Table 39.2). Advantages are their availability and simplicity in acquisition and interpretation. The ratios of peak transmitral early (E) and late (A) velocities (or their velocity time integrals [VTIs]) and the atrial filling fraction (Avti/[Evti + Avti]) estimate the relative contribution of atrial booster pump function, and the ratio of systolic (S) to diastolic (D) pulmonary venous flow estimates relative reservoir to conduit function. The magnitude and duration of reversed pulmonary flow (PVa) during atrial contraction is used to estimate atrial contractility and LV diastolic pressures.[11] Atrial ejection force accelerates blood into the LV and can be noninvasively

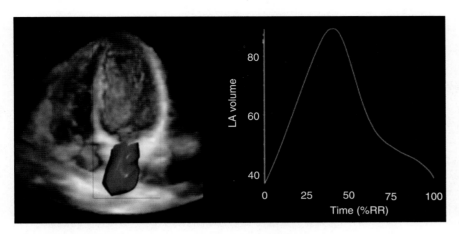

Figure 39.2. Example of left atrial (LA) volumes derived from a three-dimensional echocardiographic dataset. The volume curve for the LA *(green)* in a normal patient is shown. *RR,* interval.

TABLE 39.2 Spectral Doppler Indices of Left Atrial Function

LA Function	Transmitral Flow	Pulmonary Venous Flow	Composite Indices
Global function			LAFI
Reservoir		S vel or VTI	
Conduit	E vel or VTI, E/A	D vel or VTI	
Booster pump	A vel or VTI, E/A	PVa	Ejection force, LAKE
	AFF		
	LAA velocity		

A and *a,* Late diastole; *AFF,* atrial filling fraction; *D,* ventricular diastole; *LAFI,* left atrial functional index; *S,* ventricular systole; *E* and *e,* early diastole; *LAA,* left atrial appendage; *LAKE,* left atrial kinetic energy; *PVa,* pulmonary venous reversal velocity; *vel,* velocity; *VTI,* velocity time integral.

TABLE 39.3 Tissue Doppler and Deformational Indices of Left Atrial Function

LA Function	Tissue Velocity	Strain	Strain Rate
Reservoir	S′	ε_s, ε_{total}	SR-S
Conduit	E′	ε_e, ε_{pos}	SR-E
Booster pump	A′	ε_a, ε_{neg}	SR-A

′, Tissue velocity; *A,* late diastole; *E,* early diastole; *ε,* strain; *LA,* left atrial; *neg,* negative; *pos,* positive; *S,* systole; *SR-A,* strain rate in late diastole; *SR-E,* strain rate in early diastole; *SR-S,* strain rate in ventricular systole.

determined from the product of the mitral valve orifice area and the peak transmitral A velocity squared.[12] LA work can be expressed by LAKE (LA kinetic energy), which incorporates LA stroke volume and the transmitral Doppler peak atrial velocity.[13] LAA velocities (usually obtained from transesophageal echocardiography) reflect appendage contractile function. Interpretation of spectral Doppler indices can be difficult with sinus tachycardia, conduction system disease, and arrhythmia (especially atrial fibrillation), and obtaining high-quality pulmonary venous recordings may be difficult. A major disadvantage of spectral Doppler is its lack of specificity because changes may be caused by LV diastolic dysfunction, mitral valve disease, or abnormal loading conditions and hemodynamics.

TISSUE DOPPLER IMAGING

Pulsed-wave and color tissue Doppler imaging (TDI) of atrial contraction (A′) provide a regional snapshot of atrial systolic function, and when several sites are averaged, the view is global.[14] Reproducible data with acceptable variability is possible with proper attention to technical detail. Offline color tissue Doppler waveforms simultaneously record multiple atrial regions and demonstrate an annular to superior segment decremental gradient of atrial contraction.[15] Tissue velocities during ventricular systole (S′) and early diastole (E′) correspond to reservoir and conduit function, respectively (Table 39.3). However, tissue Doppler velocities are subject to error because of angle dependency and the effects of cardiac motion and tethering and have been superseded by deformation analysis.

DEFORMATION ANALYSIS (STRAIN AND STRAIN RATE IMAGING)

Strain and strain rates represent the magnitude and rate, respectively, of myocardial deformation; they can be assessed using

either tissue Doppler velocities (TDI) or by 2D echocardiographic (2D speckle-tracking echocardiography [2D STE]) techniques (Figs. 39.3 and 39.4; see Table 39.3). Both have been used successfully to assess LA global and regional function.[16] Although temporal resolution is excellent and ideal 2D image quality is not necessary, TDI is highly angle dependent and noisy. In contrast, 2D STE analyzes myocardial motion through frame-by-frame tracking of natural acoustic markers (speckles) that are generated without angle dependency from interactions between ultrasound and myocardial tissue within a user-defined region. Frame rates of approximately 50 to 70 Hz are needed to prevent speckle decorrelation, and good image quality is needed for accurate tracking.

An American Society of Echocardiography/European Association of Cardiovascular Imaging (ASE/EACVI) Industry Task Force has made recommendations for standardization of LA strain analysis from 2D echocardiograms.[17] The Task Force recommends reporting LA strain from an optimized LA-focused apical four-chamber view. Although biplane LA strain can be performed, it is not mandatory. The myocardial region of interest is defined by the inner and outer LA wall contours. If the width of the region of interest can be adjusted, a default width of 3 mm is suggested. In the apical four-chamber view, the tracing should start at the endocardial border of the mitral annulus with extrapolation of the contour across the pulmonary veins and the LAA orifices. Global longitudinal strain is defined by the Task Force as strain in the direction tangential to the endocardial atrial border in the apical view. Because of interpolation across the pulmonary vein orifices and LAAs and the thinness of the LA myocardium, subdivision of the LA wall into segments and assessment of radial or transverse strain are not recommended.

The zero-baseline reference used to describe atrial strain and strain rate may create confusion (Fig. 39.5). Thus, if the ventricular cycle is used, ventricular end-diastole (the QRS complex) is the zero reference, and the peak positive longitudinal strain (ε_s) corresponds to atrial reservoir function, and the strain during early and late diastole (ε_e and ε_a, respectively) correspond to conduit and atrial booster function. However, if the atrial cycle is used,

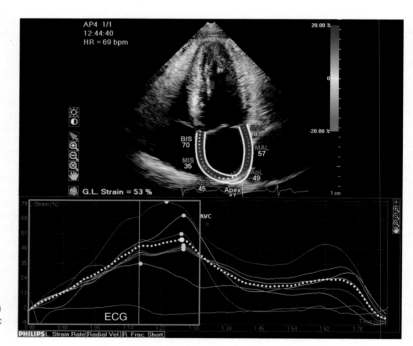

Figure 39.3. Example of left atrial strain derived from tissue Doppler imaging. Longitudinal strain curves for the septal *(purple)* and lateral segments *(yellow)* are shown. *ECG,* Electrocardiogram.

Figure 39.4. Example of left atrial strain derived from speckle tracking echocardiography. Regional strains are denoted by the *colored lines* and global longitudinal (GL) strain by the *white dotted line*. The *closed circles* on each regional strain–time curve identify peak strain. *AVC,* Aortic valve closure. *ECG,* Electrocardiogram.

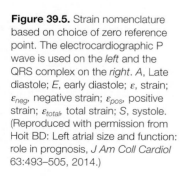

Figure 39.5. Strain nomenclature based on choice of zero reference point. The electrocardiographic P wave is used on the *left* and the QRS complex on the *right*. *A,* Late diastole; *E,* early diastole; *ε,* strain; *ε_neg,* negative strain; *ε_pos,* positive strain; *ε_total,* total strain; *S,* systole. (Reproduced with permission from Hoit BD: Left atrial size and function: role in prognosis, *J Am Coll Cardiol* 63:493–505, 2014.)

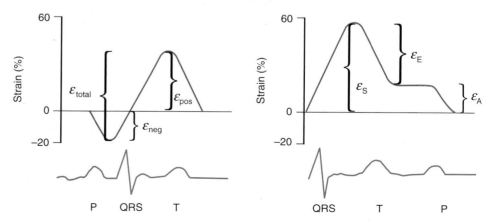

atrial end-diastole (onset of P wave) is the zero reference, and the first negative peak strain (ε_{neg}) represents the atrial booster pump function, the positive peak strain (ε_{pos}) corresponds to conduit function, and their sum (ε_{total}) represents reservoir function.[18] Strain rates in ventricular systole, early diastole, and late diastole (respectively, SR-S, SR-E, and SR-A) correspond to reservoir, conduit, and booster pump functions in both schemes. It has been reported that there are different normative values depending on whether ventricular end-diastole or the onset of atrial contraction is selected as the zero-reference point.[17] However, when viewed as scalar quantities, they are comparable, and a meta-analysis providing normal 2D LA strain values has been published.[19] The ASE/EACVI Task Force recommends that the default baseline reference for LA strain curves be at ventricular end-diastole, which should be defined by the mitral valve inflow profile.[17]

Although 2D strain and strain rate imaging overcome much of the subjectivity and variability inherent in assessing endocardial motion, these methods fail to address the complexities of 3D cardiac geometry and motion. Data suggest that 3D speckle-tracking echocardiography (3D STE) overcomes these limitations because it eliminates the effects of through-plane motion that may occur with 2D imaging.[20] 3D STE is a reproducible technique that more quickly and completely analyzes myocardial deformation. Thus, one can measure longitudinal and circumferential strains from a single 3D dataset. Moreover, the evaluation of LA endocardial area strain (ε_{area}, the product of longitudinal strain and circumferential strain) is possible. Normal values for 3D STE are available but are limited in the number of patients studied.[21,22]

CHALLENGES TO MEASUREMENT OF LEFT ATRIAL FUNCTION

It is increasingly clear that LA function provides insight into the pathophysiology of a variety of cardiovascular disorders. LA function predicts cardiovascular events in the general and referral populations and in patients with atrial fibrillation, stroke, cardiomyopathy, and ischemic and valvular heart disease.[23] It may also allow accurate classification of left ventricular diastolic dysfunction.[24] However, the methods used to measure LA function all have important limitations and indices that are needed because a specific atrial function often correlates poorly with others obtained during the same phase of the cardiac cycle. In addition, the hemodynamic and biophysical underpinnings that are responsible for the functional changes are often unknown. It is important to remember that LA dysfunction may result from an intrinsic atrial abnormality, altered load, or a compensatory response and may have different expressions at different stages of the underlying disease process. The LA offers unique challenges, such as its far-field location, reduced signal-to-noise ratio, thin walls, and the presence of the pulmonary veins and LAA. Moreover, although factors that affect LA reservoir, conduit, and booster pump function are still being studied, it is clear that LA function is affected by age, with increasing age associated with a decrease in LA reservoir and conduit function and an increase in booster pump function.[25] To date, no difference in LA function between healthy men and women has been found.[26] As to racial differences in LA function, limitations in the populations studied leave this issue unresolved with some studies indicating a difference in LA ejection fraction but not strain or strain rate.[19,27] Finally, there have been concerns that the differences between vendors seen for left ventricular strain would also be observed in LA strain analysis, but this has not been found.[19,28]

REFERENCES

1. To AC, Flamm SD, Marwick TH, et al. Clinical utility of multimodality LA imaging: assessment of size, function, and structure. *JACC Cardiovasc Imaging.* 2011;4:788–798.
2. Kuppahally SS, Akoum N, Burgon NS, et al. Left atrial strain and strain rate in patients with paroxysmal and persistent atrial fibrillation: relationship to left atrial structural remodeling detected by delayed-enhancement MRI. *Circ Cardiovasc Imaging.* 2010;3:231–239.
3. Corradi D, Maestri R, Macchi E, et al. The atria: from morphology to function. *J Cardiovasc Electrophysiol.* 2011;22:223–235.
4. Donal E, Galli E, Schnell F. Left atrial strain: a must or a plus for routine clinical practice? *Circ Cardiovasc Imag.* 2017;10:3007023.
5. Stefanadis C, Dernellis J, Stratos C, et al. Assessment of left atrial pressure-area relation in humans by means of retrograde left atrial catheterization and echocardiographic automatic boundary detection: effects of dobutamine. *J Am Coll Cardiol.* 1998;31:426–436.
6. Badano LP, Miglioranza MH, Mihaila S, et al. Left atrial volumes and function by 3D echocardiography: reference values, accuracy, reproducibility, and comparison with 2D echocardiographic measurements. *Circ Cardiovasc Imag.* 2016;9. e004229.
7. Kebed K, Kruse E, Addetia K, et al. Atrial-focused views improve the accuracy of two-dimensional echocardiographic measurements of the left and right atrial volumes: a contribution to the increase in normal values in the guidelines update. *Int J Cardiovasc Imag.* 2017;33:209–218.
8. Tsang W, Salgo IS, Medvedofsky D, et al. Transthoracic 3D echocardiographic left chamber quantification using an automated adaptive analytics algorithm. *JACC Cardiovasc Imaging.* 2016;9:769–782.
9. Kühl JT, Lønborg J, Fuchs A, et al. Assessment of left atrial volume and function: a comparative study between echocardiography, magnetic resonance imaging and multi slice computed tomography. *Int J Cardiovasc Imaging.* 2012;28:1061–1071.
10. Welles CC, Ku IA, Kwan DM, et al. Left atrial function predicts heart failure hospitalization in subjects with preserved ejection fraction and coronary heart disease: longitudinal data from the Heart and Soul Study. *J Am Coll Cardiol.* 2012;59:673–680.
11. Appleton CP, Galloway JM, Gonzalez MS, et al. Estimation of left ventricular filling pressures using two-dimensional and Doppler echocardiography in adult patients with cardiac disease: additional value of analyzing left atrial size, left atrial ejection fraction and the difference in duration of pulmonary venous and mitral flow velocity at atrial contraction. *J Am Coll Cardiol.* 1993;22:1972–1982.
12. Manning WJ, Silverman DI, Katz SE, et al. Atrial ejection force: a noninvasive assessment of atrial systolic function. *J Am Coll Cardiol.* 1993;22:221–225.
13. Boudoulas KD, Sparks EA, Rittgers SE, et al. Factors determining left atrial kinetic energy in patients with chronic mitral valve disease. *Herz.* 2003;28:437–444.
14. Khankirawatana B, Khankirawatana S, Peterson B, et al. Peak atrial systolic mitral annular velocity by Doppler tissue reliably predicts left atrial systolic function. *J Am Soc Echocardiogr.* 2004;17:353–360.
15. Thomas L, Levett K, Boyd A, et al. Changes in regional left atrial function with aging: evaluation by Doppler tissue imaging. *Eur J Echocardiogr.* 2003;4:92–100.
16. Vianna-Pinton R, Moreno CA, Baxter CM, et al. Two-dimensional speckle-tracking echocardiography of the left atrium: feasibility and regional contraction and relaxation differences in normal subjects. *J Am Soc Echocardiogr.* 2009;22:299–305.
17. Badano L, Kolias TJ, Muraru D, et al. Standardization of left atrial, right ventricular and right atrial deformation imaging using two-dimensional speckle tracking echocardiography. *Eur Heart J Cardiovasc Imag.* 2018;18:591–600.
18. Mor-Avi V, Lang RM, Badano LP, et al. Current and evolving echocardiographic techniques for the quantitative evaluation of cardiac mechanics. *J Am Soc Echocardiogr.* 2011;24:277–313.
19. Pathan F, D'Elia N, Nolan MT, et al. Normal ranges of left atrial strain by speckle-tracking echocardiography: a systematic review and meta-analysis. *J Am Soc Echocardiogr.* 2017;30:59–70.
20. Mochizuki A, Yuda S, Oi Y, et al. Assessment of left atrial deformation and synchrony by three-dimensional speckle-tracking echocardiography: comparative studies in healthy subjects and patients with atrial fibrillation. *J Am Soc Echocardiogr.* 2013;26:165–174.
21. Nemes A, Kormanyos A, Domsik P, et al. Normal reference values of three-dimensional speckle-tracking echocardiography-derived left atrial strain parameters (results from the MAGYAR-Healthy Study). *Int J Cardiovasc Imag.* 2019;35:991–998.
22. Saraiva RM, Scolin EMB, Pacheco NP, et al. 3-dimensional echocardiography and 2-d strain analysis of left ventricular, left atrial and right ventricular function in healthy Brazilian volunteers. *Arq Bras Cardiol.* 2019;113(5):935–945.
23. Hoit BD. Left atrial size and function: role in prognosis. *J Am Coll Cardiol.* 2014;63:493–505.
24. Singh A, Addetia K, Maffessanti F, et al. LA strain categorization of LV diastolic dysfunction. *JACC Cardiovasc Imaging.* 2017;10:735–743.
25. Sugimoto T, Robinet S, Dulgheru R, et al. Echocardiographic reference ranges for normal left atrial function parameters: results from the EACVI NORRE study. *Eur Heart J Cardiovasc Imag.* 2018;19(6):630–638.
26. Nikitin NP, Witte KK, Thackray SD, et al. Effect of age and sex on left atrial morphology and function. *Eur J Echocardiogr.* 2003;4:36–42.
27. Morris DA, Takeuchi M, Krisper M, et al. Normal values and clinical relevance of left atrial myocardial function analysed by speckle-tracking echocardiography: multicentre study. *Eur Heart J Cardiovasc Imag.* 2015;16:364–372.
28. Motoki H, To ACY, Bhargava M, et al. Comparison the left atrial mechanics between different techniques of two-dimensional speckle based strain in patients with atrial fibrillation. *Eur Heart J Cardiovasc Imaging.* 2011;12:ii39.

40 Ischemic Heart Disease: Which Test to Use?

Christopher B. Fordyce, Pamela S. Douglas

New-onset, stable chest pain among patients without known coronary artery disease (CAD) is a common clinical problem that results in approximately 4 million stress tests annually in the United States.[1] Significant variations in diagnostic strategies are well documented and may be related to differences in health care systems, access to testing technologies, and risk tolerance.[1,2] Furthermore, there are limited information on health-related outcomes in this stable, undiagnosed population and little consensus about which test is preferable or even when one is required.[3,4] In fact, major US and European guidelines have differed in their basic approaches and recommendations and are evolving rapidly with the availability of results from randomized trials comparing functional versus anatomical testing strategies.[5,6] The aims of this chapter are to provide a concise approach to noninvasive test selection based on recent guidelines and emerging evidence to:

1. Understand important patient characteristics and risk stratification algorithms that impact noninvasive test selection for the diagnosis of CAD.
2. Compare current guideline recommendations from the different professional organizations.
3. Incorporate recent data to enhance test selection through use of a unified approach for both functional and anatomical strategies.

PATIENT SELECTION FOR NONINVASIVE TESTING
Clinical Classification of Chest Pain

The current discussion applies specifically to stable, symptomatic patients with suspected ischemic heart disease (IHD) on the basis of a through history physical examination and laboratory data. Symptoms are classified as typical, atypical, or noncardiac to quantify the pretest probability (PTP) of underlying coronary disease.[7] Because the classic Diamond-Forrester algorithm significantly overestimates the degree of obstructive CAD,[5,6,8,9] use of the modified algorithm proposed in the 2019 European Society of Cardiology (ESC) Diagnosis and Management of Chronic Coronary Syndromes Guidelines is warranted.[10] This algorithm applies recent CAD prevalence in relevant outpatient populations to traditional DF risk categories to provide contemporary PTP (Table 40.1).

Approaches to Patient Selection

Diagnostic testing is most valuable when the PTP of IHD is intermediate because Bayesian analysis dictates that the application of a test result drives the posttest probability sufficiently lower (negative test) or higher (positive test) only in this range and thus the enhancement of future decision making. Whether the patient should proceed to cardiac catheterization is limited to those with intermediate PTP. Although there is no strict definition of intermediate PTP, 10% to 90%, first advocated in 1980,[11] has been applied in several studies and is the current definition used in the 2012 American College of Cardiology/American Heart Association (ACC/AHA) guidelines for stable IHD[12,13] and

2014 ACC Appropriate Use Criteria Task Force document.[14] In contrast, the current ESC guidelines advocate testing patients with a PTP greater than 15% (Table 40.2), and those 5% to 15% after assessing the overall clinical likelihood based on modifiers of PTP (Fig. 40.1). In contrast, the UK National Institute of Health and Care Excellence (NICE) has abandoned this probabilistic approach in favor of a symptom-focused assessment,[4] with patients having typical or atypical symptoms or an abnormal resting electrocardiogram recommended to have coronary computed tomography angiography (CCTA). The remainder are classified as nonanginal, and no further testing is recommended. This symptom-focused assessment identifies a larger group of low-risk chest pain patients potentially deriving limited benefit from noninvasive testing.[15] In fact, identifying chest pain patients based on baseline characteristics who may not receive any benefit from testing is an area of ongoing interest.[16] If the patient is unlikely to benefit from revascularization, then optimizing medical therapy with a no testing strategy is likely a reasonable approach. Similarly, a patient who is very low risk may be unlikely to benefit from testing.

SELECTING THE OPTIMAL NONINVASIVE TEST FOR ISCHEMIC HEART DISEASE DIAGNOSIS: A PROPOSED APPROACH

After the decision is made to proceed to noninvasive testing, the first decision is whether to proceed with anatomic testing (e.g., CCTA) or functional (stress) testing. The choice of modality must take into account both patient and test characteristics, cost, and local availability and expertise. The Prospective Multicenter Imaging Study for Evaluation of Chest Pain (PROMISE) and The Scottish Computed Tomography of the Heart (SCOT-HEART) trials demonstrate that an initial anatomical strategy with CCTA is a reasonable alternative to functional testing as a first-line choice, as recommended by both the UK NICE and 2019 ESC guidelines (Table 40.3).[4,10] A proposed rational approach is outlined in Fig. 40.1, which includes other imaging-specific considerations:

- Consider CCTA:
  - If needed for additional thoracic CT imaging, e.g., a triple or double rule out in suspected pulmonary embolism (d-dimer positive) and aortic dissection or if an intrathoracic pathology is suspected, such as pericardial disease[17]
  - If there is a suspected coronary anomaly[18]
  - If diagnosis of nonobstructive or obstructive CAD alone would result would result in a change in medical therapy[19–21]
- Consider stress echocardiography or cardiac magnetic resonance imaging (CMRI):
  - If evaluation of radiation-sensitive population is required; for example, gender and age or previous radiation exposure history[17]
  - If suspected valvular, pericardial, or congenital abnormality is concomitantly suspected
  - To potentially mitigate cost

TABLE 40.1 Pretest Probabilities of Obstructive Coronary Artery Disease in 15,815 Symptomatic Patients According to Age, Sex, and the Nature of Symptoms in a Pooled Analysis[41] of Contemporary Data[8,9,42]

Age	Typical		Atypical		Nonanginal		Dyspnea[a]	
	Men (%)	Women (%)	Men (%)	Women (%)	Men (%)	Women (%)	Men (%)	Women (%)
30–39	3	5	4	3	1	1	0	3
40–49	22	10	10	6	3	2	12	3
50–59	32	13	17	6	11	3	20	9
60–69	44	16	26	11	22	6	27	14
70+	52	27	34	19	24	10	32	12

[a]In addition to the classic Diamond and Forrester classification, patients with dyspnea only or dyspnea as the primary symptom are included. The regions shaded dark green denote the groups in which noninvasive testing is most beneficial (pretest probability [PTP] >15%). The *striped* regions in *light green* denote the groups with PTPs of coronary artery disease between 5% and 15%, in whom testing for diagnosis may be considered after assessing the overall clinical likelihood based on the modifiers of PTPs (Fig. 40.2).
Adapted with permission from Knuuti J, et al: 2019 ESC Guidelines for the diagnosis and management of chronic coronary syndromes, *Eur Heart J* 41:407–477, 2020.

TABLE 40.2 Selected Guideline Recommendations for the Use of Noninvasive Testing for the Diagnosis of Ischemic Heart Disease

	AHA/ACC (2012)[3]	ESC (2019)[10]	NICE (2016)[4]
PATIENT SELECTION			
Risk score to calculate PTP	Combined Diamond Forrester–CASS	Knuuti et al.[10]	Symptom based (typical or atypical chest pain)
Intermediate PTP	10%–90%	>15% 5%–15% (with modifiers)	Symptom based (typical or atypical chest pain)
TEST SELECTION			
Exercise treadmill test alone for the diagnosis of CAD[a]	Class I	Class IIb (evaluate CAD)	Second line if diagnosis is uncertain after CCTA
Stress imaging for the diagnosis of CAD[b]	Class IIa	Class I	Second line if diagnosis is uncertain after CCTA
Stress imaging if nonevaluable ECG	Class I	Class I	Second line if diagnosis is uncertain after CCTA
Stress imaging if CCTA has shown CAD of uncertain functional significance	Not specified	Class I	Second line if diagnosis is uncertain after CCTA
ANATOMICAL (CTA) TEST SELECTION			
CCTA for the diagnosis of CAD	IIb (can exercise) IIa (cannot exercise)	Class I	First line
Nonconclusive functional test or contraindications	Class IIa	Class IIa	Not applicable

[a] Able to exercise with an evaluable electrocardiogram (ECG).
[b] American College of Cardiology/American Heart Association (ACC/AHA) quantify risk as "intermediate to high."
CAD, coronary artery disease; *CASS,* Coronary Artery Surgery Study; *CCTA,* coronary computed tomography angiography; *ESC,* European Society of Cardiology; *NICE,* National Institute of Health and Care Excellence; *PTP,* pretest probability.

- Consider nuclear myocardial perfusion imaging (MPI) or positron emission tomography (PET):
  - If comparison to previous testing using these modalities is indicated
  - If cost and radiation are not significant considerations
- Consider nonimaging exercise treadmill testing:
  - If evaluation of radiation-sensitive population is required; for example, gender and age or previous radiation exposure history[17]
  - To mitigate cost

GENERAL APPROACH: FUNCTIONAL TESTING STRATEGIES

If testing is indicated and a functional strategy is selected, then the next choices are stress modality (exercise vs pharmacologic), and if exercise is used, whether additional imaging should be performed. Several stress imaging modalities currently exist, each with its advantages and disadvantages (Table 40.4), and include radionucleotide stress MPI using single-photon emission computed

tomography (SPECT) or PET, stress echocardiography, and stress CMRI (pharmacologic stress only). Decision making should proceed with a series of basic questions:

- *Can the patient exercise?* Symptom-limited exercise treadmill testing is the preferred modality (over pharmacologic) because it provides clinically useful information concerning reproducibility of symptoms, cardiovascular function, exercise capacity, and the hemodynamic response during usual activity. Furthermore, a score such as the Duke Treadmill Score can improve diagnostic certainty.[22] However, a patient may be unable to exercise because of obesity, orthopedic limitations, balance issues, vascular disease, or other impairments. A detailed discussion of exercise modalities (treadmill, upright or supine bicycle) and protocols (Bruce, Modified Bruce, Naughton) is presented elsewhere.[23]
- *Does the patient have any contraindications to exercise stress testing?* If absolute contraindications exist, then pharmacologic stress should be used; if relative contraindications exist, pharmacologic stress should be considered.[23,24]

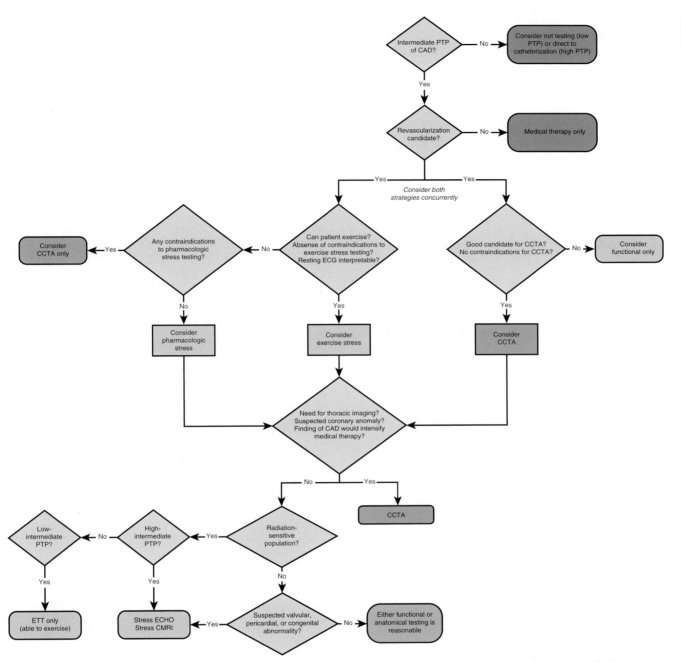

Figure 40.1. Proposed integrated approach to initial noninvasive test selection using both functional and anatomical approaches for the diagnosis of ischemic heart disease in patients with stable chest pain.[40] *CAD,* coronary artery disease; *CCTA,* coronary computed tomography angiography; *CMRI,* cardiac magnetic resonance imaging; *ECHO,* echocardiography; *ECG,* electrocardiogram; *ETT,* exercise treadmill test; *PTP,* pretest probability. (Adapted with permission from Fordyce CB, Douglas PS: Optimal non-invasive imaging test selection for the diagnosis of ischaemic heart disease, *Heart* 102:555–564, 2016.)

- *Is the resting electrocardiogram (ECG) interpretable?* Imaging should be used in the presence of conditions interfering with the ECG diagnosis of ischemia,[24] including ventricular pre-excitation (Wolff-Parkinson-White pattern), ventricular paced rhythm, left bundle branch block, 1 mm or greater ST depression at rest, digoxin use with associated ST-T abnormalities, left ventricular hypertrophy with ST-T abnormalities, or hypokalemia with ST-T abnormalities.
- *Is the patient unable to exercise to sufficient workload?* Pharmacologic stress should be considered. The decision regarding which agent to use will depend on patient factors, including

suitability of the stress agent for the chosen imaging modality; ischemic endpoints may vary accordingly.[25]
- *Does the patient have any contraindications to pharmacologic stress testing?* Vasodilator stress agents (adenosine; dipyridamole; and the selective A2A receptor agonists, including regadenoson, binodenoson, and apadenoson)[26–28] and dobutamine, a synthetic catecholamine,[29] have different mechanisms of action and different contraindications.
- *Is the patient not a candidate for exercise or pharmacologic stress testing?* An anatomical strategy with CCTA should be considered.

DIAGNOSTIC ACCURACY OF FUNCTIONAL TESTING STRATEGIES

There are distinct strengths and weaknesses of each imaging modality (see Table 40.3), and diagnostic performance varies by the prevalence of disease, the gold standard comparator used (anatomic disease vs invasive fractional flow reserve [FFR]), whether the goal is to rule in or rule out disease, and local laboratory expertise.

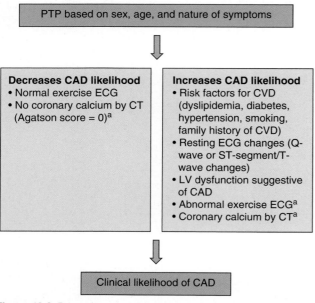

Figure 40.2. Determinants of the clinical likelihood of obstructive coronary artery disease. *CAD,* Coronary artery disease; *CT,* computed tomography, *CVD,* cardiovascular disease, *ECG,* electrocardiogram; *LV,* left ventricular; *PTP,* pretest probability. (Adapted with permission from Knuuti J, et al: 2019 ESC guidelines for the diagnosis and management of chronic coronary syndromes, *Eur Heart J* 41:407–477, 2020.)[a]

A recent meta-analysis determined the range of PTP of CAD in which stress ECG, stress echocardiography, CCTA, SPECT, PET, and CMRI could reclassify patients into a posttest probability that defines (>85%) or excludes (<15%) significant CAD both anatomically (defined by visual evaluation of invasive coronary angiography [ICA]) and functionally (defined by FFR ≤0.8) (see Table 40.4).[30] This analysis concluded (1) stress ECG has very limited diagnostic power; (2) functional imaging techniques (PET, CMRI, and SPECT), which had only moderate power in identifying anatomically significant CAD, performed much better when FFR was used as reference standard; and (3) ICA demonstrated the poorest ruling-out performance of all analyzed techniques when the reference standard was FFR. In addition, a recent controlled clinical head-to-head comparative study aiming to establish the diagnostic accuracy of CCTA, SPECT, and PET and explore the incremental value of hybrid imaging compared with FFR revealed PET to exhibit the highest accuracy for diagnosis of myocardial ischemia.[31] However, other data suggest that PET does not provide long-term clinical or cost benefit over SPECT or stress echocardiography.[32]

GENERAL APPROACH: ANATOMICAL STRATEGIES USING CORONARY COMPUTED TOMOGRAPHY ANGIOGRAPHY

Similar to functional testing, decision making when considering anatomical testing should proceed with a series of series of basic questions after the possibility of benefit from revascularization is established:

- *Is the patient a good candidate for CCTA?* According to a report from 2014 Society of Cardiovascular Computed Tomography,[17] only patients with adequate breath-holding capabilities, without severe obesity (>39 kg/m[2]), with a favorable coronary calcium score (Agatston score <400) and distribution, in sinus rhythm. and with a heart rate of 60 beats/min or less, and with normal or near normal renal function should be considered for CCTA.
- *Does the patient have any absolute contraindications to CCTA?* These include definite acute coronary syndrome, glomerular filtration rate below 30 mL/min unless on chronic dialysis,

TABLE 40.3 Advantages and Disadvantages of Stress Imaging Techniques and Coronary Computed Tomography Angiography

Technique	Advantages	Disadvantages
Stress echocardiography	• Wide access • Portability • No radiation • Low cost • Provides additional info regarding structure and function	• Echo contrast needed in patients with poor ultrasound windows • Dependent on operator skills
SPECT	• Wide access • Extensive data	• Radiation • Higher cost
PET	• Flow quantitation	• Radiation • Limited access • Highest cost
CMRI	• High soft tissue contrast • Precise imaging of myocardial scar • No ionizing radiation	• Limited access in cardiology • Contraindications • Functional analysis limited in arrhythmias • Limited 3D quantification of ischemia • High cost
CCTA	• High NPV in patients with lower PTP • Associated with improved preventive medication use and lower event rates	• Radiation • Assessment limited with extensive coronary calcium or prior stenting • Image quality limited with arrhythmias or higher heart rates that cannot be lowered • Low NPV in higher PTP

3D, Three-dimensional; *CCTA,* coronary computed tomography angiography; *CMRI,* cardiac magnetic resonance imaging; *NPV,* negative predictive value; *PET,* positron emission tomography; *PPV,* positive predictive value; *PTP,* pretest probability; *SPECT,* single-photon emission computed tomography.

TABLE 40.4 Performance of Different Tests for Anatomically and Functionally Significant Coronary Artery Disease[a]

Anatomic CAD

Test	Sensitivity (%), (95% CI)	Specificity (%), (95% CI)	+LR (95% CI)	-LR (95% CI)
Stress ECG	58 (49–69)	62 (54–69)	1.53 (1.21–1.94)	0.68 (0.49–0.93)
Stress echo	85 (80–89)	82 (72–89)	4.67 (2.95–7.41)	0.18 (0.13–0.25)
CCTA	97 (93–99)	78 (67–86)	4.44 (2.64–7.45)	0.04 (0.01–0.09)
SPECT	87 (83–90)	70 (63–76)	2.88 (2.33–3.56)	0.19 (0.15–0.24)
PET	90 (78–96)	85 (78–90)	5.87 (3.40–10.15)	0.12 (0.05–0.29)
Stress CMRI	90 (83–94)	80 (69–88)	4.54 (2.37–8.72)	0.13 (0.07–0.24)

Functionally Significant CAD

Test	Sensitivity (%), (95% CI)	Specificity (%), (95% CI)	+LR (95% CI)	-LR (95% CI)
ICA	68 (60–75)	73 (55–86)	2.49 (1.47–4.21)	0.44 (0.36–0.54)
CCTA	93 (89–96)	53 (37–38)	1.97 (1.28–3.03)	0.13 (0.06–0.25)
SPECT	73 (62–82)	83 (71–90)	4.21 (2.62–6.76)	0.33 (0.24–0.46)
PET	89 (82–93)	85 (81–88)	6.04 (4.29–8.51)	0.13 (0.08–0.222)
Stress CMRI	89 (85–92)	87 (83–91)	7.10 (5.07–9.95)	0.13 (0.09–0.18)

[a]Invasive coronary angiography (ICA) itself was used as a reference standard for the anatomically significant coronary artery disease (CAD) estimates but was included as a technique, when fractional flow reserve (FFR) was used as the reference. Not every test had enough data using FFR as reference.

CCTA, Coronary computed tomography angiography; CI, confidence interval; CMRI, cardiac magnetic resonance imaging; ECG, electrocardiogram; LR, likelihood ratio; PET, positron emission tomography; SPECT, single-photon emission computed tomography (exercise stress SPECT with or without dipyridamole or adenosine); Stress echo, exercise stress echocardiography.

Adapted with permission from Knuuti J, et al: The performance of non-invasive tests to rule-in and rule-out significant coronary artery stenosis in patients with stable angina: a meta-analysis focused on post-test disease probability, Eur Heart J 39:3322–3330, 2018.

previous anaphylaxis after iodinated contrast administration, previous episode of contrast allergy after adequate steroid or antihistamine preparation, inability to cooperate (including inability to raise the arms), or pregnancy or uncertain pregnancy status in premenopausal women.[17]

DIAGNOSTIC ACCURACY OF CORONARY COMPUTED TOMOGRAPHY ANGIOGRAPHY

Multicenter studies evaluating the diagnostic accuracy of 64-slice multidetector CCTA for detection of significant (at least 50% stenosis) CAD on quantitative ICA have found sensitivities of between 85% and 99% and specificities between 64% and 90%,[33-35] although newer equipment and scan protocols may improve the diagnostic accuracy. The variability in specificity, in particular, is strongly influenced by the baseline prevalence of CAD in the population studied and in the presence of coronary artery calcium.[33] In contrast, negative predictive values for CCTA have generally been high (95%-100%).[33,34] A recent meta-analysis (discussed earlier) confirmed that a negative CCTA excluded anatomically defined CAD independent of PTP, with moderate to good "rule in" power, with poorer performance with FFR as the reference standard (see Table 40.3).[30]

INTEGRATING FUNCTIONAL AND ANATOMICAL STRATEGIES

The association between coronary anatomy and ischemia is variable, as patients can have no ischemia in presence of significant stenosis and ischemia with only moderate stenosis.[36] Several modalities are being tested clinically, including fractional flow reserve computed tomography (FFR_{CT}) using three-dimensional mathematic modeling of coronary flow, pressure, and resistance[37]; hybrid SPECT/CCTA imaging[38]; and CMRI perfusion.[39]

SUMMARY

The prevalence of stable angina is high in the general population and increases with age in both sexes. Little consensus exists about which test is preferable when one is required for diagnosis, including significant differences in the current US and European guidelines. However, the recent PROMISE and SCOT-HEART trials incorporating the use of CCTA demonstrated that an anatomical strategy is a reasonable initial approach to use in patients with stable chest for the diagnosis of IHD. Contemporary approaches should therefore consider both functional and anatomical strategies in an integrated decision-making model.

REFERENCES

1. Ladapo JA, Blecker S, Douglas PS. Physician decision making and trends in the use of cardiac stress testing in the United States: an analysis of repeated cross-sectional data. *Ann Intern Med.* 2014;161:482–490.
2. Shaw LJ, Min JK, Hachamovitch R, et al. Cardiovascular imaging research at the crossroads. *JACC Cardiovasc Imag.* 2010;3:316–324.
3. Fihn SD, Gardin JM, Abrams J, et al. 2012. ACCF/AHA/ACP/AATS/PCNA/SCAI/STS guideline for the diagnosis and management of patients with stable ischemic heart disease. *J Am Coll Cardiol.* 2012;60:e44–e164.
4. National Institute for Health and Care Excellence. Chest pain of recent onset: assessment and diagnosis of recent onset chest pain or discomfort of suspected cardiac origin (update). *Clinical Guideline.* Vol. 95. London: NICE; 2016.
5. Scot-Heart Investigators. CT coronary angiography in patients with suspected angina due to coronary heart disease (SCOT-HEART): an open-label, parallel-group, multicentre trial. *Lancet.* 2015;385:2383–2391.
6. Douglas PS, Hoffmann U, Patel MR, et al. Outcomes of anatomical versus functional testing for coronary artery disease. *New Engl J Med.* 2015;372:1291–1300.
7. Diamond GA. A clinically relevant classification of chest discomfort. *J Am Coll Cardiol.* 1983;1(2s1):574–575.
8. Cheng VY, Berman DS, Rozanski A, et al. Performance of the traditional age, sex, and angina typicality-based approach for estimating pretest probability of angiographically significant coronary artery disease in patients undergoing coronary computed tomographic angiography: results from the multinational

9. Foldyna B, Udelson JE, Karady J, et al. Pretest probability for patients with suspected obstructive coronary artery disease: re-evaluating Diamond-Forrester for the contemporary era and clinical implications: insights from the PROMISE trial. *Eur Heart J Cardiovasc Imag.* 2019;20:574–581.
10. Knuuti J, Wijns W, Saraste A, et al. ESC Guidelines for the diagnosis and management of chronic coronary syndromes. *Eur Heart J.* 2019;41:407–477. 2020.
11. Diamond GA, Forrester JS, Hirsch M, et al. Application of conditional probability analysis to the clinical diagnosis of coronary artery disease. *J Clin Invest.* 1980;65:1210.
12. Goldman L, Cook EF, Mitchell N, et al. Incremental value of the exercise test for diagnosing the presence or absence of coronary artery disease. *Circulation.* 1982;66:945–953.
13. Melin JA, Wijns W, Vanbutsele RJ, et al. Alternative diagnostic strategies for coronary artery disease in women: demonstration of the usefulness and efficiency of probability analysis. *Circulation.* 1985;71:535–542.
14. Wolk MJ, Bailey SR, Doherty JU, et al. ACCF/AHA/ASE/ASNC/HFSA/HRS/SCAI/SCCT/SCMR/STS 2013 multimodality appropriate use criteria for the detection and risk assessment of stable ischemic heart disease. *J Am Coll Cardiol.* 2014;63:380–406.
15. Adamson PD, Newby DE, Hill CL, et al. Comparison of international guidelines for assessment of suspected stable angina: insights from the PROMISE and SCOT-HEART. *JACC Cardiovasc Imag.* 2018;11:1301–1310.
16. Fordyce CB, Douglas PS, Roberts RS, et al. Identification of patients with stable chest pain deriving minimal value from noninvasive testing: the PROMISE minimal-risk tool, a secondary analysis of a randomized clinical trial. *JAMA Cardiol.* 2017;2:400–408.
17. Raff GL, Chinnaiyan KM, Cury RC, et al. SCCT guidelines on the use of coronary computed tomographic angiography for patients presenting with acute chest pain to the emergency department. *J Cardiovasc Comput Tomogr.* 2014;8:254–271.
18. Roberts WT, Bax JJ, Davies LC. Cardiac CT and CT coronary angiography: technology and application. *Heart.* 2008;94:781–792.
19. Cheezum MK, Hulten EA, Smith RM, et al. Changes in preventive medical therapies and CV risk factors after CT angiography. *JACC Cardiovasc Imag.* 2013;6:574–581.
20. Hulten E, Bittencourt MS, Singh A, et al. Coronary artery disease detected by coronary computed tomographic angiography is associated with intensification of preventive medical therapy and lower low-density lipoprotein cholesterol. *Circulation Cardiovasc Imag.* 2014;7:629–638.
21. Pursnani A, Schlett CL, Mayrhofer T, et al. Potential for coronary CT angiography to tailor medical therapy beyond preventive guideline-based recommendations: Insights from the ROMICAT I trial. *J Cardiovasc Comput Tomogr.* 2015;9:193–201.
22. Shaw LJ, Peterson ED, Shaw LK, et al. Use of a prognostic treadmill score in identifying diagnostic coronary disease subgroups. *Circulation.* 1998;98:1622–1630.
23. Fletcher GF, Balady GJ, Amsterdam EA, et al. Exercise standards for testing and training a statement for healthcare professionals from the American Heart Association. *Circulation.* 2001;104:1694–1740.
24. Gibbons RJ, Balady GJ, Bricker JT, et al. ACC/AHA 2002 guideline update for exercise testing: summary article. *J Am Coll Cardiol.* 2002;40:1531–1540.
25. Shaw LJ, Berman DS, Picard MH, et al. Comparative definitions for moderate-severe ischemia in stress nuclear, echocardiography, and magnetic resonance imaging. *JACC Cardiovasc Imag.* 2014;7(6):593–604.
26. Trochu JN, Zhao G, Post H, et al. Selective A2A adenosine receptor agonist as a coronary vasodilator in conscious dogs: potential for use in myocardial perfusion imaging. *J Cardiovasc Pharmacol.* 2003;41:132–139.
27. Wilson RF, Wyche K, Christensen BV, et al. Effects of adenosine on human coronary arterial circulation. *Circulation.* 1990;82:1595–1606.
28. Sunderland JJ, Pan XB, Declerck J, et al. Dependency of cardiac rubidium-82 imaging quantitative measures on age, gender, vascular territory, and software in a cardiovascular normal population. *J Nucl Cardiol.* 2015;22:72–84.
29. Geleijnse ML, Elhendy A, Fioretti PM, et al. Dobutamine stress myocardial perfusion imaging. *J Am Coll Cardiol.* 2000;36:2017–2027.
30. Knuuti J, Ballo H, Juarez-Orozco LE, et al. The performance of non-invasive tests to rule-in and rule-out significant coronary artery stenosis in patients with stable angina: a meta-analysis focused on post-test disease probability. *Eur Heart J.* 2018;39:3322–3330.
31. Danad I, Raijmakers PG, Driessen RS, et al. Comparison of coronary CT angiography, SPECT, PET, and hybrid imaging for diagnosis of ischemic heart disease determined by fractional flow reserve. *JAMA Cardiol.* 2017;2:1100–1107.
32. Ma Q, Sridhar G, Power T, et al. Assessing the downstream value of first-line cardiac positron emission tomography (PET) imaging using real world Medicare fee-for-service claims data. *J Nucl Cardiol.* 2019. https://doi.org/10.1007/s12350-019-01974-8. (in press).
33. Budoff MJ, Dowe D, Jollis JG, et al. Diagnostic performance of 64-multidetector row coronary computed tomographic angiography for evaluation of coronary artery stenosis in individuals without known coronary artery disease: results from the prospective multicenter ACCURACY trial. *J Am Coll Cardiol.* 2008;52:1724–1732.
34. Meijboom WB, Meijs MF, Schuijf JD, et al. Diagnostic accuracy of 64-slice computed tomography coronary angiography: a prospective, multicenter, multivendor study. *J Am Coll Cardiol.* 2008;52:2135–2144.

35. Miller JM, Rochitte CE, Dewey M, et al. Diagnostic performance of coronary angiography by 64-row CT. *New Engl J Med.* 2008;359:2324–2336.
36. Ahmadi A, Kini A, Narula J. Discordance between ischemia and stenosis, or PINSS and NIPSS: are we ready for new vocabulary? *JACC Cardiovasc Imag.* 2015;8:111–114.
37. Precious B, Blanke P, Norgaard BL, et al. Fractional flow reserve modeled from resting coronary CT angiography: state of the science. *AJR Am J Roentgenol.* 2015;204:W243–W248.
38. Rispler S, Keidar Z, Ghersin E, et al. Integrated single-photon emission computed tomography and computed tomography coronary angiography for the assessment of hemodynamically significant coronary artery lesions. *J Am Coll Cardiol.* 2007;49(10):1059–1067.
39. Hundley WG, Bluemke DA, Finn JP, et al. ACCF/ACR/AHA/NASCI/SCMR 2010 expert consensus document on cardiovascular magnetic resonance. *Circulation.* 2010;121:2462–2508.
40. Fordyce CB, Douglas PS. Optimal non-invasive imaging test selection for the diagnosis of ischaemic heart disease. *Heart.* 2016;102:555–564.
41. Juarez-Orozco LE, Saraste A, Capodanno D, et al. Impact of a decreasing pre-test probability on the performance of diagnostic tests for coronary artery disease. *Eur Heart J.* 2019;20:1198–1207.
42. Reeh J, Therming CB, Heitmann M, et al. Prediction of obstructive coronary artery disease and prognosis in patients with suspected stable angina. *Eur Heart J.* 2019;40:1426–1435.

41 Ischemic Heart Disease: Basic Principles

Philippe B. Bertrand, Shiying Liu, Michael H. Picard

ACUTE EFFECTS OF MYOCARDIAL ISCHEMIA

Significant coronary artery stenosis results in impaired blood flow and reduced myocardial oxygen supply. When myocardial oxygen demand exceeds supply, myocardial ischemia develops. In addition, in the setting of a complete coronary artery occlusion, myocardial necrosis can occur. As a result of hypoxia, the myocardium shifts from aerobic oxidative phosphorylation to anaerobic metabolism. Consequently, both fatty acid and carbohydrate oxidation decrease, adenosine triphosphate production is impaired, and glycolysis is accelerated, which requires increased uptake of glucose by the heart.[1,2] The glucose taken up by the ischemic myocardium is not readily oxidized in the mitochondria but rather is converted to lactate, resulting in a fall in intracellular pH and a decrease in contractile work. Successful reperfusion of reversibly injured myocytes is associated with partial or complete restoration to the control state of many of the metabolic changes present in the ischemic myocytes and resumption of oxidative phosphorylation.[3,4]

ECHOCARDIOGRAPHIC DETECTION OF MYOCARDIAL ISCHEMIA AND INFARCTION

Echocardiographic detection of myocardial ischemia is based on visualizing a regional decrease in systolic endocardial motion (longitudinal and circumferential shortening) and myocardial (radial) thickening. In the presence of a flow-limiting coronary lesion, the increased myocardial blood flow that normally occurs with physiologic stress is impaired, and this results in decreased regional systolic wall thickening, or hypokinesis. Similarly, with complete coronary ligation or acute obstruction, there is an immediate loss of normal myocardial contraction in the region supplied by the affected vessel followed by regional systolic bulging.[5]

With chronic coronary artery occlusion and infarction, there can also be systolic thinning of the myocardium. Thus, regional left ventricular (LV) wall abnormalities have become the hallmark of coronary artery disease (CAD) and can be imaged on echocardiography. Studies in which progressive coronary stenoses are produced in animal models have shown a nearly linear correlation between regional wall motion (by sonomicrometry) and subendocardial blood flow,[6–9] suggesting that regional wall motion abnormality (WMA) is a sensitive marker of acute ischemic events. It has also been shown that with coronary occlusion, regional wall hypokinesis occurs earlier than the classic electrocardiographic changes.[10] Other studies have shown that a fall in regional contraction of greater than 10% is a reliable marker of regional flow deficit and reflects a defect in subendocardial perfusion.[11] Based on both experiments in dog models[10,12] and observations in

humans during percutaneous coronary angioplasty,[13,14] an ischemic cascade has been postulated (Fig. 41.1). As seen in this cascade, echocardiography allows for detection of WMAs at an earlier phase than the appearance of electrocardiographic (ECG) changes and clinical symptoms.

Experimental studies with graded coronary artery ligation to induce subendocardial ischemia indicate that in addition to dysfunction of the ischemic zone, there is also a small zone of mild hypofunction immediately adjacent to the ischemic zone, with hyperfunction beyond that zone.[15,16]

Studies have demonstrated that WMAs visualized with two-dimensional echocardiography (2DE) exceed pathologic infarct size in acute infarction.[17] This may reflect border-zone hypoperfusion, small islands of necrosis, or tethering of normal segments adjacent

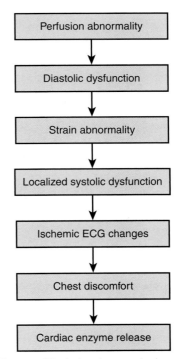

Figure 41.1. Diagram of the ischemic cascade demonstrating that localized left ventricular systolic dysfunction seen on echocardiography as a wall motion abnormality occurs before electrocardiogram (ECG) changes and chest pain symptoms.

to abnormal segments.[17,18] Wall thickening abnormalities on 2DE can be detected when necrosis involves a small (1%–20%) amount of the myocardial segment thickness.[19] When more than 20% of the transmural thickness is infarcted, the segment demonstrates a constant degree of degradation in wall thickening, and there is not a further gradual deterioration in wall thickening for larger degrees of involvement of the myocardial thickness. Thus, in addition to the effects of mechanical tethering, WMAs noted in the border zones of infarcts may reflect small amounts of necrosis.

Early experimental data showed that the resting coronary blood flow was not decreased until tight coronary stenosis greater than 90% developed.[20] Systolic dysfunction and WMAs in the setting of physiologic stress are generally perceptible in coronary artery stenoses in the range of 50% to 60%; akinesis is seen when a reduction in coronary flow that is greater than 80% is present.[21,22]

The subjective assessment of LV wall motion by echocardiography requires the interpreter to integrate both endocardial motion and transmural wall thickening during systole. Although the wall motion may be easier to assess, it does not appear to differentiate regions of ischemia and infarction as well as wall thickening does.[19] The wall thickening directly correlates with myofiber function, whereas endocardial motion is an end result of myofiber shortening. The perception of wall motion is also subject to the effects of translation and other extracardiac motions.

MYOCARDIAL DEFORMATION DURING CARDIAC ISCHEMIA

A limitation to the visual detection of both resting and stress-induced WMAs by echocardiography is the subjective nature of the assessment. Tissue Doppler echocardiography and speckle-tracking echocardiography allow a quantitative assessment of myocardial deformation (i.e., myocardial strain).[23] Strain can be quantified in the radial direction (wall thickening and thinning) as well as in the longitudinal and circumferential directions (fiber shortening and lengthening). As myocardial fiber orientation ranges from predominantly circumferential fibers in the subepicardial layers to predominantly longitudinal fibers in the subendocardium, the longitudinal deformation is the first to be affected by myocardial ischemia.[24] A decrease in both radial and longitudinal strain can be observed during acute myocardial ischemia.[25] In addition, segmental relaxation is impaired during ischemia with ongoing postsystolic thickening and shortening. The latter is detected as postsystolic strain in deformation imaging, which relates to active myocardial contraction in weakened myocardial segments but can also represent passive recoil in scarred myocardium or a combination of both phenomena[26] (Fig. 41.2).

PATTERNS OF ISCHEMIA BASED ON CORONARY ARTERY INVOLVEMENT

Clinical studies with 2DE have demonstrated a clear relationship between the location and extent of WMAs and pathologic size of infarction.[17,27,28] Although there is some variability in the branching pattern of the coronary arteries supplying the various segments of the left ventricle, the location of wall motion is reproducibly linked to the affected artery (see Fig. 25.2).[29–31] Ischemia or infarction caused by disease in the left anterior descending coronary artery results in WMAs in the anterior and anteroseptal segments at the base, midlevels, and most or all of the apex. Ischemia or infarction caused by disease in the right coronary artery results in WMAs in the inferior and inferoseptal segments at the base and mid left ventricle. Ischemia or infarction caused by disease in the left circumflex coronary artery results in WMAs in the lateral wall at the base and mid LV. The dominance of the coronary artery pattern influences whether the right coronary artery or the circumflex coronary artery supplies the inferolateral segments. Likewise, the anterolateral territory can be supplied by either the left anterior descending coronary artery or the left circumflex coronary artery.

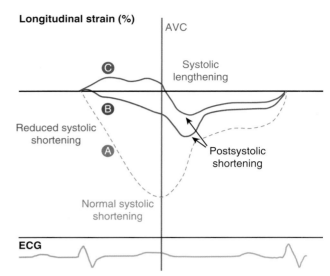

Figure 41.2. Characteristic longitudinal strain patterns of a normal myocardial segment *(dashed line)* (**A**), a segment with decreased peak systolic strain and evidence of postsystolic shortening, most likely due to active contraction (**B**), and a segment with systolic lengthening and postsystolic shortening (**C**) most likely caused by passive recoil in a segment that is potentially scarred. *AVC,* aortic valve closure; *ECG,* electrocardiogram.

Detection of isolated left circumflex CAD by stress echocardiography is much more difficult than detection of isolated left anterior or right CAD.[31] The sensitivity to detect stress-induced WMAs increases as the number of diseased vessels increases.[32]

FALSE INDICATIONS OF ISCHEMIA ON ECHOCARDIOGRAPHY

Not all LV WMAs seen on echocardiography are caused by myocardial ischemia or infarction. Other causes include septal WMAs due to left bundle branch block, right ventricular pacing, intrinsic conduction abnormality, postoperative changes, and right ventricular pressure or volume overload. In most of these situations, wall thickening is preserved, although its timing may differ from normal. That is, motion is abnormal, but thickening is normal. Nonischemic causes of cardiomyopathy (e.g., myocarditis, sarcoidosis, stress-induced cardiomyopathy) and marked hypertension are other possible causes of WMAs. In these situations, thickening is reduced. In the case of cardiomyopathy, the wall motion can reflect disruptions to normal myocyte function or extensive myocardial fibrosis. Even in the absence of significant CAD, a marked increase in blood pressure sometimes noted during stress echocardiography can prevent the development of hyperkinesis or even result in global hypokinesis. Such findings are thought to be caused by a sudden increase in myocardial oxygen demand under conditions when oxygen delivery cannot be increased because of the high pressure transmitted to the subendocardium directly from the LV cavity. False-positive WMAs perceived in the basal inferior or inferoseptal walls can be caused by off-axis imaging, poor endocardial visualization, and regional distortions in LV shape, where relatively thinner myocardium is perceived as hypokinetic.[33]

Paradoxical motion (pseudodyskinesis) of the inferior wall caused by extrinsic compression of the LV can be mistaken for inferior myocardial infarction.[34] In pseudodyskinesis, the inferior wall is flattened and the LV is noncircular at end-diastole because of external pressure; in systole, the inferior wall thickens normally, restoring a normal circular shape to the LV and creating a visual impression of dyskinesis.[34] It is important to differentiate pseudodyskinesis from true dyskinesis caused by inferior myocardial infarction. In the latter case, the inferior wall has a normally round contour at end-diastole, with outward bulging and thinning of that wall in systole.[34] Finally, in the absence of prior heart surgery and hyperdynamic mid and distal segments, an isolated basal WMA in one segment during stress echocardiography is unlikely to reflect CAD.

In the past century, the effects of myocardial ischemia and infarction on the left ventricle have been well characterized. With its excellent temporal and spatial resolution, echocardiography is an ideal modality for the assessment of the abnormalities of LV wall motion and thickening that occur with infarction and ischemia.

Acknowledgment

The authors acknowledge the contributions of Dr. Shmuel S. Schwartzenberg, MD, who was a coauthor of this chapter in the previous edition.

REFERENCES

1. Schaefer S, Schwartz GG, Wisneski JA, et al. Response of high-energy phosphates and lactate release during prolonged regional ischemia in vivo. *Circulation*. 1992;85:342–349.
2. Jennings RB, Reimer KA. The cell biology of acute myocardial ischemia. *Ann Rev Med*. 1991;42:225–246.
3. Jennings RB, Murry C, Reimer KA. Myocardial effects of brief periods of ischemia followed by reperfusion. *Adv Cardiol*. 1990;37(7–31).
4. Jennings RB, Schaper J, Hill ML, et al. Effect of reperfusion late in the phase of reversible ischemic injury. Changes in cell volume, electrolytes, metabolites, and ultrastructure. *Circ Res*. 1985;56:262–278.
5. Tennant R, Wiggers C. The effect of coronary occlusion on myocardial contraction. *Am J Physiol*. 1935;112:351.
6. Theroux P, Franklin D, Ross Jr J, Kemper WS. Regional myocardial function during acute coronary artery occlusion and its modification by pharmacologic agents in the dog. *Circ Res*. 1974;35(6):896–908.
7. Gallagher KP, Matsuzaki M, Koziol JA, et al. Regional myocardial perfusion and wall thickening during ischemia in conscious dogs. *Am J Physiol* 247. 1984:H727–H738.
8. Sasayama S, Franklin D, Ross Jr J, et al. Dynamic changes in left ventricular wall thickness and their use in analyzing cardiac function in the conscious dog. *Am J Cardiol* 38. 1976;(7):870–879.
9. Theroux P, Ross Jr J, Franklin D, et al. Coronary arterial reperfusion. III. Early and late effects on regional myocardial function and dimensions in conscious dogs. *Am J Cardiol*. 1976;38(5):599–606.
10. Battler A, Froelicher VF, Gallagher KP, et al. Dissociation between regional myocardial dysfunction and ECG changes during ischemia in the conscious dog. *Circulation*. 1980;62(4):735–744.
11. Lee JD, Tajimi T, Guth B, et al. Exercise-induced regional dysfunction with subcritical coronary stenosis. *Circulation*. 1986;73(3):596–605.
12. Pandian NG, Kieso RA, Kerber RE. Two-dimensional echocardiography in experimental coronary stenosis. II. Relationship between systolic wall thinning and regional myocardial perfusion in severe coronary stenosis. *Circulation*. 1982;66:603–611.
13. Hauser AM, Gangadharan V, Ramos RG, et al. Sequence of mechanical, electrocardiographic and clinical effects of repeated coronary artery occlusion in human beings: echocardiographic observations during coronary angioplasty. *J Am Coll Cardiol*. 1985;5:193–197.
14. Wohlgelernter D, Cleman M, Highman HA, et al. Regional myocardial dysfunction during coronary angioplasty: evaluation by two-dimensional echocardiography and 12 lead electrocardiography. *J Am Coll Cardiol*. 1986;7(8):1245–1254.
15. Gallagher KP, Gerren RA, Stirling MC, et al. The distribution of functional impairment across the lateral border of acutely ischemic myocardium. *Circ Res*. 1986;58(4):570–583.
16. Lima JA, Becker LC, Melin JA, et al. Impaired thickening of nonischemic myocardium during acute regional ischemia in the dog. *Circulation*. 1985;71:1048–1059.
17. Wilkins GT, Southern JF, Choong CY, et al. Correlation between echocardiographic endocardial surface mapping of abnormal wall motion and pathologic infarct size in autopsied hearts. *Circulation*. 1988;77(5):978–987.
18. Gillam LD, Franklin TD, Foale RA, et al. The natural history of regional wall motion in the acutely infarcted canine ventricle. *J Am Coll Cardiol*. 1986;7(6):1325–1334.
19. Lieberman AN, Weiss JL, Jugdutt BI, et al. Two-dimensional echocardiography and infarct size: relationship of regional wall motion and thickening to the extent of myocardial infarction in the dog. *Circulation*. 1981;63(4):739–746.
20. Gould KL, Lipscomb K. Effects of coronary stenoses on coronary flow reserve and resistance. *Am J Cardiol*. 1974;34:48–55.
21. Salustri A, Arnese M, Boersma E, et al. Correlation of coronary stenosis by quantitative coronary arteriography with exercise echocardiography. *Am J Cardiol*. 1995;75(4):87–90.
22. Agati L, Arata L, Luongo R, et al. Assessment of severity of coronary narrowings by quantitative exercise echocardiography and comparison with quantitative arteriography. *Am J Cardiol*. 1991;67(15):1201–1207.
23. Gorcsan J, Tanaka H. Echocardiographic assessment of myocardial strain. *J Am Coll Cardiol*. 2011;58:1401–1413.
24. Claus P, Omar AMS, Pedrizzetti G, et al. Tissue tracking technology for assessing cardiac mechanics: principles, normal values, and clinical applications. *J Am Coll Cardiol Img*. 2015;8:1444–1460.
25. Kukulski T, Jamal F, Herbots L, et al. Identification of acutely ischemic myocardium using ultrasonic strain measurements. A clinical study in patients undergoing coronary angioplasty. *J Am Coll Cardiol*. 2003;41(5):810–819.
26. Skulstad H, Edvardsen T, Urheim S, et al. Postsystolic shortening in ischemic myocardium active contraction or passive recoil? *Circulation*. 2002;106:718–724.
27. Heger J, Weyman AE, Wann LS, et al. Cross-sectional echocardiography in acute myocardial infarction: detection and localization of regional left ventricular asynergy. *Circulation*. 1979;60:531–538.
28. Crouse LJ, Harbrecht JJ, Vacek JL, et al. Exercise echocardiography as a screening test for coronary artery disease and correlation with coronary arteriography. *Am J Cardiol*. 1991;67(15):1213–1218.
29. Pellikka PA, Arruda-Olson A, Chaudhry FA, et al. Guidelines for performance, interpretation and application of stress echocardiography in ischemic heart disease: 2019 American Society of Echocardiography guidelines update. *J Am Soc Echocardiogr*. 2019 (in press).
30. Picard MH, Wilkins GT, Ray PA, Weyman AE. Natural history of left ventricular size and function after acute myocardial infarction. Assessment and prediction by echocardiographic endocardial surface mapping. *Circulation*. 1990;82(2):484–494.
31. Armstrong WF, O'Donnell J, Ryan T, Feigenbaum H. Effect of prior myocardial infarction and extent and location of coronary disease on accuracy of exercise echocardiography. *J Am Coll Cardiol*. 1997;10(3):531–538.
32. Ryan T, Vasey CG, Presti CF, et al. Exercise echocardiography: detection of coronary artery disease in patients with normal left ventricular wall motion at rest. *J Am Coll Cardiol*. 1988;11(5):993–999.
33. Bach DS, Muller DW, Gros BJ, Armstrong WF. False positive dobutamine stress echocardiograms: characterization of clinical, echocardiographic and angiographic findings. *J Am Coll Cardiol*. 1994;24(4):928–933.
34. Yosefy C, Levine RA, Picard MH, et al. Pseudodyskinesis of the inferior left ventricular wall: recognizing an echocardiographic mimic of myocardial infarction. *J Am Soc Echocardiogr*. 2007;20:1374–1379.

42 Acute Chest Pain Syndromes: Differential Diagnosis

Federico M. Asch, Neil J. Weissman

When patients present with chest pain, the clinician needs to be alert and thorough in trying to determine its cause. The patient's demographic characteristics together with a careful history should provide the initial information for understanding the likely etiologies. The addition of bedside evaluation by means of physical examination, chest radiography, and electrocardiography (ECG) should further narrow the differential diagnosis. However, more advanced diagnostic tools are frequently needed. Depending on the specific clinical scenario, the choices could range from cardiac biomarkers (e.g., troponin, and creatine kinase-MB, B-type natriuretic peptide, D-dimer) to a variety of advanced cardiac imaging tests such as cardiac computed tomography (CT), magnetic resonance imaging (MRI), stress test, and transthoracic or transesophageal echocardiograms. Although determining the likelihood of coronary artery disease as the reason for chest pain, it is of paramount importance (both for chronic and acute chest pain syndromes) for clinicians not to overlook other significant differential diagnoses (Table 42.1). Importantly, point-of-care cardiac ultrasound (POCUS)

TABLE 42.1 Differential Diagnosis for Chest Pain and Corresponding Echo Findings

Acute CP	Cardiac	ACS	WMA with coronary distribution
		Pericarditis	Pericardial effusion
		Myocarditis	WMA with: noncoronary distribution
		Takotsubo cardiomyopathy	Apical ballooning or other noncoronary WMA
	Noncardiac	Pulmonary embolism	RV strain, McConnell sign, thrombus in transit
		Aortic dissection and acute aortic syndromes	Aortic aneurysm, flap, AI, pericardial effusion
		Pneumothorax	Loss of pleural sliding and B lines
		Pleuritic syndromes	Pleural fluid
		Musculoskeletal	None
		Gastroesophageal	None
Chronic CP	Cardiac	Stable CAD	WMA with coronary distribution
		Pericarditis	Pericardial effusion
		Valvular diseases	Aortic stenosis, MV prolapse
		Cardiac tumors	LA myxoma
	Noncardiac	Gastroesophageal	None
		Musculoskeletal	None

AI, Aortic insufficiency; *CAD,* coronary artery disease; *CP,* chest pain; *LA,* left atrium; *MV,* mitral valve; *RV,* right ventricle; *WMA,* wall motion abnormality.

is becoming a tool available to newer, nontraditional users such as emergency department (ED) physicians and intensivists for a focused evaluation that will address specific clinical questions according to individual patient's needs. The role of echocardiography in this process, including POCUS, is discussed in this section with an emphasis on the differential diagnosis of acute chest pain syndromes. The use of echocardiography and stress echocardiography in stable chronic syndromes is discussed in other chapters.

Patients with acute chest pain represent a large percentage of the ED visits in the United States and worldwide and therefore incur a large burden to the health care system.[1–3] Because of its safety and easy availability, echocardiography is a very useful tool in addressing the differential diagnosis for these patients, particularly in detecting potentially life-threatening conditions. Careful evaluation of left ventricular (LV) regional and global wall motion has the highest yield in detecting acute coronary syndromes (ACSs). However, evaluation of other structures such as the right ventricle (RV), aorta, pericardium, lungs, or pleura can detect other pathologies responsible for the clinical presentation. The use of a focused POCUS in acute chest pain evaluation has been extensively embraced in recent years[4] and addressed in a joint document form the American Society of Echocardiography (ASE) and the American College of Emergency Physicians.[5]

LEFT VENTRICLE

Evaluation of the LV function, regional wall motion, and thickening as well as its morphology can be of critical significance in detecting ACSs and cardiomyopathies.

Left Ventricular Function and Acute Coronary Syndrome

As an acute coronary event occurs, coronary flow through the vessel is impaired, resulting in myocardial ischemia. The coronary arteries are not properly visualized by echocardiography; therefore, the focus is in imaging the myocardium. Classic findings in ACSs include regional wall motion abnormalities (WMAs; hypo- or akinesis) with impaired thickening of the affected regional myocardium. More recently, the use of ultrasound-enhancing agents (echo contrast) for myocardial perfusion imaging has also allowed the detection of ischemic myocardium in resting echocardiograms. Because coronary artery disease affects the myocardium in a regional manner, the distribution of such abnormalities respects the coronary territories. It should be noted, however, that coronary distribution varies on an individual basis and should only be used as a guide.[6]

Although musculoskeletal pain is the most frequent cause of chest pain upon presentation to the ED, detecting ACSs is of critical importance because adequate anti-ischemic therapies (including

revascularization) must be implemented in a timely manner. The presence of ST-segment elevation on an ECG should trigger immediate catheterization and percutaneous coronary intervention; therefore, an echocardiogram should not delay this intervention and must be postponed until the procedure is finished. However, in cases of suspected ACS without ST elevation, an echocardiogram in the ED could be of enormous value in detecting myocardial infarction (MI)[7] and predicting cardiac events.[8] Although cardiac biomarkers, particularly troponin and myoglobin, are extremely sensitive in detecting MI, the results of these tests may remain negative for a few hours after chest pain onset. Echocardiographic findings (regional WMA or thickening abnormality) of myocardial ischemia, on the other hand, are detected in almost 90% of patients scanned during or immediately after chest pain.[9] A combined approach using troponin and echocardiogram has high accuracy in detecting ACS without ST elevation, with sensitivity and specificity greater than 90%.[10,11]

Patients with chest pain and left bundle branch block represent a particular challenge in that the abnormal ECG could be masking ST elevation. Although historically this has been an indication for emergent catheterization, the concept has been challenged, and the use of biomarkers and bedside echocardiogram is being advocated to identify acute infarction: evidence of a hypokinetic or akinetic segmental WMA (lack of normal myocardial thickening in addition to myocardial excursion) in the anterior wall in the absence of evidence of a prior infarction (wall thinning, chamber dilatation) should trigger an emergent catheterization.[12,13]

The utility of contrast echocardiography in the ED to evaluate for myocardial perfusion defects has been validated in several studies and reviewed in the recent ASE guidelines.[14,15] In the setting of ischemia, typical findings are poor contrast uptake in the subendocardial myocardium (Fig. 42.1). The addition of myocardial contrast echocardiography to regional function increased the diagnostic and prognostic value of patients with chest pain and no ST elevation in the ED[16] and proved to be a cost-effective intervention by facilitating early discharge of those with normal perfusion.[17] Despite their promising potential, contrast agents for myocardial perfusion imaging have not yet been approved by the US Food and Drug Administration.

Left Ventricular Function and Cardiomyopathies

In addition to ischemic cardiomyopathy, two other myocardial diseases can present with acute-onset chest pain: myocarditis and Takotsubo cardiomyopathy (apical ballooning syndrome).

Myocarditis can present in a variety of forms, from small areas of WMA to global hypokinesis, and can be accompanied by pericardial effusion. Typically, these abnormalities do not respect a coronary territory, and frequently, wall motion patterns cannot be differentiated from the patterns of other forms of dilated cardiomyopathies.

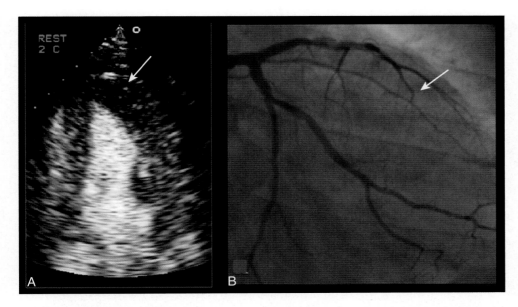

Figure 42.1. Myocardial contrast echocardiography. This patient presented with chest pain and left anterior descending (LAD) artery occlusion. **A,** A two-chamber view showing perfusion defect (minimal bubble uptake) in the mid to apical segments of the anterior wall *(arrow)*. **B,** Diffuse coronary disease with occlusion of the mid LAD *(arrow)*.

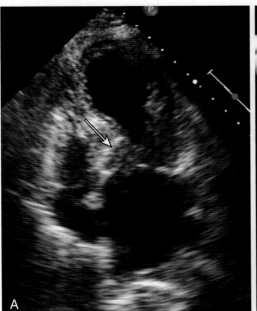
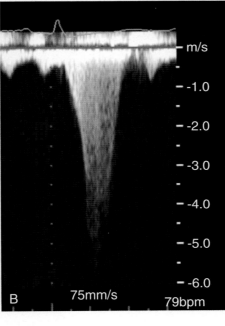

Figure 42.2. Takotsubo cardiomyopathy (apical ballooning). A 62-year-old woman with chest pain in the context of a recent stressful situation, ST-segment depression in precordial leads and normal coronaries. **A,** A five-chamber apical view in systole with classical apical ballooning caused by akinesia or dyskinesia of the apical half of the left ventricle and normally contracting basal segments. The *arrow* points at systolic anterior motion of the anterior mitral leaflet reflecting left ventricular outflow tract (LVOT) obstruction. **B,** A continuous-wave Doppler recording through the LVOT from the same window, with characteristic "dagger-shaped" spectral recording, reflecting a rapid gradual increase in the degree of obstruction as systole progress.

Takotsubo cardiomyopathy is a transient form of LV dysfunction in a characteristic pattern of apical ballooning: akinesis or dyskinesis of the apical half of the LV with normal or hyperdynamic basal segments (Fig. 42.2). It affects mostly postmenopausal women and is triggered by emotional or physical stress.[18] Although the course is generally benign and reverts within weeks, complications are common and include cardiogenic shock, ventricular tachycardia (torsade de points), atrioventricular block, apical thrombus, ventricular rupture, and LV outflow tract obstruction with systolic anterior motion of the mitral leaflets (see Fig. 42.2) and mitral regurgitation.[19] More recently, atypical forms of Takotsubo cardiomyopathy have been described, with other patterns of transient WMA triggered by stress. Importantly, apical ballooning could be indistinguishable from an anterior MI, and therefore cardiac catheterization is warranted to evaluate the left anterior descending artery.[20]

Right Ventricle

Pulmonary embolism (PE) is a critical differential diagnosis to be made in acute chest pain because specific urgent treatment is required. On rare occasions, the diagnosis of PE can be made on a transthoracic echocardiography (TTE) based on the visualization of thrombus in transit in the right cardiac chambers or a saddle embolism in the main pulmonary artery in a high short-axis view of the great vessels (Fig. 42.3). More frequently, however, indirect evidence of a PE on echocardiography include signs of RV strain such as RV dilatation and dysfunction; these echocardiography findings are not specific but are sensitive in detecting large PE. A sign described by McConnell and coworkers[21] (hypokinesis of the RV free wall with normally contracting apex) is more specific for acute RV dysfunction, which may be encountered in the setting of acute PE or RV infarction.[22] Because RV infarction almost always presents with inferior MI, the lack of LV WMAs in the presence of McConnell sign is highly specific of PE. For a more detailed description of PE, see other chapters of this book.

Aorta

Acute aortic syndromes (aortic dissection, intramural hematoma, and ulcerated plaques) present as acute chest pain and represent medical

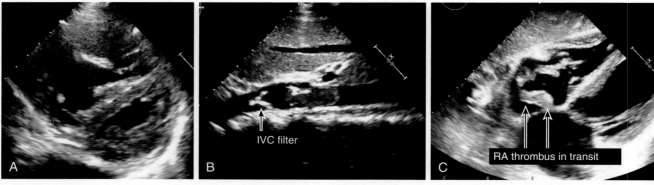

Figure 42.3. Pulmonary embolism. A 55-year-old woman with history of deep venous thrombosis and pulmonary embolism and an inferior vena cava (IVC) filter presented with chest pain, respiratory failure, and hypotension. Transthoracic echocardiography (TTE) showed a severely dilated and dysfunctional right ventricle (RV) with RV pressure and volume overload. **A,** Flattened interventricular septum during systole and diastole in a parasternal short-axis view. **B,** A large thrombus in the IVC between the IVC filter and the RA (the right atrium [RA] is on the right). **C,** A thrombus in transit in the RA on TTE (subxyphoid view) of a different patient presenting with dyspnea and chest pain.

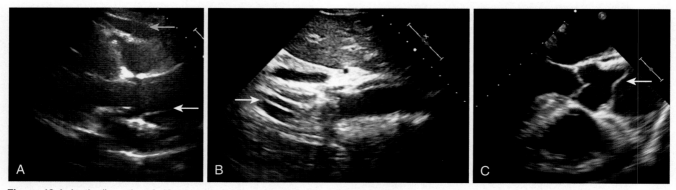

Figure 42.4. Aortic dissection. A 43-year-old woman presented with sudden onset of a lacerating chest pain, 10 of 10 in intensity from onset. **A,** Parasternal long-axis view on transthoracic echocardiography (TTE) showing a dissection flap in the ascending aorta *(white arrow)* and pericardial effusion *(blue arrow)*. **B,** A subxiphoid view with a long-axis view of the abdominal aorta shows distal extension of the dissection flap *(white arrow)*. **C,** TEE provided further details: the *arrow* shows the dissection flap extending proximally to the sinotubular junction, sparing the aortic root and the coronary ostia. In addition, a site of aortic rupture was identified in the ascending aorta.

emergencies. Therefore, although uncommon, their surveillance is critical when the clinical suspicious is present. The sensitivity of TTE for detection of aortic dissection is low because of difficulties in imaging the entire aortal but is high for the proximal ascending segment.[23,24] However, when an echocardiogram for acute chest pain is being performed, several findings should raise suspicious for aortic dissection: the presence of a dilated aortic root or ascending aorta in the parasternal long-axis view (a high probe position may be needed for proper imaging of the ascending portion), as well as a dilated arch or abdominal aorta (suprasternal notch and subxiphoid views, respectively) (Fig. 42.4). A dissection flap may be seen from any of these views, but the lack of such flap should not be assumed to rule out an aortic dissection. Detection of complications from dissection is more likely, such as acute aortic regurgitation or pericardial effusion. Whenever dissection is suspected, more advanced imaging techniques must be used such as transesophageal echocardiography (TEE), chest CT, or MRI. Their accuracy is similarly high, and the method of choice should be dependent on the availability and expertise at each center.[25]

TEE is unique in that it can be performed at the bedside when patients are hemodynamically unstable or in the operating room as the patient gets ready for surgery. In addition, a TEE does not require radiation or contrast, particularly important because the clinical situation may be complicated by acute renal injury caused by shock or renal ischemia. Although all three of these modalities have similar accuracy in detecting dissection, complications are better diagnosed and characterized by TEE: pericardial effusion and its hemodynamic consequences (impending or overt cardiac tamponade), aortic regurgitation and its underlying mechanism

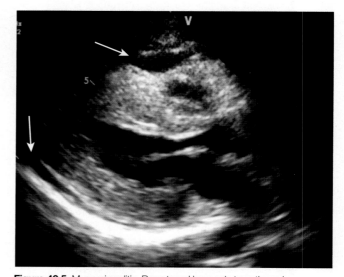

Figure 42.5. Myopericarditis. Parasternal long-axis transthoracic echocardiography view of a 42-year-old woman presenting with chest pain 2 weeks after an upper respiratory viral infection. She had ST-segment elevation in the electrocardiogram, mild troponin I elevation, and clean coronary arteries in catheterization. The echocardiogram showed a small to moderate-sized pericardial effusion *(arrows)* and left ventricular ejection fraction of 30% with moderate global hypokinesis, which subsequently improved to 50% after 2 weeks of treatment with ibuprofen and colchicine.

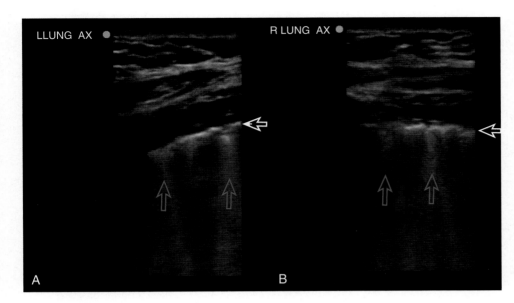

LLUNG AX • R LUNG AX •

A B

Figure 42.6. Lung congestion in a patient with heart failure. B lines *(red arrows)* are long, wide bands of hyperechoic artifact resembling a comet or flashlight. They originate at the pleural line *(white arrow)*, move with respiration, and traverse the entire ultrasound screen vertically to the bottom of the screen. They reflect edema or lung congestion, and their presence in both lungs is typical of heart failure. **A,** Left lung (LLUNG AX). **B,** Right lung (R LUNG AX).

(important in determining need for aortic valve replacement), and aortic rupture or dissection extending into the coronary ostium with subsequent acute MI (most commonly affecting the right coronary artery). A more detailed description of echocardiography in aortic aneurysms and dissection is provided in other chapters of this book.

Pericardium

The diagnosis of acute pericarditis should be made on the basis of clinical features such as the quality of the chest pain (pleuritic, worse in supine position), typical ECG findings (diffuse concave ST-segment elevation without reciprocal ST-segment depression; PR depression), and presence of a pericardial rub in auscultation. However, these features are not always evident. A pericardial effusion in TTE is frequently present (Fig. 42.5), reported in as many as 60% of patients with acute presentation. Although the effusion is usually small in size, approximately 5% present with cardiac tamponade.[26] Therefore, a careful examination for cardiac chamber compression, respiratory flow variation by pulsed-wave Doppler at the mitral and tricuspid inflow, and inferior vena cava diameter or collapsibility should be performed regardless of the size of the effusion. A more detailed description of echocardiography in pericarditis is provided on a dedicated chapter.

Lungs and Pleura

Significant progress has been made over the past 5 years in the ultrasound imaging of the pleura and lungs, particularly relevant for evaluation of patients with dyspnea and chest pain. Specific imaging of the pleura can show loss of the normal pleural sliding (visceral over parietal pleura) and of the B-line (vertical comet tails) findings that indicate loss of contact among the two layers and usually represents pneumothorax.[27] A pleural space filled with fluid represents a pleural effusion. Pulmonary edema may present in patients with ACSs and is identified by the presence of multiple B lines (Fig. 42.6; vertical lines in lung ultrasound arising from the pleura) that are present bilaterally. This finding allows differentiation of lung congestion versus chronic obstructive pulmonary disease exacerbation (B lines do not project deep in the image because of the presence of air).[28]

REFERENCES

1. Amsterdam EA, Kirk JD, Bluemke DA, et al. Testing of low-risk patients presenting to the emergency department with chest pain: a scientific statement from the American Heart Association. *Circulation.* 2010;122:1756–1776.
2. Goodacre S, Cross E, Arnold J, et al. The health care burden of acute chest pain. *Heart.* 2005;91:229–230.
3. Pitts SR, Niska RW, Xu J, et al. National hospital Ambulatory medical care Survey: 2006 emergency department summary. *Natl Health Stat Report.* 2008:1–38.
4. Buhumaid RE, St-Cyr Bourque J, Shokoohi H, et al. Integrating point-of-care ultrasound in the ED evaluation of patients presenting with chest pain and shortness of breath. *Am J Emerg Med.* 2019;37:298–303.
5. Labovitz AJ, Noble VE, Bierig M, et al. Focused cardiac ultrasound in the emergent setting: a consensus statement of the American Society of Echocardiography and American College of Emergency Physicians. *J Am Soc Echocardiogr.* 2010;23:1225–1230.
6. Pereztol-Valdes O, Candell-Riera J, Santana-Boado C, et al. Correspondence between left ventricular 17 myocardial segments and coronary arteries. *Eur Heart J.* 2005;26:2637–2643.
7. Horowitz RS, Morganroth J, Parrotto C, et al. Immediate diagnosis of acute myocardial infarction by two-dimensional echocardiography. *Circulation.* 1982;65:323–329.
8. Kontos MC, Arrowood JA, Paulsen WH, et al. Early echocardiography can predict cardiac events in emergency department patients with chest pain. *Ann Emerg Med.* 1998;31:550–557.
9. Zabalgoitia M, Ismaeil M. Diagnostic and prognostic use of stress echo in acute coronary syndromes including emergency department imaging. *Echocardiography.* 2000;17:479–493.
10. Di Pasquale P, Cannizzaro S, Scalzo S, et al. Sensitivity, specificity and predictive value of the echocardiography and troponin-T test combination in patients with non-ST elevation acute coronary syndromes. *Int J Cardiovasc Imaging.* 2004;20:37–46.
11. Mohler ER, Ryan T, Segar DS, et al. Clinical utility of troponin T levels and echocardiography in the emergency department. *Am Heart J.* 1998;135:253–260.
12. Antman EM, Anbe DT, Armstrong PW, et al. ACC/AHA guidelines for the management of patients with ST-elevation myocardial infarction—Executive summary. A report of the American College of Cardiology/American Heart Association Task Force on Practice Guidelines (Writing Committee to revise the 1999 guidelines for the management of patients with acute myocardial infarction). *J Am Coll Cardiol.* 2004;44:671–719.
13. I.J.Kontos MC, de Lemos JA. Evolving considerations in the management of patients with left bundle branch block and suspected myocardial infarction. *J Am Coll Cardiol.* 2012;60:96–105.
14. Porter TR, Mulvagh SL, Abdelmoneim SS, et al. Clinical applications of ultrasonic enhancing agents in echocardiography: 2018 American Society of Echocardiography guidelines update. *J Am Soc Echocardiogr.* 2018;31:241–274.
15. Tong KL, Kaul S, Wang XQ, et al. Myocardial contrast echocardiography versus Thrombolysis in Myocardial Infarction score in patients presenting to the emergency department with chest pain and a nondiagnostic electrocardiogram. *J Am Coll Cardiol.* 2005;46:920–927.
16. Rinkevich D, Kaul S, Wang XQ, et al. Regional left ventricular perfusion and function in patients presenting to the emergency department with chest pain and no ST-segment elevation. *Eur Heart J.* 2005;26:1606–1611.
17. Wyrick JJ, Kalvaitis S, McConnell KJ, et al. Cost-efficiency of myocardial contrast echocardiography in patients presenting to the emergency department with chest pain of suspected cardiac origin and a nondiagnostic electrocardiogram. *Am J Cardiol.* 2008;102:649–652.
18. Donohue D, Movahed MR. Clinical characteristics, demographics and prognosis of transient left ventricular apical ballooning syndrome. *Heart Fail Rev.* 2005;10:311–316.
19. Brinjikji W, El-Sayed AM, Salka S. In-hospital mortality among patients with takotsubo cardiomyopathy: a study of the National Inpatient Sample 2008 to 2009. *Am Heart J.* 2012;164:215–221.

20. Chao T, Lindsay J, Collins S, et al. Can acute occlusion of the left anterior descending coronary artery produce a typical "takotsubo" left ventricular contraction pattern? *Am J Cardiol.* 2009;104:202–204.
21. McConnell MV, Solomon SD, Rayan ME, et al. Regional right ventricular dysfunction detected by echocardiography in acute pulmonary embolism. *Am J Cardiol.* 1996;78:469–473.
22. Casazza F, Bongarzoni A, Capozi A, et al. Regional right ventricular dysfunction in acute pulmonary embolism and right ventricular infarction. *Eur J Echocardiogr.* 2005;6:11–14.
23. Cecconi M, Chirillo F, Costantini C, et al. The role of transthoracic echocardiography in the diagnosis and management of acute type A aortic syndrome. *Am Heart J.* 2012;163:112–118.
24. Evangelista A, Avegliano G, Aguilar R, et al. Impact of contrast-enhanced echocardiography on the diagnostic algorithm of acute aortic dissection. *Eur Heart J.* 2010;31:472–479.
25. Goldstein SA, Evangelista A, Abbara S, et al. Multimodality imaging of diseases of the thoracic aorta in adults: from the American Society of echocardiography and the European Association of Cardiovascular imaging: endorsed by the Society of Cardiovascular computed tomography and Society for Cardiovascular magnetic resonance. *J Am Soc Echocardiogr.* 2015;28: 119–182.
26. Imazio M, Demichelis B, Parrini I, et al. Day-hospital treatment of acute pericarditis: a management program for outpatient therapy. *J Am Coll Cardiol.* 2004;43:1042–1046.
27. Husain LF, Hagopian L, Wayman D, et al. Sonographic diagnosis of pneumothorax. *J Emerg Trauma Shock.* 2012;5:76–81.
28. Wooten WM, Shaffer LET, Hamilton LA. Bedside ultrasound versus chest radiography for detection of pulmonary edema: a prospective cohort study. *J Ultrasound Med.* 2019;38:967–973.

43 Echocardiography in Acute Myocardial Infarction

Sushil Allen Luis, Michael Y.C. Tsang, Sunil V. Mankad

Patients who have had an acute myocardial infarction (MI) are subject to a broad range of potential complications, some of which are life threatening. These complications range from cardiogenic shock caused by the loss of a critical mass of myocardium to various mechanical complications, such as the development of a left ventricular (LV) thrombus, ventricular septal rupture, free-wall rupture, papillary muscle rupture, dynamic LV outflow tract obstruction, and right ventricular infarction. Echocardiography is a valuable, noninvasive imaging tool that can be used to rapidly assess structural and hemodynamic factors and identify complications in the setting of an acute MI.

LEFT VENTRICULAR THROMBOSIS

Previous studies have demonstrated that 1.5% to 3.6% of acute myocardial infarctions (MIs) are complicated by systemic embolism,[1,2] and left ventricular (LV) mural thrombus is most often the responsible culprit. The risk of developing LV thrombus varies with location and size of the MI. A review of the GISSI-3 database revealed that 5.1% of patients treated with fibrinolytic therapy for an acute MI were diagnosed with an LV thrombus by predischarge transthoracic echocardiography (TTE).[3] Patients who sustained an anterior MI were at a higher risk of developing LV thrombosis (11.5% vs 2.3% of patients with MIs at other locations).[3] Similarly, in patients treated with percutaneous coronary intervention and dual antiplatelet therapy for an acute anterior MI, 10% and 15% were diagnosed with an LV thrombus by serial echocardiography at 1 week and 3 months, respectively.[4]

LV thrombosis in the setting of an acute MI is typically seen at the LV apex, which is often akinetic as a result of the infarction. Two-dimensional TTE is the most frequently used imaging modality for the detection of LV thrombus; the apical view is the best window to visualize an apical thrombus (Fig. 43.1A and Video 43.1A). The echocardiographic appearance of an apical thrombus is characterized by a nonhomogeneous echodensity with a margin distinct from the underlying akinetic or dyskinetic LV apex.[5] This characteristic appearance may allow differentiation of a true LV thrombus from chordae tendineae or artifacts. A protruding configuration and free mobility of LV thrombi are predictors of systemic embolization.[6]

Contrast echocardiography is particularly helpful in patients with suboptimal acoustic windows and in those with prominent LV apical muscle bands or trabeculations, which can confound the recognition of a thrombus (Fig. 43.1B and Video 43.1B). Multiple studies have demonstrated contrast echocardiography's superior sensitivity and accuracy in detecting an LV thrombus compared with noncontrast echocardiography.[7,8] For instance, in one study that examined the use of contrast in nondiagnostic transthoracic echocardiograms for the purpose of detecting LV thrombus, 90% of these studies became definitive in establishing whether an LV thrombus was present after the use of contrast.[8] Systemic anticoagulation therapy is recommended in patients who are diagnosed with an LV thrombus after an acute MI to reduce the risk of embolization.[9]

POSTINFARCTION VENTRICULAR SEPTAL RUPTURE

Rupture of the ventricular septum after an acute MI is rather uncommon, occurring in fewer than 1% of total infarcts. However,

Figure 43.1. Apical views of noncontrast (**A**) and contrast (**B**) transthoracic echocardiography. Note the anteroapical regional wall motion abnormalities and the demonstration of a filling defect at the left ventricular apex by contrast echocardiography *(right)*, consistent with a left ventricular apical thrombus measuring 1.5 × 2.3 cm. (See corresponding Video 43.1.)

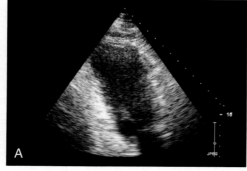
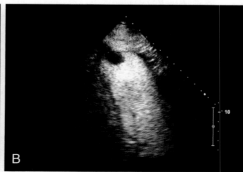

the incidence of postinfarction ventricular septal ruptures (VSRs) is higher (2%–5%) in patients with cardiogenic shock (3.9% in the SHOCK (Should We Emergently Revascularize Occluded Coronaries for Cardiogenic Shock) Trial Registry and randomized SHOCK Trial).[10] The typical clinical presentation is the development of a new holosystolic murmur and a precordial thrill along with abrupt and progressive hemodynamic deterioration. VSRs can occur as a complication of both anterior and nonanterior MIs. Apical VSRs are more commonly associated with an anterior MI, whereas VSRs associated with an inferior MI often occur in the posterobasal region of the ventricular septum. Echocardiographic examination therefore must thoroughly evaluate both of these regions of the ventricular septum (Fig. 43.2 and Video 43.2). Although visualization of the defect may be difficult, a postinfarction VSR should be suspected in the presence of severe wall motional abnormalities of the distal ventricular septum. Color Doppler imaging typically demonstrates a shunt from the LV to the right ventricle (RV). Peak flow velocity across the site of rupture measured by continuous-wave (CW) Doppler interrogation corresponds to the pressure gradient between the LV and RV and can therefore be used to estimate RV systolic pressure (RV systolic pressure = systolic blood pressure – pressure gradient between LV and RV; in the absence of LV outflow tract or aortic valve obstruction, the systolic blood pressure would equal the LV systolic pressure). In addition, CW Doppler assessment may reveal a nearly continuous shunt through the VSR except during early diastole. Pulsed-wave and CW Doppler interrogations are exceedingly sensitive in the localization of postinfarction VSRs. This diastolic left-to-right shunt is secondary to an elevated LV diastolic pressure in the setting of an acute or recent MI. It is also important to note that the magnitude of the left-to-right shunt and the intensity of the systolic murmur are inversely proportional to the size of the infarct and directly related to residual LV systolic function.[11]

LEFT VENTRICULAR FREE-WALL RUPTURE

LV free-wall rupture is the second leading cause of mortality, following cardiogenic shock, in patients with an acute MI. The incidence of free-wall rupture is estimated to be 6% (2.7% of patients in the SHOCK Trial Registry), but it accounts for 15% of in-hospital deaths after an acute MI.[10,12] LV free-wall rupture most frequently presents as a catastrophic event—electromechanical dissociation caused by cardiac tamponade. However, in some patients, rupture of the ventricular free wall takes a more stuttering course. In such patients, prompt diagnosis and surgical intervention are necessary. Echocardiography is the diagnostic modality of choice whenever there is any suspicion of free-wall rupture. Any pericardial effusion in a patient with sudden hemodynamic compromise after an acute MI should suggest the diagnosis. Enlarging pericardial effusions with echodense structures (thrombus) are characteristic and, when seen in patients with hemodynamic compromise, are greater than 98% specific for LV free-wall rupture.[13] Echocardiography is also used to locate the point of rupture, which is typically at the junction of normal and infarcted myocardium. If diagnostic uncertainty exists, microbubble contrast administration should be considered, with detection of microbubble contrast within the pericardial space confirming the diagnosis of free-wall rupture.

LV apical aneurysms may develop secondary to myocardial scar formation and thinning of the myocardium with subsequent expansion of the LV (Fig. 43.3A and Video 43.3A). In some patients, however, either the rupture occurs over time or the perforation is incomplete, resulting in the development of an LV pseudoaneurysm. Pseudoaneurysms remain somewhat contained within a limited segment of the pericardium and are commonly in the inferolateral or inferoposterior walls. As with other mechanical complications of an acute MI, LV pseudoaneurysms can also be identified by echocardiography and are typified by a pseudoaneurysm cavity that communicates with the LV chamber via a very narrow neck (diameter of entry site less than half of the maximal diameter of the pseudoaneurysm) and frequently contains thrombus (Fig. 43.3B and Video 43.3B). The characteristic to-and-fro blood flow through the site of rupture can be detected with Doppler and color-flow imaging.

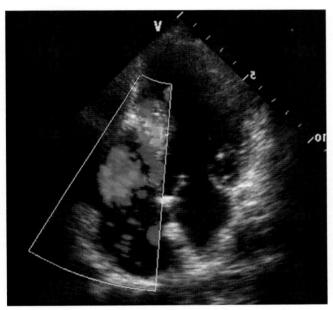

Figure 43.2. Transthoracic echocardiogram demonstrates the cause of a loud systolic murmur after myocardial infarction: a ventricular septal rupture with left-to-right shunting. (See corresponding Video 43.2.)

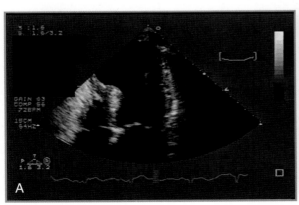
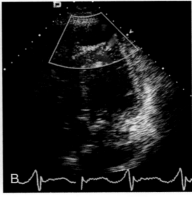

Figure 43.3. Echocardiography is useful at differentiating left ventricular (LV) aneurysm (wide entry neck) (**A**) from LV pseudoaneurysm (narrow entry neck) (B). (See corresponding Video 43.3.)

ACUTE MITRAL REGURGITATION AND PAPILLARY MUSCLE RUPTURE

Mitral regurgitation (MR) is common among patients with an acute MI. Its prevalence is up to 50%, and the presence of MR portends a worse short-and long-term prognosis.[14,15] Acute MR in the context of an acute MI can occur as a consequence of several pathophysiologic mechanisms: (1) dilatation of the mitral annulus secondary to LV dilatation, (2) papillary muscle displacement or dysfunction caused by the proximity of the insertion of the papillary muscle to the infarcted myocardium, and (3) papillary muscle or chordal rupture.[5]

Although most cases of MR are transient and asymptomatic, papillary muscle rupture is a rare but life-threatening mechanical complication of an acute MI. Previous studies have reported that papillary muscle rupture complicates approximately 1% to 3% of acute MIs with a mortality rate of 80% when treated with medical therapy alone.[16] The classic presentation of papillary muscle rupture is acute pulmonary edema and cardiogenic shock 3 to 5 days after an acute MI.[17] Physical examination may reveal a new holosystolic murmur, but it is important to note that the intensity of the systolic murmur does not necessarily correlate with the severity of MR. For instance, patients with severe acute MR have rapid equalization of pressures in the left ventricle and left atrium, thus reducing the duration and intensity of the systolic murmur.

A high index of suspicion is required for identifying patients with significant MR associated with an acute MI, and echocardiography plays an essential role in differentiating the underlying mechanism for the MR and in ruling out other etiologies for a new systolic murmur in this clinical setting. Common two-dimensional echocardiographic features of papillary muscle rupture include a flail mitral leaflet with severed chordae or papillary muscle

head moving freely within the left heart (Fig. 43.4 and Video 43.4). Complete transection of the papillary muscle is relatively rare, whereas rupture of the tip is more common.[18] Because of differences in coronary blood supply, rupture of the posteromedial papillary muscle (supplied by a single coronary artery) occurs 6 to 10 times more often than rupture of the anterolateral papillary muscle (has dual coronary supply).[5] Whereas LV chamber size is typically normal, LV function is often hyperdynamic because of a sudden decrease in afterload, and regional wall motion abnormalities may be subtle or unrecognized.[17] Color Doppler assessment typically demonstrates eccentric MR, which may lead to underestimation of the degree of MR. CW Doppler interrogation of the MR frequently shows a dense, triangular signal, reflecting a rapid early rise in left atrial pressure. Patients with papillary muscle rupture usually present with significant distress and hemodynamic compromise, resulting in suboptimal transthoracic imaging windows. Transesophageal echocardiography (TEE) may therefore be required to establish the diagnosis and to determine the severity of MR. Afterload reduction and emergent surgical intervention are the mainstays of management for these patients.

LEFT VENTRICULAR OUTFLOW TRACT OBSTRUCTION

Dynamic left ventricular outflow tract (LVOT) obstruction has traditionally been described as a hallmark of hypertrophic obstructive cardiomyopathy, and it occurs as a result of asymmetric ventricular septal hypertrophy and systolic anterior motion of the mitral valve. In recent years, dynamic LVOT obstruction that complicates an acute anterior MI has been increasingly recognized.[19–22] The common underlying mechanism for the development of acute LVOT obstruction is the compensatory hyperdynamic contraction of the basal

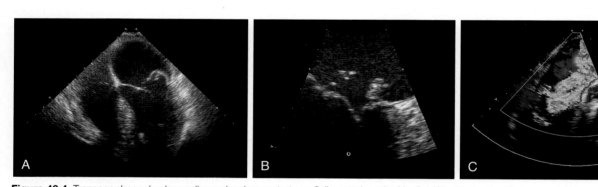

Figure 43.4. Transesophageal echocardiography demonstrates a flail posterior mitral leaflet (**A**) with the tip of a torn papillary muscle attached to it (**B**). Color Doppler assessment reveals severe anteriorly directed mitral regurgitation (**C**). (See corresponding Video 43.4.)

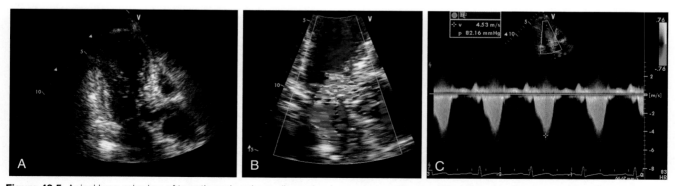

Figure 43.5. Apical long-axis view of transthoracic echocardiography demonstrates akinesis of the left ventricular apex and systolic anterior motion of mitral valve (**A**). Color Doppler assessment of the left ventricular outflow tract (LVOT) reveals turbulent flow across the LVOT and significant posteriorly directed mitral regurgitation (**B**). Late-peaking continuous wave Doppler signal is consistent with dynamic LVOT obstruction (**C**). (See corresponding Video 43.5.)

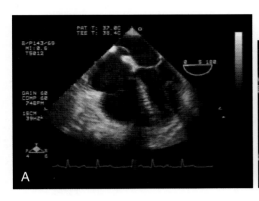 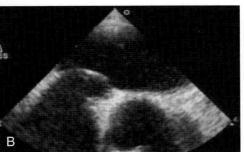

Figure 43.6. Transesophageal echocardiography demonstrates significant enlargement and systolic dysfunction of the right ventricle (**A**). Deviation of the interatrial septum toward the left side during the entire cardiac cycle suggests much elevated right atrial pressure. Color Doppler assessment of the interatrial septum reveals a right-to-left shunt through the patent foramen ovale (**B**). (See corresponding Video 43.6.)

inferolateral and inferior segments in the setting of an anteroapical MI and LV apical akinesis.[21] Hyperkinesis of the basal segments leads to a reduction in the LVOT cross-sectional area, acceleration of blood flow across the LVOT, systolic anterior motion of the mitral valve, and consequently LVOT obstruction. These patients typically present with an acute anterior MI, whereas unstable hemodynamics and a new systolic murmur are found on physical examination. Significant posteriorly directed mitral valve regurgitation secondary to systolic anterior motion of the mitral valve may also lead to acute pulmonary edema. The incidence of dynamic LVOT obstruction after an acute MI is unknown, but it is believed to be more common among women and older adult patients with a small LVOT area or basal septal hypertrophy caused by chronic hypertension.[5,23] LVOT obstruction has also been reported in up to one-third of patients with takotsubo cardiomyopathy, or apical ballooning syndrome.[5]

Urgent echocardiography should be performed in patients with a new systolic murmur and unstable hemodynamics in the setting of an acute MI. TTE should be considered the diagnostic modality of choice to assess dynamic LVOT obstruction, whereas TEE can be used in patients with suboptimal acoustic windows. Common two-dimensional echocardiographic features include regional wall motion abnormalities of the anteroapical segments, hyperkinesis of the basal ventricular segments, and systolic anterior motion of the mitral valve (Fig. 43.5 and Video 43.5). In the presence of dynamic LVOT obstruction, color Doppler imaging demonstrates turbulent blood flow across the LVOT, and posteriorly directed mitral valve regurgitation may also be present. CW Doppler examination of the LVOT from the apical imaging window reveals a late-peaking systolic (dagger-shaped) Doppler signal with a peak velocity that correlates with the degree of LVOT obstruction. Other differential diagnoses for a new murmur and hemodynamic compromise after a recent MI, such as VSR and papillary muscle rupture, can also be ruled out with echocardiography. Echocardiography plays a critical role in differentiating the previously mentioned underlying mechanisms, and a correct echocardiographic diagnosis has important implications for the management of these patients. For instance, the most appropriate treatment strategy for a patient with LVOT obstruction includes the infusion of intravenous fluids, discontinuation of vasodilators or inotropic agents, and the administration of β-blockers, α-adrenergic agonists, or both. In contrast, urgent surgical repair is recommended for patients with postinfarction VSR or papillary muscle rupture.

RIGHT VENTRICULAR INFARCTION

Up to half of acute inferior MIs are complicated by RV infarction, but significant hemodynamic compromise is relatively infrequent, and the long-term prognosis is generally favorable.[24] Data from the SHOCK Trial Registry, however, suggest that patients who develop cardiogenic shock as a result of RV infarction have similar risk of death compared with those who develop cardiogenic shock because of LV infarctions.[25]

Echocardiography is useful in the evaluation of patients with presenting symptoms of acute inferior MI and hemodynamic compromise. Echocardiographic features associated with RV infarction have been identified in a few small studies, and these include dilatation of the RV cavity, variable degrees of wall motion abnormalities of the right ventricular free wall, systolic paradoxical ventricular septal motion, plethora of the inferior vena cava, reduced right ventricular ejection fraction, and impaired tricuspid annular plane systolic excursion (TAPSE).[26,27] Other studies have also demonstrated that the tissue Doppler systolic velocity (S′) of the lateral tricuspid annulus is not only a sensitive and specific marker of RV involvement in an inferior MI but also an independent predictor of cardiovascular outcomes.[28,29] It is important to note that the specificity of the previously mentioned findings may be reduced in patients with other medical conditions that can result in RV enlargement and dysfunction, such as pulmonary hypertension and pulmonary embolism.

In patients who develop hypoxemia after sustaining an inferior MI, RV infarction and a clinically significant right-to-left shunt through a patent foramen ovale should be considered (Fig. 43.6 and Video 43.6). This occurs as a result of impaired RV compliance and elevated right atrial pressure in the setting of an RV infarction. TTE with color Doppler imaging or the injection of agitated saline (visualization of contrast medium in the left atrium after opacification of the right atrium) may help establish RV infarction. Alternatively, TEE may be the imaging test of choice in patients with suboptimal imaging windows.

Please access ExpertConsult to view the corresponding videos for this chapter.

REFERENCES

1. Vaitkus PT, Barnathan ES. Embolic potential, prevention and management of mural thrombus complicating anterior myocardial infarction: a meta-analysis. *J Am Coll Cardiol*. 1993;22:1004–1009.
2. Vaitkus PT, Berlin JA, Schwartz JS, et al. Stroke complicating acute myocardial infarction. A meta-analysis of risk modification by anticoagulation and thrombolytic therapy. *Arch Intern Med*. 1992;152:2020–2024.
3. Chiarella F, Santoro E, Domenicucci S, et al. Predischarge 2D echocardiographic evaluation of left ventricular thrombosis after acute myocardial infarction in the GISSI-3 study. *Am J Cardiol*. 1998;81:822–827.
4. Solheim S, Seljeflot I, Lunde K, et al. Frequency of left ventricular thrombus in patients with anterior wall acute myocardial infarction treated with percutaneous coronary intervention and dual antiplatelet therapy. *Am J Cardiol*. 2010;106:1197–1200.
5. Oh JK, Seward JB, Tajik AJ. Coronary artery disease and acute myocardial infarction. In: *The Echo Manual*. 3rd ed. Philadelphia: Lippincott Williams & Wilkins; 2007:154–174.
6. Visser CA, Kan G, Meltzer RS, et al. Embolic potential of left ventricular thrombus after myocardial infarction: a two-dimensional echocardiographic study of 119 patients. *J Am Coll Cardiol*. 1985;5:1276–1280.
7. Mansencal N, Nasr IA, Pilliere R, et al. Usefulness of contrast echocardiography for assessment of left ventricular thrombus after acute myocardial infarction. *Am J Cardiol*. 2007;99:1667–1670.
8. Thanigaraj S, Schechtman KB, Perez JE. Improved echocardiographic delineation of left ventricular thrombus with the use of intravenous second-generation contrast image enhancement. *J Am Soc Echocardiogr*. 1999;12:1022–1026.

9. O'Gara PT, Kushner FG, Ascheim DD, et al. ACCF/AHA guideline for the management of ST-elevation myocardial infarction. *J Am Coll Cardiol.* 2013;61:e78–e140. 2013.

10. Hochman JS, Buller CE, Sleeper LA, et al. Cardiogenic shock complicating acute myocardial infarction–etiologies, management and outcome. *J Am Coll Cardiol.* 2000;36(3 Suppl A):1063–1070.

11. Helmcke F, Mahan 3rd EF, Nanda NC, et al. Two-dimensional echocardiography and Doppler color flow mapping in the diagnosis and prognosis of ventricular septal rupture. *Circulation.* 1990;81:1775–1783.

12. Slater J, Brown RJ, Antonelli TA, et al. Cardiogenic shock due to cardiac free-wall rupture or tamponade after acute myocardial infarction: a report from the SHOCK Trial Registry. Should we emergently revascularize occluded coronaries for cardiogenic shock? *J Am Coll Cardiol.* 2000;36(3 Suppl A):1117–1122.

13. Lopez-Sendon J, Gonzalez A, Lopez de Sa E, et al. Diagnosis of subacute ventricular wall rupture after acute myocardial infarction: sensitivity and specificity of clinical, hemodynamic and echocardiographic criteria. *J Am Coll Cardiol.* 1992;19:1145–1153.

14. Lehmann KG, Francis CK, Dodge HT. Mitral regurgitation in early myocardial infarction. Incidence, clinical detection, and prognostic implications. TIMI Study Group. *Ann Intern Med.* 1992;117:10–17.

15. Picard MH, Davidoff R, Sleeper LA, et al. Echocardiographic predictors of survival and response to early revascularization in cardiogenic shock. *Circulation.* 2003;107:279–284.

16. Stout KK, Verrier ED. Acute valvular regurgitation. *Circulation.* 2009;119:3232–3241.

17. Sia YT, O'Meara E, Ducharme A. Role of echocardiography in acute myocardial infarction. *Curr Heart Fail Rep.* 2008;5:189–196.

18. Antman EA, Morrow DA. ST-segment elevation myocardial infarction: management. In: Bonow RO, Mann DL, Zipes DP, et al., eds. *Braunwald's Heart Disease: A Textbook of Cardiovascular Medicine.* 9th ed. Philadelphia: Elsevier; 2012:1111–1177.

19. Armstrong WF, Marcovitz PA. Dynamic left ventricular outflow tract obstruction as a complication of acute myocardial infarction. *Am Heart J.* 1996;131:827–830.

20. Bartunek J, Vanderheyden M, de Bruyne B. Dynamic left ventricular outflow tract obstruction after anterior myocardial infarction: a potential mechanism of myocardial rupture. *Eur Heart J.* 1995;16:1439–1442.

21. Haley JH, Sinak LJ, Tajik AJ, et al. Dynamic left ventricular outflow tract obstruction in acute coronary syndromes: an important cause of new systolic murmur and cardiogenic shock. *Mayo Clin Proc.* 1999;74:901–906.

22. Joffe II, Riley MF, Katz SE, et al. Acquired dynamic left ventricular outflow tract obstruction complicating acute anterior myocardial infarction: serial echocardiographic and clinical evaluation. *J Am Soc Echocardiogr.* 1997;10:717–721.

23. Matyal R, Warraich HJ, Karthik S, et al. Anterior myocardial infarction with dynamic left ventricular outflow tract obstruction. *Ann Thorac Surg.* 2011;91:e39–e40.

24. Kinch JW, Ryan TJ. Right ventricular infarction. *N Engl J Med.* 1994;330:1211–1217.

25. Jacobs AK, Leopold JA, Bates E, et al. Cardiogenic shock caused by right ventricular infarction: a report from the SHOCK registry. *J Am Coll Cardiol.* 2003;41:1273–1279.

26. D'Arcy B, Nanda NC. Two-dimensional echocardiographic features of right ventricular infarction. *Circulation.* 1982;65:167–173.

27. Goldberger JJ, Himelman RB, Wolfe CL, et al. Right ventricular infarction: recognition and assessment of its hemodynamic significance by 2D echocardiography. *J Am Soc Echocardiogr.* 1991;4:140–146.

28. Dokainish H, Abbey H, Gin K, et al. Usefulness of tissue Doppler imaging in the diagnosis and prognosis of acute right ventricular infarction with inferior wall acute left ventricular infarction. *Am J Cardiol.* 2005;95:1039–1042.

29. Kakouros N, Kakouros S, Lekakis J, et al. Tissue Doppler imaging of the tricuspid annulus and myocardial performance index in the evaluation of right ventricular involvement in the acute and late phase of a first inferior myocardial infarction. *Echocardiography.* 2011;28:311–319.

44 Echocardiography in Stable Coronary Artery Disease

Benjamin Byrd III, Geoff Chidsey

DIAGNOSIS

Echocardiography can show a regional wall motion abnormality (WMA) that may indicate the presence of coronary artery disease (CAD). Even in patients without established CAD, a WMA is associated with a 2.4- to 3.4-fold increase in risk of cardiac events.[1] Wall motion analysis should be done using the method recommended by the American Society of Echocardiography (ASE) in 1989, with particular attention to endocardial thickening.[2] If endocardial definition is poor, an intravenous contrast agent should be used to enhance the evaluation of wall motion. The addition of contrast has been shown to improve accuracy and decrease interobserver variability in the assessment of regional wall motion.[3] The 17-segment model recommended by the ASE should be used to describe the location of WMAs when detected.[4]

Visual wall motion analysis can be challenging, especially in smaller and subendocardial infarctions. Myocardial ischemia first affects the subendocardium, which is mostly composed of longitudinal fibers. Global longitudinal strain (GLS) is reduced in subendocardial infarctions.[5] GLS is a more sensitive method to detect subtle myocardial dysfunction than visual assessment because increased circumferential and radial shortening can mask subtle WMAs. The addition of speckle tracking software for quantitative analysis of myocardial deformation has improved the detection of myocardial infarction when combined with visual analysis.[6] But segmental strain analysis has higher variability than GLS.[7] Furthermore, there is also significant intervendor variability. With this in mind, polar strain maps can be a helpful adjunct to visual wall motion analysis (Fig. 44.1).

PROGNOSIS

Echocardiography-derived left ventricular ejection fraction (LVEF) is a very important prognostic marker in patients with CAD.[8] However, similar to wall motion evaluation, accurate determination of LVEF requires good endocardial definition. When endocardial definition is suboptimal, the addition of contrast is essential to improve the interobserver variability and accuracy of LVEF measurements.[9] GLS has recently been shown to be a better marker of prognosis in stable CAD than LVEF.[10] Furthermore, GLS measurements are highly reproducible compared with many traditional echocardiography measurements, such as wall thickness.[11]

STRESS ECHOCARDIOGRAPHY

Stress echocardiography is a very important modality in the diagnosis and prognosis of CAD. It has advantages over other imaging modalities because it does not use radiation, is less expensive, and has shorter imaging time than nuclear techniques. Furthermore, other important information may be obtained from the resting images regarding right ventricular size and function, the aortic root, the pericardium, and valvular structures. In a study of 1223 patients who had stress echocardiograms, 5% were found to have moderate mitral regurgitation by a focused Doppler examination before the stress echocardiogram.[12] Resting echocardiography can therefore provide important adjunctive clinical information that remained unrecognized before the stress echocardiogram.

Stress echocardiography relies on the principle that a WMA occurs in the distribution of a coronary lesion that limits flow when myocardial oxygen demand is increased. Side-by-side review of

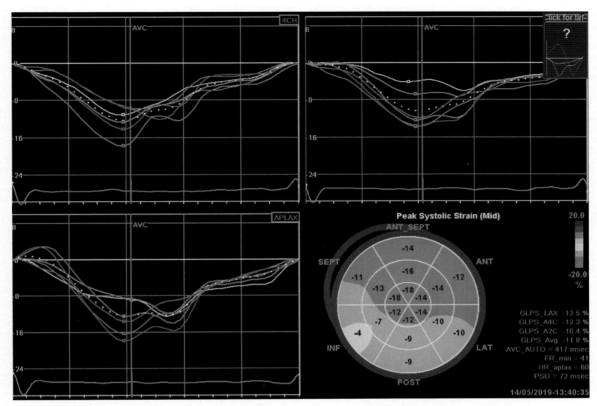

Figure 44.1. Polar strain map obtained in a patient with transmural inferior and inferior-lateral infarct.

rest and stress images is essential for optimal detection of stress-induced WMAs. Stress echocardiography is more accurate than stress electrocardiography (ECG) in the detection of CAD because WMAs occur earlier in the ischemic cascade than ECG changes. A meta-analysis of exercise echocardiography and nuclear myocardial perfusion showed similar sensitivities (85% for echocardiography, 87% for nuclear stress testing) and higher specificity for stress echocardiography (77% vs 64%) for the detection of CAD.[13] The sensitivity for the detection of CAD is higher in patients with multivessel disease than in patients with single-vessel disease. Sensitivity is lowest in the circumflex distribution because it supplies a smaller area of myocardium.[14]

Treadmill exercise echocardiography produces a higher workload than bicycle echocardiography. Supine bicycle echocardiography offers the ability to image the heart throughout the exercise protocol, not just at peak exercise. We use treadmill echocardiography for the diagnosis of CAD and bicycle echocardiography in the evaluation of valvular heart disease and hypertrophic obstructive cardiomyopathy. It is especially important to obtain the postexercise images as quickly as possible, preferably within 60 seconds, because ischemic WMAs may be transient. Apical images should be obtained first because the entire ventricle from the base to the apex is captured in these views. When the parasternal views are technically limited, the apical long-axis view should be obtained. Use of contrast agents can be very helpful and can convert a nondiagnostic examination to a diagnostic examination. In patients who cannot exercise, dobutamine stress echocardiography (DSE) is performed. Dobutamine is infused intravenously in staged increments of 10 µg/kg/min until the target heart rate is achieved, symptoms develop, or end-study indications occur, such as significant arrhythmias, hypotension, or patient intolerance. If there are no contraindications to atropine and the target heart rate is not achieved after 3 minutes of dobutamine at 40 µg/kg/min, 0.5 mg of atropine may be given intravenously and repeated once if needed to achieve target heart rate.

IMAGE INTERPRETATION

Wall motion in each left ventricular segment is scored on resting and stress images according to the following scale: 1 = normal or hyperkinetic; 2 = hypokinetic; 3 = akinetic or severely hypokinetic; 4 = dyskinetic; and 5 = aneurysmal (Fig. 44.2). Using this system, a wall motion score index can be derived at peak stress. A normal wall motion score index is 1.0. An elevated exercise wall motion score index was found to be associated with increased rates of death or nonfatal myocardial infarction in a study of 5798 patients who underwent exercise echocardiography for suspected or known CAD (Fig. 44.3).[15] This finding was also reproduced in 860 patients who had dobutamine stress echocardiography.[16] In the setting of left main CAD, left ventricular dilatation is much more commonly demonstrated by exercise echocardiography (80%) compared with DSE (12%).[17] The right ventricle should also be monitored because abnormal right ventricular wall motion at stress has prognostic value independent of left ventricular ischemia.[18]

PROGNOSTIC VALUE OF STRESS ECHOCARDIOGRAPHY

Exercise stress echocardiography has been shown to be a helpful prognostic indicator of cardiac events. In patients without known CAD, normal exercise echocardiography confers an excellent prognosis, with a cardiac event rate of 0.9% per year.[19] In patients with known or suspected CAD and good exercise capacity, the percentage of the left ventricle that shows severely abnormal wall motion after exercise is a good predictor of cardiac events.[20]

SPECKLE TRACKING WITH STRESS ECHOCARDIOGRAPHY

Currently, the clinical use of speckle tracking in stress echocardiography remains limited because of suboptimal reproducibility

Left ventricle:

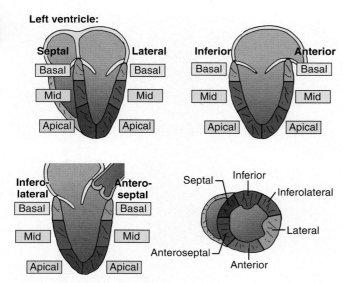

Figure 44.2. Wall motion scoring diagram. The wall motion score equals the score of all segments divided by the number of segments analyzed. A normal score is 1.0.

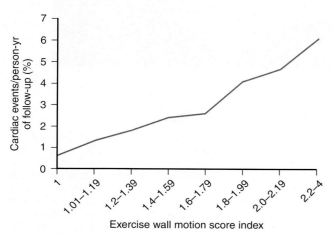

Exercise wall motion score index

Figure 44.3. Relationship between the wall motion score index and cardiac event rate. (Adapted with permission from Arruda-Olson AM, Juracan EM, Mahoney DW, et al. Prognostic value of exercise echocardiography in 5,798 patients: is there a gender difference? *J Am Coll Cardiol* 39(4):625–631, 2002.)

of segmental analysis.[7] Furthermore, intravenous echo contrast is used during many studies, which confounds the ability to track speckles accurately.

CONCLUSION

Echocardiography plays a pivotal role in the detection, management, and prognosis of stable CAD. It is the most widely used technique to assess left ventricular wall motion and LVEF. Stress echocardiography is an effective tool to diagnose CAD because it

has comparable accuracy to nuclear modalities and minimizes cost, and it does not require radiation exposure.

REFERENCES

1. Cicala S, de Simone G, Roman MJ, et al. Prevalence and prognostic significance of wall-motion abnormalities in adults without clinically recognized cardiovascular disease: the Strong Heart Study. *Circulation.* 2007;116(2):143–150.
2. Schiller NB, Shah PM, Crawford M, et al. Recommendations for quantitation of the left ventricle by two-dimensional echocardiography. *J Am Soc Echocardiogr.* 1989;2(5):358–367.
3. Hoffmann R, von Bardeleben S, Kasprzak JD, et al. Analysis of regional left ventricular function by cineventriculography, cardiac magnetic resonance imaging, and unenhanced and contrast-enhanced echocardiography: a multicenter comparison of methods. *J Am Coll Cardiol.* 2006;47(1):121–128.
4. Lang RM, Bierig M, Devereux RB, et al. Recommendations for chamber quantification: a report from the American Society of Echocardiography's Guidelines and Standards Committee and the Chamber Quantification Writing Group, developed in conjunction with the European Association of Echocardiography, a branch of the European Society of Cardiology. *J Am Soc Echocardiogr.* 2005;18(12):1440–1463.
5. Chan J, Hanekom L, Wong C, et al. Differentiation of subendocardial and transmural infarction using two-dimensional strain rate imaging to assess short-axis and long-axis myocardial function. *J Am Coll Cardiol.* 2006;48(10):2026–2033.
6. van Mourik MJW, Zaar DVJ, Smulders MW, et al. Adding speckle-tracking echocardiography to visual assessment of systolic wall motion abnormalities improves the detection of myocardial infarction. *J Am Soc Echocardiogr.* 2019;32(1):65–73.
7. Mirea O, Pagourelias ED, Duchenne J, et al. Variability and reproducibility of segmental longitudinal strain measurement: a report from the EACVI-ASE Strain Standardization Task Force. *JACC Cardiovasc Imaging.* 2018;11(1):15–24.
8. Harris PJ, Harrell FE, Lee KL, et al. Survival in medically treated coronary artery disease. *Circulation.* 1979;60(6):1259–1269.
9. Hoffmann R, von Bardeleben S, ten Cate F, et al. Assessment of systolic left ventricular function: a multi-centre comparison of cineventriculography, cardiac magnetic resonance imaging, unenhanced and contrast-enhanced echocardiography. *Eur Heart J.* 2005;26(6):607–616.
10. Stanton T, Leano R, Marwick TH. Prediction of all-cause mortality from global longitudinal speckle strain: comparison with ejection fraction and wall motion scoring. *Circ Cardiovasc Imaging.* 2009;2(5):356–364.
11. Farsalinos KE, Daraban AM, Ünlü S, et al. Head-to-head comparison of global longitudinal strain measurements among nine different vendors: the EACVI/ASE Inter-Vendor Comparison Study. *J Am Soc Echocardiogr.* 2015;28(10):1171–1181.
12. Gaur A, Yeon SB, Lewis CW, Manning WJ. Valvular flow abnormalities are often identified by a resting focused Doppler examination performed at the time of stress echocardiography. *Am J Med.* 2003;114(1):20–24.
13. Fleischmann KE, Hunink MG, Kuntz KM, Douglas PS. Exercise echocardiography or exercise SPECT imaging? A meta-analysis of diagnostic test performance. *J Am Med Assoc.* 1998;280(10):913–920.
14. Ryan T, Segar DS, Sawada SG, et al. Detection of coronary artery disease with upright bicycle exercise echocardiography. *J Am Soc Echocardiogr.* 1993;6(2):186–197.
15. Arruda-Olson AM, Juracan EM, Mahoney DW, et al. Prognostic value of exercise echocardiography in 5,798 patients: is there a gender difference? *J Am Coll Cardiol.* 2002;39(4):625–631.
16. Chuah SC, Pellikka PA, Roger VL, et al. Role of dobutamine stress echocardiography in predicting outcome in 860 patients with known or suspected coronary artery disease. *Circulation.* 1998;97(15):1474–1480.
17. Attenhofer CH, Pellikka PA, Oh JK, et al. Comparison of ischemic response during exercise and dobutamine echocardiography in patients with left main coronary artery disease. *J Am Coll Cardiol.* 1996;27(5):1171–1177.
18. Bangalore S, Yao S-S, Chaudhry FA. Role of right ventricular wall motion abnormalities in risk stratification and prognosis of patients referred for stress echocardiography. *J Am Coll Cardiol.* 2007;50(20):1981–1989.
19. McCully RB, Roger VL, Mahoney DW, et al. Outcome after normal exercise echocardiography and predictors of subsequent cardiac events: follow-up of 1,325 patients. *J Am Coll Cardiol.* 1998;31(1):144–149.
20. McCully RB, Roger VL, Mahoney DW, et al. Outcome after abnormal exercise echocardiography for patients with good exercise capacity: prognostic importance of the extent and severity of exercise-related left ventricular dysfunction. *J Am Coll Cardiol.* 2002;39(8):1345–1352.

45 Old Myocardial Infarction

Matthew Bruce, Nadia El Hangouche, Vera H. Rigolin

Myocardial infarction (MI) is characterized by acute ischemia caused by occlusion of an epicardial coronary artery causing irreversible cardiomyocyte death and subsequent cell necrosis, which results in a localized inflammatory response with recruitment and migration of macrophages, monocytes, neutrophils, and fibroblasts into the infarcted zone and eventual discrete collagen scar formation.[1,2] Within hours of the initial insult, acute dilatation and thinning of the area of infarction, also termed infarct expansion, occurs because of slippage between muscle bundles in the infarcted zone and stretching of the underlying collagen scaffold of the extracellular matrix (ECM).[1,2] As a consequence of this early remodeling caused by infarct expansion and decrease in ventricular contractility, the remote myocardium is asked to work harder, with neurohormonal-induced tachycardia and gradual left ventricular (LV) dilatation to increase preload and therefore preserve stroke volume. As an adaptive response over the following days to weeks, the noninfarcted remote myocardium undergoes compensatory hypertrophy to decrease the augmented wall stress caused by this early LV dilation. This adaptive stress response is mediated by multiple factors, including mechanical deformation from increased myocardial stretch, neurohormonal activation with increased norepinephrine producing direct and indirect activation of hypertrophic response, and renin–angiotensin–aldosterone system (RAAS) upregulation.

Despite advances in coronary reperfusion and evidence-based pharmacotherapy, approximately 30% of patients with anterior acute MI and 17% of patients with nonanterior acute MIs still experience adverse postinfarct remodeling.[3] Current estimates suggest that for patients aged 45 years or older who experience their first MI, 16% of men and 22% of women will progress to develop heart failure (HF) within 5 years post-infarct.[4] Furthermore, development of HF among patients with ST-elevation myocardial infarction (STEMI) confers a poor prognosis, with much higher long-term mortality rates compared with patients who do not develop HF.[5] Use of guideline directed medical therapy including angiotensin-converting enzyme inhibitors, angiotensin receptor blockers, β-blockers, mineralocorticoid receptor antagonists, and neprilysin inhibitors all demonstrated potential for reverse remodeling and additionally have shown mortality benefit among patients with heart failure with reduced ejection fraction (EF). As such, ventricular remodeling is an important prognostic factor after acute MI and a clear target for therapeutic intervention.[6]

The diagnosis of remodeling after infarction involves detection of morphologic changes, including LV size and shape, LV mass, LV volumes and indexes of function, extent and transmurality of scar, myocardial strain, fibrosis, and inflammatory infiltrates. Current clinical practice employs a combination of imaging modalities (echocardiography, radionuclide imaging, and cardiac magnetic resonance imaging [CMRI]) for diagnostic and prognostic assessment after MI.[7]

TIMING OF IMAGING

Data from the National Cardiovascular Data Registry (NCDR) Acute Coronary Treatment and Intervention Outcomes Network Registry—Get with the Guidelines (ACTION Registry-GWTG) showed that among 128,845 patients at 383 treatment centers with non–ST-segment elevation myocardial infarction (NSTEMI) and ST-elevation myocardial infarction (STEMI) between 2007

and 2009, 93% had in-hospital assessment of LVEF, a marked improvement compared with approximately 80% at the beginning of the decade.[8] Importantly, patients that received in-hospital LVEF assessment were more likely to be discharged on secondary prevention medical therapies compared with those that did not undergo LVEF assessment.[8] Present guidelines provide a strong recommendation for evaluation of LVEF, with preference for echocardiography rather than ventriculography given that valvular disease may influence revascularization strategy; assessment is recommended within 24-48 hours post-MI.[9,10] Follow-up postinfarct echocardiography is further recommended within the first 3 months after infarction.[3]

For CMRI, no guideline recommendations currently exist for exact timing postinfarct. Notably, clinical studies appear to demonstrate variability in CMRI quantification of infarct size, LV function, and LV volume during the first week after acute MI.[11] In a study from 2011 evaluating 57 patients with first STEMI who underwent percutaneous coronary intervention (PCI) within 12 hours of symptom onset, they found that CMRI imaging at 1 week was an independent predictor of LVEF and infarct size at 3 months, whereas imaging within the first 72 hours was not.[11]

RISK FACTORS FOR CHRONIC REMODELING

As our understanding of the mechanism leading to and propagating chronic remodeling has improved, our identification of potential risk factors for development of adverse remodeling has expanded. Well-validated determinants of LV remodeling include large infarct size, anterior location, transmurality, lack of patency of the infarct vessels, and lack of use of thrombolytic agents.[12–14] Fig. 45.1 illustrates a patient with a large acute infarct in the territory of the left anterior descending (LAD) coronary artery who underwent PCI; however, the presence of no-reflow phenomenon was revealed by microvascular obstruction seen on the CMRI. Consequently, this patient is likely to have acute and delayed complications from MI.

Infarct size may be the most important predictor of adverse LV remodeling and notably is linearly dependent on myocardial salvage by coronary reperfusion in the acute peri-infarct setting. Success of reperfusion is suggested by late patency of the infarct-related artery. Additionally, the presence of collateral circulation is associated with survival benefit and may confer better prediction of LV volume change than with infarct size.[2]

More recently, introduction of CMRI and contrast-enhanced echocardiography have elucidated a better understanding of additional biological factors affecting remodeling, particularly markers of myocardial and microvascular damage such as microvascular obstruction, myocardial salvage, intramyocardial hemorrhage, and late gadolinium enhancement.[15–17]

CHRONIC REMODELING
Left Ventricular Size, Shape, and Function

A consensus international forum has defined cardiac remodeling as a "genome expression resulting in molecular, cellular, and interstitial changes and manifested clinically as changes in size, shape, and function of the heart resulting from cardiac load or injury," with clear delineation of two types of cardiac remodeling: physiologic (adaptive)

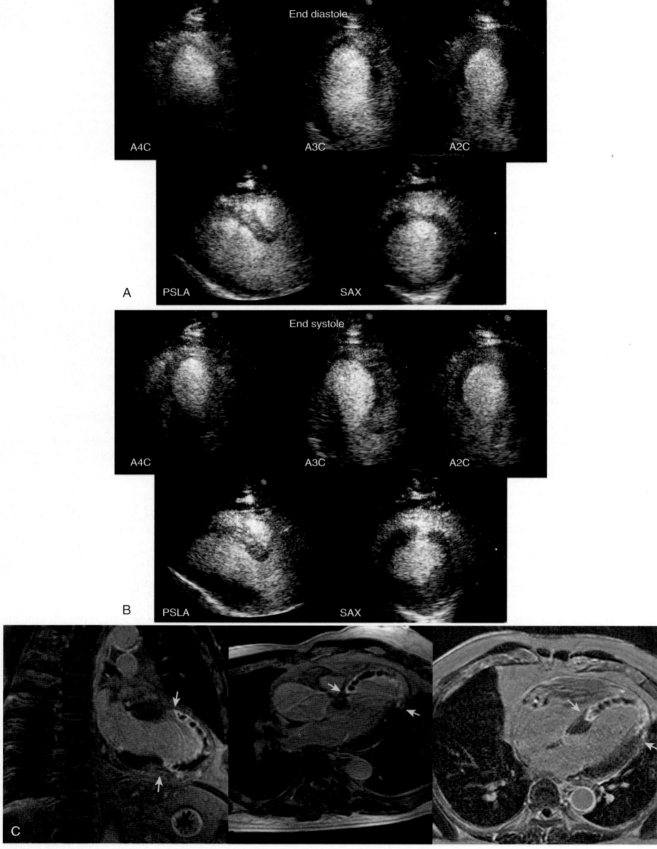

Figure 45.1. Acute left descending coronary (LAD) transmural infarct in a patient who underwent emergent revascularization with no reflow. End-diastolic (**A**) and end-systolic (**B**) transthoracic echocardiography (TTE) images show large area of akinesis in the LAD territory. Accompanying Videos 45.1A to E show the apical four-chamber (A4C), apical three-chamber 3C (A3C), apical two-chamber (A2C), parasternal long-axis (PSLA), and parasternal short-axis (SAX) TTE views, respectively. **C,** Delayed contrast-enhanced cardiac magnetic resonance image shows a transmural LAD infarct (*bright areas*) with severe microvascular obstruction (*dark endocardial areas*) extending throughout the whole thickness of the infarct (*arrows*).

and pathologic (maladaptive or adverse) remodeling.[7] Quantitatively, adverse LV remodeling has been defined as an increase in LV end-diastolic volume (LVEDV) or LV end-systolic volume (LVESV) of 20% from baseline at 6 months after MI.[3] Importantly, this definition was derived using two-dimensional (2D) echocardiography.

Two-Dimensional Echocardiography

For quantification of LV volumes and EF, the modified Simpson method with biplane LV apical imaging has been the method of choice for 2D echocardiography. LVEF, LVEDV, and LVESV are strongly associated with post-MI death, among which LVESV has the greatest predictive value for survival after acute MI.[6,18] After an acute MI and subsequent early morphologic changes (i.e., LV dilatation and remote myocardial hypertrophy), LV remodeling also leads to progressive transition from the normal prolate ellipsoid shape to a more spherical shape, with subsequent increased sphericity index, which has been defined by 2D echocardiographic parameters as the LVEDV divided by the volume of a sphere of the same circumference with the LV major end-diastolic long axis as the diameter of this sphere.[19] Fig. 45.2 demonstrates serial echocardiographic imaging of the left ventricle over time, with worsening LV dilation caused by postinfarct remodeling, also propagated by worsening ischemic mitral regurgitation (MR).

Parameters of diastolic dysfunction present on 2D echocardiography have also been suggested as potential predictive variables. Findings from a meta-analysis in 2008 that included 12 prospective studies (3396 patients) demonstrated that a restrictive mitral filling pattern on Doppler echocardiography was independently associated with increased all-cause mortality in patients after MI (hazard ratio [HR], 2.67; 95% confidence interval [CI], 2.23–3.20; $P < .001$), regardless of LVEF, end-systolic volume index, and Killip class.[20] Additionally, the ratio of transmitral flow velocity to early mitral annulus velocity (E/e′) greater than 15 has also been found to be predictive of LV adverse remodeling.[3]

Strain Imaging

Echocardiographic strain imaging offers important prognostic information in patients with acute MI. Global longitudinal strain (GLS) is an independent predictor of adverse remodeling.[21,22] Impaired baseline GLS and lack of improvement after coronary angioplasty in patients with NSTEMI is predictive for adverse remodeling at 6 months.[21,22] In patients after acute MI, both strain and strain rate correlate with all-cause mortality and a composite endpoint of reinfarction, revascularization, and HF hospitalization at 3 year follow-up; strain has also notably found to be superior to LVEF and wall motion score index for these chosen outcomes.[21]

Cardiac Magnetic Resonance Imaging

CMRI is considered the gold-standard imaging modality for infarct size, LV volumes, and LVEF.[23,24] A recent study using CMRI performed on 146 patients with revascularized STEMI has suggested the following CMRI-specific definition for adverse remodeling: 12% or greater change in LVEDV (sensitivity of 73% and specificity of 69% for detecting LVEF <50%) and 12% or greater change in LVESV (sensitivity of 89% and specificity of 62% for detecting LVEF <50%) at approximately 6 months after MI.[23] There has been a greater push toward understanding the synergism and supplementation gained when CMRI is used with echocardiography.

Other Manifestations and Sequelae of Remodeling

Left Ventricular Thrombus

The incidence of LV thrombus has been greatly reduced as a result of earlier revascularization strategies after MI. Current estimates of the incidence of thrombus are 4% among all patients after MI and higher incidence for those with anterior MI (11%). In a recent study evaluating 201 patients presenting with STEMI who underwent PCI, imaging with CMRI and echocardiography was performed within 24 hours of each other at a target of 30 days after MI. The group found an overall incidence of 8% of LV thrombus, with 94% occurring because of LAD (anterior) MI and all thrombi apically located.[25] Notably, with delayed-enhancement CMRI (DE-CMRI) as the gold standard, noncontrast and contrast echocardiography yielded limited sensitivity (35% and 64%, respectively). However, LV thrombus was associated with a higher echocardiography -measured apical wall motion score ($P < .001$), and the authors suggest use of routine noncontrast echocardiography as an effective stratification tool to identity patients who should be referred for further assessment by DE-CMRI.[25] Fig. 45.3 demonstrates evidence for LV thrombus in the same patient imaged with these three modalities (noncontrast echocardiography, contrast-enhanced echocardiography, and CMRI). Fig. 45.4 provides a direct comparison of an apical thrombus as seen with contrast echocardiography compared with CMRI.

Ischemic Mitral Regurgitation

Ischemic mitral regurgitation (IMR) has been estimated to occur in approximately 19% of patients after MI and has been implicated as a poor prognostic marker. The components of adverse LV remodeling, including LV dilation, systolic dysfunction, and myocardial scar burden, likely all contribute to development and progression of IMR.[26,27] IMR results from the restriction of the leaflet closure caused by apical displacement of the papillary muscles resulting from adverse remodeling of the LV or caused by regional tethering of a leaflet because of ischemic papillary muscle displacement. A prospective, multimodality study (echocardiography and CMRI) followed 336 patients with ischemic cardiomyopathy over a mean follow-up period of 54 months, with 154 patients revascularized and 182 medically treated to assess progression of IMR. The authors found that IMR frequently increases in severity (29% of patients demonstrated increase in effective regurgitant orifice area (EROA) ≥0.1 cm-), and progression is independently associated with adverse LV remodeling and infarct size.[27] Figs. 45.4 and 45.5 illustrate multimodal depictions of two separate patients with IMR.

VIABILITY

LV function is an important determinant of long-term outcomes in patients with CAD. A distinction should be made between "stunned" myocardium, which refers to transient postischemia dysfunction, and "hibernating" myocardium, defined as underperfused and dysfunctional myocardium that is still viable.

Present methods for assessing myocardial viability include radionuclide techniques, such as positron emission tomography for assessment of blood flow and metabolism using 18F-fluorodeoxyglucose, thallium-201 imaging for assessment of cell membrane integrity, or technetium-99m sestamibi and tetrofosmin imaging to demonstrate intact mitochondrial function; echocardiography using dobutamine for stress imaging to assess inotropic reserve; and contrast-enhanced cardiac magnetic resonance with late gadolinium enhancement for a combination of cell integrity and interstitial fibrosis. When dobutamine stress echocardiography is used to assess viability, a low-dose protocol is followed, starting at 5 mcg/kg/min and increasing at 3-minute intervals up to 20 mcg/kg/min. The low doses allow the recognition of viability, which manifest as territories with hypokinesis at rest that improve with low dose dobutamine. Higher doses of dobutamine can be used to detect ischemia, whereas territories with normal motion at rest become hypokinetic at peak. A biphasic response describes augmentation at a low dose followed by deterioration at a higher dose; this response has the highest specificity for detection of viability.[28] Video 45.6 illustrates a patient with history of infarct in the distal LAD

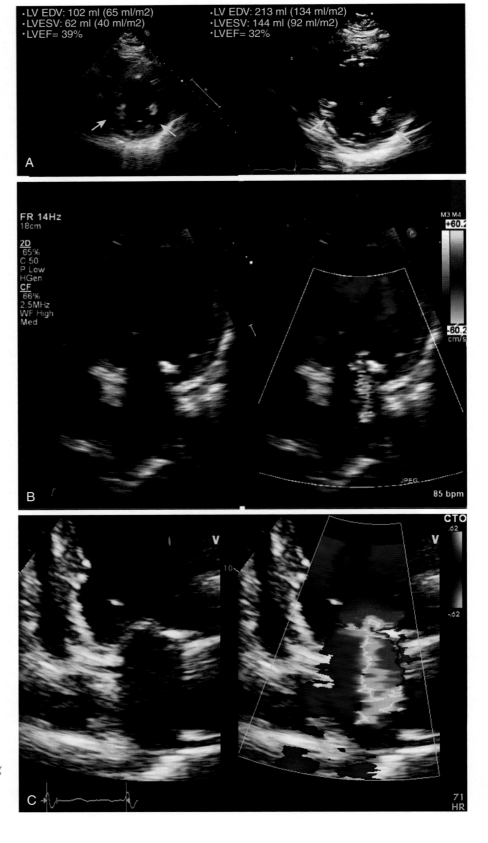

Figure 45.2. Remodeling after left circumflex infarct over 5 years. **A,** Note the thinning of the inferior and inferolateral walls and left ventricular enlargement (**A**) between the acute phase (**B** and Video 45.2A) and 5 years later (**C** and Video 45.2B). The patient also developed worsening functional mitral regurgitation that contributed to a vicious cycle of worsening left ventricle remodeling. *LV EDV,* Left ventricular end-diastolic volume; *LVEF,* left ventricular ejection fraction; *LVESV,* left ventricular end-systolic volume.

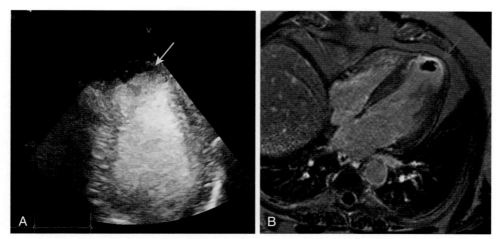

Figure 45.3. Apical thrombus complicating an old left descending coronary infarct. **A,** Contrast-enhanced transthoracic echocardiogram (TTE) revealing the thrombus in the apex of the heart *(yellow arrow)*. **B,** Delayed contrast-enhanced cardiac magnetic resonance image (CMRI) revealing the thrombus as a dark black mass, in addition to the near transmural endocardial-based bright contour of the apex caused by fibrosis of the infarcted area *(blue arrow)*. Accompanying Videos 45.3A to C show the four-chamber nonenhanced TTE, enhanced TTE, and cine CMRI views, respectively, illustrating the dyskinetic apex with the thrombus. Note the increasing sensitivity for detection of the thrombus across modalities.

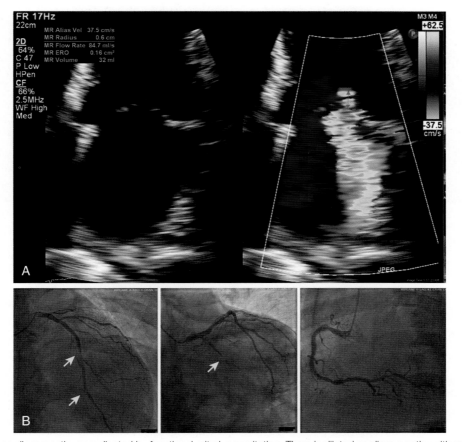

Figure 45.4. Ischemic cardiomyopathy complicated by functional mitral regurgitation. There is dilated cardiomyopathy with extensive regional wall motion abnormalities in the territory of the left anterior descending (LAD) and left circumflex (LCx) coronary arteries as shown in accompanying Videos 45.4A to C. **A,** Ischemic mitral regurgitation caused by the apical displacement of the papillary muscles resulting from the adverse remodeling. Doppler scale is baseline shifted to calculate the effective regurgitant orifice area (EROA) (see also Video 45.4D). **B,** Angiogram with tandem lesion in the LAD *(yellow arrow on the left)*, total occlusion of the left circumflex *(yellow arrow in the middle)*, and diffuse disease of the right coronary artery. The patient underwent percutaneous coronary intervention of the LAD. One year later, she presented with angina and underwent stress cardiac magnetic resonance imaging (CMRI) to assess the viability of the LCx territory and assess for ischemia in other territories.

Continued

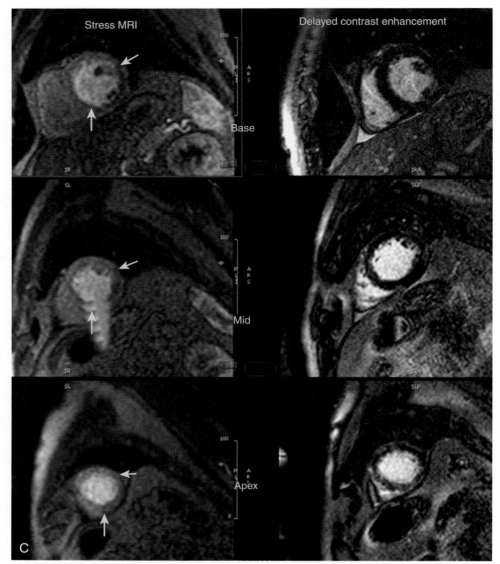

Figure 45.4, cont'd C, First-pass images of the stress CMRI on the *left* and delayed contrast enhancement sequences on the *right*. Note the hypoperfusion in the territory of the LCx *(between the yellow arrows)* with no corresponding infarct in the *right panel*. This suggests ischemia viability and no infarct in LCx territory.

territory. The infarcted territory is hypokinetic at rest and becomes akinetic at peak exercise. Exercise echocardiography combines two important features: the patient's exercise capacity and the presence of myocardial ischemia. However, it does not allow for detection of the biphasic response.

Two retrospective studies in Europe offered comparison of dobutamine echocardiography with nuclear imaging for ability to detect myocardial viability, with results suggesting dobutamine stress echocardiography conferred a higher positive predictive value (84% vs 75%) and a lower negative predictive value (69% vs 80%).[29]

The Surgical Treatment for Ischemic Heart Disease (STICH) trial, a randomized, controlled trial, was conducted to assess the relationship between viability and outcomes after revascularization. The study randomized 601 patients who underwent myocardial viability imaging to either receive medical therapy plus coronary artery bypass graft or medical therapy alone. The presence of viable myocardium conferred a significant survival benefit compared with patients without viable myocardium (HR, 0.64; 95% CI, 0.48–0.86; $P = .003$); however, after adjusting for baseline variables, the association of viability with mortality was no longer significant.[30]

SUMMARY

There have been significant advances in the treatment of acute MI in the past several decades. Such measures have resulted in improved survival and a lower incidence of HF. However, a substantial number of patients continue to experience adverse remodeling of the left ventricle after MI. Echocardiography remains the imaging procedure of choice to assess for post-MI remodeling and other complications. In more complex patients, a multimodality approach to imaging provides the most comprehensive assessment for diagnosis, prognosis, and reduction of morbidity among these individuals.

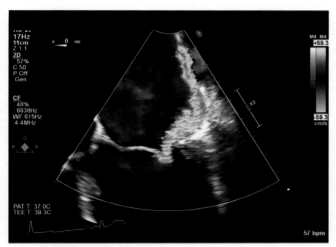

Figure 45.5. Transesophageal echocardiogram showing functional mitral regurgitation caused by local tethering of the posteromedial papillary muscle. The accompanying videos show the regional wall motion abnormalities (Video 45.5A) and restricted posterior leaflet (Video 45.5B). Video 45.5C shows the eccentric mitral regurgitation tracking along the lateral wall of the left atrium. Video 45.5D shows a color three-dimensional image of the mitral valve. Note that the jet originates from the lateral half of the valve. *MRI*, Magnetic resonance imaging.

Please access ExpertConsult to view the corresponding videos for this chapter.

REFERENCES

1. Pfeffer MA, Braunwald E. Ventricular remodeling after myocardial infarction. Experimental observations and clinical implications. *Circulation*. 1990;81:1161–1172.
2. Sutton MGSJ, Sharpe N. Left ventricular remodeling after myocardial infarction. *Circulation*. 2000;101:2981–2988.
3. Flachskampf FA, Schmid M, Rost C, et al. Cardiac imaging after myocardial infarction. *Eur Heart J*. 2010;32:272–283.
4. Benjamin EJ, Muntner P, Alonso A, et al. Heart disease and stroke statistics—2019 update: a report from the American Heart Association. *Circulation*. 2019;139:e56–e528.
5. Steg PG, Dabbous OH, Feldman LJ, et al. Determinants and prognostic impact of heart failure complicating acute coronary syndromes: observations from the Global Registry of Acute Coronary Events (GRACE). *Circulation*. 2004;109:494–499.
6. Kramer DG, Trikalinos TA, Kent DM, et al. Quantitative evaluation of drug or device effects on ventricular remodeling as predictors of therapeutic effects on mortality in patients with heart failure and reduced ejection fraction: a meta-analytic approach. *J Am Coll Cardiol*. 2010;56:392–406.
7. Cohn JN, Ferrari R, Sharpe N. Cardiac remodeling—Concepts and clinical implications: a consensus paper from an international forum on cardiac remodeling on behalf of an International Forum on Cardiac Remodeling. *J Am Coll Cardiol*. 2000;35:569–582.
8. Miller AL, Dib C, Li L, et al. Left ventricular ejection fraction assessment among patients with acute myocardial infarction and its association with hospital quality of care and evidence-based therapy use. *Circulation Cardiovasc Quality Outcomes*. 2012;5:662–671.
9. O'Gara PT, Kushner FG, Ascheim DD, et al. ACCF/AHA guideline for the management of ST-elevation myocardial infarction: a report of the American College of Cardiology Foundation/American heart association Task Force on practice guidelines. *J Am Coll Cardiol*. 2013;61:e78–e140. 2013.
10. Amsterdam EA, Wenger NK, Brindis RG, et al. AHA/ACC guideline for the management of patients with non-ST-elevation acute coronary syndromes: a report of the American College of Cardiology/American heart association Task Force on practice guidelines. *J Am Coll Cardiol*. 2014;64:e139–e228. 2014.
11. Mather AN, Fairbairn TA, Artis NJ, et al. Timing of cardiovascular MR imaging after acute myocardial infarction: effect on estimates of infarct characteristics and prediction of late ventricular remodeling. *Radiology*. 2011;261:116–126.
12. McKay RG, Pfeffer MA, Pasternak RC, et al. Left ventricular remodeling after myocardial infarction: a corollary to infarct expansion. *Circulation*. 1986;74:693–702.
13. Pirolo JS, Hutchins GM, Moore GW. Infarct expansion: pathologic analysis of 204 patients with a single myocardial infarct. *J Am Coll Cardiol*. 1986;7:349–354.
14. Leung WH, Lau CP. Effects of severity of the residual stenosis of the infarct-related coronary artery on left ventricular dilation and function after acute myocardial infarction. *J Am Coll Cardiol*. 1992;20:307–313.
15. Wu E, Ortiz JT, Tejedor P, et al. Infarct size by contrast enhanced cardiac magnetic resonance is a stronger predictor of outcomes than left ventricular ejection fraction or end-systolic volume index: prospective cohort study. *Heart*. 2008;94:730–736.
16. van Kranenburg M, Magro M, Thiele H, et al. Prognostic value of microvascular obstruction and infarct size, as measured by CMR in STEMI patients. *JACC Cardiovasc Imaging*. 2014;7:930–939.
17. Eitel I, de Waha S, Wöhrle J, et al. Comprehensive prognosis assessment by CMR imaging after ST-segment elevation myocardial infarction. *J Am Coll Cardiol*. 2014;64:1217–1226.
18. White HD, Norris RM, Brown MA, et al. Left ventricular end-systolic volume as the major determinant of survival after recovery from myocardial infarction. *Circulation*. 1987;76:44–51.
19. Ky B, Plappert T, Kirkpatrick J, et al. Left ventricular remodeling in human heart failure: quantitative echocardiographic assessment of 1,794 patients. *Echocardiography*. 2012;29:758–765.
20. Meta-Analysis Research Group in Echocardiography (MeRGE) AMI Collaborators, Møller JE, Whalley GA, et al. Independent prognostic importance of a restrictive left ventricular filling pattern after myocardial infarction: an individual patient meta-analysis. *Circulation*. 2008;117:2591–2598.
21. Singh A, Voss WB, Lentz RW, et al. The diagnostic and prognostic value of echocardiographic strain. *JAMA Cardiol*. 2019;4:580–588.
22. D'Andrea A, Cocchia R, Caso P, et al. Global longitudinal speckle-tracking strain is predictive of left ventricular remodeling after coronary angioplasty in patients with recent non-ST elevation myocardial infarction. *Int J Cardiol*. 2011;153:185–191.
23. Bulluck H, Go YY, Crimi G, et al. Defining left ventricular remodeling following acute ST-segment elevation myocardial infarction using cardiovascular magnetic resonance. *J Cardiovasc Magn Reson*. 2017;19:26.
24. Grothues F, Smith GC, Moon JC, et al. Comparison of interstudy reproducibility of cardiovascular magnetic resonance with two-dimensional echocardiography in normal subjects and in patients with heart failure or left ventricular hypertrophy. *Am J Cardiol*. 2002;90:29–34.
25. Weinsaft JW, Kim J, Medicherla CB, et al. Echocardiographic algorithm for post-myocardial infarction LV thrombus: a gatekeeper for thrombus evaluation by delayed enhancement CMR. *JACC Cardiovasc Imag*. 2016;9:505–515.
26. Grigioni F, Enriquez-Sarano M, Zehr KJ, et al. Ischemic mitral regurgitation: long-term outcome and prognostic implications with quantitative Doppler assessment. *Circulation*. 2001;103:1759–1764.
27. Kwon DH, Kusunose K, Obuchowski NA, et al. Predictors and prognostic impact of progressive ischemic mitral regurgitation in patients with advanced ischemic cardiomyopathy: a multimodality study. *Circ Cardiovasc Imag*. 2016;9:27.
28. Afridi I, Kleiman NS, Raizner AE, Zoghbi WA. Dobutamine echocardiography in myocardial hibernation: optimal dose and accuracy in predicting recovery of ventricular function after coronary angioplasty. *Circulation*. 1995;91:663–670.
29. Bax JJ, Poldermans D, Elhendy A, et al. Sensitivity, specificity, and predictive accuracies of various noninvasive techniques for detecting hibernating myocardium. *Curr Probl Cardiol*. 2001;26:147–186.
30. Bonow RO, Maurer G, Lee KL, et al. Myocardial viability and survival in ischemic left ventricular dysfunction. *N Engl J Med*. 2011;364:1617–1625.

46

End-Stage Cardiomyopathy Due to Coronary Artery Disease

Peter S. Rahko

End-stage coronary artery disease (CAD) typically manifests as a dilated cardiomyopathy, commonly termed *ischemic cardiomyopathy* (ICM). The patient has known CAD combined with significant left ventricular (LV) systolic dysfunction with an ejection fraction of 35% or less. The most common clinical presentation is that of a patient with a prior history of one or more myocardial infarctions (MIs) who now on echocardiographic evaluation has evidence of significant LV dysfunction. Occasionally (7% in one series), patients present with new symptoms of heart failure (HF) and dilated cardiomyopathy but with no prior history of CAD. These patients, on coronary angiography, typically have multivessel disease. The extent of the coronary atherosclerosis is inversely related to the long-term prognosis.

The pathophysiology of ICM is caused by ischemic damage to the myocardium. In many patients, this triggers a process called ventricular remodeling, which results in alteration of LV architecture, with changes in LV shape and increases in LV volume. The process, following a MI, is depicted in Fig. 46.1. The changes leading to the macroscopic manifestation of a dilated and dysfunctional LV are complex and are directly proportional to the size of the initial insult.[1]

After the initial infarct event, there is first an inflammatory phase that replaces necrotic myocytes with fibrotic tissue that evolves into a scar. Neovascularization occurs in an attempt to reestablish perfusion to the area and border zone where some surviving myocytes may recover function. Both at a local level within cardiac cells and in the patient's circulatory system, there is significant activation of the sympathetic nervous system, the renin–angiotensin–aldosterone system, and other regulatory mechanisms that may promote remodeling. Depending on the size of the initial insult and the repair process, there are varying levels of myocyte elongation, scar zone expansion, and thinning of the infarcted area (see Fig. 46.1). Most of these changes are adaptive to maintain cardiac output.

As the LV chamber enlarges, important changes occur in myocytes and fibrocytes outside the infarct zone. The upregulation of neuroendocrine factors and changes in loading conditions trigger changes in the myocyte causing elongation hypertrophy, cellular genetic reprogramming, loss of myofilaments, and other functional changes within the cells.[2] Fibroblast proliferation among areas of infarcted myocytes produces replacement fibrosis (see Fig. 46.1). Outside of the infarct zone, some fibroblasts are stimulated to evolve into myofibroblast cells that produce considerable fibrous material causing excessive reactive fibrosis. This can cause increased cardiac stiffness, abnormal relaxation, and reduced contractile function. The combination of all of these factors can change initial adaptive remodeling to long-term maladaptive remodeling. The end result is an ICM with secondary LV hypertrophy, chamber enlargement, LV shape changes, and diastolic dysfunction (Fig. 46.2).

A key differentiating process for ICM is to determine whether all of the remodeling changes are irreversible because of permanent changes from replacement fibrosis or if some of the dysfunction is caused by a mechanical loss of contractility in myocytes that remain viable. The discovery of "hibernating myocardium" by

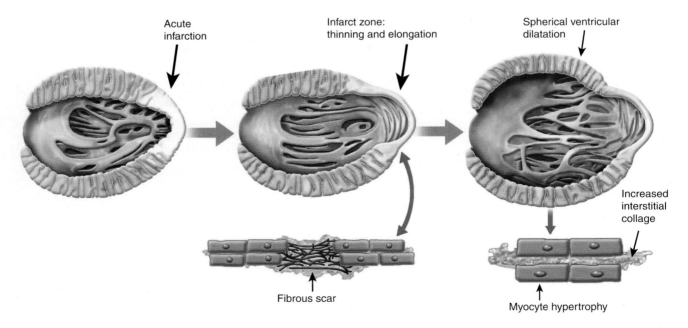

Acute infarction

Infarct zone: thinning and elongation

Spherical ventricular dilatation

Increased interstitial collage

Fibrous scar

Myocyte hypertrophy

Figure 46.1. Mechanism of progressive left ventricular remodeling after a myocardial infarction (see text). (Reproduced with permission from Konstam MA, et al: Left ventricular remodeling in heart failure: current concepts in clinical significance and assessment, *JACC Cardiovasc Imaging* 4(1):98–108, 2011.)

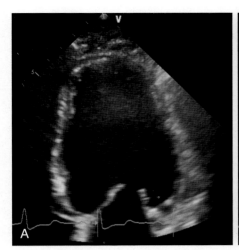 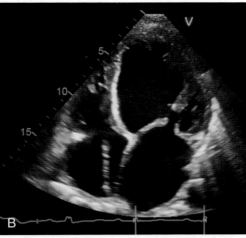

Figure 46.2. A, Ischemic cardiomyopathy (ICM) in the apical four-chamber view. Left ventricular (LV) enlargement is moderate. Some areas of the LV contract normally. **B,** ICM in the apical four-chamber view. LV enlargement is severe; all segments are akinetic or hypokinetic. (See Video 46.2.)

viability testing is a situation in which mechanical dysfunction may improve after revascularization. This can be evaluated by several types of multimodality imaging examinations, such as positron emission tomography, cardiac magnetic resonance imaging (MRI), and dobutamine stress echocardiography (see Chapter 54). Prior studies have shown that restoration of contractility in hibernating segments of the LV after revascularization may help slow down or partially reverse maladaptive remodeling.[3]

Echocardiography plays a central role in the evaluation of the left ventricle at the time of the baseline event, serially during the course of recovery from an initial MI, and onward as long-term guideline-directed medical and device therapy is initiated.

DETERMINING THE CAUSE OF VENTRICULAR DYSFUNCTION

In patients that present with new-onset HF and dilated cardiomyopathy, it is almost impossible to determine by wall motion analysis alone the underlying etiology of disease. Occasionally, patients may have specific findings that are associated with CAD, such as large discreet aneurysms or areas of discreet thinning with an end-diastolic wall thickness of less than 6 mm. Usually, a definite etiologic diagnosis is not possible without previous historical data proving the presence of CAD. When dysfunction is severe and risks are significant for CAD, current HF guidelines recommend coronary angiography for a definitive diagnosis. In younger patients expected to have less coronary artery calcium, computed tomography angiography is an alternative method. Imaging with cardiac MRI with late gadolinium enhancement can further characterize the degree of scar formation, shape alterations, and viability.[4]

CHARACTERIZATION OF LEFT VENTRICULAR SIZE AND FUNCTION

LV short-axis dimensions should be measured in all patients. This is best done using two-dimensional (2D) measurements from the parasternal long-axis view. Care should be taken to fully position the left ventricle as perpendicular to the transducer as possible to allow optimal definition of wall thickness and chamber dimensions. For serial imaging, it is important to maintain the same relative position for measurements to minimize variation because response to therapy may determine future treatment. Additional dimension measurements may be of value, such as relative wall thickness and the eccentricity index.[5] More severely affected ICMs have a greater spherical shape.

The most important measurement is calculation of the LV ejection fraction (EF). Many guidelines use EF in decision algorithms, making it important to minimize variation. Frequently, EF is

determined by visual analysis; here intraobserver variability is better than interobserver variability. When the same individual reviews serial studies, reproducibility of the EF is reasonable (±5%–10%), but variability is higher when reviewed by different individuals.[6] Image review stations that permit side-by-side comparison of the current echocardiogram with previous studies are of great value. Because the detection of change with therapy is of vital importance, it is mandatory that previous studies be reviewed before drawing conclusions regarding changes in size and function. Although image quality has markedly improved, particularly with the use of ultrasound-enhancing agents, visual analysis variability has not improved.[7] Regional function should also be reported by scoring the severity of segmental dysfunction semiquantitatively using the 17-segment model. This is important for determining the effect of not only long-term medical therapy but also reperfusion interventions.[5]

To further clinical evaluation of ICM, quantifications of LV volumes, mass, and EF have been utilized. The traditional standard has been the biplane method of discs based upon 2D apical four-chamber and two-chamber images. Although theoretically appealing, the technique has suffered from several methodologic limitations: (1) apical images are frequently foreshortened when the sonographer is unable to display the true long axis of the LV; (2) image quality degrades in freeze frame views, making it more difficult to define endocardial surfaces; (3) even when image quality is good, there is considerable variation in differentiating the compacted myocardium from trabeculations, particularly at the apex; and (4) the method is tedious and time consuming. Thus, it should not be surprising that the method of discs, although correlating reasonably well with other methods of quantification for EF, systematically underestimates LV volumes, and for all the effort expended in making the calculation, reproducibility is no better than visual assessment.[8,9] The use of ultrasound-enhancing agents has been studied and shows promise for improving volumetric calculations, EF calculations, and reproducibility.[8,10,11]

The development of three-dimensional (3D) imaging technology has greatly enhanced LV quantification and reproducibility. 3D echocardiography substantially reduces the risk of foreshortening of the LV and eliminates geometric assumptions about LV shape changes, particularly important in ICM. Comparisons with cardiac MRI show considerably better agreement for LV volumes, but systematic underestimation remains an issue.[11,12] The 3D rendering of the LV continues to be limited by slower frame rates that may miss maximum and minimum LV volumes and reduced resolution, making identification of the compacted myocardium more challenging when manual tracing algorithms are used.[9] Of great promise are recent advances in automatic 3D volume calculations of cardiac chambers using machine-based learning and artificial intelligence programming to overcome the limitations of manual semiautomatic

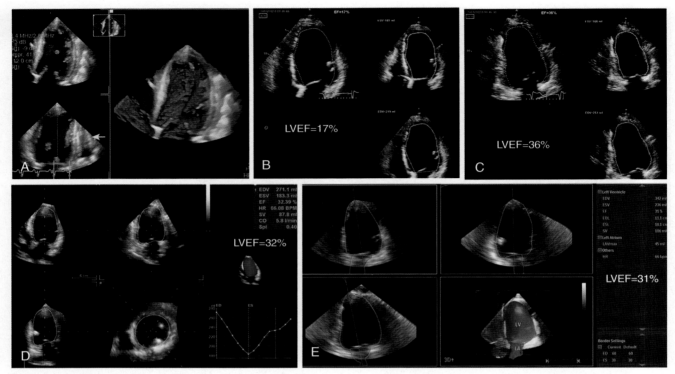

Figure 46.3. A, Three-dimensional (3D) visualization of ischemic cardiomyopathy (ICM). **B–E,** Quantification of ICM function showing heterogeneous function. In **B**, the single-plane method of discs shows a left ventricular ejection fraction (LVEF) of 17% from the apical four-chamber view and in **C** 36% from the apical two-chamber view. The biplane calculation is 27%. In **D**, the semiautomated 3D LVEF is 32%. In **E**, in the same patient using an automated calculation, the LVEF is 31%. (See Video 46.3.)

methods.[12] Automated methods process images in less than 60 seconds, which hopefully will make this quantification routine in the future. An ICM represents perhaps the greatest challenge for quantification given the marked variations in shape and regional function (Fig. 46.3).

RIGHT VENTRICLE

The size and function of the right ventricle can be highly variable in patients with ICM. Although some studies have found that for the same LVEF, the severity of right ventricular (RV) dysfunction tends to be greater in patients with nonischemic cardiomyopathy versus ICM, the relationship is complex. RV function is afterload dependent; thus, the severity of LV systolic dysfunction, LV diastolic dysfunction, and pulmonary hypertension determine RV performance over the long term. Direct ischemic injury from RV infarction also plays a role in some patients with ICM, but the relationship is complex because many patients have substantial recovery during the weeks after an RV infarction even if the coronary arteries remain persistently occluded.[13]

Because of the unique shape of the right ventricle, not only the RV free wall but also the ventricular septum plays a significant role in defining RV function. This makes it difficult for any single 2D measurement to completely represent global RV function. Given these limitations, it is important to standardize imaging views of the right ventricle to enhance reproducibility of measurements. It is important to obtain the RV-focused view by adjusting the apical four-chamber view to show the RV centered in the 2D sector, maximizing the long axis and also medial and lateral dimensions. This is usually accomplished by lateral positioning and fine rotation of the transducer to show the maximum area of the RV (Fig. 46.4) (see also Chapters 27–30).

RV function has been correlated with functional capacity, prognosis, and candidacy for placement of LV assist devices. In many clinical laboratories, RV size and function are semiquantitatively defined as normal, mildly, moderately, or severely dysfunctional. Even this is problematic when the LV is markedly enlarged because a reader tends to judge RV size in relation to LV size as a frame of reference.

Linear measurement of the RV long- and short-axis dimensions from the RV-focused view can help define RV size. A short- to long-axis linear ratio of greater than 0.6 is associated with a poor long-term outcome. An M-mode based linear measure of systolic function, tricuspid annular plane systolic excursion (TAPSE) that defines long-axis movement of the RV base in systole, is positively correlated with RVEF and has prognostic value in pulmonary hypertension and heart failure. Values greater than 17 mm are considered normal, and values less than 7.5 mm of excursion are associated with worse outcome. The measurement is angle dependent, so consistent placement of the M-mode beam to maximize linear motion is recommended.

Fractional area change is an ejection phase index analogous to EF using the percentage change of RV area in the RV focus view from end-diastole to end-systole. It is important to trace the endocardial borders, locating the compacted myocardium and keeping trabeculae within the cavity. Values greater than 35% are considered normal, but values less than 20% are associated with a particularly poor prognosis.

Similar to mitral valve tissue Doppler, motion of the lateral tricuspid valve annulus may be measured. Peak systolic velocity is of greatest value, and a value greater 9.5 cm/s has been established as normal.[5]

Application of longitudinal RV strain has been evaluated in ICM using speckle-tracking and velocity vector imaging.[14] Both techniques show promise for identification of RV dysfunction and prognosis in patients with ICM. There is good correlation with cardiac MRI, and the potential exists that strain may be superior to conventional 2D measurements of RV performance.

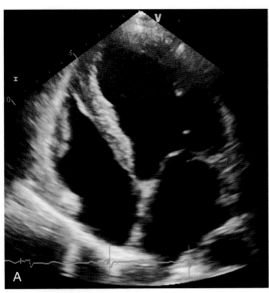
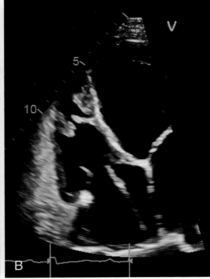

Figure 46.4. Right ventricular (RV) function. **A,** ischemic cardiomyopathy (ICM) with preserved RV function. **B,** ICM with moderately reduced RV function. (See Video 46.4.)

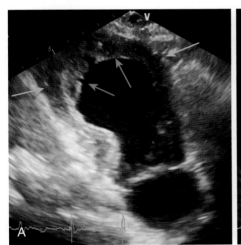
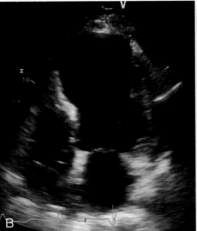
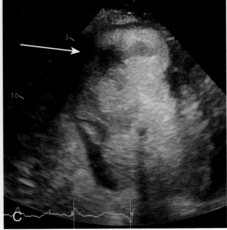

Figure 46.5. A, Example of a left ventricular (LV) apical aneurysm, apical two-chamber view *(yellow arrows)*. The LV shape remains distorted through their entire cardiac cycle. A laminated thrombus is present *(red arrows)*. **B,** Apical aneurysm four-chamber view. No thrombus. **C,** Same patient as *B*; contrast shows ineffective flow in the apex *(arrow)*. (See Video 46.5.)

LEFT VENTRICULAR ANEURYSM

An aneurysm is a discrete area of wall thinning and shape change in the LV. Aneurysms may form after large MIs in multiple locations of the LV. The aneurysm has wall motion that is either akinetic or dyskinetic. The area of the aneurysm distorts a discrete section of the LV continuously; thus, the LV never regains a normal shape in diastole. Although most commonly identified with apical shape change, it is also possible to have a significant-sized aneurysm after an inferior or inferolateral MI. In most circumstances, these aneurysms involve substantial shape changes beginning at the base of the inferior and inferolateral walls. Aneurysms are characterized by a wide opening and a continuation of the endocardial surface throughout the entire structure. Aneurysms make quantification of LV volumes, and in particular LV function, difficult. It is frequently not possible to fit an apical aneurysm into a standard 2D sector or 3D volume (Fig. 46.5). Qualitative characterization of the aneurysm and careful evaluation for the presence of thrombus are important considerations for patients with worsening ventricular function who may have progressively reduced efficiency of contraction. Off-axis views may also help fully characterize the shape of the aneurysm.

FUNCTIONAL MITRAL REGURGITATION

Determination of the severity of mitral regurgitation (MR) is an important component of the ICM examination and varies dramatically, from virtually nothing to severe. Most patients have some degree of MR, which further increases the severity of HF symptoms, reduces net cardiac output, and increases loading conditions on an already dysfunctional left ventricle. There is no primary mitral valve disease, the valve is usually anatomically normal or mildly thickened, and malfunctions are caused by LV remodeling changes. Termed *functional MR*, the effectiveness of valve coaptation is closely related to the amount of tissue available for overlap between the two leaflets. Dilatation of the annulus of the valve apparatus, secondary to both left atrial and LV enlargement, tends to distort annular shape and stretch both leaflets away from each other (Fig. 46.6). LV long-axis enlargement tethers the mitral apparatus leaflets toward the apex of the ventricle and spherical enlargement malpositions papillary muscles, restricting motion of the leaflets and moving the coaptation point of the leaflets deeper into the left ventricle. Reduced contractility of the papillary muscles, which may be asymmetric because of variable ischemic damage, further restricts valve motion and further increases the severity of regurgitation. Particularly in ICM, the MR

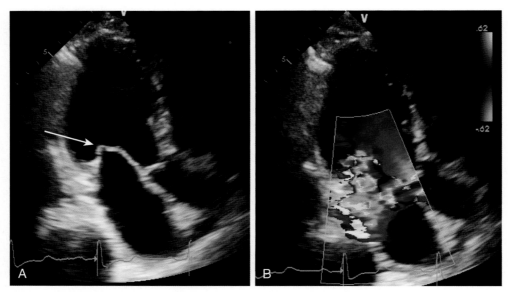

Figure 46.6. Secondary mitral regurgitation (MR). **A,** Typical changes in position and motion of the mitral valve leaflets with coaptation overlap reduced and tethered toward the apex. **B,** Color Doppler imaging of MR. (See Video 46.6.)

jet may be very eccentric because of differential movement of the two leaflets even though no part of a leaflet is flail (see Chapter 97).

Please access ExpertConsult to view the corresponding videos for this chapter.

REFERENCES

1. Konstam MA, Kramer DG, Patel AR, et al. Left ventricular remodeling in heart failure: current concepts in clinical significance and assessment. *JACC Cardiovasc Imaging.* 2011;4(1):98–108.
2. Hasenfuss G, Mann DL. Pathophysiology of heart failure. In: Zipes DP, Libby P, Bonow RO, et al, eds. *Braunwald's Heart Disease: A Textbook of Cardiovascular Medicine.* 11th ed. Philadelphia: Elsevier; 2019.
3. Carluccio E, Biagioli P, Alunni G, et al. Patients with hibernating myocardium show altered left ventricular volumes and shape, which revert after revascularization: evidence that dyssynergy might directly induce cardiac remodeling. *J Am Coll Cardiol.* 2006;47(5):969–977.
4. Patel H, Wojciech M, Williams KA, Kalra DK. Myocardial viability—State of the art: is it still relevant and how to best assess it with imaging? *Trends Cardiovasc Med.* 2018;28(1):24–37.
5. Lang RM, Badano LP, Mor-Avi V, et al. Recommendations for cardiac chamber quantification by echocardiography in adults: an update from the American Society of Echocardiography and the European Association of Cardiovascular Imaging. *J Am Soc Echocardiogr.* 2015;28(1):1–39.e14.
6. Amico AF, Lichtenberg GS, Reisner SA, et al. Superiority of visual versus computerized echocardiographic estimation of radionuclide left ventricular ejection fraction. *Am Heart J.* 1989;118(6):1259–1265.
7. Knackstedt C, Bekkers SC, Schummers G, et al. Fully automated versus standard tracking of left ventricular ejection fraction and longitudinal strain: the FAST-EFs Multicenter Study. *J Am Coll Cardiol.* 2015;66(13):1456–1466.
8. Mor-Avi V, Jenkins C, Kuhl HP, et al. Real-time 3 dimensional echocardiographic quantification of left ventricular volumes: multicenter study for validation with magnetic resonance imaging and investigation of sources of error. *JACC Cardiovasc Imaging.* 2008;1(4):413–423.
9. Lang RM, Addetia K, Narang A, Mor-Avi V. 3 dimensional echocardiography: latest developments and future directions. *JACC Cardiovasc Imaging.* 2018;11(12):1854–1878.
10. Hoffmann R, Barletta G, von Bardeleben S, et al. Analysis of left ventricular volumes and function: a multicenter comparison of cardiac magnetic resonance imaging, cine ventriculography, and unenhanced and contrast-enhanced two-dimensional and three-dimensional echocardiography. *J Am Soc Echocardiogr.* 2014;27(3):292–301.
11. Tamborini G, Piazzese C, Lang RM, et al. Feasibility and accuracy of automated software for transthoracic three-dimensional left ventricular volume and function analysis: comparisons with two-dimensional echocardiography, three-dimensional transthoracic manual method, and cardiac magnetic resonance imaging. *J Am Soc Echocardiogr.* 2017;30(11):1049–1058.
12. Medvedofsky D, Mor-Avi V, Amzulescu M, et al. Three-dimensional echocardiographic quantification of the left-heart chambers using an automated adaptive analytics algorithm: multicentre validation study. *Eur Heart J Cardiovasc Imaging.* 2018;19(1):47–58.
13. Schalla S, Jaarsma C, Bekkers SC, et al. Right ventricular function in dilated cardiomyopathy and ischemic heart disease: assessment with non-invasive imaging. *Neth Heart J.* 2015;23(4):232–240.
14. Park JH, Kusunose K, Motoki H, et al. Assessment of right ventricular longitudinal strain in patients with ischemic cardiomyopathy: head-to-head comparison between two-dimensional speckle-based strain and velocity vector imaging using volumetric assessment by cardiac magnetic resonance as a "gold standard." *Echocardiography.* 2015;32(6):956–965.

47 Coronary Artery Anomalies

Aneet Patel, Eric V. Krieger, Mariko Welch, Edward A. Gill

Congenital coronary artery (CA) anomalies (CAAs) encompass a diverse spectrum of pathology. They include both benign variations in CA anatomy as well as patterns that predispose to sudden cardiac death (SCD). Broadly speaking, congenital CA anomalies include abnormalities in (1) CA origin, (2) CA course or distribution, and (3) CA termination (fistulae). This chapter focuses on the echocardiographic evaluation of anomalous CA origin with special attention to anomalous coronary artery origin from the opposite sinus (ACAOS) of Valsalva.

ACAOS has particular clinical importance because it has been associated with SCD in asymptomatic healthy young people. ACAOS is clinically meaningful when the proximal course of the CA travels between the aorta and pulmonary artery (PA) (interarterial course). The prevalence of ACAOS with interarterial course is unknown and varies widely across reports (0.17%–1%) depending on the population studied and the imaging modality used.[1,2] Additional risk factors for sudden death are thought to include narrow ("slitlike") orifice of the anomalous CA,

TABLE 47.1 Classification of Coronary Anomalies in Human Hearts

A. Anomalies of origination and course
  1. Absent left main trunk (split origination of the LCA)
  2. Anomalous location of coronary ostium within aortic root or near proper aortic sinus of Valsalva (for each artery)
    a. High
    b. Low
    c. Commissural
  3. Anomalous location of coronary ostium outside normal "coronary" aortic sinuses
    a. Right posterior aortic sinus
    b. Ascending aorta
    c. Left ventricle
    d. Right ventricle
    e. Pulmonary artery
      (1) LCA that arises from posterior facing sinus
      (2) Cx that arises from posterior facing sinus
      (3) LAD that arises from posterior facing sinus
      (4) RCA that arises from anterior right-facing sinus
      (5) Ectopic location (outside facing sinuses) of any coronary artery from the pulmonary artery
        (a) From the anterior left sinus
        (b) From the pulmonary trunk
        (c) From the pulmonary branch
    f. Aortic arch
    g. Innominate artery
    h. Right carotid artery
    i. Internal mammary artery
    j. Bronchial artery
    k. Subclavian artery
    l. Descending thoracic aorta
  4. Anomalous location of coronary ostium at improper sinus (which may involve joint origination or "single" coronary pattern)
    a. RCA that arises from left anterior sinus, with an anomalous course
      (1) Posterior atrioventricular groove or retrocardiac
      (2) Retroaortic
      (3) Between the aorta and pulmonary artery (intramural)
      (4) Intraseptal
      (5) Anterior to pulmonary outflow
      (6) Posteroanterior interventricular groove (wraparound)
    b. LAD that arises from the right anterior sinus, with an anomalous course
      (1) Between aorta and pulmonary artery (intramural)
      (2) Intraseptal
      (3) Anterior to pulmonary outflow
      (4) Posteroanterior interventricular groove (wraparound)
    c. Cx that arises from right anterior sinus, with an anomalous course
      (1) Posterior atrioventricular groove
      (2) Retroaortic

  d. LCA that arises from right anterior sinus, with anomalous
      (1) Posterior atrioventricular groove
      (2) Retroaortic
      (3) Between aorta and pulmonary artery
      (4) Intraseptal
      (5) Anterior to pulmonary outflow
      (6) Posteroanterior interventricular groove
  5. Single coronary artery (see A4)
B. Anomalies of intrinsic coronary arterial anatomy
  1. Congenital ostial stenosis or atresia (LCA, LAD, RCA, Cx)
  2. Coronary ostial dimple
  3. Coronary ectasia or aneurysm
  4. Absent coronary artery
  5. Coronary hypoplasia
  6. Intramural coronary artery (muscular bridge)
  7. Subendocardial coronary course
  8. Coronary crossing
  9. Anomalous origination of posterior descending artery from the anterior descending branch or a septal penetrating branch
  10. Split RCA
    a. Proximal + distal PDs that both arise from RCA
    b. Proximal PD that arises from RCA, distal PD that arises from LAD
    c. Parallel PDs ×2 (arising from RCA, Cx) or "codominant"
  11. Split LAD
    a. LAD + first large septal branch
    b. LAD, double (parallel LADs)
  12. Ectopic origination of first septal branch
    a. RCA
    b. Right sinus
    c. Diagonal
    d. Ramus
    e. Cx
C. Anomalies of coronary termination
  1. Inadequate arteriolar or capillary ramifications
  2. Fistulas from RCA, LCA, or infundibular artery to:
    a. Right ventricle
    b. Right atrium
    c. Coronary sinus
    d. Superior vena cava
    e. Pulmonary artery
    f. Pulmonary vein
    g. Left atrium
    h. Left ventricle
    i. Multiple, right + left ventricles
D. Anomalous anastomotic vessels

Cx, Circumflex; *LAD*, left anterior descending coronary artery; *LCA*, left coronary artery; *PD*, posterior descending artery; *RCA*, right coronary artery.
Reproduced from Angelini P: Coronary artery anomalies: An entity in search of an identity, *Circulation* 115:1296–1305, 2007.

intramural course, and dynamic compression of the CA seen on angiography.

Accurate diagnosis of ACAOS by transthoracic echocardiography (TTE) is possible but depends on suitable acoustic windows, a protocol that is optimized for CA anatomy and highly trained sonographers. In children and thin, young adults, two separate CA ostia can be seen approximately 90% of the time using two-dimensional (2D) TTE with color Doppler, thereby excluding most important CA anomalies.[3,4] However, false-negative studies have, on rare occasion, preceded SCD.[3] In selected patients, transesophageal echocardiography (TEE) can also identify CA ostia when TTE is inadequate,[5] but increasingly, cross-sectional imaging with computed tomography (CT) or magnetic resonance imaging (MRI) is being used for definition of CA and distribution.

CLASSIFICATION OF CORONARY ARTERY ANOMALIES

Although the definition of a CAA is debated, one classification scheme by Angelini[2,6,7] defines CAA as an anatomic variation occurring in fewer than 1% of the population. Although many types of CAAs have been described (Table 47.1 and Fig. 47.1), few are clinically significant. The majorities of CAAs are clinically silent and remain undetected, so the prevalence of CAAs remains uncertain. This uncertainty is compounded by nonstandard definitions of what constitutes a coronary anomaly; differences in referral populations; and various imaging modalities including echocardiography, angiography, CT, and MRI.[1] In a prospective case series of 1950 participants referred for angiography, Angelini and coworkers[8] found CAAs in 5.64% of patients.

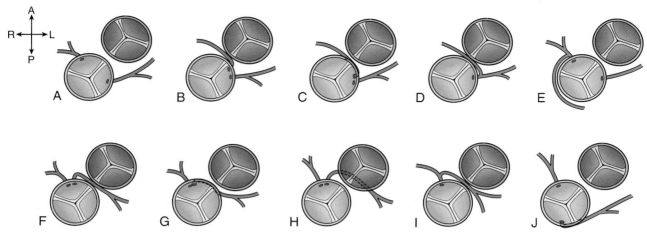

Figure 47.1. Schematic of the coronary origin and course as viewed from left ventricular apex analogous to transthoracic echocardiography images from parasternal short-axis (not surgeon's view). The coordinates anterior (A), posterior (P), left (L), and right (R) are depicted on the *top left corner* of all images. **A,** Normal coronary origin with the right coronary artery (RCA) from the right anterior-facing and left coronary artery (LCA) from the left-facing sinus of Valsalva (SOV). **B,** The RCA from the left sinus of Valsalva (LSOV) with an interarterial course. **C,** The RCA from the LSOV with an intramural course. **D,** The RCA from the LCA with an interarterial course or single coronary from the LSOV. **E,** Circumflex from the RCA with a posterior or retroaortic course. **F,** LCA from right sinus of Valsalva (RSOV) with an interarterial course. **G,** The LCA from the RSOV with an intramural course. **H,** The LCA from the RSOV with an intramyocardial, subpulmonary, intraconal, intraseptal course. **I,** The LCA from the RCA or a single coronary origin from the RSOV. **J,** The LCA from the noncoronary sinus.

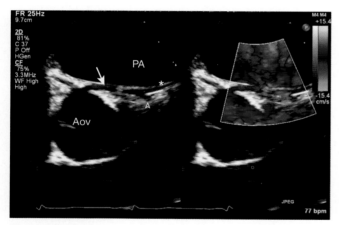

Figure 47.2. Parasternal short-axis view at the level of the aortic valve, clockwise rotated. The left coronary artery (CA) is seen arising from the right sinus of Valsalva with an interarterial course. The *arrow* is pointing at the anomalous left main CA, the *asterisk* indicates the left anterior descending CA, and the *caret* indicates the left circumflex CA. *Aov,* Aortic valve; *PA,* pulmonary artery. (See corresponding Video 47.2.)

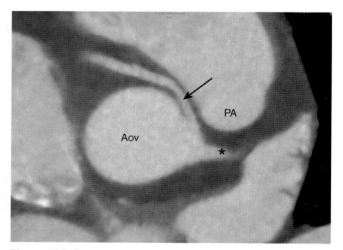

Figure 47.3. Coronary computed tomography scan demonstrates an anomalous right coronary artery (CA) arising from the left sinus of Valsalva with an interarterial course. The *arrow* is pointing at the anomalous right CA, and the *asterisk* indicates the left main CA. *Aov,* Aortic valve; *PA,* pulmonary artery.

The majority were benign, but 1.1% had ACAOS. Other authors using different modalities in dissimilar populations have found lower rates. Although the authors concede that their study is limited by referral bias, it does go to illustrate the relatively high prevalence of ACAOS, arguably the anomaly most strongly associated with SCD.[9,10]

ACAOS is the most common CAA associated with SCD in young athletes[9,10] (Figs. 47.2 and 47.3; Video 47.2). Although both anomalous right coronary artery (RCA)and left coronary artery (LCA) have been described with ACAOS, the presence of an ectopic LCA originating from the right sinus of Valsalva appears to be higher risk. The mechanism of SCD in athletes with ACAOS is not certain. It has been observed that SCD appears to be limited to patients with an interarterial course, and those with an intramural course appear to be at highest risk. For this reason,

it has been speculated that vessel compression and resultant myocardial ischemia lead to SCD in young individuals.[2,7,9] The often intramural nature and acute angle of takeoff of the anomalous artery have also been implicated in causing episodic ischemia in athletes undergoing significant physical exertion.[2,9] Indeed, controversy exists between which is more important: (1) the CA coursing between the aorta and PA, (2) the intramural course, particularly the length of intramural course, or (3) the degree of acute angle takeoff. In a review of two large registries of SCD in young competitive athletes,[9] 27 cases have been attributed to autopsy findings of ACAOS. The authors found that in all of these cases, the athletes died either during or after intense physical exertion; furthermore, 12 of the athletes (45%) experienced premonitory symptoms such as syncope or chest pain in the days to months leading up to their terminal event. Importantly, none had evidence of myocardial ischemia with treadmill stress testing. This study highlights the importance of considering ACAOS in competitive athletes presenting with exertional chest pain with normal cardiac examination and electrocardiogram findings. It also highlights the limitation of stress testing for making this diagnosis. With early detection, these athletes can be excluded from competitive sports to reduce their risk of SCD until definitive correction. Oddly, however, some victims of sudden death have been competitive athletes in their younger years and experienced sudden death at a later age.

Another CCA involving abnormalities in CA origin is anomalous origin of the right or left CA from the pulmonary artery (ALCAPA or ARCAPA) (Figs. 47.5 to 47.7; Videos 47.5 to 47.7). ALCAPA typically presents with heart failure in infancy.[11] Invariably, the CA with normal origin from the aortic root is dilated. The anomalous coronary is perfused retrograde from collaterals and drains into the PA. The most common variant of this anomaly, in which the LCA originates from PA (ALCAPA,

or Bland-White-Garland syndrome), can cause chronic myocardial ischemia caused by the LCA blood supply having decreased perfusion pressure and oxygenation because of its PA source; the presence of collateralization can also lead to coronary steal with left-to-right shunting. In a small proportion of patients with ALCAPA, robust collaterals provide adequate myocardial blood flow and delay presentation until adolescence or adulthood. They may present with ventricular arrhythmias, cardiomyopathy, ischemic mitral regurgitation, or SCD as a result of chronic left ventricular subendocardial ischemia.[12] ARCAPA generally has a more favorable prognosis.

MULTIMODALITY IMAGING FOR IDENTIFICATION OF CONGENITAL CORONARY ARTERY ANOMALIES

A multitude of imaging techniques[13] are used to detect, characterize, and potentially predict the prognosis of the known major anomalies. Coronary angiography with or without intravascular ultrasound (IVUS) has been the mainstay and can be useful for definitive diagnosis in symptomatic patients or patients with an aborted sudden death, though is not clearly acceptable as a screening tool given its invasive method, cost, and inherent risk.[14] Computed tomography angiography (CTA) offers clear spatial resolution, but it brings with it the risk of ionizing radiation and contrast in young patients.[1] Cardiac magnetic resonance imaging (CMRI) is particularly attractive because of its lack of radiation and is also optimal for anatomical definition,[2] though cost, time, noise, and claustrophobia are downsides. Furthermore, the ability of CMRI to assess for collateral vessels, coronary fistulas, or coronaries originating from the ventricle or PA is limited.[15] Transthoracic echocardiography (TTE) and to a lesser extent[16] transesophageal echocardiography (TEE) are imaging techniques with significant research history and clinical use for detection of CAA, particularly TTE for screening and TEE for more detailed confirmation of CA course. Both modalities are advantageous because of absence of radiation and widespread availability and TTE for its very noninvasive nature.

IMAGING PROTOCOL FOR TRANSTHORACIC ECHOCARDIOGRAPHY

CAAs are most reliably imaged with gated cardiac CT or MR angiography and in adults can be difficult to detect with TTE. Nonetheless, there is a critical role for echocardiography in the evaluation of patients with known CAAs. The goal of transthoracic imaging is to image the major coronaries (right, left main, left anterior descending, and circumflex) proximal course and demonstrate anterograde flow.[17,18]

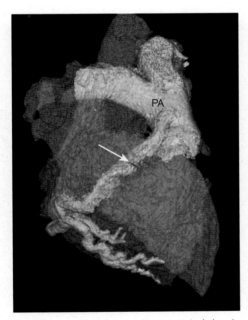

Figure 47.4. Volume-rendered computer computed showing scan a dilated anomalous right coronary artery arising from the pulmonary artery (ARCAPA). The *arrow* points at the ARCAPA. *PA,* Pulmonary artery.

Figure 47.5. A, Two-dimensional and color Doppler echocardiography at the level of the pulmonary artery (PA) showing anomalous right coronary artery arising from the pulmonary artery (ARCAPA). **B,** Note the blue diastolic coronary flow into the pulmonary artery demonstrating that the ARCAPA is perfused retrograde from collaterals from the left coronary artery and drains into the pulmonary artery. *Ao,* Aorta. (See Video 47.5.)

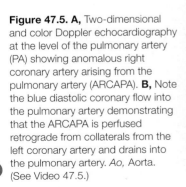

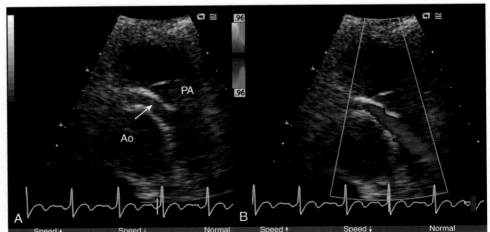

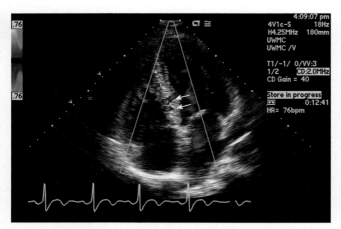

Figure 47.6. Apical four-chamber view with color Doppler in a patient with anomalous right coronary artery from the pulmonary artery (ARCAPA). *Arrows* point to diastolic color flow across the ventricular septum from dilated coronary collaterals. These can be distinguished from ventricular septal defects by their low-velocity diastolic flow. (See Video 47.6.)

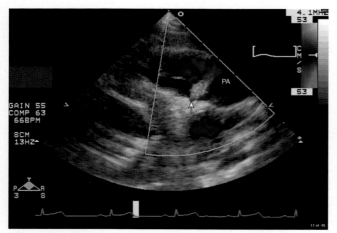

Figure 47.7. Parasternal long-axis view with color Doppler in a patient with anomalous right coronary artery from the pulmonary artery (ARCAPA). *Arrows* point to diastolic color flow across the ventricular septum from dilated coronary collaterals. These can be distinguished from ventricular septal defects by their low-velocity diastolic flow. *PA,* Pulmonary artery. (See Video 47.7.)

Coronary anomalies should be suspected in young patients with unexplained chest pain or resuscitated SCD or patients with congenital heart disease known to be associated with coronary anomalies such as tetralogy of Fallot or transposition of the great arteries.[17,18]

Basic TTE setup should include minimization of digital compression and use of harmonic imaging. In most adults and virtually all children, the ostia of the left main and the right CA can be detected by scanning in the parasternal short axis at the base of the heart, specifically at the level of the sinuses of Valsalva. The proximal left main CA can be visualized at the 4 o'clock position. Slight clockwise rotation from the short-axis view shows the bifurcation of the left anterior descending and the circumflex CAs. Sliding cephalad toward the sinotubular ridge and looking at the 11 o'clock position usually shows the RCA ostium. The right and left CA can also usually be identified from the parasternal long-axis view, and leftward angulation of the transducer shows the left CA bifurcation. Often, 2D imaging can be misleading; it may appear that a CA originates normally, but the structure may

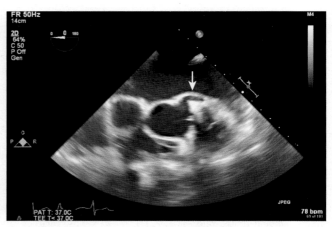

Figure 47.8. Two-dimensional transesophageal echocardiography showing the left main coronary artery arising from the left aortic sinus of Valsalva *(arrow)*. (See Video 47.8.)

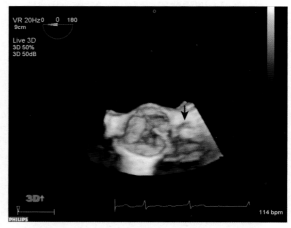

Figure 47.9. Three-dimensional transesophageal echocardiography showing the left main coronary artery (CA) arising from the left aortic sinus of Valsalva and bifurcation of the CA *(arrow)*. (See Video 47.9.)

simply represent a pericardial recess or dropout. Coronary origin is only confirmed by echocardiography when color Doppler flow from the aorta is seen entering the CA. Doppler velocity range should be set low (~15 cm/s) to record the low-velocity diastolic flow. If both ostia can be visualized arising from the appropriate anatomical locations, the likelihood of a dangerous CAA is low. However, some anomalies such as myocardial bridging and CA fistulae may still be present. Therefore, additional imaging may be warranted. A CAA should be suspected if only one ostium is located if an origin or coursing artery appears dilated or proximal course appears abnormal. Often, in adults, particularly those with unfavorable body habitus, it is not possible to convincingly demonstrate both CA origins. In this setting, the probability of coronary anomalies (and the need for additional testing to establish coronary origins) depends on the pretest probability and suspicion for important CAAs.

Many believe that an anomalous aortic origin of a CA from the opposite sinus of Valsalva is more dangerous when the course is interarterial as well as intramural in the wall of the aorta. An intramural course also facilitates surgical unroofing. Although imaging can reliably define an interarterial course, an intramural course is more difficult to determine and often requires surgical or histologic confirmation. Echocardiographic features that have been associated with an intramural course include an acute angle

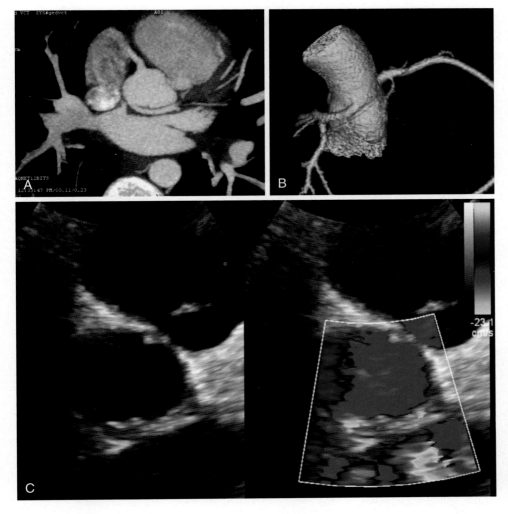

Figure 47.10. Rare condition of left coronary artery (CA) arising from the "noncoronary" sinus with a retroaortic course. **A,** Gated computed tomography (CT) angiogram using maximum-intensity projection showing the left CA arising from the posterior rightward sinus. **B,** Three-dimensional volume-rendered CT angiogram. **C,** Transthoracic echocardiographic image with color Doppler comparison. (See Video 47.10.)

of takeoff from the aortic root and diastolic color flow within the aortic wall.[19]

Markedly dilated CA can be caused by excessive flow from a CA fistula or, less commonly, ARCAPA or ALCAPA. Retrograde coronary flow in the anomalous artery or excessive low-velocity flow by color Doppler in the septum or ventricular walls can be a clue of ARCAPA and ALCAPA.[20] A detailed technique for imaging of all coronary segments is well described elsewhere.[4]

Unfortunately, institutional variability in acquisition of TTE images means that important features of CA origin, anatomy, and proximal course are missed in real-world practice. A study of the Congenital Heart Surgeons Society found that up to one third of studies of patients with anomalous CAs did not have sufficient data to make an accurate diagnosis of intraarterial or intramural course.[19]

INCIDENCE OF CORONARY ANOMALIES DIAGNOSED BY ECHOCARDIOGRAPHY

The largest prospective CAA echocardiography study examined 2388 asymptomatic children and adolescents (0–21 years of age) over a 3-year period.[1] TTE diagnosis was made by using standard TTE and color Doppler. Four children (0.17%, 2.5–18 years old) were found to have ACAOS, and all cases were confirmed with coronary angiography. The higher prevalence of ACAOS compared with autopsy studies in young athletes may have been subject to some component of selection bias due to referral for echocardiography. The sensitivity and false-negative rate of TTE was not

determined because patients with normal studies did not have additional testing. One patient thought to have normal CA origins by TTE subsequently had SCD and was found to have an anomalous coronary at autopsy, confirming that TTE does not have 100% sensitivity for the detection of ACAOS, even in children.

Direct imaging of ALCAPA can be difficult by echocardiography. However, indirect evidence of ALCAPA including left CA flow reversal, dilated right CA, and collateral flow through the septum has improved sensitivity for the diagnosis of ALCAPA; the anatomy can be subsequently confirmed by CT or MR angiography.[20] Additional indirect features that suggest ALCAPA include a dilated and dysfunctional left ventricle and mitral regurgitation; however, these findings are clearly nonspecific (Figs. 47.8 to 47.14; Videos 47.8 to 47.12).

Use of three-dimensional (3D) TEE for delineation of the course of anomalous CAs was performed by Nanda and colleagues in a series of four adult patients.[21] 2D and 3D TEE was prompted in all four cases by an angiogram that identified an anomalous CA but was unable to identify the actual course, specifically a course between the aorta and the PA. Using 2D TEE and gated reconstructive 3D TEE, including 3D color, the team was able to confirm the course between the PA and aorta in all cases. In two of the cases, both multiplane 2D TEE and 3D TEE were able to identify an anterior aortic intramural course, a feature lacking by contrast angiography. In these cases, the echocardiographic findings were essential for clinical management, even after cardiac catheterization and the 3D images were believed by the authors to improve confidence of

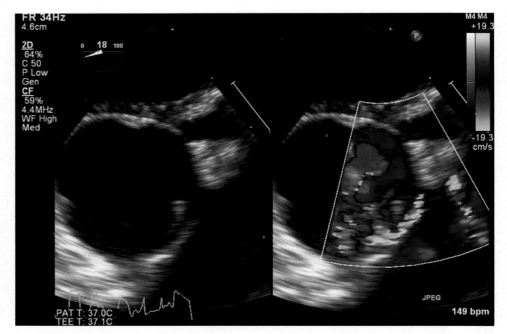

Figure 47.11. Intraoperative transesophageal echocardiography showing an anomalous left coronary artery arising from the right sinus shown with two-dimensional and color Doppler. Note the acute angle of takeoff would be typical for an intramural course, although this is not possible to determine definitively with imaging. (See Video 47.11.)

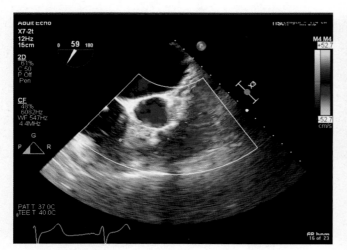

Figure 47.12. Intraoperative two-dimensional transesophageal echocardiography (TEE) image at the level of the aortic valve performed at the time of an anomalous left coronary artery from the pulmonary artery (ALCAPA) repair. The left main coronary artery (CA) could not be seen well arising from the pulmonary artery, so the main findings of the TEE image were a markedly dilated right CA. (See Video 47.12.)

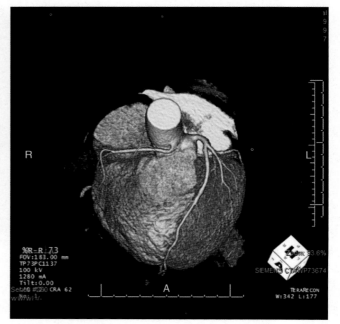

Figure 47.13. Computed tomography coronary angiogram showing an anomalous right coronary artery arising directly from the aortic wall.

the course of the artery, particularly in the case of intramural pathway. Since the advent of real-time 3D TEE, there have been precious few publications on this subject.

PERIOPERATIVE TRANSESOPHAGEAL ECHOCARDIOGRAPHY

If a diagnosis has been made by another modality, such as CTA or MRI, real-time 3D TEE has also been described for the specific use of intraoperative anatomical localization for surgical planning and perioperative monitoring before and after repair to ensure a successful outcome and absence of residual shunting. In a case described by a group from Taiwan by Jin

and colleagues,[15] a 68-year old woman was diagnosed with ALCAPA by CTA after TTE demonstrated a dilated right CA and dilated left ventricle. Because the patient was symptomatic due to coronary steal with resultant left ventricular dysfunction, she was taken to the operating room for venous bypass grafting, and 2D color Doppler was able to visualize the abnormal diastolic continuous flow at the supposed origin of the left CA in the PA. However, only with real-time 3D TEE color Doppler were they able to locate the LCA ostium. After surgical repair, the shunting was no longer visualized. Ilgenli and colleagues also describe a case[21] in which live 3D TEE full volume of the main PA with B-mode and color flow were able to assist in identifying the origin of the LCA in a patient with Eisenmenger

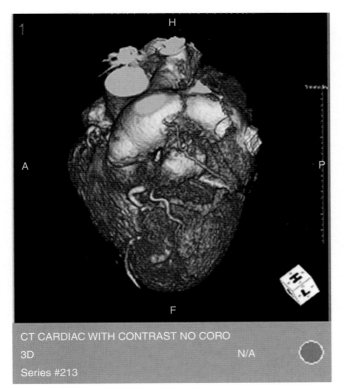

CT CARDIAC WITH CONTRAST NO CORO
3D   N/A
Series #213

Figure 47.14. Computed tomography coronary angiogram showing an anomalous circumflex coronary artery arising from the pulmonary artery.

syndrome. 2D TTE could not identify the origin. This study demonstrated that 3D TEE added to the confidence level of the patient's physicians for accurately identifying the CA ostium as well as a defect in an aortopulmonary window surgically created 13 years before the present examination.

CONCLUSIONS

CAAs, although rare, can be clinically devastating because of their propensity to cause sudden death, particularly in young athletes. Anomalous origin of CAs from the PA, although well described in pediatric population, is rare in adolescents and adults and therefore should be thought of but is unlikely to be of clinical importance, particularly in the population of young athletes. Echocardiography has the strong point of visualization of the origin and initial course of the CAs. As it turns out, this is by far the most important part of the anatomy of anomalous CAs because the majority of intermittent ischemia and causes of sudden death are related to anomalous origin, either from the opposite cusp or a very acute takeoff (or both).

To date, the bulk of the experience diagnosing coronary anomalies with echocardiography has come from standard 2D TTE, of course augmented by color Doppler. The relatively recent development within echocardiography of 3D acquisition

has dramatically improved the tomographic capabilities of this imaging modality. The ability to "crop" through the CAs allows echocardiography to follow the CA course further than previous 2D imaging. Nevertheless, the literature remains void of large prospective series evaluating the diagnosis and natural history of anomalous CA using 3D echocardiography.

Please access ExpertConsult to view the corresponding videos for this chapter.

REFERENCES

1. Davis JA, Cecchin F, Jones TK, Portman MA. Major coronary artery anomalies in a pediatric population: incidence and clinical importance. *J Am Coll Cardiol.* 2001;37:593–597.
2. Angelini P. Coronary artery anomalies: an entity in search of an identity. *Circulation.* 2007;115:1296–1305.
3. Pelliccia A, Spataro A, Maron BJ. Prospective echocardiographic screening for coronary artery anomalies in 1,360 elite competitive athletes. *Am J Cardiol.* 1993;72:978–979.
4. Zeppilli P, dello Russo A, Santini C, et al. In vivo detection of coronary artery anomalies in asymptomatic athletes by echocardiographic screening. *Chest.* 1998;114:89–93.
5. Fernandes F, Alam M, Smith S, Khaja F. The role of transesophageal echocardiography in identifying anomalous coronary arteries. *Circulation.* 1993;88:2532–2540.
6. Angelini P. Coronary artery anomalies—current clinical issues: definitions, classification, incidence, clinical relevance, and treatment guidelines. *Texas Heart Inst J.* 2002;29:271–278.
7. Angelini P, Velasco JA, Flamm S. Coronary anomalies: incidence, pathophysiology, and clinical relevance. *Circulation.* 2002;105:2449–2454.
8. Angelini P, Villason S, Chan Jr AV, Diez JG. Part 1: Historical background. In: *Normal and Anomalous Coronary Arteries in Humans.* Philadelphia: Lippincott Williams & Wilkins, 1999.
9. Basso C, Maron BJ, Corrado D, Thiene G. Clinical profile of congenital coronary artery anomalies with origin from the wrong aortic sinus leading to sudden death in young competitive athletes. *J Am Coll Cardiol.* 2000;35:1493–1501.
10. Liberthson RR. Sudden death from cardiac causes in children and young adults. *New Engl J Med.* 1996;334:1039–1044.
11. Wesselhoeft H, Fawcett JS, Johnson AL. Anomalous origin of the left coronary artery from the pulmonary trunk. Its clinical spectrum, pathology, and pathophysiology, based on a review of 140 cases with seven further cases. *Circulation.* 1968;38:403–425.
12. Yang YL, Nanda NC, Wang XF, et al. Echocardiographic diagnosis of anomalous origin of the left coronary artery from the pulmonary artery. *Echocardiography.* 2007;24:405–411.
13. Maron BJ, Thompson PD, Puffer JC, et al. Cardiovascular preparticipation screening of competitive athletes. *Circulation.* 1996;94:850–856.
14. Taylor AM, Thorne SA, Rubens MB, et al. Coronary artery imaging in grown up congenital heart disease: complementary role of magnetic resonance and x-ray coronary angiography. *Circulation.* 2000;101:1670–1678.
15. Jin YD, Hsiung MC, Tsai SK, et al. Successful intraoperative identification of an anomalous origin of the left coronary artery from the pulmonary artery using real time three-dimensional transesophageal echocardiography. *Echocardiography.* 2011;28:E149–E151.
16. Ilgenli TF, Nanda NC, Sinha A, Khanna D. Live three-dimensional transthoracic echocardiographic assessment of anomalous origin of left coronary artery from the pulmonary artery. *Echocardiography.* 2004;21:559–562.
17. Dabizzi RP, Caprioli G, Aiazzi L, et al. Distribution and anomalies of coronary arteries in tetralogy of Fallot. *Circulation.* 1980;61:95–102.
18. Kang N, Tan SY, Ding ZP, Chua YL. Abnormal origin of right coronary artery from left ventricle with bicuspid aortic stenosis. *Ann Thorac Surg.* 2013;96:e43–45.
19. Lorber R, Srivastava S, Wilder TJ, et al. Anomalous aortic origin of coronary arteries in the young: echocardiographic evaluation with surgical correlation. *JACC Cardiovasc Imag.* 2015;8:1239–1249.
20. Patel SG, Frommelt MA, Frommelt PC, et al. Echocardiographic diagnosis, surgical treatment, and outcomes of anomalous left coronary artery from the pulmonary artery. *J Am Soc Echocardiogr.* 2017;30:896–903.
21. Nanda NC, Bhambore MM, Jindal A, et al. Transesophageal three-dimensional echocardiographic assessment of anomalous coronary arteries. *Echocardiography.* 2000;17:53–60.

48 Coronary Artery Imaging

Masaaki Takeuchi

Noninvasive coronary artery imaging has become popular since it was first used to measure coronary flow velocity (CFV) of the proximal left anterior descending coronary artery (LAD) using transesophageal echocardiography in the early 1990s[1] followed by CFV measurements in the distal portion of the LAD using a transthoracic high-frequency transducer in the late 1990s.[2–4] This was followed by the recording of flow velocity of all three major coronary arteries using a standard transthoracic transducer in the past decade.[5] CFV is characterized by a biphasic flow, a small systolic forward flow, and a predominant diastolic forward flow. Although a specific pattern of systolic coronary flow sometimes provides clinically useful information regarding microvascular obstruction (systolic flow reversal) and the presence of significant coronary stenosis (predominant systolic flow), vigorous contraction of the myocardium during systole usually precludes complete visualization of the CFV envelope throughout one cardiac cycle; thus, its assessment is mainly derived from diastolic CFV, which is the main component of coronary blood flow.

INSTRUCTIONS FOR CFV RECORDING

Because the average diastolic CFV ranges from 10 to 20 cm/s, optimal measurement of CFV requires special settings for color and pulsed-wave Doppler echocardiography. Table 48.1 depicts the updated setting recommendations for CFV measurement among different ultrasound manufactures. The detailed method to record CFV has been described elsewhere.[6,7] Briefly, the LAD runs in the anterior interventricular groove, whereas the posterior descending coronary artery (PD), the terminal branch of the right coronary artery (RCA), runs in the posterior interventricular groove. Thus, visualization of these anatomical landmarks is the first step for successful recording of the LAD and PD flow. The lower parasternal long-axis view is the best plane to record flow in the middle to distal part of the LAD. The transitional view from the apical four-chamber view to the apical two-chamber view and the oblique short-axis view of the left ventricle are the ideal two-dimensional planes to visualize the PD flow. In some patients, the left circumflex coronary artery (LCX) flow can be recorded in the foreshortened apical four-chamber view. It is important to note that all these ideal views for CFV recoding are off-axis views of standard echocardiography image acquisitions (Fig. 48.1). Assessment of the CFV reserve (CFVR) in the distal LAD or PD (or both) provides reliable information on the presence or absence of proximal stenosis of the corresponding artery. Importantly, normal CFVR in the LCX does not always rule out significant stenosis of the LCX because the recording point is often at the middle portion of the LCX or a branch of the LCX, resulting in the misdiagnosis of stenosis of the middle portion of the LCX.

DIAGNOSTIC VALUE OF CORONARY FLOW VELOCITY AT REST

There are some clues for the presence of significant coronary stenosis, even for the evaluation of CFV at rest. The presence of retrograde CFV is the hallmark for the existence of total or near-total occlusion of the recording artery because this flow is reflecting the collateral flow from the ipsilateral or contralateral coronary artery (Fig. 48.2). It is important to verify that retrograde flow is a continuous decrescendo flow during the entire diastolic period to determine that this is not coronary vein flow. Anterograde CFV does not exclude the presence of total occlusion because if the main collateral input is located at the proximal portion to the recording site, flow direction should be anterograde.

TABLE 48.1 Optimal Settings for Coronary Flow Imaging in Each Ultrasound Vendor

Manufacturer	Philips		GE		Siemens		Canon	
Recoding site	LAD	PD and LCX	LAD	PD and LCX	LAD	PD and LCX	LAD	PD and LCX
Transducer	S5-1/X5-1	S5-1/X5-1	M5(4,3)S	M5(4,3)S	4Vic	4V1c	6S3	5S1, 5S2
Color Doppler								
Frequency (MHz)			2.7/2.6	2.7/2.2	3.5	2.0–2.5	3.8	2.5–3.3
Scale (cm/s)	15–25	15–25	20–24	20–24	12–22	12–26	11–17	11–19
Gain	80%	80%	0 dB	0 dB				
Persistence	2 or 3	1 or 2	3.6	3.6	2	2		
Filter[a]	High or max	High or max	8/2.8 cm	8/2.8 cm	1	1	5	5
MAP			Yellow, cyan, or mosaic		1	1	2	2
Tissue priority			0	0	2	2		
Time smooth							5	3
Spatial smooth							4	4
PW Doppler								
Frequency (MHz)			2.5/2.5	2.5/2.5	3.5	1.75	3.8	2.5–3.3
Sample volume (mm)	3	3–4	4	4	3	3–5	5	5
Gain (% or dB)	60%	45%	−10 dB	−10 dB				
Filter[a]	Low or min	Low or min	4.5/2.9 cm	4.5/4.3 cm	4 or 5	4 or 5	150	150
Power (MI)	0.4	1.0	0.5	0.5				
Reject	4	3	4.5/2.9 cm	4.5/4.3 cm				
MAP			Gray 2	Gray 2	3 or 4	3 or 4	3	3

[a]LVRej (low velocity rejection) in GE.

LAD, Left anterior descending coronary artery; *LCX,* left circumflex coronary artery; *MAP, map; MI, mechanical index; PD,* posterior descending coronary artery; *PW,* pulsed-wave.

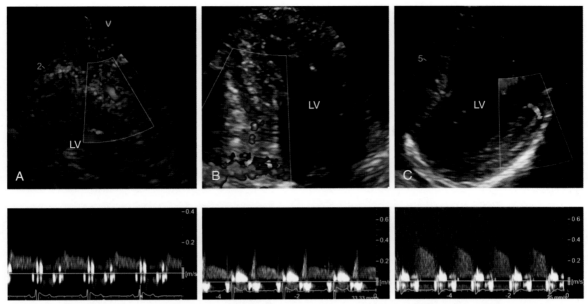

Figure 48.1. Coronary flow recordings. **A,** Coronary flow in the distal portion of the left anterior descending coronary artery. **B,** Coronary flow in the posterior descending coronary artery. This is an off-axis two-chamber view. **C,** Coronary flow in the left circumflex coronary artery. This is an off-axis four-chamber view. *LV,* Left ventricle. (See Video 48.1.)

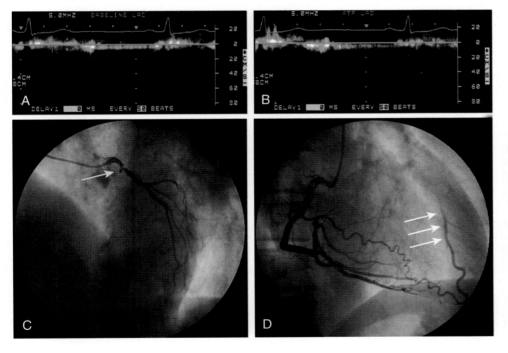

Figure 48.2. Retrograde flow. **A,** Retrograde coronary flow velocity in the distal left anterior descending coronary artery (LAD) at rest. **B,** Retrograde coronary flow velocity during adenosine infusion. Note no obvious change in coronary flow velocity, resulting in the coronary flow velocity reserve of 1.0. **C,** Coronary angiography of the left coronary artery. The proximal portion of the LAD was totally occluded *(yellow arrow).* **D,** Coronary angiography of the right coronary artery. There are well-developed collaterals *(white arrows).*

The presence of mosaic flow may reflect flow acceleration caused by severe stenosis (Fig. 48.3).[4,8,9] If flow velocity at the distal portion relative to the site of mosaic flow is low, it should be functionally significant stenosis. The presence of high flow velocity is not a specific sign for severe coronary stenosis because increased myocardial oxygen consumption enhances CFV at rest, especially in cases of severe left ventricular hypertrophy, heart failure, and anemia.

CLINICAL UTILITY OF CORONARY FLOW VELOCITY RESERVE

CFVR, which is defined as hyperemic CFV divided by baseline CFV, reflects the functional status of both epicardial coronary artery and microvascular circulation. Exercise, dobutamine, and vasodilator agents, such as dipyridamole and adenosine, could cause coronary hyperemia.[2,3,10,11] However, the most popular drug used for CFVR measurements is adenosine, mainly because of its lower cost and shorter half-life. Although coronary hyperemia increases CFV 2.5 to 4.0 times higher than baseline CFV under normal conditions, the cut-off value of CFVR for diagnosing significant stenosis is established to be 2.0 with a higher sensitivity and a good specificity.[2,3,5,10,12,13] Because the feasibility of CFVR measurements in the three major epicardial coronary arteries is 60% to 80% and not 100%, CFVR has not become a standard to diagnose significant coronary stenosis. However, CFVR measurements are quite important for making therapeutic decisions on whether to

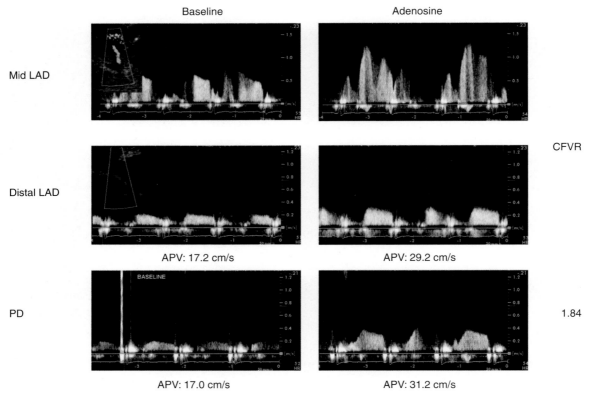

Figure 48.3. Noninvasive detection of coronary stenosis. Mosaic flow was visualized at mid left anterior descending coronary artery (LAD), and flow velocity was increased to 70 cm/s. Dark red–colored coronary flow was visualized at distal LAD, and flow velocity was 20 cm/s. Coronary flow velocity reserve (CFVR) of the distal LAD and the posterior descending coronary artery (PD) were 1.71 and 1.84, respectively, suggesting significant stenosis of both the LAD and right coronary artery (RCA). Coronary angiography showed intermediate stenosis of both the RCA and LAD. *APV,* Average peak diastolic velocity. (See Video 48.3.)

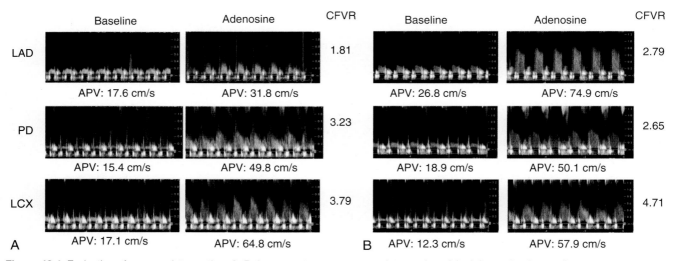

Figure 48.4. Evaluation of coronary intervention. **A,** Before percutaneous coronary intervention of the left anterior descending coronary artery (LAD), coronary flow velocity reserve (CFVR) in the LAD was 1.81. **B,** After the intervention, CFVR in the LAD was improved to 2.79. *APV,* Average peak diastolic velocity; *LCX,* left circumflex coronary artery; *PD,* posterior descending coronary artery.

proceed with percutaneous coronary intervention in patients who have intermediate coronary stenosis.[14] It is also useful to evaluate the therapeutic efficacy of coronary intervention, especially in the LAD (Fig.48.4). Not only epicardial coronary artery stenosis but also microvascular status may cause impaired CFVR. Thus, CFVR below 2.0 does not always guarantee significant epicardial coronary stenosis. Enhanced CFV at rest may produce CFVR of less than 2.0 in patients with left ventricular hypertrophy, although there

is no significant coronary stenosis (Fig. 48.5). However, impaired CFVR is associated with poor future outcomes.

Several studies verified the prognostic usefulness of CFVR measurements in patients with acute myocardial infarction, known or suspected coronary artery disease, and epicardial stenosis with intermediate severity.[15–18] In the cardiac catheterization laboratory, both fractional flow reserve (FFR) using a pressure wire and CVFR using a flow wire can be applied for the evaluation of the functional

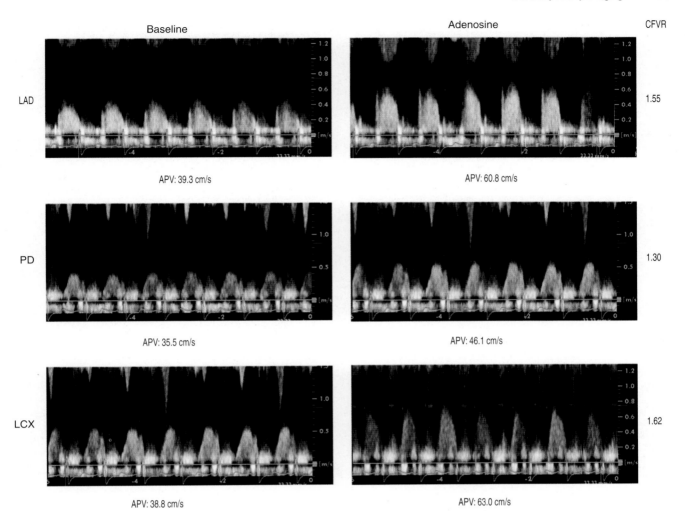

Figure 48.5. Coronary flow velocity reserve (CFVR) measurements in a patient with hypertrophic cardiomyopathy. CFVR in all three major coronary arteries was impaired. Note the high baseline coronary flow velocity in all three arteries. *APV,* Average peak diastolic velocity; *LAD,* left anterior descending coronary artery; *LCX,* left circumflex coronary artery; *PD,* posterior descending coronary artery.

significance of coronary stenosis and subsequent therapeutic management. Although concordant abnormal results of FFR and CFVR mean functionally significant coronary stenosis, and thus coronary intervention should be performed, discordant results of FFR and CFVR are observed in 30% to 40% of coronary stenosis cases. Van de Hoef and colleagues[19] performed both invasive FFR and CFVR measurements in 157 patients with intermediate coronary stenosis in whom coronary intervention was deferred. The authors found that patients who had a normal FFR but impaired CFVR, indicating predominant microvascular disease, were associated with worse prognosis than patients who had an abnormal FFR but normal CFVR, indicating predominant focal but no flow-limiting epicardial coronary stenosis. These results reinforce that coronary flow assessment is the main component of the evaluation of the functional consequences of ischemic heart disease. The finding also supports the impairment of CFVR in nonischemic dilated cardiomyopathy, and hypertrophic cardiomyopathy is a sign for poor outcome.[20]

CONCLUSIONS

CFVR is a simple and reliable method to evaluate the functional significance of coronary artery stenosis. The routine adoption of coronary artery imaging provides useful information regarding significant stenosis, even at rest in some patients.

REFERENCES

1. Iliceto S, Marangelli V, Memmola C, Rizzon P. Transesophageal Doppler echocardiography evaluation of coronary blood flow velocity in baseline conditions and during dipyridamole-induced coronary vasodilation. *Circulation.* 1991;83:61–69.
2. Hozumi T, Yoshida K, Ogata Y, et al. Noninvasive assessment of significant left anterior descending coronary artery stenosis by coronary flow velocity reserve with transthoracic color Doppler echocardiography. *Circulation.* 1998;97:1557–1562.
3. Caiati C, Montaldo C, Zedda N, et al. New noninvasive method for coronary flow reserve assessment contrast-enhanced transthoracic second harmonic echo Doppler. *Circulation.* 1999;99:771–778.
4. Hozumi T, Yoshida K, Akasaka T, et al. Value of acceleration flow and the pre-stenotic to stenotic coronary flow velocity ratio by transthoracic color Doppler echocardiography in noninvasive diagnosis of restenosis after percutaneous transluminal coronary angioplasty. *J Am Coll Cardiol.* 2000;35:164–168.
5. Hyodo E, Hirata K, Hirose M, et al. Detection of restenosis after percutaneous coronary intervention in three major coronary arteries by transthoracic Doppler echocardiography. *J Am Soc Echocardiogr.* 2010;23:553–559.
6. Meimoun P, Tribouilloy C. Non-invasive assessment of coronary flow and coronary flow reserve by transthoracic Doppler echocardiography: a magic tool for the real world. *Eur J Echocardiogr.* 2008;9:449–457.
7. Takeuchi M, Nakazono A. Coronary artery imaging with transthoracic Doppler echocardiography. *Curr Cardiol Rep.* 2016;18. 63.
8. Okayama H, Nishimura K, Saito M, et al. Significance of the distal to proximal coronary flow velocity ratio by transthoracic Doppler echocardiography for diagnosis of proximal left coronary artery stenosis, J Am Soc Echocardiogr 21:756–760.
9. Nishimura K, Okayama H, Inoue K, et al. Usefulness of the MOSAIC (measurement of stenosis by aliasing coronary flow) method using transthoracic color Doppler echocardiography in unstable angina patients. *Int J Cardiol.* 2011;151:170–174.

10. Takeuchi M, Ogawa K, Wake R, et al. Measurement of coronary flow velocity reserve in the posterior descending coronary artery by contrast-enhanced transthoracic Doppler echocardiography. *J Am Soc Echocardiogr.* 2003;17:21–27.

11. Zagatina A, Zhuravskaya N. The additive prognostic value of coronary flow velocity reserve during exercise echocardiography. *Eur Heart J Cardiovasc Imaging.* 2017;18:1179–1184.

12. Takeuchi M, Miyazaki C, Yoshitani H, et al. Assessment of coronary flow velocity with transthoracic Doppler echocardiography during dobutamine stress echocardiography. *J Am Coll Cardiol.* 2001;38:117–123.

13. Nohtomi Y, Takeuchi M, Nagasawa K, et al. Simultaneous assessment of wall motion and coronary flow velocity in the left anterior descending coronary artery during dipyridamole stress echocardiography. *J Am Soc Echocardiogr.* 2003;16:457–463.

14. Meimoun P, Benali T, Sayah S, et al. Evaluation of left anterior descending coronary artery stenosis of intermediate severity using transthoracic coronary flow reserve and dobutamine stress echocardiography. *J Am Soc Echocardiogr.* 2005;18:1233–1240.

15. Meimoun P, Benali T, Elmkies F, et al. Prognostic value of transthoracic coronary flow reserve in medically treated patients with proximal left anterior descending artery stenosis of intermediate severity. *Eur J Echocardiogr.* 2009;10:127–132.

16. Cortigiani L, Rigo F, Gherardi S, et al. Coronary flow reserve during dipyridamole stress echocardiography predicts mortality. *J Am Coll Cardiol Img.* 2012;5:1079–1085.

17. Lowenstein JA, Caniggia C, Rousse G, et al. Coronary flow velocity reserve during pharmacologic stress echocardiography with normal contractility adds important prognostic value in diabetic and nondiabetic patients. *J Am Soc Echocardiogr.* 2014;27:1113–1119.

18. Prastaro M, Pirozzi E, Gaibazzi N, et al. Expert review on the prognostic role of echocardiography after acute myocardial infarction. *J Am Soc Echocardiogr.* 2017;30:431–443. e2.

19. van de Hoef TP, van Lavieren MA, Damman P, et al. Physiological basis and long-term clinical outcome of discordance between fractional flow reserve and coronary flow velocity reserve in coronary stenoses of intermediate severity. *Circ Cardiovasc Interv.* 2014;7:301–311.

20. Tower-Rader A, Betancor J, Lever HM, Desai MY: A Comprehensive review of stress testing in hypertrophic cardiomyopathy: assessment of functional capacity, identification of prognostic indicators, and detection of coronary artery disease. *J Am Soc Echocardiogr.* 30:829–844.

49

Effects of Exercise, Pharmacologic Stress, and Pacing on the Cardiovascular System

Wojciech Kosmala, Thomas H. Marwick

The responses of the cardiovascular system to different stressors are not homogenous and vary depending on the nature of the effect sought. Although laboratories typically have expertise with one or two approaches, it is desirable to have experience with multiple stressors because not a single one suits all clinical scenarios.

HEMODYNAMIC EFFECTS

The hemodynamic effects of treadmill or bicycle exercise include an increase in heart rate (chiefly caused by sympathetic activation and partly by parasympathetic withdrawal), increase in inotropic state, increase in systolic blood pressure, decrease in systemic vascular resistance (SVR), and increased venous return (caused by sympathetic vasoconstriction of the large-capacitance veins and the pumping effect of skeletal muscles), contributing via the Frank-Starling mechanism to an increase in stroke volume.[1] Treadmill exercise permits the achievement of higher oxygen consumption than bicycle exercise. The increment of blood pressure with exertion is mainly caused by an increase in cardiac output, which outweighs the decline in peripheral resistance. The opposite changes in after- and preload are seen with isometric (handgrip) exercise, that is, SVR increases, and venous return decreases (Table 49.1).[2]

The major effects of dobutamine are mediated by β_1 adrenergic receptors. At low doses, an enhancement in myocardial contractility without tachycardia is a predominant response. At doses above 20 mcg/kg/min, there is an increase in systolic blood pressure to about 170 mm Hg (i.e., by 30–40 mm Hg) and in heart rate to about 120 beats/min (i.e., by 40–50 beats/min).[3] A decrease in blood pressure at higher doses is common, most commonly caused by the vasodilating effect of dobutamine reflecting the stimulation of β_2 adrenergic receptors. Bradycardia is less common and reflects a reflex response to blood pressure elevation or the activation of mechanoreceptors caused by myocardial hypercontractility.

The most commonly used coronary vasodilators—dipyridamole, adenosine, and regadenoson—involve the same metabolic pathway, either increasing endogenous adenosine levels (dipyridamole) or directly acting on the vasculature (exogenous adenosine or regadenoson, an A2A adenosine receptor agonist).[4] All these agents produce a small decrease in blood pressure and modest tachycardia with a minor increase in myocardial function.

Pacing represents an alternative method to increase cardiac work by the induction of tachycardia, usually of 160 beats/min. Atrial stimulation (either transvenously or by transesophageal approach) is a preferable technique because asynchronous regional contractility from ventricular pacing provides interpretive challenges. Tachycardia attained with pacing is accompanied by stable blood pressure and unchanged loading, and a major advantage of this modality is a better hemodynamic control than with other stressors.[5] The disadvantage is that the lack of a suitable blood pressure response leads to only a modest increment of the rate-pressure product.

Ergonovine stress testing is thought to be the gold standard for diagnosis of coronary artery spasm. This drug exerts coronary vasoconstricting effects by agonizing β-adrenergic, dopaminergic, and serotonin receptors. The high sensitivity of this modality, even in patients with single-vessel spasm, can be explained by the transmural nature of vasospastic ischemia leading to severe wall motion abnormalities.[6]

MECHANISMS OF ISCHEMIA

Exercise, dobutamine, and pacing can induce myocardial ischemia by an increase in cardiac work and oxygen demand exceeding the limited blood supply resulting from significant coronary stenosis. Additional mechanisms responsible for ischemia include coronary flow maldistribution with a reduction of subendocardial perfusion because of adenosine accumulation in the myocardial tissue during stress[5,7] and the "oxygen-wasting" effect evidenced for dobutamine.[8]

The use of vasoactive stressors is based in part on the development of perfusion heterogeneity. The generation of maximal vasodilation causes flow heterogeneity because the hyperemic response is limited in the territory supplied by a coronary stenosis. More controversially, it has been thought to provoke ischemia through coronary steal, implying that overperfusion of myocardial regions supplied by normal coronary arteries is at the cost of the heart muscle fed by the stenotic vessel (the so-called "reverse Robin Hood effect").[7,9] In "horizontal steal," vasodilation of distal arteriolar beds of nonstenosed coronary artery causes a decrease in perfusion pressure in the collateral circulation to the stenosed territory. In "vertical steal," the vasodilator-induced depressurization of the microcirculation in the territory of the stenotic artery produces a collapse of subendocardial vessels caused by higher extravascular pressure in this layer with a subsequent flow maldistribution favoring the subepicardium. Another contribution to the ischemic effect of vasodilators is increased oxygen demand from a reflex tachycardia in response to the decrease in blood pressure[7] or administration of atropine.

LEFT VENTRICULAR RESPONSE TO STRESS

The normal response elicited by inotropic stress includes an increase in endocardial systolic movement, systolic wall thickening, and velocity of contraction. The typical effect of dobutamine infusion is a reduction in end-diastolic and end-systolic volumes and a rise in cardiac output with a larger contribution to this from elevated heart rate than stroke volume.[10] Increased inotropic state together with the substantial decrease in loading may cause left ventricular (LV) cavity obliteration, which is a potential reason of false-negative responses, caused by reduced transmural wall stress, as well as smaller areas where wall motion abnormalities can be identified.[11]

TABLE 49.1 Physiological Responses to Different Kinds of Stressors

	Inotropic State	Heart Rate	Blood Pressure	Systemic Vascular Resistance	Venous Return
Isometric exercise (handgrip)	↑–↑↑	↑–↑↑	↑↑↑	↑	↓[a]
Supine bicycle exercise	↑↑	↑↑↑	↑↑↑	↓	↑↑↑
Upright exercise	↑↑	↑↑↑	↑↑↑	↓	↑
Dobutamine	↑↑↑	↑↑	↑–↑↑	↓↓	↓
Vasodilators	↑	↑	↓	↓↓↓	↓↓
Pacing (atrial)	0	↑↑↑	0	0	0

[a]Caused by to the Valsalva maneuver.

TABLE 49.2 Left Ventricular Response to Pharmacologic Stress With Dobutamine or Vasodilators

Diagnosis	Function at Rest	Low Dose	High Dose
Normal	Normal	Normal	Hyperkinetic (mildly with vasodilators)
Ischemic	Normal	Normal (unless severe CAD)	Reduction vs rest Reduction vs other segments Delayed contraction
Viable, patent IRA (stunning)	Hypo/akinetic	Improvement	Sustained improvement
Viable, stenosed IRA (hibernation)	Hypo/akinetic	Improvement	Reduction (vs low dose)
Infarction	A/dyskinetic	No change	No change

CAD, Coronary artery disease; *IRA,* infarct-related artery.

The decrement of regional myocardial function, both systolic excursion and wall thickening, from the resting level or after an initial augmentation of contractility represents a key marker of ischemia. The phase of transient enhancement of function is particularly important for recognition of ischemia in akinetic or dyskinetic segments, which despite their poor functional status may still include some ischemic or viable tissue. A deterioration of performance without antecedent improvement may reflect increased loading rather than ischemia.

LV cavity dilation and a decrease in ejection fraction during stress strongly suggests multivessel or left main coronary artery disease. However, these findings are much less common with pharmacologic than exercise testing, possibly because of the reduction of loading.[10] According to some observations, an abnormal end-diastolic volume response during dobutamine infusion implying severe coronary artery disease should be defined as a decrease less than 15%.[12]

Myocardium that is dysfunctional at rest, which improves in response to low-dose dobutamine (<20 mcg/kg/min) or dipyridamole (0.28–0.56 mg/kg), is considered to be viable. With dobutamine stress, the mechanism is clearly associated with adrenergic effects on contractility. However, the mechanisms behind the contractile response to dipyridamole are less obvious and possibly include sympathetic activation or systemic vasodilation causing a "local Frank-Starling effect" whereby the expansion of myocardial blood volume leads to increased tension of the myofibrils.[7]

In the presence of a patent infarct-related artery, the augmentation of function is sustained even if workload and oxygen demand increase. Generally, this is understood to signify the presence of stunned myocardium, although nontransmural infarction can also provide this "uniphasic" response. As a consequence, this is not specific for functional recovery. Initial improvement at low heart rates followed by a deterioration of regional function, as tachycardia becomes more evident and induces ischemia, is typical for viable tissue supplied by a stenosed infarct-related artery, representing hibernating myocardium.[13] However, if the region is nourished by a critically narrowed artery, the stage of conspicuous improvement may not appear because of a very early advent of ischemia. The biphasic response is strongly predictive of functional recovery after revascularization, which is an argument for proceeding to maximal stress whenever possible (Table 49.2).[13] However, it should be emphasized that the presence of severe LV dysfunction and extensive coronary artery disease necessitates a more cautious approach and early termination of the test.

COMPARISONS OF STRESSORS

Dissimilarities in hemodynamic effects of inotropic stressors account for the greater workload and, consequently, more extensive ischemia imposed by exercise than dobutamine. The rate-pressure product is higher with exercise (>25,000) than with dobutamine (~20,000) or pacing (<20,000).[1,14] The potency of exercise or dobutamine in inducing myocardial ischemia (and as a result, their diagnostic sensitivity) depends on the target heart rate, with maximal stress providing better reliability than submaximal testing.[1,14] β-Blockade may diminish the chronotropic response to dobutamine and decrease the double product to around 14,000, but this may be circumvented by the administration of atropine.[15] The combined use of dobutamine and atropine also avoids the heart rate–depressant effect of vagal activation occurring in response to hypertensive reaction or cardiac mechanoreceptor stimulation. The addition of atropine to vasodilator stress increases heart rate and myocardial oxygen demand, thereby improving diagnostic sensitivity.[16]

HYPERTENSIVE RESPONSE TO STRESS

An exaggerated systolic blood pressure response to greater than 200 mm Hg is frequent, particularly in hypertensive patients. The higher workload and greater ischemic burden caused by increased wall stress[1] may facilitate the identification of coronary artery disease. However, the scenario poses problems for specificity because global or regional (especially apical) disturbances may be caused from increased afterload.

STRESS ECHOCARDIOGRAPHY FOR NONCORONARY INDICATIONS
Mitral Regurgitation

Exercise stress echocardiography (SE) in mitral regurgitation (MR) may be helpful in the identification of patients suitable for surgical treatment. Echocardiographic findings, including increase in the extent of regurgitant jet, prominent elevation of pulmonary artery pressure, and the absence of contractile reserve, may indicate a need for intervention. This is especially relevant in case of ischemic MR, which changes dynamically according to alterations in loading conditions and inotropic state.

Supine bicycle exercise appears to be the most appropriate method to evaluate MR during stress. The hemodynamic profile of this approach, characterized by a large venous return and a moderate fall in systemic vascular resistance, contributes to unmasking the true severity of MR.[17] Compared with exercise, stress with dobutamine is not associated with an exacerbation of MR because of a more pronounced inotropic effect reducing the regurgitant orifice, greater increase in afterload, and decrease in preload produced by dobutamine, and therefore is not recommended for MR assessment.[2] Isometric exercise causes an increase in systemic resistance, but because of the Valsalva effect, it also causes a decrease in preload. Upright exercise moderately decreases venous return and is believed to have an intermediate usefulness in the verification of MR severity.[2]

Aortic Stenosis

Low-dose dobutamine echocardiography may help distinguish truly severe (low flow, low gradient) aortic stenosis (AS) from pseudo-severe stenosis in patients with a decreased LV systolic function (LV ejection fraction<50%, stroke volume index <35 mL/m[2], mean gradient <40 mm Hg, and valve area <1 cm[2]). This setting may be indicative of either severe AS with a "poor" left ventricle incapable of generating adequate force to develop higher gradients or nonsevere AS with a small valve area because of the inability of the cusps to fully open at insufficiently elevated intra-LV pressure.[18] Dobutamine-induced increase in transvalvular pressure gradient with a relatively unchanged aortic valve area indicates severe disease, whereas improvement in valve area without a significant increase in the aortic gradient indicates pseudo-severe AS. Another diagnostic benefit of stress with dobutamine is the evaluation of contractility reserve, defined as an increase in stroke volume above 20%, which provides prognostically relevant information.[19] The use of dobutamine SE in paradoxical low-flow gradient AS (reduced LV stroke volume despite preserved ejection fraction) is controversial and not uniformly recommended.[18,20] The coexistence of LV low-volume state and restrictive filling in this subset may result in failure of the LV to increase the transvalvular aortic flow and inconclusive results of the test. Besides, the infusion of dobutamine may further exacerbate disturbed LV filling, leading to cardiac decompensation.

Prosthetic Valves

In patients with prosthetic valve stenosis or patient–prosthesis mismatch (PPM), the exercise- or dobutamine-induced augmentation of blood flow results in a sizeable increase in the transvalvular gradient (>20 mm Hg for aortic and >10 mm Hg for mitral prostheses), usually paralleled by a significant elevation of pulmonary artery pressure (systolic values >60 mm Hg).[20,21] Provided that LV contractile reserve is preserved, low-dose dobutamine SE may aid in differentiating true from pseudo-severe prosthetic valve stenosis or PPM in the aortic position in participants with low LV stroke volume. In this subset, the transprosthetic flow rate at rest and, consequently, the forces exerted on the leaflets may be too low to ensure a complete valve opening. A substantial increase in valve effective orifice area (EOA) during dobutamine infusion in the absence or only a slight increase in the transvalvular gradient indicate pseudo-stenosis. Conversely, both PPM and true stenosis are characterized by a large elevation of transprosthetic gradients with a relatively unchanged EOA. Further differentiation can be accomplished by comparing calculated stress EOA with the normal reference values: a considerably smaller orifice area than that given by the manufacturer suggests true prosthesis dysfunction.[20,21]

Hypertrophic Cardiomyopathy

Exercise SE can be performed in patients with hypertrophic cardiomyopathy to evaluate inducible LV outflow tract obstruction (LVOTO), LV systolic and diastolic reserve, blood pressure response to exertion, and worsening of MR, all of which are recognized to impact the clinical risk.[22,23] The principal pathophysiological mechanism for LVOTO is systolic anterior motion of the mitral valve leaflets (SAM) that can be potentiated or unmasked by decreased LV preload and increased LV contractility. For this reason, some sites prefer upright stress (e.g., upright bike or treadmill) to amplify the effect of reduced preload. Postexertional standing gradients[20] and a delayed Doppler assessment (based on the decline in LV afterload with ongoing vasodilation during the recovery period) are two other steps that can be of value if the postexercise gradient is less than the clinically meaningful threshold of 50 mm Hg. Pharmacologic stress with dobutamine is not recommended as

a diagnostic option for LVOT gradients in hypertrophic cardiomyopathy because it can provoke LVOTO in a nonphysiological way irrespective of the underlying disease.

Nonischemic Cardiomyopathy

The assessment of LV contractile reserve by dobutamine or exercise SE can be helpful to identify the preclinical stage of myocardial impairment (e.g., early chemotherapy-induced cardiotoxicity, hypertensive or diabetic cardiomyopathy) and to obtain relevant prognostic information in the overt stage.[20] The sympathetic dysregulation with a decreased density of β-adrenergic receptors in advanced disease may require higher doses of dobutamine to invoke a contractile response, but this may be at the cost of increased arrhythmic risk.

Diastolic Dysfunction

Myocardial relaxation abnormalities provoked by ischemia may be demonstrated during each kind of stress, but measurements are more feasible using modalities with low heart rates, such as dipyridamole or pacing (after termination of stress). Alterations in diastolic function in response to stress are not specific for ischemia and may appear on account of LV hypertrophy or myocardial fibrosis. The major effect of increased myocardial and vascular stiffness on cardiovascular functioning is an exertional increase in LV filling pressure, accompanied by dyspnea. Apart from this passive component, other factors, such as impaired myocardial relaxation and LV untwisting, both affecting active LV pressure decay during early diastole, may also contribute to reduced exercise capacity.[24] The objective of diastolic exercise SE is to exacerbate these mechanisms and unmask the underlying diastolic abnormalities. Accordingly, diastolic exercise SE has been primarily dedicated to detecting impaired LV diastolic function reserve and the resulting rise in LV filling pressure; however, the use of echocardiography in the diagnostic protocol permits also the assessment of LV systolic reserve impairment, provoked LVOTO, or dynamic MR—other potential contributors to exercise intolerance.[20,25] The essential measures of diastolic exercise SE—an exertional increase in E/e′ ratio and tricuspid regurgitant velocity (TRV)—have been shown to correlate with invasively measured LV diastolic pressures. However, this is a screening test, and false-positive results have been reported.[26]

In patients unable to exercise, an alternative approach might be passive leg raise increasing venous return, which has been demonstrated to induce LV filling pressure changes analogous to exercise.[27] Another currently explored diastolic stress testis isometric handgrip echocardiography. This modality evokes an increase in E/e′ ratio comparable to dynamic exercise, although the mechanisms behind these alterations are different. Whereas in dynamic exercise, the rise in E/e′ is driven mainly by the increment in E velocity, the major reason for the stress-induced elevation of E/e′ in handgrip is the exacerbation of myocardial relaxation, as expressed by a decrease in e′.[28] The utility of pharmacologic stressors in diastolic SE remains to be established.

Pulmonary Hypertension

SE plays a role in the assessment of patients with suspected or known pulmonary hypertension (PH). Stress-induced elevation of pulmonary artery pressure and development of right ventricular (RV) dysfunction have been demonstrated to presage a poorer prognosis.[29] The preferred modality is supine exercise or, in individuals at risk for PH or high-altitude pulmonary edema, a hypoxic challenge, including the administration of a gas mixture with reduced oxygen content, triggering pulmonary artery vasoconstriction in susceptible participants.[30]

The responses of pulmonary artery pressure to exercise in normal individuals are variable, although the increase in TRV greater than 3.1 m/s usually suggests pathology, except for highly trained athletes and older persons, who may exhibit higher exertional pulmonary artery pressure in the absence of disease. The ability of RV contractility to augment to cope with increasing loading is usually impaired in patients with PH.[20] The assessment of stress-induced changes in pulmonary artery pressure, RV function, and pulmonary vascular resistance is of value in high-risk patients screened for PH. On the other hand, the clinical usefulness of SE in patients with an established diagnosis of PH is less clear, with the most relevant aspect of evaluation being RV contractile reserve.

CONCLUSIONS

The agents used for SE provide a spectrum of physiologic effects. Careful selection permits the stressor to be individualized to the clinical situation and the use of various imaging tools to examine not only wall motion but also hemodynamics, myocardial function, coronary flow, and perfusion further extend SE to new fields.

REFERENCES

1. Rallidis L, Cokkinos P, Tousoulis D, et al. Comparison of dobutamine and tread-mill exercise echocardiography in inducing ischemia in patients with coronary artery disease. *J Am Coll Cardiol.* 1997;30:1660–1668.
2. Peteiro J, Freire E, Monserrat L, et al. The effect of exercise on ischemic mitral regurgitation. *Chest.* 1998;114:1075–1082.
3. Marwick T, D'Hondt AM, Baudhuin T, et al. Optimal use of dobutamine stress for the detection and evaluation of coronary artery disease: combination with echocardiography or scintigraphy, or both? *J Am Coll Cardiol.* 1993;22:159–167.
4. Picano E, Lattanzi F. Dipyridamole echocardiography. A new diagnostic window on coronary artery disease. *Circulation.* 1991;83:III19–III26.
5. Becker L. Effect of tachycardia on left ventricular blood flow distribution during coronary occlusion. *Am J Physiol.* 1976;230:1072–1077.
6. Song JK, Picano E. Ergonovine stress echocardiography for the diagnosis of vasospastic angina. In: Picano E, ed. *Stress Echocardiography.* Berlin Heidelberg: Springer-Verlag; 2009:229–239.
7. Picano E. Stress echocardiography: from pathophysiological toy to diagnostic tool. *Circulation.* 1992;85:1604–1612.
8. Mairesse GH, Vanoverschelde JL, Robert A, et al. Pathophysiologic mechanisms underlying dobutamine-induced myocardial ischemia. *Am Heart J.* 1998;136:63–70.
9. Bin JP, Le E, Pelberg RA, et al. Mechanism of inducible regional dysfunction during dipyridamole stress. *Circulation.* 2002;106:112–117.
10. Attenhoffer CH, Pellikka PA, Oh JK, et al. Comparison of ischemic response during exercise and dobutamine echocardiography in patients with left main coronary artery disease. *J Am Coll Cardiol.* 1996;27:1171–1177.
11. Yuda S, Khoury V, Marwick TH. Influence of wall stress and left ventricular geometry on the accuracy of dobutamine stress echocardiography. *J Am Coll Cardiol.* 2002;40:1311–1319.
12. Perez JE, Waggoner AD, Davila-Roman VG, et al. On-line quantification of ventricular function during dobutamine stress echocardiography. *Eur Heart J.* 1992;13:1669–1676.
13. Afridi I, Kleiman NS, Raizner AE, et al. Dobutamine echocardiography in myocardial hibernation: optimal dose and accuracy in predicting recovery of ventricular function after coronary angioplasty. *Circulation.* 1995;91:663–670.
14. Marwick TH, D'Hondt AM, Mairesse GH, et al. Comparative ability of dobutamine and exercise stress in inducing myocardial ischaemia in active patients. *Br Heart J.* 1994;72:31–38.
15. Chen L, Ma L, de Prada VA, et al. Effects of beta-blockade and atropine on ischemic responses in left ventricular regions subtending coronary stenosis during dobutamine stress echocardiography. *J Am Coll Cardiol.* 1996;28:1866–1876.
16. Picano E, Pingitore A, Conti U, et al. Enhanced sensitivity for detection of coronary artery disease by addition of atropine to dipyridamole echocardiography. *Eur Heart J.* 1993;14:1216–1222.
17. Peteiro J, Monserrat L, Piñón P, et al: value of resting and exercise mitral regurgitation during exercise echocardiography to predict outcome in patients with left ventricular dysfunction, Rev Esp Cardiol 60:234–243.
18. Baumgartner H, Hung J, Bermejo J, et al. Recommendations on the echocardiographic assessment of aortic valve stenosis. *J Am Soc Echocardiogr.* 2017;30:372–392.
19. Levy F, Laurent M, Monin JL, et al. Aortic valve replacement for low-flow/low-gradient aortic stenosis operative risk stratification and long-term outcome: a European multicenter study. *J Am Coll Cardiol.* 2008;51:1466–1472.
20. Lancellotti P, Pellikka PA, Budts W, et al. The clinical use of stress echocardiography in non-ischaemic heart disease. *J Am Soc Echocardiogr.* 2017;30:101–138.
21. Lancellotti P, Pibarot P, Chambers JB, et al. Recommendations for the imaging assessment of prosthetic heart valves. *Eur Heart J Cardiovasc Imag.* 2016;17:589–590.
22. Argulian E, Chaudhry FA. Stress testing in patients with hypertrophic cardiomyopathy. *Prog Cardiovasc Dis.* 2012;54:477–482.
23. Maron BJ, Ommen SR, Semsarian C, et al. Hypertrophic cardiomyopathy: present and future, with translation into contemporary cardiovascular medicine. *J Am Coll Cardiol.* 2014;64:83–99.
24. Samuel TJ, Beaudry R, Sarma S, et al. Diastolic stress testing along the heart failure continuum. *Curr Heart Fail Rep.* 2018;15:332–339.
25. Nagueh SF, Smiseth OA, Appleton CP, et al. Recommendations for the evaluation of left ventricular diastolic function by echocardiography. *J Am Soc Echocardiogr.* 2016;29:277–314.
26. Obokata M, Reddy YNV, Pislaru SV, et al. Evidence supporting the existence of a distinct obese phenotype of heart failure with preserved ejection fraction. *Circulation.* 2017;136:6–19.
27. Choi EY, Shim CY, Kim SA, et al. Passive leg-raise is helpful to identify impaired diastolic functional reserve during exercise in patients with abnormal myocardial relaxation. *J Am Soc Echocardiogr.* 2010;23:523–530.
28. Samuel TJ, Beaudry R, Haykowsky MJ, et al. Diastolic stress testing: similarities and differences between isometric handgrip and cycle echocardiography. *J Appl Physiol.* 2018;125:529–535.
29. Argiento P, Chester N, Mule M, et al. Exercise stress echocardiography for the study of the pulmonary circulation. *Eur Respir J.* 2010;35:1273–1278.
30. Grünig E, Mereles D, Hildebrandt W, et al. Stress Doppler echocardiography for identification of susceptibility to high altitude pulmonary edema. *J Am Coll Cardiol.* 2000;35:980–987.

50 Diagnostic Criteria and Accuracy

Eugenio Picano, Quirino Ciampi

The main sign of ischemia during stress echocardiography (SE) is the transient regional wall motion abnormality (RWMA)[1] caused by a flow-limiting coronary artery disease (CAD). RWMA can be provoked by exercise or pharmacologic stressors, either by increased myocardial oxygen demand or decreased subendocardial myocardial oxygen supply with vasodilators determining underperfusion through horizontal and vertical steal phenomena.[2,3] All main SE modalities (exercise, dobutamine, vasodilators) have comparable diagnostic accuracy for the diagnosis of obstructive CAD, with higher specificity and slightly lower sensitivity compared with methods based on perfusion changes, such as myocardial contrast echocardiography, stress cardiac magnetic resonance imaging (CMRI) with contrast, and myocardial perfusion scintigraphy.[4] Vasodilators have the same ischemic power than exercise

and dobutamine, when appropriately high doses (state of art since 20 years) are used (0.84 mg/kg in 6 min), in presence of vulnerable coronary anatomy (flow-limiting epicardial stenosis, complex-type plaques, coronary collateral circulation favoring horizontal steal phenomena).

The higher sensitivity of perfusion changes compared with RWMA is easily understood on the basis of the ischemic cascade (Fig. 50.1), an experimental paradigm established in myocardial ischemia caused by coronary occlusion or stress-induced ischemia with coronary stenosis. Regional perfusion abnormalities are the prerequisite and an earlier event than RWMA. However, in clinical practice, this reassuring one-size-fits-all model of classical ischemic cascade is challenged because of the frequent occurrence of microvascular angina. Patients with microvascular angina

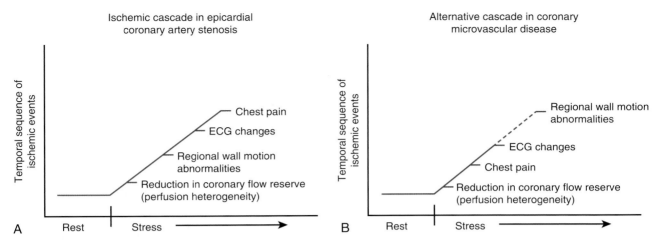

Ischemic cascade in epicardial coronary artery stenosis

Alternative cascade in coronary microvascular disease

Figure 50.1. The classic and the alternative ischemic cascades. **A,** The classic ischemic cascade, triggered by stress in presence of a flow-limiting coronary stenosis of epicardial arteries. The various markers are usually ranked according to a well-defined time sequence, with a reduction of coronary flow velocity reserve (or regional perfusion abnormalities) first followed by regional wall motion abnormalities (with impaired systolic thickening) and later appearance of ST-segment depression and chest pain. **B,** In the model of coronary microvascular disease characterized by a reduction in coronary flow reserve with normal epicardial arteries, anginal pain and ST-segment changes usually appear during stress in the absence of any detectable regional wall motion abnormality. *ECG,* Electrocardiogram.

typically have exercise-related angina, electrocardiographic (ECG) or perfusion evidence of exercise-related ischemia, and either no stenoses or mild stenoses (<50%) that are deemed functionally nonrelevant. Coronary microvascular dysfunction can be either primary (in cardiac syndrome X) or secondary to left ventricular (LV) hypertrophy (e.g., hypertrophic cardiomyopathy, aortic stenosis, and hypertensive heart disease).[5] In all these conditions, stress-induced RWMAs are the exception rather than the rule and occur in fewer than 10% of patients with perfusion changes, identifying a less favorable outcome.[6]

SE does not imply exposure to ionizing radiation associated with coronary computed tomography angiography and nuclear perfusion imaging.[7] The radiation risks are not negligible and are cumulative: exposure adds to exposure, dose to dose, and risk to risk during the lifetime.[8] This must be taken into account in the risk–benefit assessment, especially in more sensitive groups such as young individuals and women. Contraindications to contrast agents (iodine contrast for computed tomography angiography and gadolinium-based chelates for magnetic resonance), cost considerations, and environmental impact (100-fold lower for SE compared to CMRI) need also to be considered.[9] The increasing demand for SE activity posed by recent guidelines recommendations, cost considerations, growing concern about radiation exposure, and the expansion of indications and applications of SE well beyond CAD can be met by a laboratory performing a minimum of 100 studies per year, with availability of contrast agents for LV opacification, adequate knowledge of mechanisms of action and rate of complications of different physical and pharmacologic stresses, and resuscitation facilities readily available.[10] SE is a part of the core curriculum in cardiology, ultrasound machines are ubiquitously available, and the technique is used by cardiologists living an imaging experience, not by radiologists living a cardiology experience.

THE MAIN SIGN OF ISCHEMIA: REGIONAL WALL MOTION ABNORMALITIES

The response of LV function to ischemia is monotonous and independent of the stress used. Normal myocardium shows systolic thickening and endocardial movement toward the center of the cavity. The normal hyperkinetic response during stress indicates an increase in normal movement and thickening. The hallmark of transient, stress-induced myocardial ischemia is the RWMA, in its three degrees of increasing severity: hypokinesia

(decreased systolic thickening), akinesia (absent or negligible thickening), and dyskinesia (stretching). The severity of RWMA mirrors the severity of the regional subendocardial hypoperfusion. A reduction in subendocardial blood flow of about 20% produces a 20% decrease of wall thickening; a 50% reduction in subendocardial blood flow decreases regional wall thickening by about 40%, and when subendocardial blood flow is reduced by 80%, akinesia occurs. Dyskinesia appears when the flow deficit is extended to the subepicardial layer and ischemia is transmural.[11]

The 17- or 16-segments model of the left ventricle represents the anatomical background for rapid (real-time) semiquantitative assessment of wall motion (from 1 = normal, to 4 = dyskinesis). The difference between rest and stress wall motion score index provides a simple assessment of the induced ischemia, combining the horizontal extent (the number of involved segments) with the vertical depth of ischemia (the severity of abnormality of each segment, from hypo- to dyskinesia). Definition of risk is important because patients at high risk benefit from revascularization with better survival and amelioration of symptoms. High risk is defined as a cardiac mortality rate greater than 3% per year, and low risk as a cardiac mortality rate less than 1% per year. The high risk is defined as stress-induced RWMA (hypokinesia, akinesia, or dyskinesia) is 3 or more segments out of 16.[1] The low risk is defined by absence of RWMA during stress. The degree of RWMA also predicts the placebo-controlled symptomatic benefit after myocardial revascularization. The greater the downstream SE abnormality caused by the stenosis, the greater the reduction in symptoms after percutaneous coronary intervention.[12]

STRESS ECHOCARDIOGRAPHY IN FOUR EQUATIONS

Four diagnostic equations centered on RWMA describe the main SE response patterns: normal, ischemic, viable, and necrotic (Table 50.1). A normal response shows a normal-hyperkinetic, synchronous wall motion with reduced ventricular volumes at peak stress (Fig. 50.2 and Video 50.2). An abnormal response shows a RWMA of territories fed by a stenotic coronary artery (Fig. 50.3 and Video 50.3). A viable response is an akinetic segment becoming normokinetic. A necrotic or scar response is an akinetic segment with a fixed response during stress. The biphasic response is a combination of viable and ischemic responses and corresponds to a viable response at low doses (akinesia becoming normokinesia) followed by ischemic response at high doses (normokinesia becoming hypo-, a- or dyskinesia).

DIAGNOSTIC RESULTS AND ACCURACY

The diagnostic accuracy for noninvasive diagnosis of CAD is similar to other imaging functional testing techniques, with an excellent specificity (~90%) and good sensitivity (~80%) for obstructive epicardial CAD. In individual studies, the reported accuracy vary widely, as can be expected because of the many factors modulating the capability of any stress to increase diagnostic sensitivity (and, symmetrically, to reduce specificity). Higher sensitivity is observed in patients with extensive (multivessel), severe (≥90% diameter reduction) disease involving the left anterior descending artery, with complex-type morphology, compared with patients with limited (single-vessel) disease of intermediate (50%–80% diameter reduction) severity and simple-type morphology located in left circumflex or right coronary artery disease. Higher values of sensitivity balanced by a drop-off in specificity can be achieved with the assessment of myocardial perfusion by contrast SE[13] or coronary flow velocity reserve in the left anterior descending artery,[14] allowing the detection of a lower-grade coronary atherosclerosis or coronary microvascular dysfunction not linked with ischemia that go undetected with wall motion abnormalities and still contribute to prognostic vulnerability.[15]

SE data can be usefully combined with a carotid scan to rule out anatomic carotid disease[16] and with resting transthoracic echocardiography to assess cardiac calcification, based on calcification of mitral annulus, aortic valve leaflets, and ascending aorta. Both carotid disease and inappropriate cardiac calcification are markers of subclinical atherosclerosis, a predictor of subsequent events, and allow a refined risk stratification based on

SE.[17] Conceptually, cardiac calcification has a similar meaning than coronary calcification detected by with the Agatston score, and carotid scan has the same value of coronary stenosis detected by computed tomography angiography. They assess atherosclerotic disease at a prehemodynamic, and usually preclinical, stage, allowing early and aggressive intervention on risk factors with lifestyle changes and medical therapy. In the echocardiography laboratory, the detection of cardiac calcification of carotid plaque (or increased intima-media thickness) allows to image atherosclerotic disease at a very early stage, decades before the coronary flow-limiting plaque that determines stress-induced RWMA during SE.

FALSE-NEGATIVE RESULTS

Despite high diagnostic accuracy of SE in predicting obstructive epicardial CAD, anatomically significant CAD can be present in the absence of inducible RWMA ("false-negative response"), and stress-induced RWMA may occur in the absence of significant CAD ("false-positive response"). A SE false-negative result may occur for patient-, stress-, angiography-, myocardium-, reader-, and image-related reasons (Table 50.2). False-negative results with maximal tests performed off therapy are associated with good prognosis, almost comparable to true negative results.[3] Antianginal therapy with β-blockers, calcium antagonists, and nitrates lowers the sensitivity of SE and prevents stress-induced RWMA with all forms of testing. The outcome associated with a negative test result performed under anti-ischemic medical therapy is less benign than a negative test result off therapy.[3] Submaximal stresses do not test the coronary circulation efficiently, and an alternative choice test (e.g., pharmacologic after a nondiagnostic exercise test) should be used to have a diagnostic maximal result. It is more important for the patient to have a diagnostic maximal stress rather than which stress is used. Not all coronary stenoses were created equal, and when a maximal stress is administered, patients with a negative SE response more often show lesions of intermediate severity (50%–80% diameter reduction) and with preserved fractional flow reserve or coronary flow reserve, indicating that the hemodynamic severity of the lesion is more important than its anatomic severity in determining stress-induced RWMA. Conservative underreading can be a cause of low sensitivity. In some cases, true ischemia occurs but may go undetected by SE, especially in less well-imaged segments, such as the inferior or lateral walls, because of the inherent limitations of subjective analysis and lack of quantitative criteria or images of borderline quality during stress. Contrast echocardiography can be

TABLE 50.1 Stress Echocardiography in Four Patterns

Rest	Stress	Diagnosis
Normokinesis (score 1)	Normo- or hyperkinesis (score 1)	Normal
Normokinesis (score 1)	Hypo-, a-, or dyskinesis (score ≥2)	Ischemia
Akinesis (score 3)	Hypo- or normokinesis (score 1 or 2)	Viable
A- or dyskinesis (score 3 or 4)	A- or dyskinesis (score 3 or 4)	Necrosis

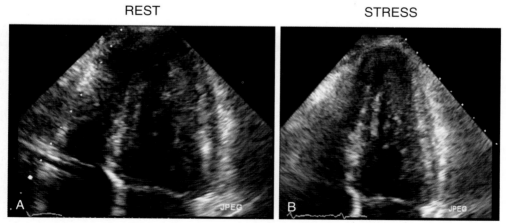

REST   STRESS

Figure 50.2. Stress echocardiogram: normal response. A normal wall thickening at rest (**A**) with hyperkinetic wall motion and reduced left ventricular cavity during stress (**B**). End-systolic frames are shown from the apical four-chamber view. A normal dipyridamole stress echocardiogram is shown in accompanying Video 50.2. (Adapted with permission from Picano E, et al: The new clinical standard of integrated quadruple stress echocardiography with ABCD protocol, *Cardiovasc Ultrasound* 16:22, 2018.)

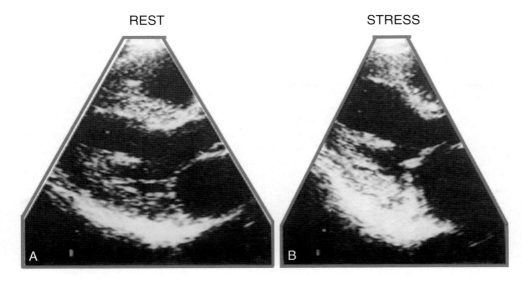

REST   STRESS

Figure 50.3. Stress echocardiogram: ischemic response. A normal wall thickening at rest (**A**) with akinetic septum and dilated left ventricular cavity during stress (**B**). End-systolic frames are shown from the parasternal long-axis view. (An abnormal dipyridamole stress is shown in accompanying Video 50.3.)

TABLE 50.2 Main Sources of False-Negative and False-Positive Results

	Reason for False-Negative Result	Reason for False-Positive Result
Patient related	Under antianginal therapy	True ischemia in HCM or AS
Stress related	Submaximal stress	Coronary vasospasm
Angiography related	Anatomically mild to intermediate (40%–70%) or functionally nonsignificant, LCX and RCA distal location	Inadequate angiographic imaging of a fixed, significant stenosis identified with reduced FFR or by ICUS
Myocardium related	Not critical ischemic mass	Occult cardiomyopathy
Image related	Inadequate segmental imaging	Inadequate segmental imaging
Reader related	Conservative reading	Aggressive reading

FFR, Fractional flow reserve; *HCM,* hypertrophic cardiomyopathy; *ICUS,* intracoronary ultrasound; *LAD,* left anterior descending coronary artery; *LCX,* left circumflex coronary artery; *RCA,* right coronary artery.

applied to achieve better wall motion assessment and is especially indicated in patients with two or more unreadable segments.[15]

FALSE-POSITIVE RESULTS

False-positive results in SE may indicate true induced ischemia and absolute subendocardial underperfusion despite angiographically nonsignificant CAD. Similar to what has been described for sources of false negativity, a false-positive response can recognize patient-, stress-, angiography-, myocardium-, reader-, and image-related reasons (see Table 50.2). False-positive results are associated with a poor prognosis, comparable to true positive results.[18] The main stress-related cause is epicardial coronary artery vasospasm, which may unpredictably occur superimposed to any degree of coronary artery stenosis (from absent to severe) during or soon after exercise, dobutamine (during or also after β-blockers administration), or dipyridamole (more frequently after the antidote aminophylline). It is a diagnosis by serendipity: coronary vasospasm is found when looking for coronary artery stenosis during testing. It is an easy diagnosis, if you think of it, and an important one because coronary vasospasm is a possible cause of chest pain, sudden cardiac death, syncope, and lack of response to medical therapy with β-blockers and coronary revascularization. It is frequent because 10% to 20% of SE positivity without coronary lesions are attributable to coronary vasospasm.[19] Specific testing for coronary vasospasm with ergonovine or hyperventilation can be safely performed in properly selected patients in the SE laboratory.[20] The main angiography-related cause is a stenosis of intermediate, subcritical severity at angiography that is, in reality, anatomically and functionally severe when verified by more accurate intracoronary ultrasound or functional assessment with

fractional flow reserve during invasive coronary angiography.[21] These patients should be considered as true positive, belong to a high risk subset, and should be treated accordingly. The myocardial revascularization cures the stress-induced RWMA and improves anginal symptoms. The main myocardium-related cause is occult cardiomyopathy or regional scar necrosis. The incipient muscle disease may not be overt at rest, but a chronotropic and afterload challenge with excessive heart rate and systolic blood pressure rise associated with stress can unmask a true regional dysfunction.

The main myocardium-related cause is any condition reducing subendocardial coronary flow reserve and determining true absolute underperfusion of the subendocardial layer during stress. This increases the rates of RWMA in conditions known to reduce profoundly the subendocardial flow reserve such as LV hypertrophy, aortic stenosis, and hypertrophic cardiomyopathy. In all these conditions, RWMAs have an excellent prognostic value. Aggressive overreading can be a cause of low specificity in images of low or borderline quality. High volumes are a necessary but not sufficient condition to achieve consistency of reading.

BEYOND REGIONAL WALL MOTION: THE ABCDE PROTOCOL OF STRESS ECHOCARDIOGRAPHY

RWMAs are essential yet underuse the unique versatility of the SE method, ideally suited to describe the different functional abnormalities underlying the same wall motion response during stress. Five parameters converge conceptually, logistically, and methodologically in the ABCDE protocol of SE,[22] assessing the many vulnerabilities of the patient above and beyond the critical coronary artery stenosis (Table 50.3): epicardial coronary artery stenosis (RWMA), pulmonary congestion and interstitial pulmonary edema (B lines), global myocardial function, coronary small vessels, and cardiac autonomic nervous system imbalance (Fig. 50.4). The five steps of the ABCDE protocol are:

- Step A: RWMA by two-dimensional echocardiography
- Step B: B lines by lung ultrasound (with the four-site simplified scan of third intercostal space) assessing the shape of lung water[23,24]
- Step C: LV contractile reserve assessed as the stress–rest ratio of force (systolic arterial pressure by cuff sphygmomanometer–end-systolic volume from 2D)[25] or more simply as LV cavity dilatation during stress[26]
- Step D: Doppler-based assessment of coronary flow velocity reserve in the left anterior descending coronary with pulsed-wave Doppler

- Step E: imaging-independent ECG-based assessment of heart rate reserve (peak/rest heart rate).

The same transducer is used for cardiac (step A and C), lung (step B), and coronary (step D) scans, while step E is imaging independent. The cutoff values are stress independent for A, C, and D but stress specific for C and E because vasodilators are a weaker inotropic and chronotropic stress than exercise and dobutamine. The abnormal cutoff value for contractile reserve is lower for vasodilators (≤1.1) compared with exercise or dobutamine stress (≤2.0). The abnormal cutoff value for chronotropic reserve is lower for vasodilators (heart rate reserve ≤1.22) compared with exercise or dobutamine stress (≤1.80). Chronotropic incompetence is associated with worse prognosis independently of induced ischemia with all forms of physical and pharmacological stresses.[27,28] The combination of these five parameters in a single test allows a more comprehensive risk stratification than RWMA alone (Fig. 50.5).

TABLE 50.3 Imaging and Non-imaging Parameters for the ABCDE Stress Echocardiography Protocol

	RWMA	B-lines	LVCR	CFVR	HRR
ABCDE	A, asynergy	B, B lines	C, contractility	D, Doppler	E, ECG
Variable	Myocardial ischemia	Lung water	Left ventricular force	Coronary	Autonomic dysfunction
Transducer	2D	LUS	2D	PWD	Not needed
Imaging time	Minutes	Seconds	Seconds	Minutes	None
Analysis time	Seconds	Seconds	Minutes	Seconds	Seconds
Feasibility (%)	>95	Almost 100	>95	>80	100

2D, Two-dimensional; CFVR, coronary flow velocity reserve; HRR, heart rate reserve; LUS, lung ultrasound; LVCR, left ventricular contractile reserve; PWD, pulsed-wave Doppler.
Adapted from Picano E, et al: The new clinical standard of integrated quadruple stress echocardiography with ABCD protocol, Cardiovasc Ultrasound 16:22, 2018.

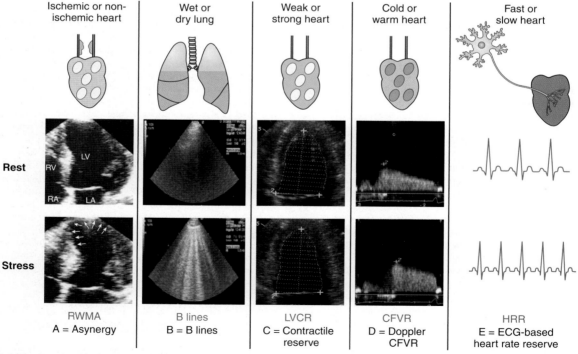

Figure 50.4. The targets of integrated ABCDE stress echocardiography (SE). The five pathophysiological targets of ABCDE SE: epicardial coronary artery stenosis (with regional wall motion abnormality [RMWA]), lung water (with B lines), myocardial function (with left ventricular end-systolic area), small vessels (with coronary flow velocity reserve [CFVR]), and cardiac autonomic balance (with heart rate reserve [HRR]). (Adapted with permission from Picano E, et al: The new clinical standard of integrated quadruple stress echocardiography with ABCD protocol, *Cardiovasc Ultrasound* 16:22, 2018.)

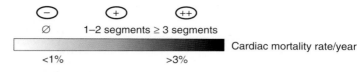

Risk stratification beyond regional wall motion abnormalities

Figure 50.5. Risk stratification with the ABCDE response. The risk stratification with stress echocardiography, from binary (*black* or *white*) response based only to regional wall motion abnormality (RMWA) endorsed by current guidelines (*upper row*) to the spectrum of responses (from *green* of lowest to *red* of highest risk) obtained by the ABCDE protocol with RWMA supplemented with B lines, left ventricular contractile reserve, coronary flow velocity reserve, and heart rate reserve. *ESC,* European Society of Cardiology. (Adapted with permission from Picano E, et al: The new clinical standard of integrated quadruple stress echocardiography with ABCD protocol, *Cardiovasc Ultrasound* 16:22, 2018.)

TOWARD QUANTITATIVE STRESS ECHOCARDIOGRAPHY

The current state-of-the-art diagnosis remains subjective by visual eyeballing, but it might be possible to corroborate the current naked eye diagnosis with quantitative assessment of regional and global myocardial deformation indices. The rationale behind strain SE is its quantitative nature, ability to differentiate tethering from surrounding segments, earlier onset than RWMA during the ischemic cascade (leading to higher diagnostic sensitivity), and longer persistence after stress interruption. At present, it cannot be used routinely in clinical practice because of limited feasibility (~80%), noisy data in high heart rate states (>100 beats/min), lack of standardization of parameters and software, and missing effectiveness studies.[29] Technological improvements are expected to allow to establish SE on a more automated and operator-independent basis, with robotic-hands off acquisition and artificial intelligence elaboration of images and data with deep learning approach.[30]

CONCLUSIONS

According to the recent 2019 European Society of Cardiology guidelines for diagnosis in chronic coronary syndromes, SE is recommended instead of exercise ECG as the initial test to diagnose obstructive CAD for a symptomatic patient (with angina or dyspnea). SE is the functional test of choice in patients with suspected or known CAD because of its widespread availability, possibility to be combined with exercise, radiation-free nature, no need to use contrast based on iodine and gadolinium, and versatility of information.[1] SE may be preferred as a first-line test in patients at the higher end of range of clinical likelihood if revascularization is likely or when patients have previously diagnosed CAD or viability assessment is also required. SE based on RWMA is essential to identify patients who will have a survival and symptomatic benefit from myocardial revascularization. Yet it underuses the unique versatility of the technique. In the ABCDE format, SE is more comprehensive and allows better functional characterization, risk stratification, and possibly a personalized tailoring of therapy.

Please access ExpertConsult to view the corresponding videos for this chapter.

REFERENCES

1. Knuuti J, Wijns W, Saraste A, et al. The task force for the diagnosis and management of chronic coronary syndromes of the European Society of Cardiology. *Eur Heart J.* 2019;00:1–71.
2. Pellikka PA, Nagueh SF, Elhendy AA, et al. American Society of Echocardiography American Society of Echocardiography recommendations for performance, interpretation, and application of stress echocardiography. *J Am Soc Echocardiogr.* 2007;20:1021–1024.
3. Sicari R, Nihoyannopoulos P, Evangelista A, et al. European Association of Echocardiography Stress echocardiography expert consensus statement. *Eur J Echocardiogr.* 2008;9:415–437.
4. Heijenbrok-Kal MH, Fleischmann KE, Hunink MG, et al. Stress echocardiography, stress single-photon-emission computed tomography and electron beam computed tomography for the assessment of coronary artery disease: a meta-analysis of diagnostic performance. *Am Heart J.* 2007;154:415–423.
5. Picano E, Pellikka PA, et al. Stress echo applications beyond coronary artery disease. *Eur Heart J.* 2014;35:1033–1040.
6. Lancellotti P, Pellikka PA, Budts W, et al. The clinical use of stress echocardiography in non-ischemic heart disease. *J Am Soc Echocardiogr.* 2017;17:1191–1229.
7. Hirschfeld Jr JW, Ferrari FA, Bengel FM, et al. 2018 ACC/HRS/NASCI/SCAI/SCCT Expert consensus document on optimal use of ionizing radiation in cardiovascular imaging: Best practices for safety and effectiveness. *J Am Coll Cardiol.* 2018;24:e286–e348.
8. Picano E, Vañó E, Rehani MM, et al. The appropriate and justified use of medical radiation in cardiovascular imaging. *Eur Heart J.* 2014;35:665–672.
9. Marwick TH, Buonocore J. Environmental impact of cardiac imaging tests for the diagnosis of coronary artery disease. *Heart.* 2011;97:1128–1131.
10. Popescu BA, Stefanidis A, Nihoyannopoulos P, et al. Updated standards and processes for accreditation of echocardiographic laboratories from the European Association of Cardiovascular Imaging. *Eur Heart J Cardiovasc Imaging.* 2014;15:717–727.
11. Picano E. *Stress Echocardiography.* 6th ed. Heidelberg, NY: Springer Verlag; 2015.
12. Al-Lamee R, Shun-Shin M, Howard J, et al. Dobutamine stress echocardiography ischemia as a predictor of placebo-controlled efficacy of percutaneous coronary intervention in stable coronary artery disease: the stress-echo stratified analysis of ORBITA. *Circulation.* 2019;140:1971–1980.
13. Gaibazzi N, Siniscalchi C, Porter T, et al. Vasodilator stress single photon emission tomography or contrast stress echocardiography association with hard cardiac events in suspected coronary artery disease. *J Am Soc Echocardiogr.* 2018;31:683–691.
14. Ciampi Q, Zagatina A, Cortigiani L, et al. Functional, coronary anatomic and prognostic correlates of coronary flow velocity reserve during stress echocardiography. *J Am Coll Cardiol.* 2019;74:2280–2293.
15. Smulders M, Jaarsma C, Nelemans P, et al. Comparison of the prognostic value of negative non-invasive cardiac investigations in patients with suspected or known coronary artery disease-a meta-analysis. *Eur Heart J Cardiovasc Imaging.* 2017;18:980–987.
16. Ahmadvazir S, Shah BN, Zacharias K, Senior R. Incremental prognostic value of stress echocardiography with carotid ultrasound for suspected coronary artery disease. *JACC Cardiovasc Imag.* 2018;11:173–180.
17. Faggiano P, Dasseni N, Gaibazzi N, et al. Cardiac calcification as a marker of subclinical atherosclerosis and predictor of cardiovascular events: a review of evidence. *Eur J Prev Cardiol.* 2019;26:1191–1204.
18. Rachwan RJ, Mshelbwala FS, Dardari Z, Batal O. False positive stress echocardiograms: predictors and prognostic relevance. *Intern J Cardiology.* 2019;296:157–163.
19. Aboukhoudir F, Rekik S. Coronary artery spasm and dobutamine echocardiography in patients without known coronary artery disease: prevalence, predictors and outcomes. *Acta Cardiol.* 2016;71:435–441.
20. Om SY, Yoo SY, Cho GY, et al. Diagnostic and prognostic value of ergonovine echocardiography for noninvasive diagnosis of coronary vasospasm. *JACC Cardiovasc Imaging.* 2020;S1936-878X(20):30262-X. https://doi.org/10.1016/j.jcmg.2020.03.008.

21. Panoulas VF, Keramida K, Boletti O, et al. Association between fractional flow reserve, instantaneous wave-free ratio and dobutamine stress echocardiography in patients with stable coronary artery disease. *Euro Intervention*. 2018;13:1959–1966.

22. Picano E, Ciampi Q, Wierzbowska-Drabik K, et al. The new clinical standard of integrated quadruple stress echocardiography with ABCD protocol. *Cardiovasc Ultrasound*. 2018;16(22).

23. Picano E, Scali MC, Ciampi Q, Lichtenstein D. Lung ultrasound for the cardiologist. *JACC Cardiovasc Imag*. 2018;12:381–390.

24. Scali MC, Ciampi Q, Zagatina A, et al. On behalf of the Stress Echo 2020 Study Group of the Italian Society of Echocardiography and Cardiovascular Imaging. Lung ultrasound and pulmonary congestion during stress echocardiography. *JACC Cardiov Imaging*. 2020;19:145–167.

25. Cortigiani L, Huqi A, Ciampi Q, et al. Integration of wall motion, coronary flow velocity and left ventricular contractile reserve in a single test: prognostic value of vasodilator stress echocardiography in diabetic patients. *J Am Soc Echocardiogr*. 2018;31:692–701.

26. Turakhia MP, McManus DD, Whooley MA, Schiller NB. Increase in end-systolic volume after exercise independently predicts mortality in patients with coronary heart disease: data from the Heart and Soul Study. *Eur Heart J*. 2009;30:2478–2484.

27. Chaowalit N, McCully RB, Callahan MJ, et al. Outcomes after normal dobutamine stress echocardiography and predictors of adverse events: long-term follow-up of 3014 patients. *Eur Heart J*. 2006;27:3039–3044.

28. Cortigiani L, Carpeggiani C, Landi P, et al. Usefulness of blunted heart rate reserve as an imaging-independent prognostic predictor during dipyridamole-echocardiography test. *Am J Cardiol*. 2019;124:972–977.

29. Gupta K, Kakar TS, Gupta A, et al. Role of left ventricle deformation analysis for significant coronary artery disease detection. *Echocardiography*. 2019;36:1084–1094.

30. Kusunose K, Abe T, Haga A, et al. A deep learning approach for assessment of regional wall motion abnormality from echocardiographic images. *JACC Cardiovasc Imaging*. 2020;13(2 Pt 1):374–381.

51 Stress Echocardiography: Methodology

Rosa Sicari

GENERAL TEST PROTOCOL

During stress echocardiography (SE), electrocardiographic leads are placed at standard limb and precordial sites, slightly displacing (upward and downward) any leads that may interfere with the chosen acoustic windows. A 12-lead electrocardiogram (ECG) is recorded in resting condition and each minute throughout the examination. An ECG lead is also continuously displayed on the echo monitor to provide the operator with a reference for ST-segment changes and arrhythmias. Cuff blood pressure is measured in resting condition and each stage thereafter. Echocardiographic imaging is typically performed from the parasternal long- and short-axis, apical long-axis, and apical four- and two-chamber views. In some cases, the subxiphoid and apical long-axis views are used. Images are recorded in resting condition from all views and captured digitally. A quad-screen format is used for comparative analysis. Echocardiography is then continuously monitored and intermittently stored. In the presence of obvious or suspected dyssynergy, a complete echo examination is performed and recorded from all employed approaches to allow optimal documentation of the presence and extent of myocardial ischemia. These same projections are obtained and recorded during the recovery phase after cessation of stress (exercise or pacing) or administration of the antidote (aminophylline for dipyridamole, β-blocker for dobutamine). An ischemic response may occasionally occur late, after cessation of drug infusion.[1] In this way, the transiently dyssynergic area during stress can be evaluated by a triple comparison: stress versus resting state, stress versus recovery phase, and at peak stress. It is critical to obtain the same views at each stage of the test. Analysis and scoring of the study are usually performed using a 16- or 17-segment model of the left ventricle[2] and a 4-grade scale of regional wall motion analysis. Regional wall motion is semiquantitatively graded from 1 to 4 as follows: 1 = normal, 2 = hypokinetic, 3 = akinetic, and 4 = dyskinetic. Wall motion score index (WMSI) is the sum of individual segment scores divided by the number of interpretable segments.[2]

Diagnostic endpoints of SE testing are maximum dose (for pharmacologic) or maximum workload (for exercise testing), achievement of target heart rate, obvious echocardiographic positivity (with akinesis of two or more left ventricular segments), severe chest pain, or obvious electrocardiographic positivity (with >2 mV ST-segment shift). Submaximal nondiagnostic endpoints of SE testing are nontolerable symptoms or limiting asymptomatic side effects such as hypertension, with systolic blood pressure greater than 220 mm Hg or diastolic blood pressure greater than 120 mm Hg; symptomatic hypotension, with a greater than 40–mm Hg drop in blood pressure; supraventricular arrhythmias, such as supraventricular tachycardia or atrial fibrillations, and complex ventricular arrhythmias, such as ventricular tachycardia or frequent, polymorphic premature ventricular beats.

SPECIFIC TEST PROTOCOLS

The most frequently used stressors for echocardiographic tests are exercise, dobutamine, and dipyridamole. Table 51.1 lists some of the advantages and disadvantages of exercise versus pharmacologic stress. Table 51.2 lists the required equipment and protocols for the various forms of SE.

EXERCISE

Exercise echocardiography can be performed using either a treadmill or bicycle protocol. When a treadmill test is performed, scanning during exercise is not feasible, so most protocols rely on immediate postexercise imaging. It is imperative to accomplish postexercise imaging as soon as possible (<1 minute from cessation of exercise). To accomplish this, the patient is moved immediately from the treadmill to an imaging bed and placed in the

TABLE 51.1 Exercise versus Pharmacologic Stress Echocardiography: Instructions for Use

Parameter	Exercise	Pharmacologic
Intravenous line required		✓
Diagnostic utility of heart rate and blood pressure response	✓	
Use in deconditioned patients		✓
Use in physically limited patients		✓
Level of echocardiography imaging difficulty	High	Low
Safety profile	High	Moderate
Clinical role in valvular heart disease	✓	
Clinical role in pulmonary hypertension	✓	
Fatigue and dyspnea evaluation	✓	
Prognostic role		✓

TABLE 51.2 Stress Echocardiography Protocols

Test	Equipment	Protocols
Exercise	Treadmill	Progressive increase in workload; many protocols
Exercise	Semi-supine bicycle ergometer	25 W × 2' with incremental loading
Dobutamine	Infusion pump	5 mcg/kg/min 10–20–30–40 + atropine (0.25 × 4) ≤1 mg
Dipyridamole	Syringe	0.84 mg/kg in 6' or 0.84 mg/kg in 10' + atropine (0.25 ×4) ≤1 mg
Adenosine	Syringe	140 mcg/kg/min in 6'
Pacing	External pacing	From 100 beats/min with increments of 10 beats/min up to target heart rate

left lateral decubitus position so that imaging may be completed within 1 to 2 minutes.[2,3] This technique assumes that regional wall motion abnormalities will persists long enough into recovery to be detected. When abnormalities recover rapidly, false-negative results occur. The advantages of treadmill exercise echocardiography are the widespread availability of the treadmill system and a greater feasibility because a number of patients are unable to cycle. Information on exercise capacity, heart rate response and rhythm, and blood pressure changes are analyzed and, together with wall motion analysis, become part of the final interpretation.

Bicycle exercise echocardiography is performed during either an upright or recumbent posture. The patient pedals against an increasing workload at a constant cadence (usually 60 rpm). The workload is escalated in a stepwise fashion while imaging is performed. Successful bicycle stress testing requires the cooperation of the patient (to maintain the correct cadence) and coordination (to perform pedaling action). The most important advantage of bicycle exercise is the chance to obtain images during the various levels of exercise (rather than relying on postexercise imaging). Although imaging can be done throughout the exercise protocol, in most cases interpretation is based on a comparison of resting and peak exercise images. In the supine posture, it is relatively easy to record images from multiple views during graded exercise. With the development of ergometers that permit leftward tilting of the patients, the ease of image acquisition has been further improved. In the upright posture, imaging is generally limited to either apical or subcostal views. By leaning the patient forward over the handlebars and extending the arms, apical images can be obtained in the majority of patients. To record subcostal views, a more lordotic position is necessary, and care must be taken to avoid foreshortening of the apex. The safety of exercise stress is witnessed by decades of experience with ECG testing and stress imaging. However, limiting side effects may occur and are related to the occurrence of myocardial ischemia. Death occurs at an average in 1 in 10,000 tests, and major life-threatening effects, including myocardial infarction (MI), ventricular fibrillation, sustained ventricular tachycardia, and stroke, were reported in about 1 in 6000 patients with exercise in the international SE registry.[4,5]

DOBUTAMINE

The standard dobutamine stress protocol usually adopted consists of continuous intravenous (IV) infusion of dobutamine in 3-minute increments, starting with 5 μg/kg/min and increasing to 10, 20, 30, and 40 μg /kg/min. If no endpoint is reached, atropine (in doses 0.25 mg up to a maximum of 1 mg) is added to the 40-μg/kg/min dobutamine infusion. Other more conservative protocols—with longer durations of steps and a peak dobutamine dosage of 20 to 30 μg/kg/min—have been proposed but are limited by unsatisfactory sensitivity. More aggressive protocols—with higher peak dosages of dobutamine up to 50 to 60 μg/kg/min and

atropine sulphate up to 2 mg—have also been proposed, but safety concern remains, and to date no advantages have been shown in larger studies. In order of frequency, limiting side effects during dobutamine stress include complex ventricular tachyarrhythmias (the most frequent complications, which are independent of ischemia in many cases and can also develop at low-dose dobutamine regimen), hypotension, atrial fibrillation, and hypertension (in some cases caused by dynamic intraventricular obstruction provoked by inotropic action of dobutamine, especially in hypertrophic hearts). A vasodepressor reflex triggered by left ventricular mechanoreceptors stimulation (Bezold-Jarisch reflex) caused by excessive inotropic stimulation may be an alternative mechanism, (through α-receptor stimulation). The rate of major complications may occur in 1 of 300 cases during dobutamine stress.[6]

DIPYRIDAMOLE

The standard dipyridamole protocol consists of an IV infusion of 0.84 mg/kg over 10 minutes in two separate infusions: 0.56 mg/kg over 4 minutes ("standard dose") followed by 4 minutes of no dose and, if still negative, an additional 0.28 mg/kg over 2 minutes. If no endpoint is reached, atropine (doses of 0.25 mg up to a maximum of 1 mg) is added. The same overall dose of 0.84 mg/kg can be given over 6 minutes—the shorter the infusion time, the higher the sensitivity.[2] Aminophylline (240 mg IV) should be available for immediate use in case of an adverse dipyridamole-related event occur and routinely infused at the end of the test independent regardless of the result. Patients should abstain from the assumption of caffeine-containing drinks (tea, coffee, cola) for 24 before the test. Patients on chronic xanthine medication should not undergo dipyridamole SE. Limiting side effects occur in 3% of patients tested with dipyridamole. In order of frequency, these side effects are hypotension, supraventricular tachycardia, general malaise, headache, dyspnea, and atrial fibrillation. Major life-threatening complications, such as MI, third-degree atrioventricular (AV) block, cardiac asystole, sustained ventricular tachycardia, or pulmonary edema, occur in about 1 in 1000 cases with high-dose dipyridamole stress.[7,8]

ADENOSINE

Adenosine can be used in a similar manner and is typically infused at a maximum dose of 140 μg/kg/min over 6 minutes. Imaging is performed before and after starting adenosine infusion. Side effects are very frequent and are limiting in up to 20% of patients investigated with adenosine SE. They include high-degree AV block, hypotension, intolerable chest pain (possibly induced for direct stimulation of myocardial A1 adenosine receptors), shortness of breath, flushing, and headache. Although side effects are frequent, the incidence of life-threatening complications, such as MI, ventricular tachycardia, and shock, has been shown to be very low, with only 1 fatal myocardial infarction in approximately 10,000 cases.[9]

PACING

The presence of a permanent pacemaker can be exploited to conduct a pacing stress test in a totally noninvasive manner by externally programming the pacemaker to increasing frequencies.[10] Pacing is started at 100 beats/min and increased every 2 minutes by 10 beats/min until the target heart rate (85% of age-predicted maximal heart rate) is achieved or until other standard endpoints are reached. The same protocol can also be followed in an accelerated fashion, with faster steps (20–30 each), up to the target heart rate. A limiting factor is, however, that several pacemakers cannot be programmed to the target heart rate. This should be checked before the patient is scheduled for such a test. Two-dimensional echocardiographic images are obtained before pacing and throughout the stress test with the final recording being obtained after 3 minutes of pacing at the highest rate reached (usually 150 beats/min) or the target heart rate.[10]

THE ROLE OF CONTRAST

Contrast for endocardial border enhancement, which should be used whenever there are suboptimal resting or peak stress images. IV contrast for LV opacification, improves endocardial border definition and may salvage an otherwise suboptimal study.[2,3]

REFERENCES

1. Cerqueira MD, Weissman NJ, Dilsizian V, et al. American heart Association Writing Group on myocardial Segmentation and Registration for cardiac imaging. Standardized myocardial segmentation and nomenclature for tomographic imaging of the heart. *A statement for healthcare professionals from the Cardiac Imaging Committee of the Council on Clinical Cardiology of the American Heart Association, Circulation.* 2002;105:539–542.
2. Pellikka PA, Nagueh SF, Elhendy AA, et al. American Society of Echocardiography recommendations for performance, interpretation, and application of stress echocardiography. *J Am Soc Echocardiogr.* 2007;20:1021–1041.
3. Sicari R, Nihoyannopoulos P, Evangelista A, et al. European Association of Echocardiography Stress echocardiography expert consensus statement. *Eur J Echocardiogr.* 2008;9:415–437.
4. Varga A, Garcia MA, Picano E. Safety of stress echocardiography (from the international stress echo complication registry). *Am J Cardiol.* 2006;98:541–543.
5. Fletcher GF, Balady GJ, Amsterdam EA, et al. Exercise standards for testing and training: a statement for healthcare professionals from the American Heart Association. *Circulation.* 2001;104:1694–1740.
6. Picano E, Mathias Jr W, Pingitore A, et al. Safety and tolerability of dobutamine-atropine stress echocardiography: a prospective, multicentre study. Echo Dobutamine International Cooperative Study Group. *Lancet.* 1994;344:1190–1192.
7. Picano E, Marini C, Pirelli S, et al. Safety of intravenous high-dose dipyridamole echocardiography. The echo-Persantine International Cooperative Study Group. *Am J Cardiol.* 1992;70:252–258.
8. Lette J, Tatum JL, Fraser S, et al. Safety of dipyridamole testing in 73,806 patients: the multicenter dipyridamole safety study. *J Nucl Cardiol.* 1995;2(3–17).
9. Cerqueira MD, Verani MS, Schwaiger M, et al. Safety profile of adenosine stress perfusion imaging: results from the Adenoscan multicenter trial registry. *J Am Coll Cardiol.* 1994;23:384–389.
10. Picano E, Alaimo A, Chubuchny V, et al. Noninvasive pacemaker stress echocardiography for diagnosis of coronary artery disease: a multicenter study. *J Am Coll Cardiol.* 2002;40:1305–1310.

52 Stress Echocardiography: Image Acquisition

Samuel Bernard, Michael H. Picard

The accuracy and reproducibility of stress echocardiography (SE) depend on attention to proper image acquisition. Although most stress echocardiograms are performed for assessment of coronary artery disease, the sonographer and physician must tailor the imaging protocol to the specific aims of the test, which may also include assessments of valvular regurgitation, valvular stenosis, pulmonary hypertension, and diastolic parameters. The American Society of Echocardiography's guidelines on SE[1] and quality operations[2] offer details on image acquisition. The ultrasound device should use electrocardiographically triggered image acquisition.[2] The echocardiography reading station should allow split- and quad-screen displays to facilitate simultaneous comparisons of images at various stages in the stress protocol.[2] This type of display (Figs. 52.1 and 52.2; Videos 52.1 and 52.2) is crucial in the assessment of subtle wall motion abnormalities (WMAs) in each segment. Tissue harmonic imaging, which enhances definition of the endocardium and reduces near-field artifacts, should be routinely used in SE.[1]

Comprehensive baseline (rest) images must include all segments of the left ventricle for comparison with postphysiologic stress images or pharmacologic stress images; whenever possible, this stage should also include a quick assessment of other structures that might cause the symptoms prompting the test (described later). When assessing for ischemia, the minimum baseline series of images should include parasternal long-axis, parasternal short-axis at the midpapillary muscle level, apical four-chamber (A4C), and apical two-chamber (A2C) views. If parasternal long-axis views are not available, apical long-axis views may be substituted.[2] Ideally, short-axis images should include views at the mitral valve, midventricle, and apical levels. Although SE display software programs allow digital acquisition and multistage comparisons for any view, typically only one short-axis view, the midventricular (midpapillary) level, is included in the SE imaging display because myocardium from all three coronary artery territories is shown in this view. However, the other short-axis images (basal

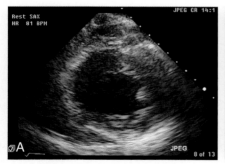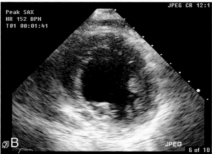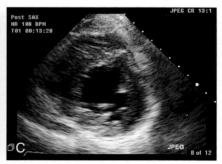

Figure 52.1. Format of a supine bicycle stress echocardiogram with simultaneous displays of the left ventricle at rest (**A**), peak stress (**B**), and post exercise (**C**). At rest, inferoposterior and posterior wall akinesis and lateral wall hypokinesis are noted. After 10 minutes of exercise, there were new wall motion abnormalities in the midseptum and anterior wall, with more prominent hypokinesis of the lateral wall. Coronary angiography revealed 90% stenosis in the proximal left anterior descending artery and 75% stenosis in the left circumflex artery. (See accompanying Video 52.1.)

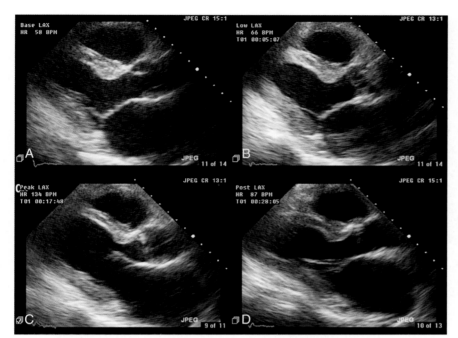

Figure 52.2. Format of a dobutamine stress echocardiogram with simultaneous displays of the left ventricle before dobutamine was administered (**A**), at low-dose dobutamine (**B**), at peak-dose dobutamine (**C**), and after dobutamine (**D**). The test result was positive for inducible wall motion abnormalities in the anterior and septal territories. In these parasternal long-axis images, inducible ischemic abnormalities at peak stress are noted in the anteroseptum. (For the full stress echocardiogram, see accompanying Video 52.2.) Coronary angiography revealed a focal 95% stenosis of the mid-left anterior descending artery.

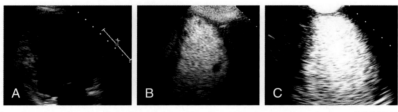

Figure 52.3. An apical two-chamber view showing the left ventricle without an ultrasound-enhancing agent (UEA) (**A**), with an UEA at low mechanical index imaging (**B**), and with an UEA at very low mechanical index (VLMI) imaging (**C**). Note the improvement in endocardial definition with contrast administration and the absence of basal segment attenuation when VLMI imaging is used (Adapted with permission from Porter TR, et al: Clinical applications of ultrasonic enhancing agents in echocardiography, *J Am Soc Echocardiogr* 31:241–274, 2018.)

and apical) can be saved in the digital archive for more detailed comparison or for use in strain analysis. Subcostal short-axis views may be substituted if the parasternal window is unavailable, but this view is more dependent on patient positioning and there may be limited time at peak stress to reposition the patient to optimize this window. In obtaining apical views, it is essential to prevent foreshortening (because these may be the only images of the left ventricular [LV] apex) while simultaneously avoiding inclusion of the left ventricular outflow tract (LVOT) because the latter may lead to misinterpretation of basal septal function. When performing the stress echocardiogram for valve disease assessments, it is also important that both diastolic and systolic images depict the four chambers (and visualize both mitral and tricuspid valves) in the apical views.

When at least two contiguous endocardial segments cannot be delineated, ultrasound-enhancing agents (i.e., contrast agents) should be used for both rest and peak images.[1] Contrast dose at peak can often be lower than the baseline dose because flow is increased. Very low mechanical index (MI) imaging (MI <0.2) is recommended with contrast administration because it achieves homogeneous LV opacification and improves the analysis of regional wall motion (Fig. 52.3).[3] Brief intermittent high-MI "flash impulses" (5–15 frames, MI >0.8) can be used to clear contrast from the myocardium to enhance endocardial borders and may be used to assess myocardial perfusion during SE.[3]

For patients who have not had a recent transthoracic echocardiogram, the baseline images should be considered as a screen for other causes of the symptoms prompting the stress

echocardiogram. A brief assessment for aortic stenosis, pulmonary hypertension, mitral regurgitation, and pericardial disease can be performed with images of aortic valve leaflet opening, continuous-wave (CW) Doppler of tricuspid regurgitation, color Doppler of the mitral valve, and assessment for the presence of pericardial effusion. If resting images demonstrate asymmetric septal hypertrophy or systolic anterior motion of the mitral valve, then the LVOT should be interrogated with CW Doppler to ensure that stress testing is not performed on a patient with unrecognized obstructive hypertrophic cardiomyopathy (especially if a resting peak late systolic pressure gradient of at least 50 mm Hg is obtained). Other findings on prestress screening that may prompt cancellation of the test include significant aortic disease, severe LV systolic dysfunction, or presence of a LV thrombus.

With treadmill exercise echocardiographic protocols, the patient must move quickly from the upright running position to the bed quickly so that imaging can be performed before WMAs resolve; the aim is for these images to be acquired within 1 minute of achieving peak exercise heart rate. During bicycle exercise stress, echocardiographic images can be taken during pedaling at peak exercise. Thus, analysis of echocardiographic images acquired during exercise protocols includes three panels: resting baseline, immediate post–peak exercise (treadmill) or peak exercise (bicycle), and recovery (see Fig. 52.1 and Video 52.1). In patients who are unable to exercise, dobutamine SE is the preferred alternative.[1] For dobutamine protocols, images of each view at four stages should be obtained and compared: baseline, low dose, peak dose, and recovery (see Fig. 52.2 and Video 52.2).

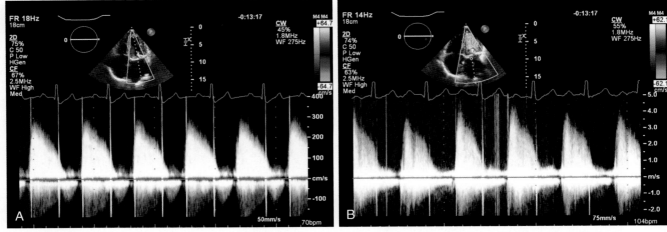

Figure 52.4. Bicycle stress echocardiogram performed for assessment of exertional dyspnea in a 40-year-old patient with a mitral valve bioprosthesis placed 13 years ago and now clinical suspicion of prosthetic valve stenosis. With 9 minutes of exercise (61% maximum predicted heart rate), dyspnea developed, and mean transmitral gradient rose from 18 mm Hg at rest, when the heart rate was 70 beats/min (**A**), to 38 mm Hg at peak exercise, when the heart rate was 104 beats/min (**B**). The right ventricular systolic pressure rose from 51 mm Hg at rest to 80 mm Hg at peak exercise.

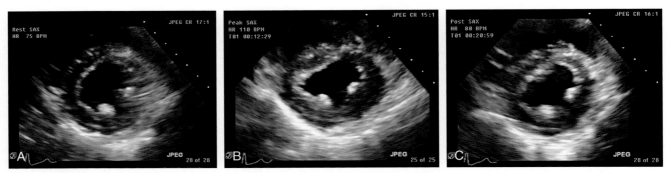

Figure 52.5. A–C, In the patient whose echocardiogram is shown in Fig. 52.4, there was evidence of systolic septal flattening at peak exercise, indicative of right ventricular systolic pressure overload. (See accompanying Videos 52.5.)

To facilitate comparisons to the resting images and promote accurate identification of WMAs, the sonographer should obtain the peak images in the same imaging planes and at the same depth as the baseline ones. This can be challenging when patients have exaggerated respiratory motion during and after exercise. Given the limited time available at peak heart rate, speed in acquisition is essential. Patients may need to be instructed to enact brief breath holds at mid-inspiration or mid-expiration to maintain the echocardiographic window. For post-treadmill imaging, the apical views should be obtained first. Certain landmarks can help ensure that the same myocardial territory is imaged both during stress and at rest. This includes visualization of a thickened valve chordae tendineae or highly reflective echoes within a specific myocardial segment. Also, if short-axis views are oblique rather than orthogonal to the long axis of the left ventricle, wall motion may be misinterpreted. Whenever possible, WMAs should be confirmed on at least one additional view. At the conclusion of image acquisition, a quality check should be conducted to ensure that the best images are used in the comparison displays. The sonographer should check that all images are labeled with the correct window name (e.g., A4C) and that the electrocardiographic waveform is the same on all images (e.g., the sonographer should exclude images acquired during ventricular ectopic beats).

Different imaging protocols are required for other applications of SE, such as for the assessment of symptoms thought to be caused by diastolic dysfunction, valvular disease, or pulmonary hypertension. For the assessment of diastolic dysfunction, bicycle exercise testing is the recommended modality because it allows for Doppler assessment of diastolic functional reserve during exercise (although treadmill testing can be used as an alternative).[4] In the A4C view, mitral E, A, e′, and right ventricular systolic pressure (RVSP) values should be obtained at rest and during exercise with subsequent calculation of E/A and E/e′. Pulsed-wave (PW) Doppler variables (E, A) are typically obtained 1 to 2 mm from the mitral valve leaflet tips and are measured in diastole. PW tissue Doppler variables (e′) are obtained at the septal or lateral (or both) mitral annulus with the Nyquist limit set to 15 to 20 cm/s. The aforementioned should be obtained when the heart rate is between 100 and 110 beats/min to avoid fusion of E and A waves.[4] This allows for integration of diastolic stress testing with ischemic testing because WMAs should be assessed first at peak stress, followed by RVSP measurements and finally the mitral valve and annular Doppler velocities.

Stress exercise echocardiography may also be used to determine the significance of asymptomatic severe valvular disease or the contribution of moderate valvular disease to patient symptoms. For this evaluation, the window for peak gradient must be established at rest because imaging through multiple windows may not be possible while at peak exercise stress. As an example, when assessing aortic valve gradients, the right parasternal window is often not available at peak bicycle stress when the patient is in the left lateral position.[5] In cases of mitral stenosis, SE can be used to determine if transmitral gradients rise[6] or RVSP significantly increases (Figs. 52.4 and 52.5; Video 52.5). In this setting, the CW Doppler is obtained across the mitral valve and tricuspid valve at both rest and peak stress (or with treadmill exercise, immediately after stress). Similarly, in patients with aortic stenosis, CW Doppler across the aortic valve and PW Doppler of the LVOT should be obtained at rest and peak stress to assess for worsening with exercise (and for calculation of aortic valve area at each of these stages using the continuity equation).[7] In cases of mitral or aortic regurgitation, SE can be used to determine if exercise ejection fraction decreases, LV cavity size increases, effective regurgitant orifice area changes, or RVSP increases.[8] In each of these scenarios, specific Doppler assessments are added to the standard images of the left ventricle at rest and peak stress. Of note, if low flow–low gradient aortic stenosis (with a reduced LV ejection fraction) requires assessment, this is performed by dobutamine infusion to a maximum of 20 mcg/kg/min.[9]

Recent studies have demonstrated the utility of strain indices (including global and regional peak systolic longitudinal strain, strain rate, and postsystolic strain index) for the assessment of ischemia and valvular heart disease (e.g., aortic stenosis and mitral regurgitation).[4] Strain data should be acquired at peak exercise (bicycle) or immediately after peak exercise (treadmill). Quantitation typically occurs using two-dimensional (2D) speckle-tracking echocardiography (STE) and has the advantage of assessing strain in multiple axes (i.e., longitudinal, radial, circumferential) with relative angle independence. The acquisition and interpretation of strain data during stress may be technically limited because of multiple factors, including poor baseline echocardiographic images, excess respiratory motion, or inadequate frame rates (which should be at least 70% of the heart rate to ensure adequate tracking of myocardial speckles). Moreover, because loading conditions influence strain values, blood pressure should be recorded at the time of analysis.[10] Finally, it should be noted that strain analysis software programs provided by different vendors use unique algorithms that may result in measurement variation if different software programs or versions are used to measure the same image.[11]

SE using real-time three-dimensional (3D) imaging has been suggested as a potential improvement over current 2D imaging techniques. Complete 3D data sets can be obtained from a single apical view (rather than multiple views) and subsequently analyzed for regional WMAs. Malalignment of myocardial segments and LV foreshortening are also obviated given that the entire left ventricle is imaged. Multibeat acquisition (typically obtained over four cycles) is limited by stitching artifacts in patients with respiratory variation and irregular heart rates, but single-beat 3D acquisitions overcome these limitations. Presently, real-time 3D imaging during SE is likely to be most valuable for pharmacologic stress testing with images obtained at baseline and peak stress.[12]

The results of SE are critically dependent on proper image acquisition and display. Each accredited echocardiography laboratory should conduct quality review and improvement initiatives. Specifically, in regard to image acquisition, for all sonographers who perform SE, a peer review of 5 to 10 studies should be conducted each year to ensure adherence to the protocol for image acquisition.[2]

Please access ExpertConsult to view the corresponding videos for this chapter.

Acknowledgment

The authors acknowledge the contributions of Dr. David Dudzinski, who was the author of this chapter in the previous edition.

REFERENCES

1. Pellikka PA, Arruda-Olson A, Chaudhry FA, et al. Guidelines for performance, interpretation and application of stress echocardiography in ischemic heart disease. *J Am Soc Echocardiogr*. 2020;33:1–41.
2. Picard MH, Adams D, Bierig SM, et al. American Society of Echocardiography recommendations for quality echocardiography laboratory operations. *J Am Soc Echocardiogr*. 2011;24:1–10.
3. Porter TR, Mulvagh SL, Abdelmoneim SS, et al. Clinical applications of ultrasonic enhancing agents in echocardiography. *J Am Soc Echocardiogr*. 2018;31:241–274.
4. Lancellotti P, Pellikka PA, Budts W, et al. The clinical use of stress echocardiography in non-ischaemic heart disease. *J Am Soc Echocardiogr*. 2017;30:101–138.
5. Pierard LA, Lancellotti P. Stress testing in valve disease. *Heart*. 2007;93:766–772.
6. Reis G, Motta MS, Barbosa MM, et al. Dobutamine stress echocardiography for noninvasive assessment and risk stratification of patients with rheumatic mitral stenosis. *J Am Coll Cardiol*. 2004;43:393–401.
7. Marechaux S, Hachicha Z, Bellouin A, et al. Usefulness of exercise-stress echocardiography for risk stratification of true asymptomatic patients with aortic valve stenosis. *Eur Heart J*. 2010;31:1390–1397.
8. Yared K, Lam KM, Hung J. The use of exercise echocardiography in the evaluation of mitral regurgitation. *Curr Cardiol Rev*. 2009;5:312–322.
9. Baumgartner H, Hung J, Bermejo J, et al. Recommendations on the echocardiographic assessment of aortic valve stenosis. *J Am Soc Echocardiogr*. 2017;30:372–392.
10. Donal E, Bergerot C, Thibault H, et al. Influence of afterload on left ventricular radial and longitudinal systolic functions: a two-dimensional strain imaging study. *Eur J Echocardiogr*. 2009;10:914–921.
11. Farsalinos KE, Daraban AM, Unlu S, et al. Head-to-head comparison of global longitudinal strain measurements among nine different vendors. *J Am Soc Echocardiogr*. 2015;28:1171–1181.
12. Berbarie RF, Dib E, Ahmad M. Stress echocardiography using real-time three-dimensional imaging. *Echocardiography*. 2018;35:1196–1203.

---

53 Stress Echocardiography: Prognosis

Jay Ramchand, Allan L. Klein

Stress echocardiography (SE), first introduced in 1979, was initially introduced for the detection of obstructive coronary artery disease (CAD). The underlying principle is that ischemic myocardium is unable to augment in function during stress. The severity and distribution of myocardial ischemia in turn determine the extent and severity of wall motion abnormalities (WMAs) detected during SE. Although initially introduced primarily for the detection of CAD, over the years, applications of SE has expanded. Beyond its role in the identification of obstructive CAD, SE can also provide prognostic information in valvular heart disease,[1,2] diastolic heart failure,[3] and after myocardial infarction (MI) and can also provide cardiovascular risk evaluation before noncardiac surgery.

EVALUATION FOR OBSTRUCTIVE CORONARY ARTERY DISEASE

In the evaluation of CAD, exercise and pharmacologic SE add incremental prognostic information to predict the occurrence of adverse cardiovascular events compared with clinical, rest echocardiographic, and exercise electrocardiographic (ECG) characteristics alone.

Exercise Echocardiography

In a cohort of 5798 individuals who underwent exercise echocardiography for evaluation of known or suspected CAD, workload

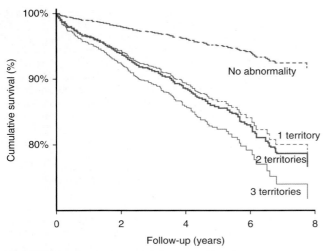

Figure 53.1. Survival curves showing worsening outcomes with increasing functional abnormalities ($P < .001$). (Reproduced with permission from Marwick TH, et al. Prediction of mortality using dobutamine echocardiography. *J Am Coll Cardiol.* 2001; 37(3):754–760.)

BOX 53.1 Variables Associated With Adverse Outcomes

- Reduced baseline LV function
- Inducible ischemia
  - Extensive
  - Low ischemic threshold
  - In LAD coronary artery territory
  - Prolonged duration of wall motion abnormality
- Poor EF response
- WMSI> 1
- Failure to reduce end-systolic volume or transient LV cavity enlargement
- RV wall motion abnormalities
- LVH hypertrophy
- Enlarged LA at baseline
- Exercise related variables
  - Exercise-induced angina
  - Low peak or fall in systolic blood pressure with exercise
  - Chronotropic incompetence
  - Slow heart rate recovery

EF, Ejection fraction; *LA,* left atrium; *LAD,* left anterior descending coronary artery; *LV,* left ventricular; *LVH,* left ventricular hypertrophy; *RV,* right ventricular; *WMSI,* wall motion score index.

---

and exercise wall motion score index had the strongest association with outcomes that included cardiac death or nonfatal MI.[4] Although other studies have shown stress testing to be less sensitive and specific in women, this study demonstrated similar prognostic value of exercise echocardiography in men and women.[4] Notably, the incremental value of SE in predicting adverse outcomes (death or nonfatal MI) has also been subsequently demonstrated across various subset of patients, including older adults (65 years of age or older),[5] after coronary bypass surgery,[6] and in those with diabetes.[7] In a study of 5375 individuals, the prognostic value of SE appeared most useful in patients with intermediate-risk Duke treadmill scores with exercise echocardiography further substratifying patients into groups with a yearly mortality rate between 2% to 7%.[8] An example of an abnormal stress echocardiogram is shown in Video 53.1.

Pharmacologic Stress Echocardiography

In a large-scale ($n = 7333$), multicenter prospective study, pharmacologic SE with either dipyridamole or dobutamine predicted a significantly better outcome for individuals with a negative pharmacologic SE test result compared with those with a positive test result (92 vs 71.2%; $P < .01$).[9] Furthermore, a negative test result was associated with an estimated mortality of less than 1% per year on long-term (200-month) follow-up. In another study of 3156 individuals who underwent dobutamine SE, individuals with both ischemic and scar or those with increasing number of functional abnormalities had an increased mortality rate (Fig. 53.1).[10]

Although pharmacologic SE has a significant prognostic role, poor exercise capacity is recognized to be one of the most powerful determinants of adverse prognosis, and hence when possible, exercise echocardiography should be performed. Furthermore, the performance of exercise rather than pharmacologic SE allows the complementary use of other exercise-related adverse risk markers such as exercise-induced angina, low peak or fall in systolic blood pressure with exercise, chronotropic incompetence, or slow heart rate recovery.

Prognosis of a Negative Stress Echocardiogram in the Current Era

Several lines of evidence confirm that normal exercise or pharmacologic stress echocardiograms confer a benign prognosis (mortality rate <1% per year) over long-term follow up. Importantly, a basic axiom of noninvasive testing is that the utility of the test depends on the pretest probability of the population tested, limiting the reliability of the aforementioned benign prognosis in those with a negative test result. Indeed, the importance of conditional probability still holds true in a seemingly low-risk population with a negative stress echocardiogram result. Increasing age and high-risk features such as the Duke treadmill score (low risk score: >= +5; moderate risk score: −10 + 4; high risk score: <= −11) still predict adverse events independent of SE findings. Thus particular care needs to be made when dealing with these three groups of patients:[11]

1. Patients with an increased pretest probability
2. Patients with a negative result at submaximal heart rate (<85% age-predicted maximum heartrate or <6 MET [metabolic equivalents]) reflecting that the heart was insufficiently stressed to become ischemic
3. Patients with a possible false-negative stress echocardiogram results in whom a wall motion may have been missed (e.g., those with angina or ischemic ECG findings)

The increasing risk profile in patients being referred for SE also begs the question of whether the changing population of patients undergoing the test has affected the prognostic value of a normal test result. Cortigiani and colleagues retrospectively analyzed outcomes of 5817 patients with no ischemia on exercise or pharmacologic SE.[12] They found an increase in mean age of patients increased across the decades, as well as increase in the rate of diabetes mellitus, hypertension, and the use of antianginal medications over the four decades from 1983 to 2016. This was accompanied by a decrease in the prognostic value of a negative SE from a mortality rate of 0.5% in the 1980s to 1.7% in the current decade.[12] Because the quality of echocardiographic images and the detection of regional WMA with the use of intravenous contrast have significantly improved over this time period, one can surmise that the decline in the prognostic value of a negative test result is mainly due to the increased risk profile of CAD in this patient population altering the negative predictive value of the test.

Multiple SE parameters have been used for risk stratification and prognosis. Box 53.1 lists some of the variables associated with adverse outcomes, though detailed discussion of individual parameters is covered elsewhere.

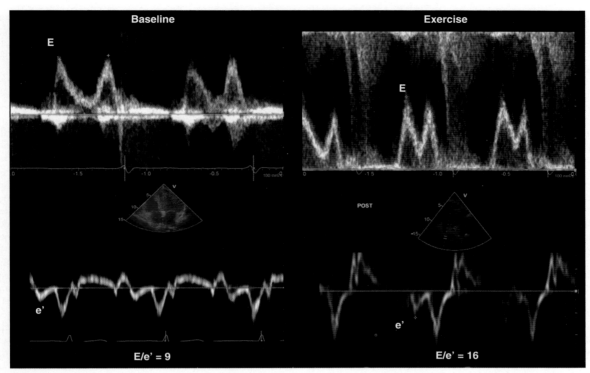

Figure 53.2. Mitral inflow and annular velocity at rest and immediately after recovery in a 66-year-old woman referred for assessment of exertional dyspnea. At baseline, the mitral inflow pattern demonstrated abnormal relaxation with normal range E/e'. After 4 minutes of exercise, E/e' increased significantly.

PROGNOSTIC IMPLICATIONS OF THE DIASTOLIC STRESS TEST

In patients with dyspnea with no other clear cause, there has been emerging interest in the assessment of exercise-induced diastolic dysfunction using diastolic SE. It is particularly useful in individuals with suspected heart failure but with preserved resting ejection fraction and no definite diastolic abnormalities at rest. Exercise using a supine bicycle is the recommended modality for diastolic SE because it allows the acquisition of Doppler recordings throughout the test and the noninvasive assessment of exercise diastolic function reserve.[13] A study is abnormal when the average E/E' is greater than 14, e' velocity is less than 7 cm/s (lateral e'<10 cm/s), and peak tricuspid regurgitant velocity is greater than 2.8 m/s.[13] Treadmill exercise SE is an alternative to supine bicycle testing because diastolic abnormalities may persist after exercise, and there is accumulating evidence between the association of SE-related diastolic abnormalities and adverse cardiovascular outcomes. An example of an abnormal diastolic stress test result is shown in Fig. 53.2.

In a prospective Australian study of 2201 individuals who underwent exercise SE, 68 patients (3%) had a nonischemic positive diastolic stress test (pretest E/e'<12, postexercise E/e' >12).[14] On Cox proportional hazards analysis, this was found to be highly predictive (hazard ratio [HR], 4.2), but a high pre-exercise E/e' was not predictive of future heart failure events. The findings suggest the diagnostic value of diastolic stress testing, though interventional trials to attenuate the adverse prognosis associated with an abnormal diastolic stress test are needed.

In another study of 522 patients who underwent diastolic SE, after a median follow-up period of 13.2 months, patients with isolated raised exercise E/e' and isolated ischemia had similar rates of cardiovascular hospitalizations.[15] In a Mayo clinic registry of 14,446 individuals who underwent treadmill SE, elevation in

exercise E/e' was a strong predictor of all-cause mortality, even in the absence of ischemia.[16]

STRESS ECHOCARDIOGRAPHY IN HYPERTROPHIC CARDIOMYOPATHY

In patients with hypertrophic cardiomyopathy (HCM), exercise SE is safe and can be useful to assess inducible left ventricular outflow tract obstruction (LVOTO) before septal-reducing therapy. Echocardiographic markers of worse prognosis or poor exercise tolerance include exercise LVOTO (>50 mm Hg), blunted systolic or diastolic reserve, dynamic increase in mitral regurgitation (MR), increase in E/e', and elevated pulmonary artery systolic pressure with exercise.[13] Despite the association of symptoms with LVOTO in HCM, there are a subset of patients with high resting intraventricular gradients at rest without significant symptoms. In a study of 107 patients with HCM, 38 had a significant gradient, 9 of whom exhibited a paradoxical reduction in gradient by at least 30 mm Hg during exercise.[17] These patients had significantly lower New York Heart Association clinical class and exhibited a trend toward lower cardiac events than patients in whom the gradient increased or did not change during SE.[17]

In a cohort of 426 individuals who were asymptomatic or minimally symptomatic, exercise capacity, not LV outflow tract gradient, was found to predict long-term outcomes that included a composite of death, appropriate internal defibrillator discharge, and admission for congestive heart failure.[18]

STRESS ECHOCARDIOGRAPHY TO GUIDE RISK EVALUATION BEFORE MAJOR NONCARDIAC SURGERY

Cardiovascular complications are an important cause of perioperative morbidity and mortality. In the nonemergent setting, the first step in perioperative cardiac assessment should include of perioperative risk on combined clinical or surgical risk evaluation of cardiovascular using a multitude of available simple risk scores. Patients undergoing low-risk surgery without high-risk factors (e.g., angina, previous MI, diabetes) are at low risk of perioperative events (<1%), and no further testing is recommended. In those with heightened risk of events (>1%), further assessment of exercise capacity is needed. In individuals with poor (<4 MET) or unknown exercise capacity, pharmacologic SE may be appropriate, particularly if it is indicated even if an individual was not having surgery.

In a cohort of 530 patients undergoing preoperative dobutamine SE before nonvascular surgery, ischemia occurring at less than 60% of age-predicted maximal heart rate was associated with highest risk of postoperative events (43%), and ischemia occurring at an ischemic threshold 60% or greater was associated with moderate risk of events (9%).[19] Importantly, in this cohort of patients with known or suspected CAD, the event rate was 0% in those with a negative test result, suggesting that further testing cannot be justified on prognostic grounds in this context.

In patients undergoing preoperative dobutamine SE, submaximal attainment of target heart rate (<85% maximum predicted) is common. In a study of 397 individuals, this occurred in 16% of individuals. Importantly, there may still be prognostic value despite this because the investigators found the overall negative predictive value for perioperative MI was high (98%) independent of attainment of target heart rate.[20]

Despite studies showing a clear relationship between the degree of myocardial ischemia found on preoperative SE majorly influences perioperative risk, there is no evidence to suggest prophylactic revascularization before surgery improves outcomes.

PROGNOSTIC ROLE OF STRESS ECHOCARDIOGRAPHY IN VALVULAR HEART DISEASE

Echocardiography in the assessment of valvular heart disease has traditionally been performed at rest. The complex interplay of heart rate, myocardial response, and loading conditions during exercise can affect the hemodynamic significance of a given valvular abnormality. Thus, SE is uniquely placed to allow the dynamic assessment of valvular function under hemodynamic stress while concurrently allowing the assessment of myocardial contractile response. The utility of stress testing is particularly valuable in those with apparent symptoms because they may be unmasked with exercise.

In patients with asymptomatic mitral stenosis, reduced compliance of the left atrium may lead to a rise in pulmonary artery pressure during exercise. The prognostic information of exercise induced pulmonary hypertension was recently assessed in 515 patients with asymptomatic patients with native or prosthetic mitral stenosis who underwent exercise SE.[2] Higher peak-stress right ventricular (RV) systolic pressure was expectedly associated with impaired exercise capacity, but importantly, it was also associated with a higher mortality rate (HR, 1.35). Furthermore, invasive mitral procedures were associated with improved survival in this seemingly asymptomatic cohort.

In apparently asymptomatic individuals with primary MR, exercise echocardiography may be used to induce symptoms and be useful to assess the systolic pulmonary artery pressure (sPAP) response and stratify risk. Exercise SE may also be reasonable in symptomatic patients with at least moderate MR. The increase in MR severity (>1 grade), dynamic pulmonary hypertension (sPAP >60 mm Hg), the absence of contractile reserve (<5% increase in ejection fraction or <2% increment in global longitudinal strain), and a limited RV contractile recruitment (quantified by tricuspid annular plane systolic excursion <18 mm) are all indicators of poor prognosis.[13]

In secondary MR, increased sPAP greater than 60 mm Hg was also a determinant (HR, 3.3) for adverse cardiovascular events (a composite of cardiac-related death, heart failure decompensation, need for cardiac resynchronization therapy or implantable cardiac defibrillator, or heart transplant).[21] Exercise-induced increase in estimated regurgitant orifice area (≥13 mm²) has also been shown to be a predictor of cardiac death.[22]

Patients with low-flow low-gradient aortic stenosis are considered to have true-severe stenosis when the mean gradient (MG) is 40 mm Hg or greater with an aortic valve area (AVA) 1 cm² or less during dobutamine SE. More recently, however, in an evaluation of 186 patients with low-flow low-gradient aortic stenosis, peak stress MG 40 mm Hg or greater, peak stress AVA 1 cm² or greater, and the combination, poorly classified AS severity compared to surgical classification or aortic valve calcium assessment by computed tomography (correctly classified in 48%, 60%, and 47% of patients, respectively).[23] Instead, calculation of the projected AVA, which is an estimate of the AVA at a standardized normal flow rate (250 mL/s), better distinguishes true-severe AS from pseudo-severe AS and was strongly associated with mortality in patients under conservative management (HR, 3.65).[23] In low-flow low-gradient aortic stenosis, absence of flow reserve (defined as <20% stroke volume increase) has in the past been associated with markedly poor outcomes. More recent studies, however, have not demonstrated any significant prognostic value of flow reserve,[23,24] and for this reason, this parameter should not be used to guide decision making.

The role of SE in the assessment of aortic insufficiency is less well established, especially because neither exercise nor pharmacologic SE can be used to reclassify aortic regurgitation severity with stress because the test-induced increase in heart rate shortens diastole and limits quantification of aortic insufficiency severity. In those without symptoms, lack of contractile reserve (<5% change in left ventricular ejection fraction) was found to predict the development of LV systolic dysfunction at follow-up or postoperatively.[25]

Please access ExpertConsult to view the corresponding videos for this chapter.

REFERENCES

1. Goublaire C, Melissopoulou M, Lobo D, et al. Prognostic value of exercise-stress echocardiography in asymptomatic patients with aortic valve stenosis. *JACC Cardiovasc Imag.* 2018;11:787–795.
2. Gentry 3rd JL, Parikh PK, Alashi A, et al. Characteristics and outcomes in a contemporary group of patients with suspected significant mitral stenosis undergoing treadmill stress echocardiography. *Circ Cardiovasc Imag.* 2019;12:e009062.
3. Kosmala W, Przewlocka-Kosmala M, Rojek A, et al. Comparison of the diastolic stress test with a combined resting echocardiography and biomarker approach to patients with exertional dyspnea: diagnostic and prognostic implications. *JACC Cardiovasc Imaging.* 2019;12:771–780.
4. Arruda-Olson AM, Juracan EM, Mahoney DW, et al. Prognostic value of exercise echocardiography in 5,798 patients: is there a gender difference? *J Am Coll Cardiol.* 2002;39:625–631.
5. Arruda AM, Das MK, Roger VL, et al. Prognostic value of exercise echocardiography in 2,632 patients > or = 65 years of age. *J Am Coll Cardiol.* 2001;37:1036–1041.
6. Arruda AM, McCully RB, Oh JK, et al. Prognostic value of exercise echocardiography in patients after coronary artery bypass surgery. *Am J Cardiol.* 2001;87:1069–1073.
7. Elhendy A, Arruda AM, Mahoney DW, et al: Prognostic stratification of diabetic patients by exercise echocardiography, *J Am Coll Cardiol.* 37:1551–1557.
8. Marwick TH, Case C, Vasey C, et al. Prediction of mortality by exercise echocardiography: a strategy for combination with the duke treadmill score. *Circulation.* 2001;103:2566–2571.
9. Sicari R, Pasanisi E, Venneri L, et al. Stress echo results predict mortality: a large-scale multicenter prospective international study. *J Am Coll Cardiol.* 2003;41:589–595.
10. Marwick TH, Case C, Sawada S, et al. Prediction of mortality using dobutamine echocardiography. *J Am Coll Cardiol.* 2001;37:754–760.
11. Marwick TH. *Stress Echocardiography.* Cham, Switzerland: Springer; 2018.
12. Cortigiani L, Urluescu ML, Coltelli M, et al. Apparent declining prognostic value of a negative stress echocardiography based on regional wall motion abnormalities in patients with normal resting left ventricular function due to the changing referral profile of the population under study. *Circ Cardiovasc Imag.* 2019;12:e008564.
13. Lancellotti P, Pellikka PA, Budts W, et al. The clinical use of stress echocardiography in non-ischaemic heart disease: recommendations from the European Association of Cardiovascular Imaging and the American Society of Echocardiography. *J Am Soc Echocardiogr.* 2017;30:101–138.

14. Fitzgerald BT, Presneill JJ, Scalia IG, et al. The prognostic value of the diastolic stress test in patients undergoing treadmill stress echocardiography. *J Am Soc Echocardiogr.* 2019;32:1298–1306.
15. Holland DJ, Prasad SB, Marwick TH. Prognostic implications of left ventricular filling pressure with exercise. *Circ Cardiovasc Imag.* 2010;3:149–156.
16. Luong CL, Padang R, Oh JK, Pellikka PA, McCully RB, Kane GC. Assessment of left ventricular filling pressure with exercise is independently associated with all-cause mortality in a cohort of 14,446 patients, B6-7; Present at the 2019 American Society of Echocardiography 30th Annual Scientific Sessions.
17. Lafitte S, Reant P, Touche C, et al. Paradoxical response to exercise in asymptomatic hypertrophic cardiomyopathy: a new description of outflow tract obstruction dynamics. *J Am Coll Cardiol.* 2013;62:842–850.
18. Desai MY, Bhonsale A, Patel P, et al. Exercise echocardiography in asymptomatic HCM: exercise capacity, and not LV outflow tract gradient predicts long-term outcomes. *JACC Cardiovasc Imag.* 2014;7:26–36.
19. Das MK, Pellikka PA, Mahoney DW, et al: Assessment of cardiac risk before nonvascular surgery: dobutamine stress echocardiography in 530 patients, J Am Coll Cardiol 35:1647–1653.
20. Labib SB, Goldstein M, Kinnunen PM, et al: Cardiac events in patients with negative maximal versus negative submaximal dobutamine echocardiograms undergoing noncardiac surgery: importance of resting wall motion abnormalities, *J Am Coll Cardiol.* 44:82–87.
21. Lancellotti P, Magne J, Dulgheru R, et al. Clinical significance of exercise pulmonary hypertension in secondary mitral regurgitation. *Am J Cardiol.* 2015;115:1454–1461.
22. Lancellotti P, Troisfontaines P, Toussaint AC, et al. Prognostic importance of exercise-induced changes in mitral regurgitation in patients with chronic ischemic left ventricular dysfunction. *Circulation.* 2003;108:1713–1717.
23. Annabi MS, Touboul E, Dahou A, et al. Dobutamine stress echocardiography for management of low-flow, low-gradient aortic stenosis. *J Am Coll Cardiol.* 2018;71:475–485.
24. Sato K, Sankaramangalam K, Kandregula K, et al. Contemporary outcomes in low-gradient aortic stenosis patients who underwent dobutamine stress echocardiography. *J Am Heart Assoc.* 2019;8:e011168.
25. Wahi S, Haluska B, Pasquet A, et al. Exercise echocardiography predicts development of left ventricular dysfunction in medically and surgically treated patients with asymptomatic severe aortic regurgitation. *Heart.* 2000;84:606–614.

54 Echocardiography for the Assessment of Myocardial Viability in Ischemic Cardiomyopathy

Federico M. Asch, Julio A. Panza

INTRODUCTION AND GENERAL CONCEPTS

There has been a dramatic change in the acute presentation, chronic consequences, and mode of death related to coronary artery disease (CAD) in the past few decades. The rapid recognition of acute coronary syndromes and increased availability and utilization of percutaneous coronary interventions have led to a reduction in sudden cardiac death and early in-hospital mortality rates, with a resulting increase in the prevalence of chronic left ventricular (LV) systolic dysfunction and in the presentation of heart failure in patients with ischemic cardiomyopathy.[1,2] Accordingly, there has been increasing interest in the mechanisms that determine LV dysfunction in these patients with a focus on the possibility of its reversal with revascularization. In this regard, impaired myocardial contraction in patients with CAD may be either a consequence of irreversibly damaged myocardium—as a result of previous infarction—or an expression of viable but dysfunctional myocardium that has the potential to recover its contractility with revascularization.

Two basic mechanisms of chronic systolic dysfunction in myocardial segments with underlying viability have been proposed.[3,4] The term *myocardial stunning* refers to myocardium that has suffered an acute ischemic insult with subsequent restoration of blood flow is still "alive" and will therefore recover its force of contraction unless another ischemic insult ensues.[5] Although typically this mechanism applies to acute coronary syndromes with rapid reperfusion, the possibility of chronic systolic dysfunction as a consequence of repeated episodes of ischemia in myocardial segments with preserved resting blood flow but critically reduced flow reserve has been described as *repetitive stunning*. The term *myocardial hibernation*, on the other hand, has been used to describe a more chronic state of decreased myocardial contraction accompanying a critical reduction in myocardial blood flow.[3] In this paradigm, systolic dysfunction is an adaptive process to reset the degree of contraction to match the level of reduced myocardial blood flow.[6] As a result, there is a steady state of matched myocardial perfusion and function that allows the myocyte to remain viable. The ischemic myocardium presents various tissue abnormalities that can result in impaired contractile function: damaged contractile apparatus, decreased myocardial metabolism, impaired mitochondrial or membrane integrity, or even replacement of myocardial tissue by fibrosis after myocardial cell death.

Importantly, both described mechanisms of chronic systolic dysfunction in the presence of viable myocardium (i.e., repetitive stunning and hibernation) are amenable to improvement with revascularization. Thus, in the case of repetitive stunning, successful revascularization would lead to increase in the coronary flow reserve, hence abating the episodes of myocardial ischemia and allowing for recovery of contractile function. On the other hand, restoration of resting myocardial blood flow with revascularization would similarly allow for restoration of systolic dysfunction in the paradigm of hibernating myocardium.

As can be surmised from the description of these proposed mechanisms, the concept of myocardial viability in ischemic cardiomyopathy is tightly linked to reduced coronary perfusion and to the potential for recovery of systolic function with successful revascularization. It is this potential that has led to the concept that unveiling myocardial viability in segments with systolic dysfunction is necessary to identify patients with ischemic cardiomyopathy that are most likely to benefit from revascularization. Because clinical and electrocardiographic criteria to detect myocardial viability have limited accuracy,[7,8] the in-depth assessment of dysfunctional but viable myocardium requires dedicated tests.

ASSESSMENT OF MYOCARDIAL VIABILITY BY ECHOCARDIOGRAPHY

Myocardial segments that are akinetic or dyskinetic, thinned (<5 mm of wall thickness), and hyperechogenic (bright by ultrasound) in a resting echocardiogram are likely to be scarred and therefore unable to recover their function. In the absence of these features, more specific testing can be done with dobutamine echocardiography (DE), myocardial strain, myocardial perfusion with ultrasound-enhancing agents, or a combination of them to distinguish myocardial scar from viable but dysfunctional myocardium.

Dobutamine Echocardiography

The evaluation of contractile response to the intravenous (IV) infusion of incremental doses of dobutamine has been the most widely used and accepted echocardiographic technique for detection of myocardial viability. In the typical DE protocol, two-dimensional echocardiographic images are obtained in the parasternal long- and short-axis views and in the apical four- and two-chamber views to properly visualize all myocardial segments at rest and during incremental doses of dobutamine, starting at 2.5 or 5 µg/kg/min and increasing to 20 and up to 40 µg/kg/min in 3- to 5-minutes stages.[9] Starting at low doses is critical because at this stage, the inotropic effect of dobutamine is more prominent than its chronotropic effect, which in turn facilitates evaluation of the contractile response without the tachycardia associated with higher doses that may lead to ischemia and thus blunt the expected increase in contraction of viable segments. This specific property, together with its short half-life (2–3 minutes) and negligible effect on β2 receptors, explains the choice of dobutamine as the adrenergic agent of choice to assess myocardial viability with echocardiography or other imaging modalities. Segmental wall motion and myocardial thickening are assessed at baseline and at each stage of dobutamine infusion and qualified as normal, hypokinesis, akinesis, or dyskinesis (Fig. 54.1A). Segments with normal baseline contractility are considered viable. Myocardial segments with baseline dysfunction (hypokinesis, akinesis, or dyskinesis) are considered viable when they show increased systolic wall thickening in response to inotropic stimulation provided by the dobutamine infusion. Three different patterns in the contractile response to dobutamine have been described as associated with myocardial viability, namely, (1) biphasic response (improvement at lower doses followed by worsening of contraction at higher doses), (2) sustained improvement (improvement at lower doses without worsening of contraction at higher doses), or (3) worsening contractility with incremental doses of dobutamine in segments with hypokinesis at rest. Accuracy for predicting contractile recovery after revascularization is highest for segments with biphasic responses.[10] Dysfunctional segments without appreciable change in contraction or thickening during infusion of dobutamine are considered not viable (Fig. 54.1B). On a per-patient level, the threshold used to define presence or absence of viability may vary, but in general, a patient with five or more dysfunctional but viable segments is considered to have significant viability. An example of DE viability assessment can be seen in Video 54.1, with a postrevascularization resting echocardiogram in Video 54.5.

Other Echocardiographic Techniques

Although not directly evaluating viability, contrast echocardiography can improve wall motion evaluation and thus enhance the performance of classic DE protocols. Myocardial contrast echocardiography has also been proposed as a method to identify viable myocardium. This technique, described in more detail in other chapters, requires IV injection of ultrasound-enhancing agents and specific imaging settings (very low ultrasound myocardial index [<0.2] and harmonic imaging, parameters that are variable and specific for each contrast manufacturer).[11] Nevertheless, its use in clinical practice has been limited.

Myocardial strain echocardiography quantifies global and segmental systolic function and has been proposed as a method to improve the sensitivity of B-mode echocardiography in detecting viability in segments with contractile dysfunction.[12] However, limited data are available to date to support its use in the evaluation of viability.

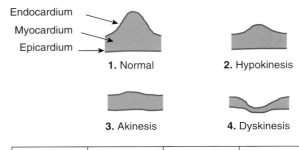

Figure 54.1. Evaluation and definition of viability by dobutamine echocardiography. *Upper panel,* Schematic of the scoring used to grade resting wall motion. *Lower panel,* Schematic of the possible myocardial thickening responses to dobutamine in myocardial segments with resting hypokinesis (responses A, C, and D could also be observed in segments with resting akinesis). Whereas segments with responses A, B, and C are considered as viable, response D is considered nonviable. A patient is considered to have significant myocardial viability if 5 or more segments are considered viable (16-segment model).

COMPARISON OF METHODS USED FOR VIABILITY TESTING

Different imaging modalities identify myocardial viability from myocardial scar based on very distinct methodological approaches. Thus, as already described, the myocardial response to dobutamine infusion visualized with echocardiography evaluates the contractile reserve to inotropic stimulation. On the other hand, nuclear tests evaluate perfusion and metabolism (in the case of positron emission tomography [PET])[13] and membrane integrity (in the case of single-photo emission computed tomography [SPECT]),[14] whereas cardiac magnetic resonance imaging (CMRI) with late gadolinium enhancement (LGE) detects increased extracellular space (specifically, scar or fibrotic replacement of necrotic myocardial tissue).[15] Despite the differences in the methodology of these techniques, previously published studies have provided strong support for the concept that dysfunctional but viable myocardium can be assessed with similar degrees of accuracy by DE, PET, and radionuclide SPECT perfusion studies, with sensitivities and specificities fluctuating in relation to the reference standard adopted.[16–18] The regional improvement of segmental ventricular dysfunction has been the most commonly used endpoint to assess viability in these studies.

Pooled data from 11 head-to-head studies showed a higher sensitivity for nuclear imaging (PET and SPECT) than for DE (90% vs 74%, respectively). However, DE had a higher specificity of 78% compared with 57% for nuclear imaging.[19] Overall, the original reports included small number of patients, with variable criteria for

TABLE 54.1 Comparison of Various Imaging Techniques for Detection of Hibernating Myocardium

Technique	Studies (n)	Patients (n)	Mean EF (%)	Sensitivity (%)	Specificity (%)
DE: total	41	1421	25–48	80	78
Low-dose DE	33	1121	25–48	79	78
High-dose DE	8	290	29–38	83	79
Myocardial contrast echocardiography: total	10	268	29–38	87	50
Thallium sonography: total	40	1119	23–45	87	54
Thallium-201	28	776	23–45	87	56
Thallium-201 reinjection	12	343	31–49	87	50
Technetium scintigraphy: total	25	721	23–54	83	65
Without nitrate protocol	17	516	23–52	83	57
With nitrate protocol	8	205	35–54	81	69
PET: total	24	756	23–53	92	63
CMRI: total	14	450	24–53	80	70
Low-dose dobutamine protocol	9	272	24–53	74	82
Late gadolinium-enhancement protocol	5	178	32–52	84	63

CMRI, Cardiovascular magnetic resonance imaging; *DE*, dobutamine echocardiography; *EF*, ejection fraction; *PET*, positron emission tomography.
Reproduced with permission from Shah BN, et al: The hibernating myocardium: current concepts, diagnostic dilemmas, and clinical challenges in the post-STICH era, *Eur Heart J* 34:1323–1336, 2013.

assessment of viability, even within the same imaging method. This latter factor may importantly influence the diagnostic and predictive accuracy of any technique. Qureshi and colleagues demonstrated that the sensitivity and specificity of both rest–redistribution thallium-201 tomography and DE depends on the criteria used to assess thallium uptake and the combination of responses used to judge the effect of dobutamine.[20] It has been shown, however, that DE predicts functional recovery after revascularization irrespective of the perfusion pattern shown on thallium scintigraphy.[21] A head-to-head study of thallium scintigraphy and DE showed that the former method detects viability in a greater number of segments compared to DE.[22] The different mechanisms of identifying viable myocardium with each technique may explain this apparent discrepancy. More specifically, the criteria used to determine myocardial viability with DE require the ability to respond to inotropic stimulation with increased contraction and therefore a relatively preserved mechanical apparatus within the myocyte. In contrast, the identification of viability with thallium scintigraphy only requires membrane integrity, thus explaining the lower threshold and, accordingly, the greater sensitivity of this method on a per-patient level to detect viable myocardium.

The use of CMRI with gadolinium (late enhancement 10–20 minutes after injection) for the evaluation of myocardial viability has a few advantages over nuclear and echocardiographic techniques and is now considered the most accurate method with increased use over the past several years because the ability to perform these studies has widely expanded. CMRI has higher spatial resolution (allows proper evaluation of transmurality) and allows for the detection of fibrotic tissue, therefore detecting scar (and by extension, considering viable any tissue that is not fibrosed). Despite its higher resolution, CMRI has similar sensitivity and specificity to that of nuclear techniques and DE (Table 54.1). Overall, contractile reserve with low-dose DE or dobutamine-CMRI offers the highest specificity for functional recovery (78 and 82% respectively), but nuclear (SPECT or PET) and CMRI with LGE have the highest sensitivity (ranging from 80%–90% for different protocols).[23] Importantly, neither head-to-head studies nor analyses of pooled data have conclusively shown the superiority of one technique over the others. Consequently, the choice of methodology for the assessment of myocardial viability in clinical practice largely rests on the local availability and expertise with a particular technique.

CLINICAL IMPLICATIONS

Previous studies have suggested that 40% to 50% of myocardial regions[24,25] and 25% to 40% of patients[26] with reduced LV

function may improve after revascularization. Several previous retrospective studies associated the presence of substantial amounts of viable myocardium with the clinical benefit of revascularization. Meta-analyses derived from data pooled from these studies advanced the concept that only patients with viable myocardium benefit from revascularization,[27] thus leading to the concept that the assessment of myocardial viability is essential for the decision regarding treatment. This tenet has formed the basis for the use of noninvasive studies to detect viable myocardium among patients with ischemic cardiomyopathy. However, studies that were prospectively designed to test the hypothesis that assessment of myocardial viability identifies patients with greater likelihood of benefiting from revascularization have consistently failed to show that this is indeed the case. In fact, a more recent meta-analysis highlights this striking difference: only the studies performed using retrospective data demonstrated that the use of methods to assess myocardial viability is critical for decision making regarding revascularization.[28]

Although determining presence or absence of myocardial viability may be a predictor of segmental and global improvement in LV systolic function, its role on clinical decision making and its impact on clinical outcomes are questionable based on the findings reported in the Positron emission tomography And Recovery following Revascularization phase 2 (PARR-2) study (using PET)[29] and the Surgical Treatment for Ischemic Heart Failure (STICH) viability substudy (using DE and SPECT).[30]

The recently published 10-year follow-up results of the STICH trial viability substudy[31] showed that the presence of viability predicted an improvement in EF regardless of the treatment arm to which patients were randomized. However, such improvement in LV function was not associated with better long-term outcomes. Most important, there was no statistically significant interaction between the presence of myocardial viability and the effect of surgical revascularization, as an addition to optimal medical therapy, on all-cause mortality.[31] Certain limitations of this study may limit the strength of its conclusions, including the relatively small number of patients that demonstrated absence of viable myocardium, the fact that only half of the overall STICH population was included in this substudy, and the lack of use of PET or CMRI that may be considered more accurate than the methods used in this study (SPECT and DE).

Whether newer imaging modalities (PET and CMRI) will provide better clinical decision-making options than "old-fashioned" viability imaging techniques is being investigated in the Alternative Imaging Modalities in Ischemic Heart Failure (AIMI-HF) trial.[32]

Please access ExpertConsult to view the corresponding videos for this chapter.

REFERENCES

1. Khera S, Kolte D, Palaniswamy C, et al. ST-elevation myocardial infarction in the elderly—Temporal trends in incidence, utilization of percutaneous coronary intervention and outcomes in the United States. *Int J Cardiol.* 2013;168:3683–3690.
2. Writing Group Members, Mozaffarian D, Benjamin EJ, et al. Heart disease and stroke statistics—2016 update: a report from the American Heart Association. *Circulation.* 2016;133:e38–360.
3. Rahimtoola SH. The hibernating myocardium. *Am Heart J.* 1989;117:211–221.
4. Rahimtoola SH. From coronary artery disease to heart failure: role of the hibernating myocardium. *Am J Cardiol.* 1995;75:16E–22E.
5. Baker CS, Rimoldi O, Camici PG, et al. Repetitive myocardial stunning in pigs is associated with the increased expression of inducible and constitutive nitric oxide synthases. *Cardiovasc Res.* 1999;43:685–697.
6. Ross J. Myocardial perfusion-contraction matching. Implications for coronary heart disease and hibernation. *Circulation.* 1991;83:1076–1083.
7. Asch FM, Shah S, Rattin C, et al. Lack of sensitivity of the electrocardiogram for detection of old myocardial infarction: a cardiac magnetic resonance imaging study. *Am Heart J.* 2006;152:742–748.
8. Haft JI, Hammoudeh AJ, Conte PJ. Assessing myocardial viability: correlation of myocardial wall motion abnormalities and pathologic Q waves with technetium 99m sestamibi single photon emission computed tomography. *Am Heart J.* 1995;130:994–998.
9. Panza JA, Curiel RV, Laurienzo JM, et al. Relation between ischemic threshold measured during dobutamine stress echocardiography and known indices of poor prognosis in patients with coronary artery disease. *Circulation.* 1995;92:2095–2101.
10. Afridi I, Kleiman NS, Raizner AE, et al. Dobutamine echocardiography in myocardial hibernation. Optimal dose and accuracy in predicting recovery of ventricular function after coronary angioplasty. *Circulation.* 1995;91:663–670.
11. Porter TR, Mulvagh SL, Abdelmoneim SS, et al. Clinical applications of ultrasonic enhancing agents in echocardiography: 2018 American Society of Echocardiography guidelines update. *J Am Soc Echocardiogr.* 2018;31:241–274.
12. Hanekom L, Jenkins C, Jeffries L, et al. Incremental value of strain rate analysis as an adjunct to wall-motion scoring for assessment of myocardial viability by dobutamine echocardiography: a follow-up study after revascularization. *Circulation.* 2005;112:3892–3900.
13. Knuesel PR, Nanz D, Wyss C, et al. Characterization of dysfunctional myocardium by positron emission tomography and magnetic resonance: relation to functional outcome after revascularization. *Circulation.* 2003;108:1095–1100.
14. Kiat H, Berman DS, Maddahi J, et al. Late reversibility of tomographic myocardial thallium-201 defects: an accurate marker of myocardial viability. *J Am Coll Cardiol.* 1988;12:1456–1463.
15. Kim RJ, Fieno DS, Parrish TB, et al. Relationship of MRI delayed contrast enhancement to irreversible injury, infarct age, and contractile function. *Circulation.* 1999;100:1992–2002.
16. Bax JJ, Wijns W, Cornel JH, et al. Accuracy of currently available techniques for prediction of functional recovery after revascularization in patients with left ventricular dysfunction due to chronic coronary artery disease: Comparison of pooled data. *J Am Coll Cardiol.* 1997;30:1451–1460.
17. Bonow RO. Identification of viable myocardium. *Circulation.* 1996;94:2674–2680.
18. Ragosta M, Beller GA, Watson DD, et al. Quantitative planar rest-redistribution 201Tl imaging in detection of myocardial viability and prediction of improvement in left ventricular function after coronary bypass surgery in patients with severely depressed left ventricular function. *Circulation.* 1993;87:1630–1641.
19. Bax JJ, Poldermans D, Elhendy A, et al. Sensitivity, specificity, and predictive accuracies of various noninvasive techniques for detecting hibernating myocardium. *Curr Problems Cardiol.* 2001;26:147–186.
20. Qureshi U, Nagueh SF, Afridi I, et al. Dobutamine echocardiography and quantitative rest-redistribution 201Tl tomography in myocardial hibernation. Relation of contractile reserve to 201Tl uptake and comparative prediction of recovery of function. *Circulation.* 1997;95:626–635.
21. Senior R, Lahiri A. Dobutamine echocardiography predicts functional outcome after revascularisation in patients with dysfunctional myocardium irrespective of the perfusion pattern on resting thallium-201 imaging. *Heart.* 1999;82:668–673.
22. Panza JA, Dilsizian V, Laurienzo JM, et al. Relation between thallium uptake and contractile response to dobutamine. Implications regarding myocardial viability in patients with chronic coronary artery disease and left ventricular dysfunction. *Circulation.* 1995;91:990–998.
23. Shah BN, Khattar RS, Senior R. The hibernating myocardium: current concepts, diagnostic dilemmas, and clinical challenges in the post-STICH era. *Eur Heart J.* 2013;34:1323–1336.
24. Brunken R, Tillisch J, Schwaiger M, et al. Regional perfusion, glucose metabolism, and wall motion in patients with chronic electrocardiographic Q wave infarctions: evidence for persistence of viable tissue in some infarct regions by positron emission tomography. *Circulation.* 1986;73:951–963.
25. Tillisch J, Brunken R, Marshall R, et al. Reversibility of cardiac wall-motion abnormalities predicted by positron tomography. *N Engl J Med.* 1986;314:884–888.
26. Elefteriades JA, Tolis G, Levi E, et al. Coronary artery bypass grafting in severe left ventricular dysfunction: excellent survival with improved ejection fraction and functional state. *J Am Coll Cardiol.* 1993;22:1411–1417.
27. Allman KC, Shaw LJ, Hachamovitch R, et al. Myocardial viability testing and impact of revascularization on prognosis in patients with coronary artery disease and left ventricular dysfunction: a meta-analysis. *J Am Coll Cardiol.* 2002;39:1151–1158.
28. Orlandini A, Castellana N, Pascual A, et al. Myocardial viability for decision-making concerning revascularization in patients with left ventricular dysfunction and coronary artery disease: a meta-analysis of non-randomized and randomized studies, *Int J Cardiol* 182:494–499.
29. Beanlands RS, Nichol G, Huszti E, et al. F-18-fluorodeoxyglucose positron emission tomography imaging-assisted management of patients with severe left ventricular dysfunction and suspected coronary disease: a randomized, controlled trial (PARR-2). *J Am Coll Cardiol.* 2007;50:2002–2012.
30. Bonow RO, Maurer G, Lee KL, et al. Myocardial viability and survival in ischemic left ventricular dysfunction. *N Engl J Med.* 2011;364:1617–1625.
31. Panza JA, Ellis AM, Al-Khalidi HR, et al. Myocardial viability and long-term outcomes in ischemic cardiomyopathy. *N Engl J Med.* 2019;381:739–748.
32. O'Meara E, Mielniczuk LM, Wells GA, et al. Alternative imaging modalities in ischemic heart failure (AIMI-HF) IMAGE HF Project I-A: study protocol for a randomized controlled trial. *Trials.* 2013;14:218.

55 Ultrasound-Enhanced Stress Echocardiography

Joan Olson, Feng Xie, Thomas R. Porter

ULTRASOUND-ENHANCING AGENTS FOR STRESS ECHOCARDIOGRAPHY

In the updated 2018 guidelines for ultrasound-enhancing agents (UEAs), it was recommended that UEAs be used whenever a coronary artery territory cannot be completely visualized on unenhanced echocardiography.[1] This becomes especially relevant during stress echocardiography (SE), when all segments must be visualized to adequately assess regional wall motion (WM) at rest and during any form of stress. Very low mechanical index (VLMI) imaging techniques (fundamental nonlinear imaging) have resulted in excellent visualization of basal, mid, and apical segments and are currently recommended for almost all UEA applications.[1,2] Use of UEAs when resting images are suboptimal has resulted in sensitivities and specificities for the detection of coronary artery disease

that are equivalent to echocardiograms performed in patients with optimal image quality.[3]

However, UEAs can also be used to examine myocardial perfusion with the same VLMI imaging techniques (available now on Philips, Siemens, Esoate, and General Electric ultrasound scanners). Perfusion imaging adds incremental value to resting WM assessment during pharmacologic SE with exercise, dobutamine, or vasodilator SE.[4] Perfusion imaging adds incremental predictive value to stress WM assessment.[5] Perfusion imaging during dobutamine or exercise SE also detects abnormalities that antedate wall motion abnormalities (WMAs) and helps delineate subendocardial wall thickening abnormalities that are induced even when overall transmural wall thickening appears normal (Table 55.1).[6] Compared with other perfusion imaging techniques, VLMI has high spatial and temporal resolution such that WM and

TABLE 55.1 Summary of Optimal Settings for Ultrasound Enhancement With Left Ventricular Opacification Versus Very Low Mechanical Index Imaging During Stress Echocardiography

	VLMI Imaging	LVO (Harmonic)
Frame rate (Hz)	20–25	>30
Mechanical index	<0.2 (very low)	<0.3 (low) but >0.2 MI or minimal contrast enhancement
Systems when available	Philips, Siemens, GE Healthcare, Esaote	All systems
Assess myocardial perfusion	Yes	No
Transmural wall motion enhancement	Yes	Yes
Subendocardial wall thickening	Yes	Not feasible
Use during treadmill or bicycle stress	Excellent (90%) Both WM and MP	Excellent (90%)
Significant CAD detection during vasodilator stress	Excellent (90%)	Reduced sensitivity (<70%)
CAD detection during dobutamine stress	Excellent (90%)	Good (80%)
Simultaneous analysis of wall motion and perfusion	Yes	No

CAD, Coronary artery disease, *LVO,* left ventricular opacification; *MP,* myocardial perfusion, *VLMI,* very low mechanical index; *WM,* wall motion.

TABLE 55.2 Perfusion Imaging Techniques

	MCE	MRI	SPECT or PET
Resolution (mm)	2–3	<2	5 (PET); 12 (SPECT)
Subendocardial Defects Detected	Yes	Yes	No
Cost	Low	High	High
Portability	Yes	Not possible	Minimal
Real-time perfusion>20 Hz frame rate	Yes	No	No
Availability	Extensive	Very limited	Limited
FDA-approved perfusion agent	Not Approved	Not approved	Approved
Radiation exposure	None	None	>10 m SV[a]

[a]Higher radiation exposure for thallium over technetium-based tracers; lower doses reported for D-single-photon emission computed tomography (SPECT) imaging and positron emission tomography (PET).

TABLE 55.3 Imaging Settings and Presets for Left ventricular Opacification and Very Low Mechanical Index Perfusion Imaging

	Presets for VLMI	Presets LVO
Depth	Depth: 140 mm	Depth: 140 mm
Focus	Focus: behind mitral valve level	Focus: behind mitral valve level
Contrast option	Contrast Option: Gen (1.5 MHz) CPS (Cadence Contrast Agent Imaging) General Electric: contrast setting Esaote: contrast key	LVO (contrast)
Gain and compression	Adjusted to ensure homogenous myocardial contrast and absence of myocardial signals after high-MI impulses	Adjusted to minimize background signals from the myocardium and valves (cavity bright and homogenous; myocardium dark)
High-MI impulse frame duration	2–5 frames at rest 5–20 frames during stress	N/A
Loop duration	Loop type: time (10 s) should include sufficient time to analyze replenishment after high-MI impulse	One cardiac cycle
High MI setting	>0.8 for high-MI impulses	All imaging at <0.3 MI but >0.2
Frame rate	20–25 Hz	>30 Hz
TGCs	TGCs are set in the middle ;on some systems, the near-field TGCs are adjusted slightly higher X5-1 on Philips requires less near-field gain adjustments	TGCs are set in the middle and adjusted slightly higher in the far field

LVO, Left ventricular opacification; *MI,* mechanical index; *N/A,* not applicable; *TGC,* time gain compensation; *VLMI,* very low mechanical index.

perfusion can be analyzed simultaneously. It also has lower cost than other perfusion imaging techniques (Table 55.2).

OPTIMIZING ULTRASOUND ENHANCEMENT DURING STRESS ECHOCARDIOGRAPHY

Optimal left ventricular opacification (LVO) during rest and SE can be achieved with either tissue harmonic imaging (THI) or real-time perfusion software on commercially available systems. For THI, the mechanical index (MI) should be set to less than 0.3

and time gain compensation (TGC) adjusted to create equivalent background contrast (Table 55.3). Tissue signals from valves and myocardium should be minimized. Real-time perfusion echocardiography (RTPE) is a VLMI imaging technique that permits real-time detection of myocardial contrast enhancement after either a small- (0.1- to 0.2-mL) bolus injection or continuous infusion of UEAs. If the MI is lowered to less than 0.2 while in THI, the contrast enhancement from microbubbles is reduced, resulting in minimal enhancement. Alternatively, RTPE is a multipulse tissue cancellation technique that is vendor specific (see Table 55.3).

Figure 55.1. Unenhanced apical four-chamber view (**A**) and enhanced image during a continuous infusion of an ultrasound-enhancing agent using fundamental nonlinear imaging (transmit, 1.8 MHz; receive, 1.8 MHz; **B**). The end-systolic images are obtained during replenishment of myocardial contrast at three seconds post high–mechanical index impulse. A basal anterolateral perfusion defect and wall thickening abnormality are evident *(arrows)*. (See corresponding Video 55.1.)

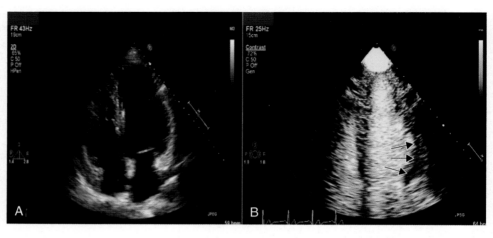

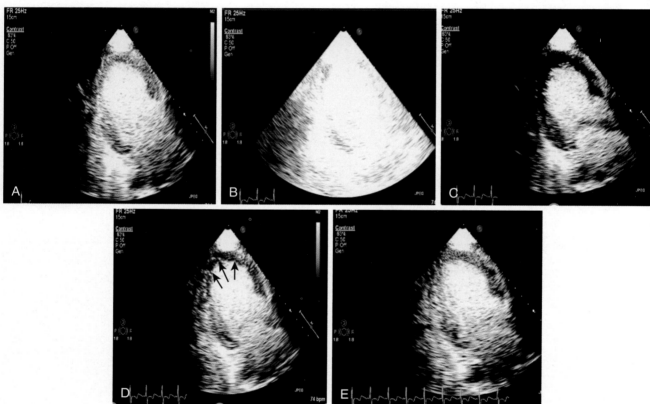

Figure 55.2. Resting images before and after high–mechanical index (MI) (flash) impulse at end-systole in a patient who had recurrent chest pain after coronary bypass surgery and was referred for stress echocardiography. The optimal high-MI impulse (**B**) results in clearance of myocardial contrast at end-systole without cavity destruction (**C**). At 2 seconds after high-MI impulse (**D**), there is a delay in replenishment in the anteroseptal, apical, and distal lateral segments *(black arrows)*. At 6 second after high-MI impulse (**E**), there is replenishment of myocardial contrast. This patient had occlusion of the graft to the left anterior descending at angiography. (See corresponding Video 55.2.)

Unlike THI, it is capable of enhancing the contrast produced from microbubbles at MIs below 0.2 and enhances both the myocardium and left ventricular (LV) cavity. It is effective for both small-bolus injections and for continuous infusions of UEAs. Because almost all RTPE systems analyze fundamental nonlinear signals, there is significantly less attenuation. A high-MI (termed "flash") impulse is delivered to clear the capillaries of microbubbles. The rate of replenishment of myocardial contrast and the plateau intensity are subsequently examined either visually or quantitatively. During the replenishment phase, regional WM in basal, mid, and distal segments can be analyzed with exquisite

sensitivity and is superior to THI techniques.[6] The VLMI imaging techniques are now the recommended imaging technique for optimal LVO and regional AM analysis.[1]

PHYSIOLOGIC BASIS FOR EXAMINING MYOCARDIAL PERFUSION WITH UEAs

Changes in myocardial blood flow can be analyzed by examining the replenishment of myocardial contrast after a high-MI impulse (Figs. 55.1 and 55.2; Videos 55.1 and 55.2). This concept was

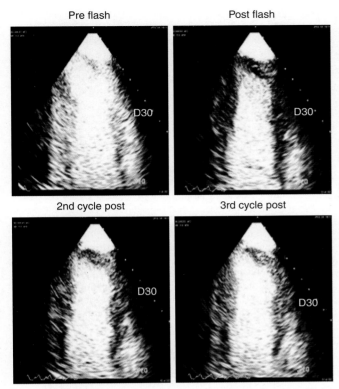

Pre flash   Post flash

D30   D30

2nd cycle post   3rd cycle post

D30   D30

Figure 55.3. Replenishment of myocardial contrast enhancement after a high–mechanical index (termed the "flash") impulse. The rate of replenishment correlates with red blood cell velocity, and the plateau intensity (at end-systole) correlates with the capillary cross-sectional area. The product of these two correlates with capillary blood flow. Because capillary blood flow is typically 1 mm/s under resting conditions and at least 2 mm/s during any form of hyperemic stress, the typical replenishment after a high-MI impulse and a two-dimensional transducer (4-mm elevation plane) should be within 4 seconds under resting conditions and within 2 seconds during stress imaging as shown in this example.

developed by Wei and coworkers.[7] The product of the rate of contrast replenishment (reflecting myocardial red blood cell velocity) and the plateau intensity (reflecting capillary cross-sectional area) correlate with myocardial blood flow. By normalizing plateau intensity to adjacent LV cavity intensity, one can compute absolute myocardial blood flow.

Most clinical applications analyze myocardial perfusion visually. A key concept is that under resting conditions with a typical diagnostic transducer having a 4-mm elevation plane, normal myocardial contrast replenishment should be within 4 seconds, but under hyperemic conditions (exercise, dobutamine, vasodilator stress), replenishment should be within 2 seconds after the high-MI impulse (Fig. 55.3).[8,9]

TECHNICAL CONSIDERATIONS AND COMPONENTS

The success of RTPE and LVO applications of contrast depend on optimizing the gain, TGC, and MI for imaging, as well as controlling the contrast infusion rate so as to obtain myocardial contrast enhancement without shadowing in the LV cavity (see Table 55.3).

ROLE OF THE PHYSICIAN

The physician is responsible for the overall quality control of the procedure, which begins by ensuring all personnel (cardiology fellows, nurses, and sonographers) are adequately educated in the concepts of

LVO or myocardial perfusion assessment with a continuous infusion of microbubble contrast. The physician needs to work with the lead sonographer and nursing team to develop a standard operating procedure to be followed whenever contrast is used to assess perfusion. Although RTPE during stress can be performed in a manner similar to standard stress procedures without contrast, the physician assigned to the laboratory needs to be level III trained in echocardiography and have been trained in the performance and interpretation of at least 50 RTPE examinations before operating independently.

ROLE OF THE IMAGING TEAM

Contrast is used to enhance images, improve border detection, and provide information on myocardial perfusion at rest and during stress echocardiographic studies. Current American Society of Echocardiography guidelines recommend that UEA administration can be by a registered nurse or other qualified allied health personnel. A continuous infusion of a saline-diluted UEA (ranging from 3% for Definity to 7.5% for Optison to 12% for Lumason/SonoVue) or small-bolus (0.1 mL for Definity, 0.2 mL for Optison and 0.5 mL for Lumason/SonoVue) injection of contrast is used both for resting, exercise, vasodilator, and dobutamine stress echocardiograms. Lower bolus doses or infusions are needed during stress imaging because of higher cardiac output. All bolus dosing should be followed by slow 10- to 20-second 5-mL flushes of saline to create an infusion of a steady concentration of microbubbles in the LV cavity.[2]

Definity is activated by agitating the vial for 45 seconds in the Vial Mix. For continuous infusions, this is then diluted by injecting 0.8 cc of Definity into 29 cc of normal saline to make a total of approximately 30 mL. Optison and Lumason/SonoVue are ready to use and do not require a Vial Mix. For Optison or Lumason/SonoVue, half of a vial can be diluted into 20 cc of saline if that is the agent desired. Do not mix until just before infusion. Two syringes should be made for stress echocardiograms. One syringe should be sufficient for resting echocardiograms. The infusion rate is approximately 4 cc per minute by hand, watching the clock. The solution should be mixed back and forth periodically so that the contrast does not settle in the bottom of the syringe. The infusion is started when the sonographer is ready to capture resting images. The nurse, physician, or sonographer starts the infusion, and the sonographer or physician starts to acquire the resting images. The infusion rate starts at 4 mL/min and can be increased or decreased if needed; this is dependent on the images. The imaging person informs the infusing person to increase or decrease the infusion rate as needed. One syringe of the mixture should be sufficient for a resting echocardiogram when looking for perfusion, LV function, WMAs, and overall ejection fraction. The second half of the UEA is needed both for exercise and pharmacologic stress echocardiograms. In addition, any leftover diluted UEA from the syringe used to obtain resting images can be used for stress images as well. The second syringe is used for the stress images. In this setting, the infusion rate is usually lower because of the higher cardiac output (2–4 cc/min). The infusion rate should remain constant unless the imaging person indicates otherwise. It is important not to mix the second syringe until the imaging person is ready to capture the intermediate images for a dobutamine stress and immediate post images for an exercise stress. For small-bolus injections of UEA, each bolus should be followed by a slow 5-mL saline or 5% dextrose flush over 10 to 20 seconds.

ADVANTAGES AND DISADVANTAGES OF REAL-TIME PERFUSION ECHOCARDIOGRAPHY VERSUS OTHER IMAGING TECHNIQUES

Ultrasound has higher spatial resolution than either radionuclide imaging (single-photo emission computed tomography [SPECT] or positron emission tomography [PET]) techniques and provides greater temporal resolution (see Table 55.2). This permits the detection of myocardial perfusion in real time along with regional function assessments, which is not possible with any other perfusion imaging technique. Despite this, SPECT and PET are the only Food and Drug Administration–approved techniques for examining myocardial perfusion. Myocardial perfusion imaging is also possible with magnetic resonance imaging (MRI). Although the spatial resolution of MRI is comparable to ultrasound, current perfusion imaging techniques with MRI are obtained after bolus injections of gadolinium and thus are subject to variable alterations in T1 and T2 times produced by the bolus injection (see Table 55.2). Functional assessments of stenosis severity are now possible with coronary computed tomography (CT-fractional flow reserve [FFR]) and appear to be reducing the need for coronary angiography.[10]

ACQUISITION OF REAL-TIME PERFUSION ECHOCARDIOGRAPHY IMAGES

The UEA infusion rate or small-bolus injection must be adjusted so as to permit homogenous myocardial opacification before application of

high-MI impulses and analysis of contrast replenishment with VLMI imaging. This usually requires that TGC potentiometers be set to slightly higher in the near field to overcome automatic reductions that typically occur in the near field. However, on the new Epiq Philips platform, this near-field adjustment is less than what has been required for earlier platforms such as iE33 (Fig. 55.4). Regardless, these settings must be such that a brief high-MI impulse (>0.8 MI) results in clearance of signals from the myocardium. Fig. 55.5 demonstrates how to adjust the near-field TGCs to create homogenous opacification. Fig. 55.6 illustrates that occasionally, the near-field TGCs (or overall gain) must be adjusted back slightly to ensure that the post–high-MI impulse adequately clears all echo signals in the apical segments (thus allowing for the analysis of replenishment in these critical segments).

The infusion rate of UEAs must be adjusted so that the high-MI impulse only clears myocardial contrast and does not excessively destroy LV cavity contrast. This results in a reduction of contrast entering the coronary circulation and creates difficulties in analyzing myocardial contrast replenishment. For small-bolus injections, the injections and flushes must be such that high-MI impulses still clear echocardiographic signals from all myocardial segments. When cavity contrast begins to wash out, a repeat bolus is necessary. Table 55.3 provides the recommended ultrasound settings and presets for RTPE and LVO. No flash imaging is needed for THI at a low MI (0.2–0.3) because it does not produce myocardial contrast, and perfusion imaging is not possible with THI.

SPECIFIC STRESS PROTOCOLS
Exercise Stress Real-Time Perfusion Echocardiography Acquisition

A two-stage Bruce protocol is used, and images are taken at rest and immediately after exercise. The correct machine settings (see Table 55.3) and protocol for myocardial contrast imaging or LVO are selected. All imaging acquisition begins with a small bolus or starts the infusion of UEA. Resting and immediate poststress images are taken after the repeated small-bolus injections or with the continuous infusion of UEA at approximately 4 cc/min for rest and 2 cc/min during stress using the dilutions described previously. The UEA injection or infusion should be started 30 seconds before treadmill termination. The myocardium should appear dark after the high-MI impulse; however, the LV cavity should remain bright. If the LV cavity is dark or exhibiting a swirling pattern, the infusion rate should be increased, or the duration of the high MI flash impulses should be adjusted (Table 55.4).

The myocardium should replenish within one to four heartbeats at rest and become bright again and during stress replenishment should be less than 2 seconds in normal myocardial blood flow responses. The high-MI impulse duration at rest should be set at around five frames and adjusted as needed depending on the

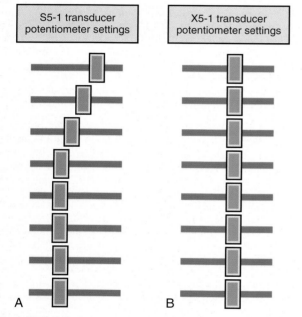

Figure 55.4. Typical time gain compensation (TGC) settings required to create homogenous myocardial contrast during real-time perfusion echocardiography on most transducers (**A**). On the X5-1 (Philips Healthcare) transducer, the TGCs can be left in a vertical position (**B**).

Figure 55.5. A time gain compensation (TGC) setting that is too low in the near field is manifest by the appearance of a pseudo-apical perfusion defect. Slightly adjusting the TGCs higher in the near field prevents this artifactual perfusion defect. These adjustments should be made with some transducers during the resting studies before stress imaging. The X5-1 (Philips Healthcare) transducer does not require this adjustment.

Corrective action

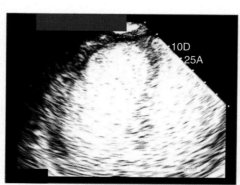
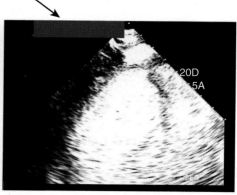

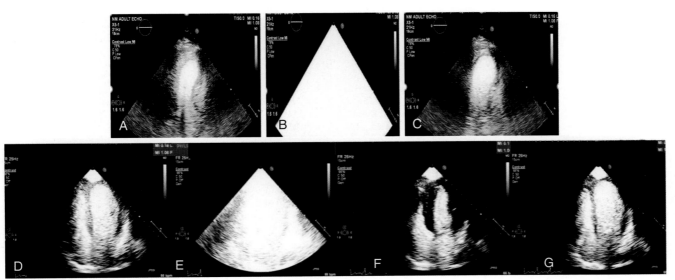

Figure 55.6. Gain settings that are too high result in unwanted tissue signals persisting in the basal, mid, and distal segments immediate after high–mechanical index (MI) images (**A–C**), preventing one from adequately analyzing myocardial contrast replenishment in these segments. Corrective action is taken in the lower panels (**D–G**) when slightly lowering the overall gain setting results in a homogenous absence of myocardial signals after the high-MI impulse that will be adequate for analyzing replenishment. Note that time gain compensations in both the near and far field are set to achieve both homogenous myocardial opacification and to ensure absence of signals from the myocardium immediately after the high-MI impulse s. All of these adjustments are required under resting conditions to prevent difficulties in interpreting peak stress images.

TABLE 55.4 Concepts Behind System Settings for Real-Time Perfusion Imaging and Left Ventricular Opacification

Key Concepts on System Settings	
Focus	Narrowest area of the beam with the greatest ultrasound intensity
	Should be placed at the most distal location for perfusion imaging
	• Allows greater resolution of the entire LV
	• Briefly adjusting to the near field may help to reduce "swirling" artifacts seen in the apex for low MI THI
Gain (overall) dynamic range	The overall gain amplifies intensity of the received echoes and uniformly increases or decreases the number of echoes displayed; should be set higher in the near field for some RTPE imaging systems
	The dynamic range boosts visibility of softer echoes from contrast
	• Both of these do not affect microbubble destruction
Mechanical index (MI)	MI set too high will cause too much bubble destruction; should be around 0.1–0.2 MI for RTPE (fundamental nonlinear imaging)
	Should be between 0.2 and 0.3 MI for THI low-MI imaging
	Should be >-0.8 MI for brief destructive impulses to clear contrast from the myocardium
Frame rate (FR)	The FR determines the repetition frequency at which pulses are received by microbubbles
	Sector size, width, and imaging depth affect the FR
	Too high a FR can disrupt microbubbles; should be around 20–25 Hertz during low-MI perfusion imaging; can be increased to 25–30 Hertz during high heart rates (exercise or dobutamine stress)
	For THI low-MI imaging, FR can run between 30–40 Hz; lower FR may reduce apical destruction swirling

LV, Left ventricle; *RTPE,* real-time perfusion echocardiography; *THI,* tissue harmonic imaging.

destruction of the microbubbles. If too many bubbles are being destroyed in the LV cavity, then the high-MI impulse duration should be reduced. Because of the higher cardiac output and cardiac motion during stress, the high-MI duration may be increased to up to 12 to 15 frames (or one to two cardiac cycles on the Siemens system) for the stress images. For all systems, the frame rate for RTPE should be around 22 to 25 Hz. The MI should be set at around 0.18 and no higher than 0.20 for RTPE. If using THI at a low MI, then the frame rates can be less than 30 Hz, and the MI typically is optimal between 0.2 to 0.3 MI (see Table 55.3).

For exercise stress with RTPE, the full-disclosure option is chosen, which indicates that each cardiac cycle is acquired after one pushes the Acquire button. The nurse needs to start infusing the contrast or administering a small bolus at about 30 seconds before the patient gets off the treadmill for immediate post images. During acquisition of images, if background echocardiographic signals are too high, then overall gain should be reduced slightly to ensure near-complete clearance of myocardial signals after the high-MI impulse (see Fig. 55.6). For THI, the myocardium should have minimal signal to optimize the endocardial border delineation with contrast within the cavity.

Exercise Stress Image Analysis

With RTPE, analysis of perfusion and WM occurs simultaneously. If you see an area of the myocardium (minimum of two contiguous segments) that does not replenish (perfusion defect) by 2 to 3 seconds after the high-MI impulse following exercise, this indicates a functionally relevant stenosis. Fig. 55.7 depicts an exercise-induced defect that occurred in both the anteroseptal segments, distal septum, apex, and anterolateral segments caused by a left main obstruction. Beware of segments that are often attenuated by rib or lung shadowing, such as the basal to midanterior and lateral segments on an apical two-chamber window. When rib or lung shadowing is preventing basal and midsegments from being visualized, it is recommended that one purposely obtain some images in a foreshortened view to reduce this attenuation or shadowing.[2] As a tip to help identify attenuation, perfusion defects are often subendocardial, but attenuation tends to involve the entire transmural extent of the segment and extends outside the segment borders.

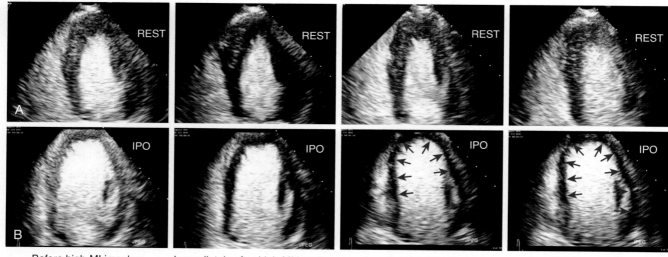

Before high-MI impulse   Immediately after high-MI impulse   2 s after high-MI impulse   4 s after high-MI impulse

Figure 55.7. Images from an exercise stress echocardiogram with real-time perfusion echocardiography. **A,** Resting end-systolic images demonstrate normal wall thickening and normal perfusion (myocardial contrast replenishment within 4 seconds of the high–mechanical index [MI] impulse). **B,** Stress images obtained within 2 seconds after a high-MI impulse demonstrate a transmural perfusion defect consistent with inducible ischemia in the mid septum, apex, and lateral segments. The patient had a significant left main obstruction. *IPO,* immediate post exercise.

DOBUTAMINE STRESS REAL-TIME PERFUSION AND LEFT VENTRICULAR OPACIFICATION PROTOCOLS
Dobutamine Stress Image Acquisition

Resting images are obtained after the infusion or bolus of Definity, Optison, or SonoVue/Lumason has been administered. The MI chosen for RTPE or THI should be kept the same as for exercise stress. When homogenous myocardial opacification is achieved (adjusting gain settings and infusion rate), then hit the acquire button. After this, a brief high-MI impulse is applied. The myocardium should appear dark after the impulse; however, the LV cavity should remain bright. If the LV cavity is dark, then you should increase the infusion rate (or bolus size) or reduce the duration of the high-MI impulse. The myocardium should replenish within 5 seconds at rest. After the myocardium has reopacified after the high-MI impulse, then hit the acquire button again to end your acquisition. A four-stage protocol is typically used, and images are taken at rest, low dose (if a resting WMA is present), intermediate stress, and peak stress (typically defined as 85% of the predicted maximum heart rate). Single breath-hold myocardial perfusions loops (consisting of a cardiac cycle before to high-MI "flash impulse" and up to 10 cardiac cycles after a high-MI impulse) are only taken in the four-, two-, and three-chamber views. This same process is repeated for low-dose, intermediate stress (70% predicted maximum heart rate), and peak stress (>85% predicted maximum heart rate) images. Low-dose dobutamine images are necessary mainly if a resting WMA is present to examine for WM recruitment as well as contrast replenishment in dobutamine nonresponsive segments.

As with exercise stress, the high-MI flash duration at rest should be set to around 3 to 5 frames and typically between 10 and 15 frames during stress imaging. As always, it is adjusted as needed depending on whether adequate clearance of microbubbles within the myocardium occurs while minimizing cavity destruction. Communication between the nurse and sonographer or physician is important to achieve the best results. The infusion rate or bolus dose may need to be altered to achieve adequate destruction of microbubbles in the myocardium. This optimal rate varies from patient to patient and from rest to peak dobutamine stress. Fig. 55.8 and Video 55.8 show an example of an inferior perfusion defect observed during the replenishment phase of contrast after a high-MI impulse at peak dobutamine stress.

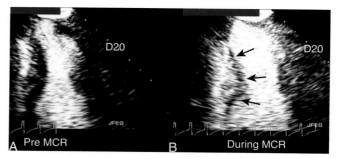

Figure 55.8. Example of an inducible perfusion defect *(arrows)* with real-time perfusion echocardiography observed during dobutamine stress contrast echocardiography. The image before myocardial contrast replenishment (MCR) obtained immediately after the high–mechanical index impulse at end-systole demonstrates good clearance of myocardial contrast (**A**). Within 2 seconds, a subsequent end systolic frame during MCR demonstrates the subendocardial perfusion defect (**B**). (See corresponding Video 55.8.)

Dobutamine Stress Image Analysis

The physician should analyze the images after all four stages have been acquired. Note that if there is a resting WMA and perfusion defect, stress images are typically compared with low-dose dobutamine images (5-μ/kg/min infusions). The same principles of replenishment rates for exercise apply to dobutamine stress as well. Subendocardial perfusion defects typically are seen within 1 to 2 seconds of the high-MI impulse application, and each coronary artery territory should be examined for this. Overall, RTPE is more sensitive than LVO or conventional stress echocardiography in detecting significant coronary artery disease than WM analysis alone and provides better prognostic data.[5,11] All analyses of perfusion should be from end-systolic or early diastolic images, which is when there is minimal interference from arterioles and predominately capillary contrast enhancement is being observed.[12] See Tables 55.4 and 55.5 for a summary of acquisition and interpretation tips for perfusion imaging with VLMI imaging.

VASODILATOR STRESS MYOCARDIAL PERFUSION IMAGING

Vasodilator Stress Image Acquisition

A two-stage protocol is used, and images are taken at rest and after infusion of the vasodilator agent. The vasodilator stress agents are listed in Table 55.6. Imaging should be with RTPE and not low-MI THI because THI just analyzes WM, which has reduced sensitivity in detecting coronary artery disease during vasodilator stress. The correct machine setting and protocol for myocardial contrast imaging are selected, and the nurse starts the 3- to 5-mL/min infusion of either diluted Definity or Optison or gives small-bolus injections of either agent or 0.5 mL boluses of Lumason/SonoVue.[13] The post images are taken during the infusion of adenosine, during and after the dipyridamole infusion, and immediately after the 400-mcg bolus of regadenoson.[14]

The UEA infusion rate or bolus dose or flush may need to be decreased or increased to achieve adequate destruction of the microbubbles in the myocardium. This varies from patient to patient similar to exercise and dobutamine stress imaging. It is important to have adequate destruction of the bubbles in the myocardium so that a perfusion defect can be identified. The perfusion defect may be transient and observable only during the first cardiac cycle of replenishment after the high-MI impulse (Fig. 55.9). If you see an area of the myocardium that does not replenish (perfusion defect) after approximately 2 to 3 heartbeats after the high-MI impulse, then this indicates a stenosis.

Vasodilator Stress Image Analysis

With vasodilator stress, WMAs are not typically induced even when a physiologically relevant stenosis is present.[13–15] Therefore, the analysis is focused mainly on perfusion. Again, the typical perfusion defects are subendocardial and occur within the first 2 seconds of myocardial contrast replenishment after the high-MI impulse. Careful comparison with resting replenishment is required to ensure defects observed during stress were not also present at rest.

PITFALLS AND CLINICAL TIPS FOR ALL REAL-TIME PERFUSION ECHOCARDIOGRAPHY STRESS ACQUISITIONS AND INTERPRETATIONS

Moving the anterior-lateral wall to the middle of the sector can reduce rib artifacts and dropout. One can purposefully foreshorten the apical windows to permit near-field visualization of the basal to midsegments and better analysis of replenishment and plateau contrast enhancement in these coronary artery territories. If there is not adequate LV cavity enhancement, infusing at a faster rate (or repeat bolus injections) may be needed. Conversely, if there is an excessive amount of cavity contrast and attenuation, reduce the administration of the contrast and wait for the attenuation to dissipate. With bolus injections, it is critical that the saline flush be administered slowly over 10 to 20 seconds to avoid wasting time and enhancing agent because of shadowing in the LV cavity.

Apical signal dropout is caused most commonly by not inadequately adjusting TGC settings when doing resting image acquisition. In addition to inadequate receiver gain in the near field, it may also be caused by an MI that is set too high, causing near field-destruction, or suboptimal placement of the focus. Transiently repositioning the focus closer to the near field reduces the near-field scan line density and helps achieve better filling in the apex. Finally, lack of myocardial contrast signal can be caused by an infusion rate that is too low. Most important, the absence of microbubble contrast in the apex may also be caused by hypoperfusion, and this is why it is critical to have the baseline set-up optimized before stress images are acquired.

If the myocardium is not dark enough after the high-MI impulse, the overall gain might need to be reduced, or the number of high-MI frames might be increased. Having the patient take a breath in and hold it may also help in this situation to reduce

TABLE 55.5 Key Set-up Points While Acquiring and Analyzing Perfusion Images

1. Optimize near-field gain.
2. Adjust contrast infusion to create homogenous myocardial opacification without shadowing.
3. Adjust duration of high-MI impulses to minimized cavity destruction.
4. Purposefully foreshorten images to analyze basal segment perfusion.
5. If resting wall motion is normal, resting myocardial perfusion should be normal. During stress, however, perfusion may be abnormal despite normal wall motion.
6. Analyze myocardial perfusion at end-systole or early diastole, when myocardial contrast enhancement reflects mainly capillary enhancement.

TABLE 55.6 Vasodilator Stress Agents Used for Real-Time Perfusion Echocardiography Pharmacologic Stress

Agent	Infusion Rate	Acquisition Time for Post Images
Regadenoson (Astellas Pharmaceuticals)	400-µg bolus ×1	Immediate after infusion
Adenosine	140-µ/kg/min for ≤6 minutes	2–4 minutes after infusion started
Dipyridamole	0.56–0.84 mg/kg over 4–6 minutes	3–7 minutes after infusion started

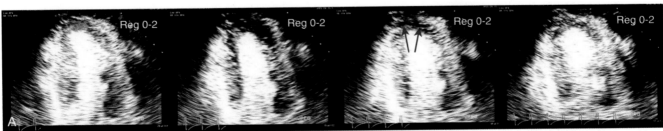

| Before high-MI impulse | Immediately after high-MI impulse | 2 s after high-MI impulse | 4 s after high-MI impulse |

Figure 55.9. A vasodilator stress study using a 400-µg bolus injection of regadenoson. **A,** Rest images in the apical two-chamber view demonstrate normal contrast replenishment within 4 seconds of the high–mechanical index (MI) impulse. After the regadenoson bolus injection (Reg 0-2), there as an anterior and apical perfusion defect evident at 2 seconds after the high-MI impulse *(arrows)*. This is not evident at plateau intensity (4 s after high-MI impulse). The patient had a collateralized left anterior descending occlusion at angiography.

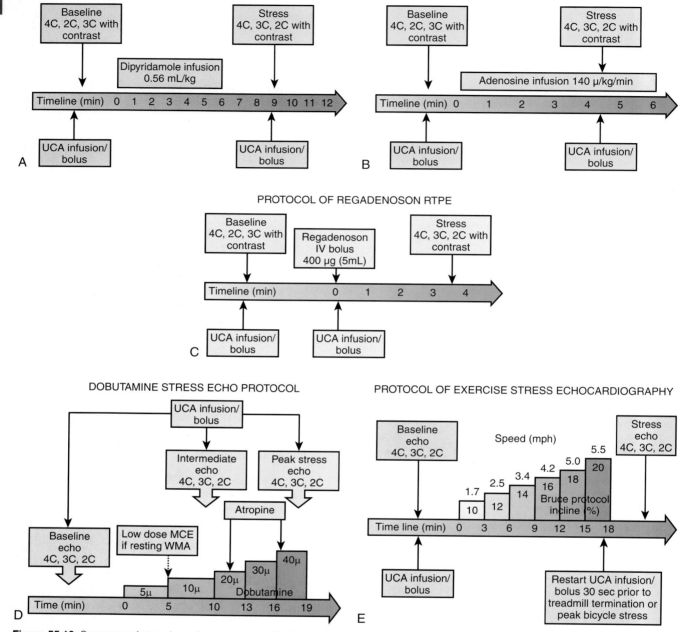

Figure 55.10. Sequence of steps in performing a treadmill, dobutamine, or vasodilator stress with real-time perfusion echocardiography (RTPE). *2C,* Two chamber; *3C,* three chamber; *4C,* four chamber; *IV,* intravenous; *MCE,* myocardial contrast echocardiography; *UCA,* ultrasound contrast agent; *WMA,* wall motion abnormality.

myocardial movement out of the plane caused by translation. Fig. 55.10 summarizes all stress protocol acquisition sequences for timing of infusions and boluses and the timing of image acquisition.

FUTURE DIRECTIONS

It has now become apparent that stenosis diameter during angiography has little predictive value in terms of predicting patient outcome and whether revascularization will improve patient outcome. Measurements of FFR or instantaneous resting measurements of pressure gradients across a stenosis have significantly more predictive value in identifying those who may benefit from

revascularization. Although abnormal capillary blood flow during demand stress with RTPE is seen in nearly all vessels with abnormal FFR, abnormal microvascular perfusion is often abnormal even when FFR is normal. This subgroup of patients (normal FFR but abnormal demand stress capillary blood flow) frequently identifies patients who will still be symptomatic if not revascularized.[16] Invasive hemodynamic studies have confirmed that abnormal microvascular perfusion measured with RTPE may correlate more closely with hyperemic microvascular resistance.[17] The predictive value of demand microvascular resistance abnormalities, even in the absence of epicardial coronary artery disease, appears to be as serious as when epicardial disease is present,[18] and RTPE provides a bedside technique that can explore the role of lifestyle, interventional, and pharmaceutical treatments in treating inducible microvascular flow abnormalities.

Please access ExpertConsult to view the corresponding videos for this chapter.

REFERENCES

1. Porter TR, Mulvagh SL, Abdelmoneim SS, et al. Clinical applications of ultrasonic enhancing agents in echocardiography. *J Am Soc Echocardiogr.* 2018;31:241–274.
2. Porter TR, Abdelmoneim S, Belcik JT, et al. Guidelines for the cardiac sonographer in the performance of contrast echocardiography. *J Am Society of Echocardiogr.* 2014;27:797–810.
3. Dolan MS, Gala SS, Dodla S, et al. Safety and efficacy of commercially available ultrasound contrast agents for rest and stress echocardiography: a multicenter experience. *J Am Coll Cardiol.* 2009;53:32–38.
4. Porter TR, Xie F. Myocardial perfusion imaging with contrast ultrasound. *J Am Coll Cardiol Cardiovasc Imag.* 2010;3:176–187.
5. Tsutsui JM, Elhendy A, Anderson JR, et al. Prognostic value of dobutamine stress myocardial contrast perfusion echocardiography. *Circulation.* 2005;112:1444–1450.
6. Thomas D, Xie F, Smith LM, et al. Prospective randomized comparison of conventional stress echocardiography and real time perfusion stress echocardiography in detecting significant coronary artery disease, J Am Soc Echocardiogr 25:1207–1214.
7. Wei K, Jayaweera AR, Firoozan S, et al. Quantification of myocardial blood flow with ultrasound-induced destruction of microbubbles administered as a constant venous infusion. *Circulation.* 1998;97:473–483.
8. Rafter P, Phillips P, Vannan MA. Imaging technologies and techniques. *Cardiol Clin.* 2004;22:181–197.
9. Peltier M, Vancraeynest D, Pasquet A, et al. Assessment of the physiologic significance of coronary disease with dipyridamole real-time myocardial contrast echocardiography. Comparison with technetium-99m sestamibi single-photon emission computed tomography and quantitative coronary angiography. *J Am Coll Cardiol.* 2004;43:257–264.
10. Cavalcante R, Onuma Y, Sotomi Y, et al. Non-invasive Heart Team assessment of multivessel coronary disease with coronary computed tomography angiography based on SYNTAX score II treatment recommendations: design and rationale of the randomized SYNTAX III Revolution trial. *Euro Intervention.* 2017;12:2001–2008.
11. Porter TR, Smith LM, Wu J, et al. Patient outcome following two different stress imaging approaches: a prospective randomized comparison. *J Am Coll Cardiol.* 2013;61:2446–2455.
12. Leong-Poi H, Le E, Rim SJ, et al. Quantification of myocardial perfusion and determination of coronary stenosis severity during hyperemia using real-time myocardial contrast echocardiography. *J Am Soc Echocardiogr.* 2001;14:1173–1182.
13. Gaibazzi N, Reverberi C, Lorenzoni V, et al. Prognostic value of high-dose dipyridamole stress myocardial contrast perfusion echocardiography. *Circulation.* 2012;126:1217–1224.
14. Porter TR, Adolphson M, High RR, et al. Rapid detection of coronary artery stenoses with real-time perfusion echocardiography during regadenoson stress. *Circ Cardiovasc Imag.* 2011;4:628–635.
15. Senior R, Moreo A, Gaibazzi N, et al. Comparison of sulfur hexafluoride microbubble (SonoVue)-enhanced myocardial contrast echocardiography with gated single-photon emission computed tomography for detection of significant coronary artery disease. *J Am Coll Cardiol.* 2013;62:1353–1361.
16. Wu J, Barton D, Xie F, et al. Comparison of fractional flow reserve assessment with demand stress myocardial contrast echocardiography in angiographically intermediate stenoses. *Circ Cardiovasc Imag.* 2016;9:e004129.
17. Barton D, Xie F, O'Leary E, et al. The relationship of capillary blood flow assessments to invasively derived microvascular and epicardial assessments. *J Am Soc Echocardiogr32.* 2019;1095. 1011.
18. Kutty S, Bisselou KS, Moukagna B, et al. The clinical outcome of patients with inducible capillary blood flow abnormalities during demand stress in the presence or absence of angiographic coronary artery disease. *Circulation Cardiovasc Imag.* 2018;11:e007483.

56 Stress Echocardiography for Valve Disease: Aortic Regurgitation and Mitral Stenosis

Patrizio Lancellotti, Alexandra Maria Chitroceanu, Simona Sperlongano, Raluca Elena Dulgheru, Adriana Postolache

Stress echocardiography (SE) has been less well validated in the context of aortic regurgitation (AR) and mitral stenosis (MS) than for coronary disease and mitral regurgitation (MR). In both these conditions, exercise stress echocardiography (ESE) represents the imaging approach of choice,[1–4] being especially useful in apparently asymptomatic patients, mainly caused by sedentary lifestyle, and in nonsevere valve disease with symptoms.[5]

STRESS ECHOCARDIOGRAPHY PROTOCOL

Either immediate after exercise (treadmill or upright bicycle ergometer) or during exercise imaging (semisupine bicycle exercise on a tilted table) can be performed. The postexercise echocardiography, although more common worldwide, can be more difficult, especially when multiple stress parameters need to be assessed in the first 1 to 2 minutes after test termination. The semisupine exercise echocardiography, which is more common in Europe, offers the advantage of a continuous evaluation of stress parameters during exercise.

The test should be performed under the supervision of an experienced physician and a nurse. Typically, the initial workload of 25 W is maintained for 2 minutes and increased every 2 minutes by 25 W, but an increase in steps of 10 W can be more appropriate in patients with a low level of physical activity. Blood pressure, heart rate, 12-lead electrocardiography, and echocardiographic parameters related to the valve, the left ventricle, and the hemodynamic consequences (i.e., pulmonary arterial pressure) are recorded in a stepwise order at baseline, low-, medium-, and high-intensity levels and immediately after exercise. The echocardiographic imaging protocol of choice varies depending on the objectives of the test (Fig. 56.1). Physicians should regularly assess any potential symptoms during the examination.

AORTIC REGURGITATION
Indications

Severe aortic regurgitation (AR) gradually leads to left ventricular (LV) dysfunction and heart failure and is associated with an increased risk of sudden death. There is a direct graded relationship between quantified AR severity and reduced survival or event-free survival.[6] Clinically, this relationship becomes evident with the dramatic change in prognosis harbored by symptom onset in severe AR. Patients with symptomatic severe AR have a yearly mortality rate of 3.4%, and even moderate AR has been shown to be associated with a 10-year cardiovascular event rate of 34% ± 6%.[6]

In both European Society of Cardiology (ESC) and American Heart Association (AHA) recommendations on valvular heart

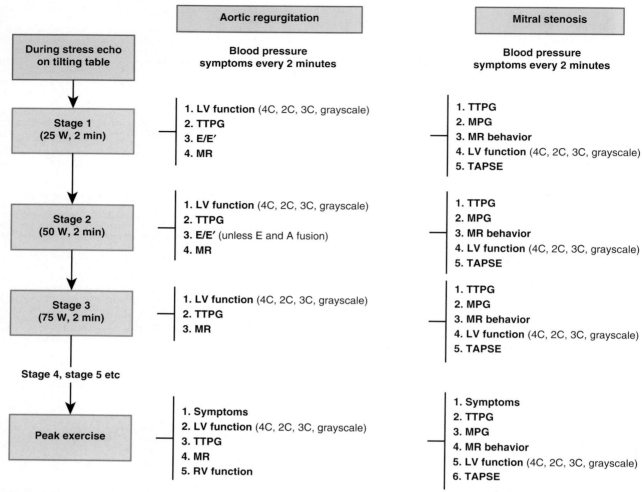

Figure 56.1. Exercise echocardiography protocol and parameters that can be assessed at each stage in aortic regurgitation and mitral stenosis. 2C, Two chamber; 3C, three chamber; 4C, four chamber; Ch, chamber; E/E′, ratio of early transmitral diastolic velocity to early tissue Doppler imaging velocity of the mitral annulus; LV, left ventricle; MPG, mean pressure gradient; MR, mitral regurgitation; RV, right ventricle; TAPSE, tricuspid annular plane systolic excursion; TTPG, transtricuspid pressure gradient. (Adapted with permission from Lancellotti P, et al: Stress echocardiography in patients with native valvular heart disease, *Heart* 104:807–813, 2018.)

disease, the presence of symptoms is a firm indication for aortic valve surgery.[1,2] Exercise echocardiography is recommended to reveal symptoms in patients with severe AR who report being asymptomatic and in symptomatic patients with nonsevere AR.[5]

Severe Aortic Regurgitation Without Symptoms

Exercise testing can unmask symptomatic patients previously classified as being asymptomatic or with equivocal symptoms, as is often the case in old or sedentary patients. ESE, comparison with a simple exercise stress test, has the advantage of evaluating at the same time the presence of subclinical systolic dysfunction based on contractile reserve and global longitudinal strain at rest.[7] The absence of contractile reserve (generally defined as a <5% increase in LV ejection fraction at exercise) seems to identify the presence of latent LV dysfunction, earlier than conventional echocardiographic parameters obtained at rest.[8]

Color tissue Doppler imaging for measuring systolic mitral annulus velocities at rest and exercise may be used as a surrogate marker of subclinical LV dysfunction.[3] Other echocardiographic indices, such as resting LV strain, resting right ventricular strain,

and exercise tricuspid annular plane systolic excursion, were independently associated with the need for earlier aortic surgery in asymptomatic patients with moderate to severe and severe AR.[9] Because of the small number of patients included in the studies cited and the sometimes contradictory results, none of these exercise parameters have been included in the guidelines of the ESC or the AHA. They could, together with other tests, such as cardiopulmonary exercise testing and brain natriuretic peptide, help anticipate surgical timing in patients approaching surgical indication (LV ejection fraction ~50%–55%, LV end-systolic dimension approaching 50 mm or 25 mm/m²) or indicate a closer follow up in some patients.

Nonsevere Aortic Regurgitation With Symptoms

SE cannot be used for regrading the severity of AR. Tachycardia-induced diastolic shortening limits the quantification of AR.[5] ESE can, on the other hand, identify other causes for the reported symptoms, such as dynamic MR, inducible ischemia, diastolic dysfunction, and pulmonary hypertension.[5]

For both indications, the minimum acquired dataset comprises LV views, tricuspid regurgitation (TR) continuous-wave (CW) Doppler for estimation of systolic pulmonary artery pressure

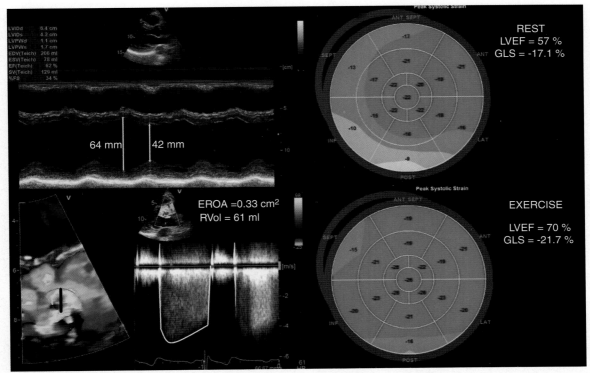

Figure 56.2. Asymptomatic patient with severe eccentric aortic regurgitation and left ventricular contractile reserve as assessed using left ventricular ejection fraction (LVEF) and global longitudinal strain (GLS). *EROA,* Effective regurgitant orifice area; *RVol,* regurgitant volume.

(sPAP), color-flow Doppler to detect MR, and evaluation of diastolic function (Figs. 56.1 and 56.2).

PROGNOSTIC VALUE OF STRESS ECHOCARDIOGRAPHY IN AORTIC REGURGITATION

Data on the prognostic value of SE in patients with AR are sparse. Whereas the absence of contractile reserve on exercise is a predictor of progressive LV dysfunction on medical treatment, the presence of contractile reserve is a predictor of improvement of LV function after aortic valve replacement.[8] This finding is, however, nonspecific, and its reliability in predicting outcome is controversial.

MITRAL STENOSIS
Indications

In patients with MS, symptoms develop insidiously over the years, and their severity strongly relates to survival.[10] Symptoms are only poorly correlated to measurements of valve area at rest.[11] This is explained by the dynamic reserve of the mitral valve orifice area that changes during exercise more with regard to mitral valve morphology (calcification, thickening, and leaflet mobility) than to resting valve area per se.[12] This dynamic reserve is also responsible for different functional New York Heart Association class and stress response variability.[13] Moreover, atrioventricular compliance seems to play an important role in specific adaptation under stress conditions in patients with severe MS.[14]

SE represents a clinically established tool for the functional assessment of MS. It is particularly indicated, when discrepancies exist between clinical and resting echocardiographic data, as is the case in severe asymptomatic disease and in nonsevere disease with discordant or equivocal symptoms (class I recommendation, level of evidence C in the American College of Cardiology/AHA guidelines from 2014).[2] Box 56.1 lists the potential indications for

> **BOX 56.1** Indications for Stress Testing in Patients With Mitral Stenosis
>
> 1. Objectify assessment of symptoms.
> 2. Determine functional capacity.
> 3. Assess hemodynamic response.
>   a. Pulmonary artery pressure (TR jet method)
>   b. Mean gradient
> 4. Evaluate discordance between symptoms and severity of MS.
>   a. Asymptomatic patient but severe MS at rest
>   b. Symptomatic patient but mild MS at rest
>
> *MS,* Mitral stenosis; *TR,* tricuspid regurgitation.

exercise testing in patients with MS. Expert opinion recommends exercise echocardiography, but in some cases, such as in patients unable to perform physical exercise, dobutamine stress test may be performed.

Severe Mitral Stenosis Without Symptoms

The severity of MS is based on valve area, with significant MS being defined as valve area smaller than 1.5 cm². In asymptomatic patients with mitral valve area smaller than 1 cm², stress testing is indicated to test for otherwise unreported symptoms.[2] When the valve area is smaller than 1.5 cm² but larger than 1 cm², SE is indicated to reveal symptoms if the valve is suitable for balloon valvotomy or when planning pregnancy or major surgery, irrespective of suitability for balloon valvotomy.[2,5]

Nonsevere Mitral Stenosis With Symptoms

A proportion of patients with MS quantified as moderate at rest develop significant exertional symptoms.[12] Moderate MS, usually

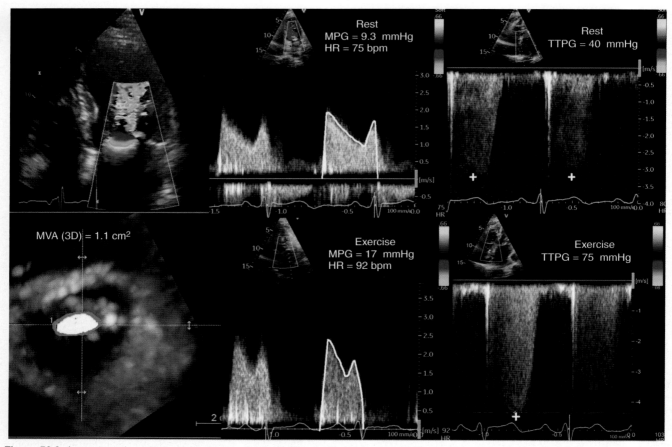

Figure 56.3. Asymptomatic patient with hemodynamically significant mitral stenosis exhibiting a marked exercise increase in transmitral mean pressure gradient (MPG) and a paralleled increase in transtricuspid pressure gradient (TTPG). MVA indicates mitral valve area calculated using three-dimensional imaging.

well compensated at rest, may be hemodynamically significant during stress as it fails to accommodate the necessary increase in flow.[15] Based on ESE, the MS is considered severe if on exertion, the mean gradient is greater than 15 mm Hg or if during dobutamine infusion the mean gradient is greater than 18 mm Hg.[18,21] An exercise sPAP greater than 60 mm Hg is also an indicator of significant MS having an important impact on survival.[16] The ability to assess the response of PAP to exercise is one of the most important aspects of SE in MS.[17,18] The main determinant of dyspnea during exercise is the rapid and early marked increase in sPAP. Patients with greater than 90% of maximal sPAP reached at or before 60 W more frequently develop excessive exercise dyspnea and an indication for percutaneous mitral valvotomy during follow-up.[20] These results suggest that instead of peak exercise sPAP, the dynamic changes in PAP during exercise and the pattern of changes may be more useful for the risk stratification and the management of patients with MS, as reported in patients with heart failure.[19,20]

Dobutamine SE is not recommended for the assessment of sPAP because of dobutamine β₂-agonist effects on pulmonary vascular resistance with a resultant decrease in systolic pulmonary artery and wedge pressures.[5,21]

For both indications, the minimum acquired dataset comprises TR CW Doppler for estimation of sPAP and mitral valve CW Doppler for gradient measurement (Figs. 56.1 and 56.3). Maximal sweep speed and minimal velocity scale should be used for mitral valve continuous Doppler acquisition. In case of atrial fibrillation, SE is better performed during continuation of rate control medication to avoid early rise in heart rate during the test.

PROGNOSTIC VALUE OF CHANGES IN TRANSMITRAL PRESSURE GRADIENT AND SYSTOLIC PULMONARY ARTERY PRESSURE

The relevance of exercise echocardiography on outcome in patients with MS has not been extensively investigated. The sole available outcome study concerned dobutamine SE. In a study by Reis and coworkers, in patients with moderate to severe MS, a mean transmitral pressure gradient greater than 18 mm Hg during dobutamine infusion was the best predictor for clinical deterioration, with a specificity of 87% and a sensitivity of 90%.[21] The recommended cut-off values for significant MS on ESE are based on consensus; an increase in mean transmitral pressure gradient greater than 15 mm Hg and an increase in sPAP greater than 60 mm Hg with exercise are markers of hemodynamically significant MS.[5]

IMPACT ON CLINICAL DECISION MAKING

The management of MS is guided by the presence of symptoms. The sole indication for intervention is considered symptomatic MS (class I indication), but suitability for percutaneous balloon valvotomy plays a central role in the final decision to treat, as mentioned earlier.[1,2] SE may unmask symptoms in patients asymptomatic at rest and may provide additional objective information for the presence of a significant MS by assessing changes in mitral gradient and PAP.[5]

REFERENCES

1. Baumgartner H, Falk V, Bax JJ, et al. ESC/EACTS Guidelines for the management of valvular heart disease. *Eur Heart J*. 2017;38:2739–2791. 2017.
2. Nishimura RA, Otto CM, Bonow RO, et al. AHA/ACC guideline for the management of patients with valvular heart disease. *J Am Coll Cardiol*. 2014:2438–2488. 2014.

3. Lancelloti P, Magne J. Stress echocardiography in regurgitant valve disease. *Circ Cardiovasc Imag.* 2013;6:840–849.
4. Magne J, Lancellotti P, Pierard LA. Stress echocardiography and mitral valvular heart disease. *Cardiol Clin.* 2013;31:311–321.
5. Lancelloti P, Pellikka PA, Co-chair F, et al. The clinical use of stress echocardiography in non-ischaemic heart disease. *J Am Soc Echocardiogr.* 2016;30:101–138.
6. Detaint D, Messika-Zeitoun D, Maalouf J, et al. Quantitative echocardiographic determinants of clinical outcome in asymptomatic patients with aortic regurgitation: a prospective study. *JACC Cardiovasc Imag.* 2008;1(1–11).
7. Lancellotti P, Dulgheru R, Go YY, et al. Stress echocardiography in patients with native valvular heart disease. *Heart.* 2018;104:807–813.
8. Wahi S, Haluska B, Pasquet A, et al. Exercise echocardiography predicts development of left ventricular dysfunction in medically and surgically treated patients with asymptomatic severe aortic regurgitation. *Heart.* 2000;84:606–614.
9. Kusunose K, Agarwal S, Marwick TH, et al. Decision making in asymptomatic aortic regurgitation in the era of guidelines. *Circ Cardiovasc Imag.* 2014;7:352–362.
10. Horstkotte D, Niehues R, Strauer BE. Pathomorphological aspects, aetiology and natural history of acquired mitral valve stenosis. *Eur Heart J.* 1991;12:55–60.
11. Cohen-Solal A, Aupetit JF, Dahan M, et al. Peak oxygen uptake during exercise in mitral stenosis with sinus rhythm or atrial fibrillation: lack of correlation with valve area. *Eur Heart J.* 1994;15:37–44.
12. Bhattacharyya S, Khattar R, Chahal N, et al. Dynamic assessment of stenotic valvular heart disease by stress echocardiography. *Circ Cardiovasc Imag.* 2013;6:583–589.
13. Grimaldi A, Olivotto I, Figini F, et al. Dynamic assessment of 'valvular reserve capacity' in patients with rheumatic mitral stenosis. *Eur Hear J Cardiovasc Imag.* 2011;13:476–482.
14. Voilliot D, Lancellotti P. Exercise testing and stress imaging in mitral valve disease. *Curr Treat Options Cardiovasc Med.* 2017;19:17.
15. Garbi M, Chambers J, Vannan MA, Lancellotti P. Valve stress echocardiography: a practical guide for referral, procedure, reporting, and clinical implementation of results from the HAVEC group. *JACC Cardiovasc Imag.* 2015;8:724–736.
16. Ward C, Hancock BW. Extreme pulmonary hypertension caused by mitral valve disease. Natural history and results of surgery. *Br Heart J.* 1975;37:74–78.
17. Schwammenthal E, Vered Z, Rabinowitz B, et al. Stress echocardiography beyond coronary artery disease. *Eur Heart J.* 1997;18:130–137.
18. Brochet E, Détaint D, Fondard O, et al. Early hemodynamic changes versus peak values: what is more useful to predict occurrence of dyspnea during stress echocardiography in patients with asymptomatic mitral stenosis? *J Am Soc Echocardiogr.* 2011;24:392–398.
19. Tolle JJ, Waxman AB, Van Horn TL, et al. Exercise-induced pulmonary arterial hypertension. *Circulation.* 2008;118:2183–2189.
20. Lewis GD, Murphy RM, Shah RV, et al. Pulmonary vascular response patterns during exercise in left ventricular systolic dysfunction predict exercise capacity and outcomes. *Circ Heart Fail.* 2011;4:276–285.
21. Reis G, Motta MS, Barbosa MM, et al. Dobutamine stress echocardiography for noninvasive assessment and risk stratification of patients with rheumatic mitral stenosis. *J Am Coll Cardiol.* 2004;43:393–401.

57 Stress Echocardiography: Comparison With Other Techniques

Amit R. Patel, Nina Rashedi

Cardiovascular disease, in particular coronary artery disease (CAD), remains the leading cause of death worldwide. There is also enormous burden on health care systems. Annually, 10 million stress tests and 1 million invasive cardiac angiograms (ICAs) are performed in the United States.[1] Management of CAD requires an accurate diagnosis. For decades, ICA has served as the gold standard for the diagnosis of CAD. However, there is a high rate of cardiac catheterizations that show normal coronary arteries at the rate of approximately 60%.[2] In patients with stable chest pain, the correlation between anatomical or stenosis severity and the physiologic significance of a lesion is only modest. The limitation may be overcome by the use of fractional flow reserve (FFR).[3] Another weakness of coronary angiography is that it cannot predict the presence of a vulnerable plaques without the use of intravascular ultrasound or other specialized catheters.[4] To avoid unnecessary procedures and risks from ICA in low- to intermediate-risk patients, myocardial stress testing has been used as a gatekeeper for the invasive procedure.

The evaluation of a patient suspected as having stable ischemic symptoms begins by assessing the pretest probability of CAD based on the patient's history and risk factors. An ideal noninvasive test is one that can determine the presence, extent, location, and functional significance of the CAD.

AIMS OF NONINVASIVE CORONARY IMAGING

With respect to the choice and role of noninvasive cardiac imaging, it is important to distinguish between patients based on the absence or presence of symptoms related to myocardial ischemia. In patients with suspected angina pectoris and acute coronary syndromes, the diagnostic objective is to identify or exclude the presence of obstructive plaques causing sufficient compromise to the blood flow or to identify an alternative etiology for the symptoms. In contrast, in the asymptomatic patient population, the goal is largely targeted at estimating the risk of future events through the identification of atherosclerotic burden, including nonobstructive disease and high-risk plaque.

Most studies performed thus far have compared noninvasive imaging testing with invasive angiography. Important data have shown that angiographic appearance of coronary atherosclerosis does not always correlate with its functional significance. The FAME (Fractional Flow Reserve versus Angiography for Multivessel Evaluation) trial showed that 20% of stenoses in the range of 70% to 90% were not severe enough to impede coronary flow.[5] The FAMOUS-NSTEMI (Fractional Flow Reserve versus Angiographically Guided Management to Optimize Outcomes in Non-ST-segment Elevation in Myocardial Infraction) trial showed there was significant discordance between angiography and FFR in 32% of cases.[6]

Given the potential discordance between the degree of a coronary stenosis and its hemodynamic significance, it may be more clinically relevant to compare noninvasive stress testing techniques that are being used to identify hemodynamically significant CAD against FFR rather than ICA as a reference standard.[7] FFR is quantified as the ratio between the maximum achievable myocardial blood flow in the case of a stenosis and the maximum achievable myocardial blood flow in the absence of stenosis.[8] It is measured during ICA by calculating the ratio between the distal and proximal stenotic coronary artery pressure during maximal myocardial hyperemia. FFR has an ischemic threshold value between 0.75 and 0.80. Multiple studies have shown that FFR 0.75 or less reliably identifies inducible myocardial ischemia, whereas FFR greater than 0.80 reliably excludes myocardial ischemia.[8] The benefits of FFR over other methods quantifying hemodynamically significant CAD are that it is not affected by changes in heart rate, blood pressure, and contractility of the heart.

Numerous cardiac imaging methods exist to diagnose ischemia causing CAD, including single-photon emission computed tomography (SPECT), positron emission tomography (PET), stress echocardiography (SE), cardiac magnetic resonance imaging

(CMRI), CT coronary angiography (CTCA), fractional flow reserved derived from CTCA (CT-FFR), CT perfusion (CTP), and ICA.

Several studies and meta-analyses have reported the accuracy of stress testing for the diagnosis of CAD as defined by the gold standard of cardiac catherization. Without imaging, the sensitivity and specificity of an exercise treadmill test for detecting CAD are modest at 70% to 80%.[9] Adding myocardial imaging to standard exercise testing increases the sensitivity for detecting CAD. SPECT and exercise testing are most commonly used in the United States.

A more recent meta-analysis by Danad and coworkers[10] showed that CMRI had the highest diagnostic performance for detecting hemodynamically significant CAD on both a per-patient and per-vessel basis compared with invasive FFR. Both CTCA and CT-FFR yielded high diagnostic sensitivity with low specificity for CTCA. Diagnostic performance of SPECT, SE, and ICA were generally poorer. Interestingly, both SE and SPECT appeared to be more accurate than ICA. Surprisingly, ICA exhibits both a low sensitivity (69%) and specificity (67%). This finding has been helpful in showing the role of noninvasive imaging to guide clinical decision making and questions the role of ICA for the initial workup of patients with suspected CAD. SPECT performed poorly on a per-vessel level (sensitivity 57% vs 70% on a per-patient basis). A significant mismatch between SPECT-defined myocardial territories and real coronary anatomy in more than half of the cases has been shown. In the presence of multivessel CAD, SPECT has the potential to miss ischemia because of the presence of balanced ischemia or underestimate the ischemic burden because only the region with the most severe ischemia is identified. Performance of SE was modest despite operator bias. CMRI and CPET have a higher diagnostic performance because of higher spatial resolution and better image quality and better endocardial definition. CTCA, on the other hand, has high diagnostic sensitivity, resulting in a high negative predictive value (NPV) to exclude hemodynamically significant CAD. The specificity of CTCA, as well as ICA, is low, which emphasizes discordance between stenosis severity and ischemia causing coronary artery lesions. CT-FFR has emerged as a new tool for the noninvasive diagnosis of ischemia causing CAD by applying computational fluid dynamics to conventional CTCA images.[11] Higher sensitivity of CT-FFR with a modest specificity was noted compared with invasive FFR. In most studies, CT-FFR was evaluated in isolation to CTCA, and therefore the combination would be expected to improve overall specificity.

ANATOMY VERSUS PHYSIOLOGY

Noninvasive imaging of the coronary arteries using CTCA allows for detailed visualization of coronary atherosclerosis and the degree of coronary stenosis. It also holds the promise of providing new insights into plaque biology and pathophysiology. Atherosclerosis is a chronic inflammatory state that is characterized by the formation of lipid-rich plaques. The hallmarks associated with high-risk plaques are characterized as either the macroscopic feature of the plaque versus the biological process within it. Histologic and imaging data have consistently demonstrated that culprit plaques responsible for myocardial infarctions (MIs) have the following characteristics: lipid-rich necrotic core, positive remodeling, microcalcification, chronic inflammation, and a thin fibrous cap. Each of these characteristics represents a potential imaging target.[12]

CORONARY ARTERY CALCIUM SCORING

Atherosclerotic calcification is a well-known process that occurs as a healing response to pathologic inflammation within the plaque. In its earliest stages, there is calcium deposition, and the resultant microcalcifications increase the likelihood of rupture of the surface of fibroatheroma. In more advanced disease by which the calcium is detected on computed tomography (CT), these microcalcifications have coalesced into a large calcific nodules.[13] The assessment of coronary artery calcification is one of the major applications of noninvasive coronary artery imaging. Coronary artery calcium (CAC) scoring is now commonly performed using noncontrast images and are obtained from multidetector CT scanners at submillisevert radiation doses. Arterial calcium is defined as the presence of a lesion with a density greater than 130 Hounsfield units across an area of at least 1 mm^2. Most commonly, these scans are described in Agatston units (AU), a semiquantitative measure that incorporates aspects of calcium density and distribution.

Calcium score has been evaluated in patients with angina and asymptomatic patients. In symptomatic patients, a CAC score greater than 0 has a diagnostic sensitivity for identifying a coronary stenosis of 50% or greater of between 0.89 and 0.99; however, specificity is low, ranging between 0.40 and 0.59.[14] Consequently, in a low-risk population with atypical symptoms in the outpatient clinic, the low positive predictive value (PPV) necessitates additional diagnostic imaging in many cases. Alternatively, in patients with high pretest probability of disease among those with positive troponin in the emergency department, the test will have an unacceptably high "false-negative" result. Therefore, calcium scoring is not recommended as a diagnostic test in patients with chest pain.

Understanding that not all plaques contain calcium, the total CAC score offers an approximate overall atherosclerotic burden for an individual. Multiple studies have confirmed the prognostic values of such scores. The St. Francis Heart Study showed an improvement in the c-statistic for clinical events from 0.69 to 0.79 when added to the Framingham risk score.[15] These findings have been confirmed in larger cohort studies, including the MESA (Multi-Ethnic Study of Atherosclerosis) trial.[16] Calcium scoring has the most clinical value in intermediate-risk patients without established cardiovascular disease when considered whether to initiate primary prevention therapy. In this context, the 2018 American College of Cardiology/American Heart Association (ACC/AHA) guidelines on the prevention of cardiovascular disease give a class IIa recommendation to calcium scoring.[17]

COMPUTED TOMOGRAPHY CORONARY ANGIOGRAPHYβ

The clinical application of CTCA for a long time was limited because of high radiation exposure and cardiac motion artifact. These problems have now mostly resolved because of advances in scanner technology and introduction of multiple dose reduction techniques. With available technology, diagnostic image quality can be obtained in 95% of scans.[18] Limiting factors in obtaining diagnostic image quality include motion artifacts at higher heart rates, presence of significant dense coronary calcification, and coronary stents. These limitations can be minimized by appropriate patient selection and preparation, including use of β-blocker and nitroglycerin therapy. Imaging is being performed on 64-slice or greater CT scanners using intravenous contrast and can be performed with radiation exposure range of 3 to 5 mSv. CTCA detect luminal narrowing 50% diameter or greater with high sensitivity and NPV. The diagnostic accuracy of CTCA for detection of 50% or greater stenosis using ICA as the reference standard has been shown to be high in a number of multicenter studies. A meta-analysis published in 2007 described a sensitivity of 93% and specificity of 96% on per segment basis for detection of CAD.[19] In symptomatic patients with an intermediate pretest probability of obstructive CAD, the NPV of a negative CTCA is more than 95%.[20] In addition to diagnosing coronary obstruction, the use of CTCA for risk stratification has been supported by a large body of literature.[21]

The clinical utility of CTCA has been rigorously evaluated in randomized trials: PROMISE (Prospective Multicenter Imaging Study for Evaluation of Chest Pain) and SCOT-HEART (Scottish Computed Tomography of the HEART). PROMISE ($n = 10,003$) randomized intermediate-risk symptomatic patients being evaluated for CAD to CTCA or noninvasive functional testing (67% nuclear stress imaging,

23% SE, 10% exercise electrocardiography [ECG]).[22] The median follow-up duration was 25 months, and no difference in the primary composite endpoint (death, MI, hospitalization for unstable angina, or major procedural complications) was shown; however, it showed downstream reduction in the rate of unnecessary coronary angiograms and apparent reduction in death or MIs at 12 months.

The SCOT-HEART trial (n = 4146) evaluated the utility of adding CTCA to standard of care (predominantly exercise ECG) in rapid access chest pain clinics across Scotland.[18] The primary endpoint of diagnostic certainty as 6 weeks was increased with CTCA. The 5-year composite clinical outcome of coronary death or nonfatal MIs reported a marked 40% relative risk reduction in the CTCA arm of the trial. These trials show a strong evidence of benefit of CT first approach for the assessment of chest pain.

COMPUTED FRACTIONAL FLOW RESERVE DERIVED FROM COMPUTED TOMOGRAPHY

The current reference standard for assessment of hemodynamically significant coronary stenosis is FFR.[8] FFR is a guide wire-based procedure performed at the time of a coronary angiogram that can accurately measure blood flow through a specific part of the coronary artery. CT-FFR is a noninvasive image postprocessing technique that enables the determination of physiologic significance of coronary artery stenosis by using acquired data from standard coronary CT angiography studies. CT-FFR involves computing FFR from CT data using the same images acquired during a standard coronary CT, and therefore it has an advantage of not using additional scan time, radiation, or more contrast amount. Using computational fluid dynamics, the myocardium and supplying coronary arteries are segmented and evaluated for coronary blood flow. CT-FFR also allows for interventional planning to visualize virtual stenting across a particular lesion to relieve ischemia. In the DISCOVER-FLOW trial (Diagnosis of Ischemia-Causing Stenosis Obtained Via Noninvasive FFR), there was a comparison between iFFR and noninvasive CT-FFR in 103 patients undergoing both CTCA and cardiac catherization. There were a per-vessel accuracy of 84%, sensitivity of 88%, specificity of 82%, PPV of 74%, and NPV of 92% for lesions causing ischemia. CT-FFR and iFFR showed good correlation (r = 0.717; P < .001) with slight underestimation by CT-FFR (0.022 ± 0.116; P = .016).[23]

The multicenter DeFACTO (Diagnostic Accuracy of Fractional Flow Reserve from Anatomic CT Angiography) study assessed the diagnostic performance of CT-FFR plus CTCA for diagnosis of hemodynamically significant coronary stenosis. Although the study did not achieve primary outcome goal for improved per-patient diagnostic accuracy, the use of noninvasive CT-FFR plus CTCA was associated with improved discrimination versus CTCA alone for the diagnosis of hemodynamically significant CAD.[24]

Initial results with CT-FFR are promising; however, prospective multicenter trials are needed to further identify its role in clinical practice. Its cost and turnaround time to receive results after being processed by an off-site computer facility are other issues that need to be resolved in the future.

MAGNETIC RESONANCE CORONARY ANGIOGRAPHY

Magnetic resonance coronary angiography (MRCA) is a widely accepted technique for imaging larger conduit vessels; however, because of spatial resolution and long scan times, coronary imaging with MRCA currently has limited indications in clinical practice except in the assessment of anomalous coronary arteries, coronary aneurysms, and coronary bypass grafts. MRCA has important potential strengths, including the ability of luminal visualization in the presence of dense calcification, absence of ionizing radiation, the possibility of concomitant functional imaging of the myocardium, and detailed tissues characterization. Advances in imaging from single-slice breath-hold sequences, free-breathing whole-heart scanning, and introduction of 3-Tesla magnets have brought a broader clinical role for MRCA. MRCA at this stage has reported to have good diagnostic accuracy with meta-analysis of 24 studies showing a pooled sensitivity and specificity for detection of greater than 50% stenosis on ICA of 89% and 72%, respectively,[25] with some evaluations suggesting a diagnostic performance comparable to that of coronary CTCA.

EXERCISE ELECTROCARDIOGRAPHY STRESS TESTING

Exercise ECG stress testing is a well-validated test for recognizing the diagnosis and prognosis of ischemic heart disease as well as assessing exercise capacity (i.e., functional capacity). It is still the initial test of choice as per ACC/AHA guidelines in low-risk patients with interpretable ECGs[26]; however, European guidelines are increasingly recommending against the use of exercise ECG as an independent test. It can be safely used for diagnostic and prognostic purposes in most patients; however, there are some relative and absolute contraindications that should be considered. Multiple studies have shown that annual event rate in patients with a low-risk exercise treadmill score are below 1%.[27] However, in patients with significant abnormalities on the rest ECG, this testing is nondiagnostic, and addition of imaging is recommended. Advantages of the ECG exercise testing over stress imaging studies include lower cost and more availability. Other advantages of exercise ECG over stress testing with imaging include less technical demand, less influence by processing, and no radiation.

When patients are unable to exercise, pharmacologic stress is recommended. Because the sensitivity of the stress ECG in patients undergoing pharmacologic stress is very low, pharmacologic stress always combines ECG testing with an imaging modality.

STRESS ECHOCARDIOGRAPHY

SE is a commonly used tool to evaluate for myocardial ischemia and has been extensively discussed elsewhere in the textbook. The reported sensitivity of SE for significant CAD detection is 88%, and specificity is 83%[28]; however, meta-analyses suggest the diagnostic performance may be worse when compared with invasive FFR as a reference standard.[10] It is important to note that both sensitivity and specificity are reduced in patients with severe left ventricular (LV) dysfunction. False-negative results are seen in those with small areas of ischemia, LV hypertrophy, or hyperdynamic states. SE is also an important prognostic tool in predicting future cardiac events. A negative SE confers an excellent 1-year prognosis with a 0.5% to 0.8% risk of cardiac death or nonfatal MI.[29] A study analyzing 32,739 patients showed an annual event rate (death or MI) of 1.2% for a normal stress echocardiogram as compared with 7% for an abnormal study.[30] Compared with stress ECG, SE is more accurate and sensitive because wall motion abnormalities (WMAs) occur earlier in the ischemic cascade. It has lower sensitivity than SPECT-MPI (myocardial perfusion imaging), as perfusion abnormalities precede WMAs.[31] Advantages and disadvantages of SE compared with other testing modalities are listed in Table 57.1.

RADIONUCLIDE STRESS MYOCARDIAL PERFUSION IMAGING

Exercise or pharmacologic stress radionuclide MPI using SPECT and PET are commonly used techniques in diagnosis and risk stratification of patients with suspected CAD. Because of the short physical half-lives of PET tracers, pharmacologic vasodilators are the preferred stress method over exercise. The most commonly used SPECT-MPI agents are technetium-99m–based (Tc-99m sestamibi, Tc-99m tetrofosmin) and less commonly thallium-201 alone or in combination with Tc-99m–based tracers (dual-isotope protocol); PET-MPI agents include rubidium-82 and N13-ammonia.

The basic feature of stress radionuclide MPI is the visual assessment of relative myocardial blood flow or perfusion between the resting and stress states. Myocardial segments that demonstrate preserved myocardial perfusion at rest but decreased myocardial perfusion during stress are considered to be ischemic, whereas matched reduced in perfusion between the rest and stress images are suggestive of MI. Other information that can be obtained with this imaging modality include cardiac size and function and regional WMAs in addition to the assessment of myocardial perfusion and viability.

A meta-analysis of numerous SPECT studies demonstrated that the sensitivity and specificity for the diagnosis of significant coronary stenosis greater than 50% was 86% and 74%, respectively.[32] However, meta-analyses suggest the diagnostic performance may be worse when compared with invasive FFR.[10]

The advantages of PET over SPECT include lower radiation and more ability for attenuation correction, which lead to a significantly higher diagnostic accuracy, especially in women and those with larger body habitus.[33]

COMPUTED TOMOGRAPHY PERFUSION

Myocardial CT perfusion can be used to assess for ischemia when CTCA images are acquired after the administration of a vasodilator. CT perfusion images can be performed in static mode, which allows for the qualitative visualization of myocardial perfusion, or in a dynamic mode, which allows for quantification of myocardial blood flow. A recent meta-analysis showed an overall sensitivity of 75% to 84% and a specificity of 78% to 95%.[34] Compared with invasive FFR, the diagnostic performance is similar to stress MRI and stress PET.[35] Currently, adoption is limited by lack of standardization and no formal mechanism for reimbursement. A disadvantage of CTP is the additional use of contrast and a second scan that adds to the total radiation dose.

CARDIOVASCULAR MAGNETIC RESONANCE PERFUSION

CMRI stress testing is performed using pharmacologic agents such as dobutamine or one of the vasodilators (e.g., regadenoson, adenosine, dipyridamole) to evaluate for ischemia. Multiple studies thus far have demonstrated high accuracy of vasodilator stress CMRI in detecting coronary stenoses and in estimating impaired flow reserve. The ACC and AHA have recommended stress CMRI as an appropriate test for evaluation of symptomatic patients with intermediate to high pretest probability of CAD[36]; however, this imaging modality is underused in the United States relative to Europe. In the SPINS (Stress CMRI Perfusion Imaging in the United States: A Society for Cardiovascular Resonance Registry Study) trial, a multicenter study of patients with chest pain, patients without CMRI evidence of ischemia or late gadolinium enhancement (LGE, a marker of myocardial scar) experienced a low incidence of cardiac events, low need for coronary revascularization, and lower spending on subsequent ischemia testing.[37] The MR-inform (Magnetic Resonance Perfusion or Fractional Flow Reserve in Coronary Disease) trial, a randomized controlled trial comparing stress CMRI-guided revascularization against invasive FFR-guided revascularization, showed that among patients with stable angina and risk factors for CAD, myocardial-perfusion CMRI was associated with a lower rate of ICA and a lower incidence of coronary revascularization compared with FFR. Importantly, the patients in the perfusion CMRI arm did not have an increased rate of major adverse cardiac events.[38] With the current focus on value-based care, these studies thus far have shown a reduced downstream rate of coronary revascularization and cost minimization.

CONCLUSIONS

Currently, there is no consensus about the optimal noninvasive approach to assessing CAD. Each of the imaging modalities has its unique strengths and weaknesses (Table 57.2). One practical

---

TABLE 57.1 Advantages and Disadvantages of Stress Echocardiography Compared With Other Testing Modalities

Advantages	Disadvantages
More specific than SPECT for diagnosis of CAD and viability	Less sensitive, particularly in patients with mild disease, submaximal stress, and antianginal treatment
More accurate in women and patients with LVH and LBBB	Less sensitive for detecting ischemia close to resting WMA
More specific for assessing myocardial viability	Less sensitive for assessing viability
Long-term prognostic value similar to SPECT	Technically difficult in patients with pulmonary disease (e.g., emphysema)
Feasible in morbidly obese patients with the aid of contrast agent; does not underestimate multivessel CAD and has no concerns of "balanced ischemia" in multivessel or left main disease	Rapid resolution of subtle wall motion abnormalities post-treadmill with submaximal exercise (not applicable to supine bicycle or pharmacologic stress)
No radiation exposure; less expensive	Highly dependent on expertise of reader for visual interpretation
Convenient; interpreted immediately; high-volume performance	
Provides information on cardiac structure and function (e.g., valvular disease, diastology, and pulmonary pressures)	

CAD, Coronary artery disease; *LBBB,* left bundle branch block; *LVH,* left ventricular hypertrophy; *SPECT,* single-photon emission computed tomography; *WMA,* wall motion abnormality.

TABLE 57.2 Advantages and Disadvantages of Different Stress Techniques

Stress techniques	Diagnostic Accuracy			Radiation	Portability	Cost	Future directions
	Sensitivity	Specificity	Prognosis				
Stress ECG	++	++	++	−	++++	+	Strategy of ECG stress + CAC
Nuclear stress/PET	++++	+++	++++	+++	−	++++	Stress only, low dose, CT correction ± CAC scoring, myocardial blood flow
Stress echocardiography	+++	++++	+++	−	++++	++	3D one-beat acquisition, perfusion, strain imaging
CTCA	++++	+++	+++	++	−	++++	CT perfusion,
Cardiac MRI perfusion	++++	+++	++	−	−	++++	Coronary artery and plaque visualization

3D, Three dimensional; *CAC,* coronary artery calcium; *CTCA,* coronary computed tomography angiography; *CT,* computed tomography; *ECG,* electrocardiogram; *FFR,* fractional flow reserve; *MRI,* magnetic resonance imaging; *PET,* positron emission tomography.

approach may be to select an anatomical test such as CTCA to assess for coronary disease in patients without a known history of CAD. Such a test would not only allow for the detection of a severe coronary artery stenosis that may explain individual patient's symptoms but also detect the presence of nonobstructive disease that might lead to the initiation of preventive medical therapy. On the other hand, a functional test such as SE, nuclear stress imaging, or CMRI might be preferred in patients with known CAD, especially those who have been previously revascularized because the key clinical question is to identify patients with hemodynamically significant CAD that might benefit from revascularization. Patient-specific characteristics and local expertise should also be considered when determining which imaging modality might be the best choice in any given situation.

REFERENCES

1. Berrington de Gonzalez A, Kim KP, Smith-Bindman R, McAreavey D. Myocardial perfusion scans: projected population cancer risks from current levels of use in the United States. *Circulation.* 2010;122:2403–2410.
2. Patel MR, Peterson ED, Dai D, et al. Low diagnostic yield of elective coronary angiography. *N Engl J Med.* 2010;362:886–895.
3. Pijls NH, Fearon WF, Tonino PA, et al. Fractional flow reserve versus angiography for guiding percutaneous coronary intervention in patients with multivessel coronary artery disease: 2-year follow-up of the FAME (Fractional Flow Reserve versus Angiography for Multivessel Evaluation) study. *J Am Coll Cardiol.* 2010;56:177–184.
4. Anderson JL, Adams CD, Antman EM, et al. ACC/AHA 2007 guidelines for the management of patients with unstable angina/non-ST-elevation myocardial infarction. *J Am Coll Cardiol.* 2007;50:e1–e157.
5. Tonino PA, Fearon WF, De Bruyne B, et al. Angiographic versus functional severity of coronary artery stenoses in the FAME study fractional flow reserve versus angiography in multivessel evaluation. *J Am Coll Cardiol.* 2010;55:2816–2821.
6. Layland J, Oldroyd KG, Curzen N, et al. Fractional flow reserve vs. angiography in guiding management to optimize outcomes in non-ST-segment elevation myocardial infarction: the British Heart Foundation FAMOUS-NSTEMI randomized trial. *Eur Heart J.* 2015;36:100–111.
7. Tonino PA, De Bruyne B, Pijls NH, et al. Fractional flow reserve versus angiography for guiding percutaneous coronary intervention. *N Engl J Med.* 2009;360(3):213–224.
8. Pijls NH, De Bruyne B, Peels K, et al. Measurement of fractional flow reserve to assess the functional severity of coronary-artery stenoses. *N Engl J Med.* 1996;334:1703–1708.
9. Gianrossi R, Detrano R, Mulvihill D, et al. Exercise-induced ST depression in the diagnosis of coronary artery disease. A meta-analysis. *Circulation.* 1989;80:87–98.
10. Danad I, Szymonifka J, Twisk JWR, et al. Diagnostic performance of cardiac imaging methods to diagnose ischaemia-causing coronary artery disease when directly compared with fractional flow reserve as a reference standard: a meta-analysis. *Eur Heart J.* 2017;38:991–998.
11. Taylor CA, Fonte TA, Min JK. Computational fluid dynamics applied to cardiac computed tomography for noninvasive quantification of fractional flow reserve: Scientific basis. *J Am Coll Cardiol.* 2013;61:2233–2241.
12. Adamson PD, Newby DE. Non-invasive imaging of the coronary arteries. *Eur Heart J.* 2019;40:2444–2454.
13. Rifkin RD, Parisi AF, Folland E. Coronary calcification in the diagnosis of coronary artery disease. *Am J Cardiol.* 1979;44:141–147.
14. Sarwar A, Shaw LJ, Shapiro MD, et al. Diagnostic and prognostic value of absence of coronary artery calcification. *JACC Cardiovasc Imag.* 2009;2:675–688.
15. Arad Y, Spadaro LA, Roth M, et al. Treatment of asymptomatic adults with elevated coronary calcium scores with atorvastatin, vitamin C, and vitamin E: the St. Francis Heart Study randomized clinical trial. *J Am Coll Cardiol.* 2005;46:166–172.
16. Brown ER, Kronmal RA, Bluemke DA, et al. Coronary calcium coverage score: determination, correlates, and predictive accuracy in the Multi-Ethnic Study of Atherosclerosis. *Radiology.* 2008;247:669–675.
17. Grundy SM, Stone NJ, Bailey AL, et al: 2018 AHA/ACC/AACVPR/AAPA/ABC/ACPM/ADA/AGS/APhA/ASPC/NLA/PCNA guideline on the management of blood cholesterol: Executive summary, Circulation 139:e1046–e1081, 2019.
18. SCOT-HEART Investigators. CT coronary angiography in patients with suspected angina due to coronary heart disease (SCOT-HEART): an open-label, parallel-group, multicentre trial. *Lancet.* 2015;385:2383–2391.
19. Vanhoenacker PK, Heijenbrok-Kal MH, Van Heste R, et al. Diagnostic performance of multidetector CT angiography for assessment of coronary artery disease: meta-analysis. *Radiology.* 2007;244:419–428.
20. Budoff MJ, Dowe D, Jollis JG, et al. Diagnostic performance of 64-multidetector row coronary computed tomographic angiography for evaluation of coronary artery stenosis in individuals without known coronary artery disease: results from the prospective multicenter ACCURACY (Assessment by Coronary Computed Tomographic Angiography of Individuals Undergoing Invasive Coronary Angiography) trial. *J Am Coll Cardiol.* 2008;52:1724–1732.
21. Min JK, Dunning A, Lin FY, et al. Age- and sex-related differences in all-cause mortality risk based on coronary computed tomography angiography findings results from the International Multicenter CONFIRM (Coronary CT Angiography Evaluation for Clinical Outcomes: an International Multicenter Registry) of 23,854 patients without known coronary artery disease. *J Am Coll Cardiol.* 2011;58:849–860.
22. Douglas PS, Hoffmann U, Patel MR, et al. Outcomes of anatomical versus functional testing for coronary artery disease. *N Engl J Med.* 2015;372:1291–1300.
23. Koo BK, Erglis A, Doh JH, et al. Diagnosis of ischemia-causing coronary stenoses by noninvasive fractional flow reserve computed from coronary computed tomographic angiograms. Results from the prospective multicenter DISCOVER-FLOW (Diagnosis of Ischemia-Causing Stenoses Obtained via Noninvasive Fractional Flow Reserve) study. *J Am Coll Cardiol.* 2011;58:1989–1997.
24. Min JK, Leipsic J, Pencina MJ, et al. Diagnostic accuracy of fractional flow reserve from anatomic CT angiography. *J Am Med Assoc.* 2012;308:1237–1245.
25. Di Leo G, Fisci E, Secchi F, et al. Diagnostic accuracy of magnetic resonance angiography for detection of coronary artery disease: a systematic review and meta-analysis. *Eur Radiol.* 2016;26:3706–3718.
26. Gibbons RJ, Balady GJ, Bricker JT, et al. ACC/AHA 2002 guideline update for exercise testing: summary article. *J Am Coll Cardiol.* 2002;40:1531–1540.
27. Rywik TM, O'Connor FC, Gittings NS, et al. Role of nondiagnostic exercise-induced ST-segment abnormalities in predicting future coronary events in asymptomatic volunteers. *Circulation.* 2002;106:2787–2792.
28. Fihn SD, Gardin JM, Abrams J, et al. ACCF/AHA/ACP/AATS/PCNA/SCAI/STS guideline for the diagnosis and management of patients with stable ischemic heart disease: Executive summary. *J Am Coll Cardiol.* 2012;60:2564–2603. 2012.
29. McCully RB, Roger VL, Mahoney DW, et al. Outcome after normal exercise echocardiography and predictors of subsequent cardiac events: follow-up of 1,325 patients. *J Am Coll Cardiol.* 1998;31:144–149.
30. Elhendy A, Mahoney DW, Khandheria BK, et al. Prognostic significance of the location of wall motion abnormalities during exercise echocardiography. *J Am Coll Cardiol.* 2002;40:1623–1629.
31. Schinkel AF, Bax JJ, Geleijnse ML, et al. Noninvasive evaluation of ischaemic heart disease: myocardial perfusion imaging or stress echocardiography? *Eur Heart J.* 2003;24:789–800.
32. Underwood SR, Anagnostopoulos C, Cerqueira M, et al. Myocardial perfusion scintigraphy: the evidence. *Eur J Nucl Med Mol Imag.* 2004;31:261–291.
33. Dilsizian V, Bacharach SL, Beanlands RS, et al: ASNC imaging guidelines/SNMMI procedure standard for positron emission tomography (PET) nuclear cardiology procedures. *J Nucl Cardiol.* 23:1187–1226.
34. Pelgrim GJ, Dorrius M, Xie X, et al. The dream of a one-stop-shop: meta-analysis on myocardial perfusion CT. *Eur J Radiol.* 2015;84:2411–2420.
35. Takx RA, Blomberg BA, El Aidi H, et al. Diagnostic accuracy of stress myocardial perfusion imaging compared to invasive coronary angiography with fractional flow reserve meta-analysis. *Circ Cardiovasc Imag.* 2015;8:1.
36. Wolk MJ, Bailey SR, Doherty JU, et al. ACCF/AHA/ASE/ASNC/HFSA/HRS/SCAI/SCCT/SCMR/STS 2013 multimodality appropriate use criteria for the detection and risk assessment of stable ischemic heart disease. *J Am Coll Cardiol.* 2014;63:380–406.
37. Kwong RY, Ge Y, Steel K, et al. Cardiac magnetic resonance stress perfusion imaging for evaluation of patients with chest pain. *J Am Coll Cardiol.* 2019;74:1741–1755.
38. Nagel E, Greenwood JP, McCann GP, et al. Magnetic resonance perfusion or fractional flow reserve in coronary disease. *N Engl J Med.* 2019;380:2418–2428.

58

Pathophysiology and Variants of Hypertrophic Cardiomyopathy

Sara Hoss, Lynne Williams, Harry Rakowski

Hypertrophic cardiomyopathy (HCM) is characterized by the presence of left ventricular (LV) hypertrophy in the absence of another cardiac or systemic etiology.[1] It is a genetic condition with an autosomal dominant inheritance, affecting 1 in 500 individuals of the general population.[2] The commonly used threshold for HCM diagnosis is unexplained maximal wall thickness of 15 mm or greater in one or more myocardial segments or 13 mm or greater in the presence of positive family history. In the setting of systemic hypertension, a ratio of septal to posterior wall thickness exceeding 1.5:1 is also strongly suggestive of the diagnosis, reflecting that one of the key features in this condition is the asymmetric nature of the hypertrophy pattern.[3] This chapter reviews the different anatomic and physiologic variants of HCM.

ANATOMIC VARIANTS

HCM is a heterogeneous condition with multiple anatomic variants, including reverse curvature, a neutral septum, a sigmoid septum, and apical hypertrophy (Figs. 58.1 and 58.2). The reverse curvature morphology involves a predominant midseptal convexity toward the LV cavity, with an overall crescent shape, whereas a sigmoid septum has an overall ovoid shape with a prominent septal bulge, and a neutral septum has a relatively straight shape.[4] Patients with HCM who are diagnosed at a young age are more likely to have the reverse curvature morphology than the sigmoid septum, which is more commonly seen in older adult patients with HCM.[5] Patients in the same family may present with more than one type of anatomic variant; the exact reason for this is unclear. It has also been shown that various anatomic forms of HCM have different genotype-positive rates. Studies from the Mayo Clinic and Toronto showed that 53% to 79% of patients with reverse septal curvature and 41% to 48% of patients with a neutral septal type were found to have an identifiable HCM-causing mutation compared with only 8% to 23% of patients with a sigmoid septum and 11% to 30% of patients with apical HCM (Fig. 58.3).[4,6]

Apart from myocardial hypertrophy, mitral valve and papillary muscles abnormalities have been well described in this condition. Elongation of mitral valve leaflets, asymmetrical enlargement of either leaflet, anterior or apical displacement of the papillary muscles, and direct insertion of the papillary muscle into the anterior mitral valve leaflet are common in this condition.[7–9] These structural changes can contribute to the degree of left ventricular outflow tract obstruction (LVOTO) and mitral regurgitation (MR) and influence the type and extent of intervention when required.[10]

PATHOPHYSIOLOGY
Diastolic Dysfunction

Diastolic dysfunction, microvascular ischemia, autonomic dysfunction, LVOTO, and MR are the key pathophysiologic mechanisms

underlying HCM (Fig. 58.4). Diastolic dysfunction is a main component in all variants of HCM. Myocardial hypertrophy is characterized by increase in muscle mass and decrease in ventricular volume, often combined with different degrees of myocardial fibrosis that cause impaired ventricular relaxation.[11] Patients with HCM have also been shown to have abnormal handling of intracellular calcium, leading to delayed inactivation, which contributes to diastolic dysfunction.[12] Typical echocardiographic findings include reduced E velocity, enhanced A velocity, increased duration and velocity of pulmonary A-wave reversal, and a higher ratio of mitral inflow to annular velocity (E/E′). In addition, patients with HCM have abnormal diastolic myocardial mechanics, with decreased peak early diastolic to peak systolic strain rates, prolonged LV untwisting time, and a lower apical reverse rotation fraction.[13] With time, left atrial remodeling and increased left atrial volume can result in atrial fibrillation and atrial flutter, which can lead to adverse long-term consequences, such as systemic embolization and heart failure symptoms.[13]

Myocardial Ischemia

Although epicardial coronary artery disease can occur in patients with HCM and has been shown to be associated with adverse clinical outcomes, myocardial ischemia in this patient population is often caused by demand–supply mismatch.[14,15] Myocardial ischemia and impaired relaxation are intimately linked, and a vicious cycle may exist in which impaired diastolic function further compromises coronary perfusion and vice versa.[16] Increased wall thickness, elevated LV filling pressure, abnormally thickened intramural coronary arteries, and increased afterload from LVOTO are all factors that contribute to myocardial ischemia and chest pain.[15,17] Patients with HCM have impaired vasodilatory capacity and blunted myocardial blood flow during stress testing, which are evident on positron emission tomography and single-photon emission computed tomography.[18,19] Chronic myocardial ischemia is considered an important reason for the development of apical infarcts and apical aneurysm in patients with apical HCM.

Autonomic Dysfunction

Another important component in the pathophysiology of HCM is autonomic dysfunction and the phenomenon of exercise-induced hypotension (lack of increase in systolic blood pressure by >20 mmHg or a decrease in blood pressure with exercise). These patients are thought to have decreased peripheral vascular resistance during exercise secondary to the activation of ventricular baroreceptor reflexes and the withdrawal of sympathetic tone to the resistant vessels.[20] Abnormal exercise blood pressure response is associated with increased risk of sudden cardiac death (SCD) in patients younger than 50 years of age.[20–22] Thus,

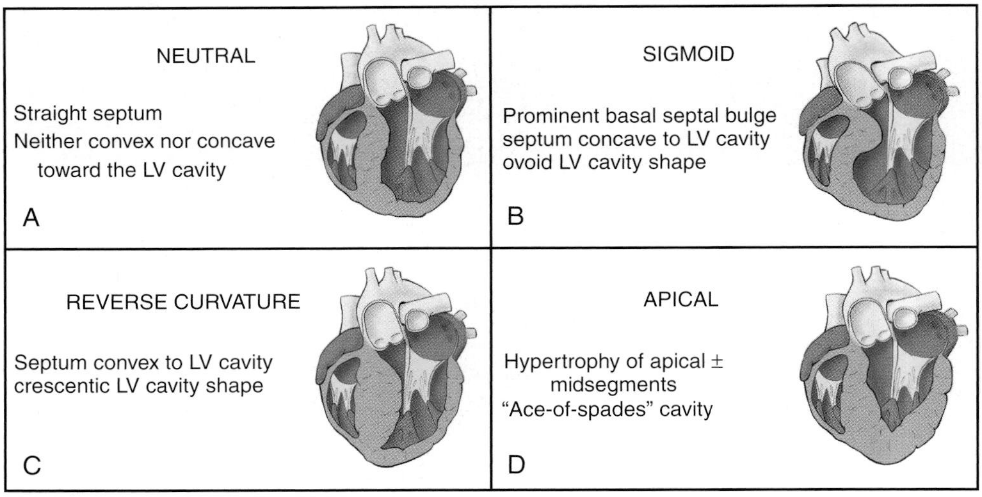

Figure 58.1. Spectrum of hypertrophic cardiomyopathy morphologies. **A,** Asymmetric septal hypertrophy with a neutral septum that is neither concave nor convex to the cavity of the left ventricle (LV). **B,** Sigmoid septum with hypertrophy confined to the basal septum. **C,** Reverse curvature pattern with a crescentic shape toward the cavity of the LV. **D,** Apical hypertrophy with hypertrophy confined to the LV apex and normal wall thickness in the basal segments.

NEUTRAL

Straight septum
Neither convex nor concave
toward the LV cavity

A

SIGMOID

Prominent basal septal bulge
septum concave to LV cavity
ovoid LV cavity shape

B

REVERSE CURVATURE

Septum convex to LV cavity
crescentic LV cavity shape

C

APICAL

Hypertrophy of apical ±
midsegments
"Ace-of-spades" cavity

D

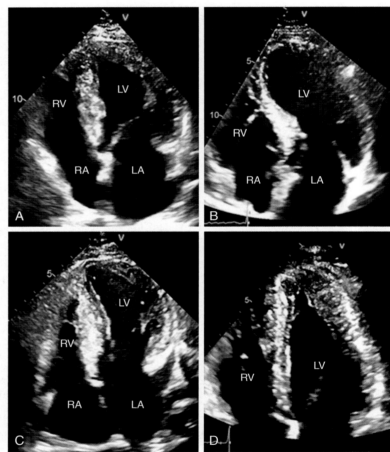

Figure 58.2. Hypertrophic cardiomyopathy morphologies in transthoracic echocardiography. Typical echocardiographic appearances of different hypertrophic cardiomyopathy morphologies including a neutral septum (**A**), a sigmoid septum (**B**), reverse curvature (**C**), and apical hypertrophy (**D**). *LA,* Left atrium; *LV,* left ventricle; *RA,* right atrium; *RV,* right ventricle.

exercise testing is recommended in young patients with HCM as part of their SCD risk stratification.[1]

PHYSIOLOGIC VARIANTS

In addition to anatomic descriptions, classification of HCM can also be based on hemodynamic features. Approximately two-thirds of patients with HCM have resting or provocable LVOTO, defined as peak gradient of 30 mmHg or greater. One-third of patients have nonobstructive HCM with a left ventricular outflow tract (LVOT) gradient of less than 30 mmHg.[23] Midventricular

obstruction (MVO) HCM is an uncommon form of the condition, defined by a midventricular gradient of 30 mmHg or greater (Fig. 58.5).

Hypertrophic Cardiomyopathy With Left Ventricular Outflow Tract Obstruction

Of all patients with obstructive HCM, half have resting LVOTO, and the other half develop LVOTO with provocation. Dynamic LVOTO is an important manifestation of HCM and a major cause of symptoms such as shortness of breath, chest pain, presyncope,

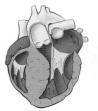 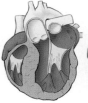 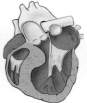 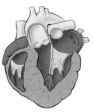

	REVERSE CURVATURE	NEUTRAL	SIGMOID SEPTUM	APICAL	OTHER
Frequency	35%*	8%	47%	10%	-
	23%**	28%	28%	17%	4%
Genotype +	79%*	41%	8%	30%	-
	53%**	48%	23%	11%	11%

Strong predictor of genopositivity

Figure 58.3. Different proportion of gene-positive patients between hypertrophic cardiomyopathy (HCM) morphologies. Studies have demonstrated a higher rate of positive genetic testing in the setting of specific morphologic subtypes. The yield from testing was highest in patients with either a neutral septum or reverse curvature morphology in comparison with low yield in patients with a sigmoid septum or apical hypertrophy. *Asterisk* and *double asterisk* represent numbers derived from two major studies.

MYOCARDIAL ISCHEMIA
- Supply–demand mismatch
- Abnormalities of coronary microvasculature
- Myocardial bridging (15–40%)

LVOT OBSTRUCTION
- Increased intracavity pressures
- Increased oxygen requirements
- Abnormal loading conditions

PATHOPHYSIOLOGY OF HYPERTROPHIC CARDIOMYOPATHY

DIASTOLIC DYSFUNCTION
- Chamber hypertrophy
- Increased muscle stiffness (myocardial disarray and fibrosis)
- Abnormal intracellular calcium handling

AUTONOMIC DYSFUNCTION
- Abnormal blood pressure response to exercise
- Decreased peripheral vascular resistance during exercise

Figure 58.4. Key pathophysiologic mechanisms underlying hypertrophic cardiomyopathy. The clinical features of hypertrophic cardiomyopathy are generally the result of a complex interplay between several pathophysiologic mechanisms. *LVOT,* Left ventricular outflow tract.

and syncope. Resting LVOTO is associated with adverse prognosis such as heart failure and death.[24]

Several anatomic abnormalities can contribute to LVOTO, including hypertrophy of the basal septum; elongation of one or both mitral valve leaflets; and papillary muscle anomalies such as anterior displacement, papillary hypertrophy, or accessory papillary muscle. These, together with rapid LV ejection caused by LV hypercontractility, cause systolic anterior movement (SAM) of the anterior mitral valve leaflet toward the septum, narrowing of the LVOT and elevated pressure gradient (see Fig. 58.5).[7–9] Additionally, SAM can cause MR with a typical posteriorly directed jet.

Nonobstructive Hypertrophic Cardiomyopathy

Nonobstructive HCM and LVOTO HCM are two phenotypes originating from the same cause, as demonstrated by a study revealing the same morphologic changes in hypertrophied myocardium of patients with and without LVOTO.[25] This was supported by recent studies showing that both obstructive and nonobstructive HCM can result from the same genetic pathogenic variant.[26] Absence of obstruction may be caused by differences in structure and intrinsic geometry of the septum, LVOT, and mitral valve apparatus.

Patients with nonobstructive HCM can experience significant chest pain and dyspnea secondary to microvascular ischemia and

abnormal vasodilatory response.[27] Symptomatic patients with no significant LVOTO or valvular abnormality pose a therapeutic challenge in the lack of target for invasive treatment, leaving medical therapy as the main option. Additionally, chronic LV diastolic dysfunction results in left atrial volumetric remodeling, which is a predictor of worse exercise capacity in patients with nonobstructive HCM.[28]

Midventricular Obstruction in Hypertrophic Cardiomyopathy

The midventricular form of obstructive HCM was first described in 1977 and is defined by a midventricular systolic gradient of 30 mmHg or greater caused by systolic apposition of the mid-LV walls, which often include the papillary muscles.[29,30] The characteristic Doppler finding is a late peaking systolic signal, which is the result of a pressure gradient formed by midseptal hypertrophy coming into contact with a hyperdynamic LV free wall, and is often aggravated by the interposition of a hypertrophied papillary muscle (see Fig. 58.5). The phenomenon of early diastole paradoxical flow has also been described, in which flow occurs from the apex toward the base of the heart during diastole.[30] In contrast to patients with LVOTO, systolic anterior motion and MR are not typical features of MVO.[11] More than a quarter of

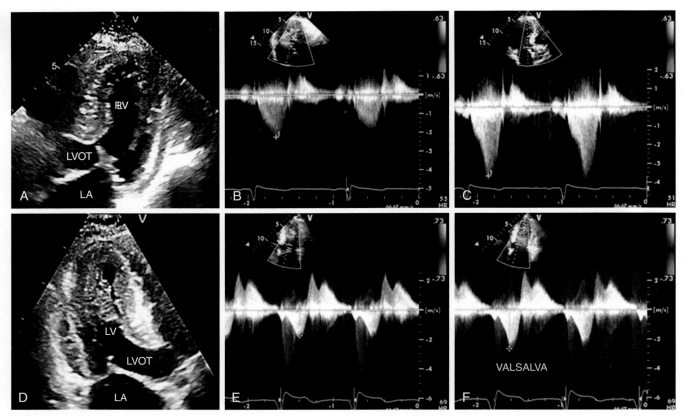

Figure 58.5. Physiological variants of hypertrophic cardiomyopathy (HCM). Patients with HCM can be grouped into three distinct categories based on the presence or absence of obstruction, either at the level of the midventricle or left ventricular outflow tract (LVOT): patients with resting gradient, patients with gradient only with provocation and patients with no obstruction. **A** demonstrates LVOT obstruction with gradients at rest (**B**) and after Valsalva maneuver (**C**). **D** demonstrates midcavity obstruction with gradients at rest (**E**) and after Valsalva maneuver (**F**). *LA,* Left atrium; *LV,* left ventricle.

patients with MVO HCM are prone to developing apical infarction and a subsequent apical aneurysm.[31] Midcavity obliteration was shown to be associated with a large pressure gradient across the midventricular level, which can lead to further hypertrophy and chronic myocardial ischemia, thus resulting in a vicious cycle.[32,33] Midventricular HCM was identified in approximately 10% of all patients with HCM based on several large cohort studies, with variations based on the ethnic background of the study patients.[31] MVO HCM was shown to be an independent predictor of adverse outcomes, such as potential lethal arrhythmic events and sudden death. It is also associated with a higher likelihood of stroke and progression to end-stage HCM.[31,34] Midventricular obstruction in the setting of an apical aneurysm is even a stronger risk factor for HCM-related death. Patients with severe symptoms despite optimal medical therapy may derive symptom relief from dual-chamber pacing and surgical myectomy.

Apical Hypertrophic Cardiomyopathy

Apical HCM is a relatively uncommon subtype of this condition, with hypertrophy predominantly involving the apex of the left ventricle resulting in a characteristic "ace of spades" configuration of the left ventricle.[35] It is more commonly seen in Asian population, with as many as 41% of patients with HCM presenting with this subtype in China and up to 15% in Japan.[36,37] Associated electrocardiographic features include the presence of giant negative T waves (>10 mm) in the precordial leads.[38] Echocardiographic diagnosis of apical HCM and apical aneurysms is challenging because of near-field artifacts.

Contrast-enhanced echocardiography and cardiac magnetic resonance imaging (CMRI) increase the diagnostic yield of apical HCM and apical aneurysms (Fig. 58.6).[39,40] Most patients with apical HCM have nonobstructive physiology, although some develop an apical gradient, which can cause chronic myocardial ischemia. Approximately 18.3% of patients with apical HCM develop apical aneurysm, a phenotype that carries prognostic implication.[41] Although the majority of patients with apical HCM have a relatively benign outcome with annual cardiovascular mortality rates of 0.1%, up to one-third of patients develop cardiovascular complications, including myocardial infarction, atrial or ventricular arrhythmia, congestive heart failure, and stroke. Some patients may experience severe diastolic dysfunction and marked reduction in the effective LV chamber size from apical cavity obliteration.[42] Apical aneurysm has been associated with adverse outcome after several studies demonstrated increased risk of arrhythmic sudden death, thromboembolic episodes, and progressive heart failure in patients with HCM with apical aneurysm.[40,43] Other predictors of adverse events include young age at diagnosis, New York Heart Association functional class II or higher, and left atrial enlargement.[42]

END-STAGE HYPERTROPHIC CARDIOMYOPATHY

Although most patients with HCM maintain a normal or high LV systolic function, some progress to end-stage hypertrophic cardiomyopathy (ES-HCM), defined by LV ejection fraction of 50% or less. ES-HCM is observed in 2% to 5% of patients with HCM and carries higher rates of morbidity and mortality.[44,45] Most patients

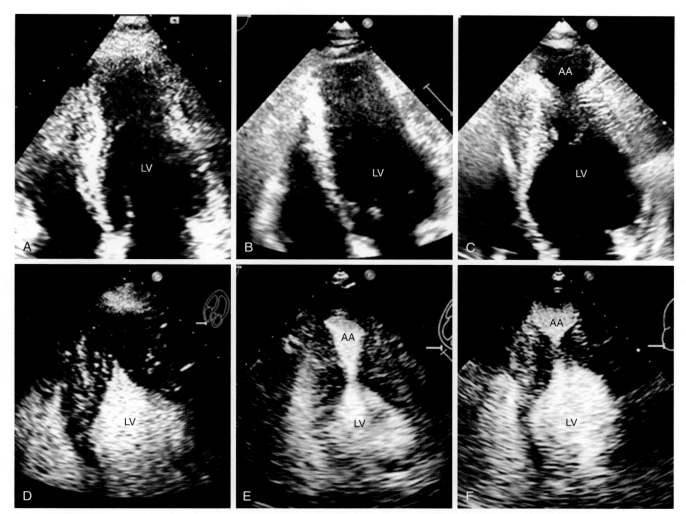

Figure 58.6. Use of contrast-enhanced echocardiography for hypertrophic cardiomyopathy diagnosis and investigation. Echocardiographic imaging of the left ventricular (LV) apex is difficult because of near-field artifacts (**A** and **B**). Contrast-enhanced echocardiography assists in diagnosis of apical hypertrophy (**D**) and apical aneurysm (AA) (**E**). Even in cases when the apical aneurysm is big and easy to identify (**C**), contrast could be used to exclude apical thrombus (**F**).

with ES-HCM gradually develop LV dilatation, myocardial wall thinning, and systolic dysfunction, sometimes accompanied by loss of previous LVOT or midventricular obstruction (Fig. 58.7). Pathology and CMRI often demonstrate extensive myocardial fibrosis, which presumably plays a pivotal role in ES-HCM pathophysiology.[44,46] Another, less frequent type of ES-HCM presents with a restrictive phenotype. These patients usually have a small LV cavity with more substantial hypertrophy and left atrial enlargement.[44,47] Cardiac MRI demonstrates fibrosis but in a lesser extent than in ES-HCM with dilated LV.[46] Patients with ES-HCM have higher rates of heart failure symptoms, atrial fibrillation, and fatal ventricular arrhythmia. Most patients are treated with standard heart failure medical therapy, and the only definite treatment is heart transplant.

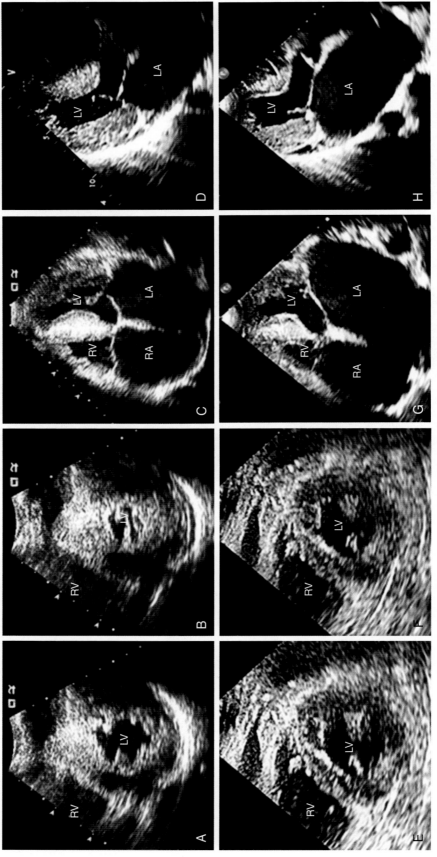

Figure 58.7. Progression to end-stage hypertrophic cardiomyopathy (ES-HCM) in transthoracic echocardiography. *Top row images* are of hypertrophic obstructive cardiomyopathy with normal systolic left ventricular (LV) function, as seen in short-axis images acquired in end-diastole (**A**) and end-systole (**B**). Apical four-chamber (**C**) and apical long-axis (**D**) images demonstrate significant septal hypertrophy with systolic anterior motion (SAM) causing left ventricular outflow tract obstruction (LVOTO). *Bottom row images* were acquired 10 years later after progression to ES-HCM. Short-axis views demonstrate decrease in septal wall thickness and very little change between end-diastole (**E**) and end-systole (**F**), indicating reduced systolic function. Apical four-chamber (**G**) and apical long-axis (**H**) images demonstrate severe left atrial (LA) enlargement and loss of SAM. *RA,* Right atrium; *RV,* right ventricle.

REFERENCES

1. Gersh BJ, Maron BJ, Bonow RO, et al. ACCF/AHA Guideline for the diagnosis and treatment of hypertrophic cardiomyopathy. *J Am Coll Cardiol.* 2011;58:e212–260. 2011.
2. Authors/Task Force m, Elliott PM, Anastasakis A, et al. ESC guidelines on diagnosis and management of hypertrophic cardiomyopathy. *Eur Heart J.* 2014;35:2733–2779. 2014.
3. Doi YL, Deanfield JE, McKenna WJ, et al. Echocardiographic differentiation of hypertensive heart disease and hypertrophic cardiomyopathy. *Br Heart J.* 1980;44:395–400.
4. Binder J, Ommen SR, Gersh BJ, et al. Echocardiography-guided genetic testing in hypertrophic cardiomyopathy: septal morphological features predict the presence of myofilament mutations. *Mayo Clin Proc.* 2006;81:459–467.
5. Lever HM, Karam RF, Currie PJ, Healy BP. Hypertrophic cardiomyopathy in the elderly. Distinctions from the young based on cardiac shape. *Circulation.* 1989;79:580–589.
6. Gruner C, Ivanov J, Care M, et al. Toronto hypertrophic cardiomyopathy genotype score for prediction of a positive genotype in hypertrophic cardiomyopathy. *Circ Cardiovasc Genet.* 2013;6:19–26.
7. Klues HG, Maron BJ, Dollar AL, Roberts WC. Diversity of structural mitral valve alterations in hypertrophic cardiomyopathy. *Circulation.* 1992;85:1651–1660.
8. Harrigan CJ, Appelbaum E, Maron BJ, et al. Significance of papillary muscle abnormalities identified by cardiovascular magnetic resonance in hypertrophic cardiomyopathy. *Am J Cardiol.* 2008;101:668–673.
9. Patel P, Dhillon A, Popovic ZB, et al. Left ventricular outflow tract obstruction in hypertrophic cardiomyopathy patients without severe septal hypertrophy: implications of mitral valve and papillary muscle abnormalities assessed using cardiac magnetic resonance and echocardiography. *Circ Cardiovasc Imag.* 2015;8. e003132.
10. Kwon DH, Smedira NG, Thamilarasan M, et al. Characteristics and surgical outcomes of symptomatic patients with hypertrophic cardiomyopathy with abnormal papillary muscle morphology undergoing papillary muscle reorientation. *J Thorac Cardiovasc Surg.* 2010;140:317–324.
11. Wigle ED, Rakowski H, Kimball BP, Williams WG. Hypertrophic cardiomyopathy. Clinical spectrum and treatment. *Circulation.* 1995;92:1680–1692.
12. Lan F, Lee AS, Liang P, et al. Abnormal calcium handling properties underlie familial hypertrophic cardiomyopathy pathology in patient-specific induced pluripotent stem cells. *Cell Stem Cell.* 2013;12:101–113.
13. Carasso S, Yang H, Woo A, et al. Diastolic myocardial mechanics in hypertrophic cardiomyopathy. *J Am Soc Echocardiogr.* 2010;23:164–171.
14. Sorajja P, Ommen SR, Nishimura RA, et al. Adverse prognosis of patients with hypertrophic cardiomyopathy who have epicardial coronary artery disease. *Circulation.* 2003;108:2342–2348.
15. Maron MS, Olivotto I, Maron BJ, et al. The case for myocardial ischemia in hypertrophic cardiomyopathy. *J Am Coll Cardiol.* 2009;54:866–875.
16. Wigle ED, Sasson Z, Henderson MA, et al. Hypertrophic cardiomyopathy. The importance of the site and the extent of hypertrophy. *Prog Cardiovasc Dis.* 1985;28(1–83).
17. Maron BJ, Wolfson JK, Epstein SE, Roberts WC. Intramural ("small vessel") coronary artery disease in hypertrophic cardiomyopathy. *J Am Coll Cardiol.* 1986;8:545–557.
18. Camici P, Chiriatti G, Lorenzoni R, et al. Coronary vasodilation is impaired in both hypertrophied and nonhypertrophied myocardium of patients with hypertrophic cardiomyopathy: a study with nitrogen-13 ammonia and positron emission tomography. *J Am Coll Cardiol.* 1991;17:879–886.
19. Yamada M, Elliott PM, Kaski JC, et al. Dipyridamole stress thallium-201 perfusion abnormalities in patients with hypertrophic cardiomyopathy: relationship to clinical presentation and outcome. *Eur Heart J.* 1998;19:500–507.
20. Sadoul N, Prasad K, Elliott PM, et al. Prospective prognostic assessment of blood pressure response during exercise in patients with hypertrophic cardiomyopathy. *Circulation.* 1997;96:2987–2991.
21. Maron BJ, Roberts WC, Epstein SE. Sudden death in hypertrophic cardiomyopathy: a profile of 78 patients. *Circulation.* 1982;65:1388–1394.
22. Olivotto I, Maron BJ, Montereggi A, et al. Prognostic value of systemic blood pressure response during exercise in a community-based patient population with hypertrophic cardiomyopathy. *J Am Coll Cardiol.* 1999;33:2044–2051.
23. Maron MS, Olivotto I, Zenovich AG, et al. Hypertrophic cardiomyopathy is predominantly a disease of left ventricular outflow tract obstruction. *Circulation.* 2006;114:2232–2239.
24. Maron MS, Olivotto I, Betocchi S, et al. Effect of left ventricular outflow tract obstruction on clinical outcome in hypertrophic cardiomyopathy. *N Engl J Med.* 2003;348:295–303.
25. Maron BJ, Ferrans VJ, Henry WL, et al. Differences in distribution of myocardial abnormalities in patients with obstructive and nonobstructive asymmetric septal hypertrophy (ASH). Light and electron microscopic findings. *Circulation.* 1974;50:436–446.
26. Weissler-Snir A, Hindieh W, Gruner C, et al. Lack of phenotypic differences by cardiovascular magnetic resonance imaging in myh7 (beta-myosin heavy chain) versus MYBPC3 (myosin-binding protein C) related hypertrophic cardiomyopathy. *Circ Cardiovasc Imag.* 2017;10.
27. Bartolomucci F, De Michele M, Kozakova M, et al. Impaired endothelium independent vasodilation in nonobstructive hypertrophic cardiomyopathy. *Am J Hypertens.* 2011;24:750–754.
28. Sachdev V, Shizukuda Y, Brenneman CL, et al. Left atrial volumetric remodeling is predictive of functional capacity in nonobstructive hypertrophic cardiomyopathy. *Am Heart J.* 2005;149:730–736.
29. Falicov RE, Resnekov L. Mid ventricular obstruction in hypertrophic obstructive cardiomyopathy. New diagnostic and therapeutic challenge. *Br Heart J.* 1977;39:701–705.
30. Nakamura T, Matsubara K, Furukawa K, et al. Diastolic paradoxic jet flow in patients with hypertrophic cardiomyopathy: evidence of concealed apical asynergy with cavity obliteration. *J Am Coll Cardiol.* 1992;19:516–524.
31. Minami Y, Kajimoto K, Terajima Y, et al. Clinical implications of midventricular obstruction in patients with hypertrophic cardiomyopathy. *J Am Coll Cardiol.* 2011;57:2346–2355.
32. Fighali S, Krajcer Z, Edelman S, Leachman RD. Progression of hypertrophic cardiomyopathy into a hypokinetic left ventricle: higher incidence in patients with midventricular obstruction. *J Am Coll Cardiol.* 1987;9:288–294.
33. Matsubara K, Nakamura T, Kuribayashi T, et al. Sustained cavity obliteration and apical aneurysm formation in apical hypertrophic cardiomyopathy. *J Am Coll Cardiol.* 2003;42:288–295.
34. Efthimiadis GK, Pagourelias ED, Parcharidou D, et al. Clinical characteristics and natural history of hypertrophic cardiomyopathy with midventricular obstruction. *Circ J.* 2013;77:2366–2374.
35. Yamaguchi H, Ishimura T, Nishiyama S, et al. Hypertrophic nonobstructive cardiomyopathy with giant negative T-waves (apical hypertrophy): ventriculographic and echocardiographic features in 30 patients. *Am J Cardiol.* 1979;44:401–412.
36. Louie EK, Maron BJ. Apical hypertrophic cardiomyopathy: clinical and two-dimensional echocardiographic assessment. *Ann Intern Med.* 1987;106:663–670.
37. Kitaoka H, Doi Y, Casey SA, et al. Comparison of prevalence of apical hypertrophic cardiomyopathy in Japan and the United States. *Am J Cardiol.* 2003;92:1183–1186.
38. Sakamoto T, Tei C, Murayama M, Ichiyasu H, Hada Y. Giant T wave inversion as a manifestation of asymmetrical apical hypertrophy (AAH) of the left ventricle. Echocardiographic and ultrasono-cardiotomographic study. *Jpn Heart J.* 1976;17:611–629.
39. Ward RP, Weinert L, Spencer KT, et al. Quantitative diagnosis of apical cardiomyopathy using contrast echocardiography. *J Am Soc Echocardiogr.* 2002;15:316–322.
40. Maron MS, Finley JJ, Bos JM, et al. Prevalence, clinical significance, and natural history of left ventricular apical aneurysms in hypertrophic cardiomyopathy. *Circulation.* 2008;118:1541–1549.
41. Hanneman K, Crean AM, Williams L, et al. Cardiac magnetic resonance imaging findings predict major adverse events in apical hypertrophic cardiomyopathy. *J Thorac Imaging.* 2014;29:331–339.
42. Eriksson MJ, Sonnenberg B, Woo A, et al. Long-term outcome in patients with apical hypertrophic cardiomyopathy. *J Am Coll Cardiol.* 2002;39:638–645.
43. Rowin EJ, Maron BJ, Haas TS, et al. Hypertrophic cardiomyopathy with left ventricular apical aneurysm: implications for risk stratification and management. *J Am Coll Cardiol.* 2017;69:761–773.
44. Harris KM, Spirito P, Maron MS, et al. Prevalence, clinical profile, and significance of left ventricular remodeling in the end-stage phase of hypertrophic cardiomyopathy. *Circulation.* 2006;114:216–225.
45. Biagini E, Coccolo F, Ferlito M, et al. Dilated-hypokinetic evolution of hypertrophic cardiomyopathy: prevalence, incidence, risk factors, and prognostic implications in pediatric and adult patients. *J Am Coll Cardiol.* 2005;46:1543–1550.
46. Cheng S, Choe YH, Ota H, et al. CMR assessment and clinical outcomes of hypertrophic cardiomyopathy with or without ventricular remodeling in the end-stage phase. *Int J Cardiovasc Imag.* 2018;34:597–605.
47. Kubo T, Gimeno JR, Bahl A, et al. Prevalence, clinical significance, and genetic basis of hypertrophic cardiomyopathy with restrictive phenotype. *J Am Coll Cardiol.* 2007;49:2419–2426.

59 Hypertrophic Cardiomyopathy: Pathophysiology, Functional Features, and Treatment of Outflow Tract Obstruction

Hassan Mir, Anna Woo

The pathophysiology of hypertrophic cardiomyopathy (HCM) involves several abnormalities that can be assessed using echocardiographic Doppler techniques. Structural and functional derangements include left ventricular (LV) hypertrophy, left ventricular outflow tract obstruction (LVOTO), mitral regurgitation (MR), diastolic dysfunction, and myocardial ischemia.[1,2] The majority of the clinical manifestations of HCM can be attributed to these structural and hemodynamic findings, along with the occurrence of atrial and ventricular arrhythmias.[1,2] Echocardiography plays a crucial role in demonstrating the underlying anatomy and pathophysiology of HCM, assessing its morphologic and hemodynamic severity, identifying patients for invasive septal reduction therapy, and evaluating

response to treatment.[3] This chapter reviews the mechanisms of LVOTO and MR in HCM.

PATHOPHYSIOLOGY OF LEFT VENTRICULAR OUTFLOW TRACT OBSTRUCTION

The combination of (1) multiple structural abnormalities and (2) hydrodynamic forces causes systolic anterior motion (SAM) of the mitral valve and the development of dynamic LVOTO in patients with HCM (Fig. 59.1 and Video 59.1). Morphologic characteristics that promote LVOTO include septal hypertrophy, narrowing of the outflow tract,[4] intrinsic abnormalities of

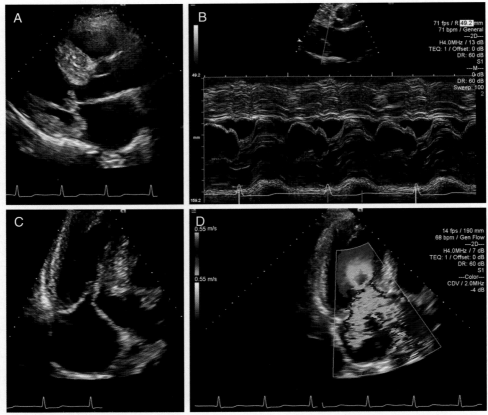

Figure 59.1. Mechanisms and functional features of obstructive hypertrophic cardiomyopathy (HCM). **A,** Parasternal long-axis view (systolic frame) in a young patient with obstructive HCM shows the asymmetric septal hypertrophy (septal thickness of 24 mm) and anterior and superior motion of the anterior mitral leaflet toward the septum during systole. **B,** Corresponding parasternal long-axis M-mode image depicts the septal hypertrophy, severe systolic anterior motion (SAM), and prolonged anterior leaflet–septal contact. **C,** Apical three-chamber view (systolic frame) provides detailed visualization of mitral leaflet elongation and morphology and leaflet motion: SAM of the anterior leaflet with septal contact in systole and, in this particular case, SAM of the posterior mitral leaflet toward the basal septum as well. The interleaflet gap between the mitral leaflets is observed. **D,** Apical three-chamber view with color Doppler imaging, which outlines the color turbulence in the left ventricular outflow tract, caused by SAM–septal contact causing left ventricular outflow tract obstruction, and the mitral interleaflet gap leading to a posteriorly directed jet of mitral regurgitation. (See accompanying Video 59.1)

the mitral leaflets,[5,6] anterior displacement of the mitral valve apparatus,[4,6] and anterior malposition of the papillary muscles.[6] Consequently, the mitral leaflets coapt in the body of the mitral leaflets rather than at the leaflet tip.[5,6] The initiation of SAM is facilitated by malposition of the papillary muscle and mitral leaflet elongation, which increase chordal-leaflet laxity.[6] During rapid ventricular ejection, the tip of the anterior mitral leaflet, distal to its point of coaptation with the posterior mitral leaflet, is susceptible to hydrodynamic forces.[3] The phenomenon of SAM was first identified by echocardiography in the late 1960s,[7] and is considered a hallmark of patients with HCM and LVOTO (Fig. 59.1B).[3] Multiple echocardiographic observations have helped to elucidate the role of Venturi[8] and drag forces[6,9,10] in drawing the anterior mitral leaflet into the outflow tract and toward the ventricular septum.[3] In typical SAM, sharp anterior and superior angulation of the anterior mitral leaflet occurs, which results in contact of the anterior mitral leaflet with the septum in early to midsystole.[5,11]

MECHANISMS OF MITRAL REGURGITATION

The unique morphologic attributes of the mitral valve and the presence of MR have long been recognized as major features of obstructive HCM.[12] The anterior and posterior mitral leaflets fail to coapt in mid to late systole because of the anterior and superior movement of the residual length of the anterior leaflet toward the outflow tract and contact of the anterior leaflet with the septum.[13] The residual lengths of the two mitral leaflets create a funnel that directs the MR posteriorly through the interleaflet gap (Fig. 59.1C and D and Video 59.1).[13] The degree of SAM-related MR has been shown to be proportional to the degree of resting LVOTO.[14] Intrinsic lesions of the mitral valve or mitral apparatus in patients with HCM include mitral valve prolapse, ruptured chordae, chordal elongation or thickening, anomalous insertion of a papillary muscle into the anterior mitral leaflet, hypertrophied papillary muscles, or leaflet thickening secondary to injury from repetitive contact with the septum.[3,15] The presence of a nonposteriorly directed jet of MR should prompt a careful evaluation of the mitral valve and mitral apparatus because it suggests the coexistence of independent mitral valve disease.[14]

FUNCTIONAL FEATURES OF OBSTRUCTIVE HYPERTROPHIC CARDIOMYOPATHY

In patients with HCM, obstruction in the left ventricular outflow tract (LVOT) causes an increase in LV systolic pressure, which in turn leads to prolongation of ventricular relaxation, elevation of LV diastolic pressure, myocardial ischemia, MR, and a decrease in forward cardiac output.[1] Symptoms attributable to LVOTO (dyspnea, angina, presyncope, syncope) are typically exacerbated during exertion or the postprandial period.[1] The presence of a resting LVOT gradient of 30 mm Hg or greater confers a twofold increase in the risk of HCM-related death.[16] Patients with HCM are generally categorized into one of three hemodynamic groups based on the LVOT gradient: (1) basal (resting) obstruction (resting LVOT gradient ≥30 mm Hg), (2) provocable (or latent) obstruction (<30 mm Hg at rest, ≥30 mm Hg with provocation), and (3) nonobstructive (<30 mm Hg at rest and with provocation) (Table 59.1).[1]

ECHOCARDIOGRAPHIC AND DOPPLER ASSESSMENT OF OBSTRUCTIVE HYPERTROPHIC CARDIOMYOPATHY

The echocardiographic techniques of M-mode, two-dimensional echocardiography, color Doppler, and continuous-wave (CW) Doppler are used to establish the presence and severity of LVOTO in patients with HCM. Distinctive M-mode findings in patients

TABLE 59.1 Hemodynamic Classification of Hypertrophic Cardiomyopathy

HCM Category	Resting LVOT Gradient (mm Hg)	Provocable LVOT Gradient (mm Hg)
Nonobstructive	<30	<30
Provocable obstruction	<30	≥30
Resting obstruction	≥30	

HCM, Hypertrophic cardiomyopathy; *LVOT,* left ventricular outflow tract.

with LVOTO include SAM of the anterior mitral valve leaflet[7,17] and midsystolic notching of the aortic valve.[18] The degree of SAM can be classified as (1) mild (anterior mitral leaflet–septal distance >10 mm), (2) moderate (anterior mitral leaflet–septal distance ≤10 mm or brief mitral leaflet–septal contact), or (3) severe (prolonged anterior leaflet–septal contact; ≥30% of echocardiographic systole).[17]

The LVOTO in patients with HCM arises secondary to mitral leaflet–septal contact and is represented on color Doppler imaging as a mosaic pattern.[3] The peak velocity at the site of obstruction can be determined using CW Doppler, with the beam directed across the outflow tract from the transthoracic apical window.[19,20] Dynamic outflow tract obstruction has a unique spectral profile, with an asymmetric leftward concave contour[3] and a late systolic peak of the maximal flow velocity (Fig. 59.2).[3,19,20] However, there may be variability in the shape of the LVOT waveform.[20] The peak LVOT gradient can be estimated using the modified Bernoulli equation, in which the peak gradient = 4 × (peak LVOT velocity)^2.[19,20] There is an excellent correlation between the pressure gradient obtained by CW Doppler and the LVOT gradient quantified by cardiac catheterization.[19,20] When measuring the peak LVOT gradient, care must be taken to avoid contamination of the LVOT signal with the mitral regurgitant jet (see Fig. 59.2).[3,19,20] In addition, spurious systolic waveforms that are different in appearance from the true LVOT velocity signal can be recorded. These waveforms generally have a late initial rise in systolic velocity and a narrow and pointed peak in end-systole.[20] They likely originate from portions of the ventricular cavity that obliterate at end-systole.[20] Finally, it is important to distinguish a dynamic LVOT gradient from fixed subaortic obstruction (caused by a congenital fibrous subaortic membrane) or from valvular aortic stenosis.[3]

In symptomatic patients with HCM and a resting LVOT gradient of less than 30 to 50 mm Hg, provocative maneuvers should be performed to determine if a higher LVOT gradient can be elicited.[1,3] Dynamic LVOTO in HCM is exacerbated by maneuvers that decrease LV preload (Valsalva maneuver, sublingual nitroglycerin, assuming an upright posture), increase LV contractility and heart rate (dobutamine, isoproterenol, upright exercise), or decrease afterload (inhalation of amyl nitrate, sublingual isosorbide dinitrate).[1,3,21] Multiple echocardiographic studies have reported on the utility of various methods of provocation to assess for inducible LVOTO.[21] Although the Valsalva maneuver is the most commonly used method of provocation in echocardiography laboratories, the magnitude of the Valsalva-induced LVOT gradient is underestimated compared with the exercise-induced LVOT gradient.[22] Therefore, exercise echocardiography is the preferred method for provoking an LVOT gradient because it best reflects the degree of outflow obstruction generated during physical activities (Fig. 59.3).[3] Dobutamine stress echocardiography is not recommended for detecting a provocable LVOT gradient unless it is performed at an experienced center because it may be difficult to distinguish cavity obliteration from a true LVOT signal.[3] In addition, dobutamine-induced intracavitary obstruction can be identified in more than 17% of tested subjects, even in those without HCM, and its presence is of unclear clinical significance.[23]

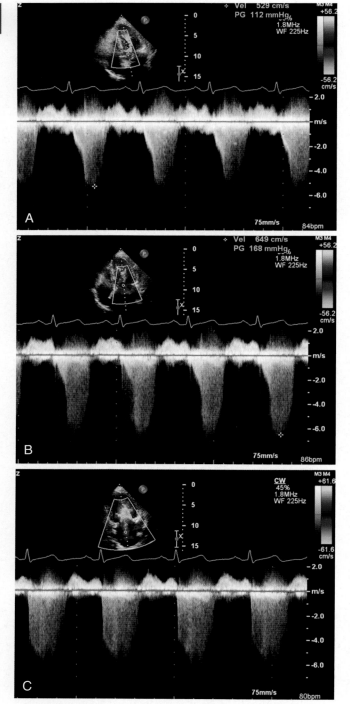

Figure 59.2. Continuous-wave Doppler assessment in a symptomatic patient with obstructive hypertrophic cardiomyopathy. **A,** Typical finding of an asymmetric concave-to-the-left contour of the Doppler spectral profile of the left ventricular outflow tract (LVOT) velocity, associated with the late systolic peak. From the apical five-chamber view, the peak velocity is 5.3 m/s, which corresponds to a peak LVOT gradient of 112 mm Hg (using the modified Bernoulli equation). **B,** Two superimposed spectral profiles can be visualized: the brighter leftward concave contour of the LVOT velocity and a fainter signal, which is wider (begins earlier in systole) and more parabolic in shape. The measured systolic velocity overestimates the actual LVOT gradient and represents contamination of the LVOT signal with the signal from the mitral regurgitant jet. **C,** The spectral profile of mitral regurgitation, which starts earlier in systole, has a more abrupt initial rise in velocity and a higher peak velocity compared with the LVOT spectral profile.

TREATMENT STRATEGIES FOR OBSTRUCTIVE HYPERTROPHIC CARDIOMYOPATHY

Medical therapy is initiated to alleviate the symptoms associated with LVOTO. The primary goal of pharmacotherapy is to decrease myocardial contractility, which results in a reduction in SAM and in the magnitude of the LVOT gradient. Beta β-blockers are the first-line agents for patients with symptomatic obstructive HCM, with benefit derived from their negative inotropic effects, attenuation of adrenergic-induced tachycardia, and prolongation of the diastolic filling period.[1] Verapamil can be prescribed to patients who are intolerant or unresponsive to β-blockade. Importantly, in the setting of a high LVOT gradient and elevated filling pressures, verapamil (or diltiazem) may generate worsened LVOTO and pulmonary edema.[1] Among patients with ongoing symptoms despite treatment with a β-blocker or verapamil, disopyramide can be safely added.[1] There is a significant improvement in symptoms and the degree of LVOTO with disopyramide.[24,25] Importantly, in patients who remain symptomatic despite maximally tolerated pharmacotherapy and who generally have a resting or provocable LVOT gradient 50 mm Hg or greater, invasive septal reduction therapy is recommended.[1]

Surgical septal myectomy acutely relieves LVOTO by widening the outflow tract, which decreases the degree of SAM and virtually eliminates the outflow tract gradient. Surgery for obstructive HCM has been performed for more than five decades.[1] There was significant variability in the early postoperative mortality of surgical cohorts published between the 1960s to 1980s.[1,26] However, more contemporary studies from experienced HCM centers have demonstrated outstanding results after surgery, with an early postoperative mortality rate of less than 1% (in patients undergoing isolated surgical myectomy)[27,28] and excellent long-term survival.[27–29] In patients with obstructive HCM and no independent mitral valve disease, the subaortic myectomy procedure is sufficient to relieve SAM and SAM-related MR, without the need for additional mitral valve procedures.[1,30] Concomitant mitral valve procedures can be performed in patients with obstructive HCM as a complementary surgical strategy.[29] The prevalence of intrinsic pathology of the mitral apparatus (mitral leaflets, chordae, or papillary muscles) and the requirement for additional mitral valve procedures (mainly mitral valve repair and not mitral valve replacement) are significantly higher in patients with a basal septal thickness of less than 2 cm.[29] Echocardiography plays a critical role in patient selection, preoperative planning, and intraoperative guidance.

Alcohol septal ablation was developed in the 1990s as a nonsurgical option. It consists of the injection of alcohol into a septal perforator branch of the left anterior descending artery to occlude the septal branch and cause a targeted infarction of the basal septum.[1] This procedure can be performed with echocardiographic guidance,[1,3] and it leads to gradual remodeling with focal septal thinning, widening of the outflow tract, and an amelioration in the LVOT gradient.[31] Alcohol septal ablation results in the relief of symptoms and a significant diminution in LVOTO.[1] Very good outcomes can be achieved when this intervention is performed at experienced centers.[24,32,33] Finally, dual-chamber permanent pacing was used to treat obstructive HCM beginning in the late 1980s.[1] However, despite initially promising reports, subsequent randomized trials showed limited benefits of pacing.[1] Therefore, dual-chamber pacing is currently only recommended in symptomatic patients who are not good candidates for either myectomy or alcohol septal ablation.[1]

The major controversy regarding the invasive treatment of obstructive HCM involves the ongoing debate regarding the relative merits of myectomy versus alcohol septal ablation.[1] In nonrandomized studies that compared the outcomes of myectomy versus alcohol septal ablation, there were no major differences in medium-term cardiac survival between the two strategies.[1,34] A meta-analysis of myectomy and alcohol septal ablation cohorts

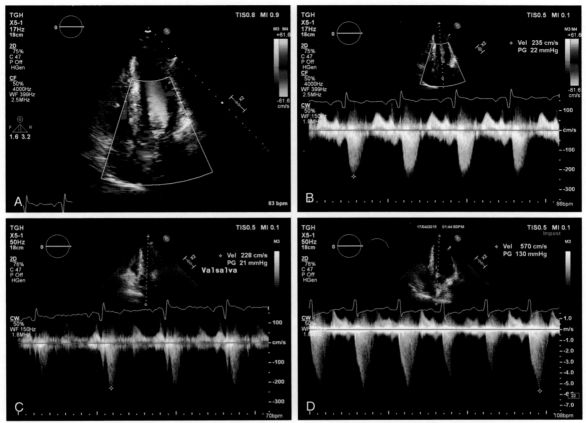

Figure 59.3. Different methods of determining the provocable left ventricular outflow tract (LVOT) gradient in a 40-year-old man with known hypertrophic cardiomyopathy and a family history of premature sudden death. **A,** Apical five-chamber view with color Doppler shows septal hypertrophy (septal thickness, 19 mm [basal level] and 21 mm [midventricular level]), flow acceleration, and color turbulence in the outflow tract. **B,** The LVOT gradient at rest is estimated at 22 mm Hg. **C,** After the Valsalva maneuver, there is no change in the LVOT gradient. **D,** After exercising for 12 minutes on the treadmill, a much higher LVOT velocity (5.7 m/s) is elicited, corresponding to an exercise-induced LVOT gradient of 130 mm Hg. Note that there may be mild respiratory variation in the LVOT signal in the early period following exercise.

revealed a higher rate of periprocedural permanent pacemaker implantation and a higher long-term risk of repeat invasive intervention in patients who undergo alcohol septal ablation.[33] Furthermore, the very long-term risks of late ventricular arrhythmias are unclear after alcohol-induced infarction.[1] Therefore, myectomy is considered the preferred treatment option for younger, healthy patients, whereas alcohol septal ablation is chosen in patients for whom surgical risks are excessive.[1] Clinical scenarios for which myectomy is particularly suitable include young patients, patients with concomitant lesions (e.g., epicardial coronary artery disease, mitral or aortic valve disease) requiring surgical correction, and the uncommon situation of cardiogenic shock, when an immediate reduction in the LVOT gradient is necessary.[35] Echocardiography provides essential information to determine the most appropriate type of invasive septal reduction therapy for individual patients (Fig. 59.4 and Video 59.4). The echocardiographic findings predictive of a good outcome after alcohol septal ablation are a septal thickness 18 mm or less (at the site of SAM) and a resting LVOT gradient less than 100 mm Hg.[36] The traditional favored morphology for candidates for alcohol septal ablation is the presence of flow acceleration proximal to the point of SAM–septal contact and focal color turbulence adjacent to the point of SAM–septal contact (and localized to the outflow tract).[37] Septal myectomy is preferred over alcohol septal ablation in cases of marked septal hypertrophy (septal thickness >30 mm) (see Fig. 59.4).[1] Patients who are eligible for either myectomy or alcohol septal ablation should be evaluated at a center experienced in the management of these challenging techniques (Fig. 59.5).[1]

Please access ExpertConsult to view the corresponding videos for this chapter.

Acknowledgment

The authors acknowledge Dr. Paul Szmitko, who was the first author of this chapter in the second edition of the textbook.

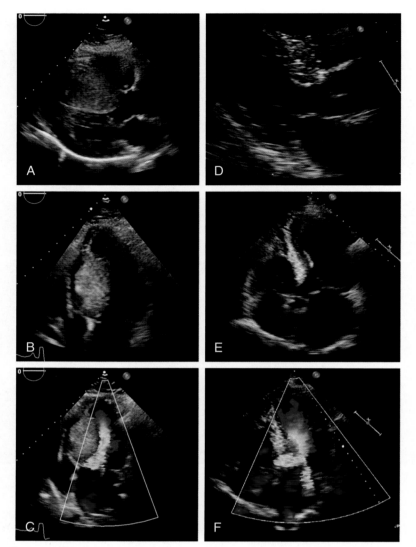

Figure 59.4. Heterogeneity of hypertrophic cardiomyopathy (HCM) causing severe obstruction. Parasternal long-axis (**A**) and apical four-chamber images (**B**) of a 41-year-old woman with advanced symptoms referred for invasive septal reduction therapy. Her echocardiogram showed diffuse and massive septal hypertrophy of the basal and midseptal segments (septal thickness, 33 mm), prominent mitral leaflets, and leaflet systolic anterior motion (SAM). **C,** Apical four-chamber view with color Doppler reveals flow acceleration beginning at the midventricular level and high-velocity color turbulence extending beyond and involving the entire outflow tract. The patient's echocardiography findings favored treatment with surgical myectomy. Parasternal long-axis (**D**) and apical five-chamber (**E**) views of a 70-year-old man with obstructive HCM caused by discrete septal hypertrophy and more focal obstruction. There is asymmetric hypertrophy of the basal septum (basal septal thickness, 17 mm) and leaflet SAM. **F,** Color Doppler imaging outlines flow acceleration in the LVOT, just proximal to the point of apposition of the anterior leaflet with the septum (point of SAM–septal contact) and color turbulence in the LVOT. Mitral regurgitation (with a posterior jet direction) develops because of the leaflet SAM. This patient underwent successful alcohol septal ablation. (See accompanying Video 59.4.)

Figure 59.5. Approach to selection of invasive septal reduction therapy (surgical myectomy or alcohol septal ablation), considering clinical and echocardiographic factors, in patients with drug-refractory symptomatic obstructive hypertrophic cardiomyopathy (HCM). See text for further details. *ASA,* Alcohol septal ablation; *LVOT,* left ventricular outflow tract.

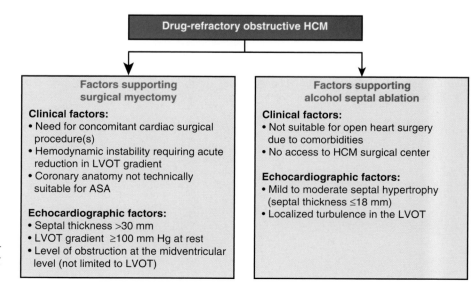

REFERENCES

1. Gersh BJ, Maron BJ, Bonow RO, et al. 2011 ACCF/AHA Guideline for the diagnosis and treatment of hypertrophic cardiomyopathy. *J Am Coll Cardiol.* 2011;58:e212–e260.
2. Maron BJ. Clinical course and management of hypertrophic cardiomyopathy. *N Eng J Med.* 2018;379:655–668.
3. Nagueh SF, Bierig SM, Budoff MJ, et al. American Society of Echocardiography clinical recommendations for multimodality cardiovascular imaging of patients with hypertrophic cardiomyopathy. *J Am Soc Echocardiogr.* 2011;24:473–498.
4. Spirito P, Maron BJ. Significance of left ventricular outflow tract cross-sectional area in hypertrophic cardiomyopathy: a two-dimensional echocardiographic assessment. *Circulation.* 1983;67:1100–1108.
5. Shah PM, Taylor RD, Wong M. Abnormal mitral valve coaptation in hypertrophic obstructive cardiomyopathy: proposed role in systolic anterior motion of mitral valve. *Am J Cardiol.* 1981;48:258–262.
6. Jiang L, Levine RA, King ME, et al. An integrated mechanism for systolic anterior motion of the mitral valve in hypertrophic cardiomyopathy based on echocardiographic observations. *Am Heart J.* 1987;113:633–644.
7. Shah PM, Gramiak R, Kramer DH. Ultrasound localization of left ventricular outflow obstruction in hypertrophic obstructive cardiomyopathy. *Circulation.* 1969;40:3–11.
8. Pollick C, Morgan CD, Gilbert BW, et al. Muscular subaortic stenosis: the temporal relationship between systolic anterior motion of the anterior mitral leaflet and the pressure gradient. *Circulation.* 1982;66:1087–1094.
9. Sherrid MV, Chu CK, Delia E, et al. An echocardiographic study of the fluid mechanics of obstruction in hypertrophic cardiomyopathy. *J Am Coll Cardiol.* 1993;22:816–825.
10. Sherrid MV, Gunsburg DZ, Moldenhauer S, et al. Systolic anterior motion begins at low left ventricular outflow tract velocity in obstructive hypertrophic cardiomyopathy. *J Am Coll Cardiol.* 2000;36:1344–1354.
11. Klues HG, Roberts WC, Maron BJ. Morphological determinants of echocardiographic patterns of mitral valve systolic anterior motion in obstructive hypertrophic cardiomyopathy. *Circulation.* 1993;87:1570–1579.
12. Woo A, Jedrzkiewicz S. The mitral valve in hypertrophic cardiomyopathy: it's a long story. *Circulation.* 2011;124:9–12.
13. Grigg LE, Wigle ED, Williams WG, et al. Transesophageal Doppler echocardiography in obstructive hypertrophic cardiomyopathy: clarification of pathophysiology and importance in intraoperative decision making. *J Am Coll Cardiol.* 1992;20:42–52.
14. Yu EH, Omran AS, Wigle ED, et al. Mitral regurgitation in hypertrophic obstructive cardiomyopathy: relationship to obstruction and relief with myectomy. *J Am Coll Cardiol.* 2000;36:2219–2225.
15. Kaple RK, Murphy RT, DiPaola LM, et al. Mitral valve abnormalities in hypertrophic cardiomyopathy: echocardiographic features and surgical outcomes. *Ann Thorac Surg.* 2008;85:1527–1535.
16. Maron MS, Olivotto I, Betocchi S, et al. Effect of left ventricular outflow tract obstruction on clinical outcome in hypertrophic cardiomyopathy. *N Engl J Med.* 2003;348:295–303.
17. Gilbert BW, Pollick C, Adelman AG, et al. Hypertrophic cardiomyopathy: subclassification by M mode echocardiography. *Am J Cardiol.* 1980;45:861–872.
18. Boughner DR, Schuld RL, Persaud JA. Hypertrophic obstructive cardiomyopathy. Assessment by echocardiographic and Doppler ultrasound techniques. *Br Heart J.* 1975;37:917–923.
19. Sasson Z, Yock PG, Hatle LK, et al. Doppler echocardiographic determination of the pressure gradient in hypertrophic cardiomyopathy. *J Am Coll Cardiol.* 1988;11:752–756.
20. Panza JA, Petrone RK, Fananapazir L, et al. Utility of continuous wave Doppler echocardiography in the noninvasive assessment of left ventricular outflow tract pressure gradient in patients with hypertrophic cardiomyopathy. *J Am Coll Cardiol.* 1992;19:91–99.
21. Chun S, Woo A. Echocardiography in hypertrophic cardiomyopathy: in with strain, out with straining? *J Am Soc Echocardiogr.* 2015;28:204–209.
22. Maron MS, Olivotto I, Zenovich AG, et al. Hypertrophic cardiomyopathy is predominantly a disease of left ventricular outflow tract obstruction. *Circulation.* 2006;114:2232–2239.
23. Luria D, Klutstein MW, Rosenmann D, et al. Prevalence and significance of left ventricular outflow tract gradient during dobutamine echocardiography. *Eur Heart J.* 1999;20:386–392.
24. Ball W, Ivanov J, Rakowski H, et al. Long-term survival in patients with resting obstructive hypertrophic cardiomyopathy: comparison of conservative versus invasive treatment. *J Am Coll Cardiol.* 2011;58:2313–2321.
25. Sherrid MV, Shetty A, Winson G, et al. Treatment of obstructive hypertrophic cardiomyopathy symptoms and gradient resistant to first-line therapy with beta-blockade or verapamil. *Circ Heart Fail.* 2013;6:694–702.
26. Woo A, Rakowski H. Does myectomy convey survival benefit in hypertrophic cardiomyopathy? *Heart Fail Clin.* 2007;3:275–288.
27. Woo A, Williams WG, Choi R, et al. Clinical and echocardiographic determinants of long-term survival after surgical myectomy in obstructive hypertrophic cardiomyopathy. *Circulation.* 2005;111:2033–2041.
28. Ommen SR, Maron BJ, Olivotto I, et al. Long-term effects of surgical septal myectomy on survival in patients with obstructive hypertrophic cardiomyopathy. *J Am Coll Cardiol.* 2005;46:470–476.
29. Desai MY, Bhonsale A, Smedira NG, et al. Predictors of long-term outcomes in symptomatic hypertrophic obstructive cardiomyopathy patients undergoing surgical relief of left ventricular outflow tract obstruction. *Circulation.* 2013;128:209–216.
30. Hong JH, Schaff HV, Nishimura RA, et al. Mitral regurgitation in patients with hypertrophic obstructive cardiomyopathy: implications for concomitant valve procedures. *J Am Coll Cardiol.* 2016;68:1497–1504.
31. Flores-Ramirez R, Lakkis NM, Middleton KJ, et al. Echocardiographic insights into the mechanisms of relief of left ventricular outflow tract obstruction after nonsurgical septal reduction therapy in patients with hypertrophic obstructive cardiomyopathy. *J Am Coll Cardiol.* 2001;37:208–214.
32. Nagueh SF, Groves BM, Schwartz L, et al. Alcohol septal ablation for the treatment of hypertrophic obstructive cardiomyopathy. A multicenter North American registry. *J Am Coll Cardiol.* 2011;58:2322–2328.
33. Liebregts M, Vriesendorp PA, Mahmoodi BK, et al. A systematic review and meta-analysis of long-term outcomes after septal reduction therapy in patients with hypertrophic cardiomyopathy. *JACC Heart Failure.* 2015;3:896–905.
34. Agarwal S, Tuzcu EM, Desai MY, et al. Updated meta-analysis of septal alcohol ablation versus myectomy for hypertrophic cardiomyopathy. *J Am Coll Cardiol.* 2010;55:823–834.
35. Maron B, Dearani JA, Ommen SR, et al. The case for surgery in obstructive hypertrophic cardiomyopathy. *J Am Coll Cardiol.* 2004;44:2044–2053.
36. Sorajja P, Binder J, Nishimura RA, et al. Predictors of an optimal clinical outcome with alcohol septal ablation for obstructive hypertrophic cardiomyopathy. *Catheter Cardiovasc Interv.* 2013;81. e58–67.
37. Faber L, Seggewiss H, Gleichmann U. Percutaneous transluminal septal myocardial ablation in hypertrophic obstructive cardiomyopathy: results with respect to intraprocedural myocardial contrast echocardiography. *Circulation.* 1998;98:2415–2421.

60 Differential of Hypertrophic Cardiomyopathy Versus Secondary Conditions That Mimic Hypertrophic Cardiomyopathy

Sara Hoss, Lynne Williams, Harry Rakowski

Left ventricular (LV) hypertrophy (LVH) can represent either a physiologic or pathologic cardiac process that can be secondary to abnormal loading conditions or a variety of cardiac and systemic diseases (Fig. 60.1). Echocardiography is not only the most commonly used method but also the most feasible method to visualize and quantify LVH in clinical practice. Although hypertrophic cardiomyopathy (HCM) is the most prevalent genetic primary cardiac disease that occurs in 0.2% of the general population,[1] several other conditions can mimic the phenotypic appearance of HCM and present with increased myocardial thickness in echocardiography. Correct identification of the underlying cause of increased myocardial thickness is of critical importance in order to distinguish between HCM, benign physiological conditions, and cardiac or systemic disorders. HCM is a genetic disease that can cause premature sudden cardiac death (SCD) and can lead to considerable morbidity. It requires proper treatment and SCD risk stratification, as well as family

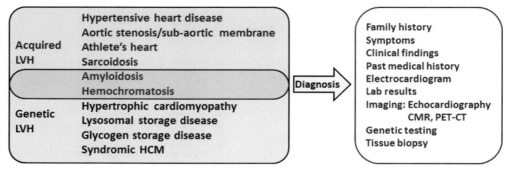

Figure 60.1. Differential diagnosis of unexplained left ventricular hypertrophy (LVH). The differential diagnosis of unexplained LVH encompasses a broad range of both primary cardiac and systemic disorders. Overall, these conditions can be broadly categorized into two groups: genetic disorders and acquired disorders. A multimodality approach is essential for an accurate diagnosis and relies on the integration of information obtained from detailed personal and family history, clinical examination, diagnostic investigations, and biochemical and genetic analysis. Diagnosis sometimes requires additional imaging methods, including cardiac magnetic resonance imaging (CMRI) and positron emission tomography scan (PET-CT). *HCM,* Hypertrophic cardiomyopathy; *LVH,* left ventricular hypertrophy.

screening. Moreover, some mimics of HCM have specific treatments with prognostic implication. The purpose of this chapter is to highlight echocardiographic features that may help to distinguish HCM from other causes of LVH. Emphasis is on the multidisciplinary and multimodality approach required for the accurate diagnosis of the underlying condition causing the LVH (see Fig. 60.1).

HYPERTENSIVE HEART DISEASE

Arterial hypertension represents a common and important health problem, with an estimated prevalence of 28% in North America and 44% in Europe.[2] With the prevalence of HCM being 1 in 500, co-existence of both disorders is common, making the diagnosis in this setting more challenging. Long-standing hypertension causes LV pressure overload and an increase in wall stress, which often results in compensatory hypertrophy. Early in the disease process, a basal septal bulge is often prominent because of the inhomogeneity of the regional LV wall stress, which is greatest in the basal septum.[3] With time, the typical concentric pattern of hypertrophy becomes more evident. An absolute wall thickness of 15 mm or greater in any myocardial segment, which is diagnostic for HCM, can also be found in hypertensive heart disease (HHD). Therefore, it is important to also consider using septal/posterior wall thickness ratio for an accurate diagnosis. Although a septal/posterior wall thickness ratio greater than 1.3:1 is supportive of HCM diagnosis in nonhypertensive patients, a ratio greater than 1.5:1 is generally applied for patients with a history of systemic hypertension. However, these data were generated from a predominantly white population and should be used with caution in other populations, especially Afro-Caribbean patients who usually display a greater propensity for LVH in response to hypertension.[4] Systolic anterior motion (SAM) of the mitral valve, which is associated with left ventricular outflow tract (LVOT) obstruction, is not pathognomonic for HCM and can also be found in patients with HHD and other conditions that cause LVH.

Advanced echocardiographic techniques, such as tissue Doppler imaging and speckle-tracking echocardiography (STE), are potentially helpful in distinguishing HHD from HCM. Global LV systolic function remains preserved in most cases of HCM and HHD, but using STE reveals changes between the two. A recent study demonstrated that although both HCM and HHD patients show decreased LV longitudinal strain compared with normal control participants, patients with HCM show lower values than those with HHD. Additionally, LV radial strain was increased in patients with HCM compared with patients with HHS and control participants.[5] Another study demonstrated changes in strain patterns of the right ventricle (RV); although HHS patients had normal RV longitudinal strain, in patients with HCM, RV longitudinal strain was significantly impaired.[6]

ATHLETES' HEARTS

The accurate diagnosis of HCM in individuals participating in competitive sports is challenging yet crucial because of the potential risk of patients with HCM for SCD. HCM has been identified as the predominant cause of SCD in young athletes. To date, the largest study showed that fewer than 2% of elite athletes had a maximal wall thickness greater than 12 mm in the interventricular septum.[7] Racial differences exist in the propensity to develop hypertrophy in response to exercise, and as many as 12% of Afro-Caribbean athletes demonstrate LV wall thickness greater than 12 mm.[8] However, the upper limit of physiologic hypertrophy in athletes of all ethnicities appears to be an absolute wall thickness of 16 mm.[7,9] Asymmetric hypertrophy is encountered rarely in athletes, with the typical distribution of LVH being concentric. Chamber dilatation found in athletes, in contrast to the normal or reduced cavity size seen in HCM, is another clue to the underlying cause. In athletes, LV end-diastolic cavity dimensions frequently exceed 55 mm, and in up to 5% of cases, these dimensions may exceed 60 mm. A practical algorithm to allow better differentiation between physiologic and pathologic hypertrophy is provided in Fig. 60.2.[10]

Accumulating evidence suggests that advanced echocardiographic techniques may play a contributory role in the differentiation between athlete's heart and HCM. Peak LV longitudinal strain and strain rate are typically normal or high-normal in athletes with physiologic hypertrophy in contrast to HCM (Fig. 60.3), in which longitudinal systolic strain (both regional and global) are impaired.[11] Moreover, diastolic function is preserved and often enhanced in athletes' hearts, demonstrated by normal diastolic tissue Doppler velocities and an increase in twist and untwist rates.[12,13] In contrast, the pathologic hypertrophy of HCM is associated with marked attenuation in diastolic tissue Doppler velocities and delayed untwist.[14] Another difference lies in the left atrium; although mild left atrial (LA) dilatation can be seen in athletes' hearts, LA function is typically preserved when measured by STE. In comparison, patients with HCM not only display an increase in LA volumes but also have a significant impairment in LA myocardial deformation, with reductions in both strain and strain rates.[15]

INFILTRATIVE DISORDERS OF THE MYOCARDIUM
Cardiac Amyloidosis

Amyloidosis is a systemic disease characterized by the deposition of extracellular interstitial misfolded proteins in various organs, including the heart. Cardiac involvement is common in hereditary transthyretin amyloidosis (ATTRm), wild-type transthyretin amyloidosis (ATTRwt), and AL (light-chain) amyloidosis. Amyloid can infiltrate the ventricles, atria, and interventricular septum and

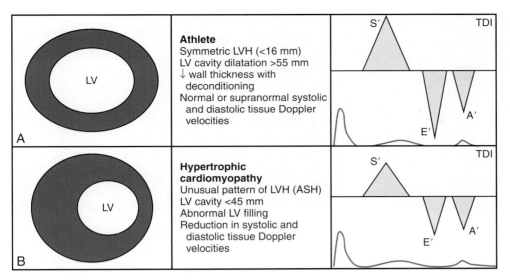

Figure 60.2. Characteristic features of left ventricular structure and function in an athlete's heart (top row) compared with hypertrophic cardiomyopathy (bottom row). Schematic representation of tissue Doppler myocardial velocities (right), demonstrating the reduction in both systolic (S′) and diastolic (E′ and A′) myocardial annular velocities in a patient with hypertrophic cardiomyopathy, compared with normal or supranormal systolic and diastolic function in an athlete's heart. *ASH,* Asymmetric septal hypertrophy; *LV,* left ventricular; *LVH,* left ventricular hypertrophy; *TDI,* tissue Doppler imaging.

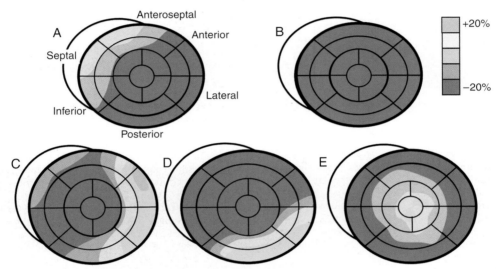

Figure 60.3. Representative peak systolic strain maps in various forms of left ventricular hypertrophy. **A,** A patient with hypertrophic cardiomyopathy and asymmetric septal hypertrophy demonstrating reduced strain in the basal and mid anteroseptal, septal, and inferior segments. **B,** An athlete with physiological hypertrophy, demonstrating normal strain values in all segments. **C,** A patient with cardiac amyloid, demonstrating reduced strain in the basal and midsegments, with relative apical sparing. **D,** A patient with Anderson-Fabry disease, demonstrating characteristic reduction in strain in the basal and mid inferolateral segments. **E,** A patient with left ventricular noncompaction cardiomyopathy demonstrating reduced strain in the mid and apical segments.

damage the ventricular function, atrial function, and valvular function as well as the conduction system. Additionally, in AL amyloidosis, light chain toxicity can contribute to cardiac dysfunction.[16] The typical echocardiographic features of cardiac amyloid are concentric hypertrophy, diastolic dysfunction, and LA enlargement (Fig. 60.4). Thickening of the RV wall and interatrial septum are also common, as well as LV systolic dysfunction, which is more prevalent in advanced cardiac amyloidosis (CA) than in HCM. Electrocardiography plays a complementary role and shows the characteristic feature of a low QRS voltage in up to 50% of patients. Although LV global systolic function is typically preserved early in the disease process, systolic longitudinal strain and strain rates are typically severely reduced in a homogenous pattern,[17] in contrast with HCM, in which the reduction in strain may be inhomogeneous and most marked in the hypertrophied segments. A distinctive pattern of regional variations in myocardial dysfunction has been described in CA, with relative sparing of the apical segments represented by better strain values. This finding could aid in the differentiation of CA from other causes of LVH (see Fig. 60.3).[18]

Cardiac Sarcoidosis

Sarcoidosis is a systemic granulomatous disease of unknown etiology which can involve different body organs. In cardiac sarcoidosis (CS) noncaseating granulomatous tissue infiltrates the heart, causing various clinical manifestations ranging from asymptomatic cardiac involvement to atrioventricular conduction disease, ventricular arrhythmia, and heart failure. Most patients with CS have extracardiac involvement, which usually includes the lungs but could also involve the skin, eyes, liver, and nerves. However, less common cases of isolated CS have been described, and therefore lack of extracardiac manifestations cannot exclude sarcoidosis. The most typical feature of CS is basal thinning of the interventricular septum. However, CS can present with different phenotypes; more commonly, it resembles dilated cardiomyopathy, but occasionally it can present with asymmetric hypertrophy mimicking HCM.[19]

Evidence of systemic sarcoidosis may point to the underlying cause in cases of extracardiac involvement. However, in cases of minimal or no extracardiac involvement, diagnosis of CS could be challenging. Using ^{18}F-fluorodeoxyglucose positron emission tomography and cardiac

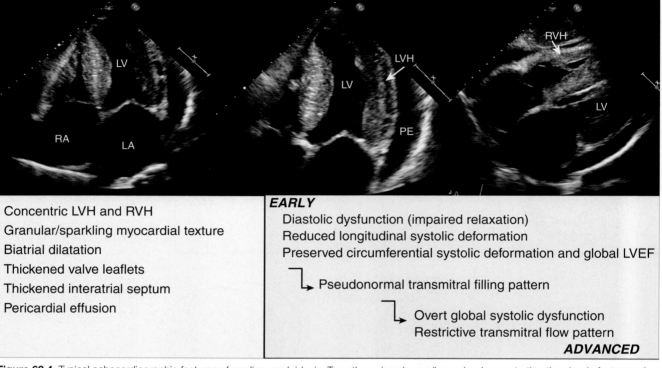

Concentric LVH and RVH	**EARLY**
Granular/sparkling myocardial texture	Diastolic dysfunction (impaired relaxation)
Biatrial dilatation	Reduced longitudinal systolic deformation
Thickened valve leaflets	Preserved circumferential systolic deformation and global LVEF
Thickened interatrial septum	Pseudonormal transmitral filling pattern
Pericardial effusion	Overt global systolic dysfunction Restrictive transmitral flow pattern **ADVANCED**

Figure 60.4. Typical echocardiographic features of cardiac amyloidosis. Transthoracic echocardiography demonstrating the classic features of cardiac amyloidosis. The progression of echocardiographic features from early to advanced disease is shown in the *lower panel*. *LA,* Left atrium; *LV,* left ventricle; *LVEF,* left ventricular ejection fraction; *LVH,* left ventricular hypertrophy; *PE,* pericardial effusion; *RA,* right atrium; *RVH,* right ventricular hypertrophy.

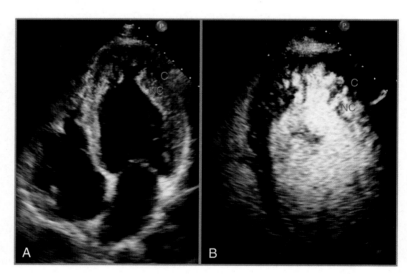

Figure 60.5. Left ventricular noncompaction cardiomyopathy. The myocardium typically displays a two-layered structure with a compacted (C) and noncompacted (NC) endocardial layer of trabecular meshwork. What appears to be myocardial hypertrophy in standard echocardiography (**A**) is proven to be deep perfused intertrabecular recesses on contrast echocardiography (**B**).

magnetic resonance imaging (CMRI) could detect both inflammation and fibrosis and is particularly helpful in clarifying the diagnosis.[20]

ISOLATED LEFT VENTRICULAR NON-COMPACTION CARDIOMYOPATHY

Isolated LV noncompaction cardiomyopathy (LVNC) is a rare primary cardiomyopathy that results from an arrest of myocardial maturation during embryogenesis. It is associated with thick, bilayered myocardium with noncompacted and compacted components, prominent trabecular outpouchings, and deep endomyocardial recesses.[21] The disease course is characterized by development of heart failure due to systolic or diastolic dysfunction (or both), ventricular and supraventricular arrhythmias, and systemic embolization.[22] LVNC can at some

stages appear similar to LVH in echocardiography, but as it has serious sequelae, making the accurate diagnosis is of great importance. Contrast echocardiography has proven to be helpful in depicting the border between the compacted and the noncompacted layers and in better demonstrating the myocardial recesses (Fig. 60.5). STE can support the diagnosis by demonstrating lower values of apical strain compared with HCM or normal hearts (see Fig. 60.3).[23]

STORAGE DISEASES

Storage diseases and syndromic cardiac hypertrophy result from genetic abnormality causing substrate accumulation in various tissues, including the heart. This may increase myocardial wall thickness and cause a cardiac phenotype that mimics HCM. Typically,

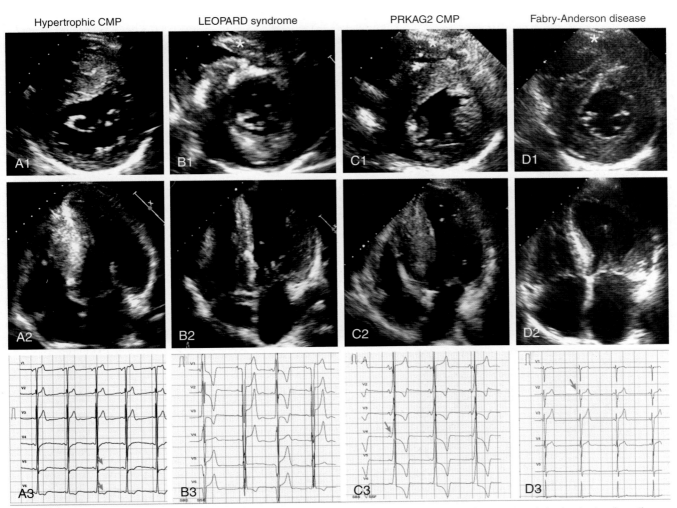

Figure 60.6. Mimics of hypertrophic cardiomyopathy. Two-dimensional echocardiographic images in the parasternal short-axis view (*row 1*), apical four-chamber view (*row 2*), and electrocardiograms (ECGs) at rest (*row 3*) from four patients with left ventricular hypertrophy (LVH). *Column A* demonstrates a classic pattern of asymmetric hypertrophy in a patient with hypertrophic cardiomyopathy (CMP), with evidence of LVH and ST-segment changes in the lateral chest leads (*arrows*). *Column B* demonstrates concentric LVH with right ventricular (RV) involvement (*asterisk*) in a patient with LEOPARD (multiple lentigines, ECG abnormalities, ocular hypertelorism, pulmonary stenosis, abnormal genitalia, retardation of growth, and sensorineural deafness) syndrome, with evidence of bundle branch block, LVH, and deep T-wave inversion on the ECG. *Column C* demonstrates a pattern of asymmetric hypertrophy with RV involvement (*asterisk*) in a patient with PRKAG2 cardiomyopathy, with evidence of LVH and pre-excitation pattern on the ECG (*arrow*). *Column D* demonstrates concentric LVH and RV involvement (*asterisk*) in a patient with Anderson-Fabry disease, with evidence of a short PR interval on the ECG (*arrow*).

these conditions present with extracardiac manifestations and require a multimodality approach for an accurate diagnosis and treatment (see Fig. 60.1). From a cardiac perspective, most storage diseases tend to present concentric LVH pattern, sometimes with right ventricular (RV) and atrial involvement. Some syndromes have distinct electrocardiographic and echocardiographic features that help determine the diagnosis, but others may present with more common imaging features, making it almost impossible to make an accurate diagnosis based on imaging alone. In recent years, genetic testing has become a pivotal tool in diagnosis of storage diseases and syndromic cardiac hypertrophy. Moreover, most HCM genetic panels today include several genes of HCM mimics, helping the diagnosis of patients with few or no extracardiac manifestations.[24]

Lysosomal Storage Disorders

Anderson-Fabry Disease

Anderson-Fabry disease (AFD) is a rare X-linked lysosomal storage disease characterized by α-galactosidase deficiency, which

leads to intracellular accumulation of glycosphingolipids. It mainly affects the kidneys, heart, central and peripheral nervous systems, skin, and gastrointestinal tract. Proper diagnosis of AFD is crucial because targeted enzyme replacement therapy is available and can slow down disease progression.[25] Patients with cardiac involvement usually present with biventricular hypertrophy, papillary muscles hypertrophy, conduction system abnormalities, valvular abnormalities, and microvascular disease (Fig. 60.6). AFD can mimic HCM by presenting with mostly concentric, but sometimes asymmetric, LVH and occasionally LVOT obstruction (LVOTO).[26] The early stage of cardiac involvement in the absence of overt LVH includes a reduction of tissue Doppler velocities. Later patients develop progressive LVH with diastolic dysfunction. LV systolic function is usually preserved but could worsen in time and lead to end-stage disease with heart failure. Although both HCM and AFD can present with asymmetric hypertrophy, studies suggest that typical patients with HCM tend to express more significant asymmetry, with an interventricular-septum–posterior-wall ratio greater than 1.3.

Two-dimensional STE imaging can be helpful distinguishing AFD from other types of LVH (see Fig. 60.3). Patients with AFD

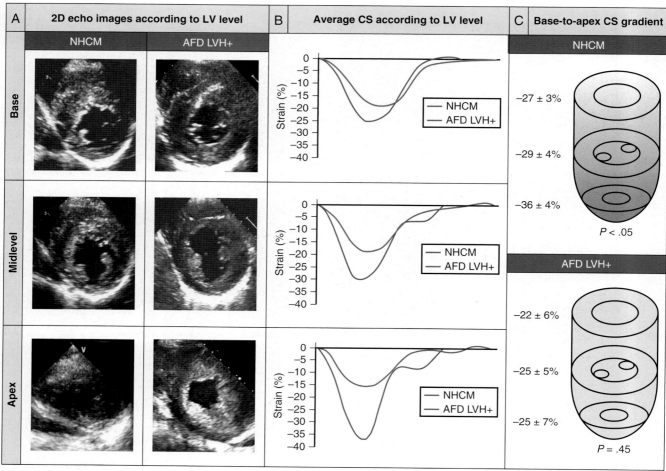

Figure 60.7. Anderson-Fabry disease (AFD). Typical examples of a patient with nonobstructive hypertrophic cardiomyopathy (NHCM) and a patient with AFD with left ventricular hypertrophy (LVH) side by side in terms of their conventional two-dimensional echocardiographic presentation at each left ventricular (LV) level (**A**) and their corresponding circumferential strain curves at each LV level (**B**). Visual and numerical summary of the LV circumferential strain and presence or absence of the base-to-apex circumferential strain gradient in patients with NHCM and in AFD, respectively (**C**). *AFD LVH +,* Anderson-Fabry disease with LVH; *CS,* circumferential strain. (Reproduced with permission from Gruner C, et al: Systolic myocardial mechanics in patients with Anderson-Fabry disease with and without left ventricular hypertrophy and in comparison to nonobstructive hypertrophic cardiomyopathy, *Echocardiography* 29:810–817, 2012.)

were found to have lower circumferential strain and demonstrate a loss of base-to-apex circumferential strain gradient compared with patients with HCM, who usually show increased circumferential strain as a compensatory mechanism for the decreased longitudinal strain (Fig. 60.7).[27] In addition, in patients with AFD, decreased segmental longitudinal strain in the inferolateral wall correlated with fibrosis in this area in CMRI, which is typical for AFD patients and is also a negative prognostic factor.[28,29]

Danon Disease

Danon disease is a rare X-linked dominant disorder caused by loss of function mutations in the lysosome-associated membrane protein 2 (LAMP2) gene. These cause LAMP2 protein deficiency, resulting in accumulation of autophagic material and glycogen in cardiac and skeletal muscle cells. Because of its X-linked inheritance, men are usually affected at a younger age and develop more severe manifestations of the disease. Clinical manifestations include cardiomyopathy, skeletal myopathy, mild intellectual difficulties, and developmental delay. An electrocardiographic (ECG) pattern of Wolff-Parkinson-White (WPW) with pre-excitation is seen in most affected men but in only 27% of affected women.[30] Patients with Danon disease most frequently develop progressive concentric LVH, but dilated

cardiomyopathy is also a possible phenotype of the disease, which is more common in women. Echocardiographic features include marked concentric LVH, which often exceeds a maximal wall thickness of 30 mm. Most patients also exhibit RV hypertrophy and LV diastolic dysfunction. Initially, systolic LV function is preserved, and the LV cavity size is normal, but disease progression can lead to LV systolic dysfunction, which is sometimes accompanied by LV dilatation. Danon disease carries a grave prognosis; men usually die before the age of 25 years, and women live approximately 10 to 15 years longer, and the only life prolonging treatment is heart transplant.[30] One should suspect Danon disease in patients with significant LVH, mostly concentric, accompanied by skeletal myopathy, intellectual impairment, and the typical ECG pattern. Definite diagnosis, however, can be made only by genetic testing.

Glycogen Storage Diseases

Glycogen storage diseases (GSDs) are a group of rare autosomal-recessive inherited disorders (all but IX, which is X-linked recessive). Inherited mutations in genes encoding enzymes that take part in glycogen metabolism cause the accumulation of glycogen in different tissues. Most GSDs are diagnosed during infancy because of various signs and symptoms, including hypoglycemia,

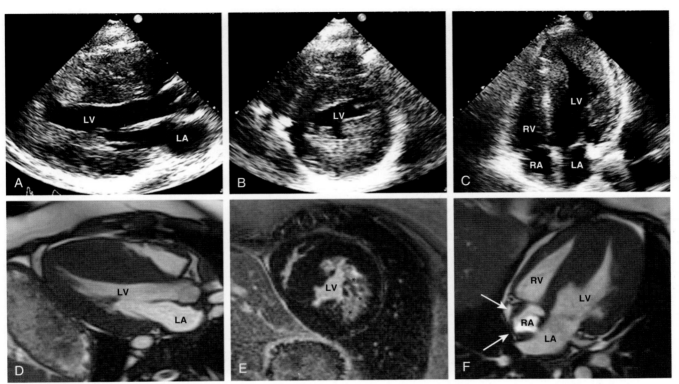

Figure 60.8. PRKAG2 syndrome. Transthoracic echocardiography (Top, **A–C**) and cardiac magnetic resonance imaging (Bottom, **D–F**) demonstrate typical findings in PRKAG2 cardiomyopathy of biventricular hypertrophy, thickening of the atrial walls (**F**, *arrows*), and diffuse late gadolinium enhancement (**E**, *asterisk*). *LA,* Left atrium; *LV,* left ventricle; *RA,* right atrium; *RV,* right ventricle.

hepatomegaly, fatigue, muscle weakness, and exercise intolerance. However, recent developments in the field of genetic testing have led to diagnosis of late-onset phenotypes which were undiagnosed previously. Several GSDs can affect the heart, but the most common is Pompe disease (GSD type II). Echocardiographic features result from glycogen deposits in the myocardium and are typically increased wall thickness with diastolic dysfunction, followed by LV systolic dysfunction in later stages.

PRKAG2 Syndrome

PRKAG2 syndrome is a genetic disorder that mostly involves the heart muscle and the conduction system. The *PRKAG2* gene encodes the γ-subunit of the AMP-activated protein kinase. Pathogenic mutations in this gene cause glycogen storage cardiac hypertrophy in the absence of significant skeletal muscle involvement. PRKAG2 is associated with ventricular pre-excitation pattern on ECG, as in WPW syndrome, as well as progressive conduction system abnormalities.[31] The echocardiographic presentation consists of LVH, mostly with a concentric hypertrophy pattern, and signs of diastolic dysfunction. RV involvement is frequent, and occasionally LVOTO can be present (see Fig. 60.6). CMRI may be helpful in demonstrating the extent of biventricular involvement, thickening of the atrial walls and interatrial septum, and the presence of myocardial scar tissue (Fig. 60.8).[32] The prognosis of patients with PRKAG2 syndrome is worse compared with classic HCM. Ventricular arrhythmias and conduction system abnormalities are the leading causes of death followed by heart failure.

Hemochromatosis

Hemochromatosis is a systemic disorder caused by abnormal iron accumulation in multiple organs, including the heart, liver, and endocrine tissue. Iron accumulation can be caused by primary hemochromatosis; a genetic disorder caused by multiple mutations that increase iron absorption in the gastrointestinal system. However, it could also be a result of secondary iron overload, which can be caused by increase in iron intake, chronic blood transfusions, and increased iron absorption seen in chronic liver failure. Accurate diagnosis is important because treatment with phlebotomy and iron chelation can improve prognosis and prevent further deterioration. Presentation with clinical symptoms is variable in both hereditary and acquired conditions, and first symptoms can appear between the ages of 15 and 80 years. Cardiac hemochromatosis usually begins with diastolic dysfunction and can involve the conduction system and cause various degrees of heart block. Cardiac hypertrophy can be seen in early stages of cardiac involvement, but progressive disease commonly leads to dilated cardiomyopathy. Diagnosis is often made following extracardiac manifestations, though if suspected, cardiac iron overload can be diagnosed by CMRI measurement of myocardial $T_2{*}$.[33]

SYNDROMIC HYPERTROPHIC CARDIOMYOPATHY
RASopathies: Noonan Syndrome and LEOPARD Syndrome

Both Noonan syndrome and LEOPARD syndrome are genetic multisystem disorders with an autosomal dominant inheritance pattern. They are caused by deleterious mutations in genes encoding the RAS-mitogen activated protein kinase pathway.[34] Because they share pathogenetic mechanisms, some clinical overlap in their phenotypes is present, including characteristic facial features, developmental delay, various cardiac manifestations, cutaneous and ocular abnormalities, and neurocognitive impairment, as well as an increased risk for developing cancer.

Noonan syndrome is typically associated with short stature, a webbed neck, hypertelorism, ptosis, low-set ears, chest deformities, bleeding disorders, and sensorineural hearing deficits.[35] More than half of the patients have at least one heart defect, including pulmonary stenosis (50%–66%), cardiac hypertrophy (20%–30%), atrial or ventricular septal defects (5%–15%), dilatation of the coronary arteries, and, rarely, coarctation of the aorta or mitral valve abnormalities.[36,37] Typical electrocardiographic findings include left-axis deviation, abnormal R/S ratio, and abnormal Q waves even in the absence of cardiac defects.

LEOPARD syndrome is an acronym that stands for multiple lentigines, ECG abnormalities, ocular hypertelorism, pulmonary stenosis, abnormal genitalia, retardation of growth, and sensorineural deafness. The most frequent cardiac finding is LVH (73%), with concomitant LVOTO in 37% followed by pulmonary stenosis (23%), mitral valve prolapse (38%), and coronary abnormalities (15%), in which mostly dilatation of the proximal vessels have been described.[38] ECG abnormalities are seen in more than 70% of patients, including signs of biventricular hypertrophy (46%), Q waves (19%), prolonged QT interval (23%), repolarization abnormalities (42%), and conduction defects (23%).

With respect to cardiac hypertrophy, both syndromes show similar features. LVH is mostly asymmetric, but it can rarely show a concentric pattern and is usually accompanied by some degree of diastolic dysfunction (see Fig. 60.6). RV involvement is present in approximately one-third of the patients, which is definitely more prevalent than in classic HCM. Moreover, both right and left ventricular outflow tracts can be obstructed.[38] Diagnosis of both syndromes is usually made by the typical extracardiac manifestations and validated using genetic testing.

Friedreich Ataxia

Friedreich ataxia is a rare (prevalence 1 in 50,000) autosomal recessive neurodegenerative disease caused by pathogenic variants in the gene encoding for the mitochondrial protein frataxin. Myocardial involvement is frequent and usually starts with concentric remodeling followed by the expression of mild concentric LVH (maximal wall thickness <15 mm) with preserved LV systolic function. End-stage disease is characterized by myocardial thinning, dilatation of the LV cavity, and a concomitant decrease in systolic function.[39] Differential diagnosis for HCM is again driven by extracardiac neurologic findings, including progressive limb and gait ataxia, and dysarthria.

Acknowledgment

The authors thank Dr. Christiane Gruner for her contribution to the previous edition of this chapter.

REFERENCES

1. Gersh BJ, Maron BJ, Bonow RO, et al. ACCF/AHA guideline for the diagnosis and treatment of hypertrophic cardiomyopathy. *J Am Coll Cardiol.* 2011;58:e212–260. 2011.
2. Wolf-Maier K, Cooper RS, Banegas JR, et al. Hypertension prevalence and blood pressure levels in 6 European countries, Canada, and the United States. *J Am Med Assoc.* 2003;289:2363–2369.
3. Baltabaeva A, Marciniak M, Bijnens B, et al. Regional left ventricular deformation and geometry analysis provides insights in myocardial remodelling in mild to moderate hypertension. *Eur J Echocardiogr.* 2008;9:501–508.
4. Doi YL, Deanfield JE, McKenna WJ, et al. Echocardiographic differentiation of hypertensive heart disease and hypertrophic cardiomyopathy. *Br Heart J.* 1980;44:395–400.
5. Sun JP, Xu TY, Ni XD, et al. Echocardiographic strain in hypertrophic cardiomyopathy and hypertensive left ventricular hypertrophy. *Echocardiography.* 2019;36:257–265.
6. Afonso L, Briasoulis A, Mahajan N, et al. Comparison of right ventricular contractile abnormalities in hypertrophic cardiomyopathy versus hypertensive heart disease using two dimensional strain imaging: a cross-sectional study. *Int J Cardiovasc Imag.* 2015;31:1503–1509.
7. Pelliccia A, Maron BJ, Spataro A, et al. The upper limit of physiologic cardiac hypertrophy in highly trained elite athletes. *N Engl J Med.* 1991;324:295–301.
8. Papadakis M, Carre F, Kervio G, et al. The prevalence, distribution, and clinical outcomes of electrocardiographic repolarization patterns in male athletes of African/Afro-Caribbean origin. *Eur Heart J.* 2011;32:2304–2313.
9. Papadakis M, Wilson MG, Ghani S, et al. Impact of ethnicity upon cardiovascular adaptation in competitive athletes: relevance to preparticipation screening. *Br J Sports Med.* 2012;46(Suppl 1). i22–28.
10. Maron BJ. Distinguishing hypertrophic cardiomyopathy from athlete's heart: a clinical problem of increasing magnitude and significance. *Heart.* 2005;91:1380–1382.
11. Afonso L, Kondur A, Simegn M, et al. Two-dimensional strain profiles in patients with physiological and pathological hypertrophy and preserved left ventricular systolic function: a comparative analyses. *BMJ Open.* 2012;2. e001390.
12. Vinereanu D, Florescu N, Sculthorpe N, et al. Differentiation between pathologic and physiologic left ventricular hypertrophy by tissue Doppler assessment of long-axis function in patients with hypertrophic cardiomyopathy or systemic hypertension and in athletes. *Am J Cardiol.* 2001;88:53–58.
13. Kovacs A, Apor A, Nagy A, et al. Left ventricular untwisting in athlete's heart: key role in early diastolic filling? *Int J Sports Med.* 2014;35:259–264.
14. Wang J, Buergler JM, Veerasamy K, et al. Delayed untwisting: the mechanistic link between dynamic obstruction and exercise tolerance in patients with hypertrophic obstructive cardiomyopathy. *J Am Coll Cardiol.* 2009;54:1326–1334.
15. Gabrielli L, Enriquez A, Cordova S, et al. Assessment of left atrial function in hypertrophic cardiomyopathy and athlete's heart: a left atrial myocardial deformation study. *Echocardiography.* 2012;29:943–949.
16. Brenner DA, Jain M, Pimentel DR, et al. Human amyloidogenic light chains directly impair cardiomyocyte function through an increase in cellular oxidant stress. *Circ Res.* 2004;94:1008–1010.
17. Bellavia D, Abraham TP, Pellikka PA, et al. Detection of left ventricular systolic dysfunction in cardiac amyloidosis with strain rate echocardiography. *J Am Soc Echocardiogr.* 2007;20:1194–1202.
18. Phelan D, Collier P, Thavendiranathan P, et al. Relative apical sparing of longitudinal strain using two-dimensional speckle-tracking echocardiography is both sensitive and specific for the diagnosis of cardiac amyloidosis. *Heart.* 2012;98:1442–1448.
19. Matsumori A, Hara M, Nagai S, et al. Hypertrophic cardiomyopathy as a manifestation of cardiac sarcoidosis. *Jpn Circ J.* 2000;64:679–683.
20. Kandolin R, Lehtonen J, Airaksinen J, et al. Cardiac sarcoidosis: epidemiology, characteristics, and outcome over 25 years in a nationwide study. *Circulation.* 2015;131:624–632.
21. Jenni R, Oechslin E, Schneider J, et al. Echocardiographic and pathoanatomical characteristics of isolated left ventricular non-compaction: a step towards classification as a distinct cardiomyopathy. *Heart.* 2001;86:666–671.
22. Oechslin E, Jenni R. Left ventricular non-compaction revisited: a distinct phenotype with genetic heterogeneity? *Eur Heart J.* 2011;32:1446–1456.
23. Haland TF, Saberniak J, Leren IS, et al. Echocardiographic comparison between left ventricular non-compaction and hypertrophic cardiomyopathy. *Int J Cardiol.* 2017;228:900–905.
24. Alfares AA, Kelly MA, McDermott G, et al. Results of clinical genetic testing of 2,912 probands with hypertrophic cardiomyopathy: expanded panels offer limited additional sensitivity. *Genet Med.* 2015;17:880–888.
25. Rombach SM, Smid BE, Bouwman MG, et al. Long term enzyme replacement therapy for Fabry disease: effectiveness on kidney, heart and brain. *Orphanet J Rare Dis.* 2013;8:47.
26. Elliott P, Baker R, Pasquale F, et al. Prevalence of Anderson-Fabry disease in patients with hypertrophic cardiomyopathy: the European Anderson-Fabry Disease survey. *Heart.* 2011;97:1957–1960.
27. Gruner C, Verocai F, Carasso S, et al. Systolic myocardial mechanics in patients with Anderson-Fabry disease with and without left ventricular hypertrophy and in comparison to nonobstructive hypertrophic cardiomyopathy. *Echocardiography.* 2012;29:810–817.
28. Kramer J, Niemann M, Liu D, et al. Two-dimensional speckle tracking as a non-invasive tool for identification of myocardial fibrosis in Fabry disease. *Eur Heart J.* 2013;34:1587–1596.
29. Weidemann F, Niemann M, Breunig F, et al. Long-term effects of enzyme replacement therapy on Fabry cardiomyopathy: evidence for a better outcome with early treatment. *Circulation.* 2009;119:524–529.
30. Boucek D, Jirikowic J, Taylor M. Natural history of Danon disease. *Genet Med.* 2011;13:563–568.
31. Arad M, Benson DW, Perez-Atayde AR, et al. Constitutively active AMP kinase mutations cause glycogen storage disease mimicking hypertrophic cardiomyopathy. *J Clin Invest.* 2002;109:357–362.
32. Poyhonen P, Hiippala A, Ollila L, et al. Cardiovascular magnetic resonance findings in patients with PRKAG2 gene mutations. *J Cardiovasc Magn Reson.* 2015;17:89.
33. Gulati V, Harikrishnan P, Palaniswamy C, et al. Cardiac involvement in hemochromatosis. *Cardiol Rev.* 2014;22:56–68.
34. Kaski JP, Syrris P, Shaw A, et al. Prevalence of sequence variants in the RAS-mitogen activated protein kinase signaling pathway in pre-adolescent children with hypertrophic cardiomyopathy. *Circ Cardiovasc Genet.* 2012;5:317–326.
35. Tartaglia M, Gelb BD. Disorders of dysregulated signal traffic through the RAS-MAPK pathway: phenotypic spectrum and molecular mechanisms. *Ann N Y Acad Sci.* 2010;1214:99–121.
36. Sharland M, Burch M, McKenna WM, Paton MA. A clinical study of Noonan syndrome. *Arch Dis Child.* 1992;67:178–183.
37. Shaw AC, Kalidas K, Crosby AH, et al. The natural history of Noonan syndrome: a long-term follow-up study. *Arch Dis Child.* 2007;92:128–132.
38. Limongelli G, Pacileo G, Marino B, et al. Prevalence and clinical significance of cardiovascular abnormalities in patients with the LEOPARD syndrome. *Am J Cardiol.* 2007;100:736–741.
39. Weidemann F, Rummey C, Bijnens B, et al. The heart in Friedreich ataxia: definition of cardiomyopathy, disease severity, and correlation with neurological symptoms. *Circulation.* 2012;125:1626–1634.

61 Hypertrophic Cardiomyopathy: Assessment of Therapy

Hanna Lee, Anna Woo

Dynamic left ventricular outflow tract obstruction (LVOTO) is an important clinical feature of hypertrophic cardiomyopathy (HCM). Resting or provocable LVOTO occurs in 70% of patients with HCM.[1] The presence of resting LVOTO (traditionally defined as an left ventricular outflow tract (LVOT) gradient of ≥30 mm Hg at rest) is associated with a significant increased risk of HCM-related death.[2] The initial treatment for symptomatic patients with obstructive HCM is pharmacotherapy with negative inotropic agents (β-blockers, verapamil, disopyramide). However, in patients who remain symptomatic and who generally have a resting or provocable LVOT gradient of at least 50 mm Hg, invasive septal reduction therapy should be considered.[3] The different invasive interventions available for the management of obstructive HCM are outlined in Chapter 59.

Medical treatment is optimized by monitoring symptom response to medications and by performing serial echocardiographic and Doppler studies to assess the LVOT gradient. The LVOT gradient can be documented by the continuous-wave (CW) Doppler technique.[3,4] If the LVOT gradient at rest is 30 to 50 mm Hg and the patient's symptoms are suggestive of underlying obstruction, then a provocative maneuver can be performed to detect for an inducible LVOT gradient.[3,4] There are numerous techniques for eliciting provocable LVOTO.[4,5] Provocation with exercise is the most physiologic method for detecting a provocable LVOT gradient.[1,3,5] Although the Valsalva maneuver is the most commonly used method of provocation, one large study has demonstrated that the Valsalva-induced LVOT gradient is underestimated compared with the exercise-induced LVOT gradient.[1]

PHARMACOTHERAPY

β-Blockers are the first-line agents in the management of symptomatic obstructive HCM.[3] By decreasing myocardial contractility, β-blockers lead to a reduction in the left ventricular (LV) ejection velocity, which causes the delayed onset of mitral leaflet systolic anterior motion (SAM), and consequently results in a decrease in the magnitude of LVOTO. Other effects of the β-blocker class of drugs include sympathetic modulation of the heart rate, relief of myocardial ischemia, and prolongation of diastole, which allows for increased passive ventricular filling.[3] Nondihydropyridine calcium channel blockers (e.g., verapamil, diltiazem) can be used in patients with HCM who have contraindications, side effects, or unresponsiveness to β-blockers.[3] Nevertheless, both verapamil and diltiazem should be used very cautiously in patients with high LVOT gradients, advanced heart failure, or sinus bradycardia.[3] In particular, in the setting of severe LVOTO, an elevated pulmonary artery wedge pressure, and low systemic blood pressure, the vasodilatation from calcium channel blockers may trigger an increase in SAM and in the severity of the LVOTO, and may precipitate pulmonary edema.[3]

Disopyramide is highly effective in the management of patients with obstructive HCM.[3,6,7] Although classified as a type IA antiarrhythmic agent, disopyramide has significant negative inotropic properties that decrease SAM and the magnitude of LVOTO.[3] If symptoms and an increased LVOT gradient persist despite monotherapy with β-blockers or verapamil, disopyramide can be introduced.[3] The addition of disopyramide results in an improvement in cardiac symptoms and a significant reduction in the resting LVOT gradient.[6,7] Data from experienced HCM centers have shown that disopyramide can be safely administered on a long-term basis.[6,7]

SURGICAL MYECTOMY

For patients with obstructive HCM and symptoms unresponsive to medical therapy, septal myectomy is considered the definitive treatment for patients who are acceptable candidates for open heart surgery.[3] Myectomy is performed using a transaortic approach and involves the resection of the hypertrophied basal (to mid) ventricular septum. Subaortic muscle resection results in the enlargement of the outflow tract, decreased SAM of the mitral valve, and abolition of the LVOTO.[3] Operative mortality rates in the contemporary era are very low for myectomy when it is performed at HCM centers with recognized expertise in the surgical management of obstructive HCM.[3,8,9] Surgical myectomy produces substantial symptomatic improvement and leads to excellent postoperative long-term survival.[3,6,8,9]

Preoperative Assessment

Preoperative echocardiographic examination includes comprehensive transthoracic imaging to characterize the degree and extent of septal hypertrophy, SAM, and the magnitude of LVOTO[3,4] (Fig. 61.1 and Video 61.1). The presence of independent mitral valve disease, structural abnormalities of the mitral apparatus, concomitant aortic valve disease, additional levels of obstruction (e.g., at the midventricle or right ventricular outflow tract), and ventricular function should also be established.[3,4] Abnormalities of the mitral valve or mitral apparatus (including the papillary muscles) have increasingly been recognized in this condition, with a higher prevalence of mitral valve surgery occurring in patients with lesser degrees of septal hypertrophy (basal septal thickness <2 cm).[9] Moreover, preoperative echocardiography provides valuable information regarding the prognosis of patients: the echocardiographic variable that is predictive of worsened postoperative long-term overall survival is the preoperative left atrial (LA) dimension (anteroposterior LA diameter ≥46 mm).[8]

Intraoperative Assessment

Intraoperative transesophageal echocardiography (TEE) improves the safety and efficacy of surgical myectomy by guiding the surgical intervention, assessing the immediate results of the muscle resection, and excluding potential complications[10] (Fig. 61.2). TEE imaging identifies the maximum thickness of the septum, the distance of the maximum septal thickness from the aortic annulus, the location of the point of contact between the anterior mitral leaflet and the septum, and the LVOT gradient.[4] The length of septal hypertrophy is measured from the base of the right coronary cusp of the aortic valve (midesophageal long-axis view), with the length of subaortic muscle resection targeted at 1 cm below the point of anterior mitral leaflet–septal contact. The LVOT gradient can be obtained by transgastric imaging with the CW Doppler beam aligned parallel to the LVOT

Figure 61.1. Transthoracic echocardiographic findings before and after surgical myectomy in a 19-year-old young man with symptomatic obstructive hypertrophic cardiomyopathy. **A,** Two-dimensional echocardiographic imaging (systolic frame) shows asymmetric septal hypertrophy (anterior septal thickness of 19 mm), severe anterior leaflet systolic anterior motion (SAM), contact of the anterior mitral leaflet with the septum in systole, and severe left atrial enlargement. **B,** Color Doppler imaging reveals color turbulence in the left ventricular outflow tract (LVOT), associated with a significant jet of posterior mitral regurgitation (MR) caused by the leaflet SAM. The LVOT gradient at rest measures 95 mm Hg. **C,** In the early postoperative setting, thinning of the basal and midanterior septum at the site of muscle resection is observed (*white arrows*), with widening of the outflow tract, and resolution of leaflet SAM. **D,** After myectomy, color Doppler imaging highlights the laminar flow in the LVOT and a marked decrease in the degree of MR. (See accompanying Video 61.1.)

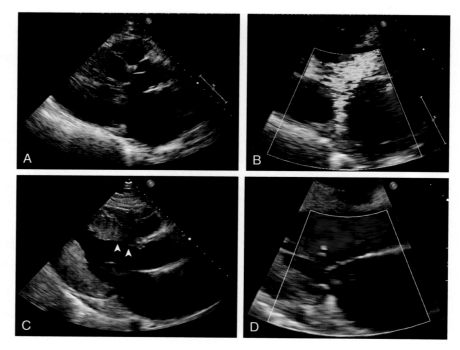

(see Fig. 61.2). Mitral regurgitation in patients with obstructive HCM is predominantly secondary to anterior mitral leaflet SAM and is characterized by a posteriorly directed jet occurring in mid to late systole (see Fig. 61.2).[10] The presence of a nonposterior jet of mitral regurgitation suggests an underlying intrinsic abnormality of the mitral leaflets or mitral apparatus (e.g., mitral valve prolapse, mitral annular calcification).[11] Mitral regurgitation due to SAM can generally be relieved with isolated myectomy without the requirement for mitral valve repair or replacement.[3,11,12] Immediately after surgical excision of the upper septum and after cardiopulmonary bypass, intraoperative TEE provides real-time feedback about the adequacy of the myectomy and ascertains if there is hemodynamically important residual obstruction or mitral regurgitation (see Fig. 61.2).[10,13] The presence of significant ongoing SAM-related mitral regurgitation can be addressed by further surgical debulking.[13] Detection of operative complications, such as iatrogenic ventricular septal defects, is also crucial to allow for additional surgical intervention.[4,13]

Postoperative Assessment

Two-dimensional echocardiographic and Doppler studies have had a long-established role in the management of patients after myectomy.[3,14] Multiple studies have demonstrated significant symptomatic improvement and a significant reduction in the LVOT gradient at rest after myectomy.[3,8,9] Specific potential findings in the postoperative setting (both in the acute and chronic period) include thinning of the basal (to mid) septum at the site of the muscle resection (Fig. 61.1C and D and Video 61.1),[14] a ventricular septal defect (in <1% of patients) (Fig. 61.3 and Video 61.3),[3] septal perforator flow, and aortic regurgitation. Septal perforator flow consists of diastolic color flow directed from the proximal septum to the LVOT and is caused by surgically incised septal perforator branches communicating with the LV cavity.[15] Finally, aortic regurgitation can develop after surgery; at least mild aortic regurgitation was been recognized in 27% of patients in the postoperative period in two different cohorts and is generally well tolerated.[16,17]

ALCOHOL SEPTAL ABLATION

Alcohol septal ablation (ASA) involves a targeted infarction of the basal interventricular septum, achieved by selective injection of ethanol into a septal perforator branch of the left anterior descending artery.[18] Developed as an alternative to surgical myectomy and indicated when surgical risk is considered excessive, the aim of the procedure is to produce a localized infarction of the hypertrophied basal septum. The targeted infarction causes focal thinning of the septum, subsequent widening of the LVOT, and a decline in the degree of LVOTO.[19] Multiple centers have demonstrated that ASA can safely and effectively reduce the LVOT gradient in patients with obstructive HCM with very good postprocedure clinical outcomes.[6,20–22]

Intraprocedure Assessment

Intraprocedural transthoracic or transesophageal echocardiography is essential for the guidance and monitoring of ASA (Fig. 61.4).[3,4] Echocardiographic contrast agent is injected into the proposed target septal branch of the left anterior descending artery, which leads to delineation of the vascular territory supplied by the septal vessel. The supplied territory demonstrates increased echo density with echocardiographic contrast administration. Alternatively, an agitated radiographic contrast agent can also be used to provide myocardial opacification.[4] The extent of myocardial opacification of both target and nontarget regions should be determined using multiple transthoracic views, including apical four- and three-chamber views and parasternal short- and long-axis views.[4] Intraprocedural TEE has also been used to guide ASA.[4] The optimal target territory of the basal septum is the site of contact between the anterior mitral leaflet and the septum, which is adjacent to the region of maximal flow acceleration and color turbulence in the LVOT (as seen by color Doppler).[4,23] The absence of opacification in any myocardial regions remote from the basal septum (nontarget sites) must also be ensured before proceeding to the injection of intracoronary alcohol. If the selected septal branch supplies other territories such as the LV free wall or apex, right ventricular free wall, or a papillary muscle, another septal perforator branch should be selected, and injection of echocardiographic contrast agent should be repeated with the new target vessel.[23] If no appropriate septal branch is found, this procedure should then be abandoned.[4]

The use of intraprocedural contrast echocardiography results in improved procedural and patient outcomes by limiting the infarct to the targeted region of interest. Advantages include

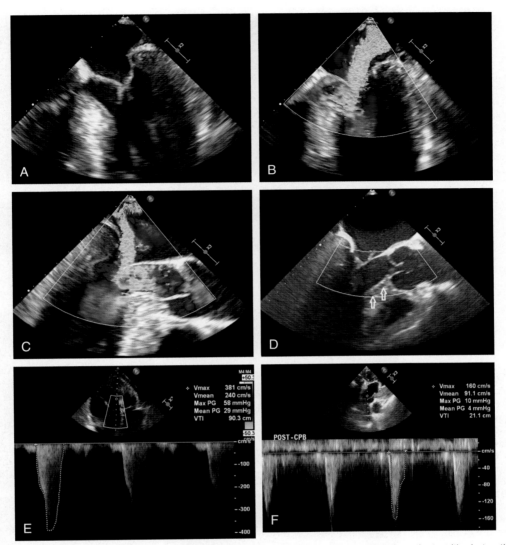

Figure 61.2. Intraoperative transesophageal echocardiographic (TEE) guidance for surgical myectomy in patients with obstructive hypertrophic cardiomyopathy. **A** and **B,** Baseline (premyectomy) TEE imaging from the midesophageal four-chamber view, with two-dimensional imaging (**A**) demonstrating asymmetric septal hypertrophy, systolic anterior motion (SAM) of the anterior mitral leaflet toward the interventricular septum, and the interleaflet gap between the anterior and posterior mitral valve leaflets. Color Doppler imaging (**B**) shows color turbulence in the left ventricular outflow tract (LVOT) caused by the anterior leaflet SAM. The interleaflet gap results in an eccentric posteriorly directed jet of mitral regurgitation (MR). **C,** Midesophageal long-axis view with two-dimensional and color Doppler imaging provides visualization of the anterior septum, LVOT, and mitral valve. The thickness and length of the hypertrophied septum (measured from the base of the right coronary cusp of the aortic valve) can be assessed. In this systolic frame, there is color turbulence in the LVOT as blood is ejected from the left ventricle and a jet of MR that is directed posteriorly into the left atrium. **D,** After subaortic muscle resection (via a transaortic approach), the site of the myectomy is denoted by the *white arrows*). The outflow tract has widened, laminar flow is seen in the outflow tract, and the leaflet SAM and SAM-related MR have resolved. There is a trace jet of residual MR. **E** and **F,** The LVOT gradient obtained from the transgastric view with continuous-wave Doppler beam parallel to the LVOT and aortic valve. Before myectomy, the LVOT gradient was 58 mm Hg at rest (**E**), and the LVOT gradient decreased to 10 mm Hg (**F**) after resection of the hypertrophied portion of the septum.

shorter intervention and fluoroscopy times, fewer occluded vessels, less ethanol use, smaller infarct size, a lower likelihood of heart block, and a higher likelihood of success.[4] Intraprocedural echocardiography also permits real-time assessment of procedural success. The area infarcted by the alcohol infusion demonstrates increased echogenicity and reflectivity, with reduced thickening and excursion (see Fig. 61.4). The degree of SAM and SAM-related mitral regurgitation and the dynamic LVOT gradient are reduced after alcohol injection.[19] Significant predictors of an unsatisfactory outcome after ASA are the presence of an ongoing LVOT gradient at rest of 25 mm Hg or more in the cardiac catheterization laboratory and a lower rise in the peak creatinine kinase level (<1300 U/L) after the procedure.[24]

Postprocedure Assessment

Serial echocardiographic and Doppler studies are an important component of the long-term follow-up of patients after ASA. Although there is generally an immediate and sustained elimination of the LVOT gradient in patients who undergo surgical myectomy,[3] there is often a triphasic hemodynamic response following ASA.[25,26] This triphasic response consists of the following: (1) an

Figure 61.3. Iatrogenic ventricular septal defect (VSD) detected after surgical myectomy. **A,** Transthoracic apical four-chamber view with color Doppler demonstrating a small iatrogenic VSD (in this case, the location of the defect was more distal than is typically seen in an iatrogenic VSD associated with a myectomy). **B,** Continuous-wave Doppler imaging documents left-to-right shunting and a gradient of 62 mm Hg across the septal defect. (See accompanying Video 61.3.)

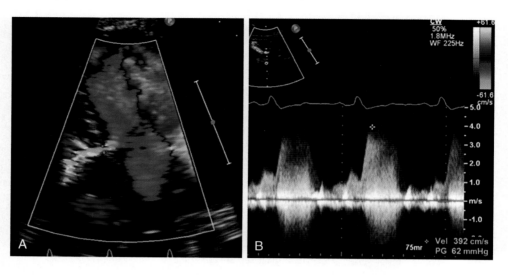

Figure 61.4. Intraprocedural transthoracic echocardiography (TTE) for guidance of alcohol septal ablation (ASA). **A,** Baseline two-dimensional TTE apical four-chamber view (systolic frame) demonstrates septal hypertrophy and anterior mitral leaflet systolic anterior motion (SAM) toward the basal septum. **B,** After the addition of echocardiographic contrast agent into the first septal perforator branch of the left anterior coronary descending (LAD) artery, contrast immediately opacifies the upper portion of the ventricular septum, in the area that involves the point of anterior mitral leaflet–septal contact. **C,** Two-dimensional apical three-chamber view with color Doppler imaging confirms accurate localization of the contrast-enhanced region (basal septum), that is, contiguous to the area of color turbulence (i.e., obstruction) in the left ventricular outflow tract (LVOT). Additional transthoracic imaging also determines that no other left ventricular wall segments opacify after the administration of contrast. **D,** Two-dimensional apical three-chamber image after intraarterial injection of ethanol into target septal branch of the LAD. Ethanol results in marked echogenicity of the upper septum. **E** and **F,** The resting LVOT gradient obtained in the cardiac catheterization laboratory before and after ASA. After the targeted infarction of the basal septum, there is a significant acute decrease in the LVOT gradient at rest from 68 mm Hg to 12 mm Hg.

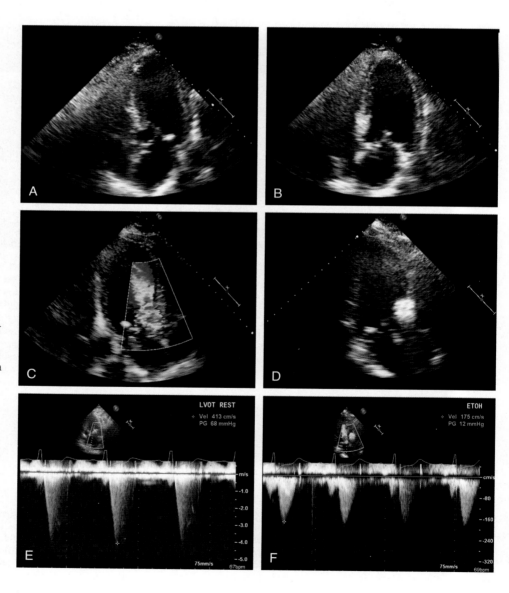

immediate reduction in the LVOT gradient after the injection of alcohol (see Fig. 61.4), (2) an early rebound increase in the LVOT gradient (a few days after the procedure), and (3) a gradual decline in the magnitude of LVOTO (with progressive reduction in both the resting and provocable LVOT gradients).[26] Longer-term benefits arise from progressive septal thinning, favorable remodeling of the outflow tract,[26,27] and an improvement in diastolic function.[28] Finally, ASA is associated with an increased need for a repeat invasive intervention (either a second ASA or referral for subsequent surgical myectomy) during long-term follow-up; it was 10% in a large European registry[21] and 8% in a meta-analysis.[22] Therefore, echocardiography is advisable for intermittent monitoring of patients following this procedure.

Dual-Chamber Pacing

Dual-chamber pacing currently has a limited role in the management of patients with obstructive HCM. It may be offered in patients with significant comorbidities for whom both surgical septal myectomy and ASA are considered to have unacceptable risk or in patients who already have an implanted dual-chamber pacing device for other reasons.[3] If a dual-chamber pacemaker is implanted, echocardiography allows for the assessment of changes to the LVOT gradient after intervention and assists with the selection of the most optimal atrioventricular delay to minimize the LVOT gradient.[4]

Acknowledgment

The authors acknowledge Dr. Paul Szmitko, who was the first author of this chapter in the second edition of the textbook.

Please access ExpertConsult to view the corresponding videos for this chapter.

REFERENCES

1. Maron MS, Olivotto I, Zenovich AG, et al. Hypertrophic cardiomyopathy is predominantly a disease of left ventricular outflow tract obstruction. *Circulation.* 2006;114:2232–2239.
2. Maron MS, Olivotto I, Betocchi S, et al. Effect of left ventricular outflow tract obstruction on clinical outcome in hypertrophic cardiomyopathy. *N Engl J Med.* 2003;348:295–303.
3. Gersh BJ, Maron BJ, Bonow RO, et al. 2011 ACCF/AHA guideline for the diagnosis and treatment of hypertrophic cardiomyopathy. *J Am Coll Cardiol.* 2011;58:e212–e260. .
4. Nagueh SF, Bierig SM, Budoff MJ, et al. American Society of Echocardiography clinical recommendations for multimodality cardiovascular imaging of patients with hypertrophic cardiomyopathy. *J Am Soc Echocardiogr.* 2011;24:473–498.
5. Chun S, Woo A. Echocardiography in hypertrophic cardiomyopathy: in with strain, out with straining? *J Am Soc Echocardiogr.* 2015;28:204–209.
6. Ball W, Ivanov J, Rakowski H, et al. Long-term survival in patients with resting obstructive hypertrophic cardiomyopathy comparison of conservative versus invasive treatment. *J Am Coll Cardiol.* 2011;58:2313–2321.
7. Sherrid MV, Shetty A, Winson G, et al. Treatment of obstructive hypertrophic cardiomyopathy symptoms and gradient resistant to first-line therapy with beta-blockade or verapamil. *Circ Heart Fail.* 2013;6:694–702.
8. Woo A, Williams WG, Choi R, et al. Clinical and echocardiographic determinants of long-term survival after surgical myectomy in obstructive hypertrophic cardiomyopathy. *Circulation.* 2005;111:2033–2041.
9. Desai MY, Bhonsale A, Smedira NG, et al. Predictors of long-term outcomes in symptomatic hypertrophic cardiomyopathy patients undergoing surgical relief of left ventricular outflow tract obstruction. *Circulation.* 2013;128:209–216.
10. Grigg LE, Wigle ED, Williams WG, et al. Transesophageal Doppler echocardiography in obstructive hypertrophic cardiomyopathy: clarification of pathophysiology and importance in intraoperative decision making. *J Am Coll Cardiol.* 1992;20:42–52.
11. Yu EH, Omran AS, Wigle ED, et al. Mitral regurgitation in hypertrophic obstructive cardiomyopathy: relationship to obstruction and relief with myectomy. *J Am Coll Cardiol.* 2000;36:2219–2225.
12. Hong JH, Schaff HV, Nishimura RA, et al. Mitral regurgitation in patients with hypertrophic obstructive cardiomyopathy: implications for concomitant valve procedures. *J Am Coll Cardiol.* 2016;68:1497–1504.
13. Ommen S, Park SH, Click RL, et al. Impact of intraoperative transesophageal echocardiography in the surgical management of hypertrophic cardiomyopathy. *Am J Cardiol.* 2002;90:1022–1024.
14. Schapira JN, Stemple DR, Martin RP, et al. Single and two-dimensional echocardiographic visualization of the effects of septal myectomy in idiopathic hypertrophic subaortic stenosis. *Circulation.* 1978;58:850–860.
15. Awasthi A, Wormer D, Heggunje PS, Obeid A. Long-term follow-up of acquired coronary artery fistula after septal myectomy for hypertrophic cardiomyopathy. *J Am Soc Echocardiogr.* 2002;15:1104–1107.
16. Sasson Z, Prieur T, Skrobik Y, et al. Aortic regurgitation: a common complication after surgery for hypertrophic cardiomyopathy. *J Am Coll Cardiol.* 1989;13:63–67.
17. Nagueh SF, Ommen SR, Lakkis NM, et al. Comparison of ethanol septal reduction therapy with surgical myectomy for the treatment of hypertrophic obstructive cardiomyopathy. *J Am Coll Cardiol.* 2001;38:1701–1706.
18. Sigwart U. Non-surgical myocardial reduction for hypertrophic obstructive cardiomyopathy. *Lancet.* 1995;346:211–214.
19. Flores-Ramirez R, Lakkis NM, Middleton KJ, et al. Echocardiographic insights into the mechanisms of relief of left ventricular outflow tract obstruction after nonsurgical septal reduction therapy in patients with hypertrophic obstructive cardiomyopathy. *J Am Coll Cardiol.* 2001;37:208–214.
20. Nagueh SF, Groves BM, Schwartz L, et al. Alcohol septal ablation for the treatment of hypertrophic obstructive cardiomyopathy. A multicenter North American registry. *J Am Coll Cardiol.* 2011;58:2322–2328.
21. Veselka J, Jensen MK, Liebregts M, et al. Long-term clinical outcome after alcohol septal ablation for obstructive hypertrophic cardiomyopathy: results from the Euro-ASA registry. *Eur Heart J.* 2016;37:1517–1523.
22. Liebregts M, Vriesendorp PA, Mahmoodi BK, et al. A systematic review and meta-analysis of long-term outcomes after septal reduction therapy in patients with hypertrophic cardiomyopathy. *JACC Heart Failure.* 2015;3:896–905.
23. Faber L, Ziemssen P, Seggewiss H. Targeting percutaneous transluminal septal ablation for hypertrophic obstructive cardiomyopathy by intraprocedural echocardiographic monitoring. *J Am Soc Echocardiogr.* 2000;13:1074–1079.
24. Chang SM, Lakkis NM, Franklin J, et al. Predictors of outcome after alcohol septal ablation therapy in patients with hypertrophic obstructive cardiomyopathy. *Circulation.* 2004;109:824–827.
25. Yoerger DM, Picard MH, Palacios IF, et al. Time course of pressure gradient response after first alcohol septal ablation for obstructive hypertrophic cardiomyopathy. *Am J Cardiol.* 2006;97:1511–1514.
26. Fifer MA, Sigwart U. Hypertrophic obstructive cardiomyopathy: alcohol septal ablation. *Eur Heart J.* 2011;32:1059–1064.
27. Mazur W, Nagueh SF, Lakkis NM, et al. Regression of left ventricular hypertrophy after nonsurgical septal reduction therapy for hypertrophic obstructive cardiomyopathy. *Circulation.* 2001;103:1492–1496.
28. Nagueh SF, Lakkis NM, Middleton KJ, et al. Changes in left ventricular diastolic function 6 months after nonsurgical septal reduction therapy for hypertrophic obstructive cardiomyopathy. *Circulation.* 1999;99:344–347.

62 Hypertrophic Cardiomyopathy: Screening of Relatives

Mina Girgis, Anna Woo

Hypertrophic cardiomyopathy (HCM) is a common genetic cardiac disorder.[1] The prevalence of overt HCM (using the threshold of a wall thickness of at least 15 mm) is 1 in 500 (0.2%) in the general adult population.[2] Because HCM has an autosomal dominant pattern of inheritance, the offspring of patients with definite HCM have a 50% chance of inheriting a mutation and developing this condition.[1] The screening of first-degree relatives (i.e., children,

siblings, parents) of patients with HCM is recommended, and it is a very important aspect of the overall management of patients.[1] The recognition of HCM in family members is particularly imperative because HCM is associated with a risk of sudden cardiac death (SCD). This devastating event occurs at a rate of approximately 1% per year in patients with HCM and is more likely to affect young individuals.[1]

EPIDEMIOLOGY OF HYPERTROPHIC CARDIOMYOPATHY

The prevalence of overt HCM of 0.2% in the adult general population is based on echocardiographic and epidemiologic studies published in the 1990s and 2000s and does not include consideration of the prevalence of HCM gene carriers.[3] The phenotypic expression of HCM is not common in children. In terms of the incidence of HCM in children, one study from Australia has reported an annual incidence of HCM of 0.32 per 100,000 in young children (younger than the 10 years of age).[4] Data from the prospective cohort of the North American Pediatric Cardiomyopathy Registry have shown an incidence of 4.7 per 1,000,000 children and adolescents (younger than 18 years of age).[5] However, the cases of HCM in both these studies also included children with malformation syndromes, neuromuscular disorders, or inborn errors of metabolism, conditions that are generally excluded from the definition of familial HCM in adult patients.[1,4,5]

GENETICS OF HYPERTROPHIC CARDIOMYOPATHY

HCM is caused by a mutation in at least one of the genes that encode cardiac sarcomeric proteins or sarcomere-associated proteins.[6] There are at least 11 causative genes associated with HCM: β-myosin heavy chain (MYH7), myosin binding protein C (MYBPC3), troponin T (TNNT2), troponin I (TNNI3), troponin C (TNNC1), α-tropomyosin (TPM1), α-actin (ACTC1), regulatory myosin light chain (MYL2), essential myosin light chain (MYL3), and Z-disc genes.[6] Over the past three decades, more than 1400 mutations (mainly missense mutations) have been detected in patients with HCM.[6] Importantly, HCM caused by a mutation of the sarcomeric proteins is distinct from other inherited causes of left ventricular hypertrophy (LVH) that are related to storage diseases (e.g., Fabry's disease) or malformation syndromes or multisystem disorders (e.g., Noonan's syndrome).[1]

Genetic Testing In Hypertrophic Cardiomyopathy

Genetic testing by automated DNA sequencing has extended beyond research settings and is now offered by commercial genetic testing services.[6] The yield of a positive genetic result in a proband (i.e., index patient with HCM) is about 50% because all genes causing HCM have not yet been identified and are absent from testing panels.[6] The type of septal morphology on echocardiography is associated with the likelihood of detecting a genetic defect: one study showed that the yield of genetic testing was 79% in patients with a reverse septal curvature morphology (i.e., predominant midseptal convexity toward the left ventricular [LV] cavity) versus 8% in patients with a sigmoid septal morphology.[7] A larger subsequent study incorporated six clinical and echocardiographic variables, determined from univariate and multivariate analyses, into a genotype predictor score. The four clinical markers in the genotype predictor score are the following: (1) age at diagnosis younger than 45 years, (2) family history of HCM, (3) family history of SCD, and (4) history of hypertension (the latter is a negative predictor of a positive genetic test result). The two echocardiographic markers in the genotype predictor score are (1) the presence of reverse-curve HCM and (2) a maximal LV wall thickness of 20 mm or greater.[8] The yield of a positive genetic test result ranged from 6% to 80%, depending on the number of positive clinical and echocardiographic markers.[8]

Genetic testing is indicated in patients with an atypical presentation of HCM or when another genetic condition (i.e., phenocopy or mimicker of HCM) is suspected.[1] In addition, it is reasonable to perform genetic testing for HCM in the index patient (proband) to facilitate the diagnosis of affected first-degree family members (i.e., cascade [generational] testing or predictive testing), particularly if relatives have negative or indeterminate results from clinical testing.[1,6] If a pathogenic mutation is documented in the proband, then first-degree relatives can be offered genetic testing. If no disease-causing mutation is found or if a sequence variant of uncertain significance is reported, then ongoing genetic screening of family members usually cannot proceed.[6] Patients who undergo genetic testing also benefit from genetic counseling.[1,6] Because of the limitations of genetic testing, the preferred initial approach to screening family members remains clinical testing with clinical assessment (history and physical examination), 12-lead electrocardiogram (ECG), and two-dimensional echocardiography.[9]

CLINICAL SCREENING IN CHILDREN AND ADOLESCENTS

Clinical screening is indicated in first-degree relatives of patients with HCM (Table 62.1). Clinical screening consists of clinical evaluation (history and physical examination), 12-lead ECG, and transthoracic echocardiography.[9] Because HCM does not usually present in childhood, screening in children younger than the age of 12 years is generally reserved for the following circumstances: (1) a malignant family history of premature HCM-related death, (2) the child is a competitive athlete in an intense training program, or (3) the child develops symptoms or other clinical suspicion of early LVH.[1,9] Screening of all first-degree relatives of probands with HCM should otherwise start at age 12 years and should be repeated every 12 to 18 months until physical maturity is achieved (generally between the ages of 18 and 21 years).[1,9]

The occurrence of HCM in the children and adolescents of patients with HCM is much greater when selected cohorts are studied. Two recent studies of children and adolescents referred for family screening at highly specialized pediatric centers in the United Kingdom and Canada detected HCM at a young age in 5% of children (defined as age 12 years or younger) in the United Kingdom cohort[10] and in 13% of children (categorized as age younger than 10 years) in the Canadian cohort.[11] Importantly, these study populations comprised high-risk families, with a family history of SCD in more than 30% of the study participants,[10,11] and a family history of childhood HCM (in 56% of phenotype-positive patients in the United Kingdom study).[10] Therefore, the findings in these studies may not be generalizable to less selected populations of patients with HCM.

CLINICAL AND ECHOCARDIOGRAPHIC SCREENING IN ADULTS

After the age of 21 years, screening should be repeated with the onset of any cardiac symptoms or at least every 5 years.[1] There is no clear age at which clinical screening should end because there may be delayed penetrance of this condition, and a significant proportion of patients with HCM are diagnosed at an older age.[1] Family members who are found to be genotype positive and remain phenotype negative should undergo the same serial clinical investigations as described above (i.e., clinical assessment, ECG, and echocardiography at 12- to 18-month intervals until end of adolescence, every 5 years in adults) to monitor for the onset of the clinical expression of HCM[1] (see Table 62.1).

Clinical and Electrocardiographic Assessment

Symptoms attributable to underlying HCM may include chest pain, dyspnea, or syncope.[1,12] Pathologic changes on the 12-lead ECG are evident in approximately 75% to 95% of patients with definite HCM.[1] The most common ECG findings in patients with overt HCM are repolarization abnormalities and ECG criteria for LVH.[13] ECG changes in relatives may appear before the onset of hypertrophy on echocardiography.[12,14] In first-degree adult

TABLE 62.1 Proposed Clinical Screening Strategies for Detection of Hypertrophic Cardiomyopathy in First-Degree Relatives

Age (years)	Clinical Screening	Comments
Younger than 12	Screening optional unless: • Malignant family history of premature death from HCM (or other adverse complications) • Patient is a competitive athlete in an intense training program • Onset of cardiac symptoms • Other clinical suspicion of early LV hypertrophy	—
12 to 18–21	Every 12–18 months	Age range takes into consideration individual variability in achieving physical maturity (in some patients may justify screening at an earlier age)
Older than 18–21	At onset of symptoms or every 5 years	More frequently if family history of malignant clinical course or late-onset HCM

HCM, Hypertrophic cardiomyopathy; *LV,* left ventricular.
Adapted from Gersh BJ, et al: 2011 ACCF/AHA guideline for the diagnosis and treatment of hypertrophic cardiomyopathy, *J Am Coll Cardiol* 58:e212–e260.

relatives, suspicious ECG results include ECG criteria for LVH, repolarization changes, prominent T-wave inversion, or abnormal Q waves.[12,15,16]

Echocardiographic Assessment

The morphologic diagnosis of overt HCM is based on the presence of a hypertrophied and nondilated left ventricle in the absence of another cardiac or systemic disease capable of producing the magnitude of hypertrophy evident in a patient (usually ≥15 mm in adults).[1] The diagnosis of HCM is made in children and adolescents in the presence of a wall thickness greater than 2 standard deviations from the mean value corrected for body surface area.[17] All myocardial segments should be assessed for evidence of hypertrophy on these screening examinations.[18] However, in affected adult family members with HCM, the magnitude of hypertrophy may be below the threshold of 15 mm.[1] Some genotyped patients may be HCM gene carriers without evidence of hypertrophy.[1,12,18]

Assessment by Cardiac Magnetic Resonance

Cardiac magnetic resonance (CMR) imaging is indicated in patients with suspected HCM when the echocardiogram is technically challenging or inconclusive for the diagnosis of HCM.[1,18] However, CMR could be considered in situations in which additional testing (e.g., ECG abnormalities) raises the suspicion of HCM despite a normal echocardiogram.[18]

FINDINGS IN HYPERTROPHIC CARDIOMYOPATHY GENE CARRIERS

Echocardiographic Studies

The era of molecular genetics has led to the recognition of a subset of individuals who have an HCM-associated mutation but who have not yet manifested hypertrophy.[1,18] These patients expand the clinical spectrum of HCM and show that any LV wall thickness can be consistent with having HCM.[1] Multiple studies have assessed echocardiographic abnormalities in these genotype-positive/phenotype-negative (or LVH-negative) patients. Using the technique of tissue Doppler imaging (TDI), Nagueh and colleagues showed that TDI systolic and early diastolic (Ea) velocities were reduced in genotype-positive/phenotype-negative patients.[19] Specific cutoff values in these TDI velocities showed 100% sensitivity and 90% or greater specificity in predicting gene-positive HCM carriers. Subsequent studies noted significant overlap in the TDI systolic and Ea velocities between the genotype-positive/LVH-negative participants and control groups.[20,21] However, these studies also demonstrated that the

combination of TDI Ea velocities and other echocardiographic findings (hyperdynamic LV function[20] and wall thickness ratio[21]) were highly specific in identifying mutation carriers. In terms of the use of strain imaging to ascertain preclinical HCM, one study has shown no difference in global longitudinal strain in genotype-positive/phenotype-negative patients compared with control participants.[22] Given these data, abnormal findings with TDI do not establish the diagnosis of HCM in family members but can be beneficial in recognizing individuals who may benefit from closer monitoring.

Other Morphologic Abnormalities in Hypertrophic Cardiomyopathy Gene Carriers

A number of findings on CMR have been reported in genotype-positive patients before the development of pathologic hypertrophy. Myocardial crypts have been documented in genotype-positive/LVH-negative patients, occurring with a prevalence ranging from 61% to 81%.[23,24] Elongated (or redundant) mitral valve leaflets have been associated with patients with HCM.[12,25] CMR has shown a longer length of the anterior mitral leaflet in genotype-positive/LVH-negative patients (compared with control participants).[26] In terms of myocardial fibrosis, as delineated by the presence of late gadolinium enhancement (LGE) on CMR, there was no LGE detected in a multicenter study that included gene-positive/LVH-negative children and adolescents (defined as age 21 years or younger).[27] However, there are published reports of LGE in gene-positive patients without overt hypertrophy.[24,28] In summary, multiple derangements (ECG features, diastolic filling abnormalities on TDI, and various CMR findings) are associated with preclinical HCM.

Acknowledgment

The authors would acknowledge Dr. Maithri Siriwardena, who was a coauthor of this chapter in the second edition of the textbook.

REFERENCES

1. Gersh BJ, Maron BJ, Bonow RO, et al. ACCF/AHA guideline for the diagnosis and treatment of hypertrophic cardiomyopathy. *Circulation.* 2011;124:e783–e831.
2. Maron BJ, Gardin JM, Flack JM, et al. Prevalence of hypertrophic cardiomyopathy in a general population of young adults. Echocardiographic analysis of 4111 subjects in the CARDIA study. *Circulation.* 1995;92:785–789.
3. Semsarian C, Ingles J, Maron MS, et al. New perspectives on the prevalence of hypertrophic cardiomyopathy. *J Am Coll Cardiol.* 2015;65:1249–1254.
4. Nugent AW, Piers EF, Chondros P, et al. The epidemiology of childhood cardiomyopathy in Australia. *N Engl J Med.* 2003;348:1639–1646.
5. Colan SD, Lipshultz SE, Lowe AM, et al. Epidemiology and cause-specific outcome of hypertrophic cardiomyopathy in children: findings from the Pediatric Cardiomyopathy Registry. *Circulation.* 2007;115:773–781.
6. Maron BJ, Maron MS, Semsarian C. Genetics of hypertrophic cardiomyopathy after 20 years, clinical perspectives. *J Am Coll Cardiol.* 2012;60:705–715.

7. Binder J, Ommen SR, Gersh BJ, et al. Echocardiography-guided genetic testing in hypertrophic cardiomyopathy: septal morphological features predict the presence of myofilament mutations. *Mayo Clin Proc.* 2006;81:459–467.

8. Bos JM, Will ML, Gersh BJ, et al. Characterization of a phenotype-based genetic test prediction score for unrelated patients with hypertrophic cardiomyopathy. *Mayo Clin Proc.* 2014;89:727–737.

9. Maron BJ, Seidman JG, Seidman CE. Proposal for contemporary screening strategies in families with hypertrophic cardiomyopathy. *J Am Coll Cardiol.* 2004;44:2125–2132.

10. Norrish G, Jager J, Field E, et al. Yield of clinical screening for hypertrophic cardiomyopathy in child first-degree relatives. *Circulation.* 2019;140:184–192.

11. Lafreniere-Roula M, Bolkier Y, Zahavic L, et al. Family screening for hypertrophic cardiomyopathy: is it time to change practice guidelines? *Eur Heart J.* 2019;40:3672–3681.

12. McKenna WJ, Spirito P, Desnos M, et al. Experience from clinical genetics in HCM: Proposal for new diagnostic criteria in adult members of affected families. *Heart.* 1997;77:130–132.

13. Savage DD, Seides SF, Clark CE, et al. Electrocardiographic findings in patients with obstructive and non-obstructive hypertrophic cardiomyopathy. *Circulation.* 1978;58:402–408.

14. Woo A, Rakowski H, Liew JC, et al. Mutations of the β-myosin heavy chain gene in hypertrophic cardiomyopathy: critical functional sites determine prognosis. *Heart.* 2003;89:1179–1185.

15. Charron P, Dubourg O, Desnos M, et al. Diagnostic value of ECG and echocardiography for familial hypertrophic cardiomyopathy in a genotyped adult population. *Circulation.* 1997;96:214–219.

16. Konno T, Shimizu M, Ino H, et al. Diagnostic value of abnormal Q waves for identification of preclinical carriers of hypertrophic cardiomyopathy based on a molecular genetic diagnosis. *Eur Heart J.* 2004;25:246–251.

17. Humez FU, Houston AB, Watson J, et al. Age and body surface area related normal upper and lower limits of M mode echocardiographic measurements and left ventricular volume and mass from infancy to early adulthood. *Br Heart J.* 1994;72:276–280.

18. Nagueh SF, Bierig M, Budoff MJ, et al. American Society of Echocardiography clinical recommendations for multi-modality cardiovascular imaging of patients with hypertrophic cardiomyopathy. *J Am Soc Echocardiogr.* 2011;24:473–498.

19. Nagueh SF, Bachinski LL, Meyer D, et al. Tissue Doppler imaging consistently detects myocardial abnormalities in patients with hypertrophic cardiomyopathy and provides a novel means for an early diagnosis before and independently of hypertrophy. *Circulation.* 2001;104:128–130.

20. Ho CY, Sweitzer NK, McDonough B, et al. Assessment of diastolic function with Doppler tissue imaging to predict genotype in preclinical hypertrophic cardiomyopathy. *Circulation.* 2002;105:2992–2997.

21. Gandjbakhch E, Gackowski A, Tezenas du Montcel S, et al. Early identification of mutation carriers in familial hypertrophic cardiomyopathy by combined echocardiography and tissue Doppler imaging. *Eur Heart J.* 2010;31:1599–1607.

22. Hoy CY, Carlsen C, Thune JJ, et al. Echocardiographic strain imaging to assess early and late consequences of sarcomere mutations in hypertrophic cardiomyopathy. *Circ Cardiovasc Genet.* 2009;2:314–321.

23. Germans T, Wilde AAM, Dijkmans PA, et al. Structural abnormalities of the inferoseptal left ventricular wall detected by cardiac magnetic resonance imaging in carriers of hypertrophic cardiomyopathy mutations. *J Am Coll Cardiol.* 2006;48:2518–2523.

24. Maron MS, Rowin EJ, Lin D, et al. Prevalence and clinical profile of myocardial crypts in hypertrophic cardiomyopathy. *Circ Cardiovasc Imag.* 2012;5:441–447.

25. Woo A, Jedrzkiewicz S. The mitral valve in hypertrophic cardiomyopathy: it's a long story. *Circulation.* 2011;124:9–12.

26. Maron MS, Olivotto I, Harrigan C, et al. Mitral valve abnormalities identified by cardiovascular magnetic resonance represent a primary phenotypic expression of hypertrophic cardiomyopathy. *Circulation.* 2011;124:40–47.

27. Axelsson Raja A, Farhad H, Valente AM, et al. Prevalence and progression of late gadolinium enhancement in children and adolescents with hypertrophic cardiomyopathy. *Circulation.* 2018;138(8):782–792.

28. Rowin EJ, Maron MS, Lesser JR, et al. CMR with late gadolinium enhancement in genotype positive-phenotype negative hypertrophic cardiomyopathy. *JACC Cardiovasc Imag.* 2012;5:119–122.

63 Apical Hypertrophic Cardiomyopathy

Steven A. Goldstein

Hypertrophic cardiomyopathy (HCM) is a primary disease of cardiac muscle characterized by a hypertrophied, nondilated left ventricle unassociated with other cardiac diseases that can reasonably account for the magnitude of hypertrophy present.[1] The distribution of left ventricular hypertrophy (LVH), the hallmark of HCM, occurs in many patterns within the ventricle.[2,3] Relatively uncommon, apical HCM is a unique subtype of HCM in which the LVH involves predominantly the apex.[4–9] Particularly common in Asia, this variant has been reported in up to 41% of HCM patients in China,[10,11] up to 30% in Japan,[12–14] and up to 38% in Korea.[15] In non-Asian populations, it has been observed in 1% to 14%[2,16–23] (Table 63.1). However, most of the epidemiologic data are derived from studies conducted in the early 1990s, and the exact prevalence of apical HCM in non-Asians may be underestimated because of diagnostic unawareness and difficulty making the diagnosis on transthoracic echocardiography (TTE), the most frequently used diagnostic modality, when the diagnosis is not suspected. The basis for the differences in the phenotypic expression of apical HCM between Asians and non-Asians is unknown.

Sakamoto and colleagues, in 1976, first described symmetrical apical hypertrophy based on the appearance of the left ventricle on M-mode echo in patients with giant negative T waves in the precordial leads[4] (Fig. 63.1). Yamaguchi and associates described its configuration on end-diastolic ventriculography in the right anterior oblique projection.[5] This configuration was nicknamed "spade-like" because the LV cavity in this projection resembled the "spade" in playing cards.

In contrast to most other forms of HCM, apical HCM was initially thought to be a benign condition, especially in Asians, in whom cardiovascular morbidity was reportedly rare.[2,5–8,16,24–28] However, early studies included relatively small sample sizes, and in recent years, especially in Western populations, this condition has been reported to be less benign than previously thought. Recent case reports have described an association of apical HCMs with ventricular arrhythmias, sudden death, and apical aneurysms.[15,17,20,22,26,29–31] Despite these complications, apical HCM is still generally characterized by a benign clinical course with a favorable long-term prognosis.

MORPHOLOGY AND ECHOCARDIOGRAPHIC FEATURES

The criteria for the diagnosis of apical HCM include the demonstration of asymmetric LVH confined to the most distal portion of the left ventricular (LV) apex below the papillary muscles, usually circumferential, with an apical wall thickness at least 15 mm and a ratio of maximal apical to posterior wall thickness of 1.5 or greater at end-diastole[16,17] (Box 63.1 and Fig. 63.2). This morphology can be identified by echocardiography, ventriculography, computed tomography, and cardiac magnetic resonance imaging (CMRI). The most readily available of these, noncontrast echocardiography, typically provides an appreciation of this unusual distribution of ventricular hypertrophy.[2,5–8,27,28,32]

The performance of TTE in apical HCM requires careful attention to the technical aspects of the examination. The parasternal long-axis view, which is critical to the diagnosis of "classic" asymmetric septal HCM, is inadequate for examining the LV apex. Apical HCM is best visualized from the apical

TABLE 63.1 Comparison of Incidence of Apical Hypertrophic Cardiomyopathy Among Patients With Hypertrophic Cardiomyopathy in Asian Versus Western Populations

	Authors	Year	Total HCM	Apical HCM	%
Japan	Sakamoto[2]	2001	—	126	15
Japan	Kitaoka et al[13]	2003	100	15	15
Japan	Nasermoaddeli et al[19]	2007	1605	532	33
Japan	Kubo et al[14]	2009	264	80	30
China	Ho et al[10]	2004	118	49	41
China	Yan et al[11]	2012	1320	208	16
Taiwan	Lee et al[23]	2006	163	40	25
Korea	Moon et al[15]	2011	1204	454	38
	Louie and Maron[16]	1987	965	23	2
	Klues et al[2]	1995	600	7	1
	Eriksson et al[17]	2002	—	105	7
	Kitaoka et al[13]	2003	361	10	3
	Gruner et al[21]	2011	429	61	14
	Klarich et al[22]	2013	2662	210	7.9

HCM, Hypertrophic cardiomyopathy.

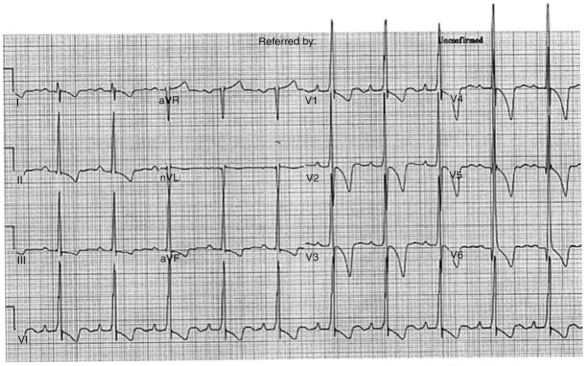

Figure 63.1. Electrocardiogram illustrating left ventricular hypertrophy with prominent T-wave inversion.

four-chamber view and apical short-axis views. Identification of apical HCM requires good endocardial definition to demonstrate the characteristic features of this disorder, thickened apical walls and obliteration of the apical cavity during systole. Apical HCM may escape echocardiographic detection because the thickness of the LV wall is not significantly increased at the basal and papillary muscle levels. The parasternal long-axis and short-axis views may appear normal. Moreover, the likelihood of overlooking this condition is increased in the face of inadequate image quality, especially when a low-frequency transducer is used for scanning.[33] Several maneuvers can be used to identify an apical HCM when it is not apparent on routine clinical examination (Box 63.2). The first is to use relatively shallow focal depths and high-frequency transducers. Second, color flow Doppler imaging from the apex, at a relatively low Nyquist limit, can demonstrate the blood pool–tissue boundary

---

BOX 63.1 Two-Dimensional Echocardiographic Criteria for Diagnosing Apical Hypertrophic Cardiomyopathy

1. Hypertrophy predominantly confined to the left ventricular (LV) apex
2. Maximal wall thickness within apical segments
3. Hypertrophy may extend from the apex to the level of the papillary muscle
4. Absence of significant hypertrophy at the basal level
5. Hypertrophy may be present in the basal septum or other basal segment if there is no evidence of LV outflow tract obstruction
6. Wall thickness ≥15 mm and ratio of apical to posterior wall thickness ≥1.5

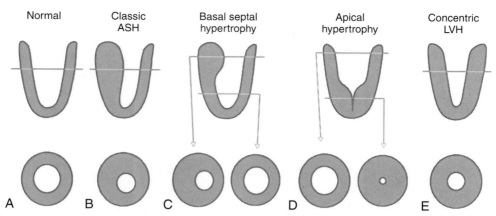

Figure 63.2. Diagram of the left ventricle in longitudinal *(upper row)* and short-axis, cross-sectional view *(lower row)* illustrating the variable distribution of hypertrophy in a normal ventricle (**A**), three subtypes of hypertrophic cardiomyopathy (**B–D**), and concentric hypertrophy (**E**). **C** and **D,** The distribution at basal and apical levels. Note the similarity of this diagram to the magnetic resonance imaging of a patient in Fig. 63.3. *ASH,* Asymmetric septal hypertrophy; *LVH,* left ventricular hypertrophy.

BOX 63.2 Echocardiographic Techniques to Improve Detection of Apical Hypertrophic Cardiomyopathy

Carefully aligned (nonforeshortened) apical images
Use of apical short-axis views
Use of color Doppler focused on the left ventricular apex
Use of high-frequency transducers with focusing at the apex
Intravenous contrast echocardiography

---

and therefore the narrowing of the LV cavity at the apex. Ultimately, contrast echocardiography, using transpulmonary agents to opacify the left ventricle, may confirm the presence of apical HCM.[12,30,34–42]

With good opacification of the LV cavity with contrast, the true extent of hypertrophy can be easily appreciated and the abnormal contour of the LV cavity documented. Because the hypertrophy is confined to the apex, dynamic LV outflow tract obstruction and systolic anterior motion (SAM) of the anterior mitral leaflet are absent. Although echocardiography usually identifies the presence of apical HCM, it can still be overlooked, particularly if adequate images of the apex are not obtained. In patients with a clinical suspicion of HCM (e.g., "giant" precordial T-wave inversions) and suboptimal echocardiographic images, the use of contrast echocardiography as mentioned, or CMRI, should be considered[22,33,43–48] (Figs. 63.3 and 63.4).

In fact, there have been reports of cases where MRI has detected apical HCM unrecognized by echocardiography. CMRI provides a large field of view and high blood-to-myocardium contrast, which is ideal for consistent and accurate imaging of the apex. In addition, CMRI can identify the presence of apical aneurysms.[20] Transesophageal echocardiography (TEE) has also been used to diagnose apical HCM when standard TTE has been suboptimal.[49] Finally, sarcomere protein gene mutations have been found in up to 47% of patients with apical HCM (Table 63.2).[18,21,50] Therefore, genetic testing may also be useful for evaluating patients with suspected apical HCM by helping to confirm the diagnosis in borderline cases, exclude disease in others, and identify family members who are carriers with a negative phenotype and may develop the disease later in life.[21,51]

Apical longitudinal strain is typically decreased as illustrated in Fig. 63.5. Paradoxical apical longitudinal strain (systolic lengthening) also has been described in apical HCM despite an apparently normal apical wall motion on conventional TEE.[52]

Apical HCM must be differentiated from apical cavity obliteration caused by thrombus, tumor, noncompaction cardiomyopathy, or hypereosinophilic syndrome. Moreover, a false-positive finding may result from hypertrophied papillary muscles or a foreshortened apical four-chamber view that produces the appearance of increased apical wall thickness because of an oblique cut (Box 63.3). Diastolic dysfunction is typically present and leads to increased filling pressures and left atrial enlargement and is central to several of the clinical manifestations of apical HCM, including dyspnea, exercise intolerance, and pulmonary edema.

SUBTYPES

Patients with apical HCM have been subdivided into two subtypes: (1) a "pure" or "isolated" form, defined as hypertrophy confined to the apical portion of the left ventricle below the papillary muscle level; and (2) a "mixed" or "distal dominant" form, in which the hypertrophy is greatest at the apex but extends to the midventricular septum, usually sparing the most basal portion of the septum.[14–17,53,54] These subgroups are illustrated in Fig. 63.6. It is important to distinguish these phenotypes of apical HCM; the mixed form is less common but is more serious.[14]

APICAL ANEURYSMS

LV apical aneurysms in the absence of epicardial coronary artery disease are present in 2% of all patients with HCM.[20] In apical HCM, the incidence of apical aneurysms has been reported to be much higher, ranging from 10% to 31%[45,55,56] (Table 63.3). These appear as a discrete, thin-walled dyskinetic or akinetic segment of cavity at the most distal portion of the LV chamber with a variable-sized communication to the main LV cavity. Fig. 63.7 illustrates a possible continuum of apical abnormalities leading to an apical aneurysm. The size of apical aneurysms may vary from very small (1–2 cm in width) to large (>5 cm).[57] Echocardiography may fail to visualize the apical cavity because of several factors, including its size and location, poor-quality images from the apical window, and foreshortened views in which the transducer is not at the true apex. Color Doppler may show systolic flow into the aneurysmal cavity and outflow from the aneurysm in diastole.

The development of an apical pouch, which still demonstrates systolic wall thickening, is thought to be an intermediate stage before formation of a larger and akinetic or dyskinetic apical aneurysm.[58] These result in a discrete apical chamber connected to the main LV

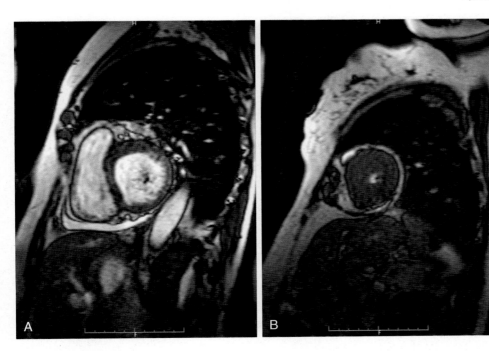

Figure 63.3. Cross-sectional views of the left ventricle by magnetic resonance imaging in a different patient illustrating the normal thickness and cavity size at the base (**A**) and the marked thickness and tiny cavity at the apex (**B**).

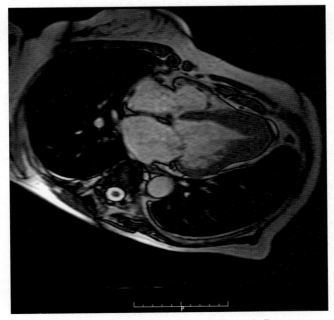

Figure 63.4. Magnetic resonance imaging (horizontal plane) illustrates the characteristic spade-like appearance of this patient (same as in Fig. 63.3) with apical hypertrophic cardiomyopathy.

TABLE 63.2 Positive Genotypes in Three Apical Hypertrophic Cardiomyopathy Cohorts

	Arad et al.[50]	Binder et al.[18]	Gruner et al.[21]
Probands with apical HCM (n)	15	37	61
Patients with a positive genotype (%)	47	30	13
Patients with a positive family history for HCM (%)	40	22	16

HCM, Hypertrophic cardiomyopathy.

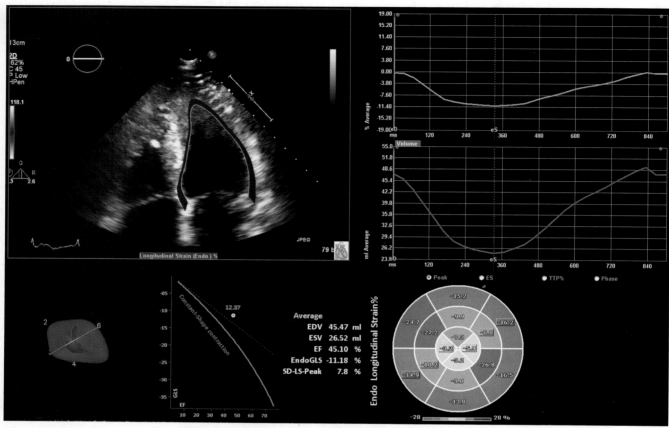

Figure 63.5. Speckle-tracking echocardiographic strain imaging from a 61-year-old woman with apical hypertrophic cardiomyopathy *(A)*. Bull's eye plot *(lower right)* illustrates decreased global longitudinal strain of −11% with the major region of decreased strain at the apex.

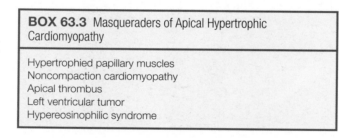

BOX 63.3 Masqueraders of Apical Hypertrophic Cardiomyopathy

Hypertrophied papillary muscles
Noncompaction cardiomyopathy
Apical thrombus
Left ventricular tumor
Hypereosinophilic syndrome

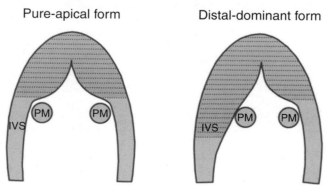

Figure 63.6. Diagram of the left ventricle illustrates the two subtypes of apical hypertrophic cardiomyopathy: pure (isolated) apical form on the *left* and distal-dominant ("mixed") form on the *right*. *IVS,* interventricular septum; *PM,* papillary muscle.

TABLE 63.3 Prevalence of Apical Aneurysms Among Patients With Apical Hypertrophic Cardiomyopathy

Author	Year	Apical HCM	Apical Aneurysm	Patients (%)
Nakamura et al.[55]	1992	198	20	10
Matsubara et al.[56]	2003	59	12	20
Fattori et al.[45]	2010	13	4	31
Chen et al.[54]	2011	47	14	30
Klarich et al.[22]	2013	193	29[a]	15

[a]Included 6 patients with apical aneurysm and 23 patients with apical "pouch" (apical dilatation and hypokinesis).
HCM, Hypertrophic cardiomyopathy.

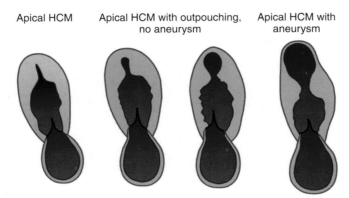

Apical HCM   Apical HCM with outpouching, no aneurysm   Apical HCM with aneurysm

Figure 63.7. Proposed continuum of morphologic features of apical hypertrophic cardiomyopathy (HCM) at end-systole from an apical slit to an outpouching at the apex to an aneurysm. *LA,* Left atrium; *LV,* left ventricle. (Modified with permission from Sanghvi NK, Tracy CM: Sustained ventricular tachycardia in apical hypertrophic cardiomyopathy, midcavitary obstruction, and apical aneurysm, *Pacing Clin Electrophysiol* 30:799–803, 2007.)

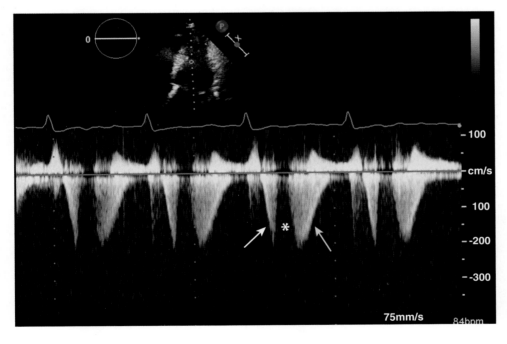

Figure 63.8. Continuous-wave Doppler tracing shows initial rapid emptying of the apical pouch in early systole *(white arrow)* followed by a void later in systole *(asterisk).* A second outflow from the incompletely emptied apical pouch into the main chamber occurs in diastole *(yellow arrow).*

cavity by a muscular neck that can disappear during contraction. These may produce a unique emptying profile consisting of an initial rapid emptying of the pouch in early systole followed by a signal void in mid to late systole caused by cessation of flow as the neck narrows during contraction obstructing flow. This signal void is followed by a second outflow from the incompletely emptied apical pouch toward the base of the main chamber. This unique flow profile is illustrated in Fig. 63.8.

CMRI appears to be superior to two-dimensional echocardiography for detecting apical aneurysms. In one study, echocardiography detected only one of four patients with apical aneurysm detected by CMRI.[45] Contrast echocardiography is also a useful diagnostic modality for detecting apical aneurysms. Apical outpouchings and aneurysms should be sought out because they are associated with adverse prognoses, including thromboembolic stroke, ventricular arrhythmias, heart failure, and sudden death.[17,20,59]

SUMMARY

Apical HCM is a variant of HCM in which the myocardial thickening occurs predominantly at the LV apex as opposed to the "classical" septal predominance. TEE is the first-line imaging technique for the diagnosis of apical HCM but requires both awareness of this entity and meticulous imaging technique. Hallmark features of apical HCM include deeply negative, "giant" T-wave inversion on electrocardiography and a "spade-like" configuration of the left ventricle in diastole on ventriculography, echocardiography, and CMRI. Involvement of the LV apex (with or without an apical aneurysm) is the sine qua non of apical HCM. Patients with apical aneurysms are an underappreciated subset of the apical HCM population. Multimodality imaging is useful for diagnosis and risk stratification. Although generally believed to be associated with a better prognosis than other forms of HCM, serious cardiac complications may occur, including progressive heart failure, myocardial infarction, stroke, ventricular arrhythmias, and sudden cardiac death.

REFERENCES

1. Maron BJ, McKenna WJ, Danielson GK, et al. ACC/ESC clinical expert consensus panel on hypertrophic cardiomyopathy. *J Am Coll Cardiol.* 2003;42:1687–1713.
2. Klues HG, Schiffers A, Maron BJ. Phenotypic spectrum and patterns of left ventricular hypertrophic cardiomyopathy: morphologic observations and significance as assessed by two-dimensional echocardiography in 600 patients. *J Am Coll Cardiol.* 1995;26:1699–1708.
3. Maron MS, Maron BJ, Harrigan C, et al. Hypertrophic cardiomyopathy phenotype revisited after 50 years with cardiovascular magnetic resonance. *J Am Coll Cardiol.* 2009;54:220–228.
4. Sakamoto T, Tei C, Murayama M, et al. Giant negative T-wave inversion as a manifestation of asymmetric apical hypertrophy (AAH) of the left ventricle. Echocardiographic and ultrasonocardiotomographic study. *Jpn Heart J.* 1976;17:611–629.
5. Yamaguchi H, Ishimura T, Nishiyama S, et al. Hypertrophic nonobstructive cardiomyopathy with giant negative T-waves (apical hypertrophy): ventriculographic and echocardiographic features in 30 patients. *Am J Cardiol.* 1979;44:401–412.
6. Maron BJ, Bonow RO, Seshagiri TNR, et al. Hypertrophic cardiomyopathy with ventricular septal hypertrophy localized to the apical region of the left ventricle. *Am J Cardiol.* 1982;49:1838–1848.
7. Varek JL, Davis WR, Bellinger RL, McKiernan TL. Apical hypertrophic cardiomyopathy in American patients. *Am Heart J.* 1984;108:1501–1506.
8. Sakamoto T, Amano K, Hada Y, et al. Asymmetric apical hypertrophy, ten years experience. *Postgrad Med J.* 1986;62:567–570.
9. Yamada M, Teraoka K, Kawade M, et al. Frequency and distribution of late gadolinium enhancement in magnetic resonance imaging of patients with apical hypertrophic cardiomyopathy: a comparative study. *Int J Cardiovasc Imaging.* 2009;25:131–138.
10. Ho HH, Lee KL, Lau CP, Tse HF. Clinical characteristics of and long-term outcome in Chinese patients with hypertrophic cardiomyopathy. *Am J Med.* 2004;116:19–23.
11. Yan L, Wang Z, Xu Z, et al. Two hundred eight patients with apical hypertrophic cardiomyopathy in China: clinical feature, prognosis, and comparison of pure and mixed forms. *Clin Cardiol.* 2012;35:101–106.
12. Sakamoto T. Apical hypertrophic cardiomyopathy (apical hypertrophy). *J Cardiol.* 2001;37(Suppl I):161–178.
13. Kitaoka H, Doi Y, Casey SA, et al. Comparison of prevalence of apical hypertrophic cardiomyopathy in Japan and the United States. *Am J Cardiol.* 2003;92:1183–1186.
14. Kubo T, Kitaoka H, Okawa M, et al. Clinical profiles of hypertrophic cardiomyopathy with apical phenotype—comparison of pure-apical form and distal-dominant form. *Circ J.* 2009;73:2330–2336.
15. Moon J, Shim CY, Ha J-W, et al. Clinical and echocardiographic predictors of outcomes in patients with apical hypertrophic cardiomyopathy. *Am J Cardiol.* 2011;108:1614–1619.
16. Louie EK, Maron BJ. Apical hypertrophic cardiomyopathy: clinical and two-dimensional echocardiography assessment. *Ann Intern Med.* 1987;106:663–670.
17. Eriksson MJ, Sonnenberg B, Woo A, et al. Long-term outcome in patients with apical hypertrophic cardiomyopathy. *J Am Coll Cardiol.* 2002;39:638–645.
18. Binder J, Ommen SR, Gersh BJ, et al. Echocardiography-guided genetic testing in hypertrophic cardiomyopathy: septal morphological features predict the presence of myofilament mutations. *Mayo Clin Proc.* 2006;81:459–467.
19. Nasermoaddeli A, Miura K, Matsumori A, et al. Prognosis and prognostic factors in patients with hypertrophic cardiomyopathy in Japan: results from a nationwide study. *Heart.* 2007;93:711–715.
20. Maron MS, Finley JJ, Bos JM, et al. Prevalence, clinical significance and natural history of left ventricular apical aneurysms in hypertrophic cardiomyopathy. *Circulation.* 2008;118:1541–1549.
21. Gruner C, Care M, Siminovitch K, et al. Sarcomere protein gene mutations in patients with apical hypertrophic cardiomyopathy. *Circ Cardiovasc Genet.* 2011;4:288–295.
22. Klarich KW, AttenhoferJost CH, Binder J, et al. Risk of death in long-term follow-up of patients with apical hypertrophic cardiomyopathy. *Am J Cardiol.* 2013;111:1784–1791.
23. Lee CH, Liu PY, Lin LJ, et al. Clinical features and outcome of patients with apical hypertrophic cardiomyopathy in Taiwan. *Cardiology.* 2006;106:29–35.
24. Webb JG, Sasson Z, Rakowski H, et al. Apical hypertrophic cardiomyopathy: clinical follow-up and diagnostic correlates. *J Am Coll Cardiol.* 1990;15:83–90.
25. Partanen J, Kupari M, Heikkila J, Keto P. Left ventricular aneurysm associated with apical hypertrophic cardiomyopathy. *Clin Cardiol.* 1991;14:936–939.
26. Chickamori T, Doi YL, Akizawa M, et al. Comparison of clinical, morphological, and prognostic features in hypertrophic cardiomyopathy between Japanese and western patients. *Clin Cardiol.* 1992;15:833–837.
27. Suzuki J, Watanabe F, Takenaka K, et al. New subtype of apical hypertrophic cardiomyopathy identified with nuclear magnetic resonance imaging as an underlying cause of markedly inverted T-waves. *J Am Coll Cardiol.* 1993;22:1175–1181.
28. Moro E, D'Angelo G, Nicolosi GL, et al. Long-term evaluation of patients with apical hypertrophic cardiomyopathy. Correlation between quantitative echocardiographic assessment of apical hypertrophy and clinical-electrocardiographic findings. *Eur Heart J.* 1995;16:210–217.
29. Wilson P, Marks A, Rostegar H, et al. Apical hypertrophic cardiomyopathy presenting with sustained monomorphic ventricular tachycardia and electrocardiographic changes simulating coronary artery disease and left ventricular aneurysm. *Clin Cardiol.* 1990;13:885–887.
30. Mitchell MA, Nath S, Thompson KA, et al. Sustained wide complex tachycardia resulting in myocardial injury in a patient with apical hypertrophic cardiomyopathy. *Pacing Clin Electrophysiol.* 1997;20:866–869.
31. Ridjab D, Koch M, Zabel M, et al. Cardiac arrest and ventricular tachycardia in Japanese-type apical hypertrophic cardiomyopathy. *Cardiology.* 2007;107:81–86.
32. Casolo GC, Trotta F, Rostagno C, et al. Detection of apical hypertrophy by magnetic resonance imaging. *Am Heart J.* 1989;117:468–472.
33. Suzuki J, Shimamoto R, Nishikawa J, et al. Morphological onset and early diagnosis in apical hypertrophic cardiomyopathy: a long-term analysis with nuclear magnetic resonance imaging. *J Am Coll Cardiol.* 1999;33:146–151.
34. Thanigaraj S, Perez JE. Apical hypertrophic cardiomyopathy echocardiographic diagnosis with the use of intravenous contrast image enhancement. *J Am Soc Echocardiogr.* 2000;13:146–149.
35. Soman P, Swinburn J, Callister M, et al. Apical hypertrophic cardiomyopathy: Bedside diagnosis by intravenous contrast echocardiography. *J Am Soc Echocardiogr.* 2001;14:311–313.
36. Maron BJ. Hypertrophic cardiomyopathy: a systematic review. *J Am Med Assoc.* 2002;287:1308–1320.
37. Ward RP, Weinert L, Spencer KT, et al. Quantitative diagnosis of apical cardiomyopathy using contrast echocardiography. *J Am Soc Echocardiogr.* 2002;15:316–322.
38. Patel J, Michaels J, Mieres J, et al. Echocardiographic diagnosis of apical hypertrophic cardiomyopathy with Optison contrast. *Echocardiography.* 2002;19:521–524.
39. Thaman R, Gimeno JR, Murphy RT, et al. Prevalence and clinical significance of systolic impairment in hypertrophic cardiomyopathy. *Heart.* 2005;91:920–925.
40. Moukarbel GV, Alam SE, Abchee AB. Contrast-enhanced echocardiography for the diagnosis of apical hypertrophic cardiomyopathy. *Echocardiography.* 2005;22:831–833.
41. Olszewski R, Timperly J, Cezary S, et al. The clinical application of contrast echocardiography. *Eur Heart J Cardiovasc Imaging.* 2007;8:513–523.
42. Walpot J, Pasteuning WH, Shivalkar B. Apical hypertrophic cardiomyopathy: elegant use of contrast-enhanced echocardiography in the diagnostic work-up. *Acta Cardiol.* 2012;67:495–497.
43. Pons-Llado G, Carreras F, Parras X, et al. Comparison of morphologic assessment of hypertrophic cardiomyopathy by magnetic resonance versus echocardiographic imaging. *Am J Cardiol.* 1997;79:1651–1656.
44. Moon JCC, Fisher NG, McKenna WJ, Pennell DJ. Detection of apical hypertrophic cardiomyopathy by cardiovascular magnetic resonance in patients with non-diagnostic echocardiography. *Heart.* 2004;90:645–649.
45. Fattori R, Biagini E, Lorenzini M, et al. Significance of magnetic resonance imaging in apical hypertrophic cardiomyopathy. *Am J Cardiol.* 2010;105:1592–1596.
46. Amano Y, Takayama M, Fukashima Y, et al. Delayed-enhancement MRI of apical hypertrophic cardiomyopathy: assessment of the intramural distribution and comparison with clinical symptoms, ventricular arrhythmias, and cine MRI. *Acta Radiol.* 2011;53:613–618.
47. Maron MS. Clinical utility of cardiovascular magnetic resonance in hypertrophic cardiomyopathy. *J Cardiovasc Magn Reson.* 2012;14:13–34.
48. Kim KH, Kim HK, Hwang IC, et al. Myocardial scarring on cardiovascular magnetic resonance in asymptomatic or minimally symptomatic patients with "pure" apical hypertrophic cardiomyopathy. *J Cardiovasc Magn Reson.* 2012;14:52–60.
49. Crowley JJ, Dardas PS, Shapiro LM. Assessment of apical hypertrophic cardiomyopathy using transesophageal echocardiography. *Cardiology.* 1997;88:189–196.
50. Arad M, Penas-Lado M, Monserrat L, et al. Gene mutations in apical hypertrophic cardiomyopathy. *Circulation.* 2005;112:2805–2811.
51. Nimura H, Patton KK, McKenna WJ, et al. Sarcomere protein gene mutations in hypertrophic cardiomyopathy of the elderly. *Circulation.* 2005;105:446–487.

52. Reddy M, Thatai D, Bernal J, et al. Apical hypertrophic cardiomyopathy: potential utility of strain imaging. *Eur J Echocardiogr.* 2008;9:560–562.
53. Choi EY, Rim SJ, Ha JW, et al. Phenotypic spectrum and clinical characteristics of apical hypertrophic cardiomyopathy: multicenter echo-Doppler study. *Cardiology.* 2008;110:53–66.
54. Chen CC, Lei MH, Hsu YC, et al. Apical hypertrophic cardiomyopathy: correlations between echocardiographic parameters, angiographic left ventricular morphology, and clinical outcomes. *Clin Cardiol.* 2011;34:233–238.
55. Nakamura T, Matsubara K, Furukowa K, et al. Diastolic paradoxic jet flow in patients with hypertrophic cardiomyopathy: evidence of concealed apical asynergy with cavity obliteration. *J Am Coll Cardiol.* 1992;19. 526–524, 526–524.
56. Matsubara K, Nakamura T, Kuribayashi T, et al. Sustained cavity obliteration and apical aneurysm formation in apical hypertrophic cardiomyopathy. *J Am Coll Cardiol.* 2003;42:288–295.
57. Olivotto I, Girolami F, Nistri S, et al. The many faces of hypertrophic cardiomyopathy: from development biology to clinical practice. *J Cardiovasc Trans Res.* 2007;2:349–367.
58. Binder J, AttenhoferJost CH, Klarich KW, et al. Apical hypertrophic cardiomyopathy: prevalence and correlates of apical outpouching. *J Am Soc Echocardiogr.* 2011;24:775–781.
59. Sanghvi NK, Tracy CM. Sustained ventricular tachycardia in apical hypertrophic cardiomyopathy, midcavitary obstruction, and apical aneurysm. *Pacing Clin Electrophysiol.* 2007;30:799–803.

64

The Role of Echocardiography in the Screening and Evaluation of Athletes

Amita Singh, Karima Addetia

In clinical practice, regular exercise is encouraged as an essential strategy in the prevention of incident coronary artery disease and heart failure. Regular, intense, and rigorous bouts of exercise, largely at a competitive level, have been associated with alterations in cardiac structure and function defined by the term "athlete's heart."[1] Echocardiography plays a pivotal role in differentiating normal physiologic adaptations from occult pathologic disease. The implications of appropriate screening are even more critical in the assessment of individuals seeking preparticipation cardiac examinations. These examinations are performed with the goal of ensuring safe involvement in athletic events and prevention of sudden cardiac death (SCD), a rare but devastating consequence associated with underlying occult cardiomyopathies.

A constellation of findings related to chamber size and systolic and diastolic function can be used to help delineate adaptive versus pathologic remodeling patterns in the hearts of athletes. Understanding what constitutes appropriate patterns of structural changes from exercise and when to consider further testing has been studied, with consensus focused around three main phenotype profiles: predominance of hypertrophy, predominantly dilated with or without dysfunction, and right ventricular (RV) involvement.

EXERCISE-ASSOCIATED CARDIAC REMODELING: THE LEFT VENTRICLE

Basic exercise physiology dictates a direct relationship between the exercise intensity and oxygen consumption. This translates to a direct relationship between oxygen uptake and cardiac output (stroke volume × heart rate) in the healthy body, in which cardiac output may increase five to sixfold with exercise. The rise in cardiac output occurs because of a combination of increased sympathetic activation resulting in an increase in heart rate and an increase in preload. To meet the demands of the rigorous exercise regimen adopted by athletes, certain adaptations are made by the cardiovascular system that are based on the nature and intensity of exercise.[2] Exercises that involve mostly static (isometric) components, characterized as short and intensive skeletal muscle contractions, are associated with a sudden rise in left ventricular (LV) afterload (pressure loading) during which the cardiac output must be maintained. Archetypal forms of static exercise include wrestling, throwing events, martial arts, and weight lifting, with adaptive changes manifesting as concentric left ventricular hypertrophy (LVH) without an ostensible increase in LV size. By comparison, dynamic (also called isotonic or endurance) exercise consists of prolonged bouts of repetitive cycles of relaxation and contraction of skeletal muscle, typified by activities such as swimming, running, and rowing. These prolonged periods of exercise are associated with increased oxygen demands of the skeletal muscle and volume loading of the LV, the needs of which are met by augmentation of cardiac output. The long-term effects of this type of exercise include LV dilatation to accommodate larger stroke volumes, and eccentric LVH in addition to more rapid diastolic filling and increased systolic contractility. An algorithmic approach to this dichotomous remodeling response has been termed the "Morganroth hypothesis," but it has faced criticism for failing to capture the effects of combined static and dynamic activity that cause combined pressure and volume loading on the LV. It is more realistic to recognize that the cumulative proportions of each types of exercise will exhibit a range of expected remodeling patterns for the individual athlete (Fig. 64.1).

Although LV dilatation and hypertrophy are prototypical effects of prolonged static and dynamic exercise, there is a spectrum of features associated with the syndrome of athlete's heart. These include an LV wall thickness that is increased but rarely exceeds 12 mm with relative symmetric involvement of the LV segments. LV dilatation may occur, with LV end-diastolic dimensions typically less than 60 mm. Degree of LV end diastolic volume increase is likely gender dependent, with three-dimensional echocardiography demonstrating greater volumes in male athletes.[3] Preservation of systolic function is a hallmark of athlete's heart, reflecting the efficiency of a highly trained cardiovascular system. Occasionally in elite athletes, lower normal systolic function has been reported, with evidence of adequate augmentation with exercise testing.[4] Additional methods for evaluation of systolic function with speckle tracking have demonstrated normal LV strain values even in athletes with LVH; thus, it stands out as an additional method for differentiating normal variants from pathology.[5]

A second component that supports the presence of athlete's heart is normal (or supranormal) diastolic function. This is caused by the ability of the highly trained and compliant LV to maintain efficient stroke volume and filling pressures even at elevated heart rates. Echocardiographic manifestations include normal mitral inflow patterns with normal E-wave deceleration time and elevated mitral e′ velocities, reflecting enhanced LV compliance and suction in early diastole. Some studies suggest tissue doppler e′ may migrate toward the normal range with increasing age in athletes.[6] Additional supportive findings include normal pulmonary vein flow patterns, and E/e′ values typically below 8, reflecting normal left atrium (LA) pressures in this population.[7]

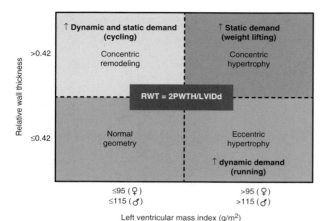

Figure 64.1. Patterns of left ventricular remodeling and wall thickness in association with exercise profile. In the equation: *RWT*, relative wall thickness; *PWTH*, posterior wall thickness; *LVIDd*, LV internal dimensions at end-diastole. (Adapted with permission from Lang RM, et al: *J Am Soc Echocardiogr* 18:1440–1463, 2005.)

Hypertrophy

As outlined earlier, wall thickness and LV mass are often increased in athletes, but significant LVH (defined by most studies as LV wall thickness >12 mm) is prevalent in only 1% to 4% of endurance athletes.[8] Demographics may play a role in the prevalence of LVH because female athletes or those younger than 16 years of age have been shown to mount lower degrees of LVH in response to exercise, whereas African American athletes have a higher prevalence and magnitude of LVH. Although isometric exercise would, in theory, generate more pronounced degrees of LVH, this has not borne out consistently in observational studies. Most often, the increased LV wall thickness seen in athletes involves the LV walls in a relatively symmetric fashion, with segment thickness variation of 2 mm or less and ratio of interventricular septal to posterior wall thickness of less than 1.5:1. Additionally, the degree of LVH is accompanied by proportionate increases in LV end-diastolic volumes, accounting for the increased pressure and volume-loading demands of the LV. Furthermore, as outlined earlier, adaptive LVH from athlete's heart typically demonstrates normal diastolic function. Findings of LV wall thickness exceeding 16 mm should be considered pathologic, particularly when accompanied by normal LV cavity dimensions, reduced mitral annular e′ or elevated E/e′ ratio, electrocardiographic (ECG) evidence of pathologic q waves or T-wave inversions, family history of cardiac disease, and any evidence of LV outflow tract obstruction; these factors all suggest the presence of hypertrophic cardiomyopathy (HCM). Cases in which the LV wall thickness falls between 13 and 16 mm constitute a clinical challenge termed the "gray zone," and diagnosis may be best adjudicated by the use of

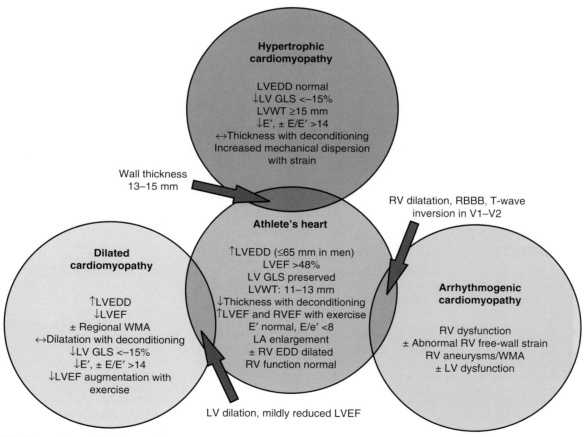

Figure 64.2. Echocardiographic features demonstrating the salient features and "gray zones" between athlete's heart and other overlapping cardiomyopathy syndromes. *EDD*, End-diastolic diameter; *GLS*, global longitudinal strain; *LA*, left atrial; *LV*, left ventricular; *LVEDD*, left ventricular end-diastolic diameter; *LVEF*, left ventricular ejection fraction; *LVWT*, left ventricular wall thickness; *RBBB*, right bundle branch block; *RV*, right ventricular; *WMA*, wall motion abnormality.

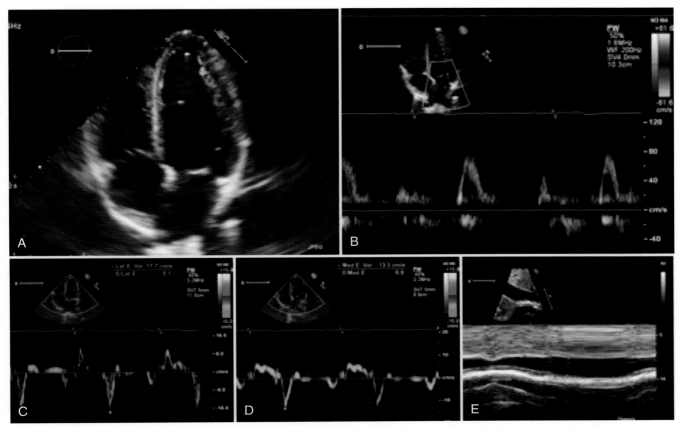

Figure 64.3. An 18-year-old male basketball player presented with atypical chest pain. Echocardiography findings notable for dilatation of the left and right heart chambers (**A**), with a normal mitral inflow pattern (**B**). Mitral annular tissue doppler e′ velocities elevated (**C** and **D**) with an enlarged but compressible inferior vena cava by M-mode echocardiography (**E**).

additional modalities. One option is the use of speckle-tracking echocardiography (STE), with limited studies indicating that athlete's heart is associated with preserved LV global longitudinal strain (GLS).[9] Mechanical dispersion (MD) by STE, defined as the segmental time to maximal shortening, is an additional echocardiographic parameter with promise in differentiating pathologic hypertrophy as seen with HCM from athlete's heart. Increasingly, MD reflects increased or heterogenic variation in systolic thickening, which may occur in regions of abnormal hypertrophy.[10] Another option for supplemental imaging comes in the form of cardiac magnetic resonance imaging (CMRI), which has the ability to detect subclinical fibrosis and asymmetric hypertrophy patterns, findings that both support a diagnosis of HCM. Ultimately, consideration of the global clinical picture, which includes resting ECG, family history, and diastolic function, are essential in contextualizing echo findings. If there is clinical equipoise regarding the true diagnosis, detraining can be implemented (Fig. 64.2).

Hypertrabeculation

LV noncompaction is an increasingly reported phenotype of inherited cardiomyopathy that can also display overlap with hypertrabeculation of the LV noted in young asymptomatic athletes.[11] This finding is distinct from the increased LV wall thickness associated with athlete's heart and characterized as a preponderance of noncompacted myocardium with increased LV trabeculation and recesses, with some studies reporting it to be present in 20% of athletes.[12] One very small case series suggests that increased trabeculation can occur as a response to exercise training, but data in this area are extremely sparse. Pathologic LV noncompaction cardiomyopathy is diagnosed

by ratios between noncompacted and compacted myocardium of more than 2.0 at end-systole on echocardiography and more than 2.3 at end-diastole on CMRI, but data have shown these criteria are present in 10% of asymptomatic athletes and thus may not be specific.[13] In cases in which LV noncompaction cardiomyopathy is of concern, the presence of family history, ventricular arrhythmias, LV dysfunction or diastolic dysfunction, and abnormal CMRI imaging should prompt concern for true pathology. Detraining has an unknown impact on trabeculation burden.

Dilatation and Dysfunction

Dilated cardiomyopathy is characterized by LV dilatation and systolic dysfunction, whereas athlete's heart is associated with modest LV dilatation with preservation of systolic function. Lower normal or even mildly reduced ejection fraction can be encountered in elite athletes. Preservation of LV GLS, normal diastolic function, and concomitant dilatation of other cardiac chambers, when present, support physiologic and not pathologic remodeling (Figs. 64.3 and 64.4). Exercise stress testing to confirm augmentation of LV ejection fraction with exercise or cardiopulmonary stress testing to document the presence of supranormal functional capacity by VO2 max assessment, are additional tests to consider because both indicate an ability to mount higher cardiac output in the face of increased metabolic demands. CMRI and genetic testing are again of use in patients with an unclear diagnosis, those with family history concerning for inherited cardiomyopathy, and in suspected myocarditis (Fig. 64.5). Detraining has a less consistent impact in the assessment of the dilated LV.

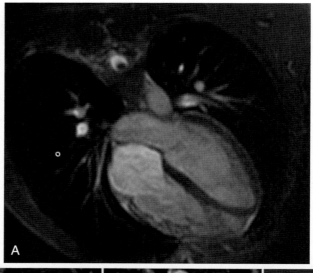

Figure 64.4. Cardiac magnetic resonance images from the same patient as in Fig. 64.2, confirming moderate four-chamber dilatation (**A**) with preserved systolic function. Late gadolinium enhancement imaging (**B–D**) with no evidence of myocardial fibrosis. Findings support the diagnosis of athlete's heart.

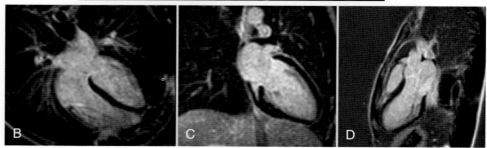

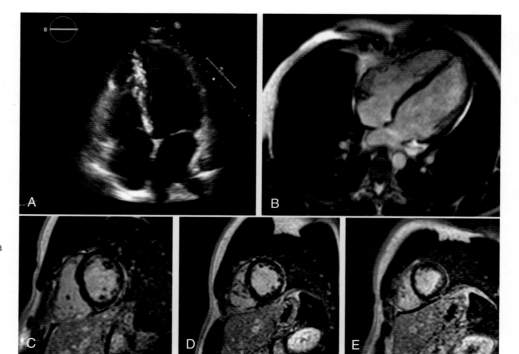

Figure 64.5. A 20-year-old male soccer player presenting with nonsustained ventricular tachycardia and abnormal ejection fraction by echocardiography (**A**). **B–E,** Cardiac magnetic resonance imaging confirmed moderate left ventricular dysfunction, with late gadolinium enhancement demonstrating epicardial fibrosis consistent with previous myocarditis.

EXERCISE-ASSOCIATED CARDIAC REMODELING: BEYOND THE LEFT VENTRICLE

Attention to chambers other than the left ventricle has yielded important information in the understanding of athlete's heart phenotypes. Limited data suggest that isometric exercises have little or no effect on the right ventricle and atria so that most of the information in this section applies to isotonic or endurance forms of training.

Right Ventricle

Remodeling patterns of the right ventricle mimic those described in the left ventricle, with increases in end-diastolic volumes and wall thickness, reflecting the results of volume and pressure overload. Interestingly, remodeling appears to spare the RV outflow tract in limited data.[14] RV chamber dilatation is usually proportional to the left ventricle, though in extreme endurance athletes, RV dilatation may exceed that seen for the LV. Systolic function is generally preserved, though cases of mild resting RV systolic dysfunction and reduced GLS have been reported, with augmentation noted with exercise.[15] Interestingly, the presence of a right bundle branch block on ECG may reflect the extent of RV dilatation.[16] Because of the complex geometry of the RV and propensity for dilatation with repetitive exercise, CMRI holds an important and supplementary role in evaluation of suspected pathologic RV dysfunction.

When findings of RV dilatation and dysfunction are present, consideration of the underlying pathology, including undiagnosed congenital heart disease, pulmonary hypertension, or arrhythmogenic right ventricular cardiomyopathy (ARVC), becomes clinically relevant, especially if RV remodeling is not accompanied by LV remodeling. Evaluation of the RV by echocardiography using the RV-focused view, meticulous chamber quantification, and assessment of systolic function is integral to a careful assessment. RV dilatation is typically proportional to the duration of exercise, with greater amounts resulting in greater dilatation; any discrepant relationship of severe dilatation with moderate amounts (<5 hours/week) of exercise should signal the possibility of true pathology. Patterns of dilatation that spare the RVOT may support exercise-associated RV dilatation. Exercise testing may also play a valuable role in such patients because it allows for simultaneous assessment of ECG with exertion for detection of arrhythmia, as well as for RV contractile reserve, which is present in athletes but absent in true RV pathologic states such as ARVC. Cardiac CMRI for the detection of regional RV wall motion abnormalities, intracardiac shunting, or myocardial fibrosis is also appropriate if testing remains equivocal. The presence of arrhythmia or family history of cardiomyopathy or SCD should also compel a thorough evaluation, with genetic testing or detraining reserved for clinical cases that remain ambiguous.

Left and Right Atrium

Atrial remodeling has also been acknowledged as a feature of athlete's heart. The LA dilates in response to chronic repetitive exercise, with increased volumes now well described in both strength and endurance training.[12,17,18] Some studies indicate this is more likely to occur with endurance athletics.[3] A hallmark of LA remodeling appears to involve preservation of LA mechanics, with volumetric function demonstrating normal or heightened reservoir function.[19] Results regarding LA strain have been mixed, with some studies indicating mild reductions in peak LA strain at rest.[20] Indeed, LA dilatation and reduced function may be a prognostic measure to follow over time because some studies indicate that LA dilatation and perturbations in LA strain denote patients at greater risk of developing atrial arrhythmia, particularly men.[21–23] Similar structural alterations have been described in the right atrium, though there are fewer data overall with regards to this chamber, with higher right atrial volumes and preservation of peak reservoir strain reported.[24,25] Last, inferior vena cava dilatation has been described in male and female athletes but is considered a reflection of repetitive volume loading of exercise rather than a signal of elevated right atrial pressures.[26]

DETRAINING

Sidelining a competitive or recreational athlete over concern for cardiomyopathy can generate downstream anxiety and uncertainty for the athlete and physician, which incentivizes securing an accurate diagnosis. The role of detraining in such cases proves valuable and hinges on the assumption that removal of repetitive or strenuous exercise and thus removal of the excessive pressure and volume loading conditions will lead to regression in the phenotypic features of athlete's heart. In contrast, true pathology will not improve

after cessation of exercise. The duration of detraining varies, with initial changes in LV mass and thickness regression seen within 6 weeks, but reductions in LV and RV chamber size may take up to 6 months (Fig. 64.6).[27] This posits detraining as a suitable strategy for "gray-zone" hypertrophy cases. Detraining for a dilated LV or RV yields less consistent results because data suggest that chamber dilatation persists for longer.[28] Less is known regarding detraining and regression in a left ventricle with hypertrabeculations when there is concern for LV noncompaction, though it is often used to help clarify the diagnosis. Interestingly, detraining appears to lead to regression in right and left atrial dimensions. Challenges to implementation include a lack of definition of optimal detraining duration and the implications of barring a competitive athlete from participation in sports.

SUDDEN CARDIAC DEATH AND SCREENING STRATEGIES

SCD etiology is largely dictated by the age of occurrence, with the majority of cases age older than 35 years because of undiagnosed coronary disease but cases occurring at younger than 35 years representing a spectrum of undiagnosed cardiomyopathy or congenital disease. Although rare, occurring in 1 in 43,770 participants per year at the collegiate level, the most common entities encountered in the younger population in the United States have traditionally been cited as HCM followed by anomalous coronary artery anatomy and less commonly ARVC.[29,30] The ultimate final common manifestation of these syndromes is fatal arrhythmic events. More contemporary data from the National Collegiate Athletic Association have highlighted a potential shifting landscape for underlying causes of SCD, with a relatively high proportion of autopsy-negative unexplained death and coronary abnormalities most frequently encountered followed by dilated cardiomyopathy and undiagnosed myocarditis, with HCM less frequently noted.[31] In Europe, ARVC is a more frequent cause of sudden death in young athletes. SCD occurs more frequently in men than women and more commonly in persons of African American descent than those of European descent. The highest risk sports include basketball and American-style football.

Whatever the underlying cause, screening programs are aimed at detecting at-risk individuals but hampered by a lack of data to support implementation of screening. The United States–based guidelines emphasize a physical examination and symptom-guided approach, with family history of sudden death or cardiomyopathy a specific inquiry that should instigate further testing.[32] In contrast, the European Society of Cardiology guidelines support the routine addition of a 12-lead resting ECG in preparticipation athletic screening examinations.[33] Imaging with either echocardiography or alternative modalities is not advocated as a first-line screening tool and should be used judiciously by consultation with sports medicine or cardiologists with expertise in this clinical setting.

CONCLUSIONS

The cumulative effects of repetitive exercise demonstrate characteristic and physiologic remodeling effects, with some variations according to underlying exercise type and duration. The typical changes associated with athlete's heart include modestly increased LV dimensions and wall thickness, with dilatation of the right ventricle and atria noted as well. In general, systolic function of the ventricles and mechanical function of the atria remain preserved. Echocardiography is indispensable in the detection and quantification of many of these adaptive responses and can distinguish cases of pronounced or asymmetric LVH, severe LV dilatation, or abnormalities in systolic and diastolic function that might suggest the presence of true cardiac pathology. Consideration of additional imaging, exercise testing, and even an interval of detraining are appropriate if cases remain undefined. Sudden death in young athletes is rare but devastating, and detection of subclinical cardiomyopathies is integral in its prevention.

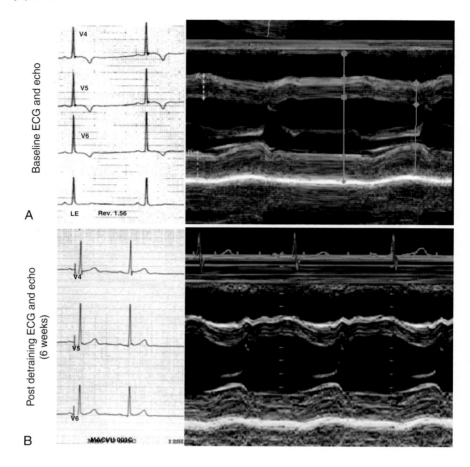

Figure 64.6. Detraining results at baseline (**A**) and after 6 months (**B**) in a young collegiate basketball player, demonstrating regression of left ventricular hypertrophy and normalization of T waves on the electrocardiogram (ECG).

REFERENCES

1. Maron BJ, Udelson JE, Bonow RO, et al. Eligibility and disqualification recommendations for competitive athletes with cardiovascular abnormalities, Task Force 3: hypertrophic cardiomyopathy, arrhythmogenic right ventricular cardiomyopathy and other cardiomyopathies, and myocarditis. *J Am Coll Cardiol.* 2015;66:2362–2371.
2. Levine BD, Baggish AL, Kovacs RJ, et al. Eligibility and disqualification recommendations for competitive athletes with cardiovascular abnormalities, Task Force 1: Classification of sports: dynamic, static, and impact. *J Am Coll Cardiol.* 2015;66:2350–2355.
3. Lakatos BK, Molnár AÁ, Kiss O, et al. Relationship between cardiac remodeling and exercise capacity in elite athletes: incremental value of left atrial morphology and function assessed by three-dimensional echocardiography. *J Am Soc Echocardiogr.* 2020;33(1):101–109. e1.
4. Pluim BM, Zwinderman AH, van der Laarse A, van der Wall EE, et al. The athlete's heart: a meta-analysis of cardiac structure and function. *Circulation.* 2000;101:336–344.
5. Richand V, Lafitte S, Reant P, et al. An ultrasound speckle tracking (two-dimensional strain) analysis of myocardial deformation in professional soccer players compared with healthy subjects and hypertrophic cardiomyopathy. *Am J Cardiol.* 2007;100:128–132.
6. Finocchiaro G, Dhutia H, D'Silva A, et al. Role of Doppler diastolic parameters in differentiating physiological left ventricular hypertrophy from hypertrophic cardiomyopathy. *J Am Soc Echocardiogr.* 2018;31:606–613.
7. Nagueh SF, Lakkis NM, Middleton KJ, et al. Doppler estimation of left ventricular filling pressures in patients with hypertrophic cardiomyopathy. *Circulation.* 1999;99:254–261.
8. Rawlins J, Bhan A, Sharma S. Left ventricular hypertrophy in athletes. *Eur J Echocardiogr.* 2009;10:350–356.
9. Butz T, van Buuren F, Mellwig KP, et al. Two-dimensional strain analysis of the global and regional myocardial function for the differentiation of pathologic and physiologic left ventricular hypertrophy: a study in athletes and in patients with hypertrophic cardiomyopathy. *Int J Cardiovasc Imaging.* 2011;27:91–100.
10. Schnell F, Matelot D, Daudin M, et al. Mechanical dispersion by strain echocardiography: a novel tool to diagnose hypertrophic cardiomyopathy in athletes. *J Am Soc Echocardiogr.* 2017;30:251–261.
11. Caselli S, Attenhofer Jost CH, et al. Left ventricular noncompaction diagnosis and management relevant to pre-participation screening of athletes. *Am J Cardiol.* 2015;116:801–808.
12. D'Ascenzi F, Anselmi F, Focardi M, Mondillo S. Atrial enlargement in the athlete's heart: assessment of atrial function may help distinguish adaptive from pathologic remodeling. *J Am Soc Echocardiogr.* 2018;31:148–157.
13. Gati S, Chandra N, Bennett RL, et al. Increased left ventricular trabeculation in highly trained athletes: do we need more stringent criteria for the diagnosis of left ventricular non-compaction in athletes? *Heart.* 2013;99:401–408.
14. D'Ascenzi F, Pelliccia A, Corrado D, et al. Right ventricular remodelling induced by exercise training in competitive athletes. *Eur Heart J Cardiovasc Imag.* 2016;17:301–307.
15. Vitarelli A, Capotosto L, Placanica G, et al. Comprehensive assessment of biventricular function and aortic stiffness in athletes with different forms of training by 3D echocardiography and strain imaging. *Eur Heart J Cardiovasc Imag.* 2013;14:1010–1020.
16. Kim JH, Noseworthy PA, McCarty D, et al. Significance of electrocardiographic right bundle branch block in trained athletes. *Am J Cardiol.* 2011;107:1083–1089.
17. Iskandar A, Mujtaba MT, Thompson PD. Left atrium size in elite athletes. *JACC Cardiovasc Imag.* 2015;8:753–762.
18. Pelliccia A, Maron BJ, Di Paolo FM, et al. Prevalence and clinical significance of left atrial remodeling in competitive athletes. *J Am Coll Cardiol.* 2005;46:690–696.
19. D'Ascenzi F, Pelliccia A, Natali BM, et al. Training-induced dynamic changes in left atrial reservoir, conduit, and active volumes in professional soccer players. *Eur J Appl Physiol.* 2015;115:1715–1723.
20. Cuspidi C, Tadic M, Sala C, et al. Left atrial function in elite athletes: a meta-analysis of two-dimensional speckle tracking echocardiographic studies. *Clin Cardiol.* 2019;42:579–587.
21. Hubert A, Galand V, Donal E, et al. Atrial function is altered in lone paroxysmal atrial fibrillation in male endurance veteran athletes. *Eur Heart J Cardiovasc Imag.* 2018;19:145–153.
22. Boraita A, Santos-Lozano A, Heras ME, et al. Incidence of atrial fibrillation in elite athletes. *JAMA Cardiol.* 2018;3:1200–1205.
23. Svedberg N, Sundström J, James S, et al. Long-term incidence of atrial fibrillation and stroke among cross-country skiers. *Circulation.* 2019;140:910–920.
24. D'Ascenzi F, Pelliccia A, Natali BM, et al. Morphological and functional adaptation of left and right atria induced by training in highly trained female athletes. *Circ Cardiovasc Imag.* 2014;7:222–229.
25. Pagourelias ED, Kouidi E, Efthimiadis GK, et al. Right atrial and ventricular adaptations to training in male Caucasian athletes: an echocardiographic study. *J Am Soc Echocardiogr.* 2013;26:1344–1352.

26. D'Ascenzi F, Cameli M, Padeletti M, et al. Characterization of right atrial function and dimension in top-level athletes: a speckle tracking study. *Int J Cardiovasc Imaging*. 2013;29:87–94.

27. Maron BJ, Pelliccia A, Spataro A, Granata M. Reduction in left ventricular wall thickness after deconditioning in highly trained Olympic athletes. *Br Heart J*. 1993;69:125–128.

28. Pelliccia A, Maron BJ, De Luca R, et al. Remodeling of left ventricular hypertrophy in elite athletes after long-term deconditioning. *Circulation*. 2002;105:944–949.

29. Harmon KG, Asif IM, Klossner D, Drezner JA. Incidence of sudden cardiac death in national collegiate athletic association athletes. *Circulation*. 2011;123:1594–1600.

30. Maron BJ, Doerer JJ, Haas TS, et al. Sudden deaths in young competitive athletes: analysis of 1866 deaths in the United States, 1980–2006. *Circulation*. 2009;119. 1085–92.

31. Harmon KG, Drezner JA, Maleszewski JJ, et al. Pathogeneses of sudden cardiac death in national collegiate athletic association athletes. *Circ Arrhythm Electrophysiol*. 2014;7:198–204.

32. Maron BJ, Thompson PD, Ackerman MJ, et al. Recommendations and considerations related to preparticipation screening for cardiovascular abnormalities in competitive athletes. *Circulation*. 2007;115. 1643–455.

33. Corrado D, Pelliccia A, Bjørnstad HH, et al. Cardiovascular pre-participation screening of young competitive athletes for prevention of sudden death: proposal for a common European protocol. *Eur Heart J*. 2005;26:516–524.

65 Echocardiographic Assessment of Myocarditis

Balaji K. Tamarappoo, Nir Flint, Robert J. Siegel

Myocarditis is a pathophysiological condition defined as infiltration of the myocardium by inflammatory cells with associated degenerative and necrotic changes not typical of ischemic injury.[1] In severe cases, myocarditis is characterized by a rapid onset of heart failure symptoms.[2] Although some patients with myocarditis may be asymptomatic, most patients present with chest pain, dyspnea, palpitations, and arrhythmias, which are symptoms seen with other cardiac diseases. Therefore, making the diagnosis of myocarditis depends on having a high index of suspicion and being able to distinguish this disease entity from other causes such as ischemic cardiac disease, infiltrative cardiomyopathy, and valvular heart disease. The definitive diagnosis of myocarditis is made by endomyocardial biopsy (EMB), in which histology identifies myocardial inflammation and cellular necrosis. However, EMB is an invasive procedure with potential risks, including cardiac perforation and tamponade, that should be done by experienced operators. EMB is often not recommended for the initial assessment of the disease.[3] Noninvasive diagnostic assessment of myocarditis largely depends on two-dimensional (2D) transthoracic echocardiography (TTE) and cardiac magnetic resonance imaging (CMRI), which are the two primary imaging modalities that are commonly used for the diagnosis of myocarditis.

CAUSE OF MYOCARDITIS

Myocarditis most often results from injury induced by a heightened immune response to infection or inflammatory stimuli. The causes include viruses, drugs, toxins, and autoimmune diseases (Table 65.1).

TRANSTHORACIC ECHOCARDIOGRAPHY

Echocardiography is important to rule out other cardiac conditions such as valve disease as well as for serial evaluation of left ventricular (LV) size and function. Although no specific echocardiographic findings are pathognomonic for myocarditis and findings often resemble those found in dilated cardiomyopathy, some features can be used to aid in diagnosis. The primary assessment of reduced LV systolic function is often performed with TTE. Evaluation of myocarditis by echocardiography primarily involves quantification of LV ejection fraction (LVEF), assessment of valvular function, evaluation of segmental wall thickening, and assessment of right ventricular function. Regional wall motion abnormalities in a noncoronary artery distribution or global LV dysfunction is often seen in myocarditis and may lead to functional mitral regurgitation (MR) (Fig. 65.1).[2,4] An increase in wall thickness resulting from myocardial edema may be observed in acute myocarditis[5] and along with infiltration of the myocardium by inflammatory cells can change the acoustic properties of the myocardium, which can manifest as increased myocardial brightness and contrast.[6] Because abnormal wall motion may also occur in ischemic disease, obstructive epicardial coronary artery disease (CAD) should be excluded by coronary computed tomography angiography (CTA) or invasive coronary angiography.[4,7]

TABLE 65.1 Causes of Myocarditis

Infection	Bacteria	*Hemophilus influenzae*, mycobacterium
	Spirochete	*Borrelia* spp., *Leptospira* spp.
	Protozoa	*Trypanosoma cruzi*
	Viral	Coxsackie A and B, echovirus, influenza A and B, respiratory syncytial virus, human immunodeficiency virus-1
		Parvovirus B19, adenovirus, cytomegalovirus, herpes simplex virus, human herpes virus-6, Epstein-Barr virus
Drugs and toxins		Immune checkpoint inhibitors, anthracyclines, fluorouracil, catecholamines, interleukin-2, trastuzumab, cyclophosphamide
		Copper, iron, lead
		Scorpion and wasp stings, snake and spider bites
		Radiation
Immune mediated		Lymphocytic, giant cell
		Systemic lupus erythematosus, rheumatoid arthritis, Churg-Strauss syndrome, Kawasaki disease, hypereosinophilic syndrome, inflammatory bowel disease, scleroderma, polymyositis, myasthenia gravis, sarcoidosis, Wegner granulomatosis
		Graft rejection

Figure 65.1. Transthoracic echocardiography image of a 33-year-old patient with no significant past medical history that presented with acute pulmonary congestion and elevated cardiac biomarkers. **A,** Long-axis view revealed a dilated left ventricle (LV) with global LV hypokinesis, LV ejection fraction (LVEF) of 25%, and a severe right ventricular dysfunction **B,** M-mode imaging showing E-point septal separation of 1.73 cm, consistent with reduced LV contractility and LVEF. **C,** Apical four-chamber view with color Doppler showing moderate to severe functional mitral regurgitation (MR) with a posteriorly directed wall-hugging MR jet. **D,** Continuous-wave (CW) spectral Doppler showing MR with a diastolic MR component (white arrow) caused by acute elevation in LV filling pressures. The patient's LV function gradually improved with medical treatment of his congestive heart failure. LVEDD, Left ventricular end-diastolic diameter; LVESD, left ventricular end-systolic diameter. (See accompanying Video 65.1.)

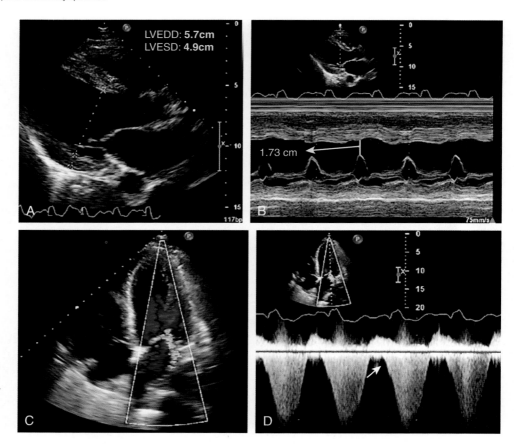

Coronary CTA, which has a high sensitivity and specificity and a high negative predictive value for obstructive CAD,[8] can serve as an excellent noninvasive test to rule out obstructive CAD as a cause of troponin elevation in patients in whom there is high suspicion for myocarditis.

Diastolic dysfunction is also commonly seen in myocarditis and can range from mild diastolic dysfunction to severe restrictive filling patterns. Persistence of diastolic dysfunction after improvement or normalization in LV systolic function is associated with worse long-term outcome.[9] Eosinophilic myocarditis (EM) is a rare and potentially life-threatening form of myocarditis, commonly presenting with peripheral eosinophilia. On echocardiography, LV hypokinesis and LV thrombus (most commonly at the apex) may be seen. (Fig. 65.2). With progression of EM, endomyocardial fibrosis and restrictive cardiomyopathy may develop. Endocardial fibrosis and thrombus formation can also involve the valve leaflets and subvalvular apparatus with thickening of these structures,[10–12] resulting in restricted leaflet motion and mitral and tricuspid regurgitation. Pericardial effusion and valvular abnormalities, which include leaflet thickening, vegetations, and valve distortion and dysfunction, may also be noted in systemic lupus erythematosus induced myocarditis.[13–15]

Strain, a dimensionless quantitative measure of myocardial deformation, is measured as the ratio of circumferential, longitudinal shortening or radial thickening of the LV to the initial length in the longitudinal, circumferential, and radial orientations.[16] Strain can be quantified using speckle-tracking echocardiography and is now routinely used for detecting subclinical myocardial injury and for prognostic purposes.[17] Global longitudinal strain (GLS) is often abnormal in patients with myocardial ischemia,[18,19] nonischemic cardiomyopathy,[20] hypertensive heart disease,[21,22] and chemotherapy-induced

cardiotoxicity.[23] Both global and regional abnormalities of longitudinal and circumferential strain have been documented in patients with myocarditis. In a small study of 28 patients with myocarditis confirmed by CMRI, GLS was abnormal, and the degree of strain impairment was proportional to the extent of myocardial injury as evaluated by CMRI.[24] In a retrospective study of 45 patients with suspected myocarditis, GLS and strain rates were reported to be abnormal compared with 83 healthy volunteers.[25] However, the routine clinical use of 2D TTE with or without strain imaging for diagnosis of myocarditis is still heavily guided by patient presentation and the use of complementary imaging with CMRI.

ELECTROCARDIOGRAM AND BIOMARKERS

Electrocardiogram (ECG) is often abnormal in myocarditis, and findings include a nonspecific ST-T changes, diffuse ST-segment elevation mimicking acute myocardial infarction, conduction abnormalities, and low ECG voltage secondary to myocardial edema or pericardial effusion. Biomarkers of myocardial damage (cardiac troponins) are often elevated in patients with acute myocarditis; however, they are nonspecific, and normal values do not exclude myocarditis.[26]

CARDIAC MAGNETIC RESONANCE IMAGING

CMRI is increasingly used as a key diagnostic test in patients with suspected myocarditis (Table 65.2). CMRI provides highly accurate assessment of LV function and segmental wall motion and enables quantitative evaluation of edema and myocardial fibrosis. CMRI diagnosis of myocarditis uses changes in T1 and T2 relaxation induced by acute inflammatory changes that occur in the

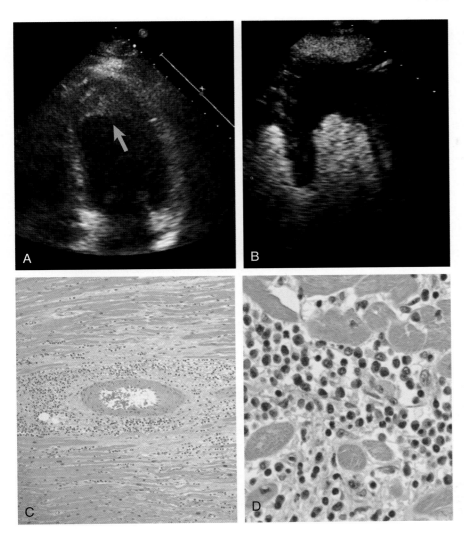

Figure 65.2. Transthoracic echocardiography image of a 65-year-old woman who presented with multiple embolic brain infarcts. Her white blood count showed a differential consisting of 58% eosinophils. **A,** Apical four-chamber view showing prominent left ventricular apical thickness consistent with a subendocardial thrombus *(arrow)* along the entire apical myocardium (**B**) also seen with the use of ultrasound-enhancing agents. **C,** Endomyocardial biopsy revealed interstitial and perivascular infiltrates with abundance of eosinophils and mononuclear cells (**D**), consistent with eosinophilic myocarditis. (See accompanying Video 65.2.) (Pathology images courtesy of Daniel Luthringer, MD.)

setting of myocarditis. The Lake Louise criteria are used as a guide for diagnosis of myocarditis and they include the following three CMRI features[27]:

1. Myocardial hyperemia in response to tissue injury is associated with increased gadolinium partitioning into the expanded interstitial space and can be detected by an increase in signal intensity of the myocardium in early postcontrast T1-weighted images compared with unaffected portions of the myocardium and muscle tissue.[27–29]
2. Tissue edema is associated with an increase in T2 of the affected myocardium. This increase in T2 is used for contrast generation and can be visualized by T2-weighted imaging (Fig. 65.3). The extent and severity of T2 abnormalities can also be detected with direct T2 quantification and T2 mapping.[30–33]
3. Late enhancement after injection of gadolinium is often observed in myocarditis because of delayed washout of gadolinium. This results from expansion of extracellular volume from interstitial edema and fibrosis.[27,34] Gadolinium enhancement in myocarditis is characterized by increased signal intensity localized to the subepicardium or extending from the subepicardium into the mid myocardium in a noncoronary distribution (Fig. 65.4). EM is an exception in that the enhancement is mostly subendocardial owing to the deposition of eosinophils in the subendocardium followed by necrosis of

the subendocardium as a result of eosinophil degradation (Fig. 65.5). It has been shown that the presence of two or more of the above-mentioned changes has high sensitivity and specificity for diagnostic of myocarditis with a diagnostic accuracy of 78%.[27] CMRI also provides prognostic information, and recent data in adults with myocarditis demonstrate a correlation between late gadolinium enhancement with subsequent cardiac events, including sudden death.[34,35] T1 and T2 mapping, which allow quantification of diffuse extracellular fibrosis and edema, respectively, have been shown to perform as well or better than the Lake Louise criteria for the diagnosis of myocarditis in adults.[31,36,37]

ROLE OF ENDOMYOCARDIAL BIOPSY

EMB is the definitive method for histopathologic diagnosis of myocarditis (Fig. 65.6). According to the European Society of Cardiology Task Force for Myocarditis consensus statement, biopsy should be obtained for a definitive diagnosis of myocarditis and to define its cause[26]; however, the sensitivity of EMB may be limited because of sampling error.[38–40] There is also poor interobserver agreement on identification of inflammatory infiltration and myocyte necrosis not characteristic of ischemic injury.[41,42]

TABLE 65.2 Cardiac Magnetic Resonance Imaging Criteria for Myocarditis

- In the setting of clinically suspected myocarditis, CMRI findings are consistent with myocardial inflammation if at least two of the following criteria are present:
    1. Regional or global myocardial signal intensity is increased in T2-weighted images with increase in global myocardial signal intensity defined as a ratio of myocardial to muscle signal intensity ≥2.
    2. Increase in global early gadolinium enhancement ratio between myocardium and skeletal muscle in gadolinium-enhanced T1-weighted images. Increase in early enhancement ratio is defined as myocardium to muscle signal intensity ≥4 or an increase of myocardial signal intensity postcontrast by ≥45% compared with signal intensity precontrast.
    3. At least one focal lesion with nonischemic regional distribution in late gadolinium inversion recovery-prepared T1-weighted images. Images should be obtained at least 5 minutes after gadolinium injection; foci typically exclude the subendocardial layer, are often multifocal, and involve the subepicardium. If the late gadolinium enhancement pattern clearly indicates myocardial infarction and is colocalized with a transmural regional edema, acute myocardial infarction is more likely and should be reported
- A CMRI study is consistent with myocyte injury or scar caused by myocardial inflammation if criterion 3 is present.
- A repeat CMRI study between 1 and 2 weeks after the initial CMRI study is recommended if:
    1. None of the criteria are present but the onset of symptoms has been very recent and there is strong clinical evidence for myocardial inflammation.
    2. One of the criteria is present.
- The presence of LV dysfunction or pericardial effusion provides additional, supportive evidence for myocarditis.

CMRI, Cardiac magnetic resonance imaging: *LV,* left ventricular.

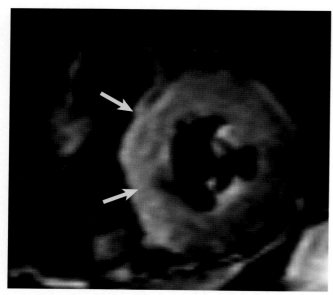

Figure 65.3. T2-weighted imaging of myocardial edema in myocarditis. A midventricular slice from a T2-weighted short-tau inversion recovery pulse sequence using cardiac magnetic resonance (CMRI) imaging in a 25-year-old man with fever, chest pain, and troponin elevation. Blood and adipose tissue appear dark, whereas regions of edema in the subepicardium and midmyocardium in the anteroseptum and inferoseptum appear hyperintense relative to the myocardium *(yellow arrows).* There was no coronary artery stenoses on invasive angiography. A diagnosis of myocarditis was made based on clinical presentation, invasive angiography, and CMRI.

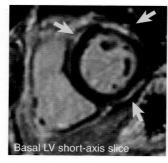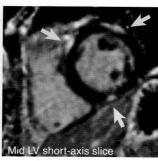

Basal LV short-axis slice   Mid LV short-axis slice

A   B

Figure 65.4. Epicardial and pericardial delayed enhancement in perimyocarditis. Late gadolinium enhancement images obtained 10 minutes after intravenous injection of gadolinium-based contrast agent in a 37-year-old man with chest pain, shortness of breath, and no coronary artery disease. **A,** A pattern of late enhancement typical for myocarditis involving the epicardium is seen in the basal anteroseptum, anterolateral wall and inferior wall *(yellow arrows).* Increased brightness of the pericardium along the basal inferior wall and the free wall of the RV represent inflammatory changes in the pericardium. **B,** Late enhancement of the epicardium and midmyocardium in the basal anteroseptum, anterolateral wall and inferior wall *(yellow arrows).*

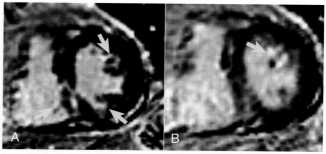

A   B

Figure 65.5. Delayed enhancement of subendocardial and papillary muscle in eosinophilic myocarditis. A 57-year-old man with hypereosinophilic syndrome who presented with dyspnea and new-onset heart failure symptoms underwent cardiac magnetic resonance imaging. Representative late gadolinium enhancement images from two contiguous midventricular slices are shown. **A,** Subendocardial enhancement in the left ventricular and right ventricular aspect of the mid-inferoseptum and mild enhancement in the anterolateral papillary muscle are indicated by the *yellow arrows.* **B,** Strong signal from delayed enhancement in the anterolateral papillary muscle is indicated by the *yellow arrow.*

CONCLUSION

There is wide heterogeneity in the cause and natural history of myocarditis with high morbidity and mortality in cases such as giant cell myocarditis, eosinophilic myocarditis, or fulminant myocarditis in which significant amount of myocardium may be affected. Diagnosis depends on echocardiographic assessment of LV function and regional myocardial dysfunction, including valvular involvement and CMRI confirmation with the use of T2-weighted early postcontrast T1 weighted and delayed postcontrast T1-weighted image acquisition. In patients suspected to have myocarditis, noninvasive imaging complements clinical and laboratory data and is an essential step for timely clinical decision making.

Please access ExpertConsult to view the corresponding videos for this chapter.

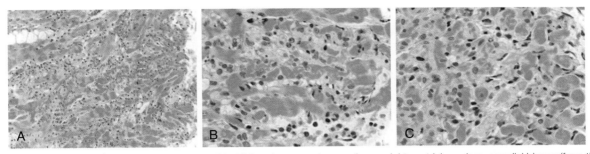

Figure 65.6. Histopathologic findings in acute myocarditis. Light microscopy images from a right ventricle endomyocardial biopsy (from the patient described in Fig. 65.1) showing active myocarditis (**A**) with diffuse infiltration of mononuclear cells (**B**) and severe myocardial degeneration with myofiber necrosis, interstitial edema, and hemorrhage (**C**) (Courtesy of Daniel Luthringer, MD.)

REFERENCES

1. Aretz HT, Billingham ME, Edwards WD, et al. Myocarditis. A histopathologic definition and classification. *Am J Cardiovasc Pathol.* 1987;1:3–14.
2. Caforio AL, Marcolongo R, Basso C, Iliceto S. Clinical presentation and diagnosis of myocarditis. *Heart.* 2015;101:1332–1344.
3. Cooper LT, Baughman KL, Feldman AM, et al. The role of endomyocardial biopsy in the management of cardiovascular disease. *J Am Coll Cardiol.* 2007;50:1914–1931.
4. Pinto YM, Elliott PM, Arbustini E, et al. Proposal for a revised definition of dilated cardiomyopathy, hypokinetic non-dilated cardiomyopathy, and its implications for clinical practice. *Eur Heart J.* 2016;37:1850–1858.
5. Felker GM, Boehmer JP, Hruban RH, et al. Echocardiographic findings in fulminant and acute myocarditis. *J Am Coll Cardiol.* 2000;36:227–232.
6. Lieback E, Hardouin I, Meyer R, et al. Clinical value of echocardiographic tissue characterization in the diagnosis of myocarditis. *Eur Heart J.* 1996;17:135–142.
7. Agewall S, Beltrame JF, Reynolds HR, et al. ESC working group position paper on myocardial infarction with non-obstructive coronary arteries. *Eur Heart J.* 2017;38:143–153.
8. Budoff MJ, Gopal A, Gopalakrishnan D. Cardiac computed tomography: diagnostic utility and integration in clinical practice. *Clin Cardiol.* 2006;29:I4–I14.
9. Escher F, Westermann D, Gaub R, et al. Development of diastolic heart failure in a 6-year follow-up study in patients after acute myocarditis. *Heart.* 2011;97:709–714.
10. Gottdiener JS, Maron BJ, Schooley RT, et al. Two-dimensional echocardiographic assessment of the idiopathic hypereosinophilic syndrome. Anatomic basis of mitral regurgitation and peripheral embolization. *Circulation.* 1983;67:572–578.
11. Kim NK, Kim CY, Kim JH, et al. A hypereosinophilic syndrome with cardiac involvement from thrombotic stage to fibrotic stage. *J Cardiovasc Ultrasound.* 2015;23:100–102.
12. Ommen SR, Seward JB, Tajik AJ. Clinical and echocardiographic features of hypereosinophilic syndromes. *Am J Cardiol.* 2000;86:110–113.
13. Cervera R, Piette JC, Font J, et al. Antiphospholipid syndrome: clinical and immunologic manifestations and patterns of disease expression in a cohort of 1,000 patients. *Arthritis Rheum.* 2002;46:1019–1027.
14. Mohammed AG, Alghamdi AA, ALjahlan MA, Al-Homood IA. Echocardiographic findings in asymptomatic systemic lupus erythematosus patients. *Clin Rheumatol.* 2017;36:563–568.
15. Tincani A, Rebaioli CB, Taglietti M, Shoenfeld Y. Heart involvement in systemic lupus erythematosus, anti-phospholipid syndrome and neonatal lupus. *Rheumatology.* 2006;45(suppl 4). iv8–13.
16. Sengupta PP, Krishnamoorthy VK, Korinek J, et al. Left ventricular form and function revisited: applied translational science to cardiovascular ultrasound imaging. *J Am Soc Echocardiogr.* 2007;20:539–551.
17. Kalam K, Otahal P, Marwick TH. Prognostic implications of global LV dysfunction: a systematic review and meta-analysis of global longitudinal strain and ejection fraction. *Heart.* 2014;100:1673–1680.
18. Dattilo G, Lamari A, Zito C, et al. 2-Dimensional strain echocardiography and early detection of myocardial ischemia. *Int J Cardiol.* 2010;145. e6-8.
19. Ng AC, Sitges M, Pham PN, et al. Incremental value of 2-dimensional speckle tracking strain imaging to wall motion analysis for detection of coronary artery disease in patients undergoing dobutamine stress echocardiography. *Am Heart J.* 2009;158:836–844.
20. Motoki H, Borowski AG, Shrestha K, et al. Incremental prognostic value of assessing left ventricular myocardial mechanics in patients with chronic systolic heart failure. *J Am Coll Cardiol.* 2012;60:2074–2081.
21. Saito M, Khan F, Stoklosa T, et al. Prognostic implications of lv strain risk score in asymptomatic patients with hypertensive heart disease. *JACC Cardiovasc Imag.* 2016;9:911–921.
22. Sun JP, Xu T, Yang Y, et al. Layer-specific quantification of myocardial deformation may disclose the subclinical systolic dysfunction and the mechanism of preserved ejection fraction in patients with hypertension. *Int J Cardiol.* 2016;219:172–176.
23. Oikonomou EK, Kokkinidis DG, Kampaktsis PN, et al. Assessment of prognostic value of left ventricular global longitudinal strain for early prediction of chemotherapy-induced cardiotoxicity: a systematic review and meta-analysis. *JAMA Cardiol.* 2019;4:1007–1018.
24. Logstrup BB, Nielsen JM, Kim WY, Poulsen SH. Myocardial oedema in acute myocarditis detected by echocardiographic 2D myocardial deformation analysis. *Eur Heart J Cardiovasc Imag.* 2016;17:1018–1026.
25. Hsiao JF, Koshino Y, Bonnichsen CR, et al. Speckle tracking echocardiography in acute myocarditis. *Int J Cardiovasc Imag.* 2013;29:275–284.
26. Caforio AL, Pankuweit S, Arbustini E, et al. Current state of knowledge on aetiology, diagnosis, management, and therapy of myocarditis. *Eur Heart J.* 2013;34:2636–2648. 2648a-2648d.
27. Friedrich MG, Sechtem U, Schulz-Menger J, et al. Cardiovascular magnetic resonance in myocarditis: a JACC white paper. *J Am Coll Cardiol.* 2009;53:1475–1487.
28. Bami K, Haddad T, Dick A, et al. Noninvasive imaging in acute myocarditis. *Curr Opin Cardiol.* 2016;31:217–223.
29. Ferreira VM, Piechnik SK, Dall'Armellina E, et al. Native T1-mapping detects the location, extent and patterns of acute myocarditis without the need for gadolinium contrast agents. *J Cardiovasc Magn Reson.* 2014;16:36.
30. Luetkens JA, Homsi R, Dabir D, et al. Comprehensive cardiac magnetic resonance for short-term follow-up in acute myocarditis. *J Am Heart Assoc.* 2016;5.
31. Luetkens JA, Homsi R, Sprinkart AM, et al. Incremental value of quantitative CMR including parametric mapping for the diagnosis of acute myocarditis. *Eur Heart J Cardiovasc Imag.* 2016;17:154–161.
32. Messroghli DR, Moon JC, Ferreira VM, et al. Clinical recommendations for cardiovascular magnetic resonance mapping of T1, T2, T2* and extracellular volume. *J Cardiovasc Magn Reson.* 2017;19:75.
33. Messroghli DR, Pickardt T, Fischer M, et al. Toward evidence-based diagnosis of myocarditis in children and adolescents: rationale, design, and first baseline data of MYKKE, a multicenter registry and study platform. *Am Heart J.* 2017;187:133–144.
34. Aquaro GD, Perfetti M, Camastra G, et al. Cardiac MR with late gadolinium enhancement in acute myocarditis with preserved systolic function: ITAMY study. *J Am Coll Cardiol.* 2017;70:1977–1987.
35. Grani C, Eichhorn C, Biere L, et al. Prognostic value of cardiac magnetic resonance tissue characterization in risk stratifying patients with suspected myocarditis. *J Am Coll Cardiol.* 2017;70:1964–1976.
36. Pan JA, Lee YJ, Salerno M. Diagnostic performance of extracellular volume, native t1, and t2 mapping versus Lake Louise criteria by cardiac magnetic resonance for detection of acute myocarditis: a meta-analysis. *Circ Cardiovasc Imag.* 2018;11. e007598.
37. Puntmann VO, Zeiher AM, Nagel E. T1 and T2 mapping in myocarditis: seeing beyond the horizon of Lake Louise criteria and histopathology. *Expert Rev Cardiovasc Ther.* 2018;16:319–330.
38. Chow LH, Radio SJ, Sears TD, McManus BM. Insensitivity of right ventricular endomyocardial biopsy in the diagnosis of myocarditis. *J Am Coll Cardiol.* 1989;14:915–920.
39. Hauck AJ, Kearney DL, Edwards WD. Evaluation of postmortem endomyocardial biopsy specimens from 38 patients with lymphocytic myocarditis: implications for role of sampling error. *Mayo Clin Proc.* 1989;64:1235–1245.
40. Shirani J, Freant LJ, Roberts WC. Gross and semiquantitative histologic findings in mononuclear cell myocarditis causing sudden death, and implications for endomyocardial biopsy. *Am J Cardiol.* 1993;72:952–957.
41. Hahn EA, Hartz VL, Moon TE, et al. The myocarditis treatment trial: design, methods and patients enrollment. *Eur Heart J.* 1995;16(Suppl O):162–167.
42. Shanes JG, Ghali J, Billingham ME, et al. Interobserver variability in the pathologic interpretation of endomyocardial biopsy results. *Circulation.* 1987;75:401–405.

66

Dilated Cardiomyopathy: Etiology, Pathophysiology, and Echocardiographic Evaluation

Mayooran Namasivayam, Michael H. Picard

Dilated cardiomyopathy (DCM) is an important cause of heart failure worldwide. The annual global prevalence of DCM is estimated at 40 cases per 100,000 persons, and the annual incidence is estimated at 7 cases per 100,000 persons.[1] Approximately 10,000 deaths and 46,000 hospitalizations per year in the United States are attributed to DCM.[2] DCM is defined as ventricular dilatation and contractile dysfunction in the absence of abnormal loading conditions or severe coronary disease.[1,3] The condition can take a variable clinical course and can be managed with medical or device therapy; however, in refractory or progressive cases, advanced heart failure therapies, including mechanical ventricular support and cardiac transplantation, may need to be considered. Echocardiography forms the mainstay of diagnosis and surveillance. This chapter briefly reviews the cause and pathophysiology of DCM and outlines key echocardiographic features in patients with DCM.

CAUSE

DCM has a spectrum of causes (Table 66.1). Genetic abnormalities encompass defects in genes encoding a variety of subcellular structures and processes, which ultimately disrupt cellular force generation and transmission, structural integrity, ion transportation, nuclear functions, and intracellular signaling (Table 66.2).[4,5] Infectious causes can span viral, bacterial, fungal, parasitic, spirochetal, and protozoal disease.[3] Cardiac dysfunction can ensue from direct effects of infection or may result from secondary effects of the immune-mediated response to infection. Autoimmune disorders, including autoimmune myocarditis, can also result in DCM. Giant cell myocarditis represents a particularly aggressive disease that can lead to rapidly declining left ventricular (LV) systolic function.[1] Toxin-mediated DCM can result from prescription drugs, recreational drugs, or environmental exposures. Alcohol abuse is an important cause of DCM. Alcohol accounts for between one-fifth and one-third of all cases of DCM in developed countries.[6] Although the initial phase of infiltrative diseases such as sarcoidosis and hemochromatosis present with normal LV cavity size, as these diseases progress, they can transform into a DCM phenotype. Endocrinopathies, nutritional deficiency, electrolyte disturbance, and uremia are other systemic causes of DCM (see Table 66.1). DCM can also be seen in neuromuscular disease, pregnancy, and tachycardia. There can be challenges in identifying the cause when DCM phenotypes may overlap with features of other cardiomyopathies. Advanced hypertrophic cardiomyopathy, arrhythmogenic right ventricular (RV) cardiomyopathy (with LV involvement), LV noncompaction, athlete's heart, and cirrhotic cardiomyopathy can share features of DCM.[3]

PATHOPHYSIOLOGY

Regardless of the cause, the underlying pathophysiology of DCM follows a final common pathway of contractile dysfunction and LV dilatation. Reduction in contractility leads to both "forward" and "backward" heart failure states. Whereas the forward failure state results in low-output physiology, the backward failure state results in elevation of LV diastolic pressure, resulting in elevation in pulmonary venous and pulmonary arterial pressure (thereby causing pulmonary edema and elevated RV afterload). Disturbances in neurohumoral response, myocardial remodeling, peripheral vascular resistance, and cardiorenal balance can exacerbate the disease and lead to vicious cycles of declining cardiovascular function.[1,7] Dilatation of the left ventricle occurs to maintain adequate stroke volume in the presence of impaired myocardial contractility, by the Frank-Starling mechanism. As the left ventricle dilates, the papillary muscles are apically displaced, impairing the closing mechanism of the mitral valve. In combination with mitral annular dilatation, this leads to secondary mitral regurgitation, which further volume loads the left ventricle and impairs forward cardiac output.[3,8] Development of ventricular fibrosis leads to ventricular arrhythmic risk.[9–11] Systemic volume overload and mitral regurgitation result in left atrial dilatation and can lead to atrial fibrillation.[12] Atrial fibrillation can further exacerbate impairment of cardiovascular performance by eliminating a key mechanism of preload (atrial systole, or "atrial kick") in the setting of LV systolic impairment. Additionally, atrial fibrillation can exacerbate mitral annular dilatation and result in worsening of mitral regurgitation (atrial functional mitral regurgitation).[13,14]

Most causes of DCM create biventricular systolic impairment, but even those with a predominance of LV systolic dysfunction can create RV systolic impairment because of secondary effects on the pulmonary circulation.[15] Additionally, in the setting of a dilated left ventricle, with walls stretched, LV compliance is reduced. Hence, markers of diastolic dysfunction are commonly seen.[16] The cascade of effects described above lead to considerable morbidity, with symptomatic fluid overload and recurrent hospitalization, multiorgan dysfunction, arrhythmias, and premature mortality. Adequate recognition of the DCM phenotype and assessment of progress over time is crucial for optimal surveillance of the efficacy of medical and device therapy and the timing of advanced interventions.

ECHOCARDIOGRAPHIC FEATURES

Chamber Size

Echocardiography is a class I indicated diagnostic modality for the evaluation of DCM.[17] One of the defining features of DCM is LV dilatation. Worsening ventricular dilatation is a sign of clinical progression (Fig. 66.1 and Video 66.1). The standard measurement of LV end-diastolic diameter should be made consistently using the guideline recommended approach (perpendicular to the LV long axis and at the level of the tips of the mitral valve) to reliably monitor ventricular dimensions over time.[18] If endocardial definition permits, the LV end-systolic or end-diastolic volume by Simpson's

TABLE 66.1 Causes of Dilated Cardiomyopathy

Infectious	Toxins	Drugs
Viral	Amphetamines	*Antineoplastic Drugs*
Adenovirus	Carbon monoxide	Alkylating agents
Coxsackie A and B	Cobalt	Anthracyclines
Cytomegalovirus	Cocaine	Antimetabolites
Epstein-Barr	Ecstasy	Hypomethylating agents
Human herpes virus 6	Ethanol	Immunomodulating agents
Human immunodeficiency virus	Iron overload	Trastuzumab
Human papilloma virus 6	Lead	Paclitaxel
Parvovirus B19	Mercury	Tyrosine kinase inhibitors
Varicella		*Psychiatric Drugs*
Bacterial	**Endocrine Diseases**	Chlorpromazine
Brucellosis	Acromegaly	Clozapine
Diphtheria	Addison's disease	Lithium
Psittacosis	Cushing's disease	Methylphenidate
Typhoid fever	Diabetes mellitus	Olanzapine
Fungal	Hypothyroidism	Phenothiazines
Spirochetal	Hyperthyroidism	Risperidone
Borreliosis (Lyme disease)	Pheochromocytoma	*Other Drugs*
Leptospirosis (Weil disease)	Takotsubo cardiomyopathy	All-trans retinoic acid
Rickettsial		Antiretroviral agents
Protozoal	**Electrolyte Disturbances**	Chloroquine
Chagas disease	Hypocalcemia	
Schistosomiasis	Hypophosphatemia	**Genetic**
Toxoplasmosis		See Table 66.2
	Neuromuscular Diseases	
Autoimmune Diseases	Dystrophinopathies	**Other**
Churg-Strauss syndrome	Duchenne muscular dystrophy	Pregnancy
Giant cell myocarditis	Becker muscular dystrophy	Tachyarrhythmia
Granulomatosis with polyangiitis	X-linked dilated cardiomyopathy	
Noninfectious myocarditis	Emery-Dreifuss muscular dystrophy	
Polyarteritis nodosa	Facioscapulohumeral muscular dystrophy	
Polymyositis/dermatomyositis	Friedrich ataxia	
Systemic lupus erythematosus	Limb-girdle muscular dystrophy	
Sarcoidosis	Myotonic dystrophy	

TABLE 66.2 Genetic Causes of Dilated Cardiomyopathy

Structure	Function	Genes
Sarcomere	Force generation and transmission	*MYH6, MYH7, TPM1, ACTC1, TNNT2, TNNC1, TNNI3, MYBPC3, TTN, TNNI3K, MYL2, MYL3, MYLK2, MYOM1, MYOZ2*
Z disk	Mechanosensing and mechanosignaling	*ACTN2, BAG3, CRYAB, TCAP, MYPN, CSRP3, NEXN, FHL1, FHL2, ANKRD1, MURC, LDB3, NEBL*
Dystrophin complex	Sarcolemma, structural integrity	*DMD, DTNA, SGCA, SGCB, SGCD, SGCG, CAV3, ILK, FKTN, FKRP*
Cytoskeleton	Mechanotransduction, mechanosignaling and structural integrity	*DES, VCL, FLNC, SYNM, PDLIM3, PLEC1*
Desmosomes	Cell–cell adhesion, mechanotransmission, mechanosignaling	*DSC2, DSG2, DSP, PKP2, CTNNA3*
Sarcoplasmic reticulum and cytoplasm	Calcium homeostasis, contractility modulation, signalling	*PLN2, RYR2, CALR3, JOH2, DOLK, MAP2K, MAP2K2, NRAS, PRKAG2, PTPN11, RAF1, RIT1, SOS1, TRDN*
Nuclear envelope	Nuclear structural integrity, mechanotransduction, mechanosignaling	*LMNA, EMD, LAP2/TMPO, SYNE1/2*
Nucleus	Transcription cofactors, gene expression	*EYA4, FOXD4, HOPX, NFKB1, PRDM16, TBX20, ZBTB17, RBM20, GATA4, GATA6, GATAD1, NKX2-5, ALSM1, ALPK3, LRRC10, NPPA, PLEKHM2, TGFB3, TMEM43*
Ion channels	Conduction	*SCN5A, ABCC9, KCNQ1, CACNA1C, HCN4*
Mitochondria	Supply and regulation of energy metabolism	*CPT2, FRDA/FXN, DNAJC19, SDHA, SOD2, TAZ/G4.5, CTF1, mtDNA, TXNRD2*
Extracellular matrix	Cell adhesion and mechanosignaling	*LAMA2, LAMA4*
Other		*LAMP2, AGL, BRAF, GAA, GLA, PSEN1, PSEN2, CHRM2, HFE, HRAS, KRAS, MIB1, SLC22A5, TTR*

biplane method can permit an alternative and more accurate measure of chamber size. It is important to consider the patient's body size when determining ventricular dilatation; hence, measurements indexed to body surface area can be of particular value.[18] Finally, three-dimensional (3D) echocardiography (Fig. 66.2), which has comparable accuracy to cardiac magnetic resonance imaging for ventricular chamber volume quantification, will undoubtedly become the standard by which chamber size is quantified and monitored in future approaches.[19]

Systolic Function

Overall LV contractile function is traditionally measured using ejection fraction (EF), the ratio of stroke volume to LV end-diastolic volume. This is done based on a volumetric approach using the biplane method of disks (Simpson's rule).[18] Increasingly, 3D measurement can permit accurate determination of LVEF.[19] Although EF is a useful marker of systolic performance, it is important to remember its dependence on loading conditions, both preload and afterload.[20] EF is a marker of ventricular-load interaction rather than an independent marker of LV contractility per se.[21] Gold-standard markers of LV contractility, including end-systolic elastance and preload recruitable stroke work, are traditionally obtained invasively, but as 3D imaging quality improves, noninvasive or semiinvasive approaches will become more feasible. Evaluation of global and regional wall motion is an important part of evaluation. Although DCM traditionally is considered to cause global

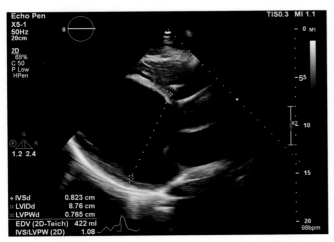

Figure 66.1. Dilated cardiomyopathy phenotype with significant ventricular dilatation as seen in the parasternal long-axis view. (See accompanying Video 66.1.)

wall motion abnormality, regional variation can occur. For instance, inferolateral regional hypokinesis or akinesis has been observed in muscular dystrophy–associated DCM and acute myocarditis.[3]

When endocardial border definition is difficult to define because of challenging imaging windows, the use of ultrasound-enhancing agents (echocardiographic contrast) can be extremely valuable (Fig. 66.3 and Video 66.3). Echocardiographic contrast can allow better visualization of left and RV endocardium and hence permit more accurate quantification of dimensions and systolic function.[22] In addition, contrast can help diagnose LV thrombus (see Secondary Findings).

The advent of myocardial strain quantification through deformation imaging has provided an enhanced means of assessing systolic performance.[23] The most robust of these strain techniques has been the global longitudinal strain (GLS) assessment (Fig. 66.4), which has been of particular value in determining subclinical LV dysfunction that might be missed by traditional echocardiographic assessment. The lower limit of normal for LV GLS is generally considered to be −18%.[23] Strain quantification has particular value in cardio-oncology for monitoring of chemotherapeutic cardiac toxicity and screening family members of patients with DCM for subclinical LV systolic dysfunction. Additional strain modalities include assessing strain at different myocardial layers (subendocardial, midmyocardial, and epicardial), radial and circumferential strain, and 3D strain. Despite the promise of strain imaging and its inevitable inclusion into routine echocardiographic assessment, it should be noted that strain assessment has shown considerable intervendor variability and even intravendor variability as software versions vary. Similar to EF, strain parameters are also subject to the confounding effect of loading conditions.[23,24]

There has been increasing value placed upon the importance of RV function in DCM. Quantification of RV function is of particular importance in patients with DCM being considered for isolated LV mechanical support with durable or percutaneous LV assist devices.[25]

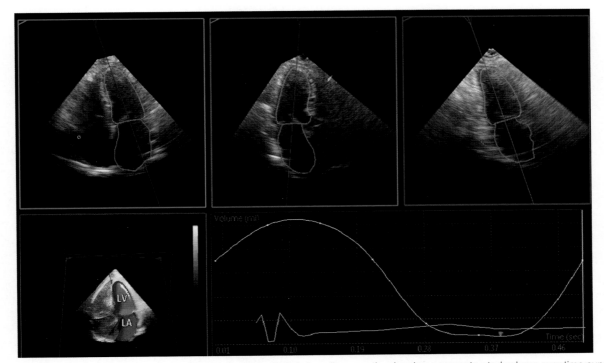

Figure 66.2. Three-dimensional quantitative volumetric imaging of dilated cardiomyopathy showing a reconstructed volume over time curve *(bottom right panel)* constructed from endocardial border tracking as displayed in the apical four- *(top left)*, three- *(top middle)*, and two- *(top right)* chamber views.

Secondary Findings

As discussed in the Pathophysiology section, in addition to LV dilation and contractile dysfunction, DCM leads to a number of secondary phenomena that can be observed on echocardiography. Secondary mitral regurgitation (Fig. 66.5 and Video 66.5), resulting from apical papillary muscle displacement and annular dilatation, is an important cause of adverse prognosis in DCM.[3,8,26] There is randomized, controlled trial evidence that supports intervention in secondary mitral regurgitation using transcatheter edge-to-edge mitral valve repair (mortality benefit).[27] Careful attention to mechanism and severity of mitral regurgitation and evaluation of potential exclusion criteria, including severe LV dilatation, RV dysfunction, pulmonary hypertension, and severe tricuspid regurgitation, are now crucial for echocardiographic assessment. Furthermore, consideration should be given for the role of transcatheter mitral repair, in comparison with or alongside mechanical circulatory supports, with individualized clinical decision making incorporating a team-based approach considering all the available options.

Severe LV dilatation and contractile dysfunction creates a nidus for LV mural thrombus (Fig. 66.6 and Video 66.6). This can be seen on standard two-dimensional imaging but can be better defined with echocardiographic contrast administration.

Atrial dilatation can follow LV dysfunction.[12] There has been increasing appreciation of the role of atrial function in DCM. Newer techniques for assessing atrial dimensions and function, including atrial strain, may permit better insights into pathophysiology and prognosis.[28]

Guidance of Therapy

In DCM, echocardiography plays a crucial role in the guidance of medical, device, interventional transcatheter, and surgical therapies. Assessment of reverse remodeling (typically assessed by reduction in LV volume and improvement in systolic function)[29] can be extremely valuable in potentially reversible DCM phenotypes, such as alcoholic cardiomyopathy. Even in cases with clinical progression, monitoring of medical therapy that can attenuate ventricular functional decline is valuable. LVEF of 35% or less is currently a central basis upon which decisions to implant cardioverter-defibrillator systems are made.[30] In addition to guiding transcatheter mitral valve repair (see Secondary Findings), transcatheter mitral valve replacement[31] and tricuspid valve intervention[32] are taking increasing roles in patients with heart failure, necessitating transthoracic and transesophageal echocardiographic (TEE) assessment. Echocardiographic assessment plays a vital role in determining timing of advanced heart failure therapy workup, including consideration of cardiac transplantation.[33] In patients with severe LV dysfunction and interventricular conduction delay (currently defined as left bundle branch block with QRS duration ≥150 ms) cardiac resynchronization therapy (CRT) can play a vital role. Although selection for therapy has been shown to be more robust in determining CRT indication using electrocardiographic

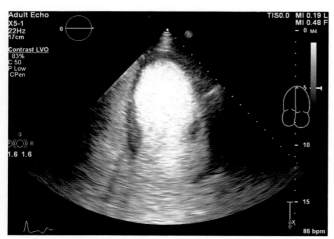

Figure 66.3. Ultrasound-enhancing agent assisting with endocardial border definition in dilated cardiomyopathy. (See accompanying Video 66.3.)

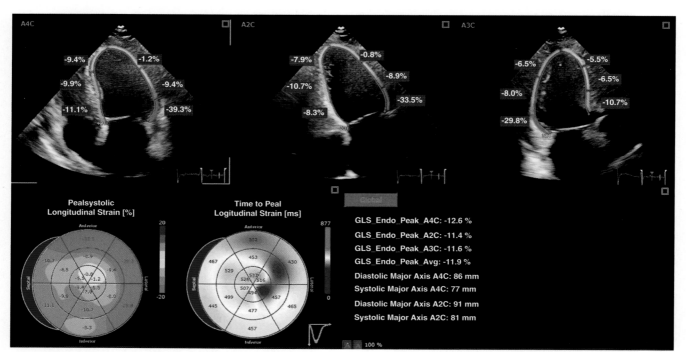

Figure 66.4. Strain imaging in dilated cardiomyopathy constructed from endocardial speckle tracking in the apical four- (top left), two- (top middle) and three- (top right) chamber views and resultant global and regional longitudinal strain and times to peak strain (bottom panels).

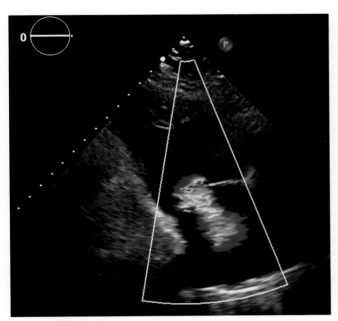

Figure 66.5. Secondary mitral regurgitation in dilated cardiomyopathy. (See accompanying Video 66.5.)

rather than echocardiographic features of dyssynchrony,[34] there remains some evidence for additional value gained by echocardiographic assessment before CRT.[35]

COMPLEMENTARY ROLE OF ALTERNATIVE MODALITIES

Although echocardiography is the most cost efficient and widely applicable method for evaluating DCM, the complementary roles of alternative diagnostic modalities should be recognized. Cardiac magnetic resonance imaging (CMRI) can provide accurate ventricular volumes, albeit this advantage of CMRI will be less relevant as 3D echocardiography technology improves. CMRI also provides valuable information about tissue characterization, including scar, by gadolinium contrast injection, and acute inflammation, from T1 and T2 mapping.[3] Fibrosis characterization on CMRI can provide additional information regarding cause and prognosis.[3,11] Positron emission tomography can be of particular value in identifying cardiac sarcoid and can also be helpful in evaluating coronary microvascular dysfunction.[36] Finally, when diagnoses are unclear, or sinister pathologies (e.g., giant cell myocarditis) need exclusion in critically ill patients, endomyocardial biopsy can be highly valuable.[1,3] Here, too, echocardiography can play a role in the guidance of safe biopsy from the interventricular septum.

FUTURE DIRECTIONS

As echocardiography technology continues to develop, the ability to better characterize the DCM phenotype will undoubtedly improve. 3D volumetric analysis will permit better assessment of chamber size and systolic function. Advanced strain methods will provide earlier detection of myocardial dysfunction. Intracardiac vortex imaging will provide detailed characterization of flow patterns, which might serve to enhance understanding of ventricular function, predisposition to thrombus, and effects of geometric change caused by ventricular dilatation. The dramatic advancements in machine learning can help enrich understanding of clinical progress in DCM, will also assist with automated chamber quantification and function assessment, and will help classify phenotypes.[37] TEE will also take on an increasingly important role in DCM for patients being considered for transcatheter interventions

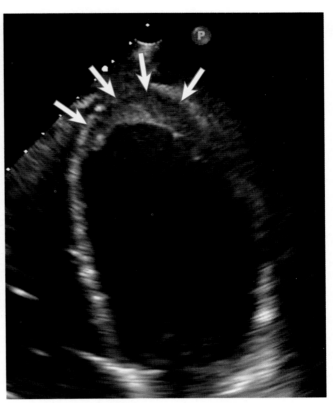

Figure 66.6. Left ventricular mural thrombus in dilated cardiomyopathy. *Arrows* show the endocardial border, with layered thrombus at the apex within the left ventricular cavity. (See accompanying Video 66.6.)

to the mitral and tricuspid valves. TEE will be important in patient selection, intraprocedural guidance, and postprocedure assessment.

CONCLUSION

DCM is an important cause of heart failure globally. Echocardiography plays a vital role in diagnosis, surveillance and monitoring, and guidance of therapy. Quantification of chamber size, systolic function, and secondary effects on the mitral valve, atria, and right heart are crucial. The advent and wider application of 3D technology, strain imaging, and ultrasound-enhancing agents will help advance the assessment of DCM. Novel techniques, including intracardiac vortex imaging and the increased application of machine learning approaches, will serve to further enhance the assessment of DCM.

ACKNOWLEDGMENT

The authors acknowledge the contributions of Dmitry Kireyev, MD, and Timothy C. Tan, MD, who were authors of this chapter in the previous edition.

Please access ExpertConsult to view the corresponding videos for this chapter.

REFERENCES

1. Weintraub RG, Semsarian C, Macdonald P. Dilated cardiomyopathy. *Lancet.* 2017;390:400–414.
2. Manolio TA, Baughman KL, Rodeheffer R, et al. Prevalence and etiology of idiopathic dilated cardiomyopathy. *Am J Cardiol.* 1992;69:1458–1466.
3. Japp AG, Gulati A, Cook SA, et al. The diagnosis and evaluation of dilated cardiomyopathy. *J Am Coll.* 2016;67:2996–3010.
4. McNally EM, Mestroni L. Dilated cardiomyopathy: genetic determinants and mechanisms. *Circ Res.* 2017;121:731–748.

5. Herschberger RE, Hedges DJ, Morales A. Dilated cardiomyopathy: the complexity of a diverse genetic architecture. *Nat Rev Cardiol*. 2013;10:531–547.

6. Laonigro I, Correale M, Di Biase M, et al. Alcohol abuse and heart failure. *Eur J Heart Fail*. 2009;11:453–462.

7. Opie LH, Commerford PJ, Gersh BJ, et al. Controversies in ventricular remodelling. *Lancet*. 2006;367:356–367.

8. Rossi A, Dini FL, Faggiano, et al. Independent prognostic value of functional mitral regurgitation in patients with heart failure. A quantitative analysis of 1256 patients with ischaemic and nonischaemic dilated cardiomyopathy. *Heart*. 2011;97:1675–1680.

9. de Leeuw N, Ruiter DJ, Balk AH, et al. Histopathologic findings in explanted heart tissue from patients with end-stage idiopathic dilated cardiomyopathy. *Transpl Int*. 2001;14:299–306.

10. Iles L, Pfluger H, Lefkovits L, et al. Myocardial fibrosis predicts appropriate device therapy in patients with implantable cardioverter-defibrillators for primary prevention of sudden cardiac death. *J Am Coll Cardiol*. 2011;57:821–828.

11. Gulati A, Jabbour A, Ismail TF, et al. Association of fibrosis with mortality and sudden cardiac death in patients with nonischemic dilated cardiomyopathy. *J Am Med Assoc*. 2013;309:896–908.

12. Gulati A, Ismail TF, Jabbour A, et al. Clinical utility and prognostic value of left atrial volume assessment by cardiovascular magnetic resonance in non-ischaemic dilated cardiomyopathy. *Eur J Heart Fail*. 2013;15:660–670.

13. Deferm S, Bertrand PB, Verburgge FH, et al. Atrial functional mitral regurgitation. *J Am Coll Cardiol*. 2019;73, 2465–2476.

14. Muraru D, Guta A, Ochoa-Jimenez RC, et al. Functional regurgitation of atrioventricular valves and atrial fibrillation: an elusive pathophysiological link deserving further attention. *J Am Soc Echocardiogr*. 2020;33:42–53.

15. Gulati A, Ismail TF, Jabbour A, et al. The prevalence and prognostic significance of right ventricular systolic dysfunction in nonischemic dilated cardiomyopathy. *Circulation*. 2013;128:1623–1633.

16. Nagueh S, Smiseth OA, Appleton CP, et al. Recommendations for the evaluation of left ventricular diastolic function by echocardiography. *J Am Soc Echocardiogr*. 2016;29:277–314.

17. Yancy C, Jessup M, Bozkurt B, et al. ACCF/AHA guideline for the management of heart failure: Executive summary. *J Am Coll Cardiol*. 2013;62:1495–1539. 2013.

18. Lang RM, Badano LP, Mor-Avi V, et al. Recommendations for cardiac chamber quantification by echocardiography in adults. *J Am Soc Echocardiogr*. 2015;29:1–39.

19. Dorosz J, Lezotte DC, Weitzenkamp DA, et al. Performance of 3-dimensional echocardiography in measuring left ventricular volumes and ejection fraction: a systematic review and meta-analysis. *J Am Coll Cardiol*. 2012;59. 1799–808.

20. Konstam MA, Abboud FM. Ejection fraction: misunderstood and overrated (changing the paradigm of categorizing heart failure). *Circulation*. 2017;135:717–719.

21. Namasivayam M, Hayward CS, Muller DWM, et al. Ventricular-vascular coupling ratio is the ejection fraction in disguise. *J Am Soc Echocardiogr*. 2019;32:791.

22. Porter TR, Mulvagh S, Abdelmoneim SS, et al. Clinical applications of ultrasonic enhancing agents in echocardiography: 2018 American Society of Echocardiography guidelines update. *J Am Soc Echocardiogr*. 2018;31:241–274.

23. Marwick TH, Shah SJ, Thomas JD. Myocardial strain in the assessment of patients with heart failure: a review. *JAMA Cardiol*. 2019;4:287–294.

24. Fredholm M, Jorgensen K, Houltz E, et al. Load-dependence of myocardial deformation variables—a clinical strain-echocardiographic study. *Acta Anaesth Scand*. 2017;61:1155–1165.

25. Hayek S, Sims DB, Markham DW, et al. Assessment of right ventricular function in left ventricular assist device candidates. *Circ Cardiovasc Imag*. 2014;7:379–389.

26. Ciarka A, Van de Viere N. Secondary mitral regurgitation: pathophysiology, diagnosis and treatment. *Heart*. 2011;97:1012–1023.

27. Stone GW, Lindenfeld, Abraham WT, et al. Transcatheter mitral-valve repair in patients with heart failure. *N Engl J Med*. 2018;379:2307–2318.

28. Kurzawski J, Janion-Sadowska A, Gackowski A, et al. Left atrial longitudinal strain in dilated cardiomyopathy patients: is there a discrimination threshold for atrial fibrillation? *Int J Cardiovasc Imaging*. 2019;35:319–325.

29. Merlo M, Cannata A, Gobbo M, et al. Evolving concepts in dilated cardiomyopathy. *Eur J Heart Fail*. 2018;20:228–239.

30. Moss AJ, Zareba W, Hall WJ, et al. Prophylactic implantation of a defibrillator in patients with myocardial infarction and reduced ejection fraction. *N Eng J Med*. 2002;346:877–883.

31. Regueiro A, Granada JF, Dagenais F, et al. Transcatheter mitral valve replacement: insights from early clinical experience and future challenges. *J Am Coll Cardiol*. 2017;69:2175–2192.

32. Asmarats L, Puri R, Latib A, et al. Transcatheter tricuspid valve interventions. *J Am Coll Cardiol*. 2019;71:2935–2956.

33. Costanzo MR, Augustine S, Bourge R, et al. Selection and treatment of candidates for heart transplantation. *Circulation*. 1995;92:3593–3612.

34. Ruschitzka F, Abraham WT, Singh JP, et al. Cardiac-resynchronization therapy in heart failure with a narrow QRS complex. *N Eng J Med*. 2013;369:1395–1405.

35. Stankovic I, Prinz C, Ciarka A, et al. Relationship of visually assessed apical rocking and septal flash to response and long-term survival following cardiac resynchronization therapy. *Eur Heart J Cardiovasc Imaging*. 2016;17:262–269.

36. Neglia D. Positron emission tomography: an additional prognostic tool in dilated cardiomyopathy? *J Nuc Cardiol*. 2016;23:768–772.

37. Przewlocka-Kosmala M, Marwick TH, Dabrowski A, et al. Contribution of cardiovascular reserve to prognostic categories of heart failure with preserved ejection fraction: a classification based on machine learning. *J Am Soc Echocardiogr*. 2019;32:604–615.

67 Echocardiographic Predictors of Outcome in Patients With Dilated Cardiomyopathy

Federico M. Asch, Neil J. Weissman

As the burden of heart failure (HF) and cardiomyopathies continues to rise, the clinical need for early detection of individuals at risk becomes critical. Identification of patients with a poor prognosis allows for early interventions (primary prevention, medications, devices) that can dramatically change the course of their disease by improving quality of life and prolonging survival. Multiple predictors of outcomes in this population have been described (Table 67.1). Although traditional clinical variables and biomarkers have been used to risk-stratify,[1,2] the addition of echocardiographic variables to clinical evaluation has shown to be of significant value.[3]

The role of cardiac imaging modalities, particularly echocardiography, has been expanding over the past decade. Historically used solely to diagnose cardiomyopathies and assess their severity, echocardiography's role in early detection, prevention, and prognostication is now well established.[4] The importance of a comprehensive echocardiographic evaluation to understand the underlying cause of the dilated cardiomyopathy (DCM; valvular, ischemic, idiopathic) cannot be overemphasized and certainly plays a role in estimating patient's prognosis. This chapter focuses on the specific variables linked to prognostic assessment. Details on echocardiographic findings for specific causes can be found in different sections of this book.

LEFT VENTRICULAR EJECTION FRACTION AND DIMENSIONS

Left ventricular ejection fraction (LVEF) is the most powerful predictor of death and cardiovascular events in patients with DCM. Quinones and colleagues demonstrated in the SOLVD trial that the mortality rate at 1 year was higher in those with LVEF below 35% (Fig. 67.1), a finding that has consistently been verified in the literature.[5] Although multiple thresholds have been evaluated, the overall concept is that prognosis worsens as LVEF decreases, even within patients with severe left ventricular (LV) dysfunction.[6] This finding holds true despite the method of evaluation of LVEF, including two-dimensional (2D) biplane Simpson's method of disks (Fig. 67.2) and three-dimensional echocardiography (Fig. 67.3).[7,8]

TABLE 67.1 Predictors of Poor Outcomes in Patients With Dilated Cardiomyopathy

Clinical predictors	Older age
	Poor functional capacity (NYHA, 6-min walk test, VO₂ max)
	S3
	Cardiac cachexia
	Poor perfusion (e.g., cold extremities, low urine output, altered mentation)
	Recurrent HF decompensation
	LBBB
	Atrial fibrillation
Biomarkers	Elevated BNP
	Hyponatremia
	BUN and creatinine (cardiorenal syndrome)
	AST, ALT, and PT (liver dysfunction)
Echocardiographic predictors	Low LVEF
	LV remodeling (large ESV, EDV)
	LV mass
	Enlarged LA (LA volume)
	Diastolic dysfunction
	Dyssynchrony
	Pulmonary hypertension
	RV dysfunction
	Severe MR
	Severe TR
	Myocardial ischemia and viability

ALT, Alanine aminotransferase; *AST,* aspartate aminotransferase; *BNP,* brain natriuretic peptide; *BUN,* blood urea nitrogen; *EDV,* end-diastolic volume; *ESV,* end-systolic volume; *HF,* heart failure; *LA,* left atrial; *LBBB,* left bundle branch block; *LV,* left ventricular; *LVEF,* left ventricular ejection fraction; *MR,* mitral regurgitation; *NYHA,* New York Heart Association; *PT,* prothrombin time; *RV,* right ventricular; *TR,* tricuspid regurgitation; *VO₂ max,* maximal oxygen uptake.

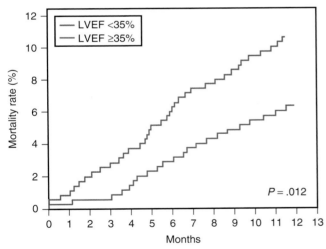

Figure 67.1. All-cause mortality according to left ventricular ejection fraction (LVEF) in the Studies of Left Ventricular Dysfunction (SOLVD) trial. (Reproduced with permission from Quinones MA, et al: Echocardiographic predictors of clinical outcome in patients with left ventricular dysfunction enrolled in the SOLVD registry and trials: significance of left ventricular hypertrophy, *J Am Coll Cardiol.* 35:1237–1244, 2000.)

LV mass has predictive value independent from other clinical variables and is additive to LVEF. In the Studies of Left Ventricular Dysfunction (SOLVD) trial and registry, patients with LVEF below 35% and LV mass greater than 298 g had the highest mortality rate.[5] Similarly, patients with larger end-systolic and end-diastolic volumes

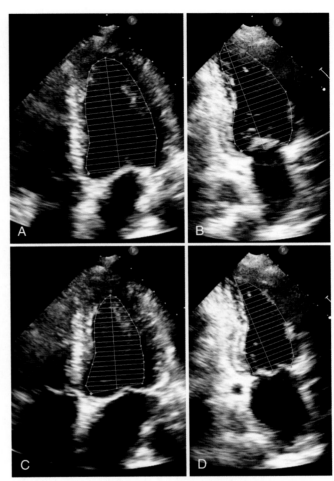

Figure 67.2. Left ventricular volumes and ejection fraction evaluation by biplane method of disks. Manual tracing of endocardial border is performed at end-systole (**C** and **D**) and diastole (**A** and **B**) in the apical two- and four-chamber views. The method uses calculation of volume of 20 disks of equal thickness to estimate ventricular volumes. The length of the left ventricle is critical for this calculation; therefore, avoiding foreshortening of the left ventricle becomes critical for its accuracy.

are at higher risks of death and cardiovascular events. However, given the close relationship with LVEF, its independent value is more difficult to prove. Reverse LV remodeling (defined as an increase in LVEF or decrease in LV diastolic dimensions) resulting from optimal medical therapy in patients with DCM has shown to predict better outcomes (specifically mortality and need for heart transplantation).[9]

LEFT VENTRICULAR DIASTOLIC DYSFUNCTION

The comprehensive evaluation of diastolic function requires recordings of flow through the mitral and tricuspid valves and pulmonary veins, tissue Doppler of the mitral annulus and left atrial (LA) size.[10] Consistently, these variables have been related to incident HF in patients with preserved HF and to increased mortality in patients with DCM. For example, analysis of the Cardiovascular Health Study shows that an E/A ratio greater than 1.5 or less than 0.7 has a high specificity in predicting development of HF during follow-up.[11] However, given the low positive predictive value and sensitivity, this information is not useful for screening purposes. Similar results were obtained from a population-based study of Olmstead County in which diastolic function evaluation included mitral inflow E and A velocities and deceleration time[12] and when LA volume, pulmonary vein flow, and tissue Doppler velocities of the mitral annulus (E/e′ ratio) were included.[13]

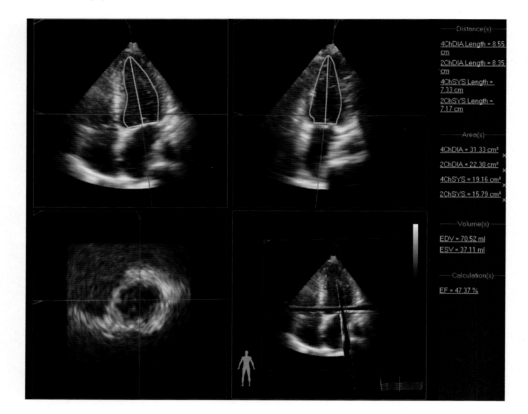

Figure 67.3. The advantage of this method over two-dimensional method of disks is that avoids foreshortening and that it uses an automated border detection that improves reproducibility.

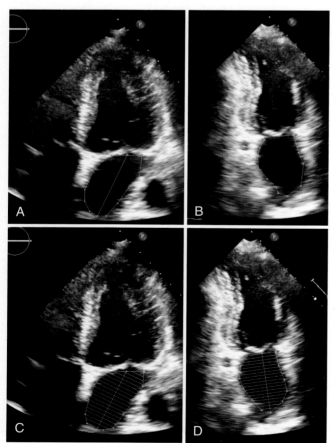

Figure 67.4. Left atrial (LA) volume evaluation. The area length method (**A** and **B**) or Simpson's method of disks (**C** and **D**) is preferred for LA volume calculation. These two methods have high agreement, as in the case illustrated, in which LA volume was 24 mL by both methods. In both cases, the maximal LA volume should be measured by tracing the LA border in four- and two- chamber views at end of ventricular systole (end of T wave on electrocardiogram or just before mitral valve opening), starting at the mitral annular level and excluding the LA appendage and pulmonary veins.

LEFT ATRIAL SIZE

Although initial reports on the clinical significance of LA size used LA dimensions by 2D or M-mode echocardiography, it is now well recognized that the morphology of the LA is asymmetric (particularly when enlarged), and therefore a single dimension is unreliable. Recent reports showed the increased accuracy and predictive value of using LA volume by biplane evaluation over LA area or dimensions.[14] LA size is a predictor of HF in patients with preserved LVEF.[15,16] Moreover, although associated with LV remodeling and diastolic dysfunction, the maximal volume of the LA has an independent and incremental prognostic value in patients with DCM[17] and in those with prior myocardial infarction.[18] It is important to note that the maximal LA volume should be measured by tracing the LA border in the four- and two-chamber views at end ventricular systole (end of T wave on the electrocardiogram [ECG] or just before mitral valve opening), starting at the mitral annular level and excluding the LA appendage and pulmonary veins (Fig. 67.4).[8]

SECONDARY MITRAL REGURGITATION

In patients with cardiomyopathy, the presence of significant secondary (functional) mitral regurgitation (MR) carries a poor prognosis, independent of other clinical and echocardiographic characteristics such as low EF and dilated ventricles.[19,20] In the recent Cardiovascular Outcomes Assessment of the MitraClip Percutaneous Therapy for Heart Failure Patients With Functional Mitral Regurgitation (COAPT) and Percutaneous Repair with the MitraClip Device for Severe Functional/Secondary Mitral Regurgitation (MITRA-FR) trials, echocardiography has played a pivotal role in selecting, among patients with cardiomyopathy and moderate to severe or severe secondary MR, patients who would[21] or would not[22] benefit from percutaneous mitral repair. In COAPT, markers of poor prognosis at 2 years were identified.[23] For patients receiving guideline-directed medical therapy, higher pulmonary systolic pressure, lower LVEF, worse TR severity, and worse MR severity (Effective Regurgitant Orifice Area (EROA) by proximal Isovelocity Surface Area (PISA)) were all independent predictors of mortality or HF hospitalizations within 2 years; for patients receiving the MitraClip, however, only the preimplant pulmonary systolic pressure remained a significant predictor. These data highlight how newer technologies are changing the prognosis of patients with HF and the importance of an in-depth echocardiographic evaluation for patient selection and prognostic assessment.

OTHER VARIABLES: MYOCARDIAL VIABILITY, ISCHEMIA, AND DYSSYNCHRONY

In patients with ischemic cardiomyopathy enrolled in the STICH trial, the absence of myocardial viability was associated with a higher risk of death. However, this trial failed to demonstrate that the presence of viability could identify patients who would benefit from coronary revascularization.[6] The recently published 10-year follow-up results of the STICH trial viability substudy showed that the presence of viability predicted an improvement in LVEF, regardless of the treatment arm (coronary artery bypass graft surgery or optimal medical therapy) to which patients were randomized.[24] However, such improvement in LV function was not associated with better long-term outcomes. Myocardial viability testing is discussed in more detail in Chapter 54 within the stress echocardiography section. On a similar analysis, the presence or absence of myocardial ischemia failed to identify patients at higher risk and patients to benefit from revascularization.[25]

The presence of LV dyssynchrony by ECG (left bundle branch block) is linked to worse prognosis in patients with depressed LVEF, and this understanding forms the basis for the indication for cardiac resynchronization therapy (CRT). More recently, efforts have been made to expand this concept by using echocardiography as a more sensitive tool to detect dyssynchrony. Although single-center studies described a multitude of parameters based on M-mode, spectral Doppler, color M-Mode, and tissue Doppler imaging,[26] their analysis has been difficult to reproduce in clinical practice and even failed to prove its utility in PROSPECT (Predictors of Response to CRT), a large multicenter trial using central readings in core laboratories.[27] Therefore, echocardiographic parameters are not currently recommended for selection of patients to receive CRT.[28,29]

REFERENCES

1. Hillege HL, Girbes AR, de Kam PJ, et al. Renal function, neurohormonal activation, and survival in patients with chronic heart failure. *Circulation.* 2000;102:203–210.
2. Likoff MJ, Chandler SL, Kay HR. Clinical determinants of mortality in chronic congestive heart failure secondary to idiopathic dilated or to ischemic cardiomyopathy. *Am J Cardiol.* 1987;59:634–638.
3. Tsang TS, Barnes ME, Gersh BJ, et al. Prediction of risk for first age-related cardiovascular events in an elderly population: the incremental value of echocardiography. *J Am Coll Cardiol.* 2003;42:1199–1205.
4. Tsang TS. Echocardiography in cardiovascular public health: the Feigenbaum Lecture 2008. *J Am Soc Echocardiogr.* 2009;22:649–656. quiz 751.
5. Quinones MA, Greenberg BH, Kopelen HA, et al. Echocardiographic predictors of clinical outcome in patients with left ventricular dysfunction enrolled in the SOLVD registry and trials: significance of left ventricular hypertrophy. *J Am Coll Cardiol.* 2000;35:1237–1244.
6. Bonow RO, Maurer G, Lee KL, et al. Myocardial viability and survival in ischemic left ventricular dysfunction. *N Engl J Med.* 2011;364:1617–1625.
7. Hung J, Lang R, Flachskampf F, et al. 3D echocardiography: a review of the current status and future directions. *J Am Soc Echocardiogr.* 2007;20:213–233.
8. Lang RM, Bierig M, Devereux RB, et al. Recommendations for chamber quantification. *J Am Soc Echocardiogr.* 2005;18:1440–1463.
9. Merlo M, Pyxaras SA, Pinamonti B, et al. Prevalence and prognostic significance of left ventricular reverse remodeling in dilated cardiomyopathy receiving tailored medical treatment. *J Am Coll Cardiol.* 2011;57:1468–1476.
10. Nagueh SF, Appleton CP, Gillebert TC, et al. Recommendations for the evaluation of left ventricular diastolic function by echocardiography. *J Am Soc Echocardiogr.* 2009;22:107–133.
11. Aurigemma GP, Gottdiener JS, Shemanski L, et al. Predictive value of systolic and diastolic function for incident congestive heart failure in the elderly: the cardiovascular health study. *J Am Coll Cardiol.* 2001;37:1042–1048.
12. Tsang TS, Barnes ME, Gersh BJ, et al. Risks for atrial fibrillation and congestive heart failure in patients >/=65 years of age with abnormal left ventricular diastolic relaxation. *Am J Cardiol.* 2004;93:54–58.
13. Al-Omari MA, Barnes ME, Fatema K, et al. Combining E/e' and indexed left atrial volume augments clinical prediction of first heart failure in elderly. *Circulation.* 2008;118(S):841.
14. Tsang TS, Abhayaratna WP, Barnes ME, et al. Prediction of cardiovascular outcomes with left atrial size: is volume superior to area or diameter? *J Am Coll Cardiol.* 2006;47:1018–1023.
15. Gottdiener JS, Kitzman DW, Aurigemma GP, et al. Left atrial volume, geometry, and function in systolic and diastolic heart failure of persons > or =65 years of age (the cardiovascular health study). *Am J Cardiol.* 2006;97:83–89.
16. Takemoto Y, Barnes ME, Seward JB, et al. Usefulness of left atrial volume in predicting first congestive heart failure in patients > or = 65 years of age with well-preserved left ventricular systolic function. *Am J Cardiol.* 2005;96:832–836.
17. Rossi A, Cicoira M, Zanolla L, et al. Determinants and prognostic value of left atrial volume in patients with dilated cardiomyopathy. *J Am Coll Cardiol.* 2002;40:1425.
18. Moller JE, Hillis GS, Oh JK, et al. Left atrial volume: a powerful predictor of survival after acute myocardial infarction. *Circulation.* 2003;107:2207–2212.
19. Rossi A, Dini FL, Faggiano P, et al. Independent prognostic value of functional mitral regurgitation in patients with heart failure. *Heart.* 2011;97:1675–1680.
20. Sannino A, Smith RL, Schiattarella GG, et al. Survival and cardiovascular outcomes of patients with secondary mitral regurgitation: a systematic review and meta-analysis. *JAMA Cardiol.* 2017;2:1130–1139.
21. Stone GW, Lindenfeld J, Abraham WT, et al. Transcatheter mitral-valve repair in patients with heart failure. *N Engl J Med.* 2018;379:2307–2318.
22. Obadia JF, Messika-Zeitoun D, Leurent G, et al. Percutaneous repair or medical treatment for secondary mitral regurgitation. *N Engl J Med.* 2018;379:2297–2306.
23. Asch FM, Grayburn PA, Siegel RJ, et al. Echocardiographic outcomes after transcatheter leaflet approximation in patients with secondary mitral regurgitation: the COAPT trial. *J Am Coll Cardiol.* 2019;74:2969–2979.
24. Panza JA, Ellis AM, Al-Khalidi HR, et al. Myocardial viability and long-term outcomes in ischemic cardiomyopathy. *N Engl J Med.* 2019;381:739–748.
25. Panza JA, Holly TA, Asch FM, et al. Inducible myocardial ischemia and outcomes in patients with coronary artery disease and left ventricular dysfunction. *J Am Coll Cardiol.* 2013;61:1860–1870.
26. Gorcsan J, Abraham T, Agler DA, et al. Echocardiography for cardiac resynchronization therapy: recommendations for performance and reporting. *J Am Soc Echocardiogr.* 2008;21:191–213.
27. Chung ES, Leon AR, Tavazzi L, et al. Results of the predictors of response to CRT. *Circulation.* 2008;117:2608–2616.
28. Brignole M, Auricchio A, Baron-Esquivias G, et al. ESC Guidelines on cardiac pacing and cardiac resynchronization therapy. *Eur Heart J.* 2013;34:2281–2329. 2013.
29. Tracy CM, Epstein AE, Darbar D, et al. ACCF/AHA/HRS focused update of the 2008 guidelines for device-based therapy of cardiac rhythm abnormalities. *Circulation.* 2012;126:1784–1800. 2012.

68 Right Ventricle in Dilated Cardiomyopathy

Nowell M. Fine, Shawn C. Pun, Lawrence G. Rudski

Dilated cardiomyopathy (DCM) encompasses a wide range of conditions in which the primary disorder is the enlargement of the ventricular chambers with normal left ventricular (LV) wall thickness, which ultimately leads to reduced LV contractile function and symptoms of heart failure.[1] Both ischemic and nonischemic causes of DCM are discussed in this chapter.

Although the prevalence of right ventricular (RV) dysfunction in patients with idiopathic DCM is variable and has been reported in as many as 65% of patients,[2] a recent cardiac magnetic resonance imaging (CMRI) study in a similar population found a prevalence of 34% using an RV ejection fraction (EF) cutoff of 45%.[3] A study of a mixed ischemic and nonischemic heart failure population with New York Heart Association (NYHA) functional class II to III symptoms identified RV dysfunction in 51% of patients using multiple echocardiographic variables.[4] Similarly, a study using gated-equilibrium radionuclide ventriculography found 52% of patients with RVEF 39% or less.[5]

Impaired RV function carries substantial prognostic significance and predicts cardiovascular death and hospitalization in patients with reduced LV systolic function.[6] It is also a predictor of impaired exercise tolerance and functional capacity,[7] cardiac cachexia, low body weight,[4] and renal dysfunction.[8,9]

In advanced heart failure, RV dysfunction adds prognostic information beyond LVEF.[10] Such prognostic information has been demonstrated, irrespective of the modality used to measure RV function and has been used in the outpatient setting,[11] during hospitalization for acute decompensated heart failure,[12] or in the context of patient referral to a specialized, advanced heart failure clinic.[13]

PATHOPHYSIOLOGY OF RIGHT VENTRICULAR DYSFUNCTION

The right ventricle is a crescent-shaped structure that wraps around the left ventricle. Although most LV contraction is circumferential, RV contraction is mainly longitudinal. Because the right ventricle and left ventricle are connected in series, they have the same stroke output; alterations in either ventricle affect the performance of the other.[14] RV failure is a clinical syndrome caused by any cardiovascular disorder that impairs the ability of the right ventricle to fill or eject blood.[15] It is recognized that left heart dysfunction is both the most common cause of RV dysfunction and the most common cause of pulmonary hypertension (PH).[15] This has been termed group 2 PH according to the 6th World symposium on Pulmonary Hypertension and is defined as a mean pulmonary artery pressure (PAP) 20 mm Hg or greater and a pulmonary wedge pressure greater than 15 mm Hg.[16] In patients with DCM or LV systolic dysfunction, RV systolic dysfunction, and ultimately, RV failure, results from several pathophysiologic mechanisms, including (1) intrinsic myocardial disease involving both ventricles; (2) increased RV afterload from increased pulmonary venous, and later, pulmonary arterial pressure, (3) increased RV preload from valvular regurgitation caused by RV dilation; and (4) reduced septal motion and ventricular interdependence.[17]

In patients with idiopathic DCM, the primary myopathy is often the cause of the RV dysfunction. This observation is supported by the fact that there is a weak relationship between elevated PAP and RV dysfunction in DCM, but there is a substantially stronger relationship between these two factors in ischemic DCM.[18] Furthermore, in idiopathic DCM, RV global longitudinal strain and regional peak myocardial RV strain are impaired compared with ischemic DCM.[19]

Elevated LV filling pressures cause pulmonary venous hypertension that results in RV hypertrophy, a process that may increase RV diastolic dysfunction.[20] Over time, these adaptations cannot overcome the chronic pressure overload and elevated wall stress, and the RV dilates and begins to fail. Initially, cardiac output is maintained through the Frank Starling mechanism, but progressive dilatation leads to decreased myocardial contraction, increased tricuspid regurgitation, and increased preload, which leads to a vicious cycle of RV dilatation, failure, and diminished cardiac output.[21] Ventricular interdependence further explains the pathophysiological link between LV and RV dysfunction.[22]

ECHOCARDIOGRAPHIC METHODS FOR EVALUATING RIGHT VENTRICULAR SIZE AND FUNCTION

Evaluation of RV size and function includes the following: (1) visual estimation of RV size (it should be less than 2/3 of the LV in a standard apical four-chamber view) and systolic function in all views (Fig. 68.1 and Video 68.1); (2) two-dimensional (2D) measurements in a RV-focused, apical four-chamber view; (3) global function assessment (Fig. 68.2) using the right index of myocardial performance (RIMP), the rate of pressure rise in the ventricles (dP/dt), and the fractional area change (FAC); and (4) regional function assessment using tricuspid annular plane systolic excursion (TAPSE) and Doppler tricuspid lateral annular systolic velocity (S′).[23] Other contemporary methods to assess RV systolic function include RVEF measurement by three-dimensional echocardiography and 2D strain, particularly of the RV free wall.

STUDIES EVALUATING RIGHT VENTRICULAR FUNCTION

Fractional Area Change

Two-dimensional FAC estimates global RV systolic function. A value below 35% indicates systolic dysfunction. Unadjusted 3-year mortality rates with an RV FAC of 35% or less, 35% to 39%, 40% to 45%, and greater than 45% were 44%, 29.2%, 11.7%, and 10.9%, respectively, in post–myocardial infarction patients with LV dysfunction, acute heart failure, or both. After adjusting for multiple clinical variables, RV FAC less than 35% and 35% to 39% had hazard ratios (HRs) of 3.56 and 2.43 for death and HRs of 2.72 and 1.78 for a composite outcome of all-cause mortality, cardiovascular death, resuscitated sudden death, recurrent myocardial infarction, hospitalization for heart failure, and stroke. Approximately 28% of the cohort had a RV FAC below 40%.[24]

Right Ventricular Index of Myocardial Performance

The RIMP provides an index of global RV function. Pulsed Doppler–derived RIMP greater than 0.40 or tissue Doppler–derived greater than 0.55 are considered abnormal. In patients with LV systolic dysfunction (LVEF <40%) and NYHA functional class II

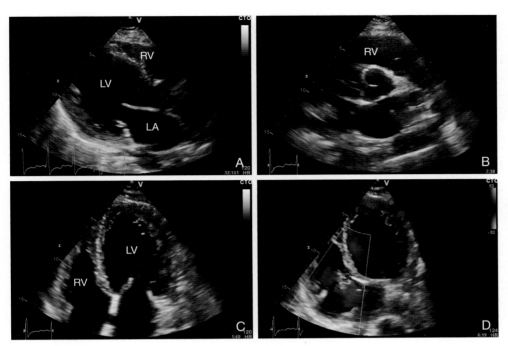

Figure 68.1. Standard echocardiographic views in a patient with a nonischemic dilated cardiomyopathy and biventricular dysfunction. **A,** Parasternal long-axis view. **B,** Parasternal short-axis view. **C,** Apical four-chamber view. **D,** Apical four-chamber view demonstrating tricuspid regurgitation. *LA,* Left atrium; *LV,* left ventricle; *RV,* right ventricle. (See accompanying Video 68.1.)

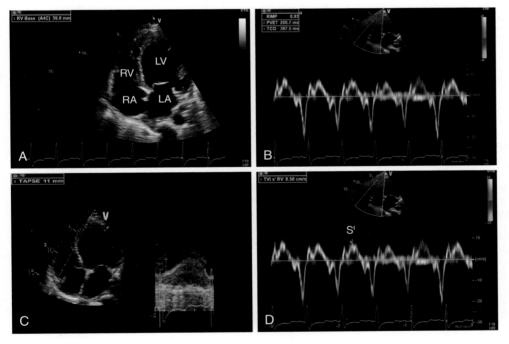

Figure 68.2. Methods to quantify right ventricular (RV) function in a patient with nonischemic dilated cardiomyopathy and biventricular dysfunction. **A,** Apical four-chamber view showing a basal RV dimension measurement. **B,** Tissue Doppler–derived RV index of myocardial performance. **C,** Tricuspid annular plane systolic excursion. **D,** Doppler S′ from pulsed tissue Doppler of the lateral tricuspid annular velocity. *LA,* Left atrium; *LV,* left ventricle; *RA,* right atrium.

symptoms, pulsed Doppler RIMP greater than 0.38 predicted cardiovascular death and hospitalization.[11] In patients with advanced heart failure referred for cardiac resynchronization therapy, LVEF less than 30% and NYHA functional class III, pulsed Doppler RIMP predicted all-cause mortality, cardiac transplantation, or ventricular assist device placement, with a HR of 1.11 for each 0.1 increase in RIMP by multivariate analysis at a median follow-up period of 21 months.[25]

Tricuspid Annular Plane Systolic Excursion

TAPSE or tricuspid annular motion measures RV longitudinal function, and a value below 16 mm suggests RV dysfunction. For a large (n = 817) unselected population of patients with heart failure and systolic dysfunction (LVEF ≤35%) who were admitted for hospitalization, TAPSE below 14 mm predicted mortality after adjustment for other risk factors for heart failure at a median of 4.1 years.[26] In patients with LV systolic dysfunction (LVEF <35%), idiopathic DCM, and NYHA functional class II heart failure, TAPSE of 14 mm or more predicted death or transplantation at 24 months and was significantly correlated with the RVEF.[27] In patients with chronic heart failure and LV dysfunction, TAPSE of 14 mm or less predicted all-cause mortality in multivariate analysis.[8] TAPSE below 18 mm predicted death and hospitalization in patients with NYHA functional class II symptoms and LV dysfunction.[11] TAPSE has proven to be similarly prognostic among patients hospitalized for acute decompensated heart failure.[28]

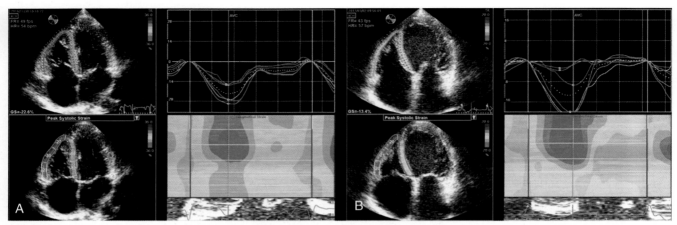

Figure 68.3. Measurement of right ventricular (RV) longitudinal systolic strain using speckle-tracking echocardiography for a patient with normal RV function (**A**) and dilated cardiomyopathy (DCM) with impaired RV function (**B**). Note that the global longitudinal strain is significantly reduced in the patient in *B* because of significant septal dysfunction, and the free-wall strain is borderline reduced.

DOPPLER S′

Pulsed tissue Doppler interrogation of the lateral tricuspid annular velocity in systole (S′) less than 10 cm/s suggests RV systolic dysfunction; this measure correlates with other measures of global RV systolic function. In patients with NYHA functional class III heart failure admitted for transplantation investigation, an S′ of less than 10.8 cm/s was a predictor of cardiac mortality in a multivariate analysis at a median 11-month follow-up.[29,30] In a similar population, S′ of 9.5 cm/s was a predictor of cardiovascular events.[31] In a population of ischemic and DCM patients admitted to the hospital with worsening symptoms (NYHA functional classes III and IV) and LVEF less than 35%, S′ less than 7.3 cm/s was an independent predictor of cardiovascular death in a multivariate analysis at 6 months.[32] The low cutoff value for S′ may have reflected overall low RV function in this cohort of patients. Prognostic value for S′ less than 9 cm/s was also found in a cohort of consecutive patients admitted with heart failure, irrespective of their LVEFs.[12]

Two-Dimensional Strain Imaging

2D strain analysis using speckle-tracking echocardiography measures myocardial deformation by tracking unique acoustic markers, or speckles, within the myocardium during the cardiac cycle and generating strain curves over either the free wall or the free wall and septum of the RV (typically from the apical four-chamber imaging window) (Fig. 68.3). In stable outpatients with NYHA functional class III or IV heart failure and a LVEF of 30% or less referred for heart transplantation, abnormal free-wall right ventricular longitudinal strain (RVLS) predicted cardiovascular events at a mean follow-up period of 1.5 ± 0.9 years; receiver-operating characteristic analysis revealed a sensitivity of 85% and specificity of 88% to predict cardiovascular events with a cut-off of −15.0%.[33] RVLS has demonstrated superior prognostic utility to both TAPSE and LVEF in stable heart failure populations[34,35] and was independently predictive of death or the need for rehospitalization in patients hospitalized with acute decompensated heart failure (HR, 1.51).[36] In a study of 200 patients with heart failure with reduced LVEF, a value of −15.3% of RVLS of the free wall was the best cutoff for predicting the outcome of all-cause mortality or heart failure hospitalization.[34] RV dysfunction as measured by RVLS was more highly predicted by noninvasively measured pulmonary artery systolic pressure (PASP) than by LVEF in a large cohort of patients with heart failure (including those with reduced and preserved

LVEF).[37] A correlation has also been demonstrated between RVLS and exercise tolerance.[19]

Multiple Parameters

Other studies have evaluated the prognostic value of multiple echocardiographic measures of RV function in a single cohort. In patients with LV systolic dysfunction who were admitted for consideration of heart transplantation or LV assist device support, LVEF less than 35%, FAC less than 36.8%, TAPSE less than 13.5 mm, and S′ less than 9.5 cm/s were all predictive of cardiovascular events (death, urgent transplantation, urgent ventricular assist device implantation, or an acute heart failure episode) on univariate analysis. However, only S′, NYHA functional class, and log brain natriuretic peptide were independent predictors on multivariate analysis.[31] TAPSE and PASP have been incorporated into the Euro Heart Failure score, a novel, echocardiography-based risk prediction score (along with LV end-systolic volume index, left atrial volume index, and mitral E-wave deceleration time) for predicting death among patients with heart failure.[38]

Pulmonary Hemodynamics

Pulmonary pressures should be assessed in all patients with DCM. PASP is estimated from the velocity of the tricuspid regurgitation jet, which is combined with an estimation of right atrial pressure from inferior vena cava size and collapsibility. Pulmonary venous hypertension is a frequent contributor to right-sided heart failure in patients with LV systolic dysfunction because elevated pulmonary pressure is initially an adaptive mechanism that reduces pulmonary edema. In early heart failure with LV dysfunction, passive PH with a normal transpulmonary pressure gradient (<12 mm Hg) and pulmonary vascular resistance, which implies no significant abnormality of the pulmonary artery structure or function may improve with diuresis and heart failure therapy. PH is classified as reactive or mixed when functional and structural alterations in the pulmonary vascular anatomy have developed.[39]

Studies have consistently demonstrated that PH is associated with increased mortality rate and hospitalization in this population. In a study of outpatients with chronic heart failure and LVEF less than 45%, who predominantly had NYHA functional class II and III symptoms, the group with PASP greater than 40 mm Hg and TAPSE 14 mm or less had the highest risk of the primary outcome (HR, 5.16) of all-cause mortality, urgent heart transplantation, and appropriately detected and treated episodes of ventricular fibrillation. Those with a normal PASP and a low TAPSE (HR, 1.50) and those with a high PASP and a preserved TAPSE (HR, 2.43) were at intermediate risk of these outcomes. It was possible to measure the PASP in 83% of patients.[40]

CONCLUSIONS AND RECOMMENDATIONS

In patients with DCM, the evaluation of RV function adds incrementally to the clinician's ability to predict death, heart failure hospitalization, transplantation, exercise capacity, and renal function. This requires an integrated approach with initial visual assessment of size and function, supplemented with quantitative measurements including FAC, RIMP, TAPSE, S′, and RVLS. The cutoff values that appear to be clinically relevant in the heart failure population are often those that are close to the lower reference limits used to define abnormal RV function. Incorporation of these parameters into standardized risk assessment tools have enhanced stratification approaches for DCM patients, including those with stable, advanced, and even decompensated heart failure.

Please access ExpertConsult to view the corresponding videos for this chapter.

REFERENCES

1. Maron BJ, Towbin JA, Thiene G, et al. Contemporary definitions and classification of the cardiomyopathies. *Circulation.* 2006;113:1807–1816.
2. La Vecchia L, Paccanaro M, Bonanno C, et al. Left ventricular versus biventricular dysfunction in idiopathic dilated cardiomyopathy. *Am J Cardiol.* 1999;83:120–122. A9.
3. Gulati A, Ismail TF, Jabbour A, et al. The prevalence and prognostic significance of right ventricular systolic dysfunction in nonischemic dilated cardiomyopathy. *Circulation.* 2013;128:1623–1633.
4. Melenovsky V, Kotrc M, Borlaug BA, et al. Relationships between right ventricular function, body composition, and prognosis in advanced heart failure. *J Am Coll Cardiol.* 2013;62:1660–1670.
5. de Groote P, Millaire A, Foucher-Hossein C, et al. Right ventricular ejection fraction is an independent predictor of survival in patients with moderate heart failure. *J Am Coll Cardiol.* 1998;32:948–954.
6. Meyer P, Filippatos GS, Ahmed MI, et al. Effects of right ventricular ejection fraction on outcomes in chronic systolic heart failure. *Circulation.* 2010;121:252–258.
7. Di Salvo TG, Mathier M, Semigran MJ, Dec GW. Preserved right ventricular ejection fraction predicts exercise capacity and survival in advanced heart failure. *J Am Coll Cardiol.* 1995;25:1143–1153.
8. Dini FL, Demmer RT, Simioniuc A, et al. Right ventricular dysfunction is associated with chronic kidney disease and predicts survival in patients with chronic systolic heart failure. *Eur J Heart Fail.* 2012;14:287–294.
9. Testani JM, Khera AV, St John Sutton MG, et al. Effect of right ventricular function and venous congestion on cardiorenal interactions during the treatment of decompensated heart failure. *Am J Cardiol.* 2010;105:511–516.
10. Ghio S, Gavazzi A, Campana C, et al. Independent and additive prognostic value of right ventricular systolic function and pulmonary artery pressure in patients with chronic heart failure. *J Am Coll Cardiol.* 2001;37:183–188.
11. Vizzardi E, D'Aloia A, Bordonali T, et al. Long-term prognostic value of the right ventricular myocardial performance index compared to other indexes of right ventricular function in patients with moderate chronic heart failure. *Echocardiography.* 2012;29:773–778.
12. Dokainish H, Sengupta R, Patel R, Lakkis N. Usefulness of right ventricular tissue Doppler imaging to predict outcome in left ventricular heart failure independent of left ventricular diastolic function. *Am J Cardiol.* 2007;99:961–965.
13. Damy T, Kallvikbacka-Bennett A, Goode K, et al. Prevalence of, associations with, and prognostic value of tricuspid annular plane systolic excursion (TAPSE) among out-patients referred for the evaluation of heart failure. *J Card Fail.* 2012;18:216–225.
14. Dell'Italia LJ. Anatomy and physiology of the right ventricle. *Cardiol Clin.* 2012;30:167–187.
15. Haddad F, Doyle R, Murphy DJ, Hunt SA. Right ventricular function in cardiovascular disease, part II: pathophysiology, clinical importance, and management of right ventricular failure. *Circulation.* 2008;117:1717–1731.
16. Simonneau G, Montani D, Celermajer DS, et al. Haemodynamic definitions and updated clinical classification of pulmonary hypertension. *Eur Respir J.* 2019;53(1).
17. Voelkel NF, Quaife RA, Leinwand LA, et al. Right ventricular function and failure. *Circulation.* 2006;114:1883–1891.
18. La Vecchia L, Zanolla L, Varotto L, et al. Reduced right ventricular ejection fraction as a marker for idiopathic dilated cardiomyopathy compared with ischemic left ventricular dysfunction. *Am Heart J.* 2001;142:181–189.
19. Salerno G, D'Andrea A, Bossone E, et al. Association between right ventricular 2D strain and exercise capacity in patients with either idiopathic or ischemic dilated cardiomyopathy. *J Cardiovasc Med.* 2011;12:625–634.
20. Brieke A, DeNofrio D. Right ventricular dysfunction in chronic dilated cardiomyopathy and heart failure. *Coron Artery Dis.* 2005;16(5–11).
21. Vitarelli A, Terzano C. Do we have two hearts? New insights in right ventricular function supported by myocardial imaging echocardiography. *Heart Fail Rev.* 2010;15:39–61.
22. Guglin M, Verma S. Right side of heart failure. *Heart Fail Rev.* 2012;17:511–527.
23. Lang RM, Badano LP, Mor-Avi V, et al. Recommendations for cardiac chamber quantification by echocardiography in adults. *J Am Soc Echocardiogr.* 2015;28:1–39. e14.
24. Anavekar NS, Skali H, Bourgoun M, et al. Usefulness of right ventricular fractional area change to predict death, heart failure, and stroke following myocardial infarction. *Am J Cardiol.* 2008;101:607–612.
25. Field ME, Solomon SD, Lewis EF, et al. Right ventricular dysfunction and adverse outcome in patients with advanced heart failure. *J Card Fail.* 2006;12:616–620.
26. Kjaergaard J, Akkan D, Iversen KK, et al. Right ventricular dysfunction as an independent predictor of short- and long-term mortality in patients with heart failure. *Eur J Heart Fail.* 2007;9:610–616.
27. Ghio S, Recusani F, Klersy C, et al. Prognostic usefulness of the tricuspid annular plane systolic excursion in patients with congestive heart failure secondary to idiopathic or ischemic dilated cardiomyopathy. *Am J Cardiol.* 2000;85:837–842.
28. Ghio S, Guazzi M, Scardovi AB, et al. Different correlates but similar prognostic implications for right ventricular dysfunction in heart failure patients with reduced or preserved ejection fraction. *Eur J Heart Fail.* 2017;19:873–879.
29. Meluzin J, Spinarova L, Dusek L, et al. Prognostic importance of the right ventricular function assessed by Doppler tissue imaging. *Eur J Echocardiogr.* 2003;4:262–271.
30. Meluzin J, Spinarova L, Hude P, et al. Prognostic importance of various echocardiographic right ventricular functional parameters in patients with symptomatic heart failure. *J Am Soc Echocardiogr.* 2005;18:435–444.
31. Damy T, Viallet C, Lairez O, et al. Comparison of four right ventricular systolic echocardiographic parameters to predict adverse outcomes in chronic heart failure. *Eur J Heart Fail.* 2009;11:818–824.
32. Bistola V, Parissis JT, Paraskevaidis I, et al. Prognostic value of tissue Doppler right ventricular systolic and diastolic function indexes combined with plasma B-type natriuretic Peptide in patients with advanced heart failure secondary to ischemic or idiopathic dilated cardiomyopathy. *Am J Cardiol.* 2010;105:249–254.
33. Cameli M, Righini FM, Lisi M, et al. Comparison of right versus left ventricular strain analysis as a predictor of outcome in patients with systolic heart failure referred for heart transplantation. *Am J Cardiol.* 2013;112:1778–1784.
34. Carluccio E, Biagioli P, Alunni G, et al. Prognostic value of right ventricular dysfunction in heart failure with reduced ejection fraction: superiority of longitudinal strain over tricuspid annular plane systolic excursion. *Circulation Cardiovasc Imag.* 2018;11:e006894.
35. Motoki H, Borowski AG, Shrestha K, et al. Right ventricular global longitudinal strain provides prognostic value incremental to left ventricular ejection fraction in patients with heart failure. *J Am Soc Echocardiogr.* 2014;27:726–732.
36. Hamada-Harimura Y, Seo Y, Ishizu T, et al. Incremental prognostic value of right ventricular strain in patients with acute decompensated heart failure. *Circulation Cardiovasc Imag.* 2018;11. e007249.
37. Bosch L, Lam CSP, Gong L, et al. Right ventricular dysfunction in left-sided heart failure with preserved versus reduced ejection fraction. *Eur J Heart Fail.* 2017;19:1664–1671.
38. Carluccio E, Dini FL, Biagioli P, et al. The 'Echo Heart Failure Score': an echocardiographic risk prediction score of mortality in systolic heart failure. *Eur J Heart Fail.* 2013;15:868–876.
39. Georgiopoulou VV, Kalogeropoulos AP, Borlaug BA, et al. Left ventricular dysfunction with pulmonary hypertension: part 1: epidemiology, pathophysiology, and definitions. *Circulation Heart Fail.* 2013;6:344–354.
40. Ghio S, Temporelli PL, Klersy C, et al. Prognostic relevance of a non-invasive evaluation of right ventricular function and pulmonary artery pressure in patients with chronic heart failure. *Eur J Heart Fail.* 2013;15:408–414.

69 Restrictive Cardiomyopathy: Classification

Sherif F. Nagueh

RCM is characterized by normal left ventricular (LV) volumes, usually normal LV ejection fraction (EF), and abnormal LV filling. Morphologic features include increased or normal LV wall thickness and biatrial enlargement.[1] There are rare familial cases in which the disease is caused by sarcomeric protein mutations (troponin I, troponin T, α-actin, and β myosin heavy chain mutations).[2] Other reasons include secondary myocardial infiltrative and storage disorders as well as other diseases associated with increased interstitial fibrosis. These disorders are not considered among the primary cardiomyopathic diseases. Myocardial infiltrative diseases include an infiltrative process that occurs in the interstitial space as cardiac amyloidosis, whereas storage diseases are characterized by deposits in the myocytes (Table 69.1). The differential diagnosis for RCM includes pericardial constriction. Restrictive LV filling should be distinguished from RCM because restrictive LV filling can be present in other diseases, including DCM and hypertrophic cardiomyopathy. Furthermore, depending on the stage of the disease, a number of patients with myocardial infiltrative disorders do not manifest restrictive LV filling.

Excluding systemic manifestations of diseases that affect other organs, the clinical presentation is usually characterized by symptoms of pulmonary and systemic congestion and increased serum brain natriuretic peptide (BNP) level. Findings of low cardiac output, as fatigue and increased BUN-to-creatinine ratio, may be present in patients with advanced disease. Noninvasive imaging is of value in the initial evaluation and can reveal abnormal LV and right ventricular (RV) filling. As already noted, early findings may include an impaired LV relaxation pattern that progresses to grade III diastolic dysfunction in patients with advanced disease (Figs. 69.1 to 69.3 and Videos 69.1 to 69.3). Doppler echocardiography is an important diagnostic modality that can help distinguish this condition from constrictive pericarditis.[3,4] Recent studies have shown abnormal LV systolic function detected by reduced deformation parameters in patients with RCM. Abnormal systolic function as detected by myocardial strain appears to have the highest prevalence in symptomatic patients.[5] Invasive hemodynamics show evidence of increased LV chamber and myocardial stiffness (shift to the left in the pressure–volume relationship) with elevated LV end-diastolic pressure, left atrial pressure, pulmonary hypertension, and elevated RV filling pressures. Frequently, a "dip and plateau" pattern can be noted in LV diastolic pressure recordings, reflecting the rapid rise in LV early diastolic pressure upon mitral valve opening. Pathologically, variable degrees of hypertrophy and fibrosis are observed in addition to specific findings based on the disease (e.g., amyloid deposits). Treatment options are often limited to diuretics and salt restriction and, when the disease is advanced, cardiac transplantation. The latter option may be limited, however, in the presence of systemic disease. Patients can develop conduction disturbances and tachycardia, which necessitates the use of rate slowing medications. The latter drugs have the adverse effect of decreasing cardiac output because of slowing heart rate at a time when LV filling and thus stroke volume are fixed because of cardiac disease, and heart rate is needed to maintain cardiac output.[2] The use of angiotensin-converting enzyme inhibitors or angiotensin receptor blockers is accompanied by hypotension and is not needed in these patients.

Loeffler endocarditis is one of the diseases causing RCM and is seen in patients with hypereosinophilic syndrome. Patients have an elevated eosinophil count (>1500 eosinophils/mL) in the absence of other reasons that can cause eosinophilia. It is characterized by multiple organ involvement, including the heart. There are increased eosinophil counts with degranulation causing endocardial damage with initial necrosis followed by and culminating in fibrosis. Thrombus formation is common and can occur in the left ventricle and the right ventricle. Two-dimensional echocardiography shows reduced LV volumes and biatrial enlargement because of biventricular diastolic dysfunction. Treatment with steroids is possible in patients with early disease. Other therapeutic approaches include chemotherapy and the tyrosine kinase inhibitor imatinib.[6] Surgery for the removal of fibrotic plaques is considered in late cases. Endocardial fibroelastosis is another condition that leads to LV diastolic dysfunction and is common in the tropical region of Africa, where it is an important cause of heart failure. Fibrosis involves the LV and RV apexes and extends to the chordae and posterior mitral leaflet tissue as well as the tricuspid valve. Surgery can be performed for removal of fibrotic lesions and for valvular repair, but the outcome remains poor.

Please access ExpertConsult to view the corresponding videos for this chapter.

TABLE 69.1 Classification of Restrictive Cardiomyopathy

Primary Disease	Infiltrative Disorders	Storage Disorders	Other
Idiopathic	Amyloidosis Sarcoidosis	Fabry Hemochromatosis Glycogen storage disease Mucopolysaccharidosis Niemann-Pick disease	Loeffler endocarditis Endocardial fibroelastosis Carcinoid Post radiation Post chemotherapy Lymphoma Scleroderma Churg-Strauss disease Pseudoxanthoma elasticum

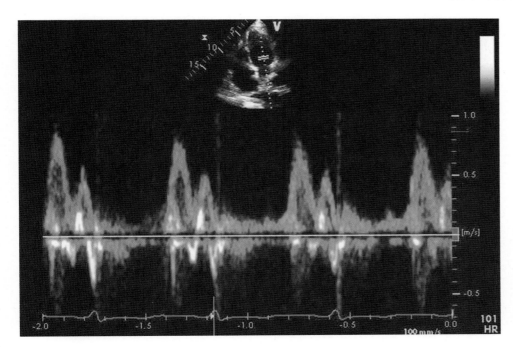

Figure 69.1. Mitral inflow from a patient with Loeffler endocarditis. Notice the presence of predominant early diastolic left ventricular (LV) filling consistent with increased left atrial pressure in this patient with increased chamber stiffness. (See corresponding Video 69.1.)

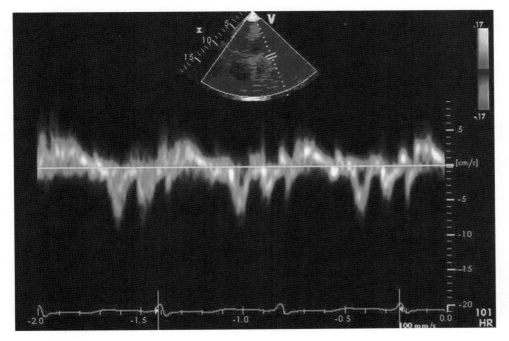

Figure 69.2. Tissue Doppler signals at the lateral side of the mitral annulus. Notice the reduced systolic and diastolic velocities. (See corresponding Video 69.2.)

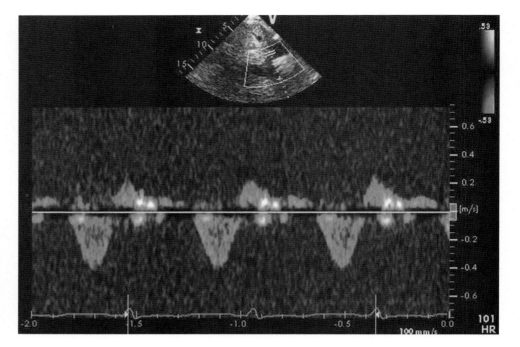

Figure 69.3. Hepatic vein flow from the same patient with Loeffler endocarditis. Notice the presence of forward flow only in diastole, which is consistent with markedly elevated right atrial (RA) pressure. The elevated RA pressure in this patient is caused by right ventricular diastolic dysfunction due to increased chamber stiffness. (See corresponding Video 69.3.)

REFERENCES

1. Ammash NM, Seward JB, Bailey KR, et al. Clinical profile and outcome of idiopathic restrictive cardiomyopathy. *Circulation.* 2000;101:2490–2496.
2. Muchtar E, Blauwet LA, Gertz MA. Restrictive cardiomyopathy: genetics, pathogenesis, clinical manifestations, diagnosis, and therapy. *Circ Res.* 2017;121:819–837.
3. Nagueh SF, Appleton CP, Gillebert TC, et al. Recommendations for the evaluation of left ventricular diastolic function by echocardiography. *J Am Soc Echocardiogr.* 2009;22:107–133.
4. Hatle LK, Appleton CP, Popp RL. Differentiation of constrictive pericarditis and restrictive cardiomyopathy by Doppler echocardiography. *Circulation.* 1989;79:357–370.
5. Mor-Avi V, Lang RM, Badano LP, et al. Current and evolving echocardiographic techniques for the quantitative evaluation of cardiac mechanics. *J Am Soc Echocardiogr.* 2011;24:277–313.
6. Cools J, DeAngelo DJ, Gotlib J, et al. A tyrosine kinase created by fusion of the PDGFRA and FIP1L1 genes as a therapeutic target of imatinib in idiopathic hypereosinophilic syndrome. *N Engl J Med.* 2003;348:1201–1214.

70 Echocardiographic Diagnosis of Left Ventricular Noncompaction Cardiomyopathy

Ferande Peters, Bijoy K. Khandheria

Left ventricular noncompaction (LVNC) is characterized by the presence of prominent left ventricular (LV) trabeculae with adjacent deep intertrabecular recesses overlying a thin compacted layer of myocardium. There are several controversies relating to LVNC, including whether LVNC is a genetic disorder or merely a remodeling phenomenon.[1,2] A second major controversy relates to whether this process occurs exclusively as an arrest during embryologic development or whether postnatal factors (e.g., volume overload) may cause the development of the LVNC phenotype. The initial reports that described LVNC were associated with a dilated dysfunctional left ventricle, which often had an adverse clinical course characterized by heart failure, atrial and ventricular arrhythmia, and cardioembolism. This clinical scenario was documented as LVNC cardiomyopathy. In more recent years, the LVNC phenotype has been identified in several clinical scenarios, which include normal individuals, athletes, pregnant women, and people with several neuromuscular disorders, and is associated with other myocardial diseases.[3–5] This has supported the postulate that LVNC is merely an epiphenomenon.

CLINICAL SPECTRUM OF LEFT VENTRICULAR NONCOMPACTION CARDIOMYOPATHY

A more pragmatic approach maybe to view the phenotype of LVNC to be to that of LV hypertrophy, which can occur in a spectrum ranging from clinical scenarios characterized by physiological adaptive changes to primary genetic cardiomyopathy. The diagnosis of LVNC relies on imaging to identify a specific phenotype that is different to that normally visualized in the myocardium of humans. After a phenotype of LVNC is identified, it is imperative that the phenotype be integrated with the clinical scenario and functional state of the heart. Based on this, one should decide if this constitutes a normal variant, physiological adaptation, or primary myocardial pathology.

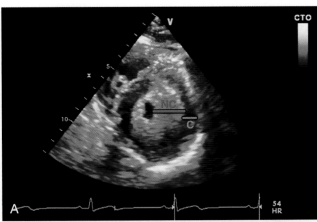

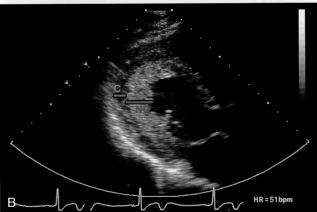

Figure 70.1. A, Parasternal short-axis view of the left ventricular apex demonstrating compacted (C) and noncompacted (NC) myocardium. **B,** Modified parasternal view of the left ventricle demonstrating C and NC myocardium. (See accompanying Video 70.1)

The definitions "LVNC-like phenotype" or "prominent trabeculations not meeting the criteria for LVNC" have been proposed by some and should refer to the scenario in which prominent trabeculations are identified but the structure of the heart is normal with normal ejection fraction (EF).[6] The significance of this scenario is not clearly elucidated but thought to represent a normal variant. Whether this normal variant will transition to LVNC cardiomyopathy remains an enigma. Several physiological states are characterized by volume overload of the left ventricle in which the LVNC phenotype has been described. These include anemia, pregnancy, and athletes.[3,4,7] This physiological adaptive change maybe reversible as documented in the experience of Gati and coworkers, who found that the LVNC phenotype reverses after pregnancy in certain individuals.[4]

Pathological LVNC may occur if there is associated congenital heart disease; neuromuscular disease; or other myocardial disease such as hypertrophic cardiomyopathy (HCM), myocarditis, or Fabry disease. The screening of family members of individuals with known genetic myocardial disorders such as HCM and less commonly familial dilated cardiomyopathy (DCM) may results in cases of LVNC cardiomyopathy being identified.

DIAGNOSIS

There are several proposed echocardiographic and cardiac magnetic resonance imaging (CMRI) criteria for diagnosing LVNC.[8–13] CMRI has superior spatial resolution compared with echocardiography and thus has the advantage of detecting the LVNC phenotype

in scenarios in which echocardiographic imaging is suboptimal and is superior at imaging the apex and apicolateral walls. Additional advantages of CMRI include the detection of concomitant late gadolinium enhancement suggestive of myocardial scar and detection of myocarditis. Thus, CMRI should be used ideally in addition to echocardiography, although its major limitations include its cost and availability. Furthermore, it appears that CMRI tends to result in overdiagnosis of LVNC compared with echocardiography with one large study detecting the phenotype in 43% of normal individuals. Thus, detection of the LVNC phenotype in isolation by CMRI does not constitute a diagnosis. Instead, as mentioned previously, detection of the phenotype of LVNC must be integrated with several key clinical features to improve diagnosis.

ECHOCARDIOGRAPHY

Echocardiography is safe, widely available, cost-effective imaging that maybe used to diagnose the distinct morphology of LVNC and should be based on the phenotype detected in LVNC cardiomyopathy. The pathognomonic echocardiographic features in individuals affected by LVNC cardiomyopathy include a thick, bilayered (noncompacted [NC] and compacted [C]) myocardium, prominent ventricular trabeculations, and deep intertrabecular recesses (Fig. 70.1 and Video 70.1).[3]

Current echocardiographic imaging definitions for the diagnosis of LVNC cardiomyopathy vary regarding the morphologic definitions used and quantitative methods proposed. The lack of a true gold standard makes it difficult to know which criteria are the most sensitive and specific. The available diagnostic criteria are all limited because of the complexity involved in validating them and poor reproducibility.

The diagnostic criteria used by Jenni and colleagues[9] included a bilayered myocardium that consists of a thin C layer and a NC layer with deep myocardial recesses; specifically, this is a NC/C ratio greater than 2 measured at end-systole in the apical short-axis view. Chin and colleagues[8] defined LVNC cardiomyopathy as C/(NC + C) less than 0.5 at end-diastole in the parasternal short-axis view. Stöllberger and Finsterer[10] defined LVNC cardiomyopathy as four or more trabeculations protruding from the LV wall located apically to the papillary muscles and visible in one imaging plane. Paterick and coworkers[11] used the ratio of NC to C greater than 2 at end-diastole as diagnostic of LVNC cardiomyopathy. This modification was based on the observation that measurements of the C and NC layers are more precise during end-diastole. This approach is consistent with the American Society of Echocardiography's convention of measuring chamber wall thickness at end-diastole rather than at end-systole (Fig. 70.2).

Several technical and analytic pitfalls should be avoided (Box 70.1) when acquiring echocardiographic data and performing qualitative and quantitative analysis that is required when using any of the aforementioned echocardiographic methods. This rigorous detail is required to improve the accuracy of diagnosis in all instances. In some instances, contrast can be used to opacify the LV apex and allow more precise delineation of the C layer, which allows for improved precision in measurements. There is a role for three-dimensional (3D) echocardiography with full-volume acquisition to characterize the C and NC myocardium (Fig. 70.3). The imaging specialist must meet the challenge of considering all mimickers of pathological LVNC. It can be challenging to distinguish pathological LVNC from apical HCM, apical thrombus, false tendons, aberrant chords, cardiac fibromas, eosinophilic heart disease, endomyocardial fibrosis, and cardiac metastases.[14]

The most common pathological LVNC phenotype is that of the dilated LV with low EF, which resembles the phenotype of DCM. However, LVNC is characterized by focal morphologic abnormality despite the possible presence of more generalized functional

Figure 70.2. Diagnostic criteria for left ventricular noncompaction (LVNC). **A,** Jenni and coworkers[9] (Zurich) criteria: LVNC is defined by a ratio of noncompacted (NC) to compacted (C) myocardium greater than 2, measured at end-systole. **B,** Chin and coworkers[8] (California) criteria: LVNC is defined by a ratio of the distance from the epicardial surface to the trough of the trabecular recesses (X) to the distance from the epicardial surface to the peak of the trabeculations (Y) at 0.5 or less, measured at end-diastole. **C,** Stöllberger and Finsterer[10] (Vienna) criteria: LVNC is defined by trabeculations (four or more) protruding from the left ventricular wall, located apically to the papillary muscles and visible in one imaging plane. **D,** Paterick and coworkers[11] (Wisconsin) criteria (not validated): LVNC is defined by an NC-to-C ratio greater than 2, measured at end-diastole. (Reproduced with permission from Paterick TE, et al: Left ventricular noncompaction: A 25-year odyssey, *J Am Soc Echocardiogr* 25:363–375, 2012.)

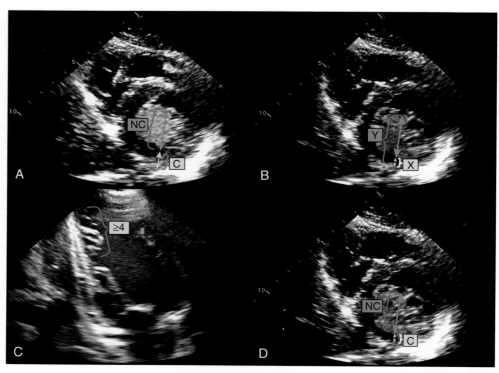

BOX 70.1 Technical and Analysis Tips

TECHNICAL TIPS

1. Comprehensive imaging of the left ventricle is essential with the acquisition of all views.
2. The highest transducer frequencies, with adjustment of beam focus, gain, and reject settings, are recommended to obtain well-defined images.
3. Meticulous technique with avoidance of foreshortening in the long-axis views and avoidance of off-axis views of short-axis planes is essential.
4. Short-axis images should be perpendicular to the ventricular long-axis views such that a circular LV cavity image should be obtained and maintained in all short-axis views.
5. Imaging of the true apex requires using the intercostal space either 1 or 2 spaces below where the normal short axis is obtained with rotation of the probe to obtain an accurate image
6. To accurately differentiate trabeculae from false tendons and bands, the use of live multiplane 2D imaging or 3D imaging maybe required to map out the entire anatomical spatial extent of structures.
7. Imaging of the compacta is best done using the zoom mode and using a focus enhancement function that maybe available on certain vendors.
8. The color scale should be reduced to demonstrate flow from the LV cavity into the intertrabecular spaces.
9. Adequate acquisition of basal and apical images preferably end expiration with an adequate frame rate should be done if rotational parameters such as LV twist is to be evaluated.

ANALYSIS TIPS

1. Ensure that the images are obtained in a technically appropriate manner.
2. Identify true trabeculae; they should be distal to the papillary muscles with no attachments to the septum.
3. There should be four or more trabeculae with accompanying intertrabecular spaces that demonstrate color flow from the LV cavity with no flow into the compacta.
4. Measurements of the trabeculae and compacta should be performed at the same site and at the same time of the cardiac cycle depending on the criteria used.

2D, Two-dimensional; *3D,* three-dimensional; *LV,* left ventricular.

---

abnormality. Therefore, a systematic regional myocardial wall evaluation is required to detect the phenotype, which is most commonly detected in the apex, apicolateral, and mid lateral walls. Speckle tracking can be used to identify the absence of LV twist-termed rigid body rotation, which may be more commonly found in LVNC compared to DCM.

The accurate measurement of EF in LVNC can be challenging in certain instances. Exclusion of all trabeculae is mandatory, and the boundary tracing should be performed at the junction of the C and NC areas. Attention to detail is required to obtain an accurate measurement of LVEF because some guidelines advocated the insertion of an implantable cardioverter-defibrillator as a primary

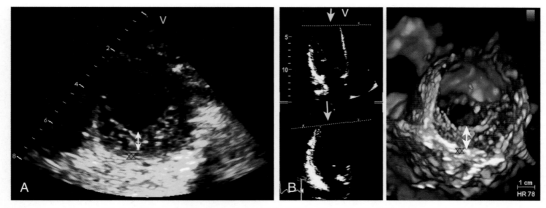

Figure 70.3. Images of a 15-year-old male high school track and football player with a family history of sudden cardiac death; his father died at 42 years of age. The father's autopsy was consistent with left ventricular noncompaction cardiomyopathy. **A,** Demonstration of compacted (C; *green bullet*) and noncompacted (NC; *white arrow*) myocardium at end-diastole, with an NC-to-C ratio of 2:1 (using Paterick and coworkers6 criteria). **B,** Three-dimensional echocardiogram (with full-volume acquisition) demonstrating the NC *(white arrow)* and C *(green bullet)* myocardium from the apex toward the mitral valve. (Reproduced with permission from Paterick TE, et al: Left ventricular noncompaction: A 25-year odyssey, *J Am Soc Echocardiogr* 25:363–375, 2012.)

preventative strategy if the LVEF is below 30%. After LVNC with a low EF is detected, a systematic evaluation for known complication such as functional mitral regurgitation, pulmonary hypertension, right ventricular dysfunction, and LV thrombus should be systematically performed. Multiple echocardiographic views, off-axis imaging, and 3D echocardiography maybe required to detect LV thrombus and differentiate it from trabecular in certain instances.

CONCLUSION

Accurate diagnosis of the LVNC phenotype requires a rigorous technical and analytic approach. Integration of the detection of the LVNC phenotype with the appropriate clinical scenario allows for more accurate clinical diagnosis. Identification of LVNC cardiomyopathy is important because its major complications alter prognosis and may offer benefit from certain therapies in some instances.

Please access ExpertConsult to view the corresponding video for this chapter.

REFERENCES

1. Maron BJ, Towbin JA, Thiene G, et al. Contemporary definitions and classification of the cardiomyopathies. *Circulation.* 2006;113:1807–1816.
2. Elliott P, Andersson B, Arbustini E, et al. Classification of the cardiomyopathies. *Eur Heart J.* 2008;29:270–276.
3. Gati S, Chandra N, Bennett RL, et al. Increased left ventricular trabeculation in highly trained athletes: do we need more stringent criteria for the diagnosis of left ventricular non-compaction in athletes? *Heart.* 2013;99:401–408.
4. Gati S, Papadakis M, Papamichael ND, et al. Reversible de novo left ventricular trabeculations in pregnant women: implications for the diagnosis of left ventricular noncompaction in low-risk populations. *Circulation.* 2014;130:475–483.
5. Kohli SK, Pantazis AA, Shah JS, et al. Diagnosis of left-ventricular non-compaction in patients with left-ventricular systolic dysfunction: time for a reappraisal of diagnostic criteria. *Eur Heart J.* 2008;29:89–95.
6. Klem I, Goyal A. Left ventricular noncompaction: Meglio solo che mal accompagnati: Italian proverb: "Better alone than in bad company." *JACC Cardiovasc Imaging.* 2019;12:2152–2154.
7. Gati S, Papadakis M, Van Niekerk N, et al. Increased left ventricular trabeculation in individuals with sickle cell anaemia: physiology or pathology. *Int J Cardiol.* 2013;168:1658–1660.
8. Chin TK, Perloff JK, Williams RG, et al. Isolated noncompaction of left ventricular myocardium. A study of eight cases. *Circulation.* 1990;82:507–513.
9. Jenni R, Oechslin E, Schneider J, et al. Echocardiographic and pathoanatomical characteristics of isolated left ventricular non-compaction: a step towards classification as a distinct cardiomyopathy. *Heart.* 2001;86:666–671.
10. Stöllberger C, Finsterer J. Left ventricular hypertrabeculation/noncompaction. *J Am Soc Echocardiogr.* 2004;17:91–100.
11. Paterick TE, Umland MM, Jan MF, et al. Left ventricular noncompaction: a 25-year odyssey. *J Am Soc Echocardiogr.* 2012;25:363–375.
12. Petersen SE, Selvanayagam JB, Wiesmann F, et al. Left ventricular non-compaction: insights from cardiovascular magnetic resonance imaging. *J Am Coll Cardiol.* 2005;46:101–105.
13. Jacquier A, Thuny F, Jop B, et al. Measurement of trabeculated left ventricular mass using cardiac magnetic resonance imaging in the diagnosis of left ventricular non-compaction. *Eur Heart J.* 2010;31:1098–1104.
14. Paterick TE, Gerber TC, Pradhan SR, et al. Left ventricular noncompaction cardiomyopathy: what do we know? *Rev Cardiovasc Med.* 2010;11:92–99.

71 Hereditary and Acquired Infiltrative Cardiomyopathy

Ferande Peters, Bijoy K. Khandheria

Infiltrative cardiomyopathies (ICMOs) are a form of restrictive cardiomyopathy that may be caused by either hereditary or acquired diseases. They are characterized by the deposition of abnormal substances within the myocardium that cause stiffening of the left ventricular (LV) walls. These disorders can be caused by conditions that cause abnormal substances to deposit within the myocyte, referred to as storage disorders, or abnormal deposition of substances within the interstitium (Table 71.1). The 2006 American College of Cardiology/American Heart Association guidelines state that conditions that cause ICMO may be classified as diseases of either hereditary or mixed pathology.[1] The purpose of this chapter is to accentuate the salient features of ICMO and highlight some conditions that manifest as ICMO. Some of these disorders are elaborated upon in greater detail in other parts of this book.

TABLE 71.1 Disorders Causing Infiltrative Cardiomyopathy

Storage Disorders	Infiltrative Disorders
Fabry disease	Amyloid
Glycogen storage diseases	Sarcoid
Hemochromatosis	Hurler syndrome
Danon disease	Gaucher disease
Oxalosis	

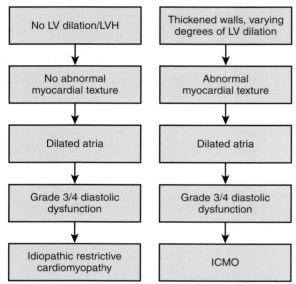

Figure 71.1. Echocardiographic features of idiopathic restrictive cardiomyopathy versus infiltrative cardiomyopathy (ICMO). *LV,* Left ventricular; *LVH,* left ventricular hypertrophy.

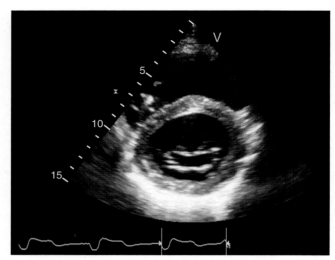

Figure 71.2. Basal short-axis view of the left ventricle demonstrating speckling of the myocardium in the inferior wall and anterior septum in contrast to the normal appearance of the anterior wall.

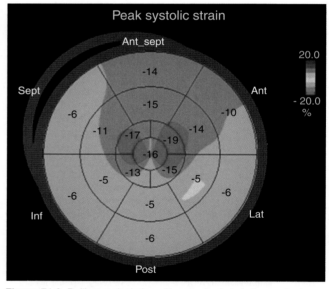

Figure 71.3. Bull's eye depiction of longitudinal strain in a patient with Fabry disease and a normal ejection fraction. The global strain is decreased, and there is lower strain in the basal regions compared with the apex.

CLINICAL SPECTRUM

ICMOs are characterized by noncompliant LV walls that impede normal diastolic filling. Thus, varying degrees of diastolic dysfunction can occur, with the classic presentation being that of heart failure with a preserved ejection fraction (EF) accompanied by severe restrictive diastolic dysfunction, biatrial enlargement, and often pulmonary hypertension. In some instances of more advanced disease, significant impairment of the EF occurs. There is a diverse spectrum of phenotypic manifestations, ranging from left ventricles with small-volume cavities associated with markedly thickened walls to dilated thin-walled dysfunctional ventricles.[2] ICMOs can be differentiated from idiopathic restrictive cardiomyopathy despite some similar clinical and echo-Doppler features (Fig. 71.1).

DIAGNOSIS

When hereditary disorders are suspected, a detailed family history with a third-generation pedigree should be obtained. This information must be integrated with the ethnic background and age of the patient because certain disorders are more common in certain populations. In both hereditary and acquired disorders, detailed systemic evaluation is of paramount importance, particularly of the neurologic, renal, and reticuloendothelial systems.

The electrocardiogram (ECG) has traditionally been an important diagnostic tool to ascertain the presence of ICMO. A discrepancy of low QRS voltages and thickened myocardial walls has traditionally been suggestive of ICMO, with amyloidosis being the most common and widely studied condition. However, the sensitivity and specificity for this combination vary greatly. Currently, this model is inadequate because many patients with

ICMO can have thick or thin walls, variable QRS voltages, and either a normal or an abnormal EF.

The provisional diagnosis can be narrowed down considerably by integrating data from the clinical evaluation, ECG findings, and the use of multimodality imaging (echocardiography and cardiac magnetic resonance imaging [CMRI]). This can be diagnostic if accompanied by an abnormality in the appropriate biochemical or disease markers. Tissue diagnosis may still be needed, and thus, cardiac biopsy remains the gold standard to provide an accurate diagnosis.

ECHOCARDIOGRAPHY

The role of echocardiography is to exclude other pathophysiologic states that simulate the clinical presentation at hand, to assess the anatomy and the function of the cardiac chambers of patients with ICMO, and to provide clues to the diagnosis of the underlying cause. The first step involves a thorough evaluation of the regional anatomy of the left ventricle focusing on identifying wall hypertrophy, wall motion abnormality, and the presence of altered myocardial texture or speckling. The latter has also been termed "sparkling or granular myocardium" (Fig. 71.2 and Video 71.2); the term "speckling" will be used in this text. At the outset, it is imperative for the echocardiographer to avoid several pitfalls related to inappropriate gain settings and tissue harmonic imaging that may cause inaccurate diagnosis of speckling. Most reports in the literature of increased echogenicity of the myocardium with speckling refer to ICMO, in particular, amyloid, but this pattern may also uncommonly occur in LV hypertrophy (LVH). Using the 17-segment model of the American Society of Echocardiography as the basis of analysis from multiple views provides a comprehensive assessment of the three key features.

Assessment of the EF and diastolic function is the next step. In most instances, the EF is preserved early on, whereas a restrictive filling pattern (grade 3 diastolic dysfunction) is present. These findings are associated with marked dilatation of the atria and pulmonary hypertension. As opposed to the hemodynamics of constrictive pericarditis, interrogation of mitral and tricuspid inflow velocities using pulsed-wave Doppler reveals no marked expiratory or inspiratory increment in velocities, whereas hepatic vein Doppler reveals an increment in the atrial reversal wave with inspiration and not with expiration.[3,4] Tissue Doppler imaging of the mitral annulus depicts a depressed E′, in keeping with abnormal myocardial relaxation.[5,6] Furthermore, the medial E′ is usually less than the lateral E′, unlike constrictive pericarditis.[7] Using both the calculated E/E′ ratio and the left atrial volume index provides insight into acute and chronic filling pressures. A careful interrogation of these important echocardiographic features aids in differentiating restrictive cardiomyopathy from constrictive pericarditis, which is the most frequent clinical scenario that mimics these hemodynamics. LV systolic function, as estimated by the EF, is usually normal until the late stages of disease progression.

SPECKLE TRACKING

This technique has emerged as a robust technique to assess regional and global myocardial mechanics. It has been applied to several conditions; cardiac amyloidosis is the most common condition. The most important clinical caveat is that although most patients with ICMOs have normal EFs, it does not imply that they have normal systolic function. Impairment of longitudinal function, both regionally and globally, is often found despite a normal EF (Fig. 71.3). These techniques may detect an abnormality before overt phenotypic or functional abnormalities on echocardiography and thus may detect subclinical hereditary ICMO or even cardiac involvement in systemic disease.[8]

Another possible application for this technique is that the site and distribution of pathological involvement in different ICMOs vary, and therefore, varying patterns of abnormal mechanics can occur. Apical sparing is a pattern of regional differences in deformation; longitudinal strain in the basal and middle segments of the left ventricle is more severely impaired compared with strain values in apical segments. Phelan and coworkers[9] were the first to demonstrate the clinical relevance of this strain pattern in patients with cardiac amyloidosis. In their study, apical sparing differentiated cardiac amyloidosis from other causes of LVH with high sensitivity and specificity. This apical-sparing pattern was also described recently with oxalosis.[10] Liu and coworkers[11] used the ratio of systolic longitudinal strain at the apex to systolic longitudinal strain measured at the base in combination with deceleration time to accurately differentiate cardiac amyloid from hypertension and Fabry disease.

TABLE 71.2 Cardiac Magnetic Resonance Imaging Features of Infiltrative Cardiomyopathy

Disease	Cardiac Magnetic Resonance Abnormality
Amyloid	Patchy focal or global subendocardial LGE
Sarcoid	Patchy subendocardial, midmyocardial, or subepicardial LGE
Fabry disease	Patchy basolateral subepicardial or midmyocardial LGE Reduced noncontrast myocardial T1 values
Danon disease	Subendocardial LGE
Hemochromatosis	Reduced T2 values

LGE, Late gadolinium enhancement.

CARDIAC MAGNETIC RESONANCE

The CMRI technique has superior spatial resolution to echocardiography and is the gold standard for establishing information on ventricular volumes, mass, and EF. Its most important use is in detecting the presence and anatomical extent of late gadolinium enhancement (LGE) within the myocardium. Gadolinium causes magnetic hyperenhancement in conditions in which extracellular space is expanded (e.g., myocyte necrosis, myocardial edema, scar formation, and protein infiltration).[12] The pattern of LGE may suggest a potential diagnosis (Table 71.2).[13–15]

ENDOMYOCARDIAL BIOPSY

Endomyocardial biopsy (EMB) is frequently required to obtain a definitive diagnosis, usually when no other anatomic sites can be used for tissue diagnosis. Recent reports suggest that EMB can be safely performed from both ventricles with a low complication rate.[16] The diagnostic yield was very high in the largest series of EMBs when echocardiography demonstrated abnormalities of the left or right ventricle. If echocardiography revealed no abnormality of the right ventricle in the face of LV abnormality, the diagnostic yield of right ventricular (RV) EMB was much lower than that of LV EMB in these patients, suggesting that echocardiography is important in guiding EMB strategy.[16] The use of CMRI to guide EMB has been anecdotal, but its use is promising. In one series, EMB resulted in 18% of patients who were presumed to have hypertrophic cardiomyopathy (HCM) to be reclassified as having either infiltrative or storage myocardial disease.[17]

Thus, a contemporary approach to the diagnosis of ICMO requires integration of clinical and ECG data, as well as multimodality data from echocardiography and CMRI to guide diagnosis or select patients for EMB. A practical approach we advocate to improving the diagnostic algorithm is to integrate these data with a morphologic classification, as outlined by Seward and Casaclang-Verzosa.[2] This morphologic classification distinguishes ICMO based on LV wall morphology and identifies two major categories of patients, namely those with thickened LV walls and those with a dilated phenotype.

Infiltrative Cardiomyopathy With Thick Walls

Thick-walled ICMO disorders have a phenotype that may mimic hypertensive heart disease or HCM. Disorders that produce this phenotype include amyloid, Fabry disease, Danon disease, mucopolysaccharidosis, and oxalosis. When evaluating this phenotype, mimickers of ICMO with thick walls must be excluded by systematic echocardiography in conjunction with relevant clinical scenarios, such as cardiac tumors, LV noncompaction, mitochondriopathies, infiltrative eosinophilic myocarditis, carnitine deficiency, and Friedreich

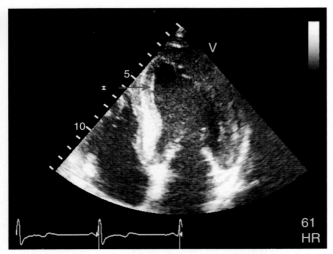

Figure 71.4. Apical four-chamber view demonstrating the altered myocardial texture in the inferoseptum and the bilayered endocardium *(red arrow).*

ataxia.[18,19] The latter two disorders do not usually cause restrictive hemodynamics. Cardiac amyloidosis is the most frequent of these disorders encountered in clinical practice and is covered in greater detail elsewhere in this book. Fabry disease is perhaps the one disorder that, if recognized early, allows for clinical intervention. An important caveat when assessing these disorders is that an integrated approach based on identifying relevant systemic abnormalities, ECG abnormalities, and patterns of LGE on CMRI should be used. QRS voltage is reduced in amyloid and diminished or increased in mucopolysaccharidosis, whereas the QRS interval is normal or increased in the other pathologies within this category.

Fabry Disease

Fabry disease is an X-linked autosomal recessive disease caused by a deficiency of the lysosomal enzyme, α-galactosidase. The pathophysiology is not clearly delineated, but it is related to the accumulation of glycolipids within the lysozymes of organs, which ultimately results in fibrosis. Systemic involvement includes the skin, kidneys, and neurologic abnormalities that may coexist.[20] Homozygous males develop clinical manifestations by the second decade, with cardiac involvement occurring in the third decade of life; these patients have a poorer prognosis compared with heterozygous females, who may have a normal life expectancy and are often asymptomatic with mildly thickened LV walls.[21]

Echocardiography maybe used for diagnostic purposes in three clinical scenarios. The first entails evaluating a patient with a classical presentation for Fabry disease for cardiac abnormality, the second scenario is the patient in whom unexplained thick LV walls are detected, and the third is the patient who undergoes evaluation as part of family screening for Fabry disease.

The hallmark of myocardial abnormality is that of symmetrical thickened LV walls, which can mimic nonobstructive HCM and has presented in this manner in some series.[22–24] Importantly, the EF is usually preserved, with diastolic dysfunction being present, although severe restrictive diastolic dysfunction is uncommon. The detection of a binary endocardial layer has been suggested to be an important echocardiographic feature in differentiating Fabry disease from HCM or hypertensive heart disease (Fig. 71.4 and Video 71.4).[25] Identifying a binary endocardial layer has a sensitivity of 94% and a specificity of 100% for distinguishing the diagnosis of Fabry disease from HCM and hypertensive heart disease. The binary endocardial layer is thought to be caused by endomyocardial glycosphingolipid compartmentalization.[25]

Speckle tracking may show reduced strain and strain rate in the basal inferolateral wall that correlates with CMRI which typically shows focal inferolateral midwall LGE sparing of the subendocardium.[26] An additional sign that maybe detected using speckle tracking is that of a decrement in the global CS accompanied by loss of the normal base-to-apex gradient.[27] This sign maybe present in individuals with or without LVH. The abnormalities in myocardial mechanics together with symmetry of the basal septum thickening with that of the basal inferolateral wall are diagnostic pointer for Fabry disease as opposed to HCM.

Enzyme replacement offers the opportunity to attenuate the disease process especially in cases that present early.[28] Echocardiography can be used to monitor therapy. The key variables to be evaluated are LV wall thickness and mass, LV diastolic function, and either tissue Doppler imaging or speckle tracking. The response of wall thickness is variable, with women being more likely then men to have regression of wall thickness.[29]

Danon Disease

Danon disease is a rare X-linked disorder caused by lysosome-associated membrane protein 2 deficiency.[2] It affects men at an early age (their teens) and women in later years (their 20s). Males may present with the triad of intellectual abnormality, myopathy, and cardiomyopathy (phenotype mimicking HCM), whereas females tend to present only with cardiomyopathy (either mimicking HCM or dilated cardiomyopathy [DCM]). The echocardiographic phenotype is characterized by marked symmetrical LVH, a depressed EF, and, frequently, thickening of the RV walls, independent of the degree of pulmonary hypertension. Pre-excitation and tachyarrhythmias satisfying the diagnosis of Wolff-Parkinson-White syndrome can occur. CMRI reveals subendocardial LGE. Genetic testing for lysosome-associated membrane protein 2 gene mutation is definitive and is the major diagnostic criterion in women.

Oxalosis

Oxalosis is an autosomal-recessive disorder characterized by increased production of oxalic acid, with involvement affecting the kidneys, liver, and heart. Echocardiography reveals thickening of both the LV and RV walls with speckling. The latter may be most prominent in the papillary muscles. Initially, the EF is preserved with severe diastolic dysfunction, and elevated filling pressure is typical. Renal and liver transplantation have been attempted with no overt success in terms of regressing the cardiac abnormality.

Mucopolysaccharidoses

Mucopolysaccharidoses are autosomal recessive disorders that cause deficiencies in the lysosomal enzymes that break down glycosaminoglycans. Cardiac involvement occurs in most of these disorders. Hurler syndrome is the classic example and is often the most severe disease. Myocardial involvement can be either symmetrical or asymmetrical thickening with a preserved EF. Valvular abnormalities and coronary narrowing can occur in these disorders. Diagnosis entails integrating clinical features with serum analysis for enzyme deficiencies and urine analysis for excess mucopolysaccharidosis.

Glycogen Storage Disease

Cardiac involvement has been documented in types 2, 3, 4, and 5 of glycogen storage disease. Type 3 is the most commonly encountered scenario in adults and is characterized by thickened walls with a preserved EF. Rarely, some patients present with a DCM phenotype.

Gaucher Disease

Gaucher disease is an autosomal recessive disorder characterized by a defect of the lysosomal enzyme, β-glucocerebrosidase. The consequence of this deficiency is the accumulation of glucocerebroside in various organs, in particular, the reticuloendothelial system, which results in hepatosplenomegaly. Orthopedic manifestations such as severe bone pain, avascular necrosis of the head of the femur, and pathological fractures may occur. This disorder can manifest in early childhood with neurologic abnormalities or in adults with no neurologic abnormalities. In the latter scenario, cardiac abnormalities include ICMO and hemorrhagic pericarditis. Valvular involvement occurs with the juvenile presentation of this disorder. Diagnosis is usually made by biopsy of the reticuloendothelial organs or bone marrow analysis.

INFILTRATIVE CARDIOMYOPATHY WITH THE DILATED PHENOTYPE

ICMO may manifest with a dilated left ventricle with no overtly thickened walls, varying degrees of speckling, and a low EF. These disorders mimic nonischemic DCM and ischemic cardiomyopathy. Sarcoid, hemochromatosis, Wegener granulomatosis, and amyloid are less commonly present, with these features as well.[2]

Hemochromatosis

Hemochromatosis is an autosomal recessive condition most frequently caused by two gene abnormalities, C282Y and H63D, which are point mutations on chromosome 6. This disorder is characterized by excessive iron absorption from the intestine, which consequently leads to increased iron deposition in the liver, pancreas, joints, pituitary gland, and heart.

Echocardiography detects functional consequences of iron overload, and in its most overt form, speckling of the myocardium may be detected. LV wall thickness is not increased, and early in the disease course only diastolic dysfunction may be documented, which may cause shortness of breath. As the disease progresses, more commonly, a DCM phenotype that can cause severe heart failure occurs. Uncommonly, some patients may develop a restrictive phenotype characterized by preserved EF, severe diastolic dysfunction, and pulmonary hypertension.[30] Speckle tracking may reveal abnormal longitudinal strain and torsion in instances when the heart appears structurally and functionally normal. However, the earliest detection of iron overload of the heart is detected with CMRI. This is important because there is some evidence to suggest that therapeutic strategies such as phlebotomy or chelation therapy may reverse this process if initiated early on. A second scenario in which CMRI may be useful is in patients who are scheduled to undergo liver transplantation. Diagnosis is facilitated by serological evidence of T2-weighted iron overload in the heart and liver as seen on CMRI and tissue diagnosis. Therapy with phlebotomy and chelating agents can improve cardiac manifestations, whereas cardiac transplantation has been performed for advanced heart failure in selected cases.

CONCLUSIONS

ICMO commonly presents as heart failure with a preserved EF and thickened walls with severe restrictive diastolic dysfunction or as a phenocopy of DCM. Integration of clinical, echocardiographic, and CMRI findings are key in the diagnostic algorithm of these rare hereditary or acquired disorders.

Please access ExpertConsult to view the corresponding videos for this chapter.

REFERENCES

1. Maron BJ, Towbin JA, Thiene G, et al. Contemporary definitions and classification of the cardiomyopathies. *Circulation.* 2006;113:1807–1816.
2. Seward JB, Casaclang-Verzosa G. Infiltrative cardiovascular diseases: cardiomyopathies that look alike. *J Am Coll Cardiol.* 2010;55:1769–1779.
3. Hatle LK, Appleton CP, Popp RL. Differentiation of constrictive pericarditis and restrictive cardiomyopathy by Doppler echocardiography. *Circulation.* 1989;79:357–370.
4. Reuss CS, Wilansky SM, Lester SJ, et al. Using mitral "annulus reversus" to diagnose constrictive pericarditis. *Eur J Echocardiogr.* 2009;10:372–375.
5. Garcia MJ, Rodriguez L, Ares M, et al. Differentiation of constrictive pericarditis from restrictive cardiomyopathy: assessment of left ventricular diastolic velocities in longitudinal axis by Doppler tissue imaging. *J Am Coll Cardiol.* 1996;27:108–114.
6. Sohn DW, Kim YJ, Kim HS, et al. Unique features of early diastolic mitral annulus velocity in constrictive pericarditis. *J Am Soc Echocardiogr.* 2004;17:222–226.
7. Ha JW, Ommen SR, Tajik AJ, et al. Differentiation of constrictive pericarditis from restrictive cardiomyopathy using mitral annular velocity by tissue Doppler echocardiography. *Am J Cardiol.* 2004;94:316–319.
8. Gruner C, Verocai F, Carasso S, et al. Systolic myocardial mechanics in patients with Anderson-Fabry disease with and without left ventricular hypertrophy and in comparison to nonobstructive hypertrophic cardiomyopathy. *Echocardiography.* 2012;29:810–817.
9. Phelan D, Collier P, Thavendiranathan P, et al. Relative apical sparing of longitudinal strain using two-dimensional speckle-tracking echocardiography is both sensitive and specific for the diagnosis of cardiac amyloidosis. *Heart.* 2012;98:1442–1448.
10. Lagies R, Beck BB, Hoppe B, et al. Apical sparing of longitudinal strain, left ventricular rotational abnormalities, and short-axis dysfunction in primary hyperoxaluria type 1. *Circ Heart Fail.* 2013;6:e45–47.
11. Liu D, Hu K, Niemann M, et al. Effect of combined systolic and diastolic functional parameter assessment for differentiation of cardiac amyloidosis from other causes of concentric left ventricular hypertrophy. *Circ Cardiovasc Imag.* 2013;6:1066–1072.
12. Vöhringer M, Mahrholdt H, Yilmaz A, et al. Significance of late gadolinium enhancement in cardiovascular magnetic resonance imaging. *Herz.* 2007;32:129–137.
13. Rudolph A, Abdel-Aty H, Bohl S, et al. Noninvasive detection of fibrosis applying contrast-enhanced cardiac magnetic resonance in different forms of left ventricular hypertrophy relation to remodeling. *J Am Coll Cardiol.* 2009;53:284–291.
14. Srinivasan G, Joseph M, Selvanayagam JB. Recent advances in the imaging assessment of infiltrative cardiomyopathies. *Heart.* 2013;99:204–213.
15. Thompson RB, Chow K, Khan A, et al. T_1 mapping with cardiovascular MRI is highly sensitive for Fabry disease independent of hypertrophy and sex. *Circ Cardiovasc Imag.* 2013;6:637–645.
16. Chimenti C, Frustaci A. Contribution and risks of left ventricular endomyocardial biopsy in patients with cardiomyopathies: a retrospective study over a 28-year period. *Circulation.* 2013;128:1531–1541.
17. Frustaci A, Russo MA, Chimenti C. Diagnostic contribution of left ventricular endomyocardial biopsy in patients with clinical phenotype of hypertrophic cardiomyopathy. *Hum Pathol.* 2013;44:133–141.
18. Lee GY, Kim WS, Ko YH, et al. Primary cardiac lymphoma mimicking infiltrative cardiomyopathy. *Eur J Heart Fail.* 2013;15:589–591.
19. Thebault C, Ollivier R, Leurent G, et al. Mitochondriopathy: a rare aetiology of restrictive cardiomyopathy. *Eur J Echocardiogr.* 2008;9:840–845.
20. Desnick RJ, Astrin KH, Bishop DF. Fabry disease: Molecular genetics of the inherited nephropathy. *Adv Nephrol Necker Hosp.* 1989;18:113–127.
21. Nelis GF, Jacobs GJ. Anorexia, weight loss, and diarrhea as presenting symptoms of angiokeratoma corporis diffusum (Fabry-Anderson's disease). *Dig Dis Sci.* 1989;34:1798–1800.
22. Colucci WS, Lorell BH, Schoen FJ, et al. Hypertrophic obstructive cardiomyopathy due to Fabry's disease. *N Engl J Med.* 1982;307:926–928.
23. Sachdev B, Takenaka T, Teraguchi H, et al. Prevalence of Anderson-Fabry disease in male patients with late onset hypertrophic cardiomyopathy. *Circulation.* 2002;105:1407–1411.
24. Chimenti C, Pieroni M, Morgante E, et al. Prevalence of Fabry disease in female patients with late-onset hypertrophic cardiomyopathy. *Circulation.* 2004;110:1047–1053.
25. Pieroni M, Chimenti C, De Cobelli F, et al. Fabry's disease cardiomyopathy: echocardiographic detection of endomyocardial glycosphingolipid compartmentalization. *J Am Coll Cardiol.* 2006;47:1663–1671.
26. Krämer J, Niemann M, Liu D, et al. Two-dimensional speckle tracking as a noninvasive tool for identification of myocardial fibrosis in Fabry disease. *Eur Heart J.* 2013;34:1587–1596.
27. Labombarda F, Saloux E, Milesi G, et al. Loss of base-to-apex circumferential strain gradient: a specific pattern of Fabry cardiomyopathy. *Echocardiography.* 2017;34:504–510.
28. Frustaci A, Chimenti C, Ricci R, et al. Improvement in cardiac function in the cardiac variant of Fabry's disease with galactose-infusion therapy. *N Engl J Med.* 2001;345:25–32.
29. Lin HY, Liu HC, Huang YH, et al. Effects of enzyme replacement therapy for cardiac-type Fabry patients with a Chinese hotspot late-onset Fabry mutation (IVS4+919G>A). *BMJ Open.* 2013;3:e003146.
30. Gujja P, Rosing DR, Tripodi DJ, et al. Iron overload cardiomyopathy: better understanding of an increasing disorder. *J Am Coll Cardiol.* 2010;56:1001–1012.

72 Endomyocardial Fibrosis

Beatriz Ferreira, Ferande Peters

Endomyocardial fibrosis (EMF) is a restrictive cardiomyopathy that was first described as an independent pathological entity in 1948 by John N.P. Davies of Makerere University in Uganda. At necropsy, he found a series of hearts that had dense scarring of the mural endocardium. The fibrosis predominated at the apices and crept up toward the inflow tract. These cases presented with what he described as the "heart of Africa," a dilated right atrium and a depressed rugose sulcus over the retracted apex of the right ventricle, which resembled a rough outline of Africa as seen on a map.[1,2] Subsequent work in the following three decades defined the epidemiology, clinical features, hemodynamics, and surgical experience with EMF.[3–9]

CAUSE

More than 60 years after its first description, the cause of EMF is still a mystery. The concentration of the disease in tropical and subtropical regions led to searches for infectious or nutritional causes. The similarity of the lesions with Loeffler endocarditis and carcinoid heart disease suggested a relation to eosinophil toxicity and serotonin.[10,11] Because EMF is prevalent in countries close to the equator, which endemic for worm infestation and parasitic diseases such as malaria, filariasis, and schistosomiasis, research led to the suggestion that parasite-induced eosinophilia precipitated the disease.[12] An autoimmune etiology was postulated when increased levels of antimalaria antibodies and antiheart antibodies were found, together with a hyperimmune malaria splenomegaly.[13] A geochemical hypothesis related EMF to cerium and thorium has also been postulated.[14] Investigations into nutritional factors focused on a possible connection with cassava toxicity. In some countries, an association between EMF and poverty, low protein, and a cassava-based diet were found. Some suggested that cerium-mediated cassava toxicity in the setting of protein deficiency played a role in pathogenesis of the disease.[15] Familial occurrence[16] suggested a genetic susceptibility. The finding of a preponderance of the *HLA-B*58* gene in patients with severe disease favored an immunogenetic predisposition.[17]

EPIDEMIOLOGY

EMF is prevalent worldwide, but it is more endemic in parts of tropical and subtropical Africa. The disease also occurs in South American countries such as Brazil, Colombia, and Venezuela and in Asia in India, Thailand, Ceylon, and Malaysia. Sporadic cases have been described in other countries.[18] There have been several reports of EMF in Europeans who resided in tropical Africa for several years.[19] In endemic areas such as Uganda, 20% of the cases referred for echocardiography are EMF.[20] In Mozambique, two epidemiologic studies found prevalence in rural areas of 8.9% and 19.8%.[21,22] Different rates were found among regions within Mozambique (18.3 vs 3.2 per 100,000).[23] In some countries, such as India, the incidence of EMF is declining.[24] This reduction seems to be related to improved living conditions in these populations.

PATHOPHYSIOLOGY, KEY CLINICAL MANIFESTATIONS, AND DISEASE COURSE

The initial stage seems to present with febrile episodes, hypereosinophilia, pancarditis, edema, effort dyspnea, palpitations, itching,

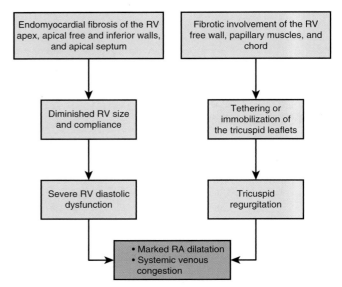

Figure 72.1. Pathogenesis of predominant right-sided endomyocardial fibrosis. *RV,* Right ventricular.

and urticaria. After the initial stage, the disease alternates between stable periods and active episodes. For some patients, the disease can be rapidly progressive, with death occurring in 2 years. For others, there is 70% of survival rate at 5 years. Death is caused by heart failure, thromboembolism, or arrhythmia.

The pathophysiology of advanced right-sided EMF relates to the degree and sites of RV EMF and its ensuing two key abnormalities, right ventricular (RV) diastolic dysfunction and tricuspid regurgitation (TR) (Fig. 72.1). In severe forms, the RV apex is completely obliterated, and the right ventricle is reduced to the inflow tract and infundibulum. The right atrium is often aneurysmal secondary to the combination of severe RV diastolic dysfunction and severe (TR. This imposes both a pressure and volume overload on the right atrium.

In the left forms, fibrosis affects the apex and inflow tract, particularly the posterior papillary muscle. The posterior mitral leaflet is immobile and absorbed by the fibrosis, which results in mitral regurgitation (MR). Both ventricles and atria can present with organized thrombi. Endocardial calcification and pericardial effusion can be present.

PHYSICAL EXAMINATION

In the right forms, patients present with growth retardation, delayed secondary sexual characteristics, swollen face, exophthalmos, cyanosis, elevated jugular venous pressure, a third sound of the right ventricle, a pansystolic murmur of TR, hepatosplenomegaly, and voluminous ascites that can lead to an inguinal hernia (Fig. 72.2) in the absence of significant pedal edema. Patients with the left forms present with signs of pulmonary congestion with progressive levels of dyspnea. A pansystolic murmur and a third heart sound are often heard, which is related to MR. When

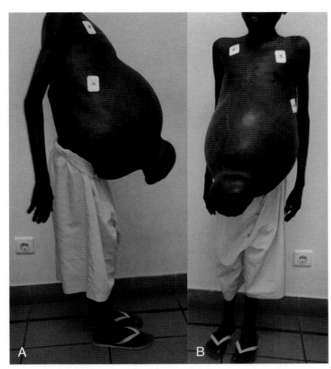

Figure 72.2. A and **B,** Advanced right ventricular endomyocardial fibrosis with voluminous ascites and inguinal hernia.

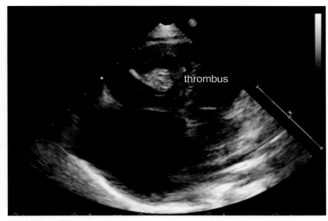

Figure 72.3. Endomyocardial fibrosis acute phase–thrombi at tricuspid subvalvular apparatus in a 2-year-old child.

BOX 72.1 Technical Tips

1. Ensure that the gain is standardized to avoid artifactual diagnosis of hyperechoic abnormality versus true hyperechoic abnormality caused by pathology.
2. When the image quality in the far field is poor, it may be caused by apical scarring and calcification of the apex preventing optimal transmission of the ultrasound beam beyond this area.
3. Systematic evaluation of the entire right ventricle in numerous views is required to identify pathology that alters the normal architecture of the ventricle in particular areas of fibrosis and scarring that cause retraction of the apex and apical obliteration.
4. Differentiation of organized chronic calcific thrombus from fibrosis with calcification is important. A clue to the latter is that the movement of the underlying myocardium may be normal when there is no obliteration of the area.
5. The mitral valve and subvalvular apparatus require careful evaluation to identify fibrotic thickening, chordal thickening, and retraction and posterior leaflet restriction.
6. Differentiation of valvular abnormality from rheumatic heart disease is occasionally needed. Clues to the diagnosis of EMF are accompanying abnormalities in the apical regions and the marked diastolic abnormality often seen.
7. In predominant RV EMF, the diastolic overload of the right ventricle secondary to severe diastolic dysfunction can be best observed by the abnormal septal motion noted.
8. LV involvement maybe subtle in some instances and maybe best recognized by careful evaluation of the endocardium for thickening and hyper echoic abnormality suggestive of fibrosis. TDI may be required to identify lower than expected E′ suggestive of concomitant abnormal relaxation.

EMF, endomyocardial fibrosis; *LV,* left ventricular; *RV,* right ventricular; *TDI,* tissue Doppler imaging.

---

both ventricles are involved, the clinical features of RV EMF are dominant.

Diagnostic testing

Electrocardiography can reveal supraventricular arrhythmia and, in the advanced forms, atrial fibrillation. In sinus rhythm, signs of dilatation of the right or left atrium can be seen. In the advanced right forms, a QR interval in leads V1 and V4R are typical. Incomplete right or left bundle brunch block and ST-segment depression associated with T-wave inversion are frequent.[25] When there is pericardial effusion, a globular heart shadow can be seen on chest radiography. In the right forms, there is dilatation of the right atrium and the infundibulum. The lungs are clear. In the left forms, there is dilatation of the left ventricle and atrium with prominent pulmonary artery and pulmonary congestion. Pleural effusions are frequent at the end stage of the disease.[26]

Echocardiography

Echocardiography is the diagnostic procedure of choice for the diagnosis of EMF. The key to making an accurate diagnosis depends on performing a systematic evaluation to integrate the key morphologic and functional abnormalities that are detected. This information is used to determine the stage of the disease (acute phase or more commonly the chronic phase) and the degree of involvement of each ventricle (biventricular, pure right sided or left sided) and to detect complications. It is imperative that attention to the following technical tips be undertaken when performing echocardiography (Box 72.1)

Active Phase: Key Morphology to be Identified by Echocardiography

Only a few cases are found in the acute phase. EMF is a disease of the apex, the admission chamber, and the atrioventricular valves of both ventricles. The outflow tract and semilunar valves are spared. In the acute phase, the walls may appear to be thickened because of diffuse soft echogenic infiltrates that may be associated with thrombi (thrombotic phase), which are usually detected at the apex or in the subvalvular apparatus (Fig. 72.3 and Video 72.3).

The Chronic Phase: Key Right-Sided Morphologic Features

On the right side, the advanced lesions present with thick patches of hyperechogenic fibrosis that involve the apex, the free wall, and the interventricular septum. The apical fibrosis is associated with varying degrees of obliteration or retraction of the apex, reducing its distance to the tips of the tricuspid leaflets. The RV outflow tract is dilated and hyperkinetic. Shrinkage of the right apex results in a characteristic apical notch. Obliteration of the papillary muscles and chordae may immobilize the tricuspid valve, which remains open throughout the cardiac cycle. There is an important dilatation of the right atrium in which dynamic intracavitary echoes or even large thrombi can be seen (Fig. 72.4 and Video 72.4). The inferior vena cava is dilated.

Key Right-Sided Hemodynamic Features

As outlined previously, the key hemodynamic changes are related to the presence of severe RV diastolic dysfunction, often severe TR, and consequent high right atrial (RA) pressures. Features of severe diastolic dysfunction include a restrictive pattern of tricuspid inflow with a short deceleration time and abnormal interventricular septal motion on M-mode echocardiography, and on pulsed-wave Doppler, the pulmonary valve shows presystolic opening; forward flow is seen in systole and diastole (Fig. 72.5). Doppler color-flow mapping reveals low-velocity TR. The hepatic veins can show a systolic reversal of flow (Fig. 72.6) or a prominent reversal flow during atrial systole (Fig. 72.7). These hepatic Doppler findings are also influenced by the severity of TR, the presence of atrial fibrillation, and the stage of the disease and its degree of diastolic dysfunction.

Key Left-Sided Morphological Abnormalities

Left ventricular (LV) EMF presents with increased apical and admission tract echogenicity, particularly in the posterior wall. The posterior mitral leaflet is frequently tethered down or plastered to the LV posterior wall. Mitral stenosis can be seen rarely. The papillary muscles can be highly echogenic (Fig. 72.8 and Video 72.8). Apical obliteration is seen in advanced cases. Areas of calcification can be present. When the apical obliteration is severe, the long axis of the left ventricle is reduced, whereas its diameter is increased. As in RV EMF, the outflow tract is spared. The left atrium is enlarged, and there may be evidence of prethrombotic smoke or thrombus.

On M-mode echocardiography, restricted motion of the posterior mitral leaflet is noted. There is a rapid early diastolic posterior motion of the LV posterior wall that flattens out in the remainder of diastole. Similarly, the interventricular septum shows a steep anterior displacement in early diastole, with an abrupt cessation of diastolic anterior movement.[1] It can present as an M movement (Fig. 72.9). Doppler studies reveal rapid E acceleration and deceleration slopes with a shortening of the rapid filling phase (Fig. 72.10). MR is almost always present and can be severe. The Doppler tracings of the pulmonary veins may show dominance of the D wave and a broad

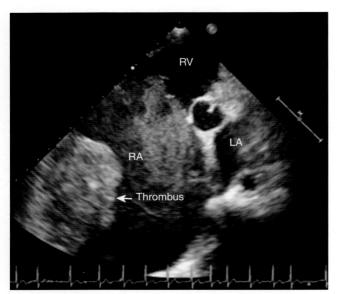

Figure 72.4. Advanced right ventricular (RV) endomyocardial fibrosis with small RV cavity, right atrial (RA) dilatation, voluminous thrombus, and dynamic intracavitary echoes. *LA,* Left atrial.

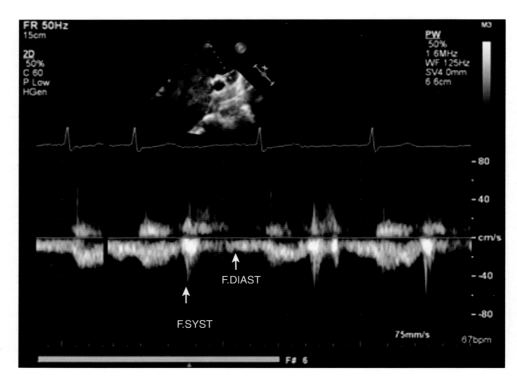

Figure 72.5. Diastolic forward flow on the pulmonary artery.

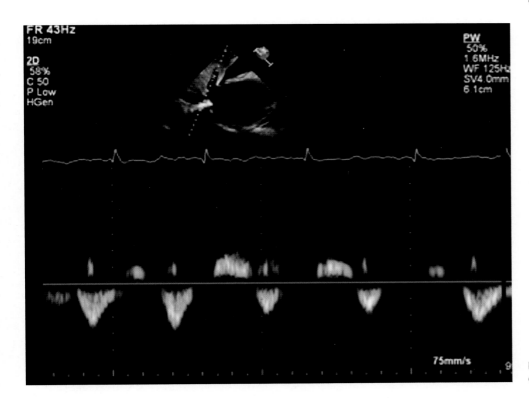

Figure 72.6. Systolic reversal flow of the hepatic veins.

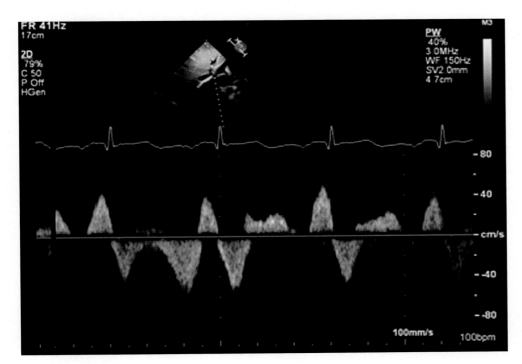

Figure 72.7. Prominent reversal flow during atrial systole in the hepatic veins.

reversal of the A wave in keeping with the high left atrial pressures. Evidence of pulmonary hypertension is frequent and should be detected by careful quantitative analysis of pulmonary and tricuspid regurgitant Doppler traces. In biventricular advanced EMF (Fig. 72.11 and Video 72.11), there is a typical inversion of the normal ventricular-to-atrial size ratio, with obliterated small ventricles and dilated atria. Systolic function is normal until the very advanced stages of the disease.

Three-dimensional transthoracic echocardiography has a complementary role to two-dimensional transthoracic echocardiography, adding information regarding distribution of the fibrotic lesions and characteristics of the thrombus (Fig. 72.12 and Video 72.12).[27] Magnetic resonance imaging with late gadolinium enhancement characterizes the fibrotic tissue distribution, which is the hallmark of the disease.[28]

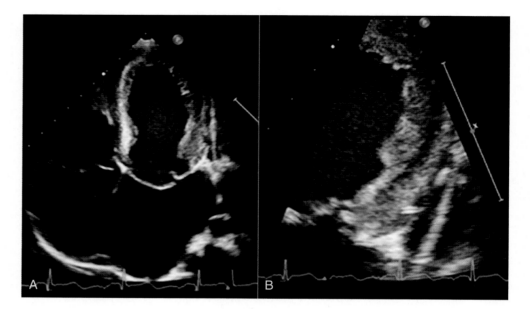

Figure 72.8. A and **B,** Posterior papillary muscle plastered to the wall.

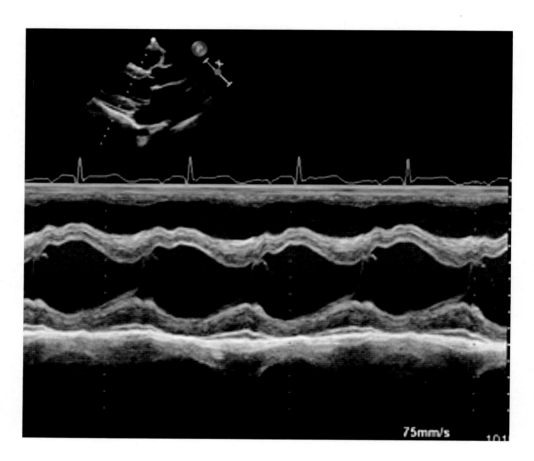

Figure 72.9. Septal M movement in left ventricular endomyocardial fibrosis.

Detection of Complications

Atrial thrombi form frequently and may be a source for cardioembolism to the systemic circulation or pulmonary embolism, and thus must be carefully and systematically excluded by the imager. These thrombi form because of stasis of blood in the markedly enlarged atrium independent of the presence of atrial fibrillation.

Both right and left EMF present with different grades of pericardial effusion, varying from minimal to large (Fig. 72.13), with a thin pericardium. A large pericardial effusion may be present in advanced stages and may worsen the clinical right-sided congestion noted. Tamponade maybe less common because of the very high RV diastolic pressure and high RA

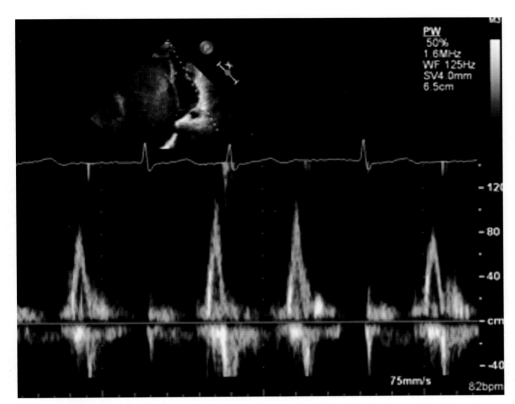

Figure 72.10. Mitral flow with a restrictive pattern.

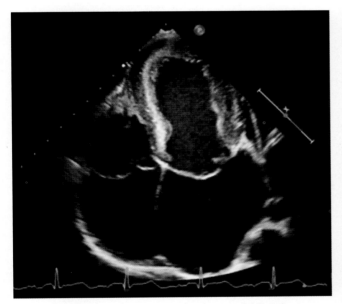

Figure 72.11. Biventricular endomyocardial fibrosis.

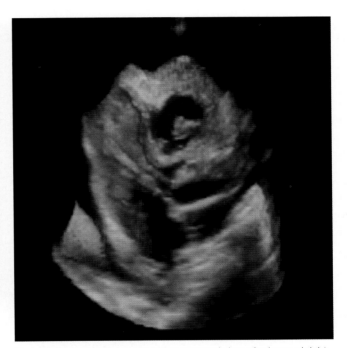

Figure 72.12. Three-dimensional parasternal view of advanced right ventricular endomyocardial fibrosis.

pressures caused by EMF. Consequently, the classic features of tamponade do not occur. However, drainage of the effusion maybe required to improve the right heart congestion of the patients or occasionally to exclude another endemic illness such as tuberculosis.

TR is often severe with predominate right-sided or biventricular EMF and adds to the hemodynamic burden of the severe RV diastolic dysfunction and RA overload. The TR jet is often low velocity with no overt mosaic pattern and can be noted by the classic continuous-wave Doppler features. These Doppler findings are related to the fact that the pressure difference between the right ventricle and right atrium are often minimal and that there is usually no leaflet coaptation in severe cases.

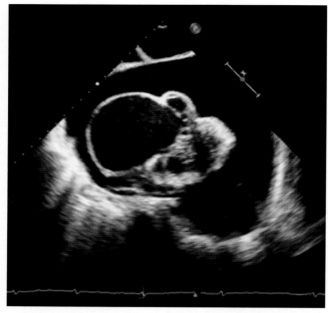

Figure 72.13. Important pericardial effusion in right ventricular endomyocardial fibrosis.

Management

Medical therapy is limited to the treatment of heart failure symptoms. Eosinophilia is suppressed with short courses of corticosteroids. Surgical treatment consists of endocardial resection and atrioventricular valve repair or replacement and improves survival, but most patients in endemic areas may not have access to surgery.[29]

Please access ExpertConsult to view the corresponding videos for this chapter.

REFERENCES

1. Davies JNP. EMF—the beginning. In: Valiathan MS, Somers K, Kartha CC, eds. *Endomyocardial Fibrosis*. Oxford, UK: Oxford University Press; 1993.
2. Davies JNP. Endomyocardial fibrosis in Uganda. *East Afr Med J*. 1948;25:10–16.
3. Williams AW, Somers K. The electrocardiogram in endomyocardial fibrosis. *Br Heart J*. 1960;22:311–315.
4. Somers K, Williams AW. The phonocardiogram in endomyocardial fibrosis. *Br Heart J*. 1960;22:546–550.
5. Shillingford JP, Somers K. Clinical and haemodynamic patterns in endomyocardial fibrosis. *Br Heart J*. 1961;23:433–446.
6. Van der Geld H, Peetom F, Somers K, et al. Immunohistological and serological studies in endomyocardial fibrosis. *Lancet*. 1966;2:1210–1213.
7. Falase AO. Endomyocardial fibrosis in Africa. *Postgrad Med J*. 1983;59:170–178.
8. Bertrand E. *Comite OMS d'Experts des Myocardiopathies*; April 1983. CVD/CMP/EC/83.
9. Metras D, Coulibaly AO, Ouattara K, et al. Endomyocardial fibrosis: early and late results of surgery in 20 patients. *J Thorac Cardiovasc Surg*. 1982;83:52–64.
10. Brockington IF, Olsen EGJ. Loeffler's endocarditis and Davies' endomyocardial fibrosis. *Am Heart J*. 1973;85:308–322.
11. Ball JD. Endomyocardial fibrosis. *Proc R Soc Med*. 1957;50:43–46.
12. Andy JJ. Helminthiasis, the hypereosinophilic syndrome and endomyocardial fibrosis: some observations and a hypothesis. *Afr J Med Sci*. 1983;12:155–164.
13. Shaper AG, Kaplan MH, Mody NJ, et al. Malarial antibodies and autoantibodies to heart and other tissues in the immigrant and indigenous peoples of Uganda. *Lancet*. 1968;1:1342–1346.
14. Valiathan MS, Kartha CC, Panday VK, et al. A geochemical basis for endomyocardial fibrosis. *Cardiovasc Res*. 1986;20:679–682.
15. Sezi CL. Effect of protein deficient cassava diet on Cercopithecus aethiops hearts and its possible role in the aetiology and pathogenesis of endomyocardial fibrosis in man. *East Afr Med J*. 1996;73:S11–S16.
16. Patel AK, Ziegler JL, D'Arbela PG, et al. Familial cases of endomyocardial fibrosis in Uganda. *BMJ*. 1971;4:331–334.
17. Mocumbi AO. *Epidemiology, Pathogenesis and Management of Endomyocardial Fibrosis. PhD Thesis, Imperial College of Science, Technology and Medicine*. NHL Institute; 2008.
18. Shaper AG. The geographical distribution of endomyocardial fibrosis. *Pathol Microbiol*. 1970;35:26–35.
19. Somers K, D'Arbela PG, Patel AK. Endomyocardial fibrosis. In: Shaper AG, Kibukamusoke JW, Hutt MSR, eds. *Medicine in a Tropical Environment*. London: British Medical Association; 1972:348–363.
20. Brockington IF, Olsen EGJ, Goodwin JF. Endomyocardial fibrosis in Europeans resident in tropical Africa. *Lancet*. 1967;1:583–588.
21. Ferreira MB. *Endomyocardial Fibrosis in Mozambique. PhD Thesis*. Faculté de Médicine Université Paris V France; 2001.
22. Mocumbi AO, Ferreira MB, Sidi D, et al. A population study of endomyocardial fibrosis in a rural area of Mozambique. *N Engl J Med*. 2008;359:43–49.
23. Ferreira MB, Matsika-Claquin MD, Mocumbi AO, et al. Geographic origin of endomyocardial fibrosis treated at the central hospital of Maputo (Mozambique) between 1987 and 1999. *Bull Soc Pathol Exot*. 2002;95:276–279.
24. Vijayaraghavan G, Sivasankaran S. Tropical endomyocardial fibrosis in India: a vanishing disease! *Indian J Med Res*. 2012;136:729–738.
25. Adenle AD, Awotedu AA. Specificity of right ventricular QR waves in endomyocardial fibrosis. *Trop Cardiol*. 1983;9:155–158.
26. Cockshott WP, Saric S, Ikeme AC. Radiological findings in endomyocardial fibrosis. *Circulation*. 1967;35:913–922.
27. Kharwar BR, Sethi R, Narain VS. Right-sided endomyocardial fibrosis with a right atrial thrombus: T-dimensional transthoracic echocardiographic evaluation. *Echocardiography*. 2013;10:E322–E325.
28. Salemi VM, Rochitte CE, Shiozaki AA, et al. Late gadolinium enhancement magnetic resonance imaging in the diagnosis and prognosis of endomyocardial fibrosis patients. *Circ Cardiovasc Imag*. 2011;4:304–311.
29. Dubost C, Chapelon C, Deloche A, et al. Surgery of endomyocardial fibrosis. Apropos of 32 cases. *Arch Mal Cœur Vaiss*. 1990;83:481–486.

73 Restriction Versus Constriction

Manish Bansal, Partho P. Sengupta

Constrictive pericarditis (CP) and restrictive cardiomyopathy (RCM) are both characterized by impairment of ventricular filling and manifest predominantly as so-called diastolic heart failure. However, the underlying pathophysiology in these two conditions is vastly different, which allows us to distinguish between these two conditions even though their clinical presentation may be quite similar. The distinction between CP and RCM is crucial because whereas CP is surgically curable, there are currently no curative therapies for most forms of RCM, with cardiac transplantation remaining the only potential option.

CAUSE

CP is usually a consequence of long-standing pericardial inflammation that ultimately leads to pericardial scarring, fibrosis, and calcification. Myocardial involvement may also occur but usually in the late stages. There are two main forms of CP: (1) the fibroelastic form (acute or subacute) in which the patients present with subtle signs and symptoms and (2) the rigid shell form (chronic) in which the pericardium is usually calcified and the patients present with advanced heart failure, hepatic dysfunction, and so on.[1] In developed countries, CP is mostly idiopathic in origin or secondary to viral pericarditis, cardiac surgery, or radiotherapy. In contrast, tuberculosis remains the leading cause of CP in developing nations (Table 73.1).[2]

Unlike CP, RCM is primarily a myocardial or endomyocardial disorder characterized by a nondilated stiff ventricle(s) with severe diastolic dysfunction. There may be predominant involvement of the left ventricle, right ventricle, or both. A number of primary cardiac or systemic disorders can give rise to RCM. In the United States, the most common cause of RCM is amyloidosis (primary, familial, and senile amyloidosis), whereas in the tropics (especially in Africa), endomyocardial fibrosis is quite common (see Table 73.1).

HEMODYNAMICS IN CONSTRICTION AND RESTRICTION

The primary pathology in CP is the loss of pericardial elasticity with its replacement with a rigid fibrocalcific shell that prevents ventricular filling (Fig. 73.1). Characteristically, there is no

TABLE 73.1 Common Underlying Causes of Constrictive Pericarditis and Restrictive Cardiomyopathy

Constrictive Pericarditis	Restrictive Cardiomyopathy
• Idiopathic	• Infiltrative cardiomyopathy and storage diseases (e.g., amyloid heart disease, mucopolysaccharidoses, sarcoidosis, hemochromatosis, glycogen storage diseases, Fabry disease)
• Cardiac surgery	
• Radiation therapy	
• Postinfectious (tuberculous, bacterial, or viral pericarditis)	
• Collagen vascular disease	
• Miscellaneous causes (e.g., malignancy, trauma, drug induced, uremic pericarditis)	• Idiopathic
	• Familial or genetic
	• Eosinophilic endomyocardial disease, endomyocardial fibrosis
	• Scleroderma
	• Post medical irradiation
	• Carcinoid heart disease
	• Medications causing fibrous endocarditis (e.g., serotonin, methysergide maleate, ergotamine tartrate, busulfan)
	• Doxorubicin or daunorubicin toxicity

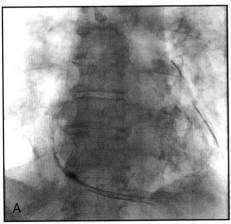
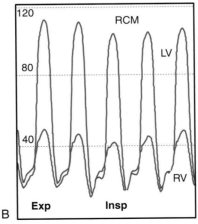
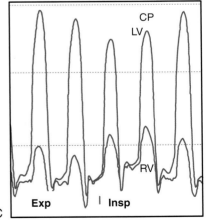

Figure 73.1. A, Fluoroscopy showing calcified pericardium *(arrow)* in a patient with constrictive pericarditis (CP). **B** and **C,** Pressure tracings recorded with high-fidelity manometer-tipped catheters in the left ventricle (LV) and right ventricle (RV) during the respiratory cycle in two different patients: one with restrictive cardiomyopathy (RCM) and the other with CP. **B,** In this patient with RCM, there are concordant changes in left and right ventricular pressures during inspiration (Insp) and expiration (Exp). This indicates that the elevation of ventricular filling pressures is caused by a myocardial restrictive disease. **C,** In this patient with CP, there is ventricular discordance, with an increase in right ventricular pressure and a decrease in left ventricular pressure during inspiration and vice versa during expiration. This is caused by the enhancement of ventricular interaction and dissociation of intrathoracic and intracardiac pressures.

TABLE 73.2 Differentiating Features of Constrictive Pericarditis and Restrictive Cardiomyopathy

Feature	Constrictive Pericarditis	Restrictive Cardiomyopathy
Jugular venous waveform	Prominent X and Y descents (Y descent is of brief duration); Kussmaul sign often present	Prominent Y descent but not X descent; Kussmaul sign less common
Cardiac auscultation	S3 with high-pitched pericardial knock; no S4; mitral and tricuspid regurgitation usually absent	Increased S2 and S3 with low-pitched triple rhythm; S4 often present; mitral and tricuspid regurgitation common
Chest radiograph	Pericardial calcification (20%–30% prevalence); mild cardiomegaly and pulmonary venous congestion; bilateral pleural effusion less common	Pericardial calcification rare; mild cardiomegaly with biatrial enlargement, pulmonary venous congestion; bilateral pleural effusion more common
Electrocardiogram	Low amplitude (<50%); atrial fibrillation; P wave usually wide and notched	High or low amplitude (amyloidosis), atrial fibrillation, depolarization abnormalities (BBB), pathologic Q waves, and impaired atrioventricular conduction; P wave may be wide and increased in amplitude
Echocardiogram: gray-scale imaging	Increased pericardial thickness; normal wall thickness; septal bounce and respirophasic septal deviation	Increased wall thickness; thickened cardiac valves (amyloid); granular sparkling texture (amyloid); biatrial enlargement; apical obliteration (endomyocardial fibrosis)
Doppler studies	Significant respiratory variation in mitral and tricuspid inflow velocities; exaggerated medial mitral annular early diastolic velocity; expiratory augmentation of hepatic vein diastolic flow reversal	No significant respiratory variation in mitral and tricuspid inflow velocities; inspiratory augmentation of hepatic vein diastolic flow reversal; mitral and tricuspid regurgitation common
Cardiac catheterization	RVEDP and LVEDP usually equal; ventricular filling pressure waveforms show "square-root" sign; RV systolic pressure <50 mm Hg; RVEDP more than one-third of RV systolic pressure	LVEDP often >5 mm Hg greater than RVEDP; "square-root" sign is variable; RV systolic pressure usually >50 mm Hg; RVEDP less than one-third of RV systolic pressure
CT or cardiac MRI	Demonstrate a thickened pericardium in most cases; pericardial hyperenhancement after gadolinium contrast injection denotes inflammation	Pericardium usually of normal thickness; myocardial LGE seen in various inflammatory or infiltrative forms of RCM
Endomyocardial biopsy	May be normal or may demonstrate nonspecific hypertrophy or myocardial fibrosis	May reveal specific cause of RCM, especially in infiltrative conditions
BNP	Normal or minimally elevated BNP	Significantly elevated BNP

BBB, Bundle branch block; *BNP,* brain natriuretic peptide; *CT,* computed tomography; *LGE,* late gadolinium enhancement; *LVEDP,* left ventricular end-diastolic pressure; *MRI,* magnetic resonance imaging; *RCM,* restrictive cardiomyopathy; *RV,* right ventricular; *RVEDP,* right ventricular end-diastolic pressure; *S,* heart sound.

impediment to ventricular filling during early diastole, but as soon as the total cardiac volume reaches the limit set by the rigid pericardium, further ventricular filling is suddenly halted. Second, because the total cardiac volume is now constrained by the pericardium, any filling of one ventricle occurs at the expense of the other ventricle. This is known as ventricular interdependence. Although, to some extent, it is present in normal ventricles as well, it is greatly exaggerated in CP. Third, thickened, calcific pericardium shields the cardiac chambers from changes in intrathoracic pressures, a phenomenon known as dissociation of intracardiac and intrathoracic pressures. As a consequence of this, the reduction in intrathoracic pressure and subsequent pulmonary venous pressure during inspiration is not accompanied by an equivalent reduction in left ventricular (LV) diastolic pressure, and consequently, the pressure gradient between the pulmonary veins and LV diastolic pressure is markedly reduced. This results in reduced transmitral filling during inspiration and vice versa during expiration (see Fig. 73.1). Finally, the inflamed pericardium leads to tethering of the underlying myocardium, resulting in impairment of its contractile function. This tethering effect affects mainly the free walls of the atria and ventricles; the interatrial and interventricular septae are relatively spared. These hemodynamic and functional abnormalities result in several characteristics findings (Tables 73.2 and 73.3) that are helpful in distinguishing between these two conditions, as discussed later.[2–6]

In RCM, on the other hand, impairment to ventricular filling occurs throughout diastole. Additionally, because the stiffness is intrinsic to the myocardium and there is no external constraint, ventricular interdependence is not exaggerated, and there is no dissociation of intracardiac and intrathoracic pressures. Furthermore, because RCM is a myocardial disease, myocardial dysfunction is invariably present and is generally global, with no specific predilection for free walls or septae.

ECHOCARDIOGRAPHIC DIFFERENTIATION OF CONSTRICTION AND RESTRICTION
Respiratory Variation in Intracardiac Velocities

In CP, because of the combined effects of exaggerated ventricular interdependence and dissociation of intracardiac and intrathoracic pressures, transmitral filling is significantly reduced, and transtricuspid filling is augmented during inspiration. Reciprocal changes occur during expiration (Fig. 73.2). These changes manifest as significant respiratory variation in mitral and tricuspid inflow velocities and can be recorded within the first cardiac cycle after the onset of inspiration and expiration. More than 25% increase in early diastolic mitral velocity (E) during expiration and a more than 40% increase in transtricuspid velocity during inspiration is considered significant.[2,7,8] Similar respiratory variations can also be noted in pulmonary venous and LV outflow velocities. However, these changes may be absent in some patients with constriction with extremely elevated filling pressures.[7,9,10] Conversely, significant respiratory variations in mitral and tricuspid inflow velocities may also be present in conditions other than CP, such as any disease associated with exaggerated respiratory effort.[11] In patients with RCM, there is usually no significant respiratory variation in mitral and tricuspid inflow velocities, with mitral E velocity increasing by less than 10% during expiration (see Fig. 73.2).

Abnormal Septal Motion

The exaggerated ventricular interdependence in CP results in two forms of abnormal septal movements (Fig. 73.3 and Video 73.3). These septal abnormalities are not seen in RCM. During each cardiac cycle, as the ventricles fill in, temporal heterogeneity in filling of the two ventricles leads to phasic differences between the pressures in the two ventricles. This results in abrupt, to-and-fro movement of

TABLE 73.3 Distinctive Echocardiographic Findings in Constrictive Pericarditis and Restrictive Cardiomyopathy

Parameter	Constrictive Pericarditis	Restrictive Cardiomyopathy
Septal bounce	Yes	No
Respirophasic septal deviation	Yes	No
Mitral inflow respiratory variation	≥25%	None (<10%)
Tricuspid inflow respiratory variation	>40%	None
LV isovolumic relaxation time	Decreases during expiration, increases during inspiration	No change
Mitral annular e′	Relatively preserved or even exaggerated, medial e′ ≥ lateral e′	Markedly attenuated, medial e′ < lateral e′
Mitral E/e′	<8–10	>15
Hepatic vein flow reversal	Diastolic reversal with expiration	Significant reversal during both inspiration and expiration but more pronounced during inspiration
Myocardial mechanics	• Relatively preserved LV longitudinal strain with decreased LV circumferential strain, apical rotation, and net-twist angle • LV free-wall longitudinal strain lower than interventricular septal longitudinal strain • LA free-wall reservoir strain reduced, atrial septal reservoir strain relatively preserved or exaggerated	• Significantly reduced LV longitudinal strain, relatively preserved circumferential strain and twist mechanics • LV free wall and interventricular septal longitudinal strain equally impaired • LA free wall and septal strain equally impaired
Other findings	Thickened pericardium with or without calcification; tethering of RV free wall; distortion of LV and/or RV contours	Increased LV and/or RV wall thickness; thickened cardiac valves (amyloid); granular sparkling texture (amyloid); biatrial enlargement; apical obliteration (endomyocardial fibrosis)

E, Peak transmitral early diastolic flow velocity; *e′,* peak early diastolic mitral annular velocity; *LV,* left ventricular; *RV,* right ventricular

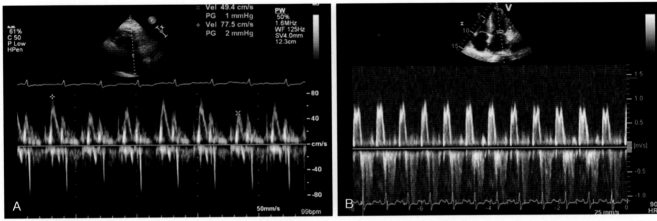

Figure 73.2. A, Significant respiratory variation in mitral inflow velocities in a patient with constrictive pericarditis. **B,** Lack of respiratory variation in mitral inflow velocities in a patient with restrictive cardiomyopathy.

ventricular septum as it responds to these changes in the intraventricular pressures. This is known as septal shudder or septal bounce and can be best appreciated on M-mode imaging (see Fig. 73.3).[12–14]

The second form of abnormal septal motion is the shift in its position with respiration. As discussed previously, during inspiration, the RV filling is augmented, whereas LV filling is compromised. This leads to an increase in RV size with displacement of the interventricular septum toward the left ventricle; the reverse happens during expiration (see Fig. 73.3). Such respirophasic septal deviation is reported to have high sensitivity (93%) for diagnosing CP.[15] However, it is not very specific for CP because any condition associated with increased respiratory effort such as severe obstructive lung disease may lead to a similar ventricular septal motion with respiration.

Annulus Paradoxus and Reversus

In CP, early diastolic filling is unimpeded. Additionally, because the radial expansion is limited by thickened pericardium, most of the ventricular filling occurs by expansion along the long-axis of the ventricle. As a result, early diastolic mitral annular velocity (e′) becomes paradoxically increased. This exaggerated, or at least preserved, mitral e′ despite elevated LV filling pressure, is known as annulus paradoxus (Fig. 73.4). The increase in e′ velocity is more marked at the medial mitral annulus because the pericardial tethering interferes with LV free wall excursion with consequent reduction in lateral mitral annular e′. Because this pattern is opposite to that seen in normal ventricles, it is designated as annulus reversus. In contrast, in RCM, which is a myocardial disease, mitral annular velocities are invariably and globally reduced (Fig. 73.5). In a recent study from the Mayo Clinic, comparing CP with RCM, medial e′ greater than 9 cm/s had an 83% sensitivity and 81% specificity, and the ratio of medial e′ to lateral e′ 0.91 or greater had a 75% sensitivity and 85% specificity for diagnosing CP.[15]

Hepatic Venous Flow Pattern

In CP, hepatic venous return to the right side of the heart is significantly compromised during expiration because of deviation of the

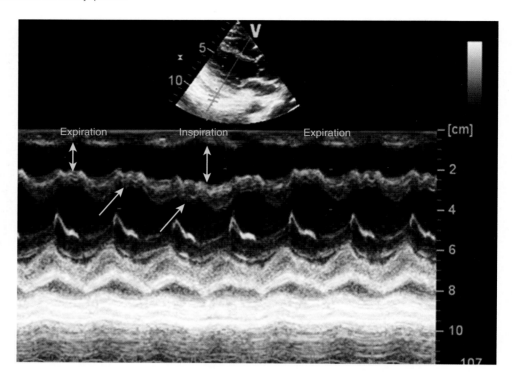

Figure 73.3. Abnormal ventricular septal motion in a patient with constrictive pericarditis. The septum moves toward the right ventricle during expiration and toward the left ventricle during inspiration *(double-headed arrows)*. Additionally, there is brisk oscillatory movement of the septum during diastole in each cardiac cycle, known as septal bounce *(open arrows)*. (See accompanying Video 73.3.) (Reproduced with permission from Mahmoud A, et al: New cardiac imaging algorithms to diagnose constrictive pericarditis versus restrictive cardiomyopathy, *Curr Cardiol Rep* 19:43, 2017.)

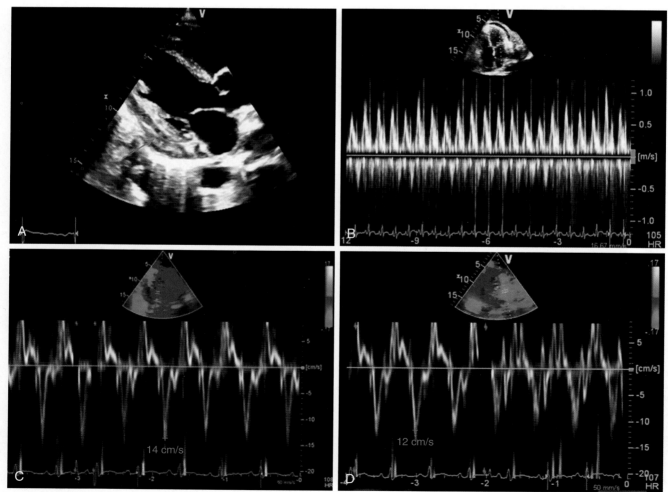

Figure 73.4. Annulus paradoxus and annulus reversus in a patient with constrictive pericarditis. **A,** Markedly thickened pericardium *(arrow)* posterior to the left ventricle. **B,** Increased early diastolic mitral inflow velocity with significant respiratory variation. **C,** Exaggerated medial mitral annular early diastolic velocity (annulus paradoxus). **D,** Lateral mitral annular velocity is lower than the medial mitral annular velocity (annulus reversus).

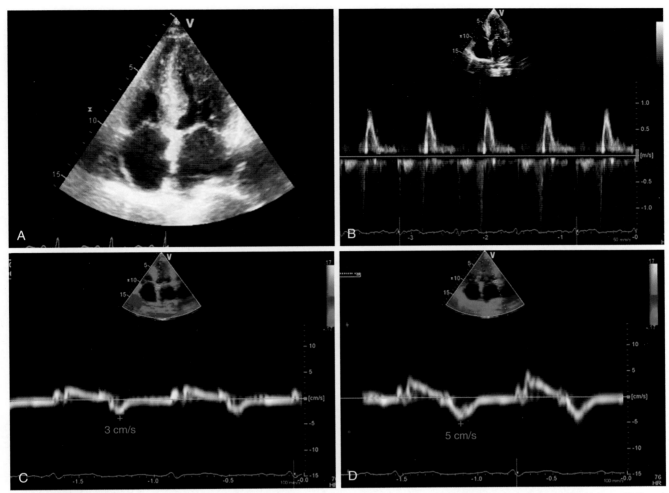

Figure 73.5. Mitral valve and mitral annular velocities in a patient with amyloid-related restrictive cardiomyopathy. **A,** Markedly thickened left and right ventricular walls with biatrial enlargement. **B,** Restrictive mitral inflow pattern with lack of respiratory variation. Both medial (**C**) and lateral (**D**) mitral annular early diastolic velocities are markedly reduced, but lateral velocity is still higher than the medial annular velocity (i.e., absence of annulus paradoxus and annulus reversus).

ventricular septum toward the right ventricle (which occurs secondary to exaggerated LV filling). As a result, hepatic venous reversal increases during expiration. In contrast, in RCM, reversal is more marked during inspiration because the right atrium is unable to accommodate extra venous return triggered by the fall in intrathoracic pressure (Fig. 73.6). Thus, the ratio of the hepatic venous diastolic reversal velocity to the diastolic forward flow velocity during expiration may help in distinguishing between CP and RCM. A cutoff value of 0.79 or greater for this ratio has been shown to have 76% sensitivity and 88% specificity for diagnosing CP.[15]

Myocardial Deformation Abnormalities

In CP, as the disease process affects the heart from outside, LV subepicardial fibers are preferentially affected, whereas the subendocardial fibers are relatively spared. As a result, LV circumferential and torsion mechanics are significantly attenuated, whereas longitudinal mechanics remain relatively preserved, at least during the early stages (Fig. 73.7). Furthermore, just as with the annular velocities, the long-axis contraction of the septum is exaggerated compared with that of LV or RV free walls.[16,17] Thus, a reduced ratio of lateral wall to septal longitudinal strain is highly suggestive of underlying constriction and is even superior to the ratio of medial to lateral e′ velocity for differentiating CP from RCM (areas under the curve, 0.91 and 0.76, respectively; $P = .011$).[17] Unlike

in CP, in RCM, there is marked attenuation of LV longitudinal mechanics. The circumferential strain and rotational mechanics are less affected and may even be normal during the early stages.[17,18]

Other Echocardiographic Findings

Echocardiography may reveal pericardial thickening with or without calcification in CP. Transthoracic echocardiogram is less sensitive for this purpose, but transesophageal echocardiogram has good sensitivity.[19] When appreciable, a thickness of greater than 3 mm has high specificity for CP, especially if combined with septal bounce.[11,19] However, the absence of pericardial thickness does not rule out CP because the pericardial thickness is reported to be normal in roughly 20% patients undergoing pericardiectomy for CP.[20] Pericardial calcification is much less common, seen only in 20% to 40% patients with CP, mostly in those with tuberculosis.[6] Pericardial thickening may also result in tethering of RV free-wall motion, which can be appreciated on subcostal imaging.[15] There may also be distortion of LV or RV contours, especially in the region of atrioventricular grooves (Fig. 73.8).

In RCM, the LV wall thickness is usually increased, and echo texture may be abnormal suggestive of cardiac infiltration. In amyloidosis, there may be additional findings such as increase thickness of valve leaflets, interatrial septum, and RV free wall; atrial arrest; and so on. In hypereosinophilic syndrome, apical thrombi are common and there

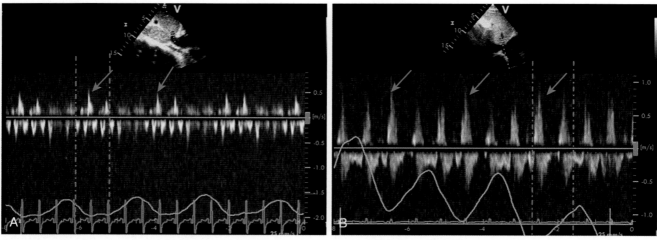

Figure 73.6. Hepatic vein flow patterns in constrictive pericarditis and restrictive cardiomyopathy. **A,** In constrictive pericarditis, reversal occurs mainly during expiration *(arrows)*. **B,** In restrictive cardiomyopathy, there is exaggerated hepatic venous reversal, which is more pronounced during inspiration *(arrows)*.

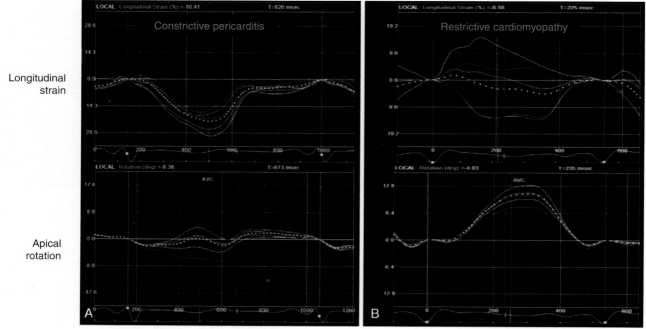

Figure 73.7. A, Preserved left ventricular longitudinal strain but markedly reduced apical rotation in a patient with constrictive pericarditis. **B,** The opposite pattern is seen in restrictive cardiomyopathy.

is often involvement of posterobasal region of the left ventricle with eccentric, posteriorly directed mitral regurgitation. In endomyocardial fibrosis, there is fibrotic obliteration of LV and RV apices caused by organized thrombi. In carcinoid heart disease, there are fibrous plaque-like deposits on the endocardium of cardiac chambers and valves, mainly on the right side of the heart. There may be other distinctive echocardiographic findings in various other forms of RCM.

Integrating Echocardiographic Findings

No single echocardiographic finding is accurate enough to distinguish CP from RCM; therefore, all the findings need to be viewed together. In the previously mentioned study from the Mayo Clinic, respirophasic ventricular shift had 93% sensitivity for CP, but the specificity (69%) was suboptimal.[15] Combining it with either

medial e′ 9 cm/s or greater or hepatic vein expiratory diastolic reversal ratio 0.79 or greater yielded an optimum combination of sensitivity (87%) and specificity (91%). Combining all the three resulted in even better specificity (97%), but sensitivity was compromised (64%).

Artificial intelligence using machine-learning algorithms has also been applied to integrate various clinical, conventional echocardiographic, and speckle-tracking echocardiography findings for the differentiation between CP and RCM. It has been demonstrated to yield a high degree of diagnostic accuracy and could be particularly helpful for less experienced readers.[21]

Acknowledgment

The authors thank Dr. Karen Modesto for her contribution to the previous edition of this chapter.

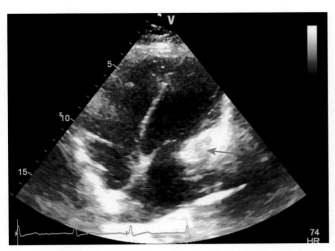

Figure 73.8. Dense calcification and pericardial thickening in the left atrioventricular groove *(arrow)* with distortion of left ventricular contour in a patient with constrictive pericarditis.

Please access ExpertConsult to view the corresponding video for this chapter.

REFERENCES

1. Hancock EW. On the elastic and rigid forms of constrictive pericarditis. *Am Heart J.* 1980;100:917–923.
2. Klein AL, Abbara S, Agler DA, et al. American Society of Echocardiography clinical recommendations for multimodality cardiovascular imaging of patients with pericardial disease. *J Am Soc Echocardiogr.* 2013;26:965–1012.
3. Dal-Bianco JP, Sengupta PP, Mookadam FC, et al. Role of echocardiography in the diagnosis of constrictive pericarditis. *J Am Soc Echocardiogr.* 2009;22:24–33.
4. Geske JB, Anavekar NS, Nishimura RA, et al. Differentiation of constriction and restriction: complex cardiovascular hemodynamics. *J Am Coll Cardiol.* 2016;68:2329–2347.
5. Mahmoud A, Bansal M, Sengupta PP. New cardiac imaging algorithms to diagnose constrictive pericarditis versus restrictive cardiomyopathy. *Curr Cardiol Rep.* 2017;19:43.
6. Garcia MJ. Constrictive pericarditis versus restrictive cardiomyopathy? *J Am Coll Cardiol.* 2016;67:2061–2076.
7. Oh JK, Hatle LK, Seward JB, et al. Diagnostic role of Doppler echocardiography in constrictive pericarditis. *J Am Coll Cardiol.* 1994;23:154–162.
8. Hatle LK, Appleton CP, Popp RL. Differentiation of constrictive pericarditis and restrictive cardiomyopathy by Doppler echocardiography. *Circulation.* 1989;79:357–370.
9. Oh JK, Tajik AJ, Appleton CP, et al. Preload reduction to unmask the characteristic Doppler features of constrictive pericarditis. A new observation. *Circulation.* 1997;95:796–799.
10. Ha JW, Oh JK, Ommen SR, et al. Diagnostic value of mitral annular velocity for constrictive pericarditis in the absence of respiratory variation in mitral inflow velocity. *J Am Soc Echocardiogr.* 2002;15:1468–1471.
11. Cosyns B, Plein S, Nihoyanopoulos P, et al. Multimodality imaging in pericardial disease. *Eur Heart J Cardiovasc Imag.* 2015;16:12–31.
12. Himelman RB, Lee E, Schiller NB. Septal bounce, vena cava plethora, and pericardial adhesion: informative two-dimensional echocardiographic signs in the diagnosis of pericardial constriction. *J Am Soc Echocardiogr.* 1988;1:333–340.
13. Engel PJ, Fowler NO, Tei CW, et al. M-mode echocardiography in constrictive pericarditis. *J Am Coll Cardiol.* 1985;6:471–474.
14. Candell-Riera J, Garcia del Castillo H, Permanyer-Miralda G, Soler-Soler J. Echocardiographic features of the interventricular septum in chronic constrictive pericarditis. *Circulation.* 1978;57:1154–1158.
15. Welch TD, Ling LH, Espinosa RE, et al. Echocardiographic diagnosis of constrictive pericarditis: mayo Clinic criteria. *Circ Cardiovasc Imag.* 2014;7:526–534.
16. Negishi K, Popovic ZB, Negishi T, et al. Pericardiectomy is associated with improvement in longitudinal displacement of left ventricular free wall due to increased counterclockwise septal-to-lateral rotational displacement. *J Am Soc Echocardiogr.* 2015;28:1204–1213.
17. Kusunose K, Dahiya A, Popovic ZB, et al. Biventricular mechanics in constrictive pericarditis comparison with restrictive cardiomyopathy and impact of pericardiectomy. *Circ Cardiovasc Imaging.* 2013;6:399–406.
18. Sengupta PP, Krishnamoorthy VK, Abhayaratna WP, et al. Disparate patterns of left ventricular mechanics differentiate constrictive pericarditis from restrictive cardiomyopathy. *JACC Cardiovasc Imag.* 2008;1:29–38.
19. Ling LH, Oh JK, Tei C, et al. Pericardial thickness measured with transesophageal echocardiography: feasibility and potential clinical usefulness. *J Am Coll Cardiol.* 1997;29:1317–1323.
20. Talreja DR, Edwards WD, Danielson GK, et al. Constrictive pericarditis in 26 patients with histologically normal pericardial thickness. *Circulation.* 2003;108:1852–1857.
21. Sengupta PP, Huang YM, Bansal M, et al. Cognitive machine-learning algorithm for cardiac imaging: a pilot study for differentiating constrictive pericarditis from restrictive cardiomyopathy. *Circ Cardiovasc Imag.* 2016;9:e0043309.

74 Echocardiography in Arrhythmogenic Right Ventricular Cardiomyopathy

Mayooran Namasivayam, Samuel Bernard, Danita M. Yoerger Sanborn

Arrhythmogenic right ventricular cardiomyopathy (ARVC) is an inherited disorder causing fibrofatty replacement of the right ventricular myocardium.[1,2] This pathological change results in right ventricular (RV) dilatation and dysfunction, myocardial scarring, and risk of sudden cardiac death (SCD) caused by ventricular arrhythmia.[2] Increasingly, there is appreciation of left heart involvement in ARVC, to the extent that some authors suggest excluding the RV specification and renaming the disease "arrhythmogenic cardiomyopathy."[1,2]

Desmosomal mutations in plakophilin 2, desmoplakin, desmoglein 2, desmocollin 2, and plakoglobin can result in the phenotype of ARVC.[1] Most mutations follow autosomal dominant transmission with variable penetrance, although recessive variants exist. Desmosome mutations result in abnormalities in cell–cell adhesion, cellular signaling (intra- and intercellular), and gene expression related to adipogenesis and fibrogenesis. Fibrofatty scarring of the myocardium then provides the substrate for scar reentry based ventricular arrhythmias.[1] Nondesmosomal mutations that are also important include transmembrane protein 43, lamin A/C, desmin, titin, alpha-T-catenin, N-cadherin, and phospholamban.[3]

The diagnosis of ARVC is multifaceted, but cardiac imaging plays a central role. Although there is an increasing focus on cardiac magnetic resonance imaging (CMRI), echocardiography is widely considered the first-line diagnostic imaging modality in light of its availability and cost efficiency. This chapter outlines the echocardiographic approach to the assessment of ARVC, including a description of traditional techniques and a discussion about emerging methods, including strain quantification. The role of nonechocardiographic imaging modalities in establishing the diagnosis is subsequently reviewed.

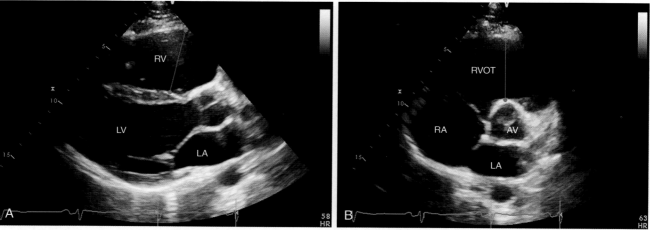

Figure 74.1. Measurement of right ventricular outflow tract (RVOT) dimensions on two-dimensional echocardiography in arrhythmogenic right ventricular cardiomyopathy in the parasternal long-axis (**A**) and parasternal short-axis (**B**) views. *AV,* Aortic valve; *LA,* left atrium; *LV,* left ventricle; *RA,* right atrium.

TWO-DIMENSIONAL ECHOCARDIOGRAPHY

Size

RV dilatation is almost uniformly noted in ARVC (Fig. 74.1). All patients in the original descriptions of the disease had either local or global RV dilatation.[4] RV outflow tract (RVOT) dilatation was found in 100% of probands from the North American Multidisciplinary Study of ARVC.[5] According to the 2010 revised Task Force Criteria (Table 74.1), a major criterion for ARVC is fulfilled when there is RVOT dilatation seen in the parasternal long-axis (PLAX) view 32 mm or greater or parasternal short-axis (PSAX) view 36 mm or greater in conjunction with impaired RV systolic function or localized aneurysms (akinesia or dyskinesia).[6] Sensitivity and specificity for the diagnosis of ARVC are 75% and 95% for the PLAX view and 62% and 95% for the PSAX views, respectively.

Systolic Function

Either global or regional RV systolic impairment is commonly seen in ARVC, particularly in more advanced stages of the disease. A total of 79% of probands in the North American Multidisciplinary Study had qualitative abnormalities in regional RV systolic function.[5] The anterior wall and apex were most commonly affected. Because of the asymmetric geometry of the right ventricle and difficulty visualizing the entire RV endocardium, estimation of RV volume (and hence RV ejection fraction) by two-dimensional (2D) echocardiography is challenging. In cases in which endocardial definition is poor, the administration of an ultrasound-enhancing agent can facilitate assessment of global and regional RV systolic function.[3]

RV fractional area change (FAC) from the apical four-chamber view has been shown to be a useful correlate of RV systolic function and is decreased in individuals with ARVC compared with control participants (Fig. 74.2). In the proposed Task Force Criteria modification, the optimal cutpoint for FAC (≤33%) was determined using data from the Multidisciplinary Study coupled with a large group (*n* = 450) of normal individuals.[6] In the presence of regional wall motion abnormality, an FAC of 33% or less had a sensitivity of 55% and specificity of 95% for the diagnosis of ARVC. Importantly, FAC also has prognostic value, predicting an increase in major adverse cardiac events in this population.[7,8] Although measuring FAC can be difficult without adequate RV endocardial delineation, given its importance in diagnosis and prognosis, it should be quantified whenever possible.

TABLE 74.1 2010 Revised Task Force Criteria for Echocardiography

Global or Regional Dysfunction and Structural Alterations
Major
1. Regional RV akinesia, dyskinesia, or aneurysm and one of the following:
a. PLAX ≥32 mm (≥19 mm/m²)
b. PSAX ≥36 mm (≥21 mm/m²)
c. FAC ≤33%
Minor
1. Regional RV akinesia or dyskinesia and one of the following:
a. PLAX: 29–32 mm
b. PSAX: 32–36 mm
c. RV FAC: 33%–40%

FAC, Fractional area change; *PLAX,* parasternal long-axis view; *RV,* right ventricular.

Adapted from Marcus FI, et al: Diagnosis of arrhythmogenic right ventricular cardiomyopathy/dysplasia: proposed modification of the Task Force Criteria, *Circulation* 121:1533–1541, 2010.

Conventional measurements of RV systolic function, such as tricuspid annular plane systolic excursion and RV peak systolic annular velocity (RV S′), tend to become abnormal only in advanced stages of disease.[9] They are also limited by angle dependency of this measurement relative to longitudinal contraction. This can be problematic late in the course of disease when dilatation and displacement of the tricuspid annulus alter the plane of annular motion.

Structural Features

RV structural abnormalities have also been noted with increased frequency in ARVC. These include prominent trabeculae, focal aneurysms or sacculations, and a hyperreflective moderator band (Fig. 74.3). Trabecular derangement was the most frequent abnormality in a subgroup of probands from the North American Multidisciplinary Study. In this group, 54% of probands had trabecular derangement compared with none of matched control participants.[5]

Mimics

It is well established that RV dilatation and remodeling (including prominent trabeculations and hyperreflective moderator bands) occur in response to high-intensity exercise.[10–12] As a result, the

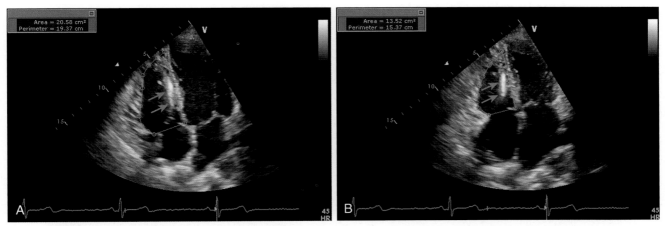

Figure 74.2. Measurement of fractional area change (FAC) of the right ventricle in a patient with known arrhythmogenic right ventricular cardiomyopathy using end-diastolic (**A**) and end-systolic (**B**) areas. FAC is calculated as the ratio of the difference between end-diastolic area (EDA) and end-systolic area (ESA) to EDA (i.e., FAC = [EDA-ESA]/EDA). It is important to carefully delineate pacemaker or implantable cardioverter-defibrillator wires *(arrows)* from the endocardial border of the right ventricle.

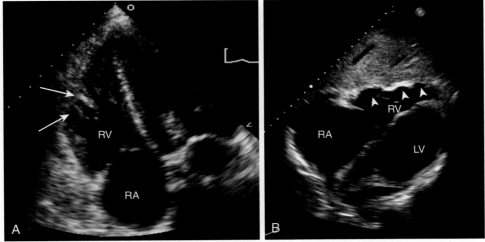

Figure 74.3. Structural changes noted on two-dimensional echocardiography with increased frequency in arrhythmogenic right ventricular cardiomyopathy, including (a) trabecular derangement (**A,** *arrows*) and localized aneurysms (**B,** *arrowheads*) in the right ventricular free wall. *LV,* Left ventricle; *RV,* right ventricle; *RA,* right atrium. (See accompanying Video 74.3.)

diagnosis of ARVC may be delayed or unrecognized in younger patients and athletes. Indeed, a prospective analysis of sudden death in patients younger than 30 years of age in the Veneto region of Italy demonstrated that 20% of fatal events were caused by undiagnosed ARVC.[13] Given the difficulty in diagnosing this disease in young patients and highly trained athletes, it is essential to obtain detailed medical and family history and use Task Force Criteria (exclusive of RV structure and function) to distinguish ARVC from physiologic adaptation.[14] Strain quantification (see later) also holds promise in better delineating these two entities.

Similarly, RV dilatation and dysfunction in the setting of congenital heart disease; ischemic, infiltrative, valvular, or dilated cardiomyopathy; and pulmonary arterial hypertension can be difficult to differentiate from ARVC.[3] As noted, physicians should integrate echocardiographic findings with the patient's clinical history, family history, electrocardiogram, and other cardiac imaging (e.g., CMRI, cardiac catheterization) to establish the appropriate diagnosis.[14]

STRAIN QUANTIFICATION

Tissue deformation imaging (strain quantification) has permitted further insights into RV mechanical function in ARVC (Fig. 74.4).

Abnormalities in RV strain occur before overt RV dysfunction, thereby making it a promising avenue for screening individuals with genetic abnormalities or family history in the absence of Task Force Criteria disease phenotype. Normal RV longitudinal strain using the average of a six-segment model (apical, basal, and mid free wall and septum) is less than −20% in healthy men and women.[15] A cutoff of −18% has been shown to differentiate normal from abnormal segments in ARVC.[7] Mechanical dispersion, a metric of variation (commonly standard deviation) in time to peak systolic strain of RV segments, is also diagnostically and prognostically useful in ARVC.[16] In patients with known disease, strain abnormalities have been correlated to disease severity and malignant arrhythmias.[17,18] Particular emphasis has been placed on mechanical dysfunction in the subtricuspid RV basal region in both established and preclinical stages of ARVC.[19,20]

Pathological data have suggested that the particular areas of the right ventricle that are most commonly affected in ARVC occur within a "triangle of dysplasia" encompassing the apex, subpulmonic anterior wall, and inferoposterior RV wall.[3,4] More recently, this concept has been revised to consider a "quadrangle of dysplasia" that additionally involves the inferolateral left ventricular (LV) wall (see the Emerging Concepts regarding Left Ventricular Involvement, section).[14] Fibrofatty change occurs in an

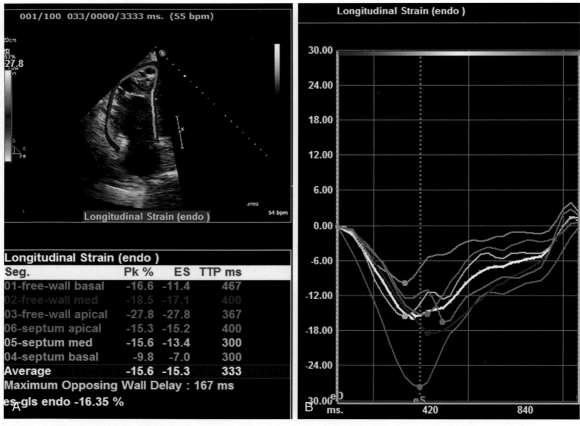

Figure 74.4. Longitudinal strain of the right ventricle measured by speckle tracking in a patient with arrhythmogenic right ventricular cardiomyopathy. **A,** A reduction of global right ventricular strain (−16.4%) and segmental variation with the interventricular septum and basal right ventricular free wall most prominently affected. **B,** Increased mechanical dispersion across the segments is also noted. Note that prominent trabeculations should be excluded for strain analysis, with the focus primarily on endocardial contraction. (See accompanying Video 74.4.)

epicardial-to-endocardial direction in ARVC. These observations provide a mechanistic basis to regional variations in tissue deformation and suggest a possible role for evaluation of epicardial strain rather than endocardial strain in ARVC. Even within endocardial strain, however, the best metric of strain evaluation (e.g., free-wall strain, global longitudinal strain, segmental strain) has yet to be clarified.

THREE-DIMENSIONAL ECHOCARDIOGRAPHY

Three-dimensional (3D) imaging of the RV is attractive because it can overcome the planar limitations of 2D imaging, which can confound quantification of RV size by 2D imaging.[21,22] With this said, 3D imaging of the RV can be more challenging than that of the left ventricle.[22] Issues related to image quality, cropping, and measurement generally require considerable experience with the technique. Despite this, early data have shown that RV volume calculated from 3D echocardiography can have less variability compared with2D echocardiography.[23,24] Clinical studies have substantiated these early studies by demonstrating a promising role for 3D echocardiographic assessment in suspected ARVC.[25,26] A promising avenue for further investigation is 3D speckle-tracking imaging.[27,28] In the future, 3D analysis of regional and global RV function, including volumetric assessment and tissue deformation quantification, might be the norm.

OTHER IMAGING MODALITIES

Although echocardiography is the most cost-efficient, resource-efficient, and widely available imaging modality, alternative modalities

are essential in the assessment of ARVC. CMRI has developed an increasingly important role because of its ability to visualize the 3D RV structure and function at higher spatial (but less temporal) resolution than echocardiography. RV dilatation, RV volumes, and global and regional dysfunction (dyskinesia, akinesia, or asynchronous contraction) are highly reproducible and well characterized by CMRI. Initially, there was hope that visualization of fibrofatty change would be an important feature on MRI, but this approach has limitations. Fibrosis can be technically difficult to detect in the thin RV wall, and both fibrosis and fat deposition in the RV are not specific to ARVC. Current CMRI sequencing also precludes the simultaneous assessment of fat and fibrosis, complicating this evaluation.[3] It is worth noting that CMRI for ARVC requires particular technical expertise in acquisition and interpretation and hence should be performed in centers with experience in ARVC evaluation. Computed tomography was not included in the 2010 Task Force Criteria, but studies have shown good spatial and temporal resolution and ability to identify fatty epicardial deposition and trabecular enlargement. Fewer data are available than for echocardiography and CMRI. Radiation dose, which is a concern, can be brought to a minimum (as low as 1–2 mSv).[3] Finally, it is worth noting that the Task Force Criteria do include RV angiography features; however, this technique is less frequently performed than the noninvasive methods described.

EMERGING CONCEPTS REGARDING LEFT VENTRICULAR INVOLVEMENT

There is increasing appreciation for involvement of the LV in a significant proportion of patients with ARVC. Pathologic data from the

United Kingdom have shown that 87% of patients with SCD caused by ARVC had LV histopathologic involvement on postmortem assessment.[29] There have been calls to alter the disease nomenclature such that ARVC would be termed "arrhythmogenic cardiomyopathy."[30] The most commonly involved LV territory is the inferolateral wall, leading to its incorporation into the "quadrangle of dysplasia" concept (described earlier).[15] There are two key benefits of reducing the emphasis on RV involvement. First, it would broaden the assessment of ventricular function for clinicians evaluating patients with ARVC. Second, it would reduce misclassification of ARVC cases as dilated cardiomyopathy in those with biventricular involvement. In the future, patients being assessed for ARVC should have a thorough echocardiographic assessment of LV as well as RV function in addition to strain analysis and 3D imaging when possible.

SUMMARY

Echocardiography is an important tool in the evaluation of ARVC. RV dilatation, global and regional systolic dysfunction, and abnormal structural features, including trabecular disarrangement, hyperreflective moderator bands, and sacculations, can help identify the phenotype of disease. Newer imaging methods, including strain analysis, can help identify earlier stages of disease and predict adverse outcomes. As the first line of imaging in patients with ARVC, echocardiography will undoubtedly continue to play an important role in the evaluation of this serious disease.

Please access ExpertConsult to view the corresponding videos for this chapter.

REFERENCES

1. Calkins H, Corrado D, Marcus F. Risk stratification in arrhythmogenic right ventricular cardiomyopathy. *Circulation.* 2017;136:2068–2082.
2. Corrado D, Link MS, Calkins H. Arrhythmogenic right ventricular cardiomyopathy. *N Engl J Med.* 2017;376:61–72.
3. Gandjbakhch E, Redheuil A, Pousset F, et al. Clinical diagnosis, imaging, and genetics of arrhythmogenic right ventricular cardiomyopathy/dysplasia. *J Am Coll Cardiol.* 2018;72:784–804.
4. Marcus FI, Fontaine GH, Guiraudon G, et al. Right ventricular dysplasia: a report of 24 adult cases. *Circulation.* 1982;65:384–398.
5. Yoerger DM, Marcus F, Sherrill D, et al. Echocardiographic findings in patients meeting Task Force Criteria for arrhythmogenic right ventricular cardiomyopathy. *J Am Coll Cardiol.* 2005;45. 86–865.
6. Marcus FI, McKenna WJ, Sherrill D, et al. Diagnosis of arrhythmogenic right ventricular cardiomyopathy/dysplasia: proposed modification of the Task Force Criteria. *Circulation.* 2010;121:1533–1541.
7. Corrado D, Wichter T, Link MS, et al. Treatment of arrhythmogenic right ventricular cardiomyopathy/dysplasia: an International Task Force consensus statement. *Circulation.* 2015;132:441–453.
8. Saguner AM, Vechhiati A, Baldinger SH, et al. Different prognostic value of functional right ventricular parameters in arrhythmogenic right ventricular cardiomyopathy/dysplasia. *Circ Cardiovasc Imag.* 2014;7. 230–230.
9. Prakasa KR, Wang J, Tandri H, et al. Utility of tissue Doppler and strain echocardiography in arrhythmogenic right ventricular dysplasia/cardiomyopathy. *Am J Cardiol.* 2007;100:507–512.
10. D'Ascenzi F, Pelliccia A, Solari M, et al. Normative reference values of right heart in competitive athletes: a systematic review and meta-analysis. *J Am Soc Echocardiogr.* 2017;30:845–858.
11. La Gerche A, Burns AT, D'Hooge J, et al. Exercise strain rate imaging demonstrates normal right ventricular contractile reserve and clarifies ambiguous resting measures in endurance athletes. *J Am Soc Echocardiogr.* 2012;25:253–262.
12. Churchill TW. The right heart: acute and chronic issues. *Curr Treat Options Cardio Med.* 2017;19:83.
13. Thiene G, Nava A, Corrado D, et al. Right ventricular cardiomyopathy and sudden death in young people. *N Engl J Med.* 1988;318:129–133.
14. Corrado D, van Tintelen PJ, McKenna WJ, et al. Arrhythmogenic right ventricular cardiomyopathy: evaluation of the current diagnostic criteria and differential diagnosis. *Eur Heart J.* 2019;41:1414–1429.
15. Muraru D, Onciul S, Peluso D, et al. Sex- and method-specific reference values for right ventricular strain by 2-dimensional speckle-tracking echocardiography. *Circ Cardiovasc Imag.* 2016;9:e003866.
16. Haugaa KH, Basso C, Badano LP, et al. Comprehensive multi-modality imaging approach in arrhythmogenic cardiomyopathy. *Eur Heart J.* 2017;18:237–253.
17. Teske AJ, Cox MG, De Boeck BW, et al. Echocardiographic tissue deformation imaging quantifies abnormal regional right ventricular function in arrhythmogenic right ventricular dysplasia/cardiomyopathy. *J Am Soc Echocardiogr.* 2009;22:920–927.
18. Sarvari SI, Haugaa KH, Anfinsen OG, et al. Right ventricular mechanical dispersion is related to malignant arrhythmias: a study of patients with arrhythmogenic right ventricular cardiomyopathy and subclinical right ventricular dysfunction. *Eur Heart J.* 2011;32:1089–1096.
19. Mast TP, Taha K, Cramer MJ, et al. The prognostic value of right ventricular deformation imaging in early arrhythmogenic right ventricular cardiomyopathy. *J Am Coll Cardiol Imag.* 2019;12:446–455.
20. Haugaa KH, Lie OH. Reveal the concealed: the quest for early disease detection in family members at risk of developing arrhythmogenic cardiomyopathy. *J Am Coll Cardiol Imag.* 2019;12:456–457.
21. Addetia K, Maffessanti F, Muraru D, et al. Morphologic analysis of the normal right ventricle using three-dimensional echocardiography-derived curvature indices. *J Am Soc Echocardiogr.* 2018;31:614–623.
22. Fernandez-Golfin C, Zamorano JL. Three-dimensional echocardiography and right ventricular function: the beauty and the beast? *Circ Cardiovasc Imag.* 2017;10:e006099.
23. Jiang L, Handschumacher MD, Hibberd MG, et al. Three-dimensional echocardiographic reconstruction of right ventricular volume: in vitro comparison with two-dimensional methods. *J Am Soc Echocardiogr.* 1994;7:150–158.
24. Jiang L, Siu SC, Handschumacher MD, et al. Three-dimensional echocardiography. In vivo validation for right ventricular volume and function. *Circulation.* 1994;89:2342–2350.
25. Kjaergeaard J, Hastrup Svendsen J, Sogaard P, et al. Advanced quantitative echocardiography in arrhythmogenic right ventricular cardiomyopathy. *J Am Soc Echocardiogr.* 2007;20:27–35.
26. Prakasa KR, Dalal D, Wang J, et al. Feasibility and variability of three-dimensional echocardiography in arrhythmogenic right ventricular dysplasia/cardiomyopathy. *Am J Cardiol.* 2006;87:703–709.
27. Muraru D, Niero A, Rodriguez-Zanella H, et al. Three-dimensional speckle-tracking echocardiography: benefits and limitations in integrating myocardial mechanics with three-dimensional imaging. *Cardiovasc Diagn Ther.* 2018;8:101–117.
28. Atsumi A, Seo Y, Ishizu T, et al. Right ventricular deformation analyses using a three-dimensional speckle-tracking echocardiographic system specialized for the right ventricle. *J Am Soc Echocardiogr.* 2016;29:402–411.
29. Miles C, Finocchiaro G, Papadakis M, et al. Sudden death and left ventricular involvement in arrhythmogenic cardiomyopathy. *Circulation.* 2019;139:1786–1797.
30. Bennett RG, Haqqani H, Berruezo A, et al. Arrhythmogenic cardiomyopathy in 2018-2019: ARVC/ALVC or both? *Heart Lung Circ.* 2019;28:164–177.

75   Takotsubo Cardiomyopathy

Nozomi Watanabe

Takotsubo-like transient left ventricular (LV) dysfunction (Takotsubo cardiomyopathy, Takotsubo syndrome) was first reported in Japan in 1990. The mysterious myocardial disease, which was known as *apical ballooning syndrome*, is characterized by an expansion of the apical segments with basal hyperkinesis. *Takotsubo* is the Japanese word for octopus trap, which has traditionally been used by Japanese fishermen (from *tako,* meaning "octopus," and *tsubo* meaning "pot").

Japanese investigators originally coined the name because of the unique shape of the left ventricle during systole (ballooned apex with narrow base; Fig. 75.1).

The majority of patients presenting with this condition are older women, with Asians being the largest group affected followed by whites. The symptoms of chest pain and dyspnea are frequently preceded by emotional or physical stress.[1,2] Interestingly, the

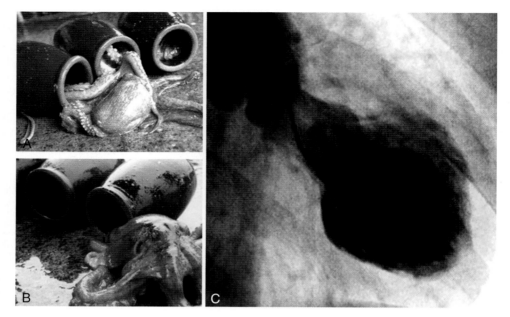

Figure 75.1. A and **B,** A Japanese octopus trap, or Takotsubo (Tako = octopus, Tsubo = pot). **C,** Left ventriculography of a patient with Takotsubo cardiomyopathy (systole). (Parts A and B courtesy of Ushibuka Suisan Co., Ltd.)

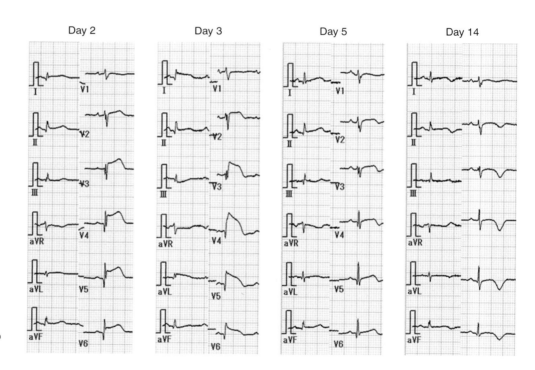

Figure 75.2. Follow-up electrocardiograms of Takotsubo cardiomyopathy.

incidence of Takotsubo cardiomyopathy dramatically increased after a major earthquake in Nigata, Japan, in 2004; 69% of patients developed symptoms on the same day as the earthquake.[3] There have also been some case reports of this stress-induced cardiomyopathy related to the Great East Japan earthquake in 2011.

The clinical findings of Takotsubo cardiomyopathy mimic an acute myocardial infarction (AMI), including sudden onset of chest pain, ST-T elevation followed by T-wave inversion, and apical wall motion abnormality.[4,5] Hence, this relatively benign disease is often diagnosed as an AMI but with normal epicardial coronary arteries found on emergent coronary angiography. Despite the extensive wall motion abnormality, which goes beyond the territory of a single coronary artery, the elevation

of biomarker levels (creatine kinase myocardial band, troponin) is usually modest compared with the elevations of biomarkers in AMI. LV wall motion abnormalities spontaneously improve within 3 months on average. T-wave inversion after initial ST-T elevation is generally deeper than that in AMI, and the characteristic changes persist for several months and then recover to normal (Figs. 75.2 to 75.4 and Video 75.1). Other than the typical apical ballooning, subtypes of this unique stress-induced cardiomyopathy have been recognized, including midventricular type; inverted, reverse, or basal type; focal type; and atypical type including right ventricular (RV) involvement (Fig. 75.5).[6–10] A study using magnetic resonance imaging (MRI) depicted biventricular Takotsubo cardiomyopathy with RV involvement in

34% of 239 cases.[11] MRI has demonstrated myocardial edema without gadolinium enhancement as a characteristic findings of the acute phase of Takotsubo cardiomyopathy.[11,12]

Prognosis has been considered to be generally good, with complete recovery in most patients. However, fatal complications have been rarely reported (e.g., cardiogenic shock or ventricular rupture), and recent studies have shown that Takotsubo cardiomyopathy may be associated with considerable in-hospital mortality rates, which could be similar to that of AMI.[13] Tentative LV outflow obstruction with or without mitral regurgitation can be seen in the acute phase (Fig. 75.6),[14] and initial echocardiographic screening is useful to identify systolic anterior motion of the mitral leaflets along with a hyperkinetic basal left ventricle. Doppler echocardiography can demonstrate accelerated flow signal in the LV outflow with mitral regurgitation.[15] Risk factors for cardiac rupture are persistent ST-segment elevation, female gender, older age, higher systolic or diastolic blood pressure, and a lower LV ejection fraction (Table 75.1).[16] Recently published meta-analysis of 53 published articles (>4600 cases) regarding long-term mortality rates of patients with Takotsubo cardiomyopathy has shown that in-hospital death occurred in 1.8%.[17] Long-term death after discharge occurred in 10.2%, but only 22% of the long-term deaths were from cardiac causes. The annual rate of long-term total mortality was 3.5%, and older age, physical stressor, and atypical ballooning were significantly associated with an unfavorable long-term prognosis. Intraventricular thrombus formation in the acute phase of Takotsubo syndrome has been reported; therefore, careful screening using echocardiography is crucial (Fig. 75.7).[13]

The underlying mechanisms of Takotsubo cardiomyopathy have not been elucidated. Catecholamine-induced myocardial injury is one of the possible mechanisms.[18] Because this disease is explicitly related to emotional or physical stress, this supports this theory. Norepinephrine concentration has been reported to be elevated in more than 70% of patients with Takotsubo cardiomyopathy.[2] Nevertheless, more recent reports have shown similar plasma catecholamine and cortisol level in both Takotsubo and AMI, and the diagnostic role of serum catecholamine remains uncertain. Vasospasm has also been considered to be a cause of this disease. Some recent studies using optical coherence tomography have suggested the presence of coronary plaque in patients with Takotsubo syndrome. A study using Doppler guidewires reported decreased coronary flow velocity reserve in patients with Takotsubo cardiomyopathy in the acute phase, which improved 3 weeks later.[19] Coronary microvascular dysfunction probably exists in this disease, but the cause still remains unclear. Transthoracic coronary Doppler echocardiography can help to determine the preserved coronary flow velocity in the distal left anterior descending artery in Takotsubo syndrome with apical ballooning.[20]

Please access ExpertConsult to view the corresponding video for this chapter.

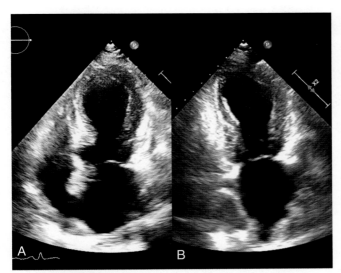

Figure 75.3. A and **B,** Echocardiographic images in a patient with Takotsubo cardiomyopathy (apical four- and two-chamber views by 3D bi-plane images).

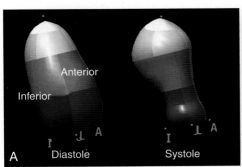
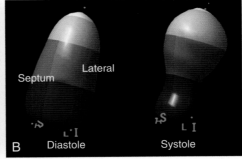
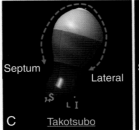
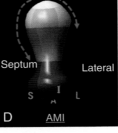

Figure 75.4. Left ventricular volumetric images by three-dimensional echocardiography in an apical ballooning type of Takotsubo cardiomyopathy **(A,B)**. Comparison between apical ballooning **(C)** and acute myocardial infarction (AMI) in the left anterior descending artery (LAD) territory **(D)**. Wall motion abnormality (red dotted arrows) is seen beyond LAD territory in the Takotsubo cardiomyopathy.

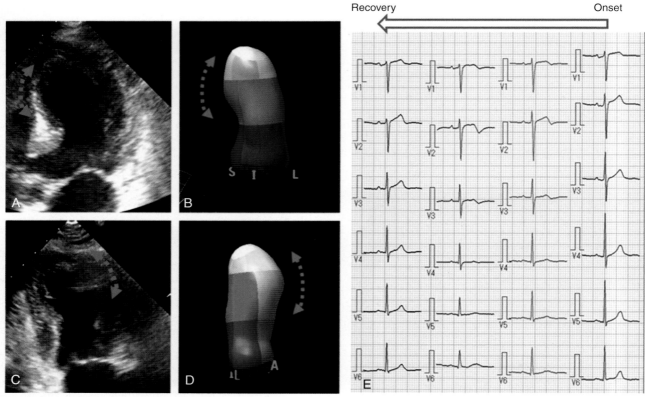

Figure 75.5. Uncommon type (partial) of Takotsubo cardiomyopathy. Two-and three-dimensional echocardiography **(A-D)** shows regional wall motion abnormality in the midanteroseptal region *(red dotted arrows)* with minor ST-T changes.

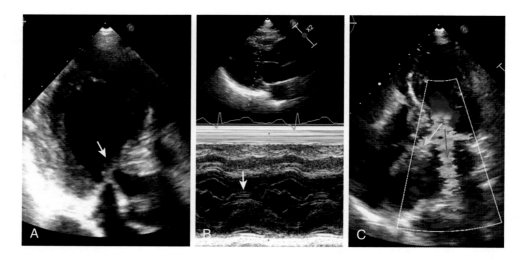

Figure 75.6. Systolic anterior movement of the mitral valve leaflet *(white arrows)* along with a hyperkinetic basal left ventricle **(A** and **B)**. Color Doppler echocardiography reveals left ventricular outflow obstruction *(yellow arrow)* and severe mitral regurgitation *(red arrow)* **(C)**.

TABLE 75.1 Presentation and Findings of Takotsubo Cardiomyopathy

Sex	Female (>90%)
Symptoms	Sudden-onset chest pain > dyspnea
ECG	ST-T elevation followed by deep T-wave inversion
Creatine kinase MB and troponin levels:	Modest elevation or within normal range
Echocardiography	Decreased EF with apical expansion and basal hyperkinesis; wall motion abnormalities recover to normal within several months; tentative LV outflow obstruction with or without mitral regurgitation can be seen in the acute phase
	Uncommon types of regional wall motion abnormality have been reported
Angiography	No significant abnormalities in epicardial coronary arteries
Doppler flow wire	Reduced coronary flow velocity reserve in three major vessels
Complications	Apical thrombus, congestive heart failure, cardiogenic shock, arrhythmia, ventricular rupture (rare)

ECG, Electrocardiography; *EF,* ejection fraction; *LV,* left ventricular; *MB,* myocardial band.

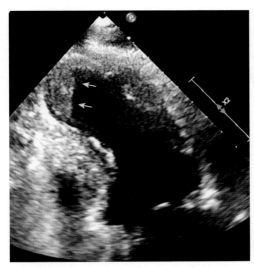

Figure 75.7. Left ventricular apical thrombus formation in the acute phase of apical ballooning type (*yellow arrows*).

REFERENCES

1. Donohue D, Movahed MR. Clinical characteristics, demographics and prognosis of transient left ventricular apical ballooning syndrome. *Heart Fail Rev.* 2005;10:311–316.
2. Gianni M, Dentali F, Grandi AM, et al. Apical ballooning syndrome or takotsubo cardiomyopathy: a systematic review. *Eur Heart J.* 2006;27:1523–1529.
3. Sato M, Fujita S, Saito A, et al. Increased incidence of transient left ventricular apical ballooning (so-called "Takotsubo" cardiomyopathy) after the mid-Niigata Prefecture earthquake. *Circ J.* 2006;70:947–953.
4. Kurisu S, Sato H, Kawagoe T, et al. Tako-Tsubo-like left ventricular dysfunction with ST-segment elevation: a novel cardiac syndrome mimicking acute myocardial infarction. *Am Heart J.* 2002;143:448–455.
5. Abe Y, Kondo M, Matsuoka R, et al. Assessment of clinical features in transient left ventricular apical ballooning. *J Am Coll Cardiol.* 2003;41:737–742.
6. Steen H, Merten C, Katus HA, Giannitsis E. Images in cardiovascular medicine. A rare form of midventricular Tako-Tsubo after emotional stress followed up with magnetic resonance imaging. *Circulation.* 2006;114:e248.
7. Blessing E, Steen H, Rosenberg M, et al. Recurrence of Takotsubo cardiomyopathy with variant forms of left ventricular dysfunction. *J Am Soc Echocardiogr.* 2007;20(439):e11–e12.
8. Hurst RT, Prasad A, Askew 3rd JW, et al. Takotsubo cardiomyopathy: a unique cardiomyopathy with variable ventricular morphology. *JACC Cardiovasc Imag.* 2010;3:641–649.
9. Dias A, Nunez Gil IJ, Santoro F, et al. Takotsubo syndrome: State-of-the-art review by an expert panel—part 1. *Cardiovasc Revasc Med.* 2019;20:70–79.
10. Kagiyama N, Okura H, Tamada T, et al. Impact of right ventricular involvement on the prognosis of takotsubo cardiomyopathy. *Eur Heart J Cardiovasc Imag.* 2016;17:210–216.
11. Eitel I, von Knobelsdorff-Brenkenhoff F, Bernhardt P, et al. Clinical characteristics and cardiovascular magnetic resonance findings in stress (Takotsubo) cardiomyopathy. *J Am Med Assoc.* 2011;306:277–286.
12. Dawson DK, Neil CJ, Henning A, et al. Tako-Tsubo cardiomyopathy: a heart stressed out of energy? *JACC Cardiovasc Imag.* 2015;8:985–987.
13. Templin C, Ghadri JR, Diekmann J, et al. Clinical features and outcomes of Takotsubo (stress) cardiomyopathy. *N Engl J Med.* 2015;373:929–938.
14. Dawson DK. Acute stress-induced (Takotsubo) cardiomyopathy. *Heart.* 2018;104:96–102.
15. Citro R, Rigo F, D'Andrea A, et al. Echocardiographic correlates of acute heart failure, cardiogenic shock, and in-hospital mortality in Tako-Tsubo cardiomyopathy. *JACC Cardiovasc Imag.* 2014;7:119–129.
16. Kurisu S, Inoue I. Cardiac rupture in Tako-Tsubo cardiomyopathy with persistent ST-segment elevation. *Int J Cardiol.* 2012;158:e5–e6.
17. Pelliccia F, Pasceri V, Patti G, et al. Long-term prognosis and outcome predictors in Takotsubo syndrome: a systematic review and meta-regression study. *JACC Heart Fail.* 2019;7:143–154.
18. Ueyama T, Senba E, Kasamatsu K, et al. Molecular mechanism of emotional stress-induced and catecholamine-induced heart attack. *J Cardiovasc Pharmacol.* 2003;41:S115–S118.
19. Kume T, Akasaka T, Kawamoto T, et al. Assessment of coronary microcirculation in patients with takotsubo-like left ventricular dysfunction. *Circ J.* 2005;69:934–939.
20. Watanabe N. Noninvasive assessment of coronary blood flow by transthoracic Doppler echocardiography: basic to practical use in the emergency room. *J Echocardiogr.* 2017;15:49–56.

76 Familial Cardiomyopathies

Grace Hsieh, Jennifer Hellawell, Frederick L. Ruberg, Omar K. Siddiqi, Ravin Davidoff

This chapter reviews four of the most common familial neuromuscular diseases that have significant cardiac manifestations: Friedreich ataxia (FA), myotonic dystrophy (DM), Duchenne muscular dystrophy (DMD), and Becker muscle dystrophy (BMD). These syndromes vary significantly in their inheritance patterns, epidemiology, and cardiac manifestations (Table 76.1).

FRIEDREICH ATAXIA

FA is an autosomal recessive disease characterized by spinocerebellar degeneration that leads to progressive ataxia, diabetes mellitus, and cardiac abnormalities. FA is the most prevalent of all spinocerebellar ataxias and occurs in an estimated 1 in 50,000 whites.[1] It was originally described in 1863 by the German neurologist and pathologist Nikolaus Friedreich and is caused by the expansion of glutamic acid (GAA) trinucleotide repeats in the gene encoding frataxin, a protein that plays a central role in mitochondrial iron transport. GAA triplet expansion results in transcriptional gene silencing and loss of frataxin expression.[2] Frataxin deficiency is thought to cause mitochondrial iron accumulation in neurons, cardiomyocytes, and other cell types, which results in cellular and subsequent organ dysfunction, manifesting in the first or second decade of life.[3]

Cardiac Manifestations

Up to 90% of patients with FA have cardiac involvement, which is characterized microscopically by cardiomyocyte hypertrophy, focal necrosis, and diffuse fibrosis. There are two different cardiac phenotypes. The most common form is hypertrophic cardiomyopathy, which can be further subdivided into asymmetric hypertrophy, which predominantly involves the septum, or concentric left ventricular (LV) hypertrophy. The other observed phenotype is a dilated cardiomyopathy (DCM) with global hypokinesis.[4] There is no apparent relationship between the degree of neurologic and cardiac involvement. Cardiac involvement is not only common in FA but is also a frequent cause of death. In one retrospective study of patients with FA, death from a cardiac cause was the most frequent cause of death (59%), with most mechanisms being congestive heart failure and supraventricular arrhythmias.[5] Compared with noncardiac deaths, cardiac deaths occurred earlier in the disease course (median, 17 years vs 29 years, respectively).[5]

TABLE 76.1 Characteristics of Familial Cardiomyopathies

Familial Cardiomyopathy	Genetics	ECG Findings	Echo Findings	CMRI Findings
Friedreich ataxia (FA)	Autosomal recessive Triplet repeat ~90% have cardiac involvement	Repolarization abnormalities Inferolateral T-wave inversions Mismatch between increased LV mass and absence of LVH by voltage	Concentric LVH with no intracavitary gradient Asymmetric septal hypertrophy Globally decreased LV systolic function	Subendocardial perfusion abnormality in stress CMRI with LGE on LGE CMRI
Myotonic dystrophy (DM)	Autosomal dominant Clinical anticipation ~37%–80% have cardiac involvement	Atrial fibrillation and flutter Varying degrees of AV block and bundle branch block	Often normal Rare systolic dysfunction	Focal fibrosis usually involving midmyocardium to epicardium with endocardial sparing on LGE CMRI
Duchenne muscular dystrophy (DMD)	X-linked ~100% have cardiac involvement	Sinus tachycardia Right axis Posterior and inferolateral pseudo-infarct pattern with deep inferolateral Q waves, tall R wave in lead V_1	Focal hypokinesis basal inferolateral wall MR when involving posterior papillary muscle	Subepicardial and midmyocardial fibrosis involving inferolateral and anterolateral segments on LGE CMRI
Becker muscular dystrophy (BMD)	X-linked ~60%–70% have cardiac involvement	Same as with DMD	Same as with DMD	Same as with DMD

CMRI, Cardiac magnetic resonance imaging; *ECHO*, echocardiogram; *ECG*, electrocardiogram; *LGE*, late gadolinium enhancement; *LV*, left ventricular; *LVH*, left ventricular hypertrophy; *MR*, mitral regurgitation.s

Imaging

The classic echocardiographic finding in FA is increased LV wall thickness, which most commonly involves the septum (Fig. 76.1).[6] Although the degree of overall cardiac involvement does not correlate with the degree of neuromuscular dysfunction, the degree of septal thickening on echocardiography has been correlated with the number of GAA triplet repeats in some studies.[7] Unlike the asymmetric septal hypertrophy associated with other conditions, such as hypertrophic obstructive cardiomyopathy, intracavitary gradient is not typically seen in FA cardiomyopathy. In addition, in one natural history study, a large majority of FA patients had evidence of diastolic dysfunction, and age did not predict its presence or severity, suggesting that diastolic dysfunction may be an early or intrinsic component of FA cardiomyopathy that correlates more strongly with genetic severity than neurologic disability.[8] Cardiac magnetic resonance imaging (CMRI) in FA similarly reveals the hypertrophy seen on echocardiography.[9] Myocardial perfusion studies using CMRI with an adenosine stress modality have demonstrated a reduced myocardial perfusion reserve index, which appears to parallel development of the metabolic syndrome in these patients (Fig. 76.2).[3] Because impaired perfusion reserve does not appear to correlate with the degree of hypertrophy or fibrosis, this may represent a new therapeutic target in patients with FA.[3]

Management

Although guidelines for screening in FA are lacking, a consensus is emerging that patients with this diagnosis benefit from cardiac screening with an annual electrocardiogram (ECG), echocardiogram, and/or CMRI, with follow-up imaging dictated by symptoms and/or changes on the ECG.[1] Treatment of the cardiomyopathy involves early initiation of agents that reduce afterload and that may also reduce fibrosis (e.g., angiotensin-converting enzyme inhibitors and angiotensin receptor blockers).[10] Other treatment modalities, including antioxidants and iron chelation, are under investigation.[11] Preclinical studies have also shown reversal of LV dysfunction in mouse FA models by gene therapy, establishing a proof of concept for the potential of gene therapy in treating FA cardiomyopathy.[12] More recently, cardiomyocytes derived from induced pluripotent stem cells from FA patients were used to demonstrate correction of the frataxin gene and associated cardiomyocyte defects, by

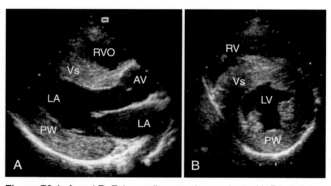

Figure 76.1. A and **B,** Echocardiograms in a patient with Friedreich ataxia. The myocardium, including the papillary muscles, is diffusely increased in thickness and has a granular texture. *AV,* Aortic valve; *LA,* left atrium; *LV,* left ventricle; *PW,* posterior wall; *RV,* right ventricle; *RVO,* right ventricular outflow; *Vs,* ventricular septum.

zinc-finger nuclease mediated editing of the GAA repeats, thus establishing a target for gene therapy in the future.[13]

Myotonic Dystrophy

DM is the most common form of muscular dystrophy that presents in adult life, with an estimated prevalence of 1 in 8000. It is a multisystem and heterogeneous inherited disease that manifests in an autosomal- dominant inheritance pattern with variable penetrance; not all carriers of the gene express the characteristic phenotype. DM also displays clinical anticipation, a phenomenon in which symptoms manifest at an earlier age and often with greater severity in subsequent generations.[14] The disease manifests in three different forms—congenital, classical, and minimal—and is also classified into DM1 and DM2 based on the mutated gene. Classic DM, which is also referred to as Steinert disease or DM1, was first described in 1909 by Hans Steinert. It results from expansion of a trinucleotide CTG repeat in the gene DM protein kinase (*DMPK*).[15] Classic DM onset begins between the second and sixth decades of life and usually presents with myotonia or muscle weakness, cataracts, and cardiac involvement. Congenital

DM (also DM1) is symptomatic within the first year of life and usually presents with respiratory and feeding problems, maternal polyhydramnios, and diffuse muscle weakness. Minimal DM (also DM2) is a milder form of the disease that results from expansion of a tetranucleotide CCTG repeat in the gene *ZNF9*.

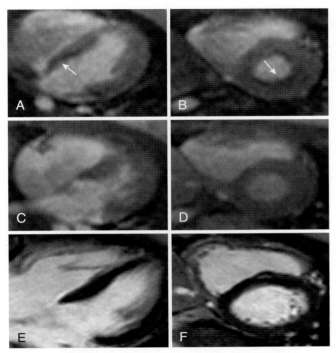

Figure 76.2. Friedreich ataxia stress perfusion cardiac magnetic resonance imaging. Stress perfusion (**A** and **B**), resting perfusion (**B** and **C**), and late postgadolinium imaging shows a significant subendocardial perfusion abnormality, which is most prominent along the basal inferoseptum as seen in the horizontal long-axis (**A, C,** and **E**) and basal short-axis (**B, D,** and **F**) planes. Corresponding late gadolinium enhancement images show no late gadolinium enhancement in the region of perfusion abnormalities that are consistent with absence of infarct scar or fibrosis.

Minimal DM presents later in life, with clinical manifestations of cataracts and mild muscle weakness.

Cardiac Manifestations

Cardiac involvement is observed in both subtypes of DM, but patients with DM1 often have a more complex and aggressive cardiac phenotype. Increased risk of conduction system disturbances, arrhythmias, and compromised systolic and diastolic functions are frequently observed in DM1. The overall incidence of ECG abnormalities in these patients ranges from 37% to 80%.[16] The histopathology involves fibrosis and fatty infiltration of the conduction system and nodal tissue. The most common conduction abnormalities are a slowing of conduction, such as atrioventricular block or bundle branch block, but up to 25% of patients can also have tachyarrhythmias, with atrial fibrillation being the most common. Sudden death represents 2% to 30% of fatalities in patients with DM1, with proposed mechanisms of ventricular asystole and ventricular arrhythmias.[17] Although much less frequent than the electrophysiologic manifestations, DCM may also occur in DM. Though cardiomyopathy is less prevalent, LV systolic dysfunction and heart failure are associated with a poor prognosis in DM1.

Imaging

In keeping with the previously described manifestations, patients with DM may have DCM with increased wall thickness and decreased systolic function. In one study that characterized echocardiographic findings in 382 patients with DM1, 20% of patients had LV hypertrophy, 19% had LV dilatation, 14% had LV systolic dysfunction, and 11% had regional wall motion abnormalities.[17] Studies have additionally demonstrated that significant impairment of LV apical global longitudinal strain seen in DM1, despite preserved LV ejection fraction, may be a potential imaging biomarker to help screen high-risk patients.[18] CMRI can identify focal fibrosis, as identified by late gadolinium enhancement (LGE), in a midmyocardial pattern with occasional extension into the epicardium and notable endocardial sparing (Fig. 76.3).[19] CMRI studies have also shown a high prevalence of reduced LV mass, impaired right ventricular contractility, and LV noncompaction in patients with DM without cardiac symptoms, suggesting a role for CMRI in detecting subclinical cardiac dysfunction.[20]

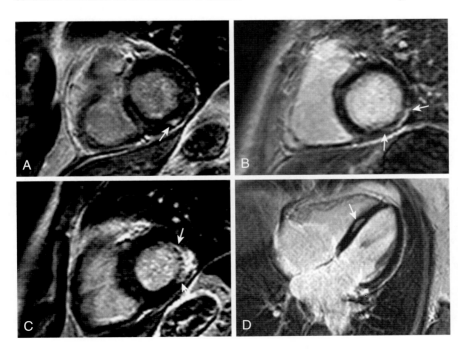

Figure 76.3. Myotonic dystrophy cardiac magnetic resonance imaging with late gadolinium enhancement. Late gadolinium enhancement images in short-axis (**A–C**) and four-chamber long-axis views (**D**) of four patients with myotonic dystrophy type 1. Regions of increased signal intensity are between the *arrows*, which indicates focal fibrosis, and is visible as midmyocardial enhancement to epicardial enhancement with endocardial sparing.

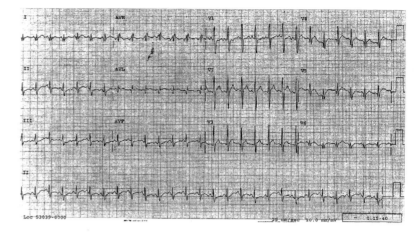

Figure 76.4. Electrocardiogram in a patient with Duchenne muscular dystrophy. Sinus tachycardia at rest, deep inferolateral Q waves, tall R wave in lead V_1, and right-axis deviation. (Courtesy of Dr. Phillip Podrid, VA Boston Medical Center, Boston, MA.)

Management

Diagnosis of cardiac involvement involves careful review of cardiac symptoms and an annual ECG, with a low threshold for ambulatory monitoring in appropriate patients. Many patients are asymptomatic from their cardiac disease because of exertional limitations from neuromuscular involvement. Management of manifest conduction system problems in these patients is no different than in other patients and should be guided by American College of Cardiology/American Heart Association (ACC/AHA) guidelines.[21] However, because studies show that patients experience a high burden of asymptomatic bradyarrhythmias and tachyarrhythmias, maintaining a low threshold for invasive electrophysiological testing and device implantation may be appropriate.[22]

DYSTROPHIN RELATED CARDIOMYOPATHIES
Duchenne Muscular Dystrophy and Becker Muscular Dystrophy

DMD and BMD are caused by X-linked mutations that result in complete or near-complete loss of the dystrophin protein (at locus Xp21) in the case of DMD or in the production of an abnormal truncated dystrophin protein in the case of BMD. DMD has an estimated incidence of 1 in 3500 males. The incidence of BMD is about 1 in 1850 males.[23] Dystrophin is a high-molecular-weight structural protein that links the internal cytoskeleton to the extracellular matrix, allowing for mechanical support during myocyte cellular contraction.

Loss of this protein in DMD results in intracellular mechanical destabilization that weakens the sarcolemma and causes progressive cellular degeneration, with muscle loss and skeletal muscle weakness beginning in the second decade of life, and ultimately, cardiopulmonary failure and subsequent death between ages 20 and 40 years. It was first described in 1836 as a syndrome with both skeletal muscle and cardiac involvement.[24]

In contrast to DMD, patients with BMD express an abnormal but functional dystrophin or a reduced amount of the dystrophin protein. BMD is characterized by skeletal muscle weakness. Because this disease is marked by distorted dystrophin protein rather than an absence of dystrophin as in DMD, the prognosis of BMD is more favorable, with patients living until their fourth to fifth decade of life, with survival to the 80s being described as well.[25]

Cardiac Manifestations

Cardiomyopathy is a prominent feature of DMD. In an observational study of more than 300 patients with DMD, clinically apparent cardiomyopathy was first seen at age 10 years and apparent in all patients by age 20 years. DMD cardiomyopathy was first

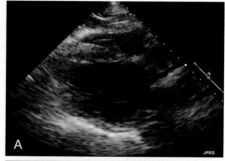

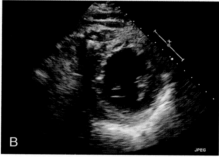

Figure 76.5. Electrocardiogram in a patient with Duchenne muscular dystrophy . Focal wall motion abnormality is seen in the basal inferolateral wall in the absence of significant coronary disease. Findings apparent in the parasternal long-axis (**A**) and parasternal short-axis (**B**) views. (See also Video 75.5.)

described in autopsy studies in the 1930s; the pathognomonic histologic finding of focal myocardial fibrosis that develops first in the inferolateral base and progressively affects the entire LV.[24,26] Scintigraphic and magnetic resonance imaging studies suggest that abnormalities in glucose and fat metabolism in the posterolateral wall segments may contribute to the characteristic focal wall motion abnormality seen in DMD.[27,28]

Cardiac manifestations are common in BMD, affecting 60% to 70% of patients, and cardiac disease is the leading cause of death in these patients.[29] Cardiac involvement is typically manifest at a median age of 29 years.[30] Similar to DMD, cardiac involvement in BMD most commonly consists of a DCM, conduction defects, and arrhythmias.[31] LV hypertrophy is rare. About one-third of patients may develop symptoms of heart failure, but most patients with BMD have asymptomatic cardiac involvement.[23] Female carriers may develop cardiac manifestations without skeletal muscle involvement, although this is not thought to affect overall life expectancy.[32]

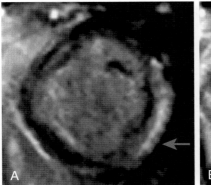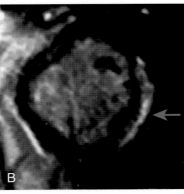

Figure 76.6. Cardiac magnetic resonance imaging of a patient with Duchenne muscular dystrophy (DMD). Basal (**A**) and midcavity (**B**) slices of subepicardial and midmyocardial fibrosis involving the inferolateral and anterolateral segments in a patient with DMD. The *white* late gadolinium enhancement region *(arrows)* is fibrosis, and the *black region* represents the normal myocardium.

Imaging

The ECGs of patients with DMD and BMD typically reveal a pseudo-myocardial infarction pattern of the posterolateral walls characterized by inferolateral Q waves and a tall R wave in lead V_1 (Fig. 76.4). By echocardiography, a concordant wall motion abnormality is observed in the basal inferolateral wall (Fig. 76.5 and Video 76.5). Over time, the fibrosis can also extend into the lateral wall and may involve the posterolateral papillary muscle, which results in secondary mitral regurgitation. Fibrosis can be visualized by LGE CMRI and is also seen in the inferior, inferolateral, and anterolateral segments.[33] LGE usually begins in the subepicardium and can then extend into the midmyocardium or become transmural (Fig. 76.6).[34] The presence of transmural LGE in conjunction with LV systolic dysfunction is associated with increased adverse cardiac events.[35] More recently, native T1 mapping has been shown to be more sensitive in detecting early myocardial scar.[36]

Management

In DMD, the guidelines for screening for cardiac involvement in known male carriers of the dystrophin mutation include ECG and transthoracic echocardiography in children younger than 10 years of age as a baseline study and then yearly thereafter.[22] For asymptomatic female carriers, ECG and transthoracic echocardiography should be performed every 5 years after the age of 16 years.[22] Screening of patients with BMD has historically consisted of ECG and echocardiogram monitoring at the time of diagnosis and every 5 years thereafter. However, with the recognition that CMRI may allow for early diagnosis of cardiac involvement, it is now recommended that patients with BMD undergo a screening CMRI at diagnosis followed by repeat CMRI testing every 2 years.[37]

It is crucial that pharmacologic treatment be initiated before LV dysfunction is detected to delay the onset of heart failure. Corticosteroids are the most relevant class of drugs in the treatment of DMD and BMD, with a profound impact on the natural history of the disease. CMRI imaging studies have showed that steroid treatment results in decreased LV fibrosis burden and a positive impact on LV function though the mechanism is unknown.[38,39] Unfortunately, the cardiomyopathy of DMD and BMD does not respond as well to conventional therapies for heart failure, such as β-blockade and afterload reduction, though early use of angiotensin-converting enzyme inhibitor therapy may slow the progression of myocardial fibrosis.[40] However, it is reasonable to introduce these therapies and titrate to symptomatic benefit. In addition, patients with DMD and BMD with severe systolic dysfunction should also be considered for implantable cardiac defibrillators for primary prevention of sudden cardiac death according to 2008 ACC/AHA/Health Resources and Services Administration guidelines.[21]

SUMMARY

FA, DM, DMD, and BMD are uncommon familial cardiomyopathies that vary significantly in their mode of transmission, epidemiology, and cardiac manifestations, with characteristic associated findings on ECG, echocardiography, and CMRI (Table 76.1). The syndromes themselves were described before the era of genetic identification; the reported clinical phenotypes, ages of onset, and disease severity can be difficult to categorize. One unifying feature of these inherited diseases is that cardiac involvement is unpredictable and often unrelated to the duration of diagnosis or the severity of neurologic or skeletal muscular disease. In addition, life expectancy in patients with cardiac involvement in these diseases is considerably reduced, either due to arrhythmic complications or heart failure. The risk of sudden cardiac death can be mitigated with appropriate electrophysiology studies or device implantation and heart failure therapy. For this reason, early consideration of cardiac involvement and assessment with appropriate imaging modalities is essential to diagnose and treat cardiac manifestations of these neuromuscular syndromes. Ongoing studies are needed to help identify imaging biomarkers for risk-stratification and provide insights into potential therapeutic targets.

Please access ExpertConsult to view the corresponding videos for this chapter.

REFERENCES

1. Weidemann F, Rummey C, Bijnens B, et al. The heart in Friedreich ataxia: definition of cardiomyopathy, disease severity, and correlation with neurological symptoms. *Circulation.* 2012;125:1626–1634.
2. Arbustini E, Di Toro A, Giuliani L, et al. Cardiac phenotypes in hereditary muscle disorders. *J Am Coll Cardiol.* 2018;72:2485–2506.
3. Raman SV, Dickerson JA, Al-Dahhak R. Myocardial ischemia in the absence of epicardial coronary artery disease in Friedreich's ataxia. *J Cardiovasc Magn Reson.* 2008;10:15.
4. Child JS, Perloff JK, Bach PM, et al. Cardiac involvement in Friedreich's ataxia: a clinical study of 75 patients. *J Am Coll Cardiol.* 1986;7:1370–1378.
5. Tsou AY, Paulsen EK, Lagedrost SJ, et al. Mortality in Friedreich ataxia. *J Neurol Sci.* 2011;307:46–49.
6. Alizad A, Seward JB. Echocardiographic features of genetic diseases: part 1. Cardiomyopathy. *J Am Soc Echocardiogr.* 2000;13:73–86.
7. Dutka DP, Donnelly JE, Nihoyannopoulos P, et al. Marked variation in the cardiomyopathy associated with Friedreich's ataxia. *Heart.* 1999;81:141–147.
8. Regner SR, Lagedrost SJ, Plappert T, et al. Analysis of echocardiograms in a large heterogeneous cohort of patients with Friedreich ataxia. *Am J Cardiology.* 2012;109:401–405.
9. Meyer C, Schmid G, Gorlitz S, et al. Cardiomyopathy in Friedreich's ataxia—assessment by cardiac MRI. *Mov Disord.* 2007;22:1615–1622.
10. Payne RM. The heart in Friedreich's ataxia: basic findings and clinical implications. *Prog Pediatr Cardiol.* 2011;31:103–109.
11. Velasco-Sanchez D, Aracil A, Montero R, et al. Combined therapy with idebenone and deferiprone in patients with Friedreich's ataxia. *Cerebellum.* 2011;10:1–8.
12. Perdomini M, Belbellaa B, Monassier L, et al. Prevention and reversal of severe mitochondrial cardiomyopathy by gene therapy in a mouse model of Friedreich's ataxia. *Nat Med.* 2014;20:542–549.
13. Li J, Rozwadowska N, Clark A et al. Excision of the expanded GAA repeats corrects cardiomyopathy phenotypes of iPSC-derived Friedreich's ataxia cardiomyocytes. *Stem Cell Res.* 2019;40:101529.

14. Melacini P, Villanova C, Menegazzo E, et al. Correlation between cardiac involvement and CTG trinucleotide repeat length in myotonic dystrophy. *J Am Coll Cardiol.* 1995;25:239–245.
15. Phillips MF, Harper PS. Cardiac disease in myotonic dystrophy. *Cardiovasc Res.* 1997;33:13–22.
16. Pelargonio G, Dello Russo A, Sanna T, et al. Myotonic dystrophy and the heart. *Heart.* 2002;88:665–670.
17. Mathieu J, Allard P, Potvin L, et al. A 10-year study of mortality in a cohort of patients with myotonic dystrophy. *Neurology.* 1999;52:1658–1662.
18. Garcia R, Labarre Q, Degand B, et al. Apical left ventricular myocardial dysfunction is an early feature of cardiac involvement in myotonic dystrophy type 1. *Echocardiography.* 2017;34:184–190.
19. Hermans MC, Faber CG, Bekkers SC, et al. Structural and functional cardiac changes in myotonic dystrophy type 1: a cardiovascular magnetic resonance study. *J Cardiovasc Magn Reson.* 2012;14:48.
20. Choudhary P, Nadakumar R, Greig H, et al. Structural and electrical cardiac abnormalities are prevalent in asymptomatic myotonic dystrophy. *Heart.* 2016;102:1472–1478.
21. Epstein AE, Dimarco JP, Ellenbogen KA, et al. ACC/AHA/HRS 2008 guidelines for device-based therapy of cardiac rhythm abnormalities: executive summary. *Heart Rhythm.* 2008;5:934–955.
22. Bouhouch R, Elhouari T, Oukerraj L, et al. Management of cardiac involvement in neuromuscular diseases: review. *Open Cardiovasc Med J.* 2008;2:93–96.
23. Yilmaz A, Sechtem U. Cardiac involvement in muscular dystrophy: advances in diagnosis and therapy. *Heart.* 2012;98:420–429.
24. Nigro G, Comi LI, Politano L, et al. The incidence and evolution of cardiomyopathy in Duchenne muscular dystrophy. *Int J Cardiol.* 1976;26:271–277.
25. van den Bergen JC, Schade van Westrum SM, Dekker L, et al. Clinical characterisation of Becker muscular dystrophy patients predicts favourable outcome in exon-skipping therapy. *J Neurol Neurosurg Psychiatry.* 2014;85:92–98.
26. Fayssoil A, Abasse S, Silverston K. Cardiac involvement classification and therapeutic management in patients with Duchenne muscular dystrophy. *J Neuromuscul Dis.* 2017;4:17–23.
27. Perloff JK, Henze E, Schelbert HR. Alterations in regional myocardial metabolism, perfusion, and wall motion in Duchenne muscular dystrophy studied by radionuclide imaging. *Circulation.* 1984;69:33–42.
28. Suttie JJDS, Karamitsos TD, Holloway CJ, et al. Becker and Duchenne muscular dystrophy (BMD, DMD) are associated with myocardial fibrosis and abnormal cardiac energetics even in the presence of normal left ventricular ejection fraction. *J Cardiovasc Magn Reson.* 2010;12:1–4.
29. Rajdev A, Groh WJ. Arrhythmias in the muscular dystrophies. *Card Electrophysiol Clin.* 2015;7:303–308.
30. Groh WJ. Arrhythmias in the muscular dystrophies. *Heart Rhythm.* 2012;9:1890–1895.
31. Vidal-Pérez R, Diaz-Villanueva J, Arzanauskaite M, et al. Cardiac involvement in Becker muscular dystrophy: role of cardiovascular magnetic resonance. *Eur Heart J Cardiovasc Imag.* 2013;14:1038.
32. Holloway SM, Wilcox DE, Wilcox A, et al. Life expectancy and death from cardiomyopathy amongst carriers of Duchenne and Becker muscular dystrophy in Scotland. *Heart.* 2008;94:633–636.
33. Verhaert D, Richards K, Rafael-Fortney JA, et al. Cardiac involvement in patients with muscular dystrophies: magnetic resonance imaging phenotype and genotypic considerations. *Circ Cardiovasc Imag.* 2011;4:67–76.
34. Bilchick KC, Salerno M, Plitt D, et al. Prevalence and distribution of regional scar in dysfunctional myocardial segments in Duchenne muscular dystrophy. *J Cardiovasc Magn Reson.* 2011;13:20.
35. Poonja S, Power A, Mah JK, Fine N, et al. Current cardiac imaging approaches in Duchenne Muscular dystrophy. *J Clin Neuromusc Dis.* 2018;20:85–93.
36. Soslow JH, Damon BM, Saville BR, et al. Evaluation of post-contrast myocardial T1 in Duchenne muscular dystrophy using cardiac magnetic resonance imaging. *Pediatr Cardiol.* 2015;36:49–56.
37. Ho R, Nguyen ML, Mather P. Cardiomyopathy in Becker muscle dystrophy: overview. *World J Cardiol.* 2016;8:356–361.
38. D'Amario D, Amodeo A, Adorisio R, et al. A current approach to heart failure in Duchenne muscular dystrophy. *Heart.* 2017;103:1770–1779.
39. Tandon A, Villa CR, Hor KN, et al. Myocardial fibrosis burden predicts left ventricular ejection fraction and is associated with age and steroid treatment duration in Duchenne muscular. *J Am Heart Assoc.* 2015;26:4.
40. Silva MC, Magalhaes TA, Meira ZMA, et al. Myocardial fibrosis progression in Duchenne and Becker muscular dystrophy. *JAMA Cardiol.* 2017;2:190–199.

77 Echocardiography in Cor Pulmonale and Pulmonary Heart Disease

Brent White, Nadia El Hangouche, Andrew C. Peters, Benjamin H. Freed

Cor pulmonale refers to right ventricular (RV) hypertrophy and enlargement caused by disorders of the lung parenchyma or vasculature. This excludes RV dysfunction from left heart failure or congenital heart disease.[1] Cor pulmonale results from pulmonary hypertension (PH), which causes increased RV afterload and preload because of elevated central venous pressure leading to RV failure. The Sixth World Symposium on Pulmonary Hypertension in 2018 revised the definition of PH as having a pulmonary vascular resistance (PVR) greater than 3 Woods units (WU) and a mean pulmonary artery pressure (mPAP) greater than 20 mm Hg from the previous definition of a mPAP greater than 25 mm Hg.[2] It can be subdivided hemodynamically into precapillary (pulmonary capillary wedge pressure [PCWP] <15 mm Hg and PVR >3 WU caused by dysfunction of the pulmonary vasculature or parenchyma) and postcapillary disease (PCWP >15 mm Hg, PVR <3 WU) caused by transmission of elevated left-sided cardiac pressures to the pulmonary circulation.[2] PH is further classified into five groups according to clinical presentation, hemodynamics, disease mechanism, and treatment algorithm (Table 77.1).[2–4]

The most common respiratory cause of chronic cor pulmonale is chronic obstructive pulmonary disease (COPD). A large number of other diseases can lead to cor pulmonale, including (but not limited to) cystic fibrosis, interstitial lung disease, sickle cell anemia, sarcoidosis, obstructive sleep apnea, alveolar hypoventilation disorders, and neuromuscular and chest wall disorders.[4] Typically, PH worsens insidiously over years causing chronic cor pulmonale

but can also occur rapidly. The causes of acute cor pulmonale are limited and include massive pulmonary embolism or acute respiratory distress syndrome (ARDS) in which major insult to the pulmonary vasculature or parenchyma causes acute PH, leading to rapid RV pressure and volume overload.

Echocardiography is the cornerstone of noninvasive imaging in the diagnosis and assessment of cor pulmonale and PH. Echocardiography is advantageous because it is low cost and readily available and has an excellent safety profile with no ionizing radiation. Guidelines recommend assigning a probability of PH based on echocardiography findings with the main criteria being an elevated tricuspid regurgitant (TR) velocity and supporting criteria including RV, pulmonary artery (PA), right atrial (RA), and inferior vena cava size; interventricular septal contour; and PA Doppler characteristics.[3] Asymptomatic individuals at high risk for PH, such as those with systemic sclerosis, a known genetic mutation, a first-degree relative with familial PAH, or portal hypertension, are recommended to undergo yearly screening echocardiography to diagnose PH early before the development of cor pulmonale.[4] When long-standing PH is suspected or known, patients with cor pulmonale will manifest more advanced RV dysfunction such as flattening of the interventricular septum (IVS), RV dilatation, and RV systolic dysfunction. This chapter highlights the essential role of echocardiography in diagnosis, prognosis, disease monitoring, and treatment evaluation in patients with PH and cor pulmonale.

TABLE 77.1 Classification of Pulmonary Hypertension

	HEMODYNAMICS	CLINICAL GROUP	CAUSE
Precapillary PH	Mean PAP >20 mm Hg PCWP <15 mm Hg PVR >3 WU	Group 1: PAH	Idiopathic PAH Heritable PAH Connective tissue disease HIV associated Portal hypertension Drugs
		Group 3: lung disease	COPD ILD Sleep-disordered breathing Alveolar hypoventilation Chest wall abnormalities
		Group 4: CTEPH	Chronic thromboembolic PH
		Group 5: unclear or multifactorial	Hematologic disorders Pulmonary sarcoidosis Langerhans cell histiocytosis Neurofibromatosis Vasculitis
Postcapillary PH	Mean PAP >20 mm Hg PCWP >15 mm Hg PVR <3 WU	Group 2: left heart disease	LV systolic dysfunction LV diastolic dysfunction Valvular heart disease
		Group 5: unclear or multifactorial	Hematologic disorders Pulmonary sarcoidosis Langerhans cell histiocytosis Neurofibromatosis Vasculitis

COPD, Chronic obstructive pulmonary disease; *CTEPH,* chronic thromboembolic pulmonary hypertension; *ILD,* interstitial lung disease; *LV,* left ventricular; *PAH,* pulmonary arterial hypertension; *PAP,* pulmonary artery pressure; *PCWP,* pulmonary capillary wedge pressure; *PH,* pulmonary hypertension; *PVR,* pulmonary vascular resistance.

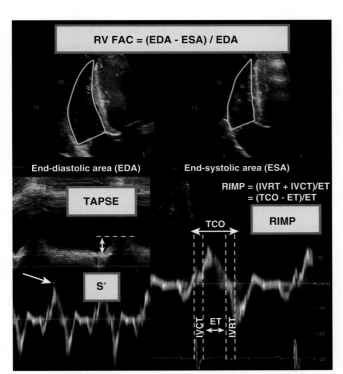

Figure 77.1. Standard two-dimensional echocardiographic methods of assessing right ventricular (RV) systolic function, including fractional area change (FAC), tricuspid annular plane systolic excursion (TAPSE), S′ tissue Doppler, and right ventricular index of myocardial performance (RIMP). *ET,* Ejection time; *IVCT,* isovolumic contraction time; *IVRT,* isovolumic relaxation time; *TCO,* tricuspid closure-open time.

STRUCTURAL ABNORMALITIES

One of the earliest changes that occurs in the setting of chronic pressure overload is RV chamber dilatation.[5] This can be assessed with two-dimensional (2D) echocardiography, most commonly by measuring the diameter of the RV base in the RV-focused apical four-chamber view, with a diameter greater than 41 mm indicating dilatation.[6] As PH progresses, RV contractility becomes impaired, which manifests as reduced systolic function.[5] There are several methods to assess RV systolic function on 2D echocardiography, including tricuspid annular plane systolic excursion (TAPSE), S′, fractional area change, and the RV index of myocardial performance (RIMP) (Fig. 77.1).[6] Bossone and coworkers studied a population of patients referred to a tertiary care center with known or suspected pulmonary arterial hypertension (PAH), finding that 98% had RV dilatation and 78% had reduced RV systolic function.[7] Systolic flattening of the IVS is a common finding when the PA systolic pressures are significantly elevated.[7,8] This is best seen from the parasternal short-axis view of the ventricles (Fig. 77.2 and Video 77.2). The impact of RV pathology on the IVS in both end-systole and end-diastole can be further characterized by calculating the eccentricity index, defined as the ratio of D2 to D1, in which D2 is the minor-axis dimension of the left ventricle parallel to the septum and D1 is the minor-axis dimension perpendicular to and bisecting the septum (Fig. 77.3).[9]

Pericardial effusions have also been described in the setting of chronic elevation of pulmonary pressures (see Fig. 77.2).[7,10,11] The exact mechanism is unknown but may be caused by elevation of lymphatic and venous or RA pressures (or both), which results in reduced drainage of the pericardium. Patent foramen ovale, with shunting identified by agitated saline contrast, has also been described with increased frequency,[7] which may be related to the opening of an existing patent foramen ovale tunnel in the setting of elevated RA pressures.

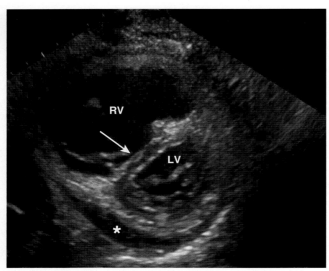

Figure 77.2. Basal parasternal short-axis view of a patient with severe pulmonary arterial hypertension. Note the severe dilatation of the right ventricle (RV), septal flattening *(arrow)*, and presence of a pericardial effusion *(asterisk)*. *LV,* Left ventricle. (See accompanying Video 77.2.)

DOPPLER FINDINGS

TR is frequently noted in individuals with PAH, with moderate to severe TR occurring in up to 80% of individuals in some series.[7] The TR jet can be used to estimate PA systolic pressure using the modified Bernoulli equation plus the estimated RA pressure (Fig. 77.4).[12] Elevated PA systolic pressures are a hallmark feature in cor pulmonale, with estimates commonly being greater than 60 mm Hg.[7,8]

The current PH guidelines recommend using the peak TR velocity without the RA pressure estimate for initial assessment, with a peak velocity of 3.4 m/s or greater conferring a high probability of PH.[3] It is also worth noting important demographic differences in PA systolic pressure. A large study in normal participants found that PA systolic pressure increases with age and body mass index, and that males have a slightly higher PA systolic pressure than females.[13]

Mean and diastolic PA pressures can be calculated by using the pulmonic regurgitation Doppler signal (Fig. 77.5). Using the modified Bernoulli equation, the peak and end pulmonary regurgitant velocities plus the RA pressure have been show to correlate well with mean and diastolic pulmonary pressures, respectively.[14,15] A midsystolic notch in the RV outflow tract (RVOT) Doppler signal and a shortening of the acceleration time have both been described in the setting of significant elevation in PA systolic pressure (Fig. 77.6).[16] Assessment of PVR is also important in PH, and the ratio of peak TR to the RVOT velocity time integral

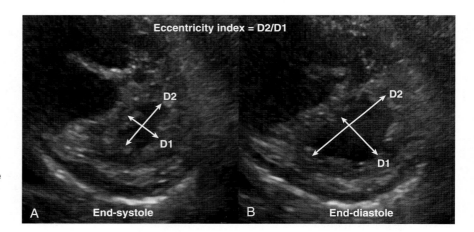

Figure 77.3. Basal parasternal short-axis cine of a patient with severe pulmonary arterial hypertension. The eccentricity index (D2/D1), measured in both end-systole (**A**) and end-diastole (**B**).

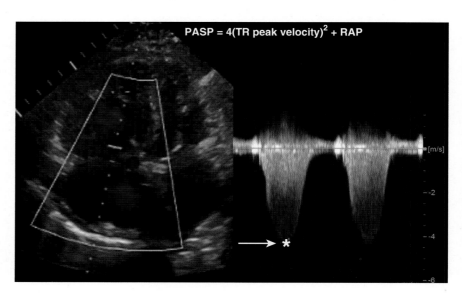

Figure 77.4. Continuous wave Doppler showing an elevated peak tricuspid regurgitation gradient *(arrow and asterisk)* and calculation of the pulmonary artery systolic pressure (pulmonary artery systolic pressure). *RAP,* Right atrial pressure; *TR,* tricuspid regurgitation.

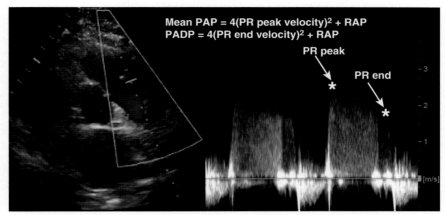

Figure 77.5. Continuous-wave Doppler of the pulmonic valve revealing a pulmonic regurgitation Doppler signal. Calculation of the mean and diastolic pulmonary artery pressures using the peak and end-pulmonic regurgitation velocities, respectively (*arrows* and *asterisks*). *PA,* Pulmonary artery pressure; *PADP,* pulmonary artery diastolic pressure; *PR,* pulmonic regurgitation; *RAP,* right atrial pressure.

has been shown to correlate well with invasively-derived PVR.[17] Finally, when assessing for PH, it is critical to differentiate PAH from pulmonary venous hypertension (PVH) (Fig. 77.7). This can be done by evaluating for echocardiographic evidence of left-sided heart disease, which includes left atrial enlargement, bowing of the interatrial septum to the right, decreased tissue Doppler velocity (e′), and a high E/e′ ratio.[18]

THREE-DIMENSIONAL ECHOCARDIOGRAPHY

The RV has a complex crescent shape with a thin wall and prominent trabeculations, which makes the assessment of its volume and ejection fraction limited by the classical 2D echocardiographic measures. Three-dimensional (3D) echocardiography offers a more reliable assessment that is independent of geometric assumptions. Compared with magnetic resonance imaging, 3D-derived RV volumes are similar with a slight tendency to underestimate stroke volume and ejection fraction.[19] The main limitation of this technique is related to the suboptimal imaging windows in patients with chronic lung disease, in addition to their limited ability to perform the breath holds required for multibeat acquisitions.

MYOCARDIAL STRAIN

Strain is a novel nonvolumetric parameter used to assess myocardial deformation of the ventricles (Fig. 77.8 and Video 77.8). It is independent from the respiratory translational motion of the heart or the clockwise rotation of the apex that affects TAPSE or S′.[20,21] An absolute value less than 20% is likely abnormal for RV free wall strain,[22] but lower absolute values have been used for prognosis.[23] RV free wall strain has been studied more extensively than global RV strain, but it does not take into consideration the potential dyssynchronous contraction of opposing wall that is present with various degrees of ventricular dysfunction.[24]

ECHOCARDIOGRAPHY AND PROGNOSIS

In addition to its importance in diagnosing PH and subsequent cor pulmonale, echocardiography is also central in informing prognosis and treatment for these patients. The most common cause of death from cor pulmonale historically has been attributed to right heart failure, although this has been decreasing in the age of PH-specific therapies.[25,26] Echocardiography findings such as moderate to severe TR and a pericardial effusion are independent risk factors for death in PH.[27] Reduced TAPSE is a risk factor for mortality in acute cor pulmonale caused by ARDS.[28] In a prospective study of patients with known or suspected PH, a TAPSE below 18

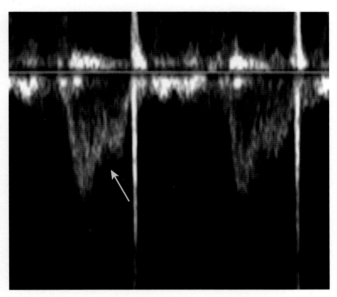

Figure 77.6. Pulsed-wave Doppler of the right ventricular outflow tract showing the characteristic midsystolic notching in pulmonary hypertension *(arrow)*.

mm was associated with a 5.7-fold increased risk of death over a mean follow-up period of 19.3 months.[29] In the treatment algorithm for acute pulmonary embolism, RV dysfunction on echocardiography is associated with a higher risk of early death and plays an important role in triaging a patient to more aggressive care.[30] In cor pulmonale, peak TR velocity has been shown to predict exercise tolerance and prognosis in moderate to severe COPD.[31,32]

RV strain provides incremental prognostic value over conventional clinical and echocardiographic variables in patients with PH. In a study of 575 patients, RV strain predicted outcome across pulmonary pressures and groups of PH. Eighteen-month survival rates were 92%, 88%, 85%, and 71% according to RV strain quartile (< .001), with a 1.46 higher risk of death per 6.7% decline in RV strain.[22] In another study of 150 patients with PH, patients with RV free-wall strain worse than −19% had a threefold risk of all-cause mortality, and every 1% decrease in strain correlated with a 13% increase in risk of death.[33]

3D echocardiography is also emerging as an important prognostic tool in patients with PH.[34] In a study of 228 patients with PH, 3D-derived RV volumes and ejection fraction correlated

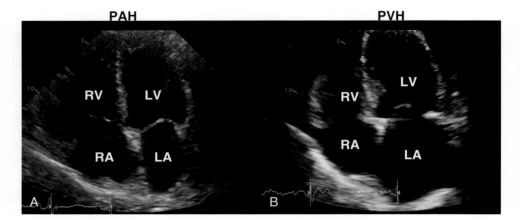

Figure 77.7. Apical four-chamber views of a patient with pulmonary arterial hypertension (PAH; **A**) and a patient with pulmonary venous hypertension (PVH; **B**). *LA,* Left atrium; *LV,* left ventricle; *RA,* right atrium; *RV,* right ventricle.

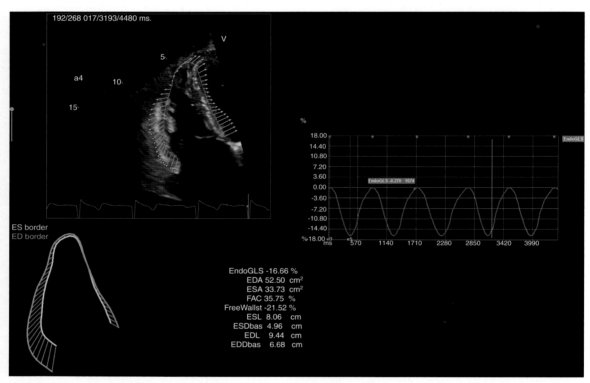

Figure 77.8. Apical four-chamber focused view of the right ventricle with strain overlay and associated right ventricular strain curve. The global longitudinal strain is −16.7%, and the free-wall strain is −21.5%. *ED,* End diastolic; *EDA,* end-diastolic area; *EDDbas,* end-diastolic diameter base; *EDL,* end-diastolic length; *EndoGLS,* right ventricular global longitudinal strain; *ES,* end-systolic; *ESA,* end-systolic area; *ESDbas,* end-systolic diameter base; *ESL,* end-systolic length; *FAC,* fractional area change; *FreeWallst,* free wall strain;. (See accompanying Video 77.8.)

better than the usual 2D parameters with the primary endpoint defined as death, hospitalization, and lung surgery (transplantation or endarterectomy).[35] In this study, an RV end-systolic volume index of 114 mL/m^2 was described as the cutoff distinguishing patients with RV adaptation from RV adverse remodeling with worse short-term outcome.

ECHOCARDIOGRAPHY TO MONITOR RESPONSE TO THERAPY

Echocardiography has been used to monitor response to therapy in PH and cor pulmonale. Hinderliter and coworkers studied PAH patients treated with a 12-week intravenous infusion of epoprostenol and found a reduction in the maximal TR velocity, less RV dilatation, and an improved curvature of the IVS.[36] Tonelli and colleagues retrospectively studied PAH patients being treated with

parenteral prostacyclin therapy who had echocardiograms performed at baseline and 12 months after therapy. They found that a decrease in RV end-diastolic area, decrease in peak TR velocity, increase in the RVOT velocity time integral, and improvement in RV systolic function were all associated with decreased mortality rates.[26] Finally, two recent studies both found that having a higher TAPSE after initiating therapy for PAH was associated with decreased mortality rates.[37,38]

RV strain was also shown to improve in patients responsive to PH treatment and to correlate with outcome. In a small cohort of 50 patients treated for PH by prostacyclin, calcium channel inhibitor, or combination, authors found that patients with a 5% improvement or greater in RV free-wall systolic strain had a greater than sevenfold lower mortality risk at 4 years.[39] RV strain at rest and after exercise as well as RV 3D volumes were also studied in a small cohort of PH patients before and after pulmonary endarterectomy.[40] This study showed reverse remodeling of the RV at 12 months and increased contractile reserve after exercise.

CONCLUSION

Echocardiography is the primary noninvasive test of choice to evaluate patients with PH. Elevated RV pressures on spectral Doppler and patterns of RV pressure–volume overload such as midsystolic notching of the RVOT Doppler signal and IVS flattening are hallmarks of disease. RV chamber quantification with 2D echocardiography have been the mainstay of a thorough evaluation but are problematic because of the irregular geometry of the RV. Newer techniques such as the 3D volumetric assessment of RV size and function as well as speckle tracking–derived strain may improve accuracy of diagnosis, prognosis, and serial assessment in patients with PH and cor pulmonale.

Please access ExpertConsult to view the corresponding videos for this chapter.

Acknowledgment

The authors acknowledge the contributions of Dr. Danita M. Yoerger Sanborn, who was the author of this chapter in the previous edition.

REFERENCES

1. Budev MM, Arroliga AC, Wiedemann HP, Matthay RA. Cor pulmonale: an overview. *Semin Respir Crit Care Med*. 2003;24:233–244.
2. Frost A, Badesch D, Gibbs JSR, et al. Diagnosis of pulmonary hypertension. *Eur Respir J*. 2019;53.
3. Galie N, Humbert M, Vachiery JL, et al. 2015 ESC/ERS Guidelines for the diagnosis and treatment of pulmonary hypertension. *Eur Heart J*. 2016;37:67–119.
4. Bossone E, D'Andrea A, D'Alto M, et al. Echocardiography in pulmonary arterial hypertension: from diagnosis to prognosis. *J Am Soc Echocardiogr*. 2013;26:1–14.
5. Bogaard HJ, Abe K, Vonk Noordegraaf A, Voelkel NF. The right ventricle under pressure: cellular and molecular mechanisms of right-heart failure in pulmonary hypertension. *Chest*. 2009;135:794–804.
6. Lang RM, Badano LP, Mor-Avi V, et al. Recommendations for cardiac chamber quantification by echocardiography in adults. *J Am Soc Echocardiogr*. 2015;28:1–39.
7. Bossone E, Duong-Wagner TH, Paciocco G, et al. Echocardiographic features of primary pulmonary hypertension. *J Am Soc Echocardiogr*. 1999;12:655–662.
8. Raymond RJ, Hinderliter AL, Willis PW, et al. Echocardiographic predictors of adverse outcomes in primary pulmonary hypertension. *J Am Coll Cardiol*. 2002;39:1214–1219.
9. Ryan T, Petrovic O, Dillon JC, et al. An echocardiographic index for separation of right ventricular volume and pressure overload. *J Am Coll Cardiol*. 1985;5. 918–27.
10. Hinderliter AL, Willis PW, Long W, et al. Frequency and prognostic significance of pericardial effusion in primary pulmonary hypertension. *Am J Cardiol*. 1999;84:481–484. A10.
11. Fenstad ER, Le RJ, Sinak LJ, et al. Pericardial effusions in pulmonary arterial hypertension: characteristics, prognosis, and role of drainage. *Chest*. 2013;144:1530–1538.
12. Yock PG, Popp RL. Noninvasive estimation of right ventricular systolic pressure by Doppler ultrasound in patients with tricuspid regurgitation. *Circulation*. 1984;70:657–662.
13. McQuillan BM, Picard MH, Leavitt M, Weyman AE. Clinical correlates and reference intervals for pulmonary artery systolic pressure among echocardiographically normal subjects. *Circulation*. 2001;104:2797–2802.
14. Abbas AE, Fortuin FD, Schiller NB, et al. Echocardiographic determination of mean pulmonary artery pressure. *Am J Cardiol*. 2003;92:1373–1376.
15. Masuyama T, Kodama K, Kitabatake A, et al. Continuous-wave Doppler echocardiographic detection of pulmonary regurgitation and its application to noninvasive estimation of pulmonary artery pressure. *Circulation*. 1986;74:484–492.
16. Kitabatake A, Inoue M, Asao M, et al. Noninvasive evaluation of pulmonary hypertension by a pulsed Doppler technique. *Circulation*. 1983;68:302–309.
17. Abbas AE, Fortuin FD, Schiller NB, et al. A simple method for noninvasive estimation of pulmonary vascular resistance. *J Am Coll Cardiol*. 2003;41:1021–1027.
18. Willens HJ, Chirinos JA, Gomez-Marin O, et al. Noninvasive differentiation of pulmonary arterial and venous hypertension using conventional and Doppler tissue imaging echocardiography. *J Am Soc Echocardiogr*. 2008;21:715–719.
19. Knight DS, Grasso AE, Quail MA, et al. Accuracy and reproducibility of right ventricular quantification in patients with pressure and volume overload using single-beat three-dimensional echocardiography. *J Am Soc Echocardiogr*. 2015;28:363–374.
20. Motoji Y, Tanaka H, Fukuda Y, et al. Association of apical longitudinal rotation with right ventricular performance in patients with pulmonary hypertension: Insights into overestimation of tricuspid annular plane systolic excursion. *Echocardiography*. 2016;33:207–215.
21. Collier P, Xu B, Kusunose K, et al. Impact of abnormal longitudinal rotation on the assessment of right ventricular systolic function in patients with severe pulmonary hypertension. *J Thorac Dis*. 2018;10:4694–4704.
22. Fine NM, Chen L, Bastiansen PM, et al. Outcome prediction by quantitative right ventricular function assessment in 575 subjects evaluated for pulmonary hypertension. *Circ Cardiovasc Imag*. 2013;6:711–721.
23. Lee K, Kwon O, Lee EJ, et al. Prognostic value of echocardiographic parameters for right ventricular function in patients with acute non-massive pulmonary embolism. *Heart Ves sels*. 2019;34:1187–1195.
24. Lamia B, Muir JF, Molano LC, et al. Altered synchrony of right ventricular contraction in borderline pulmonary hypertension. *Int J Cardiovasc Imag*. 2017;33:1331–1339.
25. D'Alonzo GE, Barst RJ, Ayres SM, et al. Survival in patients with primary pulmonary hypertension. Results from a national prospective registry. *Ann Intern Med*. 1991;115:343–349.
26. Tonelli AR, Conci D, Tamarappoo BK, et al. Prognostic value of echocardiographic changes in patients with pulmonary arterial hypertension receiving parenteral prostacyclin therapy. *J Am Soc Echocardiogr*. 2014;27:733–741.
27. Grapsa J, Pereira Nunes MC, Tan TC, et al. Echocardiographic and hemodynamic predictors of survival in precapillary pulmonary hypertension: seven-year follow-up. *Circ Cardiovasc Imag*. 2015;8.
28. Shah TG, Wadia SK, Kovach J, et al. Echocardiographic parameters of right ventricular function predict mortality in acute respiratory distress syndrome. *Pulm Circ*. 2016;6:155–160.
29. Forfia PR, Fisher MR, Mathai SC, et al. Tricuspid annular displacement predicts survival in pulmonary hypertension. *Am J Respir Crit Care Med*. 2006;174:1034–1041.
30. Konstantinides SV, Barco S, Lankeit M, Meyer G. Management of pulmonary embolism: an update. *J Am Coll Cardiol*. 2016;67:976–990.
31. Schoos MM, Dalsgaard M, Kjaergaard J, et al. Echocardiographic predictors of exercise capacity and mortality in chronic obstructive pulmonary disease. *BMC Cardiovasc Disord*. 2013;13:84.
32. Sims MW, Margolis DJ, Localio AR, et al. Impact of pulmonary artery pressure on exercise function in severe COPD. *Chest*. 2009;136:412–419.
33. Haeck ML, Scherptong RW, Marsan NA, et al. Prognostic value of right ventricular longitudinal peak systolic strain in patients with pulmonary hypertension. *Circ Cardiovasc Imag*. 2012;5:628–636.
34. Jone PN, Schafer M, Pan Z, et al. 3D echocardiographic evaluation of right ventricular function and strain: a prognostic study in paediatric pulmonary hypertension. *Eur Heart J Cardiovasc Imag*. 2018;19:1026–1033.
35. Ryo K, Goda A, Onishi T, et al. Characterization of right ventricular remodeling in pulmonary hypertension associated with patient outcomes by 3-dimensional wall motion tracking echocardiography. *Circ Cardiovasc Imag*. 2015;8.
36. Hinderliter AL, Willis PW, Barst RJ, et al. Effects of long-term infusion of prostacyclin (epoprostenol) on echocardiographic measures of right ventricular structure and function in primary pulmonary hypertension. *Circulation*. 1997;95:1479–1486.
37. Ghio S, Pica S, Klersy C, et al. Prognostic value of TAPSE after therapy optimisation in patients with pulmonary arterial hypertension is independent of the haemodynamic effects of therapy. *Open Heart*. 2016;3:e000408.
38. Mazurek JA, Vaidya A, Mathai SC, et al. Follow-up tricuspid annular plane systolic excursion predicts survival in pulmonary arterial hypertension. *Pulm Circ*. 2017;7:361–371.
39. Hardegree EL, Sachdev A, Villarraga HR, et al. Role of serial quantitative assessment of right ventricular function by strain in pulmonary arterial hypertension. *Am J Cardiol*. 2013;111:143–148.
40. Waziri F, Mellemkjaer S, Clemmensen TS, et al. Long-term changes of resting and exercise right ventricular systolic performance in patients with chronic thromboembolic pulmonary hypertension following pulmonary thromboendarterectomy. *Echocardiography*. 2019;36:1656–1665.

78   Aortic Stenosis Morphology

Steven A. Goldstein

CONGENITAL AORTIC STENOSIS
Bicuspid Aortic Valve

Congenital aortic valve malformation reflects a phenotypic continuum of unicuspid valve (severe form), bicuspid valve (moderate form), tricuspid valve (normal, but may be abnormal), and the rare quadricuspid forms. Bicuspid aortic valves (BAVs) are the result of abnormal cusp formation during the complex developmental process. In most cases, adjacent cusps fail to separate, resulting in one larger conjoined cusp and a smaller one. Therefore, BAV (or bicommissural aortic valve) has partial or complete fusion of two of the aortic valve leaflets, with or without a central raphe, resulting in partial or complete absence of a functional commissure between the fused leaflets.[1]

The generally accepted prevalence of BAV in the general population is 1% to 2%, making it the most common congenital heart defect. Information on the prevalence of BAV comes primarily from pathology centers.[1–7] Valvular aortic stenosis (AS), a chronic progressive disease, usually develops over decades. Box 78.1 lists the most common causes of valvular AS, as illustrated in Fig. 78.1. The majority of cases of AS are acquired and result from degenerative (calcific) changes in an anatomically normal trileaflet aortic valve that becomes gradually dysfunctional over time. Congenitally abnormal valves may be stenotic at birth but usually become dysfunctional during early adolescence or early adulthood. A congenitally BAV is now the most common course of valvular AS in patients younger than the age of 65 years. Rheumatic AS is now much less common than in prior decades and is virtually always accompanied by mitral valve disease. Other forms of nonvalvular left ventricular (LV) outflow obstruction (e.g., discrete subvalve AS, hypertrophic cardiomyopathy, and supravalve AS) are discussed in other chapters.

The most reliable estimate of BAV prevalence is often considered to be the 1.37% reported by Larson and Edwards.[4] These authors have a special expertise in aortic valve disease and amassed 21,417 consecutive autopsies with 293 BAVs. An echocardiographic survey of primary school children demonstrated a BAV in 0.5% of males and 0.2% of females.[8] A more recent study detected 0.8% BAVs in nearly 21,000 men in Italy who underwent echocardiographic screening for the military.[9] Table 78.1 summarizes data on the prevalence of bicuspid valves. BAV is seen predominantly in males, with a 2 to 1 male-to-female ratio.[10–12] Although BAV may occur in isolation, it may also be associated with other congenital cardiovascular malformations, including coarctation, patent ductus arteriosus, supravalvular AS, atrial septal defect, ventricular septal defect, sinus of Valsalva aneurysm, and coronary artery anomalies.[1,13–16] There are also several syndromes in which BAV is a part of left-sided obstructive lesions of LV inflow and outflow obstruction, including Shone syndrome (multiple left-sided lesions of inflow and outflow obstruction), Williams syndrome (supravalvular stenosis), and Turner syndrome (coarctation).

Natural History of Bicuspid Aortic Valves

Although a few patients with BAV may go undetected or without clinical consequences for a lifetime, most develop complications. The most important clinical consequences of BAV are valve stenosis, valve regurgitation, infective endocarditis, and aortic complications such as dilatation, dissection, and rupture (Box 78.2). Estimates of the prevalence of these complications and outcomes have varied depending on the era of the study, the cohort selected, and the method used to diagnose BAV (clinical examination, cardiac catheterization, or echocardiography). Several large recent studies have helped better define the unoperated clinical course in the modern era.[17–19]

Isolated AS is the most frequent complication of BAV, occurring in approximately 85% of all BAV cases.[10,18–20] BAV accounts for the majority of patients aged 15 to 65 years with significant AS. The progression of the congenitally deformed valve to AS presumably reflects its propensity for premature fibrosis, stiffening, and calcium deposition in these structurally abnormal valves.

Aortic regurgitation (AR), present in approximately 15% of patients with BAV,[10] is usually caused by dilatation of the sinotubular junction of the aortic root, preventing cusp coaptation. It may also be caused by cusp prolapse, fibrotic retraction of the leaflet(s), or damage to the valve from infective endocarditis. Compared with AS, AR tends to occur in younger patients.

Why some patients with a BAV develop stenosis and others regurgitation is unclear. As mentioned, rarely, patients may not develop hemodynamics consequences. Roberts and colleagues reported three congenital BAVs in nonagenarians who underwent surgery for AS.[21] Why some patients with a congenital BAV do not become symptomatic until they are in their 90s and why others become symptomatic early in life is also unclear.

Echocardiographic Features of Bicuspid Aortic Valves

The roles of echocardiography in the detection and evaluation are listed in Box 78.3. The diagnosis of a BAV can usually be made by transthoracic echocardiography (TTE). When adequate images are obtained, sensitivities and specificities of up to 92% and 96%, respectively, have been reported for detecting BAV.[22–24] The most reliable and useful views are the parasternal short-axis (PSAX) and long-axis (PLAX) views. The echocardiographic features and their respective views are summarized in Table 78.2. The PAX view extremely useful to examine the number and position of the commissures, the opening pattern, the presence of a raphe, and the leaflet mobility. In contrast to the normal tricuspid aortic valve (TAV), which opens in a triangular fashion with straightening of the leaflets (Figs. 78.1 and 78.2A), the BAV opens in an elliptical ("fishmouth" or "football") shape with curvilinear leaflets (Figs. 78.1, 78.3, and 78.4). There is typically a raphe, a fibrous ridge that represents the region where the cusps failed to separate.[10,25] The raphe is usually distinct and generally extends from the free margins to the base of the leaflet. Calcification commonly occurs first along this raphe, ultimately hindering the motion of the conjoined cusp.[26] Rarely, the leaflets are symmetric, and there is no raphe—a "pure" or "true" bicuspid valve. Note that a false-negative diagnosis may occur when the raphe gives the appearance of a third coaptation line. In diastole, the normal trileaflet aortic valve appears like a Y (inverted "Mercedes-Benz" sign), with the commissures at 10, 2, and 6 o'clock positions (see Figs. 78.1 and 78.2B). When the commissures are deviated from those clock-face position, one should suspect a BAV and evaluate carefully. An additional short-axis (SAX) feature is a variable degree of leaflet redundancy. In patients with very little redundancy of the leaflet margins, the development of stenosis is likely, whereas a significantly redundant leaflet with associated prolapse is more likely to lead to regurgitation.

The morphologic patterns of BAV vary according to which commissures have fused, and a number of classifications have been devised that pertain to the orientation of the leaflets[1,10,27,28] (Fig. 78.5 and Table 78.2). Fusion of the right and left cusps is the most common morphologic type.[28,29] In an echocardiographic study by Brandenburg and colleagues,[23] the posterior commissure was located at the 4 or 5 o'clock position, and the anterior commissure was located at the 9 or 10 o'clock position when the valve is viewed in a PSAX view. The second most frequent type, fusion of the right and noncoronary cusps, has been linked to aortic arch involvement[30–33] and may also be related to an increased risk of AS and regurgitation compared with the other anatomic types.[29] The least common type is fusion of the left and noncoronary cusps.[28] Michelena and colleagues similarly classified BAVs as *typical* (right–left coronary cusp fusion) if the commissures were at the 4 and 10 o'clock, 5 and 11 o'clock, or 3 to 9 o'clock (anterior–posterior cusps) positions and *atypical* (right-noncoronary cusp fusion) if the commissures were at the 1 and 7 o'clock or 12 and 6 o'clock positions.[19]

The PLAX view typically shows systolic doming (Figs. 78.4B; and 78.6) caused by the limited valve opening. In a normal TAV, the leaflets open parallel to the aortic walls. In diastole, one of the leaflets (the larger, conjoined cusp) may prolapse. The PLAX view

---

BOX 78.1 Causes of Aortic Stenosis

1. Congenital (unicuspid, bicuspid, quadricuspid)
2. Degenerative (sclerosis of previously normal valve)
3. Rheumatic

---

with color Doppler is also useful to evaluate for AR (the diastolic aortic regurgitant jet is usually eccentric) and AS (turbulence in the aortic root and ascending aorta in systole). Last, the PLAX view is also important for sizing the sinus of Valsalva, sinotubular junction, and ascending aorta. With increasing age, as the leaflets become thickened, fibrotic, and calcified, systolic doming may no longer be evident, and the typical SAX appearance of the BAV may be difficult to distinguish from calcific AS of a TAV. In fact, there is an inverse association between the degree of valve stenosis and accuracy of echocardiographically determined valve structure and cause.[34] The elliptical systolic opening in the SAX view is not easily appreciated in a severely stenotic valve. M-mode echocardiography of a BAV may demonstrate an eccentric closure line (Fig. 78.7), but this sign is not reliable, and approximately 25% of patients with a BAV have a relatively central closure line. Moreover, occasionally TAVs can also appear to have an eccentric closure line depending on image quality and orientation of the echocardiography beam.

Common reasons that lead to misclassification or misdiagnosis of BAV include shadowing due to calcium, oblique axis imaging, and poor or suboptimal image quality.[35] The diagnosis of BAV becomes more difficult in older individuals (older than 65 years) because of fibrosis or sclerosis. In such instances, transesophageal echocardiography (TEE) may improve visualization of the leaflets and may be helpful for accurate evaluation of the aortic valve anatomy and confirmation of a BAV.[35,36] However, studies have noted that even with TEE sensitivity and specificity for detecting BAV are reduced in the presence of more than moderate aortic valve calcification.[37] In some instances, alternative cardiac imaging, such as computed tomography (CT) or magnetic resonance imaging (MRI), may help confirm BAV anatomy. More commonly, these imaging modalities are used to visualize the thoracic aorta.

The mechanism(s) of ascending aortic dilatation in BAV has long been debated, and this controversy remains. Two hypotheses include (1) abnormal hemodynamics causing increases wall stress related to eccentric turbulent blood flow and (2) genetic pathological (cellular) structural deficits in the aortic wall. In fact, evidence for each aspect of this "flow versus fate" controversy is not overwhelming.

The advent of time-resolved phase contrast four-dimensional magnetic resonance imaging (4D flow MRI) has shed some light on this controversy. 4D flow MRI has demonstrated abnormal three-dimensional flow patterns and hemodynamic forces that act on the aortic wall that may be implicated in aortic dilatation.[32,38–41] Flow through the aortic valve is normally laminar with little force

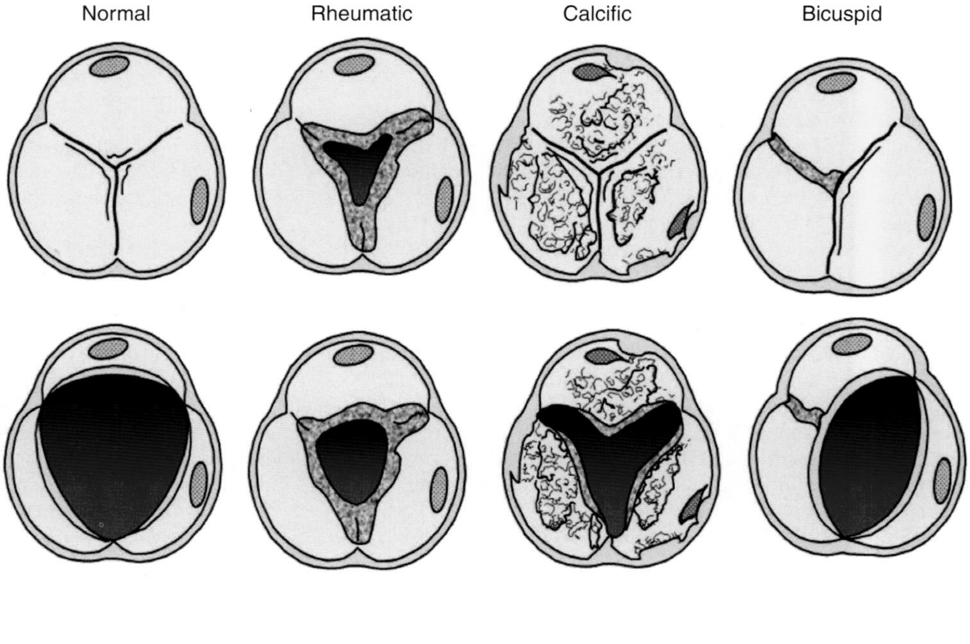

Normal Rheumatic Calcific Bicuspid

Figure 78.1. Diagram illustrating the diastolic *(top row)* and systolic *(bottom row)* appearances of a normal aortic valve and the three common causes of valvular aortic stenosis. (Modified from Baumgartner H, et al: Echocardiographic assessment of valve stenosis: EAE/ASE recommendations for clinical practice, *Eur J Echocardiogr* 10:1–25, 2009.)

TABLE 78.1 Prevalence of Bicuspid Aortic Valves

Author	Year	Patients (n)	Bicuspid Aortic Valve Prevalence	Method
Wauchope.[2]	1928	9996	0.5	Autopsy
Gross.[3]	1937	5000	0.56	Autopsy
Larson and Edwards.[4]	1984	21,417	1.37	Autopsy
Datta et al.[5]	1988	8800	0.59	Autopsy
Pauperio et al.[6]	1999	2000	0.65	Autopsy
Basso et al.[8]	2004	817	0.5	2D echo
Nistri et al.[9]	2005	20,946	0.8	2D echo

2D, Two-dimensional.

BOX 78.2 Complications of Bicuspid Aortic Valves

Valve complications
- Stenosis
- Regurgitation
- Infection (endocarditis)

Aortic complications
- Dilatation
- Aneurysm
- Dissection
- Rupture

BOX 78.3 The Role of Echocardiography in Bicuspid Aortic Valve

- Detection of bicuspid aortic valve
- Evaluation for aortic stenosis or regurgitation
- Careful measurements of the aortic root and ascending aorta
- Search for coarctation
- Screening first-degree family members
- Surveillance: following valve dysfunction and aortopathy

TABLE 78.2 Distinctive Echocardiographic Features of Bicuspid Aortic Valves

	View
Systolic doming	PLAX
Eccentric valve closure	PLAX
Single commissural line in diastole	SAX
Two cusps, two commissures	SAX
Raphe	SAX
Oval opening (football-shaped; fish-mouth, elliptical; "CBS eye")	SAX
Unequal cusp size	PLAX, SAX

PLAX, Parasternal long-axis; *SAX,* parasternal short-axis.

---

directed toward the aortic wall. However, in the presence of a BAV (even with normal function), blood flow is abnormal with spiral or helical flow patterns impinging the outer curvature of the proximal aorta resulting in increased shear stress as shown in Fig. 78.8.[32,39,42,43] Furthermore, several groups using a similar imaging approach have demonstrated that the BAV cusp fusion pattern (i.e., right-left cusp fusion vs right noncusp fusion) impacts the type of flow eccentricity and helicity and the type and degree of wall shear stress.[32,44] If validated, the determination of the various transvalvular blood flow patterns by MRI may identify patients at risk for aortography progression and may enable the development of individualized approach to the management of BAV-related aortic disease beyond the traditional diameter-based guidelines.

Coarctation

BAV may occur in isolation or in association with other forms of congenital heart disease. There is a well-documented association of BAV with coarctation.[7,20,24,45–50] An autopsy study found coexisting coarctation of the aorta in 6% of cases of BAV,[1] and an echocardiographic study found coarctation in 10% of patients with BAV.[48] On the other hand, as many as 30% to 70% of patients with coarctation have a BAV.[7,20,29,47,50] Therefore, when a BAV is detected on an echocardiogram, coarctation of the aorta should always be sought.

Infective Endocarditis

Patients with BAVs are particularly susceptible to infective endocarditis. Although the exact incidence of endocarditis remains controversial, the population risk, even in the presence of a functionally normal valve, may be as high as 3% over time.[1] The estimated incidence is 0.16% per year in unoperated children and adolescents.[51] In adults, the two large case series by Tzemos and Michelena and their colleagues[18,19] suggest that the incidence is 0.3% and 2% per year, respectively. In a series of 128 microbiologically proven episodes of endocarditis, the commonest predisposing risk factor was BAV (16.7%).[52] In another series of 50 patients with native valve endocarditis, 12% had BAV.[53]

In many cases of BAV, endocarditis is the first indication of structural heart disease. This fact emphasizes the importance of either clinical or echocardiographic screening for the diagnosis of BAV. Unexplained systolic ejection sounds (clicks) should prompt echocardiographic evaluation. Surprisingly, bacterial endocarditis prevention is no longer recommended by the most recent American College of Cardiology/American Heart Association (ACC/AHA) Guideline for BAV.[54]

Aortic Complications

BAV is associated with several additional abnormalities, including displaced coronary ostia, left coronary artery dominance, and a shortened left main coronary artery; coarctation of the aorta; aortic interruption; Williams syndrome; and, most important, aortic dilatation, aneurysm, and dissection. Given these collective findings, it can be suggested that BAV is the result of a developmental disorder involving the entire aortic root and arch. Although the pathogenesis is not well understood, these associated aortic malformations suggest a genetic defect.[14]

Although less well understood, these aortic complications of BAV disease can cause significant morbidity and mortality. As listed in Box 78.2, BAV may be associated with progressive dilatation, aneurysmal formation, and dissection (Tables 78.3 and 78.4). These vascular complications may occur independent of valvular dysfunction[9,11,15,55–57] and can manifest in patients without significant stenosis or regurgitation. According to Nistri and colleagues, 50% or more of young patients with normally functioning BAVs have echocardiographic evidence of aortic dilatation.[9] Therefore, the size and shape of the aortic root and dimensions should be carefully evaluated and followed serially. Aortic root dimensions should be performed at the level of the annulus, sinuses of Valsalva, sinotubular junction (STJ), and proximal ascending aorta (Fig. 78.9). In BAV (unlike Marfan syndrome, in which the dilatation is usually more pronounced at the sinus level), the sinuses are usually normal or mildly dilated, and the aortic dilatation is often most pronounced in the ascending aorta distal to the STJ[58,59] (Figs. 78.10 and 78.11). Therefore, effort should be made to image this portion of the aorta. The midportion of the ascending aorta may not be easily imaged

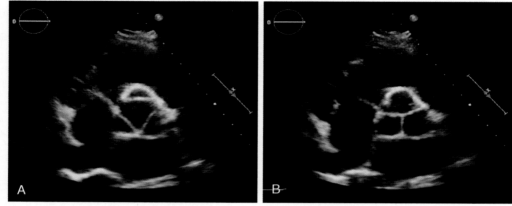

Figure 78.2. Transthoracic echocardiogram (short-axis view) of a normal tricuspid aortic valve. **A,** In diastole, the normal trileaflet valve appears like a Y with the commissures at the 10, 2, and 6 o'clock positions. **B,** In systole, the valve opens in a triangular fashion with straightening of the leaflets.

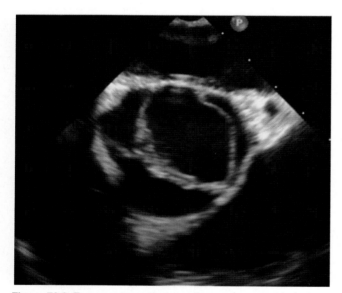

Figure 78.3. Transesophageal echocardiogram (cross section) of a bicuspid aortic valve illustrating the elliptical ("fish-mouth" or "football") shape with curvilinear leaflets in systole.

with echocardiography, and evaluation with CT or MRI may be required.[60] The aortic arch and descending thoracic aorta may also become dilated. Recently, it has been reported that patients with BAV are also at increased risk for intracranial aneurysms compared with the general population.[61]

Although BAV aortopathy may share similarities with the Marfan syndrome, and aortic aneurysms are common in both conditions, a recent retrospective cohort study of 416 consecutive patients with definite BAV provides evidence that their clinical outcomes are different and that aortic dissection is more common in Marfan syndrome.[18] The risk of aortic dissection in this BAV cohort was approximately eight times higher than in the general population, but despite the high relative risk, the absolute incidence of aortic dissection was very low (given the BAV prevalence of 1.3% of the general population).[17]

Transcatheter Aortic Valve Implantation in Bicuspid Aortic Valves

Transcatheter aortic valve implantation (TAVR) has been demonstrated to be a viable treatment for inoperable, high-risk,

intermediate-risk,[62–64] and even low-risk[65–67] older adult patients with severe AS. The treatment of younger AS populations is already in the pipeline.[68] Although TAVR has now become a standard procedure, there remain a few areas of controversy, one of which is the role of TAVR in patients with BAVs. The landmark randomized trials of TAVR versus surgical aortic valve replacement that established TAVR as the preferred treatment for patients with severe AS who are at high, intermediate, or low surgical risk systematically excluded patients with BAVs. However, despite the absence of supportive randomized trial data, TAVR is being done off label for patients with BAV. BAVs have a high prevalence in younger patients, but even in older adults (i.e., older than 80 years of age), bicuspid valves comprise approximately 20% of the surgical cases.[69] Early experience with TAVR in BAVs demonstrated that this anatomic variant has several adverse features that make the outcomes of TAVR less predictable and often suboptimal, including a more elliptical annulus shape, unequal leaflet size, heavy and uneven calcification of the leaflets, and the presence of calcified raphes[70] (Box 78.4).

From a technical standpoint, selection of an appropriately sized TAVR device in bicuspid AS is similar to tricuspid AS because both are based on annular properties. However, cusp morphology and calcium pattern are more complex in BAVs, which might interfere with optimal transcatheter heart valve (THV) deployment or lead to malpositioning, aortic injuries, and suboptimal hemodynamics with increased paravalvular leak (PVL). Bicuspid valve anatomy may also have effects on TAVR expansion. Two recent studies on early generation TAVR devices showed a higher incidence of THV malposition requiring multiple THVs implantation (7.2%) and moderate or severe PVL that was found in 28.4%.[71] In a large multicenter propensity-based analysis comparing TAVR outcomes in BAVs versus TAVs, Yoon and colleagues[72] showed that among the early generation THV group, TAVR in patients with bicuspid AS was complicated more frequently with aortic root injury and moderate or severe paravalvular regurgitation. Among the group treated with new-generation devices, however, there were no significant differences in procedural outcomes between BAVs and TAVs. This study suggests that advancements incorporated by the new-generation TAVR devices may partially overcome some of the limitations encountered in treating patients with bicuspid valve,[72,73] in which operators and researches still need to reach definitive conclusions.

Surveillance (Serial Assessment of Patients With Bicuspid Aortic Valve)

Because of the risk of progressive aortic valve disease (stenosis, regurgitation, or both) and aortopathy, all patients with BAV should undergo annual imaging, even when asymptomatic. The 2008 focused

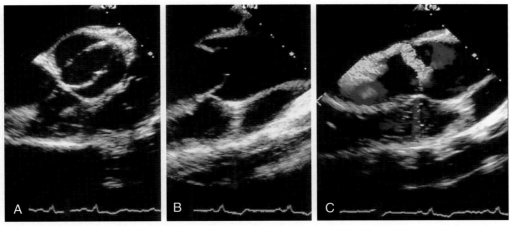

Figure 78.4. Bicuspid aortic valve. **A,** Short-axis view shows "fish-mouth" or football-shaped opening. **B,** Long-axis view shows systolic doming. **C,** Color Doppler shows eccentric aortic regurgitant jet (typical of bicuspid aortic valve).

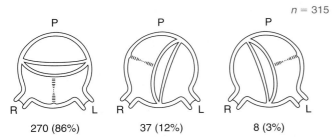

$n = 315$

270 (86%)   37 (12%)   8 (3%)

Figure 78.5. Variations in bicuspid valves. Relative positions of raphe and conjoined cusp. *L,* Left; *P,* Posterior; *R,* right. (Adapted from Sabet HY, et al: Congenital bicuspid aortic valves: a surgical pathology study of 542 cases and a literature review of 2,715 additional cases, *Mayo Clin Proc* 74:14–26, 1999.)

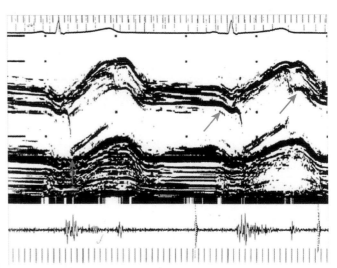

Figure 78.7. M-mode echocardiogram (echo) and phonocardiogram (phono) from a patient with a bicuspid aortic valve. The echo illustrates an eccentric closure line *(green arrows)* in both late and early diastolic; the phono illustrates an aortic ejection sound (indicated by the bottom of the *red arrow*) that occurs at the maximal abrupt opening of the aortic valve (indicated by the *red arrowhead*).

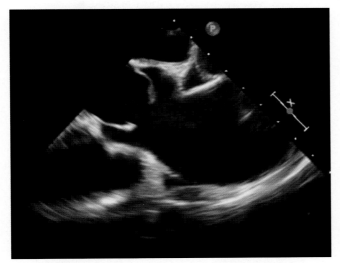

Figure 78.6. Transesophageal echocardiographic longitudinal view of the aortic root and ascending aorta illustrating the systolic doming of a bicuspid aortic valve.

update of the 2006 ACC/AHA guidelines recommended monitoring adolescents and young adults, older patients with AS, and patients with a BAV and dilatation of the aortic root or ascending aorta.[74] TTE can be used for serial imaging follow-up of the ascending aorta when the dimensions measured by TTE and CT or MRI have been confirmed. After identification of ascending aortic enlargement in a patient with BAV, repeat imaging at 6 months is recommended. If the aorta remains stable at 6 months and is less than 45 mm in size and if there is no family history of aortic dissection, annual imaging is recommended. Patients who do not meet these criteria should have repeat aortic imaging with TTE every 6 months. If the aortic root is poorly visualized on echocardiography, cardiac CT and MRI are excellent substitutes. TEE is generally not used for serial follow-up of BAV-related aortopathy because of its semi-invasive nature and the difficulty of comparing dimensions over time.

Family Screening of Patients With Bicuspid Aortic Valve

BAV appears inheritable and was present in 9.1% of first-degree relatives in one study.[48] Although the current ACC/AHA guidelines on valve disease[74] do not recommend screening for relatives of individuals with BAV, the ACC/AHA guidelines on congenital heart disease[75] and thoracic aortic disease[76] do recommended echocardiographic screening of first-degree relatives (class I; level of evidence: C).

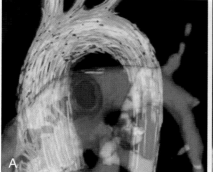 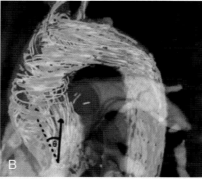 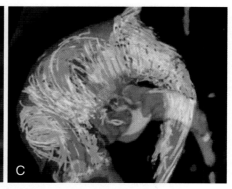

Figure 78.8. Flow patterns in bicuspid aortic valve disease. **A,** Normal flow pattern. **B,** Right-handed helical flow. **C,** Left-handed helical flow. The systolic flow angle (θ) is demonstrated in *B*: the angle between the aortic midline *(dashed)* and the instantaneous mean flow vector at peak systole *(arrow)*. (From Bissell MM, et al: Aortic dilatation in bicuspid aortic valve disease: flow pattern is a major contributor and differs with valve fusion type, *Circ Cardiovasc Imag* 6(4):499–507, 2013; with permission from Elsevier.)

TABLE 78.3 Frequency of Aortic Dissection in Persons With a Bicuspid Aortic Valve

Author(s)	Year	Frequency of Aortic Dissection in Bicuspid Aortic Valves	Population
Fenoglio et al.[121]	1977	8 of 152 (5%)	Autopsy, older than 20 years old
Larsen and Edwards.[4]	1984	18 of 293 (6%)	Autopsy, all ages
Roberts and Roberts.[122]	1991	14 of 328 (4%)	Autopsy, older than 15 years old
Michelena et al.[19]	2011	2 of 416 (0.4%)	Echocardiography by population-based community cohort

TABLE 78.4 Frequency of Bicuspid Aortic Valve in Aortic Dissection (Spontaneous, Noniatrogenic Dissection at Autopsy).

Author(s)	Year	Number of Bicuspid Aortic Valves per Dissection
Gore and Seiwert[123]	1952	11 of 85 13%
Edwards et al.[124]	1978	11 of 119 9%
Larson and Edwards[4]	1984	18 of 161 11%
Roberts and Roberts[122]	1991	14 of 186 7.5%
Totals	—	54 of 551 = 10%

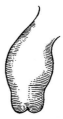

Figure 78.10. Diagram of a thoracic aorta illustrating the most common type of aortopathy associated with bicuspid aortic valves—normal aortic root with dilatation beginning at and above the sinotubular junction.

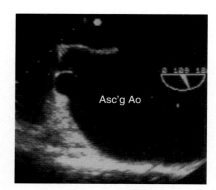

Figure 78.11. Transesophageal echocardiographic longitudinal view that shows a markedly dilated ascending aorta (Asc'g Ao) that spares the aortic root, the typical type of aortopathy associated with bicuspid aortic valve.

Unicuspid Aortic Valve

Other, less common congenital abnormalities of the aortic valve include the unicuspid valve and quadricuspid valve. The unicuspid aortic valve (UAV) is a rare congenital malformation seen in approximately 0.002% of patients referred for echocardiography but in as many as 4% to 6% of patients undergoing surgery for "pure" (isolated) AS.[77] Two forms of UAV are recognized: One has no commissures or lateral attachments to the aorta at the level of the orifice (acommissural), and the second has one lateral attachment to the aorta at the level of the orifice (unicommissural).[78] Both of these types, like the BAV, produce a dome-shaped opening in systole[79] (Fig. 78.12). The latter is the more common of the two. AS of an acommissural UAV is quite severe, presents in infancy, and is seldom, if ever, seen in adults.[80] An acommissural type of

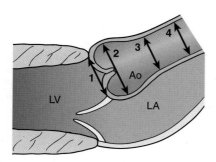

Figure 78.9. Diagram of a parasternal long-axis view illustrating where aortic dimension measurements should be made: *1,* aortic annulus; *2,* midpoint of the sinuses of Valsalva level; *3,* sinotubular junction level; *4,* mid ascending aorta. Measurements should be made perpendicular to the long axis of the aorta. *Ao,* Aortic root; *LA,* left atrium; *LV,* left ventricle.

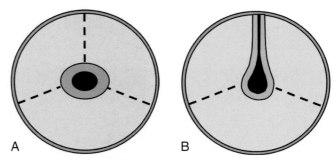

Figure 78.13. Diagram illustrating the two types of unicuspid aortic valves. **A,** Unicommissural valve has a teardrop opening and a lateral attachment. **B,** Acommissural valve illustrating a central round or oval opening at the top of a conical or dome-shaped valve.

BOX 78.4 Bicuspid Aortic Valves: Adverse Anatomic Features for Transcatheter Aortic Valve Replacement

Left ventricular outflow tract size (larger than tricuspid valve)
Annular eccentricity
Asymmetrical calcification
Calcified raphe
Unequally sized leaflets
Commissural fusion
Concomitant aortopathy

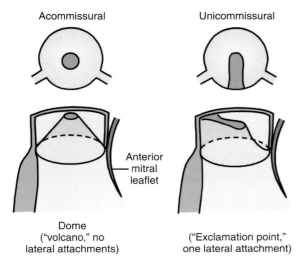

Figure 78.12. Diagram of the two types of unicuspid aortic valves (see text).

UAV has a central round, oval, or triangular opening caused by underdevelopment of all three cusps, resulting in a "volcano-like" structure with a small, central orifice (see Fig. 78.12A). Stenosis of an acommissural valve is typically very severe and occurs during infancy. In a unicommissural type of UAV, there is usually an eccentric "teardrop"-shaped opening (Figs. 78.13B and 78.14; Box 78.5). The most common position of the single commissural attachment zone in this type is posterior[81] (Video 78.1). This configuration results in a relatively larger orifice than the acommissural type. As a result, some patients with a unicommissural UAV live into adulthood before manifesting valvular obstruction. Similar to the case with BAV patients with UAV are more often male.[81] Compared with patients undergoing surgery for BAV and TAV disease, unicommissural UAV patients present about two decades earlier than patients with BAV[82] and three decades earlier than patients with TAV.[83] Unicommissural UAV patients usually require surgery in the third decade of life.

In a UAV, the coronary arteries are generally in the normal position.[80] As is the case for the more prevalent BAV, the unicuspid valve is also associated with aortopathy. This aortopathy not only involves the aortic root and ascending aorta but may also involve the aortic arch and descending thoracic aorta.[84] Therefore, all segments of the aorta should be assessed in patients with unicuspid valves. Unicuspid aortic valves usually have severe, diffuse calcification, and distinguishing a UAV from a BAV can be challenging (see Fig. 78.12). TEE is more accurate for making this distinction.[79,85,86]

Quadricuspid Aortic Valve

Quadricuspid aortic valve (QAV) is a rare congenital cardiac abnormality with a prevalence that ranges from 0.008% to 0.043%, according to autopsy and echocardiography series (Table 78.5).[87,88]

A much higher incidence was reported by Olson and colleagues in a review of 225 patients undergoing surgery for pure AR.[89] Most cases historically were discovered incidentally at surgery or postmortem examination. However, the majority of cases are now diagnosed antemortem by echocardiography.[90,91] Because of further advances in imaging, including TEE, CT, and MRI, more cases are being detected, which is likely to alter the incidence of QAV.[92,93]

Based on the relative size of the cusps and their equality, Hurwitz and Roberts delineated seven morphologic subtypes of QAV (types A–G), ranging from four cusps of equal size to four unequal cusps.[94] The most common configuration appears to be that of four equal or nearly equal cusps (Table 78.6).[95,96]

The QAV may function normally, most commonly when the cusps are relatively equal in size.[85,94] In general, valve dysfunction is seldom present or minimal during childhood or adolescence.[85,85,95,97] Aortic valve dysfunction is usually caused by AR (Table 78.7) and tends to occur later in life, a consequence of progressive leaflet thickening with resultant incomplete coaptation (Video 78.2). Unlike BAV, the association of ascending aortic aneurysm is extremely rare.

The characteristic echocardiographic finding is an X-shaped pattern in diastole in SAX views (formed by the commissural lines of the closed QAV), compared with the Y in normal trileaflet valves (Fig. 78.15). Because valve dysfunction may occur with advancing age, clinical and echocardiographic follow-up is recommended.

Although QAV is usually an isolated anomaly,[85,94,95] various cardiac and noncardiac anomalies have been reported in association with it (Box 78.6).[98–100] The most prevalent cardiac malformations associated with QAV are coronary artery anomalies, which have been reported in 10% of cases.[90,101–105]

In summary, QAV is a rare congenital disorder, usually diagnosed in adulthood, with a potential for complications, mainly AR. QAVs often require surgery, usually in the fifth and sixth decades of life, and therefore need close follow-up.

CALCIFIC (DEGENERATIVE) AORTIC STENOSIS

Calcific AS is the most common cause of valvular AS in older adult patients. The prevalence of calcific AS increases with age.[106] AS has a prevalence of about 5% in individuals age 65 years or older and about 10% in individuals age 80 years or older. AS is the most common indication for valve replacement surgery and the second most common indication for surgery in older adults, surpassed only by coronary artery bypass grafting.[107] Calcific AS affects men and women equally.

Because the prevalence of AS increases with age and because calcification occurs in regions of mechanical stress, AS was previously thought to be a degenerative disorder caused by passive "wear and tear." However, the view that aortic valve calcification is a passive consequence of cellular aging has been challenged. AS

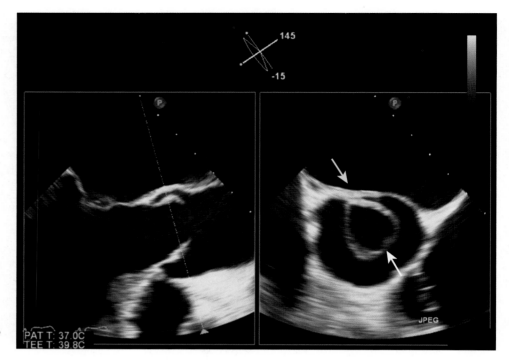

Figure 78.14. Biplane transesophageal echocardiographic images of a unicuspid, unicommissural aortic valve in a 36-year old woman. *Left panel* illustrates systolic doming. *Right panel* illustrates a teardrop opening in systole, a single commissural zone of attachment *(yellow arrow)*, and a rounded free-edge of the leaflet on the opposite side of the commissural attachment zone *(white arrow)*.

BOX 78.5 Echocardiographic Features of Unicuspid Unicommissural Aortic Valve

- Single commissural zone of attachment (usually posterior)
- Eccentric circular or teardrop-shaped orifice during systole
- Rounded free edge of leaflet on the opposite side of the commissural attachment zone

TABLE 78.5 Quadricuspid Aortic Valve Prevalence

Author	Year	Method	Patients (n)	Patients (%)
Simonds[87]	1923	Autopsy	0 of 2000	0.000%
Simonds[87]	1923	Autopsy	2 of 25,666	0.008%
Feldman et al.[88]	1990[a]	(literature review)	8 of 60,446	0.013%
	1990[b†]		6 of 13,805	0.043%
Feldman et al.[88]	1984	2D echo	2 of 225	1%
Olson et al.[89]		2D echo Surgery for pure AR		

[a]1982–1988.
[b]1987–1988.
2D, Two-dimensional; *AR,* aortic regurgitation.

TABLE 78.6 Quadricuspid Aortic Valves: Morphologic Types.

Anatomic Variation—Cusps	Patients (n)
4 equal	51
3 equal, 1 smaller	43
2 equal larger and 2 equal smaller	10
1 large, 2 intermediate, 1 small	7
3 equal and 1 larger	4
2 equal, 2 unequal smaller	4
4 unequal	5

From Hurwitz LE, Roberts WC: Quadricuspid semilunar valve, *Am J Cardiol* 31:623–626, 1973 and Davia JE, et al: Quadricuspid semilunar valves, *Chest* 72:186–189, 1977.

TABLE 78.7 Function of Quadricuspid Aortic Valves

Valve Function	Patients (n)	Patients (%)
AR	115	75%
AS + AR	13	8%
AS	1	1%
Normal	25	16%

AR, Aortic regurgitation; *AS,* aortic stenosis.
From Tutarel: The quadricuspid aortic valve: a comprehensive review, *J Heart Valve Dis* 13:534–537, 2004; Olson LJ, et al: Surgical pathology of pure aortic insufficiency: a study of 725 cases, *Mayo Clin Proc* 59:835–841, 1984.

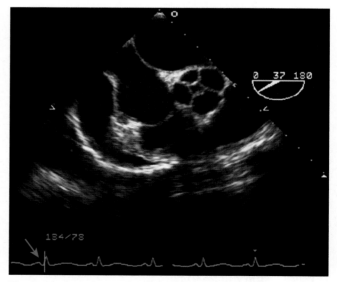

Figure 78.15. Quadricuspid aortic valve. Transesophageal echocardiographic short-axis view (37 degrees) illustrates failure of leaflet coaptation in diastole *(arrow)* with a square central opening and typical X-shaped configuration of the four commissures.

is now considered to be an active process with some similarities to atherosclerosis, including inflammation, lipid infiltration, and dystrophic calcification.[108–113] Therefore, the term *calcific* AS seems more appropriate than degenerative AS. Currently, the pathology of calcific aortic valve disease is an area of active research.[114,115]

BOX 78.6 Cardiac and Noncardiac Abnormalities Associated With Quadricuspid Valve

1. Patent ductus arteriosus
2. Hypertrophic cardiomyopathy
3. Subaortic stenosis
4. Ehlers-Danlos syndrome
5. Coronary ostium displacement
6. Ventricular septal defect

TABLE 78.8 Grading the Severity of Aortic Stenosis

Characteristic	Mild	Moderate	Severe
Aortic jet velocity (m/s)	2.6–2.9	3.0–4.0	>4.0
Mean gradient[a] (mm Hg)	<20	20–40	>40
Mean gradient[b] (mm Hg)	<30	30–50	>50
Aortic valve area (cm²)	>1.5	1.0–1.5	<1.0
Dimensionless index	—	—	<0.25

[a]According to American Heart Association/American College of Cardiology guidelines.[7]
[b]According to European Society of Cardiology guidelines.[6]

Calcific AS results from slowly progressing fibrosis and calcification, which occurs over several decades, leading to variable degrees of thickening and rigidity of the aortic valve cusps. This process begins with aortic valve sclerosis that does not limit flow through the aortic orifice. The morphologic hallmark is the formation of calcified masses along the aortic side of the cups. The earliest deposits occur at the cusp attachments and along the line of cusp coaptation—the sites of greatest bending and unbending during valve opening and closing.[116] Irregular leaflet thickening and focal increased echogenicity (calcifications) are the echocardiographic hallmarks of calcific AS. These focal areas of thickening are typically seen in the center of the valve cusps. The degree of calcification is best assessed in the PSAX view. The degree of calcification can be qualitatively classified as mild (small isolated spots or nodules), moderate (multiple larger nodules), and severe (extensive thickening and calcification of all of the cusps).[112,116]

The degree of leaflet calcification is a marker of disease progression and should be reported.[117,118] As the leaflets become more sclerotic, they become progressively more rigid and less mobile and begin to obstruct flow. Increases in aortic transvalvular flow velocity mark the progression from aortic sclerosis to AS (Table 78.8). In the most severe cases, the aortic root appears to be filled with dense, amorphous echoes that have little or no motion. In some patients, one of the leaflets may become immobile while the others move freely. When only one leaflet is immobile, there is usually only a mild increase in transaortic velocity (mild AS). Unlike rheumatic AS, commissural fusion is usually absent or only minimal in calcific AS. The valve orifice tends to be triradiate—three slitlike openings in systole (Figs. 78.16E and 78.17).[119] Calcification often extends onto the base of the anterior mitral leaflet. Calcification may also extend from the valve cusps into the ventricular septum and may induce conduction abnormalities.

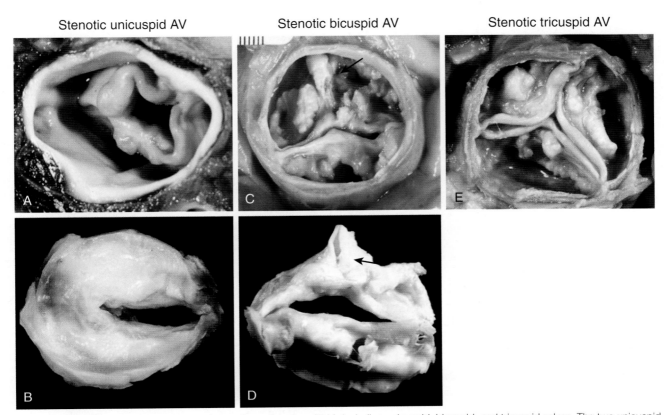

Stenotic unicuspid AV   Stenotic bicuspid AV   Stenotic tricuspid AV

Figure 78.16. Gross pathology specimens of stenotic aortic valves (AVs), including unicuspid, bicuspid, and tricuspid valves. The two unicuspid AVs (**A** and **B**) are unicommissural with lateral attachments; the two bicuspid valves (**C** and **D**) have raphes *(arrows)*. The tricuspid valve (**E**) does not have fused commissures and shows the slitlike orifices resulting from bulky calcific deposits that restrict leaflet motion. (Courtesy of Dr. Renu Virmani, CVPath Institute, Gaithersburg, MD.)

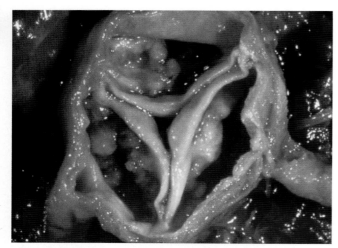

Figure 78.17. Gross pathology specimen of a calcific (degenerative) trileaflet aortic valve illustrating the absence of commissural fusion and a triradiate orifice, each of which is slitlike. (Courtesy of Dr. Renu Virmani, CVPath Institute, Gaithersburg, MD.)

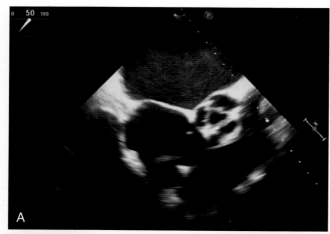

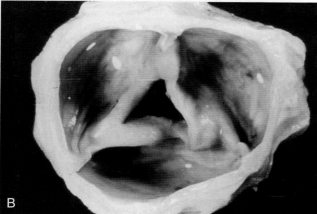

Figure 78.18. A, Typical rheumatic aortic stenosis with commissural fusion resulting in a central triangular (as shown here) or oval or circular (not shown) orifice as shown in the transesophageal echocardiogram. **B,** A pathologic specimen from a different patient.

RHEUMATIC AORTIC STENOSIS

Rheumatic AS has become uncommon in the developed world, although it remains a significant cause of AS worldwide. In adults undergoing aortic valve replacement for symptomatic AS in the United States, calcific tricuspid AS accounts for 51% of cases, bicuspid AS for 36%, and rheumatic AS for 9%.[119] Aortic rheumatic valve disease is never isolated but is virtually always associated with rheumatic mitral valve disease. Rheumatic valvular dysfunction may affect not only an anatomically normal TAV but also a congenital BAV.

Similar to rheumatic mitral valve disease, rheumatic aortic valve deformities are characterized by diffuse cuspal thickening that extends to their free edges and by commissural fusion. These features contrast with the morphologic features of degenerative (calcific) AS, which depicts basal calcific nodules, minimal or no involvement of the free edges, and no commissural fusion. The acquired commissural fusion in rheumatic AS may affect one, two, or all three commissures and is usually distinguishable from the commissural fusion of congenital valve abnormalities. The commissural fusion, which begins at the annulus and progresses toward the center, often affects each commissure equally, producing a small, central, circular or triangular orifice (Figs. 78.1 and 78.18). Subsequent calcium deposition occurs secondarily. Commissural fusion is the primary lesion of AS, as opposed to fibrosis or sclerosis, shortening, and retraction of the cusps, which produce rheumatic AR. Interestingly, the sole pathognomonic feature of rheumatic valve disease, the Aschoff granuloma, is virtually never found in aortic valve tissue.[120]

Please access ExpertConsult to view the corresponding videos for this chapter.

REFERENCES

1. Roberts WC. The congenitally bicuspid aortic valve. A study of 85 autopsy cases. *Am J Cardiol.* 1970;26:72–83.
2. Wauchope GM. The clinical importance of variations in the number of cusps forming the aortic and pulmonary valves. *Q J Med.* 1928;21:383–399.
3. Gross L. So-called congenital bicuspid aortic valve. *Arch Pathol.* 1937;23:350–362.
4. Larson EW, Edwards WD. Risk factors for aortic dissection: a necropsy study of 161 cases. *Am J Cardiol.* 1984;53:849–855.
5. Datta BN, Bhusnurmah B, Khatri HN, et al. Anatomically isolated aortic valve disease. Morphologic study of 100 cases at autopsy. *Jpn Heart J.* 1988;29:661–670.
6. Pauperio HM, Azevedo AC, Ferreira C. The aortic valve with two leaflets. A study in 2000 autopsies. *Cardiol Young.* 1999;9:488–498.
7. Ward C. Clinical significance of the bicuspid aortic valve. *Heart.* 2000;83:81–85.
8. Basso C, Boschello M, Perrone C, et al. An echocardiographic survey of primary school children for bicuspid aortic valve. *Am J Cardiol.* 2004;93:661–663.
9. Nistri S, Basso C, Marzari C, et al. Frequency of bicuspid aortic valve in young male conscripts by echocardiogram. *Am J Cardiol.* 2005;96:718–721.
10. Sabet HY, Edwards WD, Tazelaar HD, et al. Congenital bicuspid aortic valves: a surgical pathology study of 542 cases and a literature review of 2,715 additional cases. *Mayo Clin Proc.* 1999;74:14–26.
11. Keane MG, Wiegers SE, Plappert T, et al. Bicuspid aortic valves are associated with dilatation out of proportion to coexistent valvular lesions. *Circulation.* 2000;102(Suppl III):III 35–III 39.
12. Chan KL, Ghani M, Woodend K, et al. Case-controlled study to assess risk factors for aortic stenosis in congenitally bicuspid aortic valve. *Am J Cardiol.* 2001;88:690–693.
13. Jureidini SB, Singh GK, Marino CJ, et al. Aberrant origin of the left coronary artery from the right aortic sinus: surgical intervention based on echocardiographic diagnosis. *J Am Soc Echocardiogr.* 2000;13:1117–1120.

14. Fedak PW, Verma S, David TE, et al. Clinical and pathophysiological implications of a bicuspid aortic valve. *Circulation.* 2002;106:900–904.

15. Doty DB. Anomalous origin of the left circumflex coronary artery association with bicuspid aortic valve. *J Thorac Cardiovasc Surg.* 2001;122:842–843.

16. Ko SM, Song MG, Hwang HK. Bicuspid aortic valve: spectrum of imaging findings at cardiac MDCT and cardiovascular MRI. *AJR Am J Roentgenol.* 2012;198:89–97.

17. Michelena HI, Desjardins VA, Avierinos JF, et al. Natural history of asymptomatic patients with normally functioning or minimally dysfunctional bicuspid aortic valve in the community. *Circulation.* 2008;117:2776–2784.

18. Tzemos N, Therrien J, Yip J, et al. Outcomes in adults with bicuspid aortic valve. *J Am Med Assoc.* 2008;300:1317–1325.

19. Michelena HI, Khanna AD, Mahoney D, et al. Incidence of aortic complications in patients with bicuspid aortic valves. *J Am Med Assoc.* 2011;306:1104–1113.

20. Siu SC, Silversilles CK. Bicuspid aortic valve disease. *J Am Coll Cardiol.* 2010;55:2789–2800.

21. Roberts WC, Ko JM, Matter GJ. Isolated aortic valve replacement without coronary bypass for aortic valve stenosis involving a congenitally bicuspid valve in a nonagenarian. *Am Geriatr Cardiol.* 2006;15:389–391.

22. Zema MJ, Caccavano M. Two-dimensional echocardiographic assessment of aortic valve morphology: feasibility of bicuspid aortic valve detection. Prospective study of 100 adult patients. *Br Heart J.* 1982;48:428–433.

23. Brandenburg RO, Tajik AJ, Edwards WD, et al. Accuracy of 2 dimensional echocardiographic diagnosis of congenitally bicuspid aortic valve: echocardiographic-anatomic correlation in 115 patients. *Am J Cardiol.* 1983;51:1469–1473.

24. Chan KL, Stinson WA, Veinot JP. Reliability of transthoracic echocardiography in the assessment of aortic valve morphology: pathological correlations in 178 patients. *Can J Cardiol.* 1999;15:48–52.

25. Pomerance A. Pathogenesis of aortic stenosis and its relation to age. *Br Heart J.* 1972;334:569–574.

26. Waller BF, Carter JB, Williams Jr HJ, et al. Bicuspid aortic valve. Comparison of congenital and acquired types. *Circulation.* 1973;48:1140–1150.

27. Angelini A, Ho SY, Anderson RH, et al. The morphology of the normal aortic valve as compared with the aortic valve having 2 leaflets. *J Thorac Cardiovasc Surg.* 1989;98:362–367.

28. Sievers HH, Schmidtke C. A classification system for the bicuspid aortic valve from 304 surgical specimens. *J Thorac Cardiovasc Surg.* 2007;133:1226–1233.

29. Fernandes SM, Sanders SP, Khairy P, et al. Morphology of bicuspid aortic valve in children and adolescents. *J Am Coll Cardiol.* 2004;44:1648–1651.

30. Schaefer BM, Lewin MB, Stout KK, et al. The bicuspid aortic valve: an integrated phenotypic classification of leaflet morphology and aortic root shape. *Heart.* 2008;94:1634–1638.

31. Della Corte A, Cortufo M. Bicuspid aortopathy or bicuspid aortopathies? The risk in generalizing. *J Thorac Cardiovasc Surg.* 2008;136:1604.

32. Hope MD, Meadows AK, Hope TA, et al. Evaluation of bicuspid aortic valve and aortic coarctation with 4D flow magnetic resonance imaging. *Circulation.* 2008;117:2818–2819.

33. Giradauskas E, Borger MA, Secknus MA, et al. Is aortopathy in bicuspid aortic valve disease a congenital defect or a result of abnormal hemodynamics? A critical appraisal of one-sided argument. *Eur J Cardio Thorac Surg.* 2011;39:809–814.

34. Ayad RF, Grayburn PA, Ko JM, et al. Accuracy of two-dimensional echocardiography in determining aortic valve structure in patients>50 years of age having aortic valve replacement for aortic stenosis. *Am J Cardiol.* 2011;108:1589–1599.

35. Jain R, Ammar KA, Kalvin L, et al. Diagnostic accuracy of bicuspid aortic valve by echocardiography. *Echocardiography.* 2018;35:1932–1938.

36. Yousry M, Rickenlund A, Petrini J, et al. Aortic valve type and calcification as assessed by transthoracic and transesophageal echocardiography. *Clin Physiol Funct Imag.* 2015;35:306–313.

37. Makkar A, Siddiqui TS, Stoddard MF, et al. Impact of valvular calcification on the diagnostic accuracy of transesophageal echocardiography for the detection of congenital aortic valve malformation. *Echocardiography.* 2007;24:745–749.

38. Barker AJ, Markl M, Burk J, et al. Bicuspid aortic valve is associated with altered wall shear stress in the ascending aorta. *Circ Cardiovasc Imag.* 2012;5:457–466.

39. Bissell MM, Hess AT, Biasiolli L, et al. Aortic dilatation in bicuspid aortic valve disease: flow pattern is a major contributor and differs with valve fusion type. *Circ Cardiovasc Imag.* 2013;6(4):499–507.

40. Meierhofer C, Schneider EP, Lyko C, et al. Wall shear stress and flow patterns in the ascending aorta in patients with bicuspid aortic valve differs significantly from tricuspid aortic valves: a prospective study. *Eur Heart J Cardiovasc Imag.* 2013;14:797–804.

41. Mahadevia R, Barker AJ, Schnell S, et al. Bicuspid aortic cusp fusion morphology alters three-dimensional outflow patterns, wall shear stress, and expression of aortopathy. *Circulation.* 2014;129:673–682.

42. Kimura N, Nakamura M, Komiya K, et al. Patient-specific assessment of hemodynamics by computational fluid dynamics in patients with bicuspid aortopathy. *J Thorac Cardiovasc Surg.* 2017;153:S52–S62.

43. Shan Y, Li J, Wang Y, et al. Aortic shear stress in patients with bicuspid aortic valve with stenosis and insufficiency. *J Thorac Cardiovasc Surg.* 2017;153(6):1263–1272.

44. Youssefi P, Gomez A, He T, et al. Patient-specific computational fluid dynamics assessment of aortic hemodynamics in a spectrum of aortic valve pathologies. *J Thorac Cardiovasc Surg.* 2017;153:8–20.

45. Litherson RR, Pennington DG, Jacobs ML, et al. Coarctation of the aorta: review of 234 patients and clarification of management problem. *Am J Cardiol.* 1979;43:835–840.

46. Folger Jr GM, Stein PD. Bicuspid aortic valve morphology associated with coarctation of the aorta. *Cathet Cardiovasc Diagn.* 1984;10:17–25.

47. Nihoyannopoulos P, Karas S, Sapsford RN, et al. Accuracy of two-dimensional echocardiography in the diagnosis of aortic arch obstruction. *J Am Coll Cardiol.* 1987;10:1072–1077.

48. Huntington K, Hunter A, Chan K. A prospective study to assess the frequency of familial clustering of congenital bicuspid aortic valve. *J Am Coll Cardiol.* 1997;30:1809–1812.

49. Warnes CA. Bicuspid aortic valve and coarctation: two villains part of a diffuse problem. *Heart.* 2003;89:965–966.

50. Oliver JM, Gallego P, Gonzalez A, et al. Risk factors for aortic complications in adults with coarctation of the aorta. *J Am Coll Cardiol.* 2004;44:1641–1647.

51. Gersony WM, Hayes CJ, Driscoll DJ, et al. Bacterial endocarditis in patients with aortic stenosis. Pulmonary stenosis, or ventricular septal defect. *Circulation.* 1993;87(suppl 2):I 121–I 126.

52. Dyson C, Barnes RA, Harrison GA. Infective endocarditis: an epidemiological review of 128 episodes. *J Infect.* 1999;38:87–93.

53. Lamas CC, Eykyn SJ. Bicuspid aortic valve—a silent danger: analysis of 50 cases of infective endocarditis. *Clin Infect Dis.* 2000;30:336–341.

54. Wilson W, Taubert KA, Gewitz M, et al. Prevention of infective endocarditis: a guideline from the American Heart Association. *Circulation.* 2007;116:1736–1754.

55. Niwa K, Perloff JK, Bhuta SM, et al. Structural abnormalities of great arterial walls in congenital heart disease: light and electron microscopic analyses. *Circulation.* 2001;103:393–400.

56. Ferencik M, Pape LA. Changes in size of ascending aorta and aortic valve function with time in patients with congenitally bicuspid aortic valves. *Am J Cardiol.* 2003;92:43–46.

57. Plaisance BR, Winkler MA, Attili AK, et al. Congenital aortic valve first presenting as an aortic aneurysm. *Am J Med.* 2012;125:e5–e7.

58. Della Corte A, Bancone C, Quarto C, et al. Predictors of ascending aortic dilatation with bicuspid aortic valve: a wide spectrum of disease expression. *Eur J Cardio Thorac Surg.* 2007;31:397–404.

59. Braverman AC. Aortic involvement in patients with a bicuspid aortic valve. *Heart.* 2011;97:506–513.

60. Isselbacher EM. Thoracic and abdominal aortic aneurysms. *Circulation.* 2005;111:816–828.

61. Schievink WI, Raissi SG, Maya MM, et al. Screening for intracranial aneurysms in patients with bicuspid aortic valve. *Neurology.* 2010;74:1430–1433.

62. Mack MJ, Leon MB, Smith CR, et al. 5-year outcomes of transcatheter aortic valve replacement or high surgical risk patients with aortic stenosis (PARTNER 1): a randomised controlled trial. *Lancet.* 2015;385(9986):2477–2484.

63. Leon MB, Smith CR, Mack MJ, et al. Transcatheter or surgical aortic-valve replacement in intermediate-risk patients. *N Engl J Med.* 2016;374(17):1609–1620.

64. Reardon MJ, Van Mieghem NM, Popma JJ, et al. Surgical or transcatheter aortic-valve replacement in intermediate-risk patients. *N Engl J Med.* 2017;376(14):1321–1331.

65. Waksman R, Rogers T, Torguson R, et al. Transcatheter aortic valve replacement in low-risk patients with symptomatic severe aortic stenosis. *J Am Coll Cardiol.* 2018;72(18):2095–2105.

66. Mack MJ, Leon MB, Thourani VH, et al. Transcatheter aortic-valve replacement with a balloon-expandable valve in low-risk patients. *N Engl J Med.* 2019;380(18):1695–1705.

67. Popma JJ, Deeb GM, Yakubov ST, et al. Transcatheter aortic-valve replacement with a self-expanding valve in low-risk patients. *N Engl J Med.* 2019;380(18):1706–1715.

68. Capodanno D, Leon MB. Upcoming TAVI trials: rationale, design, and impact on clinical practice. *Eur Intervention.* 2016;12:51–55. Y.

69. Roberts WC, Janning KG, Ko JM, et al. Frequency of congenitally bicuspid aortic valves in patients ≥80 years of age undergoing aortic valve replacement for aortic stenosis (with or without aortic regurgitation) and implications for transcatheter aortic valve implantation. *Am J Cardiol.* 2012;109(11):1632–1636.

70. Jilaihawi H, Chen M, Webb J, et al. A bicuspid aortic valve imaging classification for the TAVR era. *JACC Cardiovasc Imag.* 2016;9:1145–1158.

71. Mylotte D, Lefevre T, Sondergaard L, et al. Transcatheter aortic valve replacement in bicuspid aortic valve disease. *J Am Coll Cardiol.* 2014;64(22):2330–2339.

72. Yoon SH, Bleiziffer S, De Backer O, et al. Outcomes in transcatheter aortic valve replacement for bicuspid versus tricuspid aortic valve stenosis. *J Am Coll Cardiol.* 2017;69:2579–2589.

73. Perlman GY, Blanke P, Dvir D, et al. Bicuspid aortic valve stenosis: favorable early outcomes with a next-generation transcatheter heart valve in a multicenter study. *JACC Cardiovasc Interv.* 2016;9(8):817–824.

74. Bonow RO, Carabello BA, Chatterjee K, et al. Focused update incorporated into the ACC/AHA 2006 guidelines for the management of patients with valvular heart disease. *Circulation.* 2008;118:e523–e564. 2008.

75. Warnes CA, Williams RG, Bashore TM, et al. ACC/AHA 2008 guidelines for the management of adults with congenital heart disease. *Circulation.* 2008;118(1):e714–e833.

76. Hiratzka LF, Bakris GL, Beckman JA, et al. 2010 ACCF/AHA/AATS/ACR/SCA/SCAI/SIR/SVM guidelines for the diagnosis and management of patients with thoracic aortic disease. *Circulation.* 2010;121:e266–e369.

77. Roberts WC, Ko JM. Frequency by decades of unicuspid, bicuspid, and tricuspid aortic valves in adults having isolated aortic valve replacement for aortic stenosis, with or without associated aortic regurgitation. *Circulation.* 2005;111:920–925.

78. Tempe DK, Garg M, Tower AS, et al. Unicuspid aortic valve: transesophageal echocardiographic features. *J Cardiothorac Vasc Anesth.* 2012;26:277–279.

79. Osman K, Nanda NC, Kim K-S, et al. Transesophageal echocardiographic features of a unicuspid aortic valve. *Echocardiography.* 1994;11:469–473.

80. Sniecinski RM, Shanewisc JS, Glas KE. Transesophageal echocardiography of a unicuspid aortic valve. *Anesth Analg.* 2009;108:788–789.

81. Novaro GM, Tiong IY, Pearce GL, et al. Features and predictors of ascending aortic dilatation in association with a congenital bicuspid aortic valve. *Am J Cardiol.* 2003;92:99–101.

82. Yotsumoto G, Moriyama Y, Toyohira H, et al. Congenital bicuspid aortic valve: analysis of 63 surgical cases. *J Heart Valve Dis.* 1998;7:500–503.

83. Passik CS, Ackerman DM, Pluth JR, et al. Temporal changes in the cases of aortic stenosis: a surgical pathology study of 646 cases. *Mayo Clin Proc.* 1987;62:119–123.

84. Michelena HI, Della Corte A, Prakash SK, et al. Bicuspid valve aortopathy in adults: incidence, etiology, and clinical significance. *Int J Cardiol.* 2015;201:400–407.

85. Chu JW, Picard MH, Agnihotri AK, et al. Diagnosis of congenitally unicuspid aortic valve in adult population: the value and limitation of transesophageal echocardiography. *Echocardiography.* 2010;27:1107–1112.

86. Brantley HP, Nekkanti R, Anderson CA, et al. Three-dimensional echocardiographic features of unicuspid aortic valve stenosis correlate with surgical findings. *Echocardiography.* 2012;29:E204–E207.

87. Simonds JP. Congenital malformation of the aortic and pulmonary valves. *Am J Med Sci.* 1923;166:584–595.

88. Feldman BJ, Khandheria BK, Warnes CA, et al. Incidence description, and functional assessment of isolated quadricuspid aortic valves. *Am J Cardiol.* 1990;65:937–938.

89. Olson LJ, Subramannian MB, Edwards WD. Surgical pathology of pure aortic insufficiency: a study of 725 cases. *Mayo Clin Proc.* 1984;59:835–841.

90. Tutarel O. The quadricuspid aortic valve: a comprehensive review. *J Heart Valve Dis.* 2004;13:534–537.

91. Zacharaki AA, Patrianakos AP, Parthenakos FI, et al. Quadricuspid aortic valve associated with non-obstructive sub-aortic membrane: a case report and review of the literature. *Hellenic J Cardiol.* 2009;50:544–547.

92. Hunt GB. Congenital quadricuspid aortic valve detected on chest CT. *J Med Imag Radiol Oncol.* 2009;53:380–381.

93. Chapman CB, Kohmoto T, Kelly AF, et al. Cardiac computed tomography and quadricuspid aortic valve: a case report. *Wis Med J.* 2010;109:219–221.

94. Davia JE, Fenoglio JJ, De Castro CM, et al. Quadricuspid semilunar valves. *Chest.* 1977;72:186–189.

95. Hurwitz LE, Roberts WC. Quadricuspid semilunar valve. *Am J Cardiol.* 1973;31:623–626.

96. Barbosa MM, Motta MS. Quadricuspid aortic valve and aortic regurgitation diagnosed by Doppler echocardiography. Report of two cases and a review of the literature. *J Am Soc Echocardiogr.* 1991;4:69–74.

97. Peretz DI, Changfoot GH, Gourlay RH. Four-cusped aortic valve with significant insufficiency. *Am J Cardiol.* 1969;23:291–293.

98. Janssens U, Klues HG, Hanrath P. Congenital quadricuspid aortic valve anomaly associated with hypertrophic nonobstructive cardiomyopathy: a case report and review of the literature. *Heart.* 1997;78:83–87.

99. Brouwer MHJ, de Graaf JJ, Ebels T. Congenital quadricuspid aortic valve. *Int J Cardiol.* 1993;38:196–198.

100. Dotti MT, De Stefano N, Mondillo S, et al. Neurologicalinvolvement and quadricuspid aortic valve in a patient with Ehlers-Danlos syndrome [letter]. *J Neurol.* 1999;246:612–613.

101. Robicsek F, Sanger PW, Daughtery HK, et al. Congenital quadricuspid aortic valve with displacement of the left coronary orifice. *Am J Cardiol.* 1969;23:288–290.

102. Korosawa H, Wagenaar SS, Becker AZ. Sudden-death in a youth. A case of quadricuspid aortic valve with isolation of original left coronary artery. *Br Heart J.* 1981;46:211–215.

103. Rosenkranz ER, Murphy Jr DJ, Cosgrove 3rd DM. Surgical management of left coronary ostial atresia and supravalvular aortic stenosis. *Am Thorac Surg.* 1992;94:779–781.

104. Lanzillo G, Breccia PA, Intonti F. Congenital quadricuspid aortic valve with displacement of the right coronary orifice. *Scand J Thorac Cardiovasc Surg.* 1981;15:149–151.

105. Okmen AS, Okmen E. Quadricuspid aortic valve without severe dysfunction despite advanced age. *Texas Heart Inst J.* 2009;36:486–488.

106. Lindroos M, Kupari M, Heikkila J, et al. Prevalence of aortic valve abnormalities in the elderly: an echocardiographic study of a random population sample. *J Am Coll Cardiol.* 1993;21:1220–1225.

107. Rajamannan NM, Bonow RO, Rahimtoola SH. Calcific aortic stenosis: an update. *Nat Clin Pract Cardiovasc Med.* 2007;4:254–262.

108. Stewart BF, Siscovick D, Lind BK, et al. Clinical factors associated with calcific aortic valve disease: cardiovascular health study. *J Am Coll Cardiol.* 1997;29:630–634.

109. Agmon Y, Khandheria BK, Meissner I, et al. Aortic valve sclerosis and aortic atherosclerosis: different manifestations of the same disease? Insights from a population-based study. *J Am Coll Cardiol.* 2001;38:827–834.

110. O'Brien KD. Pathogenesis of calcific aortic valve disease: a disease process comes of age (and a great deal more). *Arterioscler Thromb Vasc Biol.* 2006;26:1721–1728.

111. Otto CM. Calcific aortic stenosis—time to look more closely at the valve. *N Engl J Med.* 2008;359:1395–1398.

112. Owens DS, Katz R, Takasu J, et al. Incidence and progression of aortic valve calcium in the Multi-Ethnic Study of Atherosclerosis (MESA). *Am J Cardiol.* 2010;105:701–708.

113. Owens DS, Otto CM. Is it time for a new paradigm in calcific aortic valve disease? *JACC Cardiovasc Imag.* 2009;2:928–930.

114. Marincheva-Savcheva G, Subramannian S, Qadir S, et al. Imaging of the aortic valve using fluorodeoxyglucose positron emission tomography. Increased valvular fluorodeoxyglucose uptake in aortic stenosis. *J Am Coll Cardiol.* 2011;57:2507–2915.

115. Thubrikar MJ, Aouad J, Nolan SP. Patterns of calcific deposits in operatively excised stenotic or purely regurgitant aortic valves and their relation to mechanical stress. *Am J Cardiol.* 1986;58:304–308.

116. Rosenhek R, Binder T, Porenta G, et al. Predictors of outcome in severe, asymptomatic aortic stenosis. *N Engl J Med.* 2000;343:611–617.

117. Owens DS, Budoff MJ, Katz R, et al. Aortic valve calcium independently predicts coronary and cardiovascular events in a primary prevention population. *JACC Cardiovasc Imag.* 2012;5:619–625.

118. Adegunsoye A, Mundkur M, Nanda NC, et al. Echocardiographic evaluation of calcific aortic stenosis in the older adult. *Echocardiography.* 2011;28:117–129.

119. Dare AJ, Veinot JP, Edwards WD, et al. New observations on the etiology of aortic valve disease: a surgical pathologic study of 236 cases from 1990. *Hum Pathol.* 1993;24:1330–1338.

120. Wallby L, Steffensen T, Jonasson L, Broqvist. Inflammatory characteristics of stenotic aortic valves: a comparison between rheumatic and nonrheumatic aortic stenosis. *Cardiol Research and Practice* 2013 (2): 895215.

121. Fenoglio JJ, McAllister HA, DeCastro CM, et al. Congenital bicuspid aortic valve after age 20. *Am J Cardiol.* 1977;39:164–169.

122. Roberts CS, Roberts WC. Dissection of the aorta associated with congenital malformation of the aortic valve. *J Am Coll Cardiol.* 1991;17:712–716.

123. Gore I, Seiwert VJ. Dissecting aneurysm of the aorta, pathologic aspects: an analysis of eighty-five fatal cases. *Arch Pathol.* 1952;53:121–141.

124. Edwards WD, Leaf DS, Edwards JE. Dissecting aortic aneurysm associated with congenital bicuspid aortic valve. *Circulation.* 1978;57:1022–1025.

79 Quantification of Aortic Stenosis Severity

Steven A. Goldstein

Aortic stenosis (AS) is the most common cardiac valve lesion in developed countries, including North America and Europe, with an incidence of 2% to 9% in patients older than 65 years of age.[1] Moreover, the incidence is increasing as the population ages. Aortic sclerosis, the precursor of AS, is present in nearly one-third of patients older than age 65 years.

AS is suspected clinically when a harsh systolic ejection murmur is heard, a delayed carotid upstroke is palpated, or typical symptoms (angina pectoris, exertional dyspnea, or exertional syncope) occur. However, the clinical diagnosis of AS can be challenging. Clinical signs and symptoms are limited for distinguishing critical AS from noncritical AS, and these signs have reduced sensitivity and specificity in older adults.[2,3] Cardiac catheterization, once considered the gold standard for quantitation of AS, is invasive, and the frequency of complications increases with age.[4] Omran and coworkers demonstrated evidence of acute, focal embolic events on magnetic resonance imaging (MRI) in 22% of 152 patients who underwent retrograde catheterization.[5]

In contrast, echocardiography provides noninvasive assessment of both valve morphology and hemodynamics. Because of its versatility, noninvasiveness, reproducibility, and accuracy, current guidelines endorse echocardiography as the diagnostic method of choice for the assessment and management of AS.[6,7] Cardiac catheterization is no longer recommended and is only performed in a limited subset of patients in whom echocardiography is nondiagnostic or discrepant with clinical parameters.[6,7] In most situations, transthoracic echocardiography (TTE) is sufficient, and it is the current standard procedure for assessing both severity and serial evaluations of AS. Moreover, the prediction of clinical outcomes of patients with AS has been studied mainly using TTE.[8–10]

Precise assessment of AS severity is necessary for clinical decision making. The primary hemodynamic parameters recommended for the quantitation of AS severity are peak jet velocity, transaortic gradients, and aortic valve area (AVA) calculated by the continuity equation.[11] Box 79.1 lists the echocardiographic and Doppler parameters that should be evaluated in patients with valvular AS. These are subsequently discussed in the following.

NORMAL AORTIC VALVE
Two-Dimensional Echocardiography

The normal aortic valve is composed of three leaflets or cusps (the left, right, and noncoronary cusps [NCCs]) of equal or nearly equal size. Two-dimensional (2D) TTE of the normal aortic valve in the parasternal long-axis (PLAX) view shows two leaflets: (1) the right coronary cusp, which is the most anterior cusp, and (2) either the noncoronary cusp [NCC] (most commonly) or the left coronary cusp. Normal aortic valve cusps appear thin and delicate. In the PLAX view, the cusps open rapidly in systole and appear as parallel lines close to the aortic walls (Fig. 79.1). In diastole, the leaflets come together and appear as a linear density in the center of the aortic root, parallel to the aortic walls. The aortic leaflets are seldom seen during the opening and closing because their motion is very rapid relative to the frame rate of the 2D ultrasound system. In the short-axis (SAX) view, the three thin leaflets open in systole to form a triangular or circular orifice (Fig. 79.2). During diastole, the closure lines of the three leaflets form a Y shape (an inverted Mercedes Benz sign). Sometimes there is a slight thickening of the midportion of each closure line formed by nodules known as the *nodules of Arantius*. In the SAX view, the NCC is located posteromedially. The atrial septum always points to the NCC. The left coronary cusp is located posterolaterally.

M-Mode Echocardiography

M-mode echocardiography of the aortic valve is formed by directing the M-mode echo beam through the aortic leaflets. This can be done from both the PLAX and SAX views. At the onset of systole, the leaflets open rapidly and become parallel to, and nearly oppose, the walls of the aortic root (Fig. 79.3). They remain open throughout systole and rapidly close again at end-systole, forming a box or parallelogram. Normally, these leaflets show fine, regular vibrations during systole. These fine vibrations actually indicate that the leaflets are thin and are able to luff, like a sail, because of the rapid flow through them on one side (their ventricular surface) and eddy currents swirling behind the leaflets on the aortic side, resulting in

---

BOX 79.1 Echo Doppler Parameters to Evaluate in Aortic Valve Stenosis

1. Two-dimensional (2D) measurement of the left ventricular outlet tract (LVOT) diameter and aortic annulus
2. LVOT velocity (V1)—by pulsed-wave Doppler
3. Velocity across the aortic valve (V2 or Vmax) by continuous wave Doppler (from apex, right parasternal view, suprasternal notch, subxiphoid view)
4. Calculation of peak instantaneous gradient and mean gradient
5. Calculation of aortic valve area by the continuity equation
6. Dimensionless index
7. M-mode or 2D measurements of left ventricular size
8. Calculation of LV mass
9. Assessment of aortic insufficiency
10. Assessment of other cardiac defects

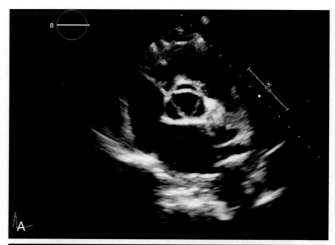

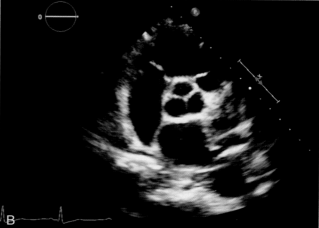

Figure 79.2. Transthoracic echocardiogram (short-axis view) of a normal tricuspid aortic valve. **A**, In systole, the valve opens in a triangular fashion with straightening of the leaflets. **B**, In diastole, the normal trileaflet valve appears like a Y, with the commissures at the 10 o'clock, 2 o'clock, and 6 o'clock positions.

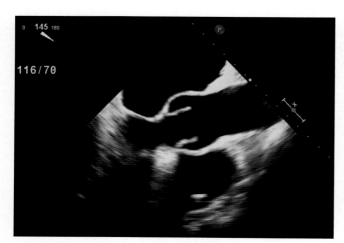

Figure 79.1. Transesophageal echocardiogram, longitudinal view (similar to transthoracic parasternal long-axis view) of a normal tricuspid aortic valve illustrates normal opening with the leaflets parallel to the aortic root walls.

opposing forces that cause these vibrations. During diastole, the coapted leaflets form a single (or sometimes multiple parallel) central closure line(s) midway between the aortic walls (see Fig. 79.3). The left ventricular (LV) ejection time can be measured from the point of the cusp opening to the point of the cusp closing.

A rough estimate of the severity of AS can be obtained by noting the maximal degree of separation of the leaflets at the onset of systole. In patients with valvular AS, the thickened leaflets (caused by fibrosis, calcium, or both) appear as dense echoes in both systole and diastole. In systole, the thickened rigid leaflets fail to open widely. The distance between the anterior cusp (right coronary cusp) and the posterior cusp (usually the NCC; sometimes, the left coronary cusp) is reduced or not even visible, which suggests moderate or severe AS (Fig. 79.4). In the absence of a bicuspid valve, a maximal opening of the leaflets of at least 1.5 cm virtually excludes significant valvular AS.[12,13] When any of the three leaflets opens normally or maximally, regardless of the degree of limitation of the other two, the degree of AS is not more than mild.

QUANTITATIVE DIAGNOSIS OF AORTIC STENOSIS

With the development of acquired AS, the cusps become thickened, and their motion is restricted. The degree of thickening and restriction

progresses as the severity of AS increases. In severe AS, the leaflets become markedly thickened and calcified, and there is nearly a total lack of mobility. Identification of individual cusps is often difficult or impossible. Moreover, attempts to planimeter the aortic valve orifice by TTE have been largely unsuccessful.[14] Nevertheless, a qualitative estimation of AS severity should be attempted and correlated with quantitative methods. If leaflet separation is at least 15 mm or if at least one cusp moves normally, critical AS is unlikely. However, as will be discussed later, planimetry is possible in the majority of patients using transesophageal echocardiography (TEE).

QUANTITATIVE DOPPLER ASSESSMENT OF SEVERITY OF AORTIC STENOSIS

The previously mentioned, 2D and M-mode features are useful for detecting AS, but they are unreliable for quantitating AS. The severity of AS is determined by a combination of 2D and Doppler echocardiography. As the aortic valve becomes stenotic and obstruction to blood flow occurs, a pressure gradient develops across the valve. This obstruction is associated with an increase in transaortic jet velocity. The primary routine parameters used to quantitate AS include the peak aortic jet velocity, the mean pressure gradient, and the AVA.

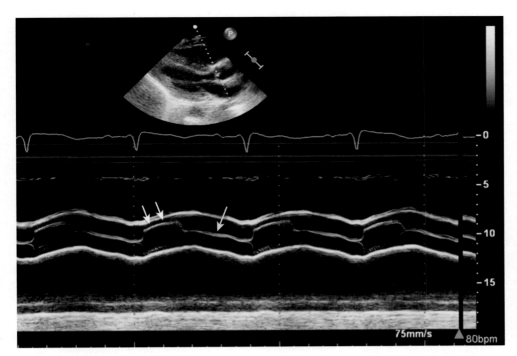

Figure 79.3. M-mode echocardiogram of an aortic valve illustrating the rapid opening slope of the aortic leaflets at the onset of systole, the leaflets aligned parallel to the aortic walls throughout systole *(white arrows)*, and the central closure line in diastole *(yellow arrow)*.

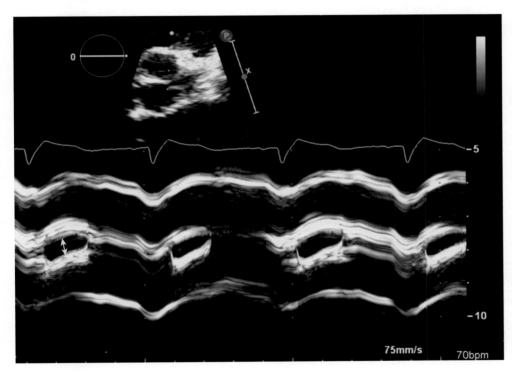

Figure 79.4. M-mode echocardiogram from a patient with moderate aortic stenosis. The maximal opening between the anterior (right coronary cusp) leaflet and a posterior leaflet (noncoronary cusp) *(yellow arrow)* is less than 5 mm.

Transaortic Velocities

Transaortic jet velocities are directly obtained using a continuous-wave (CW) Doppler probe. To obtain the highest velocity, the angle of interrogation should be as parallel to flow as possible. Therefore, multiple transducer windows should be used to obtain the Doppler signal that is aligned most parallel to the direction of the stenotic jet. These windows include the apical three- and five-chamber views, the right sternal border, the suprasternal notch (SSN), and subxiphoid views. A careful, thorough, meticulous manipulation of the transducer is necessary to achieve optimal alignment and to determine the highest velocity possible (Fig. 79.5). The highest velocity obtained from any window is used in the calculation of the gradient and the AVA. Lower values from the other windows are ignored. Using a nonimaging CW Doppler probe (so-called *Pedoff probe* or *pencil probe*) is recommended because it is smaller, easier to manipulate between the ribs and in the SSN, and has a higher signal-to-noise ratio.

Pressure Gradients

The highest transaortic jet velocity (Vmax) measured by Doppler reflects the pressure gradient according to the Bernoulli equation. The maximum pressure gradient (ΔPmax) across the stenotic aortic

Apical 3-ch, 5-ch, Rt. sternal border
Supra Sternal Notch, subxiphoid

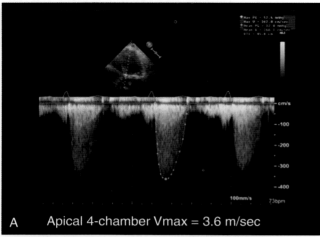

A Apical 4-chamber Vmax = 3.6 m/sec

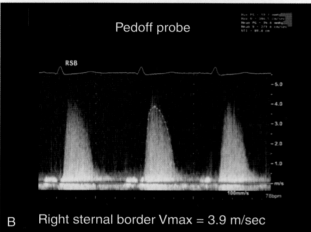

B Right sternal border Vmax = 3.9 m/sec

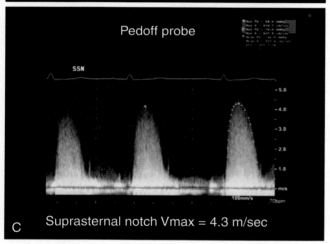

C Suprasternal notch Vmax = 4.3 m/sec

Figure 79.5. Continuous-wave Doppler tracings from a patient with severe aortic stenosis illustrate the importance of using multiple transducer positions to obtain the highest (maximal) transaortic velocity. **A,** Apical four-chamber view using imaging probe detects a velocity of 3.6 m/s. **B,** A slightly higher velocity (3.9 m/s) is obtained from the right sternal border using a nonimaging (Pedoff) probe. **C,** The highest velocity (4.3 m/s) was obtained from the suprasternal notch using a non-imaging probe.

TABLE 79.1 Recommendations for Grading the Severity of Aortic Stenosis

	Aortic Sclerosis	Mild	Moderate	Severe
Peak velocity (m/s)	≤2.5	2.6–2.9	3.0–4.0	≥4.0
Mean gradient (mm Hg)	—	<20	20–40	≥40
AVA (cm²)	—	>1.5	1.0–1.5	<1.0
Indexed AVA (cm²/m²)	—	>0.85	0.60–0.85	<0.6
Velocity ratio	—	>0.50	0.25–0.50	<0.25

AVA, Aortic valve area.
From Baumgartner H, et al: Recommendations on the echocardiographic assessment of aortic valve assessment: a focused update from the European Association of Cardiovascular Imaging and the American Society of Echocardiography, *J Am Soc Echocardiogr* 30:372–392, 2017. With permission from the European Society of Cardiology and the American Society of Echocardiography.

valve can be calculated by using the simplified Bernoulli equation that ignores viscous losses and the effects of flow acceleration. These can be neglected in the usual clinical setting:

$$\Delta Pmax = 4(Vmax)^2$$

However, when the proximal or left ventricular outflow tract (LVOT) velocity (V_{LVOT}) exceeds 1.5 m/s, the modified Bernoulli ejection should be used:

$$\Delta Pmax = 4\left(Vmax^2 - V_{LVOT^2}\right)$$

The mean pressure gradient is obtained by a manual tracing of the Doppler velocity envelope. The ultrasound machine's software integrates the instantaneous velocities throughout systole and provides a mean value. Both peak and mean gradients should be reported. A mean gradient more than 40 to 50 mm Hg is consistent with severe AS (Table 79.1). However, because calculated pressure gradients depend not only on the degree of stenosis but also on (flow stroke volume and/or cardiac) output, higher gradients than those outlined in Box 79.1 may occur in patients with altered volume flow rates. Examples of increased flow rates occur in aortic regurgitation (AR), anemia, and pregnancy. In these situations, relatively high-pressure gradients may be present, although the degree of AS may only be mild. In contrast, patients with significant LV systolic dysfunction, small left ventricles, high systemic vascular resistance, or mitral regurgitation (MR) may have relatively low gradients despite severe AS. The accuracy of Doppler-derived peak instantaneous maximal and mean pressure gradients has been validated with simultaneous cardiac catheterization data[15,16] (Figs. 79.6 and 79.7). It is important to recognize that the peak instantaneous systolic pressure gradient measured by Doppler is higher than the peak-to-peak gradient obtained during cardiac catheterization (Fig. 79.8). Potential sources of error in the Doppler assessment of transaortic gradients are listed in Box 79.2.

Doppler measurement of gradients may be limited by TEE because of the difficulty in aligning the echo beam parallel to the stenotic jet from standard esophageal views. However, in the majority of cases, the deep transgastric view can be used to obtain accurate maximal velocities and gradients (Fig. 79.9). A second useful view can be obtained by slight clockwise rotation of the TEE probe from a standard gastric longitudinal view of the left ventricle (Fig. 79.10).

Aortic Valve Area by the Continuity Equation

Echo Doppler assessment of the severity of AS includes the calculation of AVA using the continuity equation. The continuity principle, based on the conservation of mass, states that the flow volumes (Q) at different sites in a closed system, like the heart, are identical:

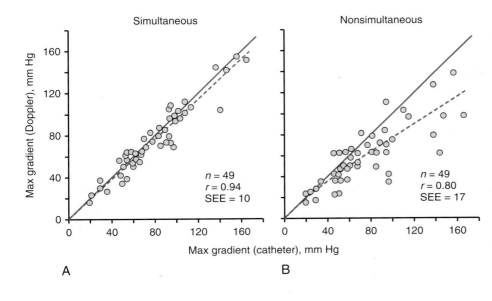

Figure 79.6. Good correlation between Doppler- and catheter-derived peak instantaneous gradients (Max gradient) when performed simultaneously (**A**) versus nonsimultaneously (**B**). The *dotted lines* represent the regression lines, and the *solid lines* represent the lines of identity. (Modified from Currie PJ, et al: Instantaneous pressure gradient: a simultaneous Doppler and dual catheter study, *J Am Coll Cardiol* 7:800–806, 1986.)

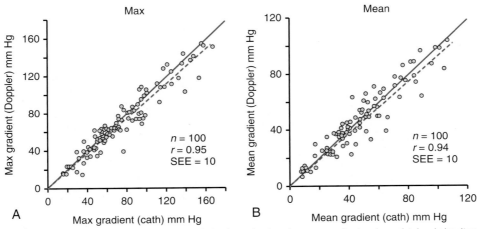

Figure 79.7. Good correlation between Doppler- and catheter-derived maximal and mean gradients when obtained simultaneously in 100 patients. The *dotted lines* represent the regression line, and the *solid lines* represent the line of identity. (Modified from Currie PJ, et al: Continuous-wave Doppler echocardiographic assessment of severity of calcific aortic stenosis, *Circulation* 71:1162–1169, 1985.)

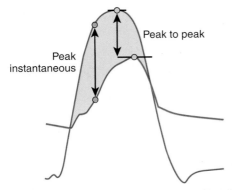

Figure 79.8. Simultaneous left ventricular *(white trace)*–aortic *(yellow trace)* pressures. The *gray-hatched area* between these two tracings represents the pressure gradient throughout systole. Note that the peak instantaneous gradient measured by Doppler *(green arrow)* is higher than the peak-to-peak gradient measured by catheterization *(yellow arrow)*. Also note that the peak-to-peak gradient is artificial (the peak left ventricular pressure and the peak aortic pressures occur at different times).

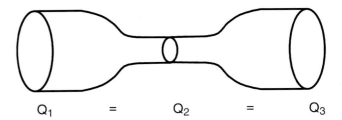

In the case of AS, the stroke volume proximal to the aortic valve in the LVOT, or Q_1, must equal the stroke volume through the stenotic aortic valve (Q_2). Because stroke volume is the product of the cross-sectional area (CSA) and the time velocity integral (TVI) at that point, the continuity equation can be stated as:

$$Q_1 - CSA_1 \times TV_1 = CSA_2 \times TVI_2$$

The continuity equation can be rearranged as follows:

$$CSA = \frac{CSA_1 \times TVI_1}{TVI_2}$$

BOX 79.2 Sources of Error in Doppler Assessment of Transvalvular Gradient Overestimation Compared With Catheter Gradient

- Failure to account for increased subvalvular velocity
- Recording the wrong gradient (mitral regurgitation)
- Nonrepresentative selection of velocity (arrhythmias—highest velocity often incorrectly selected)
- Pressure recovery in patients with small aorta (<3.0 cm)

In the case of AS, site 1 is the LVOT, and site 2 is the stenotic aortic orifice. Thus, the continuity equation can be restated as:

$$AV\ area = \frac{CSA_{LVOT} \times TVI_{LVOT}}{TVI_{AS}}$$

Therefore, to calculate the AVA, three measurements must be obtained (Fig. 79.11):

1. CSA of the LVOT (CSA_{LVOT})
2. TVI of the LVOT (TVI_{LVOT})
3. TVI of the aortic stenotic jet (TVI_{AS})

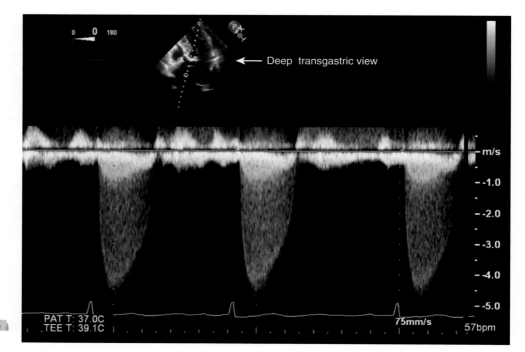

Figure 79.9. Continuous Doppler tracing from a deep transgastric transesophageal echocardiographic view, which detects a transaortic velocity (V2) of 4.5 m/s in a patient with severe aortic stenosis.

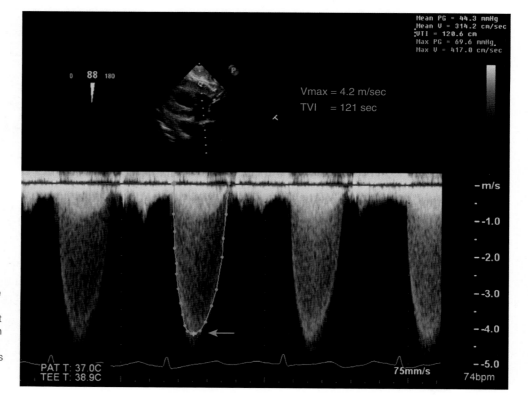

Figure 79.10. Transesophageal echocardiogram continuous-wave Doppler tracing from a standard gastric longitudinal view with slight clockwise rotation in a patient with severe aortic stenosis revealing a maximal velocity (Vmax) of 4.2 m/s and time velocity integral (TVI) of 121 s.

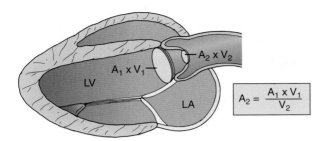

Figure 79.11. The continuity equation as applied to valvular aortic stenosis: $A_1 \times V_1$ = the flow volume in the left ventricular outflow tract and $A_2 \times V_2$ = the flow volume across the stenotic aortic valve. The stenotic aortic valve area (A_2) can be calculated from the continuity equation.

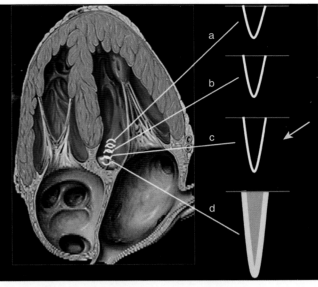

Figure 79.12. The method used to obtain the optimal left ventricular outflow tract (LVOT) velocity (V1) for the continuity equation. The pulsed-wave Doppler sample volume is initially placed in the LVOT *(a)*, serially moved toward the aortic valve *(b* and *c)* until the sample volume enters the flow convergence region *(d)*, and the spectral display demonstrates spectral broadening. The sample volume should then be moved back (apically) slightly until spectral broadening disappears. This is the optimal LVOT velocity *(c; yellow arrow)*.

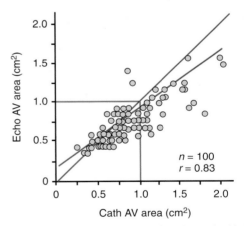

Figure 79.13. Good correlation between catheterization (cath)-derived aortic valve (AV) area and Doppler echocardiography (Echo)-derived area using left ventricular outflow tract and transaortic valve time-velocity integral ratio in 100 patients. Mean SEE was 0.19 cm². (Modified from Oh JK, et al: Prediction of the severity of aortic stenosis by Doppler aortic valve area determination, *J Am Coll Cardiol* 11:1227–1234, 1988.)

Calculation of the AVA relies on the measurement of these three parameters. Although measurement error may occur in all three, the main source of error for the calculation of AVA is that of the CSA of the LVOT. The CSA of the LVOT is obtained from the PLAX view. The LVOT region should be zoomed, and the maximum inner-edge to inner-edge diameter should be measured just below the insertion of the aortic valve leaflets in midsystole. There is still ongoing debate as to whether the LVOT diameter should be measured at the level of the leaflet insertion (i.e., the aortic annulus) versus more apically (i.e., 1–10 mm below the annulus). The recent recommendation from the American Society of Echocardiography (ASE) and the European Association of Cardiovascular Imaging (EACVI) does not provide a definitive answer.[17]

The TVI_{LVOT} is obtained from an apical window (apical five- or three-chamber view), using pulsed-wave Doppler, placing the sample volume (use a small sample volume) just proximal to the stenotic aortic valve, and tracing the waveform. This waveform should yield the highest-velocity laminar flow immediately proximal to the flow acceleration that occurs as the sample volume approaches the stenotic valve. This can be accomplished by placing the sample volume in the LVOT (beneath the stenotic valve), slowly inching toward the stenotic valve, and recording the enveloped (laminar) velocity profiles at each step until flow acceleration (spectral broadening) occurs. The sample volume should then be backed up (i.e., moved apically) until a smooth, laminar velocity curve without spectral broadening is detected, which indicates a position proximal to the flow acceleration zone (Fig. 79.12). This represents the correct LVOT velocity tracing. Next, using CW Doppler from multiple transducer positions (as discussed in the previous section), the maximal TVI_{AS} is obtained. The highest transaortic velocity and TVI from any of the transducer positions should be used to calculate the AVA. Although TVI is preferred, the peak velocity can also be used in the continuity equation. The use of velocity is more practical in patients with atrial fibrillation, when 5 to 10 consecutive beats should be measured and averaged.[11] A sample calculation of the AVA using the continuity equation and velocity instead of TVI is as follows:

- LVOT diameter: 2.0 cm
- LVOT velocity: 1.0 m/s
- AS peak jet velocity: 4.0 m/s

$$AV \ area = CSA_{LVOT} \times \frac{V_{LVOT}}{VAo}$$

$$AV \ area = \frac{(3.14)(1.0)^2 (1.0)}{4.0} = 0.8 \ cm^2$$

LIMITATIONS AND PITFALLS IN THE ECHO DOPPLER QUANTITATION OF AORTIC STENOSIS

Calculation of the AVA by the continuity equation requires painstaking attention to detail in the measurement of the three previously mentioned parameters. Good correlation between echocardiography and catheter-derived valve area has been demonstrated[17–19] (Fig. 79.13). As mentioned earlier, the primary cause of inaccuracy with the continuity equation is error in the measurement of the LVOT diameter. Because the square of the radius is used in the continuity equation, even minor errors in the measurement of the LVOT diameter may result in substantial

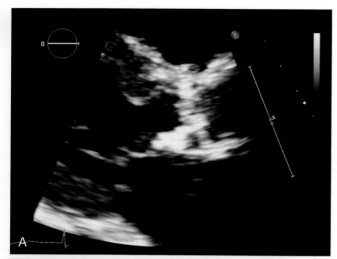

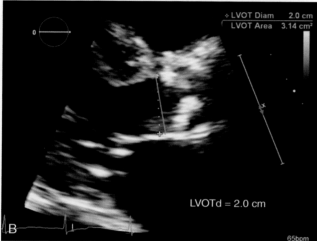

Figure 79.14. A, Zoomed parasternal long-axis view of the left ventricular outflow tract (LVOT) illustrates a chunk of calcium protruding into the LVOT. This view might yield an incorrectly small LVOT diameter (LVOTd) because the calcium does not represent the entire perimeter of the orifice. **B,** A slightly altered view misses this chunk of calcium and yields a larger and more accurate diameter of 2.0 cm.

error in the calculation of the AVA. There is a tendency to underestimate the LVOT for several reasons. First, the LVOT may be elliptical rather than circular, and in such instances, the smallest diameter is usually measured in the PLAX view.[20–24] Second, in patients with calcific AS, blooming and reverberations from the calcified aortic annulus, and often from the extension of calcium onto and/or into the base of the anterior mitral leaflet, can artificially make the LVOT appear smaller than its actual size, especially when using low-frequency transducers and high-gain settings (Fig. 79.14). Technical tips to avoid this potential problem include using as high a frequency transducer as possible, imaging the LVOT as close to the center of the sector as possible (axial resolution is superior to lateral resolution), and using relatively low-gain settings. Last, especially in older adult patients, the upper (basal) septum may bulge into the LVOT, making this measurement difficult.

Three-dimensional (3D) imaging techniques have demonstrated that the LVOT is often elliptical rather than circular. The anteroposterior diameter (sagittal) as obtained from the transthoracic echocardiographic (TTE) PLAX view is smaller than the

larger medial-lateral (coronal) diameter. Therefore, the LVOT cross-sectional area as obtained by TTE may lead to underestimation of AVA. To overcome this pitfall of 2D echocardiography for the measurement of LVOT area used in the continuity equation, some investigators have proposed using a so-called hybrid approach (or "fusion data") in which LVOT area is planimetered by multidetector computed tomography (MDCT), cardiac magnetic resonance imaging (CMRI), or 3D echocardiography, and the LVOT and aortic velocities and TVIs are determined using Doppler echocardiography.[25–28,29] However, the hybrid methods are also subject to a number of pitfalls and limitations. They are more cumbersome and more expensive than echocardiography because they require the performance of two different imaging examinations to measure a single stenotic parameter (i.e., AVA). In addition, these "hybrid" AVAs have not been validated or proven to better predict outcomes compared with conventional 2D echocardiography. Moreover, no reference value ("gold standard") was used in these studies combining computed tomography (CT) and echocardiography.

Theoretically, the LVOT diameter (LVOTd) should be measured in midsystole at the same time in the cardiac cycle that the LVOT velocity is measured. However, sometimes the image quality is suboptimal in mid-systole and the outflow tract is imaged more clearly at end-diastole. Skjaerpe and coworkers suggested that the LVOTd could be measured at end-diastole.[17] When accurate measurement of the LVOTd is not possible, one should not guess or use an assumed diameter (e.g., 2.0 cm), as some have recommended. In this situation, the dimensionless index (DI), or velocity ratio, may be used as an alternative to the AVA. This simplified parameter avoids the necessity to accurately measure LVOTd and is independent of cardiac output. This Doppler-only method uses the following equation:

$$DI = \frac{TVI_{LVOT}}{TVI_{AS}}$$

A DI less than 0.25 is consistent with severe AS (see Table 79.1). The accuracy of DI in assessing AS severity may be affected by extremes in LVOT size.[30,31] The second parameter subject to limitations is the LVOT velocity (so-called *V1*). The method recommended to measure this parameter has been discussed. However, this parameter may not be measurable in several situations. The most common pitfall occurs when there is associated subaortic stenosis that may cause high-velocity turbulent flow in the LVOT, precluding accurate measurement of V1. The strut of a bioprosthetic mitral valve may protrude into the LVOT, creating turbulence, which occurs less commonly.

Other parameters used for quantitating AS are the transaortic velocity (Vmax, or so-called *V2*) and the transaortic pressure gradient derived from V2. Underestimation of this velocity and pressure may occur if there is poor alignment of the Doppler beam (not parallel to the stenotic aortic jet). This potential problem can be minimized by using multiple transducer positions, as discussed earlier. Overestimation of the true velocity and pressure gradient is less common than underestimation. This may be due to mistaking a MR jet (or rarely at tricuspid regurgitant [TR] jet) for the aortic stenotic jet, especially when using a nonimaging probe. These three jets are similar in direction as seen from apical views. Sweeping the transducer back and forth to distinguish which jet is which may help to avoid this pitfall. A second clue to help distinguish these jets is their duration. MR and TR jets are always longer than the AS jet because they include isovolumic contraction and isovolumic relaxation. In addition, the MR jet has a higher velocity because the LV–left atrial (LA) gradient is higher than the left ventricular–aortic gradient in systole. Another method to distinguish the AS jet from the MR jet is the associated diastolic signals in the tracing. The MR jet is associated with mitral flow, whereas the AS jet is not and may be associated with AR if AR is present (Table 79.2).

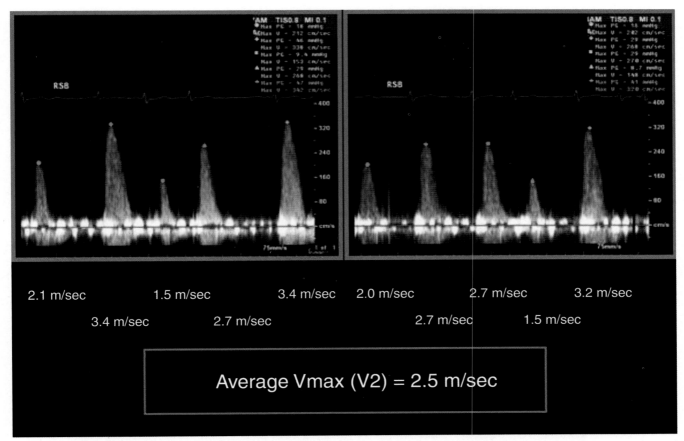

2.1 m/sec   1.5 m/sec   3.4 m/sec   2.0 m/sec   2.7 m/sec   3.2 m/sec

3.4 m/sec   2.7 m/sec   2.7 m/sec   1.5 m/sec

Average Vmax (V2) = 2.5 m/sec

Figure 79.15. Continuous-wave Doppler tracings using a nonimaging probe from the right sternal border illustrating the beat-to-beat variability of the transaortic velocities. Ten consecutive beats were averaged (average Vmax = 2.5 m/s).

TABLE 79.2 Factors Helping to Differentiate an Aortic Stenotic Jet From Mitral Regurgitant Jet

Characteristic	AS	MR
Shape	Early systolic peak when AS is less than severe but parabolic in severe AS	Parabolic Peaks in mid to late systole (exception acute, severe MR)
Duration	AS shorter than MR (no flow during isovolumic periods)	MR longer than AS (includes IVCT and IVRT)
Diastolic signals	Gap between end of AS and mitral inflow (IVRT)	End of MR jet is continuous with mitral inflow
Velocity	AS < MR	MR > AS

AS, Aortic stenosis; *IVCT,* isovolumic contraction time; *IVRT,* isovolumic relaxation time; *MR,* mitral regurgitation.

BOX 79.3 Potential Pitfalls of Doppler-Derived Gradients in Aortic Stenosis

- Poor alignment of Doppler beam (improper intercept angle between the aortic stenosis jet and Doppler beam)
- Left ventricular outlet tract (LVOT) velocity may be important (cannot be ignored if >1.4 m/s)
- Mitral regurgitant jet may be mistaken for aortic jet
- Subaortic obstruction may preclude measurement of LVOT velocity
- Comparison with catheter gradients (peak instantaneous vs peak to peak)
- Beat-to-beat variability (atrial fibrillation, premature ventricular contractions)

A rare situation may occur when a high-velocity jet from a stenotic arch vessel is mistaken for an AS jet from the SSN transducer position. These potential pitfalls are summarized in Box 79.3. In the presence of atrial fibrillation or frequent premature ventricular contractions, averaging the velocity from 5 to 10 consecutive beats is recommended (Fig. 95.15). The use of the highest velocity alone results in overestimating the gradient and underestimating the AVA calculated by the continuity equation. The effect of systemic blood pressure on the assessment of the mean pressure gradient and AVA remains controversial.[25,32]

Recommendations for measuring and recording valve morphology and echo Doppler parameters in patients with AS are listed in Table 79.3. Given the potential therapeutic and prognostic importance of these echocardiographic parameters and their potential limitations, they should only be reported when imaging is adequate and there is a high level of confidence in their accuracy. If the level of confidence of these measurements is reduced or if there is a discrepancy between the echo Doppler and clinical or catheterization data, the raw data of all of the echocardiographic measurements should be reviewed carefully and critically. Other

TABLE 79.3 Recommendations for Date Recording and Measurement for Aortic Stenosis Quantitation

Date Element	Recording	Measurement
LVOT diameter	2D parasternal long-axis view Zoom mode Adjust gain to optimize the blood–tissue interface	Inner edge to inner edge Midsystole Parallel and adjacent to the aortic valve or at the site of velocity measurement (see text) Diameter is used to calculate a circular CSA
LVOT velocity	PW Doppler Apical long axis or five-chamber view Sample volume positioned just on LV side of valve and moved carefully into the LVOT is required to obtain laminar flow curve Velocity baseline and scale adjusted to maximize size of velocity curve Time axis (sweep speed), 100 mm/s Low wall filter setting Smooth velocity curve with a well-defined peak and a narrow velocity range at peak velocity	Maximum velocity from peak of dense velocity curve VTI traced from modal velocity
AS jet velocity	CW Doppler (dedicated transducer) Multiple acoustic windows (e.g., apical, suprasternal, right parasternal) Decrease gains, increase wall filter, adjust baseline, and scale to optimize signal Grayscale spectral display with expanded time scale Velocity range and baseline adjusted so velocity signal fits and fills the vertical scale	Maximum velocity at peak of dense velocity curve Avoid noise and fine linear signals VTI traced from outer edge of dense signal curve Mean gradient calculated from traced velocity curve
Valve anatomy	Parasternal long- and short-axis views Zoom mode	Identify number of cusps in systole, raphe if present Assess cusp mobility and commissural fusion Assess valve calcification

2D, Two-dimensional; *AS*, aortic stenosis; *CSA*, cross-sectional area; *CW*, continuous wave; *LV*, left ventricular; *LVOT*, left ventricular outflow tract; *PW*, pulsed-wave; *VTI*, velocity time integral.
With permission from the European Society of Cardiology and the American Society of Echocardiography.

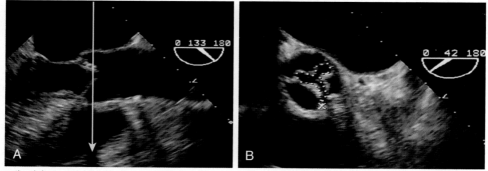

Figure 79.16. The methodology used for planimetry of the aortic valve orifice by transesophageal echocardiogram. **A,** In a longitudinal (long-axis) view, the aortic valve should be placed as close to the center of the sector as possible (to take advantage of axial resolution). **B,** The image plane *(arrow)* should then be rotated 90 degree to obtain a short-axis view and the plane moved cranially and caudally to obtain the smallest orifice. The aortic valve can then be planimetered.

diagnostic modalities may be considered to further assess the morphology and hemodynamics of the stenotic aortic valve. These may include TEE, MRI, and, rarely, cardiac catheterization as outlined in the ASE/EACVI guidelines.[6,7,11]

PLANIMETRY OF AORTIC VALVE ORIFICE

Theoretically, the aortic valve orifice can be measured by planimetry using TTE in a manner similar to that used for assessing the orifice area in mitral stenosis. However, this method is unreliable in calcific AS for several reasons: (1) the inability to determine whether the plane of imaging is at the leaflet tips where maximum stenosis occurs and is parallel to the orifice; and (2) planimetry is difficult because of poor cusp definition from heavy calcium deposition, acoustic shadowing, and reverberation artifact.[26]

Because of its superior resolution and unobstructed visualization, TEE provides excellent views of the aortic valve leaflets as they open and close throughout the cardiac cycle. Therefore, unlike with TTE, direct measurement of the AVA by TEE planimetry can be performed with excellent correlation with cardiac catheterization using the Gorlin equation and with echo Doppler using the continuity equation.[27–30] Planimetry by TEE has also been shown to correlate well with planimetry by CT.[31] To measure the AVA accurately, the image plane must be located at the tips of the aortic valve leaflets. This measurement requires a careful technique to produce the correct imaging angle and plane. It is useful to begin with a longitudinal view (usually between 110 and 150 degrees) to align the aortic root perpendicular to the echo beam and to place the aortic valve at or near the center of the sector (Fig. 79.16A). This takes advantage of the axial resolution and provides the optimal plane parallel to the aortic annulus and valve. Subsequently, the image plane can be rotated 90 degrees to view the aortic valve in a precise SAX view (Fig. 79.16B). Alternately, the biplane function of newer ultrasound machines can be used to achieve this view. Slight withdrawal and advancement of the

TEE probe cranially and caudally is useful to find the smallest orifice at the maximal leaflet tip separation. The smallest systolic orifice is frequently found at a plane slightly higher than the "Mercedes Benz sign" visualized in diastole. The view should image all three cusps simultaneously. Color Doppler may aid in determining the stenotic orifice. Adjusting the gain settings (reducing gain without losing definition of the leaflet and commissural edges) may help delineate the true margins of the orifice for planimetry. The smallest orifice area at the time of maximal opening in early to midsystole should then be planimetered.

THREE-DIMENSIONAL ASSESSMENT OF THE AORTIC VALVE AREA

Real-time three-dimensional TTE (RT3D TTE) has the potential to overcome a shortcoming of 3D-TTE by providing imaging at any plane. The cropping plane in the 3D dataset can provide a true en face view aligned exactly to image the smallest stenotic aortic valve orifice for planimetry. Several studies have documented superior accuracy of planimetry by RD3D TTE compared with conventional 2D-TTE.[22,33–37] Therefore, RT3D TTE can, in some situations, overcome some of the limitations of the continuity equation; the AVA can be reliably evaluated when valvular AS coexists with hypertrophic obstructive cardiomyopathy, discrete subaortic stenosis, or supravalvular AS. In addition, the evaluation of AS severity by the continuity equation may be enhanced by using a RT3D TTE approach for the measurement of the LVOT diameter or CSA.[37]

OTHER METHODS OF MEASURING AORTIC STENOSIS SEVERITY

Several additional echocardiographic parameters have been proposed to better define the severity of AS and its risk. Those include valve resistance,[38–42] the energy loss index,[43–45] stroke work loss,[46–48] and valvuloarterial impedance.[49–52] However, their utility and prognostic significance remain to be proven in large-scale prospective trials, and their clinical relevance has not yet been established.

CMRI[53] and CT[31,54,55] have also been used to evaluate AVA. However, these methods have not been fully validated and are subject to some of the same limitations of echocardiography (e.g., heavily calcified valve).

Aortic valve CT calcium scoring (Agatston method) has emerged as an alternative method for assessing the severity of AS, especially when echocardiographic parameters are inconclusive and in evaluating disease progression.[29] Strengths of CT assessment include independence from flow, geometric assumptions, and the presence of other cardiovascular conditions such as hypertension and mitral regurgitation. The latest recommendation from the EACVI and the ASE have set categorical cutoffs for very likely, likely, and unlikely severe AS of 3000 or greater, ≥2000 or greater, and less than 1600 AU, respectively, in men and 1600 or greater, 1200 or greater, and less than 800 AU, respectively, in women.[17]

NEW CLASSIFICATION SCHEME FOR AORTIC STENOSIS

Despite all of the standard and new methods for quantitating AS and all of the newly defined entities of AS (described in Chapter 78), the definition of severe AS has become challenging in recent years. Therefore, the current guidelines have emphasized that the clinical diagnosis must be based on an integrated approach that includes transvalvular velocity and gradient, valve area, valve morphology, flow rate, LV morphology and function, blood pressure, and symptoms.[56,57] Correspondingly, the recent focused update has proposed a new classification scheme consisting of an integrated, stepwise approach to grading AS severity shown in Fig. 79.17.[17]

SERIAL EVALUATION OF AORTIC STENOSIS

Valvular aortic stenosis is a progressive disease, and an increase is severity is inevitable; however, the rate of progression is variable among individuals with AS. Because of the inability to predict this individual variability, serial clinical and echocardiographic follow-up is recommended in all patients with AS, as outlined in Table 79.4.

PHYSIOLOGIC CONSEQUENCES OF AORTIC STENOSIS

For complete assessment of a patient with AS, not only the appearance of the valve and its area and gradient but also the physiologic consequences of the stenosis should be evaluated and reported. These include the degree of hypertrophy (i.e., LV mass), systolic and diastolic dysfunction, degree of LA enlargement, and pulmonary hypertension (PH).

Left Ventricular Systolic Dysfunction

The chronic pressure overload imposed by valvular AS leads to concentric left ventricular hypertrophy (LVH). This increase in wall thickness is an adaptive process that maintains normal wall stress. However, as the stenosis progresses, this initially adoptive process eventually becomes deleterious. The progressive LVH, increasing afterload, and increasing wall stress lead to compromised coronary flow reserve and subendocardial ischemia.[58,59] Even in the absence of significant epicardial coronary artery narrowing, the increased muscle mass, the increased wall stress, and the result of ventricular pressure compressing the microcirculation will ultimately lead to myocardial fibrosis and gradually cause reduced systolic and diastolic function.[60] The development of diffuse myocardial fibrosis is believed to be an essential step in the transition from cardiac adaptation to cardiac failure.[61]

LV systolic dysfunction usually occurs late in the disease course of AS. Early, the left ventricular ejection fraction (LVEF) is preserved by the increased wall thickness that maintains wall stress and is therefore an insensitive measure of the early maladaptive process within the myocardium. However, there is recent awareness of subclinical LV dysfunction in AS that can be detected by global LV longitudinal strain (GLS).[62–67] Furthermore, impaired GLS has been independently associated with poor long-term outcome.[66,67] Lancellotti and colleagues have demonstrated that the presence of impaired GLS in asymptomatic patients with moderate to severe AS is independently associated with the development of symptoms, need for aortic valve replacement, and death.[68]

Left Ventricular Diastolic Dysfunction

In patients with AS, diastolic dysfunction begins at an earlier stage than the decrease in the LVEF.[69] Abnormal measures of diastolic function are common in patients with AS. At an early stage, the compensatory LVH of AS is associated with impaired relaxation. This filling pattern is common in mild and moderate AS. As the degree of AS progresses, the degree of diastolic dysfunction also increases. The dyspnea that often accompanies severe AS is typically attributed to the outflow obstruction; however, diastolic dysfunction likely also contributes to this symptom. These patients often have pseudonormal or restrictive filling patterns, suggesting an elevated filling pressure.[69–71] In addition, the early diastolic Doppler tissue velocity of the mitral annulus (e′) is decreased and may increase after aortic valve replacement.[72]

Preliminary data from the Mayo Clinic demonstrated that among asymptomatic patients with severe AS, those with an enlarged left atrium were more likely to develop symptoms than those with a smaller left atrium. Moreover, LA diameter was a strong independent prediction of all-cause mortality after adjusting

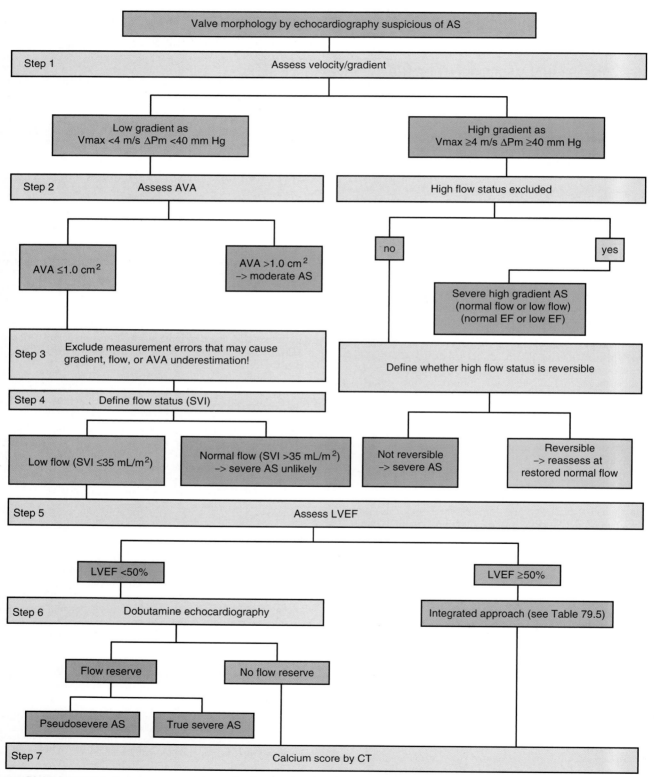

Figure 79.17. Integrated, stepwise approach to grading the severity of aortic stenosis (AS). *AVA,* Aortic valve area; *CT,* computed tomography; *EF,* ejection fraction; *LVEF,* left ventricular ejection fraction; *SVI,* stroke volume index.

TABLE 79.4 Serial Echocardiography in Asymptomatic Patients With Valvular Aortic Stenosis with Normal Left Ventricular Systolic Function

Aortic Velocity	Serial Echocardiography[a]
2.0–2.9 m/s	Every 3–5 years
3.0–3.9 m/s	Every 1–2 years
>4.0 m/s	6 months to 1 year

[a]Echocardiography should be performed more frequently if there is a change in signs or symptoms.

Adapted from Nishimura RA, et al: 2014 AHA/ACC guideline for the management of patients with valvular heart disease: a report of the American College of Cardiology/American Heart Association Task Force on Practice Guidelines, *J Am Coll Cardiol* 63:e57–e185, 2014.

for age, AVA, peak aortic valve velocity, and mean gradient. Their findings support the importance of diastolic function in these patients, and they recommend comprehensive assessment of diastolic function, including LA size.[73]

Pulmonary Hypertension

Severe PH is an expected finding in patients with mitral valve disease, especially mitral stenosis. However, severe PH is not widely associated with severe AS. Nevertheless, it has been reported in up to 34% of patients before aortic valve replacement for AS.[74–76] Although the cause of PH in severe AS remains unclear, it is associated with systolic and diastolic dysfunction.[77,78] Moderate or severe mitral regurgitation may also contribute to elevated LA and pulmonary artery pressure. When present, severe PH portends a poor prognosis and significantly increases morbidity and mortality.[79]

AORTIC VALVE SCLEROSIS

Aortic valve thickening (fibrosis, sclerosis, or both) without stenosis (i.e., without pressure gradient) is common in older adults. AS is present in approximately 25% to 30% of adults older than age 65 years and in nearly 50% of adults older than age 85 years.[80–82] Aortic valve sclerosis is generally defined as focal or diffuse thickening of the aortic cusps with minimal or no restriction of leaflet motion and a peak transvalvular velocity by Doppler of les than 2 m/s. The focal areas of thickening are usually irregular and non-uniform and involve the base and center of the valve cusps rather than the leaflet edges and commissures.

Aortic sclerosis is an asymptomatic condition that is usually detected either as a short, systolic ejection murmur or as an incidental finding on echocardiography performed for other indications. Until recently, aortic valve sclerosis was considered to be a physiologic result of aging without clinical relevance. However, aortic valve sclerosis may be important as a marker for increased cardiovascular risk, including progression to AS.[83–86]

REFERENCES

1. Iung B, Baron G, Butchart EG, et al. A prospective survey of patients with valvular heart disease in Europe. *Eur Heart J*. 2003;24:1231–1243.
2. Eddleman Jr EE, Frommeyer WB, Lyle DP, et al. Critical analysis of clinical factors in estimating severity of aortic valve disease. *Am J Cardiol*. 1973;31:686–695.
3. Rajamannan NM, Bonow RO, Rahimtoola SH. Calcific aortic stenosis: an update. *Nat Clin Pract Cardiovasc Med*. 2007;4:254–262.
4. Mallavarapu RK, Mankad S, Nanda NC. Echocardiographic assessment of aortic stenosis in the elderly. *Am J Geriatr Cardiol*. 2007;16:343–348.
5. Omran H, Schmidt H, Hackenbroch M, et al. Silent and apparent cerebral embolism after retrograde catheterization of the aortic valve in valvular aortic stenosis. *Lancet*. 2003;361:1241–1246.
6. Vahanian A, Baumgartner H, Bax JJ, et al. Guidelines on the management of valvular heart disease. *Eur Heart J*. 2007;28:230–268.
7. Bonow RO, Carabello BA, Chatterjee K, et al. Focused update incorporated into the ACC/AHA 2006 guidelines for the management of patients with valvular heart disease. *J Am Coll Cardiol52:el*. 2008;192:2008.
8. Otto CM, Burwash IG, Legget ME, et al. Prospective study of asymptomatic valvular aortic stenosis. Clinical echocardiography and exercise predictors of outcome. *Circulation*. 1997;45:2262–2270.
9. Rosenhek R, Binder T, Porenta G, et al. Predictors of outcome in severe, symptomatic aortic stenosis. *N Engl J Med*. 2000;343:611–617.
10. Pellikka PA, Sarano ME, Nishimura RA, et al. Outcome of 622 patients with asymptomatic, hemodynamically significant aortic stenosis during prolonged follow-up. *Circulation*. 2005;111:3290–3295.
11. Baumgartner H, Hong J, Bermejo J, et al. Echocardiographic assessment of valve stenosis: EAE/ASE recommendations for clinical practice. *Eur J Echocardiogr*. 2009;10:1–25.
12. DeMaria AN, Joye JA, Bommer W. Sensitivity and specificity of cross-sectional echocardiography in the diagnosis and quantification of valvular aortic stenosis (abstr). *Circulation*. 1978;57(Suppl II):232.
13. Godley RW, Green D, Dillon JC, et al. Reliability of two-dimensional echocardiography in assessing the severity of valvular aortic stenosis. *Chest*. 1981;79:657–662.
14. DeMaria AN, Bommer W, Jaye J, et al. Value and limitation of cross-sectional echocardiography of the aortic valve in the diagnosis of valvular aortic stenosis. *Circulation*. 1980;62:304–312.
15. Currie PJ, Seward JB, Reeder GS, et al. Continuous-wave Doppler echocardiographic assessment of severity of calcific aortic stenosis. *Circulation*. 1985;71:1162–1169.
16. Currie PJ, Hagler DJ, Seward JB, et al. Instantaneous pressure gradient: a simultaneous Doppler and dual catheter study. *J Am Coll Cardiol*. 1986;7:800–806.
17. Baumgartner H, Hung J, Bermejo J, et al. Recommendations on the echocardiographic assessment of aortic valve assessment: a focused update from the European Association of Cardiovascular Imaging and the American Society of Echocardiography. *J Am Soc Echocardiogr*. 2017;30:372–392.
18. Skjaerpe T, Hegreraes L, Hatle L. Noninvasive estimation of valve area in patients with aortic stenosis by Doppler ultrasound and two-dimensional echocardiography. *Circulation*. 1985;72:810–818.
19. Zoghbi WA, Farmer KL, Soto IG, et al. Accurate noninvasive quantification of stenotic aortic valve area by Doppler echocardiography. *Circulation*. 1986;73:452–459.
20. Oh JK, Taliercio CP, Holmes Jr DR, et al. Prediction of the severity of aortic stenosis by Doppler aortic valve area determination. *J Am Coll Cardiol*. 1988;11:1227–1234.
21. Baumgartner H, Kratzer K, Helmreich G, et al. Determination of aortic valve area by Doppler echocardiography using the continuity equation: a critical evaluation. *Cardiology*. 1990;77:101–114.
22. Baumgartner H. Hemodynamic assessment of aortic stenosis: are there still lessons to learn? *J Am Coll Cardiol*. 2006;47:138–140.
23. Doddamani S, Bella R, Friedman MA, et al. Demonstration of left ventricular outflow tract eccentricity by real time 3D echocardiography. *Echocardiography*. 2007;24:860–866.
24. Burgstahler C, Kunze M, Loffler C, et al. Assessment of left ventricular outflow tract geometry in non-stenotic and stenotic aortic valves by cardiovascular magnetic resonance. *J Cardiovasc Magn Res*. 2006;8:825–829.
25. Clavel M-A, Malouf J, Messika-Zeitoun D, et al. Aortic valve area calculation in aortic stenosis by CT and Doppler echocardiography. *JACC Cardiovasc Imag*. 2015;8:248–257.
26. Mehrotra P, Flynn AW, Jansen K, et al. Differential left ventricular outflow tract remodeling and dynamics in aortic stenosis. *J Am Soc Echocardiogr*. 2015;28:1259–1266.
27. Pibarot P, Clavel M-A. Doppler echocardiographic quantitation of aortic valve stenosis: a science in constant evolution. *J Am Soc Echocardiogr*. 2016;29:1019–1022.
28. Jander N, Wienecke S, Dorfs S, et al. Anatomic estimation of aortic stenosis severity vs "fusion" of data from computed tomography and Doppler echocardiography. *Echocardiography*. 2018;35:777–784.
29. Chin CW, Pawade TA, Newby DE, Dweck MR. Risk stratification in patients with aortic stenosis using novel imaging approaches. *Circ Cardiovasc Imag*. 2015;8:e003421.
30. Rusinaru D, Malaquin D, Marechaux S, et al. Relation of dimensionless index to long-term outcome in aortic stenosis with preserved ejection fraction. *JACC Cardiovasc Imag*. 2015;8(7):766–775.
31. Zoghbi WA. Velocity acceleration in aortic stenosis revisited. *JACC Cardiovasc Imag*. 2015;8:776–778.
32. Jander N, Minners J, Holme I, et al. Outcome of patients with low-gradient "severe" aortic stenosis and preserved ejection fraction. *Circulation*. 2011;123:887–895.
33. Kadem L, Dumesnil JG, Rieu R, et al. Impact of systemic hypertension on the assessment of aortic stenosis. *Heart*. 2005;91:354–361.
34. Little SH, Chan KL, Burwash IF. Impact of blood pressure on the Doppler echocardiographic assessment of the severity of aortic stenosis. *Heart*. 2007;93:848–855.
35. Gilon D, Cape EG, Handschumacher MD, et al. Effect of three-dimensional shape on the hemodynamics of aortic stenosis. *J Am Coll Cardiol*. 2002;40:1479–1486.
36. Stoddard MF, Aree J, Liddell NE, et al. Two-dimensional transesophageal echocardiographic determination of aortic valve area in adult with aortic stenosis. *Am Heart J*. 1991;122:1415–1422.
37. Kim CJ, Berglund H, Nishioka T, et al. Correspondence of aortic valve area determination from transesophageal echocardiography, transthoracic echocardiography, and cardiac catheterization. *Am Heart J*. 1996;132:1163–1172.

38. Cormier B, Iung B, Porte JM, et al. Value of multiplane transesophageal echocardiography in determining aortic valve area in aortic stenosis. *Am J Cardiol.* 1996;77:882–885.

39. Klass O, Walker MJ, Olszewski ME, et al. Quantification of aortic valve area at 256–slice computed tomography: comparison with transesophageal echocardiography and cardiac catheterization in subjects with high-grade aortic valve stenosis prior to percutaneous valve replacement. *Eur J Radiol.* 2011;80:151–157.

40. Vengala S, Nanda NC, Dod SH, et al. Images in geriatric cardiology. Usefulness of live three-dimensional transthoracic echocardiography in aortic valve stenosis evaluation. *Am J Geriatr Cardiol.* 2004;13:279–284.

41. Blot-Souletie N, Hebrand A, Acar P, et al. Comparison of accuracy of aortic valve area assessment in aortic stenosis by real time three-dimensional echocardiography in biplane mode versus two-dimensional transthoracic and transesophageal echocardiography. *Echocardiography.* 2007;24:1065–1072.

42. Goland S, Trento A, Iida K, et al. Assessment of aortic stenosis by three-dimensional echocardiography: an accurate and novel approach. *Heart.* 2007;93:801–807.

43. Gutierrrez-Chico JL, Zamorano JL, Prieto-Moriche E, et al. Real-time three-dimensional echocardiography in aortic stenosis: a novel, simple, and reliable method to improve accuracy in area calculation. *Eur Heart J.* 2008;29:1296–1306.

44. Poh KK, Levine RA, Solis J, et al. Assessing aortic valve area in aortic stenosis by continuity equation: a novel approach using real-time three-dimensional echocardiography. *Eur Heart J.* 2008;29:2526–2535.

45. Cannon JD, Zile MR, Crawford FA, et al. Aortic valve resistance as an adjunct to the Gorlin formula in assessing the severity of aortic stenosis in symptomatic patients. *J Am Coll Cardiol.* 1992;20:1517–1523.

46. Ho PP, Paulis GL, Lamberton DF, et al. Doppler derived aortic valve resistance in aortic stenosis: its hemodynamic validation. *J Heart Valve Dis.* 1994;3:283–287.

47. Bermejo J, Antoranz JC, Burwash IG, et al. In vivo analysis of the instantaneous transvalvular pressure difference—flow relationship in aortic valve stenosis: implications of unsteady fluid-dynamics for the clinical assessment of disease severity. *J Heart Valve Dis.* 2002;11:557–566.

48. Kadem JJ, Freyer S, Weisser G, et al. Correlation of degree of aortic valve stenosis by Doppler echocardiogram to quantity of calcium in the valve by election beam tomography. *Am J Cardiol.* 2002;90:554–557.

49. Otto CM. Valvular aortic stenosis: disease severity and timing of intervention. *J Am Coll Cardiol.* 2006;47:2141–2151.

50. Garcia D, Pibarot P, Dumesnil JG, et al. Assessment of aortic valve stenosis severity: a new index based on the energy loss concept. *Circulation.* 2000;101:765–771.

51. Garcia D, Dumesnil JG, Durand LG, et al. Discrepancies between catheter and Doppler estimates of valve effective orifice area can be predicted from the pressure recovery phenomenon: practical implications with regard to quantification of aortic stenosis severity. *J Am Coll Cardiol.* 2003;041:435–442.

52. Bahlmann E, Cramariuc D, Gredts E, et al. Impact of pressure recovery on echocardiographic assessment of asymptomatic aortic stenosis: a SEAS substudy. *JACC Cardiovasc Imag.* 2010;3:555–562.

53. Tobin JR, Rahimtoola SH, Blundell PE, et al. Percentage of left ventricular stroke work loss. A single hemodynamic concept for estimation of severity in valvular aortic stenosis. *Circulation.* 1967;35:868–879.

54. Bermejo J, Odreman R, Feijoo J, et al. Clinical efficacy of Doppler-echocardiographic indices of aortic valve stenosis: a comparative test-based analysis of outcome. *J Am Coll Cardiol.* 2003;41:142–151.

55. Turto H, Lommi J, Ventila M, et al. Doppler echocardiography markedly underestimates left ventricular stroke work loss in severe aortic valve stenosis. *Eur J Echocardiogr.* 2007;8:341–345.

56. Nishimura RA, Otto CM, Bonow RO, et al. 2014 AHA/ACC guideline for the management of patients with valvular heart disease: a report of the American College of cardiology/American heart association Task force on practice guidelines. *J Am Coll Cardiol.* 2014;63:e57–e185.

57. Vahanian A, Alfieri O, Andreotti F, et al. Guidelines on the management of valvular heart disease. *European Heart J.* 2012;33:2451–2496.

58. Briand M, Dumesnil JG, Kadem L, et al. Reduced systemic arterial compliance impacts significantly on left ventricular afterload and function in aortic stenosis: implications for diagnosis and treatment. *J Am Coll Cardiol.* 2005;46:291–298.

59. Hachicha Z, Dumesnil JG, Pibarot P. Usefulness of the valvuloarterial impedance to predict adverse outcome in asymptomatic aortic stenosis. *J Am Coll Cardiol.* 2009;54:1003–1011.

60. Levy F, Monin JL, Rusinaru D, et al. Valvuloarterial impedance does not improve risk stratification in low-ejection fraction, low-gradient aortic stenosis: results from a multicentre study. *Eur J Echocardiogr.* 2011;12:358–363.

61. Lancellotti P, Magne J. Valvuloarterial impedance in aortic impedance in aortic stenosis: look at the load, but do not forget the flow. *Eur J Echocardiogr.* 2011;12:354–357.

62. Reant P, Lederlin M, Lafitte S, et al. Absolute assessment of aortic valve stenosis by planimetry using cardiovascular magnetic resonance imaging: comparison with transesophageal echocardiography, transthoracic echocardiography, and cardiac catheterization. *Eur J Radiol.* 2006;59:276–283.

63. Bouvier E, Logeart D, Sablarolles JL, et al. Diagnosis of aortic valvular stenosis by multislice cardiac computed tomography. *Eur Heart J.* 2006;27:3033–3038.

64. Abdulla J, Silvertsen J, Kofoed KF, et al. Evaluation of aortic valve stenosis by cardiac multislice computed tomography compared with echocardiography: a systematic review and meta-analysis. *J Heart Valve Dis.* 2009;18:634–643.

65. Rajappan K, Rimoldi OE, Dutka DP, et al. Mechanisms of coronary microcirculatory dysfunction in patients with aortic stenosis and angiographically normal coronary arteries. *Circulation.* 2002;105:470–476.

66. Rajappan K, Rimoldi OE, Camici PG, et al. Functional changes in coronary microcirculation after valve replacement in patients with aortic stenosis. *Circulation.* 2003;107:3170–3175.

67. Tzivoni D. Effect of transient ischaemia on left ventricular function and prognosis. *Eur Heart J.* 1993;14(Suppl A):2–7.

68. Creemers EE, Pinto YM. Molecular mechanisms that control interstitial fibrosis in the pressure-overload heart. *Cardiovasc Res.* 2011;89:265–272.

69. Poulsen SH, Sogaard P, Nielsen-Kudsk JE, et al. Recovery of left ventricular systolic longitudinal strain after valve replacement in aortic stenosis and relation to natriuretic peptides. *J Am Soc Echocardiogr.* 2007;20:877–884.

70. Weidemann F, Herrmann S, Stork S, et al. Impact of myocardial fibrosis in patients with symptomatic severe aortic stenosis. *Circulation.* 2009;120:577–584.

71. Delgado V, Tops LV, van Bommel RJ, et al. Strain analysis in patients with severe aortic stenosis and preserved left ventricular ejection fraction undergoing surgical valve replacement. *Eur Heart J.* 2009;30:3037–3047.

72. Geyer H, Caracciolo G, Abe H, et al. Assessment of myocardial mechanics using speckle tracking echocardiography: fundamentals and clinical applications. *J Am Soc Echocardiogr.* 2010;23:351–369.

73. Herrmann S, Stork S, Niemann M, et al. Low-gradient aortic valve stenosis myocardial fibrosis and its influence on function and outcome. *J Am Coll Cardiol.* 2011;58:402–412.

74. Ng AC, Delgado V, Bertini M, et al. Alternations in multidirectional myocardial function in patients with aortic stenosis and preserved ejection fraction: a two-dimensional speckle tracking analysis. *Eur Heart J.* 2011;32:1542–1550.

75. Miyazaki S, Daimon M, Miyazaki T, et al. Global longitudinal strain in relation to the severity of aortic stenosis: a two-dimensional speckle-tracking study. *Echocardiography.* 2011;28:703–708.

76. Dahl JS, Videbaek L, Poulsen MK, et al. Global strain in severe aortic valve stenosis. Relation to clinical outcome after aortic valve replacement. *Circ Cardiovasc Imag.* 2012;5:613–620.

77. Kearney LG, Lu K, Ord M, et al. Global longitudinal strain is a strong independent predictor of all-cause mortality in patients with aortic stenosis. *Eur Heart J Cardiovasc Imag.* 2012;12:827–833.

78. Lancellotti P, Donal E, Magne J, et al. Impact of global left ventricular afterload on left ventricular function in asymptomatic severe aortic stenosis: a two-dimensional speckle-tracking study. *Eur J Echocardiogr.* 2010;11:637–643.

79. Lund O, Flo C, Jensen FT, et al. Left ventricular systolic and diastolic function in aortic stenosis. Prognostic value after valve replacement and underlying mechanisms. *Eur Heart J.* 1997;18:1977–1987.

80. Hess OM, Villari B, Krayenbuehl HP. Diastolic dysfunction in aortic stenosis. *Circulation.* 1993;87(Suppl IV):73–76.

81. Villari B, Campbell SE, Hess OM, et al. Influence of collagen network on left ventricular systolic and diastolic function in aortic valve disease. *J Am Coll Cardiol.* 1993;22:177–184.

82. Casaclang-Verzosa G, Ommen SR, Oh JK. Effects of aortic valve replacement on annular tissue Doppler velocities (abstr). *J Am Soc Echocardiogr.* 2005;18:41.

83. Casaclang-Verzosa G, Malouf JP, Scott CG, et al. Does left atrial size predict mortality in asymptomatic patients with severe aortic stenosis? *Echocardiography.* 2010;27:105–109.

84. Silver K, Aurigemma G, Krendel S, et al. Pulmonary artery hypertension in severe aortic stenosis: incidence and mechanism. *Am Heart J.* 1993;125:146–150.

85. Ben-Dor I, Goldstein SA, Pichard AD, et al. Clinical profile, prognostic implication, and response to treatment of pulmonary hypertension in patients with severe aortic stenosis. *Am J Cardiol.* 2011;107:1046–1051.

86. Zlotnick DM, Ouellette ML, Malenka DJ, et al. Effect of preoperative pulmonary hypertension on outcomes in patients with severe aortic stenosis following surgical aortic valve replacement. *Am J Cardiol.* 2013;142:1635–1640.

87. Aragam JR, Folland ED, Lapsley, et al. Cause and impact of pulmonary hypertension in isolated aortic stenosis on operative mortality for aortic valve replacement in men. *Am J Cardiol.* 1992;69:1365–1367.

88. Faggiano P, Antanini-Canterin F, Ribichini F, et al. Pulmonary artery hypertension in adult patients with symptomatic valvular aortic stenosis. *Am J Cardiol.* 2000;85:204–208.

89. Malouf JF, Enriquez-Sarano M, Pellikka PA, et al. Severe pulmonary hypertension in patients with severe aortic valve stenosis: clinical profile and prognostic implications. *J Am Coll Cardiol.* 2002;40:789–795.

90. Lindroos M, Kupari M, Heikkila J, et al. Prevalence of aortic valve abnormalities in the elderly: an echocardiographic study of a random population sample. *J Am Coll Cardiol.* 1993;21:1220–1225.

91. Otto CM, Lind BK, Kitzman DM, et al. Association of aortic valve stenosis with cardiovascular mortality and morbidity in the elderly. *N Engl J Med.* 1999;341:142–147.

92. Stewart BF, Siscovick D, Lind BK, et al. Clinical factors associated with calcific aortic valve disease. *J Am Coll Cardiol.* 1997;29:630–634.

93. Freeman RV, Otto CM. Spectrum of calcific aortic valve disease: pathogenesis, disease progression, and treatment strategies. *Circulation.* 2005;111:3316–3326.

94. Agmon Y, Khandheria BK, Meissner I, et al. Aortic valve sclerosis and aortic atherosclerosis: different manifestations of the same disease? Insights from a population-based study. *J Am Coll Cardiol.* 2001;38:827–834.

95. Cosmi JE, Kort S, Tunick PA, et al. The risk of the development of aortic stenosis in patients with "benign "aortic valve thickening. *Arch Intern Med.* 2002;162:2345–2347.

96. Carabello BA, Paulus WJ. Aortic stenosis. *Lancet.* 2009;373:956–966.

80 Asymptomatic Aortic Stenosis

Vedant A. Gupta, Vincent L. Sorrell

Aortic stenosis (AS) is the most commonly encountered valvular degenerative pathology in the world, affecting between 2% and 5% of the general population.[1] The prevalence of AS increases with age and can be as high as 4% to 13% in those older than 75 years of age. Although the overall incidence of AS has not dramatically changed over time, the burden of disease has increased because of increased longevity of the population.[2] Even though mitral regurgitation may be more common in population-based studies, the clinical impact of AS is higher. In some registries, it represents about one-third of all patients followed for valvular heart disease but represents nearly half of all patients undergoing valve procedures.[3] The pathogenesis of calcific aortic valve disease is complex and involves an interplay of genetics, lipoprotein processing, inflammation, oxidation, and ossification rates of valve leaflets.[1] This complex and dynamic interaction of causes helps explain some of the variance seen in the rates of progression, hemodynamics, and the effect on ventricular function. Given the heterogeneity of affected patients, guideline documents have largely focused on therapeutic interventions on more advanced disease states.

The importance of symptoms in AS is well-established. Patients with severe symptomatic AS have a median survival of less than 3 years, with early hazard as high as 3% to 6% in the first 6 months.[4,5] This is the primary reason why current guidelines emphasize symptoms as the primary indication for aortic valve replacement (AVR).[6,7] However, some observational studies have suggested that a strategy that awaits for symptoms may be suboptimal compared with strategies that recommend early presymptomatic intervention.[8] Reliable markers that predict those who would benefit from an early intervention are not known and some parameters, such as global left ventricular (LV) systolic dysfunction, may be too late in the disease progression and represent an irreversible finding (Fig. 80.1). Finally, therapeutic interventions have historically been limited to surgical aortic valve replacement (SAVR) and its higher initial risks. With the rapidly evolving and lower risk therapeutic intervention now commonly available in transcatheter aortic valve replacement (TAVR), the understanding of overall risk of an early invasive strategy will continue to be reassessed in asymptomatic severe (and potentially even moderate) AS. This individualized risk–benefit analysis will evolve with future clinical trial results and a better understanding of the long-term durability of TAVR versus SAVR valves.

NATURAL HISTORY OF SEVERE AORTIC STENOSIS

The rate of progression of AS is variable patient to patient. However, certain factors are known to be associated with a more rapid progression. Male gender, smoking, renal failure, hyperlipidemia, coronary artery disease, previous radiation exposure, age, and baseline degree of AS are all associated with more rapid progression of gradients.[9] Among patients with severe AS, the peak velocity increases on average 0.3 m/s every year with an estimated decrease in aortic valve area (AVA) of about 0.1 cm^2/year. Aortic valve calcification on multidetector computed tomography (MDCT) is one of the biggest predictors of progression.[10]

RISK OF DEFERRING INTERVENTION

The reported survival in asymptomatic patients with severe AS who were not offered AVR initially is highly variable and ranges from 67% to 97% at 1 year.[4] In the largest cohort reported of just over 1500 patients, Taniguchi and colleagues showed 1- and 5-year survival rates of about 93% and 74%, respectively.[11] It is important to understand that many of these patients at risk were not truly asymptomatic and developed symptoms before dying, but for various reasons, were not offered a therapeutic intervention. The risk of symptom development and mortality is related to the degree of hemodynamic impact (gradient across the valve). Other studies included the need for AVR and mortality as a combined endpoint given the frequency of symptom development even though a delayed intervention is always more common with an initial conservative strategy.

Perhaps more important is the inherent risk to the patient from the underlying disease in an initial conservative or active monitoring strategy. It has long been appreciated that asymptomatic severe AS is not an entirely benign disease, with a risk of sudden cardiac death ranging from 1.0% to 1.5% per year.[4,11] This risk is also associated with the hemodynamic impact of the stenosis and increases dramatically with the onset of symptoms. This provides a significant impetus to identify at-risk cohorts before the development of symptoms.

FEATURES THAT PREDICT INCREASED RISK

Whereas some variables are associated with the progression of the degree of stenosis, which is directly related to risk, other factors have been independently and directly associated with risk (Table 80.1).

Clinical

Concomitant heart failure has been associated with an increased risk of death in patients with AS. However, this can be difficult to distinguish as independent from or as a result of the valve disease by clinical examination alone. Advanced age, end-stage renal disease, and previous radiation exposure are each associated with an increased risk of death and a need for AVR.[4] Most likely, a part of this risk is due to progression of valve disease. Obesity is also associated with worse outcomes in asymptomatic severe AS, but at least in the Simvastatin Ezetimibe Aortic Stenosis (SEAS) study, was not caused solely by the progression of AS.[12] Obesity had a greater impact on changes in LV geometry and impairment of mid-wall fractional shortening at all hemodynamic gradients, which suggests a concurrent or exaggerated effect on the left ventricle.

Biomarkers

Cardiac biomarkers are routinely being used in the assessment of patients presenting with cardiovascular symptoms but may have an emerging role in asymptomatic patients with AS. Most of the research to date has been focused on natriuretic peptides and has been associated with hemodynamic progression, symptom development, and death before AVR. Unfortunately, clinical studies have used different optimal cut points for brain natriuretic peptide (BNP) and N-terminal pro-brain natriuretic peptide (NT-proBNP), making it challenging to apply in clinical practice even though there is an appreciation that higher overall levels portend worse outcomes.[13] The recent 2017 European Society of Cardiology (ESC)/European Association for Cardio-Thoracic Surgery (EACTS)

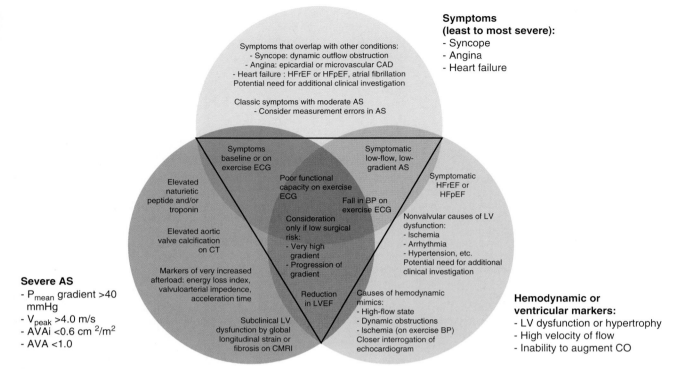

Symptoms (least to most severe):
- Syncope
- Angina
- Heart failure

Symptoms that overlap with other conditions:
- Syncope: dynamic outflow obstruction
- Angina: epicardial or microvascular CAD
- Heart failure : HFrEF or HFpEF, atrial fibrillation
Potential need for additional clinical investigation

Classic symptoms with moderate AS
- Consider measurement errors in AS

Symptoms baseline or on exercise ECG

Poor functional capacity on exercise ECG

Symptomatic low-flow, low-gradient AS

Symptomatic HFrEF or HFpEF

Elevated naturietic peptide and/or troponin

Fall in BP on exercise ECG

Consideration only if low surgical risk:
- Very high gradient
- Progression of gradient

Nonvalvular causes of LV dysfunction:
- Ischemia
- Arrhythmia
- Hypertension, etc.
Potential need for additional clinical investigation

Elevated aortic valve calcification on CT

Markers of very increased afterload: energy loss index, valvuloarterial impedence, acceleration time

Reduction in LVEF

Causes of hemodynamic mimics:
- High-flow state
- Dynamic obstructions
- Ischemia (on exercise BP)
Closer interrogation of echocardiogram

Severe AS
- P_{mean} gradient >40 mmHg
- V_{peak} >4.0 m/s
- AVAi <0.6 cm^2/m^2
- AVA <1.0

Subclinical LV dysfunction by global longitudinal strain or fibrosis on CMRI

Hemodynamic or ventricular markers:
- LV dysfunction or hypertrophy
- High velocity of flow
- Inability to augment CO

Figure 80.1. The interplay between aortic stenosis (AS), symptoms, hemodynamics, and ventricular function underlying some of the challenges in the assessment of AS. In the *center of the triangle* are the current indications for valve replacement, although many other features around the classic indications, especially in the severe AS section, may portend higher risk and benefit from intervention. *BP*, Blood pressure; *CAD*, coronary artery disease; *CMRI*, cardiac magnetic resonance imaging; *CO*, cardiac output; *CT*, computed tomography; *ECG*, electrocardiography; *HFpEF*, heart failure with preserved ejection fraction; *HFrEF*, heart failure with reduced ejection fraction; *LV*, left ventricular; *LVEF*, left ventricular ejection fraction.

guidelines offer a threefold increase in BNP or NT-proBNP over age- and gender-matched control participants as a IIa indication for AVR in asymptomatic patients with severe AS; however, a similar recommendation was not made in the 2014 American College of Cardiology (ACC)/American Heart Association (AHA) guideline document.

There is significantly less published experience with cardiac troponin in AS, and the guideline documents do not specifically mention their role. Recent studies looking at high-sensitivity troponin (both TnT and TnI) found an independent association with worse clinical outcomes beyond hemodynamic impact and clinical variables.[14,15] Further research is warranted, but troponin may be helpful in identifying early negative impact on the left ventricle before conventional imaging findings demonstrate LV dysfunction.

Valve Features
Gradients and Rate of Progression

Although the pioneering work on AS used peak velocity across the aortic valve, a more comprehensive assessment of the hemodynamics of valve stenosis involves consideration of all gradients, rates of AS "progression" (rate of change of pressure gradients over time), relative flow rates, and calculated AVA or area indices. It is important to recognize that peak velocity remains independently associated with clinical outcomes and is still one of the only hemodynamic variables that is an isolated indication for intervention (along with rate of AS progression). A peak velocity of greater than 5.0 m/s or less than 5.5 m/s is an indication for therapeutic intervention in the ACC/AHA and ESC/EACTS guidelines, respectively (Fig. 80.2).

Furthermore, although all of the aforementioned variables associated with hemodynamic impact of the stenosis are associated with worse outcomes, only rate of progression greater than 0.3 m/s per year is currently an indication for therapeutic intervention in the guideline documents.

Acceleration Time

With more severe AS, there is a progressive delay in achieving peak velocity, resulting in a late peaking murmur on cardiac auscultation and a prolonged acceleration slope of the continuous wave Doppler spectrum. This delay in acceleration time (AT) is measured precisely from the start of ejection to the peak velocity, and greater than 112 ms has been associated with worse clinical outcomes.[16] Because the AT is affected by heart rate, adjusting for ejection time (ET) helps to minimize underestimation of risk from tachycardia (Fig. 80.3). The role of this measure was initially identified in prosthetic valve assessment but has been shown to be of value in native valves as well. Griguer and coworkers found that an AT-to-ET ratio of 0.36 or greater conferred a 2.5-fold increased risk of mortality compared with an AT-to-ET ratio less than 0.36.

Energy Loss Index and Valvuloarterial Impedance

Valvular impedance is an assessment of the load exerted by the valvular stenosis as a function of flow across the valve. It is routinely assessed, even if not identified in those specific terms. The cumulative effect of valvular and arterial impedance (valvuloarterial impedance, Zva) is thought to be a more comprehensive measure of the total afterload on the left ventricle. Valvuloarterial impedance is

TABLE 80.1 Markers of Increased Risk in Asymptomatic Aortic Stenosis Patients Not Currently Incorporated Into the American College of Cardiology/American Heart Association Guidelines

Variable	Significant Value
BIOMARKERS	
• NT proBNP[6,13]	>3 times upper limit of normal
• Troponin[14,15]	hsTnI >9.5 ng/L
	hsTnT>10 ng/L
ECHOCARDIOGRAPHY FEATURES	
• Energy loss index[19]	<0.76 cm^2/m^2
• Valvuloarterial impedance[17,18]	>4.7 mm Hg/mL/m^2
• Acceleration time (AT) and ejection time (ET)[16]	AT >112 ms
	AT-to-ET ratio >0.36
• LVEF[21,22]	<55% (maybe even <60%)
• Global longitudinal strain[17,22]	<−16.0%
EXERCISE HEMODYNAMICS	
• Symptoms[6,7,20]	Any inducible symptoms typical of aortic stenosis
• Functional capacity[6,7,20]	<80% of age and gender predicted
• BP response[6,7,20]	<20 mm Hg rise in BP with peak exertion
• AoV gradients on echcardiogram[6]	Increase in mean gradient by >20 mm Hg
• PA systolic pressure[6,20]	PASP >60 mm Hg
MULTIMODALITY IMAGING FEATURES	
• Aortic valve calcification[10]	Female: >1274 Agatston units (AU)
	Male: >2065 AU
• Aortic valve calcium density[10]	Female: >292 AU/cm^2
	Male: >476 AU/cm^2
• Fibrosis on CMRI[14,23,24]	Midwall LGE or diffuse fibrosis by extracellular volume or T1 values

AoV, Aortic valve; *BP,* blood pressure; *CMRI,* cardiac magnetic resonance imaging; *hsTnI,* high-sensitivity troponin I; *hsTnT,* high-sensitivity troponin T; *LGE,* late gadolinium enhancement; *LVEF,* left ventricular ejection fraction; *NT proBNP,* N-terminal pro-brain natriuretic peptide; *PASP,* pulmonary artery systolic pressure.

Vpeak 4.6 m/sec
Δp mean 54 mm Hg

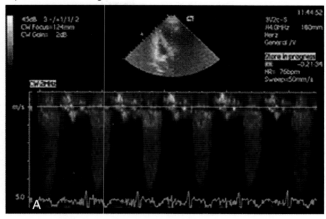

Vpeak 5.3 m/sec
Δp mean 75 mm Hg

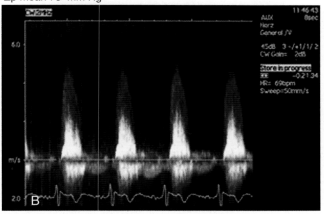

Figure 80.2. Continuous-wave Doppler recordings of an asymptomatic patient with severe aortic stenosis. Note that the recording from a right parasternal approach (**A**) yielded significantly higher velocities (peak velocity, 5.3 m/s; mean gradient, 75 mm Hg) than those obtained from an apical approach (**B**; peak velocity, 4.6 m/s; mean gradient, 54 mm Hg).

measured using the following equation: Zva = (mean gradient$_{AVA}$ + systolic arterial pressure)/stroke volume indexed to body surface area (BSA). Zito and coworkers showed that a Zva greater than 4.7 mm Hg/mL/m^2 was highly sensitive and specific for identifying patients who developed symptoms and required an AVR or died at 2 years.[17,18]

Building on knowledge obtained on pressure recovery, the energy loss index (ELI) tries to adjust for the impact of the aortic root on the conversion of kinetic energy to additional pressure gradient in the aortic root, which can lead to overestimation of AS severity by AVA alone. ELI is calculated using the following equation: ELI = (AVA × Aa)/(Aa − AVA)/BSA, in which Aa is the aortic area at the sinotubular junction. A lower ELI suggested more severe disease and a two- to sixfold increase in AVR and a twofold increase in mortality.[19] In this study, ELI was a better predictor than AVA but not of AVA indexed to BSA consistent with the concept that pressure recovery is largely caused by aortic root size, which is associated with body size.

Aortic Valve Morphology

Aortic valve morphology has classically been assessed with echocardiography and still remains the most important initial tool (Fig. 80.4). However, aortic valve calcification by gated MDCT has an emerging role in the assessment of morphology. Aortic valve calcification on MDCT is traditionally used to help identify the severity of valve stenosis, especially in low-gradient, low-flow symptomatic

severe AS patients. Clavel and associates showed an independent association of both severity of aortic valve calcification (AVC, reported in Agatston units) and aortic valve density (aortic valve calcification over cross-sectional area of the aortic annulus) with outcomes, even when controlling for gradients LV function, and routine clinical variables.[10] The 2017 ESC/EACTS guidelines included severe aortic valve calcification as a IIa indication for AVR. Given the integral role of gated MDCT in the workup and planning for TAVR, AVC can be readily assessed and offers the potential to identify asymptomatic patients who may benefit from early intervention.

Exercise Hemodynamics

Exercise stress testing is contraindicated in symptomatic patients with severe AS but is an integral part of the workup for patients with asymptomatic severe AS. Carefully monitored exercise stress testing provides important information on functional capacity, occult symptoms because of the gradual nature of the disease, and the ability to appropriately augment cardiac output. The definition of an abnormal ECG response to exercise ranges from 2 to 5 mm of ST-segment depression considering the influence of the highly prevalent LV hypertrophy; therefore, the guideline documents have largely avoided ST-segment depression as an indication for AVR. Inducible symptoms (angina, dyspnea, or altered cognition), less than 80% of age-predicted functional capacity, or a decrease in blood pressure with exercise are considered independent indications for AVR in both guideline documents.[6,7] Even an insufficient rise in systolic blood pressure of 20 mm Hg or greater is associated with poor outcomes.[20]

The role of exercise Doppler echocardiography is debated, and the 2014 ACC/AHA guideline document does not believe there is any additive value to support it, but the 2017 ESC/EACTS guideline did identify specific stress echocardiography factors that

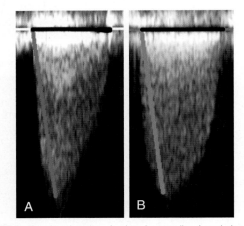

Figure 80.3. Acceleration time (*red* and *green lines*) and ejection time *(black lines)* measurements for two patients with peak velocities greater than 4 m/s. **A,** Acceleration time (AT) of 110 ms and ejection time (ET) of 300 ms with an AT-to-ET ratio of 0.37 (high clinical risk). **B,** AT of 100 ms and ET of 340 ms with an AT-to-ET ratio of 0.30 (low clinical risk).

would warrant AS intervention. An increase in exercise-induced mean gradients by more than 20 mm Hg, exercise-induced reduction in LV function, and exercise-induced pulmonary hypertension (systolic pulmonary artery pressure >60 mm Hg) are each associated with worse outcomes in asymptomatic patients with severe AS.[6]

Impact on the Left Heart

Finally, the true impact of AS cannot be assessed without a comprehensive understanding on the impact on the myocardium, specifically of the left ventricle. Resting assessment of LV function, chamber size, and hypertrophy were recognized early as markers of poor outcomes. In the SEAS trial, LV hypertrophy on ECG conferred a 2.5-fold increase risk of major adverse cardiovascular events.[29] The functional assessment of the left ventricle is still the cornerstone of echocardiography, but waiting for a reduction in global LV systolic function frequently results in a lower likelihood of function recovery. Guideline documents have used less than 50% as a marker for intervention. However, multiple studies have suggested that a higher cutoff ought to be used.[21,22] Bohbot and colleagues assessed 1678 patients with asymptomatic severe AS and identified that the optimal cutoff for left ventricular ejection fraction (LVEF) may be any reduction (<55%) to identify those at higher risk of clinical events.[21]

Other echocardiographic measures of LV systolic function identify patients with a preserved LVEF who are at risk for adverse events. Global longitudinal strain (GLS) has been integrated into guideline recommendations for other conditions, and multiple studies have assessed its role in AS. Patients with a reduced GLS below the lower limit of normal are consistently shown to be at a higher risk for worse clinical outcomes, although optimal cutoff values for determining this risk in asymptomatic AS is unclear.[17,18]

Given the importance of the left ventricle in the assessment of severity of AS, cardiac magnetic resonance imaging (CMRI) is a potentially vitally important tool as the reference standard for ventricular size and function as well as myocardial tissue characterization. Myocardial fibrosis is the hallmark of irreversible

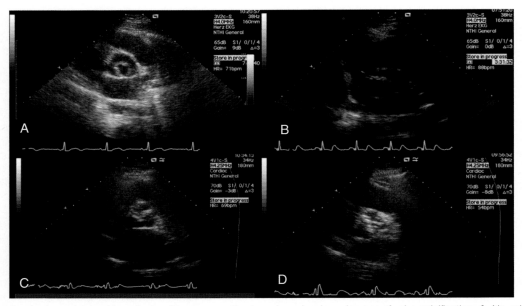

Figure 80.4. Short-axis views obtained in patients with severe aortic stenosis and various degrees of valve calcification. **A,** No calcification. **B,** Mild calcification. **C,** Moderate calcification. **D,** Severe calcification.

myocardial damage and can be assessed either by late gadolinium enhancement (LGE) or by extracellular volume assessment with T1 maps. Both have been associated with increased risk and can rapidly progress once identified, often before a drop in LVEF.[14,23,24] More important, both are associated with an increase in an increased risk for adverse clinical events.

EVOLVING UNDERSTANDING OF THE RISK OF THE INTERVENTION

Intrinsic to the risk–benefit discussion on an active monitoring and structured surveillance approach is the inherent risk of the intervention. SAVR has been the primary therapeutic modality tested in observational studies that suggest a risk-based approach to AVR is better than a symptom-based one. However, assessing superiority of this approach would largely require the outcomes be limited to mortality or heart failure hospitalizations and not including downstream AVR. SAVR as a routine strategy in either all or selected high-risk patients with asymptomatic severe AS has not been studied in a randomized controlled fashion. Without a standard risk stratification schema, conducting a randomized clinical trial for high-risk patients remains difficult.

Proposed new sentence: SAVR has an operative surgical risk that remains higher than the procedural risks from TAVR despite outstanding developments with anesthesia and circulatory support. As procedural risk decreases, the risk–benefit analysis favors early intervention. With the progressive shift to TAVR in lower risk patients, the natural question becomes whether TAVR in the routine management of patients with asymptomatic severe AS would improve outcomes. Although appealing in the short to midterm, there continues to be a question regarding long-term durability of TAVR valves that only time will resolve. Recent trials, such as those from the UK Transcatheter Aortic Valve Intervention (UK TAVI)

and Nordic Aortic Valve Intervention (NOTION) registries, show some promise out to approximately 10 years, but valve durability becomes extremely relevant when considering intervention in these lower risk, younger populations.[25,26]

FUTURE DIRECTIONS

Even with the growing data on risk stratification, the implementation of a more aggressive, risk-based approach to valve replacement needs to be studied. Multiple clinical trials are planned or actively enrolling to answer this question. The Evaluation of Transcatheter Aortic Valve Replacement Compared to SurveilLance for Patients With AsYmptomatic Severe Aortic Stenosis (EARLY TAVR) trial is looking at the early use of TAVR in severe asymptomatic AS. The Early Valve Replacement Guided by Biomarkers of LV Decompensation in Asymptomatic Patients With Severe AS (EVoLVeD) trial is looking at risk stratification using midwall LGE on CMRI with randomization of therapeutic interventions or monitoring frequency based on risk stratification.[5] One area not clearly addressed is the role of imaging to identify those at risk of progression. 18F-Sodium fluoride positron emission tomography may be able to identify individuals likely to have progression of aortic valve calcification.[27] Finally, given coexistent renal failure, imaging strategies that do not expose patients to risk of gadolinium will be clinically beneficial. Studies evaluating the use of echocardiographic correlates of fibrosis have an important role in the future.[28] With these tools, a more comprehensive risk stratification schema would help guide therapeutic trials in the hopes of improving outcomes in patients with asymptomatic severe AS (Fig. 80.5).

Acknowledgment

The authors acknowledge the contributions of Dr. Smith, who was the author of this chapter in the previous edition.

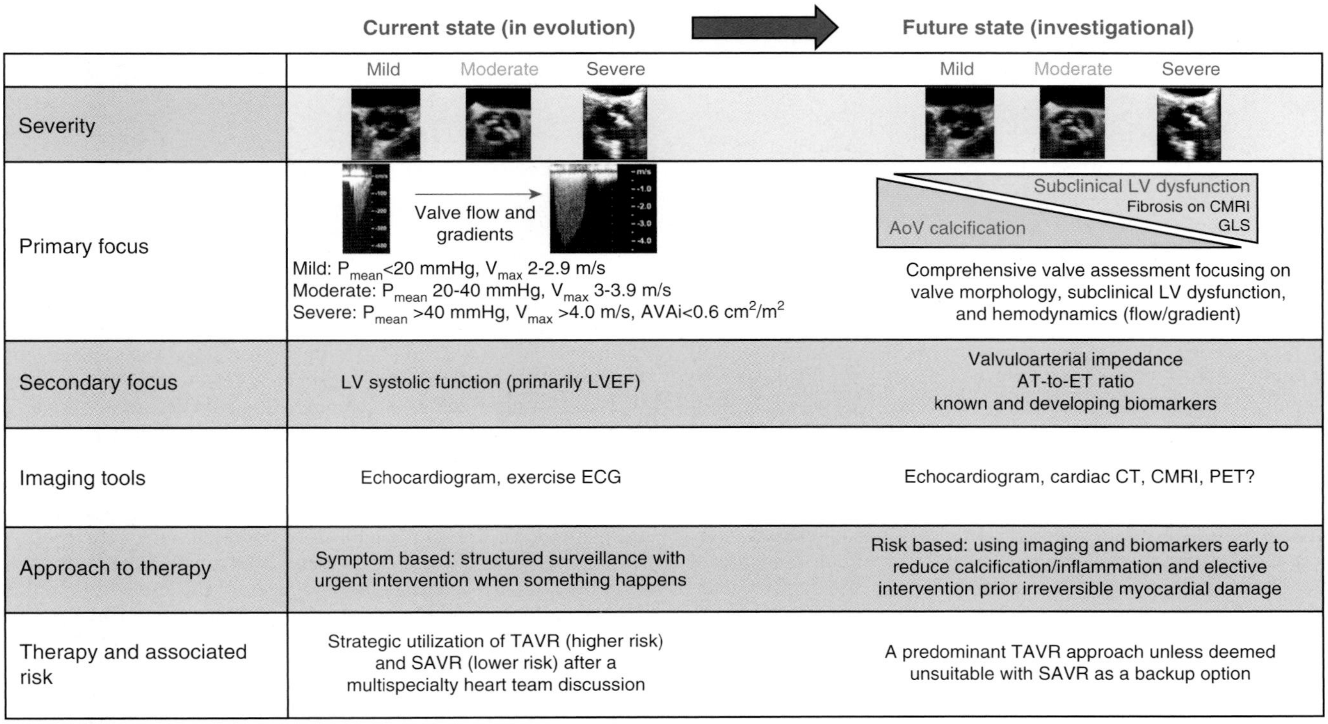

Figure 80.5. Current and proposed future state in the evaluation of aortic stenosis, including the tools for evaluation, the focus of therapeutic interventions, and the valve replacement strategies available. *AoV,* Aortic valve; *AT,* acceleration time; *CMRI,* cardiac magnetic resonance imaging; *CT,* computed tomography; *ECG,* electrocardiography; *ET,* ejection time; *GLS,* global longitudinal strain; *LV,* left ventricular; *LVEF,* left ventricular ejection fraction; *PET,* positron emission tomography; *SAVR,* surgical aortic valve replacement; *TAVR,* transcatheter aortic valve replacement.

REFERENCES

1. Lindman BR, Clavel MA, Mathieu P, et al. Calcified aortic stenosis. *Nat Rev Dis Primers*. 2016;2:16006.
2. Bonow RO, Greenland P. Population-wide trends in aortic stenosis incidence and outcomes. *Circulation*. 2015;131:969–971.
3. Nikomo VT, Gardin JM, Skelton TN, et al. Burden of valvular heart diseases: a population-based study. *Lancet*. 2006;368:1005–1011.
4. Généreux P, Stone G, O'Gara PT, et al. Natural history, diagnostic approaches, and therapeutic strategies for patients with asymptomatic severe aortic stenosis. *J Am Coll Cardiol*. 2016;67:2263–2288.
5. Lindman BR, Dweck MR, Lancellotti P, et al. Management of asymptomatic severe aortic stenosis: evolving concepts in timing of valve replacement. *J Am Coll Cardiol Imag*. 2019 (in press).
6. Baumgartner H, Falk V, Bax JJ, et al. 2017 ESC/EACTS Guidelines for the management of valvular heart disease. *Eur Heart J*. 2017;38(36):2739–2791.
7. Nishimura RA, Otto CM, Bonow RO, et al. 2017 AHA/ACC guideline for the management of patients with valvular heart disease: Executive summary: a report of the 2017 American College of Cardiology/American Heart Association Task Force on Practice Guidelines. *J Am Coll Cardiol*. 2014;63:2438–2488.
8. Campo J, Tsoris A, Kruse J, et al. Prognosis of severe asymptomatic aortic stenosis with and without surgery. *Ann Thorac Surg*. 2019;108:74–80.
9. Ersboll M, Schulte PJ, Alenezi F, et al. Predictors and progression of aortic stenosis in patients with preserved left ventricular ejection fraction. *Am J Cardiol*. 2015;115:86–92.
10. Clavel MA, Pibarot P, Messika-Zeitoun D, et al. Impact of aortic valve calcification, as measured by MDCT, on survival in patients with aortic stenosis: results of an international registry study. *J Am Coll Cardiol*. 2014;64:1202–1213.
11. Taniguchi T, Morimoto T, Shiomi H, et al. Initial surgical versus conservative strategies in patients with asymptomatic severe aortic stenosis. *J Am Coll Cardiol*. 2015;66:2827–2838.
12. Rogge BP, Cramariuc D, Lonnebakkan MT, et al. Effect of overweight and obesity on cardiovascular events in asymptomatic aortic stenosis: a SEAS Substudy (Simvastatin Ezetimibe in aortic stenosis). *J Am Coll Cardiol*. 2013;62:1683–1690.
13. Parikh V, Kim C, Siegel RJ, Arsanjani R, Rader F. Natriuretic peptides for risk stratification of patients with valvular aortic stenosis. *Circulation Heart Failure*. 2015;8:373–380.
14. Chin C, Shah A, McAllister DA, et al. High-sensitivity troponin I concentrations are a marker of an advanced hypertrophic response and adverse outcomes in patients with aortic stenosis. *European Heart J*. 2014;35:2312–2321.
15. Ferrer-Sistach E, Lupón J, Cediel G, et al. High-sensitivity troponin T in asymptomatic severe aortic stenosis. *Biomarkers*. 2019;24:334–340.
16. Griguer AR, Tribouilloy C, Truffier A, et al. Clinical significance of ejection dynamic parameters in patients with severe aortic stenosis: an outcomes study. *J Am Soc Echocardiogr*. 2018;31(5):551–560.
17. Lancellotti P, Donal E, Magne E, et al. Risk stratification in asymptomatic moderate to severe aortic stenosis: the importance of the valvular, arterial, and ventricular interplay. *Heart*. 2010;96:1364–1371.
18. Zito C, Salvia J, Cusma-Piccione M, et al. Prognostic significance of valvulo-arterial impedance and left ventricular longitudinal function in asymptomatic severe aortic stenosis involving three-cuspid valves. *Am J Cardiol*. 2011;108:1463–1469.
19. Bahlmann E, Gerdts E, Cramariuc D, et al. Prognostic value of energy loss index in asymptomatic aortic stenosis. *Circulation*. 2013;127:1149–1157.
20. Redfors B, Pibarot P, Gillam L, et al. White paper: stress testing in asymptomatic aortic stenosis. *Circulation*. 2017;135:1956–1976.
21. Bohbot Y, de Ravenstein C, Chadha G, et al. Relationship between left ventricular ejection fraction and mortality in asymptomatic and minimally symptomatic patients with severe aortic stenosis. *J Am Coll Cardiol Imag*. 2019;12:38–48.
22. Lancellotti P, Magne J, Dulgheru R, et al. Outcomes of patients with asymptomatic aortic stenosis followed up in heart valve clinics. *JAMA Cardiol*. 2018;3(11):1060–1068.
23. Chin C, Everett RJ, Kwiecinski J, et al. Myocardial fibrosis and cardiac decompensation in aortic stenosis. *J Am Coll Cardiol Imag*. 2017;10:1320–1333.
24. Dweck MR, Joshi S, Murigu T, et al. Midwall fibrosis is an independent predictor of mortality in patients with aortic stenosis. *J Am Coll Cardiol*. 2011;58:1271–1279.
25. Blackman DJ, Saraf S, MacCarthy PA, et al. Long-term durability of transcatheter aortic valve prostheses. *J Am Coll Cardiol*. 2019;73:537–545.
26. Søndergaard L, Ihlemann N, Capodanno D, et al. Durability of transcatheter and surgical bioprosthetic aortic valves in patients at lower surgical risk. *J Am Coll Cardiol*. 2019;73:546–553.
27. Dweck MR, Jenkins W, Vesey AT, et al. 18F-sodium fluoride uptake is a marker of active. *Circulation Cardiovasc Imag*. 2014;7:371–378.
28. Gaibazzi N, Bianconcini M, Marziliano N, et al. Scar detection by pulse-cancellation echocardiography: Validation by CMR in patients with recent STEMI. *J Am Coll Cardiol Imag*. 2016;9:1239–1251.
29. Greve AM, Boman K, Gohlke-Baerwolf C, et al. Clinical implications of electrocardiographic left ventricular strain and hypertrophy in asymptomatic patients with aortic stenosis: The Simvastatin and Ezetimibe in Aortic Stenosis Study. *Circulation*. 2012;125:346–353.

81 Aortic Stenosis: Risk Stratification and Timing of Surgery

Linda D. Gillam, Yash Patel

Echocardiography plays a pivotal role in decision making in patients with aortic stenosis (AS) and contributes to decision making for aortic valve replacement (AVR), as guided by the 2014 American Heart Association (AHA)/American College of Cardiology (ACC) Guideline for the Management of Patients with Valvular Heart Disease[1] and its 2017 Focused Update,[2] as well as the 2017 American College of Cardiology Appropriate Use Criteria Task Force/American Association for Thoracic Surgery/American Heart Association/American Society of Echocardiography/ European Association for Cardio-Thoracic Surgery/Heart Valve Society/Society of Cardiovascular Anesthesiologists/Society for Cardiovascular Angiography and Interventions/Society of Cardiovascular Computed Tomography/Society for Cardiovascular Magnetic Resonance/Society of Thoracic Surgeons (ACC/AATS/ AHA/ASE/EACTS/HVS/SCA/SCAI/SCCT/SCMR/STS) 2017 Appropriate Use Criteria for the Treatment of Patients With Severe Aortic Stenosis.[3] AS is relentlessly progressive. Although there is a long period when patients remain asymptomatic as disease progresses, when symptoms occur, AS becomes a malignant disease. The classic symptoms are those of heart failure, typically dyspnea and, to a lesser degree, evidence of low cardiac output, angina, and syncope or presyncope, the latter typically with exertion. The negative prognostic impact of symptoms was first described by Ross and Braunwald in 1968[4] in a group of patients with predominantly rheumatic and bicuspid AS whose symptoms onset in the patients' early 60s. Importantly, this observation was subsequently confirmed in the Partner I (Placement of Aortic Transcatheter Valves I) trial, in which inoperable patients who did not undergo transcatheter aortic valve replacement (TAVR) had a 1-year all-cause mortality rate greater than 50%. A survival benefit with surgical aortic valve replacement (SAVR) or TAVR has been a consistent finding. Thus, risk stratification and appropriate selection of patients for intervention is clinically important. The role of echocardiography is in identifying patients who are candidates for AVR. First, it establishes the diagnosis of severe AS, a topic covered in Chapters 78 and 79. The focus of this chapter is on patients with classical severe high-gradient AS (mean gradient ≥40 mm Hg, peak velocity ≥4 m/s, AVA ≤1.0 cm^2).

ASSESSMENT OF LEFT VENTRICULAR SYSTOLIC FUNCTION

The guidelines (Table 81.1) assign a class I indication for patients with severe AS and left ventricular (LV) systolic dysfunction defined as a left ventricular ejection fraction (LVEF) less than 50%. Echocardiographic methods for calculating LVEF are discussed in Chapters 23 and 24 along with the ASE Recommendations for Cardiac Chamber Quantitation with Echocardiography in Adults.[5] However, it has been noted that reduced LVEF (<50%)

is uncommon in AS (0.4%)[6] in the absence of symptoms that also carry a class I indication for intervention. It has been shown that patients with LVEFs of 50% to 59% are at increased risk versus those with LVEFs 60% or greater, and it has therefore been argued that a cutoff of 60% would be more appropriate.

Furthermore, since global longitudinal strain (GLS) was recognized to be a more sensitive index of LV systolic dysfunction than LVEF, a number of studies have explored its value in AS. Indeed, although abnormal LV strain has not yet transitioned to a guideline indication for intervention, it is important to note the expanding literature that speaks to the prognostic value of GLS in patients with severe AS. In a recent meta-analysis of 10 studies with 1067 individual participants with severe AS, all asymptomatic and with LVEF greater than 50%, Magne and coworkers reported that abnormal GLS was predictive of survival at 2- and 4-year follow-up (Fig. 81.1). An empiric cut-off of −14.7% best identified low- and high-risk groups, and the prognostic importance of GLS was particularly strong in those with LVEF of 60% or greater.[7] An example of this is shown in Fig. 81.2 in a patient with severe AS and LVEF of 62% with an abnormal GLS. These data support the general concept that LVEF below 50% is an insensitive marker of LV decompensation and that GLS has incremental value as a tool for risk stratification and perhaps identifying those who would benefit from intervention.[8]

UNMASKING SYMPTOMS IN "ASYMPTOMATIC" PATIENTS

Given the slow progression of AS, it is not surprising that symptoms may be insidious and that patients subconsciously slow down or otherwise restrict activity to avoid symptoms. Additionally, symptoms of AS may be erroneously attributed to aging or a comorbid condition. Thus, exercise stress testing, preferably with echocardiography is considered an essential step in the evaluation of patients with severe "asymptomatic" AS. Indeed it carries a class IIA indication in the current ACC/AHA guidelines for patients with classic severe AS (peak velocity ≥4 m/s and mean gradient ≥40 mm Hg)[1] and is an important consideration in many of the high-gradient AS scenarios in the appropriate use criteria.[3]

TABLE 81.1 Summary of Recommendations for Intervention for Aortic Stenosis: Timing of Intervention

Recommendation	Class of Recommendation /Level of Evidence
AVR is recommended for symptomatic patients with severe AS	I/B
AVR is recommended for asymptomatic patients severe AS (stage C2) when LVEF <50%	I/B
AVR is reasonable for asymptomatic patients with very severe AS (stage C1) (aortic velocity ≥5 m/s) and low surgical risk	IIa/B
AVR is reasonable in symptomatic patients with low-flow/low-gradient severe AS with reduced LVEF (stage D2) with a positive low-dose dobutamine stress study (increase in aortic velocity ≥4 m/s and aortic mean gradient ≥40 mm Hg, with a valve area <1 cm²)	IIa/B
AVR is reasonable in symptomatic patients with low-flow/low-gradient severe AS (stage D3) with LVEF ≥50% if clinical, hemodynamic, and anatomic data support AS as the most likely cause of symptoms	IIa/C
AVR is reasonable for patients with moderate AS (stage B) who are undergoing other cardiac surgery	IIa/C

AVR, Aortic valve replacement; *AS,* aortic stenosis; *LVEF,* left ventricular ejection fraction.
Modified with permission from Nishimura RA, et al. 2014 AHA/ACC guideline for the management of patients with valvular heart disease. *J Am Coll Cardiol* 2014; 63:e57–e85.

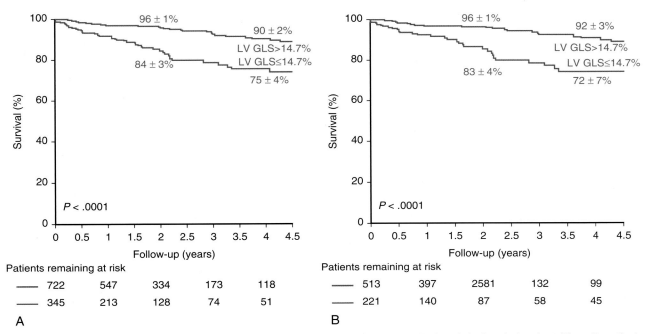

Figure 81.1. Kaplan-Meier survival curves stratified according to left ventricular global longitudinal strain in the whole cohort (**A**) and in patients with left ventricular ejection fraction of 60% (**B**). Percentage in the graphs are survival rate at 2- and 4-year follow-up. *LV GLS,* Left ventricular global longitudinal strain (Reproduced with permission from Magne J, et al. Distribution and prognostic significance of left ventricular global longitudinal strain in asymptomatic significant aortic stenosis. *JACC Cardiovasc Imag* 2019; 12:84.)

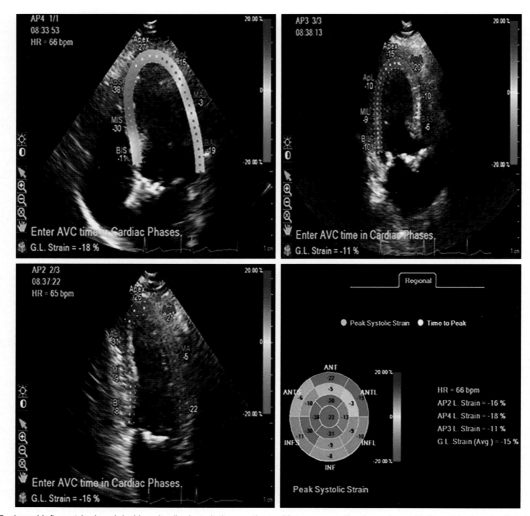

Figure 81.2. Reduced left ventricular global longitudinal strain in a patient with severe aortic stenosis and left ventricular ejection fraction of 62%. *AVC,* Aortic valve closure; *GL,* global longitudinal; *HR,* heart rate.

The implication of an exercise stress echocardiography (ESE) result that is positive, as defined by symptoms, is that the patient is considered to be symptomatic and therefore a candidate for AVR. Thus, exercise-induced symptoms carry class I indications for surgery in both the ACC/AHA[1] and ESC/EACTS Guidelines.[9] Other ESE outcomes including a decrease or a less than 20 mmHg increase in systolic blood pressure (BP),[10,11] mean gradient increase of greater than 18[10] or 20[12] mmHg, ventricular arrhythmias,[11,12] 2 mm or greater ST-segment depression,[10,11] and exercise-induced decrease in LVEF[13] have also been shown to be predictive of spontaneous symptom onset,[10-13] symptom-driven AVR,[10,12] and sudden cardiac death.[10-12] However, the link between ESE results other than symptoms and outcomes has not been entirely consistent,[14] and death has been a rare event typically occurring only after patients have become symptomatic.[11,12] In particular, electrocardiographic (ECG) changes have been reported to be inadequately discriminating,[14] particularly in women. ECG ST-segment changes are not specific when AS is present, with significant ST-segment depression seen in 80% of adults with AS regardless of whether coronary artery disease is present. Thus, these ESE measures of test positivity carry no (ECG changes, decrease in EF, ventricular arrhythmias) or only class IIA (decrease in BP)[1,2,9] or IIB (>20 mm Hg rise in gradient)[9] indications for AVR.

Although exercise-induced chest pain, presyncope, and syncope are fairly clear-cut, the interpretation of dyspnea is more difficult. For example, the dyspnea of patients with AS and concomitant lung disease may be caused by pulmonary rather than cardiac limitations, and even healthy individuals become short of breath with high-intensity or prolonged exercise, making the workload at which dyspnea occurs an important consideration. Indeed, Masri and colleagues[15] reported the incremental prognostic utility of reduced exercise tolerance (as defined by <85% age-gender predicted metabolic equivalents [METs] achieved) and slower 1-minute postexercise heart rate recovery after symptom-limited treadmill ESE with a primary outcome of all-cause mortality.

Although the authors used age- and gender-predicted METS achieved using the approaches of Morris and coworkers[16] for men and Gulati and coworkers[17] for women, it is worth noting that these references include few participants in the very old (older than 80 years) age groups in whom AS is typically encountered. Indeed, the nomograms provided in these references do not extend beyond age cut-offs of 70 to 75 years. Thus, there are challenges in establishing benchmarks for normal exercise performance in the typical patient with AS.

Recognizing the advanced age of many patients with AS, Naughton, modified Bruce, or manual protocols are often used. Physician presence for test supervision is essential. BP must be monitored carefully, and failure to augment BP is considered a positive response. Although concomitant coronary artery disease is not unusual, the default would be to attribute the chest pain to AS pending coronary angiography, although regional wall motion abnormalities and localizing ST-segment elevation may be helpful.

One-third of patients with severe AS who are "asymptomatic" in fact have exercise-limiting symptoms detected during exercise testing. Although exercise testing has been found to be relatively safe in asymptomatic patients, symptomatic patients with severe AS should not undergo exercise testing because of the high risk of complications, including syncope, ventricular tachycardia, and death.

OTHER ELEMENTS OF ECHOCARDIOGRAPHY-BASED RISK STRATIFICATION
Severity of Stenosis: Severe versus Very Severe

The prognostic importance of peak transvalvular velocity (Vmax) with an inflection point at 4 m/s helps form the foundation for the working definition of severe AS. However, there have been reports that even higher gradients (>5 m/s or >5.5 m/s) are additionally predictive of reduced event-free survival. Rosenhek and colleagues[18] first introduced the concept of very severe AS in a study of 116 asymptomatic patients with Vmax of 5 m/s or greater reporting high event rates, the majority undergoing aortic valve intervention but with a small number of deaths. Those with Vmax of 5.5 m/s or greater had statistically higher event rates versus those with Vmax of 5 to 5.49 m/s, and this provided the basis for a class IIA indication for surgical AVR in asymptomatic patients with preserved LVEF and Vmax of 5.5 m/s or greater in the European guidelines.[9]

More recently Bohbot and colleagues[19] revisited this topic in a study of more than 1000 total patients with severe AS (AVA ≤1 cm[2], Vmax ≥4 m/s) and preserved LVEF. After adjustment for covariates that included surgery, they reported similar all-cause mortality in those with velocities of 4 to 4.49 m/s and 4.5 to 4.99 m/s. However, those with peak velocities of 5 to 5.49 m/s and 5.5 m/s or greater exhibited a significant excess mortality rate compared with those with peak velocities of 4 to 4.49 m/s. However, risk was comparable between the two higher velocity groups. The authors argue that the European guidelines should lower the 5.5 m/s definition of very severe AS and adopt the 5-m/s cutoff used in the American guidelines in which surgery is considered reasonable (class IIA)[1] in those at low surgical risk and SAVR or TAVR are considered appropriate regardless of surgical risk in the appropriate use criteria.[3]

The likelihood of symptom onset increases as aortic velocity increases, with symptom onset within 1 year in 36% of those with an aortic velocity greater than 5 m/s and in 66% of those with a velocity greater than 5.5 m/s.

Valve Calcification

Although Agatston scoring with computed tomography is the preferred quantitative approach for assessing valve calcification, calcium burden and distribution may be assessed semiquantitatively with echocardiography. Severe calcification has been identified as a marker of increased risk of symptom onset and disease progression but has not been demonstrated to pose an increased risk of sudden death in the absence of symptoms. In the appropriate use criteria guidelines, this high-risk feature is associated with an appropriate indication for intervention, although medical management is identified as a "may be appropriate" alternative. At a minimum, the presence of heavy calcification may justify more frequent clinical and echocardiographic monitoring.

Rate of Progression

AS is a progressive disease with, on average, an increase in aortic jet velocity of 0.3 m/s per year or a decrease in valve area of 0.1 cm[2] per year.[20] More rapid disease progression is considered a high-risk feature with intervention deemed appropriate per appropriate use criteria guidelines, although ongoing medical management until symptom onset considered "may be appropriate." The presence of rapid disease progression may again justify more frequent clinical and echocardiographic monitoring.

Diastolic Function

Impaired diastolic function has been reported to be prognostically important in outcomes following AVR, a concept that has been best studied in the TAVR population. Additionally, patterns of diastolic function have been correlated with symptom type. However, there has, to date, been no suggestion that diastolic dysfunction per se should be a trigger for intervention or more frequent monitoring. However, the newly proposed classification system for AS based on cardiac damage may open additional study of diastolic dysfunction and associated pulmonary hypertension.[21]

CONCLUSION

After the severity is confirmed in a patient with AS, echocardiography can identify LV systolic dysfunction that provides a class I indication for AVR. Stress echocardiography is used to unmask symptoms that provide another class I indication for intervention with gradient and BP responses predictive of symptom onset. Other predictors of symptom onset include very high gradients (>5 m/s), calcium burden, and rapid progression.

Accordingly, the role of echocardiography extends beyond that of making the diagnosis of AS to identifying risks and triggers for valve replacement.

REFERENCES

1. Nishimura RA, Otto CM, Bonow RO, et al. AHA/ACC guideline for the management of patients with valvular heart disease. *J Am Coll Cardiol.* 2014;63:e57–e85. 2014.
2. Nishimura RA, Otto CM, Bonow RO, et al. AHA/ACC focused update of the 2014 AHA/ACC guideline for the management of patients with valvular heart disease. *J Am Coll Cardiol.* 2017;70:252–289. 2017.
3. Bonow RO, Brown AS, Gillam LD, et al. ACC/AATS/AHA/ASE/EACTS/HVS/SCA/SCAI/SCCT/SCMR/STS 2017 appropriate use criteria for the treatment of patients with severe aortic stenosis. *J Am Coll Cardiol.* 2017;70:2566–2598.
4. Ross J, Braunwald E. Aortic stenosis. *Circulation.* 1968;38:V–61.
5. Lang RM, Badano LP, Mor-Avi V, et al. Recommendations for cardiac chamber quantification by echocardiography in adults. *J Am Soc Echocardiogr.* 2007;28:1–39.
6. Henkel DM, Malouf JF, Connolly H, et al. Asymptomatic left ventricular systolic dysfunction in patients with severe aortic stenosis: characteristics and outcomes. *J Am Coll Cardiol.* 2012;60:2325–2329.
7. Magne J, Cosyns B, Popescu BA, et al. Distribution and prognostic significance of left ventricular global longitudinal strain in asymptomatic significant aortic stenosis. *JACC Cardiovasc Imag.* 2019;12:84.
8. Dahl JS, Magne J, Pellikka PA, et al. Assessment of subclinical left ventricular dysfunction in aortic stenosis. *JACC Cardiovasc Imag.* 2019;12:163.
9. Baumgartner H, Falk V, Bax JJ, et al. ESC/EACTS Guidelines for the management of valvular heart disease. *Eur Heart J.* 2017;38:2739–2791. 2017.
10. Lancellotti P, Lebois F, Simon M, et al. Prognostic importance of quantitative exercise Doppler echocardiography in asymptomatic valvular aortic stenosis. *Circulation.* 2005;112(9 suppl):I–377.
11. Amato MC, Moffa PJ, Werner KE, Ramires JA. Treatment decision in asymptomatic aortic valve stenosis: role of exercise testing. *Heart.* 2001;86:381–386.
12. Marechaux S, Hachicha Z, Bellouin A, et al. Usefulness of exercise-stress echocardiography for risk stratification of true asymptomatic patients with aortic valve stenosis. *Eur Heart J.* 2010;31:1390–1397.
13. Marechaux S, Ennezat PV, LeJemtel TH, et al. Left ventricular response to exercise in aortic stenosis: an exercise echocardiographic study. *Echocardiography.* 2007;24:955–959.
14. Das P, Rimington H, Chambers J. Exercise testing to stratify risk in aortic stenosis. *Eur Heart J.* 2005;26:1309–1313.
15. Masri A, Goodman A, Barr T, et al. Predictors of long-term outcomes in asymptomatic patients with severe aortic stenosis and preserved left ventricular systolic function undergoing exercise echocardiography. *Circ Cardiovasc Imag.* 2016;9. e004689.
16. Morris CK, Myers J, Froelicher VF, et al. Nomogram based on metabolic equivalents and age for assessing aerobic exercise capacity in men. *J Am Coll Cardiol.* 1993;22:175–182.
17. Gulati M, Black HR, Shaw LJ, et al. The prognostic value of a nomogram for exercise capacity in women. *New Engl J Med.* 2005;353:468–475.
18. Rosenhek R, Zilberszac R, Schemper M, et al. Natural history of very severe aortic stenosis. *Circulation.* 2010;121:151–156.
19. Bohbot Y, Rusinaru D, Delpierre Q, et al. Risk stratification of severe aortic stenosis with preserved left ventricular ejection fraction using peak aortic jet velocity. *Circ Cardiovasc Imag.* 2017;10. e006760.
20. Otto CM, Burwash IG, Legget ME, et al. Prospective study of asymptomatic valvular aortic stenosis: clinical, echocardiographic, and exercise predictors of outcome. *Circulation.* 1997;95:2262–2270.
21. Genereux P, Pibarot P, Redfors B, et al. Staging classification of aortic stenosis based on the extent of cardiac damage. *Eur Heart J.* 2017;38:3351–3358.

82 Low-Flow, Low-Gradient Aortic Stenosis With Reduced Left Ventricular Ejection Fraction

Mohamed-Salah Annabi, Marie-Annick Clavel, Philippe Pibarot, Jean G. Dumesnil

Low-flow, low-gradient (LF-LG) aortic stenosis (AS) with reduced left ventricular ejection fraction (LVEF) occurs in approximately 5% to 10% of patients with AS.[1-3] This entity is characterized by a small aortic valve area (AVA) compatible with severe AS (i.e., ≤1.0 cm^2 and/or ≤0.6 cm^2/m^2) combined with low mean transvalvular gradient (MG i.e., less than 40 mm Hg), a low LVEF (i.e., <50 %), and a low-flow state (i.e., stroke volume index [SVI] <35 mL/m^2; Video 82.1).[4,5] It is also commonly referred to as classical LF-LG or stage D2 AS and represents one of the most challenging subsets of patients in terms of diagnosis and treatment.[4] The left ventricular (LV) systolic dysfunction and ensuing low-flow state could result from an afterload mismatch[6,7] caused by the AS or from the combination of a preexistent myocardial disease and AS. The main diagnostic challenge in LF-LG AS with low-LVEF is to distinguish true-severe from pseudo-severe (i.e., incomplete opening of a moderately stenotic valve caused by a low-flow state) stenosis. The distinction between these two entities is crucial for therapeutic decision making. Patients with true-severe AS generally benefit from aortic valve replacement (AVR), whereas those with pseudo-severe AS may not. The prognosis is usually poor (3-year survival rates <50%) in patients with LF-LG treated medically, and operative mortality after surgical aortic valve replacement (SAVR) is high, ranging between 6% and 33% depending on the presence or the absence of LV flow reserve and other comorbidities.[8-15] Precise assessment of both the severity of AS and the degree of myocardial impairment is crucial for optimal risk stratification and therapeutic management in patients with LF-LG AS and reduced LVEF.

USEFULNESS OF DOBUTAMINE STRESS ECHOCARDIOGRAPHY FOR ASSESSMENT OF AS SEVERITY AND DEGREE OF MYOCARDIAL IMPAIRMENT

Low-dose (5–20 μg/kg/min) dobutamine stress echocardiography (DSE) has been shown to be useful to distinguish true-severe from pseudo-severe AS (Fig. 82.1).[16-19] For this purpose, it is recommended to use longer DSE stages (5–8 minutes) with infusion of dobutamine during 3 to 5 minutes and then acquisition of images once heart rate and hemodynamics have reached a steady state.[18] The LV outflow tract diameter is considered constant during DSE.[18,20] Assessing the severity of LV dysfunction usually relies on the magnitude of contractility improvement during DSE (i.e., contractile reserve).

ASSESSING STENOSIS SEVERITY

Some patients with mildly to moderately reduced LVEF and a large LV cavity may nonetheless generate a normal LV stroke volume (SV) and flow rate. However, the vast majority of patients with reduced LVEF are in low-flow state (SVI <35 mL/m^2 and mean flow rate <200 mL/s). In low-flow conditions, the AVA may overestimate and the gradient may underestimate the true stenosis severity. DSE is helpful in this context to reconcile the AVA–gradient discordance and thereby corroborate stenosis severity. The distinction between true versus pseudo-severe stenosis is essentially based

on the changes in AVA and gradients that occur with increasing flow rate during DSE (see Fig. 82.1). Typically, pseudo-severe AS shows a marked increase in AVA and little or no increase in gradients in response to increasing flow (case 1, Fig. 82.2A), whereas true-severe AS shows little or no increase in AVA and a marked increase in gradients which is congruent with the relative increase in flow (case 2, Fig. 82.2B). True-severe AS is generally defined by an AVA of 1.0 cm^2 or less and a MG of 40 mm Hg or greater at any stage during DSE.[4] However, only a minority of patients reaches a MG of 40 mm Hg or more during DSE, and the sensitivity of this criterion was recently reported to be as low as 35%,[19] whereas the prevalence of true-severe AS is reported as being between 65% and 80%.[18,19,21] Alternatively, a peak stress MG less than 30 mm Hg or a more sensitive peak stress AVA threshold of greater than 1.2 cm^2 have been proposed to rule out true severe AS.[16,17] Nevertheless, AVA and MG are flow dependent and are thus difficult to interpret without considering the relative changes in mean systolic flow rate (i.e., SV/LV ejection time). According to the Gorlin formula

$$\left(AVA = \frac{\text{Mean flow rate}}{44.3 * \sqrt{\text{Mean gradient}}}\right),$$ for a fixed AVA of 1.0 cm^2, a

normal flow rate of 250 to 280 mL/s is required to generate an MG of 40 mm Hg. In practice, 20% to 30% of the patients do not reach normal flow, and AVA and MG thus often remain discordant (e.g., patients 3 and 4, Fig. 82.2, C and E). Another 20% to 30% reach supranormal flow rates (>300 mL/s) during DSE, which may lead to a MG greater than 40 mm Hg but with an AVA greater than 1.0 cm^2; this situation is referred to as inverted discordant grading.

To overcome the inherent flow-dependency of MG and AVA, a new parameter derived from DSE, i.e., the projected AVA at normal flow rate (AVA$_{Proj}$) has been proposed (Fig. 82.2 D). Using the linear relationship between flow rate and AVA during DSE, it is possible to predict the AVA at a normal flow rate of 250 mL/s (which is approximately the median of the range of normal flow rate).[18,20] For example, in the case illustrated in Fig. 82.2C, the flow increased significantly with dobutamine but not enough to reach normal range. The AVA was 0.64 cm^2 at rest and increased up to 0.69 cm^2 (thus remaining "severe") at DSE, whereas the peak and mean gradients increased from 36/21 to 50/29 mm Hg (thus remaining "moderate"). In this patient, the calculation of the AVA$_{Proj}$ (0.79 cm^2) permits us to reconcile this AVA–gradient discordance that persists with DSE and thereby confirms that the AS is truly severe (see Fig. 82.2D).

AVA$_{Proj}$ 1.0 cm^2 or less, which is consistent with the AVA threshold proposed in the guidelines for severe stenosis in patients with normal LVEF, has been shown to be more accurate than traditional DSE criteria for the diagnosis of true AS severity. AVA$_{Proj}$ is also a predictor of mortality with conservative management unlike traditional DSE criteria.[11,18-20,22,23]

In about 10% of patients with LF-LG AS, the increase in mean flow rate induced by low-dose DSE is not sufficient (i.e., <15%) to induce significant changes in AVA or gradient and to obtain reliable estimate of AVA$_{Proj}$ (case 4, Fig. 82.2E). In this situation, DSE would be nondiagnostic and quantification of aortic valve calcification load by multidetector computed tomography (MDCT), a highly accurate and flow-independent parameter of anatomic AS may be

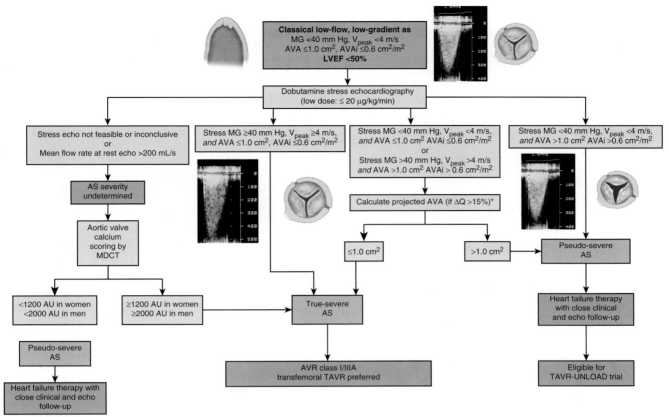

Figure 82.1. Algorithm for the diagnostic and therapeutic management of patients with low-flow, low-gradient aortic stenosis and reduced left ventricular ejection fraction (LVEF). *AU,* Arbitrary unit using the Agatston calcium scoring method; *AVA,* aortic valve area; *AVR,* aortic valve replacement; *MG,* mean transvalvular gradient; *projected AVA,* projected aortic valve area at normal flow rate (250 mL/s); *MDCT,* multidetector computed tomography; *TAVR,* transcatheter aortic valve replacement; *TAVR-UNLOAD trial,* Transcatheter Aortic Valve Replacement to UNload the Left Ventricle in Patients With ADvanced Heart Failure randomized trial; *ΔQ,* relative increase in mean flow rate (stroke volume/left ventricular ejection time); V_{Peak}, peak transvalvular velocity.

used to distinguish true-severe from pseudo-severe AS (Fig. 82.2F). Recommended cut-off values of aortic valve calcium load to identify severe AS are 1200 AU or greater in women and 2000 AU or greater in men (see Fig. 82.1).[24,25] In patients with normal flow rate at rest (>200 mL/s), that is, with normal-flow, low-gradient AS, it has been suggested that the AVA measured at rest reflects the true severity of AS and that DSE is thus not necessary.[26] It may, however, be preferable to corroborate AS severity by MDCT in these patients.[27]

ASSESSING THE DEGREE OF LV MYOCARDIAL IMPAIRMENT

Contractile reserve can be defined as the myocardial contractility that can be restored after AVR, the absence of which would suggest advanced LV myocardial impairment caused by terminal and extensive fibrotic remodeling. Given the high operative risk of low-LVEF, LF-LG AS,[9] assessing LV contractile reserve was proposed to estimate the surgical risk for AVR. LV flow reserve defined by a 20% or greater increase in SV during DSE, has been proposed and widely used as a surrogate of contractile reserve. According to a French multicenter study, patients with no LV flow reserve had much higher operative mortality rate (33%) than those with flow reserve (6%).[9] However, the postoperative improvement in LVEF as well as the late survival benefit are similar and good in both patients with flow reserve and those without flow reserve[12] and much better than in those with no flow reserve treated medically.[15] Hence, LV flow reserve by DSE may be useful to estimate operative risk for SAVR but not to predict recovery of LV function,

improvement in symptomatic status, or late survival after operation.[11–13,17] Importantly, the association between absence of flow reserve on DSE and surgical risk was not replicated in other studies.[13,18,23] More recently, absence of flow reserve on DSE did not correlate with the volume of LV myocardial diffuse fibrosis as assessed by magnetic resonance imaging in patients with LFLG AS[28] and did not associate with 30-day or 1-year mortality following transcatheter aortic valve replacement (TAVR)[29,30] or contemporary surgical AVR.[23] Hence, the assessment of LV flow reserve by DSE has limited utility in the current era, and the absence of LV flow reserve should not preclude consideration for AVR.[9,15,27,28]

Studies suggest that more precise assessment of the LV contractile reserve can be achieved by measuring the changes in global longitudinal myocardial strain and strain rate by speckle tracking imaging during DSE.[31] Others proposed the use of brain natriuretic peptide (BNP) to assess the extent of myocardial impairment, and this biomarker appears to be superior to flow reserve in predicting outcomes.[13] Further studies in larger number of patients are needed to determine the incremental prognostic value of these novel surrogates of LV impairment in patients with low LVEF, LF-LG AS.

THERAPEUTIC MANAGEMENT OF LOW-LVEF LOW-FLOW, LOW-GRADIENT AORTIC STENOSIS

According to American College of Cardiology and American Heart Association guidelines, AVR is a class IIa (level of evidence B) for symptomatic patients with low-LVEF, LF-LG AS showing a high gradient (MG >40 mm Hg) during DSE.[4] The 2017 European Society

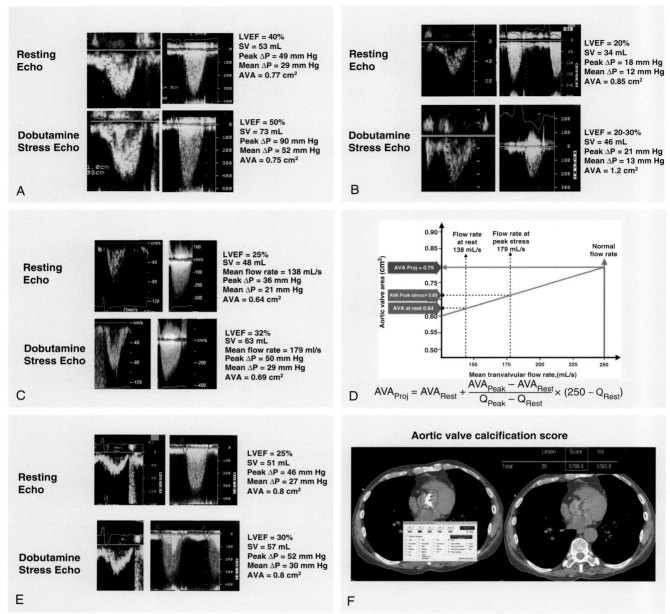

Figure 82.2. Illustrative cases of patients with low-flow, low-gradient aortic stenosis (AS) and reduced left ventricular ejection fraction (LVEF). **A,** Case 1: a patient with true severe AS, that is, with findings consistent with concordant severe stenosis (mean gradient >40 mm Hg and <1.0 cm^2) at flow normalization. **B,** Case 2: a patient with pseudo-severe stenosis, that is, with findings consistent with concordant moderate stenosis (mean gradient <40 mm Hg and aortic valve area [AVA] >1.0 cm^2) at peak stress. **C,** Case 3: a patient with persisting discordant AS grading (i.e., AVA <1.0 cm^2 and mean gradient <40 mm Hg at peak stress). **D,** Determination of AS severity in case 3 using projected AVA at a normal flow rate. Using the linear relation between AVA and mean flow rate, it is possible to determine the value of AVA had the patient reached a normal flow rate of 250 mL/s. **E,** Case 4: a patient with persisting discordant AS grading and insufficient flow rate increase to reliably calculate projected AVA. **F,** Aortic valve calcium score measured in case 4 by multidetector computed tomography. The high calcium score (6788 AU) suggests the presence of a true-severe aortic stenosis in this patient. *AV,* Aortic valve; *AVA$_{Rest}$* and *Q$_{Rest}$,* AVA and Q at rest; *AVAi,* aortic valve area indexed to body surface area; *Echo,* echocardiogram; *ΔP,* transvalvular gradient; *Q,* mean transvalvular flow rate (Q is calculated with the formula, $Q = SV/LVET$ *(mL/s),* in which *SV,* stroke volume and *LVET,* left ventricular ejection time); *SV,* stroke volume.

of Cardiology/European Association for Cardio-Thoracic Surgery guidelines[25] give a class I indication (level of evidence: C) to the consideration of AVR in the subset of patients with LV flow reserve and evidence of true-severe AS (as defined by peak stress AVA <1.0 cm^2) and a class IIa (level of evidence: C) in the absence of flow reserve if true-severe AS is confirmed by aortic valve calcium scoring by MDCT.

TAVR is a valuable alternative to surgical aortic valve replacement (SAVR), especially in patients with high or intermediate surgical risk (see Fig. 82.1).[32] TAVR was reported to be associated with lower incidence of severe prosthesis patient mismatch, which may be more detrimental in patients with LF-LG AS[2] and better LVEF improvement compared with SAVR.[33,34] With late generations of transcatheter heart valves, the incidence of moderate to severe paravalvular regurgitation is low. Nevertheless, even mild paravalvular regurgitation can be detrimental in patients with low-LVEF LF-LG AS.[35] Further studies are needed to determine whether TAVR provides better outcome than surgical AVR in patients with low LVEF, LF-LG AS.

Patients with pseudo-severe AS (case 2; see Fig. 82.2B) should be managed with optimal heart failure therapy and followed closely (see Fig. 82.1). However, several studies suggest that less stringent cut-off values (e.g., AVA or $AVA_{Proj} \leq 1.2$ cm^2 vs 1.0 cm^2) would be more appropriate for patients with reduced LVEF, suggesting that a certain proportion of patients with pseudo-severe AS may likely benefit from AVR.[11,16,19,20] This is consistent with the concept that the increased LV afterload imposed by a moderate AS may be well tolerated by a healthy ventricle but poorly tolerated by a failing ventricle. Recent studies suggest that patients with systolic heart failure and moderate AS have poor outcomes despite optimal heart failure therapy.[36] The benefit and safety of early transfemoral TAVR in patients with moderate AS and systolic heart failure are currently being tested in the context of the Transcatheter Aortic Valve Replacement to UNload the Left Ventricle in Patients With ADvanced Heart Failure (TAVR-UNLOAD) trial.

CONCLUSIONS

LF-LG AS with reduced LVEF is among the most challenging conditions encountered in patients with valvular heart disease. DSE greatly aids clinical decision making in these patients by allowing the differentiation of true versus pseudo-severe stenosis. The calculation of AVA_{Proj} may be useful to corroborate stenosis severity in patients with persisting AVA–gradient discordance at DSE. Aortic valve calcium quantification by MDCT can differentiate true versus pseudo-severe stenosis in patients with no significant increase in flow rate and in whom DSE remains inconclusive. In patients with low-LVEF, LFLG and confirmed true-severe AS, AVR is recommended, and transfemoral TAVR may be preferred. The absence of flow reserve during DSE should not preclude AVR especially when considering TAVR. Patients with pseudo-severe AS should be followed closely because even a moderate AS may be detrimental in patients with depressed LVEF.

Please access ExpertConsult to view the corresponding video for this chapter.

REFERENCES

1. Pibarot P, Gertz Z, Herrmann H, et al. Outcomes of the different flow/gradient patterns of aortic stenosis after aortic valve replacement: insights from partner 2A trial. *J Am Coll Cardiol.* 2017;69(11 suppl):1036.
2. Kulik A, Burwash IG, Kapila V, et al. Long-term outcomes after valve replacement for low-gradient aortic stenosis: impact of prosthesis-patient mismatch. *Circulation.* 2006;114:I5553–I5558.
3. Lauten A, Figulla HR, Mollmann H, et al. TAVI for low-flow, low-gradient severe aortic stenosis with preserved or reduced ejection fraction: a subgroup analysis from the German Aortic Valve Registry (GARY). *EuroIntervention.* 2014;10:850–859.
4. Nishimura RA, Otto CM, Bonow RO, et al. AHA/ACC focused update of the 2014 AHA/ACC guideline for the management of patients with valvular heart disease. *J Am Coll Cardiol.* 2017;70:252–289. 2017.
5. Baumgartner H, Hung J, Bermejo J, et al. Recommendations on the echocardiographic assessment of aortic valve stenosis. *J Am Soc Echocardiogr.* 2017;30:372–392.
6. Carabello BA, Green LH, Grossman W, et al. Hemodynamic determinants of prognosis of aortic valve replacement in critical aortic stenosis and advanced congestive heart failure. *Circulation.* 1980;62:42–48.
7. Ito S, Miranda WR, Nkomo VT, et al. Reduced left ventricular ejection fraction in patients with aortic stenosis. *J Am Coll Cardiol.* 2018;71:1313–1321.
8. Connolly HM, Oh JK, Schaff HV, et al. Severe aortic stenosis with low transvalvular gradient and severe left ventricular dysfunction. Result of aortic valve replacement in 52 patients. *Circulation.* 2000;101:1940–1946.
9. Monin JL, Quere JP, Monchi M, et al. Low-gradient aortic stenosis: operative risk stratification and predictors for long-term outcome: a multicenter study using dobutamine stress hemodynamics. *Circulation.* 2003;108:319–324.
10. Schwammenthal E, Vered Z, Moshkowitz Y, et al. Dobutamine echocardiography in patients with aortic stenosis and left ventricular dysfunction: predicting outcome as a function of management strategy. *Chest.* 2001;119:1766–1777.
11. Clavel MA, Fuchs C, Burwash IG, et al. Predictors of outcomes in low-flow, low-gradient aortic stenosis: results of the multicenter TOPAS Study. *Circulation.* 2008;118:S234–S242.
12. Quere JP, Monin JL, Levy F, et al. Influence of preoperative left ventricular contractile reserve on postoperative ejection fraction in low-gradient aortic stenosis. *Circulation.* 2006;113:1738–1744.
13. Bergler-Klein J, Mundigler G, Pibarot P, et al. B-type natriuretic peptide in low-flow, low-gradient aortic stenosis: relationship to hemodynamics and clinical outcome. *Circulation.* 2007;115:2848–2855.
14. Pai RG, Varadarajan P, Razzouk A. Survival benefit of aortic valve replacement in patients with severe aortic stenosis with low ejection fraction and low gradient with normal ejection fraction. *Ann Thorac Surg.* 2008;86:1781–1789.
15. Tribouilloy C, Levy F, Rusinaru D, et al. Outcome after aortic valve replacement for low-flow/low-gradient aortic stenosis without contractile reserve on dobutamine stress echocardiography. *J Am Coll Cardiol.* 2009;53:1865–1873.
16. Fougères F, Tribouilloy C, Monchi M, et al. Outcomes of pseudo-severe aortic stenosis under conservative treatment. *Eur Heart J.* 2012;33:2426–2433.
17. Nishimura RA, Grantham JA, Connolly HM, et al. Low-output, low-gradient aortic stenosis in patients with depressed left ventricular systolic function: the clinical utility of the dobutamine challenge in the catheterization laboratory. *Circulation.* 2002;106:809–813.
18. Blais C, Burwash IG, Mundigler G, et al. Projected valve area at normal flow rate improves the assessment of stenosis severity in patients with low flow, low-gradient aortic stenosis: the multicenter TOPAS (Truly or Pseudo Severe Aortic Stenosis) study. *Circulation.* 2006;113:711–721.
19. Annabi MS, Touboul E, Dahou A, et al. Dobutamine stress echocardiography for management of low-flow, low-gradient aortic stenosis. *J Am Coll Cardiol.* 2018;71:475–485.
20. Clavel MA, Burwash IG, Mundigler G, et al. Validation of conventional and simplified methods to calculate projected valve area at normal flow rate in patients with low flow, low gradient aortic stenosis: the multicenter TOPAS (True or Pseudo Severe Aortic Stenosis) study. *J Am Soc Echocardiogr.* 2010;23:380–386.
21. Fischer-Rasokat U, Renker M, Liebetrau C, et al. 1-year survival after TAVR of patients with low-flow, low-gradient and high-gradient aortic valve stenosis in matched study populations. *JACC Cardiovasc Interv.* 2019;12:752–763.
22. Kusunose K, Yamada H, Nishio S, et al. Preload stress echocardiography predicts outcomes in patients with preserved ejection fraction and low-gradient aortic stenosis. *Circ Cardiovasc Imag.* 2017;10.
23. Sato K, Sankaramangalam K, Kandregula K, et al. Contemporary outcomes in low-gradient aortic stenosis patients who underwent dobutamine stress echocardiography. *J Am Heart Assoc.* 2019;8:e011168.
24. Clavel MA, Messika-Zeitoun D, Pibarot P, et al. The complex nature of discordant severe calcified aortic valve disease grading: new insights from combined Doppler-echocardiographic and computed tomographic study. *J Am Coll Cardiol.* 2013;62:2329–2338.
25. Baumgartner H, Falk V, Bax JJ, et al. ESC/EACTS Guidelines for the management of valvular heart disease. *Eur Heart J.* 2017;38:2739–2791. 2017.
26. Chahal NS, Drakopoulou M, Gonzalez-Gonzalez AM, et al. Resting aortic valve area at normal transaortic flow rate reflects true valve area in suspected low-gradient severe aortic stenosis. *JACC Cardiovasc Imag.* 2015;8:1133–1139.
27. Clavel MA, Guzzetti E, Annabi MS, et al. Normal-flow low-gradient severe aortic stenosis: Myth or reality? *Structural Heart.* 2018;2:180–187.
28. Rosa VEE, Ribeiro HB, Sampaio RO, et al. Myocardial fibrosis in classical low-flow, low-gradient aortic stenosis. *Circ Cardiovasc Imag.* 2019;12:e008353.
29. Ribeiro HB, Lerakis S, Gilard M, et al. Transcatheter aortic valve replacement in patients with low-flow, low-gradient aortic stenosis: the TOPAS-TAVI registry. *J Am Coll Cardiol.* 2018;71:1297–1308.
30. Buchanan KD, Rogers T, Steinvil A, et al. Role of contractile reserve as a predictor of mortality in low-flow, low-gradient severe aortic stenosis following transcatheter aortic valve replacement. *Catheter Cardiovasc Interv.* 2019;93:707–712.
31. Dahou A, Bartko PE, Capoulade R, et al. Usefulness of global left ventricular longitudinal strain for risk stratification in low ejection fraction, low-gradient aortic stenosis: results from the multicenter True or Pseudo-Severe Aortic Stenosis study. *Circ Cardiovasc Imag.* 2015;8:e002117.
32. Herrmann HC, Pibarot P, Hueter I, et al. Predictors of mortality and outcomes of therapy in low flow severe aortic stenosis: a PARTNER trial analysis. *Circulation.* 2013;127:2316–2326.
33. Clavel MA, Webb JG, Rodés-Cabau J, et al. Comparison between transcatheter and surgical prosthetic valve implantation in patients with severe aortic stenosis and reduced left ventricular ejection fraction. *Circulation.* 2010;122:1928–1936.
34. Clavel MA, Webb JG, Pibarot P, et al. Comparison of the hemodynamic performance of percutaneous and surgical bioprostheses for the treatment of severe aortic stenosis. *J Am Coll Cardiol.* 2009;53:1883–1891.
35. Chrysohoou C, Hayek SS, Spilias N, Lerakis S. Echocardiographic and clinical factors related to paravalvular leak incidence in low-gradient severe aortic stenosis patients post-transcatheter aortic valve implantation. *Eur Heart J Cardiovasc Imag.* 2015;16:558–563.
36. van Gils L, Clavel MA, Vollema EM, et al. Prognostic implications of moderate aortic stenosis in patients with left ventricular systolic dysfunction. *J Am Coll Cardiol.* 2017;69:2383–2392.

83 Low-Flow, Low-Gradient Aortic Stenosis With Preserved Left Ventricular Ejection Fraction

Ezequiel Guzzetti, Florent Le Ven, Marie-Annick Clavel, Philippe Pibarot, Jean G. Dumesnil

Low-flow, low-gradient (LF-LG) aortic stenosis (AS) is characterized by a small aortic valve area (AVA<1.0 cm^2), a low gradient (mean <40 mm Hg), and a low-flow state (stroke volume index [SVI] <35 mL/m^2). The LF-LG AS pattern may occur in the context of either a reduced (i.e., "classical" low-flow; see Chapter 82) or preserved (i.e., "paradoxical" low-flow) left ventricular ejection fraction (LVEF).[1–3] Besides classical and paradoxical LF-LG AS, there is another entity called normal-flow, low-gradient AS that is characterized by a small AVA and low gradient but with a normal SVI and a preserved LVEF (Fig. 83.1).[4] In these patients with normal-flow, low-gradient AS, the SVI is normal, but the mean flow rate (stroke volume [SV]/left ventricular [LV] ejection time) is generally low (<200 mL/s). The purpose of this chapter is to provide an update on the Doppler echocardiographic assessment of paradoxical LF-LG AS.

CLINICAL PRESENTATION AND PATHOPHYSIOLOGY OF PARADOXICAL LOW-FLOW, LOW-GRADIENT AORTIC STENOSIS

Paradoxical LF-LG AS is defined as a small AVA (i.e., AVA<1.0 cm^2 and indexed AVA<0.6 cm^2/m^2), a low gradient (i.e., <40 mm Hg), a low flow (i.e., SVI <35 mL/m^2), and a preserved LVEF (i.e., ≥50%). The reported prevalence of this entity includes 5% to 25% of AS patients and has been shown to increase with age, female gender, and concomitant presence of systemic arterial hypertension, metabolic syndrome, or diabetes.[3] The cumulative effect of one or more of these factors contributes to more pronounced or exaggerated LV concentric remodeling, the development of myocardial fibrosis, and, as a result, reduction in the size, compliance, and filling of the LV

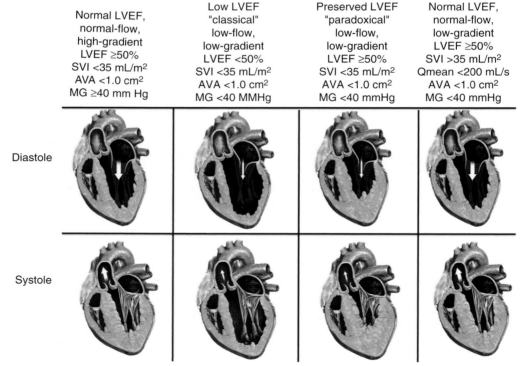

| Normal LVEF, normal-flow, high-gradient LVEF ≥50% SVI <35 mL/m^2 AVA <1.0 cm^2 MG ≥40 mm Hg | Low LVEF "classical" low-flow, low-gradient LVEF <50% SVI <35 mL/m^2 AVA <1.0 cm^2 MG <40 MMHg | Preserved LVEF "paradoxical" low-flow, low-gradient LVEF ≥50% SVI <35 mL/m^2 AVA <1.0 cm^2 MG <40 mmHg | Normal LVEF, normal-flow, low-gradient LVEF ≥50% SVI >35 mL/m^2 Qmean <200 mL/s AVA <1.0 cm^2 MG <40 mmHg |

Figure 83.1. Different patterns of severe aortic stenosis (AS) according to flow, gradient, and left ventricular (LV) geometry in cases of preserved left ventricular ejection fraction (LVEF). The majority of patients with severe AS develop LV hypertrophy with normal LV cavity size (*left*), which allows maintenance of normal LV pump function. These patients with severe AS and normal transvalvular flow generally exhibit a high gradient. In contrast, patients with low LVEF, "classical" low-flow, low-gradient AS (*middle*) are characterized by a dilated left ventricle with markedly decreased LV systolic function most often caused by ischemic heart disease or afterload mismatch. On the other hand, normal LVEF, "paradoxical" low-flow, low-gradient AS (*right*) is characterized by pronounced LV concentric remodeling, leading to impaired filling and reduced pump function. Because of the low flow state, the patients in the two latter categories may present with a low gradient despite presence of severe stenosis. *AVA,* Aortic valve area; *MG,* mean transvalvular gradient; *SVI,* stroke volume index. (Adapted with permission from Pibarot P, Dumesnil JG: Low-flow, low-gradient aortic stenosis with normal and depressed left ventricular ejection fraction, *J Am Coll Cardiol* 2012;60:1845–1853.)

TABLE 83.1 Clinical and Doppler Echocardiographic Features of Paradoxical Low-Flow, Low-Gradient Aortic Stenosis

CLINICAL CHARACTERISTICS

Older age

Predominantly women

Frequent comorbidities: systemic hypertension, metabolic syndrome, diabetes

Atrial fibrillation

Doppler Echocardiographic Features

Aortic Valve

Severely thickened and calcified valve with reduced opening

AVA <1.0 cm^2, AVAi <0.6 cm^2/ m^2, DVI <0.25

Mean transvalvular gradient <40 mm Hg

Valvuloarterial impedance >4.5 mm Hg.mL^{-1}.m^2

Left Ventricle

Ejection fraction ≥50%

Small cavity size:

• End-diastolic diameter <47 mm[a]

• End-diastolic volume <55 mL.m^{-2a}

Relative wall thickness ratio >0.5

Impaired LV filling

Impaired GLS: <15%[a]

SVI <35 mL/m^2

Transvalvular flow rate <200 mL/s[a]

Other Valves

Mitral regurgitation or stenosis

Tricuspid regurgitation

[a]Values based on initial retrospective studies[1,7,12,30] and are given as an indication. Further investigations are needed to determine more precise cut points.

AVA, Aortic valve area; *AVAi,* aortic valve area indexed to body surface area; *DVI,* Doppler velocity index; *GLS,* global longitudinal strain; *LV,* left ventricular; *SVI,* stroke volume index.

cavity (see Fig. 83.1).[1,5,6] Moreover, LV systolic function, which is apparently normal when only observing the LVEF, is, in fact, substantially reduced when considering global LV longitudinal strain. Longitudinal strain has been shown to be more sensitive to detect subclinical alterations of intrinsic myocardial systolic function.[6,7] Hence, decreased SV in paradoxical LF-LG AS is predominantly caused by impaired LV filling but also in part by abnormal LV emptying. Table 83.1 summarizes the main clinical and Doppler echocardiographic features of paradoxical LF-LG AS, and Fig. 83.2 and Video 83.2 present an example of a patient with this entity. It is also important to emphasize that several other factors, besides the restrictive LV physiology, may also contribute to the reduction of LV forward SV in patients with AS and preserved LVEF, including reduced arterial compliance, atrial fibrillation, concomitant mitral regurgitation, mitral stenosis, or tricuspid regurgitation.[1,8–10]

The presence of a low-flow state in the context of preserved LVEF complicates the assessment of stenosis severity and therapeutic decision making. Patients with paradoxical LF-LG severe AS have a 40% to 50% lower referral to surgery compared with patients with the expected normal-flow, high-gradient pattern of AS, likely because of underestimation of stenosis severity consequently to the relatively low gradient.[2,11] Yet several studies have demonstrated that these patients have worse prognosis compared with those with normal-flow, high-gradient AS and have much better prognosis when treated surgically than medically.[2,5,6,9,12–16]

Assessment of Flow and Stenosis Severity

The main pitfall associated with the echocardiographic diagnosis of paradoxical LF-LG AS is an error in the calculation of the Doppler SV caused by inaccurate measurement of LV outflow tract (LVOT) diameter or misplacement of pulsed-wave Doppler sample volume.[3,17,18] Indeed, an underestimation of SV may lead to the erroneous conclusion that the patient has paradoxical LF-LG severe AS, whereas, in fact, the stenosis is moderate with normal flow (referred to as pseudo-severe AS). Conversely, an overestimation of SV may lead to the misidentification and gross underestimation of the prevalence of the entity.[11]

Hence, when confronted with a patient with discordant AVA-gradient finding and preserved LVEF, the first step in the diagnostic and therapeutic management algorithm presented in Fig. 83.3 should be to rule out measurement errors in the estimation of SV and thereby confirm the presence of low flow.[10] The most frequent cause of error in the measurement of the Doppler SV is underestimation of the LVOT diameter. The LVOT cross-section is often elliptical and the diameter measured by two-dimensional (2D) echocardiography in the parasternal long-axis view is the anteroposterior diameter, which is generally the smaller diameter of the ellipse. To attenuate this limitation, it is preferable to measure the LVOT diameter at the base of the aortic valve cusps (where the LVOT is more circular) rather than 5 to 10 mm below the aortic annulus.[17] Also, three-dimensional (3D) transthoracic or transesophageal echocardiography or multidetector computed tomography (MDCT) may be used to obtain a more accurate estimation of the LVOT cross-sectional area. Hybrid methods (i.e., using LVOT area measured by MDCT 3D echocardiography and velocity time integral [VTI] from Doppler echocardiography) may be helpful in these patients but are also subject to significant pitfalls.[10] Indeed, hybrid methods measure systematically larger AVAs compared with standard Doppler echocardiography, and as a consequence, one should apply a larger AVA threshold for defining severe AS (≤1.2 vs ≤1.0 cm^2) when using hybrid methods.[19] Another option to rule out a possible error in the measurement LVOT diameter is to use the Doppler velocity index (i.e., the ratio between the VTI in the LVOT divided by the VTI in the aorta). This parameter should be in accordance with AVA regarding AS severity: if AVA is 1 cm^2 or less, the VTI ratio should be 0.25 or less. A discordance between AVA and DVI should raise the concern of error in the measurement of LVOT diameter.

When paradoxical LF-LG AS is suspected, measurements of LV geometry and function should first be reviewed with the expectation of finding typical echocardiographic features characterizing this entity: pronounced concentric remodeling, small LV cavity size, reduced global longitudinal strain, and so on (see Table 83.1 and Fig. 83.3). Second, the measurement of LVOT SV by the Doppler method should be systematically corroborated by other means such as comparisons of LVEF estimated by the Dumesnil method (Doppler SV/LV end-diastolic volume calculated with the Teichholz formula) with the LVEF obtained by the biplane Simpson or visual method. If the LVEF by the Dumesnil method is substantially lower than the LVEF estimated to be right, then one should strongly suspect that the Doppler SV has been underestimated. On the other hand, overestimation by the Dumesnil method may be caused by overestimation of SV but is less specific since the Dumesnil's LVEF may overestimate the true LVEF in the case of very small ventricles.[20] 2D volumetric methods can also be used but with caution because the images of the LV are frequently foreshortened and may lead to gross underestimations of volumes. Third, it is important to also identify other potential causes of low flow such as concomitant systemic arterial hypertension, mitral regurgitation or stenosis, tricuspid regurgitation, or atrial fibrillation. If these conditions are present, the antegrade stoke volume may be reduced despite the absence of some of the typical features of paradoxical low-flow gradient described in Table 83.1.

The second step in the algorithm (see Fig. 83.3) is to assess the presence of symptoms. In patients who claim to be asymptomatic or in those with equivocal symptoms (frequent in the older adult AS population), exercise testing may be considered to confirm the symptomatic status.[21] "Truly" asymptomatic patients should be managed with close follow-up, and no additional diagnostic tests are required. In symptomatic patients, the third step of the algorithm is to assess the presence of concomitant hypertension (see Fig. 83.3). Hypertension may indeed contribute to the low-flow state and to the symptoms.[8] In this context, patients with paradoxical LF-LG often have reduced arterial compliance, increased vascular resistance, or both.[1,6,8] However, because of the low-flow state, the blood pressure may be lower than expected or "pseudo-normalized," similar to what may occur in the case of the transvalvular gradient, and as a consequence, the presence and severity of hypertension may be underestimated in these patients.[11,22] Hence, blood pressure should be systematically measured at the time of the echocardiographic examination,[10] and arterial compliance as well as vascular resistance should be calculated.[1] If the presence of hypertension is confirmed, antihypertensive therapy should be instituted or optimized, and the echocardiographic parameters and symptoms should then be reassessed after normalization of arterial hemodynamics (i.e., systolic blood pressure ≤140 mm Hg) (see Fig. 83.3).

The fourth and last step of the algorithm is to confirm the stenosis severity (see Fig. 83.3). Indeed, given that transvalvular flow rate is reduced in these patients, it cannot be excluded that the AVA may be pseudo-severe. The flow may not be high enough to fully open a moderately stenotic valve, such as described in the patients with "classical" low-flow and reduced LVEF (see Chapter 82). Exercise stress echocardiography can be useful in patients with no or equivocal symptoms to confirm the

symptomatic status and assess the response of AVA and gradient with increasing flow rate and to calculate the projected AVA at a normal flow rate (see Chapter 82).[23] Low-dose dobutamine-stress echocardiography (starting at 2.5 µg/kg/min and up to a maximum of 20 µg/kg/min) may also be considered in symptomatic patients (e.g., patient in Fig. 83.2), but it should be used with caution and with close monitoring of blood pressure and LVOT velocity (i.e., watch for LVOT acceleration and development of a significant intraventricular gradient, especially in patients with asymmetric septal hypertrophy or a prominent septal bulge) and is contraindicated in patients with severe restrictive physiology. A multicenter study has reported that stress echocardiography is in fact safe and clinically useful in selected patients with paradoxical LF-LG AS, and projected AVA was better than standard echocardiographic measurements to assess AS severity and predict outcome.[23] The measurement of aortic valve calcification load and density by noncontrast MDCT to assess anatomical AS severity is a flow-independent technique that allows determination of anatomical severity and that has been recently incorporated in AS guidelines.[21] It has the advantage of being a fast and straightforward technique, with low radiation (~1 mSv) and no intravenous contrast. As opposed to echocardiography that gives a qualitative assessment of valve calcification but with limited ability to quantify calcium, MDCT is an accurate technique to

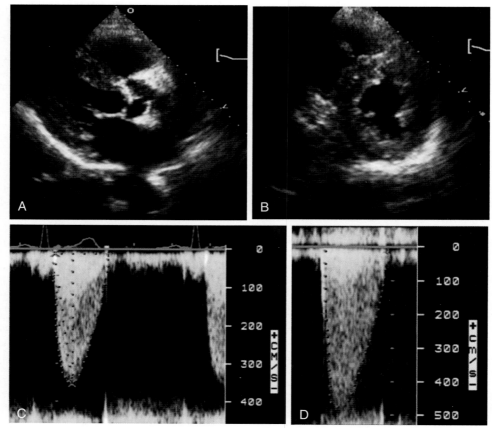

Figure 83.2. Patient with paradoxical low-flow, low-gradient aortic stenosis (AS). This is the case of a 78-year-old woman with a history of calcific AS who is in New York Hear Association functional class III. The parasternal long- and short-axis views show a small left ventricular cavity with pronounced concentric remodeling and preserved left ventricular ejection fraction (LVEF) and a calcified and thickened aortic valve with restricted opening (**A** and **B**; see Video 83.2). This patient underwent low-dose dobutamine stress echocardiography up to 15 µg/kg/min. The LVEF increased from 60% to 70%, the stroke volume increased from 42 to 52 mL, the peak/mean gradient increased from 51/29 to 94/57 mm Hg (**C** and **D**), and the aortic valve area increased slightly from 0.70 to 0.77 cm². This is a case of paradoxical low-flow, low-gradient severe AS. This patient underwent a successful aortic valve replacement.

quantify calcium load using the Agatston method (Fig. 83.4). Furthermore, the sex-specific thresholds of 2000 Agatston units or greater and 1200 Agatston units greater in men and women, respectively, have shown excellent sensitivity and specificity for defining severe AS and provide powerful independent prognostic information of incremental value to echocardiographic assessments.[24–26] A similar four-step algorithm may also be used in the subset of patients with normal-flow, low-gradient AS.

Therapeutic Management

The 2014 American Heart Association/American College of Cardiology[27] and 2017 European Society of Cardiology (ESC)/European Association for Cardio-Thoracic Surgery guidelines[21] have acknowledged paradoxical LF-LG AS as an important entity which requires careful evaluation.[18] Moreover, a class IIa (level of evidence: C) indication for transcatheter aortic valve replacement (TAVR) has been included in both guidelines, provided that stenosis severity is carefully confirmed by a comprehensive evaluation (including aortic valve calcium scoring by MDCT in the ESC guidelines) (see Fig. 83.3). Multiple studies have provided further support for this recommendation.[6,9,13–16] Paradoxical LF-LG AS is associated with several factors (i.e., pronounced concentric remodeling, small LV cavity, myocardial fibrosis, impaired myocardial function, small aortic annulus) that may increase the risk of operative mortality as well as prosthesis–patient mismatch.[2,28] Some studies suggest that TAVR may provide a valuable alternative to surgical AVR in patients with paradoxical LF-LG AS[13,29] (see Fig. 83.3).

CONCLUSION

Doppler echocardiography plays a crucial role for (1) the differential diagnosis between true paradoxical LF-LG AS and other situations associated with small AVA and low gradient (i.e., classical LF-LG and normal-flow, low-gradient) and (2) the confirmation of stenosis severity and thus the indication for AVR if the patient is symptomatic. A particular effort should be made to rule out measurement errors in AS patients with discordant AVA–gradient findings. Symptomatic patients with true paradoxical LF-LG require further investigations (i.e., stress echocardiography, MDCT, or both) to confirm the stenosis severity and the need for AVR. TAVR may provide a valuable alternative to surgical AVR in patients with paradoxical LF-LG AS. Optimization of antihypertensive therapy should be considered in these patients regardless of whether the patient is to be treated conservatively or with surgical or transcatheter valve replacement.

Please access ExpertConsult to view the corresponding videos for this chapter.

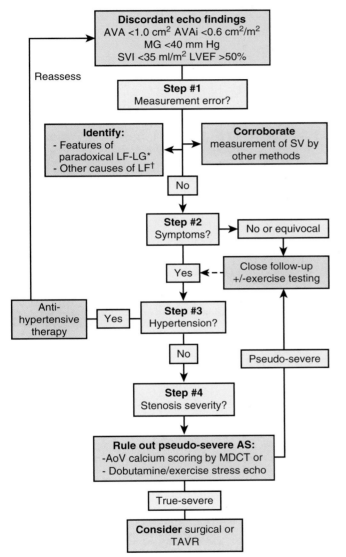

Figure 83.3. Algorithm for the diagnostic and therapeutic management of patients with preserved left ventricular ejection fraction (LVEF) presenting with a small aortic valve area but a low gradient. *AoV,* Aortic valve; *AS,* aortic stenosis; *AVA,* aortic valve effective orifice area; *AVAi,* aortic valve area indexed to body surface area; *AVR,* aortic valve replacement; *LF,* low-flow; *LF-LG,* low-flow, low-gradient; *MDCT,* multidetector computed tomography; *MG,* mean transvalvular gradient; *SV,* stroke volume; *SVI,* stroke volume index; *TAVR,* transcatheter aortic valve replacement. *Asterisk:* See Table 83.1 for the clinical and Doppler echocardiographic features of paradoxical low-flow, low-gradient AS. *Dagger:* These other potential causes of low flow include reduced arterial compliance, atrial fibrillation, and concomitant mitral regurgitation, mitral stenosis, or tricuspid regurgitation.

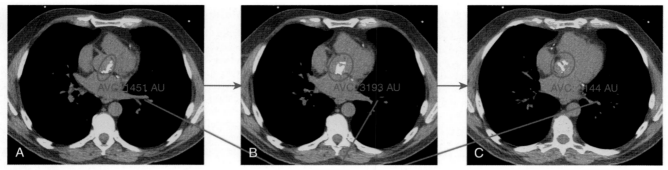

Figure 83.4. Aortic valve calcium quantification using multidetector computed tomography (MDCT). Using axial stacks of electrocardiography-gated, noncontrast MDCT cardiac scans, the software automatically detects calcium (voxels with >130 Hounsfield units of attenuation). **A**, **B**, and **C** are showing different slices of calcified aortic valve. The Agatston score method is used for each lesion, and the sum of values for all lesions is used to determine the total Agatston score of the valve. In this symptomatic patient with a mean gradient of 32 mm Hg, the Agatston score of 6788 AU definitely confirmed presence of severe aortic stenosis, and the patient was referred to aortic valve replacement.

REFERENCES

1. Hachicha Z, Dumesnil JG, Bogaty P, Pibarot P. Paradoxical low flow, low gradient severe aortic stenosis despite preserved ejection fraction is associated with higher afterload and reduced survival. *Circulation.* 2007;115:2856–2864.
2. Dumesnil JG, Pibarot P, Carabello B. Paradoxical low flow and/or low gradient severe aortic stenosis despite preserved left ventricular ejection fraction: implications for diagnosis and treatment. *Eur Heart J.* 2010;31:281–289.
3. Pibarot P, Dumesnil JG. Low-flow, low-gradient aortic stenosis with normal and depressed left ventricular ejection fraction. *J Am Coll Cardiol.* 2012;60:1845–1853.
4. Clavel M-A, Guzzetti E, Annabi M-S, et al. Normal-flow low-gradient severe aortic stenosis: myth or reality? *Structural Heart.* 2018;2:180–187.
5. Barasch E, Fan D, Chukwu EO, et al. Severe isolated aortic stenosis with normal left ventricular systolic function and low transvalvular gradients: pathophysiologic and prognostic insights. *J Heart Valve Dis.* 2008;17:81–88.
6. Mehrotra P, Jansen K, Flynn AW, et al. Differential left ventricular remodelling and longitudinal function distinguishes low flow from normal-flow preserved ejection fraction low-gradient severe aortic stenosis. *Eur Heart J.* 2013;34:1906–1914.
7. Adda J, Mielot C, Giorgi R, et al. Low-flow, low-gradient severe aortic stenosis despite normal ejection fraction is associated with severe left ventricular dysfunction as assessed by speckle tracking echocardiography: a multicenter study. *Circ Cardiovasc Imag.* 2012;5:27–35.
8. Eleid MF, Nishimura RA, Sorajja P, Borlaug BA. Systemic hypertension in low gradient severe aortic stenosis with preserved ejection fraction. *Circulation.* 2013;128:1349–1353.
9. Eleid MF, Sorajja P, Michelena HI, et al. Flow-gradient patterns in severe aortic stenosis with preserved ejection fraction: clinical characteristics and predictors of survival. *Circulation.* 2013;128:1781–1789.
10. Clavel MA, Burwash IG, Pibarot P. Cardiac imaging for assessing low-gradient severe aortic stenosis. *JACC Cardiovasc Imag.* 2017;10:185–202.
11. Pibarot P, Dumesnil JG. Paradoxical low-flow, low-gradient aortic stenosis: new evidences, more questions. *Circulation.* 2013;128:1729–1732.
12. Lancellotti P, Magne J, Donal E, et al. Clinical outcome in asymptomatic severe aortic stenosis: insights from the new proposed aortic stenosis grading classification. *J Am Coll Cardiol.* 2012;59:235–243.
13. Herrmann HC, Pibarot P, Hueter I, et al. Predictors of mortality and outcomes of therapy in low flow severe aortic stenosis: a PARTNER trial analysis. *Circulation.* 2013;127:2316–2326.
14. Clavel MA, Dumesnil JG, Capoulade R, et al. Outcome of patients with aortic stenosis, small valve area and low-flow, low-gradient despite preserved left ventricular ejection fraction. *J Am Coll Cardiol.* 2012;60:1259–1267.
15. Le Ven F, Freeman M, Webb J, et al. Impact of low flow on the outcome of high risk patients undergoing transcatheter aortic valve replacement. *J Am Coll Cardiol.* 2013;62:782–788.
16. Ozkan A, Hachamovitch R, Kapadia SR, et al. Impact of aortic valve replacement on outcome of symptomatic patients with severe aortic stenosis with low gradient and preserved left ventricular ejection fraction. *Circulation.* 2013;128:622–631.
17. Hahn RT, Pibarot P. Accurate measurement of left ventricular outflow tract diameter: comment on the updated recommendations for the echocardiographic assessment of aortic valve stenosis. *J Am Soc Echocardiogr.* 2017;30:1038–1041.
18. Baumgartner H, Hung J, Bermejo J, et al. Recommendations on the echocardiographic assessment of aortic valve stenosis. *J Am Soc Echocardiogr.* 2017;30:372–392.
19. Clavel MA, Malouf J, Messika-Zeitoun D, et al. Aortic valve area calculation in aortic stenosis by CT and Doppler echocardiography. *JACC Cardiovasc Imag.* 2015;8:248–257.
20. Dumesnil JG, Dion D, Yvorchuk K, et al. A new, simple and accurate method for determining ejection fraction by Doppler echocardiography. *Can J Cardiol.* 1995;11:1007–1014.
21. Baumgartner H, Falk V, Bax JJ, et al. 2017 ESC/EACTS guidelines for the management of valvular heart disease. *Eur Heart J.* 2017;38:2739–2791.
22. Mohty D, Pibarot P, Echahidi N, et al. Reduced systemic arterial compliance measured by routine Doppler echocardiography: a new and independent predictor of mortality in patients with type 2 diabetes mellitus. *Atherosclerosis.* 2012;225:353–358.
23. Clavel MA, Ennezat PV, Maréchaux S, et al. Stress echocardiography to assess stenosis severity and predict outcome in patients with paradoxical low-flow, low-gradient aortic stenosis and preserved LVEF. *J Am Coll Cardiol Imag.* 2013;6:175–183.
24. Clavel MA, Messika-Zeitoun D, Pibarot P, et al. The complex nature of discordant severe calcified aortic valve disease grading: new insights from combined Doppler-echocardiographic and computed tomographic study. *J Am Coll Cardiol.* 2013;62:2329–2338.
25. Clavel MA, Pibarot P, Messika-Zeitoun D, et al. Impact of aortic valve calcification, as measured by MDCT, on survival in patients with aortic stenosis. *J Am Coll Cardiol.* 2014;64:1202–1213.
26. Pawade T, Clavel MA, Tribouilloy C, et al. Computed tomography aortic valve calcium scoring in patients with aortic stenosis. *Circ Cardiovasc Imag.* 2018;11:e007146.
27. Nishimura RA, Otto CM, Bonow RO, et al. AHA/ACC guideline for the management of patients with valvular heart disease. *J Am Coll Cardiol.* 2014;63:e57–185. 2014.
28. Herrmann S, Stork S, Niemann M, et al. Low-gradient aortic valve stenosis: myocardial fibrosis and its influence on function and outcome. *J Am Coll Cardiol.* 2011;58:402–412.
29. Fischer-Rasokat U, Renker M, Liebetrau C, et al. 1-year survival after TAVR of patients with low-flow, low-gradient and high-gradient aortic valve stenosis in matched study populations. *JACC Cardiovasc Interv.* 2019;12:752–763.
30. Vamvakidou A, Jin W, Danylenko O, et al. Low transvalvular flow rate predicts mortality in patients with low-gradient aortic stenosis following aortic valve intervention. *JACC Cardiovasc Imag.* 2019;12:1715–1724.

84 Asymptomatic Severe Aortic Stenosis

Thomas F. O'Connell, Amr E. Abbas

According to the guidelines, there are four stages of aortic stenosis (AS), which are differentiated by valve anatomy, hemodynamics, left ventricular (LV) dysfunction, and patient symptoms:[1]

A. Stage A: at-risk anatomy, such as aortic sclerosis or bicuspid aortic valve
B. Stage B: progressive hemodynamic obstruction with mild or moderate AS
C. Stage C: severe asymptomatic AS
D. Stage D: severe symptomatic AS

Symptoms from AS include exertional dyspnea, angina, heart failure, presyncope, and syncope. Patients with symptomatic severe AS do poorly, and aortic valve replacement (AVR) whether surgical (SAVR) or transcatheter aortic valve replacement (TAVR), is indicated to improve survival, reduce symptoms, and improve exercise capacity.[1–3] Currently, in asymptomatic severe AS, SAVR is recommended when:

1. Left ventricular ejection fraction (LVEF) <50%
2. "Very severe AS" with low surgical risk
3. Rapidly progressing AS with low surgical risk
4. The patient is undergoing another cardiac surgery

An outline of current guidelines recommendations for SAVR in asymptomatic AS can be found in Table 84.1.[1–3] Currently, there is no indication in the guidelines for TAVR in patients with asymptomatic severe AS. However, with the availability of less invasive techniques to treat patients with AS, including TAVR and minimally invasive AVR, and with reported poor outcomes associated with asymptomatic patients with AS, the decision of whether or not to undergo AVR is often debated.[4] For patients with asymptomatic severe AS without another reason for AVR, stress testing is an important tool that can guide decision making on whether or not to perform AVR.

NATURAL HISTORY OF ASYMPTOMATIC SEVERE AORTIC STENOSIS

Of more than 3800 patients analyzed in the Contemporary Outcomes After Surgery and Medical Treatment in Patients With Severe Aortic Stenosis (CURRENT AS) Registry, approximately 50% were asymptomatic when diagnosed with severe AS.[5] Although patients with asymptomatic severe AS have a low risk of sudden cardiac death at 1% to 1.5% per year, AS is a chronic and progressive disease that does not carry a benign prognosis.[5,6] On average:

1. Aortic jet velocity increases 0.3 m/s/year.
2. Mean gradient increases 7 mm Hg per year.
3. AVA decreases 0.1 cm^2 per year.

However, hemodynamic progression has been shown to be highly variable, and death in this population is associated with the severity and rate of AS progression.[6,7] Retrospective database analysis demonstrated rates of AVR or cardiac death to be 20%, 37%, and 75% at 1, 2, and 5 years, respectively.[6] Zilberszac and colleagues[8] prospectively followed 103 patients with asymptomatic severe AS older than 70 years of age with transthoracic echocardiography (TTE) and clinical evaluation of symptoms. Indications for AVR or cardiac death were observed in 27%, 57%, 77%, and 84% of patients at 1, 2,

3, and 4 years, respectively. Of the patients who developed symptoms during follow-up, 43% experienced severe onset of symptoms (New York Heart Association Class III or IV). The patients with severe symptom onset had a higher postoperative mortality rate than the patients with mild onset of symptoms. Twenty-nine percent of patients had a medical comorbidity limiting mobility, which highlights the difficulty in determining AS symptoms in this patient population.[8] This data confirms the poor prognosis of AS in asymptomatic patients.

STRESS TESTING

AS is a chronic and progressive disease that is mostly found in older adults. Many patients do not recognize or underestimate their symptoms because of unknowingly decreasing their activity level. Medical comorbidities and deconditioning can make it difficult for patients and physicians when seeking to determine if symptoms are related to AS. Stress testing is an important tool to assess for symptoms while also providing prognostic insight and helping determine whether to proceed with AVR.[9]

Stress testing can be performed by exercise or with a pharmacologic agent, but exercise is preferred because it is more physiologic and better supported in the literature.[9]

1. Modalities of exercise: Whereas the treadmill test is the most common exercise test in the North America and the United Kingdom, the upright bicycle test is the most common exercise test in European Union countries.
2. Modalities of assessment of cardiac function: Stress electrocardiography (ECG), stress echocardiography, longitudinal strain during exercise, and cardiopulmonary exercise testing (CPET) have been studied.

Stress testing can safely be performed in patients with asymptomatic severe AS. A meta-analysis of seven studies with close to 500 patients did not report complications during or after stress testing.[10] Despite guideline recommendations and data confirming safety, performance of exercise stress testing remains low in this patient population.[11] Exercise stress testing carries a class III recommendation in patients with symptomatic severe AS.[1] Contraindications include an established indication for AVR, symptomatic or hemodynamically significant cardiac arrhythmias, uncontrolled hypertension, and physical disability prohibiting safe and adequate testing.[12]

Exercise Stress Electrocardiography

More than 20 studies have assessed exercise ECG stress testing in the setting of asymptomatic severe AS. The majority of studies evaluating treadmill exercise testing used a Bruce protocol. The semisupine position was most commonly used when studying the bicycle exercise test, but supine and upright bicycles have been studied as well. Symptom-limited testing was most commonly performed in bicycle exercise testing, but other protocols have used age-related maximal heart rate and peak oxygen consumption when CPET was part of the protocol.[9]

The American Heart Association/American College of Cardiology (AHA/ACC) Guidelines for the Management of Patients with Valvular Heart Disease defines an exercise stress test as abnormal if:

TABLE 84.1 Guidelines Comparison of American Heart Association/American College of Cardiology and European Society of Cardiology/European Association for Cardio-Thoracic Surgery

RECOMMENDATIONS FOR SAVR IN PATIENTS WITH ASYMPTOMATIC SEVERE AS	AHA/ACC 2014/2017 COR	ESC/EACTS 2017 COR
Severe AS and LVEF ≤50% not due to other cause	I	I
Severe AS when undergoing other cardiac surgery	I	I
Abnormal exercise test showing symptoms related to AS	I	I
Very severe AS (aortic velocity ≥5.0 m/s) and low surgical risk	IIa	
Very severe AS (aortic velocity ≥5.5 m/s) and low surgical risk		IIa
Exercise test showing exercise decrease in BP	IIa	IIa
Exercise test showing decreased exercise tolerance	IIa	
Rapid disease progression (V_{max} ≥0.3 m/s/year) and low surgical risk	IIb	IIa
Elevated BNP (>3 times age- and sex-corrected normal range) confirmed by repeated measurements without further explanation		IIa
Severe pulmonary hypertension (PASP at rest >60 mm Hg on invasive measurement) without other explanation		IIa

AHA/ACC, American Heart Association/American College of Cardiology; *AS,* aortic stenosis; *BP,* blood pressure; *BNP,* B-type natriuretic peptide; *COR,* Class of Recommendation; *ESC/EACTS,* European Society of Cardiology/European Association for Cardio-Thoracic Surgery; *LVEF,* left ventricular ejection fraction; *PASP,* pulmonary artery systolic pressure; *SAVR,* surgical aortic valve replacement; V_{max}, maximum transvalvular flow velocity.

1. the patient experiences typical symptoms of AS,
2. the patient experiences a decrease in exercise tolerance in comparison to age and sex normal standards, or
3. the patient's systolic blood pressure decreases or fails to increase at least 20 mm Hg.[1]

There is no consistent definition for a positive exercise stress test result in the literature as outlined in Table 84.2. In more than 20 studies reviewed, all studies specified angina or chest pain and dizziness, presyncope, and syncope as symptoms that qualified as a positive test result. Most studies included dyspnea as a symptom signaling a positive test result, but only a few studies counted fatigue as a positive symptom. About half the studies defined an abnormal blood pressure response as a decrease in systolic blood pressure by a specific threshold below baseline; the remaining defined it as failure of the systolic blood pressure to increase by at least 20 mm Hg with exercise.[9]

Almost every study had ECG criteria for ST-segment depression and arrhythmias that qualified the test result as positive. Most studies used a cutoff greater than 2 mm of ST-segment depression to qualify as a positive study result. All of the studies identified ventricular arrhythmias as a criteria for an abnormal test result with the definition ranging from greater than 3 premature ventricular contractions to sustained ventricular arrythmias.[9]

The results of up to half of the stress tests ordered for asymptomatic severe AS are positive.[4] Multiple studies have shown that a positive exercise stress test result is associated with an increased event and death rate.[9] A meta-analysis found that at 1 year follow-up, there were no sudden cardiac deaths in patients with a normal exercise stress test result and a 5% risk of sudden cardiac death with positive test results. The same meta-analysis found that exercise stress testing had 75% sensitivity and 71% specificity in predicting adverse cardiac events.[10] It remains a challenge to determine if symptoms experienced during exercise testing are due to AS or other causes, especially in older patients. The specificity of symptoms during an exercise stress test predicting onset of spontaneous symptoms over the course of 12 months was shown to be 93% in patients less than 70 years old compared with 78% in the entire patient population.[13] A positive test due to AS symptoms carries greater prognostic significance than blood pressure or ST-segment endpoints. However, it is unclear which symptom is the best predictor of adverse cardiac events or death.[12]

Other data: Metabolic equivalents and heart rate recovery have also been used to predict outcomes. One study showed that patients unable to achieve at least 85% of age- and sex-predicted metabolic equivalents were more likely to die on long-term follow-up than patients able to achieve 85%. Slow heart rate recovery, measured as a decrease in heart rate from peak to 1-minute after exercise, is associated with death.[14]

Exercise Stress Echocardiography

Stress echocardiography has been used to gather additional information during exercise stress testing in patients with asymptomatic severe AS. Most of the studies also included patients with moderate AS:[9,15,16]

1. Stress modalities for stress echocardiogram: Although dobutamine stress echocardiography is recommended in patients with a severely low AVA, low-gradient, and reduced ejection fraction, exercise is the recommended stress modality for asymptomatic severe AS with a preserved LVEF.[1]
2. Exercise modalities for stress echocardiogram: Bicycle exercise is preferred over treadmill exercise because it allows echocardiography to be recorded continuously.[9]
3. Stress echocardiogram protocol: Almost every study evaluated symptom-limited graded bicycle exercise testing in a semisupine position. Testing protocols started with a workload of 20 to 30 Watts (W), which is increased 20 to 30 W every 2 to 3 minutes.[9,15,16] Exercise stress echocardiography requires a high level of expertise with coordination between the stress laboratory and sonographers.[9]
4. Stress echocardiogram parameters: Parameters measured during exercise stress echocardiogram include LVEF, AVA, change in the aortic valve mean pressure gradient (MPG), and change in the pulmonary artery systolic pressure (PASP).[9]

The most studied parameter in exercise stress echocardiography is the increase in MPG with exercise as demonstrated in Fig. 84.1.[9,15,16] Large increases in the MPG with exercise are concerning for a stiffer, less compliant aortic valve that is restricted despite exercise. A study of patients with moderate and severe AS demonstrated that patients with an increase in MPG 20 mm Hg or greater with exercise had a faster progression of AS on follow-up TTE.[15] Rapid progression of AS has previously been associated with poor outcomes.[7] Three key studies have investigated the prognostic value of changes in the MPG with exercise in patients with asymptomatic severe AS:

1. Lancellotti and colleagues[16] prospectively studied 69 patients with asymptomatic AS with an AVA less than 1.0 cm² and preserved LVEF showing that an increase in MPG 18 mm Hg or greater with exercise and an AVA less than 0.75 cm² during exercise both independently predicted cardiac events.
2. Maréchaux and colleagues[17] extended this work prospectively, studying 135 patients with asymptomatic moderate to severe AS

TABLE 84.2 Criteria for Abnormal Exercise Electrocardiography Testing in Asymptomatic Severe Aortic Stenosis

GUIDELINES ON EXERCISE ECG IN ASYMPTOMATIC SEVERE AS	EXERCISE ECG ABNORMALITIES PER GUIDELINES
AHA/ACC	1. Typical symptoms of AS 2. Systolic blood pressure decreases or fails to increase by ≥20 mm Hg 3. Decrease in exercise tolerance compared with age and sex normal standards
ESC/EACTS	1. Typical symptoms of AS 2. Decrease in blood pressure below baseline
LITERATURE ON EXERCISE ECG IN ASYMPTOMATIC SEVERE AS	**EXERCISE ECG ABNORMALITIES PER LITERATURE**
Symptoms	• All studies considered chest pain and presyncope or syncope as positive symptoms • Most studies considered dyspnea as a positive symptom • A few studies considered fatigue as a positive symptom
ECG	• ST-segment depression: all studies considered ST-segment depression abnormal with most considering >2 mm a positive test result • Ventricular arrhythmias: whereas all studies considered ventricular arrhythmias abnormal, the threshold for a positive test result ranged from >3 PVCs to sustained VT
METS	• One study demonstrated achieving ≥85% of age- and sex-predicted METs was associated with a mortality benefit
Heart rate recovery	• One study demonstrated slow heart rate recovery (peak to 1-minute after exercise) was associated with mortality

AHA/ACC, American Heart Association/American College of Cardiology; *AS,* aortic stenosis; *ECG,* electrocardiogram; *ESC/EACTS,* European Society of Cardiology/European Association for Cardio-Thoracic Surgery; *MET,* metabolic equivalent; *PVC,* premature ventricular contraction; *VT,* ventricular tachycardia

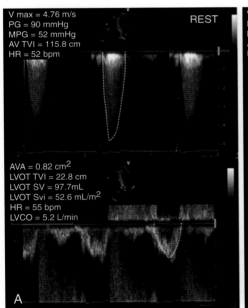 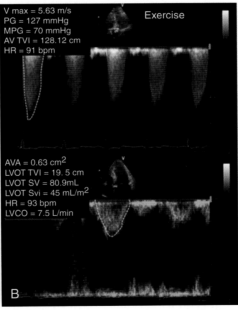

Figure 84.1. Change in the aortic valve (AV) mean pressure gradient (MGP) from rest (**A**) to exercise (**B**) transthoracic echocardiography. The MGP across the AV increases from 52 to 70 mm Hg with exercise, and the aortic valve area (AVA) decreases from 0.82 to 0.63 cm^2. *HR,* Heart rate; *LVCO,* left ventricular cardiac output; *LVOT,* left ventricular outflow tract; *PG,* peak pressure gradient; *SV,* stroke volume; *Svi,* stroke volume index; *TVI,* time velocity integral; *Vmax,* maximum transvalvular flow velocity.

and normal exercise stress test results. The increase in MPG with exercise was not associated with the rest gradient or any other parameters from the rest TTE. Greater increases in MPG with exercise were associated with younger patients, larger increases in heart rate and stroke volume, and smaller increases in AVA. In multivariate analysis, an increase in MPG 20 mm Hg or greater with exercise predicted cardiovascular death or future indication for AVR. Patients with an increase in MPG greater than 20 mm Hg with exercise and rest gradient greater than 35 mm Hg had a hazard ratio of 9.6, whereas patients with a change in MPG 20 mm Hg or less with exercise and rest gradient greater than 35 mm Hg had a hazard ratio of 2.5.[17]

3. Goublaire and colleagues[18] performed a similar study of 112 patients with asymptomatic moderate and severe AS and normal exercise stress test results. Contrary to the previous studies, an increase in the MPG with exercise did not predict events related to AS or future AVR. This also held true in subgroup analysis of patients with severe AS.[18]

Some of the factors that may have contributed to different outcomes in the aforementioned studies are that the studies were small, single center, had different follow-up lengths, and included patients with moderate AS.[15–18] The additive value of measuring changes in MPG with stress echocardiography compared with exercise stress ECG testing remains uncertain. This is highlighted by the fact that the European Society of Cardiology/European Association for Cardio-Thoracic Surgery (ESC/EACTS) guidelines from 2012 stated an increase in MPG greater than 20 mm Hg with

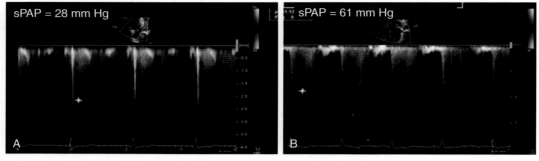

Figure 84.2. Systolic pulmonary artery pressure (sPAP) with exercise transthoracic echocardiography. Continuous-wave Doppler across the pulmonary valve demonstrates a sPAP of 28 mm Hg with rest (**A**) and 61 mm Hg (**B**) with exercise.

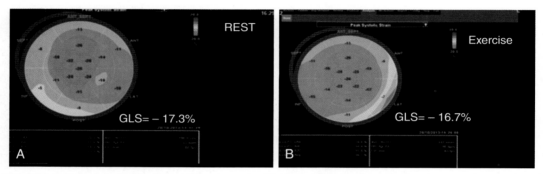

Figure 84.3. Global longitudinal strain (GLS) with rest (**A**) and exercise (**B**). GLS with rest and exercise has been used as a tool to detect early left ventricular dysfunction in patients with aortic stenosis.

exercise in patients with asymptomatic severe AS was a class IIb recommendation for SAVR in patients with low surgical risk, whereas the ESC/EACTS guidelines from 2017 listed an increase in the MPG greater than 20 mm Hg as predictor of symptom development and adverse outcomes but removed it as a criterion for SAVR.[3,19] There is no guidelines recommendation for AVR based on MPG with exercise from the AHA/ACC.[1,2]

Pulmonary hypertension has been shown to be a predictor of death as well as major adverse cardiovascular and cerebrovascular events after SAVR.[20] The ESC/EACTS guidelines give a class IIa recommendation for AVR in patients with asymptomatic severe AS with preserved LVEF and severe pulmonary hypertension without other explanation. Severe pulmonary hypertension is defined as a PASP greater than 60 mm Hg measured invasively.[3] Studies have hypothesized that severe pulmonary hypertension that develops during exercise is an early form of disease that portends a poor prognosis and warrants early AVR.[17,20] One study found that a PASP greater than 60 mm Hg (Fig. 84.2) on stress echocardiography in asymptomatic patients with severe AS predicted cardiac events on follow-up with a sensitivity of 70% and specificity of 62%.[20] However, this was not able to be reproduced in other studies.[17,21]

Exercise Longitudinal Strain

LV pressure overload from AS leads to subendocardial stress, reduction in coronary flow reserve, and ventricular hypertrophy before progressing to concentric remodeling and myocardial fibrosis, which cannot be reversed. The LVEF can be normal until late in the disease process, which has led to the study of longitudinal strain for early detection of LV dysfunction.[9,21] Resting global and basal longitudinal strain has been shown to be lower in patients with severe AS and positive exercise stress test results compared with patients with severe AS and normal exercise stress test results (Fig. 84.3). In patients with asymptomatic moderate and severe AS, peak exercise basal longitudinal strain was found to independently predict a combined endpoint of cardiovascular death, cardiovascular hospitalization, and future AVR.[21] There is a growing body of literature exploring the best ways to use longitudinal strain analysis to evaluate patients with AS.

Cardiopulmonary Exercise Testing

CPET measures respiratory gas exchange and calculates maximum oxygen uptake (VO_2), which reflects the heart's ability to deliver oxygen to the body. Maximum VO_2 has been used in the heart failure population to predict adverse events.[9,22] Severe valvular heart disease has been listed as an absolute contradiction to CPET. However, Le and colleagues demonstrated the test could be performed safely in patients with severe AS.[22,23]

1. CPET to determine the cause of dyspnea symptoms: In patients with dyspnea of undetermined cause, CPET respiratory gas exchange patterns can distinguish between cardiac disease, lung disease, pulmonary vascular disease, obesity, deconditioning, and suboptimal effort.[22]

2. CPET and survival outcomes: Le and colleagues studied 101 patients with severe AS and preserved LVEF who were asymptomatic, had equivocal symptoms, or had mild symptoms from AS. Patients were managed conservatively when there was abnormal peak oxygen consumption or peak oxygen pulse, but the CPET pattern pointed to a cause other than AS. The conservatively managed patients had survival rates comparable to an age- and gender-matched population.[23]

Although further research is needed in CPET, the potential incremental value compared with exercise stress testing is the ability to differentiate symptoms in complex patients while also offering further prognostication.

OUTCOMES AND FUTURE RESEARCH

The CURRENT AS registry was used to retrospectively review more than 1800 patients with asymptomatic severe AS of whom more than 80% were managed conservatively. Among the remaining patients

TABLE 84.3 Ongoing Trials Assessing Early Intervention for Severe Asymptomatic Aortic Stenosis

TRIALS	SAVR	TAVR	RANDOMIZED BY CARDIAC MRI
ESTIMATE	✓		
AVATAR	✓		
EVoLVeD	✓	✓	✓
EARLY TAVR		✓	

AVATAR, Aortic Valve Replacement Versus Conservative Treatment in Asymptomatic Severe Aortic Stenosis; *EARLY TAVR,* Evaluation of Transcatheter Aortic Valve Replacement Compared to Surveillance for Patients with Asymptomatic Severe Aortic Stenosis; *ESTIMATE,* Early Surgery for Patients with Asymptomatic Aortic Stenosis; *EVoLVeD,* Early Valve Replacement Guided by Biomarkers of LV Decompensation in Asymptomatic Patients with Severe AS; *MRI,* magnetic resonance imaging; *SAVR,* surgical aortic valve replacement; *TAVR,* transcatheter aortic valve replacement

managed with AVR, 98% of patients had SAVR performed. After propensity-score matching, patients in the initial AVR cohort were younger, had lower Society of Thoracic Surgeons (STS) scores, and had greater AS severity. Patients in the initial AVR group were found to have a lower risk of all-cause death and heart failure hospitalizations in final propensity score-matched analysis.[5] These data have made it worrisome that a watchful waiting strategy in patients with asymptomatic severe AS may increase morbidity and mortality.[4] A recent study of 145 asymptomatic patients demonstrated that patients with very severe AS, as defined by AVA 0.75 cm^2 or less plus an aortic jet velocity of 4.5 m/s or greater or a mean transaortic gradient of 50 mm Hg or greater, had significantly had less composite operative mortality and death from cardiovascular causes with early SAVR compared with those undergoing conservative care.[24] There are currently four other trials evaluating watchful waiting versus an early intervention strategy with TAVR or SAVR (Table 84.3). One of the studies is investigating an early intervention strategy based on cardiac magnetic resonance imaging midwall fibrosis.

Acknowledgment

The authors acknowledge the contributions of Dr. Patrizio Lancellotti, who was the author of this chapter in the previous edition.

REFERENCES

1. Nishimura RA, Otto CM, Bonow RO, et al. 2014 AHA/ACC guideline for the management of patients with valvular heart disease: a report of the American College of Cardiology/American heart association task force on Practice guidelines. *Circulation.* 2014;129:e521. 64.
2. Nishimura RA, Otto CM, Bonow RO, et al. 2017 AHA/ACC focused update of the 2014 AHA/ACC guideline for the management of patients with valvular heart disease: a report of the American College of Cardiology/American Heart Association Task Force on Clinical Practice Guidelines. *Circulation.* 2017;135(25):1159. 1159.
3. Baumgartner H, Falk V, Bax JJ, et al. 2017 ESC/EACTS guidelines for the management of valvular heart disease. *Eur Heart J.* 2017;38(36):2739–2791.
4. Genereux P, Stone GW, O'Gara PT, et al. Natural history, diagnostic approaches, and therapeutic strategies for patients with asymptomatic severe aortic stenosis. *J Am Coll Cardiol.* 2016;67(19):2263–2288.
5. Taniguchi T, Morimoto T, Shiomi H, et al. Initial surgical versus conservative strategies in patients with asymptomatic severe aortic stenosis. *J Am Coll Cardiol.* 2015;66(25):2827–2838.
6. Pellikka PA, Sarano ME, Nishimura RA, et al. Outcome of 622 adults with asymptomatic, hemodynamically significant aortic stenosis during prolonged follow-up. *Circulation.* 2005;111(24):3290–3295.
7. Otto CM, Burwash IG, Legget ME, et al. Prospective study of asymptomatic valvular aortic stenosis: clinical, echocardiographic, and exercise predictors of outcomes. *Circulation.* 1997;95(9):2262–2270.
8. Zilberszac R, Gabriel H, Schemper M, et al. Asymptomatic severe aortic stenosis in the elderly. *JACC Cardiovasc Imag.* 2017;10(1):43–50.
9. Redfors B, Pibarot P, Gillam L, et al. Stress testing in asymptomatic aortic stenosis. *Circulation.* 2017;135(20):1956–1976.
10. Rafique AM, Biner S, Ray I, et al. Meta-analysis of prognostic value of stress testing in patients with asymptomatic severe aortic stenosis. *Am J Cardiol.* 2009;104(7):972–977.
11. Iung B, Baron G, Butchart EG, et al. A prospective survey of patients with valvular heart disease in Europe: the Euro heart Survey on valvular heart disease. *Eur Heart J.* 2003;24(13):1231–1243.
12. Fletcher GF, Ades PA, Klingfield P, et al. Exercise standards for testing and training: a scientific statement from the American Heart Association. *Circulation.* 2013;128(8):873–934.
13. Das P, Rimington H, Chambers J. Exercise testing to stratify risk in aortic stenosis. *Eur Heart J.* 2005;26(13):1309–1313.
14. Masri A, Goodman AL, Barr T, et al. Predictors of long-term outcomes in asymptomatic patients with severe aortic stenosis and preserved left ventricular systolic function undergoing exercise echocardiography. *Circulation Cardiovasc Imag.* 2016;9(7):e004577. 9.
15. Ringle A, Levy F, Ennezat PV, et al. Relationship between exercise pressure gradient and haemodynamic progression of aortic stenosis. *Arch Cardiovasc Dis.* 2017;110(8):466–474.
16. Lancellotti P, Lebois F, Simon M, et al. Prognostic importance of quantitative exercise Doppler echocardiography in asymptomatic valvular aortic stenosis. *Circulation.* 2005;112(9 Suppl). I-377-I-382.
17. Maréchaux S, Hachicha Z, Bellouin A, et al. Usefulness of exercise-stress echocardiography for risk stratification of true asymptomatic patients with aortic valve stenosis. *Eur Heart J.* 2010;31(11):1390–1397.
18. Goublaire C, Melissopoulou M, Lobo D, et al. Prognostic value of exercise-stress echocardiography in asymptomatic patients with aortic valve stenosis. *JACC Cardiovasc Imag.* 2018;11(6):787–795.
19. Vahanian A, Alfieri O, Andreotti F, et al. Guidelines on the management of valvular heart disease (version 2012): the joint task force on the management of valvular heart disease of the European Society of Cardiology (ESC) and the European Association for Cardio-Thoracic Surgery (EACTS). *Eur Heart J.* 2012;33:2451–2496.
20. Lancellotti P, Magne J, Donal E, et al. Determinants and prognostic significance of exercise pulmonary hypertension in asymptomatic severe aortic stenosis. *Circulation.* 2012;126(7):851–859.
21. Levy-Neuman S, Meledin V, Gandelman G, et al. The association between longitudinal strain at rest and stress and outcome in asymptomatic patients with moderate and severe aortic stenosis. *J Am Soc Echocardiogr.* 2019;32(6):722–729.
22. Datta D, Normandin E, ZuWallack R. Cardiopulmonary exercise testing in the assessment of exertional dyspnea. *Ann Thorac Med.* 2015;10(2):77–86.
23. Le VD, Jensen GV, Kjøller-Hansen L. Prognostic usefulness of cardiopulmonary exercise testing for managing patients with severe aortic stenosis. *Am J Cardiol.* 2017;120(5):844–849.
24. Kang D, Park S, Lee S, et al: Early surgery or conservative care for asymptomatic aortic stenosis, N Engl J Med 382(2), 2020.

85 Subaortic Stenosis

Daniel A. Daneshvar, Itzhak Kronzon

EPIDEMIOLOGY

Subaortic stenosis (SAS) is rarely found in infants and is responsible for 10% of cases of left ventricular outflow (LVOT) obstruction in children.[2] Although it can be diagnosed at any age, the most common presentation is in the first decade of life.[3] Similar to valvular aortic stenosis, SAS is more common in males, with a male-to-female ratio of 2 to 1.[4] Up to 50% of all cases are associated with other congenital abnormalities, including ventricular septal defect (VSD), aortic coarctation, atrioventricular septal defect, patent ductus arteriosus, bicuspid aortic valve, and often the Shone complex.[5]

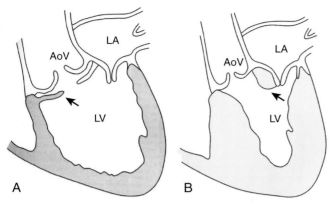

Figure 85.1. A, Subaortic discrete membrane. **B,** Tunnel-like subaortic stenosis showing subaortic stenosis *(arrow)*. *AoV,* Aortic valve; *LA,* left atrium; *LV,* left ventricle. (Courtesy of V. Lennie and JL Zamorano-Gomez.)

MORPHOLOGY

There are two main morphologies seen in SAS. In 90% of cases, a focal membrane or ridge is found, which is also known as discrete SAS (Fig. 85.1A). The circumferential ring may extend from the anterior septum to the anterior mitral leaflet, encircling the LVOT below the aortic valve.[6,7] The less common muscular, tunnel-type lesion is associated with a greater degree of stenosis caused by the diffuse thickening and narrowing of the LVOT (Fig. 85.1B).[8] Patients with this form more commonly have concentric left ventricular hypertrophy (LVH). Other anatomic variants of obstruction exist, including abnormal mitral valve attachments and accessory endocardial cushion tissue. These forms of subaortic obstruction may represent a spectrum of morphology, with discrete SAS as a milder form and tunnel-type as the severe form.

CAUSE AND PATHOPHYSIOLOGY

SAS is more commonly an acquired lesion with a genetic predisposition that develops over time. Previous reports have described families with multiple affected members with SAS, which supports its being a genetic disease.[9,10] Abnormal LVOT geometry with altered flow patterns has been postulated to increase fluid shear stress on the interventricular septum. Subsequently, the embryonic cells are differentiated into a fibrotic tissue variant, which causes a subaortic membrane to develop.[11,12] The theory that SAS is an acquired condition is substantiated by the fact that SAS is rarely found in infants. The turbulent flow may be caused by an apical septal ridge, malalignment of the septum, an elongated or hypoplastic LVOT, or an apical muscular band.[13] The resulting fibrous or muscular structure in the LVOT may then cause clinical and hemodynamic compromise. The hypothesis of chronic turbulence is further supported by the considerable rate of recurrence of disease even after surgical removal of the subvalvular membrane.[14]

The natural history of SAS is variable and unpredictable. SAS is commonly found as a secondary lesion in patients with VSDs or other congenital abnormalities. The clinical features of SAS are determined by the severity of the pressure gradient. Patients may remain asymptomatic for some time with mild gradients, but they may also develop symptoms of LVOT obstruction with disease progression. Rapid hemodynamic worsening of symptoms and obstruction may occur during early childhood.[15] Adults may more commonly remain asymptomatic, with a slow course over several decades when presenting with mild stenosis, especially in patients with isolated disease.[4] Certain risk factors portend a faster progression of disease, including a higher initial peak pressure gradient, lesions closer to the aortic valve or involving the mitral

valve, long and narrow LVOT, and a steep aortoventricular septal angle (>130 degrees).[16] The delayed progression of disease in adults is likely caused by decreased disease severity. Like aortic stenosis (AS), patients with SAS develop LVH to reduce wall stress caused by the elevated afterload. With development of LVOT obstruction, the most common presentation is limited exercise tolerance, but syncope, angina pectoris, and dyspnea have also been described.[17]

Aortic regurgitation (AR) is present in half of patients with SAS, but it is usually mild in severity. The mechanism is thought to be thickened aortic valve leaflets from the high-velocity systolic jet caused by the membrane.[18] The damaged aortic valve is then more susceptible to clots and vegetations. Although bicuspid aortic valves are present in 23% of patients with SAS, the frequency of AR is not increased in this population.[8] Surgical repair in children does not prevent the development of AR in adults. Significant AR is more likely to be found in patients who have undergone surgical intervention or balloon dilatation attempts than those who have not had surgery.[4] The highest risk for progressive AR after surgery is in patients with a preoperative peak instantaneous gradient of 80 mmHg or more.[19] VSDs, which are typically perimembranous, are found in 65% of patients with SAS, and malalignment of the infundibular septum is seen.[20] Infective endocarditis that affects the aortic valve may be seen, especially with more severe LVOT gradients and significant AR.[21]

DIAGNOSIS

SAS is often diagnosed when proceeding to surgery of another congenital defect.

On physical examination, SAS is usually first identified by a murmur that is characterized by a harsh systolic ejection murmur, which is heard best at the left sternal border; an occasional thrill; and delayed and diminished peripheral pulses. The absence of a systolic ejection click differentiates the murmur from valvular AS. The diagnosis by physical examination remains a challenge because this feature can also be found in other causes of LVOT obstruction. The Valsalva maneuver may be used to differentiate SAS from hypertrophic cardiomyopathy (HCM). The murmur in SAS decreases with the Valsalva maneuver, but it is intensified with HCM. A blowing diastolic murmur may also be present in cases of AR. The electrocardiogram is typically abnormal, with nonspecific findings, including LVH, strain patterns, and left atrial enlargement. Chest radiographic findings are often normal.

The echocardiogram is the cornerstone of diagnosis of SAS. It defines the anatomy and type of defect, as well as functioning of the LVOT. Associated cardiac defects can also be diagnosed with this imaging technique. The objective measurements of systolic Doppler pressure gradient, AR, or mitral regurgitation are vital to establishing patient treatment and follow-up. The parasternal long-axis and apical long-axis views are informative; these views allow visualization of the relationship of the membrane to the aortic valve and the dimensions of the aortic annulus (Fig. 85.2 and Video 85.2). On M-mode echocardiography, the characteristic midsystolic partial closure and coarse fluttering of the aortic valve cusps are seen, indicating a subvalvular pressure gradient (Fig. 85.3). Color Doppler imaging is essential for finding the site of onset of the turbulent jet and for the presence of AR. The apical five-chamber view allows the best site for measurement of the peak pressure gradient across the membrane using pulsed- or continuous-wave Doppler (Fig. 85.4). If surgery has already been performed, the echocardiogram should help the physician to determine the type of intervention (simple resection, myotomy, myectomy, Konno intervention, valve prosthesis) and to rule out the existence of an iatrogenic VSD.

Two-dimensional transthoracic echocardiography (TTE) and transesophageal echocardiography (TEE) are the standard techniques for diagnosis of SAS. However, these methods are often limited in their ability to visualize the details of SAS and the LVOT.[22]

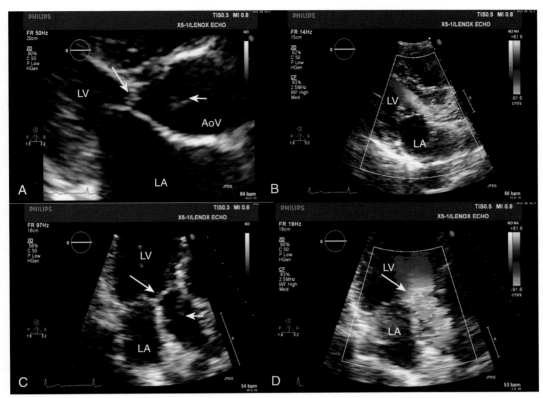

Figure 85.2. A, Parasternal long-axis view, magnified view of left ventricular outflow tract (LVOT), with subaortic membrane *(arrow)* and aortic valve *(arrowhead)*. **B,** Color Doppler demonstrating turbulent flow in LVOT. **C,** Apical three-chamber view again showing subaortic membrane *(arrow)* and aortic valve *(arrowhead)*, with color Doppler flow in **D,** *AoV,* Aortic valve; *LA,* left atrium; *LV,* left ventricle. (Also see Video 85.2.)

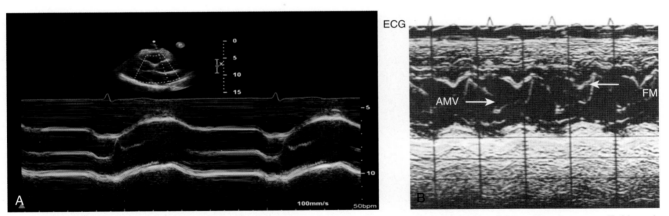

Figure 85.3. A, M-mode echocardiography demonstrating midsystolic partial closure and coarse fluttering of the aortic valve cusps. **B,** M-mode echocardiography showing distinct echo from the discrete, fibrous membrane in the left ventricular outflow tract. *AMV,* Anterior leaflet of the mitral valve; *ECG,* electrocardiogram; *FM,* fibrous membrane.

Three-dimensional (3D) TEE can accurately diagnose and measure SAS; 3D TEE also is a useful tool for guiding transcatheter interventions or evaluating intraoperative gradients (Fig. 85.5 and Video 85.5).[23] The aortotomy view below the plane of the aortic valve provides an excellent perspective for assessing the entire SAS and quantifying the LVOT obstruction by planimetry.[24] Cardiac magnetic resonance imaging (CMRI) and cardiac computed tomography (CT) angiography are emerging techniques to further evaluate the anatomy and flow quantification in SAS.[25,26] The limitation with CMRI remains the difficulty to visualize the thin SAS membrane.[27] Cardiac CT drawbacks are the exposure to radiation and contrast as well as the cost.[28]

Cardiac catheterization was the previously preferred technique before the development of the current gold standard of echocardiography. Although catheterization provides anatomic and hemodynamic data, it lacks the definition of small anatomic structures and assessment of the mitral apparatus. Catheterization for SAS involves calculating the intraventricular gradient, as opposed to AS, in which the transvalvular gradient is measured between the aorta and left ventricle. A single end-hole catheter, as opposed to a pigtail catheter, is used for pull-back traces of the gradient. The measurement of the peak-to-peak gradient at catheterization is often lower than the maximum instantaneous gradient seen in echocardiography, and therefore, it is difficult to

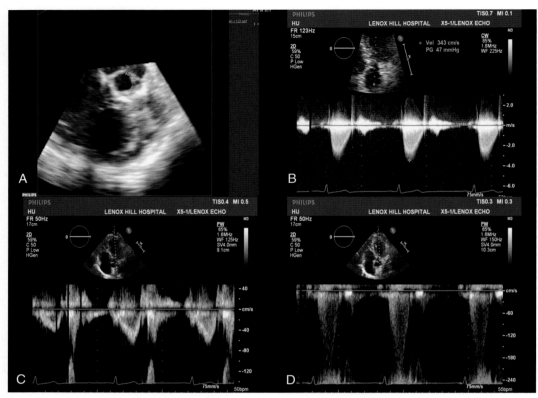

Figure 85.4. A, Multiplanar view of three-dimensional volume set. Planimetry measurement of the orifice in the subaortic membrane yielded 1.2 cm². **B,** Continuous-wave Doppler recording obtained from the apical five-chamber view, displaying a peak instantaneous gradient of 47 mmHg. **C,** Pulsed-wave Doppler demonstrating normal velocities proximal to the obstruction, with high, turbulent velocities in the left ventricular outflow tract (**D**).

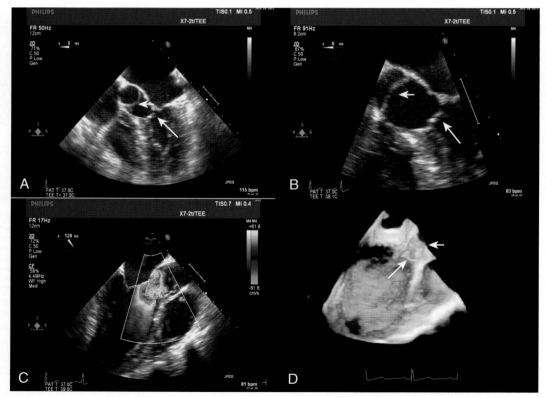

Figure 85.5. A, Midesophageal transesophageal echocardiography, five-chamber view, demonstrating the subaortic membrane *(arrow)* and the aortic valve *(arrowhead)*. **B,** Magnified view on the subaortic membrane *(arrow)* and the aortic valve *(arrowhead)* in a five-chamber view. **C,** Color-flow Doppler demonstrating mosaic pattern and flow acceleration at the orifice in the left ventricular outflow tract. **D,** Live real-time, three-dimensional image demonstrating the subaortic membrane *(arrow)* and the aortic valve *(arrowhead)*. (Also see Video 85.5.)

compare.[29] However, the Doppler mean pressure gradient measured by Doppler echocardiography and catheterization correlate well.[30] Both echocardiography and catheterization may underestimate the LVOT gradient in patients with decreased left ventricular ejection fractions (LVEFs) or a nonrestrictive VSD with left-to-right shunting.[25]

TREATMENT

Definitive management for patients with SAS is surgical repair and correction of the obstruction. The operation has been performed with low surgical mortality and minimal complications.[31] The timing of surgery should be based on the LVEF, presence of LVH, LVOT obstruction severity, AR, and patient age. The optimal timing still remains controversial, especially with the high rate of recurrence.

Surgery is the recommended option in patients with severe obstruction with a peak instantaneous pressure gradient greater than 50 mmHg and a mean gradient greater than 30 mmHg.[32,33] Consideration for earlier intervention should be given to patients with lower gradients but who have significant AR, a depressed ejection fraction, or a VSD. For equivocal cases, stress testing can be done to determine exercise capacity, symptoms, or increase in LVOT gradient.[32] Patients with symptoms attributed to SAS, such as angina, dyspnea, or syncope, should also undergo surgical evaluation. Both children and adults with mild gradients require close follow-up to monitor progression.

The specific operation depends on the type of SAS, but it is typically performed through a transaortic approach. Patients with discrete SAS may require membrane removal or ring resection with focal myomectomy. The tunnel-type variation is a technically more difficult surgery and often requires a myomectomy or the Konno procedure (aortic valve replacement with widening of the ventricular septum) for LVOT reconstruction.[34] There has been some consideration of performing selective myectomy at the time of surgery for relief of the LVOT obstruction; however, the data have not demonstrated a reduction in recurrence.[35]

A high rate of restenosis after surgery, up to 30%, has also been reported. Risk factors associated with restenosis include older age at diagnosis, tunnel-type morphology, and early surgery.[36,37] Reoperation rates vary from 4% to 35%, with higher rates found in those with the most severe preoperative gradient and in women.[8,38] The simple resection of the ridge renders it more likely to develop restenosis because the geometry in the ventricle remains the same with continued turbulent flow and hemodynamics. However, a large multicenter study that evaluated the utility of additional myectomy to enucleation did not demonstrate lower rates of restenosis or reoperation.[38] The rates of complete atrioventricular block were also significantly increased with the added myectomy. Performing interventions earlier has not demonstrated any clinical benefit in patients with mild gradients.[39] Percutaneous balloon dilatation has been performed as a less invasive alternative to surgical repair. Balloon tearing of SAS was first described in 1985 for the treatment of discrete thin membranes.[40] Although balloon dilatation is not widely used, study results have demonstrated that the procedure may be more than just a short-term option for nonsurgical candidates.[41]

The postoperative prognosis for patients with SAS is dependent on the morphology of SAS and the complexity of the disease. Altogether, the course is favorable, with long-term survival similar to the normal population.[38] Like preoperative patients, however, close follow-up is necessary with echocardiography after surgery to monitor for worsening gradients and AR.[32] The previously mentioned higher-risk groups should be evaluated more frequently for the need of reoperation.

ACKNOWLEDGMENTS

The author acknowledges the contributions of Dr. Lennie and Dr. Zamorano-Gomez, who were the authors of this chapter in the previous edition and who provided Fig. 85.1.

Please access ExpertConsult to view the corresponding videos for this chapter.

REFERENCES

1. Choi JY, Sullivan ID. Fixed subaortic stenosis: anatomical spectrum and nature of progression. *Br Heart J.* 1991;65:280–286.
2. Liu CW, Hwang B, Lee BC, et al. Aortic stenosis in children: 19-year experience. *Yi Xue Za Zhi (Taipei).* 1997;59:107–113.
3. Sigfusson G, Theresa TA, Vanauker MD, Cape EG. Abnormalities of the left ventricular outflow tract associated with discrete subaortic stenosis in children: an echocardiographic study. *J Am Coll Cardiol.* 1997;30:255–259.
4. Oliver JM, González A, Gallego P, et al. Discrete subaortic stenosis in adults: increased prevalence and slow rate of progression of the obstruction and aortic regurgitation. *J Am Coll Cardiol.* 2001;38:835–842.
5. Cilliers AM, Gewillig M. Rheology of discrete subaortic stenosis. *Heart.* 2002;88:335–336.
6. Katz NM, Buckley MJ, Liberthson RR. Discrete membranous subaortic stenosis. Report of 31 patients, review of the literature, and delineation of management. *Circulation.* 1977;56:1034–1038.
7. Brown JW, Stevens LS, Holly S, et al. Surgical spectrum of aortic stenosis in children: a thirty-year experience with 257 children. *Ann Thorac Surg.* 1988;45:393–403.
8. Brauner R, Laks H, Drinkwater D, et al. Benefits of early surgical repair in fixed subaortic stenosis. *J Am Coll Cardiol.* 1997;30:1835–1842.
9. Fatami SH, Ahmad U, Javed MA, et al. Familial membranous subaortic stenosis: review of familial inheritance patterns and a case report. *J Thorac Cardiovasc Surg.* 2006;132:1484–1486.
10. Abdallah H, Toomey K, O'Riordan AC, et al. Familial occurrence of discrete subaortic membrane. *Pediatr Cardiol.* 1994;15:198–200.
11. Leichter DA, Sullivan I, Gersony WM. "Acquired" discrete subvalvular aortic stenosis: natural history and hemodynamics. *J Am Coll Cardiol.* 1989;14:1539–1544.
12. Rosenquist GC, Clark EB, McAllister HA, Bharati S, Edwards JE. Increased mitral-aortic separation in discrete subaortic stenosis. *Circulation.* 1979;60:70–74.
13. Pyle R, Patterson D, Chacko S. The genetics and pathology of discrete subaortic stenosis in the Newfoundland dog. *Am Heart J.* 1976;92:324–334.
14. Gewillig M, Daenen W, Dumoulin M, Van der Hauwaert L. Rheologic genesis of discrete subvalvular aortic stenosis: a Doppler echocardiographic study. *J Am Coll Cardiol.* 1992;19:818–824.
15. Freedom RM, Pelech A, Brand A, et al. The progressive nature of subaortic stenosis in congenital heart disease. *Int J Cardiol.* 1985;8:137–148.
16. Bezold LI, Smith EO, Kelly K, et al. Development and validation of an echocardiographic model for predicting progression of discrete subaortic stenosis in children. *Am J Cardiol.* 1998;81:314–320.
17. Darcin OT, Yagdi T, Atay Y, et al. Discrete subaortic stenosis. *Tex Heart Inst J.* 2003;30:286–292.
18. McMahon CJ, Gauvreau K, Edwards JC, Geva T. Risk factors for aortic valve dysfunction in children with discrete subvalvar aortic stenosis. *Am J Cardiol.* 2004;94:459–464.
19. Rizzoli G, Tiso E, Mazzucco A, et al. Discrete subaortic stenosis: operative age and gradient as predictors of late aortic valve incompetence. *J Thorac Cardiovasc Surg.* 1993;106:95–104.
20. Kitchiner D, Jackson M, Malaiya N, et al. Morphology of left ventricular outflow tract structures in patients with subaortic stenosis and a ventricular septal defect. *Br Heart J.* 1994;72:251–260.
21. Pentousis D, Cooper J, Rae AP. Bacterial endocarditis involving a subaortic membrane. *Heart.* 1996;76:370–371.
22. Miyamoto K, Nakatani S, Kanzaki H, et al. Detection of discrete subaortic stenosis by 3-dimensional transesophageal echocardiography. *Echocardiography.* 2005;22:783–784.
23. Ge S, Warner Jr JG, Fowle KM, et al. Morphology and dynamic change of discrete subaortic stenosis can be imaged and quantified with three-dimensional transesophageal echocardiography. *J Am Soc Echocardiogr.* 1997;10:713–716.
24. Agrawal GG, Nanda NC, Htay T, et al. Live three-dimensional transthoracic echocardiographic identification of discrete subaortic membranous stenosis. *Echocardiography.* 2003;20:617–619.
25. Aboulhosn J, Child JS. Left ventricular outflow obstruction: subaortic stenosis, bicuspid aortic valve, supravalvar aortic stenosis, and coarctation of the aorta. *Circulation.* 2006;28:2412–2422.
26. Takx R, Schoepf UJ, Friedman B, et al. Recurrent subaortic membrane causing subvalvular aortic stenosis 13 years after primary surgical resection. *J Cardiovasc Comput Tomogr.* 2011;5:127–128.
27. Krieger EV, Stout KK, Grosse-Wortmann L. How to image congenital left heart obstruction in adults. *Circ Cardiovasc Imag.* 2017;10:e004271.

28. Mun HS, Wann LS. Noninvasive evaluation of membranous subaortic stenosis: complimentary roles of echocardiography and computed tomographic angiography. *Echocardiography.* 2010;27:E34–E35.

29. Currie PJ, Hagler DJ, Seward JB, et al. Instantaneous pressure gradient: a simultaneous Doppler and dual catheter correlative study. *J Am Coll Cardiol.* 1986;7:800–806.

30. Bengur AR, Snider AR, Serwer GA, et al. Usefulness of the Doppler mean gradient in evaluation of children with aortic valve stenosis and comparison to gradient at catheterization. *Am J Cardiol.* 1989;64:756–761.

31. van Son JA, Schaff HV, Danielson GK, et al. Surgical treatment of discrete and tunnel subaortic stenosis: late survival and risk of reoperation. *Circulation.* 1993;88:159–169.

32. Warnes CA, Williams RG, Bashore TM, et al. ACC/AHA 2008 guidelines for the management of adults with congenital heart disease: a report of the American College of Cardiology/American heart association task force on practice guidelines (Writing Committee to develop guidelines on the management of adults with congenital heart disease) developed in collaboration with the American Society of Echocardiography, Heart Rhythm Society, International Society for Adult Congenital Heart Disease, Society for Cardiovascular Angiography and Intervention. *J Am Coll Cardiol.* 2008;52:e143–263.

33. The task force on the management of grown-up congenital heart disease of the European Society of Cardiology (ESC): ESC guidelines for the management of grown-up congenital heart disease. *Eur Heart J.* 2010;31:2915–2957.

34. Konno S, Imai Y, Lida Y, et al. A new method for prosthetic valve replacement in congenital aortic stenosis associated with hypoplasia of the aortic valve ring. *J Thorac Cardiovasc Surg.* 1975;70:909–917.

35. Hirata Y, Chen JM, Quaegebeur JM, Mosca RS. The role of enucleation with or without septal myectomy for discrete subaortic stenosis. *J Thorac Cardiovasc Surg.* 2009;137:1168–1172.

36. Serraf A, Zoghby J, Lacour-Gayet F, et al. Surgical treatment of subaortic stenosis: a seventeen-year experience. *J Thorac Cardiovasc Surg.* 1999;117:669–678.

37. Dodge-Khatami A, Schmid M, Rousson V, et al. Risk factors for reoperation after relief of congenital subaortic stenosis. *Eur J Cardio Thorac Surg.* 2008;33:885–889.

38. van der Linde D, Roos-Hesselink JW, Rizopoulos D, et al. Surgical outcome of discrete subaortic stenosis in adults: a multicenter study. *Circulation.* 2013;127:1184–1191.

39. Kitchiner D. Subaortic stenosis: still more questions than answers. *Heart.* 1999;82:647–648.

40. Rao PS, Wilson AD, Chopra PS. Balloon dilatation for discrete subaortic stenosis: immediate and intermediate-term results. *J Invasive Cardiol.* 1990;2:65–71.

41. de Lezo JS, Romero M, Segura J, et al. Long-term outcome of patients with isolated thin discrete subaortic stenosis treated by balloon dilatation: a 25-year study. *Circulation.* 2011;124:1461–1468.

86 Aortic Regurgitation: Etiologies and Left Ventricular Responses

Roosha K. Parikh, William A. Zoghbi

ANATOMY OF THE AORTIC VALVE

The aortic valve is a semilunar valve, which typically has three cusps that are attached to the aortic wall to form the sinuses of Valsalva. The highest point of attachment at the leaflet commissures defines the sinotubular junction, and the most ventricular point (i.e., the nadir of the cusps) defines the annular plane. Note that the aortic annulus is not a real (physical) structure but rather a virtual "structure" defined by the bottom of the aortic cusps. The coaptation zone of the leaflets may include slight thickening or prominences at the central contact point (midpoint) of each cusp known as nodules of Arantius.[1] Fenestrations at the free edges of the cusps are common but seldom cause aortic regurgitation (AR) because they are above the closure line. Large fenestrations or torn fenestrations, however, can lead to AR. Normally, the integrity of the aortic orifice during diastole is maintained by an intact aortic root and firm apposition of the coaptation zone. The proper functioning of the valve depends on the proper relationship between the leaflets within the aortic root.

ETIOLOGY OF AORTIC REGURGITATION

AR is caused by a variety of disorders affecting the valve cusps, aortic root, or both (Table 86.1). With rheumatic heart disease becoming less common, nonrheumatic causes currently account for the majority of the underlying causes of aortic insufficiency, including congenitally malformed aortic valves, infective endocarditis, and connective tissue diseases.[2,3] Disorders affecting the aortic root also account for a large number of patients with AR. These conditions include cystic medial necrosis, Marfan syndrome, aortic dissection, and inflammatory diseases. At the tissue level, the aorta shows cystic medial necrosis, loss of elastic fibers, increased apoptosis, and altered smooth muscle cell alignment.[4] Note that the term "cystic medial necrosis" is actually a misnomer because this form of medial degeneration contains neither true cysts nor necrosis. Bicuspid aortic valve (BAV) is the most common congenital cardiac abnormality and is a common cause of AR (Fig. 86.1 and Video 86.1). Most BAVs consist of one free leaflet and two leaflets that are conjoined (or have failed to separate during embryonic development) instead of the typical three leaflets. The term "raphe" defines the conjoined area of the two underdeveloped leaflets turning into a malformed commissure between both leaflets.[5] Raphe may be complete, incomplete, or absent. Various causes have been suggested to explain the mechanism of AR in BAV, including cusp prolapse, endocarditis, dilated aortic root, and myxoid degeneration of the valve.[4] Less common types of congenital aortic valves include unicuspid and quadricuspid valves. These are discussed in greater detail in Chapter 78.

Calcific aortic valve disease can cause calcification spots or more extensive calcification of all the cusps, interfering with cusp motion and resulting in AR. Even in the absence of any obvious pathology of the aortic valve or root, severe systemic hypertension has been reported to cause significant AR.

MECHANISM OF AORTIC REGURGITATION

Evaluation of the mechanisms of AR, following the same principles as for the mitral valve's Carpentier classification, can help understand the mechanism of AR (Fig. 86.2). This classifies dysfunction based on the aortic root and leaflet morphology.

Type I dysfunction is identified when the leaflet motion is normal. However, there is enlargement of dimensions of any component of the aortic root, and no other cause of AR is identified. In type Ia, there is enlargement of the ascending aorta; in type Ib, there is enlargement of the sinuses of Valsalva and the sinotubular junction (Fig. 86.3 and Video 86.3); in type Ic, there is enlargement of the ventriculo-arterial junction (i.e., the aortic annulus); and in type Id, there is cusp perforation or fenestration, with preserved aortic root dimensions. Fenestration of a cusp free edge is considered in the presence of an eccentric AR jet, with normal leaflet motion (i.e., no prolapse).[6] There is disruption of the aortic root in aortic dissection, which may be a combination of all the types of dysfunction described (Fig. 86.4 and Video 86.4).

Type II dysfunction is considered when the leaflets have increased motion with cusp prolapse or commissural disruption. There are three subtypes of cusp prolapse—cusp flail, whole-cusp prolapse, and partial-cusp prolapse. Cusp prolapse occurs when the free edge of one or more the aortic cusps overrides the plane of the aortic annulus with some billowing. Cusp flail is defined as the complete eversion of a cusp into the LV outflow tract in the long-axis views (Fig. 86.5 and Video 86.5). Partial cusp prolapse is considered when the distal part of a cusp prolapses into the left ventricular (LV) outflow tract.[6]

Type III dysfunction is considered when the cusp tissue is restricted with reduced motion. This category includes congenitally abnormal valves, thickened and rigid valves, valves whose leaflet tissue have been destroyed by endocarditis, and severely calcified valves as described earlier.

LEFT VENTRICULAR REMODELING

The presentation and findings in patients with AR depend on its severity and rapidity of onset. The hemodynamic effects of acute severe AR are entirely different from the chronic type, and the two will be discussed separately.

Chronic Aortic Regurgitation

In response to the LV volume overload associated with AR, progressive LV dilatation occurs. This results in a higher wall stress that stimulates ventricular hypertrophy that in turn tends to normalize wall stress. Patients with severe AR may have the largest end-diastolic volumes of any other heart disease (so-called "bovine heart"), yet their end-diastolic pressures are not uniformly elevated. In keeping with

TABLE 86.1 Causes and Mechanisms of Aortic Regurgitation

MECHANISM	SPECIFIC CAUSE
Congenital or leaflet abnormalities	• Bicuspid, unicuspid, or quadricuspid aortic valve • Ventricular septal defect
Acquired leaflet abnormalities	• Senile calcification • Infective endocarditis • Rheumatic disease or inflammatory: systemic lupus erythematous, rheumatoid arthritis, Behcet syndrome • Radiation-induced valvulopathy • Toxin-induced valvulopathy: anorectic drugs, 5-hydroxytryptamine (carcinoid) • Trauma or iatrogenic • Leaflet damage caused by subaortic stenosis
Congenital or genetic aortic root abnormalities	• Annuloaortic ectasia • Connective tissue disease: Loeys-Dietz syndrome, Ehlers-Danlos syndrome, Marfan syndrome, osteogenesis imperfecta
Acquired aortic root abnormalities	• Idiopathic aortic root dilatation • Systemic hypertension • Autoimmune disease: systemic lupus erythematosus, ankylosing spondylitis, Reiter syndrome, relapsing polychondritis, • Aortitis: syphilitic, Takayasu arteritis, other infections, idiopathic • Aortic dissection • Trauma

Modified from Zoghbi WA, Adams D, Bonow RO, et al. Recommendations for non-invasive evaluation of native valvular regurgitation: a report from the American Society of Echocardiography developed in collaboration with the Society of Cardiovascular Magnetic resonance. J Am Soc Echocardiogr 2017; 30:303-71.

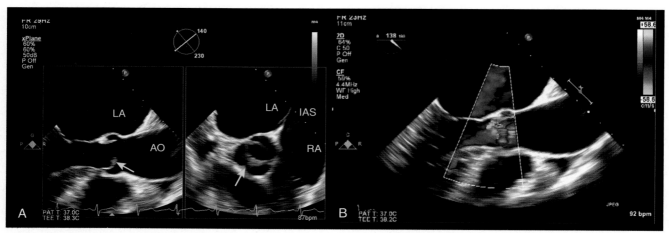

Figure 86.1. Two-dimensional and color Doppler images of a bicuspid aortic valve. Midesophageal transesophageal echocardiography (TEE) long-axis view with X-plane at the level of the aortic valve (**A**) demonstrates doming of the leaflet *(arrow)*, and the X-plane short-axis view demonstrates a bicuspid aortic valve with fusion of the right and left coronary cusp with a raphe *(arrow)* with fish-mouth appearance of valve orifice. TEE long-axis view of the aortic valve with color Doppler (**B**). The aortic regurgitation jet is eccentric *(arrow)*. *AO,* Aorta; *IAS,* interatrial septum; *LA,* left atrium; *RA,* right atrium. (See accompany Video 86.1).

the Frank-Starling mechanism, the stroke volume is also increased. Thus, despite the presence of regurgitation, a normal effective forward cardiac output can be maintained. Chronic severe AR results in a state of gradual LV volume overload with resultant progressive and eccentric hypertrophy and an increase in LV dimensions to counter high wall stress, thus initially keeping the LV diastolic pressure low.[7] This state persists for several years, keeping patients asymptomatic. Gradually, LV diastolic properties and contractile function start to decline. The adaptive dilatation and hypertrophy can no longer match the loading conditions. The LV end-diastolic pressure begins to rise, and the ejection fraction drops with a decline in effective forward output and development of heart failure.[8]

In patients with chronic isolated AR, echocardiographic analysis of LV longitudinal deformation and deformation rate with speckle-tracking echocardiography is useful for the detection of clinically relevant LV systolic and diastolic dysfunction. Both the systolic and the early diastolic myocardial deformation are impaired early in the disease course in AR (Fig. 86.6 and Video 86.6). A strong

relationship of this with reduced functional status shows that the impairment of the global longitudinal strain may be clinically relevant.[7,9]

Acute Aortic Regurgitation

When sudden severe AR occurs, there is no time for the left ventricle to undergo adaptation. This is in contrast to chronic AR. Therefore, the acute ventricular volume overload results in a small increase in end-diastolic volume and severe elevation of end-diastolic pressure, which is transmitted to the left atrium and pulmonary veins culminating in acute pulmonary edema. Because the ventricular end-diastolic volume is normal, the total stroke volume is not increased, and the effective forward cardiac output drops. To compensate for the low-output state, sympathetic stimulation occurs, which produces tachycardia and peripheral vasoconstriction, the latter further worsening AR.

Please access ExpertConsult to view the corresponding videos for this chapter.

Aortic regurgitation

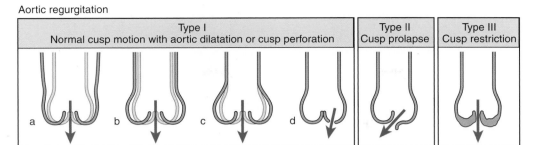

Figure 86.2. Suggested classification of aortic regurgitation (AR) morphology[1,10] depicting the various mechanisms of AR. Type Ia is sinotubular junction enlargement and dilatation of the ascending aorta. Type Ib is dilatation of the sinuses of Valsalva and sinotubular junction. Type Ic is dilatation of the ventriculoarterial junction (annulus). Type Id is aortic cusp perforation. Types II and III are also illustrated.

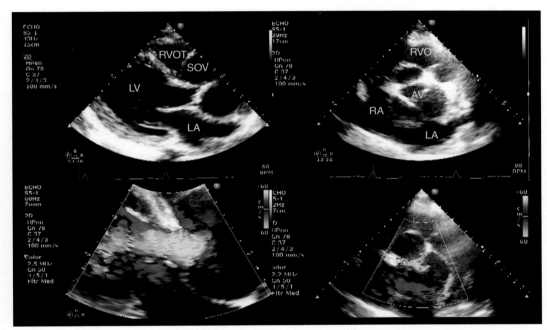

Figure 86.3. Transthoracic echocardiography two-dimensional *(top panel)* and color Doppler *(bottom panel)* images in parasternal long-axis *(left panel)* and parasternal short-axis views at the level of the aortic valve *(right panel)*. The aortic root is dilated at the level of sinus of Valsalva and measures 7.2 cm. This is classified as Ib with normal leaflet motion and a dilated aortic root. There is severe aortic regurgitation as demonstrated in the *bottom panel* on color Doppler. *AV,* Aortic valve; *LA,* left atrium; *LV,* left ventricle; *RVOT,* right ventricular outflow tract; *SOV,* sinus of Valsalva. (See accompanying Video 86.3.)

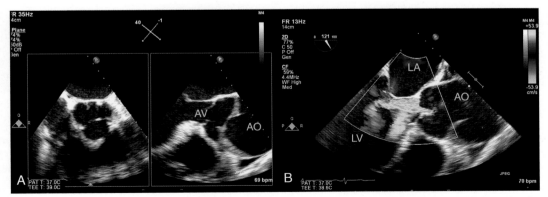

Figure 86.4. Midesophageal short-axis transesophageal echocardiography (TEE) view of the aortic valve (AV) with X-plane showing the long axis of the AV and the ascending aorta (**A**). There is an ascending aorta aneurysm with a dissection flap *(arrow)*. There is also AV cusp prolapse *(arrow)* noted with billowing of the cusp into the left ventricular outflow tract. Color Doppler image of the midesophageal long-axis TEE view of the AV and ascending aorta (**B**) demonstrates an eccentric aortic regurgitation jet directed to the anterior mitral valve leaflet. *AO,* Aorta; *LA,* left atrium; *LV,* left ventricle. (See accompanying Video 86.4.)

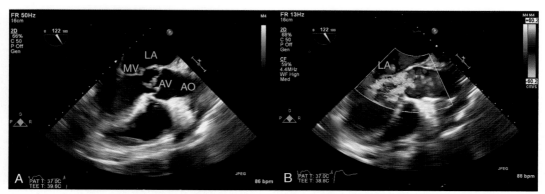

Figure 86.5. Two-dimensional and color Doppler images of the aortic valve (AV). **A,** Midesophageal transesophageal echocardiography (TEE) long-axis view at the level of the AV demonstrates large mobile echodensity measuring 1.5 × 1.5 cm on the AV leaflet with a flail leaflet *(arrow)*. **B,** The mitral valve is involved here with a small aneurysm that is perforated, and the same view with color Doppler added shows severe aortic regurgitation and eccentric mitral regurgitation (on the video). *AO,* Aorta; *LA,* left atrium; *MV,* mitral valve. (See accompanying Video 86.5).

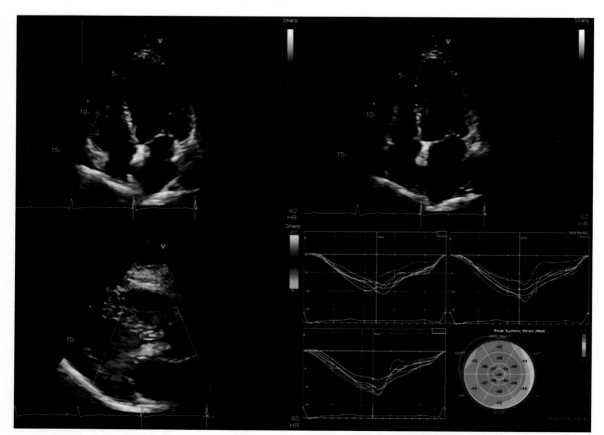

Figure 86.6. Two-dimensional (2D) transthoracic four-chamber view showing a mildly enlarged left ventricle (LV) with the LV at end-diastole *(left)* and end-systole *(right)* with a biplane left ventricular ejection fraction of 56%. *Top,* 2D transthoracic parasternal long-axis view with color Doppler demonstrating mild to moderate aortic regurgitation. (See accompanying Video 86.6). *Bottom right,* Left ventricular longitudinal strain values from transthoracic four-, two-, and three-chamber (long-axis) views for each wall segment and the average peak systolic longitudinal strain values of each left ventricular myocardial segment are reported in a bull's eye plot. As illustrated on the *colored strain bars*, segments with normal strain values are depicted in *dark red*, and other colors indicate progressive degrees of systolic dysfunction. The average global longitudinal strain here is reduced at −14.6% *(bottom right)*.

REFERENCES

1. Zoghbi WA, Adams D, Bonow RO, et al. Recommendations for noninvasive evaluation of native valvular regurgitation. *J Am Soc Echocardiogr.* 2017;30:303–371.
2. Guiney TE, Davies MJ, Parker DJ, et al. The aetiology and course of isolated severe aortic regurgitation: a clinical, pathological, and echocardiographic study. *Br Heart J.* 1987;58:358–368.
3. Turri M, Thiene G, Bortolotti U, et al. Surgical pathology of aortic valve disease. A study based on 602 specimens. *Eur J Cardiothorac Surg.* 1990;4:556–560.
4. Lewin MB, Otto CM. The bicuspid aortic valve: adverse outcomes from infancy to old age. *Circulation.* 2005;111:832–834.
5. Koenraadt WM, Grewal N, Gaidoukevitch OY, et al. The extent of the raphe in bicuspid aortic valves is associated with aortic regurgitation and aortic root dilatation. *Neth Heart J.* 2016;24:127–133.
6. Gallego Garcia de Vinuesa P, et al. Functional anatomy of aortic regurgitation. Role of transesophageal echocardiography in aortic valve-sparing surgery. *Rev Esp Cardiol.* 2010;63:536–543.
7. Alashi A, Mentias A, Abdallah A, et al. Incremental prognostic utility of left ventricular global longitudinal strain in asymptomatic patients with significant chronic aortic regurgitation and preserved left ventricular ejection fraction. *JACC Cardiovasc Imag.* 2018;11:673–682.
8. Levine HJ. Left ventricular function after correction of chronic aortic regurgitation. *Circulation.* 1988;78:1319–1321.
9. Olsen NT, Sogaard P, Larsson HB, et al. Speckle-tracking echocardiography for predicting outcome in chronic aortic regurgitation during conservative management and after surgery. *JACC Cardiovasc Imag.* 2011;4:223–230.
10. Boodhwani M, de Kerchove L, Glineur D, et al. Repair-oriented classification of aortic insufficiency: impact on surgical techniques and clinical outcomes. J Thor Cardiovasc Surg. 2009;137:286–294.

87 Aortic Regurgitation: Pathophysiology

Nir Flint, Roy Beigel, Robert J. Siegel

Aortic regurgitation (AR) results from reflux of blood from the aorta into the left ventricle during diastole, caused by aortic valve or aortic root disease. The pathophysiology of AR depends whether the AR is acute or chronic. Acute AR is a medical emergency characterized by abrupt left ventricular (LV) volume overload, leading to rapid increase in left ventricular end-diastolic pressures (LVEDPs). Conversely, chronic AR is a slowly progressing condition in which adaptive changes occur in the LV to accommodate for the increase in preload and afterload. LV filling pressures can remain normal for a long period. As chronic AR progresses, wall stress increases because LV dilatation and hypertrophy cannot compensate for the volume overload. Myocardial fibrosis develops, LV filling pressures increase, and symptoms of heart failure and coronary hypoperfusion may appear. Timely repair of AR, usually by surgical or percutaneous aortic valve replacement (AVR) and sometimes by surgical repair, may lead to improvement in LV size and function.

AORTIC REGURGITATION PATHOPHYSIOLOGY

AR results from incomplete coaptation or closure of the aortic valve cusps during diastole, leading to reflux of blood from the aorta into the left ventricle. AR results from various causes involving the aortic valve cusps or aortic root. AR can also result from a paravalvular leak originating around the circumference of a prosthetic valve or from structural deterioration of a bioprosthetic valve. The pathophysiology, hemodynamics, and clinical presentation of AR depend on its severity and differ whether AR develops abruptly (acute AR) or progresses over time (chronic AR). Table 87.1 lists the main differences between these two distinct scenarios.

ACUTE AORTIC REGURGITATION

Acute severe AR is a potentially catastrophic condition with several causes, including endocarditis, aortic dissection, trauma, or iatrogenic. Acute severe AR is characterized by abrupt LV volume overload leading to a rapid increase in LVEDP because the LV has not had the time to dilate and adapt to the rapid increase in preload. In acute AR, the LV size is often normal. The high preload and afterload (increased LV wall stress) result in an acute increase in LVEDP, and consequently a reduction in left ventricular ejection fraction (LVEF) and LV stroke volume, despite a relatively maintained myocardial contractility.[1] The acute rise in LV filling pressures leads to an acute increase in left atrial (LA) pressure, and subsequently, an increase in the pulmonary capillary wedge pressure. Thus, patients often present with pulmonary edema and even cardiogenic shock. Reflex tachycardia reduces diastolic filling time and AR, which helps maintain cardiac output.

Acute volume overload shifts the LV hemodynamics to operate at the extreme of the pressure–volume curve (Fig. 87.1). In severe cases, the LVEDP can exceed the LA pressure and lead to premature, presystolic closure of the mitral valve with or without diastolic mitral regurgitation (MR) (Fig. 87.2). This is commonly seen in patients with preexisting LV hypertrophy (e.g., in patients with hypertension or aortic stenosis), in whom acute AR begets an "exaggerated" hemodynamic response because these patients often have concentric hypertrophy with a small, noncompliant LV. When the diastolic aortic pressure approaches the LVEDP, reduced myocardial perfusion pressure (defined as diastolic aortic pressure – LVEDP) may develop, leading to subendocardial hypoperfusion. This may result in myocardial ischemia and further deterioration in LV function and stroke volume. Acute AR can also lead to distention and dilatation of the LV as well as dilatation and distortion of the mitral annulus, resulting in functional MR, which further increases LA and pulmonary capillary wedge pressures. Optimally, acute severe AR should be treated with emergent AVR. Depending on the AR mechanism, replacement of the aortic root and possibly the ascending aorta may also be required. Stabilization with vasodilators to reduce LV filling pressures and inotropes to improve forward stroke volume can sometimes serve as a temporary bridge to surgery.

CHRONIC AORTIC REGURGITATION

The most common causes of chronic AR in industrialized countries are calcific aortic valve degeneration and congenital bicuspid aortic valve (with or without concomitant aortic stenosis).[2,3] In the early phase of chronic AR, compensatory mechanisms maintain the LVEF and forward stroke volume within the normal range. Over time, the LV dilates and hypertrophies to maintain a normal ratio of ventricular wall thickness to cavity radius, and consequently, a normal LV end-diastolic wall stress. These adaptive mechanisms are responsible for the slow progression and long asymptomatic phase of chronic AR by allowing the LV to accommodate large stroke volumes, with only a mild increase in LV filling pressures.

The AR regurgitant volume is proportional to the effective regurgitant orifice (ERO) and, to a lesser extent, the diastolic pressure gradient between the aorta and the LV. Bradycardia, which prolongs diastole, may increase the regurgitant volume[4] and is not well tolerated in patients with significant AR. With the progression of AR over time, left ventricular end-diastolic volume (LVEDV) increases. When all the sarcomeres within the LV are maximally distended, the preload reserve is reached, and any further increase in the LV afterload will result a reduction in LV stroke volume.[1]

Although both AR and MR are conditions associated with volume overload, in MR, the regurgitant volume flows retrograde into the low-pressure LA, whereas in AR, the sum of the regurgitant volume and the forward stroke volume is ejected into the high-pressure aorta during systole. The large total forward stroke volume may induce systolic hypertension (increased afterload). This is usually associated with low diastolic pressure, caused by the regurgitation of blood back

from the aorta into the LV during diastole, resulting in a wide pulse pressure.[5] In AR, end-diastolic dimensions are generally larger compared with MR; hence, LVEF is low-normal in AR, whereas it is preserved or supranormal in MR. Although both MR and AR are associated with a mechanical overload of the left ventricle, the systolic wall stress is higher in patients with AR than in those with MR. Wall stress may reach a level similar to that found in patients with aortic stenosis.[6] The law of Laplace expresses systolic wall stress as $p \times r/2h$ (p = LV pressure; r = LV radius; h = LV wall thickness). In patients with AR, both p and r are increased, and although h is also increased, it is generally not sufficient to compensate for the combined increase of both p and r.[7] Consequently, the increase in systolic wall stress and LV afterload in AR, increases the energy requirements of the left ventricle.[8] In AR, modest reduction in LVEF is likely a reflection of increased afterload and not necessarily contractile

TABLE 87.1 Major Differences Between Acute and Compensated Chronic Severe Aortic Regurgitation (AR)

	Acute AR	Chronic AR
Clinical presentation	Pulmonary edema, refractory heart failure	Often asymptomatic
Left ventricular size	Normal to slightly enlarged	Markedly enlarged
Left ventricular end-diastolic pressure	Markedly elevated	Normal to slightly elevated
Systolic aortic pressure	Normal or slightly decreased	Elevated
Diastolic aortic pressure	Normal or slightly decreased	Decreased
Pulse pressure	Normal or slightly increased	Increased
Cardiac output	Decreased	Normal
Heart rate	Elevated	Normal or slightly elevated

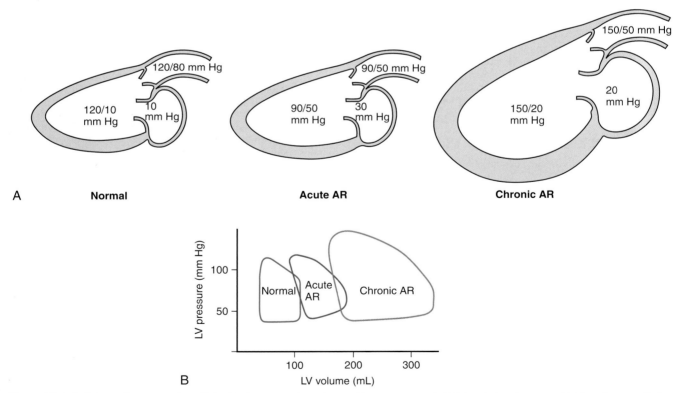

Figure 87.1. A, Schematic presentation of left-sided pressures in patients with acute severe *(middle)* and chronic severe *(right)* aortic regurgitation (AR) compared with a normal heart *(left)*. In acute severe AR, there is a dramatic rise in end-diastolic pressure and as a result an increase in left atrial pressure. Total stroke volume is increased, but the effective forward stroke volume is reduced. In compensated chronic AR, there are left ventricular (LV) dilatation and eccentric hypertrophy, which help reduce wall stress and maintain total and forward stroke volume. LV filling pressures are normal. **B,** Pressure volume loops of acute AR *(middle)* and chronic AR *(right)* compared with a normal heart *(left)*. In acute AR, volume and pressure overload are acting on an unconditioned, noncompliant left ventricle; thus, there is a large change in pressure per volume. In chronic AR, the adapted LV can sustain markedly higher volumes with a more modest change in pressure per volume. See text for details.

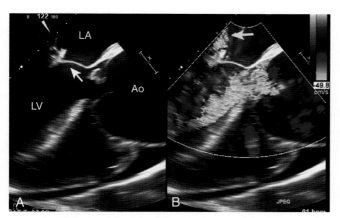

Figure 87.2. Transesophageal echocardiography (TEE) images of a patient with severe aortic regurgitation (AR) caused by infective endocarditis and aortic root aneurysm. **B,** Wide color flow jet in the LV outflow tract consistent with severe aortic regurgitation. Diastolic mitral regurgitation jet is present *(yellow arrow).* **A,** The same view, without color Doppler, showing a dilated aortic root and a vegetation on the noncoronary cusp. There is diastolic preclosure of the mitral valve *(white arrow). Ao,* Aorta; *LA,* left atrium; *LV,* left ventricle.

dysfunction, compared with MR, in which decreased LVEF often reflects some degree of myocyte damage.[5] However, with the progression of chronic severe AR, if wall thickening fails to keep up with the volume overload, the elevated wall stress can lead to myocyte damage and contractile dysfunction.[9] Early evidence of myocardial damage can be evident by myocardial fibrosis in the context of AR, which precedes the development of heart failure.[4] A subclinical decrease in LV function can be detected by reduced LV global longitudinal strain, which is superior to LVEF as a prognostic marker after surgical AVR.[10] Table 87.2 summarizes the differences in the pathophysiologic features affecting the LV during the chronic phase of aortic and mitral regurgitation.

Volume overload associated with chronic AR triggers a series of pathophysiologic events (Figs. 87.1 and 87.3). Initially, the increase in LVEDV increases LV compliance to accommodate the volume overload while maintaining normal filling pressures. The chronic LV volume overload results in chamber enlargement along with an eccentric pattern of hypertrophy with an increase in LV mass, permitting the ventricle to eject a large stroke volume to maintain a normal forward stroke volume.[11]

Patients with chronic severe AR can have the largest LVEDVs that occur in patients with heart failure. The resultant cardiomegaly in this setting has been termed *cor bovinum* (Fig. 87.4). In chronic severe AR, LVEDVs can increase by as much as

TABLE 87.2 Differences in Left Ventricular (LV) Pathophysiology and Hemodynamics During the Chronic Phase of Aortic and Mitral Regurgitation

	Aortic Regurgitation (AR)	Mitral Regurgitation (MR)
Pathophysiological mechanism	Volume and pressure overload	Volume overload
LV afterload	Increased	Decreased
LV wall stress[8]	Higher than MR	Lower than AR
LV geometry	Eccentric hypertrophy with modest concentric hypertrophy[16]	Enlarged LV
LV mass to volume ratio	1[16]	<1[5]
LV ejection fraction	Can be lower before myocyte damage and contractile dysfunction have developed	Greater than normal in compensated phase Normal or lower in decompensated phase or when contractile dysfunction has developed
Mechanism of reduced LV contractility	Increased afterload[6]	A reduction in EF signifies loss of contractile elements[17]
Mechanism of LV hypertrophy	Increase in protein synthesis[18]	Reduced rate of protein degradation[19,20]
LV radius to thickness	Lower than MR	Higher than AR
Reversibility with treatment	Mostly reversible	Mostly reversible

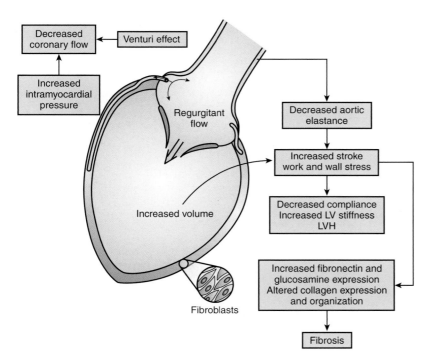

Figure 87.3. Severe chronic aortic regurgitation increases the volume load on the left ventricle (LV), which, combined with decreasing aortic distensibility over time, increases stroke work and wall stress. These maladaptations lead to LV hypertrophy and decreasing LV compliance. As a result of these stressors, the expression of collagen and certain proteins in fibroblasts changes, promoting myocardial fibrosis. *LVH,* Left ventricular hypertrophy (Reproduced with permission from Carabello BA: Progress in mitral and aortic regurgitation, *Prog Cardiovasc Dis* 43:457–475, 2001.)

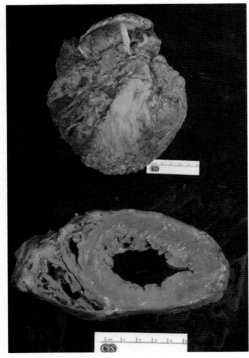

Figure 87.4. Postexplant images from a patient with chronic severe aortic regurgitation. In this explanted heart weighing 860 g (normal, 350–400 g), there are pronounced cardiomegaly *(top)* along with left ventricular hypertrophy *(bottom)* and moderately increased interstitial and endocardial fibrosis (not shown).

three to four times normal, which allows these patients to sustain high cardiac outputs. LV compliance is usually also increased, so the LVEDP may be only slightly elevated. These compensatory mechanisms enable patients to remain stable for years even in the presence of severe AR. However, this is a progressive condition, and the combination of increased preload and afterload results in an increase in end-systolic dimensions and eventually, a reduction in LVEF.

As LV filling pressure rise, symptoms of fatigue and dyspnea may appear. Low aortic diastolic pressures, shorter diastolic time (caused by increased heart rate), and elevated LVEDP lead to decreased coronary perfusion pressure.[12] Angina may develop even in the presence of normal coronary arteries because of the combination of reduced coronary blood flow and high O_2 requirements from increased wall tension and LV mass.[13] As in acute severe AR, in chronic AR, the distention and dilatation of the LV can also result in secondary (functional) MR. This pathophysiological cycle leads

to subsequent decompensation manifested by a decrease in cardiac output, increased LVEDP and LVEDV, and symptoms of heart failure.

Current guidelines recommend surgical AVR in symptomatic patients with severe AR or in asymptomatic patients when LVEF is below 50% or when there is progressive LV dilatation (LV endsystolic dimension >50 mm or end-diastolic dimension >65 mm).[14] Appropriately timed AVR will lead to improvement in LVEF, LV chamber volume, and wall thickness.[15]

REFERENCES

1. Ross Jr J. Afterload mismatch in aortic and mitral valve disease: implications for surgical therapy. *J Am Coll Cardiol.* 1985;5:811–826.
2. Enriquez-Sarano M, Tajik AJ. Clinical practice. Aortic regurgitation. *N Engl J Med.* 2004;351:1539–1546.
3. Nishimura RA, Otto CM, Bonow RO, et al. AHA/ACC guideline for the management of patients with valvular heart disease. *J Am Coll Cardiol.* 2014;63:e57–185. 2014.
4. Goldbarg SH, Halperin JL. Aortic regurgitation: disease progression and management. *Nat Clin Pract Cardiovasc Med.* 2008;5:269–279.
5. Carabello BA. Progress in mitral and aortic regurgitation. *Prog Cardiovasc Dis.* 2001;43:457–475.
6. Sutton M, Plappert T, Spiegel A, et al. Early postoperative changes in left ventricular chamber size, architecture, and function in aortic stenosis and aortic regurgitation and their relation to intraoperative changes in afterload: a prospective two-dimensional echocardiographic study. *Circulation.* 1987;76:77–89.
7. Carabello BA. Aortic regurgitation. A lesion with similarities to both aortic stenosis and mitral regurgitation. *Circulation.* 1990;82:1051–1053.
8. Wisenbaugh T, Spann JF, Carabello BA. Differences in myocardial performance and load between patients with similar amounts of chronic aortic versus chronic mitral regurgitation. *J Am Coll Cardiol.* 1984;3:916–923.
9. Rigolin VH, Bonow RO. Hemodynamic characteristics and progression to heart failure in regurgitant lesions. *Heart Fail Clin.* 2006;2:453–460.
10. Smedsrud MK, Pettersen E, Gjesdal O, et al. Detection of left ventricular dysfunction by global longitudinal systolic strain in patients with chronic aortic regurgitation. *J Am Soc Echocardiogr.* 2011;24. 1253–129.
11. Grossman W, Jones D, McLaurin LP. Wall stress and patterns of hypertrophy in the human left ventricle. *J Clin Invest.* 1975;56:56–64.
12. Tamborini G, Barbier P, Doria E, et al. Coronary flow and left ventricular diastolic function in aortic regurgitation. *Coron Artery Dis.* 1995;6:635–643.
13. Nitenberg A, Foult JM, Antony I, et al. Coronary flow and resistance reserve in patients with chronic aortic regurgitation, angina pectoris and normal coronary arteries. *J Am Coll Cardiol.* 1988;11:478–486.
14. Nishimura RA, Otto CM, Bonow RO, et al. AHA/ACC guideline for the management of patients with valvular heart disease. *J Thorac Cardiovasc Surg.* 2014;148:e1–e132. 2014.
15. Chaliki HP, Mohty D, Avierinos JF, et al. Outcomes after aortic valve replacement in patients with severe aortic regurgitation and markedly reduced left ventricular function. *Circulation.* 2002;106:2687–2693.
16. Feiring AJ, Rumberger JA. Ultrafast computed tomography analysis of regional radius-to-wall thickness ratios in normal and volume-overloaded human left ventricle. *Circulation.* 1992;85:1423–1432.
17. Urabe Y, Mann DL, Kent RL, et al. Cellular and ventricular contractile dysfunction in experimental canine mitral regurgitation. *Circ Res.* 1992;70:131–147.
18. King RK, Magid NM, Opio G, Borer JS. Protein turnover in compensated chronic aortic regurgitation. *Cardiology.* 1997;88:518–525.
19. Imamura T, McDermott PJ, Kent RL, et al. Acute changes in myosin heavy chain synthesis rate in pressure versus volume overload. *Circ Res.* 1994;75:418–425.
20. Matsuo T, Carabello BA, Nagatomo Y, et al. Mechanisms of cardiac hypertrophy in canine volume overload. *Am J Physiol.* 1998;275:H65–H74.

88 Quantitation of Aortic Regurgitation

Hari P. Chaliki, Minako Katayama, Vuyisile T. Nkomo

Aortic regurgitation (AR), either acute or chronic, can be caused by valvular pathology, aortic root pathology, or a combination of the two. In developed countries, chronic isolated AR is predominantly caused by aortic root disease or congenital aortic valve disease, but rheumatic fever still remains the leading cause of chronic AR in developing countries.[1] Surgery is frequently needed for patients

with acute AR, and the timing of surgery for chronic AR depends on regurgitation severity, the patient's symptoms, and left ventricular (LV) size and function.[2] Therefore, accurate determination of cause and severity of AR is crucial when managing patients with AR. Semiquantitative and quantitative techniques should be used in an integrated fashion to assess the severity of AR.

QUANTITATION OF AORTIC REGURGITATION
Semiquantitative Methods

Currently, Doppler color flow imaging is widely used to determine the severity of AR despite its limitations and semiquantitative nature.[3] Parasternal long-axis, short-axis, and apical views can demonstrate the color Doppler recording of the AR well. Maximal length and area of the aortic regurgitant jet show poor correlation with aortic angiography. Short-axis jet area at the high left ventricular outflow tract (LVOT) relative to the LVOT area correlates well with angiography. The proportion of either jet area or jet width compared with LVOT area or width in excess of 65% indicates severe AR.[3,4] Although appealing, it is important to note that this method requires careful attention to gain settings and Nyquist limits to avoid over- or underestimating the severity of regurgitation. In general, this method only provides a rough estimate of the severity of AR. This method is of limited utility in patients with eccentric jets, diffuse jets, and jets originating along the entire coaptation line.[4]

Both continuous-wave (CW) and pulsed-wave (PW) Doppler techniques are useful for the semiquantitative assessment of AR. Whereas dense CW Doppler signal implies greater quantity of regurgitation, faint signals generally represent mild regurgitation. Pressure halftime, the time for the pressure gradient to drop by half of its original value, is another measure of severity of AR obtained by CW Doppler.[5,6] It is expected that the pressure halftime is shorter (<200 msec) in patients with severe AR because of the rapid rise in LV pressure from a large amount of regurgitant volume (RV), especially in patients with acute AR. Conversely, in patients with mild AR, the pressure halftime is longer (>500 msec) because of a more gradual rise in LV pressure. Pressure halftime cannot be used alone to determine the severity of AR because it is dependent on chronicity of the regurgitation, systolic blood pressure, and LV compliance.[4] For example, pressure halftime may be short because of underlying severe LV diastolic dysfunction. Another frequently used Doppler technique involves PW Doppler of the proximal descending thoracic aorta. Significant holodiastolic flow reversal in the descending thoracic aorta, diastolic velocity time integral similar to systolic velocity time integral, and relatively high end-diastolic velocity (>18 cm/s) are indicative of moderate to severe or severe AR (Fig.88.1 and Video 88.1).[7] In some older patients, diastolic flow reversal is a less reliable indicator of the severity of AR because of a stiff aorta.[4]

It has been proposed that the smallest area of the aortic regurgitant jet hydrodynamically represents VC.[8] From parasternal views, using the zoom function, one can visualize the proximal flow convergence zone, flow at the aortic valve, and flow below the aortic valve.[9] In early to mid-diastole, VC is then measured, which is defined as the width of the narrowest portion of the aortic regurgitant jet that occurs immediately distal to the anatomic orifice. A VC width greater than 6 mm is indicative of severe AR with a sensitivity of 81% and specificity of 94%.[9] In some patients, a right parasternal transthoracic window[10] or transesophageal echocardiography (TEE) may be required to obtain adequate VC measurements (Fig. 88.2 and Video 88.2).

Quantitative Methods

The continuity method uses the principle of conservation of mass for determination of AR. Assuming there is no or minimal mitral regurgitation (MR), the volume of AR can be precisely calculated by subtracting the flow through the mitral valve from the LVOT flow.[11,12] This method uses the combination of two-dimensional information and Doppler technique. Flow through the mitral annulus and LVOT can be calculated by multiplying mitral annular area and LVOT areas with their corresponding time velocity integrals (TVIs). Assuming a circular mitral annulus and LVOT, the following formulae are used to determine the mitral flow, LVOT flow, and aortic RV:[11]

$$\text{Mitral flow} = \text{Mitral annulus area} \times \text{TVI at the mitral annulus level}$$

$$\text{LVOT flow} = \text{LVOT area} \times \text{TVI at the LVOT level}$$

$$\text{RV} = \text{LVOT flow} - \text{Mitral flow}$$

RV 60 mL or greater is considered severe. In selected cases, LV volume measurements using biplane method of disks (modified Simpson rule)[13] without foreshortening the LV (using contrast if needed) or three-dimensional (3D) LV volumes is necessary to verify the stroke volume. This method has the advantage of being useful in case of multiple AR jets. Even though this technique is based on solid principles, it is a challenging technique to master, and attention to detail is mandatory. A small error in mitral annular measurement or LVOT measurement can greatly impact the calculations. Similarly, if the modal mitral inflow velocity (brightest signal) is not traced, this can result in an erroneous estimate of RV.[4]

Similar to continuity method, the proximal isovelocity surface area (PISA) method or the flow convergence method is based on the conservation-of-mass principle. Unlike the continuity method, the presence of MR does not affect the quantitation of AR. As the flow approaches a regurgitant orifice, there is flow acceleration with resultant isovelocity surfaces proximal to the regurgitant

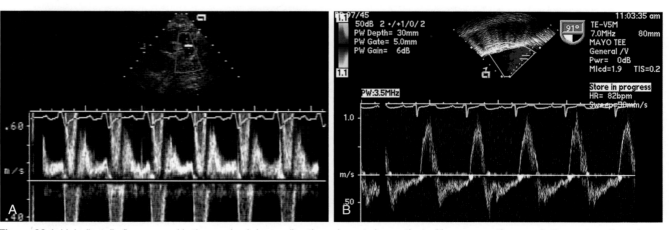

Figure 88.1. Holodiastolic flow reversal in the proximal descending thoracic aorta in a patient with severe aortic regurgitation on transthoracic study (**A**) and transesophageal study (**B**).

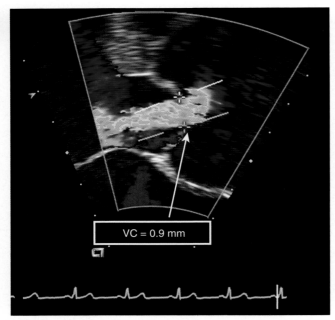

Figure 88.2. Vena contracta (VC) width (9 mm) measurement in a patient with chronic severe aortic regurgitation on transesophageal study.

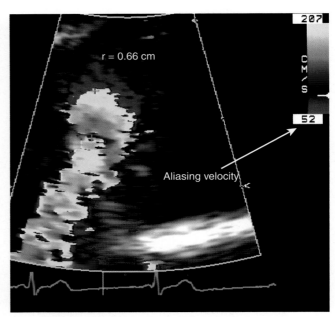

Figure 88.3. Proximal isovelocity surface area (PISA). PISA is visualized by shifting the baseline. PISA r is the radius (0.66 cm) of the proximal flow convergence, and Vr is the aliasing velocity (52 cm/s).

orifice. Using the conservation-of-mass principle, effective regurgitant orifice area (EROA)[14] and finally RV can be calculated by assuming a hemispheric shape of the proximal isovelocity. By baseline shifting the color scale in the direction of the jet, the isovelocity surface can be viewed, and resultant flow convergence radius and velocity can be obtained (Fig. 88.3 and Video 88.3).[14] The zoom feature in combination with either parasternal view or apical long-axis view is used to optimize the images. The AR flow rate is calculated as: $2\pi \times r^2 \times Vr$ in which r is the radius of the flow convergence measured in early diastole and Vr is the corresponding aliasing velocity. All units are centimeters. Doppler tracing of the aortic regurgitant jet can then be used to calculate EROA and RV as follows:[14]

$$EROA = \text{Regurgitant flow rate/Peak aortic regurgitant velocity in early diastole}$$

$$RV = EROA \times TVI \text{ of the AR}$$

EROA 0.3 cm^2 or greater and RV 60 mL or greater are considered severe. Selected ranges for grading of the severity of AR are shown in Table 88.1. In a few patients who have dilated ascending aorta, flow convergence zone may occupy greater than 220 degrees around the aortic valve leaflets and leads to underestimation of EROA and RV by this method.[14]

Left Ventricular Measurements

The chronicity and severity of AR determine the LV response to volume overload. In acute severe AR, one would not expect the left ventricle to be large in the absence of other causes. On the contrary, in chronic severe AR, the left ventricle is dilated. One should measure the LV end-diastolic and systolic dimensions using either a two-dimensional (2D) method or 2D-targeted M-mode echocardiography at or below the level of the mitral valve leaflet tips[13] because the current guidelines for surgery in asymptomatic patients are based on these measurements.[2] More recent studies indicating the need for earlier surgical intervention[15] for patients with chronic asymptomatic severe AR are also based on 2D echocardiographic measurements indexed to body

surface area; therefore, extreme care need to be taken when making these 2D measurement, especially as they apply to serial studies. It is likely that future guidelines will be based on 3D volumetric measurements as more outcome data become available. Although LV ejection fraction and end-systolic dimension are reasonable measures of LV systolic function, recent studies indicate that global longitudinal strain may be better in predicting optimal timing of surgery and prognosis in patients with chronic severe AR.[16,17]

Role of Transesophageal Echocardiography

In some patients, TEE may be necessary if the cause and extent of aortic valve or root pathology causing AR are not fully discernible from transthoracic imaging. This is especially true in cases of aortic valve endocarditis, dissection, and prosthetic aortic valves. Imaging of the mechanical and bioprosthetic valve regurgitation can be challenging by 2D transthoracic echocardiography (TTE) and TEE because of acoustic shadowing from the sewing rings, stents, calcification, and occluder mechanisms. In some cases, eccentric AR may be overestimated if there is broadening of the jet soon after VC, which may not be visible because of acoustic shadowing, especially in the case of mechanical aortic valves. Similarly, eccentric regurgitation can be underestimated as well if the jet courses along the anterior septum or anterior mitral leaflet.[18] The role of TEE in the assessment of AR after transcatheter aortic valve replacement is discussed elsewhere in this book and is not covered in this chapter.

Role of Three-Dimensional Echocardiography

Current advancements in 3D echocardiography now make it possible to not only visualize the aortic valve anatomy better but also measure the VC area (Fig. 88.4) and PISA without the need for geometric assumptions.[19–21] Some studies have demonstrated that VC area measurement using 3D color Doppler TTE improved quantitation of AR compared with 2D EROA by PISA method or conventional echo Doppler methods when magnetic resonance imaging was used as the gold standard.[22,23] Although attractive, measuring 3D VC area requires exceptional care in acquisition of

TABLE 88.1 Semiquantitative and Quantitative Measures for the Assessment of the Severity of Aortic Regurgitation

Aortic Regurgitation	Mild	Moderate		Severe
STRUCTURAL PARAMETERS				
LV size	Normal[a]	Normal or dilated		Usually dilated[b]
Aortic leaflets	Normal or abnormal	Normal or abnormal		Abnormal or flail or wide coaptation defect
DOPPLER PARAMETERS				
Jet width in LVOT: color flow[c]	Small in central jets	Intermediate		Large central jets; variable in eccentric jets
Jet density: CW	Incomplete or faint	Dense		Dense
Jet deceleration rate: CW (PHT, ms)[d]	Slow >500	Medium, 500–200		Steep <200
Diastolic flow reversal in descending aorta: PW	Brief, early diastolic reversal	Intermediate		Prominent holodiastolic reversal
QUANTITATIVE PARAMETERS[E]				
VC width, cm[c]	<0.3	0.3–0.60		>0.6
Jet width/LVOT width, %[c]	<25	25–45	46–64	≥65
Jet CSA/LVOT CSA, %[c]	<5	5–20	21–59	≥60
R Vol, mL/beat	<30	30–44	45–59	≥60
RF, %	<30	30–39	40–49	≥50
EROA, cm²	<0.10	0.10–0.19	0.20–0.29	≥0.30

[a]Unless there are other reasons for left ventricular (LV) dilatation. Normal two-dimensional measurements: LV minor axis ≤2.8 cm/m², LV end-diastolic volume ≤82 mL/m².
[b]Exception: acute aortic regurgitation (AR), in which chambers have not had time to dilate.
[c]At a Nyquist limit of 50–70 cm/s.
[d]Pressure halftime (PHT) is shortened with increasing LV diastolic pressure and vasodilator therapy and may be lengthened in chronic adaptation to severe AR.
[e]Quantitative parameters can subclassify the moderate regurgitation group into mild to moderate and moderate to severe regurgitation as shown.
Reproduced with permission from Zoghbi WA, et al: Recommendations for noninvasive evaluation of native valvular regurgitation, *J Am Soc Echocardiogr* 30:303–371, 2017.
CSA, Cross-sectional area; CW, continuous-wave Doppler; EROA, effective regurgitant orifice area; LVOT, left ventricular outflow tract; PW, pulsed-wave Doppler; R Vol, regurgitant volume; RF, regurgitant fraction; VC, vena contracta.

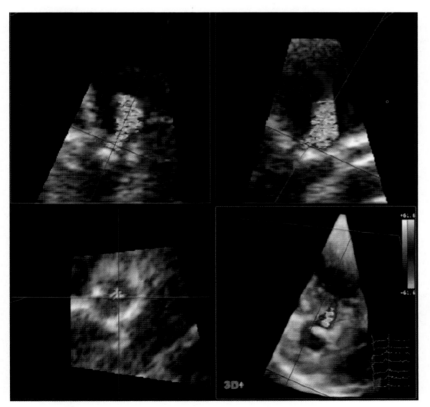

Figure 88.4. Demonstration of the proper plane for the measurement of three-dimensional (3D) color Doppler vena contracta area measurement using a 3D data set. (Reproduced with permission from Perez de Isla L, et al: 3D color-Doppler echocardiography and chronic aortic regurgitation: a novel approach for severity assessment, *Int J Cardiol* 166:640–645, 2013).

the data set as well as measurements so that the cropped plane is perpendicular to the VC area and not the expanding regurgitant jet, which can result in overestimation of AR. Temporal and spatial resolution of the 3D data set, shadows from calcification, reverberation and blooming artifacts, and machine gain settings can result in nonoptimal visualization of the 3D VC jet area. In addition, the proposed cut-off values of 3D VC area for determining severe AR have been variable,[23,24] and thus further validation studies are needed for native aortic valve regurgitation assessment.

Similar to VC, real-time 3D color Doppler PISA methods also theoretically improve the AR quantitation.[25] Real-time 3D peak and integrated PISA[26] measurement improved quantification of mitral and tricuspid valvular regurgitation compared with 2D methods, which can be adapted to AR as well in the future.[21] With rapid dissemination of technology, better operator experience, and novel solutions to technological limitations related to 3D echocardiography such as frame rates and stitch artifacts, it is expected that in the very near future, quantitation of AR will be much improved.

Role of Cardiovascular Magnetic Resonance Imaging

Although TTE and TEE can accurately determine the severity of AR in most cases, cardiovascular magnetic resonance imaging (CMRI) may be needed in selected cases. Specifically, CMRI is useful when (1) echocardiographic images are suboptimal, (2) there is discrepancy between LV size and severity of AR, (3) there is discordance between clinical findings and severity of AR as assessed by echocardiography, and (4) the ascending aorta is not well visualized by echocardiography.[27] However, a recent article has demonstrated the agreement between CMRI and echocardiography was modest in the assessment of AR severity.[28] Therefore, caution needs to be exercised in the interpretation of CMRI results.

CONCLUSIONS

Assessment of AR requires an integrative and comprehensive approach with attention to anatomy and physiology. One should use both semiquantitative and quantitative techniques (see Table 88.1) to arrive at the final determination of the severity of AR. TEE and CMRI may be necessary in some patients. Ongoing scientific advances in 3D echocardiography and CMRI techniques will make it possible in the near future to further improve the quantitation of AR.

Please access ExpertConsult to view the corresponding videos for this chapter.

REFERENCES

1. Enriquez-Sarano M, Tajik AJ. Clinical practice. Aortic regurgitation. *N Engl J Med*. 2004;351:1539–1546.
2. Nishimura RA, Otto CM, Bonow RO, et al. AHA/ACC Guideline for the management of patients with valvular heart disease. *Circulation*. 2014;129:e521–e643. 2014.
3. Perry GJ, Helmcke F, Nanda NC, et al. Evaluation of aortic insufficiency by Doppler color flow mapping. *J Am Coll Cardiol*. 1987;9:952–959.
4. Zoghbi WA, Adams D, Bonow RO, et al. Recommendations for noninvasive evaluation of native valvular regurgitation. *J Am Soc Echocardiogr*. 2017;30:303–371.
5. Griffin BP, Flachskampf FA, Siu S, et al. The effects of regurgitant orifice size, chamber compliance, and systemic vascular resistance on aortic regurgitant velocity slope and pressure halftime. *Am Heart J*. 1991;122:1049–1056. 1991.

6. Teague SM, Heinsimer JA, Anderson JL, et al. Quantification of aortic regurgitation utilizing continuous wave Doppler ultrasound. *J Am Coll Cardiol*. 1986;8:592–599.
7. Tribouilloy C, Avinee P, Shen WF, et al. End diastolic flow velocity just beneath the aortic isthmus assessed by pulsed Doppler echocardiography: a new predictor of the aortic regurgitant fraction. *Br Heart J*. 1991;65:37–40.
8. Yoganathan AP, Cape EG, Sung HW, et al. Review of hydrodynamic principles for the cardiologist: Applications to the study of blood flow and jets by imaging techniques. *J Am Coll Cardiol*. 1988;12:1344–1353.
9. Tribouilloy CM, Enriquez-Sarano M, Bailey KR, et al. Assessment of severity of aortic regurgitation using the width of the vena contracta: a clinical color Doppler imaging study. *Circulation*. 2000;102:558–564.
10. Shiota T, Jones M, Agler DA, et al. New echocardiographic windows for quantitative determination of aortic regurgitation volume using color Doppler flow convergence and vena contracta. *Am J Cardiol*. 1999;83:1064–1068.
11. Enriquez-Sarano M, Bailey KR, Seward JB, et al. Quantitative Doppler assessment of valvular regurgitation. *Circulation*. 1993;87:841–848.
12. Rokey R, Sterling LL, Zoghbi WA, et al. Determination of regurgitant fraction in isolated mitral or aortic regurgitation by pulsed Doppler 2D echocardiography. *J Am Coll Cardiol*. 1986;7:1273–1278.
13. Lang RM, Badano LP, Mor-Avi V, et al. Recommendations for cardiac chamber quantification by echocardiography in adults. *J Am Soc Echocardiogr*. 2015;28: 1–39 e14.
14. Tribouilloy CM, Enriquez-Sarano M, Fett SL, et al. Application of the proximal flow convergence method to calculate the effective regurgitant orifice area in aortic regurgitation. *J Am Coll Cardiol*. 1998;32:1032–1039.
15. Yang LT, Michelena HI, Scott CG, et al. Outcomes in chronic hemodynamically significant aortic regurgitation and limitations of current guidelines. *J Am Coll Cardiol*. 2019;73:1741–1752.
16. Alashi A, Khullar T, Mentias A, et al. Long-term outcomes after aortic valve surgery in patients with asymptomatic chronic aortic regurgitation and preserved left ventricular ejection fraction: impact of baseline and follow-up global longitudinal strain. *JACC Cardiovasc Imag*. 2020;13:12–21.
17. Alashi A, Mentias A, Abdallah A, et al. Incremental prognostic utility of left ventricular global longitudinal strain in asymptomatic patients with significant chronic aortic regurgitation and preserved left ventricular ejection fraction. *JACC Cardiovasc Imag*. 2018;11:673–682.
18. Zoghbi WA, Chambers JB, Dumesnil JG, et al. Recommendations for evaluation of prosthetic valves with echocardiography and Doppler ultrasound. *J Am Soc Echocardiogr*. 2009;22:975–1014. quiz 1082–1084.
19. Lang RM, Mor-Avi V, Sugeng L, et al. Three-dimensional echocardiography: the benefits of the additional dimension. *J Am Coll Cardiol*. 2006;48:2053–2069.
20. Sugeng L, Mor-Avi V, Weinert L, et al. Quantitative assessment of left ventricular size and function: side-by-side comparison of real-time three-dimensional echocardiography and computed tomography with magnetic resonance reference. *Circulation*. 2006;114:654–661.
21. Thavendiranathan P, Liu S, Datta S, et al. Quantification of chronic functional mitral regurgitation by automated 3D peak and integrated proximal isovelocity surface area and stroke volume techniques using real-time 3D volume color Doppler echocardiography: in vitro and clinical validation. *Circ Cardiovasc Imag*. 2013;6:125–133.
22. Ewe SH, Delgado V, van der Geest R, et al. Accuracy of three-dimensional versus two-dimensional echocardiography for quantification of aortic regurgitation and validation by three-dimensional three-directional velocity-encoded magnetic resonance imaging. *Am J Cardiol*. 2013;112:560–566.
23. Perez de Isla L, Zamorano J, Fernandez-Golfin C, et al. 3D color-Doppler echocardiography and chronic aortic regurgitation: a novel approach for severity assessment. *Int J Cardiol*. 2013;166:640–645.
24. Sato H, Ohta T, Hiroe K, et al. Severity of aortic regurgitation assessed by area of vena contracta: a clinical two-dimensional and three-dimensional color Doppler imaging study. *Cardiovasc Ultrasound*. 2015;13:24.
25. Pirat B, Little SH, Igo SR, et al. Direct measurement of proximal isovelocity surface area by real-time three-dimensional color Doppler for quantitation of aortic regurgitant volume: an in vitro validation. *J Am Soc Echocardiogr*. 2009;22: 306–313.
26. de Agustin JA, Viliani D, Vieira C, et al. Proximal isovelocity surface area by single-beat three-dimensional color Doppler echocardiography applied for tricuspid regurgitation quantification. *J Am Soc Echocardiogr*. 2013;26:1063–1072.
27. Zoghbi WA, Adams D, Bonow RO, et al. Recommendations for noninvasive evaluation of native valvular regurgitation. *J Am Soc Echocardiogr*. 2017;30:303–371.
28. Kammerlander AA, Wiesinger M, Duca F, et al. Diagnostic and prognostic utility of cardiac magnetic resonance imaging in aortic regurgitation. *JACC Cardiovasc Imag*. 2019;12:1474–1483.

Risk Stratification: Timing of Surgery and Percutaneous Interventions for Aortic Regurgitation

Muhamed Saric

Aortic regurgitation (AR) may lead to serious morbidity and excess mortality. As noted in the preceding chapters, the diagnosis of AR should be based on the guidelines for native valvular regurgitation by the American Society of Echocardiography and other international organizations.[1,2] The role of medical, percutaneous, and surgical options for the treatment of AR is discussed in this chapter. The recommendations for AR treatment follow the latest joint American Heart Association (AHA) and American College of Cardiology (ACC) valvular heart disease guidelines.[3] Surgery remains the only definitive means of treating AR in appropriate patients. There is a fundamental difference between acute and chronic AR. Acute severe AR is a medical emergency that rapidly progresses from an asymptomatic to a symptomatic stage resulting in severe heart failure. In contrast, chronic AR progresses through four stages (A–D) as described in 2014 ACC/AHA guidelines (Table 89.1).

MEDICAL THERAPY

No medical therapy has been shown to alter the natural progression or to improve survival in patients with AR. The role of medical therapy is primarily to alleviate the symptoms and to treat associated conditions such as systemic hypertension and heart failure.

Acute Aortic Regurgitation

There are limited medical management options for patients with acute AR. Surgical aortic valve replacement (AVR) remains the primary form of treatment. β-Blockers are used in the treatment of AR associated with type A aortic dissection. When acute AR is associated with other causes, β-blockers should be used with caution, if at all, because their use prevents compensatory tachycardia and may lead to hypotension. In hemodynamically unstable patients with acute AR, intravenous (IV) arterial dilators can be used to decrease afterload and improve forward flow. IV diuretics may be given to relieve congestion. If the patient is in cardiogenic shock, then IV inodilators, such as dobutamine, may be used.

Chronic Aortic Regurgitation

In chronic severe AR, there is no proven disease-modifying medical therapy. Systolic hypertension (systolic blood pressure >140 mm Hg) in patients with chronic AR should preferably be treated with vasodilators (dihydropyridine calcium channel blockers, angiotensin-converting enzyme [ACE] inhibitors, and/or angiotensin receptor blockers [ARBs]). If the left ventricular ejection fraction (LVEF) is diminished, the used of β-blockers, ACE inhibitors, and/or ARBs is recommended.[4] In contrast, vasodilator therapy has not been shown to be beneficial in asymptomatic patients with chronic AR and normal LVEF.[5] Surgery is the only definitive therapy for severe chronic AR.

PERCUTANEOUS INTERVENTIONAL THERAPY
Percutaneous Aortic Valves

In contrast to aortic stenosis, percutaneously implantable aortic prosthetic valves are not approved for the treatment of native AR at present in the United States. However, a percutaneous Jena valve specifically designed for isolated AR (JenaValve Technology GmbH) has been approved in Europe.[6] The percutaneous aortic valve-in-valve procedure is becoming the primary means of treating failed aortic surgical bioprostheses (implantation of a transcatheter aortic valve [AV] inside a stenosed and/or regurgitant aortic surgical bioprosthesis).

Intraaortic Balloon Pump

The use of intraaortic pump is contraindicated in patients with AR.[7]

LEFT VENTRICULAR ASSIST DEVICES

LV mechanical support with a percutaneous LV assist device may provide hemodynamic support in patients with severe AR.

SURGICAL THERAPY

In appropriate patients, AV surgery remains the only definitive treatment for AR. AVR is the primary form of surgical therapy for AR. AV repair (valve-sparing surgery) is feasible in some instances, provided that the leaflets are not deformed, scarred, or calcified. Indications for AV repair include (1) bicuspid valve with prolapsed of a single leaflet, (2) tricuspid valve with prolapsed of one leaflet, and (3) normal aortic leaflets with dilated sinotubular junction. Limited cusp destruction caused by infective endocarditis may also be amenable to repair in select instances. However, such repair should preferably be done at centers with specialized expertise. The timing of surgery for AR is dependent on the following five decision points: severity of AR, symptoms, left ventricular (LV) systolic function, LV size, and the need for other cardiac surgery (Fig. 89.1). It should be mentioned that progression of AR occurs in patients with all degrees of AR and at variable rates. It is difficult,

TABLE 89.1 Staging of Chronic Aortic Regurgitation According to the 2014 American College of Cardiology/American Heart Association Guidelines

Patients With Aortic Regurgitation	Class of Recommendation	Level of Evidence
Symptomatic Severe AR	I	B
Asymptomatic Severe AR		
LVEF <50%	I	B
LVESD >50 mm or indexed LVESD >25 mm/m²	IIa	B
LVEDD >65 mm and low surgical risk	IIb	C
Undergoing other cardiac surgery	I	C
Severe AR	I	C
Moderate AR	IIa	C

AR, Aortic regurgitation; *LVEDD*, left ventricular end-diastolic diameter; *LVEF*, left ventricular ejection fraction; *LVESD*, left ventricular end-systolic diameter.

Stage		AR Severity	Symptoms	LV Remodeling	LVEF	Surgery Indicated
A		None or trivial	Asymptomatic	None	≥50%	No
B		Mild or moderate				
C	**C1**	Severe		• Mild to moderate LV dilatation (LVESD ≤50 mm)		
	C2			• Severe LV dilatation • LVESD >50 mm or • Indexed LVESD >25 mm/m^2 or • LVEDD > 65 mm	<50%[a]	Yes
D			Symptomatic	Absent or present	Any	

[a] In stage C2, either LV remodeling or LVEF criteria should be met for surgical intervention.

Figure 89.1. Algorithm for surgical treatment of chronic aortic regurgitation (AR). *LV,* Left ventricular; *LVEF,* left ventricular ejection fraction; *LVEDD,* left ventricular end-diastolic diameter; *LVESD,* left ventricular end-systolic diameter.

if not impossible, to predict which individuals will progress and at what rate. Therefore, echocardiographic follow-up is indicated in all patients with AR.

Severity of Aortic Regurgitation

Surgery is performed typically only for severe AR; moderate AR is treated surgically only when the patient is already undergoing cardiac or aortic surgery for other indications.

Acute Versus Chronic Aortic Regurgitation

Severe acute AR is typically a medical emergency requiring prompt surgical intervention. The leading causes of acute severe AR include type A AR, infective endocarditis, blunt chest trauma, iatrogenic complications of aortic catheterization, and spontaneous rupture of a congenitally fenestrated AV. Surgery in patients with acute AR is necessary both to reverse the hemodynamic instability (pulmonary edema, hypotension, low cardiac output) and to provide the definitive therapy for AV pathology, especially in cases of type A aortic dissection. Several studies have demonstrated improved survival in patients with acute severe AR who were treated with prompt AV surgery.[8] The timing of surgical intervention for chronic AR is dependent on symptoms, LV systolic function, and LV size.

Symptoms

Clinical presentations of severe AR include angina (even in the presence of angiographically normal coronary arteries), exertional dyspnea, and other signs and symptoms of heart failure. If the nature of symptoms is unclear, exercise testing can be used to objectively assess exercise capacity and symptom status. Symptomatic severe chronic AR is an indication for surgery irrespective of LV size and LV systolic function.[9]

Left Ventricular Systolic Function

Chronic AR leads to a progressive increase in LV size and a progressive decrease in LV systolic function. Surgery is typically indicated in the asymptomatic C2 stage and the symptomatic D stage.

In asymptomatic patients with severe chronic AR, surgery is indicated when (1) LVEF is diminished (<50%)[10] or (2) LVEF is normal (>50%) but there is LV dilatation (LV end-systolic diameter [LVESD] >50 mm or LV end-diastolic diameter [LVEDD] >65 mm).

The evidence for the use of the end-systolic diameter cutoff value[11] is stronger than that for the end-diastolic diameter. Symptomatic patients with severe chronic AR should be considered for AV surgery irrespective of LVEF and LV size. When these criteria for surgery have been met, surgery should not be delayed significantly because progression to a more advance stage is associated with a more adverse long-term postoperative outcome than in patients operated sooner.

Need for Other Cardiac Surgery

If the patient is undergoing cardiac surgery for other indications, AV surgery should be considered in all patients with moderate or severe AR irrespective of symptoms, LVEF, or LV size.

DECISION ALGORITHMS FOR SURGICAL TREATMENT OF AORTIC REGURGITATION
Level of Evidence

In general, there is a relative paucity of studies evaluating the effectiveness of therapies for AR; therefore, no AHA/ACC treatment recommendation has the level of evidence A, the highest level that is based on multiple randomized trials or meta-analyses. The recommendations for AR treatment are based on single randomized trials and nonrandomized studies (level of evidence: B) or consensus opinions of experts (level of evidence: C).

Strength of Recommendations

As with other treatment recommendations, class I indication implies that the treatment should be administered. Class IIa implies that it is reasonable to administer the treatment, whereas class IIb implies that the treatment may be considered. Recommendations for AR fall into class I, IIa, and IIb. There are no class III recommendations for AR (treatments that have no proven benefits or are harmful).

SEVERE ACUTE AORTIC REGURGITATION

As previously noted, severe acute AR is a medical emergency requiring prompt AV surgery. LVEF as well as LV end-systolic and end-diastolic cutoff values discussed earlier do not apply to severe acute AR because LVEF and LV size are typically normal if the heart is otherwise healthy.

SEVERE CHRONIC AORTIC REGURGITATION

Class I Indications: Aortic Valve Surgery Should Be Performed

- Severe chronic AR in symptomatic patients irrespective of LV size or systolic function (level of evidence: B)[12,13]
- Severe chronic AR with LV systolic dysfunction (LVEF <50%) irrespective of symptoms (level of evidence: B)[14,15]
- Severe chronic AR in patients undergoing cardiac surgery for other indications irrespective of symptoms and LV systolic function (level of evidence: C)

Class IIa Indications: Aortic Valve Surgery Is a Reasonable Option

- Asymptomatic severe chronic AR with normal LVEF (>50%) but with severe LV dilatation as defined by LVESD greater than 50 mm (level of evidence: B)[16,17]
- Moderate chronic AR in patients undergoing cardiac surgery for other indications irrespective of symptoms and LV systolic function (level of evidence: C)

Class IIb Indication: Aortic Valve Surgery May Be Considered

- Asymptomatic severe chronic AR with normal LVEF (>50%) but with severe LV dilatation as defined by LVEDD greater than 65 mm if surgical risk is low (level of evidence: C) (Table 89.1)

REFERENCES

1. Zoghbi WA, Adams D, Bonow RO, et al. Recommendations for Noninvasive evaluation of native valvular regurgitation. *J Am Soc Echocardiogr.* 2017;30:303–371.
2. Baumgartner H, Falk V, Bax JJ, et al. ESC/EACTS guidelines for the management of valvular heart disease the Task Force for the management of valvular heart disease of the European Society of Cardiology (ESC) and the European association for Cardio-Thoracic surgery (EACTS). *Euro Heart J.* 2017;38:2739–2791. 2017.
3. Nishimura RA, Otto CM, Bonow RO, et al. AHA/ACC guideline for the management of patients with valvular heart disease. *J Am Coll Cardiol.* 2014;129:2440–2492. 2014.
4. Elder DH, Wei L, Szwejkowski BR, et al. The impact of renin-angiotensin-aldosterone system blockade on heart failure outcomes and mortality in patients identified to have aortic regurgitation. *J Am Coll Cardiol.* 2011;58:2084–2091.
5. Sondergaard L, Aldershvile J, Hildebrandt P, et al. Vasodilatation with felodipine in chronic asymptomatic aortic regurgitation. *Am Heart J.* 2000;139:667–674.
6. Seiffert M, Diemert P, Koschyk D, et al. Transapical implantation of a second-generation transcatheter heart valve in patients with noncalcified aortic regurgitation. *J Am Coll Cardiol Interv.* 2013;6:590–597.
7. Trost JC, Hillis LD. Intra-aortic balloon counter-pulsation. *Am J Cardiol.* 2006;97:1391–1398.
8. Lalani T, Cabell CH, Benjamin DK, et al. Analysis of the impact of early surgery on in-hospital mortality of native valve endocarditis: use of propensity score and instrumental variable methods to adjust for treatment-selection bias. *Circulation.* 2010;121:1005–1013.
9. Greves J, Rahimtoola SH, McAnulty JH, et al. Preoperative criteria predictive of late survival following valve replacement for severe aortic regurgitation. *Am Heart J.* 1981;101:300–308.
10. Forman R, Firth BG, Barnard MS. Prognostic significance of preoperative left ventricular ejection fraction and valve lesion in patients with aortic valve replacement. *Am J Cardiol.* 1980;45:1120–1125.
11. Bonow RO, Dodd JT, Maron BJ, et al. Long-term serial changes in left ventricular function and reversal of ventricular dilatation after valve replacement for chronic aortic regurgitation. *Circulation.* 1988;78:1108–1120.
12. Tornos P, Sambola A, Permanyer-Miralda G, et al. Long-term outcome of surgically treated aortic regurgitation: Influence of guideline adherence toward early surgery. *J Am Coll Cardiol.* 2006;47:1012–1017.
13. Dujardin KS, Enriquez-Sarano M, Schaff HV, et al. Mortality and morbidity of aortic regurgitation in clinical practice. A long-term follow-up study. *Circulation.* 1999;99:1851–1857.
14. Klodas E, Enriquez-Sarano M, Tajik AJ, et al. Optimizing timing of surgical correction in patients with severe aortic regurgitation: role of symptoms. *J Am Coll Cardiol.* 1997;30:746–752.
15. Chaliki HP, Mohty D, Avierinos JF, et al. Outcomes after aortic valve replacement in patients with severe aortic regurgitation and markedly reduced left ventricular function. *Circulation.* 2002;106:2687–2693.
16. Bhudia SK, McCarthy PM, Kumpati GS, et al. Improved outcomes after aortic valve surgery for chronic aortic regurgitation with severe left ventricular dysfunction. *J Am Coll Cardiol.* 2007;49:1465–1471.
17. Van Rossum AC, Visser FC, Sprenger M, et al. Evaluation of magnetic resonance imaging for determination of left ventricular ejection fraction and comparison with angiography. *Am J Cardiol.* 1988;62:628–633.
18. Gaasch WH, Carroll JD, Levine HJ, et al. Chronic aortic regurgitation: prognostic value of left ventricular end-systolic dimension and end-diastolic radius/thickness ratio. *J Am Coll Cardiol.* 1983;1:775–782.

89

90   Rheumatic Mitral Stenosis

Muhamed Saric, Roberto M. Lang, Itzhak Kronzon

Worldwide, rheumatic heart disease (RHD) is the predominant cause of mitral stenosis (MS) but is rare in developed countries. Most cases of rheumatic mitral stenosis (RMS) in developed countries are found among immigrants from less developed parts of the world where the prevalence of rheumatic fever may be as high as 150 cases per 100,000 people. Acute rheumatic fever is triggered by rheumatogenic group A β-hemolytic *Streptococcus pyogenes* infection, typically pharyngitis ("strep throat"). RMS may be considered an autoimmune disease triggered by streptococcal infection mediated by cross-reactivity between the streptococcal M antigen (mucoid surface protein) and human epitopes in the heart, skin, and connective and nerve tissues. The index streptococcal infection and subsequent reinfections trigger lifelong progressive fibrosis and calcifications leading to MS. In this chapter, we concentrate on transthoracic (TTE) and transesophageal echocardiographic (TEE) analysis of mitral valve morphology and secondary cardiac changes in RMS.

CAUSE OF MITRAL STENOSIS

MS may result from a variety of congenital and acquired conditions. Worldwide, rheumatic heart disease is the predominant cause of MS but is rare in developed countries.

Nonrheumatic Mitral Stenosis

Congenital MS is very rare (~1% of all patients with MS) and may be caused by cor triatriatum, a supravalvular mitral ring, or a parachute mitral valve (typically as a part of the Shone syndrome).[1] Nonrheumatic causes of acquired MS include lupus erythematosus, carcinoid, rheumatoid arthritis, radiation valvulitis, and age-related degenerative mitral annular calcifications. They are all rare except for mitral annular calcification, which is becoming the leading cause of acquired MS in developed countries.

Rheumatic Mitral Stenosis

The disease typically starts in childhood with a bout of acute rheumatic fever and is followed by lifelong progressive valvular damage. Acute rheumatic fever is triggered by rheumatogenic group A β-hemolytic *Streptococcus pyogenes* infection, typically pharyngitis ("strep throat"). Rheumatic heart disease may be considered an autoimmune disease triggered by streptococcal infection mediated by cross-reactivity between the streptococcal M antigen (mucoid surface protein) and human epitopes in the heart, skin, and connective and nerve tissues. Streptococci do not invade and are not present in the affected tissues. The index streptococcal infection and subsequent reinfections trigger lifelong progressive fibrosis and calcifications.

Clinically, acute rheumatic fever is characterized by five major findings: (1) pancarditis (endocarditis, myocarditis, and pericarditis), (2) migrating arthritis of large joints, (3) subcutaneous nodules, (4) skin rash (erythema marginatum), and (5) Sydenham chorea (random rapid dancelike movements of the face and the extremities). Minor (nonspecific) signs of inflammation include fever, leukocytosis, and an elevated erythrocyte sedimentation rate.

The so-called Jones criteria (first published in 1944) are used to establish the clinical diagnosis of acute rheumatic fever. In addition to evidence of a recent group A β-hemolytic streptococcal infection (such as antistreptococcal antibody titers), two major criteria or one major criterion plus two minor criteria are required for the diagnosis.[2]

Although any cardiac valve may be involved, the mitral valve is virtually always affected, and MS with or without concomitant mitral regurgitation (MR) is the predominant chronic form. MS results primarily from commissural fusion along leaflet edges, with an additional contribution from chordal fusion and shortening. In general, leaflet thickening and calcification proceed from the leaflet tips toward the leaflet bases. This contrasts with MS caused by age-related mitral annular calcification, in which the process starts at the base of the posterior mitral leaflet.

EPIDEMIOLOGY

The prevalence of acute rheumatic fever and RMS reflects the overall socioeconomic development and access to medical care. Because of introduction of antistreptococcal antibiotics and improvement in living standard, the incidence of rheumatic fever has declined dramatically since World War II in developed countries to fewer than 1 case to 100,000 people.[3] Most cases of RMS in developed countries are found among immigrants from less developed parts of the world where the prevalence of rheumatic fever may be as high as 150 cases per 100,000 people.[4]

In developed countries, MS becomes symptomatic 20 to 30 years after the onset of rheumatic fever. In contrast, RMS progresses more rapidly in developing countries and may be observed even in children and adolescents because of frequent streptococcal reinfections.

Rheumatic fever occurs exclusively in humans because there are no known animal reservoirs. Acute rheumatic fever affects both sexes equally, but women are at least twice as likely as men to develop RMS. This may reflect the generally higher prevalence of autoimmune disorders in women compared with men.

PATHOPHYSIOLOGY

Clinical manifestations of RMS, first described in 1668 by the English physician John Mayow,[5] reflect progressive decrease in mitral valve area, development of atrial fibrillation, and thrombus formation in the left atrium and left atrial appendage (LAA). They included elevation of left atrial (LA) pressure, pulmonary edema and other signs of left heart failure, pulmonary hypertension, right ventricular (RV) hypertrophy and dilatation, secondary tricuspid regurgitation, and right heart failure.

The blood crosses the normal mitral valve (area ~4–6 cm² in adults) without an appreciable transvalvular pressure gradient during diastole. When the valve area drops below 2 cm², an abnormal diastolic pressure gradient develops between the left atrium and the left ventricle, leading to an elevated LA pressure, dyspnea on exertion, or frank pulmonary edema at rest. This gradient is inversely proportional to the valve area and directly proportional to transvalvular flow. An increase in cardiac output or heart rate during exercise, fever, pregnancy, or atrial fibrillation augments the transmitral blood flow and pressure gradient.

Elevated LA pressure in significant RMS may typically leads to pulmonary venous hypertension with normal pulmonary vascular resistance (PVR). For unknown reasons, a subset of patients may also develop superimposed pulmonary arterial hypertension with elevated PVR because of arteriolar spasm, medial hypertrophy, and intimal thickening. Occasionally, pulmonary artery pressure may reach or even exceed systemic levels, leading to low cardiac output, fatigue, poor organ perfusion, and cardiac cachexia. Pulmonary hypertension may increase RV afterload, leading to RV dilatation, secondary tricuspid regurgitation, elevation of RV diastolic and right atrial (RA) pressures, and signs of right heart failure: venous engorgement, leg edema, cardiac cirrhosis, ascites, and protein-losing enteropathy.

Patients with RMS are at high risk for development of valvular atrial fibrillation and systemic thromboembolism. This risk is not directly proportional to the severity of MS and depends on concomitant atrial myocarditis and patient's age.[6] Pathophysiology of MS is summarized in Fig. 90.1. MS quantification is discussed in another chapter.

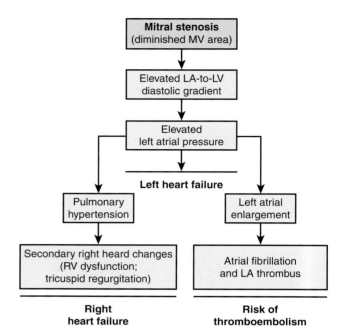

Figure 90.1. Pathophysiology of mitral stenosis. *LA*, Left atrium; *LV*, left ventricle; *MV*, mitral valve; *RV*, right ventricle.

PHYSICAL EXAMINATION

Precordial thrill: By placing the palm of one's hand on the precordium of a patient with RMS, one can feel the diastolic thrill. It was first reported in France at the beginning of the 19th century as *bruissement* by Jean-Nicolas Corvisart and later as *frémissement cataire* (cat purr in English or *sussurus felinus* in Latin) by René Laënnec.[7] The invention of the stethoscope by Laënnec and others gradually led to the description of the characteristic heart sounds and murmurs.

Auditory findings: Typical finding of RMS on auscultation and phonocardiography include a loud first heart sound (S_1), an opening snap (OS; *claquement d'ouverture*) after the second heart sound (S_2), and a diastolic rumble. The S_1 is often loud. An OS is frequently heard after the S_2. The duration of the S_2–OS interval (between the aortic component of the S_2 and the OS) is inversely proportional to the severity of MS. In severe MS, the S_2–OS interval is typically less than 80 ms. The S_2–OS interval is roughly equivalent to the isovolumic relaxation time.[8] The S_2–OS interval can be measured on M-mode echocardiography of the aortic valve and the left atrium (Fig. 90.2). Although of historic significance, this M-mode technique is not a part of the current MS guidelines.[9]

A characteristic diastolic rumble is frequently heard best at the apex. In patients with normal sinus rhythm, there is also an end-diastolic ("presystolic") accentuation of the rumble. When the cardiac output declines, the murmur may become softer. The pulmonic component of S_2 is loud in cases of pulmonary hypertension.

Other physical signs: These include malar flush and signs of low cardiac output and left and right heart failure. Massive LA enlargement may compress the left recurrent laryngeal nerve and cause hoarseness (Ortner syndrome).[10] A combination of atrial septal defect and RMS is referred as *Lutembacher syndrome*.[11]

ELECTROCARDIOGRAPHY

Electrocardiography (ECG) may demonstrate (1) signs of LA enlargement (*P mitrale*) with wide, saddle-shaped P wave in leads I and II, and late, deep P-wave inversion in lead V1; (2) RV hypertrophy; and (3) atrial fibrillation. In 1749, the French physician Jean-Baptiste de Sénac noted a correlation between RMS and the irregular pulse of "rebellious palpitations" or *delirium cordis*.[12] This irregular rhythm was first described on ECG 1909 by the British physician Thomas Lewis.[13]

CHEST RADIOGRAPHY

Chest radiography usually demonstrate with straightening of the left cardiac silhouette because of LA enlargement. Mitral valve calcifications, pulmonary venous congestion, pulmonary edema, and RV enlargement may also be seen.

TRANSTHORACIC ECHOCARDIOGRAPHY

In the 1950s, RMS was the very first heart disease visualized by the inventors of echocardiography, Inge Edler and Carl Hertz.[14] In this section, we concentrate on echocardiographic analysis of mitral valve morphology and secondary cardiac changes in RMS (Fig. 90.3 and Video 90.3). Quantification of mitral valve area and pressure gradients is discussed in another chapter of this book.

During bouts of acute rheumatic fever, which are exceedingly rare in developed countries, MR is the primary echocardiographic finding. In contrast, during the chronic phase, RMS with or without concomitant MR is the norm. Leaflet thickening, leaflet calcifications, decreased leaflet mobility, and commissural fusions are the hallmarks of RMS together with chordal fusion and shortening. Leaflet thickening and calcification start at the leaflet tips and extends toward the leaflet bases over time. Similarly, chordal thickening and fusion start at the leaflet tips and then extend distally toward the papillary muscles. This orderly progression in the leaflet tip-to-base direction and the chordal tip-to-papillary muscle direction is pathognomonic and allows for determining the severity of RMS and eligibility for percutaneous mitral balloon valvuloplasty (see Treatment later).

Two-dimensional (2D) parasternal long-axis view: Mitral leaflet thickness is typically measured in this view. Decreased mobility of the posterior mitral leaflet and the characteristic doming

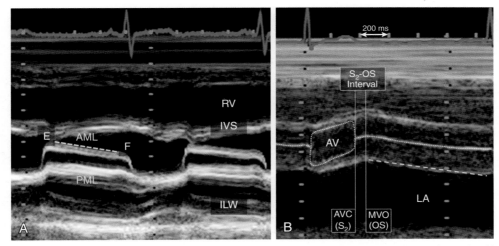

Figure 90.2. M-mode echocardiography of rheumatic mitral stenosis (RMS). **A,** M-mode recording through the mitral valve. Note marked thickening and increased echogenicity of both mitral leaflets and a very flat ejection fraction slope indicative of significant mitral stenosis. **B,** M-mode recording through the aortic valve (AV) and left atrium (LA). Note a very short S_2–OS interval (~80 ms) and markedly diminished rate of LA emptying *(broken yellow line)* after mitral valve opening (MVO). *AML,* Anterior mitral leaflet; *AVO,* aortic valve opening; *ILW,* inferolateral wall; *IVS,* interventricular septum; *OS,* opening snap; *PML,* posterior mitral leaflet; *RV,* right ventricle; S_2, second heart sound.

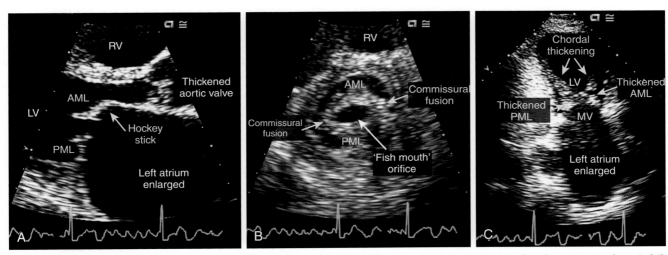

Figure 90.3. Transthoracic echocardiography (TTE) of rheumatic mitral stenosis (RMS). **A,** Parasternal long-axis view demonstrates characteristic hockey-stick appearance of the anterior mitral leaflet (AML), decreased mobility of the posterior mitral leaflet (PML), and markedly enlarged left atrium (LA) consistent with RMS. Note also the rheumatic aortic valve thickening. **B,** Parasternal short-axis view at the level of the mitral valve. Note the commissural fusion resulting in mitral stenosis with the characteristic fish-mouth appearance of the mitral orifice. **C,** Apical two-chamber view demonstrates marked chordal thickening and chordal fusion as well as thickening of both mitral leaflet and marked left atrial enlargement. *AML,* Anterior mitral leaflet; *LV,* left ventricle; *MV,* mitral valve; *PML,* posterior mitral leaflet; *RV,* right ventricle. (See corresponding Video 90.3.)

resulting in a hockey-stick appearance of the anterior leaflet may be seen (see Fig. 90.3 and Video 90.3A).

2D parasternal short-axis view at the level of the mitral valve: Commissural fusions results in a fish-mouth appearance of the mitral orifice (see Fig. 90.3 and Video 90.3B). It is in this view that 2D planimetry of the mitral orifice is performed, with the caveat that on 2D, one may not be able to identify true leaflet tips because in RMS, the orifice may be eccentric and separate from the 2D short-axis plane. The eccentricity of the orifice can often be appreciated in 2D apical views of the mitral valve. Three-dimensional (3D) echocardiography, especially multiplane reconstruction techniques, overcomes the limitations of 2D echocardiography and allow for precise orifice planimetry exactly at leaflet tips as described in the chapter on quantification of MS.

Apical views: Chordal involvement is best seen in the apical transthoracic views, especially the apical two-chamber view or its TEE equivalents, such as the transgastric two-chamber view (see Fig. 90.3 and Video 90.3C).

RMS may lead to an often mark LA enlargement (which may not be proportional to MS severity), aortic and tricuspid regurgitation, right heart enlargement, and elevation of LA and right heart pressures. The left ventricle typically has a normal size and systolic function.

M-mode echocardiography: Many of the previously mentioned changes can also be seen on M-mode echocardiography. The severity of MS can be assessed semiquantitatively by measuring either the EF slope of the mitral valve (see Fig. 90.2A) or the rate of LA emptying (see Fig. 90.2B). Normally, the EF slope is steep (>8 cm/s). The flatter the EF slope, the more severe the MS. Similarly, the slower the rate of diastolic LA emptying, the more severe the MS. Although of historical importance, these M-mode techniques are imprecise and no longer supported by valvular stenosis guidelines.

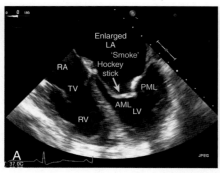
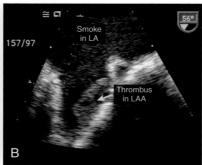
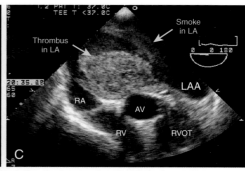

Figure 90.4. Two-dimensional transesophageal echocardiography (TEE) of rheumatic mitral stenosis (RMS). **A,** Midesophageal four-chamber view demonstrates findings typical of RMS: thickening and calcifications of both anterior (AML) and posterior mitral leaflet (PML), hockey-stick appearance of the AML, and marked enlargement of the left atrium (LA). **B,** TEE demonstrates a large thrombus in the left atrial appendage (LAA) as well as smoke in the body of the LA. **C,** TEE shows a very large thrombus in the body of the LA as well as smoke in the LA and LAA. (See corresponding Video 90.4.)

TRANSESOPHAGEAL ECHOCARDIOGRAPHY

TEE is typically not required for routine evaluation of RMS. However, TEE should be considered when the image quality is poor, Doppler information is suboptimal or TTE finding do not correlate with the clinical impression (Fig. 90.4 and Video 90.4A). TEE is especially useful in evaluating complications of RMS (e.g., LA clot or endocarditis) and in guiding percutaneous mitral balloon valvuloplasty. Patients with RMS are at a high risk for developing intracardiac thrombus. Although those in atrial fibrillation are at a high risk of developing LA stasis with smoke, sludge, and thrombus formation, such findings may be seen even when patients with RMS are in sinus rhythm.

In RMS, most thrombi develop in the LAA (Fig. 90.4 and Video 90.4B); however, a substantial proportion occurs in the body of the left atrium (Fig. 90.4 and Video 90.4C). According to one surgical series, 57% of thrombi were in the LAA versus 43% in the left atrium.[15] This is contrast to nonvalvular atrial fibrillation, in which thrombi outside the LAA are unusual.

THERAPY

RMS is a progressive lifelong disease. Without treatment, the 10-year survival rate is less than 15% when significant symptoms develop, and in those who develop severe pulmonary hypertension, mean survival drops to less than 3 years.

Medical Therapy

There is no effective medical therapy that alters the progression of RMS except for long-term antibiotic prophylaxis of recurrent streptococcal pharyngitis in endemic areas. Medical therapy with diuretics and heart rate–controlling agents (β-blockers, calcium channel blockers, and digoxin) provides symptomatic relief. The very first clinical use of digoxin was in patients with atrial fibrillation and RMS, as reported in 1785 by the British physician William Withering who discovered digitalis.[16]

Management of atrial fibrillation (including chemical and electrical cardioversion) should follow standard guidelines. Chronic anticoagulation to prevent thromboembolism is recommended in patients with atrial fibrillation and may be considered even in patients with sinus rhythm. In contrast to nonvalvular atrial fibrillation, the efficacy of anticoagulation in RMS has not been proven in a randomized trial; nonetheless, anticoagulation is recommended based on several retrospective studies.[17] Although patients with RMS are at risk for mitral valve endocarditis, current guidelines do not recommend routine antibiotic prophylaxis for endocarditis. Significant RMS is a mechanical disorder that requires a mechanical treatment for effective symptom relief and improvement in survival.

Percutaneous Mitral Balloon Valvuloplasty

In eligible patients, percutaneous mitral balloon valvuloplasty (PMBV) is the treatment of choice; surgery is reserved for those who cannot undergo valvuloplasty. Currently, approximately 1500 PMBVs are performed in the United States annually. The PMBV technique was perfected in the 1980s by Kanji Inoue of Japan, who developed the Inoue Balloon (Toray Industries), which remains the preferred balloon for PMBV.[18]

The Wilkins score, originally developed by TTE in the 1980s, is often used to determine eligibility for valvuloplasty using four parameters: three related to mitral leaflets (thickening, mobility, and calcification) and one related to the degree of chordal involvement.[19] Because each parameter is scored on a scale from 0 (normal) to 4 (severe), the Wilkins score ranges from 0 (normal valve) to 16 (poorly mobile, severely calcified leaflets with severe chordal fusion and shortening). Good PMV candidates should have a Wilkins score of 10 or less, preferably 8 or less (Table 90.1).

Recently, a different RMS grading scheme, referred as the Nunes score, has been proposed. It consists of four parameters: mitral valve area, maximal leaflet displacement, commissural fusion asymmetry, and subvalvular involvement.[20]

TEE plays an essential role in the refinement of patient selection (Fig. 90.5 and Video 90.5A), guidance of PMBV (Fig. 90.5 and Video 90.5B), and assessment of post-PMBV results (Fig. 90.5 and Video 90.5C and D). In the absence of contraindications, PMBV is recommended in the following instances: (1) in symptomatic patients with moderate or severe MS, (2) in asymptomatic patients with moderate or severe MS when pulmonary artery systolic pressure is greater than 50 mm Hg at rest or greater than 60 mm Hg with exercise or when there is new-onset atrial fibrillation, and (3) in symptomatic patients with mild stenosis (valve area >1.5 cm²) when pulmonary artery systolic pressure is greater than 60 mm Hg, pulmonary artery wedge pressure is greater than 25 mm Hg, or mean mitral valve gradient is greater than 15 mm Hg during exercise. Contraindications for PMBV include an unfavorable Wilkins score (≥10), more than moderate MR, and the presence of intracardiac thrombus.

TEE also plays a key role in guiding PMBV, including guidance of transseptal puncture, visualization of wires and catheters, and proper placement of the valvuloplasty balloon across the mitral orifice, as well as in the assessment of procedure outcomes. A favorable outcome is characterized by leaflet separation along commissural lines with a concomitant increase in mitral valve area and a decrease in transvalvular gradient (see Fig. 90.5 and Video 90.5C). Leaflet tear is the most feared complication of PMBV because it may lead to severe acute MR, necessitating urgent mitral valve surgery (see Fig. 90.5 and Video 90.5C).

TABLE 90.1 Wilkins Criteria for Assessment of Mitral Valve Anatomy Before Percutaneous Balloon Valvuloplasty[a]

Grade	0	1	2	3	4
Leaflet mobility	Normal	Highly mobile with only leaflet tip restricted	Leaflet mid and base portions have normal mobility	Valve continues to move in diastole, mainly from the base	No or minimal forward leaflet motion in diastole
Valve thickness	Normal	Near-normal thickness (4–5 mm)	Mid leaflets normal; thickened leaflet tips (5–8 mm)	Entire leaflet thickened (5–8 mm)	Marked thickening of entire leaflet (>8–10 mm)
Leaflet calcification	None	Single area of echo brightness	Scattered areas of brightness at leaflet margins	Brightness extends to mid leaflets	Extensive brightness throughout leaflets
Subvalvular thickening	None	Minimal chordal thickening just below leaflet tips	Thickening from leaflet tips to up to one-third of chordal length	Thickening extending to the distal third of chordae	Extensive chordal thickening down to papillary muscle

[a]The Wilkins score ranges from 0 (normal valve) to 16 (poorly mobile, severely calcified leaflets with severe chordal fusion and shortening). Good valvuloplasty candidates should have a Wilkins score of 10 or less, preferably 8 or less.

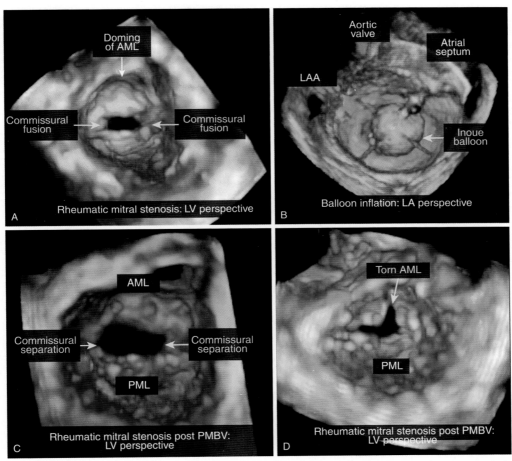

Figure 90.5. Three-dimensional transesophageal echocardiography (3D TEE) in guidance of percutaneous mitral balloon valvuloplasty (PMBV) of rheumatic mitral stenosis (RMS). **A,** Before PMBV, there is typical appearance of RMS from left ventricular (LV) perspective. Note the commissural fusion, the doming of the anterior mitral leaflet (AML), and the fish-mouth appearance of the mitral orifice. **B,** During PMBV, 3D TEE is used to properly place the balloon across the mitral orifice. **C,** In this patient, PMBV had a favorable outcome: the mitral orifice increased in size as a result of commissural separation. **D,** This patient had a complication of PMBV, tearing of the AML *(arrow)*, which resulted in severe acute mitral regurgitation. *AML,* Anterior mitral leaflet; *LAA,* left atrial appendage; *PML,* posterior mitral leaflet. (See corresponding Video 90.5.)

Mitral Valve Surgery

Surgical options include closed or open commissurotomy, mitral valve replacement, and occasionally mitral valve repair. In the 1920s, Henry Souttar in England and Elliot Cutler in the United States led the first attempts to perform surgical relief of RMS using what would later be termed *closed commissurotomy.* Their technique was improved soon after World War II by the American surgeons Charles Bailey and Dwight Harken. Bailey called the procedure "mitral commissurotomy," whereas Harken called it "mitral valvuloplasty."[21] In developed countries, open commis- surotomy requiring cardiac arrest and cardiopulmonary bypass is preferred over closed commissurotomy, which is performed on a beating heart. Because of its simplicity, closed commissurotomy is still widely performed in developing countries. In the 1960s, RMS was the first valvular disease to be treated with a prosthetic valve replacement using the mechanical mitral valve developed by Albert Starr and Lowell Edwards.[22] For further discussion of surgical options in RMS, readers are referred to the appropriate treatment guidelines.[23]

Please access ExpertConsult to view the corresponding videos for this chapter.

REFERENCES

1. Shone JD, Sellers RD, Anderson RC, et al. The developmental complex of "parachute mitral valve," supravalvular ring of left atrium, subaortic stenosis, and coarctation of aorta. *Am J Cardiol*. 1963;11:714–725.
2. Jones TD. The diagnosis of rheumatic fever. *J Am Med Assoc*. 1944;126:481–484.
3. Denny Jr FW. A 45-year perspective on the streptococcus and rheumatic fever: the Edward H. Kass Lecture in infectious disease history. *Clin Infect Dis*. 1994;19:1110–1122.
4. Stollerman GH. Rheumatic fever. *Lancet*. 1997;349:935–942.
5. Mayow J. *Tractatus Quinque Medico-Physic*. Oxford, UK: Oxford University Press; 1674:373–377.
6. Carabello BA. Modern management of mitral stenosis. *Circulation*. 2005;112:432–437.
7. Corvisart JN. *Essai sur les maladies et les lésions organiques du coeur et des gros vaisseaux*. Paris: Migneret; 1806:231–242.
8. Kalmanson D, Veyrat C, Bernier A, et al. Opening snap and isovolumic relaxation period in relation to mitral valve flow in patients with mitral stenosis. Significance of A2–OS interval. *Br Heart J*. 1976;38:135–146.
9. Baumgartner H, Hung J, Bermejo J, et al. Echocardiographic assessment of valve stenosis: EAE/ASE recommendations for clinical practice. *J Am Soc Echocardiogr*. 2009;22(1–23).
10. Ortner N. Recurrenslähmung bei Mitralstenose. *Wien Klin Wochenschr*. 1897;10:753–755.
11. Lutembacher R. De la sténose mitrale avec communication interauriculaire. *Arch Mal Coeur Vaiss*. 1916;9:237–250.
12. De Sénac JB. *Traité de la structure du coeur, de son action, et de ses maladies*. Paris: Jacque Vincent; 1749:509–514.
13. Lewis T, Report CXIX. Auricular fibrillation: a common clinical condition. *Br Med J*. 1909;2:1528.
14. Edler I, Hertz CH. The use of ultrasonic reflectoscope for the continuous recording of movements of heart walls, *Kungl Fysiogr Sallsk i Lund Forhandl* 24:5, 1954. *Reproduced in Clin Physiol Funct Imag*. 2004;24:118–136.
15. Blackshear JL, Odell JA. Appendage obliteration to reduce stroke in cardiac surgical patients with atrial fibrillation. *Ann Thorac Surg*. 1996;61:755–759.
16. Withering W. *An Account of the Foxglove and Some of its Medical Uses: With Practical Remarks on Dropsy and Other Diseases*. London: J and J Robinson; 1785.
17. Pérez-Gómez F, Salvador A, Zumalde J, et al. Effect of antithrombotic therapy in patients with mitral stenosis and atrial fibrillation: a sub-analysis of NASPEAF randomized trial. *Eur Heart J*. 2006;27:960–967.
18. Inoue K, Owaki T, Nakamura T, et al. Clinical application of transvenous mitral commissurotomy by a new balloon catheter. *J Thorac Cardiovasc Surg*. 1984;87:394–402.
19. Wilkins GT, Weyman AE, Abascal VM, et al. Percutaneous balloon dilatation of the mitral valve: an analysis of echocardiographic variables related to outcome and the mechanism of dilatation. *Br Heart J*. 1988;60:299–308.
20. Nunes MC, Tan TC, Elmariah S, et al. The echo score revisited: impact of incorporating commissural morphology and leaflet displacement to the prediction of outcome for patients undergoing percutaneous mitral valvuloplasty. *Circulation*. 2014;129:886–895.
21. Saric M, Benenstein R. Three-dimensional echocardiographic guidance of percutaneous procedures. In: Nanda NC, ed. *Comprehensive Textbook of Echocardiography*. New Delhi, India: Jaypee Brothers; 2013.
22. Starr A, Herr RH, Wood JA. The present status of valve replacement. Special issue on the VII Congress of the International Cardiovascular Society. Philadelphia. *J Cardiovasc Surg*. 1965:95–103.
23. Bonow RO, Carabello BA, Chatterjee K, et al. ACC/AHA 2006 guidelines for the management of patients with valvular heart disease. *J Am Coll Cardiol*. 2006;48(3):e1–e148.

91 Quantification of Mitral Stenosis

Muhamed Saric, Roberto M. Lang, Itzhak Kronzon

Echocardiography is the modality of choice for the diagnosis of mitral stenosis (MS). The joint American Society of Echocardiography and European Association of Echocardiography guidelines for native valvular stenosis feature an exhaustive review of echocardiographic methods for quantitative assessment of MS.[1] Full echocardiographic evaluation of MS includes the following triad: (1) MVA; (2) mean diastolic transmitral pressure gradient; and (3) secondary changes, including measurements of relevant chamber sizes and estimation of right heart pressures. Most modern ultrasound systems contain built-in software packages for determining these parameters. Major methods for quantification of MS are presented in Figs. 91.1 and 91.2. In most instances, evaluation of MS by invasive methods of cardiac catheterization is not necessary unless there is a discrepancy between clinical and echocardiographic findings.

A major change in MS quantification occurred with the publication of the 2014 American Heart Association (AHA)/American College of Cardiology (ACC) valvular heart disease guidelines.[2] The changes were threefold: (1) MS, like other valvular disorders, was given stages A through D; (2) MVA cutoff values for the severity of MS were changed; and (3) the role of transmitral pressure gradients is no longer considered the major determinant of MS severity (Table 91.1).

MITRAL VALVE AREA MEASUREMENTS

Normal MVA in an adult is approximately 4.0 to 6.0 cm². MVA can be calculated using a variety of noninvasive and invasive methods, none of which is considered a true gold standard. Historically, severe MS was defined as MVA less than 1.0 cm², moderate when MVA is 1.0 to 1.5 cm², and mild when MVA is greater than 1.5 cm². However, in the 2014 AHA/ACC valvular heart disease guideline, severe MS was defined as MVA 1.5 cm² or less and very severe MS as MVA 1.0 cm² or less (see Table 91.1). Indexing of MVA for body surface area has not been validated.

INVASIVE METHOD

The most common invasive method for estimating MVA is based on the Gorlin equation[3] published in 1951:

$$MVA = \frac{Q}{44.3 * c * \sqrt{\Delta P}}$$

in which Q is the diastolic transmitral flow rate (in mL/min), c is a constant (0.85 for MV), and ΔP is the mean diastolic transmitral gradient (in mm Hg).

This method requires invasive measurements of both the cardiac output and the diastolic transmitral pressure gradient. Ideally, the gradient should be measured directly as the difference between left ventricular (LV) and left atrial (LA) diastolic pressure, typically after a transseptal puncture. However, pulmonary artery wedge pressure is often used in lieu of LA pressure; this typically overestimates the transmitral gradient (and thus the severity of MS) compared with direct LA pressure measurements.[4]

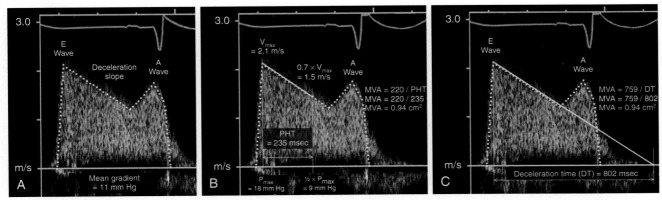

Figure 91.1. Quantitative assessment of mitral stenosis (MS) by spectral Doppler. **A,** Assessment of the mean diastolic mitral gradient. This patient has severe MS (mean gradient, 11 mm Hg at a heart rate of 70 beats/min). **B,** Mitral valve area (MVA) by pressure halftime (PHT). This patient has severe MS (MVA, 0.94 cm²). Note that a 50% drop in initial pressure (from 18 to 9 mm Hg) corresponds to a 70% drop in initial velocity (from 2.1 to 1.5 ms). (See Video 91.1B , which conceptually corresponds to this panel, albeit in a different patient.) **C,** MVA by deceleration time (DT). Because PHT is approximately 0.29 × DT, the formula MVA = 220/PHT may be expressed as MVA = 759/DT.

ECHOCARDIOGRAPHY METHODS

By echocardiography, MVA can either be measured directly (anatomic orifice area) or estimated from Doppler measurements (effective orifice area).

Pressure Halftime Method

Pressure halftime (PHT) is defined as the length of time required for the maximal early diastolic transmitral gradient to reach half its value (see Fig. 91.1B and Video 91.1B). PHT is inversely related to MVA. PHT is quite short in patients without significant MS because the transmitral (LA to LV) diastolic pressure gradient declines rapidly as the pressures in these two chambers quickly equalize. On the other hand, with severe MS, the pressure gradient declines very slowly, resulting in a long PHT.

A semiquantitative method for estimating MVA from PHT was originally a cardiac catheterization technique using direct pressure measurements (thus the PHT name).[5] The technique was later adapted for quantitative MVA assessments from noninvasive Doppler measurements. Historically, pulsed-wave (PW) spectral Doppler was first used to measure PHT; continuous-wave (CW) Doppler is now preferred.

Using the simplified Bernoulli equation:

$$\Delta P = 4 * V^2$$

in which ΔP is the transmitral gradient (in mm Hg) and V is the velocity of blood (in m/s). One can demonstrate that PHT is reached when the initial maximal velocity of blood across the MV during diastole drops to 70% of its initial value. Hatle and colleagues[6] developed an empirical equation for calculating MVA from PHT:

$$\mathrm{MVA}\left(\mathrm{cm}^2\right) = 220/\mathrm{PHT}\ (\mathrm{ms})$$

Thus, in a patient with PHT of 220 ms, the MVA is calculated to be 1.0 cm². Because of its simplicity, PHT is the most used Doppler technique for estimating MVA.

It is important to emphasize that the 220/PHT formula was developed for rheumatic MS and should not be used for, for example, senile MS related to mitral annular calcification.

For patients in atrial fibrillation, an average value of PHT derived from (typically) five cardiac cycles should be used. Short cardiac cycles should be avoided because they may be too brief for the pressure to drop to half its value. In some instances, the spectral Doppler velocity decay has not one but two slopes; this may be seen in patients with both MS and mitral regurgitation (MR). In such instances, the initial slope (occurring typically within the first 300 ms of transmitral flow) can be ignored; subsequent (mid-diastolic) slope should be used to measure PHT.[7]

Occasionally, the PHT method may not accurately calculate MVA (e.g., when the changes in LA and/or LV pressures are independent of MS, when the initial transmitral pressure gradient is very high, or after percutaneous mitral balloon valvuloplasty [PMBV]).[8] The PHT method overestimates MVA in patients with large atrial septal defects, significant aortic regurgitation (AR), or LV diastolic dysfunction and when the initial transmitral pressure gradient is very high.

In patients with both MS and atrial septal defect (referred to as Lutembacher syndrome),[9] a significant left-to-right shunt decompresses the leaf atrium, decreases the transmitral gradient, and shortens the PHT, leading to overestimation of MVA. Significant AR and/or LV diastolic dysfunction may lead to increased LV diastolic pressure; this in turn diminishes the transmitral gradient, shortens the PHT, and leads to overestimation of MVA.

In patients with LV diastolic dysfunction (who tend to be older adults), abnormal LV relaxation leads to either prolongation or shortening of PHT independent of MS. Abnormal LV relaxation prolongs PHT (leading to underestimation of MVA), whereas abnormal LV compliance shortens PHT (leading to overestimation of MVA). Thus, the PHT method should be used with caution in older adult patients with MS. One should not use PHT to estimate MVA after PMBV because LV diastolic pressure may rise significantly as the relatively noncompliant left ventricle experiences an abrupt increase in transmitral flow after balloon-mediated relief of MS.[10] When PHT is unavailable, one can use mitral deceleration time (DT) instead.

Mitral Deceleration Time Method

The DT of the mitral E wave is defined as the length of time from the peak velocity of early diastolic mitral flow (E wave V_{max}) to the end of antegrade transmitral flow (V = 0). Like PHT, the length of DT is also inversely related to the MVA (i.e., longer DT indicates smaller MVA). Because DT is related to PHT according to:

$$\mathrm{PHT}\ (\mathrm{ms}) = 0.29 \times \mathrm{DT}\ (\mathrm{ms})$$

MVA can then be calculated from DT (see Fig. 91.1C) from the following equation:

$$\mathrm{MVA}\left(\mathrm{cm}^2\right) = 759/\mathrm{DT}\ (\mathrm{ms})$$

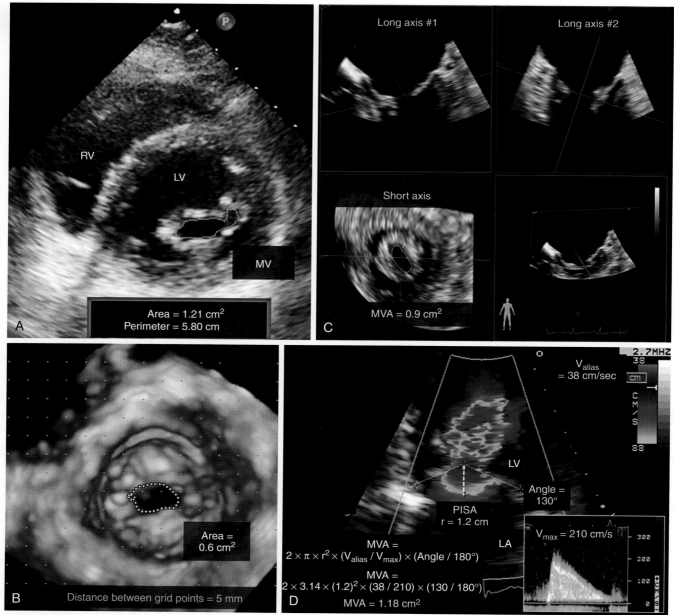

Figure 91.2. Quantitative assessment of mitral stenosis (MS) by mitral valve area (MVA) methods. **A,** MVA by two-dimensional planimetry at mitral leaflet tips in the transthoracic short axis. The patient has mild to moderate MS (MVA = 1.21 cm^2) (see Video 91.2A). **B,** MVA by three-dimensional (3D) planimetry in this patient with severe MS. The panel demonstrates the left ventricular aspect of the mitral valve (MV). On newer systems, MVA can be planimetered directly on a 3D image (0.6 cm^2 in this patient). On older systems, a grid is used to calculate MVA. Each rectangle on the grid corresponds to 0.25 cm^2 (5 × 5 mm) (see Video 91.2B). **C,** MVA by multiplane reconstruction (MPR) of a 3D transesophageal echocardiography clip. MPR allows for localizing true tips of mitral leaflets; thus, this method allows for most accurate assessment of anatomic MVA. **D,** MVA by proximal isovelocity surface area (PISA) method. Both color and continuous-wave spectral Doppler are required. Note that when the color Doppler baseline is shifted, the aliasing velocity used to calculate MVA is the one in the direction of blood flow (38 cm/s in this case). This patient has moderate MS (MVA = 1.12 cm^2). *LA,* Left atrium; *LV,* left ventricle; *RA,* right atrium.

Mitral Valve Area by Planimetry

Anatomic MVA can be measured by either two-dimensional (2D) or three-dimensional (3D) planimetry; measurements should be done in mid-diastole at leaflet tips. For 2D planimetry, a short axis at the level of the mitral leaflet tips is obtained, and a mid-diastolic frame with maximal opening of mitral leaflets is chosen (see Fig. 91.2A and Video 91.2A). MVA is then planimetered using standard ultrasound-system quantitative tools. The major shortcoming of 2D planimetry is its inability to accurately determine the location of the true leaflet tips because they are often eccentrically located outside the short-axis plane.

3D planimetry overcomes these limitations and is now considered the echocardiographic gold standard for calculation of MVA.[11] 3D planimetry may be done using a variety of methods such as multiplane reconstruction, on-image planimetry, or estimation of MVA using a rectangular reference grid (see Fig. 91.2B and C; Video 91.2B).

TABLE 91.1 Staging of Mitral Stenosis by 2014 American Heart Association/American College of Cardiology Guidelines[a]

Stage	Definition	Symptoms	MS Severity	MVA	PHT	LA Dilatation	PASP
A	At risk of MS	None	None or trivial	4–6 cm^2		None	Normal
B	Progressive MS		Mild or moderate	>1.5 cm^2	<150 ms	Mild to moderate	Normal at rest
C	Asymptomatic severe MS		Severe	Severe MS: ≤1.5 cm^2	Severe MS: ≥150 ms	Severe	>30 mm Hg
D	Symptomatic severe MS	Exertional dyspnea		Very severe MS: ≤1.0 cm^2	Very severe MS: ≤220 ms		

[a]The transmitral mean pressure gradient should be obtained to further determine the hemodynamic effect of the mitral stenosis (MS) and is usually >5 to 10 mm Hg in severe MS; however, because of the variability of the mean pressure gradient with heart rate and forward flow, it has not been included in the criteria for severity

LA, Left atrium; *MVA*, mitral valve area; *PASP*, pulmonary artery systolic pressure; *PHT*, pressure halftime.

Mitral Valve Area by Doppler Techniques

Doppler methods for calculated MVA include pressure halftime, continuity equation, and proximal isovelocity surface area (PISA).

Mitral Valve Area by Continuity-Equation Method

The continuity equation method assumes that a stroke volume (SV_1) across one orifice equals the stroke volume (SV_2) across another orifice in the same closed circulatory system. In the absence of significant MR or AR, *diastolic* stroke volume across the MV is equal to the *systolic* stroke volume across the LV outflow tract (LVOT):

$$SV_{MV} = SV_{LVOT}$$

Using echocardiography, SV across any orifice can be calculated as a product of the orifice area and the flow velocity time integral (VTI):

$$\text{LVOT area} \times \text{LVOT VTI} = \text{MVA} \times \text{MV VTI}$$

Solving for MVA, one obtains the following equation:

$$\text{MVA} = \text{LVOT area} * \frac{\text{LVOT VTI}}{\text{MV VTI}}$$

Systolic LVOT VTI and diastolic MV VTI are measured by PW and CW Doppler, respectively. LVOT area is typically calculated after measuring the systolic LVOT diameter (d) in the parasternal long-axis view and assuming a circular LVOT shape:

$$\text{LVOT area} = \pi * \left(\frac{d}{2}\right)^2$$

Thus, using the continuity equation, MVA can be calculated as follows:

$$\text{MVA} = \pi * \left(\frac{d}{2}\right)^2 * \frac{\text{LVOT VTI}}{\text{MV VTI}}$$

Aside from significant MR and AR, a miscalculation of LVOT area is the major limitation of estimating MVA by the continuity equation method. This occurs because of either mismeasurement of LVOT diameter or frequent noncircularity of LVOT area. In general, the continuity equation method for estimating MVA should not be used in atrial fibrillation.

Mitral Valve Area by Proximal Isovelocity Surface Area Method

The PISA method is also based on the continuity principle. The method is described in detail in another chapter.[12] Briefly, blood flow progressively accelerates as it approaches an orifice (e.g., a stenotic MV). This then ideally leads to formation of a series of hemispheric isovelocity surfaces whose areas become progressively smaller and their velocities progressively faster as the flow approaches the orifice.

According to the continuity principle, the amount of flow at the level of any of the hemispheres should equal the flow across the stenotic MV.[13] Using Doppler methods and the PISA method, MVA area can be calculated using the following formula:

$$\text{MVA} = 2 * \pi * r^2 * \frac{V_{alias}}{V_{max}}$$

in which r is the radius of the hemisphere (PISA radius) in centimeters, V_{alias} is the aliasing velocity of color Doppler flow (in cm/s), and V_{max} is the maximal transmitral velocity (also in cm/s).

The basic PISA method assumes that the orifice is a planar structure (i.e., at a 180-degree angle). Typically, this is not the case with MS, in which the orifice is funnel shaped (i.e., at an angle that is <180 degrees). Consequently, as the flow approaches a stenosed mitral orifice, PISA shells are not full hemispheres but partial hemispheres. Thus, to properly calculate MVA by the PISA method, the earlier equation needs to be modified to include an angle correction factor:

$$\text{MVA} = 2 * \pi * r^2 * \frac{V_{alias}}{V_{max}} * \frac{\vartheta}{180}$$

in which ϑ is the angle between the two mitral leaflets in diastole (see Fig. 91.2D).

The PISA method for MVA calculation is valid even in the presence of concomitant MR because increased diastolic flow caused by MR equally affects the flow at the level of both isovelocity hemispheres and mitral leaflet tips.

Semiquantitative Mitral Valve Area Assessment by M-Mode Echocardiography

M-mode echocardiography has high sensitivity and specificity for the diagnosis of MS. It may demonstrate thickened, calcified, and abnormally moving mitral leaflets. The smaller posterior leaflet, which is fused with the larger anterior leaflet, demonstrates an abnormal anterior motion on M-mode echocardiography during diastole.

The severity of MS can be roughly estimated from the EF slope of the anterior leaflet. In MS, after initial opening (E point), the anterior leaflet does not travel posteriorly toward the closing position fast enough because the elevated transmitral pressure gradient maintains the valve in the opened position longer than normal. The more severe the MS, the flatter the EF slope.

Similarly, the rate of emptying of the left atrium visualized by M-mode echocardiography can be used to roughly estimate the severity of MS. Normally, most atrial emptying (or LV filling) occurs promptly in early diastole, whereas in MS, LA emptying is gradual and lasts throughout diastole.

MEAN PRESSURE GRADIENT MEASUREMENTS

Mean diastolic pressure gradient is inversely related to MVA; that is, the more severe the MS, the higher the mean diastolic pressure gradient across the MV. This gradient can be easily measured by PW and CW Doppler.[14] The best approach for transmitral flow evaluation and gradient determination should be with the transducer at the apex, imaging in four- or two-chamber views. Color-flow imaging can be helpful for the assessment of the exact direction of the transmitral flow. The angle between the interrogating beam and the transmitral jet should be 0 degrees.

Gradient can be assessed by PW Doppler with the sample volume at the tips of the leaflets or by CW Doppler. By tracing the spectral Doppler-derived diastolic transmitral flow velocity envelope and with the use of built-in algorithms available in most modern ultrasound imaging systems, one can obtain the mean MV gradient (see Fig. 91.1A). To calculate the mean gradient, the system first calculates instantaneous pressure gradients using the simplified Bernoulli equation and then averages them out:

$$\Delta P = \frac{\sum_{i=0}^{n} Vi^2}{n}$$

in which ΔP is the mean diastolic transmitral pressure gradient, V is the instantaneous transmitral velocity, and n is the number of instantaneous gradients measured.

In the presence of atrial fibrillation, mean diastolic gradient should be averaged from multiple (typically five) cardiac cycles. When the MV is normal, there is no significant diastolic transmitral pressure gradient.

It is important to emphasize that these cutoff values assume a normal transmitral flow (a normal stroke volume and a normal heart rate). Mean diastolic gradient is strongly influenced by changes in transmitral flow:

$$\Delta P \approx \left(Flow^2\right)$$

Thus, exercise, fever, anemia, and pregnancy may lead to marked increases in transmitral pressure gradients and worsening of patients' symptoms. For instance, during pregnancy, cardiac output may increase 1.7-fold; this theoretically translates to a 1.7^2 or 2.9-fold increase in transmitral pressure gradient.[15]

According to the 2019 AHA/ACC valvular disease guidelines, because of the variability of the mean pressure gradient with heart rate and forward flow, it has not been included in the criteria for severity of MS; the mean gradient is typically greater than 5 to 10 mm Hg in severe MS.

Stress testing may provide additional information on hemodynamic significance of MS; transmitral pressure gradients and right heart pressures are measured during exercise or dobutamine stress echocardiography. Stress testing in MS may be used to assess patients' symptoms or to evaluate for PMBV. For instance, in asymptomatic patients with moderate or severe MS, PMBV is indicated when pulmonary artery systolic pressure is greater than 50 mm Hg at rest or greater than 60 mm Hg with exercise or when there is new-onset atrial fibrillation. PMBV may also be considered in symptomatic patients with moderate MS (valve area >1.5 cm²) when pulmonary artery systolic pressure is greater than 60 mm Hg, pulmonary artery wedge pressure is greater than 25 mm Hg, or mean MV gradient is greater than 15 mm Hg during exercise.[16]

Unlike the mean gradient, the peak diastolic mitral gradient is not a good measure of MS severity because it is often markedly influenced by other factors such as the LA compliance and LV diastolic function.

SECONDARY CHANGES CAUSED BY MITRAL STENOSIS

MS may lead to chronic LA pressure overload, potentially resulting in LA enlargement, pulmonary hypertension, right heart dilatation, and functional tricuspid regurgitation. Techniques for estimating chamber sizes and right heart pressures are discussed in other chapters.

In patients with MS, a wide range of pulmonary artery pressures has been observed for a given MVA. Elevated LA pressure leading to pulmonary venous congestion is the primary reason for pulmonary hypertension in patients with MS. For unclear reasons, a subset of

patients may also develop pulmonary arterial hypertension, which, unlike pulmonary venous hypertension, may not resolve after percutaneous or surgical correction of MS.

Noninvasive assessment of pulmonary vascular resistance (PVR) by echocardiography may help differentiate between pure pulmonary venous hypertension (normal PVR) and superimposed pulmonary arterial hypertension (high PVR). In general, PVR is directly related to transpulmonary pressure gradient and inversely related to the transpulmonary blood flow. Noninvasively, PVR can be calculated from spectral Doppler tracings of tricuspid regurgitant jet and the flow across the right ventricular outflow tract using the so-called Abbas[17] equation:

$$PVR = 0.16 + 10 * \frac{Vmax \text{ of TR Jet}}{RVOT \text{ VTI}}$$

in which V_{max} of the tricuspid regurgitant (TR) jet is in meters per second, right ventricular outflow tract (RVOT) VTI in centimeters, and PVR in Wood units. In principle, echocardiographic PVR measurements should be confirmed by invasive methods.

The routine echocardiographic evaluation of MS does not require transesophageal echocardiography (TEE). However, TEE should be considered when the image quality and Doppler information are suboptimal or do not correlate with the clinical impression. TEE is also useful in the evaluation of complications of MS, such as LA clot or endocarditis. TEE is also frequently used before and during MV balloon valvuloplasty.[18]

Please access ExpertConsult to view the corresponding videos for this chapter.

REFERENCES

1. Baumgartner H, Hung J, Bermejo J, et al. Echocardiographic assessment of valve stenosis: EAE/ASE recommendations for clinical practice. *J Am Soc Echocardiogr.* 2009;22(1):1–23. erratum in J Am Soc Echocardiogr 2009;22:442.
2. Nishimura RA, Otto CM, Bonow RO, et al. 2014 AHA/ACC Guideline for the management of patients with valvular heart disease. *J Am Coll Cardiol.* 2014;63:2489.
3. Gorlin R, Gorlin SG. Hydraulic formula for calculation of the area of the stenotic mitral valve, other cardiac valves, and central circulatory shunts. *Am Heart J.* 1951;41:1–29.
4. Nishimura RA, Rihal CS, Tajik AJ, Holmes Jr DR. Accurate measurement of the transmitral gradient in patients with mitral stenosis: a simultaneous catheterization and Doppler echocardiographic study. *J Am Coll Cardiol.* 1994;24:152–158.
5. Libanoff AJ, Rodbard S. Atrioventricular pressure halftime: measure of mitral valve orifice area. *Circulation.* 1968;38:144–150.
6. Hatle L, Angelsen B. *Doppler Ultrasound in Cardiology: Physical Principles and Clinical Applications.* Philadelphia: Lea and Febiger; 1985:118.
7. Gonzalez MA, Child JS, Krivokapich J. Comparison of two-dimensional and Doppler echocardiographic and intracardiac hemodynamics for quantification of mitral stenosis. *Am J Cardiol.* 1987;60:327–332.
8. Thomas JD, Weyman AE. Mitral pressure halftime: a clinical tool in search of theoretical justification. *J Am Coll Cardiol.* 1987;10:923–929.
9. Lutembacher R. De la sténose mitrale avec communication interauriculaire. *Arch Mal Coeur Vaiss.* 1916;9:237–250.
10. Thomas JD, Wilkins GT, Choong CY, et al. Inaccuracy of mitral pressure halftime immediately after percutaneous mitral valvotomy. Dependence on transmitral gradient and left atrial and ventricular compliance. *Circulation.* 1988;78:980–993.
11. Schlosshan D, Aggarwal G, Mathur G, et al. Real-time 3D transesophageal echocardiography for the evaluation of rheumatic mitral stenosis. *JACC Cardiovasc Imag.* 2011;4:580–588.
12. Recusani F, Bargiggia GS, Yoganathan AP, et al. A new method for quantification of regurgitant flow rate using color flow imaging of the flow convergence region proximal to a discrete orifice: an in vitro study. *Circulation.* 1991;83:594–604.
13. Rodriguez L, Thomas JD, Monterroso V, et al. Validation of the proximal flow convergence method. Calculation of orifice area in patients with mitral stenosis. *Circulation.* 1993;88:1157–1165.
14. Hatle L, Brubakk A, Tromsdal A, Angelsen B. Noninvasive assessment of pressure drop in mitral stenosis by Doppler ultrasound. *Br Heart J.* 1978;40:131–140.
15. Carabello BA. Modern management of mitral stenosis. *Circulation.* 2005;112:432–437.
16. Bonow RO, Carabello BA, Kanu C, et al. ACC/AHA 2006 guidelines for the management of patients with valvular heart disease. *Circulation.* 2006;114:e84–e231.
17. Abbas AE, Fortuin FD, Schiller NB, et al. A simple method for noninvasive estimation of pulmonary vascular resistance. *J Am Coll Cardiol.* 2003;41:1021–1027.
18. Perk G, Ruiz C, Saric M, Kronzon I. Real-time three-dimensional transesophageal echocardiography in transcutaneous, catheter-based procedures for repair of structural heart diseases. *Curr Cardiovasc Imag Rep.* 2009;2:363–374.

92 Nonrheumatic Etiologies of Mitral Stenosis: Situations That Mimic Mitral Stenosis

Steven A. Goldstein

MITRAL ANNULAR CALCIFICATION

Rheumatic mitral stenosis (MS) is, by far, the most common cause of left ventricular (LV) inflow obstruction. Less common cause are listed in Box 92.1. Among these, a heavily calcified mitral annulus is the most often encountered. Calcium deposits in the mitral annulus are extremely common,[1] mainly in older persons or "prematurely" in patients with chronic renal disease on long-term dialysis.[2,3] Mitral annulus calcium (MAC) is commonly asymptomatic and an incidental finding. Despite the frequency with which such deposits are encountered, hemodynamic consequences are relatively uncommon. Large deposits, however, may produce mild or moderate degrees of mitral regurgitation (MR) and uncommonly severe MR.[1,4] The valvular MR results from splinting of the physiologic contraction of the mitral annulus during systole and by stiffening of the leaflets. MS caused by severe MAC is much less common.[2–11] The mechanisms by which MAC contributes to degenerative mitral stenosis (DMS) include (1) reduced normal annular dilatation during diastole, (2) impaired mobility of the anterior mitral leaflet because the leaflet's hinge point is displaced toward its free margin because of calcium, and (3) large posterior mitral annular deposits narrowing the annulus.[3,5,6,8] This is especially true in patients with valvular aortic stenosis (AS) because of calcium extending from the aortic annulus into the base of the anterior mitral leaflet.[12] Elevated LV pressure (as is the case in significant AS) increases mitral annular stress and, if present, may lead to trauma and annular micro cracks. These sites of annular damage are thought to undergo further degenerative calcification, leading to MAC.[13]

Gross pathologic differences exist between rheumatic mitral stenosis (RMS) and MS associated with MAC (Boxes 92.2 and 92.3). Likewise, the echocardiographic appearance of the mitral apparatus can distinguish these entities. The echocardiographic features of MS caused by MAC can be seen in Fig. 92.1 and Video 92.1 and are summarized as follows: Calcification is prominent in the basal portion of both mitral leaflets with sparing of the free edges of the leaflets. This is precisely the opposite of the pattern seen in RMS where the tips or free edges are the thickest portion of the leaflets.[14] In addition, unlike RMS, in which the mitral leaflets move in tandem ("parallel") because of commissural fusion, the leaflets in MAC have qualitatively normal ("antiparallel") diastolic motion, although the amplitude of leaflet motion is reduced. These features are best imaged in the parasternal long-axis and apical four-chamber views. Last, in rheumatic MS, there is commissural fusion best imaged in the short-axis view. Commissural fusion is absent in MS because of MAC. This feature has important clinical relevance, because these patients do not benefit from percutaneous balloon mitral valvotomy, which derives its benefit from splitting the fused commissure(s).

There are no standardized echocardiographic criteria to grade the severity of MAC. The classic echocardiographic techniques used for rheumatic MS (mitral valve [MV] area planimetry, pressure halftime, proximal isovelocity surface area, and continuity equation) lack validation for DMS. The limiting orifice of mitral inflow in DMS is typically located at the base of the mitral leaflets. Thus, planimetry at the level of the leaflet tips does not represent the true stenotic orifice. Moreover, severe calcification and blooming artifacts may interfere with visualizing the limiting orifice. Three-dimensional (3D) echocardiography, with transthoracic (TTE) or transesophageal echocardiography (TEE), may overcome these limitations be cause of its ability to obtain an en face view of the mitral orifice. 3D-echocardiography can also be helpful in demonstrating the absence of commissural fusion.

The treatment of calcific MS has been challenging for several reasons, including the unavailability of medical therapies to prevent progression and the lack of role for balloon mitral valvuloplasty or surgical commissurotomy. In addition, surgical MV replacement is limited by technical difficulties and complications related to trying to remove heavy MAC, placing sutures, and seating prosthetic valves, especially in older adult high-risk patients with comorbidities.

BOX 92.1 Causes of Mitral Stenosis

- Rheumatic heart disease
- Nonrheumatic acquired mitral stenosis
  - Massive mitral annular calcification
  - Ergotamine induced and methysergide induced
  - Infective endocarditis with obstructive vegetations
  - Radiation-induced valve disease
  - Systemic lupus erythematosus
  - Antiphospholipid antibody syndrome
  - Carcinoid heart disease
  - Rheumatoid arthritis
  - Whipple disease
  - Pseudoxanthoma elasticum
  - Left atrial myxoma and other tumors
  - Mitral valve repair (e.g., undersized annuloplasty rings)
- Cor triatriatum
- Other congenital causes of mitral stenosis
  - Supravalve stenosing ring
  - Parachute mitral valve
  - Double orifice mitral valve

BOX 92.2 Cardinal Anatomic Changes in Rheumatic Mitral Valve Stenosis

Leaflet thickening (diffuse, especially free edges)
Commissural fusion
Shortening, thickening, and fusion of chordae
Oval or slitlike orifice ("fish mouth")

BOX 92.3 Anatomic Changes in Nonrheumatic Mitral Stenosis Caused by Mitral Annular Calcification

Leaflet thickening (focal, avoids free edges)
No commissural fusion
No chordal shortening, thickening, or fusion
Calcium deposition in other intracardiac sites (aortic valve, aortic annulus, sinotubular junction, papillary muscles)

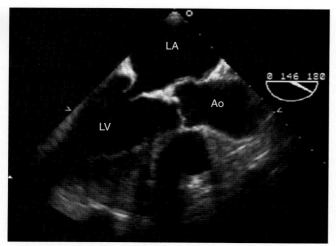

Figure 92.1. Transesophageal echocardiography from a 78-year-old woman with mild mitral stenosis caused by mitral annular and leaflet calcification that illustrates differences from rheumatic mitral stenosis. Calcification is present in the basal portion of both leaflets and spares the free edges (tips) of the leaflets. There is also lack of commissural fusion (not shown in this view). *Ao,* Ascending aorta; *LA,* left atrium; *LV,* left ventricle.

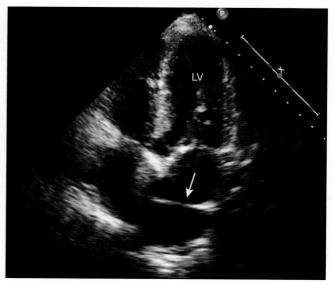

Figure 92.2. Transthoracic echocardiographic apical four-chamber view from a patient with cor triatriatum that illustrates a linear echodensity that traverses the left atrium *(arrow). LV,* Left ventricle.

Recent innovations in transcatheter interventional procedures for MV disease has been aimed predominantly at MR. Nevertheless, procedures such as transcatheter MV replacement may provide an option for these patients. Initial results have been promising.[15–17]

OTHER NONRHEUMATIC FORMS OF ACQUIRED MITRAL STENOSIS

Valve dysfunction caused by infective endocarditis is nearly always regurgitation, often new. The occurrence of an obstructive or "functionally" stenotic MV caused by endocarditis is rare.[18–20] Tiong and colleagues reviewed the literature from 1966 to 2002 and found only 20 cases of significant native valve obstruction secondary to endocarditis.[20] Although fungal endocarditis is usually suspected in this setting, bacterial endocarditis also causes obstruction.

The overuse of ergot alkaloids (e.g., ergotamine and methysergide) may cause plaquelike lesions on the MV, leading to MS.[21,22] In addition, appetite suppressants can cause lesions that resemble those associated with ergot alkaloids.[23] Carcinoid syndrome is a rare disease that usually involves only the valves on the right side of the heart. However, left-sided involvement can occur (presumably caused by either bronchial metastases[24] or patent foramen ovale). Carcinoid valvular disease can cause either regurgitant or stenotic lesions.[25]

Large left atrial (LA) myxomas (and less commonly sarcomas) can prolapse into the MV "funnel" in diastole and produce inflow obstruction because of their bulk. Malignant neoplasms such as sarcomas and lymphomas can mechanically deform and obstruct the MV. Lung tumors that invade the pulmonary veins can also be a rare cause of MS.[26]

Mediastinal radiation may result in fibrocalcific valve disease and either MR or MS.[27] MS is an infrequent complication of systemic lupus erythematosus or the antiphospholipid syndrome.[28–30] MS has been reported in patients with familial pseudoxanthoma elasticum, in which histologic sections of the valve shows irregular, coarse-fibered, abnormally fragmented elastic fibers similar to those seen in skin lesions.[31]

Cor Triatriatum

Cor triatriatum is a rare congenital anomaly in which a perforated fibrous or fibromuscular membrane divides the left atrium into two chambers. The posterior-superior (common pulmonary venous chamber) chamber receives the pulmonary veins, and the anterior-inferior (true left atrium) chamber receives the left atrial appendage (LAA). One or more openings in the fibrous membrane permit flow of blood from the pulmonary veins into the true left atrium. The opening(s) may be small, producing obstruction to flow, or large with little or no obstruction. The extent of obstruction determines the age of onset and severity of symptoms. Cor triatriatum may become manifest at any time from infancy to adulthood but usually becomes apparent in childhood, either as an isolated abnormality or associated with other congenital heart defects.[32,33] The clinical manifestations depend on the size of the opening of the membrane and are similar to MS. In adults, perforations are usually large, and nonobstructive or fenestrated membranes may be detected fortuitously in asymptomatic patients who undergo echocardiography for an unrelated indication as illustrated by Video 92.2. Two-dimensional echocardiography, including TEE, has become the procedure of choice for diagnosing cor triatriatum.[34–37] The echocardiographic features are characteristic and consist of a linear echo-density that stretches across the left atrium at a level midway between the mitral annulus and the superior border (or roof) of the left atrium[38] (Figs. 92.2 and 92.3). This membrane may show phasic motion, moving inferiorly toward the mitral orifice in diastole and superiorly toward the superior LA border during systole.[38] The membrane can be seen in multiple views, including the parasternal long-axis, the subcostal long-axis, or the apical four-chamber or long-axis views. The four-chamber view is usually preferable because it places the membrane perpendicular to the echo beam. The perforation is most often posterior and, as stated, can be multiple. Color Doppler aids in demonstrating the number, location, and size of the openings in the membrane. Spectral Doppler (either pulsed or continuous wave) provides hemodynamic assessment.[39] Peak instantaneous and mean gradients can be calculated using the modified Bernoulli equation and the size of the orifice(s) by the continuity equation. If the turbulent jet produced by the midcavitary obstruction strikes the MV, it can produce fluttering of the mitral leaflets, best seen on M-mode echocardiography.

When the transthoracic study is suboptimal, TEE may be used to evaluate cor triatriatum.[35,40] 3D echocardiography has also been used to evaluate cor triatriatum.[41]

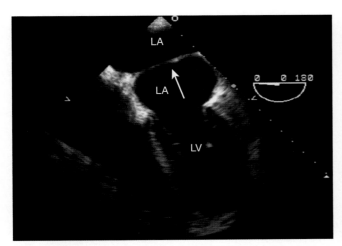

Figure 92.3. Transthoracic echocardiographic four-chamber view from a different patient with cor triatriatum that illustrates a linear echo density *(arrow)* that traverses the left atrium (LA). *LV,* Left ventricle.

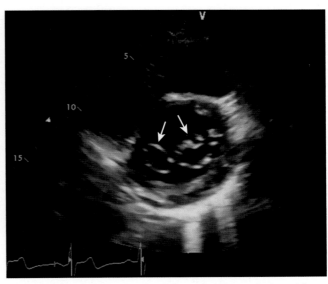

Figure 92.4. Transthoracic echocardiography short-axis view at the level of the mitral valve that illustrates a double-orifice mitral valve *(arrows).*

Other Congenital Causes of Mitral Stenosis

Cor triatriatum must be distinguished from a mitral supravalvular stenosing ring, another rare cause of MS.[42,43] In contrast to cor triatriatum, these membranes are closer to the MV (and may actually adhere to the valve leaflets) and are characterized by their position inferior to the LAA. The proximity of the membrane to the valve can lead to leaflet damage resulting from high-velocity turbulent flow. Leaflet thickening and MR can develop as a consequence. Color Doppler is useful to identify flow acceleration and turbulence at the level of the annulus rather than at the leaflet tips (like rheumatic MV stenosis). Continuous-wave Doppler can be used to assess the severity of the obstruction. Caution must be used when diagnosing a supravalvular stenosing ring. Differentiating this entity from a calcified mitral annulus may be difficult, leading to both false-positive and false-negative diagnoses.[44]

A parachute MV, another congenital cause of MS,[42,43,45,46] results when only one papillary muscle is present (or two that are very close together). As a consequence, interchordal spaces are narrowed, producing subvalvular obstruction. This abnormality may be associated with other congenital cardiac anomalies or may occur as an isolated lesion. Parachute MV may be part of the Shone syndrome, which also includes subaortic stenosis and coarctation of the aorta.[40,41,43,45,46]

A double-orifice mitral valve (DOMV) is an uncommon anomaly that is characterized by a MV with a single fibrous annulus with two orifices that open into the left ventricle as depicted in Fig. 92.4. Subvalvular structures usually show various degrees of abnormality. Although DOMV may allow normal blood flow between the left atrium and the left ventricle, it can produce either obstruction or regurgitation.[47–49]

Please access ExpertConsult to view the corresponding videos for this chapter.

REFERENCES

1. Roberts WC, Perloff JK. Mitral valve disease. A clinicopathologic survey of the conditions causing the mitral valve to function abnormally. *Ann Intern Med.* 1972;77:939–975.
2. Schott CR, Kotler MN, Parry WR, et al. Mitral annular calcification: clinical and echocardiographic correlations. *Arch Intern Med.* 1977;133:1143–1152.
3. Hammer WJ, Roberts WC, de Leon AC. Mitral stenosis secondary to combined "massive" mitral annular calcific deposits and small, hypertrophied left ventricles. Hemodynamic documentation in four patients. *Am J Med.* 1978;64:371–376.
4. Perloff K, Roberts WC. The mitral apparatus. Functional anatomy of mitral regurgitation. *Circulation.* 1972;46:227–239.
5. Korn D, DeSanctis RW, Sell S. Massive calcification of the mitral annulus. A clinicopathologic study of fourteen cases. *N Engl J Med.* 1962;257:900–909.
6. Osterberger LE, Goldstein S, Khaja F, et al. Functional mitral stenosis in patients with massive mitral annular calcification. *Circulation.* 1981;64:472–746.
7. Theleman KP, Grayburn PA, Roberts WC. Mitral "annular" calcium forming a complete circle "O" causing mitral stenosis in association with a stenotic congenitally bicuspid aortic vale and severe coronary artery disease. *Am J Geriatr Cardiol.* 2006;1558–1561.
8. Hakki AH, Iskandrian AS. Obstruction to left ventricular inflow secondary to combined mitral annular calcification and idiopathic subaortic stenosis. *Cathet Cardiovasc Diagn.* 1980;6:191–196.
9. D'Cruz IA, Madu EC. Progression to calcific mitral stenosis in end-stage renal disease. *Am J Kidney Dis.* 1995;26:956–959.
10. De Pace NL, Rohrer AH, Kotler MN, et al. Rapidly progressing, massive mitral annular calcification: occurrence in a patient with chronic renal failure. *Arch Intern Med.* 1981;141:1663–1665.
11. Straumann E, Misteli M, Blumberg A, et al. Aortic and mitral valve disease in patients with end-stage renal failure on long-term hemodialysis. *Br Heart J.* 1992;67:236–239.
12. Iwataki M, Takeuchi M, Otani K, et al. Calcific extension towards the mitral valve causes non-rheumatic mitral stenosis in degenerative aortic stenosis: real-time 3D transesophageal echocardiography study. *Open Heart.* 2014;1. e000136.
13. Sud K, Agarwal S, Parashar A, et al. Degenerative mitral stenosis. *Circulation.* 2016;133:1594–1604.
14. Madu EC, D'Cruz IA, Wall B, et al. Transesophageal echocardiographic spectrum of calcific mitral abnormalities in patients with end-stage renal disease. *Echocardiography.* 2000;17:29–35.
15. Puri R, Abdul-Jawad O, del Trigo M, et al. Transcatheter mitral valve implantation for inoperable severely calcified native mitral valve disease: a systematic review. *Catheter Cardiovasc Interv.* 2016;87:540–548.
16. Guerrero M, Dvir D, Himbert D, et al. Transcatheter mitral valve replacement in native mitral valve disease with severe mitral annular calcification: results from the first multicenter global registry. *J Am Coll Cardiol Interv.* 2016;9:1361–1371.
17. Guerrero M, Urena M, Himbert D, et al. 1-year outcomes of transcatheter mitral valve replacement in patients with severe mitral annular calcification. *J Am Coll Cardiol.* 2018;71:1841–1853.
18. Ghosh PK, Miller HI, Vidne BA. Mitral obstruction in bacterial endocarditis. *Br Heart J.* 1985;53:341–344.
19. Prasad TR, Valiathan MS, Venkitachalam CG, et al. Unusual manifestation of valvular vegetations. *Thorac Cardiovasc Surg.* 1988;36:171–180.
20. Tiong IY, Novaro GM, Jefferson B, et al. Bacterial endocarditis and functional mitral stenosis. A report of two cases and brief literature review. *Chest.* 2002;122:2259–2262.
21. Hauck AJ, Edwards WD, Danielson GK, et al. Mitral and aortic valve disease associated with ergotamine therapy for migraine. *Arch Pathol Lab Med.* 1990;114:62–64.
22. Redfield MM, Nicholson WJ, Edwards WD, et al. Valve disease associated with ergot alkaloid use: echocardiographic and pathologic correlations. *Ann Intern Med.* 1992;117:50–52.
23. Connolly HM, Crary JL, McGoon MD, et al. Valvular heart disease associated with fenfluramine-phentermine. *N Engl J Med.* 1997;337:581–588.

24. Himelman RB, Schiller NB. Clinical and echocardiographic comparison of patients with the carcinoid syndrome with and without carcinoid heart disease. *Am J Cardiol.* 1989;63:347–352.
25. Horstkotte D, Niehues R, Strauer BE. Pathomorphologic aspects aetiology and natural history of acquired mitral valve disease. *Eur Heart J.* 1991;12(Suppl B):55–60.
26. Reddy YNV, Sundaram, Stamler JS. An unusual case of peripartum pulmonary oedema. *BMJ Case Rep 1–.* 2013;3.
27. Veinot JP, Edwards WD. Pathology of radiation-induced heart disease: a surgical and autopsy study of 27 cases. *Hum Pathol.* 1996;27:766–773.
28. Alameddine AK, Schoen FJ, Yanagi H, et al. Aortic or mitral valve replacement in systemic lupus erythematosus. *Am J Cardiol.* 1992;70:955–956.
29. Hojnik M, George J, Ziporen L, et al. Heart valve involvement (Libman-Sacks endocarditis) in the antiphospholipid syndrome. *Circulation.* 1996;93:1579–1587.
30. Yusuf S, Madden BP, Pumphrey CW. Left atrial thrombus caused by the primary antiphospholipid syndrome causing critical functional mitral stenosis. *Heart.* 2003;89:262.
31. Fukuda K, Uno K, Fujii T, et al. Mitral stenosis in pseudoxanthoma elasticum. *Chest.* 1992;101:1706–1707.
32. Marin-Garcia J, Tandon R, Lucas RV, et al. Cor triatriatum: study of 20 cases. *Am J Cardiol.* 1975;35:54–66.
33. van Son JAM, Danielson GK, Schaff HV, et al. Cor triatriatum: diagnosis, operative approach, and late results. *Mayo Clin Proc.* 1993;68:854–859.
34. Ostman-Smith I, Silverman NH, Oldershaw P, et al. Cor triatriatum sinistrum: diagnostic features on cross sectional echocardiography. *Br Heart J.* 1984;51:211–219.
35. Seward JB, Tajik AJ. Transesophageal echocardiography in congenital heart disease. *Am J Cardiac Imag.* 1990;4:215–222.
36. Lengyel M, Arvay A, Biro V. Two-dimensional echocardiographic diagnosis of cor triatriatum. *Am J Cardiol.* 1987;59:484–485.
37. Fagan LE, et al. Two-dimensional, spectral Doppler and color flow imaging in adults with acquired and congenital cor triatriatum. *J Am Soc Echocardiogr.* 1991;4:177–184.
38. Snider AR, Roge CH, Schiller NB, et al. Congenital left ventricular inflow obstruction evaluated by two-dimensional echocardiography. *Circulation.* 1980;61:848–855.
39. Radhakrishnan S, Shrivastava S. Doppler echocardiography in the diagnosis of divided left atrium (cor triatriatum sinister). *Int J Cardiol.* 1988;21:183–187.
40. Vuocolo L, Stoddard M, Longaker R. Transesophageal two-dimensional and Doppler echocardiographic diagnosis of cor triatriatum in the adult. *Am Heart J.* 1992;124:791–794.
41. Bartel T, Muller S, Geibel A. Preoperative assessment of cor triatriatum in an adult by dynamic three-dimensional echocardiography was more informative than transesophageal echocardiography or magnetic resonance imaging. *Br Heart J.* 1994;72:498–499.
42. Ruckman RN, Van Praagh R. Anatomic types of congenital mitral stenosis: report of 49 autopsy cases with consideration of diagnosis and surgical implications. *Am J Cardiol.* 1978;42:592.
43. Shone JD, Sellers RD, Anderson RC, et al. The developmental complex of "parachute mitral valve" supravalve ring of left atrium, subaortic stenosis, and coarctation of aorta. *Am J Cardiol.* 1963;11:714–725.
44. Feigenbaum H, Armstrong WF, Ryan T. Congenital heart diseases. In: Feigenbaum H, Armstrong WF, Ryan T, eds. *Feigenbaum's Echocardiography.* 6th ed. Philadelphia: Lippincott Williams & Wilkins; 2005.
45. Tandon R, Moller JH, Edwards JE. Anomalies associated with the parachute mitral valve: a pathologic analysis of 52 cases. *Can J Cardiol.* 1986;2:278–281.
46. Bolling SF, Iannettoni MD, Rosenthal A, et al. Shone's anomaly: operative results and late outcome. *Ann Thorac Surg.* 1990;49:887–893.
47. Trowitzsch E, Bano-Rodrigo A, Burger BM, et al. Two-dimensional echocardiographic findings in double orifice mitral valve. *J Am Coll Cardiol.* 1985;6:383–387.
48. Bano-Rodrigo A, Van Praagh S, Trowitzsch E, et al. Double orifice mitral valve: a study of 27 postmortem cases with developmental, diagnostic, and surgical considerations. *Am J Cardiol.* 1988;61:152–160.
49. Anwar AM, McGhie JS, Meijboom FJ, et al. Double orifice mitral valve by real-time three dimensional echocardiography. *Eur J Echocardiogr.* 2008;9:731–732.

93   Role of Hemodynamic Stress Testing in Mitral Stenosis

Neda Dianati-Maleki, Smadar Kort

Mitral valve (MV) stenosis causes a fixed obstruction in the left ventricular (LV) inflow and decreases the LV preload, thus leading to decreased cardiac output (CO). When severe enough, it can result in elevated pulmonary artery pressures (PAP) and right ventricular (RV) failure. The severity of clinical symptoms directly correlates with the pressure gradient across the MV and left atrial (LA) pressure. Percutaneous mitral balloon commissurotomy or MV surgery is a class I recommendation for patients with severe symptomatic mitral stenosis (MS) (American College of Cardiology [ACC]/American Heart Association [AHA] 2014 and European Society of Cardiology [ESC]/European Association for Cardio-Thoracic Surgery [EACTS] 2017 guidelines).[1,2] Echocardiography has a pivotal role in diagnosis and grading of the severity of MS as well as assessment of potential hemodynamic consequences.

Most patients with severe MS present with clinical symptoms of exertional shortness of breath. However, some individuals may complain of nonspecific and equivocal symptoms or may completely be unaware of their symptoms and subjectively feel asymptomatic. This could be because of the insidious rate of progression of MS leading to a sedentary lifestyle from limited functional capacity with no evident symptoms. Echocardiographic assessment of mean mitral gradients and systolic PAP during hemodynamic stress testing can help differentiate this high risk group who would benefit from MV intervention from truly asymptomatic individuals with MS. On the other hand, patients with apparently less severe MS may present with significant exertional symptoms that are not proportional to the severity of MS, as assessed by echocardiography at rest. In this clinical scenario, hemodynamic stress testing is indicated to assess the changes in pulmonary pressures with exercise as a possible cause of the exertional symptoms. In asymptomatic patients with severe MS, the atrioventricular compliance dictates which patients will develop elevated mean mitral gradients and systolic PAP with stress testing.

During the echocardiography examination, the mean mitral gradient can be accurately and reproducibly measured using a continuous-wave (CW) Doppler interrogation across the MV in an apical four-chamber view during supine exercise or immediately post-treadmill exercise. Color Doppler can be used to direct the CW signal to avoid underestimation of the mean gradient. Atrial fibrillation is common in patients with MS, and in these patients, hemodynamic variables should be averaged over 5 to 10 cardiac cycles. Examples of mean pressure gradient across the MV at rest and postexercise are seen in Figs. 93.1 and 93.2. Similarly, the systolic PAP, estimated based on the tricuspid regurgitation jet velocity at rest and postexercise, are demonstrated in Figs. 93.3 and 93.4.

INDICATIONS FOR HEMODYNAMIC STRESS TESTING IN MITRAL STENOSIS ACCORDING TO THE MOST RECENT GUIDELINES:

The 2014 AHA/ACC Guideline for the Management of Patients with Valvular Heart Disease, recommends exercise stress echocardiography (ESE) with Doppler or invasive hemodynamic assessment to evaluate the response of the mean mitral gradient and systolic PAP in patients with MS when there is a discrepancy between resting Doppler echocardiographic findings and clinical symptoms or signs (class I; level of evidence: C).[1]

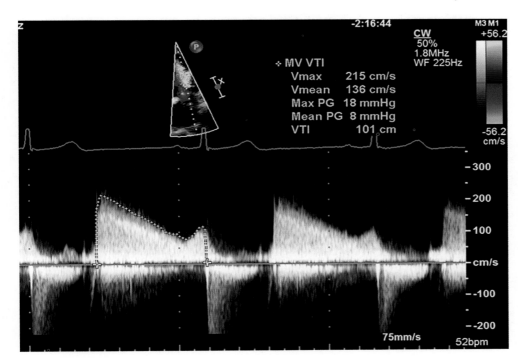

Figure 93.1. Resting mitral valve mean gradient. This 38-year-old woman with no prior medical history originally from South America presented with exertional dyspnea. Baseline transthoracic echocardiography demonstrates a rheumatic mitral valve with mild mitral regurgitation and moderate mitral stenosis, with no other abnormalities. Exercise stress echocardiography is performed. *CW,* Continuous wave; *MV,* mitral valve; *PG,* peak gradient; *Vmax,* maximal (peak) velocity; *Vmean,* mean velocity; *VTI,* velocity time integral.

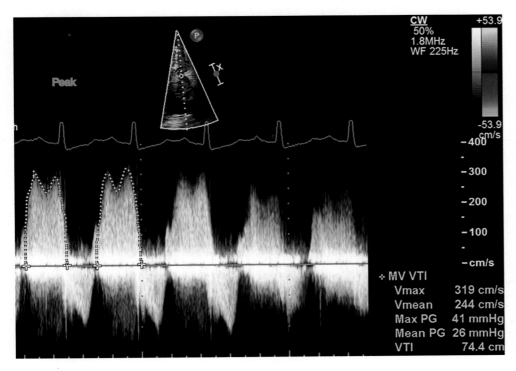

Figure 93.2. Postexercise mean transmitral gradient. She exercised for 11 minutes and 10 seconds of a modified Bruce protocol, achieving 7 METs. Peak heart rate was 132 beats/min (77% of predicted), and peak blood pressure during stress was 120/60 mmHg, from a baseline of 92/56 mmHg. The study was terminated secondary to severe dyspnea. No electrocardiographic changes or wall motion abnormalities were noted with stress. The patient remained in sinus rhythm. Her mean forward flow gradient rose to 26 mmHg. *CW,* Continuous wave; *MV,* mitral valve; *PG,* peak gradient; *Vmax,* maximal (peak) velocity; *Vmean,* mean velocity; *VTI,* velocity time integral.

This is supported by the American College of Cardiology Appropriate Use Criteria Task Force/American Association for Thoracic Surgery/American Heart Association/American Society of Echocardiography/European Association for Cardio-Thoracic Surgery/Heart Valve Society/Society of Cardiovascular Anesthesiologists/Society for Cardiovascular Angiography and Interventions/Society of Cardiovascular Computed Tomography/Society for Cardiovascular Magnetic Resonance/Society of Thoracic Surgeons (ACC/AATS/AHA/ASE/EACTS/HVS/SCA/SCAI/SCCT/SCMR/STS) 2017 Appropriate Use Criteria for Multimodality Imaging in Valvular Heart Disease. According to this document, ESE is deemed appropriate to "evaluate mean mitral gradient and PAP, in case of discrepancy between resting Doppler echocardiographic findings and clinical symptoms or signs."[3]

According to 2017 ESC/EACTS guidelines for the management of valvular heart disease, asymptomatic patients with significant MV stenosis, defined as mitral valve area (MVA)1.5 cm² or less who are not identified as high risk for embolism or hemodynamic

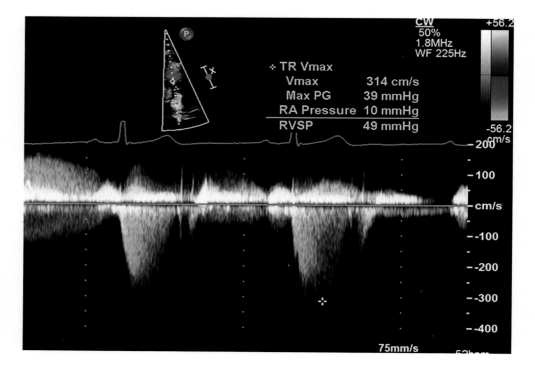

Figure 93.3. Resting pulmonary artery systolic pressure measurement. *CW,* Continuous wave; *MV,* mitral valve; *PG,* peak gradient; *RA,* right atrial; *RVSP,* right ventricular systolic pressure; *TR,* tricuspid regurgitation; *Vmax,* maximal (peak) velocity.

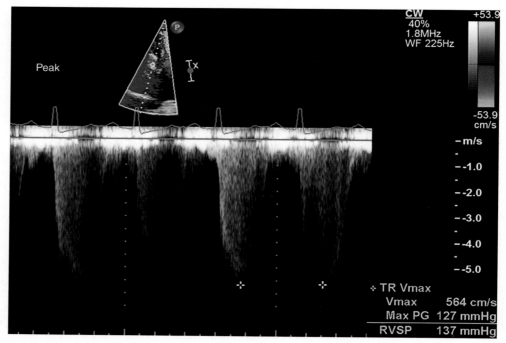

Figure 93.4. Postexercise pulmonary artery systolic pressure measurement. A marked increase in pulmonary artery pressure is noted with exercise. *CW,* Continuous wave; *PG,* peak gradient; *RVSP,* right ventricular systolic pressure; *TR,* tricuspid regurgitation; *Vmax,* maximal (peak) velocity.

decompensation, should undergo stress testing for further risk stratification. MV intervention, including surgical valve replacement or percutaneous mitral balloon commissurotomy, is indicated when the stress test is positive with symptoms. High-risk features for thromboembolism risk include a history of systemic embolism, dense spontaneous echo contrast in the left atrium, or new-onset atrial fibrillation. High-risk characteristics for hemodynamic compromise includes those with systolic PAP greater than 50 mmHg, need for major noncardiac surgery or patients desire for pregnancy. All asymptomatic patients with these high-risk features should directly undergo evaluation for MV intervention without the need for stress testing.

VALVULAR STRESS ECHOCARDIOGRAPHY

Valvular stress echocardiography can be performed as ESE or dobutamine stress echocardiography (DSE) depending on the patient's clinical status, severity, and type of valve disease.[2]

EXERCISE STRESS ECHOCARDIOGRAPHY

A comprehensive clinical evaluation to identify any potential contraindications is essential before undergoing exercise testing. A symptom-limited exercise test performed under direct supervision with the goal of reaching at least 85% of the age-predicted heart rate is recommended. Patients should continue taking their usual medication(s). Treadmill or semisupine bicycle exercise testing can be performed. In North America, treadmill exercise is more commonly performed using the modified Bruce protocol and allows imaging after exercise. In Europe, semisupine ergocycle with a tilting table is the preferred approach for valvular stress testing and permits image acquisition during each step of exercise testing.[4]

The main parameters assessed in ESE include mean mitral gradient and systolic PAP, which are estimated through CW Doppler interrogation of MV and tricuspid regurgitation signals, respectively. These parameters are compared at baseline and at peak stress.[4] An exercise-induced rise in mean mitral gradient to greater than 15 mmHg or an exercise-induced rise in systolic PAP to greater than 60 mmHg indicates hemodynamically significant MS requiring MV intervention. Other important parameters to assess during a ESE include development of symptoms, blood pressure response, new wall motion abnormalities, and potential decrease in LV ejection fraction.[5]

DOBUTAMINE STRESS ECHOCARDIOGRAPHY

The safety and feasibility of DSE in assessment of asymptomatic severe MS has been evaluated and DSE may be performed instead of ESE. DES seems to lead to similar hemodynamic changes in mean mitral gradient and systolic PAP as ESE. DSE protocol is started at 10 mcg/kg/min for 5 minutes and increased by 10 mcg/kg/min every 3 minutes to a maximal dose of 40 mcg/kg/min. It is important to note that the threshold for severe mean gradient is 18 mmHg during DSE (90% sensitivity and 87% specificity), which is slightly higher than the cut-off for ESE.[6]

SUMMARY

Hemodynamic stress echocardiography is indicated for risk stratification of asymptomatic patients with significant MS (MVA <1.5 cm^2) or when there is a discrepancy between the level of MS and the patient's symptoms. According to current multisocietal guidelines, asymptomatic patients with significant MS and exercise-induced pulmonary hypertension (systolic PAP >60 mmHg) or exercise-induced rise in mean mitral gradient to greater than 15 mmHg benefit from early MV intervention.

Acknowledgments

We thank Kathleen Stergiopoulos, MD, PhD, and Fabio Lima, MPH, for their contributions to the previous edition of this chapter.

REFERENCES

1. Nishimura RA, Otto CM, Bonow RO, et al. 2014 AHA/ACC guideline for the management of patients with valvular heart disease: a report of the American College of Cardiology/American heart Association Task Force on Practice guidelines. *J Thoracic Cardiovasc Surg.* 2014;148:e1–e132.
2. Baumgartner H, Falk V, Bax JJ, et al. 2017 ESC/EACTS Guidelines for the management of valvular heart disease. *Eur Heart J.* 2017;38:2739–2791.
3. Doherty JU, Kort S, Mehran R, et al. ACC/AATS/AHA/ ASE/ASNC/HRS/SCAI/SCCT/SCMR/STS 2017 Appropriate use criteria for multimodality imaging in valvular heart disease : a report of the American College of Cardiology Appropriate Use Criteria Task Force. *American Association for Thoracic Surgery, American Heart Association, American Society of Echocardiography, American Society of Nuclear Cardiology.* Heart Rhythm Society, Society for Cardiovascular Angiography and Interventions, Society of Cardiovascular Computed Tomography, Society for Cardiovascular Magnetic Resonance, and Society of Thoracic Surgeons, *J Nucl Cardiol.* 2017;24:2043–2063.
4. Henri C, Pierard LA, Lancellotti P, et al. Exercise testing and stress imaging in valvular heart disease. *Can J Cardiol.* 2014;30:1012–1026.
5. Lancellotti P, Dulgheru R, Go YY, et al. Stress echocardiography in patients with native valvular heart disease. *Heart.* 2018;104:807–813.
6. Reis G, Motta MS, Barbosa MM, et al. Dobutamine stress echocardiography for noninvasive assessment and risk stratification of patients with rheumatic mitral stenosis. *J Am Coll Cardiol.* 2004;43:393–401.

---

94 Consequences of Mitral Stenosis

Wendy Tsang, Roberto M. Lang

Mitral stenosis (MS) results from obstruction of blood flow from the left atrium into the left ventricle at either the valve or the subvalvular level (Fig. 94.1 and Videos 94.1 to 94.4). Complications from MS include pulmonary edema, pulmonary hypertension (PH), right heart failure, atrial arrhythmias, and low cardiac output (Fig. 94.2). In addition to these complications, this chapter also discusses the need to assess the involvement of other valves in patients with rheumatic heart disease and the impact of MS during pregnancy.

PULMONARY EDEMA

Symptoms of MS typically begin when the normal mitral valve (MV) area (4.0–5.0 cm^2) is reduced to less than 2.5 cm^2. When the valve area reaches less than 1.5 cm^2, patients can develop symptoms at rest (see Fig. 94.2).[1,2] However, symptoms may occur in valves with larger areas when patients exercise or experience emotional stress, infection, pregnancy, or atrial fibrillation (AF). Under these circumstances, there is an increase in transmitral flow or a decrease in the diastolic filling period, which results in a rise in left atrial (LA) pressure and the development of dyspnea and eventually pulmonary edema. This pathway also explains why patients' exercise tolerance decreases as MS progresses.

The mechanism for dyspnea in patients with MS results from a decrease in blood flow from the left atrium into the left ventricle during diastole (Figure 94.3 A, B). To compensate, there is an increase in LA pressures to drive blood forward into the left ventricle. This augmentation in LA pressures also results in increased pulmonary venous pressure and distention of the pulmonary veins and capillaries. When the pulmonary venous pressure exceeds the plasma oncotic pressure, pulmonary edema results. However, in patients with chronic MS, pulmonary edema may not occur even when the stenosis is severe and pulmonary venous pressures are very high. This is because there may be an associated decrease in pulmonary microvascular permeability.[2]

In patients in whom symptoms do not correlate with measured valve parameters, there is a role for exercise stress testing. If stress echocardiography is used, the development of B lines indicating the development of pulmonary edema after stress may be of diagnostic value and corroborate with echocardiographic parameters and clinical findings. Additionally, significant increases to pulmonary pressures and diastolic MV gradients would be supportive of symptomatic disease with exertion.

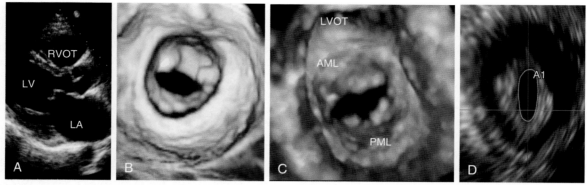

Figure 94.1. A, Transthoracic two-dimensional echocardiographic image of a stenotic mitral valve (MV) with the "hockey stick" appearance of the anterior mitral leaflet during diastole. **B,** Transesophageal three-dimensional echocardiographic image of a stenotic MV visualized from the left atrial perspective and **C,** the left ventricular perspective. Note the thickened leaflet tips. **D,** Measurement of the MV area from a three-dimensional echocardiographic dataset with the planes placed at the smallest orifice. *AML,* Anterior mitral valve leaflet; *LA,* left atrium; *LAA,* left atrial appendage; *LV,* left ventricle; *PML,* posterior mitral valve leaflet; *RVOT,* right ventricular outflow tract.

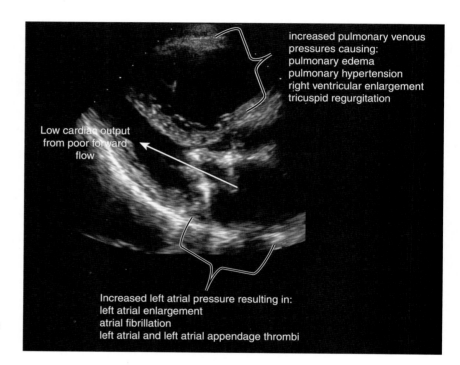

Figure 94.2. Schematic summarizing the effects of mitral stenosis on cardiac hemodynamics, function, and structure.

increased pulmonary venous pressures causing:
pulmonary edema
pulmonary hypertension
right ventricular enlargement
tricuspid regurgitation

Low cardiac output from poor forward flow

Increased left atrial pressure resulting in:
left atrial enlargement
atrial fibrillation
left atrial and left atrial appendage thrombi

PULMONARY HYPERTENSION

In addition to pulmonary edema, patients with MS may develop PH. The degree of pulmonary vascular disease is an important determinant of PH in patients with MS. Initially, PH associated with MS is known as passive or obligatory when it is caused by the elevated LA pressures needed to drive blood across the stenotic MV. There are no abnormalities in the pulmonary arterial bed at this stage. Moderate PH occurs when the right ventricle needs to generate high systolic pressure to ensure adequate cardiac output. When this occurs, elevated pulmonary capillary wedge pressure (PCWP) and mean pulmonary arterial pressure with minimal elevation in transpulmonary gradient (<12 mm Hg) and normal pulmonary vascular resistance are found on right heart catheterization.

Chronically elevated PCWP results in functional and structural abnormalities in the pulmonary vascular bed, leading to the development of pulmonary vascular disease and eventually severe PH. This form of PH is known as reactive PH. Initially this begins

with increased capillary endothelial basement membrane thickness due to excessive deposition of type IV collagen.[3] This increase in interstitial connective tissue as well as increased production of extracellular matrix components increases extravascular fluid storage capacity as an adaptive reaction to protect the lungs from pulmonary edema. In conjunction with the elevated venous pressure, disruption of the endothelium leads to activation of vascular serine elastase and matrix metalloproteinases and growth factors that result in migration of smooth muscle and hypertrophy and fibrosis from elastin synthesis. The consequences of these changes are enlarged, thickened pulmonary veins; pulmonary capillary dilatation; capillary dilatation; alveolar hemorrhage; and lymphatic vessel and lymph node enlargement.[4] However, plexiform lesions are not present in these patients. It must be noted that not all these changes are seen in patients with elevated pulmonary venous pressures, and there may be a genetic predisposition. In addition, reversible obstruction may develop at the level of the pulmonary veins.[5,6]

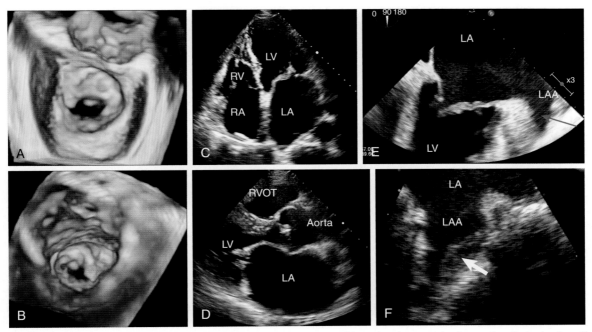

Figure 94.3. Complications of mitral stenosis. 3D transesophageal echocardiographic en face images of a rheumatic mitral valve from the left atrial (**A**) and left ventricular perspectives (**B**). On transthoracic imaging, enlargement of the left atrium can be seen in the apical 4-chamber view (**C**) and in the parasternal long-axis view (**D**). The dilated left atrium can result in atrial arrhythmias with "smoke" in the left atrial appendage (**E**) or thrombus (**F**). *LA,* Left atrium; *LV,* left ventricle; *RA,* right atrium; *RV,* right ventricle; *RVOT,* right ventricular outflow tract.

Patients with reactive PH have increased mean pulmonary arterial pressure, transpulmonary gradient, and pulmonary vascular resistance. As well, treatments to lower the PCWP may not normalize the pulmonary arterial pressure, as seen in passive PH.

RIGHT HEART FAILURE

Right heart failure occurs in MS from stress on the right ventricle to generate the forces necessary to drive blood across the stenotic MV. Initially, this stress results in right ventricular pressure overload. However, the development of PH from MS-related pulmonary vasoconstriction and LA hypertension compounds the stress and leads to the development of right heart failure. Right heart failure is associated with right ventricular dilatation and tricuspid regurgitation (TR), which is discussed later. Right heart failure also results in elevated jugular venous pressure, liver congestion, and peripheral edema. Note that left ventricular (LV) function can be normal in isolated MS.

ATRIAL ARRHYTHMIAS

In response to increased LA pressure, the left atrium adversely remodels and enlarges (Fig. 94.3 C and D). Patients with MS and LA enlargement may develop atrial arrhythmias such as flutter or fibrillation. In addition, and particularly with rheumatic MS, fibrosis of the internodal and interatrial tracts as well as damage to the sinoatrial node may occur.

In patients with symptomatic MS, 30% to 40% will develop AF, which is associated with a poor prognosis.[1] Those with AF have a 10-year survival rate of 25% compared with 46% in those who remain in sinus rhythm.[7] One important predictor for the development of atrial fibrillation is older age.[1,8] In addition to prognosis, the development of AF may have significant consequences for patients' hemodynamic stability and their risk of systemic embolic events. In acute AF with a rapid ventricular rate, patients may become hemodynamically unstable. This is because the rapid ventricular rate will result in a short diastolic filling period, reducing cardiac output and elevating LA pressure, resulting in pulmonary edema. Treatment of AF includes anticoagulation with warfarin and control of the heart rate response through pharmacologic or direct current cardioversion. Currently, the use of direct oral anticoagulants is not recommended in patients with AF in the setting of rheumatic MS.

ATRIAL THROMBUS

MS is associated with LA thrombus in up to 17% of patients, and this risk doubles when AF is present.[9] The majority of thrombi are located in the LA appendage, but in 2%, the thrombus extends into the LA cavity (Fig. 94.3F and Video 94.5).[10] Note that thrombus may be present in the LA cavity without involvement of the LA appendage.

Previous studies have demonstrated that LA clots and systemic thromboembolization are associated with spontaneous echo contrast in the left atrium on transesophageal echocardiography, and the incidence of spontaneous echo contrast in MS varies from 21% to 67%.[11] In addition to the presence of clot in the left atrium, spontaneous echo contrast has also been found to be an important independent factor for predicting systemic embolization in patients with rheumatic heart disease.[11]

Patients with MS and atrial thrombi have a higher chance of experiencing systemic embolization. Risk factors for this complication include increasing age and the presence of AF.[12] It must be noted that factors such as MS severity, cardiac output, size of the left atrium, and the presence of symptoms of heart failure do not affect the rate of embolic events (see Fig. 94.2).[1,13,14] For those who develop AF, studies have reported that one-third of embolic events occur within 1 month of the onset of AF and two-thirds within 1 year. For patients who have experienced an embolic event, the frequency of a recurrent event is as high as 15 to 40 events per 100 patient-months.[15]

Although no specific randomized trial has been conducted on the efficacy of anticoagulation in patients with MS, retrospective studies have demonstrated a 4- to 15-fold decrease in the incidence of systemic and pulmonic embolic events with anticoagulation in

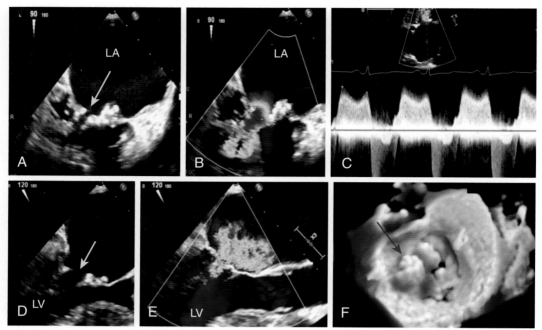

Figure 94.4. Transesophageal echocardiographic images demonstrating a rheumatic valve with significant calcification restriction motion during diastole (**A** and **B**) and systole (**C** and **D**), resulting in significant stenosis, as seen on this Doppler tracing (**E**), and regurgitation. Transesophageal three-dimensional echocardiographic image with photorealistic rendering demonstrating the calcium on the leaflets as viewed from the left atrial perspective. *LA,* Left atrium; *LV,* left ventricle.

these patients.[13] Randomized trials for anticoagulation in AF have demonstrated that those who benefit the most are patients who have had prior embolic events and those with paroxysmal or persistent AF.[1,8] It must be emphasized that although embolic events are believed to be caused by thrombi in the left atrium, studies have not found such a correlation. The frequency of LA thrombus in patients with MS is similar between those who have experienced an embolic event and those who have not.[8,12] Nonetheless, anticoagulation should be used if LA thrombus is identified. Conversely, patients with MS who do not have AF or an embolic event should not receive anticoagulation because there are no data to support such practice.[16] As mentioned previously, the use of direct oral anticoagulants in these patients is not recommended.

Finally, it has been suggested that percutaneous mitral valvotomy be performed in patients with new-onset AF with moderate to severe MS. However, this approach may not resolve the AF because age and LA size are stronger predictors of the development of AF.[16] Also, others advocate that surgical commissurotomy be performed to reduce the incidence of future embolic events.[17] Overall, the literature is inconclusive about this approach. No randomized trials have been performed to address this issue, and retrospective and prospective trials have resulted in conflicting conclusions.[17–19]

LOW CARDIAC OUTPUT

As MS progresses, there is a reduction in cardiac output caused by poor LV filling (Fig. 94.4). Frequently, this is secondary to increased pulmonary vascular resistance. It is believed that LV contractility is normal in most cases of MS; however, some believe that there is LV contractile damage from the rheumatic fever.[20] The development of any rapid arrhythmia that reduces ventricular filling times may cause a further deterioration in cardiac output, thereby resulting in hemodynamic instability. Under such conditions, electrical cardioversion should be considered. If the patient is stable, medications that slow conduction of the atrioventricular node should be considered.

OTHER VALVE INVOLVEMENT

In patients with MS secondary to rheumatic heart disease, the other cardiac valves should be evaluated for involvement. Specifically, the aortic and tricuspid valves should be examined (see Fig. 94.3). Although the aortic valve is more commonly affected, involvement of the tricuspid valve is not rare. When the aortic valve is involved, aortic stenosis (AS) typically results. In patients with MS and AS, careful evaluation of the severity of the AS is warranted. Stenosis severity may be underestimated under these circumstances because of decreased stroke volume from the MS, resulting in low transaortic gradients.[21] Ideally, the aortic valve area should be quantified using planimetry. When the tricuspid valve is affected, either stenosis or regurgitation may result. The treatment of choice for patients with tricuspid stenosis is balloon or surgical commissurotomy over replacement if possible.

In addition to rheumatic tricuspid valve disease, TR may be secondary to RV failure secondary to PH. Quantification of the severity of TR should be performed with attention to the patient's hemodynamic status, which may affect the evaluation. Last, with MS from degenerative calcific disease, the aortic valve may be involved in addition to the MV

PREGNANCY

MS in pregnancy is associated with significant morbidity, even in patients with mild to moderate disease. For those with mild, moderate, or severe disease, complication rates are 26%, 38%, and 67%, respectively.[22] Those with New York Heart Association (NYHA) class I/II symptoms at baseline can worsen during pregnancy, and the development of complications is strongly correlated with NYHA class.[22] During pregnancy, symptoms of MS and the transvalvular gradient may increase because of increased intravascular volume, increased cardiac output, and tachycardia associated with pregnancy. The timing of symptoms is related to the physiologic changes that occur during different stages of pregnancy and delivery. One group presents before 28 weeks' gestation. This is

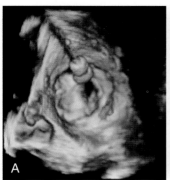
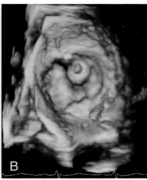
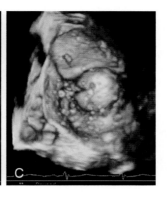

Figure 94.5. Transesophageal three-dimensional echocardiographic images of balloon placement (**A** and **B**) and inflation (**C**) during percutaneous mitral valvotomy.

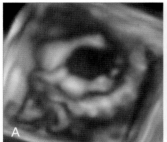
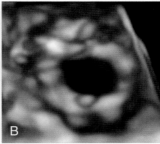
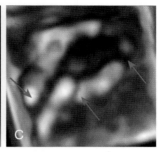

Figure 94.6. Transesophageal three-dimensional echocardiographic image of a rheumatic mitral valve from the left atrial perspective before balloon valvuloplasty (**A**), after the first inflation (**B**) with no significant leaflet tears, and after a second inflation (**C**) when there are significant tears at the commissure and leaflet edge *(red arrows)*. (Reproduced with permission from Mahía P, et al: Valvuloplastia mitral percutánea guiada por ecocardiografía tridimensional [Percutaneous mitral valvuloplasty guided by three-dimensional echocardiography]. *Rev Esp Cardiol* 2003;56:1016.)

because early in pregnancy, there is a decrease in systemic vascular resistance caused by progesterone-induced peripheral vasodilation. Cardiac compensation occurs through an increase in cardiac output from 20% at 8 weeks' gestation to a "maximum predelivery" increase of 40% to 50% at 20 to 28 weeks' gestation. This increase in cardiac output results from an associated increase in stroke volume and heart rate. Thus, women with MS who are unable to increase their cardiac output may decompensate early in pregnancy.

Women who tolerate this increase in stroke volume during pregnancy may still develop problems during delivery and in the immediate postpartum period. During labor, there is a need to further increase cardiac output by 15% during the first stage and 50% during the second stage because of autotransfusion of blood back into the circulation with each uterine contraction and sympathetic stimulation from pain. Immediately after delivery, there is a further 60% to 80% increase in cardiac output caused by autotransfusion from uterine contraction and relief of aortocaval compression. Cardiac output normalizes to prelabor values within 1 hour of delivery. This need to increase cardiac output is worsened by an increase in preload resulting from the administration of excessive intravenous fluids or increase in pulmonary capillary permeability from preeclampsia. Overall, maternal mortality is between 0% to 3% in western countries. For maternal morbidity one-half of mothers with a valve area less than or equal to 1.5 cm² will experience heart failure, even in the absence of symptoms before pregnancy.[23] These women also experience fetal death rates of 1% to 5%, premature birth rates of 20% to 30%, and fetal intrauterine growth retardation of 5% to 20%.[22] The risk of these adverse fetal outcomes is higher in women with NYHA III or IV symptoms during pregnancy. Given these risks, follow-up during pregnancy should be through a specialized multidisciplinary team with cardiologist and obstetricians. Even patients with mild MS should be evaluated every trimester before delivery.[23] Management

includes diuresis, heart rate control with β-blockers, and, if necessary, percutaneous mitral valvuloplasty. Mitral valvuloplasty can be performed during pregnancy with excellent clinical and hemodynamic results and few to no complications to both the mother and fetus.[23] Anticoagulation should be used in women with paroxysmal or permanent AF, LA thrombus or previous embolism and should be considered in women in sinus rhythm with significant stenosis and spontaneous LA echocardiographic contrast, a left atrium larger than or equal to 60 mL/m², or congestive heart failure.[23]

COMPLICATIONS FROM PERCUTANEOUS MITRAL VALVOTOMY

Typically, the immediate results of percutaneous mitral valvotomy are similar to those of mitral commissurotomy, with a doubling of mitral valve area and a 50% to 60% reduction in transmitral gradient.[16] Because there is a steep learning curve with this procedure, centers with high volumes have high success rates and low complication rates. Success is defined as achieving a MV area greater than 1.5 cm² and a LA pressure of less than 18 mmHg in the absence of complications. The most commonly reported complications are acute severe mitral regurgitation, which occurs in 2% to 10% of patients, and residual atrial septal defect. The use of three-dimensional echocardiography has improved not only the evaluation of patients for percutaneous mitral valvotomy but also procedural performance and postprocedural monitoring (Figs. 94.5 and 94.6; Video 94.6).[24]

VALVE REPAIR SURGERY

There is a growing body of literature and experience with MV repair in patients with rheumatic MV disease. This is in part due to the recognition that there are differences between patients with rheumatic MV disease who undergo surgery in developed countries compared with less developed nations.[25] Patients with rheumatic valve disease undergoing surgery in developed countries tend to be older with quiescent rheumatic disease, whereas those in developing countries tend to be younger with active, progressive, or recurrent rheumatic disease. Because of the active nature of their disease, those in developing countries tend to require reoperation. Despite these differences, it is thought that both groups of patients would benefit from valve repair. However, the literature supporting this is mixed with some studies demonstrating no difference in outcomes between valve repair and replacement but others suggesting better outcomes with valve repair.[26,27]

SUMMARY

Because of lack of forward blood flow, MS results in low cardiac output, as well as increased LA size, atrial arrhythmias, and systemic embolic events. In addition, pulmonary edema and PH may develop, leading to right ventricular enlargement or failure and TR. If the MS is secondary to rheumatic heart disease, other valves such as the aortic and tricuspid should also be evaluated. Similarly, degenerative calcific disease can affect the aortic as well as the MV. However, quantitation of severity of valvular involvement should be performed carefully because of the effects of the patient's hemodynamic status and poor stroke volume from MS.

Please access ExpertConsult to view the corresponding videos for this chapter.

REFERENCES

1. Rowe JC, Bland EF, Sprague HB, White PD. The course of mitral stenosis without surgery: ten- and twenty-year perspectives. *Ann Intern Med*. 1960;52:741–749.
2. Hugenholtz PG, Ryan TJ, Stein SW, Abelmann WH. The spectrum of pure mitral stenosis. Hemodynamic studies in relation to clinical disability. *Am J Cardiol*. 1962;10:773–784.
3. Kay JM, Edwards FR. Ultrastructure of the alveolar-capillary wall in mitral stenosis. *J Pathol*. 1973;111:239–245.
4. Adir Y, Amir O. Pulmonary hypertension associated with left heart disease. *Semin Respir Crit Care Med*. 2013;34:665–680.
5. Halperin JL, Brooks KM, Rothlauf EB, et al. Effect of nitroglycerin on the pulmonary venous gradient in patients after mitral valve replacement. *J Am Coll Cardiol*. 1985;5:34–39.
6. Halperin JL, Rothlauf EB, Brooks KM, et al. Effect of nitroglycerin during hemodynamic estimation of valve orifice in patients with mitral stenosis. *J Am Coll Cardiol*. 1987;10:342–348.
7. Olesen KH. The natural history of 271 patients with mitral stenosis under medical treatment. *Br Heart J*. 1962;24:349–357.
8. Wood P. An appreciation of mitral stenosis. I: clinical features. *Br Med J*. 1954;1:1051–1063.
9. Shrestha NK, Moreno FL, Narciso FV, et al. Two-dimensional echocardiographic diagnosis of left-atrial thrombus in rheumatic heart disease. A clinicopathologic study. *Circulation*. 1983;67:341–347.
10. Rost C, Daniel WG, Schmid M. Giant left atrial thrombus in moderate mitral stenosis. *Eur J Echocardiogr*. 2009;10:358–359.
11. Goswami KC, Yadav R, Rao MB, et al. Clinical and echocardiographic predictors of left atrial clot and spontaneous echo contrast in patients with severe rheumatic mitral stenosis. *Int J Cardiol*. 2000;73:273–279.
12. Coulshed N, Epstein EJ, McKendrick CS, et al. Systemic embolism in mitral valve disease. *Br Heart J*. 1970;32:26–34.
13. Abernathy WS, Willis 3rd PW. Thromboembolic complications of rheumatic heart disease. *Cardiovasc Clin*. 1973;5:131–175.
14. Stroke prevention in atrial fibrillation study: Final results. *Circulation*. 1991;84:527–539.
15. Adams GF, Merrett JD, Hutchinson WM, Pollock AM. Cerebral embolism and mitral stenosis: survival with and without anticoagulants. *J Neurol Neurosurg Psychiatry*. 1974;37:378–383.
16. Bonow RO, Carabello BA, Chatterjee K, et al. Focused update incorporated into the ACC/AHA 2006 guidelines for the management of patients with valvular heart disease. *J Am Coll Cardiol*. 2008;52:e1–e142. 2008.
17. Munoz S, Gallardo J, Diaz-Gorrin JR, Medina O. Influence of surgery on the natural history of rheumatic mitral and aortic valve disease. *Am J Cardiol*. 1975;35:234–242.
18. Chiang CW, Lo SK, Ko YS, et al. Predictors of systemic embolism in patients with mitral stenosis. A prospective study. *Ann Intern Med*. 1998;128:885–889.
19. Deverall PB, Olley PM, Smith DR, et al. Incidence of systemic embolism before and after mitral valvotomy. *Thorax*. 1968;23:530–536.
20. Carabello BA. Modern management of mitral stenosis. *Circulation*. 2005;112:432–437.
21. Unger P, Lancellotti P, de Cannière D. The clinical challenge of concomitant aortic and mitral valve stenosis. *Acta Cardiol*. 2016;71:3–6.
22. Chandrashekhar Y, Westaby S, Narula J. Mitral stenosis. *Lancet*. 2009;374:1271–1283.
23. Regitz-Zagrosek V, Roos-Hesselink JW, Bauersachs J, et al. ESC guidelines for the management of cardiovascular diseases during pregnancy. *Eur Heart J 7*. 2018;39(34):3165–3241. 2018.
24. Gupta A, Lokhandwala YY, Satoskar PR, Salvi VS. Balloon mitral valvotomy in pregnancy: maternal and fetal outcomes. *J Am Coll Surg*. 1998;187:409–415.
25. Antunes MJ. Repair for rheumatic mitral valve disease. *The controversy goes on! Heart*. 2018;104:796–797. https://doi.org/10.1136/heartjnl-2017-312674.
26. Yakub MA, Dillon J, Krishna Moorthy PS, et al. Is rheumatic aetiology a predictor of poor outcome in the current era of mitral valve repair? Contemporary long-term results of mitral valve repair in rheumatic heart disease. *Eur J Cardio Thorac Surg*. 2013;44:673–681.
27. Dillon J, Yakub MA, Kong PK, et al. Comparative long-term results of mitral valve repair in adults with chronic rheumatic disease and degenerative disease: is repair for "burnt-out" rheumatic disease still inferior to repair for degenerative disease in the current era? *J Thorac Cardiovasc Surg*. 2015;149:771–779.

95 | Etiologies and Mechanisms of Mitral Valve Dysfunction

Benjamin H. Freed, Wendy Tsang, Roberto M. Lang

Mitral valve (MV) disease may best be described by defining the *cause* of the disease, the *specific lesions* caused by the disease, and the *dysfunction* it creates in the MV apparatus. This "pathophysiologic triad," first described by Carpentier and coworkers in the early 1980s, is still useful today in characterizing different types of MV disorders.[1]

CAUSES OF MITRAL VALVE DISEASE

MV disease is caused by either primary (direct) abnormalities of the MV apparatus or secondary (indirect) causes due to cardiac disease not involving the valve. Examples of diseases that directly affect the MV include congenital malformations such as valve clefts, rheumatic disease, infective endocarditis, trauma, MV annular calcification, valvular tumors, and degenerative diseases. Cardiac diseases that indirectly affect the MV include ischemic and nonischemic dilated cardiomyopathy, hypertrophic cardiomyopathy, and myocardial infiltrative diseases.

Rheumatic MV disease is uncommon in developed countries but continues to be a significant cause of MV disease worldwide. Rheumatic heart disease accounts for about a quarter of all patients with heart failure in endemic countries.[2] Chronic valve disease occurs after one or more episodes of acute rheumatic fever and tends to affect females more than males. Although the MV is involved in almost every case, the aortic and tricuspid valves can also be affected. Younger patients tend to develop pure mitral regurgitation (MR), middle-aged patients more frequently develop mitral stenosis, and older patients usually develop a combination of stenosis and regurgitation.[3]

Degenerative MR, usually associated with mitral valve prolapse (MVP), is the most common cause of MR in developed countries.[4] MVP is an abnormal systolic valve motion of the mitral leaflet into the left atrium (≥2 mm beyond the annulus). Three-dimensional echocardiography (3DE) technology has considerably improved the ability of physicians to both diagnose and treat MVP,[5] which results primarily from two distinctive types of degenerative diseases: Barlow disease and fibroelastic deficiency.

Ischemic MR is the pathophysiologic outcome of ventricular remodeling arising from ischemic heart disease and is also a very common cause of MR in developed countries. Ischemic MR occurs in approximately 20% to 25% of patients with myocardial infarction even in the era of reperfusion, and these patients have significantly worse outcomes irrespective of the degree or MR.[6] The resultant volume overload caused by MR worsens myocardial contractility, which in turn worsens ventricular dysfunction, eventually leading to heart failure and death.[7–10]

MITRAL VALVE LESIONS

No matter the cause of the MV disease, each disease process frequently results in one or more lesions. For example, dilated cardiomyopathy can result in mitral annular dilatation in what is commonly referred to as functional MR. Degenerative diseases such as Barlow disease and fibroelastic deficiency result in multiple types of lesions, including excess myxomatous leaflet tissue and chordal elongation, thinning, and rupture. Rheumatic heart disease results in commissural fusion, leaflet thickening, and chordal fusion, whereas myocardial infarction can lead to lesions such as papillary muscle displacement, leaflet tethering, and mitral annulus dilatation.[11]

Barlow disease results from an excess of myxomatous tissue, which is an abnormal accumulation of mucopolysaccharides in one or both of the leaflets and many or only few of the chordae.[12] This myxoid infiltration results in thick, bulky, redundant billowing leaflets and elongated chordae, which often lead to bileaflet, multisegmental prolapse. Barlow disease is usually diagnosed in young adulthood, and patients are typically followed for many decades with well-preserved left ventricular (LV) size until indications for surgery are met in the fourth or fifth decade of life.

In contrast, fibroelastic deficiency results from acute loss of mechanical integrity caused by abnormalities of connective tissue structure or function (or both).[12] It usually results in a localized or unisegmental prolapse caused by elongated chordae or flail leaflet caused by ruptured chordae. Patients most commonly present in the sixth decade of life with a relatively short history of MR. This entity is the most common form of organic MV disease for which MV repair surgery is required.

Recent work with 3DE shows that mitral annular disjunction—the decoupling of the atrial wall-MV junction and LV attachment—might contribute to the blunted annular dynamics observed in degenerative MV disease.[13] Patients with MVP and mitral annular disjunction have a larger regurgitant orifice and more severe regurgitation caused by paradoxical systolic expansion and flattening of the annulus.

There is considerable overlap between Barlow disease and fibroelastic deficiency, and it is difficult to reliably distinguish them based on either the gross or histologic appearance of the valve. One way to differentiate these two entities is by leaflet distensibility. Patients with Barlow disease have increased mitral tissue distensibility during mid to late systole, whereas patients with fibroelastic deficiency have little tissue reserve.[14] This might explain how patients with Barlow disease have a similar degree of regurgitation despite a greater degree of prolapse. Some valves may represent a forme fruste of Barlow disease and demonstrate myxoid infiltration on subsequent histologic examination (Fig. 95.1).[15]

Classically, ischemic MR was thought to develop because of posteromedial papillary muscle dysfunction given this muscle's dependence on a single blood supply. Multiple 3DE studies have shown that papillary muscle dysfunction is, in fact, not responsible for ischemic MR. In fact, there is a wide spectrum of geometric distortions secondary to LV remodeling that result in this type of

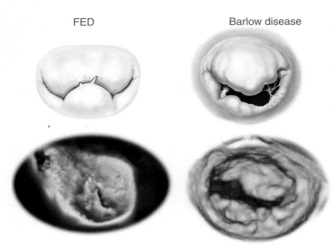

FED   Barlow disease

Figure 95.1. Three-dimensional echocardiography images and corresponding illustrations showing examples of degenerative mitral valve disease, from fibroelastic deficiency (FED) with P2 flail *(left)* to Barlow disease with multisegmental prolapse *(right)*.

valve dysfunction. The observations provided by 3DE have helped reshape our understanding of ischemic MR.

The MV is dynamic and changes from a saddle shape (hyperbolic paraboloid) during systole to a flatter configuration during diastole. During systole, competing forces act on the MV leaflets. Increased LV pressure acts to push the leaflets toward the left atrium while tethering forces from the chordae act to pull the leaflets in the direction of the left ventricle. The saddle-shape morphology is believed to balance these forces by optimizing leaflet curvature and thus minimizing mitral leaflet stress.[16] In the setting of a myocardial infarction and resultant LV remodeling, an outward and apical displacement of the posteromedial papillary muscle occurs, which tethers the MV leaflets into the left ventricle, restricting their ability to coapt effectively at the level of the mitral annulus.[17]

This mitral leaflet tethering is a major contributing factor to the development of ischemic MR. Two-dimensional echocardiography has been extensively used to calculate the MV tenting area and tenting length; however, studies have shown that the asymmetry of these single-plane measurements is commonly inaccurate compared with intraoperative findings.[18] 3DE overcomes this limitation by providing more accurate and reproducible measurements.

In one of the first studies to examine leaflet tethering with 3DE, patients with severe MR were shown to have significantly larger tethering lengths and tenting volumes than control patients.[19] Furthermore, this study found that the leaflet site where peak-tenting occurred was different in each individual. This suggests that different chordae are involved in the disease process.

More recent 3DE studies confirm previous findings and provide further detail on pathologic changes that occur with ischemic MR. In 66 patients with ischemic MR undergoing MV surgery, 3DE identified specific regional MV changes, including lengthening of the middle portion of the anterior annulus, a larger nonplanarity angle, and increased tenting angle of the posteromedial scallop of the posterior leaflet compared with control participants.[20] 3DE also provides insight into the impact of asymmetric vs symmetric tethering patterns on degree of MR. Patients with asymmetric tethering develop less annular dilatation, greater annular height, and smaller tenting volume with more posterior displacement of the coaptation line compared with patients with symmetric tethering.[21] Despite less overall tethering, an asymmetric pattern results in greater MR.

Conformational changes of the MV annulus also contribute to the development of ischemic MR. Multiple studies have shown that the annulus dilates and flattens, becoming essentially adynamic throughout the cardiac cycle.[17,19] In addition, 3DE imaging has revealed more subtle anatomic changes such as greater dilatation in the anteroposterior dimension and greater overall dilatation and flattening in anterior compared with inferior infarcts.[18,22] This is in contrast to degenerative MV disease in which the mitral annulus dilates in all directions and retains its dynamics during the cardiac cycle.[5,14,23] The annular-ventricular disjunction discussed earlier is thought to contribute greatly to the significant regurgitation in these patients.

One of the most intriguing findings by 3D echocardiography is that whereas leaflet tethering and annular geometric changes drive the development of ischemic MR, leaflet growth occurs in an attempt to compensate for the decrease in leaflet coaptation.[24] In one of the earliest studies to examine this phenomenon, Chaput and colleagues found that leaflet area increased by 35% in patients with LV dysfunction.[25] Studies using molecular histopathology showed that this leaflet growth might be caused by an increase in α-smooth muscle actin in tethered leaflets indicating endothelial–mesenchymal transdifferentiation.

In a recent 3DE study examining patients with both mild and severe ischemic MR, all patients showed a loss of mitral annular motility and nonplanarity, but only patients with severe regurgitation showed annular dilatation and a significant reduction in active posterior leaflet area in early systole.[26] Furthermore, the compensatory augmentation of active anterior leaflet area in patients with severe MR was delayed into late systole. The authors speculate that this spatial-temporal alteration likely contributes to the severity of regurgitation and underscores the importance of treatment targeting leaflet growth.

The adaptive changes in leaflet size likely explain the differences between acute and chronic ischemic MR as well. Although the degree of tethering and annular dilatation is less in patients with acute versus chronic MR, the failure to appropriately augment leaflet size contributes greatly to the significant degree of regurgitation witnessed in these patients.[27]

MITRAL VALVE DYSFUNCTION

All of these lesions lead to MV dysfunction. Instead of classifying this dysfunction as simply MV stenosis or regurgitation, Carpentier developed a classification scheme to aid in the surgical strategy based on the type of leaflet motion (Fig. 95.2).[28] Patients with mitral annular dilatation, clefts (Fig. 95.3), or leaflet perforation usually have normal leaflet motion and are categorized as type I dysfunction (Fig. 95.4). Type II dysfunction includes patients with prolapse and flail (excessive motion of the leaflet margin above the plane of the annulus) caused by excessive and redundant leaflet tissue or chordal rupture, respectively (see Fig. 95.4). Leaflet restriction during valve closure caused by fusion of various components of the MV apparatus is defined as type IIIa dysfunction (Fig. 95.5), whereas leaflet restriction during valve opening resulting from leaflet tethering is defined as type IIIb dysfunction (Fig. 95.6).

It is important to emphasize that the different components of the pathophysiologic triad are not mutually exclusive and can be clinically combined in different ways. For example, the typical lesions seen in type IIIa dysfunction can also occur in conjunction with the lesions of type II dysfunction. Type IIIb dysfunction is the result of ventricular remodeling, with the primary lesion being leaflet tethering caused by papillary muscle displacement as occurs in ischemic MR. Associated annular dilatation is a common finding in patients with chronic degenerative MR, but the classification of dysfunction should differentiate the primary lesion causing the regurgitation (i.e., chordal rupture) from secondary lesions (i.e., annular dilatation).

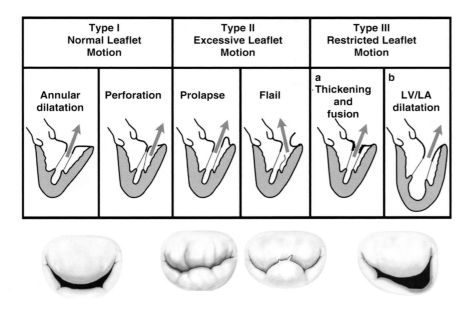

Type I Normal Leaflet Motion		Type II Excessive Leaflet Motion		Type III Restricted Leaflet Motion	
Annular dilatation	Perforation	Prolapse	Flail	a Thickening and fusion	b LV/LA dilatation

Figure 95.2. Carpentier classification of mitral valve dysfunction based on leaflet motion. *LA,* Left atrium; *LV,* left ventricle.

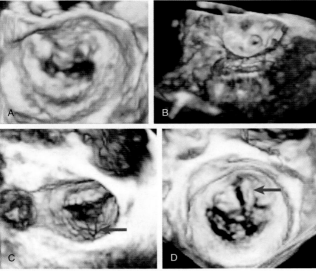

Figure 95.3. Type I dysfunction. Three-dimensional echocardiography (3DE) images show that although the leaflet motion is normal, the annulus is clearly stretched and dilated (**A**). Leaflet perforation is considered type I dysfunction. 3DE shows the perforation as a large crater-like structure in the posterior leaflet (**B**). 3DE is especially useful in identifying clefts *(blue arrows)* usually between leaflet scallops in both the posterior (**C**) and anterior (**D**) leaflets. (See accompanying Video 95.3.)

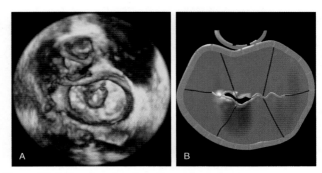

Figure 95.4. Type II dysfunction. Three-dimensional echocardiography image of the mitral valve demonstrating P2 flail of the posterior leaflet (**A**) and its corresponding parametric map (**B**). P2 flail with multiple ruptured chords. (See accompanying Video 95.4.)

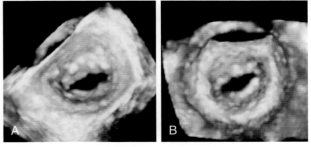

Figure 95.5. Type IIIA dysfunction. Three-dimensional echocardiography of the mitral valve as visualized from the left atrium (**A**) and left ventricle (**B**) reveals thickened leaflets with fused commissures consistent with rheumatic valve disease.

MR is a very common disease that can lead to substantial morbidity and mortality. Understanding the multiple underlying causes of this disease and their respective mechanisms of valvular disturbance is crucial to choosing the appropriate treatment.

Please access ExpertConsult to view the corresponding videos for this chapter.

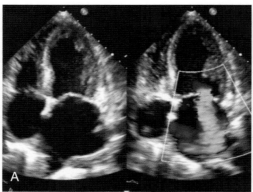
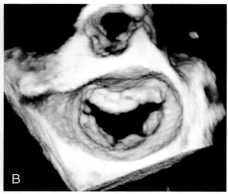

Figure 95.6. Type IIIB dysfunction. Two-dimensional echocardiography with Doppler revealing severe mitral regurgitation due to ischemic mitral valve disease (**A**). Corresponding three-dimensional echocardiography image of the mitral valve from the left atrial view depicting tethering and a dilated annulus that is flat (has lost its saddle shape) (**B**). (See accompanying Video 95.6.)

REFERENCES

1. Carpentier A, Adams DH, Filsoufi F. Pathophysiology, preoperative valve analysis, and surgical indications. In: carpentier A, Adams DH, Filsoufi F, eds. *Reconstructive Valve Surgery: From Valve Analysis to Valve Reconstruction.* Maryland Heights, MD: Saunders; 2010:43–53.
2. Ntusi NB, Mayosi BM. Epidemiology of heart failure in Sub-Saharan Africa. *Expert Rev Cardiovasc Ther.* 2009;7:169.
3. Bocchi EA, Guimaraes G, Tarasoutshi F, et al. Cardiomyopathy, adult valve disease and heart failure in South America. *Heart.* 2009;95:181.
4. Krishnaswamy A, Griffin BP. Myxomatous mitral valve disease. In: Otto CM, Bonow RO, eds. *Valvular Heart Disease.* Philadelphia: Saunders; 2014:278–294.
5. Antoine C, Mantovani F, Benfari G, et al. Pathophysiology of degenerative mitral regulation: new 3D imaging insights. *Circ Cardiovasc Imag.* 2018;11. e005971.
6. Foster E, Rao RK. Secondary mitral regurgitation. In: Otto CM, Bonow RO, eds. *Valvular Heart Disease.* Philadelphia: Saunders; 2014:295–297.
7. Lamas GA, Mitchell GF, Flaker GC, et al. Clinical significance of mitral regurgitation after acute myocardial infarction. *Circulation.* 1997;96:827–833.
8. Bursi F, Enriquez-Sarano M, Nkomo VT, et al. Heart failure and death after myocardial infarction in the community: the emerging role of mitral regurgitation. *Circulation.* 2005;111:295–301.
9. Grigioni F, Detaint D, Avierinos JF, et al. Contribution of ischemic mitral regurgitation to congestive heart failure after myocardial infarction. *J Am Coll Cardiol.* 2005;45:260–267.
10. Grigioni F, Enriquez-Sarano M, Zehr KJ, et al. Ischemic mitral regurgitation: long-term outcome and prognostic implications with quantitative Doppler assessment. *Circulation.* 2001;103:1759–1764.
11. Enriquez-Sarano M, Akins CW, Vahanian A. Mitral regurgitation. *Lancet.* 2009;373:1382–1394.
12. Anyanwu AC, Adams DH. Etiologic classification of degenerative mitral valve disease: Barlow's disease and fibroelastic deficiency. *Semin Thorac Cardiovasc Surg.* 2007;19:90–96.
13. Lee AP, Jin CN, Fan Y, et al. Functional implication of mitral annular disjunction in mitral valve prolapse: a quantitative dynamic 3D echocardiographic study. *JACC Cardiovasc Imag.* 2017;10:1424–1433.
14. Clavel MA, Mantovani F, Malouf J, et al. Dynamic phenotypes of degenerative myxomatous mitral valve disease: quantitative 3-dimensional echocardiographic study. *Circ Cardiovasc Imag.* 2015;8:5.
15. Adams DH, Anyanwu AC, Sugeng L, et al. Degenerative mitral valve regurgitation: surgical echocardiography. *Curr Cardiol Rep.* 2008;10:226–232.
16. Salgo IS, Gorman 3rd JH, Gorman RC, et al. Effect of annular shape on leaflet curvature in reducing mitral leaflet stress. *Circulation.* 2002;106:711–717.
17. Otsuji Y, Levine RA, Takeuchi M, et al. Mechanism of ischemic mitral regurgitation. *J Cardiol.* 2008;51:145–156.
18. Daimon M, Shiota T, Gillinov AM, et al. Percutaneous mitral valve repair for chronic ischemic mitral regurgitation: a real-time three-dimensional echocardiographic study in an ovine model. *Circulation.* 2005;111:2183–2189.
19. Watanabe N, Ogasawara Y, Yamaura Y, et al. Mitral annulus flattens in ischemic mitral regurgitation: geometric differences between inferior and anterior myocardial infarction: a real-time 3D echocardiographic study. *Circulation.* 2005;112(9 Suppl):I458–I462.
20. Mahmood F, Knio ZO, Yeh L, et al. Regional heterogeneity in the mitral valve apparatus in patients with ischemic mitral regurgitation. *Ann Thorac Surg.* 2017;103:1171–1177.
21. Zeng X, Nunes MC, Dent J, et al. Asymmetric versus symmetric tethering patterns in ischemic mitral regurgitation: geometric differences from three-dimensional transesophageal echocardiography. *J Am Soc Echocardiogr.* 2014;27:367–375.
22. Vergnat M, Jassar AS, Jackson BM, et al. Ischemic mitral regurgitation: a quantitative three-dimensional echocardiographic analysis. *Ann Thorac Surg.* 2011;91:157–164.
23. Grewal J, Suri R, Mankad S, et al. Mitral annular dynamics in myxomatous valve disease: New insights with real-time 3D echocardiography. *Circulation.* 2010;121:1423–1431.
24. Lang RM, Tsang W, Weinert L, et al. Valvular heart disease: the value of 3D echocardiography. *J Am Coll Cardiol.* 2011;58:1933–1944.
25. Chaput M, Handschumacher MD, Tournoux F, et al. Mitral leaflet adaptation to ventricular remodeling: Occurrence and adequacy in patients with functional mitral regurgitation. *Circulation.* 2008;118:845–852.
26. Morbach C, Bellavia D, Stork S, Sugeng L. Systolic characteristics and dynamic changes of the mitral valve in different grades of ischemic mitral regurgitation: insights from 3D transesophageal echocardiography. *BMC Cardiovasc Disord.* 2018;18:93.
27. Nishino S, Watanabe N, Kimura T, et al. Acute versus chronic ischemic mitral regurgitation: an echocardiographic study of anatomy and physiology. *Circ Cardiovasc Imag.* 2018;11. e007028.
28. Carpentier A. Cardiac valve surgery—the "French correction. *J Thorac Cardiovasc Surg.* 1983;86:323–337.

96 Mitral Valve Prolapse

Wendy Tsang, Benjamin H. Freed, Roberto M. Lang

Mitral valve prolapse (MVP) is the most common cause of mitral regurgitation (MR) in developed countries.[1] It is also known as degenerative or myxomatous mitral valve (MV) disease and consists of a spectrum, with its mildest form known as fibroelastic deficiency and its most severe as Barlow disease (Table 96.1). In this chapter, will discuss the etiology, diagnosis, and management of MVP.

ETIOLOGY

The form of MVP known as fibroelastic deficiency occurs when there is a loss of mechanical tissue integrity caused by deficiencies in the MV connective tissue structure and function.[2] This typically results in a localized, single-segment prolapse from elongated chordae or a flail leaflet secondary to ruptured chordae (Fig. 96.1A and Video 96.1A). Patients most commonly present in the sixth decade of life with a relatively short history of MR.

In contrast, Barlow disease results from an excess of myxomatous tissue, secondary to abnormal accumulation of mucopolysaccharides in multiple scallops of one or both leaflets and the chordae.[2] This myxoid infiltration leads to thick, bulky, redundant billowing leaflets and elongated chordae. Overall, Barlow disease is best recognized by imaging and at surgery as

TABLE 96.1 Differences Between Barlow Disease and Fibroelastic Deficiency

Differentiating Characteristics	Barlow Disease	Fibroelastic Deficiency
Pathology	Excess leaflet tissue caused by accumulation of mucopolysaccharides	Loss of mechanical integrity caused by impaired production of connective tissue
Typical age at diagnosis	Younger (younger than 40 years old)	Older (older than 60 years old)
Duration of disease	Years to decades	Days to months
Physical exam	Midsystolic click and late systolic murmur	Holosystolic murmur
Leaflet involvement	Multisegmental	Unisegmental
Leaflet lesions	Leaflet billowing and thickening	Thin leaflets with thickened involved segment
	Moderately increased length and area	Severely increased length and area
	Smaller prolapse volume compared with patients with Barlow disease	Larger prolapse volume compared with patients with fibroelastic deficiency
	Minimal distensibility during systole	Significant distensibility during mid and late systole
Chordal lesions	Chordal thickening and elongation	Chordal elongation and chordal rupture
Annulus	Severely dilated	Moderately dilated
	Flattened shape	Preserved shape
	Loss of systolic accentuation of the saddle shape	Relatively preserved contraction
	Annular–ventricular decoupling	
Carpentier classification	Type II	Type II
Type of dysfunction	Bileaflet prolapse	Prolapse, flail, or both
Complexity of valve repair	More complex	Less complex

bileaflet, multisegmental prolapse (Fig. 96.1C and Video 96.1C). Because this is a chronic process, Barlow disease is usually diagnosed in young adulthood, and patients are typically followed for many decades with mild MR and well-preserved left ventricular size until indications for surgery are frequently met in the fourth or fifth decade of life.

ARRHYTHMOGENIC MITRAL VALVE PROLAPSE

Patients with MVP are at risk for ventricular arrhythmias and sudden cardiac death. There has been recent recognition that these arrhythmic issues related to MVP may require management separate to that for regurgitation.[3,4] Patients with MVP who have experienced ventricular arrhythmias and sudden death have been reported to have papillary muscle fibrosis with extension to the inferobasal walls on cardiac magnetic resonance imaging (CMR). It is believed that this scarring occurs from the mechanical stretch of the inferobasal papillary muscle and wall by the billowing leaflets (Fig. 96.2A–C).[5,6] This scarring is postulated to provide the substrate for ventricular arrhythmias, which are triggered by ventricular ectopy that are caused by acute stretch forces (Fig. 96.2F).

These ventricular arrhythmias may be modulated by transient factors such as autonomic dysfunction. Notably, patients do not need to have significant MR to develop papillary or ventricular muscle fibrosis, and even a small burden of late gadolinium enhancement on CMR imaging can be associated with sudden cardiac death. The lack of clinically significant MR also makes it challenging to determine the true incidence of sudden death attributable to MVP because it is hard to attribute the cause of death to MVP identified at autopsy. Overall, it is believed that the risk of sudden cardiac death in MVP is underestimated and some contemporary studies report that it may be the third most common cause of sudden death in people younger than 35 years of age.

Patient and imaging features associated with higher risk of developing sustained ventricular arrhythmias and sudden cardiac death in patients with MVP are presented in Table 96.2 and Fig. 96.2F. Echocardiographic features that could be used to identify these patients include the presence of mitral annular disjunction, systolic curling of the posterior leaflet, or the presence of a spiked lateral mitral annular velocity of greater than 16 cm/s (Pickelhaube sign; see Fig. 96.2D).[7,8] Mitral annular disjunction is an anatomic abnormality of the mitral annulus due to separation of the MV annulus and the left atrial wall (see Fig. 96.2A–C and Video 96.2).

It results in functional decoupling of the mitral annulus from the ventricle, resulting in paradoxical annular dynamics with systolic expansion and flattening (see Fig. 96.2E). Although mitral annular disjunction has been mainly noted in patients with myxomatous valve disease, it is also present in those with fibroelastic deficiency and may be a normal mitral annular variant found in normal patients. Thus, the use of mitral annular disjunction to identify those at risk for arrhythmic complications requires additional study because the value of its presence is unclear.

DIAGNOSIS

The specific diagnosis of fibroelastic deficiency versus Barlow disease is often difficult to definitively determine by either the gross or histologic appearance of the MV because of the overlap of these diseases. Some valves that appear to be secondary to fibroelastic deficiency may actually represent a forme fruste of Barlow disease and demonstrate myxoid infiltration on subsequent histologic examination.[9] However, preoperative differentiation of the extent and location of mitral involvement is crucial for surgeon-specific referral, determination of optimal surgical strategy, and postoperative outcome. The lesions resulting from Barlow disease are complex and frequently require superb surgical skills to achieve a successful repair, whereas lesions resulting from fibroelastic deficiency are more localized and can typically be undertaken with simple repair techniques by most cardiothoracic surgeons. Poor presurgical planning or referral may lead to either unsuccessful repair or conversion to valve replacement with less favorable long-term outcomes in patients with complex valvular diseases.[10,11]

Three-dimensional echocardiography (3DE) has greatly improved the ability to diagnose and treat MVP.[12] Multiple studies have shown that 3DE is superior to two-dimensional echocardiography (2DE) in accurately diagnosing MVP compared with surgical findings.[10,13–15] 3DE is less operator dependent and more reproducible than 2DE at any expertise level. As well, 3D transesophageal echocardiography (TEE) has been shown to correctly identify prolapse in 92% of patients versus 78% of patients using 2D TEE. 3DE also improves quantification of the associated regurgitation. The development of new 3D volume renderings such as photorealistic transillumination will only improve lesion identification (see Fig. 96.1).

3DE has also increased appreciation of the presence and frequency of MV cleftlike indentations or pseudoclefts in patients with myxomatous MV disease. Pseudoclefts are deep folds in the

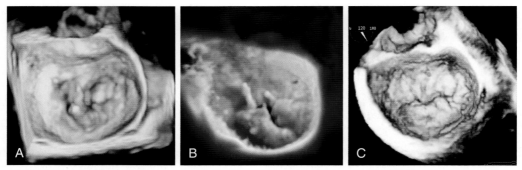

Figure 96.1. A, Three-dimensional (3D) transesophageal echocardiographic (TEE) zoomed image of a patient with fibroelastic deficiency resulting in P2 scallop prolapse and flail. **B,** 3D TEE zoomed image with photorealistic transillumination mode of a patient with P2 and P3 leaflet flail. **C,** 3D TEE zoomed image of a patient with Barlow disease with bileaflet prolapse with greater involvement of the posterior leaflet. *AL,* Anterolateral; *An,* anterior; *Av,* aortic valve; *LA,* left atrium; *LV,* left ventricle; *PM,* posteromedial; *Po,* posterior. (See accompanying Videos 96.1A and 96.1C.)

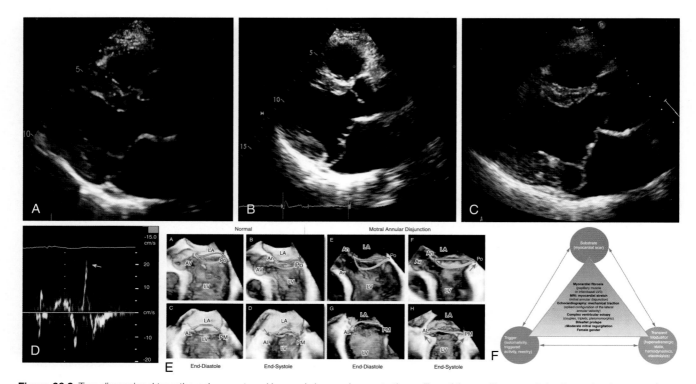

Figure 96.2. Two-dimensional transthoracic parasternal long-axis image demonstrating pulling of the papillary muscle by the prolapsing posterior mitral valve leaflet with no valvular–annular dysfunction (**A**), mild valvular–annular disjunction (**B**), and severe valvular–annular disjunction (**C**). **D,** Example of the Pickelhaube sign, which is the presence of a spiked lateral mitral annular velocity of greater than 16 cm/s *(arrow)*. **E,** The paradoxical annular dynamics in patients with mitral annular disjunction. **F,** The complex interactions that may result in ventricular arrhythmias and sudden cardiac death in patients with mitral valve prolapse. (See accompanying Video 96.2.) (Part E from Lee AP-W, et al: Functional implication of mitral annular disjunction in mitral valve prolapse: A quantitative dynamic 3D echocardiographic study, *JACC Cardiovasc Imag* 10:1424–33, 2017. Part F from Miller MA, et al: Arrhythmic mitral valve prolapse: JACC review topic of the week, *J Am Coll Cardiol* 72:2904–2914, 2018.)

MV leaflets that appear similar to clefts (see Fig. 96.3 and Video 96.3A). Recognition of these pseudoclefts is important because they can unfold and be sources of residual regurgitation after valve repair or clip. These pseudoclefts must also be differentiated from true clefts, which are true breaks in the leaflets that reach the annulus (Video 96.3B).

Parametric maps transform the 3DE images of the MV into color-encoded topographic displays of MV anatomy (Fig. 96.4). The color gradations on the parametric maps indicate the distance of the leaflet from the mitral annular plane toward the left atrium. The use of these maps has been demonstrated to improve the diagnostic accuracy and reproducibility of interpretation by novice readers compared to lesion identification with 2DE.[14] More recently, these

maps have been reported to improve the differentiation of mitral leaflet billowing from prolapse while accounting for the saddle shape of the mitral annulus.[15]

On 2DE, MVP is identified if the mitral leaflet tip is above the annular plane at end-systole. In contrast, MV billowing is identified if the leaflet body protrudes above the annular plane, but the leaflet tip remains at or below the annulus at end-systole. With 3DE, leaflet billowing can be identified from 3D parametric maps, when the line of coaptation between the anterior and posterior leaflets is intact and the region of maximal leaflet excursion into the left atrium does not extend to the coaptation zone. Similarly, leaflet prolapse is identified when the line of coaptation is disrupted by gaps and the region of maximal leaflet excursion extends to the zone of coaptation.

In addition to improving visual assessment of the valve, these maps also allow quantitation of MV parameters, such as leaflet height and annular area. This has provided additional factors for consideration in differentiating Barlow disease from fibroelastic deficiency. 3DE quantification of billowing height with a cutoff value of 1.0 mm can differentiate between normal valves and MVP without overlap, whereas 3DE billowing volume with a cutoff value of 1.15 mL can differentiate between Barlow disease and fibroelastic deficiency.[16] Of note, these measurements were found to be highly reproducible.

TABLE 96.2 Risk Factors for Sudden Death in Mitral Valve Prolapse

Factors	Findings
Patient	Young females
Echocardiogram	Bileaflet prolapse
	Mitral annular disjunction
	Systolic curling of the posterior leaflet
	"Pickelhaube sign": peak systolic lateral mitral annular velocity >16 cm/s
	Moderate or great mitral regurgitation
Electrocardiogram	Frequent premature ventricular complexes
	Complex (multiform) premature ventricular complexes as couplets or nonsustained ventricular tachycardia
	Premature ventricular complexes originate from the papillary muscle region and the outflow tract
	Biphasic or inverted T waves in the inferior leads
CMR	Late gadolinium enhancement of the papillary muscles or inferobasal LV wall
	Myocardial scarring
	Mitral annular disjunction

CMR, Cardiac magnetic resonance imaging; *LV,* left ventricular.

Patients with Barlow disease also differ from those with fibroelastic deficiency with respect to mitral annular and leaflet distensibility.[17,18] Patients with Barlow disease have annular dynamics that are blunted greater than what would be expected from the amount of ventricular and atrial remodeling observed, and this may be related to mitral annular disjunction.[19] Patients with Barlow disease also have greater mitral tissue distensibility during mid to late systole that may explain how patients with Barlow disease with greater prolapse severity and annular enlargement have quantitatively similar regurgitation severity as patients with fibroelastic deficiency. Patients with fibroelastic deficiency have reduced systolic leaflet area change and so experience greater regurgitation with "fewer" morphologic changes. These differences in annular and leaflet tissue dynamics suggests that Barlow disease and fibroelastic deficiency would respond differently to different MV repair techniques.

RISK STRATIFICATION FOR SURGERY

It is recognized that there is an underreferral of patients with significant MR for surgery and of those who are sent to surgery too many received valve replacement instead of repair.[20,21] This may be caused by underestimation of patient risks for surgery and referral of complex repair patients to non-MV repair specialist surgeons. To address these issues, scores have been developed to help risk stratify patients.

The Mitral Regurgitation International Database (MIDA) score was developed for use at the time of diagnosis of severe MR from a flail leaflet to help improve risk stratification for continuation of medical therapy or referral to surgery (Table 96.3).[22] The MIDA score has been shown to provide incremental prognostic predictive value over the European System for Cardiac Operative Risk Evaluation (EuroSCORE) II and has been validated in a population with severe MR from either MVP or flail leaflets. However, it does not include measurements from 3DE, global longitudinal strain, the

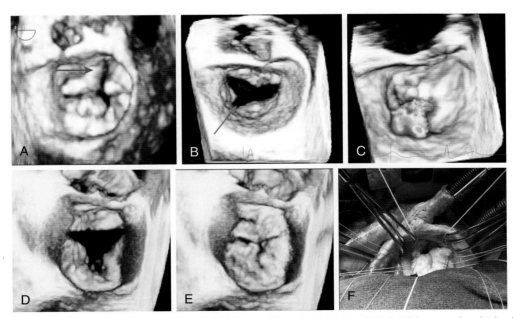

Figure 96.3. A, En face three-dimensional echocardiographic (3DE) image of the mitral valve from the left atrial perspective obtained via transesophageal echocardiography demonstrating the presence of an anterior cleft *(blue arrow)* pointing at the left ventricular outflow tract. **B,** En face 3DE TEE image of the mitral valve from the left atrial perspective during diastole demonstrating the presence of a cleftlike indentation or pseudocleft *(red arrow).* **C,** En face 3DE TEE color Doppler image of the mitral valve from the left atrial perspective during systole demonstrating that this patient's mitral regurgitation originated through the cleftlike indentation. 3D transesophageal echocardiographic image of a mitral pseudocleft or deep fold in the posterior leaflet of a myxomatous valve during diastole (**D**) and systole (**E**) and in the operative room (**F**). (See accompanying Videos 96.3A and 96.3B.)

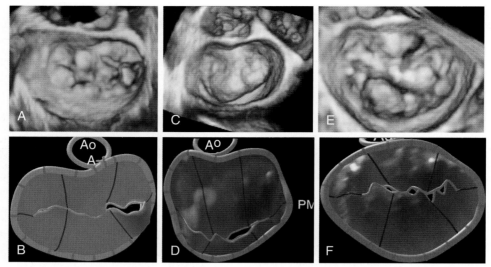

Figure 96.4. A, Three-dimensional transesophageal echocardiographic (3D TEE) zoomed image of the mitral valve with P3 flail. **B,** The parametric map of this valve clearly demonstrates the location of the prolapse segment *(red)* and resultant gap in leaflet coaptation. **C,** 3D TEE zoomed image of the mitral valve with anterior leaflet prolapse. **D,** The parametric map demonstrates the location of the prolapsing anterior leaflet segments *(red)* and resultant gap in leaflet coaptation. **E,** 3D TEE zoomed image of a patient with Barlow disease and bileaflet multisegmental prolapse. **F,** The parametric map of this valve clearly demonstrates the multisegmental bileaflet prolapsing segments *(red)*. *A,* anterior; *Ao,* aorta; *PM,* posteromedial.

TABLE 96.3 MIDA Score for Risk Stratification With Myxomatous Mitral Valve Disease

	Points
Age older than 65 years	3
Symptoms	3
Right ventricular systolic pressure >50 mm Hg	2
Atrial fibrillation	1
Left atrial diameter >55 mm	1
Left ventricular end-systolic diameter >40 mm	1
Left ventricular ejection fraction <60%	1

presence of fibrosis on CMR, peptides, or exercise testing, all of which could improve the score.

Stratification of patients by MV lesion complexity may assist in directing those with complex causes or lesions to surgeons with greater expertise and volumes with the intent of improving repair rates. Standardization of assessment of MV reparability complexity was been proposed in the 2017 Expert Consensus paper published by the American College of Cardiology (ACC). The ACC expert based decision-making tool classifies the feasibility of repair as ideal, challenging, or contraindicated based on anatomic factors (Table 96.4).[23] However, its use is limited because it does not recognize the spectrum and combination of abnormalities that may be present.

A second proposed score (Table 96.5) grades valves on a scale from 1 to 5, in which a value of 1 is considered a simple repair, 2 to 4 is considered intermediate, and 5 or more is complex.[24] This score allows consideration for the spectrum of changes to the valve and is easy to use, especially compared with the ACC tool, but the weight attributed to each factor or abnormality was arbitrarily assigned. Also, this score was developed in a center with a high repair rate and has not been prospectively validated. Further work in this area is warranted.

SURGICAL MITRAL VALVE REPAIR

3DE quantification has also been applied in MVP patients undergoing MV repair.[25] Prolapsing height and anterior leaflet surface area derived from 3DE parametric maps can accurately predict surgical repair complexity, irrespective of the cause of MR.[26] Also, with 3D quantification, it was found that (1) 3DE mitral annular dimensions were accurate and reproducible compared with direct intraoperative measurements; (2) patients with MVP have significantly larger annular dimensions than control participants during diastole; (3) control participants have early-systolic anteroposterior and area contraction, increased annular height, larger saddle shape depth, and unchanged intercommissural diameter, whereas patients with MVP have mostly unchanged annular dimensions, albeit with significant intercommissural dilatation; and (4) after repair, the annulus is smaller in MVP patients but continues to lack systolic saddle-shape accentuation.

Overall, 3D TEE provides in greater detail information regarding the pathomorphologic changes to the MV, allowing a tailored rather than standard approach, in which a preestablished operation is performed according to the Carpentier classification system. This is an especially important change in the surgical approach to myxomatous MV disease because patients often have more than a single mechanism of MR, which limits the utility of the Carpentier classification system.

3DE has also highlighted the different conformational changes that occur between Barlow disease and fibroelastic deficiency after MV repair. Not surprisingly, the annular diameters and MV area were significantly reduced for both disease entities after repair. However, the MV annulus was found to be larger in patients with Barlow disease, which is consistent with the different mean sizes of the implanted prosthetic rings.[27] In addition, the greater reduction in posterior leaflet area in patients with Barlow disease compared with fibroelastic deficiency is in agreement with the higher rate of posterior leaflet resection and sliding performed for this type of degenerative disease.

The propensity for developing systolic anterior motion after MV repair is, in part, dependent on the degree of aortomitral and septoaortic angles, presence of excess tissue, and displacement of mitral coaptation line toward the posterior leaflet, all of which can be well characterized by 3DE.[28–31] By quantifying the extent of the excess anterior and posterior leaflet length, surface area, and billowing volume before and after surgery, 3DE analysis helps identify patients who are most at risk for developing systolic anterior motion.

TABLE 96.4 Feasibility of Mitral Valve Repair From the American College of Cardiology 2017 Expert Consensus Decision Pathway on the Management of Mitral Regurgitation[23]

	Ideal Pathoanatomy	Challenging Pathoanatomy	Contraindicated Pathoanatomy
Primary lesion location	Posterior leaflet only	Anterior leaflet or bileaflet	None
Leaflet calcification	None	Mild	Moderate to severe
Annular calcification	None	Mild to moderate with minimal leaflet encroachment	Severe or with significant leaflet encroachment
Subvalvular apparatus	Thin, normal	Mild diffuse thickening or moderate focal thickening	Severe and diffuse thickening with leaflet retraction
Mechanism of mitral regurgitation	Type II fibroelastic deficiency or focal myxomatous prolapse or flail	Type II forme fruste or bileaflet myxomatous disease Type I healed or active endocarditis Type IIIA/B with mild restriction or leaflet thickening	Type IIIB with severe tethering and inferobasal aneurysm Type IIIA with severe bileaflet calcification Type I active infection with severe leaflet or annular tissue destruction
Unique anatomic complexities	None	Redo cardiac operation or mitral re-repair; anatomic predictors of systolic anterior motion, adult congenital anomalies; focal papillary muscle rupture	Mitral valve reoperation with paucity of leaflet tissue; diffuse radiation valvulopathy; papillary muscle rupture with shock

From O'Gara PT, et al: 2017 ACC expert consensus decision pathway on the management of mitral regurgitation, *J Am Coll Cardiol* 70:2421–2449, 2017.

TABLE 96.5 Risk Stratification of Complexity for Repair of Myxomatous Mitral Valves

	Points
Segment prolapse	
P1	1
P2	1
P3	1
A1	2
A2	2
A3	2
Anterolateral commissure prolapse	2
Posteromedial commissure prolapse	2
Any leaflet restriction	2
Papillary muscle or leaflet calcification without annular involvement	2
Annular calcification	3
Previous mitral valve repair	3

PERCUTANEOUS MITRAL VALVE REPAIR

Although there are many transcatheter MV repair techniques in development, only edge-to-edge repair through the MitraClip procedure has become widely adopted in routine clinical practice. The MitraClip procedure has low procedural mortality and is therefore performed in patients with symptomatic regurgitation who have limited surgical treatment options. 2DE and 3DE remain the main technique used to assess patients before and after the procedure and to guide the procedure. For patients with MVP, the clip is ideal for those where the main regurgitant jet is located between the A2 andP2 segments and the flail segment height is less than 1 cm and the gap is less than 3 mm. Patients may require more than one clip to reduce the MR, especially if the prolapsing or flailing segment is wide. The additional clips may also provide stability given the greater leaflet mobility because of the prolapsing leaflets. Other percutaneous techniques such as percutaneous chordal placements and annuloplasty are still in a testing phase but ultimately may offer a more complete repair approach, similar to surgical repair. The use of multiple devices may also improve long-term durability, but the costs of using multiple devices in a single individual would need to be addressed.

SUMMARY

MVP is a spectrum that ranges from fibroelastic deficiency to Barlow disease. 3DE has improved diagnosis by improving not only accuracy of lesion localization but also quantification of the associated annular and leaflet changes. This knowledge may improve clinical outcomes with respect to arrhythmic complication. It may also lead to improvements in MV surgical repair techniques and new developments in percutaneous interventions.

Please access ExpertConsult to view the corresponding videos for this chapter.

REFERENCES

1. Griffin BP. Myxomatous mitral valve disease. In: Otto CM, Bonow RO, eds. *Valvular Heart Disease*. Philadelphia: Saunders Elsevier; 2009:243–259.
2. Anyanwu AC, Adams DH. Etiologic classification of degenerative mitral valve disease: Barlow's disease and fibroelastic deficiency. *Semin Thorac Cardiovasc Surg*. 2007;19:90–96.
3. Basso C, Perazzolo Marra M, Rizzo S, et al. Arrhythmic mitral valve prolapse and sudden cardiac death. *Circulation*. 2015;132:556–566.
4. Han Y, Peters DC, Salton CJ, et al. Cardiovascular magnetic resonance characterization of mitral valve prolapse. *JACC Cardiovasc Imag*. 2008;1:294–303.
5. Edwards NC, Moody WE, Yuan M, et al. Quantification of left ventricular interstitial fibrosis in asymptomatic chronic primary degenerative mitral regurgitation. *Circ Cardiovasc Imag*. 2014;7:946–953.
6. Bui AH, Roujol S, Foppa M, et al. Diffuse myocardial fibrosis in patients with mitral valve prolapse and ventricular arrhythmia. *Heart*. 2017;103:204–209.
7. Perazzolo Marra M, Basso C, de Lazzari M, et al. Morphofunctional abnormalities of mitral annulus and arrhythmic mitral valve prolapse. *Circ Cardiovasc Imag*. 2016;9. e005030.
8. Dejgaard LA, Skjølsvik ET, Lie ØH, et al. The mitral annulus disjunction arrhythmic syndrome. *J Am Coll Cardiol*. 2018;72:1600–1609.
9. Adams DH, Anyanwu AC, Sugeng L, Lang RM. Degenerative mitral valve regurgitation: surgical echocardiography. *Curr Cardiol Rep*. 2008;10:226–232.
10. Gillinov AM, Cosgrove DM, Blackstone EH, et al. Durability of mitral valve repair for degenerative disease. *J Thorac Cardiovasc Surg*. 1998;116:734–743.
11. Lee EM, Shapiro LM, Wells FC. Superiority of mitral valve repair in surgery for degenerative mitral regurgitation. *Eur Heart J*. 1997;18:655–663.
12. Sugeng L, Shernan SK, Salgo IS, et al. Live 3D transesophageal echocardiography initial experience using the fully-sampled matrix array probe. *J Am Coll Cardiol*. 2008;52:446–449.
13. Chandra S, Salgo IS, Sugeng L, et al. Characterization of degenerative mitral valve disease using morphologic analysis of real-time three-dimensional echocardiographic images: objective insight into complexity and planning of mitral valve repair. *Circ Cardiovasc Imag*. 2011;4:24–32.
14. Tsang W, Weinert L, Sugeng L, et al. The value of three-dimensional echocardiography derived mitral valve parametric maps and the role of experience in the diagnosis of pathology. *J Am Soc Echocardiogr*. 2011;24(8):860–867.

15. La Canna G, Arendar I, Maisano F, et al. Real-time three-dimensional transesophageal echocardiography for assessment of mitral valve functional anatomy in patients with prolapse-related regurgitation. *Am J Cardiol.* 2011;107:1365–1374.
16. Addetia K, Mor-Avi V, Weinert L, et al. A new definition for an old entity: improved definition of mitral valve prolapse using three-dimensional echocardiography and color-coded parametric models. *J Am Soc Echocardiogr.* 2014;27(8–16).
17. Clavel M-A, Mantovani F, Malouf J, et al. Dynamic phenotypes of degenerative myxomatous mitral valve disease: quantitative 3D echocardiographic study. *Circ Cardiovasc Imag.* 2015;8. e002989.
18. Antoine C, Mantovani F, Benfari G, et al. Pathophysiology of degenerative mitral regurgitation: new 3D imaging insights. *Circ Cardiovasc Imag.* 2018;11. e005971.
19. Lee AP-W, Jin C-N, Fan Y, et al. Functional implication of mitral annular disjunction in mitral valve prolapse: a quantitative dynamic 3D echocardiographic study. *JACC Cardiovasc Imagi.* 2017;10:1424–1433.
20. Bach DS, Awais M, Gurm HS, et al. Failure of guideline adherence for intervention in patients with severe mitral regurgitation. *J Am Coll Cardiol.* 2009;54:860–865.
21. Chikwe J, Toyoda N, Anyanwu AC, et al. Relation of mitral valve surgery volume to repair rate, durability, and survival. *J Am Coll Cardiol.* 2017;24. S0735-1097(17)30677-0.
22. Grigioni F, Clavel M-A, Vanoverschelde J-L, et al. The MIDA Mortality Risk Score: development and external validation of a prognostic model for early and late death in degenerative mitral regurgitation. *Eur Heart J.* 2018;39:1281–1291.
23. O'Gara PT, Grayburn PA, Badhwar V, et al. ACC expert consensus decision pathway on the management of mitral regurgitation. *J Am Coll Cardiol 2017.* 2017;70:2421–2449.
24. Anyanwu AC, Itagaki S, Chikwe J, et al. A complexity scoring system for degenerative mitral valve repair. *J Thorac Cardiovasc Surg.* 2016;151:1661–1670.
25. Grewal J, Suri R, Mankad S, et al. Mitral annular dynamics in myxomatous valve disease: new insights with real-time 3- dimensional echocardiography. *Circulation.* 2010;121:1423–1431.
26. Chikwe J, Adams DH, Su KN, et al. Can three-dimensional echocardiography accurately predict complexity of mitral valve repair? *Eur J Cardio Thorac Surg.* 2012;41:518–524.
27. Maffessanti F, Marsan NA, Tamborini G, et al. Quantitative analysis of mitral valve apparatus in mitral valve prolapse before and after annuloplasty: a three-dimensional intraoperative transesophageal study. *J Am Soc Echocardiogr.* 2011;24:405–413.
28. Lee KS, Stewart WJ, Lever HM, et al. Mechanism of outflow tract obstruction causing failed mitral valve repair. Anterior displacement of leaflet coaptation. *Circulation.* 1993;88:II24–II29.
29. Carpentier A, Chauvaud S, Fabiani JN, et al. Reconstructive surgery of mitral valve incompetence: ten-year appraisal. *J Thorac Cardiovasc Surg.* 1980;79:338–348.
30. Flameng W, Meuris B, Herijgers P, Herregods MC. Durability of mitral valve repair in Barlow disease versus fibroelastic deficiency. *J Thorac Cardiovasc Surg.* 2008;135:274–282.
31. Jebara VA, Mihaileanu S, Acar C, et al. Left ventricular outflow tract obstruction after mitral valve repair. Results of the sliding leaflet technique. *Circulation.* 1993;88:II30–II34.
32. Miller MA, Dukkipati SR, Turagam M, et al. Arrhythmic mitral valve prolapse: JACC review topic of the week. *J Am Coll Cardiol.* 2018;72:2904–2914.

97 Secondary Mitral Regurgitation

Philippe B. Bertrand, Jacqueline S. Danik, Judy Hung

Mitral regurgitation (MR) is a frequent complication of myocardial infarction (MI), severe coronary artery disease, and congestive heart failure that is associated with an adverse prognosis independent of underlying left ventricular (LV) dysfunction.[1–3] In the medical literature, several terms have been used to describe this type of MR. *Ischemic MR* is a commonly used but ill-defined term because nonischemic cardiomyopathy is equally relevant. *Functional MR* refers to the presence of MR without any structural abnormality of the mitral valve (MV) leaflets or chordal apparatus. *Secondary MR* is the more encompassing term, referring to the mechanism that is secondary to nonvalvular pathology (as opposed to *primary MR*), typically in the setting chamber dilatation caused by coronary artery disease, nonischemic cardiomyopathy, or congestive heart failure.[4]

In a majority of patients, the initial insult in secondary MR is *ventricular*. In ischemic heart disease, it is primarily the remodeling that follows MI or ischemia that causes the MR rather than being caused by active or reversible ischemia. Acute ischemia can sometimes cause fluctuating MR or severe acute MR because of papillary muscle rupture, yet this is not prevalent. Alternatively, *atrial functional MR* in the setting of atrial fibrillation or heart failure with preserved ejection fraction is increasingly recognized as a distinct form of secondary MR, with different mechanistic basis and different management options.[5] Isolated annular dilatation, annular flattening, and impaired annular dynamics are thought to be the culprit cause of the regurgitation, whereas LV size and function are typically normal in atrial functional MR.

There is clinical heterogeneity of secondary MR in various clinical situations. The following sections focus on the unifying mechanisms in secondary MR, the echocardiographic diagnosis, and the implications for prognosis and management.

MECHANISMS

Mitral Regurgitation Secondary to Geometric Changes (Remodeling) of the Left Ventricle

Mitral leaflet morphology is essentially normal in secondary MR. The primary cause of MR is ventricular distortion of the normal spatial relationship of the MV apparatus and the left ventricle. With adverse LV remodeling (dilatation and change of shape), one or both mitral leaflets are pulled apically into the left ventricle and radially away from the center of the left ventricle because of the outward displacement of the papillary muscles that results from remodeling. This results in incomplete mitral leaflet closure, in which the leaflet coaptation point is apically displaced (Fig. 97.1). This pattern is best seen in the apical four-chamber view. The leaflets are apically displaced and tethered and may restrict mobility, especially of the posterior leaflet (Fig. 97.2).

Quantification of Tethering

There are a number of methods to quantify the degree of tethering.

Tenting area. The most common is a simple area measurement from the leaflets to the annular plane (tenting area), which is typically performed at midsystole, when the area is at a minimum.

Coaptation depth (height). Another measure is coaptation depth or height, which measures the maximal distance from the leaflet tips to the annular plane, which appears to correlate with the presence and severity of MR.

Tethering distance and tenting volume. Three-dimensional (3D) echocardiography can be used to quantify leaflet tethering by measuring the tethering distance from the papillary muscle tip to the mitral annulus and to measure the tenting volume (volume from leaflets to annular plane), which may provide additional data to assess tethering.

Although this appears to be the primary mechanism of secondary MR, other factors may play a role. Tethering of the anterior leaflet by the secondary (basal or strut) chordae can result in a *seagull* deformation of the body of the anterior leaflet, which further impairs coaptation (Fig. 97.3).

Annular Dilatation

Mitral annulus dilatation (primarily anteroposterior and to a lesser degree medial-lateral) may also be a contributing factor of secondary MR. However, the degree of annular dilatation can vary and does not necessarily correlate with the degree of MR.[6] In addition, there is evidence that the nonplanar saddle shape of the annulus is

important to minimize stress on the valve leaflets and contributes to valve competence; this shape can be altered in secondary MR.[7] In addition to the simple geometry of the annulus, the actual kinetics of the mitral annulus during the cardiac cycle may play a role.[8] Normally, the mitral annulus changes size throughout the cardiac cycle, and this may be altered in the presence of distorted LV geometry and regional wall motion abnormalities. Last, intraventricular dyssynchrony may contribute to secondary MR. In this setting, uncoordinated contraction of the papillary muscles or posterobasal wall (or both) of the left ventricle may result in LV malalignment of the MV leaflets, thus interfering with leaflet coaptation.[9]

Characteristic echocardiographic features of secondary MR are listed in Box 97.1. It is generally stated that the valve leaflets are normal in secondary MR. However, there may be minor abnormalities, such as nonspecific thickening caused by the mitral regurgitant jet or aging. Moreover, although the leaflets are initially "innocent bystanders," structural changes in leaflet architecture

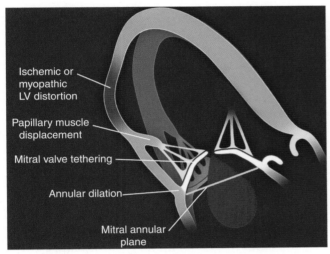

Figure 97.1. Secondary mitral regurgitation caused by ventricular distortion of the mitral valve apparatus. Note the apical and lateral displacement of the papillary muscles caused by left ventricular (LV) remodeling, which results in apical displacement of both mitral valve leaflets relative to the mitral annular plane, that is, "tenting." (© American Society of Echocardiography.)

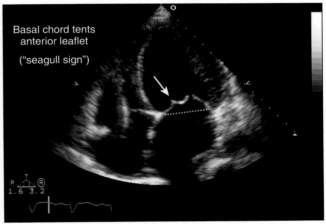

Figure 97.3. The seagull sign. Transthoracic echocardiogram (apical four-chamber view) illustrating tethering of the anterior mitral leaflet *(arrow)* caused by a basal chord (not shown). This has been referred to as the "seagull sign" (or leaflet bend) because the anterior leaflet resembles the schematic of a flying bird. The *yellow dotted line* indicates the plane of the mitral annulus; an increased tenting area is seen above.

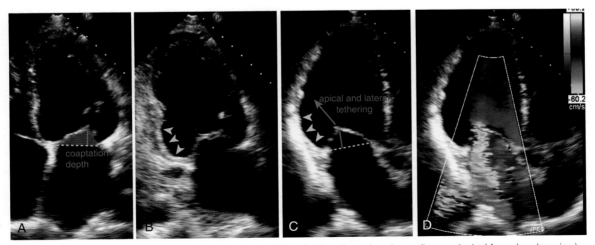

Figure 97.2. Mitral leaflet tethering caused by left ventricular remodeling. **A,** Transthoracic echocardiogram (apical four-chamber view) illustrating tethering of both the anterior and posterior mitral leaflet due to inferolateral left ventricular wall motion abnormality and remodeling. The coaptation is apically displaced (coaptation depth, *red line*) above the annular plane *(dashed line)*. A tenting area can be measured as well *(shaded area)*. **B,** Apical two-chamber view shows inferobasal wall motion abnormality *(arrowheads)* with severe leaflet tethering. **C,** Apical long-axis view demonstrates apical and lateral leaflet tethering with increased tenting of the valve (i.e., increased coaptation depth; *red line*). **D,** There is severe secondary mitral regurgitation by color Doppler. (See accompanying Video 97.2.)

BOX 97.1 Echocardiographic Features of Secondary Mitral Regurgitation

- Absence of organic mitral valve abnormalities
- Apical tethering or restriction of the mitral leaflets, especially the posterior leaflet
- Increased coaptation depth and decreased overlap of leaflet contact
- Dilated mitral annulus
- Left ventricular wall motion abnormalities, especially the inferior or inferolateral (posterior) wall
- Central or posteriorly directed mitral regurgitant jet

TABLE 97.1 Differences Between Asymmetric (Regional) Versus Symmetric (Global) Remodeling Patterns

	Asymmetric	Symmetric
Leaflet tethering	PML tethered toward posterior wall	Both tethered toward apex
MR jet direction	Eccentric, posterior	Usually central
Tenting area	Increased	Greatest
Annulus	Minor change	Dilated and flattened
LV remodeling	Regional	Global
MI site	Inferior	Anterior or multiple
CAD extent	RCA or LCx	Multivessel

CAD, Coronary artery disease; *LCx,* left circumflex; *LV,* left ventricular; *MI,* myocardial infarction; *MR,* mitral regurgitation; *PML,* posterior mitral leaflet; *RCA,* right coronary artery.

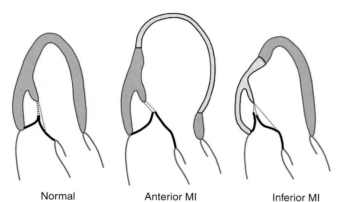

Normal   Anterior MI   Inferior MI

Figure 97.4. Different tethering patterns relate to regional or global remodeling patterns (or both). Normal coaptation and the differences in coaptation resulting from an anterior myocardial infarction (MI) and an inferior MI. An inferior MI usually results in an asymmetric tethering pattern in which the coaptation line is shifted posteriorly because of restriction of the posterior leaflet. Global remodeling in nonischemic cardiomyopathy has a tethering pattern similar to the anterior MI group, with more symmetric apical tethering.

over time caused by abnormal stretching have been described and may further impair coaptation.[10,11]

Regional Versus Global Left Ventricular Remodeling

Although both regional and global remodeling may lead to MR, the specific site of remodeling is relevant. Inferior MIs are more likely to be associated with significant MR compared with anterior MI.[12] Differences between regional versus global remodeling typically result in different tethering patterns[13] (Fig. 97.4 and Table 97.1). A symmetric tethering pattern is characterized by apical tethering of both leaflets to a similar degree, resulting in symmetric coaptation and a centrally directed MR jet. An asymmetric tethering pattern has posterior tethering of both leaflets, but tethering occurs predominantly in the posterior leaflet, which results in a posterior shift of the coaptation line and restriction of the posterior leaflet, which leads to asymmetric coaptation and a posteriorly directed MR jet.

Patients with a symmetric tethering pattern (as seen after anterior MIs or in nonischemic dilated cardiomyopathy) usually have worse ejection fractions, more global wall motion abnormalities, greater dilatation of the mitral annulus, and a decrease in the normal nonplanar (saddle-shaped) annulus shape.[14] Nevertheless, the degree of MR tends to be less in this group of patients. Patients with asymmetric tethering tend to have a more preserved saddle shape of the annulus and less significant global remodeling. Therefore, the degree of MR may not correlate with LV volumes or the degree of global LV dysfunction.

Echocardiographic findings in secondary MR depend on LV function and contractility. In normal ventricles, a delicate balance

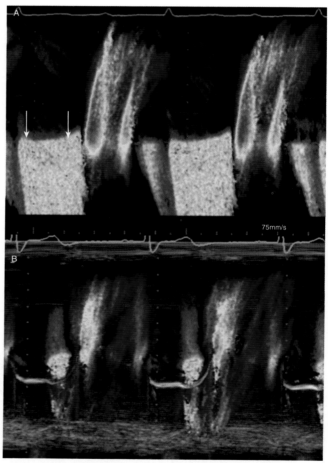

Figure 97.5. Dynamics of the mitral regurgitant orifice area. **A,** Color M-mode echocardiography of a patient with secondary mitral regurgitation (MR) showing holosystolic regurgitation with early and late flow peaks. **B,** Color M-mode echocardiography in a patient with mitral valve prolapse and mostly late systolic MR.

is maintained between closing forces acting on the MV during systole and the tethering forces that prevent leaflet prolapse into the left atrium. In secondary MR, systolic LV contraction forces are typically decreased against more pronounced opposing tethering forces.[15] The closing force is strongest in midsystole, so that secondary MR is greatest in early and late systole when the opposing tethering forces predominate.[16,17] The more severe the MR, the more holosystolic is the duration of regurgitant flow during systole (Fig. 97.5). Cardiac resynchronization therapy can

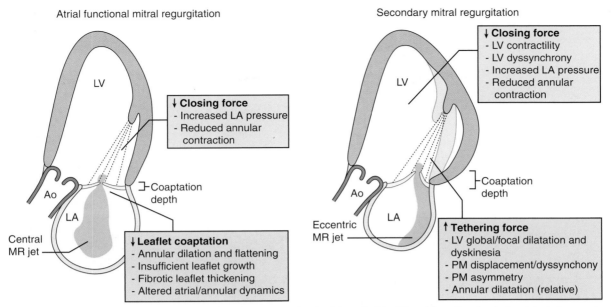

Atrial functional mitral regurgitation

LV

↓ **Closing force**
- Increased LA pressure
- Reduced annular contraction

Ao

LA

⊐-Coaptation depth

Central MR jet —

↓ **Leaflet coaptation**
- Annular dilation and flattening
- Insufficient leaflet growth
- Fibrotic leaflet thickening
- Altered atrial/annular dynamics

Secondary mitral regurgitation

↓ **Closing force**
- LV contractility
- LV dyssynchrony
- Increased LA pressure
- Reduced annular contraction

LV

Ao

LA

⊐-Coaptation depth

Eccentric MR jet —

↑ **Tethering force**
- LV global/focal dilatation and dyskinesia
- PM displacement/dyssynchrony
- PM asymmetry
- Annular dilatation (relative)

Figure 97.6. Atrial functional mitral regurgitation (MR) has a distinct pathophysiology that is different from the classic "ventricular" secondary MR. *Ao,* Aorta; *LA,* left atrium; *LV,* left ventricle; *PM,* papillary muscle.

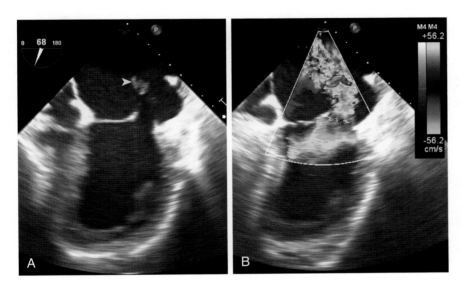

Figure 97.7. Mitral regurgitation (MR) caused by ischemic papillary muscle rupture. **A** and **B,** Two-dimensional transesophageal echocardiography in midesophageal bicommissural view (68 degrees) shows the large torn papillary muscle tip in the left atrium (*arrowhead*) causing severe MR. (See accompanying Video 97.7)

reduce secondary MR by prolonging the time during each cardiac cycle when LV closure force effectively opposes tethering.[18]

Atrial Functional Mitral Regurgitation

In patients with atrial fibrillation or heart failure with preserved ejection fraction, different mechanisms can cause functional MR.[5] Left atrial (LA) dilatation or dysfunction is the culprit, whereas LV size and function are grossly normal. There is minimal to no apical tethering of the leaflets. Instead, incomplete closure of the (structurally normal) MV leaflets relates to mitral annular dilatation (relative to the leaflet length), annular flattening (loss of the non-planar saddle shape), and insufficient atrial or annular dynamics to enhance leaflet coaptation (Fig. 97.6). Of note, posterior leaflet tethering can sometimes be observed in atrial functional MR. It has been hypothesized that this is related to outward displacement of the posterior mitral annulus, leading to so called atriogenic leaflet tethering.[19] Restoration of sinus rhythm, when successful and durable, has shown to decrease the severity of MR.[20]

Papillary Muscle Rupture

The most acute and catastrophic form of secondary (ischemic) MR is papillary muscle rupture. When papillary muscle rupture occurs, acute severe MR, pulmonary edema, and cardiogenic shock typically ensue. The left atrium is usually normal in size, and the sudden increase in LA pressure is reflected backward into the pulmonary veins, causing pulmonary edema. Absence of previous LV remodeling and dilatation prevents maintenance of forward stroke volume, which results in cardiogenic shock.

MI causes sufficient tissue necrosis to avulse the papillary muscle head, which may result in a partially or completely flail leaflet. The papillary muscle head appears as a bullet-shaped (or bell-shaped) mass flailing from the left ventricle to the left atrium in systole (Fig. 97.7). Less severe MR may be seen with rupture of only a papillary muscle tip. Compared with the lateral papillary muscle with its dual coronary artery blood supply (left anterior descending, left circumflex artery, or both), the medial papillary muscle more commonly ruptures because of its single coronary artery supply (right coronary artery).[21]

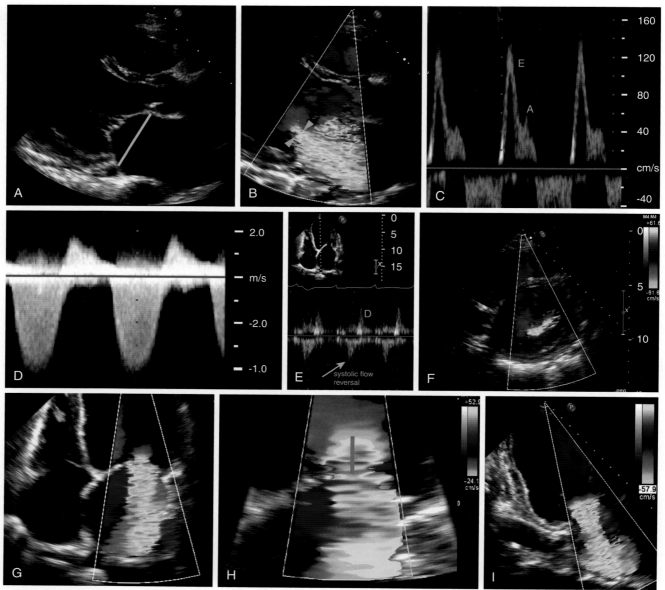

Figure 97.8. The echocardiographic assessment of secondary mitral regurgitation (MR) severity. **A,** Two-dimensional transthoracic echocardiography in parasternal long-axis view demonstrates tenting of the leaflets above the annular plane. **B,** Vena contracta width *(arrowheads)* to estimate MR severity. Indirect signs of MR severity include E-wave predominance on pulsed-wave Doppler inflow (**C**), dense MR continuous-wave Doppler signal (**D**), and evidence of systolic flow reversal in the pulmonary veins (**E**). **F,** In the parasternal short-axis view the slitlike regurgitant orifice can be observed. **G,** Apical four-chamber view of the MR jet area. **H,** Measurement of the proximal isovelocity surface area method in a zoomed apical four-chamber view can be used to quantify secondary MR, although the hemispherical assumption is not strictly applied to this situation. **I,** Apical two-chamber view showing the wide MR orifice. (See accompanying Video 97.8.).

The echocardiographer must be alert to papillary muscle rupture in a hyperdynamic left ventricle after MI because the necrotic zone may be limited, and by itself, hard to discern.

ECHOCARDIOGRAPHIC ASSESSMENT OF SECONDARY MITRAL REGURGITATION

Echocardiographic assessment of secondary MR should include careful assessment of LV function and quantitation of the degree of MR. Color Doppler usually reveals a central or posteriorly directed MR jet. Measurement of LV function should include the ejection fraction, LV dimensions, assessment of wall motion abnormalities, and structural abnormalities of the MV chordae and papillary muscles. An integrative approach to the quantitation of MR should

be performed, including Doppler techniques for direct quantitation and supportive echo data (LA size, LV chamber size, pattern of pulmonary vein flow) in the overall assessment.[22]

Echocardiographic quantification of the regurgitant MR volume is important for prognosis and can help guide therapy. The major obstacles are spatial (elliptical vs spherical flow convergence region) and temporal (early and late systole). Routine echocardiographic assessment of two-dimensional (2D) or 3D vena contracta can rapidly differentiate between mild or less MR and more than mild MR (Fig. 97.8). Although the orifice area varies, typically the largest vena contracta is used to scale the orifice, and care must be taken not to confuse a brief early systolic orifice with a nearly holosystolic one. Despite its limitations, jet area, for the typically central jets, remains a useful and rapid visual clue. Overall severity assessment, for MR in general, integrates LV size and function and LA size and has an impact on Doppler flows and predicted pressures. Quantification of MR volume may be attempted with 2D or 3D flow convergence methods, bearing in mind the typical slitlike orifice and therefore the hemielliptical proximal flow convergence surface area; the hemispherical assumption is not strictly applied to this situation (see Fig. 97.8).[23]

MR may also occur with active or reversible myocardial ischemia and may disappear after the ischemia resolves. Furthermore, if the patient's clinical presentation and symptoms seem out of proportion to the echocardiographic MR findings, stress echocardiography can unmask the dynamic nature of the lesion by demonstrating increased MR during exertion.[4]

PROGNOSIS

Secondary MR is associated with significant morbidity and mortality. The presence of MR in patients with coronary artery disease, even when only mild, is associated with an increased mortality rate independent of other predictors of outcome.[1,2] Similar prognostic impact of secondary MR is observed in patients with chronic heart failure.[3] Remarkably, the most prominent prognostic impact of MR is observed in a subgroup with intermediate LV dysfunction, in which the presence of severe secondary MR is likely a driving force of progressive heart failure more than a mere marker of the LV dysfunction.[24] In this setting, assessing the regurgitant fraction of MR on top of the effective regurgitant orifice area and volume could be particularly useful to address whether the MR is disproportionate to the severity of LV disease (i.e., driving heart failure) or proportionate (i.e., marker of disease).[25,26]

Moreover, the degree of MR is central to the prognostic impact and the decision making. Characterization of the severity of valve regurgitation is among the most difficult problems in valvular heart disease. Preoperative transthoracic echocardiography by experienced laboratories is preferred to intraoperative transesophageal echocardiography to reflect the true degree of MR because secondary MR is often underestimated by the altered hemodynamics in anesthetized patients. Moreover, as recommended by the American Society of Echocardiography, a comprehensive, multifaceted, integrated approach to quantitating MR should be performed (see Chapter 98).

MANAGEMENT OF ISCHEMIC MITRAL REGURGITATION

The optimal management of secondary MR remains controversial despite improved understanding of its mechanisms. It is important to identify and address potentially reversible LV dysfunction by optimal medical therapy, revascularization, and cardiac resynchronization therapy. Surgical treatment options for (ischemic) secondary MR include coronary artery bypass grafting alone or with concomitant MV annuloplasty or replacement. In the multicenter randomized trial by the Cardiothoracic Surgical Trials Network, the most common technique to repair ischemic MR by placement of an undersized annuloplasty ring (restrictive annuloplasty) did not result in better LV remodeling or clinical outcome than MV replacement.[27] Moreover, the rate of MR recurrence after restrictive annuloplasty was up to 30% at 1 year, increasing to almost 60% at 2 years.[28] MR recurrence occurs because MV repair with an undersized annuloplasty ring does not address the fundamental ventricular pathology, and ongoing adverse remodeling can continue to occur.[29]

Aside from revascularization, percutaneous MV repair can be considered to treat severe secondary MR in patients with symptomatic heart failure despite optimal heart failure management. The COAPT (Cardiovascular Outcomes Assessment of MitraClip Percutaneous Therapy for Heart Failure Patients With Functional Mitral Regurgitation) trial, as a first, demonstrated that targeting secondary MR with percutaneous MV repair (MitraClip, Abbott

Vascular) significantly reduces heart failure hospitalizations and mortality at 2 years in symptomatic patients on optimized heart failure treatment.[30] However, the importance of patient selection—and the central role of echocardiography in this patient selection—is highlighted by the marked differences in outcome with a similar contemporary prospective trial (MITRA-FR, Percutaneous Repair with the MitraClip Device for Severe Functional/Secondary Mitral Regurgitation).[30,31] Other percutaneous devices for MV repair or replacement in secondary MR are currently under investigation, and their relevance will become clear in the near future. What is clear at this point, however, is the central role of echocardiography in the assessment, quantification, and procedural guidance of these percutaneous interventions for secondary MR.

Please access ExpertConsult to view the corresponding videos for this chapter.

Acknowledgments

The authors acknowledge the contributions of Drs. Jacob Dal-Bianco, Robert Levine, and Steven Goldstein, who were the authors of this chapter in the previous edition.

REFERENCES

1. Lamas GA, Mitchell GF, Flaker GC, et al. Clinical significance of mitral regurgitation after acute myocardial infarction. *Circulation.* 1997;96:827–833.
2. Grigioni F, Enriquez-Sarano M, Zehr KJ, et al. Ischemic mitral regurgitation: long-term outcome and prognostic implications with quantitative Doppler assessment. *Circulation.* 2001;103:1759–1764.
3. Rossi A, Dini FL, Faggiano P, et al. Independent prognostic value of functional mitral regurgitation in patients with heart failure: a quantitative analysis of 1256 patients with ischaemic and non-ischaemic dilated cardiomyopathy. *Heart.* 2011;97:1675–1680.
4. Bertrand PB, Schwammenthal E, Levine RA, et al. Exercise dynamics in secondary mitral regurgitation: pathophysiology and therapeutic implications. *Circulation.* 2017;135:297–314.
5. Deferm S, Bertrand PB, Verbrugge FH, et al. Atrial functional mitral regurgitation: JACC review topic of the week. *J Am Coll Cardiol.* 2019;73:2465–2476.
6. Otsuji Y, Kumanohoso T, Yoshifuku S, et al. Isolated annular dilatation does not usually cause important functional mitral regurgitation: comparison between patients with lone atrial fibrillation and those with idiopathic or ischemic cardiomyopathy. *J Am Coll Cardiol.* 2002;39:1651–1656.
7. Kaji S, Nasu M, Yamamuro A, et al. Annular geometry in patients with chronic ischemic mitral regurgitation: 3D magnetic resonance imaging study. *Circulation.* 2005;112:I409–I1414.
8. Daimon M, Gillinov AM, Liddicoat JR, et al. Dynamic change in mitral annular area and motion during percutaneous mitral annuloplasty for ischemic mitral regurgitation: preliminary animal study with real-time 3D echocardiography. *J Am Soc Echocardiogr.* 2007;20:381–388.
9. Bartko PE, Arfsten H, Heitzinger G, et al. Papillary muscle dyssynchrony-mediated functional mitral regurgitation: mechanistic insights and modulation by cardiac resynchronization. *JACC Cardiovasc Imag.* 2019;12:1728–1737.
10. Dal-Bianco JP, Aikawa E, Bischoff J, et al. Active adaptation of the tethered mitral valve: insights into a compensatory mechanism for functional mitral regurgitation. *Circulation.* 2009;120:334–342.
11. Dal-Bianco JP, Aikawa E, Bischoff J, et al. Myocardial infarction alters adaptation of the tethered mitral valve. *J Am Coll Cardiol.* 2016;67:275–287.
12. Gorman 3rd JH, Gorman RC, Plappert T, et al. Infarct size and location determine development of mitral regurgitation in the sheep model. *J Thorac Cardiovasc Surg.* 1998;115:615–622.
13. Watanabe N, Ogasawara Y, Yamaura Y, et al. Geometric differences of the mitral valve tenting between anterior and inferior myocardial infarction with significant ischemic mitral regurgitation: quantitation by novel software system with transthoracic real-time 3D echocardiography. *J Am Soc Echocardiogr.* 2006;19:71–75.
14. Zeng X, Nunes MC, Dent J, et al. Asymmetric versus symmetric tethering patterns in ischemic mitral regurgitation: geometric differences from three-dimensional transesophageal echocardiography. *J Am Soc Echocardiogr.* 2014;27:367–375.
15. Otsuji Y, Handschumacher MD, Schwammenthal E, et al. Insights from 3D echocardiography into the mechanism of functional mitral regurgitation: direct in vivo demonstration of altered leaflet tethering geometry. *Circulation.* 1997;96:1999–2008.
16. Hung J, Otsuji Y, Handschumacher MD, et al. Mechanism of dynamic regurgitant orifice area variation in functional mitral regurgitation: physiologic insights from the proximal flow convergence technique. *J Am Coll Cardiol.* 1999;33:538–545.
17. Schwammenthal E, Chen C, Benning F, et al. Dynamics of mitral regurgitant flow and orifice area. Physiologic application of the proximal flow convergence method: clinical data and experimental testing. *Circulation.* 1994;90:307–322.
18. Breithardt OA, Sinha AM, Schwammenthal E, et al. Acute effects of cardiac resynchronization therapy on functional mitral regurgitation in advanced systolic heart failure. *J Am Coll Cardiol.* 2003;41:765–770.

19. Silbiger JJ. Does left atrial enlargement contribute to mitral leaflet tethering in patients with functional mitral regurgitation? Proposed role of atriogenic leaflet tethering. *Echocardiography.* 2014;31:1310–1311.
20. Gertz ZM, Raina A, Saghy L, et al. Evidence of atrial functional mitral regurgitation due to atrial fibrillation: reversal with arrhythmia control. *J Am Coll Cardiol.* 2011;58:1474–1481.
21. Harari R, Bansal P, Yatskar L, et al. Papillary muscle rupture following acute myocardial infarction: anatomic, echocardiographic, and surgical insights. *Echocardiography.* 2017;34:1702–1707.
22. Zoghbi WA, Adams D, Bonow RO, et al. Recommendations for noninvasive evaluation of native valvular regurgitation. *J Am Soc Echocardiogr.* 2017;30:303–371.
23. Yosefy C, Levine RA, Solis J, et al. Proximal flow convergence region as assessed by real-time 3-dimensional echocardiography: challenging the hemispheric assumption. *J Am Soc Echocardiogr.* 2007;20:389–396.
24. Goliasch G, Bartko PE, Pavo N, et al. Refining the prognostic impact of functional mitral regurgitation in chronic heart failure. *Eur Heart J.* 2018;39:39–46.

25. Bartko PE, Arfsten H, Heitzinger G, et al. A unifying concept for the quantitative assessment of secondary mitral regurgitation. *J Am Coll Cardiol.* 2019;73:2506–2517.
26. Grayburn PA, Sannino A, Packer M. Proportionate and disproportionate functional mitral regurgitation: a new conceptual framework that reconciles the results of the MITRA-FR and COAPT trials. *JACC Cardiovasc Imag.* 2019;12:353–362.
27. Acker MA, Gelijns AC, Kron IL. Surgery for severe ischemic mitral regurgitation. *N Engl J Med.* 2014;370:1463.
28. Goldstein D, Moskowitz AJ, Gelijns AC, et al. Two-year outcomes of surgical treatment of severe ischemic mitral regurgitation. *N Engl J Med.* 2015;374:344–353.
29. Hung J, Papakostas L, Tahta SA, et al. Mechanism of recurrent ischemic mitral regurgitation after annuloplasty: continued LV remodeling as a moving target. *Circulation.* 2004;110:II85–II90.
30. Stone GW, Lindenfeld J, Abraham WT, et al. Transcatheter mitral-valve repair in patients with heart failure. *N Engl J Med.* 2018;379:2307–2318.
31. Obadia JF, Messika-Zeitoun D, Leurent G, et al. Percutaneous repair or medical treatment for secondary mitral regurgitation. *N Engl J Med.* 2018;379:2297–2306.

98   Quantification of Mitral Regurgitation

Mohammed A. Chamsi-Pasha, Stephen H. Little

Mitral regurgitation (MR) is the most common valvular disease in the developed world and is expected to increase with the aging population.[1] Primary MR is caused by an intrinsic valve abnormality (usually degenerative mitral valve [MV] disease), whereas secondary (functional) MR occurs in the setting of left ventricular (LV) remodeling, mitral annular dilatation, or both. Numerous studies have shown that untreated, severe MR is associated with poor outcomes because of adverse remodeling of the left ventricle. Among patients with flail MVs and severe MR, 90% were dead or required surgery at 10 years follow-up in a multicenter study.[2]

ECHOCARDIOGRAPHIC ASSESSMENT OF MR

Transthoracic echocardiography (TTE) with Doppler is the initial recommended modality for MR evaluation. The role of TTE is to identify the cause of MR, quantify the lesion severity, assess the response of the LV to volume overload, and determine the feasibility of durable repair.[3] Detailed assessment of the MV anatomy, including annular and subvalvular structures (chordae and papillary muscles), need to be well described on TTE. Severe MR rarely occurs when the MV leaflets or apparatus or LV structure or function are normal.

The most recent 2017 American Society of Echocardiography (ASE) guidelines for native valvular regurgitation[4] recommend integrating multiple parameters because all of the proposed indices have intrinsic limitations, mainly because of the complex geometry of the mitral orifice. It is important to recognize that the data obtained from imaging studies need to be interpreted in the context of the clinical presentation and physical examination.

Semiquantitative methods. There are multiple semiquantitative parameters derived from TTE when assessing the severity of MR. These parameters include color-flow Doppler (with its three components: flow convergence, vena contracta, and jet area) (Fig. 98.1), MR signal intensity, transmitral flow, and pulmonary venous flow pattern.

Quantitative methods. Quantitative assessment uses either the proximal isovelocity surface area (PISA)–derived effective regurgitant orifice area (EROA) or the Doppler-volumetric method. The development of three-dimensional echocardiography (3DE) has improved the assessment of MR by measuring the

vena contracta area (VCA the narrowest, highest-velocity region of the jet flow), which is a direct measure of the EROA, although data relating different cutoffs to outcomes are not yet available. Its advantages lie in overcoming the limitations that can be posed by a noncircular orifice.

Impact of hemodynamics on MR evaluation. Hemodynamic condition such as blood pressure and the duration of MR can have significant effect on the accuracy of MR severity assessment.[5] This is particularly relevant when using color-flow Doppler as a solo method for assessing MR severity. The high driving pressure of a hypertensive LV can lead to a larger jet area without increase in MR volume because color Doppler displays velocity and not flow (Fig. 98.2).

MR duration. The duration of MR is also important, especially in the setting of MV prolapse, in which predominant late systolic MR may occur with a large regurgitant jet that is only present for a fraction of systole. A large jet that appears late in systole may result in a larger EROA but with a small regurgitant volume (Fig. 98.3). All single-frame measurements such as jet area, vena contracta width, or PISA should be used only cautiously when MR is not holosystolic.

TWO-DIMENSIONAL PROXIMAL ISOVELOCITY SURFACE AREA METHOD

As flow approaches a circular orifice, concentric hemispheric shells of increasing velocity and decreasing surface area form proximal to the orifice. With color Doppler imaging, the hemispheric shells proximal to the regurgitant orifice area can be identified and the radius (r) measured at appropriate aliasing velocity (Va). An important consideration is that the measurement of the PISA radius should be performed at the time of the peak MR velocity by continuous-wave (CW) Doppler. The squared radius is then used to calculate the surface area ($2 \pi r^2$) of the hemisphere. Thereafter, the mitral regurgitant flow (MRF, in mL/s) can be calculated by multiplying the area of the shell by the aliasing velocity:

$$\text{MRF} = 2 \pi r^2 \times \text{Va}$$

The maximum effective regurgitant orifice area (EROA, in cm²) can then be derived by dividing the mitral regurgitant flow by the corresponding peak MR velocity (in cm/s) based on the conservation of mass law.[5] If the regurgitant orifice area is constant throughout

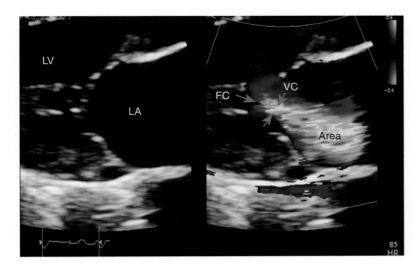

Figure 98.1. Depiction of the three components of a color flow regurgitant jet of mitral regurgitation: flow convergence (FC), used for the proximal isovelocity surface area method, vena contracta (VC), and jet area. *LA,* Left atrium; *LV,* left ventricle.

Effect of Pressure Difference on Regurgitation Severity

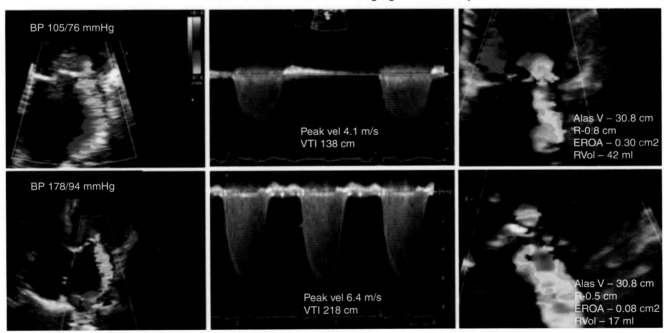

Figure 98.2. The images are from two patients with functional ischemic mitral regurgitation (MR) caused by posterior leaflet restriction, left ventricular ejection fraction of 30%, and similar appearance of eccentric MR jets directed laterally but different regurgitant volumes. The patient in the *top panels* has a low MR velocity (4.1 m/s) consistent with low blood pressure (BP) and/or elevated left atrial pressure, with moderate MR (regurgitant volume [RVol], 42 m). The patient in the *lower panels* has a peak MR velocity of 6.4 m/s because of hypertension but with mild MR (RVol,17 mL). *Alas V,* Aliasing velocity; *EROA,* effective regurgitant orifice area; *vel,* velocity. (Reproduced with permission from Zoghbi WA, et al: Recommendations for noninvasive evaluation of native valvular regurgitation, *J Am Soc Echocardiogr* 30:303–371, 2017.)

systole, the regurgitant volume can be calculated as the product of EROA and the velocity time integral (VTI) of the MR jet (Fig. 98.4).

One caveat to this method is that it assumes a hemispheric shape. When the orifice is noncircular (as is typically seen with functional MR), the PISA method may underestimate EROA.[6] In addition, proper CW Doppler alignment with the MR jet is needed because poor alignment can result in underestimation of the peak velocity and an overestimation of EROA. This method has been widely used and validated in numerous studies, with a cutoff of 40 mm^2 or greater carrying an independent prognostic marker for poor outcomes in asymptomatic patients.[7]

TWO-DIMENSIONAL VOLUMETRIC METHOD

Quantitative Doppler method. Flow rate and stroke volume of the mitral and aortic valve annuli can be obtained using pulse Doppler VTI recordings and two-dimensional (2D) measurements (Fig. 98.5). This is derived by measuring the diameter of the annulus and VTI of the mitral inflow velocity using pulsed-wave (PW) Doppler at the mitral annulus. In the presence of regurgitation of one valve, the flow through the affected valve will be larger than that through a competent valve. MR regurgitant volume can then be calculated as the stroke volume difference

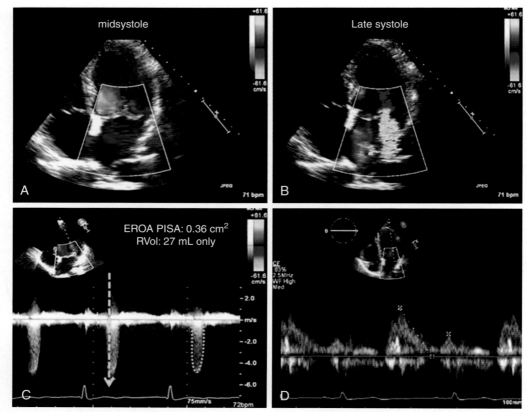

Figure 98.3. Late systolic mitral regurgitation (MR) in mitral valve prolapse (MVP). **A,** Midsystolic frame shows no MR by color Doppler. **B,** Late systolic frame shows an eccentric MR jet with a large flow convergence. **C,** Continuous-wave Doppler profile of MR jet demonstrates that MR is confined to late systole (onset at *yellow arrow*, small velocity time integral of jet, *dotted contour*). **D,** Pulsed-wave Doppler of mitral inflow shows an E wave velocity of 75 cm/s with normal E/e′ ratio consistent with normal left atrial pressure. Calculation of effective regurgitant orifice area (EROA) overestimates the severity of regurgitation when the quantitation of regurgitation should rely on regurgitant volume (RVol) by either proximal isovelocity surface area (PISA) or volumetric measures (RVol, 27 mL). (Reproduced with permission from Zoghbi WA, et al: Recommendations for noninvasive evaluation of native valvular regurgitation, *J Am Soc Echocardiogr* 30:303–371, 2017.)

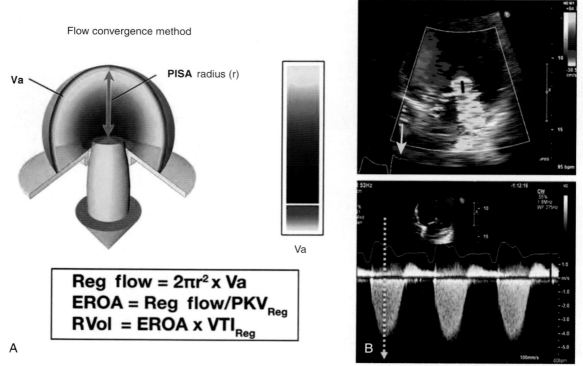

Figure 98.4. A, Schematic representation of the flow convergence method (PISA). **B,** Measurement of PISA radius and timing of the selection of the color frame for measurement *(solid yellow arrow)*, corresponding to the maximal jet velocity by continuous-wave Doppler *(dashed arrow)*. *EROA,* Effective regurgitant orifice area; *PKV,* peak velocity; *Reg,* regurgitant; *RVol,* regurgitant volume; *VTI,* velocity time interval. (Reproduced with permission from Zoghbi WA, et al: Recommendations for noninvasive evaluation of native valvular regurgitation, *J Am Soc Echocardiogr* 30:303–371, 2017.)

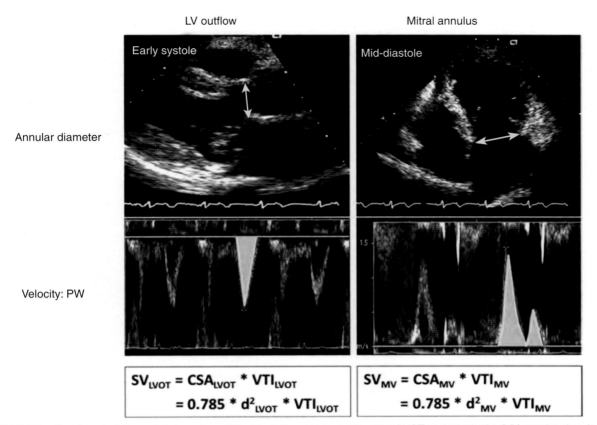

LV outflow   Mitral annulus

Early systole   Mid-diastole

Annular diameter

Velocity: PW

$$SV_{LVOT} = CSA_{LVOT} * VTI_{LVOT}$$
$$= 0.785 * d^2_{LVOT} * VTI_{LVOT}$$

$$SV_{MV} = CSA_{MV} * VTI_{MV}$$
$$= 0.785 * d^2_{MV} * VTI_{MV}$$

Figure 98.5. Echo Doppler calculations of stroke volume (SV) at the left ventricular outflow tract (LVOT) and mitral valve (MV) annulus sites. In this example of severe mitral regurgitation, SV at MV was 183 mL (d = 3.5 cm, VTI = 19 cm). and SV at the LVOT was 58 mL (d = 2.3 cm, VTI = 14 cm). This yielded a regurgitant volume (RVol) of 125 mL and a regurgitant fraction (RF) of 125/183 or 68%. *CSA,* Cross-sectional area; *d,* diameter of the annulus; *PW,* pulsed-wave Doppler.

between mitral flow and left ventricular outflow tract (LVOT) flow. This method is especially recommended in early and late systolic MR and eccentric and multiple jets (Video 98.1).[4]

To reduce errors in the calculation, the sample volume should be placed at the level of the annulus, tracing of the PW Doppler envelope should be done at the modal velocity, and the annulus should be properly measured. Limitations of this method include errors in mitral annular diameter measurement, noncircular annular dimension, and inapplicability of this method in the presence of concomitant aortic regurgitation.[3]

Alternative method. An alternative method is to subtract the LVOT volume from the 2D total LV stroke volume (derived using the Simpson's biplane method of discs to measure LV end-diastolic and end-systolic volume). One limitation to this technique is that TTE tends to underestimate stroke volume because of LV foreshortening of the apex and because of difficulties delineating the entire endocardial border. Use of LV opacification agents reduces this limitation. A recent study assessed the use of 3D full-volume color Doppler to quantify mitral inflow and aortic outflow stroke volumes and compared each with a cardiac magnetic resonance imaging (CMRI) reference standard. This showed better accuracy and agreement than the conventional 2D method, especially in multijet MR.[8]

THREE-DIMENSIONAL ECHOCARDIOGRAPHY

3D transesophageal echocardiography (TEE) has been the cornerstone for evaluating MV morphology and provide high-resolution imaging to accurately localize lesions. The technique has been instrumental over the years to delineate the mechanism of MR but also to allow more accurate assessment of MR severity (Video 98.2). Direct assessment of the vena contracta by 3DE revealed significant asymmetry of the VCA in MR. This is best demonstrated in patients with ischemic MR, in whom 3DE frequently depicts the VCA to be eccentric rather than circular (Fig. 98.6). This highlights why EROA is underestimated by single-plane vena contracta width measurement. Studies comparing VCA by 3DE with other quantitative parameters show better reproducibility and accuracy.[9] In one study, A 3D VCA cutoff of 0.41 cm[2] was 82% sensitive and 97% specific in differentiating moderate from severe MR, regardless of whether the cause of MR is ischemic or degenerative.[10]

SUPPORTIVE FINDINGS

Other findings that support the presence of severe MR include density of the CW Doppler signal of the MR jet, the presence of pulmonary hypertension, the profile of pulsed Doppler tracing of the mitral inflow, and the pattern of pulmonary vein flow.

MR jet density. The intensity of the CW spectral Doppler signal of the MR jet reflects the number of red blood cells in the jet and the regurgitant volume. Very dense signal, at least equal to that of antegrade flow, suggest that the degree of MR is moderate or severe. A faint or incomplete signal suggests a mild degree of MR. These generalizations require that the CW cursor passes through the vena contracta. Another indicator of severe MR is the so-called cutoff sign. In cases of acute, severe MR, the contour of the CW spectral Doppler may be asymmetric, truncated, or triangular, with early peaking of the maximal velocity. The

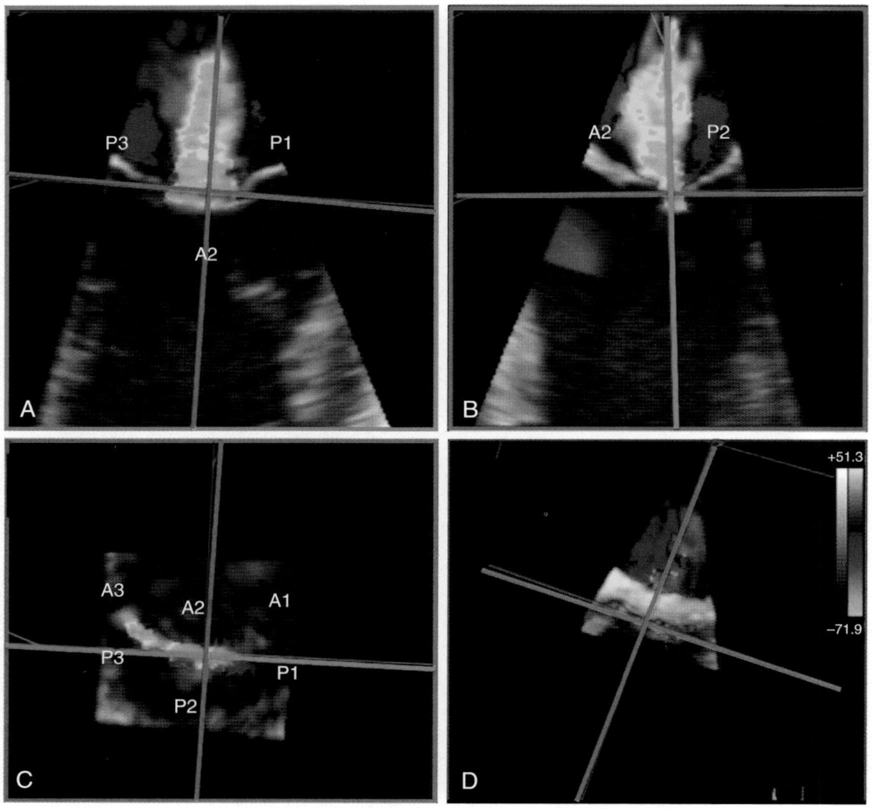

Figure 98.6. Multiplanar reconstruction analysis of a three-dimensional (3D) transesophageal echocardiography color Doppler data set of a patient with ischemic mitral regurgitation. The *green* (**A**), *red* (**B**), and *blue* (**C**) *frames* are orthogonal cut planes through the 3D color Doppler data set (**D**). The *blue plane* (**C**) is an en face view through which the *green* (**A**) and *red* (**B**) cut planes through the mitral valve or regurgitant jet can be visualized. Note that in this en face view, the vena contracta area is not circular but crescent. Also, from the en face view, the differences in the vena contracta width seen in the *green* (**A**) and *red* (**B**) cut planes can be understood.

CW Doppler signal of chronic MR is usually symmetric and parabolic. Low velocity less than 4 m/s suggests markedly elevated left atrial (LA) pressure or low LV systolic pressures (or both).

Mitral inflow velocities. When there is severe MR with large regurgitant volume, the antegrade flow across the MV is increased. Thus, severe MR is suggested when the pulse Doppler tracing of mitral inflow at the mitral leaflet tips demonstrated a velocity of greater than 1.2 m/s. In contrast, severe MR is effectively excluded when an A-wave dominant mitral inflow pattern is present.

Pulmonary veins. The presence of systolic flow reversal in the pulmonary veins is a specific finding of severe MR. With TEE, both a right and left pulmonary vein should be sampled because eccentric jets may enter only right- or left-sided veins.

Chamber dilatation. Enlargement of the LV and LA nearly always accompany chronic, severe MR. Normal LA and LV virtually excludes chronic, severe MR. Moreover, the LV size has prognostic significance. However, enlargement of the left atrium or left ventricle may be caused by other pathologies and are not specific for severe MR.

CARDIAC MAGNETIC RESONANCE IMAGING ROLE IN MITRAL REGURGITATION ASSESSMENT

CMRI has been the gold standard for assessment of LV size and systolic function. Consistently, CMRI has been shown to be accurate and reproducible and is able to indirectly assess severity of MR by quantifying the difference in LV stroke volume and forward flow (aortic stroke volume).[4] Few studies have compared the quantitation of MR using a TTE-derived integrative approach compared with volumetric assessment with CMRI, which at best is modest. An absolute agreement varies widely from 47% to 87% based on the studies.[11] Most of these differences were noted in patients with late systolic or multiple jets. Discordant findings (CMRI severe with echo moderate or CMRI moderate with echo severe) were

seen in 24% among 258 asymptomatic patients with moderate or severe MR.[12] The mean echo-derived regurgitant volume was about 17 mL larger than the CMRI derived regurgitant volume. When looking at all-cause mortality and indications for MV surgery, CMRI regurgitant volumes had the largest area under the curve to predict these endpoints. Another study looked at 109 patients with asymptomatic severe MR with mean duration follow-up of 8 years. A total of 91% of subjects with regurgitant volume 55 mL or less survived to 5 years without surgery versus 21% with a regurgitant volume greater than 55 mL.[13]

One advantage of CMRI is the ability to detect replacement fibrosis using late gadolinium enhancement (LGE). In patients with MV prolapse, a higher prevalence of LGE in the posteromedial papillary muscle has been described and interpreted as being an incremental predictor of arrhythmic events (sudden cardiac death, ventricular arrhythmias).[14] One of the few limitations of CMRI is that it is not widely available compared with echocardiography. In addition, there are no established CMRI-derived regurgitant volume threshold values to establish independent cutoffs of MR severity or predictors of surgical benefit.

SUMMARY

Assessment of MR severity is challenging for a variety of reasons, including the complexity of the MR orifice and the resulting jet. The sole reliance on the visual assessment of MR color jet area should be discouraged. Multiple 2D echocardiographic methods should be integrated into routine assessment. The strengths and weaknesses of each of these methods should be appreciated. Obviously, the accurate assessment of MR may not be feasible in every case. Hence, the ASE guidelines emphasize the need for additional testing when the echocardiographic examination is inadequate or with discordant parameters between Doppler findings and clinical assessment.[4] This can be done with either TEE or CMRI[4] (Fig. 98.7).

98

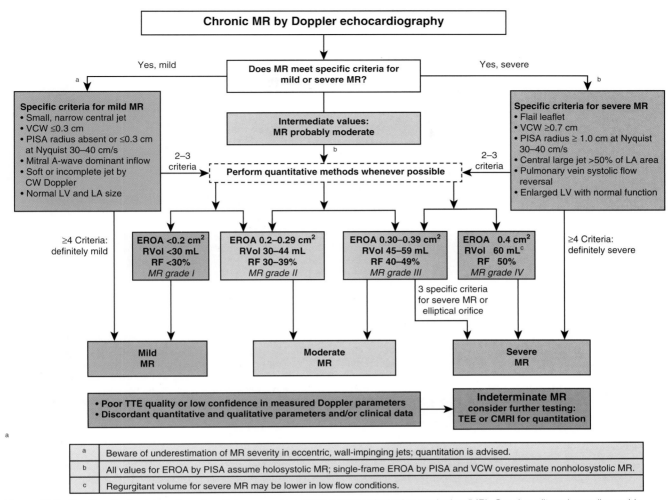

Figure 98.7. Algorithm for the integration of multiple parameters of the severity of mitral regurgitation (MR). Good-quality echocardiographic imaging and complete data acquisition are assumed. If imaging is technically difficult, consider transesophageal echocardiography (TEE) or cardiac magnetic resonance imaging (CMRI). The severity of MR is indeterminate because of poor image quality, technical issues with data, internal inconsistency among echo findings, or discordance with clinical findings. *CW,* Continuous wave; *EROA,* effective regurgitant orifice area; *LA,* left atrium; *LV,* left ventricle; *PISA,* proximal isovelocity surface area; *RF,* regurgitant fraction; *RVol,* regurgitant volume; *VCW,* vena contracta width. (Reproduced with permission from Zoghbi WA, et al: Recommendations for noninvasive evaluation of native valvular regurgitation, *J Am Soc Echocardiogr* 30:303–371, 2017.)

Acknowledgments

The authors acknowledge the contributions of Drs. Wendy Tsang, Benjamin Freed, and Roberto Lang, who were the authors of this chapter in the previous edition.

Please access ExpertConsult to view the corresponding videos for this chapter.

REFERENCES

1. Nishimura RA, Otto CM, Bonow RO, et al. 2017 AHA/ACC focused update of the 2014 AHA/ACC guideline for the management of patients with valvular heart disease. *J Am Coll Cardiol.* 2017;70:252–289.
2. Grigioni F, Tribouilloy C, Avierinos JF, et al. Outcomes in mitral regurgitation due to flail leaflets a multicenter European study. *JACC Cardiovasc Imag.* 2008;1:133–141.
3. Essayagh B, Antoine C, Benfari G, et al. Prognostic implications of left atrial enlargement in degenerative mitral regurgitation. *J Am Coll Cardiol.* 2019;74:858–870.
4. Zoghbi WA, Adams D, Bonow RO, et al. Recommendations for noninvasive evaluation of native valvular regurgitation. *J Am Soc Echocardiogr.* 2017;30:303–371.
5. El-Tallawi KC, Messika-Zeitoun D, Zoghbi WA. Assessment of the severity of native mitral valve regurgitation. *Prog Cardiovasc Dis.* 2017;60:322–333.
6. Chandra S, Salgo IS, Sugeng L, et al. A three-dimensional insight into the complexity of flow convergence in mitral regurgitation: adjunctive benefit of anatomic regurgitant orifice area. *Am J Physiol Heart Circ Physiol.* 2011;301:H1015–H1024.
7. Enriquez-Sarano M, Avierinos JF, Messika-Zeitoun D, et al. Quantitative determinants of the outcome of asymptomatic mitral regurgitation. *N Engl J Med.* 2005;352:875–883.
8. Heo R, Son JW, Ó Hartaigh B, et al. Clinical implications of three-dimensional real-time color Doppler transthoracic echocardiography in quantifying mitral regurgitation: a comparison with conventional two-dimensional methods. *J Am Soc Echocardiogr.* 2017;30:393–403.
9. Little SH, Pirat B, Kumar R, et al. Three-dimensional color Doppler echocardiography for direct measurement of vena contracta area in mitral regurgitation: in vitro validation and clinical experience. *JACC Cardiovasc Imag.* 2008;1:695–704.
10. Zeng X, Levine RA, Hua L, et al. Diagnostic value of vena contracta area in the quantification of mitral regurgitation severity by color Doppler 3D echocardiography. *Circ Cardiovasc Imag.* 2011;4:506–513.
11. Uretsky S, Argulian E, Narula J, Wolff SD. Use of cardiac magnetic resonance imaging in assessing mitral regurgitation: Current evidence. *J Am Coll Cardiol.* 2018;71:547–563.
12. Penicka M, Vecera J, Mirica DC, et al. Prognostic implications of magnetic resonance-derived quantification in asymptomatic patients with organic mitral regurgitation: comparison with Doppler echocardiography-derived integrative approach. *Circulation.* 2018;137:1349–1360.
13. Myerson SG, d'Arcy J, Christiansen JP, et al. Determination of clinical outcome in mitral regurgitation with cardiovascular magnetic resonance quantification. *Circulation.* 2016;133:2287–2296.
14. Kitkungvan D, Nabi F, Kim RJ, et al. Myocardial fibrosis in patients with primary mitral regurgitation with and without prolapse. *J Am Coll Cardiol.* 2018;72:823–834.

99 Asymptomatic Severe Mitral Regurgitation

Mohammed A. Chamsi-Pasha, Stephen H. Little

Mitral regurgitation (MR) may result from primary abnormalities of the mitral valve (MV) apparatus (primary or degenerative MR) or from left ventricular (LV) dysfunction and remodeling (functional or secondary MR). The current American College of Cardiology (ACC)/American Heart Association (AHA) guidelines recommend surgery in symptomatic patients with chronic severe MR; ACC/AHA stage D in all patients with primary (degenerative) MR and only in selected patients with secondary (functional) MR (those with persistent marked heart failure symptoms).

The severity of either primary or secondary MR is based on the presence of an effective regurgitant orifice area (EROA) 0.4 cm^2 or greater, regurgitant volume 60 mL or greater, and regurgitant fraction 50% or greater, which applies for both primary or secondary MR.[1] One should keep in mind that in secondary MR, EROA and regurgitant volume can be lower because of the crescent shape of the flow convergence (when using the Proximal Isovelocity Surface Area (PISA) method) or low-flow conditions. Per the American Society of Echocardiography guidelines on valvular regurgitation, when multiple parameters are concordant, MR severity can be determined with high probability, especially for mild or severe MR.[2]

APPROACH TO ASYMPTOMATIC SEVERE MITRAL REGURGITATION

The paucity of high-quality studies in asymptomatic patients with chronic severe MR makes management controversial between watchful waiting versus early surgery. Indications for surgical treatment of MR are summarized in Table 99.1. Historically, the defendants of the *primum non nocere* concept suggest that a watchful waiting strategy is reasonable given the overall low annual mortality rate in this group. Recent growing evidence (albeit consisting only of observational studies) shows better outcomes in surgically treated asymptomatic patients, specifically in the setting of flail leaflets when the operative mortality rate is low in experienced valve centers. One study has shown that in asymptomatic MR patients with normal ventricular function, the 5-year combined incidence of atrial fibrillation, heart failure, or cardiovascular death was 42% ± 8%.[3]

SURGICAL INDICATIONS IN ASYMPTOMATIC PATIENTS

In MR, loading conditions on the heart with typically reduced afterload alter the left ventricular ejection fraction (LVEF); hence, hyperdynamic function is expected in significant MR. The main indications for surgery in asymptomatic patients are based on data showing that dysfunctional myocardium in the setting of severe MR is associated with impaired postoperative survival.[4] The current ACC/AHA guidelines recommend surgery for asymptomatic patients with severe primary MR (ACC/AHA stage C) when the LVEF is 60% or less or the left ventricular end-systolic dimension (LVESD) is above 40 mm (signs of impending irreversible LV dysfunction).[1] In asymptomatic patients with severe primary MR with preserved LVEF who have a high likelihood of having MV repair (>95%) and a very low operative mortality rate, the ACC/AHA gives a class IIa indication for surgery. This is in contrast to the European Society of Cardiology (ESC)[5] guidelines, which consider surgical treatment when the LVESD is 40 to 44 mm in the presence of either a flail leaflet or significant left atrial (LA) dilatation (volume index ≥60 mL/m^2).

WATCHFUL WAITING VERSUS EARLY SURGERY

The data supporting the watchful waiting strategy in patients with chronic severe primary MR come from multiple studies. Rosenhek and colleagues[6] prospectively followed 132 asymptomatic patients with severe MR with serial examination and referred to surgery only when class I or class II criteria (as described in the guidelines) were fulfilled. Freedom from all-cause mortality was not significantly different from the expected survival. Data in favor of early surgery come from the Mitral Regurgitation International Database registry showing that MV repair was associated with survival benefit in patients with flail leaflets compared with watchful waiting (freedom from all-cause mortality, 89% ± 2% vs, 85% ± 2%, respectively).[7] In a recent contemporary cohort by Kang and colleagues,[8] 610 patients with asymptomatic severe MR were evaluated with early surgery versus watchful waiting. In a propensity-matched cohort, significant reduction in cardiac mortality rate and events was noted in the surgical arm, particularly in patients older than 50 years of age.

A recent systematic review looking at five observational studies published to date comparing management plans for asymptomatic severe MR[9] found a significant reduction in long-term mortality with an early surgery strategy (hazard ratio [HR], 0.38; 95% confidence interval [CI], 0.1–0.71) versus watchful waiting. Inherent limitations of this analysis involve the observational nature of those studies, significant heterogeneity of the demographics, and selection bias because these studies were conducted at tertiary care centers. Per guideline recommendations, asymptomatic patients with severe asymptomatic MR and preserved LV function are to be followed on a yearly basis with serial echocardiographic examinations. The active surveillance strategy proved efficacious in a single-center study involving 280 patients prospectively enrolled with severe MR.[10] Event-free survival rates were 78% at 2 years, 52.2% at 6 years, 35.5% the 10 years, and 18.7% at 15 years. Long-term survival and surgical outcomes were excellent. In summary, most patients with severe MR require surgery over the next 6 to 10 years after diagnosis, mostly because of symptoms or LV dysfunction.

If patients are asymptomatic, exercise stress testing may be performed to unmask symptoms or demonstrate elevated pulmonary artery systolic pressure, worsening MR, or failure of LV systolic function to augment normally.[11] Recent data show that exercise-induced pulmonary hypertension (systolic pulmonary pressure ≥60 mm Hg) can predict the need for surgery.[5] Other markers that can influence decision making is LA dilatation. This has been incorporated in the ESC guidelines as a surrogate to early intervention. A recent study by Essayagh and coworkers.[12] showed that severe LA enlargement (LA volume index ≥60 mL/m^2) in patients with primary MR was an independent predictor of increased mortality rate and that it was partially reversed by surgery versus medical management. Indeed, these patients had the most severe MR, larger LV volumes, and higher prevalence of atrial fibrillation, pulmonary hypertension, and tricuspid regurgitation, which can introduce a source of bias.

TABLE 99.1 Indications for Surgery in Asymptomatic Severe Mitral Regurgitation

	ESC 2017	ACC/AHA 2017
LV dysfunction (LVESD ≥45 mm and/or LVEF ≤60%)	Class I; LOE: B	
LV dysfunction (LVESD ≥40 mm and/or LVEF ≤60%)		Class I; LOE: B
Preserved LVEF >60% and LVESD <45 mm with atrial fibrillation or pulmonary hypertension (PASP >50 mm Hg)	Class IIa; LOE: B	Class IIa; LOE: B
Preserved LVEF >60% and LVESD 40–44 mm when durable repair is likely, surgical risk is low, and repair is performed in a heart valve center with at least flail leaflet or significant LA dilatation (LA volume index ≥60 mL/m²)	Class IIa; LOE: C	
Preserved LVEF >60% and LVESD <40 mm when successful and durable repair likelihood is >95% and low mortality		Class IIa, LOE: B
Preserved LVEF >60% and LVESD <40 mm with a progressive increase in LV size or decrease in EF on serial imaging studies		Class IIa; LOE: C

ACC, American College of Cardiology; *AHA,* American Heart Association; *EF,* ejection fraction; *ESC,* European Society of Cardiology; *LA,* left atrial; *LV,* left ventricular; *LVESD,* left ventricular end-systolic diameter; *LVEF,* left ventricular ejection fraction; *LOE,* level of evidence; *PASP,* pulmonary artery systolic pressure.

GLOBAL LONGITUDINAL STRAIN AND SEVERE MITRAL REGURGITATION

Global longitudinal strain (GLS) is a sensitive marker for subclinical LV dysfunction with growing role in cardio-oncology and patients with valvular heart disease and cardiomyopathy. In asymptomatic severe MR patients, few studies have shown that the impaired LV GLS predicts a decrease in LVEF shortly after surgery and is independently associated with an increased mortality rate (HR, 1.6; 95% CI, 1.47–1.73) for strain values below a median of 21.7%.[13]

REFERENCES

1. Nishimura RA, Otto CM, Bonow RO, et al. 2017 AHA/ACC Focused update of the 2014 AHA/ACC guideline for the management of patients with valvular heart disease. *J Am Coll Cardiol.* 2017;70:252–289.
2. Zoghbi WA, Adams D, Bonow RO, et al. Recommendations for noninvasive evaluation of native valvular regurgitation. *J Am Soc Echocardiogr.* 2017;30:303–371.
3. Grigioni F, Tribouilloy C, Avierinos JF, et al. Outcomes in mitral regurgitation due to flail leaflets a multicenter European study. *Cardiovasc Imag.* 2008;1:133–141.
4. Enriquez-Sarano M, Tajik AJ, Schaff HV, et al. Echocardiographic prediction of left ventricular function after correction of mitral regurgitation: results and clinical implications. *J Am Coll Cardiol.* 1994;24:1536–1543.
5. Baumgartner H, Falk V, Bax JJ, et al. 2017 ESC/EACTS Guidelines for the management of valvular heart disease. *Eur Heart J.* 2017;38:2739–2791.
6. Rosenhek R, Rader F, Klaar U, et al. Outcome of watchful waiting in asymptomatic severe mitral regurgitation. *Circulation.* 2006;113:2238–2244.
7. Suri RM, Vanoverschelde JL, Grigioni F, et al. Association between early surgical intervention vs watchful waiting and outcomes for mitral regurgitation due to flail mitral valve leaflets. *J Am Med Assoc.* 2013;310:609–616.
8. Kang DH, Park SJ, Sun BJ, et al. Early surgery versus conventional treatment for asymptomatic severe mitral regurgitation: a propensity analysis. *J Am Coll Cardiol.* 2014;63:2398–2407.
9. Goldstone AB, Patrick WL, Cohen JE, et al. Early surgical intervention or watchful waiting for the management of asymptomatic mitral regurgitation: a systematic review and meta-analysis. *Ann Cardiothorac Surg.* 2015;4:220–229.
10. Zilberszac R, Heinze G, Binder T, et al. Long-term outcome of active surveillance in severe but asymptomatic primary mitral regurgitation. *JACC Cardiovasc Imag.* 2018;11:1213–1221.
11. O'Gara PT, Grayburn PA, Badhwar V, et al. 2017 ACC expert consensus decision pathway on the management of mitral regurgitation. *J Am Coll Cardiol.* 2017;70:2421–2449.
12. Essayagh B, Antoine C, Benfari G, et al. Prognostic implications of left atrial enlargement in degenerative mitral regurgitation. *J Am Coll Cardiol.* 2019;74:858–8570.
13. Mentias A, Naji P, Gillinov AM, et al. Strain echocardiography and functional capacity in asymptomatic primary mitral regurgitation with preserved ejection fraction. *J Am Coll Cardiol.* 2016;68:1974–1986.

100 Role of Exercise Stress Testing in Mitral Regurgitation

Patrizio Lancellotti, Simona Sperlongano, Alexandra Maria Chitroceanu, Adriana Postolache, Raluca Elena Dulgheru

Mitral regurgitation (MR) is a load-dependent valvular disease, and its increase in severity during exercise has been reported irrespective of cause.[1–7] The evaluation of MR limited to resting conditions risks may underestimate the full clinical impact of the lesion. Exercise stress testing (EST) can be a useful tool to identify the dynamic nature of MR. Indeed, EST is recommended by the guidelines on the management of heart valve disease in patients with severe primary MR who claim to be asymptomatic or have nonspecific symptoms, with the purpose to objectively unmask their symptoms.[8] Exercise stress echocardiography (ESE) is accepted by the current guidelines as a useful tool to identify the cardiac origin of dyspnea, and its use can provide diagnostic and prognostic information. Other EST modalities, such as treadmill exercise electrocardiography (ECG) or cardiopulmonary exercise testing (CPET), can be useful in the evaluation of patients with severe MR, not fulfilling other criteria for surgery, and claiming to be asymptomatic.

For patients with severe secondary MR, who are inherently symptomatic, treadmill exercise ECG does not provide information that would help managing the valve disease itself. However, EST is useful in assessing the full clinical impact of this valve lesion, namely increase or decrease of MR during exercise, rapid development of pulmonary hypertension during exercise, and its relation to symptoms. CPET can be used in all patients with

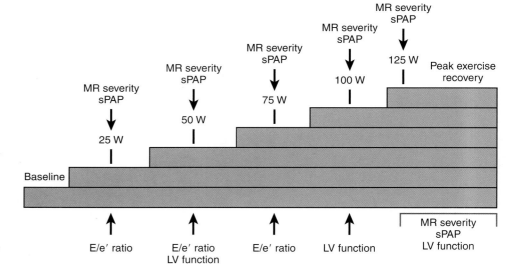

Figure 100.1. Stepwise Doppler echocardiography image acquisition in patients with mitral regurgitation (MR). *E/e´ ratio,* An estimate of left ventricular filling pressure; *LV,* left ventricular; *sPAP,* systolic pulmonary arterial pressure.

secondary MR, especially for its prognostic role in patients with heart failure. This chapter focuses on the use of ESE in patients with primary and secondary MR and discusses briefly other EST modalities in these patients.

EXERCISE STRESS ECHOCARDIOGRAPHY PROTOCOL

Images should be acquired at baseline and immediately postexercise when using a treadmill, or at baseline, low workload and peak exercise when using a semisupine bicycle ergometer. Exercise imaging allows quantification of changes in valvular regurgitation severity, left ventricular (LV) function, and pulmonary arterial pressure. A symptom-limited graded exercise test is recommended (patients should be encouraged to exercise until exhaustion), and at least 80% of the age-predicted upper heart rate should be reached in absence of symptoms.[3] The test should be performed under the supervision of an experienced physician. Typically, the initial workload of 25 W is maintained for 2 minutes, and the workload is increased every 2 minutes by 25 W (Fig. 100.1). An increase in steps of 10 W seems more appropriate in patients with a low level of physical activity (i.e., secondary MR in heart failure). In practice, image recordings are obtained in a stepwise fashion at baseline; at low, medium, and high levels of exercise; and at peak test (see Fig. 100.1). Images and loops are stored and analyzed offline after the test; often no measurements are done during image acquisition. Usually the following imaging sequence is used:

1. Two-dimensional (2D) grayscale loops (frame rate >50–70/s) of the left ventricle in four-, two-, and three-chamber views for global and regional LV systolic function assessment
2. Mitral annulus tissue Doppler velocities (~95–105 beats/min, before e´- and a´-wave fusion) and mitral inflow with pulsed-wave Doppler (close to e´ recording) to evaluate LV filling pressures
3. Color-flow Doppler of the MR for quantification of severity by the proximal isovelocity surface area (PISA) method and vena contracta and continuous-wave Doppler on the MR for quantification of severity by the PISA method
4. Continuous-wave (CW) Doppler of the tricuspid regurgitant jet to assess the transtricuspid pressure gradient and estimate the systolic pulmonary artery pressure (sPAP). To better identify patients with a rapid increase in pulmonary artery pressure at first stages of the exercise, CW Doppler of the tricuspid regurgitant jet should be the first parameter to be acquired before each level of exercise.

5. Dobutamine stress echocardiography is rarely used to assess MR dynamic behavior because of its nonphysiologic effect on the severity of regurgitation; the only exception is when ischemia is the suspected mechanism of MR.[1]

PRIMARY MITRAL REGURGITATION
Indications For Stress Echocardiography

In patients with severe MR, symptoms predict poor outcome after valve repair or replacement.[9] Reduced LV ejection fraction (LVEF) and LV dilatation are also important predictors of postoperative LV dysfunction[10] and subsequent cardiac morbidity and mortality.[11] Therefore, when patients with severe MR become symptomatic or develop LV dysfunction or dilatation (decrease in LVEF or increase in LV end-systolic diameter), mitral valve (MV) surgery, especially repair, is mandatory[8,12,13] (Fig. 100.2). American and European guidelines consider reasonable to perform an exercise Doppler echocardiography in symptomatic patients when there is a discrepancy between symptoms and severity of MR at rest or when LV and left atrial (LA) enlargement seem out of proportion to the severity of resting MR.[8,12] In such cases, the increase of MR severity or sPAP during exercise and the absence of LV contractile reserve may explain symptoms and justify mitral surgery. Moreover, stress echocardiography is recommended in patients who claim to be asymptomatic to objectively evaluate exercise tolerance and symptoms because symptoms may be unrecognized by the patient (e.g., progressive disease, patient who unconsciously limit physical activity to avoid symptoms).[12]

Clinical and Prognostic Value of Stress Echocardiography Parameters (Table 100.1)

Symptom evaluation. Exercise capacity is a predictor of the development of symptoms or LV dysfunction in asymptomatic patients with MR.[14,15] An increase in MR severity by one grade (effective regurgitant orifice increase by >10 mm²) is observed in about one-third of patients with degenerative MR and appears to correlate with a poor prognosis.[16,17]

sPAP evaluation. Important changes in MR severity are often associated with exercise-induced changes in sPAP. It has been shown that exercise-induced pulmonary hypertension (SPAP >60 mm Hg) is more accurate than resting SPAP in predicting the occurrence of symptoms and cardiovascular events during follow-up and that it is also associated with an increased risk of adverse cardiac events after MV surgery in patients with primary

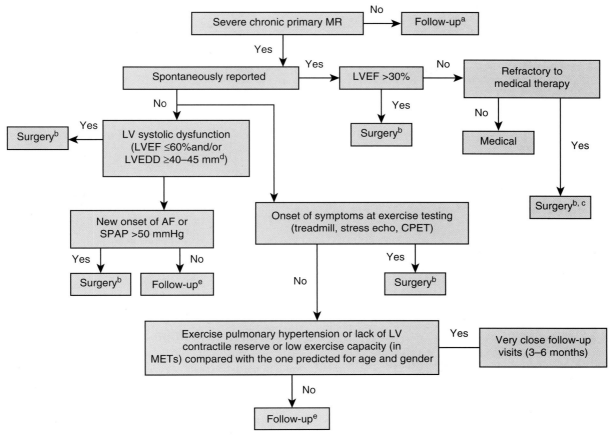

Figure 100.2. Decisional algorithm for the management of patients with primary severe mitral regurgitation (MR). [a]In case of moderate MR and symptoms, consider stress echocardiography. [b]Mitral valve (MV) repair should be preferred to MV replacement whenever possible, and results are expected to be durable. [c]In case of high surgical risk, a therapy for end-stage heart failure (including cardiac resynchronization therapy [CRT], left ventricular assist device [LVAD], heart transplantation) is needed and a percutaneous edge-to-edge MV repair can be considered. [d]The American guidelines put a cutoff at 40 mm; in contrast, the European guidelines put a cut off at 45 mm, 40 mm only in case of flail leaflet or significant left atrial dilatation (indexed volume ≥60 mL/m²). [e]The follow-up includes clinical examination, electrocardiography, echocardiography, and exercise testing. *AF,* Atrial fibrillation; *CPET,* cardiopulmonary exercise testing; *LV,* left ventricular; *LVEDD,* left ventricular end-diastolic diameter; *LVEF,* left ventricular ejection fraction; *sPAP,* systolic pulmonary artery pressure.

TABLE 100.1 Exercise Echocardiography in Primary Mitral Regurgitation

Clinical Condition	Major Parameters to Be Measured	Diagnostic Parameters	Prognostic Parameters
Primary MR	Symptoms	Dyspnea at low level exercise	Dyspnea at low level of exercise predicts poor spontaneous outcome and the need for MVR
	MR severity	• Increase in severity • Stable or decreased MR degree	• Increase in MR severity explains symptoms • Increase in MR severity of one grade at least explains symptoms and predicts decreased event-free survival
	LV function (LVEF, LVGLS)	• Increased: presence of contractile reserve • Stable or decreased: absence of contractile reserve	• Increase in LVEF <5% or in GLS <2% predicts decreased event-free survival, postoperative LV dysfunction, and morbidity
	Transtricuspid pressure gradient	• Increased >60 mm Hg: elevated sPAP • Rapid increase in sPAP: low pulmonary compliance and markedly increase pulmonary resistance	sPAP >60 mm Hg predicts reduced cardiac event–free survival
	Mitral E/e′ ratio	Increased: elevated LV filling pressure	Explains symptoms

E/e′ ratio, An estimate of left ventricular filling pressure; *GLS,* global longitudinal strain; *LV,* left ventricular; *LVEF,* left ventricular ejection fraction; *LVGLS,* left ventricular global longitudinal strain; *MR,* mitral regurgitation; *MVR,* mitral valve replacement or repair; *sPAP,* systolic pulmonary arterial pressure.

TABLE 100.2 Exercise Echocardiography in Secondary Mitral Regurgitation

Clinical Condition	Major Parameters to Be Measured	Diagnostic Parameters	Prognostic Parameters
Secondary MR	Symptoms	Dyspnea at low level exercise	Dyspnea at low level of exercise predicts the need to adapt the treatment
	MR severity	• Increase in severity • Stable or decreased MR degree	• Increase in MR severity explains symptoms • Increase in EROA >13 mm² predicts decreased event-free survival, cardiac mortality, episode of pulmonary edema
	LVEF	• Increased: presence of contractile reserve • Stable or decreased: absence of contractile reserve	Increase in LVEF fraction by 5% predicts global LV contractile recovery after revascularization
	Regional LV function	Worsening in wall motion or in global function: indicates ischemia	Ischemia predicts the presence of limited coronary flow reserve and poor outcome
	Transtricuspid pressure gradient	• Increased >60 mm Hg: elevated sPAP • Rapid increase in sPAP: low pulmonary compliance and markedly increase pulmonary resistance	• sPAP >60 mm Hg predicts higher risk of cardiac-related death during follow-up
	Mitral E/e′ ratio	Increased: elevated LV filling pressure	Explains symptoms

E/e′ ratio, An estimate of left ventricular filling pressure; *EROA,* effective regurgitant orifice area; *LV,* left ventricular; *LVEF,* left ventricular ejection fraction; *MR,* mitral regurgitation; *sPAP,* systolic pulmonary arterial pressure.

MR.[18–22] The level of increase in SPAP depends on the ability to successfully recruit the pulmonary vasculature to accommodate the increase in blood flow that occurs with exercise, the contribution (or proportion) of the reduction in the cross-sectional area of the pulmonary circulation, the changes in pulmonary vascular compliance, resistance and impedance, and the increase in LA pressure, each of which may be abnormal at rest.

Right ventricular (RV) function. In addition to exercise pulmonary hypertension, exercise-induced RV dysfunction, as assessed by tricuspid annular plane systolic excursion (TAPSE) less than 17.6 mm, has been shown to be an independent predictor of survival free from surgery. Indeed, patients with both exercise-induced pulmonary hypertension and RV dysfunction had the worst prognosis.[21]

LV function. LV contractile function may be impaired even in the setting of preserved LVEF. Lack of contractile reserve (<5% increase in ejection fraction) is an early marker of impaired myocyte contractility and predicts postoperative LV dysfunction after MV surgery.[23] Preliminary results suggest that 2D strain obtained during exercise could be useful to better identify contractile reserve in asymptomatic patients with severe degenerative MR.[24–26] An increase in global longitudinal strain (GLS) during exercise of less than 1.9% predicts postoperative LV dysfunction as well as impairment in LV function in medically treated patients with a better sensitivity and specificity than an inadequate increase in LVEF.[26] More recently, it has been shown that the absence of LV contractile reserve, assessed using 2D speckle-tracking analysis (<2% GLS increase during exercise), is associated with a greater than twofold increase in risk of cardiovascular event in asymptomatic patients with degenerative MR and preserved LVEF at rest.[27] Hence, myocardial deformation imaging is a more sensitive marker of LV contractile function than LVEF.

Impact on Clinical Decision Making

No specific recommendation has been provided in the last American and European guidelines, regarding the need for surgery in relation to exercise echocardiographic parameters.[8–12] Patients with increasing MR during exercise, exercise-induced pulmonary hypertension, and lack of contractile reserve should be treated medically and closely followed (every 3–6 months), preferably in a dedicated heart valve clinic,[28] to assess for the onset of symptoms and LV systolic dysfunction.

SECONDARY (ISCHEMIC) MITRAL REGURGITATION
Indications to Perform Stress Echocardiography

ESE is widely accepted as important diagnostic and prognostic tool in the assessment of ischemic heart disease. In patients with LV systolic dysfunction, the results of ESE (viability, ischemia, LV dyssynchrony, worsening MR) have the potential to influence revascularization strategies and possible concomitant MV repair versus resynchronization therapy.[29] The European and American societies of echocardiography provide the circumstances in which ESE is indicated for secondary MR (SMR).[1] ESE can be useful in patients with SMR and dyspnea out of proportion when compared with the MR severity, the degree of LV diastolic dysfunction, and the extent of LV dyssynchrony at rest. The usefulness of ESE has also been shown in patients with SMR who develop recurrent and unexplained acute pulmonary edema. In addition, ESE may be indicated in patients with moderate MR before surgical revascularization to identify those who may benefit from a combined coronary artery bypass grafting and MV repair. Finally, ESE may also be useful in cases of persistent pulmonary hypertension after restrictive MV annuloplasty.[19,30]

Clinical and Prognostic Value of Stress Echocardiography Parameters (Table 100.2)

SMR is dynamic and affected by changes in hemodynamic conditions, which occur during exercise (Fig. 100.3), and which can be reliably quantified by the PISA method during semisupine exercise echocardiography.[31,32] Exercise-induced changes in SMR severity (increase in effective regurgitant orifice area [EROA]), are not related to the degree of SMR at rest but to changes in MV deformation (increase in systolic tenting area, coaptation distance or mitral annulus diameter) or in basal LV dyssynchrony.[33–36] Rarely, exercise-induced increase in MR occurs as a consequence of acute transient myocardial ischemia.

An increase in mitral regurgitant volume during exercise correlates well with elevation of SPAP.[32] The magnitude of rise in both MR severity and SPAP is more pronounced in patients with exercise-limiting dyspnea and in those hospitalized for an acute pulmonary edema.[37] Dynamic changes in SMR provide additional prognostic information compared with resting evaluation and unmask patients at high risk for poor outcome.[38,39] In particular, a large exercise-induced increase in SMR, defined as a 13 mm² or greater increase in EROA, is associated with increased mortality

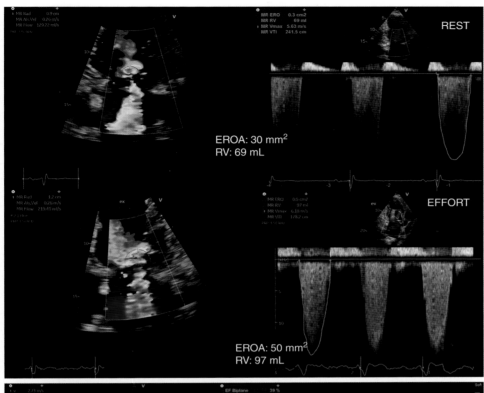

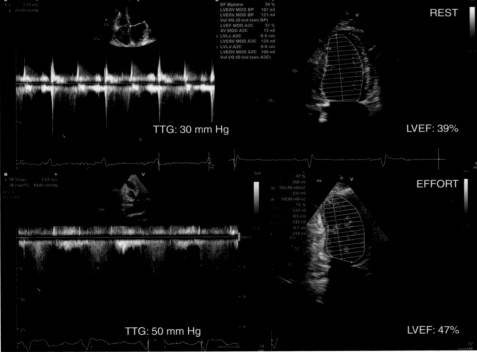

Figure 100.3. Dynamic secondary mitral regurgitation (MR). Exercise-induced increase in the severity of MR in a patient with chronic ischemic left ventricular systolic dysfunction. *EROA,* Effective regurgitant orifice area; *LVEF,* left ventricular ejection fraction; *RV,* regurgitant volume; *TTG,* transtricuspid gradient.

and morbidity rates.[39] Dynamic pulmonary hypertension (SPAP ≥60 mm Hg) is also a powerful predictor of poor prognosis, being associated with a higher risk of cardiac-related death during follow-up.[40] Conversely, the presence of viable myocardium predicts LV reverse remodeling and a better outcome after revascularization, β-blocker therapy, and cardiac resynchronization therapy.[29] LV reverse remodeling and reduced mitral apparatus deformation after cardiac resynchronization therapy are associated with a reduction in both resting and exercise-induced MR and an improvement in cardiopulmonary performance.[41] Moreover, SMR

decreases more significantly in patients with viability in the region of the pacing lead after cardiac resynchronization therapy.[42]

Impact on Clinical Decision Making

According to the European and American guidelines on the management of heart valve diseases, severe SMR should be corrected at the time of bypass surgery.[8–12] Much more controversial is the management of chronic SMR in patients without a revascularization solution. Optimal medical treatment should be ensured in all patients. Cardiac resynchronization therapy should be performed according to current recommendations. The presence of exercise dyssynchrony or viability in the potential pacing lead region may be used as incentive to determine the most appropriate site of implantation of biventricular pacing. However, both American and European guidelines do not at this time recommend interventions based on exercise-induced changes in the severity of SMR.

OTHER EXERCISE TESTING IN MITRAL REGURGITATION

European and American guidelines propose treadmill exercise testing and CPET as alternative tools to establish symptom status and functional capacity in asymptomatic patients with severe MR.[8–12] Asymptomatic patients with chronic severe nonischemic MR and good exercise tolerance on treadmill testing show a relatively benign course compared with those with poorer exercise tolerance.[43] Conversely, ST-segment depression does not seem to have prognostic value in asymptomatic patients with primary MR and preserved resting LVEF. It has been recently demonstrated that an impaired LV GLS is associated with a lower exercise capacity and a combination of abnormal resting LV GLS and percentage of age and sex-predicted METs less than 100% correlates to higher mortality rates.[44,45] Moreover, patients who achieve less than 100% of their age- and gender-predicted METs seem to have worse outcomes even after MV surgery.[46]

Reduced peak oxygen consumption (VO_2) on CPET is considered an important prognostic factor in patients with significant degenerative MR.[47–49] The usefulness of CPET becomes stronger when associated with ESE. Recently, reduced values in pulmonary vascular reserve evaluated by PAPm cardiac output slope, and in RV contractile reserve expressed by TAPSE or PAPs changes between rest and peak effort, were found to predict a lower peak VO_2 response during effort.[50]

REFERENCES

1. Lancellotti P, Pellikka PA, Budts W, et al. The clinical use of stress echocardiography in non-ischaemic heart disease. *J Am Soc Echocardiogr.* 2017;30:101–138.
2. Lancellotti P, Fattouch K, La Canna G. Therapeutic decision-making for patients with fluctuating mitral regurgitation. *Nat Rev Cardiol.* 2015;12:212–219.
3. Lancellotti P, Magne J. Stress echocardiography in regurgitant valve disease. *Circ Cardiovasc Imag.* 2013;6:840–849.
4. Izumo M, Suzuki K, Moonen M, et al. Changes in mitral regurgitation and left ventricular geometry during exercise affect exercise capacity in patients with systolic heart failure. *Eur J Echocardiogr.* 2011;12:54–60.
5. Yamano T, Nakatani S, Kanzaki H, et al. Exercise-induced changes of functional mitral regurgitation in asymptomatic or mildly symptomatic patients with idiopathic dilated cardiomyopathy. *Am J Cardiol.* 2008;102:481–485.
6. Giga V, Ostojic M, Vujisic-Tesic B, et al. Exercise-induced changes in mitral regurgitation in patients with prior myocardial infarction and left ventricular dysfunction: relation to mitral deformation and left ventricular function and shape. *Eur Heart J.* 2005;26:1860–1865.
7. Lebrun F, Lancellotti P, Pierard LA. Quantitation of functional mitral regurgitation during bicycle exercise in patients with heart failure. *J Am Coll Cardiol.* 2001;38:1685–1692.
8. Baumgartner H, Falk V, Bax JJ, et al. ESC/EACTS Guidelines for the management of valvular heart disease. *Eur Heart J.* 2017;38:2739–2791. 2017.
9. Tribouilloy C, Enriquez-Sarano M, Schaff H, et al. Impact of preoperative symptoms on survival after surgical correction of organic mitral regurgitation: rationale for optimizing surgical indications. *Circulation.* 1999;99:400–405.
10. Enriquez-Sarano M, Tajik A, Schaff H, et al. Echocardiographic prediction of left ventricular function after correction of mitral regurgitation: results and clinical implications. *J Am Coll Cardiol.* 1994;24:1536–1543.
11. Tribouilloy C, Grigioni F, Avierinos JF, et al. Survival implication of left ventricular end-systolic diameter in mitral regurgitation due to flail leaflets a long-term follow-up multicenter study. *J Am Coll Cardiol.* 2009;54:1961–1968.
12. Nishimura RA, Otto CM, Bonow RO, et al. AHA/ACC guideline for the management of patients with valvular heart disease. *J Am Coll Cardiol.* 2014;63:e57–185. 2014.
13. Nishimura RA, Otto CM, Bonow RO, et al. AHA/ACC focused update of the 2014 AHA/ACC guideline for the management of patients with valvular heart disease. *Circulation.* 2017;135:e1159–e1195. 2017.
14. Supino PG, Borer JS, Schuleri K, et al. Prognostic value of exercise tolerance testing in asymptomatic chronic nonischemic mitral regurgitation. *Am J Cardiol.* 2007;100:1274–1281.
15. Messika-Zeitoun D, Johnson BD, Nkomo V, et al. Cardiopulmonary exercise testing determination of functional capacity in mitral regurgitation: physiologic and outcome implications. *J Am Coll Cardiol.* 2006;47:2521–2527.
16. Magne J, Lancellotti P, Pierard LA. Exercise-induced changes in degenerative mitral regurgitation. *J Am Coll Cardiol.* 2010;56:300–309.
17. Coisne A, Levy F, Malaquin D, et al. Feasibility of Doppler hemodynamic evaluation of primary and secondary mitral regurgitation during exercise echocardiography. *Int J Cardiovasc Imag.* 2015;31:291–299.
18. Magne J, Lancellotti P, Pierard LA. Exercise pulmonary hypertension in asymptomatic degenerative mitral regurgitation. *Circulation.* 2010;122:33–41.
19. Magne J, Pibarot P, Sengupta PP, et al. Pulmonary hypertension in valvular disease: a comprehensive review on pathophysiology to therapy from the HAVEC Group. *JACC Cardiovasc Imag.* 2015;8:83–99.
20. Suzuki K, Izumo M, Yoneyama K, et al. Influence of exercise-induced pulmonary hypertension on exercise capacity in asymptomatic degenerative mitral regurgitation. *J Cardiol.* 2015;66:246–252.
21. Kusunose K, Popovic ZB, Motoki H, et al. Prognostic significance of exercise induced right ventricular dysfunction in asymptomatic degenerative mitral regurgitation. *Circ Cardiovasc Imag.* 2013;6:167–176.
22. Magne J, Donal E, Mahjoub H, et al. Impact of exercise pulmonary hypertension on postoperative outcome in primary mitral regurgitation. *Heart.* 2015;101:391–396.
23. Lee R, Haluska B, Leung DY, et al. Functional and prognostic implications of left ventricular contractile reserve in patients with asymptomatic severe mitral regurgitation. *Heart.* 2005;91:1407–1412.
24. Mascle S, Schnell F, Thebault C, et al. Predictive value of global longitudinal strain in a surgical population of organic mitral regurgitation. *J Am Soc Echocardiogr.* 2012;25:766–772.
25. Donal E, Mascle S, Brunet A, et al. Prediction of left ventricular ejection fraction 6 months after surgical correction of organic mitral regurgitation: the value of exercise echocardiography and deformation imaging. *Eur Heart J Cardiovasc Imag.* 2012;13:922–930.
26. Lancellotti P, Cosyns B, Zacharakis D, et al. Importance of left ventricular longitudinal function and functional reserve in patients with degenerative mitral regurgitation: assessment by two-dimensional speckle tracking. *J Am Soc Echocardiogr.* 2008;21:1331–1336.
27. Magne J, Mahjoub H, Dulgheru R, et al. Left ventricular contractile reserve in asymptomatic primary mitral regurgitation. *Eur Heart J.* 2014;35:1608–1616.
28. Lancellotti P, Rosenhek R, Pibarot P, et al. ESC working group on valvular heart disease position paper—heart valve clinics: organization, structure, and experiences. *Eur Heart J.* 2013;34:1597–1606.
29. Moonen M, O'Connor K, Magne J, et al. Stress echocardiography for selecting potential responders to cardiac resynchronisation therapy. *Heart.* 2010;96:1142–1146.
30. Magne J, Sénéchal M, Mathieu P, et al. Restrictive annuloplasty for ischemic mitral regurgitation may induce functional mitral stenosis. *J Am Coll Cardiol.* 2008;51:1692–1701.
31. Magne J, Senechal M, Dumesnil JG, et al. Ischemic mitral regurgitation: a complex multifaceted disease. *Cardiology.* 2009;112:244–259.
32. Lebrun F, Lancellotti P, Pierard LA. Quantitation of functional mitral regurgitation during bicycle exercise in patients with heart failure. *J Am Coll Cardiol.* 2001;38:1685–1692.
33. Lancellotti P, Lebrun F, Pierard LA. Determinants of exercise-induced changes in mitral regurgitation in patients with coronary artery disease and left ventricular dysfunction. *J Am Coll Cardiol.* 2003;42:1921–1928.
34. Giga V, Ostojic M, Vujisic-Tesic B, et al. Exercise-induced changes in mitral regurgitation in patients with prior myocardial infarction and left ventricular dysfunction: relation to mitral deformation and left ventricular function and shape. *Eur Heart J.* 2005;26:1860–1865.
35. Ennezat PV, Marechaux S, Le Tourneau T, et al. Myocardial asynchronism is a determinant of changes in functional mitral regurgitation severity during dynamic exercise in patients with chronic heart failure due to severe left ventricular systolic dysfunction. *Eur Heart J.* 2006;27:679–683.
36. Voilliot D, Lancellotti P. Exercise testing and stress imaging in mitral valve disease. *Curr Treat Options Cardio Med.* 2017;19:17.
37. Pierard LA, Lancellotti P. The role of ischemic mitral regurgitation in the pathogenesis of acute pulmonary edema. *N Engl J Med.* 2004;351:1627–1634.
38. Lancellotti P, Troisfontaines P, Toussaint AC, et al. Prognostic importance of exercise-induced changes in mitral regurgitation in patients with chronic ischemic left ventricular dysfunction. *Circulation.* 2003;108:1713–1717.
39. Lancellotti P, Gerard PL, Pierard LA. Long-term outcome of patients with heart failure and dynamic functional mitral regurgitation. *Eur Heart J.* 2005;26:1528–1532.
40. Lancellotti P, Magne J, Dulgheru R, et al. Clinical significance of exercise pulmonary hypertension in secondary mitral regurgitation. *Am J Cardiol.* 2015;115:1454–1461.
41. Madaric J, Vanderheyden M, Van Laethem C, et al. Early and late effects of cardiac resynchronization therapy on exercise-induced mitral regurgitation: relationship with left ventricular dyssynchrony, remodelling and cardiopulmonary performance. *Eur Heart J.* 2007;28:2134–2141.
42. Senechal M, Lancellotti P, Magne J, et al. Impact of mitral regurgitation and myocardial viability on left ventricular reverse remodeling after cardiac resynchronization therapy in patients with ischemic cardiomyopathy. *Am J Cardiol.* 2010;106:31–37.
43. Supino PG, Borer JS, Shuleri K, et al. Prognostic value of exercise treadmill testing in asymptomatic chronic nonischemic mitral regurgitation. *Am J Cardiol.* 2013;111:1625–1630.

44. Mentias A, Naji P, Gallinov M, et al. Strain echocardiography and functional capacity in asymptomatic primary mitral regurgitation with preserved ejection fraction. *J Am Coll Cardiol*. 2016;68:1974–1986.

45. Mentias A, Alashi A, Naji P, et al. Exercise capacity in asymptomatic patients with significant primary mitral regurgitation: independent effect of global longitudinal left ventricular strain. *Cardiovasc Diagn Ther*. 2018;8:460–468.

46. Naji P, Griffin BP, Barr T, et al. Importance of exercise capacity in predicting outcomes and determining optimal timing of surgery in significant primary mitral regurgitation. *J Am Heart Assoc*. 2014;3:e001010.

47. Santoro C, Sorrentino R, Esposito R, et al. Cardiopulmonary exercise testing and echocardiographic exam: an useful interaction. *Cardiovasc Ultrasound*. 2019;17:29.

48. Naji P, Griffin BP, Asfahan F, et al. Predictors of long-term outcomes in patients with significant myxomatous mitral regurgitation undergoing exercise echocardiography. *Circulation*. 2014;129:1310–1319.

49. Mentias A, Naji P, Gillinov AM, et al. Strain echocardiography and functional capacity in asymptomatic primary mitral regurgitation with preserved ejection fraction. *J Am Coll Cardiol*. 2016;68:1974–1986.

50. Utsunomiya H, Hidaka T, Susawa H, et al. Exercise-stress echocardiography and effort intolerance in asymptomatic/minimally symptomatic patients with degenerative mitral regurgitation combined invasive-non invasive hemodynamic monitoring. *Circ Cardiovasc Imag*. 2018;11:e007282.

100

101 Tricuspid Valve Complex: Anatomy by Two-Dimensional and Three-Dimensional Echocardiography

Miriam Shanks, Jeroen J. Bax, Victoria Delgado

TRICUSPID VALVE ANATOMY

The tricuspid valve (TV) is the largest of the four cardiac valves, with a normal valve area of 7 to 9 cm^2.[1] The TV lies between the right atrium and the right ventricle and is placed in a more apical position than the mitral valve. The TV functional anatomy can be divided into four components: the leaflets, annulus (with attached right atrium and ventricle), papillary muscles, and chordae tendineae (Fig. 101.1).

Tricuspid Leaflets

The number of TV leaflets is highly variable, with the trileaflet valve being the most common configuration.[2,3] Typically, the three leaflets are referred to as the septal, anterior, and posterior leaflets (see Fig. 101.1A). Tricuspid leaflets are significantly different in circumferential and radial size.[1] The anterior leaflet is the longest in the radial direction with the largest area and the greatest motion. The posterior leaflet is the shortest circumferentially and may have multiple scallops. It may not be clearly separated from the anterior leaflet in approximately 10% of patients.[3] The septal leaflet is the shortest in the radial direction and is the least mobile. It is attached to the tricuspid annulus directly above the interventricular septum, 10 mm or less apically to the septal insertion of the anterior mitral leaflet.[3] It has many third-order chordae that may be attached directly to the septum.[2–4] The commissure between the septal and posterior leaflets is usually located near the entrance of the coronary sinus to the right atrium. The commissure between the septal and anterior leaflets is the longest and is adjacent to the noncoronary sinus of Valsalva of the aortic root and 3 to 5 mm anterior to the atrioventricular node.[1] Coaptation of the TV is located at the level of the annulus or just below it with a coaptation length of 5 to 10 mm, allowing some dilatation of the annulus before malcoaptation occurs.[5] The TV is separated from the pulmonary valve by the ventriculoinfundibular fold (see Fig. 101.1B).

Tricuspid Annulus

The tricuspid annulus is typically triangular or D-shaped and nonplanar with two distinct segments: a larger C-shaped segment that corresponds to the free wall of the right atrium and right ventricle and a shorter, relatively straight segment that corresponds to the ventricular septum.[1] In addition, the tricuspid annulus is saddle shaped with the anterior and posterior aspects displaced toward the right atrium. This saddle shape becomes progressively more circular and flatter with worsening of secondary tricuspid regurgitation. The tricuspid annulus lies closer (≤1 cm) to the apex than

the mitral annulus. The tricuspid annulus plane is nearly vertical and about 45° from the sagittal plane and is superiorly (atrially) displaced in the anteroseptal portion and inferiorly (apically) displaced in the posteroseptal portion.[4] Unlike the mitral valve, there is no fibrous continuity with the corresponding semilunar valve.[6,7] There appears to be very little fibrous tissue or collagen in the tricuspid annulus; rather, the right ventricular (RV) free wall segment is composed of epicardium and endocardium, with the coronary artery and veins surrounded by adipose tissue in the atrioventricular groove.[1] In some hearts, the base of the TV consists entirely of atrial tissue.[8] The tricuspid annulus is dynamic and can change up to approximately 30% in its area during the cardiac cycle. Normal tricuspid annular circumference and area are 12 ± 2 cm and 11 ± 2 cm^2, respectively, with an increase in annular area during atrial systole and late systole or early diastole.[7,9]

Papillary Muscles and Chordae Tendineae

Papillary muscles and chordae form the tensor apparatus of the TV (see Fig. 101.1B).[10] There are two distinct anterior and posterior papillary muscles and a highly variable septal papillary muscle. The largest anterior papillary muscle provides chordal support to the anterior and posterior leaflets and is often joined by the moderator band. The posterior papillary muscle is often bifid or trifid and lends chordal support to the posterior and septal leaflets. The septal papillary muscle may be small or multiple or even absent in up to 20% of normal patients.[1] Chordae may arise directly from the septum to the anterior and septal leaflets or may attach to the RV free wall as well as to the moderator band as accessory chordae.[1] Chordae tendineae are fibrous chords that are highly variable in their number, morphology, and mode of insertion into the leaflet tissue (see Fig. 101.1B).[5] True chordae typically originate from the papillary muscle but can originate from the ventricular walls, as is often seen in the septal leaflets. In addition, false chordae can connect two papillary muscles or a papillary muscle to the ventricular wall, or they may connect points on the ventricular wall.[1] TV chords consist of fairly straight collagen bundles and thus exhibit less extensibility than normal mitral valve chordae.[11] This may explain marked tethering that occurs with displacement of the papillary muscles or dilatation of the right ventricle.[1]

IMAGING OF TRICUSPID VALVE WITH TWO-DIMENSIONAL ECHOCARDIOGRAPHY

TV anatomy can be assessed using transthoracic and transesophageal echocardiography (TTE and TEE, respectively). Because it is

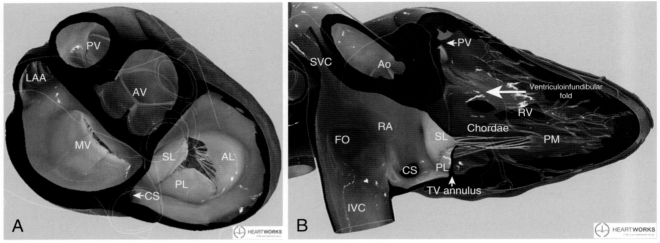

Figure 101.1. Tricuspid valve (TV) anatomy. **A,** En face view of the TV from the right atrial side. **B,** Sagittal view of the right atrium (RA) and right ventricle (RV) with the TV and its spatial relationships with atrial and ventricular structures. The septal leaflet (SL) and posterior leaflet (PL) are shown with the chordae tendineae raising from papillary muscle (PM). The ventriculoinfundibular fold is shown. *AL,* Anterior leaflet; *Ao,* aorta; *AV,* aortic valve; *CS,* coronary sinus; *FO,* fossa ovale; *IVC,* inferior vena cava; *LAA,* left atrial appendage; *MV,* mitral valve; *PV,* pulmonic valve; *SVC,* superior vena cava.

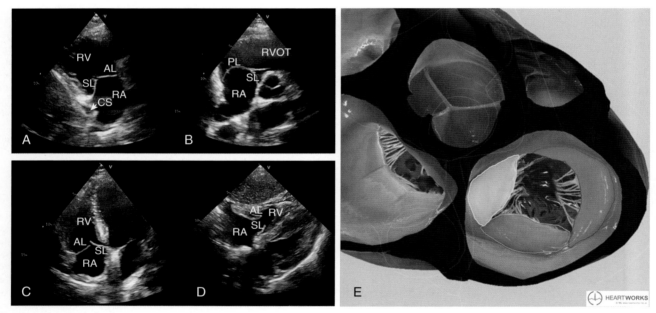

Figure 101.2. Analysis of the tricuspid valve (TV) with two-dimensional transthoracic echocardiography (TTE). The parasternal long-axis (**A**), short-axis (**B**), four-chamber apical (**C**), and subcostal (**D**) views are presented. **E,** The three-dimensional (3D) reconstruction of the TV and the septal leaflet (SL; *yellow*), anterior leaflet (AL; *blue*), and posterior leaflet (PL; *green*) are indicated. The different TTE views show the tricuspid leaflets color coded as in the 3D reconstruction. *CS,* Coronary sinus; *RA,* right atrium; *RV,* right ventricle; *RVOT,* right ventricular outflow tract.

difficult to visualize all three TV leaflets in a single two-dimensional plane and there is a great variability as to which leaflets are visualized in a given view, multiple TTE and TEE views should be used for comprehensive assessment of the valve.

Transthoracic Echocardiography

Fig. 101.2 demonstrates the standard TTE imaging planes from which the TV can be visualized. The RV inflow view is obtained from the parasternal long-axis plane by inferior (toward the right hip) angulation of the transducer such as the ultrasound beam is directed beneath the sternum. In this view, the right atrium and right ventricle as well as two leaflets of the TV can be clearly seen. The near field leaflet is always the anterior leaflet. The far field leaflet

may be the septal leaflet (typically seen together with the muscular interventricular septum and/or the coronary sinus ostium) (see Fig. 101.2A) or the posterior leaflet (more extreme rightward and inferior tilt of the transducer with interventricular septum is no longer in view).[3,12] The short-axis view is obtained from the parasternal window by rotating the transducer clockwise 90 degrees and then angulating it superiorly to obtain imaging plane at the aortic valve level. In this view, the leaflet adjacent to the aorta is either anterior or septal, and the leaflet adjacent to the RV free wall is usually the posterior leaflet (see Fig. 101.2B).[13,14] An extreme anterior angulation may result in imaging of a single large anterior leaflet (Fig. 101.3). From the apical four-chamber (see Fig. 101.2C) and subcostal views (Fig. 101.2D), typically the septal and anterior leaflets are visualized, although the posterior leaflet may be imaged if

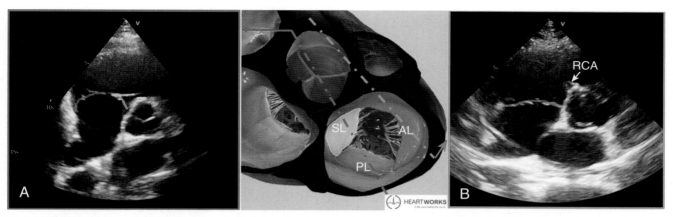

Figure 101.3. Visualization of the tricuspid valve leaflets from the parasternal short-axis view. **A,** Septal leaflet (SL; *yellow*) and posterior leaflet (PL; *green*) when the angulation of the probe is tilted posteriorly *(red axis)*. **B,** Entire anterior leaflet (AL) when the probe is tilted anteriorly *(blue axis)*. Note the visualization of the right coronary artery in that plane (RCA).

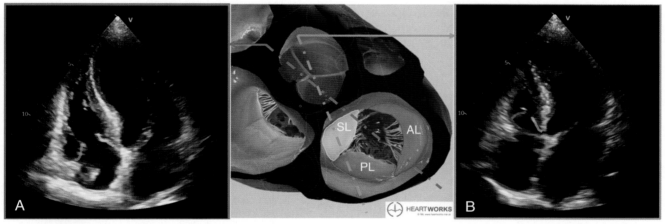

Figure 101.4. Visualization of the tricuspid valve leaflets from the four-chamber apical view. **A,** Septal (SL; *yellow*) and anterior (AL; *blue*) leaflets when the angulation of the probe is tilted anteriorly *(red axis)*. **B,** Posterior leaflet (PL; *green*) and SL *(yellow)* when the probe is tilted posteriorly *(blue axis)*.

posterior angulation of the transducer is used (Fig. 101.4).[15–17] The sepal-lateral diameter of the tricuspid annulus is traditionally measured in the apical four-chamber view focused on the right ventricle at end-diastole (Fig. 101.5). The normal tricuspid annulus diameter in adults is 28 ± 5 mm; however, it is known that 2D echocardiography may underestimate the tricuspid annulus maximal dimensions compared with measurements obtained by three-dimensional (3D) imaging modalities (see Fig. 101.5).[18–21]

Transesophageal Echocardiography

The imaging of the TV using TEE may be more challenging because of the anterior position of the valve and should be used if transthoracic windows are suboptimal.[22] Comprehensive assessment of the TV with TEE should include imaging from several depths (midesophageal, distal esophageal, shallow transgastric, and deep transgastric views) and multiple rotation angles (Fig. 101.6).[23] At the midesophageal depth, the TV is visualized in the following views: four-chamber view (0-degree angle with rightward probe rotation), RV inflow–outflow view (50- to 7-degree angle with slight advancement of the probe), and modified bicaval view (90- to 110-degree angle with clockwise rotation) (see Fig. 101.6A–C). After advancing the probe to the distal esophagus just proximal to the gastroesophageal junction, the TV, right atrium, and coronary sinus are visualized without the left heart structures in the view (see

Fig. 101.6D). Further advancement of the probe into the stomach produces transgastric views that often provide superb visualization of the TV as well. From this position, the following views are imaged: RV inflow–outflow view (0- to 20-degree angle with right flexion), RV basal short-axis view (0- to 20-degree angle with anteflexion), and RV inflow view (90- to 110-degree with clockwise rotation) (see Fig. 101.6E and G). The RV basal short-axis view is the only 2D view that demonstrates all three TV leaflets simultaneously. Advancing the probe further into the stomach along with rightward maximal anterior flexion and return to a 0-degree angle produces a deep transgastric view of the TV (see Fig. 101.6H).

IMAGING OF TRICUSPID VALVE WITH THREE-DIMENSIONAL ECHOCARDIOGRAPHY
Transthoracic Echocardiography

The proximity of the TV to the chest wall facilitates the imaging of this valve with 3D TTE. There is no specific view to acquire 3D transthoracic data of the TV. However, the apical RV-focused view or a foreshortened four-chamber view usually provides the best image quality, allowing the inclusion of the entire TV. Alternatively, the parasternal long-axis view of the RV can be used to acquire the 3D dataset and provides better spatial resolution than the apical views. On TTE, the full-volume (single- or multibeat) display is the

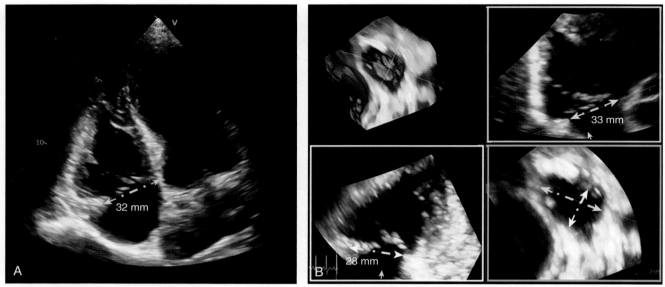

Figure 101.5. Measurement of the tricuspid valve (TV) annulus on two- and three-dimensional (3D) transthoracic echocardiography. **A,** The diameter of the TV annulus is measured on a systolic frame in the apical four-chamber view. **B,** Multiplanar reformation planes from a 3D acquisition of the TV. The *yellow* and *white planes* show two orthogonal longitudinal views of the right ventricle, and the *green plane* shows the short-axis view of the TV annulus where the maximum and minimum diameter can be measured.

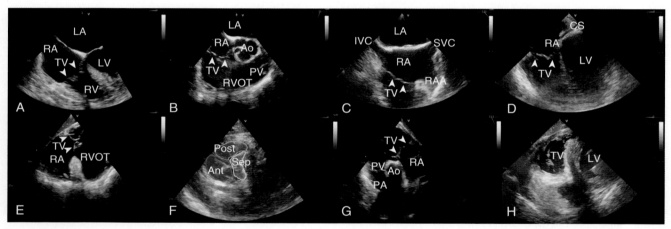

Figure 101.6. Analysis of the tricuspid valve (TV) anatomy with two-dimensional transesophageal echocardiography. From the midesophageal depth, the four-chamber view (**A**), right ventricular inflow–outflow view (**B**), and modified bicaval view (**C**) are shown. From the distal esophagus, the TV, right atrium (RA), and coronary sinus are visualized (**D**). From transgastric views, the right ventricular inflow–outflow view (**E**), right ventricular basal short-axis view (**F**), and right ventricular inflow view (**G**) are presented. Advancing the probe farther into the stomach the deep transgastric view of the TV can be obtained (**H**). *Ant,* Anterior leaflet; *Ao,* aortic valve; *LA,* left atrium; *LV,* left ventricle; *PA,* pulmonary artery; *Post,* posterior leaflet; *PV,* pulmonic valve; *RV,* right ventricle; *RVOT,* right ventricular outflow tract; *Sep,* septal leaflet.

most frequently used to acquire the 3D dataset of the TV and appreciate the anatomy of this valve. From biplane views that permit visualization of the TV from two orthogonal planes, the region of interest is usually positioned to include the leaflets and their attachments to the annulus as well as surrounding structures that permit orientation an identification of the components of the TV (i.e., the aortic valve because it is a central structure and the noncoronary sinus is in relation with the commissure between the septal and anterior leaflets or the interventricular septum) (Fig. 101.7). By activating the 3D visualization, an "en face" view of the TV will be displayed and can be subsequently postprocessed to appreciate the anatomy from the 3D volume renderings (see Fig. 101.7 and Video 101.7) or from multiplanar reformation planes (Fig. 101.8), which allow the measurement of the length of the leaflets, the tricuspid annulus dimensions, and the coaptation gap when there is tricuspid regurgitation. Advances in postprocessing software allow the TV to

be modeled to provide automated measurement of the TV annulus and leaflet areas. 3D TTE permits characterization of the leaflet tissue characteristics and may help to refine the diagnosis of the mechanism of tricuspid regurgitation or stenosis (i.e., location of pacemaker leads entrapping or perforating the leaflets or thickening of the leaflets caused by carcinoid syndrome).

Transesophageal Echocardiography

Visualization of the TV anatomy with 3D TEE has become key during the guidance of transcatheter TV interventions. However, acquisition of good-resolution datasets is more challenging compared with TTE because on TEE, the TV is in the far field. When using distal esophageal views, the TV can frequently be well visualized because the right atrium and the shadowing that the interatrial septum may cause are eliminated from the plane. Similar to

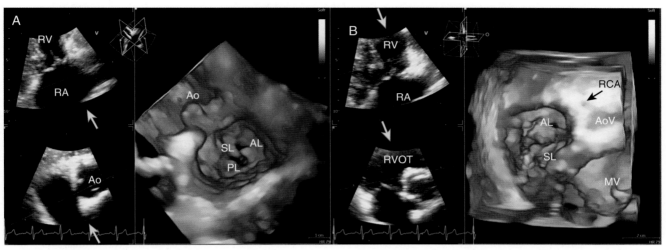

Figure 101.7. Analysis of the tricuspid valve (TV) with three-dimensional (3D) transthoracic echocardiography. **A,** Orthogonal two-dimensional apical views of the TV from where the 3D volume is obtained. The *yellow arrow* indicate that the TV is visualized from the right atrium (RA). The aortic valve (AoV) is anteriorly located (at 12 o'clock). **B,** The TV from the right ventricle (RV). *AL,* Anterior leaflet; *MV,* mitral valve; *PL,* posterior leaflet; *RCA,* right coronary artery; *SL,* septal leaflet. (See accompanying Video 101.7.)

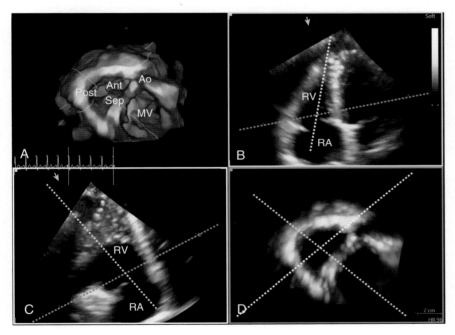

Figure 101.8. Multiplanar reformation planes of three-dimensional (3D) volume rendering of the tricuspid valve (TV). **A,** 3D volume of the TV visualized from the right ventricle (RV); note the *yellow arrows* on the orthogonal longitudinal planes of the RV. **B** *(yellow plane)* and **C** *(white plane)* show the orthogonal longitudinal planes of the RV. **C** *(green plane),* Short-*axis* view of the SV. *Ant,* Anterior leaflet; *Ao,* aortic valve; *MV,* mitral valve; *Post,* posterior leaflet; *RA,* right atrium; *Sep,* septal leaflet.

TTE, the region of interest is set to include the entire TV ensuring visualization of the leaflets and insertion points into the annulus in two orthogonal views (Fig. 101.9). In addition, inclusion of the aortic valve and the coronary sinus is advisable to facilitate orientation during offline analysis. Alternatively, from the midesophageal bicaval view at 110 to 120 degrees focusing on the TV, the 3D dataset of the TV can be also acquired. Subsequently, the 3D volume rendering can be displayed on multiplanar reformation planes to analyze the components of the TV (see Fig. 101.9 and Video 101.9). However, when using TEE transgastric views of the TV, the biplane mode acquisition can provide important information when the 3D volume renderings are noisy or the spatial resolution is not appropriate. The short-axis view of the TV on transgastric views is used as a reference view and biplane views can be used across the desire structures to visualize the perpendicular views (Fig. 101.10 and Video 101.10). Using this technique, the posterior and septal leaflets and the posterior and anterior leaflets can be readily visualized and identified during the procedure. This mode of visualization is very helpful during transcatheter procedures because it permits accurate guidance of catheters.

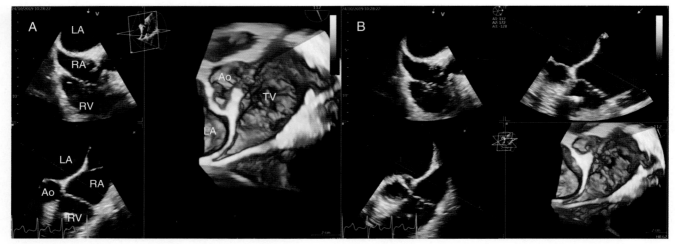

Figure 101.9. Visualization of the tricuspid valve (TV) with three-dimensional (3D) TEE. **A,** Two-dimensional orthogonal planes from where the 3D volume of the TV is obtained. **B,** Visualization of the TV on three orthogonal planes. *AL,* Anterior leaflet; *Ao,* aortic valve; *LA,* left atrium; *RA,* right atrium; *RV,* right ventricle. (See accompanying Video 101.9.)

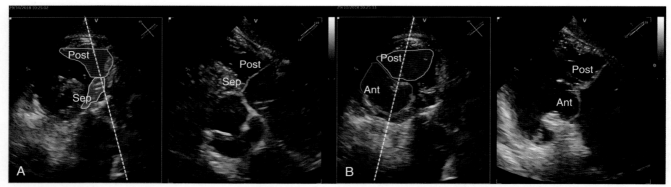

Figure 101.10. Biplane visualization of the tricuspid valve from the transgastric short-axis view. **A,** Posterior (Post; *green*) and septal (Sep; *yellow*) leaflets on the short-axis view. The *dotted line* indicates the orthogonal view that is displayed simultaneously on the right, allowing the analysis of the coaptation of the leaflets. **B,** Short-axis and longitudinal views of the anterior (Ant; *blue*) and posterior (Post; *green*) leaflets. (See accompanying Video 101.10.)

REFERENCES

1. Dahou A, Levin D, Reisman M, Hahn RT. Anatomy and physiology of the tricuspid valve. *JACC Cardiovasc Imag*. 2019;12:458–468.
2. Xanthos T, Dalivigkas I, Ekmektzoglou KA. Anatomic variations of the cardiac valves and papillary muscles of the right heat. *Ital J Anat Embryol*. 2011;116:111–126.
3. Hahn RT. State-of-the-art review of echocardiographic imaging in the evaluation and treatment of functional tricuspid regurgitation. *Circ Cardiovasc Imag*. 2016;9. e005332.
4. Martinez RM, O'Leary PW, Anderson RH. Anatomy and echocardiography of the normal and abnormal tricuspid valve. *Cardiol Young*. 2006;16(suppl 3):4–11.
5. Silver MD, Lam JHC, Ranganathan N, Wigle ED. Morphology of the human tricuspid valve. *Circulation*. 1971;43:333–334.
6. Rogers JH, Bolling SF. The tricuspid valve: Current perspective and evolving management of tricuspid regurgitation. *Circulation*. 2009;119:2718–2725.
7. Fukuda S, Saracino G, Matsumura Y, et al. Three-dimensional geometry of the tricuspid annulus in healthy subjects and in patients with functional tricuspid regurgitation: a real-time, 3D echocardiographic study. *Circulation*. 2006;114(1 Suppl):I492–I498.
8. Messer S, Moseley E, Marinescu M, et al. Histologic analysis of the right atrioventricular junction in the adult human heart. *J Heart Valve Dis*. 2012;21:368–373.
9. Ton-Nu TT, Levine RA, Handschumacher MD, et al. Geometric determinants of functional tricuspid regurgitation: insights from 3D echocardiography. *Circulation*. 2006;114:143–149.
10. Tretter JT, Sarwark AE, Anderson RH, Spicer DE. Assessment of the anatomical variation to be found in the normal tricuspid valve. *Clin Anat*. 2016;29:399–407.
11. Lim KO. Mechanical properties and ultrastructure of normal human tricuspid valve chordae tendineae. *Jpn J Physiol*. 1980;30:455–464.
12. Chan K-L, Veinot JP. *Anatomic Basis of Echocardiographic Diagnosis*. London: Springer; 2011.
13. Zoghbi WA, Adams D, Bonow RO, et al. Recommendations for non-invasive evaluation of native valvular regurgitation. *J Am Soc Echocardiogr*. 2017;30:305–312.
14. Anwar AM, Geleijnse ML, Soliman OI, et al. Assessment of normal tricuspid valve anatomy in adults by real-time three-dimensional echocardiography. *Int J Cardiovasc Imag*. 2007;23:717–724.
15. Addetia K, Yamat M, Mediratta A, et al. Comprehensive two-dimensional interrogation of the tricuspid valve using knowledge derived from three-dimensional echocardiography. *J Am Soc Echocardiogr*. 2016;29:74–82.
16. Stankovic I, Daraban AM, Jasaityte R, et al. Incremental value of the en-face view of the tricuspid valve by two-dimensional and three-dimensional echocardiography for accurate identification of tricuspid valve leaflets. *J Am Soc Echocardiogr*. 2014;27:376–384.
17. Otto CM. *Textbook of Clinical Echocardiography*. 5th ed. Philadelphia: Elsevier/Saunders; 2013.
18. Dreyfus J, Durand-Viel G, Raffoul R, et al. Comparison of 2D, 3D, and surgical measurements of the tricuspid annulus size: Clinical implications. *Circ Cardiovasc Imag*. 2015;8. e003241.
19. Anwar AM, Soliman OI, Nemes A, et al. Value of assessment of tricuspid annulus: real-time three dimensional echocardiography and magnetic resonance imaging. *Int J Cardiovasc Imag*. 2007;23:701–705.
20. Anwar AM, Geleijnse ML, Ten Cate FJ, Meijboom FJ. Assessment of tricuspid valve annulus size, shape and function using real-time three-dimensional echocardiography. *Interact Cardiovasc Thorac Surg*. 2006;5:683–687.
21. van Rosendael PJ, Joyce E, Katsanos S, et al. Tricuspid valve remodeling in functional tricuspid regurgitation: Multidetector row computed tomography insights. *Eur Heart J Cardiovasc Imag*. 2016;17:96–105.
22. Khalique OK, Cavalcante JL, Shah D, et al. Multimodality imaging of the tricuspid valve and right heart anatomy. *JACC Cardiovasc Imag*. 2019;12:516–531.
23. Hahn RT, Abraham T, Adams MS, et al. Guidelines for performing a comprehensive transesophageal echocardiographic examination. *J Am Soc Echocardiogr*. 2013;26:921–964.

102 Epidemiology, Etiology, and Natural History of Tricuspid Regurgitation

Luigi P. Badano, Denisa Muraru

Tricuspid regurgitation (TR) is characterized by a variable amount of blood regurgitating from the right ventricle (RV) into the right atrium (RA) during systole, eventually leading to excess mortality and cardiac morbidity. Several studies showed that the prevalence of clinically significant (i.e., moderate or severe) TR in the general population is around 0.5% to 0.8% and is more common in women and older adults.[1,2] Although minimal or trivial TR may be considered a normal variant in structurally normal tricuspid valves, which may be detected in 80% to 90% of normal participants undergoing a state-of the-art echocardiographic examination, moderate to severe TR is pathological and can be caused by annular dilatation and/or tethering of anatomically normal valve leaflets (secondary or functional TR) and/or intrinsic abnormalities of the tricuspid valve apparatus (primary or organic TR).

The clinical importance of TR and its impact on patients' mortality and morbidity have long been underestimated and led to undertreatment of patients with severe TR.[3,4]

EPIDEMIOLOGY

Using echocardiography, the Framingham Heart study investigators found a prevalence of moderate or severe TR of 0.8% and an increased prevalence with aging.[1] In 2000, the worldwide population of persons aged older than 65 years was an estimated to be 420 million.[5] From 2000 to 2030, the worldwide population aged older than 65 years is projected to increase by approximately 550 million to 973 million, increasing from 6.9% to 12.0% worldwide, from 15.5% to 24.3% in Europe, from 12.6% to 20.3% in North America, from 6.0% to 12.0% in Asia, and from 5.5% to 11.6% in Latin America and the Caribbean.[5] The largest increases in absolute numbers of older persons will occur in developing countries. From 2000 to 2030, the number of persons in developing countries aged older than 65 years is projected to almost triple, from approximately 249 million in 2000 to an estimated 690 million in 2030, and the developing countries' share of the world's population aged older than 65 years is projected to increase from 59% to 71%.[5] Thus, the already notable prevalence of significant TR will most likely increase dramatically in the near future.

Overall, the prevalence of significant TR was 4.3 times greater in women than in men.[1] Recently, in a retrospective, observational study including 16,380 echocardiograms performed at Mayo Clinic over a 10-year interval, Topilsky and coworkers[2] found that the prevalence of isolated TR of moderate or greater severity among the inhabitants of the Olmsted County was 0.4%, seen more commonly in women and elderly persons. Moderate or severe TR accompanied around 25% of all left-side heart valve diseases. The most common cause of moderate or severe TR in community residents diagnosed by Doppler echocardiography was functional TR secondary to left valvular disease (49.5%) followed by functional TR associated with pulmonary hypertension unrelated to any heart disease (23.0%), functional TR related to left ventricular dysfunction (12.9%), functional isolated TR (8.1%), organic TR (4.8%), and congenital (1.7%).[2] When the severity of isolated TR was moderate or greater, survival was worse than for matched control participants with trivial or less TR. Notably, atrial fibrillation is increasingly more recognized as an important factor in the cause of functional TR,[6–10] and its prevalence in the so-called "isolated functional TR" group of the Olmsted county study was 68%.[2]

TR is frequently present in patients with mitral valve disease, and more than one-third of patients with mitral stenosis have at least moderate.TR[11] Severe TR has been reported in 23% to 37% of patients after mitral valve replacement for rheumatic valve disease.[12] In the majority of patients, TR is not related to primary valve pathology and is defined as "functional." Functional TR is frequently observed in the advanced stage of left-sided valvular heart disease or myocardial disease.[13,14]

In 14% of patients, TR may occur in the absence of structural tricuspid valve alterations, pulmonary hypertension, or left heart dysfunction.[12,15]

Finally, the development of hemodynamically significant TR has been reported in 27% of patients who had only mild TR at the time of left-sided valve surgery.[16] In most cases, TR is diagnosed late after mitral valve replacement.[12,17]

CAUSE AND MECHANISMS OF TRICUSPID REGURGITATION

The cause of TR is generally divided into primary (or intrinsic) valve disease and secondary (or functional) valve dysfunction (Table 102.1). Primary TR results from structural abnormalities of

TABLE 102.1 Cause of Tricuspid Regurgitation

Functional (Morphologic Normal Leaflets With Annular Dilatation) (75%)
- Left heart diseases (LV dysfunction or valve diseases) resulting in pulmonary hypertension
- Primary pulmonary hypertension
- Secondary pulmonary hypertension (e.g., chronic lung disease, pulmonary thromboembolism, left-to-right shunt)
- RV dysfunction from any cause (e.g., myocardial diseases, ischemic heart disease)
- Atrial fibrillation
- Cardiac tumors (particularly right atrial myxomas)Structural Abnormality of the Tricuspid Valve (25%)
- Rheumatic
- Prolapse
- Congenital
  - Ebstein anomaly
  - Tricuspid valve dysplasia
  - Tricuspid valve hypoplasia
  - Tricuspid valve cleft
  - Double orifice tricuspid valve
  - Unguarded tricuspid valve orifice
- Endocarditis
- Endomyocardial fibrosis
- Carcinoid disease
- Traumatic (blunt chest injury, laceration)
- Iatrogenic
  - Pacemaker or defibrillator lead interference
  - Right ventricular biopsy
  - Drugs (e.g., exposure to fenfluramine–phentermine or methysergide)
  - Radiation

LV, Left ventricular; *RV,* right ventricular.

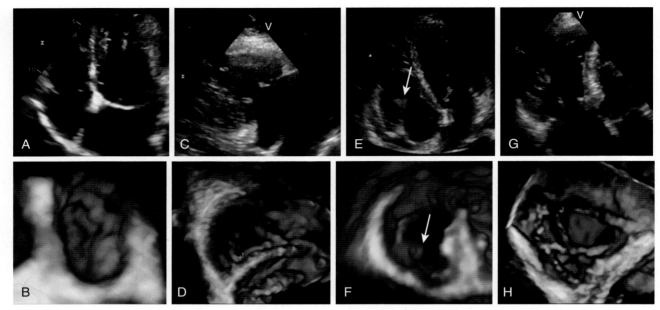

Figure 102.1. Various causes of organic tricuspid regurgitation illustrated by two- (**A, C, E,** and **G**) and three-dimensional (**B, D, F,** and **H**) echocardiography (3DE). Prolapse of anterior and posterior leaflets in Barlow disease suspected in four-chamber view (**A**) and visualized with 3DE from the "surgical view" of tricuspid valve (**B**); rheumatic tricuspid valve disease with characteristic leaflet thickening (**C**), reduced diastolic opening (orifice area planimetry 2.5 cm^2) and commissural fusion (**D**); and endocarditis vegetation (*arrow,* **E**) attached to the posterior leaflet (**F**); carcinoid disease, with typical thickening and stiffness of tricuspid leaflets, fixed in semi-open position (**G**), resulting in free regurgitation and mild stenosis (**H**).

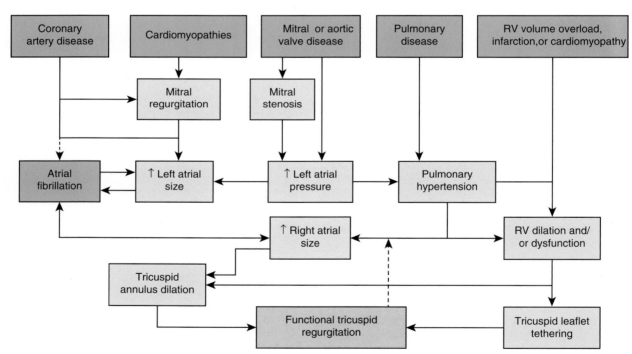

Figure 102.2. Mechanisms of functional tricuspid regurgitation (TR). Flow chart summarizing the main causes and mechanisms leading to secondary or functional TR. *RV,* Right ventricular.

valve apparatus, may be congenital or acquired, and accounts for only 8% to 10% of all severe TRs[8,18,19] (Fig. 102.1). Secondary or functional TR is usually caused by tricuspid annulus dilatation that may be primary (atrial fibrillation) or secondary to RV dilatation or dysfunction most frequently caused by pulmonary hypertension that may be either pre- or postcapillary (i.e., secondary to diseases affecting the left heart) (Fig. 102.2).[20] However, even though pulmonary arterial hypertension from any cause is known

to be associated with the occurrence of secondary or functional TR, not all patients with pulmonary hypertension develop significant TR because its mechanisms are multifactorial. Mutlak and coworkers[21] assessed the determinants of TR severity in a large cohort (2139 patients) with mild (<50 mmHg), moderate (50–70 mmHg), or severe (>70 mmHg) elevation of pulmonary artery systolic pressure (PASP). In this population, elevated PASP was associated with more severe TR (odds ratio, 2.26 per 10–mmHg

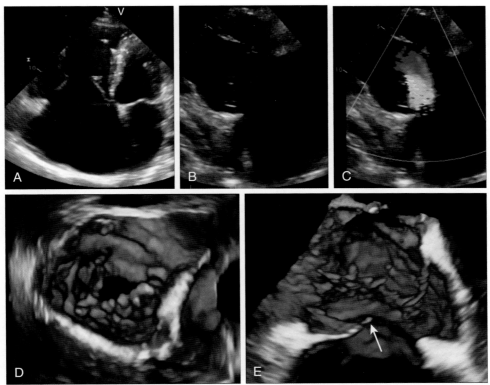

Figure 102.3. Traumatic organic tricuspid regurgitation (TR). **A** to **C,** Standard two-dimensional echocardiography shows characteristic changes suggestive for a severe functional TR (severely dilated right heart chambers and tricuspid annulus; severe leaflet tenting with lack of coaptation and no apparent structural abnormality). **D,** Because its ability to display all leaflets in a single view, real-time three-dimensional echocardiography reveals in addition a flail of the anterior leaflet with ruptured chord (**E,** *arrow*), which in the context of severe blunt chest trauma in patient history was interpreted as having a traumatic cause.

increase). However, a large number of patients with elevated PASP showed only mild TR (65.4% of patients with moderate and 45.6% of patients with severe pulmonary hypertension). Authors showed that other factors such as atrial fibrillation, pacemaker leads, and RV remodeling were also significant determinants of the severity of TR. Among them, remodeling of the right heart in response to the increase in PASP was the most powerful predictor of TR. These data confirm earlier observations that annular dilatation, RV dilatation, and tricuspid valve tenting and not pulmonary hypertension itself are the main determinants of functional TR[22,23] (see Fig. 102.2).

Even in the absence of pulmonary hypertension, tricuspid annular dilatation may cause significant regurgitation.[23,24] In patients with chronic pulmonary thromboembolic hypertension and in patients with mitral stenosis in whom TR resolved after successful pulmonary thromboendoarterectomy or mitral balloon valvuloplasty, there was no change in tricuspid annulus diameter after the resolution of pulmonary hypertension.[25,26] These observations suggest that tricuspid annulus dilatation could be irreversible and might be the mechanism of late TR encountered in mitral valve diseases. When TR has become significant, progressive RA and/or RV remodeling and dysfunction caused by chronic volume overload result in further annulus dilatation, papillary muscle displacement, and leaflet tethering, which worsen TR and lead to further RA and RV dilatation.

Particular cases of TR are those developing after blunt chest trauma or as a consequence of pacemaker or defibrillator leads (see also Chapter 106), which may directly interfere with leaflet coaptation while crossing the valve from the RA to the RV. TR is a rare complication of blunt chest trauma, most frequently of high-impact road traffic accidents. If the acute rise in right

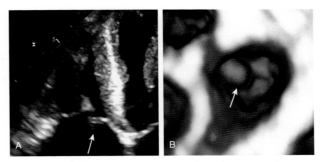

Figure 102.4. Iatrogenic tricuspid valve flail in a heart transplant patient. **A,** Two-dimensional four-chamber view shows a leaflet with the free edge completely reversed into the right atrium (RA), causing lack of coaptation *(arrow).* **B,** Three-dimensional rendering ("surgical view") shows a bulging of septal leaflet into the RA *(arrow).*

intraventricular cavity pressure happens when the valve is closed, it may result in chordal rupture (Fig. 102.3); however, both anterior papillary muscle rupture or leaflet tears (primarily the anterior leaflet) have also been reported.[27] In the acute phase of the injury, the traumatic lesion can go undetected. In the chronic phase, many patients remain asymptomatic, but others exhibit symptoms and signs of right heart failure.

TR caused by endocardial lead implantation or removal of permanent pacemakers or implantable cardioverter defibrillators is a known complication of these procedures (see Chapter 106).[28]

Another cause of iatrogenic, traumatic TR is represented by repeated endomyocardial biopsies (Fig. 102.4). TR is the most frequent valvular abnormality that occurs after cardiac

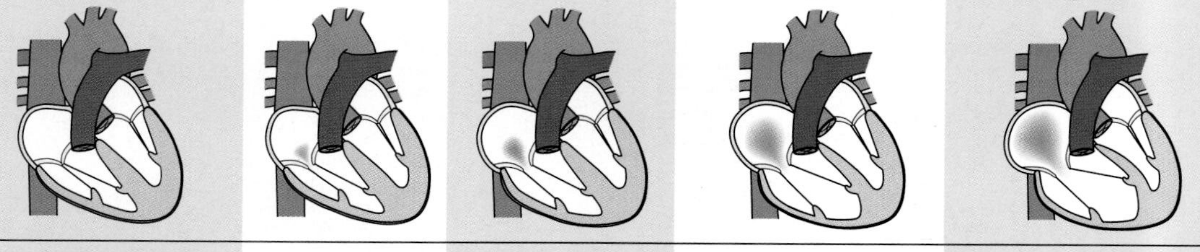

	Stage 1	Stage 2	Stage 3	Stage 4	Stage 5
Clinical picture	Asymptomatic patient at risk (pulmonary hypertension, chronic atrial fibrillation, post-mitral valve surgery etc)	Asymptomatic	No or aspecific symtoms	Episodes of RV heart failure	RV heart failure and/or end-organ damage due to chronic RV overload
RA remodeling	Mild or no dilation	Dilatation	Severe dilatation	Severe dilatation	Severe dilatation
TR severity	Trivial or mild	≧Moderate	Severe	Severe	Torrential or massive
Annular size	Normal	Dilated	Dilated	Severely dilatation	Severely dilatation
Leaflet tethering	None	None or mild (<8 mm)	Mild (<8 mm)	>8 mm	>8 mm
Leaflet coaptation	Normal	Mildly abnormal	Abnormal	Coaptation gap	Large coaptation depth
RV function and remodeling	Normal	Normal function, no remodeling	Mild RV dilatation, normal function	Moderate remodeling, varying degrees of RV dysfunction according to the cause of TR	Severe RV dilatation with varying degrees of RV dysfunction according to the cause of TR

Figure 102.5. Staged scheme of the idealized natural clinical history of patients with functional tricuspid regurgitation (TR). The evolution structural and functional alterations of the right heart structures that can be detected with echocardiography, and their relationships with the severity of functional TR are also reported. *RA,* Right atrial; *RV,* right ventricular.

transplantation.[29] Chordal damage at the time of endomyocardial biopsy leading to tricuspid valve prolapse is the cause of TR in these patients. In 101 patients who underwent orthotopic cardiac transplantation and survived more than 1 year, Nguyen and colleagues[29] reported that 25% developed severe TR (4% required valve replacement for refractory right-sided heart failure). In their series, there were no cases of severe TR in those patients who underwent fewer than 18 biopsies. Conversely, the incidence of severe TR was 60% in those who underwent more than 31 endomyocardial biopsies.

NATURAL HISTORY

The presence of significant TR has been associated with increased mortality and morbidity,[30–32] and there is a clear relationship between outcomes and the degree of severity of TR[18,33,34] that may also extend beyond the conventional definition of severe.[35] However, a recent retrospective study of 5886 consecutive patients followed for 10 years reported that even though in patients with moderate/severe TR without left heart disease, there was an increased risk for heart failure (hazard ratio [HR], 3.10; 95% confidence interval [CI], 1.41–6.84, $P = .005$) and heart failure hospitalization and cardiovascular mortality (HR, 2.75; 95% CI, 1.34–5.63, $P = .006$), after rigorous propensity matching of the entire cohort, there was no significant difference in outcomes between patients with moderate or severe TR and trivial or mild TR. These results are contradictory to most of the available literature and should be viewed with caution considering the limitations of the study, including its retrospective nature, selection bias of the patients who were followed, and the lack of quantitative assessment of TR severity.[3]

The idealized natural clinical and echocardiographic history of patients with functional TR is summarized in Fig. 102.5. Although the proposed scheme implies a linear progression of TR, the relationships between morphologic and functional alterations of the right heart structures and the severity of TR are quite variable and depend largely on the etiology of functional TR.[24] In patients with "atriogenic" TR (i.e., patients with atrial fibrillation), there is little tethering of the leaflet and RV remodeling, whereas the main structural abnormality is the severe annular dilatation. Conversely, in patients with "ventriculogenic" TR (i.e., patients with pulmonary hypertension), there is less annular dilatation, and the main structural abnormalities are RV dilatation and dysfunction with severe tethering of the leaflet. In most of the patients, particularly in the advanced stages of the disease, all reported morphologic and functional abnormalities coexist to variable extent. The increase of the pulmonary artery pressure and permanent atrial fibrillation have been reported as the most powerful determinant of the progression of the severity of TR.[21,36]

REFERENCES

1. Singh JP, Evans JC, Levy D, et al. Prevalence and clinical determinants of mitral, tricuspid, and aortic regurgitation: the Framingham Heart Study. *Am J Cardiol.* 1999;83:897–902.
2. Topilsky Y, Maltais S, Medina Inojosa J, et al. Burden of tricuspid regurgitation in patients diagnosed in the community setting. *JACC Cardiovascular Imag.* 2019;12:433–442.
3. Hahn RT. Avoiding mistakes of the past with tricuspid regurgitation. *J Am Soc Echocardiogr.* 2019;32:1547–1550.
4. Agarwal S, Tuzcu EM, Rodriguez ER, et al. Interventional cardiology perspective of functional tricuspid regurgitation. *Circ Cardiovasc Interv.* 2009;2:565–573.
5. Centers for Disease C, Prevention. Trends in aging—United States and worldwide. *MMWR Morb Mortal Wkly Rep.* 2003;52:101–106.
6. Utsunomiya H, Itabashi Y, Mihara H, et al. Functional tricuspid regurgitation caused by chronic atrial fibrillation: a real-time 3-dimensional transesophageal echocardiography study. *Circ Cardiovasc Imag.* 2017;10.
7. Muraru D, Guta A-C, Ochoa-Jimenez RC, et al. Functional regurgitation of atrioventricular valves and atrial fibrillation: an elusive pathophysiological link deserving further attention. *J Am Soc Echocardiogr.* 2020;33:42–53.

8. Mutlak D, Lessick J, Reisner SA, et al. Echocardiography-based spectrum of severe tricuspid regurgitation: the frequency of apparently idiopathic tricuspid regurgitation. *J Am Soc Echocardiogr.* 2007;20:405–408.

9. Najib MQ, Vinales KL, Vittala SS, et al. Predictors for the development of severe tricuspid regurgitation with anatomically normal valve in patients with atrial fibrillation. *Echocardiography.* 2012;29:140–146.

10. Yamasaki N, Kondo F, Kubo T, et al. Severe tricuspid regurgitation in the aged: atrial remodeling associated with long-standing atrial fibrillation. *J Cardiol.* 2006;48:315–323.

11. Boyaci A, Gokce V, Topaloglu S, et al. Outcome of significant functional tricuspid regurgitation late after mitral valve replacement for predominant rheumatic mitral stenosis. *Angiology.* 2007;58:336–342.

12. Izumi C, Iga K, Konishi T. Progression of isolated tricuspid regurgitation late after mitral valve surgery for rheumatic mitral valve disease. *J Heart Valve Dis.* 2002;11:353–356.

13. Bruce CJ, Connolly HM. Right-sided valve diseases deserves a little more respect. *Circulation.* 2009;119:2726–2734.

14. Badano LP, Muraru D, Enriquez-Sarano M. Assessment of functional tricuspid regurgitation. *Eur Heart J.* 2013;34:1875–1885.

15. Topilsky Y, Khanna A, Le Tourneau T, et al. Clinical context and mechanism of functional tricuspid regurgitation in patients with and without pulmonary hypertension. *Circ Cardiovasc Imag.* 2012;5:314–323.

16. Dreyfus GD, Corbi PJ, Chan KM, Bahrami T. Secondary tricuspid regurgitation or dilatation: which should be the criteria for surgical repair. *Ann Thorac Surg.* 2005;79:127–132.

17. Matsunaga A, Duran CM. Progression of tricuspid regurgitation after repaired functional ischemic mitral regurgitation. *Circulation.* 2005;112:I453–I1457.

18. Nath J, Foster E, Heidenreich PA. Impact of tricuspid regurgitation on long-term survival. *J Am Coll Cardiol.* 2004;43:405–409.

19. Ong K, Yu G, Jue J. Prevalence and spectrum of conditions associated with severe tricuspid regurgitation. *Echocardiography.* 2014;31:558–562.

20. Muraru D, Surkova E, Badano LP. Revisit of functional tricuspid regurgitation: current trends in the diagnosis and management. *Korean Circ J.* 2016;46:443–455.

21. Mutlak D, Aronson D, Lessick J, et al. Functional tricuspid regurgitation in patients with pulmonary hypertension: is pulmonary artery pressure the only determinant of regurgitation severity? *Chest.* 2009;135:115–121.

22. Sagie A, Schwammenthal E, Padial LR, et al. Determinants of functional tricuspid regurgitation in incomplete tricuspid valve closure: Doppler color flow study of 109 patients. *J Am Coll Cardiol.* 1994;24:446–453.

23. Porter A, Shapira Y, Wurzel M, et al. Tricuspid regurgitation late after mitral valve replacement: clinical and echocardiographic evaluation. *J Heart Valve Dis.* 1999;8:57–62.

24. Badano LP, Hahn RT, Zanella-Rodriguez H, et al. Morphological assessment of the tricuspid apparatus and grading regurgitation severity in patients with functional tricuspid regurgitation. Thinking outside the box. *JACC Cardiovascular Imag.* 2019;12:652–664.

25. Song H, Kang DH, Kim JH, et al. Percutaneous mitral valvuloplasty versus surgical treatment in mitral stenosis with severe tricuspid regurgitation. *Circulation.* 2007;116:1246–1250.

26. Sadeghi HM, Kimura BJ, Raisinghani A, et al. Does lowering pulmonary arterial pressure eliminate severe functional tricuspid regurgitation? Insights from pulmonary thromboendarterectomy. *J Am Coll Cardiol.* 2004;44:126–132.

27. Franceschi F, Thuny F, Giorgi R, et al. Incidence, risk factors, and outcome of traumatic tricuspid regurgitation after percutaneous ventricular lead removal. *J Am Coll Cardiol.* 2009;53:2168–2174.

28. Chang JD, Manning WJ, Ebrille E, Zimetbaum PJ. Tricuspid valve dysfunction following pacemaker or cardioverter-defibrillator implantation. *J Am Coll Cardiol.* 2017;69:2331–2341.

29. Nguyen V, Cantarovich M, Cecere R, Giannetti N. Tricuspid regurgitation after cardiac transplantation: how many biopsies are too many. *J Heart Lung Transplant.* 2005;24:S227–S231.

30. Chorin E, Rozenbaum Z, Topilsky Y, et al. Tricuspid regurgitation and long-term clinical outcomes. *Eur Heart J Cardiovasc Imag.* 2019.

31. Wang N, Fulcher J, Abeysuriya N, et al. Tricuspid regurgitation is associated with increased mortality independent of pulmonary pressures and right heart failure: a systematic review and meta-analysis. *Eur Heart J.* 2019;40:476–484.

32. Benfari G, Antoine C, Miller WL, et al. Excess mortality associated with functional tricuspid regurgitation complicating heart failure with reduced ejection fraction. *Circulation.* 2019;140:196–206.

33. Bartko PE, Arfsten H, Frey MK, et al. Natural history of functional tricuspid regurgitation: implications of quantitative Doppler assessment. *JACC Cardiovascular Imag.* 2019;12:389–397.

34. Shiran A, Sagie A. Tricuspid regurgitation in mitral valve disease incidence, prognostic implications, mechanism, and management. *J Am Coll Cardiol.* 2009;53:401–448.

35. Santoro C, Marco Del Castillo A, et al. Mid-term outcome of severe tricuspid regurgitation: are there any differences according to mechanism and severity? *Eur Heart J Cardiovasc Imag.* 2019;20:1035–1042.

36. Shiran A, Najjar R, Adawi S, Aronson D. Risk factors for progression of functional tricuspid regurgitation. *Am J Cardiol.* 2014;113:995–1000.

---

103 Quantification of Tricuspid Regurgitation

Luigi P. Badano, Denisa Muraru

Two- and three-dimensional echocardiography (2DE and 3DE, respectively), combined with spectral and color-flow Doppler evaluation, provides the most accurate laboratory test in detection and quantification of tricuspid regurgitation (TR).[1] "Physiologic" TR is associated with normal valve leaflet morphology and normal right ventricular and atrial size (Fig. 103.1). When "pathologic" TR is suspected on color Doppler, a complete understanding of leaflet morphology and of the pathophysiological mechanisms underlying TR is mandatory (see Chapter 101). In these cases, a more comprehensive assessment of the morphology of the tricuspid valve (TV) apparatus using transthoracic 2DE and 3DE (see Chapter 101) provides important clues on the underlying etiology and mechanisms of TV dysfunction.[2–4]

Current guidelines[1] recommend a multiparametric approach to assess the severity of TR (Table 103.1), taking into account qualitative, semiquantitative, and quantitative parameters. Even though the echo Doppler parameters used to assess TR are the same used to assess left-sided valve regurgitation, several critical factors should be taken into account when using them to grade the severity of TR. The most important ones are (1) the anatomic differences between the TV (three-leaflet) and the mitral valve (two-leaflet); (2) except in patients with severe pulmonary hypertension, the TR

jet has lower velocity and lower pressure than the mitral one; and (3) the severity of TR varies during the respiratory cycle.[5]

COLOR JET AREA

When looking at the color jet area to estimate the severity of a regurgitant jet, we need to take into account that the color jet area is not related to regurgitant volume, but it is determined by conservation of jet momentum (roughly defined as flow × velocity or Q × v) and technical factors (Box 103.1). Accordingly, the same color jet area can be seen for completely different regurgitant orifice areas (EROA) and volumes (Fig. 103.2). Because flow (Q) = EROA × v and momentum (M) = Q × v or EROA × v², it is clear that, for the same EROA, a 6-m/s mitral regurgitant jet will create a jet area that is four times larger than a 3-m/s TR jet.

In addition to jet momentum, several instrument settings affect the jet size by color Doppler; the most important among them is the color scale (see Chapters 88 and 98). Finally, the displayed jet size is also affected by constraint of the right atrium (RA) and the direction of the jet. Eccentric jets, directed against the RA wall, are, on average, 75% smaller that central jets of similar severity that are free to expand in the RA cavity.[6]

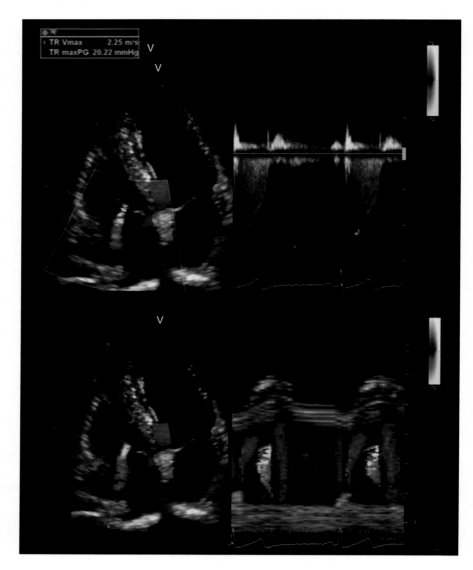

Figure 103.1. Physiological tricuspid regurgitation (TR). The color jet is localized in a small region adjacent to valve closure (<1 cm), is thin and central, and often does not extend throughout systole as shown by the color M-mode tracing *(lower right)*. Continuous-wave Doppler spectral tracing is faint and peak velocity is between 1.7 and 2.3 m/s *(upper right)*.

Accordingly, when assessing TR color Doppler jets to estimate the severity of TR, some key points should be taken into consideration: (1) the color Doppler jet area depends on jet momentum, which is lower for TR than for mitral regurgitation (MR); (2) reducing the color scale enlarges the color jet area; and (3) usually, the severity of TR is overestimated with centrally directed jets and underestimated with eccentric jets that run along the RA wall.

The jet-to-RA area ratio is another commonly reported parameter to estimate the severity of TR. However, RA size increases with the severity of TR,[7] and particularly in patients with atrial fibrillation, enlargement of RA size itself is involved in the pathophysiology of TR.[3,8,9] Therefore, using a fixed jet-to-RA area ratio threshold value would lead to underestimation of the severity of TR with progressive enlargement of the RA.

VENA CONTRACTA WIDTH

Vena contracta (VC) represents the cross-sectional area of the blood column as it leaves the regurgitant orifice; it should thus reflect thus the regurgitant orifice area. The VC of the TR jet is typically imaged in the apical four-chamber view using a careful probe angulation to optimize the flow image, an adapted Nyquist limit (color Doppler scale, 40–70 cm/s) to perfectly identify the neck of the jet, and a narrow sector scan coupled with the zoom mode to maximize temporal resolution and measurement accuracy

(Fig. 103.3). Averaging measurements over at least two to three beats is recommended. A VC diameter larger than 6.5 mm is usually associated with severe TR. Intermediate values are not accurate for distinguishing moderate from mild TR.

The basic geometric assumptions in using the diameter of the VC of the regurgitant jet to estimate The severity of TR are that (1) the proximal portion of the jet has a circular cross section, and (2) the 2DE view used to measure VC diameter is passing though the actual diameter of its cross-sectional area. Because of the noncircular and nonplanar shape of the TR jet, both of those assumptions are unlikely to occur in clinical practice (Fig. 103.4). Moreover, VC width is affected by the lateral resolution of the probe, flow rate, and machine settings. In vitro tests have shown that VC diameter measured by color Doppler can be more than twice the actual size of directly visualized orifices.[10]

The diameter of the VC of the TR jet was validated by Tribouilloy and associates[11] in 71 patients with various degrees of TR. They measured it from a single four-chamber apical view and used the 2DE Doppler EROA and hepatic venous flow as reference. Both of them having suboptimal accuracy and a number of limitations in patients with TR.[1,4] They found that a VC diameter greater than 6.5 mm identified severe TR with 88.5% sensitivity and 93.3% specificity. However, they tested the accuracy of the parameter on the same study population from which the parameter was derived.

TABLE 103.1 Echocardiographic Assessment of Tricuspid Regurgitation Severity

Parameter	Mild	Moderate	Severe
RIGHT HEART STRUCTURES			
TV leaflets	Normal or mildly abnormal	Moderately abnormal	Flail leaflets, severe tethering or retraction with large coaptation defect, perforation
RV and RA size	Usually normal	Normal or mild dilatation	Usually dilated
Inferior vena cava	Normal (<2 cm)	Normal or mildly dilated (2.1–2.5 cm)	Usually dilated[1]
QUALITATIVE DOPPLER			
Color flow jet area[a]	Small, narrow, central	Moderate central	Large central or eccentric wall-impinging jet of variable size
Flow convergence zone	Not visible, transient or small	Intermediate in size and duration	Large throughout systole
Continuous-wave Doppler spectral tracing	Faint, incomplete, parabolic	Dense, parabolic or triangular	Dense, often triangular with early peaking
SEMIQUANTITATIVE DOPPLER			
Color-flow jet area (cm^2)[b]	Not defined	Not defined	>10
VC width (cm)[b]	<0.3	0.3–0.69	≥7
PISA radius (cm)[c]	≤0.5	0.6–0.9	≥1
Hepatic vein flow[d]	Systolic dominance	Systolic blunting	Systolic flow reversal
Tricuspid inflow[d]	A-wave dominant	Variable	E-wave >1 m/s
QUANTITATIVE DOPPLER			
EROA (cm^2)	<0.2	0.2–0.39[e]	≥0.4
Regurgitant volume (mL)	<30	30–44[e]	≥45
Regurgitant fraction (%)	Not defined	Not defined	Not defined

[a]Right ventricular (RV) and atrial (RA) size can be within the "normal" range in patients with acute severe tricuspid regurgitation.
[b]With Nyquist limit >50 to 70 cm/s.
[c]With baseline Nyquist limit shift of 28 cm/s.
[d]Signs are nonspecific and are influenced by many other factors (RV diastolic function, atrial fibrillation, RA pressure).
[e]There are few data to support further separation of these values.
Modified from Zoghbi WA, et al: Recommendations for noninvasive evaluation of native valvular regurgitation, *J Am Soc Echocardiogr* 30:303–371, 2017.
EROA, Effective regurgitant orifice area; *PISA,* proximal isovelocity surface area *TV,* tricuspid valve; *VC,* vena contracta.

BOX 103.1 Technical Factors That Can Affect Color Jet Area

- Gain
- Scale
- Frame rate
- Transducer
- Color-flow algorithms
- Ultrasound machine

However, recent studies using the Doppler volumetric method to quantitate EROA and regurgitant volume showed that the threshold value of VC diameter (calculated either as an average of the diameters measured between two orthogonal planes obtained from multiplane imaging or the diameters measured in apical four-chamber view and the parasternal inflow view) to identify severe TR was 9 mm.[12] Finally, in a study that used clinical outcome as a reference, higher values of VC diameter (i.e., ≥5 mm) were associated with an increased mortality rate.[13]

Accordingly, when looking at VC diameter to estimate the severity of TR, some key points should be taken into consideration: (1) the diameter of the VC is affected by the resolution of probe and by machine settings; (2) because of the noncircularity and nonplanarity of the regurgitant orifice, it is unlikely that a single diameter may be representative of actual EROA; and (3) currently reported threshold values for grading the severity of TR lack of validation.

Three-dimensional echocardiography (3DE) color Doppler studies have shown the highly variable cross-sectional shape of the VC[5] and a planimetry of the area of the VC obtained with 3DE color Doppler has been proposed as a parameter of the severity of TR that may overcome the geometrical assumptions inherent to VC

diameter. Recent studies report a threshold value around 0.6 cm^2 to identify patients with severe TR.[12,14]

CONTINUOUS-WAVE DOPPLER SPECTRAL TRACING

Both the shape and the density (but not the velocity!) of the continuous-wave Doppler spectral tracing have been used to estimate the severity of TR. When TR is mild, there are a limited number of red cells passing from the right ventricle (RV) to the RA, and the jet is not holosystolic. Therefore, the tracing is weak and incomplete (Fig. 103.5A). Conversely, when TR is severe, the spectra is dense and complete.

In patients with mild or moderate TR, the shape of the tracing is usually parabolic, reflecting the typical change of atrioventricular gradients during systole (Fig. 103.5B). In patients with severe TR, there is a large regurgitant orifice with a reduced atrioventricular gradient. Consequently, maximal TR velocity is usually lower, and the RA pressure rises rapidly with early pressure equalization, resulting in a spectral tracing characterized by early peaking of the velocity and a dense and triangular shape (Fig. 103.5C).

PULSED-WAVE DOPPLER FLOW IN THE HEPATIC VEIN

Severe TR is often associated with systolic flow reversal in the hepatic vein (Fig. 103.6) detected by pulsed-wave spectral Doppler using a subcostal view.[15] However, there is no fixed regurgitant volume threshold over which systolic flow reversal occurs because it depends also on the size and compliance of the RA and on right ventricular function. When the RA is small, systemic venous pressure is high, or right ventricular function (and tricuspid annular descent) is reduced, a smaller amount of regurgitant volume will be enough to raise the pressure in inferior vena and reverse the flow in the hepatic veins.

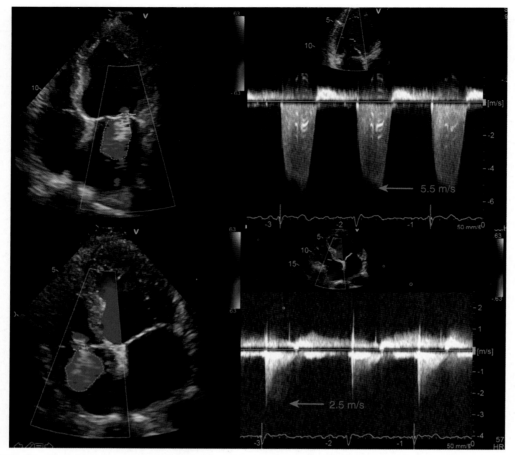

Figure 103.2. Misleading effect of jet area size to quantitate tricuspid regurgitation severity. The areas of the mitral *(upper left)* and tricuspid *(lower left)* regurgitant jets are similar in size (8.2 cm² and 7.6 cm², respectively), but the driving forces (Vmax) across the two regurgitant orifices are quite different (5.5 m/s and 2.5 m/s, respectively) *(right)*. Accordingly, the regurgitant volume across the tricuspid valve is much larger than the one crossing the mitral valve

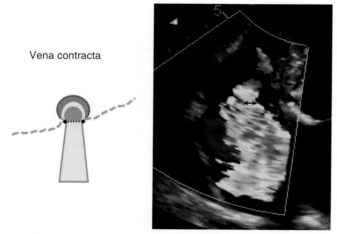

Vena contracta

Figure 103.3. Measurement of the vena contracta of the tricuspid regurgitation jet with two-dimensional color Doppler. The baseline Nyquist limit shift has been reduced too 28 cm/s, and the image has been zoomed.

PROXIMAL ISOVELOCITY SURFACE AREA ANALYSIS

One of the semiquantitative (proximal isovelocity surface area [PISA] radius) and all quantitative (EROA and regurgitant volume) parameters recommended to assess the severity of TR are obtained from the analysis of the proximal convergence zone of the regurgitant

jet (see Chapter 98). The PISA radius is the simplest of these parameters (Fig. 103.7). Qualitatively, a TR PISA radius larger than 9 mm at a Nyquist limit of 28 cm/s has been associated with the presence of significant TR (corresponding to an effective regurgitant orifice area ≥40 mm² and a regurgitant volume ≥45 mL, the quantitative thresholds for severe TR), whereas a radius smaller than 5 mm suggests mild regurgitation. However, the PISA method is based on several geometric assumptions, such as when flow approaches a point-like orifice in a flat plate, a series of concentric hemispheric shells with decreasing surface area and increasing velocities is formed. This concept is particularly challenging when applied to TR.[5]

Regurgitant orifices are never point-like orifices but finite openings (that are particularly large in case of significant TR) within the valve. Consequently, shell contours flatten as they get closer to the regurgitant orifice. This leads to underestimation of regurgitant flow and EROA by a factor equivalent to the ratio of the aliasing velocity divided by the peak orifice velocity (or v_a/v_p). For high-velocity MR jets, this underestimation is usually negligible (e.g., using 40 cm/s aliasing velocity with a 5 m/s regurgitation jet velocity will end in 8% underestimation inflow). Conversely, with the much lower TR jet velocity this underestimation is much more significant.[16] Moreover, according to the anatomy of the TV, the regurgitant orifice in functional TR is star-like or elliptical (i.e., not rounded), with the largest dimension in the anteroposterior direction (see Fig. 103.4). Thus, the PISA generated by this regurgitant jet would likely be hemielliptical and not hemispheric (Fig. 103.8), leading to underestimation of severity of TR when using the PISA radius as a sole parameter of the severity of TR. Finally, even if both the PISA radius and EROA were accurate estimates of the

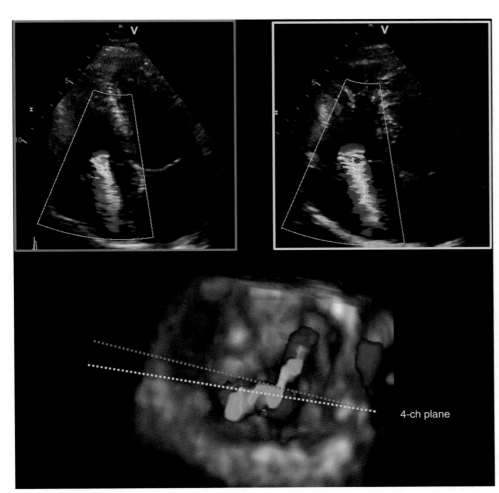

Figure 103.4. Effects of little changes of probe rotation on the measurement of tricuspid regurgitation (TR) vena contracta width using two-dimensional color Doppler imaging. Three-dimensional color flow imaging of the tricuspid valve from the ventricular perspective allows appreciation of the complex slitlike shape of the vena contracta in functional TR. *Red* and *yellow dashed lines* show the orientation of the two-dimensional views of the same color shown in the *upper panels*.

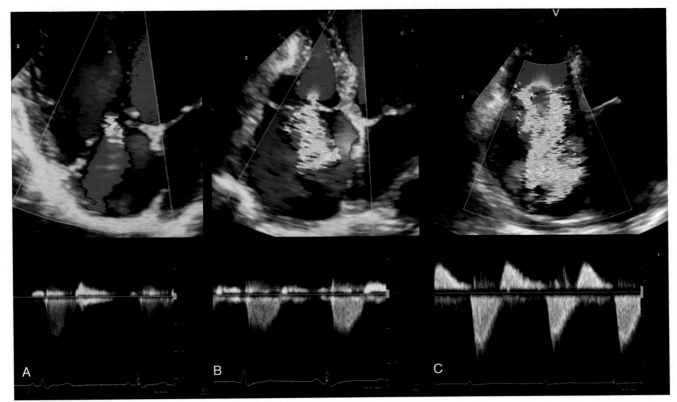

Figure 103.5. Color and continuous-wave Doppler appearance of mild (**A**), moderate (**B**), and severe (**C**) tricuspid regurgitation. See text and Table 103.1 for details.

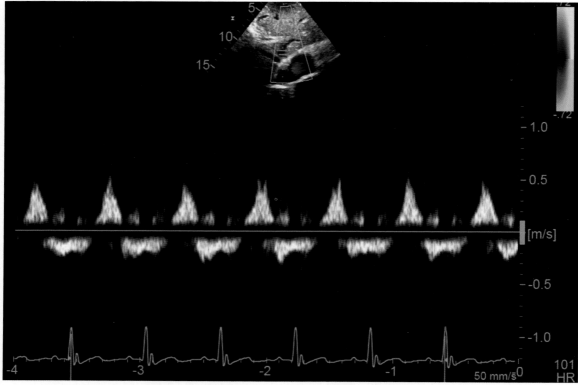

Figure 103.6. Systolic flow reversal in the hepatic vein in a patient with severe tricuspid regurgitation.

PISA radius

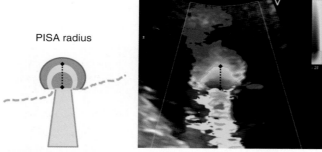

Figure 103.7. Measurement of the proximal isovelocity surface area (PISA) radius of the tricuspid regurgitation jet with two-dimensional color Doppler. The apical four-chamber view and the parasternal long- and short-axis views are classically recommended for an optimal visualization of the PISA. The area of interest is optimized by reducing imaging depth and Nyquist limit to approximately 30 cm/s. The PISA radius is measured at midsystole using the first aliasing.

severity of TR in the frame they are calculated, it should be taken into account that TR is not constant, but it varies continuously throughout systole (Fig. 103.9); therefore, a measurement taken in a single frame does not seem to be the ideal parameter to assess the severity of TR. Furthermore, both the EROA and the regurgitant volume across the TV are influenced by the respiratory cycle (Fig. 103.10). Compared with expiration, during inspiration, TR presents a decrease in driving forces while the size of the regurgitant orifice increases by 69%.[17] During inspiration, as venous return to the right side of the heart increases, the RV and RA expand their widths to accommodate a higher volume, without significantly changing their longitudinal dimensions. The increase in widths of the RA and the RV result in an increase of the tricuspid annulus dimension.

Moreover, the horizontal displacement of the papillary muscles and the anatomic particularities of the TV (with the insertion of chordae tendinae to multiple papillary muscles and the right ventricular free wall) determine an increase in leaflet coaptation distance and tenting volume.[18] Consequently, TR orifice area increases, ultimately resulting in an average increase in 20% of regurgitant volume during inspiration.[17] Currently, it remains to be determined which is the best moment to quantitate TR: during inspiration, during expiration, during halted respiration, or integrating the regurgitant volume over time through the respiratory cycle.

Another geometric assumption that affects calculations using the PISA method is the position of the orifice on a flat plane. In patients with significant functional TR, the TV leaflets are often severely tethered toward the RV (Fig. 103.11), and the outer angle formed by these should be accounted for in the calculation of regurgitant flow.[16] The issue of the nonplanar geometry of the regurgitant orifice is not a major problem in assessing MR (more planar geometry), but it significantly affects calculations of TR regurgitant flow by using $2\pi(\alpha/180)$, in which α is the solid angle subtended by the tricuspid leaflets.[16]

Finally, when assessing the severity of TR, we should also take into account the extreme load dependency of the TR volume. Changes in patient's position, diuretic therapy, and lack of standardization of timing in measuring severity of TR are among the most frequent causes of intertechnique and day-to-day variability of the severity of TR.

Apart from the limitations and technical challenges of the currently recommended parameters, the current grading system has been challenged, too. This issue raised during the assessment of the results of early percutaneous tricuspid intervention trials which showed that patients enrolled in those trials had the severity of TR up to two grades above the current severe thresholds of EROA (40 mm²), regurgitant volume (45 mL), and VC diameter (7 mm). Despite a significant reduction of the severity of TR and clinical improvement after

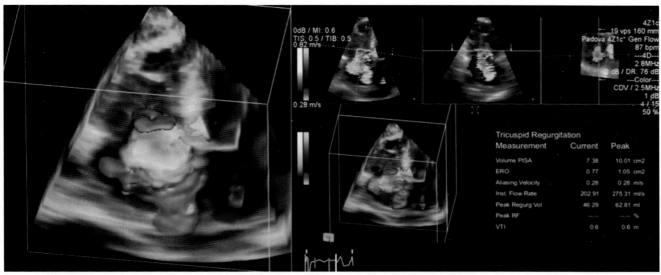

Figure 103.8. Three-dimensional reconstruction of the isovelocity surface area (*left, green surface*) and a transversal cut plane at the level of the proximal part of the jet *(upper right)* show that the assumptions about the hemispheric shape of the isovelocity surface area and the round shape of the regurgitant orifice that are the bases for calculation of effective orifice area with two-dimensional color Doppler echocardiography are not met in the case of tricuspid regurgitation. Accordingly, caution should be used in calculations based on measurement of a single linear dimension (proximal isovelocity surface area [PISA] radius) to obtain the effective regurgitant orifice area and volume. *ERO*, Effective regurgitant orifice area.

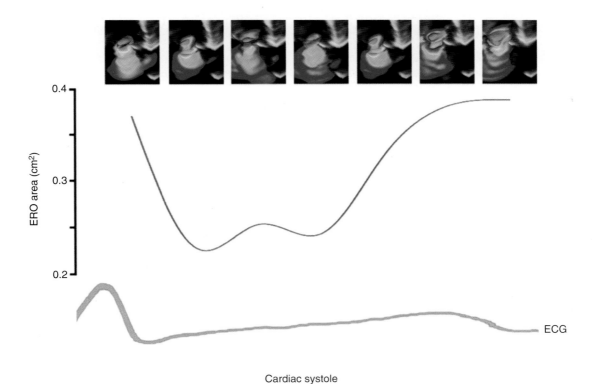

Figure 103.9. Plot showing the effective regurgitant orifice area (EROA) variations during systole in a patient with moderate tricuspid regurgitation. EROA is larger at early and late systole and decreases significantly in midsystole when the contraction of the right ventricle pushes the tricuspid valve leaflets toward the annulus. *ECG,* Electrocardiography.

transcatheter tricuspid interventions, using the current grading system, the severity of TR was reduced from severe to "severe." Accordingly, two new grades were proposed to expand the TR grading scheme beyond severe and take into account this clinical need.[19] The proposed grade of "massive" has been defined by an EROA of 60 to 79 mm^2, a regurgitant volume of 60 to 74 mL, and a VC diameter of 14 to 20 mm,

whereas "torrential" was defined by an EROA of 80 mm^2 or greater, a regurgitant volume 75 mL or greater, and a VC diameter of 21 mm or larger.[19] Even though the threshold values used to define massive and torrential TR are just a mathematical transposition of the differences in the considered parameters between current moderate and severe grades (without no hemodynamic or clinical validation), they may be

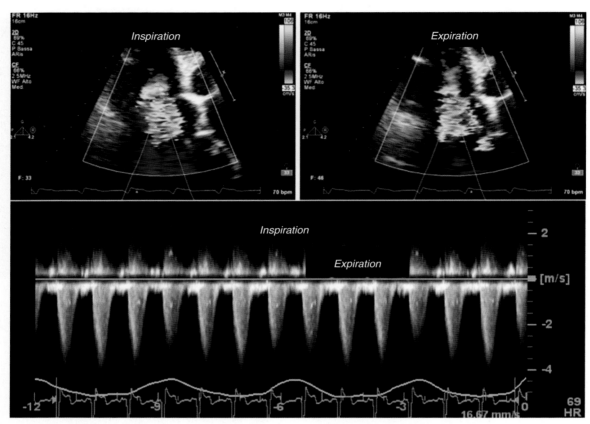

Figure 103.10. Color Doppler *(upper panels)* and continuous-wave Doppler recordings *(lower panels)* of tricuspid regurgitation (TR) showing significant respiratory variations of its severity. The severity of TR increases during inspiration and decreases during expiration (i.e., the Rivero Carvallo sign).

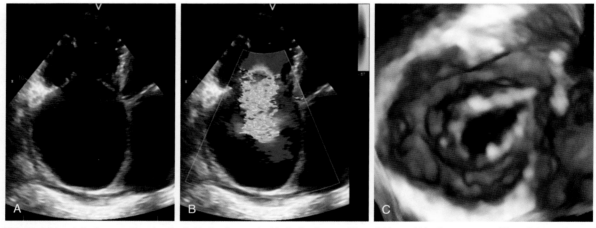

Figure 103.11. Midsystolic frames showing leaflet tethering and wide lack of apposition of tricuspid leaflets on two- (**A**) and three-dimensional (**C**) echocardiography in a patient with severe functional tricuspid regurgitation (**B**).

instrumental to determine the efficacy of new transcatheter treatments of TR, and they have been shown to be predictive of cardiovascular death in a recent outcome study.[20]

REFERENCES

1. Zoghbi WA, Adams D, Bonow RO, et al. Recommendations for noninvasive evaluation of native valvular regurgitation. *J Am Soc Echocardiogr.* 2017;30:303–371.
2. Muraru D, Hahn RT, Soliman OI, et al. Three-dimensional echocardiography in imaging the tricuspid valve. *JACC Cardiovasc Imag.* 2019;12:500–515.
3. Muraru D, Guta AC, Ochoa-Jimenez RC, et al. Functional regurgitation of atrioventricular valves and atrial fibrillation: an elusive pathophysiological link deserving further attention. *J Am Soc Echocardiogr.* 2020;33:42–53.
4. Hahn RT, Thomas JD, Khalique OK, et al. Imaging assessment of tricuspid regurgitation severity. *JACC Cardiovasc Imag.* 2019;12:469–490.
5. Badano LP, Hahn RT, Zanella-Rodriguez HA, et al. Morphological assessment of the tricuspid apparatus and grading regurgitation severity in patients with functional tricuspid regurgitation. Thinking outside the box. *JACC Cardiovasc Imag.* 2019;12 (in press).
6. Rivera JM, Vandervoort PM, Vazquez de Prada JA, et al. Which physical factors determine tricuspid regurgitation jet area in the clinical setting. *Am J Cardiol.* 1993;72:1305–1309.

7. Nemoto N, Lesser JR, Pedersen WR, et al. Pathogenic structural heart changes in early tricuspid regurgitation. *J Thorac Cardiovasc Surg*. 2015;150:323–330.
8. Utsunomiya H, Itabashi Y, Mihara H, et al. Functional tricuspid regurgitation caused by chronic atrial fibrillation: a real-time 3-dimensional transesophageal echocardiography study. *Circ Cardiovasc Imag*. 2017;10.
9. Najib MQ, Vinales KL, Vittala SS, et al. Predictors for the development of severe tricuspid regurgitation with anatomically normal valve in patients with atrial fibrillation. *Echocardiography*. 2012;29:140–146.
10. Mascherbauer J, Rosenhek R, Bittner B, et al. Doppler echocardiographic assessment of valvular regurgitation severity by measurement of the vena contracta: an in vitro validation study. *J Am Soc Echocardiogr*. 2005;18:999–1006.
11. Tribouilloy C, Enriquez-Sarano M, Bailey K, et al. Quantification of tricuspid regurgitation by measuring the width of the vena contracta with Doppler color flow imaging: a clinical study. *J Am Coll Cardiol*. 2000;36:472–478.
12. Dahou A, Ong G, Hamid N, et al. Quantifying tricuspid regurgitation severity: a comparison of proximal isovelocity surface area and novel quantitative Doppler methods. *JAC, Cardiovasc Imag*. 2019;12:560–562.
13. Bartko PE, Arfsten H, Frey MK, et al. Natural history of functional tricuspid regurgitation: implications of quantitative Doppler assessment. *JACC Cardiovasc Imag*. 2019;12:389–397.
14. Utsunomiya H, Harada Y, Susawa H, et al. Comprehensive evaluation of tricuspid regurgitation location and severity using vena contracta analysis: a color Doppler three-dimensional transesophageal echocardiographic study. *J Am Soc Echocardiogr*. 2019;32:1526–1537. e2.
15. Fadel BM, Vriz O, Alassas K. Manifestations of cardiovascular disorders on Doppler interrogation of the hepatic veins. *JACC Cardiovasc Imag*. 2019;12:1872–1877.
16. Rivera JM, Vandervoort PM, Mele D, et al. Quantification of tricuspid regurgitation by means of the proximal flow convergence method: a clinical study. *Am Heart J*. 1994;127:1354–1362.
17. Topilsky Y, Tribouilloy C, Michelena HI, et al. Pathophysiology of tricuspid regurgitation. Quantitative Doppler echocardiographic assessment of respiratory dependence. *Circulation*. 2010;122:1505–1513.
18. van Rosendael PJ, Joyce E, Katsanos S, et al. Tricuspid valve remodelling in functional tricuspid regurgitation: multidetector row computed tomography insights. *Eur Heart J Cardiovasc Imag*. 2016;17:96–105.
19. Hahn RT, Zamorano JL. The need for a new tricuspid regurgitation grading scheme. *Eur Heart J Cardiovasc Imag*. 2017;18:1342–1343.
20. Santoro C, Marco Del Castillo A, et al. Mid-term outcome of severe tricuspid regurgitation: are there any differences according to mechanism and severity. *Eur Heart J Cardiovasc Imag*. 2019;20:1035–1042.

104   Indications for Tricuspid Valve Intervention

Adam M. Dryden, Stanton K. Shernan, A. Stephane Lambert

Tricuspid valve (TV) surgery has one of the highest morbidity and mortality rates of all cardiac surgical procedures.[1,2] This is not necessarily because TV repair (TVr) or TV replacement (TVR) is particularly difficult technically, but rather because the presence of tricuspid regurgitation (TR) often reflects advanced cardiac disease, right ventricular (RV) dysfunction, chronic heart failure, and generally poor functional state.[3]

The evolution of two- and three-dimensional (2D and 3D, respectively) intraoperative transesophageal echocardiography (TEE) over the past two decades has enabled routine and comprehensive evaluation of the TV and consideration for intervention at the time of surgery for left-sided valvular disorders. In that context, conventional wisdom is that TVr adds little to the overall risk of the procedure. Consequently, attitudes have been shifting toward considering TV surgery for less than severe TR or even toward prophylactic interventions on valves with a high potential for future dysfunction.[2]

A recent analysis of more than 88,000 cases in the Society of Thoracic Surgeons (STS) database by Badhwar and colleagues revealed that between 2011 and 2014, TVr was performed in 14.3% of all mitral valve (MV) repair or replacement surgeries: 3.5% of patients with none to mild TR, 30.6% with moderate TR, and 75.6% with severe TR.[4] These authors reported that adding a TVr to MV surgery with or without coronary bypass grafting (CABG) was associated with an increased morbidity rate, including ventilation longer than 24 hours, renal failure, stroke, deep sternal wound infection, and reoperation, but not 30-day mortality rate. They also noted that the frequency of patients requiring a permanent pacemaker after isolated MV surgery was 6.2%, and this increased to 14.5% when TVr was added to the procedure.[4] This report suggests that there may be tangible morbidity risks associated with adding a TV procedure on to a left-sided valve procedure.

Most TR is *functional*, as a result of leaflet tethering and annular dilatation from RV remodeling in patients with left-sided ventricular or valvular disease (Fig. 104.1 and Video 104.1).

Table 104.1 compares the latest American College of Cardiology/ American Heart Association (AHA/ACC) and European Society

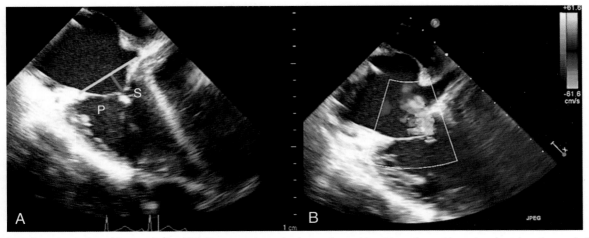

Figure 104.1. Functional tricuspid regurgitation (TR). Transesophageal echocardiographic midesophageal four-chamber view demonstrating tricuspid valve leaflet tethering (**A**) from the annulus *(yellow line)* toward the right ventricular apex *(red line)*, leading to functional TR (**B**). *P,* Posterior leaflet; *S,* septal leaflet. (See accompanying Video 104.1.)

TABLE 104.1 Comparison of American College of Cardiology (ACC)/ American Heart Association Guidelines (AHA) and European Society of Cardiology (ESC) Guidelines

	AHA/ACC 2014	ESC 2012
ISOLATED TRICUSPID VALVE SURGERY (PRIMARY)		
Symptomatic severe TR unresponsive to medical therapy	Class IIa	Class I[a]
Asymptomatic severe TR with RV dilatation or dysfunction	Class IIb	Class II
Reoperation (after left-sided procedure) for severe symptomatic TR	Class IIb	Class IIa
TRICUSPID VALVE SURGERY WITH CONCOMITANT LEFT-SIDED SURGERY (SECONDARY)		
Severe TR at the time of MV surgery (regardless of symptoms)	Class I	Class I
MILD OR MODERATE, PRIMARY OR SECONDARY TR		
Regardless of other considerations	No mention	Class IIa
With TV annular dilatation	Class IIa	Class IIa[b]
PH without annular dilatation	Class IIb	Class IIa[b]

[a]Without severe right ventricular (RV) dysfunction.
[b]This level of recommendation is not explicitly mentioned in the ESC guidelines, but it is implied by the comment "regardless of other considerations."
MV, Mitral valve; PH, pulmonary hypertension; TR, tricuspid regurgitation.

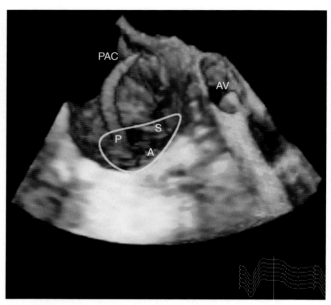

Figure 104.2. Saddle-shaped tricuspid valve annulus, demonstrated from a three-dimensional transesophageal echocardiographic full-volume dataset using offline software. *A,* Anterior leaflet; *AV,* aortic valve; *P,* posterior leaflet; *PAC,* pulmonary artery catheter; *S,* septal leaflet.

of Cardiology (ESC) guidelines for the management of TR in various clinical situations.[5,6] The decision of *whether* and *when* to recommend a TVr depends on the patient's symptoms, severity of TR, RV function, size of the annulus, and presence of pulmonary hypertension (PH) or atrial fibrillation.[6,7]

SEVERITY OF TRICUSPID REGURGITATION

The severity of functional TR graded by echocardiography can be influenced by RV preload, afterload, and contractile state, all of which may be significantly affected by general anesthesia and positive-pressure ventilation.[8] Thus, functional TR severity can change acutely and repeatedly during the course of cardiac surgery. The ACC/AHA and ESC universally recognize severe TR as an indication for TVr at the time of MV surgery (class I indication). The addition of a corrective TV procedure to the planned MV procedure is associated with a relatively significant long-term clinical benefit. In a recent meta-analysis of 15 studies including 2840 patients, Pagnesi and colleagues[9] reported that the addition of TV surgery to mitral or aortic valve surgery was associated with a significant decrease in the risk of cardiac-related mortality at a mean follow-up of 6 years (odds ratio [OR], 0.38). The addition of TVr also resulted in a lower risk of developing more than moderate TR (OR, 0.16). Most of the studies included in this meta-analysis were observational.[9] In another retrospective analysis of nearly 24,000 patients between 1990 and 2014, Kelly and colleagues[10] found a correlation between the severity of TR diagnosed by intraoperative preprocedural TEE and postcardiac surgical mortality rate for all cardiac surgical procedures. When adjusted for confounders, moderate TR (hazard ratio [HR], 1.24) and severe TR (HR, 2.02) were associated with an increased risk of mortality. On the other hand, patients who underwent TV surgery had a statistically lower chance of death regardless of the grade of TR (HR, 0.74).[10]

The ACC/AHA and ESC guidelines are less committed to providing recommendations on valve repair for severe TR in the context of procedures that do not involve an open cardiotomy, such as CABG. In the case of symptomatic TR associated with RV failure and liver congestion, the ESC guidelines recommend TVr as a class

I indication, whereas this is considered a class IIa indication in the ACC/AHA guidelines.[5] When less than severe TR is present, the decision to repair the TV is even more controversial and depends on the presence of other factors such as RV dysfunction or annular dilatation.

RIGHT VENTRICULAR FUNCTION

Although serial measurements of left ventricular ejection fraction can guide the timing of MV surgery, it is more difficult to objectively quantify RV ejection fraction accurately by echocardiography because the assessment is most often qualitative. Consequently, recommendations pertaining to the timing of TV surgery based on RV function remain less definite.[5,6]

The TV annulus is a complex 3D saddle-shaped structure that plays an important role in TV competence (Fig. 104.2).[11] Tricuspid annular dilatation appears to be a strong predictor for the development of TR and an important prognostic factor, whether or not MV disease is corrected.[12,13] Therefore, the approach of simply "fixing the primary left-sided lesion and letting the right-sided disease take care of itself" is likely inappropriate in many cases.

Both the AHA/ACC and the ESC guidelines recommend TV annuloplasty at the time of MV repair if the TR is less than severe and there is significant annular dilatation (class IIa recommendation).[5,6] Based on Dreyfus and coworkers'[8] definition, the AHA/ACC guidelines define abnormal annular dilatation as 40 mm or 21 mm/m^2 as measured in the transthoracic echocardiographic (TTE) apical four-chamber view or greater than 70 mm in the anteroseptal to anteroposterior commissural diameter measured directly in the surgical field.

There remains controversy about what size of TV annulus should prompt consideration of TVr. Dreyfus and colleagues reported in 2005 on 311 patients undergoing MV surgery between 1989 and 2001.[8] TV annular diameter was directly measured by the surgeon, from the anteroseptal to the anteroposterior commissures. TV annuloplasty was performed when the annular diameter was more than twice normal at a dimension greater than 70 mm (Fig. 104.3 and Video 104.3). During a mean follow-up period of 4.8 years, the patients who underwent TVr demonstrated significantly less TR

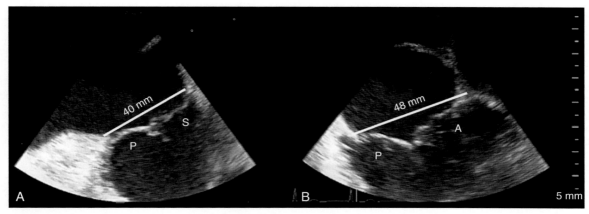

Figure 104.3. Tricuspid valve annular dilatation. Transesophageal echocardiographic midesophageal views at 0 degrees (**A**) and 90 degrees of multiplane rotation (**B**). Note the significant difference in dimensions between the two orthogonal views. *A,* Anterior leaflet; *P,* posterior leaflet; *S,* septal leaflet. (See accompanying Video 104.3.)

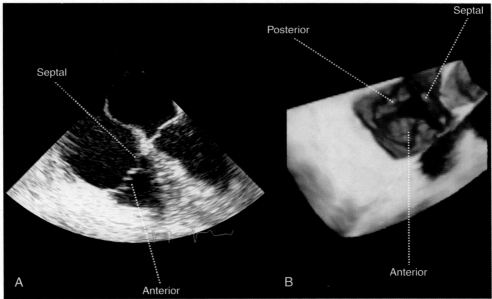

Figure 104.4. Two-dimensional (2D) versus three-dimensional (3D) transesophageal echocardiography views of the tricuspid valve. **A,** A midesophageal four-chamber view that typically demonstrates the septal and posterior leaflets. However, in this example, as confirmed by the corresponding 3D pyramidal volume, (**B**) the septal and anterior leaflets are shown. Thus, care must be taken with 2D echocardiography not to rely solely on pattern recognition when obtaining views.

and improved perioperative morbidity and survival compared with the patients who did not undergo TV annuloplasty.

Traditionally, the TV annular diameter is measured in the four-chamber TTE view or the equivalent TEE) midesophageal four-chamber view.[14,15] It is important to remember that the correlation between direct physical intercommissural diameter and measurements made in the four-chamber TTE or TEE view may not always be consistent, in part because the TV annulus is not circular, and the typical 2D TEE four-chamber view is not aligned with either the long or the shore axes.[16] Slight changes in probe position, as well as anatomic changes caused by RV remodeling and loading conditions, may result in unpredictable variability in measurement of the TV annulus. Because 3D echocardiography relies a lot less on scanning accuracy, pattern recognition, and geometric assumptions, it is more reliable for depicting and measuring the true size of the TV annulus[17] (see Figs. 104.3 and 104.4). It remains unclear in which exact plane on a multiple plane

reconstruction of a 3D image the TV annulus should be measured and what corresponds to normal values, TR progression, or, most important, clinical outcomes.[18–20]

Based on the foregoing discussion, patients with significant TV annular dilatation at the time of MV surgery, especially if PH is present, should be considered for prophylactic annuloplasty to reduce or prevent further expansion of the annulus, and 40 mm in the apical four-chamber TTE midview currently remains the generally accepted threshold to intervene. Past studies suggested that patients whose dilated TV annulus underwent repair at the time of MV surgery demonstrated significant reverse RV remodeling and no TR progression.[21]

This practice was recently challenged by David and colleagues, however, who reported on a cohort of 312 patients followed for 6 years after surgery for isolated MV disease: there was no significant difference in the rate of TR in patients who had a TV annular diameter greater than 40 mm versus those whose TV annular diameter was less than 40mm.[22]

LATE DEVELOPMENT OF TRICUSPID REGURGITATION AFTER MITRAL VALVE SURGERY

More than mild TR after MV surgery is usually associated with worse outcome. Untreated TR at the time of MV surgery has a negative impact on perioperative morbidity, functional status, and survival.[23] Moreover, the development of late severe TR as a marker of significant cardiac disease is invariably associated with a poor prognosis. Generally accepted risk factors for TR progression include atrial fibrillation and recurrent MR.[24]

When a patient develops late, severe, symptomatic TR, however, the approach is controversial. Whereas the ESC guidelines consider this a class IIa indication for TVr, the ACC/AHA guidelines consider it a class IIb indication, perhaps because a reoperation to correct late severe TR after MV repair has been associated with an increased surgical mortality rate of 10% to 25%.[5] Recent advances in percutaneous valve interventions, well developed for aortic and MV disorders, may change this reality in the future.[25] Indeed, the lower mortality rates of percutaneous procedures compared with open surgery, as seen with the mitral and aortic valves, may mean that the threshold to percutaneously intervene on *isolated* TR may be different from those suggested by current guidelines.

Please access ExpertConsult to view the corresponding videos for this chapter.

REFERENCES

1. Rankin H, Hamill B, Ferguson T, et al. Determinants of operative mortality in valvular heart surgery. *J Thorac Cardiovasc Surg.* 2006;131:547–557.
2. Rogers J, Bolling S. Valve repair for functional tricuspid valve regurgitation: anatomical and surgical considerations. *Semin Thorac Cardiovasc Surg.* 2010;22:84–89.
3. Kundi H, Popma JJ, Cohen DJ, et al. Prevalence and outcomes of isolated tricuspid valve surgery among medicare beneficiaries. *Am J Cardiol.* 2019;123:132–1382.
4. Badhwar V, Rankin JS, He M, et al. Performing concomitant tricuspid valve repair at the time of mitral valve operations is not associated with increased operative mortality. *Ann Thorac Surg.* 2016;103:587–594.
5. Nishimura RA, Otto CM, Bonow RO, et al. AHA/ACC guideline for the management of patients with valvular heart disease: executive summary. *J Am Coll Cardiol.* 2014;63:2438–2488.
6. Vahanian A, Alfieri O, Andreotti F, et al. Guidelines on the management of valvular heart disease. *Eur J Cardio Thoracic Surg.* 2012;42:S1–S44.
7. Najib MQ, Vittala SS, Challa S, et al. Predictors of severe tricuspid regurgitation in patients with permanent pacemaker or automatic implantable cardioverter-defibrillator leads. *Texas Heart Inst J.* 2012;40:529–533.
8. Dreyfus G, Corbi P, Chan K, et al. Secondary tricuspid regurgitation or dilatation: which should be the criteria for surgical repair? *Ann Thorac Surg.* 2005;79:127–132.
9. Pagnesi M, Montalto C, Mangieri A, et al. Tricuspid annuloplasty versus a conservative approach in patients with functional tricuspid regurgitation undergoing left-sided heart valve surgery: a study-level meta-analysis. *Int J Cardiol.* 2017;240:138–144.
10. Kelly BJ, Luxford JMH, Butler CG, et al. Severity of tricuspid regurgitation is associated with long term mortality. *J Thorac Cardiovasc Surg.* 2018;155:1032–1038.
11. Spinner E, Buice D, Yap C, Yoganathan A. The effects of a three-dimensional saddle-shaped annulus on anterior and posterior leaflet stretch and regurgitation of the tricuspid valve. *Ann Biomed Eng.* 2012;40:996–1005.
12. Benedetto U, Melina G, Angeloni E, et al. Prophylactic tricuspid annuloplasty in patients with dilated tricuspid annulus undergoing mitral valve surgery. *J Thorac Cardiovasc Surg.* 2012;143:632–638.
13. Navia J, Brozzi N, Klein A, et al. Moderate tricuspid regurgitation with left-sided degenerative heart valve disease to repair or not to repair? *Ann Thorac Surg.* 2012;93:59–67.
14. Lancellotti P, Moura L, Pierard L, et al. European Association of Echocardiography recommendations for the assessment of valvular regurgitation. Part 2: mitral and tricuspid regurgitation (native valve disease). *Eur J Echocardiogr.* 2010;11:307–332.
15. Hahn R, Abraham T, Adams M, et al. Guidelines for performing a comprehensive transesophageal echocardiographic examination. *J Am Soc Echocardiogr.* 2013;26:921–964.
16. Rehfeldt K. Two-dimensional transesophageal echocardiographic imaging of the tricuspid valve. *Anesth Analg.* 2012;114:547–550.
17. Lang R, Badano L, Tsang W, et al. EAE/ASE Recommendations for image acquisition and display using three-dimensional echocardiography. *J Am Soc Echocardiogr.* 2012;25:3–46.
18. Hahn RT. State-of-the-art review of echocardiographic imaging in the evaluation and treatment of functional tricuspid regurgitation. *Circ Cardiovasc Imag.* 2016;9. e005332.
19. Dreyfus J, Durand-Viel G, Raffoul R, et al. Comparison of 2-dimensional, 3-dimensional, and surgical measurements of the tricuspid annulus size clinical implications. *Circ Cardiovasc Imag.* 2015;8. e003241.
20. Volpato V, Lang R, Yamat M, et al. Echocardiographic assessment of the tricuspid annulus: the effects of the third dimension and measurement methodology. *J Am Soc Echocardiogr.* 2019;32:238–247.
21. Chikwe J, Itagaki S, Anyanwu A, et al. Impact of concomitant tricuspid annuloplasty on tricuspid regurgitation, right ventricular function, and pulmonary artery hypertension after repair of mitral valve prolapse. *J Am Coll Cardiol.* 2015;65. 1931–8.
22. David TE, David CM, Manlhiot C. Tricuspid annulus diameter does not predict the development of tricuspid regurgitation after mitral valve repair for mitral regurgitation due to degenerative diseases. *J Thorac Cardiovasc Surg.* 2018;155:2429–2436.
23. Nath J, Foster E, Heidenreich P. Impact of tricuspid regurgitation on long-term survival. *J Am Coll Cardiol.* 2004;43:405–409.
24. Ito H, Mizumoto T, Sawada Y, et al. Determinants of recurrent tricuspid regurgitation following tricuspid valve annuloplasty during mitral valve surgery. *J Card Surg.* 2017;32:237–244.
25. Taramasso M, Alessandrini H, Latib A, et al. Outcomes after current transcatheter tricuspid valve intervention: mid-term results from the International TriValve Registry. *JACC Cardiovasc Interv.* 2019;28:155–165.

105 Imaging for Surgical and Percutaneous Tricuspid Valve Procedures

Rebecca T. Hahn

Tricuspid valve (TV) disease or dysfunction is classified as primary (i.e., intrinsic) valve pathology or secondary.[1,2] Secondary or functional tricuspid regurgitation (TR) is the most common cause of TR and represents an important unmet treatment need given its prevalence, adverse prognostic impact, and symptom burden associated with progressive right heart failure.[3,4] Indications for intervening on TR are dependent first on determining valve morphology (primary or secondary), TR severity, and right heart size and function, as well as pulmonary artery pressures.[5,6] Assessment of these parameters is covered in other chapters. The specific role of imaging in TV interventions is reviewed in this chapter.[7]

CURRENT GUIDELINES: INDICATIONS FOR SURGICAL INTERVENTION AND OUTCOMES

Although current class I recommendations for surgical treatment of severe, symptomatic functional TR is at the time of left heart surgery, isolated treatment of the TV is a class IIa indication for treatment.[6,8] Multiple studies have shown that the majority of TV surgeries are performed with concomitant left heart surgery with as few as 15% performed as isolated interventions.[9,10] A recent 10-year study of 5005 patients in the Unites States National Inpatient Sample showed that isolated TV surgeries increased from 290 in 2004 to 780 in 2013;

TABLE 105.1 Summary of Main Considerations for Type of Tricuspid Valve Surgical Approach

TV Repair

- Tricuspid annuloplasty is more often used for initial stages of annulus dilatation (>40 mm) with TR that is less than severe.
- Tricuspid ring annuloplasty is typically preferred over suture annuloplasty
- Tricuspid annuloplasty may be used for pacemaker lead-induced TR when factors for failure of TR repair are absent. (Note: Concomitant removal of leads and epicardial implantation for reducing the risk of recurrent TR should be considered.)
- When predictors of recurrence of TR are present (i.e., advanced leaflet tethering and RV remodeling), repair with adjunctive techniques (i.e., anterior leaflet augmentation) may be considered for increasing coaptation.

TV Replacement

- TV replacement is more often used for treatment of primary TR with severe leaflet pathology.
- TV replacement should be considered with functional TR or pacemaker lead–induced TR when risk of recurrence after repair is high.
- TV replacement has been associated with a worse prognosis than TV repair, but this is likely because of baseline differences in treated populations.

RV, Right ventricular; *TR,* tricuspid regurgitation; *TV,* tricuspid valve.
Adapted with permission from Taramasso M, et al: Tricuspid regurgitation: predicting the need for intervention, procedural success, and recurrence of disease, *JACC Cardiovasc Imag* 12:605–621, 2019.

TABLE 105.2 Risk Factors Associated With Recurrence of Tricuspid Regurgitation After Tricuspid Annuloplasty[a]

Risk Factors for Recurrence of Significant TR After Repair	Impact on Early TR Recurrence	Impact on Mid and Late TR Recurrence
Echocardiographic Predictors		
• Preoperative TR severity	++	+
• Larger annular diameter	+	−
• Advanced leaflet tethering	+++	+++
• Presence or persistence of severe PH after TV repair	+	++
• Reduced LV function (<40%)	+	++
Clinical Predictors		
• Female gender	+	+
• Chronic atrial fibrillation	+	++
• Presence of ischemic coronary disease	+	+
• Presence of intraannular pacemaker leads	−	+++
• Kidney dysfunction	+	+++
• Concomitant COPD	+	+
Surgical or Procedural Predictors		
• Repair technique (suture vs ring annuloplasty; flexible vs rigid or semirigid ring)	+	+++
• Concomitant MV replacement rather than repair	+	+

[a]+ and - represent the presence or absence, respectively, of evidence supporting that data, with more than one + indicating strength of evidence to support it.
COPD, Chronic obstructive pulmonary disease; *LV,* left ventricular; *MV,* mitral valve; *PH,* pulmonary hypertension; *PM,* pacemaker; *TR,* tricuspid regurgitation; *TV,* tricuspid valve.
Adapted with permission from Taramasso M, et al: Tricuspid regurgitation: predicting the need for intervention, procedural success, and recurrence of disease, *JACC Cardiovasc Imag* 12:605–621, 2019.

however, the in-hospital mortality rate remained constant at 8.8%.[11] Compared with patients receiving concomitant left and right valve surgery, patients undergoing isolated TV surgery are older with a higher risk profile and had high rates of postoperative morbidities as well as protracted hospitalizations.

SURGICAL TRICUSPID VALVE INTERVENTION

The complex anatomy of the TV has been described in a previous chapter as well as a number of reviews.[12,13] Echocardiography is the imaging modality of choice for the initial evaluation of the TV and right heart morphology and function.[13–15] The surgical TV annulus can be segmented in four regions: aortic, anterior, posterior, and septal. The aortic segment is adjacent to the noncoronary sinus of Valsalva and formed by the hinge lines of the anteroseptal commissure. For both surgical and transcatheter devices, identification of this segment is important to avoid injuring or perforating the aorta but also to anchor annular devices because this region of the annulus contains the most fibrous tissue and has the greatest "pull-through" strength.[16] The atrioventricular (AV) node and the bundle of His cross the septal leaflet attachment 3 to 5 mm posterior to the anteroseptal commissure and should be avoided for both surgical and transcatheter repair procedures. The anterior segment is demarcated by the remaining anterior leaflet hinge line, the posterior segment by the posterior leaflet hinge line and the septal segment by the septal leaflet hinge line. The coronary sinus enters the right atrium consistently near the commissure between the septal and posterior leaflets. Importantly, the anterior and the septal leaflets have the longest circumferential hinge line, so the commissure between these leaflets is also the longest. The septal leaflet, however, is the shortest radial leaflet with chordal attachments to multiple small septal papillary muscles or direct chordal attachments to the septum.

Choosing between surgical TV repair or replacement may be based on a number of factors (Table 105.1).[17–28] In patients undergoing concomitant TR repair at the time of mitral surgery, persistent severe TR is still present in 11% at 3 months and 17% at 5 years.[29] Reintervention for recurrent TR carries an in-hospital mortality rate of up to 37%.[21] Several clinical, echocardiographic,

and procedural risk factors have been associated with failed tricuspid repair at follow-up (Table 105.2).[21,23–25,27,30–36] These parameters should help inform procedure choice at the time of surgery, including the use of adjunctive procedures.

Tricuspid Valve Repair Techniques

The two principal surgical methods used to perform tricuspid annuloplasty are suture and ring annuloplasty. Suture annuloplasty methods reduce the size of the tricuspid annulus with a continuous suture to cinch the annulus. With ring annuloplasty, a rigid or semirigid prosthetic, undersized ring is sewn to the tricuspid annulus. Tricuspid annuloplasty rings are incomplete to preserve the native annulus at the site of the AV node and reduce the risk of postoperative heart block. Durability and clinical outcomes of tricuspid repair for secondary TR have been improved with the use of rigid prosthetic ring annuloplasty over suture annuloplasty methods.[23,29]

In the presence of high risk for failure with annuloplasty and advanced leaflet tethering, adjunctive repair techniques may be considered. Leaflet coaptation can be increased by means of anterior leaflet augmentation with the use of an autologous pericardial patch. Leaflet coaptation may also be achieved with double orifice stitch techniques approximating the anterior and septal leaflets[37] or the "clover" technique, which approximates the free edges of the three leaflets, producing a clover-shaped valve opening.[28]

Tricuspid Valve Replacement

TV replacement should be performed when valve repair is not technically feasible in the setting of leaflet pathology or when valve

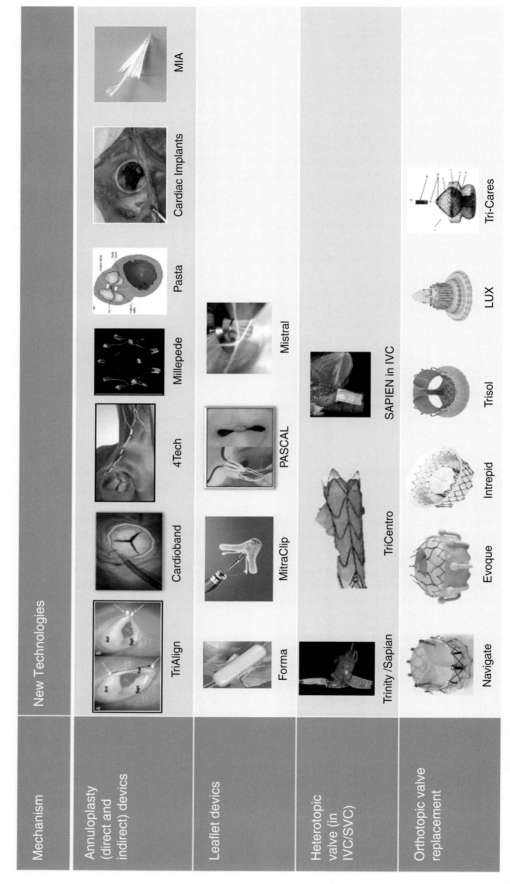

Figure 105.1. Examples of transcatheter tricuspid valve devices under development or in early trials. *IVC,* Inferior vena cava; *SVC,* superior vena cava.

repair carries high risk for early and late recurrence of TR according to known risk factors.[38] The choice of prosthesis type should be individualized,[39] and although bioprostheses are currently favored, there are no differences in survival or adverse events at long-term follow-up in patients receiving mechanical or biological valves.[40]

TRANSCATHETER TRICUSPID VALVE INTERVENTIONS

Interest in the transcatheter solutions for TR has increased in recent years with the recognition of the impact of secondary TR on outcomes[41-44] and the high in-hospital mortality rate associated with isolated TV surgery.[10,11] Important lessons from the surgical literature could be applied to the transcatheter TR population with predictors of recurrence after surgical annular repair identifying patients who may also have less benefit from transcatheter annular repair.

Transcatheter TV devices currently under investigation or development (Fig. 105.1) can be roughly divided into those treating annular dilatation (i.e., Trialign, Cardioband, TriCinch, Millipede, DaVingi), those approaching leaflet malcoaptation (i.e., TriClip, PASCAL, FORMA), heterotopic valve implantation (i.e., Cavi, Tricentro), and orthotopic transcatheter TV replacements (i.e., Navigate, EVOQUE). The list of devices continues to expand however procedural guidance with transesophageal echocardiography (TEE) or intracardiac echocardiography (ICE) remains a nuanced and often a limitation to procedural success.

Access to the Tricuspid Valve

A number of access sites can be considered for delivery of a transcatheter TV device: transvenous (superior vena cava or inferior vena cava), transapical, or transatrial. The optimal approach primarily depends on (1) the size of the delivery system, (2) the position of the intended device, and (3) the anatomy of the access route. The transvenous route clearly has significant advantages. Transjugular access, obtained either percutaneously or surgically, offers a relatively straight angle of approach to the TV, with a delivery system that may require less steering. The smaller venous caliber and focal narrowing under the clavicle may limit this approach for sheaths larger than 35 Fr. The femoral vein, on the other hand, is a large-caliber vessel; however, the angle between the inferior vena cava and posterior TV annulus is acute and thus requires extensive guide torque. The transatrial or transapical approaches are minimally invasive and require either a right or left thoracotomy. For the Navigate system, transatrial access has been used in the majority of cases because of the large delivery sheath (currently 40-Fr).[45] The EVOQUE transcatheter tricuspid valve replacement system is deployed via a transfemoral approach using a 28-Fr sheath and the early feasibility trial (ClinicalTrials.gov Identifier: NCT04221490) is currently enrolling.

Method of Device Anchoring

Because the tricuspid annulus is nonfibrotic and does not calcify, annular devices should anchor in the thickest portion of annular tissue while avoiding the right coronary artery within the AV groove. Anchoring into the RV myocardium beneath the annulus is another option. The Cardioband Tricuspid Valve Reconstruction System (Edwards Lifesciences) uses up to 17 corkscrew anchors implanted around about 60% to 75% of the annulus. The TriCinch system (4Tech Cardio) uses a single anchor through the lateral annulus and RV free wall. The DaVingi TR System (Cardiac Implants LLC) creates its own annulus in a two-stage procedure, in which an annular plication suture is initially positioned using small barb-like anchors with no force applied. After the suture is fibrosed to the annular tissue, essentially forming a new fibrous annulus, the suture is plicated to reduce the annular area.

Devices that attach directly to the leaflets must rely on leaflet and chordal tensile strength to anchor. The TriClip (Abbott) or PASCAL (Edwards Lifesciences) devices have small tines either along the clip arms or at the top of the clip arms to attach to the leaflets. Both devices have been shown to reduce TR and improve functional status in early registries or single site studies.[46-48] The Triluminate Pivotal Trial (ClinicalTrials.gov Identifier: NCT03904147) test the safety and effectiveness of the TriClip device in improving clinical outcomes in symptomatic patients with severe TR, who are at intermediate or greater estimated risk for mortality with TV surgery. This randomized controlled trial will compare the investigational device (TriClip device) with control (medical therapy). A similar pivotal trial using the PASCAL device is currently enrolling (ClinicalTrials.gov Identifier: NCT04097145).

The challenge of anchoring a transcatheter TV replacement device is similar to the mitral side.[49] Valve prostheses used to treat TR in native valves need to be anchored into a dynamic, D-shaped noncalcified structure; however, the systolic forces acting on the tensor apparatus is a fraction of that on the mitral side. Mechanisms for anchoring thus may include (1) ventricular anchors to grasp the free margins of the native leaflets, (2) atrial and ventricular flanges that engage the TV annulus and leaflets or chordae, (3) a series of anchors around the edge of the valve that either pierce the TV tissue or provides friction with radial interference, and (4) use of oversizing and radial force along of the valve stent along the annular rim. TV specific devices are currently being developed.[50,51]

EXAMPLES OF PROCEDURAL GUIDANCE FOR SPECIFIC DEVICES

Edwards Cardioband Tricuspid Valve Reconstruction System

Imaging for each device focuses on the target for repair and the mechanism of anchoring.[52] The surgical predicate for the Cardioband Tricuspid Valve Reconstruction System[53,54] is an annular repair with an incomplete, flexible ring. Preprocedural planning is performed using computed tomography (CT) with device-specific software to implant a virtual device (Fig. 105.2). The implant consists of a contraction wire within a polyester fabric sleeve that is attached to an adjustment mechanism. The polyester sleeve is marked with radiopaque markers at set distances along the implant. Stainless steel anchors are placed through the polyester cover and into the tricuspid annulus at intervals between these markers. Starting at the anteroseptal commissure, up to 17 anchors deployed, ending at ideally beyond the posteroseptal commissure. The contraction wire is then gradually shortened, effective cinching the annulus and reducing both septolateral and anteroposterior dimensions. Fluoroscopy is used to position the catheters and monitor the advancement of the device around the annulus; however, imaging of each anchor deployment is performed with TEE or ICE (Fig. 105.3). Early feasibility studies have shown significant reduction in tricuspid annular area and TR (Fig. 105.4) with associated improvement in functional status.[55] Although three-dimensional (3D) imaging is essential for gross anatomic positioning, two-dimensional (2D) imaging allows for optimal spatial and temporal resolution of anchor position and deployment.

Tricuspid Edge-to-Edge Device

Edge-to-edge repair has emerged as the most frequently performed interventional procedure for severe mitral regurgitation, mostly using the TriClip device.[56] Imaging of the leaflets is essential for device success; however, this may be limited by the thin leaflet structure, shallow angles of insonation, and significant shadowing by left heart structures. Preprocedural planning is performed using TEE imaging and usually does not require CT imaging. All four levels of TV imaging be performed (midesophageal, distal esophageal, transgastric, and deep transgastric) to ensure at least

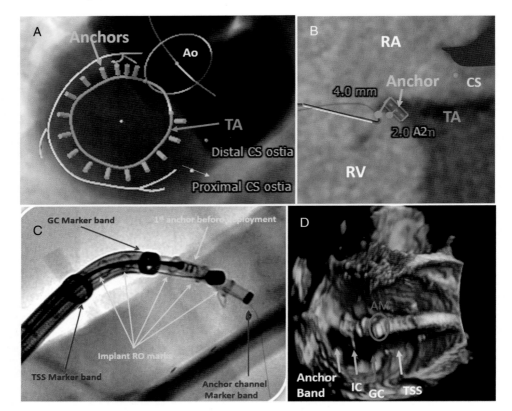

Figure 105.2. Cardioband planning and device components. Planning for direct annuloplasty devices is commonly performed using computed tomography using device-specific software (**A**). Virtual annular anchors can be positioned to understand the adjacent anatomy (**B**). An understanding of the fluoroscopic (**C**) and three-dimensional echocardiographic (**D**) appearance of the device is important for intraprocedural guidance. *Ao,* Aorta; *AM,* adjustment mechanism; *CS,* coronary sinus; *GC,* guide catheter; *IC,* implant catheter; *RA,* right atrium, *RO,* radiopaque; *RV,* right ventricle; *TA,* tricuspid annulus. *TSS,* transseptal steerable sheath.

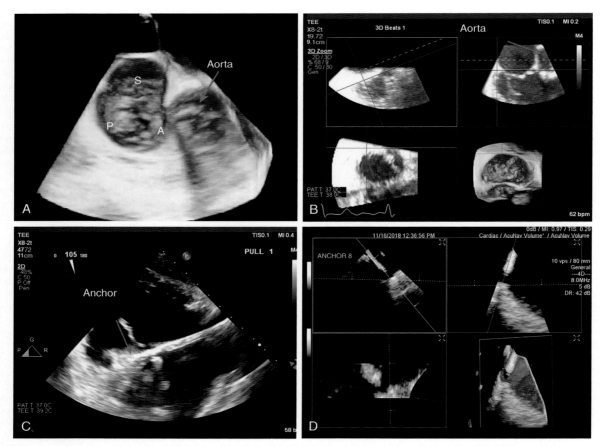

Figure 105.3. An en face three-dimensional (3D) view of the tricuspid valve obtained from a midesophageal view (**A**). 3D live multiplanar reconstruction of valve, which may be instrumental in guiding the placement of the anchors around the annulus (**B**). However, two-dimensional imaging (**C**) may provide higher-resolution images and is frequently required. When transesophageal views of the anchors are acoustically shadowed by the guide catheter, 3D live multiplanar imaging by intracardiac echocardiography imaging may be used (**D**). *A,* Anterior; *P,* posterior; *S,* septal.

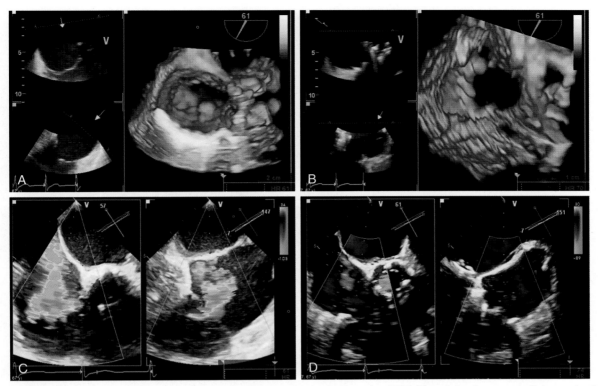

Figure 105.4. Baseline and final echocardiographic imaging. The baseline three-dimensional (3D) (**A**) and simultaneous multiplane color Doppler systolic phase (**B**) images of a patient with torrential tricuspid regurgitation are shown. After Cardioband placement and cinching, the 3D (**C**) and color Doppler (**D**) imaging shows significant reduction in tricuspid annular dimensions, with no significant residual tricuspid regurgitation.

two adequate levels of leaflet imaging. To determine whether the patient is a candidate for this procedure, the following anatomy should be defined (Fig. 105.5): (1) location and extent of the leaflet malcoaptation, (2) leaflet length at the proposed region of device placement, and (3) chordal and papillary muscle morphology relative to the grasping zone.

For controlled advancement of the clip delivery system (CDS) and navigation of the CDS to the TV, a midesophageal bicaval view should be used. Single-plane, simultaneous biplane, or live 3D imaging from this view (Fig. 105.6) may be useful to image and orient the device to the tricuspid annular plane. During continuous imaging, advancing the system without contact with native structures can be accomplished, with gradual guidance of the clip toward the annular plane (Fig. 105.7A). Aligning the trajectory of the CDS is accomplished using imaging planes that align the entire curved guide and CDS with the long axis of the right atrium and ventricle. This can be accomplished typically using 2D imaging (either single plane at 0–30 degrees) or using the 60 to 80 degrees "commissural" with simultaneous biplane imaging (Fig. 105.7B). Using 3D en face views of the TV, the clip arm orientation and positioning of the clip over the target zone are easily accomplished (Fig. 105.7C). In addition, after being advanced across the annular plane, the orientation of the device can be confirmed from the same 3D views with reduced gain settings. Depending on the 3D image quality and the temporal and spatial resolution achieved, clip orientation may require confirmation from transgastric windows.

Grasping and securing leaflet insertion require a mid- to distal esophageal windows with the primary plane adjusted perpendicular to the clip arms showing the clip position along the commissure (Fig. 105.8). Again, live 3D multiplanar reconstruction may be used if resolution is adequate. Essential to achieving procedural success, adequate leaflet capture in each clip arm must be imaged. Knowing the leaflet length before clip

grasp and subtracting the leaflet length outside the clip arms give a confirmatory calculation of adequate leaflet capture. Continuous imaging on color Doppler during clip closure should demonstrate reduction in TR. After complete clip closure, a comprehensive evaluation of the TV should include color Doppler for residual TR, pulsed-wave Doppler of the hepatic vein to document resolution of systolic flow reversal, and continuous-wave Doppler across the TV to assess peak and mean gradients. If the mean gradient is greater than 3 mmHg, repositioning the clip or even partial opening of the clip arms could be considered. If more than moderate TR remains, a second clip could also be considered if mean gradients allow. This same evaluation is performed after final clip release (Fig. 105.9). Analysis of 3D volumes (with and without color) would provide a more quantitative assessment of residual TR and effective orifice area.

FUTURE PERSPECTIVE

In this early stage of transcatheter device development, feasibility and safety have been the focus of current trials. Determining efficacy has been limited by the known pitfalls of echocardiographic assessment of native valve TR severity[15] with even greater difficulty and little validation for assessing TR after devices are implanted. Nonetheless, the reduction in TR with most devices is modest, yet patients show clinically significant improvements in symptoms and quality of life.[48,57–59] The lack of efficacy is in part explained by the late presentation with not only end-stage changes in valvular and ventricular morphology but also multiple comorbidities. This results in a very heterogeneous group of patients in which choosing the correct treatment may be challenging. A more comprehensive understanding of TV disease and the relationship to the right ventricle and pulmonary circulation, as well as how to best evaluate the pathophysiology, should lead to earlier diagnosis and improved timing of intervention. Importantly, if devices

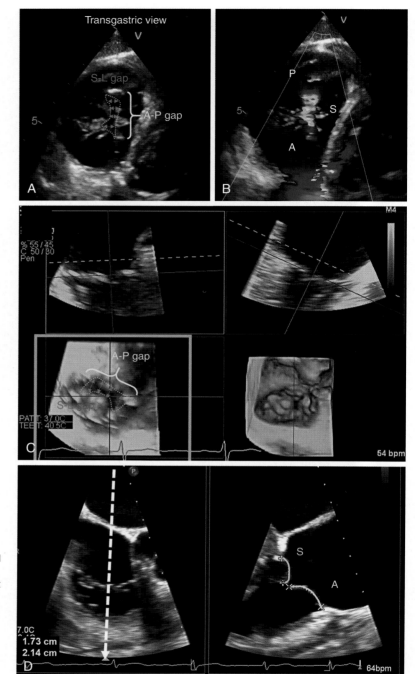

Figure 105.5. Preprocedural transesophageal echocardiographic. The transgastric view (**A** and **B**) allows imaging of all three leaflet tips and should be used to measure the septolateral (S-L) gaps as well as the anteroposterior (A-P) gap. If on-axis imaging of the leaflet tips cannot be achieved using two-dimensional imaging, three-dimensional reconstruction of the short-axis at the tips of the leaflets (**C**) will also allow for measurements, with the caveat that resolution on these images may not be ideal. Adequate leaflet length must also be determined (**D**) to help determine procedural feasibility and device choice. *A,* Anterior; *S,* septal.

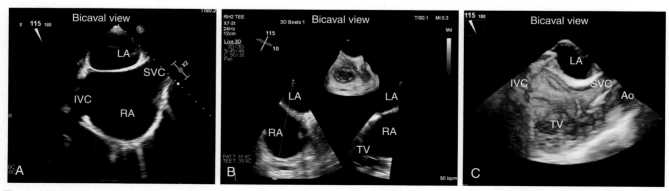

Figure 105.6. Bicaval views. Single-plane (**A**), simultaneous biplane (**B**), or live three-dimensional imaging from this view (**C**) may be useful to image and orient the device to the tricuspid annular plane. *Ao,* Aorta; *IVC,* inferior vena cava; *LA,* left atrium; *RA,* right atrium; *SVC,* superior vena cava; *TV,* tricuspid valve.

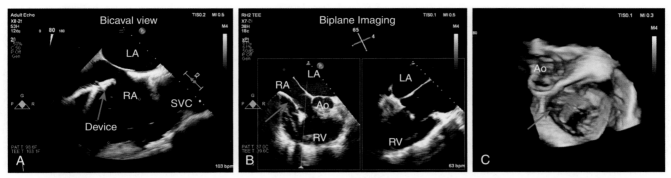

Figure 105.7. Clip delivery. During continuous imaging, the clip delivery system (CDS) *(red arrow)* is advanced avoiding contact with native structures (**A**). Aligning the trajectory of the CDS is accomplished using imaging planes that align the entire curved guide and CDS with the long axis of the right atrium (RA) and right ventricle (RV; **B**). Using three-dimensional (3D) en face views of the tricuspid valve (**C**), the clip arm orientation and positioning of the clip arms *(red opaque outline)* over the target zone is performed. *Ao,* Aorta; *LA,* left atrium; *SVC,* superior vena cava.

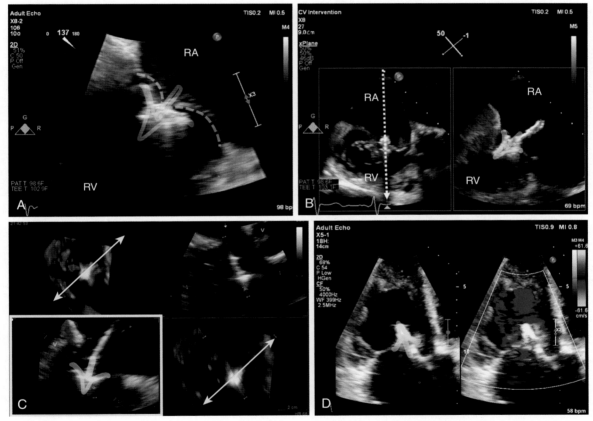

Figure 105.8. Grasping views. When imaging leaflet capture, multiple different modalities can be used. Single-plane transesophageal imaging may optimize resolution for imaging of leaflet extension to the base of the clip arms (**A**, *blue dashed lines*). If a single-plane image of the two clip arms cannot be obtained, using the orthogonal image from the commissural view (**B**) may optimize imaging of simultaneous leaflet grasp. Real-time three-dimensional (3D) multiplanar reconstruction (**C**) reorients the two-dimensional images using the 3D en face view of the tricuspid valve and can be used from any imaging plane that optimized tricuspid leaflet imaging. Transthoracic imaging (**D**) has also been used for imaging of leaflet grasp when transesophageal imaging is limited. *RA,* Right atrium; *RV,* right ventricle.

have a high safety profile, then the trade-off of efficacy for functional improvement may tip the balance in favor of transcatheter therapies.

CONCLUSIONS

Secondary or functional TR represents an important unmet treatment need given its prevalence, adverse prognostic impact, and symptom burden associated with progressive right heart failure. Imaging plays an integral role in the assessment of TV morphology and TR severity, as well as ventricular size and function and pulmonary vascular hemodynamics. Surgical intervention has been associated with high mortality rates, paving the way for less invasive treatment options. Numerous devices using different tricuspid apparatus targets, methods of access, and anchoring, are under development.

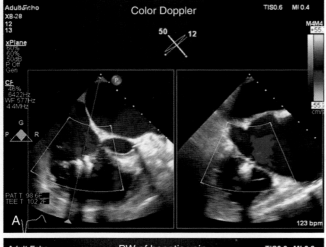

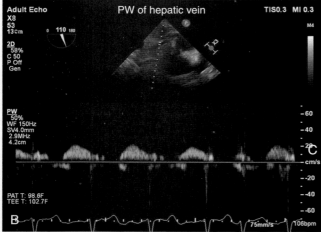

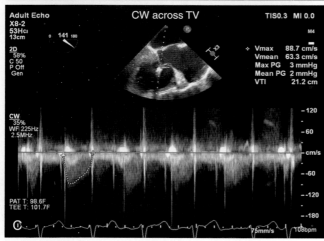

Figure 105.9. Evaluation after edge-to-edge device. After device placement, color Doppler imaging from multiple views (**A**) should be performed. In the setting of significant reduction of tricuspid regurgitation, systolic reversal of flow in the hepatic vein may no longer be seen (**B**) or may be significantly reduced. Peak and mean gradients across the tricuspid orifice using continuous-wave (CW) Doppler (**C**) ensure that tricuspid stenosis has not been created with a reduction in diastolic valve area after edge-to-edge tricuspid valve (TV) repair. *PW,* Pulsed wave.

REFERENCES

1. Nishimura RA, Otto CM, Bonow RO, et al. AHA/ACC guideline for the management of patients with valvular heart disease. *J Am Coll Cardiol.* 2014;63:e57–e185. 2014.
2. Shah PM, Raney AA. Tricuspid valve disease. *Curr Probl Cardiol.* 2008;33:47–84.
3. Dreyfus GD, Martin RP, Chan KM, et al. Functional tricuspid regurgitation: a need to revise our understanding. *J Am Coll Cardiol.* 2015;65:2331–2336.
4. Rodes-Cabau J, Taramasso M, O'Gara PT. Diagnosis and treatment of tricuspid valve disease: current and future perspectives. *Lancet.* 2016;388:2431–2442.
5. Hahn RT, Delhaas T, Denti P, Waxman AB. The tricuspid valve relationship with the right ventricle and pulmonary vasculature. *JACC Cardiovasc Imag.* 2019;12:564–565.
6. Nishimura RA, Otto CM, Bonow RO, et al. AHA/ACC focused update of the 2014 AHA/ACC guideline for the management of patients with valvular heart disease. *J Am Coll Cardiol.* 2017;70:252–289. 2017.
7. Taramasso M, Gavazzoni M, Pozzoli A, et al. Tricuspid regurgitation: predicting the need for intervention, procedural success, and recurrence of disease. *JACC Cardiovasc Imag.* 2019;12:605–621.
8. Baumgartner H, Falk V, Bax JJ, et al. ESC/EACTS Guidelines for the management of valvular heart disease. *Eur Heart J.* 2017;38:2739–2791. 2017.
9. Kilic A, Saha-Chaudhuri P, Rankin JS, Conte JV. Trends and outcomes of tricuspid valve surgery in North America. *Ann Thorac Surg.* 2013;96:1546–1552.
10. Alqahtani F, Berzingi CO, Aljohani S, et al. Contemporary trends in the use and outcomes of surgical treatment of tricuspid regurgitation. *J Am Heart Assoc.* 2017;6.
11. Zack CJ, Fender EA, Chandrashekar P, et al. National trends and outcomes in isolated tricuspid valve surgery. *J Am Coll Cardiol.* 2017;70:2953–2960.
12. Dahou A, Levin D, Reisman M, Hahn RT. Anatomy and physiology of the tricuspid valve. *JACC Cardiovasc Imag.* 2019;12:458–468.
13. Faletra FF, Leo LA, Paiocchi VL, et al. Imaging-based tricuspid valve anatomy by computed tomography, magnetic resonance imaging, two and three-dimensional echocardiography: correlation with anatomic specimen. *Eur Heart J Cardiovasc Imag.* 2019;20:1–13.
14. Lang RM, Badano LP, Mor-Avi V, et al. Recommendations for cardiac chamber quantification by echocardiography in adults. *J Am Soc Echocardiogr.* 2015;28:1–39. e14.
15. Hahn RT. State-of-the-art review of echocardiographic imaging in the evaluation and treatment of functional tricuspid regurgitation. *Circ Cardiovasc Imag.* 2016;9. e005332.
16. Singh-Gryzbon S, Siefert AW, Pierce EL, Yoganathan AP. Tricuspid valve annular mechanics: interactions with and implications for transcatheter devices. *Cardiovasc Eng Tech.* 2019;10:193–204.
17. Chidambaram M, Abdulali SA, Baliga BG, Ionescu MI. Long-term results of DeVega tricuspid annuloplasty. *Ann Thorac Surg.* 1987;43:185–188.
18. McGrath LB, Gonzalez-Lavin L, Bailey BM, et al. Tricuspid valve operations in 530 patients. Twenty-five-year assessment of early and late phase events. *J Thorac Cardiovasc Surg.* 1990;99:124–133.
19. Breyer RH, McClenathan JH, Michaelis LL, et al. Tricuspid regurgitation: a comparison of nonoperative management, tricuspid annuloplasty, and tricuspid valve replacement. *J Thorac Cardiovasc Surg.* 1976;72:867–874.
20. Moraca RJ, Moon MR, Lawton JS, et al. Outcomes of tricuspid valve repair and replacement: a propensity analysis. *Ann Thorac Surg.* 2009;87:83–88.
21. King RM, Schaff HV, Danielson GK, et al. Surgery for tricuspid regurgitation late after mitral valve replacement. *Circulation.* 1984;70:I193–I197.
22. Rizzoli G, Vendramin I, Nesseris G, et al. Biological or mechanical prostheses in tricuspid position? A meta-analysis of intra-institutional results. *Ann Thorac Surg.* 2004;77:1607–1614.
23. Onoda K, Yasuda F, Takao M, et al. Long-term follow-up after Carpentier-Edwards ring annuloplasty for tricuspid regurgitation. *Ann Thorac Surg.* 2000;70:796–799.
24. McCarthy PM, Bhudia SK, Rajeswaran J, et al. Tricuspid valve repair: Durability and risk factors for failure. *J Thorac Cardiovasc Surg.* 2004;127:674–685.
25. Min SY, Song JM, Kim JH, et al. Geometric changes after tricuspid annuloplasty and predictors of residual tricuspid regurgitation: a real-time three-dimensional echocardiography study. *Eur Heart J.* 2010;31:2871–2880.
26. Fukuda S, Gillinov AM, Song JM, et al. Echocardiographic insights into atrial and ventricular mechanisms of functional tricuspid regurgitation. *Am Heart J.* 2006;152:1208–1214.
27. Fukuda S, Gillinov AM, McCarthy PM, et al. Determinants of recurrent or residual functional tricuspid regurgitation after tricuspid annuloplasty. *Circulation.* 2006;114:I582–I587.
28. Lapenna E, De Bonis M, Verzini A, et al. The clover technique for the treatment of complex tricuspid valve insufficiency: midterm clinical and echocardiographic results in 66 patients. *Eur J Cardio Thorac Surg.* 2010;37:1297–1303.
29. Navia JL, Nowicki ER, Blackstone EH, et al. Surgical management of secondary tricuspid valve regurgitation: annulus, commissure, or leaflet procedure? *J Thorac Cardiovasc Surg.* 2010;139:1473–1482.
30. Tei C, Pilgrim JP, Shah PM, et al. The tricuspid valve annulus: study of size and motion in normal subjects and in patients with tricuspid regurgitation. *Circulation.* 1982;66:665–671.
31. Vassileva CM, Shabosky J, Boley T, et al. Tricuspid valve surgery: the past 10 years from the Nationwide Inpatient Sample (NIS) database. *J Thorac Cardiovasc Surg.* 2012;143:1043–1049.

32. Fukuda S, Song JM, Gillinov AM, et al. Tricuspid valve tethering predicts residual tricuspid regurgitation after tricuspid annuloplasty. *Circulation.* 2005;111:975–979.

33. Kabasawa M, Kohno H, Ishizaka T, et al. Assessment of functional tricuspid regurgitation using 320-detector-row multislice computed tomography: risk factor analysis for recurrent regurgitation after tricuspid annuloplasty. *J Thorac Cardiovasc Surg.* 2014;147:312–320.

34. Sagie A, Schwammenthal E, Padial LR, et al. Determinants of functional tricuspid regurgitation in incomplete tricuspid valve closure: Doppler color flow study of 109 patients. *J Am Coll Cardiol.* 1994;24:446–453.

35. Sukmawan R, Watanabe N, Ogasawara Y, et al. Geometric changes of tricuspid valve tenting in tricuspid regurgitation secondary to pulmonary hypertension quantified by novel system with transthoracic real-time 3D echocardiography. *J Am Soc Echocardiogr.* 2007;20:470–476.

36. Park YH, Song JM, Lee EY, et al. Geometric and hemodynamic determinants of functional tricuspid regurgitation: a real-time 3D echocardiography study. *Int J Cardiol.* 2008;124:160–165.

37. Hetzer R, Komoda T, Delmo Walter EM. How to do the double orifice valve technique to treat tricuspid valve incompetence. *Eur J Cardio Thorac Surg.* 2013;43:641–642.

38. Chang BC, Lim SH, Yi G, et al. Long-term clinical results of tricuspid valve replacement. *Ann Thorac Surg.* 2006;81:1317–1323.

39. Kaplan M, Kut MS, Demirtas MM, et al. Prosthetic replacement of tricuspid valve: bioprosthetic or mechanical. *Ann Thorac Surg.* 2002;73:467–473.

40. Cho WC, Park CB, Kim JB, et al. Mechanical valve replacement versus bioprosthetic valve replacement in the tricuspid valve position. *J Cardiac Surg.* 2013;28:212–217.

41. Nath J, Foster E, Heidenreich PA. Impact of tricuspid regurgitation on long-term survival. *J Am Coll Cardiol.* 2004;43:405–409.

42. Lee JW, Song JM, Park JP, et al. Long-term prognosis of isolated significant tricuspid regurgitation. *Circ J.* 2010;74:375–3780.

43. Ohno Y, Attizzani GF, Capodanno D, et al. Association of tricuspid regurgitation with clinical and echocardiographic outcomes after percutaneous mitral valve repair with the MitraClip system: 30-day and 12-month follow-up from the GRASP Registry. *Eur Heart J Cardiovasc Imag.* 2014;15:1246–1255.

44. Lindman BR, Maniar HS, Jaber WA, et al. Effect of tricuspid regurgitation and the right heart on survival after transcatheter aortic valve replacement: insights from the Placement of Aortic Transcatheter Valves II inoperable cohort. *Circulation Cardiovasc Interv.* 2015;8.

45. Hahn RT, Kodali SK, Fam N, et al. Early multinational experience of transcatheter tricuspid valve replacement for treating severe tricuspid regurgitation. *JACC Cardiovasc Interv.* 2020;13(21):2482–2493.

46. Orban M, Besler C, Braun D, et al. Six-month outcome after transcatheter edge-to-edge repair of severe tricuspid regurgitation in patients with heart failure. *Eur J Heart Fail.* 2018;20:1055–1062.

47. Praz F, Spargias K, Chrissoheris M, et al. Compassionate use of the PASCAL transcatheter mitral valve repair system for patients with severe mitral regurgitation: a multicentre, prospective, observational, first-in-man study. *Lancet.* 2017;390:773–780.

48. Nickenig G, Kowalski M, Hausleiter J, et al. Transcatheter treatment of severe tricuspid regurgitation with the edge-to-edge MitraClip technique. *Circulation.* 2017;135:1802–1814.

49. Regueiro A, Granada JF, Dagenais F, Rodes-Cabau J. Transcatheter mitral valve replacement: insights from early clinical experience and future challenges. *J Am Coll Cardiol.* 2017;69:2175–2192.

50. Navia JL, Kapadia S, Elgharably H, et al. First-in-human implantations of the navigate bioprosthesis in a severely dilated tricuspid annulus and in a failed tricuspid annuloplasty ring. *Circ Cardiovasc Interv.* 2017;10. e005840.

51. Demir OM, Regazzoli D, Mangieri A, et al. Transcatheter tricuspid valve replacement: Principles and design. *Front Cardiovasc Med.* 2018;5:129.

52. Hahn RT, Nabauer M, Zuber M, et al. Intraprocedural imaging of transcatheter tricuspid valve interventions. *JACC Cardiovasc Imag.* 2019;12:532–553.

53. Schueler R, Malasa M, Hammerstingl C, Nickenig G. Transcatheter interventions for tricuspid regurgitation: MitraClip. *EuroIntervention.* 2016;12:Y108–Y109.

54. Kuwata S, Taramasso M, Nietlispach F, Maisano F. Transcatheter tricuspid valve repair toward a surgical standard: first-in-man report of direct annuloplasty with a cardioband device to treat severe functional tricuspid regurgitation. *Eur Heart J.* 2017;38:1261.

55. Nickenig G, Weber M, Schueler R, et al. 6-month outcomes of tricuspid valve reconstruction for patients with severe tricuspid regurgitation. *J Am Coll Cardiol.* 2019;73:1905–1915.

56. Taramasso M, Hahn RT, Alessandrini H, et al. The International Multicenter TriValve Registry: which patients are undergoing transcatheter tricuspid repair? *JACC Cardiovasc Interv.* 2017;10:1982–1990.

57. Hahn RT, Meduri CU, Davidson CJ, et al. Early feasibility study of a transcatheter tricuspid valve annuloplasty: SCOUT Trial 30-Day Results. *J Am Coll Cardiol.* 2017;69:1795–1806.

58. Perlman G, Praz F, Puri R, et al. Transcatheter tricuspid valve repair with a new transcatheter coaptation system for the treatment of severe tricuspid regurgitation: 1-year clinical and echocardiographic results. *JACC Cardiovasc Interv.* 2017;10:1994–2003.

59. Schueler R, Hammerstingl C, Werner N, Nickenig G. Interventional direct annuloplasty for functional tricuspid regurgitation. *JACC Cardiovasc Interv.* 2017;10:415–416.

106 Device Lead–Associated Tricuspid Regurgitation

Karima Addetia, Roberto M. Lang

According to the American Heart Association (AHA) heart disease and stroke statistics, in the year 2014, more than 300,000 pacemakers (PMs) and 60,000 intracardiac defibrillators (ICDs) were implanted in United States.[1] As the population continues to age, the number of cardiac implantable electronic device (CIED) leads, which includes PMs, ICDs, and cardiac resynchronization therapy (CRT), will most likely increase. The first reports of device lead–mediated interference with the tricuspid valve (TV) apparatus were published in the late 1900s. Subsequently, multiple case reports, case series, and retrospective cohort studies have shown an association between the presence of a device lead and worsening tricuspid regurgitation (TR). With the recent surge in percutaneous options for valvular dysfunction and the realization that TR is not a benign condition,[1a,2] the interest in this topic has soared among both echocardiographers and interventionalists. All currently available device leads have been documented to interfere with the TV apparatus, and the resultant TR is classified as primary (organic) TV dysfunction. This chapter reviews the existing evidence behind CIED-mediated TR, discusses the potential mechanisms of CIED-mediated interference of the TV apparatus, and provides an overview on how to diagnose CIED-mediated interference using echocardiography.

CARDIAC IMPLANTABLE ELECTRONIC DEVICES AND TRICUSPID REGURGITATION

The reported frequency of significant TR after CIED placement is variable, ranging anywhere from 7% to 45% in selected studies.[3–16] Initial studies using two-dimensional (2D) echocardiography reported conflicting results[17] with early studies being mostly negative, showing no difference in TR severity before and after right ventricular (RV) lead implantation, while later studies suggested an increase in TR severity after CIED implantation.[4–6,14,18,19] Some studies even suggested an improvement in TR after CIED implantation. This was in part believed to be attributable to improvement in right heart hemodynamics with pacing.[4,14] One might ask why reports of CIED-related TR were so conflicting in the early studies. In part, this could be caused by limitations of study design. Many of these studies were retrospective and observational and without control groups, and minimal data were reported on outcomes. Furthermore, the assessment of TR severity was largely qualitative instead of objective, based on measured parameters. These limitations are further compounded by the challenges associated with TR

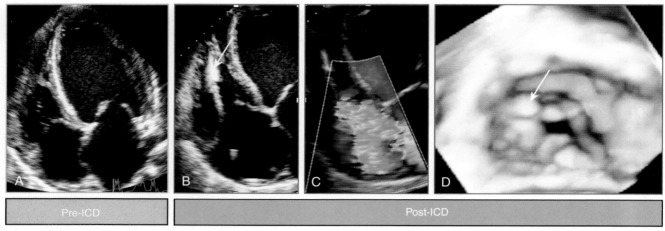

Figure 106.1. Pre- and post–intracardiac defibrillator (ICD) implantation echocardiograms performed in a patient with nonischemic cardiomyopathy. Before ICD implantation, the right ventricular size was normal, and tricuspid regurgitation (TR) was minimal (**A**). After ICD lead implantation, the right ventricle was dilated, and TR was severe (**B** and **D**). On careful examination of the two-dimensional images, it appears that the lead moves with one of the tricuspid valve (TV) leaflets (**B**). The three-dimensional zoomed view from the right ventricular perspective with the septal leaflets in the six o'clock position suggests that the ICD lead is indeed interfering with the posterior leaflet of the TV.

assessment on 2D echocardiography. Comparison of TR degree before and after device lead implantation is frequently confounded by the strong reflectivity of the device lea das well as lead-generated acoustic artifact, both of which may lead to underestimation of TR severity by color Doppler.[20] Device leads are fully visualized as they traverse the TV annulus in only 15% of cases on 2D echocardiography.[21] Finally, many of these patients (at least those with ICD and CRT devices) have underlying left ventricular (LV) dysfunction, which, over time may lead to RV enlargement, tricuspid annular dilatation, and functional TR, a situation that may confound the underlying cause of TR in a cross-sectional study. More recently, studies have incorporated outcomes into their methods and have shown that CIED-induced TR is associated with a poorer prognosis.[4,8,10] One single-center study examined the prevalence of significant TR in 634 consecutive patients over a 6-year period. PM leads were associated with a higher risk of developing significant TR and higher likelihood of death even after adjustment for LV dysfunction and pulmonary hypertension.[8]

NATURAL HISTORY OF CARDIAC IMPLANTABLE ELECTRONIC DEVICE–INDUCED TRICUSPID REGURGITATON

CIED-related TR has been shown to result in adverse remodeling, including dilatation of the right heart cavities and worsened RV function.[5,10] The degree of TR has been shown to increase over time in patients with CIEDs. In one of the largest retrospective studies on this topic,[4] which included 1596 patients with early (1-month postimplant) and late (4-year) follow-up, there was a small but significant increase in the prevalence of moderate and severe TR, both acutely and chronically. In the worst-case scenario, lead-related TR may manifest clinically with right heart failure symptoms, including hepatomegaly, ascites, and peripheral edema. In a series of patients with severe lead-related TR requiring TV surgery, approximately 50% presented primarily with severe right heart failure.[20] In another report, severe lead-related TR was associated with more heart failure–related events (i.e., heart failure hospitalization, TV surgery, or upgrade to CRT) and worsening long-term survival.[10] When specifically looking at the impact of TR on survival in patients with

CIED,[4,8,10] there was 40% to 75% excess mortality rate attributed to severe TR after multivariate adjustment. CIED-induced TR should be suspected whenever a patient with a device lead has significant TR, especially when an echocardiogram acquired before device lead implantation had little or no TR (Fig. 106.1).

MECHANISMS OF CARDIAC IMPLANTABLE ELECTRONIC DEVICE–INDUCED TRICUSPID REGURGITATON

CIED-induced TR can be classified as (1) implantation-related, (2) pacing mediated, and (3) device mediated. There are reportedly certain technical factors related to the implantation procedure that can be associated with an increased likelihood of damage to the TV apparatus, although there are limited data. A higher pacing burden has not been shown to correlate with worsening TR.[4,6,9,13] Nevertheless, a number of studies have associated RV pacing with worsening TR degree. The suggested mechanism for this is the alteration in RV geometry with pacing.[22] Postmortem examinations of hearts with device leads have shown that leads can interfere with the TV apparatus by impinging on a leaflet; adhering to a leaflet; interfering with the subvalvular apparatus; perforating or lacerating a leaflet; or leaflet avulsion, which may uncommonly happen, for instance, during lead extraction or RV biopsy. It has been shown on postmortem examinations in patients with device leads and during open heart surgery that a fibrotic process can entrap the device lead within the TV leaflet or subvalvular apparatus, resulting in varying degrees of leaflet malalignment and malcoaptation. A case series of 41 patients with CIED and severe TR who were undergoing surgery to repair or replace the TV reported on the following mechanisms of TR according to intraoperative findings: lead entrapment in the subvalvular apparatus, leaflet perforation, lead impingement of a TV leaflet, and adherence to the TV leaflet.[20]

Lead extraction can also result in damage to the TV apparatus, thus becoming an additional mechanism of lead-mediated TV dysfunction. Newer methods for lead extraction, including laser-assisted dissection of the lead from adherent material, have been shown to result in lower incidence of complications such as worsening TR (0%–6%).[6,23–25] Furthermore, if a lead is found to be resistant to extraction, it may be left in the chest cavity or

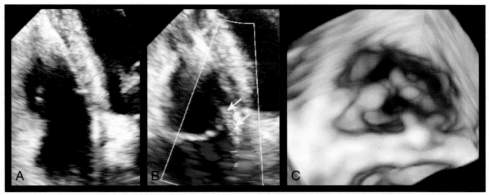

Figure 106.2. Cardiac implantable electronic device–induced tricuspid regurgitation (TR) may be suspected if the lead is seen to move with the septum or septal leaflet or otherwise appear attached to septal leaflet or the septum (A, *yellow arrows*) on the right ventricular side. Additionally, there may be "hugging" of the TR jet to the device lead as noted here (B, *white arrows*). In this patient, as seen on the three-dimensional zoom image, the device lead was impinging on the septal leaflet of the tricuspid valve, preventing valve closure and resulting in TR (**C**).

alternatively surgically extracted if necessary. It has been shown that older leads are more likely to be encapsulated and require laser extraction tools than newer leads.[23]

ECHOCARDIOGRAPHY IN THE DIAGNOSIS OF CARDIAC IMPLANTABLE ELECTRONIC DEVICE–INDUCED TRICUSPID REGURGITATON

The TV can be imaged from both the transthoracic and transesophageal perspective using both 2D and three-dimensional (3D) echocardiography. Because the TV is anteriorly located in the mediastinum, it is often more easily accessible with the transthoracic rather that the transesophageal probe. With 3D echocardiography, all three leaflets can be visualized simultaneously from both the right atrial and RV perspectives, and the location of the device lead can often be seen in reference to the TV leaflets and annulus. Visualization of the device lead in this manner may help determine whether there is device lead–mediated interference with the TV leaflets in patients with suspected device lead–mediated TR. With full-volume datasets of the RV, it is also often possible to follow the trajectory of the device lead in the RV to establish the relationship between the CIED and the tricuspid subvalvular apparatus.

To reliably identify the mechanism of CIED interference with the TV apparatus on 2D echocardiography, it is important to interrogate the TV using a protocol that allows the image to determine with near certainty the specific TV leaflet combinations being imaged. Recent data suggest that it is impossible to know with certainty which pair of leaflets are being imaged in each of the standard views.[26,27] This is further confounded by the extreme variability of the leaflet sizes, as well as the number of tricuspid leaflets. Although the TV is typically described as being composed of three leaflets of unequal size, in many cases, two (bicuspid) or more than three leaflets can be seen.[28,29] Accordingly, targeted 2D imaging of the TV leaflets with attention to specific adjacent anatomic landmarks has been suggested as a manner to identify TV anatomy accurately.[26,30] For instance, in the RV inflow view, when the septum is visualized, the septal leaflet is imaged in the far field with the anterior leaflet imaged in the near field. In the apical four-chamber view, if the aortic valve is brought into view, the anterior and septal tricuspid leaflets are being imaged. However, when the coronary sinus is seen in this imaging plane, the septal and posterior leaflets are being imaged. In the parasternal short-axis view, if a single leaflet is visualized, this

leaflet is always the anterior leaflet, which is the largest of all three TV leaflets. Targeted interrogation of the TV leaflets is important to localize TR and hence TV pathology to a specific leaflet and to understand the mechanism of TR in patients with CIEDs. The information provided by these views must be integrated to isolate the TR jet and connect it with the CIED. An echocardiogram before device insertion may help, especially if it was normal and no new pathology affecting the right heart occurred in the interim. Sometimes CIED-induced TR can be suspected if the origin of the TR color Doppler jet is higher than the coaptation point of the TV leaflets, suggesting that TR may be caused by CIED-induced interference with the tricuspid subvalvular apparatus. "Hugging" of the TR jet to the device lead, leaflet malcoaptation, and movement of the lead with the subvalvular apparatus may also suggest device lead interference with the tricuspid apparatus (Fig. 106.2). Sometimes the CIED is seen to "move with" or appear attached to the septal leaflet or the septum itself on the RV side; this also may suggest interference.[13]

On 2D echocardiography, the trajectory of the device lead is visualized in only 17% of cases.[15] Identification of device lead–mediated interference of the TV as a cause of TV dysfunction is likewise relatively low (~12% of cases).[15,20] With 3D echocardiography, visualization of the lead was more reliable with a feasibility of 74% (153 of 207 patients) in one study that used 3D zoom views together with RV full-volume datasets (both four-beat gated acquisitions in suspended respiration).[31] CIEDs can be visualized in a number of different positions relative to the tricuspid annulus and leaflets using 3D echocardiography. They can be found in the commissures (anteroseptal, posteroseptal, or anteroposterior), against, impinging, or adherent to a leaflet or in the middle of the valve.[15,31] Leads labeled as "impinging" or "adherent" were associated with greater degrees of TR according to one retrospective, single-center, high-volume referral tertiary care center (Fig. 106.3). Leads located in commissural positions or in the "center of the valve" were less likely to be associated with significant TR.[16] An "impinging" lead directly interferes with leaflet coaptation. An adherent lead, on the other hand, is stuck to the leaflet–tricuspid apparatus but still moves along with it. In a multivariable analysis of patients with device leads and pre- and postimplantation echocardiography, preimplantation vena contracta width and the presence of an interfering lead were independently associated with postdevice TR.[32]

CIED-associated TR, if not recognized and treated promptly, is associated with excess mortality rate, which has been estimated to be around 40% to 75%,[8,10] and significant morbidity. Management

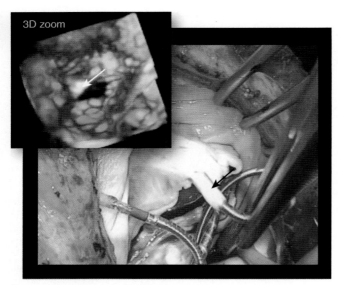

Figure 106.3. Example of device lead adherence to the tricuspid valve (TV) anterior leaflet. The *top right* shows a three-dimensional (3D) zoom as displayed from the right ventricular perspective in which the device lead moves with the anterior leaflet. The *bottom image* shows the same patient in the operating room. The device lead *(white arrow)* is attached to the anterior leaflet of the TV. This patient has severe tricuspid regurgitation.

strategies include medical therapy, consideration for transvenous lead extraction, and TV repair or replacement.

FUTURE DIRECTIONS

Although it is clear that CIED-mediated TV dysfunction occurs, it is not always possible to recognize it on echocardiography. Careful interrogation of the device lead using 2D or 3D echocardiography and color Doppler imaging and comparison with prior studies performed before lead implantation might be helpful.

REFERENCES

1. Benjamin EJ, Muntner P, Alonso A, Bittencourt MS, Callaway CW, , et al. American Heart Association Council on Epidemiology and Prevention Statistics Committee and Stroke Statistics Subcommittee. Heart disease and stroke statistics—2019 update: a report from the American Heart Association. *Circulation*. 2020;141(2):e33. PMID: 30700139.
1a. Dreyfus GD, Corbi PJ, Chan KM, Bahrami T. Secondary tricuspid regurgitation or dilatation: which should be the criteria for surgical repair? *Ann Thorac Surg*. 2005;79:127–132.
2. Nath J, Foster E, Heidenreich PA. Impact of tricuspid regurgitation on long-term survival. *J Am Coll Cardiol*. 2004;43:405–409.
3. Al-Bawardy R, Krishnaswamy A, Bhargava M, et al. Tricuspid regurgitation in patients with pacemakers and implantable cardiac defibrillators: a comprehensive review. *Clin Cardiol*. 2013;36:249–254.
4. Al-Bawardy R, Krishnaswamy A, Rajeswaran J, et al. Tricuspid regurgitation and implantable devices. *PACE (Pacing Clin Electrophysiol)*. 2015;38:259–266.
5. Arabi P, Ozer N, Ates AH, et al. Effects of pacemaker and implantable cardioverter defibrillator electrodes on tricuspid regurgitation and right sided heart functions. *Cardiol J*. 2015;22:637–644.
6. Chang JD, Manning WJ, Ebrille E, Zimetbaum PJ. Tricuspid valve dysfunction following pacemaker or cardioverter-defibrillator implantation. *J Am Coll Cardiol*. 2017;69:2331–2341.
7. de Cock CC, Vinkers M, Van Campe LC, et al. Long-term outcome of patients with multiple (> or = 3) noninfected transvenous leads: a clinical and echocardiographic study. *PACE (Pacing Clin Electrophysiol)*. 2000;23:423–426.
8. Delling FN, Hassan ZK, Piatkowski G, et al. Tricuspid regurgitation and mortality in patients with transvenous permanent pacemaker leads. *Am J Cardiol*. 2016;117:988–992.
9. Fanari Z, Hammami S, Hammami MB, et al. The effects of right ventricular apical pacing with transvenous pacemaker and implantable cardioverter defibrillator on mitral and tricuspid regurgitation. *J Electrocardiol*. 2015;48:791–797.
10. Hoke U, Auger D, Thijssen J, et al. Significant lead-induced tricuspid regurgitation is associated with poor prognosis at long-term follow-up. *Heart*. 2014;100:960–968.
11. Kim JB, Spevack DM, Tunick PA, et al. The effect of transvenous pacemaker and implantable cardioverter defibrillator lead placement on tricuspid valve function: an observational study. *J Am Soc Echocardiogr*. 2008;21:284–287.
12. Klutstein M, Balkin J, Butnaru A, et al. Tricuspid incompetence following permanent pacemaker implantation. *PACE (Pacing Clin Electrophysiol)*. 2009;32(suppl 1):S135–S137.
13. Lee RC, Friedman SE, Kono AT, et al. Tricuspid regurgitation following implantation of endocardial leads: incidence and predictors. *PACE (Pacing Clin Electrophysiol)*. 2015;38:1267–12674.
14. Paniagua D, Aldrich HR, Lieberman EH, et al. Increased prevalence of significant tricuspid regurgitation in patients with transvenous pacemakers leads. *Am J Cardiol*. 1998;82:1130–1132. A9.
15. Seo Y, Ishizu T, Nakajima H, et al. Clinical utility of 3D echocardiography in the evaluation of tricuspid regurgitation caused by pacemaker leads. *Circulation J*. 2008;72:1465–1470.
16. Webster G, Margossian R, Alexander ME, et al. Impact of transvenous ventricular pacing leads on tricuspid regurgitation in pediatric and congenital heart disease patients. *J Interv Card Electrophysiol*. 2008;21:65–68.
17. Greenspon AJ, Patel JD, Lau E, et al. Trends in permanent pacemaker implantation in the United States from 1993 to 2009: increasing complexity of patients and procedures. *J Am Coll Cardiol*. 2012;60:1540–1545.
18. Lee ME, Chaux A, Matloff JM. Avulsion of a tricuspid valve leaflet during traction on an infected, entrapped endocardial pacemaker electrode. The role of electrode design. *J Thorac Cardiovasc Surg*. 1977;74:433–435.
19. Ong LS, Barold SS, Craver WL, et al. Partial avulsion of the tricuspid valve by tined pacing electrode. *Am Heart J*. 1981;102:798–799.
20. Lin G, Nishimura RA, Connolly HM, et al. Severe symptomatic tricuspid valve regurgitation due to permanent pacemaker or implantable cardioverter-defibrillator leads. *J Am Coll Cardiol*. 2005;45:1672–1675.
21. Al-Mohaissen MA, Chan KL. Prevalence and mechanism of tricuspid regurgitation following implantation of endocardial leads for pacemaker or cardioverter-defibrillator. *J Am Soc Echocardiogr*. 2012;25:245–252.
22. Vaturi M, Kusniec J, Shapira Y, et al. Right ventricular pacing increases tricuspid regurgitation grade regardless of the mechanical interference to the valve by the electrode. *Eur J Echocardiogr*. 2010;11:550–553.
23. Byrd CL, Wilkoff BL, Love CJ, et al. Intravascular extraction of problematic or infected permanent pacemaker leads: 1994–1996. *PACE (Pacing Clin Electrophysiol)*. 1999;22:1348–1357.
24. Coffey JO, Sager SJ, Gangireddy S, et al. The impact of transvenous lead extraction on tricuspid valve function. *PACE (Pacing Clin Electrophysiol)*. 2014;37:19–24.
25. Rodriguez Y, Mesa J, Arguelles E, Carrillo RG. Tricuspid insufficiency after laser lead extraction. *PACE (Pacing Clin Electrophysiol)*. 2013;36:939–944.
26. Addetia K, Yamat M, Mediratta A, et al. Comprehensive two-dimensional interrogation of the tricuspid valve using knowledge derived from three-dimensional echocardiography. *J Am Soc Echocardiogr*. 2016;29:74–82.
27. Stankovic I, Daraban AM, Jasaityte R, et al. Incremental value of the en face view of the tricuspid valve by two-dimensional and three-dimensional echocardiography for accurate identification of tricuspid valve leaflets. *J Am Soc Echocardiogr*. 2014;27:376–384.
28. Wafae N, Hayashi H, Gerola LR, Vieira MC. Anatomical study of the human tricuspid valve. *Surg Radiol Anat*. 1990;12:37–41.
29. Xanthos T, Dalivigkas I, Ekmektzoglou KA. Anatomic variations of the cardiac valves and papillary muscles of the right heart. *Ital J Anatomy Embryol*. 2011;116:111–126.
30. Hahn RT. State-of-the-art review of echocardiographic imaging in the evaluation and treatment of functional tricuspid regurgitation. *Circulation Cardiovasc Imag*. 2016;9.
31. Mediratta A, Addetia K, Yamat M, et al. 3D echocardiographic location of implantable device leads and mechanism of associated tricuspid regurgitation. *JACC Cardiovascular Imag*. 2014;7:337–347.
32. Addetia K, Maffessanti F, Mediratta A, et al. Impact of implantable transvenous device lead location on severity of tricuspid regurgitation. *J Am Soc Echocardiogr*. 2014;27:1164–1175.

107 Pulmonic Regurgitation: Etiology and Quantification

Kelly Axsom, Muhamed Saric

Trivial or mild degrees of pulmonic regurgitation (PR) are common in structurally normal hearts, and the presence of pathologic PR is rare in adults.[1] Some degree of PR is present in between 5% and 78% in echocardiograms of patients with normal pulmonic valves (PVs) and structurally normal hearts.[2] Echocardiographic evaluation of the degree PR is much less well defined than for the other heart valves and is either descriptive or semiquantitative. This is primarily because of the low prevalence of clinically severe PR. In one series, only 1.6% of all severe valvular regurgitation was caused by PR.[3]

PULMONIC REGURGITATION EVALUATION OVERVIEW

As with other valve lesions, assessment of PR includes three basic elements: (1) establishing the mechanism of PR, (2) determining the severity of PR, and (3) assessing the impact of PR on cardiac chambers, primarily the right ventricle (RV) and the pulmonary artery (PA). Whereas the severity of PR is best assessed by Doppler echocardiography, the mechanism of PR and its impact on cardiac chambers is evaluated by two- and three-dimensional echocardiography (2DE and 3DE, respectively).

The American College of Cardiology and the American Heart Association guidelines on valvular heart disease address the issue of PR only briefly.[4] The American Society of Echocardiography recommendations for evaluation of severity of PR include evaluation of anatomical structure of the pulmonary valve, right ventricular (RV) size, color Doppler pulmonic regurgitant jet size, spectral Doppler jet density, duration, and deceleration rate as well as a comparison echocardiography and magnetic resonance imaging in PR diagnosis.[5] Other parameters of PR severity include timing of tricuspid valve (TV) closure and PV opening, holodiastolic flow reversal in the PA, low peak velocity of PR jet, and laminar retrograde flow.[3] Echocardiographic markers of PR severity are summarized in Table 107.1 and shown in Figs. 107.1 and 107.2.

CAUSE AND MECHANISM OF PULMONIC REGURGITATION

A normal pulmonary valve is semilunar, trileaflet valve located anterior, superior, and slightly to the left of the aortic valve. The valve leaflets are very thin and highly pliable, making the PV the most challenging valve to image. In addition, visualization of the PV is often limited because only one or two posterior leaflets are imageable. Moreover, because of rapid opening, the leaflets are difficult to visualize in systole. PR can be either congenital or acquired. The most common causes of severe PR included carcinoid disease and status post surgically repaired pulmonic stenosis of tetralogy of Fallot (Fig. 107.3).[6] Endocarditis rarely affects the native PV. Box 107.1 lists the majority of causes of PR.

The primary mechanisms of PR include distorted or absent leaflets, annular dilatation, or both. When assessing PR, it is best to evaluate the right ventricular outflow tract (RVOT), PV, and PA together. Imaging of the PV is often better by transthoracic echocardiography (TTE) than transesophageal echocardiography (TEE) given the anterior location of the valve, which is in the far field by TEE. 2D TTE and TEE imaging typically allows for visualization of only long-axis views of the PV. On TTE, PR is best visualized on the parasternal short-axis view at the level of the aortic valve and from the subxiphoid view. On TEE, the PV and PA can be imaged in the midesophageal and transgastric views using approximately the 60-degree acquisition angle. The short axis of the PV can be obtained by 3D TTE and TEE imaging.[7]

SEMIQUANTITATIVE ASSESSMENT OF THE SEVERITY OF PULMONIC REGURGITATION

Color and spectral Doppler echocardiography are the primary means of quantifying the degree of PR. As with other valvular regurgitations, the severity of PR depends on the interplay between the regurgitant orifice size, the amount of regurgitant volume, and

TABLE 107.1 Markers of Severe Pulmonic Regurgitation

	Parameter	Moderate to Severe PR	Severe PR
Color Doppler	Jet length and area	Increased	May be short
	Jet turbulence	Turbulent jet	Laminar jet
	Vena contracta	Wide	Very wide
CW Doppler	Jet density	Dense	Very dense
	Deceleration slope	Short	Very short
	Premature cessation of retrograde flow	May be absent	Typically present
	To-and-fro flow	Absent	Present
	Peak PR velocity	Normal	Low
	Premature opening of the pulmonic valve	Absent	Present
	Premature closure of the tricuspid valve	Absent	Present
PW Doppler	Regurgitant volume	<60 mL/beat	≥60 mL/beat
	Regurgitant fraction	<50%	(50%
	Holodiastolic flow reversal in PA	Absent	Present
Additional Signs	RV and PA size	Progressively increases with the severity and chronicity of PR	

CW, Continuous-wave; *PR,* pulmonic regurgitation; *PW,* pulsed-wave; *RV,* right ventricular.

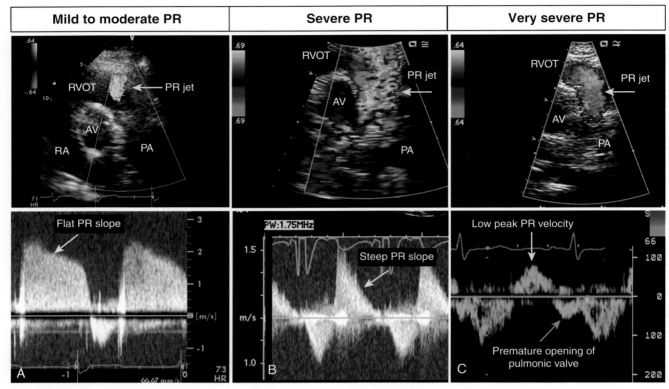

Figure 107.1. Color and spectral Doppler markers of pulmonic regurgitation (PR). Transthoracic short-axis view at the level of the aortic valve demonstrate color Doppler *(top)* and spectral Doppler *(bottom)* findings in mild to moderate, severe, and very severe PR. **A.** Mild to moderate PR. On color Doppler, the jet is small *(arrow)*, and vena contracta at the jet origin is narrow. On spectral Doppler, the slope of PR jet is relatively flat *(arrow)*. **B,** Severe PR. On color Doppler, the jet is large and turbulent *(arrow)*, but on spectral Doppler, the PR slope is steep *(arrow)*. **C,** Very severe PR. On color Doppler, the jet is laminar *(arrow)* and of short duration. On spectral Doppler, there is a low peak velocity of PR jet *(yellow arrow)*, and there is premature opening of pulmonic valve with abnormal antegrade flow in late diastole. *AV,* Aortic valve; *RA,* right atrium; *RVOT,* right ventricular outflow tract. (See accompanying Video 107.1.)

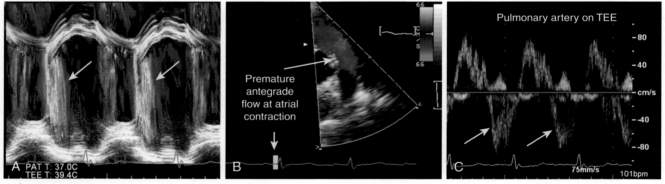

Figure 107.2. Additional markers of severe pulmonic regurgitation (PR). **A,** Color M-mode echocardiography demonstrates that PR jet terminates abnormally in early diastole *(arrows)*. This is in contrast to less severe forms of PR in which the PR jet lasts throughout the diastole. **B,** Color Doppler on a transthoracic short-axis view at the level of the aortic valve demonstrates abnormal antegrade flow across the pulmonic valve at the time of atrial contraction indicative of premature pulmonic valve opening resulting from elevated right ventricular pressures in severe PR. **C,** Transesophageal echocardiography (TEE) spectral Doppler tracing demonstrates abnormal holodiastolic flow reversal in the pulmonary artery indicative of severe PR.

the transvalvular pressure gradient (the diastolic pressure gradient between the PA and the RV in the case of PR).

To a certain point, as the regurgitant volume and the severity of PR increase, so do the size and the turbulence of the regurgitant jet. However, when the regurgitant orifice becomes very large, a rapid equalization of pressures may lead to a smaller and more laminar regurgitant jet that terminates prematurely (before the end of diastole). It is important to bear in mind that the degree of PR is not the only determinant of the rate

of pressure equalization; rapid equalization of pressures may also be mediated by a low diastolic PA pressure or high RV diastolic pressure. Collectively, all these phenomena form the basis of semiquantitative PR assessment by both color and spectral Doppler imaging.

Historically, angiography has been the primary means of validating echocardiographic methods for PR. However, angiography has recently been supplanted by cardiac magnetic resonance imaging (CMRI).

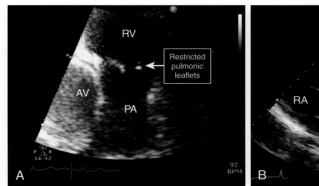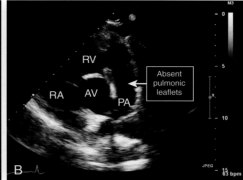

Figure 107.3. Causes of severe pulmonic regurgitation (PR). **A,** Carcinoid disease of the pulmonic valve. **B,** Severe PR occurring decades after surgical repair of tetralogy of Fallot. *AV,* Aortic valve; *PA,* pulmonary artery; *RA,* right atrium; *RV,* right ventricle. (See accompanying Video 107.3.)

BOX 107.1 Causes of Pulmonic Regurgitation

- Pulmonary hypertension (dilatation of the pulmonary artery)
- Congenital (e.g., bicuspid or quadricuspid)
- Status post pulmonic valvotomy (surgical or balloon)
- Rheumatic heart disease
- Infective endocarditis
- Marfan syndrome
- Carcinoid (stenosis or regurgitation)
- Trauma (including injury from a pulmonary artery catheter)

COLOR DOPPLER

Color Doppler is the most widely accepted method for assessing PR. The typical PR jet is seen in the RVOT during diastole. PR jets in the normal heart are usually narrow or "spindle-like" and originate centrally from the pulmonary leaflet coaptation site.

Jet length. Original studies suggested that a jet length of less than 10 mm implies trivial regurgitation.[1] Theoretically, more severe PR should be associated with longer jets. However, jet length is not considered a reliable index of PR severity because abrupt cessation of diastolic flow in severe PR may lead to relatively short PR jets. Furthermore, the more severe the PR, the less likely a full jet length can be appreciated on the parasternal TTE window.

Jet area. Planimetry of the jet area indexed for body surface area has been shown to correlate well with angiographic grades of PR severity in patients with tetralogy of Fallot repair.[6] However, there are no well-validated criteria on what jet area defines severe PR. Again, it is important to emphasize that with very severe PR, when equalization of the PA to RV gradient takes place early in diastole, the color Doppler jet area can be small and brief; this seemingly paradoxical diminution of jet area size should not be misinterpreted as less than severe PR.

Turbulent vs laminar regurgitant jet. Lesser degrees of PR are typically characterized by turbulent jets. When PR is very severe and when there is rapid equalization of pressure between the PA and the RV in diastole, the PR jet may become laminar. This seemingly paradoxical finding is an important semiquantitative marker of PR severity.

Vena contracta. The use of vena contracta width for determining severity of regurgitation is generally reserved for the other valves and has not been validated for PR. Semiquantitatively, a wide vena contracta in the setting of a brief and small color Doppler jet area supports the diagnosis of severe PR.

CONTINUOUS-WAVE SPECTRAL DOPPLER

Continuous-wave (CW) spectral Doppler of the PR jet should be attempted on all echocardiographic examinations. Semiquantitative measures of PR severity include signal density, deceleration slope, and the timing of jet cessation.

Jet density. Theoretically, more severe PR should be associated with more dense spectral tracings. However, there is no accepted method for fully quantifying PR using spectral density.

Deceleration slope. A rapid deceleration slope of the diastolic Doppler signal is only a rough estimate of PR severity because there are no well-validated deceleration cutoff values for various degrees of PR. Although severe PR leads to a rapid declaration slope of PR jet, not all instances of rapid deceleration slope are indicative of severe PR. This is because the deceleration slope depends on both the size of the regurgitant orifice and the pressure gradient of the diastolic PA to the right atrium. Thus, in patients with low PA diastolic pressures or elevated RV diastolic pressures, a rapid slope may be seen in the absence of severe PR (Fig. 107.1).

Premature cessation of retrograde flow. Severe PR is characterized by premature cessation of retrograde spectral Doppler flow; instead of end-diastole, the flow ends in mid to late diastole (see Fig. 107.1). However, not all instances of premature PR jet cessation are indicative of severe PR because the phenomenon may also be seen in patients with low PA diastolic pressures or elevated RV diastolic pressures in the absence of severe PR.

To-and-fro flow. In patients with very severe PR, there may be little net antegrade flow across the PV; the bulk of flow simply recirculates across the PV (retrograde in diastole then antegrade in systole). This gives rise to a characteristic sinusoid "to-and-fro" velocity pattern on CW Doppler in patients with severe PR.

Low peak PR velocity. Another marker of severe PR is a low peak PR velocity. It is typically seen with the to-and-fro flow pattern.

Premature tricuspid and PV events. Premature closure of the TV and premature opening of the PV are markers of severe PR seen on Doppler echocardiography and reflect elevated RV pressures.

PULSED-WAVE SPECTRAL DOPPLER

When PR jet is not aliased, spectral pulsed-wave (PW) Doppler recordings can be used to assess the severity of PR in the same manner as described for CW.

Regurgitant fraction by PV PW. Spectral PW Doppler recordings can be used to roughly estimate the regurgitant fraction of PR by tracing retrograde and antegrade flow velocity profiles individually to obtain respective velocity time integrals (VTIs). Assuming a constant PV diameter in systole and diastole, a ratio of retrograde VTI (a measure of regurgitant volume) to antegrade VTI (a measure of total stroke volume) represents the regurgitant fraction.[8] Theoretically, a ratio of 0.5 or more would indicate severe PR (i.e., a regurgitant fraction of ≥50%). However, there are no empirically validated cutoff values for grading PR severity using this method. Furthermore, this method cannot be used in patients with concomitant pulmonic stenosis because of the poststenotic turbulence.

Regurgitant volume and fraction by comparing pulmonic to systemic flow. Systolic antegrade flow across a RVOT in a patient with PR represents the total stroke volume (TSV). If the patient does not have significant aortic regurgitation and no shunt, then systolic antegrade flow across the left ventricular outflow tract (LVOT) represents the net stroke volume (NSV). A difference between TSV and NSV represents the regurgitant volume.

RVOT and LVOT stroke volumes (TSV and NSV, respectively) can be calculated using the standard echocardiographic method of measuring the outflow tract diameter (d) in systole; calculating the cross-sectional outflow tract area (A), assuming a circular shape [A = (0.5*d)^2 * π]; and then multiplying the area by the systolic VTI. Thereafter, regurgitant volume and fraction can be calculated as:

$$\text{Regurgitant volume} = \text{TSV} - \text{NSV}$$

$$\text{Regurgitant fraction} = \text{Regurgitant volume/TSV}$$

Although these calculations are feasible, the cutoff values have not been validated for PR. The major limitation to this method is the frequent inability to measure the RVOT diameter accurately. It has been shown that regurgitant fraction calculation by echocardiography only moderately correlates with measurements obtained with CMRI.[9]

Holodiastolic flow reversal in PA. Normally, the PW spectral Doppler profile in the PA contains a large antegrade component in systole and a very small retrograde component confined to early diastole. As the severity of PR increase, so does the duration of retrograde flow in the PA. In severe PR, there is typically a holodiastolic flow reversal in the PA spectral Doppler tracings. This is analogous to holodiastolic flow reversal in the thoracic and abdominal aorta in the setting of severe aortic regurgitation. This diastolic flow reversal needs to be differentiated from diastolic flow caused by patent ductus arteriosus.

M-MODE ECHOCARDIOGRAPHY

Many aspects of PR assessment by M-mode echocardiography have only historic value. However, with its excellent temporal resolution, M-mode echocardiography allows for very precise timing of cardiac events. For instance, one can easily demonstrate by color M-mode echocardiography the short, early diastolic nature of jet in severe PR.

Moreover, recently a PR index by M-mode echocardiography (PRIME) to estimate the pulmonary regurgitation fraction (PRF) using a nonlinear regression was developed. M-mode tracings of the right PA from the suprasternal notch are used to measure the maximal systolic and minimum diastolic dimensions. PRIME values of 1.21 or greater identified patients with a PRF of 25% or greater. Compared with PRF calculated by CMRI, this measurement was accurate. It remains unknown if this method can be replicated by other investigators.[10]

IMPACT OF PULMONIC REGURGITATION ON CARDIAC CHAMBERS

Chronic PR is associated with PA and RV dilatation. PA dilatation may both lead to and be the result of severe PR. RV dilatation and interventricular septal flattening in diastole (a marker of RV volume overload) are nonspecific signs of severe chronic PR. Conversely, a normal RV size excludes severe chronic PR.

Please access ExpertConsult to view the corresponding videos for this chapter.

REFERENCES

1. Takao S, Miyatake K, Izumi S, et al. Clinical implications of pulmonary regurgitation in healthy individuals: detection by cross sectional pulsed Doppler echocardiography. *Br Heart J.* 1988;59:542–550.
2. Choong CY, Abascal VM, Weyman J, et al. Prevalence of valvular regurgitation by Doppler echocardiography in patients with structurally normal hearts by two-dimensional echocardiography. *Am Heart J.* 1989;117:636–642.
3. Jhaveri RR, Saric M, Kronzon I. Uncommon Doppler echocardiographic findings of severe pulmonic insufficiency. *J Am Soc Echocardiogr.* 2010;23:1071–1075.
4. Nishimura RA, Otto CM, Bonow RO, et al. AHA/ACC guideline for the management of patients with valvular heart disease: a report of the American College of Cardiology/American Heart Association Task Force on practice guidelines. *J Am Coll Cardiol.* 2014;63:2489. 2014.
5. Zoghbi WA, Adams D, Bonow RO, et al. Recommendations for noninvasive evaluation of native valvular regurgitation: a report from the American Society of Echocardiography developed in collaboration with the Society for Cardiovascular Magnetic Resonance. *J Am Soc Echocardiogr.* 2017;30:303–371.
6. Kobayashi J, Nakano S, Matsuda H, et al. Quantitative evaluation of pulmonary regurgitation after repair of tetralogy of Fallot using real-time flow imaging system. *Jpn Circ J.* 1989;53:721–727.
7. Anwar AM, Nosir YF, Zainal-Abidin SK, et al. Real-time three-dimensional transthoracic echocardiography in daily practice: initial experience. *Cardiovasc Ultrasound.* 2012 26;10:14.
8. Goldberg SJ, Allen HD. Quantitative assessment by Doppler echocardiography of pulmonary or aortic regurgitation. *Am J Cardiol.* 1985;56:131–135.
9. Mercer-Rosa L, Yang W, Kutty S, et al: Quantifying pulmonary regurgitation and right ventricular function in surgically repaired tetralogy of Fallot: a comparative analysis of echocardiography and magnetic resonance imaging, Circ Cardiovasc Imag 5:637–643.
10. Festa P, Ait-Ali L, Minichilli F, et al. A new simple method to estimate pulmonary regurgitation by echocardiography in operated Fallot: comparison with magnetic resonance imaging and performance test evaluation. *J Am Soc Echocardiogr.* 2010;23:496–503.

108 Tricuspid and Pulmonic Stenosis

Priti Mehla, Jennifer Conroy, Itzhak Kronzon

TRICUSPID STENOSIS
Cause

Tricuspid stenosis (TS) is the least common stenotic valvulopathy. TS is most commonly the result of rheumatic heart disease (RHD). Isolated involvement of the tricuspid valve (TV) is seen in congenital TS or in carcinoid heart disease. Other causes include metabolic or enzymatic abnormalities such as Fabry and Whipple disease.[1]

1. *Rheumatic TS.* RHD, although infrequent in developed countries, accounts for the majority (>90%) of all cases. Approximately 3% to 5% of patients with rheumatic mitral disease have concomitant TS.[2,3] Large majority of patients with rheumatic TS have coexisting mitral valve involvement.[4] Diffuse fibrous leaflet thickening with commissural fusion, especially the anteroseptal commissure, is typical. Chordal involvement in TS is less pronounced than in rheumatic mitral stenosis (MS).[1]

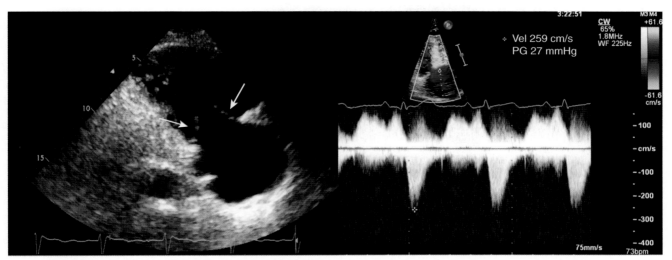

Figure 108.1. The *left panel* illustrates a two-dimensional echocardiographic image of a tricuspid valve (TV) in a patient with carcinoid syndrome, obtained in a right ventricular inflow view in systole. Note the frozen appearance of the tricuspid leaflets *(white arrows)*. The *right panel* shows a continuous-wave (CW) Doppler recording through the TV. Note the presence of elevated diastolic gradient with significant tricuspid regurgitation. *PG,* Pressure gradient; *Vel,* velocity. (Accompanying Video 108.1 corresponds to the *left panel.*)

2. *Congenital TS.* Isolated TV involvement is usually caused by congenital lesions. Although rare, Ebstein anomaly can result in TS.[5]
3. *Carcinoid heart disease.* Carcinoid heart disease affects more than 50% of those with carcinoid tumor and almost exclusively involves the right heart.[6] TV involvement can result in tricuspid regurgitation (TR), TS, or mixed disease. Vasoactive amines produced by the carcinoid tumor result in thick and rigid leaflets giving a frozen appearance. Chordae and papillary muscles may also be affected (Fig. 108.1).
4. *Miscellaneous.* Right atrial (RA) tumors or clots or infective endocarditis with vegetations may cause tricuspid obstruction mimicking TS. Rare cases of iatrogenic TS secondary to pacemaker leads have been reported. External right chamber compression from loculated pericardial effusion can result in elevated tricuspid gradients mimicking TS.
5. *Prosthetic TS.* Compared with left-sided bioprosthetic valves, TV prostheses generally have less durability. Prosthetic valve dysfunction may result in stenosis, regurgitation, or a combination of both. Common causes of prosthetic dysfunction include leaflet degeneration, valve thrombosis, endocarditis, and pannus formation.[7]

PATHOPHYSIOLOGY

TS severity is defined by the diastolic pressure gradient between the right-sided chambers. Mean gradients of 4 mmHg and above generally lead to high RA pressure and systemic venous congestion.[8] Simultaneously, the right ventricle is underfilled, leading to low cardiac output. As a result, patients with concurrent MS may not exhibit significant elevation of left atrial, pulmonary artery (PA), or right ventricular (RV) systolic pressures.

DIAGNOSIS
Physical Examination and Clinical Manifestations

Patients with hemodynamically significant TS present with signs and symptoms of elevated venous pressures, including fatigue, edema, anasarca, and congestive hepatomegaly. Patients have relatively little dyspnea for the degree of systemic venous congestion. Jugular venous pulsations may show a prominent A wave with a slow Y descent (reflecting delayed emptying of the RA). In atrial fibrillation, a positive CV systolic wave with a slow Y descent can

be seen.[9] On auscultation, TS may produce a soft opening snap followed by a middiastolic rumbling murmur with presystolic accentuation at the parasternal border in the fourth intercostal space. The murmur intensity (and the diastolic pressure gradient) increases with maneuvers that increase venous return such as leg raising, inspiration, squatting, and exercise.[10]

Imaging

Echocardiography is the primary noninvasive tool for the initial diagnosis and evaluation of TS. A comprehensive evaluation includes assessment of valve anatomy, stenosis severity, and associated lesions. Upstream dilatation of cardiac chambers should be assessed as well. Multiple windows (parasternal RV inflow, short-axis, apical four-chamber, subcostal views) with multiparametric assessment with two- and three-dimensional imaging with spectral and color Doppler should be performed.

The normal TV orifice area is 7 to 9 cm². The TV is typically composed of three unequal leaflets, namely the septal, anterior, and posterior. The anterior leaflet is the largest, with greater mobility compared with the septal leaflet, which has the least mobility. Approximately 10% of patients do not exhibit clear demarcation between the anterior and posterior leaflets.[11]

Peak diastolic velocities across the normal TV are usually less than 1 m/s with a mean gradient of less than 2 mmHg. Stenosis severity is determined using continuous-wave (CW) Doppler with heart rates less than 100 beats/min. Because of respiratory variation, inflow velocities throughout the respiratory cycle should be averaged or recorded at end-expiration. At least five beats should be averaged in patients with atrial fibrillation.[10] The mean transvalvular pressure gradient is calculated by measuring the individual maximal velocities throughout diastole (Fig. 108.2). Table 108.1 summarizes the recommended European Association of Echocardiography (EAE)/American Society of Echocardiography (ASE) guidelines for grading the severity of TS.

Valve area is determined either by the pressure halftime (PHT) method or by the continuity equation. PHT is the time required for the maximal pressure to decrease by half. The constant 190 (as opposed to 220 for the mitral valve) is then divided by the PHT to derive valve area.[12] This method, however, has not been widely validated for TV area calculation.[13]

The continuity equation, using pulsed-wave (PW) and CW Doppler, can also be used to calculate valve area. TV area can be

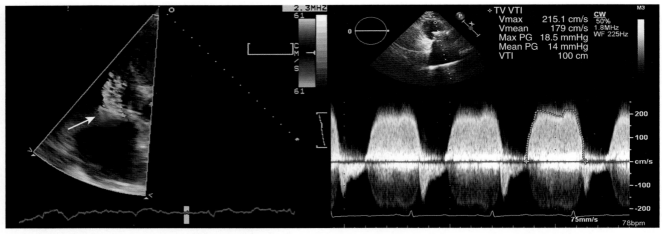

Figure 108.2. The *left panel* illustrates a two-dimensional echocardiographic image with color Doppler flow across a stenotic tricuspid valve (TV) obtained in an apical four-chamber view during diastole. Note the turbulent flow across the TV. The *right panel* shows a continuous-wave (CW) Doppler recording through the TV. Note the elevated peak diastolic velocity of 2.2 m/s. The diastolic velocity time in (100 cm) and mean gradient (14 mm Hg) are listed. *PG,* Pressure gradient; *Vmax,* peak velocity; *Vmean,* mean velocity; *VTI,* velocity time integral. (Accompanying Video 108.2 corresponds to the *left panel*.)

TABLE 108.1 How to Grade Tricuspid Stenosis: European Association of Echocardiography/American Society of Echocardiography Guidelines[11]

	Mild	Moderate	Severe
Valve area (cm²)	>1.5	1–1.5	<1
Mean gradient (mm Hg)	<5	5–10	>10
Pulmonary artery pressure (mm Hg)	<30	30–50	>50

TABLE 108.2 Findings Indicative of Hemodynamically Significant Tricuspid Stenosis per European Association of Echocardiography/American Society of Echocardiography Recommendations[11]

Specific Findings	
Mean pressure gradient	≥5 mm Hg
Inflow time velocity integral	>60 cm
$T_{1/2}$ (pressure halftime)	≥190 ms
Valve area by continuity equation	≤1 cm²
Supportive Findings	
Enlarged right atrium ≥ moderate	
Dilated inferior vena cava	

TABLE 108.3 Doppler Parameters of Prosthetic Tricuspid Valve Function[15]

	Consider Valve Stenosis
Peak velocity	>1.7 m/s
Mean gradient	≥6 mm Hg
Pressure halftime	≥230 ms
EOA and VTI$_{PrTV}$	No data available yet for tricuspid prosthesis

EOA, Effective orifice area; *PrTV,* prosthetic tricuspid valve; *VTI,* velocity time integral.

obtained by dividing stroke volume (SV) by velocity time integral (VTI) of the TV.[14]

One of the key limitations of the continuity equation is the assumption of a circular, rather than elliptical, shape of the outflow tract, which can underestimate the cross-sectional area. Another challenge is obtaining accurate inflow volumes, particularly in the setting of concomitant TR. As TR increases, valve area is underestimated by the continuity equation. Despite its use, robust data are not available for the application of the continuity equation in assessing TVs.[13] Findings supportive of significant TS are listed in Table 108.2. Invasive hemodynamic assessment of TS may be considered in symptomatic patients with discordant clinical and noninvasive data.

Just like native TV, prosthetic TV evaluation is primarily done by echocardiography. Prosthetic valve function is assessed by recording Doppler parameters such as peak E and A velocity, PHT, mean gradient, and VTI. Despite scarce data for the TV, prosthetic effective orifice area (EOA) can be calculated

using the continuity principle by dividing the LV outflow SV by prosthesis VTI. LV outflow SV can be substituted by RV outflow SV in the presence of significant aortic regurgitation, given pulmonic valve (PV) regurgitation is no more than mild. Analogous to native TV, regardless of the cardiac rhythm, at least five cardiac cycles should be averaged when recording tricuspid prosthetic velocity.[15] Elevated gradients across a dysfunctional prosthesis may be due to stenosis or insufficiency. Prolonged PHT is suggestive of stenosis rather than regurgitation.[7] PHT, however, should not be used to determine EOA because this method overestimates the valve area.[16] Doppler parameters suggestive of valve stenosis as recommended by ASE are listed in Table 108.3.

Alternatively, a large retrospective series examining tricuspid prostheses early after implantation found other benchmarks that may be used to determine prosthetic stenosis. This study proposes a peak E velocity greater than 2.1 m/s, mean gradient greater than 8.8 mm Hg, PHT greater than 193 m/s, VTI of the TV prosthesis greater than 66 mm, and ratio of the TV prosthesis VTI to the left ventricular outflow tract (LVOT) VTI greater than 3.3 as abnormal parameters suggestive of stenosis.[16]

MANAGEMENT

TV surgery is recommended for patients with isolated symptomatic severe TS or in those with significant TS undergoing surgery on left-sided valves.[17] Valve anatomy and available surgical expertise determines the type of surgical intervention—repair versus replacement.

Echocardiographic evaluation of valvular and subvalvular anatomy helps determine valve reparability. One of the main limitations of repair strategy is the lack of pliable leaflet tissue. In patients deemed suitable for valve replacement, biological prostheses are preferred over mechanical because of the high risk of thrombosis with mechanical valves.[18] Patients with dysfunctional prostheses have significant risks associated with redo sternotomies, making surgical intervention prohibitive. Prosthetic TV reinterventions are associated with significant mortality rates ranging from 17% to 37%.[7]

Percutaneous balloon tricuspid commissurotomy can be considered in isolated symptomatic severe TS in anatomically suitable valves.[17] Novel transcatheter percutaneous therapies are emerging as an effective alternative to repeat surgical approach in patients with prohibitive surgical risk. Stenosed TV prosthesis have been treated with TV in-valve implantation with good hemodynamic and clinical outcomes.[19]

PULMONIC VALVE STENOSIS
Cause

PS is the most common form of right ventricular outflow tract (RVOT) obstruction.[20] The majority of PS cases (~95% of cases) are congenital or associated with congenital conditions such as Tetralogy of Fallot (ToF), double-outlet RV, univentricular atrioventricular connection, and atrioventricular canal defects. PS and peripheral PA stenosis are also often encountered in genetic syndromes such as Noonan and Williams syndrome.

Acquired causes of PS include carcinoid disease, RHD, infective endocarditis, and iatrogenic causes.[21] The most common cause of acquired PS is carcinoid disease. RHD generally involves additional valves. Compression from a tumor or a vascular structure may result in functional PS.

Pathophysiology

PS leads to RV pressure overload, resulting in increased wall stress and compensatory RV hypertrophy. The resulting decline in RV compliance is manifested by elevated RV end-diastolic pressure and RA pressure. With significant PS, these changes ultimately lead to diastolic and systolic RV dysfunction.[22]

Diagnosis
Physical Examination

On inspection, a prominent jugular venous A wave may be appreciated. In significant PS, on palpation of the precordium, a parasternal systolic thrill at the upper left sternal border or a RV lift or heave may be appreciated. During auscultation, a widely split S2 (caused by prolonged pulmonic ejection time and delayed closure of the PVs) can be heard. An ejection click is commonly audible in mild PS. With increasing PS severity, the click approximates the first heart sound, but in severe cases, the click may become inaudible. At the left upper sternal border, a harsh crescendo–decrescendo ejection murmur can be heard, which increases in intensity with inspiration. With RV failure and hypertrophy, a right-sided fourth heart sound may be audible.[23]

Clinical Manifestations

The majority of patients with mild or moderate PS are asymptomatic. In significant disease, the right ventricle cannot appropriately augment cardiac output, and this may lead to dyspnea, exertional chest pain, dizziness, and syncope. Increased RV mass can cause supply–demand mismatch, resulting in ischemia and arrhythmias. Patients with an underlying interatrial communication can exhibit right-to-left shunting and oxygen desaturation. Advanced untreated cases can progress to right heart failure.[22]

Imaging

The normal PV is trileaflet with thin pliable cusps. Stenotic valves always have anatomic abnormalities with fibrous thickening and may rarely have calcific deposits.[24] Distinct morphologic types of valvular PS[21,24] are:

1. *Dome shaped.* In about 40% to 60% of cases, the valve is dome shaped and acommissural, with a central or eccentric opening and preserved valve mobility. A variable number of ridges representing rudimentary raphe extend from the cusp tips toward the base of the leaflets. PS may result in PA dilatation caused by eccentric flow through the valve aperture. Intrinsic pulmonary trunk connective tissue abnormalities such as medial wall degeneration may play a role as well. There is a predilection for involvement of left PA because of its relatively obtuse take-off from the main PA.
2. *Dysplastic.* About 20% of cases exhibit this morphology. The valve is tricuspid with no commissural fusion. The leaflets are thick and myxomatous with reduced mobility. The valve annulus is usually small and hypoplastic. Dysplastic valves are usually seen in Noonan syndrome and are associated with supravalvular stenosis.
3. *Bicuspid or multicuspid.* Bicuspid valves are frequently seen in association with ToF. Quadricuspid valves generally present with pulmonic regurgitation (PR).

Uniquely, carcinoid disease produces carcinoid plaques, rendering the pulmonic cusps rigid with whitish colored leaflets.[24]

Echocardiography

Echocardiography is essential in detecting the precise site of stenosis, quantifying severity, determining the cause, identifying coexisting pathology, and selecting the appropriate management strategy. Transthoracic echocardiography is recommended for both initial and follow-up examinations. Imaging the PV is challenging because of its retrosternal location. Multiple windows should be used allowing for parallel Doppler alignment (particularly the parasternal short-axis view, subcostal views, and a modified apical five-chamber view bringing the RVOT into plane).[25]

M-mode echocardiography may aid in diagnosis by providing information on leaflet motion. In the setting of decreased RV compliance, RV end-diastolic pressure exceeds PA pressure with RA contraction causing presystolic opening of the PV. This is reflected on the M mode as exaggerated "A" wave (representing posterior motion of the valve cusp following the P wave of the electrocardiogram).[26]

The severity of stenosis is determined by CW and PW Doppler (Fig. 108.3). The simplified Bernoulli equation is used to calculate the systolic gradient across the PV. Transpulmonic pressure gradient is the main discriminator of the severity of PS (Table 108.4). The highest obtained velocity determines the transpulmonic gradient. Doppler gradient-based PS severity has been derived from catheterization data. Doppler-derived peak gradients have been shown to correlate well with the catheter-derived peak-to-peak pressure gradient, though with a tendency to overestimate the peak-to-peak gradient.[27] Alternatively, one study has shown mean Doppler gradients to have superior correlation and agreement with invasive peak-to-peak gradients.[28]

In the presence of concomitant subvalvular stenoses, the simplified Bernoulli equation cannot be used. It is difficult to determine the exact contribution of individual lesions in such cases. PW Doppler with careful sample volume placement should be used to identify different sites of obstruction. As in LVOT tracings in cases of hypertrophic cardiomyopathy, patients with RV muscular infundibular obstruction demonstrate a late peaking systolic jet, signifying dynamic obstruction as opposed to an early peaking systolic jet more typical of fixed obstructions.

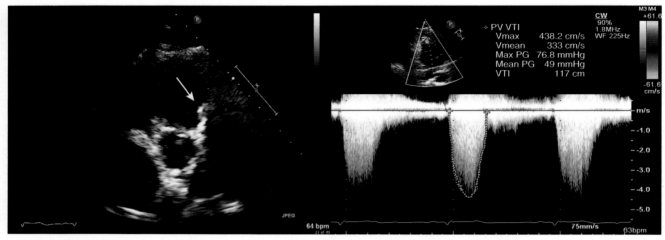

Figure 108.3. The *left panel* illustrates a two-dimensional echocardiographic image of a stenotic pulmonic valve (PV) obtained in a parasternal short-axis view. Note the thickened valve cusps *(white arrow)*. The *right panel* shows a continuous-wave (CW) Doppler recording through the pulmonic valve with an elevated peak systolic velocity of 4.4 m/s. *PG,* Pressure gradient; *Vmax,* peak velocity; *Vmean,* mean velocity; *VTI,* velocity time integral. (Accompanying Video 108.3 corresponds to the *left panel*.)

TABLE 108.4 Grading of Pulmonic Valve Stenosis: European Association of Echocardiography/American Society of Echocardiography Recommendations

	Mild	Moderate	Severe
Peak velocity (m/s)	<3	3–4	>4
Peak gradient (mm Hg)	<36	36–64	>64

PV area calculation via planimetry is often not feasible. Alternative quantitative methods such as the continuity equation and proximal isovelocity surface area method have not been validated in PS.[10]

In patients with suboptimal images, transesophageal echocardiography can be performed. Transgastric views of the PV are mainly used to align RVOT flow with the Doppler beam. The upper esophageal aortic arch short-axis view usually shows the long-axis view of the main PA and the PV. The midesophageal RV inflow-outflow view allows visualization of at least two cusps.[29]

The hemodynamic consequences of PS such as RV hypertrophy, right-sided chamber enlargement, and RV dysfunction are thoroughly assessed by echocardiography. A bubble study using agitated saline can help assess for the presence of interatrial shunt.

Patients with history of isolated PS and subsequent valvular intervention require regular follow up for monitoring of PR and RV size and function. Significant PR in the setting of normal PA pressure should be assessed carefully as PA end-diastolic pressure may be only slightly greater than the RV end-diastolic pressure. This minimal diastolic gradient may produce laminar flow making color Doppler evaluation difficult.[22] Any evidence of pulmonary arterial hypertension in isolated PS cases should raise a suspicion of associated peripheral PA stenosis.

Cardiac catheterization is rarely necessary for diagnosis and is usually performed before balloon valvotomy. Gradients above, at, and below the PV should be obtained. Cardiac magnetic resonance (CMRI) or computed tomography (CT) may be used as confirmatory tests in uncomplicated valvular PS cases. CT, which uses radiation, is excellent for the assessment of branch pulmonary arteries and proximity of coronary arteries to the valve annulus. CT can also be used to assess RV size and function. CMRI can help distinguish serial stenosis such as valvular and dynamic subvalvular infundibular stenosis. Additionally, the transpulmonic gradient may be determined via velocity mapping. This method, however, may underestimate severity, and for this reason, gradients obtained by echocardiography are generally preferred.[22,30] Postoperative PV function, grading of PR severity, and assessment of RV size and function are well evaluated by CMRI.

MANAGEMENT

Most patients with moderate or less pulmonic stenosis are asymptomatic with survival similar to the general population.[31] Severe PS often requires intervention in infancy or childhood. Medical therapy is not specific and usually includes diuretics for right heart failure symptoms. Significant PS is treated with either percutaneous balloon valvuloplasty or surgical valvotomy.[32]

Surgical therapy is recommended in patients with a hypoplastic pulmonary annulus, severe PR, sub- or supravalvular stenosis, dysplastic valves associated with severe TR, or a coexisting need for a surgical Maze procedure. For patients with acquired PS secondary to carcinoid or rheumatic involvement, balloon valvuloplasty is generally not recommended because of the often concomitant presence of PR and involvement of other cardiac valves.[23]

Both pulmonic valvuloplasty and valvotomy can result in hemodynamically significant PR, requiring PV replacement. Consequently, close follow-up is warranted to evaluate symptoms, functional capacity, and hemodynamic consequences on RV size and function.

The 2018 American College of Cardiology (ACC)/American Heart Association (AHA) guidelines for management of pulmonic stenosis are summarized in Table 108.5.

Classification of recommendation and level of evidence expressed as listed in the ACC/AHA format as follows:

- Class I: Strength of recommendation is strong.
- Class IIa: Strength of recommendation is moderate.
- Level B-NR: moderate-quality evidence from one or more well-designed, well-executed nonrandomized studies, observational studies, and registry studies
- Level C-EO: consensus of expert opinion based on clinical experience

Please access ExpertConsult to view the corresponding videos for this chapter.

TABLE 108.5 American College of Cardiology/American Heart Association Congenital Heart Disease Guidelines for Management of Pulmonic Valve Stenosis[32]

Class of Recommendation	Level of Evidence	Recommendations
I	B-NR	In adults with moderate or severe valvular PS and otherwise unexplained symptoms of HF, cyanosis from interatrial right-to-left communication, and/or exercise intolerance, balloon valvuloplasty is recommended.
I	B-NR	In adults with moderate or severe valvular PS and otherwise unexplained symptoms of HF, cyanosis, and/or exercise intolerance who are ineligible for or who failed balloon valvuloplasty, surgical repair is recommended.
IIa	C-EO	In asymptomatic adults with severe valvular PS, intervention is reasonable.

B-NR, Moderate-quality evidence from one or more well-designed, well-executed nonrandomized studies, observational studies, and registry studies; *C-EO,* consensus of expert opinion based on clinical experience; *HF,* heart failure; *PS,* pulmonic stenosis.

REFERENCES

1. Waller BF, Howard J, Fess S. Pathology of tricuspid valve stenosis and pure tricuspid regurgitation—Part I. *Clin Cardiol.* 1995;18(2):97–102.
2. Kitchin A, Turner R. Diagnosis and treatment of tricuspid stenosis. *Br Heart J.* 1964;26:354–379.
3. Roberts WC, Ko JM. Some observations on mitral and aortic valve disease. *Proc - Bayl Univ Med Cent.* 2008;21(3):282–299.
4. Watkins DA, Beaton AZ, Carapetis JR, et al. Rheumatic heart disease worldwide: JACC scientific expert panel. *J Am Coll Cardiol.* 2018;72(12):1397–1416.
5. Anderson KR, Lie JT. Pathologic anatomy of Ebstein's anomaly of the heart revisited. *Am J Cardiol.* 1978;41(4):739–745.
6. Lundin L, Norheim I, Landelius J, et al. Carcinoid heart disease: relationship of circulating vasoactive substances to ultrasound-detectable cardiac abnormalities. *Circulation.* 1988;77(2):264–269.
7. Praz F, George I, Kodali S, et al. Transcatheter tricuspid valve-in-valve intervention for degenerative bioprosthetic tricuspid valve disease. *J Am Soc Echocardiogr.* 2018;31(4):491–504.
8. O'Gara PT, Loscalzo J. Tricuspid valve disease. In: Jameson JL, Fauci AS, Kasper DL, Hauser SL, Longo DL, Loscalzo J, eds. *Harrison's Principles of Internal Medicine.* New York: McGraw-Hill; 2018.
9. el-Sherif N. Rheumatic tricuspid stenosis. A haemodynamic correlation. *Br Heart J.* 1971;33(1):16–31.
10. Baumgartner H, Hung J, Bermejo J, et al. Echocardiographic assessment of valve stenosis: EAE/ASE recommendations for clinical practice. *Eur J Echocardiogr.* 2009;10(1):1–25.
11. Dahou A, Levin D, Reisman M, Hahn RT. Anatomy and physiology of the tricuspid valve. *JACC Cardiovasc Imag.* 2019;12(3):458–468.
12. Fawzy ME, Mercer EN, Dunn B, et al. Doppler echocardiography in the evaluation of tricuspid stenosis. *Eur Heart J.* 1989;10(11):985–990.
13. Quinones MA, Otto CM, Stoddard M, et al. Recommendations for quantification of Doppler echocardiography: a report from the Doppler Quantification Task Force of the Nomenclature and Standards Committee of the American Society of echocardiography. *J Am Soc Echocardiogr.* 2002;15(2):167–184.
14. Karp K, Teien D, Eriksson P. Doppler echocardiographic assessment of the valve area in patients with atrioventricular valve stenosis by application of the continuity equation. *J Intern Med.* 1989;225(4):261–266.
15. Zoghbi WA. Recommendations for evaluation of prosthetic valves with echocardiography and Doppler ultrasound. *J Am Soc Echocardiogr.* 2009;22(9):975–1014.
16. Blauwet LA, Danielson GK, Burkhart HM, et al. Comprehensive echocardiographic assessment of the hemodynamic parameters of 285 tricuspid valve bioprostheses early after implantation. *J Am Soc Echocardiogr.* 2010;23(10):1045–1059.
17. Nishimura RA, Otto CM, Bonow RO, et al. AHA/ACC guideline for the management of patients with valvular heart disease: a report of the American College of Cardiology/American Heart Association Task Force on practice guidelines. *Circulation.* 2014;129(23):2440–2492. 2014.
18. Baumgartner H, Falk V, Bax JJ, et al. ESC/EACTS guidelines for the management of valvular heart disease. *Eur Heart J.* 2017;38(36):2739–2791. 2017.
19. McElhinney DB, Cabalka AK, Aboulhosn JA, et al. Transcatheter tricuspid valve-in-valve implantation for the treatment of dysfunctional surgical bioprosthetic valves: an international, multicenter registry study. *Circulation.* 2016;133(16):1582–1593.
20. Margey R, Inglessis-Azuaje I. Percutaneous therapies in the treatment of valvular pulmonary stenosis. *Interv Cardiol Clin.* 2012;1(1):101–119.
21. Fathallah M, Krasuski RA. Pulmonic valve disease: review of pathology and current treatment options. *Curr Cardiol Rep.* 2017;19(11):108.
22. Ruckdeschel E, Kim YY. Pulmonary valve stenosis in the adult patient: pathophysiology, diagnosis and management. *Heart.* 2018;105:414–422.
23. Lin G, Bruce C, Connolly HM. Diseases of the tricuspid and pulmonic valves. In: Otto C, Bonow RO, eds. *Valvular Heart Disease: A Companion to Braunwald's Heart Disease.* St. Louis: Elsevier; 2013:375–395.
24. Waller BF, Howard J, Fess S. Pathology of pulmonic valve stenosis and pure regurgitation. *Clin Cardiol.* 1995;18(1):45–50.
25. Frantz EG, Silverman NH. Doppler ultrasound evaluation of valvar pulmonary stenosis from multiple transducer positions in children requiring pulmonary valvuloplasty. *Am J Cardiol.* 1988;61(10):844–849.
26. Heger JJ, Weyman AE. A review of M-mode and cross-sectional echocardiographic findings of the pulmonary valve. *J Clin Ultrasound.* 1979;7(2):98–107.
27. Aldousany AW, DiSessa TG, Dubois R, et al. Doppler estimation of pressure gradient in pulmonary stenosis: maximal instantaneous vs peak-to-peak, vs mean catheter gradient. *Pediatr Cardiol.* 1989;10(3):145–149.
28. Silvilairat S, Cabalka AK, Cetta F, et al. Outpatient echocardiographic assessment of complex pulmonary outflow stenosis: Doppler mean gradient is superior to the maximum instantaneous gradient. *J Am Soc Echocardiogr.* 2005;18(11):1143–1148.
29. Hahn RT, Abraham T, Adams MS, et al. Guidelines for performing a comprehensive transesophageal echocardiographic examination: recommendations from the American Society of Echocardiography and the Society of Cardiovascular Anesthesiologists. *J Am Soc Echocardiogr.* 2013;26(9):921–964.
30. Saremi F, Gera A, Ho SY, et al. CT and MR imaging of the pulmonary valve. *Radiographics.* 2014;34(1):51–71.
31. Hayes CJ, Gersony WM, Driscoll DJ, et al. Second natural history study of congenital heart defects. Results of treatment of patients with pulmonary valvar stenosis. *Circulation.* 1993;87(2 Suppl):I28–I137.
32. Stout KK, Daniels CJ, Aboulhosn JA, et al: 2018 AHA/ACC guideline for the management of adults with congenital heart disease: a report of the American College of Cardiology/American Heart Association Task Force on clinical practice guidelines, *J Am Coll Cardiol* 73(12):e81–e192, 2019.

109 Classification of Prosthetic Valve Types and Fluid Dynamics

Erwan Salaun, Marie-Annick Clavel, Philippe Pibarot

More than 300,000 patients per year require valve replacement in the world, and this number is estimated to triple to more than 850,000 by 2050.[1] The ideal valve substitute should mimic the characteristics of a normal native valve with excellent hemodynamics, long durability, high thromboresistance, and excellent implantability. Unfortunately, this ideal valve substitute does not exist, and each of the currently available prosthetic valves has inherent limitations. Despite the marked improvements in prosthetic valve designs and procedures over the past decades, valve replacement does not provide a definitive cure to the patient, and the patient's prognosis may be affected by prosthesis-related complications. However, many of these complications can be prevented or their impact minimized through optimal prosthesis selection in the individual patient and careful medical management and follow-up after implantation. In this regard, Doppler echocardiography is the method of choice for the evaluation and follow-up of prosthetic valve function. This evaluation follows the same basic principles used for the evaluation of native valves with some important particularities and caveats because of significant differences between the fluid dynamics of prosthetic valve and those of native valves.

DIFFERENT TYPES OF PROSTHETIC VALVES

Surgical valve replacement is the standard therapy for patients with severe nonrepairable mitral and tricuspid valvular heart disease as well as for patients with severe aortic valve disease. Among the surgical prosthetic valves, there are two main categories: the mechanical valves and the tissue valves. The stented bioprosthetic valves are by far the most frequently used tissue valves followed by stentless bioprostheses, homografts, and autografts (Fig. 109.1). During the past decade, there has been a dramatic shift toward the use of bioprosthetic valves rather than mechanical valves for surgical aortic valve replacement in the United States.[2] Furthermore, transcatheter aortic valve implantation (TAVI) has emerged as a valuable alternative to surgical valve replacement in patients with severe aortic stenosis (AS) and with high, intermediate, or low surgical risk.[3] In 2019, transcatheter bioprosthetic valves implantation in the aortic position worldwide was estimated at 144,000 and is expected to double by 2025.[4]

Surgical Prosthetic Valves

Mechanical Valves

The three basic types of mechanical valves are ball-cage, tilting-disk, and bileaflet valves (see Fig. 109.1). Given that there are major differences in the design of these three types of valves, their flow pattern and hemodynamics differ markedly (Fig. 109.2). Furthermore, all these types of mechanical valves have a normal regurgitant volume that includes a backflow related to the backward motion of the occluder(s) (i.e., the closing volume) and leakage backflow through the components of the prosthesis (leakage volume) (Fig. 109.3). This "built-in" regurgitation theoretically prevents blood stasis and thrombus formation by a washing effect. As opposed to the pathologic regurgitant jets, the normal regurgitant jets are characterized by being short in duration, narrow, and symmetrical.

Ball-Cage Valves

The only ball-cage valve that is still encountered nowadays in patients is the Starr-Edwards 1260, which consists of a silastic ball with a circular sewing ring and a cage formed by three metal arches located at 120-degree intervals around the sewing ring (see Fig. 109.1). Antegrade blood flows around the ball, and a large wake is generated in the central part (see Fig. 109.2). Large regions of flow separation are responsible for thrombogenicity of the valves and the obstruction to flow caused by the valve results in high pressure gradients. The normal regurgitant flow is composed mainly of the closing volume (2–6 mL per beat) that can be visualized on color-flow Doppler imaging[5] (see Fig. 109.3). This type of valve is no longer implanted, but owing to its relatively good durability, several thousands of patients still have ball-cage valves.

Monoleaflet Valves

Monoleaflet or tilting-disk valves use a single circular disk that rotates within a rigid annulus to occlude or open the valve orifice (see Fig. 109.1). The disk is secured by lateral or central metal struts. The opening angle of the disk relative to the valve annulus ranges from 60 to 80 degrees, resulting in two orifices of different size (see Fig. 109.3). The jet through the major orifice is semicircular in cross-section and flow through the minor orifice consists of one, two, or three jets. Depending on the number of struts, minor orifice jet velocities are 30% to 40% lower than those of major orifice (see Fig. 109.2). The nonperpendicular opening angle of the valve occluder tends to slightly increase the resistance to blood flow, particularly in the major orifices.

To minimize flow turbulence, the preferred orientation of monoleaflet valves in the aortic position is with the major orifice toward the right posterior aortic wall and in the mitral position is with the major orifice oriented toward the left ventricular free wall as opposed to the septum. Because of the eccentricity of the jet in the major orifice, it is also crucial to use multiwindow interrogation with continuous-wave (CW) Doppler to get the maximum transvalvular velocity. Normal regurgitant volume is low (5–9 mL per beat) and includes the closing volume as well leakage backflow through small gaps around the perimeter of the valve, and with the Medtronic Hall valves, there is a small amount of regurgitation around the central strut (see Fig. 109.3; Videos 109.1 and 109.2).

Mechanical Prostheses

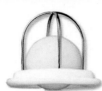

**Starr-Edwards
Ball-and-Cage**
(Edwards Lifesciences
Corp., Irvine, CA, USA)

**Medtronic-Hall
Tilting Disc**
(Medtronic, Inc.,
Minneapolis, MN, USA)

**St Jude
Bileaflet valve**
(St. Jude Medical,. Inc.,
St. Paul, MN, USA)

Human Tissue Valves

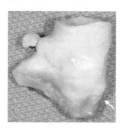

Aortic Homograft

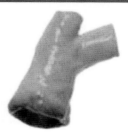

Pulmonary Autograft

Stented Bioprostheses

**Medtronic
Mosaic**
(Medtronic, Inc.,
Minneapolis, MN, USA)

**Carpentier-
Edwards Magna**
(Edwards Lifesciences
Corp., Irvine, CA, USA)

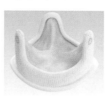

**Metronic
Hancock II**
(Medtronic, Inc.,
Minneapolis, MN, USA)

Sutureless Bioprostheses

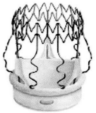

Perceval valve
(LivaNova, London, UK)

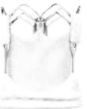

3f®-Enable valve
(Medtronic, Inc.,
Minneapolis, MN, USA)

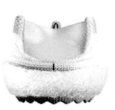

INTUITY valve
(Edwards Lifesciences
Corp., Irvine, CA, USA)

Stentless Bioprostheses

**Metronic
Freestyle**
(Medtronic, Inc.,
Minneapolis, MN, USA)

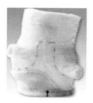

**Edwards Prima
Plus**
(Edwards Lifesciences
Corp., Irvine, CA, USA)

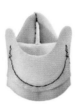

**Sorin Pericarbon
Freedom**
(Sorin Group, Saluggia,
Italy)

Transcatheter Bioprostheses

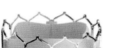
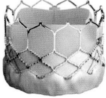

SAPIEN 3 valve
(Edwards Lifesciences
Corp., Irvine, CA, USA)

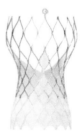

Evolut R
(Medtronic, Inc.,
Minneapolis, MN, USA)

New Generation of Surgical Bioprostheses

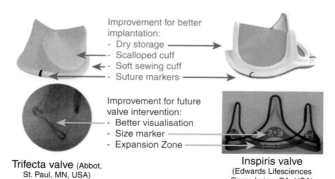

Improvement for better
implantation:
- Dry storage
- Scalloped cuff
- Soft sewing cuff
- Suture markers

Improvement for future
valve intervention:
- Better visualisation
- Size marker
- Expansion Zone

Trifecta valve (Abbot,
St. Paul, MN, USA)

Inspiris valve
(Edwards Lifesciences
Corp., Irvine, CA, USA)

Figure 109.1. Prosthetic valve types and design.

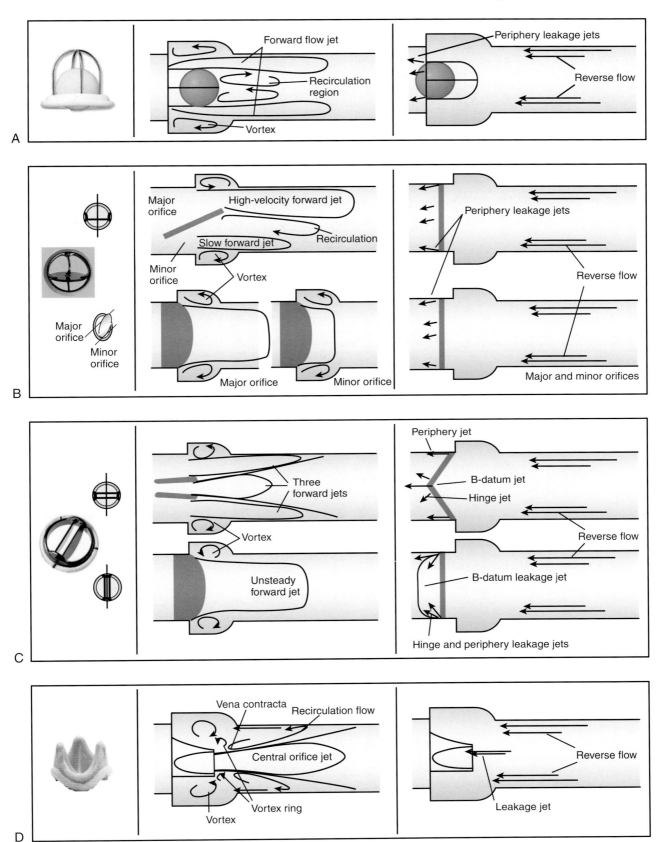

Figure 109.2. Flow patterns downstream of selected prosthetic valve designs during the forward flow phase *(left)* and the leakage flow phase *(right).* **A,** Ball-cage valve. **B,** Monoleaflet valve. **C,** Bileaflet valve. **D,** Stented bioprosthetic valve. (Adapted with permission from Dasi LP, Simon HA, Sucosky P, Yoganathan AP: Fluid mechanics of artificial heart valves, *Clin Exp Pharmacol Physiol* 36:225–237, 2009.)

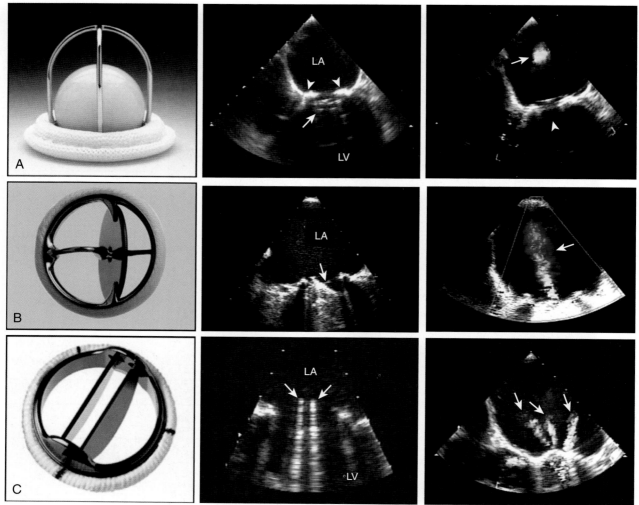

Figure 109.3. Examples of caged-ball (**A**), monoleaflet (**B**), and bileaflet (**C**) mechanical valves and stented (**D**), stentless (**E**), and transcatheter (**F**) bioprosthetic valves and their transesophageal echocardiographic characteristics taken in the mitral (**A, B, C, and D**) or aortic (**E** and **F**) positions in diastole *(middle)* and in systole *(right)*. For mechanical valves (**A, B,** and **C**), the *arrows* in diastole point to the occluder mechanism of the valve, and in systole to the characteristic physiologic regurgitation. In the transcatheter valve (**F**), the *arrow* shows a mild paravalvular aortic regurgitation. *LA,* Left atrium; *LV,* left ventricle.

Bileaflet Valves

These valves consist of two pyrolytic carbon semicircular leaflets attached to a rigid valve ring by small hinges (see Fig. 109.1). The opening angle of the leaflets relative to the annulus plane ranges from 75 to 90 degrees, with the open valve consisting of three orifices: a smaller, slitlike central orifice between the two open leaflets and two larger semicircular orifices laterally (see Figs. 109.2 and 109.3). The pattern of the antegrade transvalvular flow is thus characterized by three separate jets, and because the central orifice is smaller than the two lateral orifices, higher flow velocities may be recorded within the central orifice (see Figs. 109.2 and 109.3). For a given valve annulus size, the effective orifice areas (EOAs) are generally larger for the bileaflet mechanical valves than for the monoleaflet valves (Tables 109.1 and 109.2). Bileaflet valves typically have a small amount (5–10 mL per beat) of normal regurgitation. On Doppler color-flow imaging, two converging regurgitant jets originating from the pivot points of the valve disks and a smaller central jet are often seen. Smaller jets around the closure rim of the leaflets may also be appreciated (see Fig. 109.3; Videos 109.3 and 109.4). When implanted in the aortic position,

there is no clear advantage to a specific orientation of the leaflet opening plane relative to the aortic root. For the mitral position, it is suggested that an orientation perpendicular to the normal plane of mitral valve opening may be optimal. Available bileaflet valves include the St. Jude Medical and Carbomedics valves, the On-X and ATS valves.

TISSUE VALVES

Tissue valves include stentless or stented (porcine or bovine) bioprostheses made of porcine or bovine tissues, homografts from human cadaveric sources, and autografts of pericardial or pulmonary valve origin (see Fig. 109.1).

Stented Bioprostheses

The traditional design of a heterograft valve consists of three biologic leaflets made from the porcine aortic valve or bovine pericardium treated with glutaraldehyde to reduce its antigenicity (see Fig. 109.1). The leaflets are mounted on a metal or polymeric stented ring; they open to a circular orifice in systole, resembling the

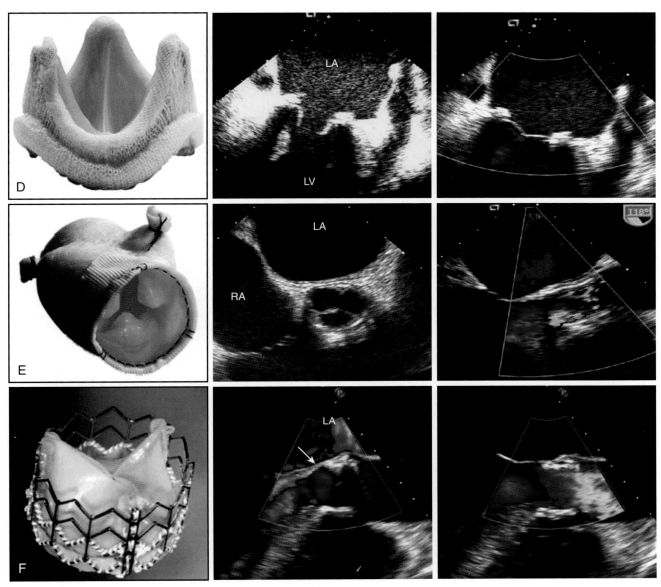

Figure 109.3, cont'd.

anatomy of the native aortic valve (see Figs. 109.2 and 109.3). The vast majority of bioprosthetic valves are treated with anticalcifying agents or processes. A circular central flow field with a relatively flat flow velocity profile characterizes the normal flow pattern in stented bioprostheses (Figs. 109.2 and 109.4). In vitro studies show that flow stagnation occurs on the outflow surfaces of the bioprosthetic leaflets during systole (see Fig. 109.2). Although bioprosthetic valves are considered to be relatively nonthrombogenic, flow turbulence and stagnation that are confined to the perimeter of flow stream may increase the likelihood of thromboembolic events.

For a given valve annulus size, the EOAs are generally smaller for the stented bioprostheses compared with the bileaflet mechanical valves (see Tables 109.1 and 109.2). However, the hemodynamic performance of stented bioprosthetic valves has improved substantially with the newer valve generations.

A small degree of central regurgitation (<1 mL) is also often observed in bioprosthetic valves and more frequently in bovine pericardial valves (see Fig. 109.2; Videos 109.5 and 109.6). The available stented bioprostheses include the Carpentier-Edwards Perimount, Magna, and S.A.V. valves and the Epic, Biocor, Hancock II, Mitroflow, Mosaic, and Trifecta bioprostheses.

Several new technologies are continuously being developed to improve implantation, the durability, and the management of stented bioprostheses. For example, the INSPIRIS valve combines a novel integrity preservation technology of the bovine pericardial tissue, allowing dry storage without requirement of rinse procedure as well as a VFit technology, which facilitates a future valve-in-valve therapy by the presence of size marker visible on fluoroscopy and expansible stent (see Fig. 109.1).

Stentless Bioprostheses

In an effort to improve valve hemodynamics and durability while retaining the advantages of a bioprosthetic valve, several types of stentless bioprosthetic valves have been developed. Stentless bioprostheses are manufactured from intact porcine aortic valves or from bovine pericardium (see Fig. 109.1). Stentless bioprosthetic valves have been used only in the aortic position, and they may be implanted in the subcoronary position as an inclusion cylinder, a miniroot, or a total root replacement with the most frequently used techniques being the subcoronary and the total root techniques. The advantage of a subcoronary implantation is to avoid the

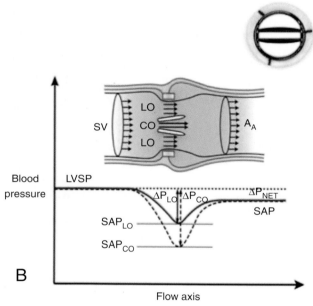

Figure 109.4. Schematic representation of velocity and pressure changes from the left ventricular outflow tract (LVOT) to the ascending aorta (A_A) in the presence of a stented bioprosthesis *(left)* and a bileaflet mechanical valve *(right)* illustrating the phenomena of pressure recovery and localized high gradient. Because of pressure recovery, velocities are lower, and systolic arterial pressure (SAP) is higher at the distal aorta than at the level of the vena contracta (VC). This phenomenon may occur in both bioprosthetic and mechanical valves (*solid dark red line* for blood pressure in **A** and **B**). Furthermore, in bileaflet mechanical valves, the velocity is locally higher in the central orifice (CO), and thus the pressure gradient (ΔP) is higher at that level. Doppler gradients are estimated from maximal velocity at the level of the vena contracta and represent the maximal pressure gradient, whereas invasive estimation of gradients usually reflect net pressure difference (ΔP_{NET}) between LV systolic pressure (LVSP) and ascending aorta. *LO,* Lateral orifice; *SV,* stroke volume in the LVOT. (Adapted with permission from Zoghbi WA, et al: Recommendations for evaluation of prosthetic valves with echocardiography and doppler ultrasound, *J Am Soc Echocardiogr* 22:975–1014, 2009.)

reimplantation of the coronary arteries, but on the other hand, there is a risk of central valvular insufficiency in the late postoperative course caused by the continued dilatation of the aortic root. The first-generation of stentless bioprostheses include the Medtronic Freestyle, the Toronto SPV, and the Prima-Edwards. New generations of stentless valves (Shelhigh Super Stentless aortic valve, Sorin Pericarbon Freedom valve) are easier to implant because they require only one layer of suture.

The echocardiographic appearance mimics a normal aortic valve with increased echogenicity in the annulus and the aortic root from the surgical procedure and the layer of fabric supporting the graft (Videos 109.7 and 109.8). The flow accelerates uniformly through the valve, and downstream the flow has a relatively flat profile (see Fig. 109.3). The EOAs are generally higher and gradients lower in stentless valves than in stented valves (see Table 109.1). The hemodynamic performance of the stentless valves often improve within the first 3 to 6 months of follow-up because of remodeling of the aortic root.

Sutureless Bioprostheses

The sutureless stent-mounted bioprosthetic valves are designed to replace a diseased native or malfunctioning prosthetic aortic valve via open heart surgery with sutureless positioning and anchoring at the implantation site (see Fig. 109.1; Videos 109.9 and 109.10). These valves can be implanted with minimally invasive cardiac surgery either through a partial sternotomy or right minithoracotomy. This type of valve allows substantial reduction of aortic cross-clamp time. The sutureless valves include the Perceval, the 3F Enable valve, and the Intuity.

Aortic Homografts

Aortic valve homografts are harvested from human cadavers within 24 hours of death as blocks of tissue comprising the ascending aorta, aortic valve, a portion of interventricular septum, and the anterior mitral valve leaflet (see Fig. 109.1). They are treated with antibiotics and cryopreserved at −196 degrees. They are now most commonly implanted in the form of a total root replacement with reimplantation of the coronary arteries. Homografts have excellent hemodynamics with antegrade velocities similar to those of a native valve. Regurgitation is rare with the root replacement technique. However, with subcoronary implantation, nearly 25% of patients develop moderate or severe aortic regurgitation by 2 years, and up to 5% require reoperation for significant aortic regurgitation. Long-term durability beyond 10 years is not superior to that of current-generation pericardial bioprostheses.

Pulmonary Autografts (Ross Procedure)

The native pulmonary valve is harvested as a small cylinder consisting of the pulmonary valve, annulus, and proximal main pulmonary artery (see Fig. 109.1). Autografts are most often implanted as complete root replacement with reimplantation of the coronaries. The pulmonary valve and right ventricular outflow tract are then replaced with a pulmonary homograft. Two separate valve interventions are required within the Ross procedure, meaning a longer cardiopulmonary bypass time and a steep learning curve. The hemodynamics of the pulmonary autografts are similar to those of a normal native aortic valve both at rest and with exercise.[6] However, the pulmonary homograft is subject to early degeneration and failure. Autografts have the ability to increase in size during childhood growth and are usually reserved for children and young adults. They are also nonthrombogenic and resistant to infections. However, the autograft may fail in some patients because of dilatation of the autograft and ensuing aortic regurgitation.

TABLE 109.1 Normal Reference Values of Effective Orifice Areas for the Prosthetic Aortic Valves

Surgical Prosthetic Valve Size (mm)	19	21	23	25	27	29
STENTED BIOPROSTHETIC VALVES						
Mosaic	1.1 ± 0.2	1.2 ± 0.3	1.4 ± 0.3	1.7 ± 0.4	1.8 ± 0.4	2.0 ± 0.4
Hancock II	—	1.2 ± 0.2	1.3 ± 0.2	1.5 ± 0.2	1.6 ± 0.2	1.6 ± 0.2
Carpentier-Edwards Perimount	1.1 ± 0.3	1.3 ± 0.4	1.5 ± 0.4	1.8 ± 0.4	2.1 ± 0.4	2.2 ± 0.4
Carpentier-Edwards Magna	1.3 ± 0.3	1.5 ± 0.3	1.8 ± 0.4	2.1 ± 0.5	—	—
Biocor (Epic)	1.0 ± 0.3	1.3 ± 0.5	1.4 ± 0.5	1.9 ± 0.7	—	—
Mitroflow	1.1 ± 0.2	1.2 ± 0.3 ·	1.4 ± 0.3	1.6 ± 0.3	1.8 ± 0.3	—
Trifecta[a]	1.41	1.63	1.8	2.02	2.20	2.35
STENTLESS BIOPROSTHETIC VALVES						
Medtronic Freestyle	1.2 ± 0.2	1.4 ± 0.2	1.5 ± 0.3	2.0 ± 0.4	2.3 ± 0.5	—
St. Jude Medical Toronto SPV	—	1.3 ± 0.3	1.5 ± 0.5	1.7 ± 0.8	2.1 ± 0.7	2.7 ± 1.0
Prima Edwards	—	1.3 ± 0.3	1.6 ± 0.3	1.9 ± 0.4	—	—
MECHANICAL VALVES						
Medtronic-Hall	1.2 ± 0.2	1.3 ± 0.2	—	—	—	—
St. Jude Medical Standard	1.0 ± 0.2	1.4 ± 0.2	1.5 ± 0.5	2.1 ± 0.4	2.7 ± 0.6	3.2 ± 0.3
St. Jude Medical Regent	1.6 ± 0.4	2.0 ± 0.7	2.2 ± 0.9	2.5 ± 0.9	3.6 ± 1.3	4.4 ± 0.6
MCRI On-X	1.5 ± 0.2	1.7 ± 0.4	2.0 ± 0.6	2.4 ± 0.8	3.2 ± 0.6	3.2 ± 0.6
Carbomedics Standard and Top Hat	1.0 ± 0.4	1.5 ± 0.3	1.7 ± 0.3	2.0 ± 0.4	2.5 ± 0.4	2.6 ± 0.4
ATS Medical[b]	1.1 ± 0.3	1.6 ± 0.4	1.8 ± 0.5	1.9 ± 0.3	2.3 ± 0.8	—

Transcatheter Prosthetic Valve Size (mm)	20	23	26	29	31	
SAPIEN	—	1.6 ± 0.4	1.8 ± 0.5	—	—	—
SAPIEN XT	—	1.4 ± 0.30	1.7 ± 0.4	2.1 ± 0.5	—	—
SAPIEN 3[a]	1.2 ± 0.2	1.5 ± 0.3	1.7 ± 0.4	1.9 ± 0.4	—	—
CoreValve	—	1.1 ± 0.4	1.7 ± 0.5	2.0 ± 0.5	2.2 ± 0.7	—
Evolut R[a]	—	1.10 ± 0.3	1.7 ± 0.4	2.0 ± 0.5	2.6 ± 0.8	—

[a]Effective orifice area is expressed as mean values available in the literature. Further studies are needed to validate these reference values, in particular for the newer models such as the Trifecta and the transcatheter SAPIEN 3 and CoreValve Evolut R valves.
[b]For the ATS medical valve, the label valve sizes are: 18, 20, 22, 24, and 26 mm.
These normal reference values of EOAs were obtained from Lancellotti P, et al: Recommendations for the imaging assessment of prosthetic heart valves, *Eur Heart J Cardiovasc Imag* 17:589–590, 2016; and Hahn RT, et al: Comprehensive echocardiographic assessment of normal transcatheter valve function, *JACC Cardiovasc Imag* 12:25–34, 2019.

TABLE 109.2 Normal Reference Values of Effective Orifice Areas for the Prosthetic Mitral Valves[a]

Prosthetic Valve Size (mm)	25	27	29	31	33
STENTED BIOPROSTHETIC VALVES					
Medtronic Mosaic	1.5 ± 0.4	1.7 ± 0.5	1.9 ± 0.5	1.9 ± 0.5	—
Hancock II	1.5 ± 0.4	1.8 ± 0.5	1.9 ± 0.5	2.6 ± 0.5	2.6 ± 0.7
Carpentier-Edwards Perimount	1.6 ± 0.4	1.8 ± 0.4	2.1 ± 0.5	—	—
MECHANICAL VALVES					
St. Jude Medical Standard	1.5 ± 0.3	1.7 ± 0.4	1.8 ± 0.4	2.0 ± 0.5	2.0 ± 0.5
MCRI On-X[b]	2.2 ± 0.9	2.2 ± 0.9	2.2 ± 0.9	2.2 ± 0.9	2.2 ± 0.9

[a]Effective orifice area is expressed as mean values available in the literature. Further studies are needed to validate these reference values.
[b]The ON-X valve has just 1 size for 27 to 29 and 31 to 33 mm prostheses. In addition, the strut and leaflets are identical for all sizes (25- to 33-mm); only the size of the sewing cuff is different.
The normal reference values of EOAs were obtained from Lancellotti P, et al: Recommendations for the imaging assessment of prosthetic heart valves, *Eur Heart J Cardiovasc Imag* 17:589–590, 2016; and Hahn RT, et al: Comprehensive echocardiographic assessment of normal transcatheter valve function, *JACC Cardiovasc Imag* 12:25–34, 2018.

TRANSCATHETER BIOPROSTHETIC VALVES

Initially, TAVI was performed in patients with symptomatic AS considered to be at high or prohibitive operative risk for surgical aortic valve replacement. Currently, TAVI is an alternative to surgery in patients with intermediate risk,[7] and randomized trials report noninferiority or superiority of transcatheter versus surgical aortic valve replacement in patients with low surgical risk.[8,9] Two main types of transcatheter aortic valves are currently used: balloon-expandable valves and self-expanding valves.

Balloon-Expandable Valves

The first two generations of the Edwards balloon-expandable valves comprised three leaflets fabricated with equine pericardium (Cribier-Edwards) or bovine pericardium (Edwards SAPIEN) mounted in a stainless-steel frame, available in two sizes (23 and 26 mm). The valves were implanted using 22- and 24-Fr delivery catheters. The third generation, named Edwards SAPIEN XT, introduced two new sizes, 20 and 29 mm, and required a reduced delivery system using 18-, 19-and 22-Fr delivery catheters. The

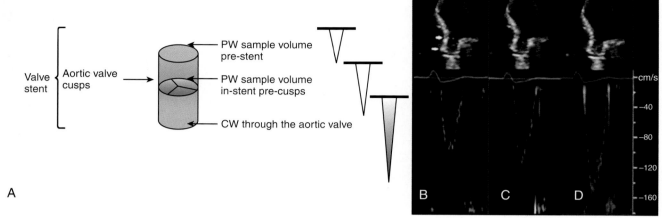

Figure 109.5. Flow velocity pattern in transcatheter valves. **A,** Schematic presentation of echocardiographic pulsed-wave (PW) Doppler patterns when the sample volume is placed prestent, in-stent but pre-cusps, and continuous wave (CW) through the aortic valve. **B,** The PW Doppler pattern of a sample volume placed before stent. *White arrows* show the extent of the transcatheter heart valve in the aortic root. *Red arrow* shows the level of the prosthetic aortic cusps. **C,** The PW Doppler pattern of sample volume placed within the stent but before cusps. **D,** The PW Doppler pattern of a sample volume placed at the level of the cusps. (Reproduced with permission from Bloomfield GS, et al: A practical guide to multimodality imaging of transcatheter aortic valve replacement, *JACC Cardiovasc Imag* 5:441–455, 2012.)

last iteration SAPIEN 3 valve is currently available in the four sizes (20, 23, 26, and 29 mm) and requires a smaller delivery system (14 Fr). SAPIEN 3 has also a polyethylene terephthalate outer skirt that functions as a blood-soaked sponge to reduce paravalvular regurgitation (see Fig. 109.1). The most often used approach nowadays is the transfemoral retrograde approach consisting of entering through the femoral artery and backtracking through the aorta to the aortic valve. An accurate evaluation of the iliofemoral anatomy by contrast-enhanced computed tomography helps to determine the appropriateness of the transfemoral approach for each patient. If the iliofemoral arteries are too small, diseased, or tortuous, a transapical, transaortic, transcarotid, or transcaval approach may be used. The transapical approach requires a small left lateral thoracotomy and a direct puncture of the left ventricular apex and thus leads to a greater degree of myocardial injury. The transcarotid vascular access is associated with clinical benefit compared with the more invasive transapical or transaortic strategies.

The normal EOAs of the SAPIEN valves are between 1.3 to 2.0 cm[2].[10–12] As opposed to surgical prostheses, the EOA of a given prosthesis size varies significantly depending on the size of patient's aortic annulus[12] (see Fig. 109.3). Several studies, including the randomized trial PARTNER-I Cohort A, have demonstrated that for a given aortic annulus size, first generations of balloon-expandable valves have larger EOAs and lower gradients compared with surgical bioprosthetic valves.[10,12] On the other hand, unlike surgical bioprosthetic valves, paravalvular regurgitation is common after TAVI (see Fig. 109.3). Mild to moderate regurgitation occurs in 30% to 80% of cases with 5% to 20% being moderate to severe with the first generations of Edwards SAPIEN valves (Video 109.11).[10,13,14] Moderate to severe paravalvular regurgitation is associated with a two- to threefold increase in mortality.[15] Paravalvular leak can also cause high blood shear stress and thereby damage to blood cells and coagulation factors, which could increase the risk of hemolysis, thromboembolic events, or bleeding.[16] The SAPIEN 3, which includes a skirt to reduce paravalvular regurgitation, harbors a markedly decreased rate of moderate or greater paravalvular regurgitation between 0% and 5%. However, SAPIEN 3 has somewhat higher aortic mean gradient and smaller EOAs compared with SAPIEN XT.

Self-Expanding Valves

The first generation of the CoreValve system consisted of a self-expanding nitinol frame with a bovine pericardial heart valve and was implanted using a 25-Fr delivery catheter. The second generation of the CoreValve system consisted of three leaflets of porcine pericardium seated higher in the nitinol frame to provide true supra-annular placement and is implanted using a 21-Fr delivery catheter. The next generation, named Evolut R, included a shorter stent and a sealing skirt to reduce paravalvular regurgitation, available in 23-, 26-, 29-, and 31-mm sizes and implanted using a 14-Fr delivery catheter (see Fig. 109.3). The last generation, named the Evolut Pro, includes an external pericardial wrap to further reduce paravalvular regurgitation. The CoreValve is mostly implanted using the transfemoral approach. However, the subclavian and transaxillary approaches can also be used if the transfemoral access is not feasible. Some studies suggest that the CoreValve has slightly larger EOAs and lower gradients compared with the SAPIEN valves but a higher incidence of paravalvular regurgitation.[17]

The flow pattern of transcatheter valves differs from that of surgical bioprostheses in the sense that there are two levels of flow acceleration at the inflow aspect of the valve: a first level when the flow enters the apical portion of the stent and a second level when the flow passes through the prosthetic valve leaflets (Fig. 109.5). For this reason, it is generally recommended to measure the left ventricular outflow tract (LVOT) diameter and velocity immediately proximal to the apical end of the stent when measuring the stroke volume and EOA of transcatheter valves.[18,19] However, if the stent sits low in the LVOT, which may occur more frequently with the self-expanding prostheses, it may be preferable to measure the LVOT diameter and velocity within the proximal portion of the stent below the bioprosthetic leaflets.

PRESSURE RECOVERY

Doppler echocardiography is the method of choice for the evaluation of prosthetic valve function. However, several studies have reported that Doppler may overestimate the gradient across native, mechanical, or bioprosthetic aortic valves compared with catheter measurements.[20,21] As blood flow velocity decelerates between the aortic valve and the ascending aorta, part of the kinetic energy

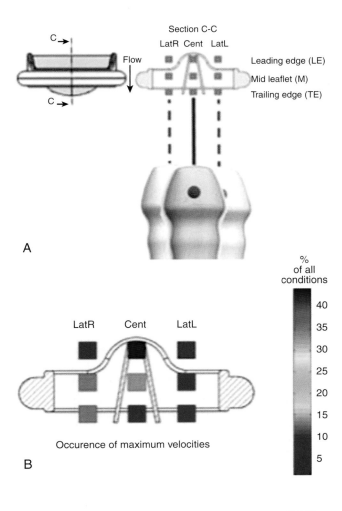

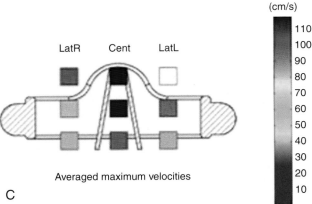

Figure 109.6. Location of maximum flow velocity in bileaflet mechanical valves. **A,** In this in vitro study, the flow velocity was measured by pulsed-wave Doppler at nine locations (three levels for each of the three orifices) **B,** The color scale represents the percentage of occurrence of maximum velocity at the different sample volume locations for the 81 test conditions. **C,** The color scale represents the averaged value of the maximum velocities recorded at each sampling volume location. *Cent,* Central orifice; *LatL,* lateral orifice located along the distal and left pulmonary veins; *LatR,* lateral orifice of the prosthesis located along the atrial septum and right pulmonary veins. (Reproduced with permission from Evin M, et al: Localized transvalvular pressure gradients in mitral bileaflet mechanical heart valves and impact on gradient overestimation by Doppler, *J Am Soc Echocardiogr* 26:791–800, 2013.)

is reconverted back to static energy (i.e., pressure) because of a phenomenon called pressure recovery, and hence the net gradient between the left ventricle and the ascending aorta (i.e., the gradient measured by catheter) is less than the maximum pressure gradient measured by Doppler at the level of the vena contracta (see Fig. 109.4).[21–25] The extent of pressure recovery is determined by the ratio between the valve EOA and the cross-sectional area of the downstream chamber (i.e., the ascending aorta in the case of native or prosthetic aortic valves). Hence, pressure recovery generally becomes clinically relevant in patients with smaller aortas (i.e., with an aorta diameter at the sinotubular junction $\leq$30 mm).[23,24] In these patients, it is thus appropriate to account for pressure recovery by using the simple formula proposed by Garcia and colleagues[22] to calculate the energy loss coefficient: ELC = (EOA $\times$ A_A/A_A − EOA), in which A_A is the cross-sectional area of the aorta measured at about 1 cm downstream of the sinotubular junction. The energy loss coefficient should be indexed for body surface area (i.e., energy loss index) to account for the change in cardiac output related to body size. An energy loss index less than 0.55 to 0.6 cm^2/m^2 is suggestive a significant prosthetic valve stenosis or patient–prosthesis mismatch (PPM; see later discussion).[22] Not accounting for pressure recovery in patients with small aortas (i.e., <30 mm) may cause overestimation of prosthetic valve stenosis or PPM by Doppler echocardiography and lead to unwarranted investigations or interventions. The pressure recovery is generally negligible in the case of mitral prostheses because the size of the downstream chamber (i.e., the left ventricle) is large relative to the EOA of the prosthesis.

LOCALIZED HIGH GRADIENT IN BILEAFLET MECHANICAL VALVES

Significant pressure recovery, which may occur downstream of aortic valves regardless of their type (i.e., native, bioprosthetic, or mechanical), should not be mistaken with the phenomenon of localized high gradient that is specific of bileaflet mechanical valves[26] (Figs. 109.4 and 109.6). A localized high gradient may indeed be recorded through the central orifice of bileaflet mechanical valves, and this phenomenon may yield to overestimation of gradient and underestimation of EOA regardless of the position (aortic or mitral) of the prosthesis. Because the central orifice is smaller than the lateral orifices, the blood flow velocity may be locally higher within the inflow aspect of the central orifice, and CW Doppler may record this high velocity[26] (see Figs. 109.4 and 109.6). The prevalence, magnitude, and predictors of this phenomenon are not fully understood but are probably related to prosthetic valve size and design (ratio of the size of the central orifice to that of lateral orifices) and flow conditions.[25,27] Also, given that the localized high-velocity region is very small and located at the inflow of the central orifice (see Fig. 109.6), the recording of this velocity is highly inconsistent and may vary from one patient to the other and even from one visit to another in a given patient, depending on the direction and angulation of the Doppler beam.[26]

PROSTHESIS–PATIENT MISMATCH

PPM occurs when the EOA of a normally functioning prosthesis is too small in relation to the patient's body size (and thus cardiac output requirements), resulting in abnormally high postoperative gradients. Hence, PPM is not an intrinsic prosthesis dysfunction per se. The most widely accepted and validated parameter for identifying PPM is the indexed EOA, that is, the EOA of the prosthesis divided by the patient's body surface area.[28–32] The use of the body surface area for the normalization of EOA may overestimate the prevalence and severity of PPM in obese patients. For this reason, it has been suggested to use lower cut-off values of indexed EOA to define PPM in patients with a body mass index 30 kg/m^2 or greater. Table 109.3 shows the cut-off values of indexed EOA generally used to

TABLE 109.3 Criteria of Indexed Prosthetic Valve Effective Orifice Area (EOA) for the Identification and Quantitation of Prosthesis–Patient Mismatch (PPM)[a]

	Indexed EOA, cm²/m²		
	Not Clinically Significant or Mild PPM	Moderate PPM	Severe PPM
Aortic position	>0.85 (0.8–0.9) >0.70[b]	≤0.85 (0.8–0.9) ≤0.70[b]	≤0.65 (0.6–0.7) ≤0.55[b]
Mitral position	>1.2 (1.2–1.3) >1.0[b]	≤1.2 (1.2–1.3) ≤1.0[b]	≤0.9 (0.9) ≤0.80

[a]Numbers in parentheses represent the range of threshold values that have been used in the literature.
[b]Cut-off values for patients with body mass index ≥30 kg/m².

identify PPM and quantify its severity. Moderate PPM may be quite frequent both in the aortic (20%–70%) and mitral (30%–70%) positions, whereas the prevalence of severe PPM ranges from 2% to 10% in both positions.[30,31] PPM is associated with worse hemodynamics, less regression of left ventricular hypertrophy and pulmonary hypertension, worse functional class, worse exercise capacity, worse quality of life, more cardiac events, higher risk of structural valve deterioration, and lower survival.[31] PPM can largely be prevented by using a prospective strategy at the time of operation consisting in systematically calculating the "projected" indexed EOA of the prosthesis to be inserted (projected indexed EOA is derived from the normal reference values of EOA provided in the literature for the different types and sizes of prostheses) (see Tables 109.1 and 109.2) and in the case of anticipated PPM, to consider alternate procedures such as insertion of a better performing valve substitute (e.g., newer generation of supraannular bioprostheses or mechanical valves, stentless bioprostheses, homografts, or transcatheter valves) or insertion of a larger prosthesis by means of aortic root enlargement. The prevention of PPM in the mitral position represents a much greater challenge than in the aortic position. Indeed, mitral valve surgery does not allow annular enlargement, and the implantation of a homograft or a stentless prosthesis is technically more demanding and associated with poor long-term durability. Hence, the only alternative at present is the implantation of a prosthesis having a larger EOA for a given annulus size, which unfortunately may not be sufficient to completely avoid PPM in some cases.

CONCLUSION

Several prosthetic valve designs are currently available for valve replacement procedures, and many new models will be introduced in the future owing to the rapidly growing expansion of transcatheter valve therapy. Optimal Doppler echocardiographic evaluation of prosthesis structure and function requires a good knowledge of the specifics of each type of prosthesis in terms of valve design, implantation technique, and fluid dynamics.

Please access ExpertConsult to view the corresponding videos for this chapter.

Acknowledgments

The authors thank Drs. Jean G. Dumesnil and Haifa Mahjoub for their contributions to this chapter in the previous edition.

REFERENCES

1. Yacoub MH, Takkenberg JJ. Will heart valve tissue engineering change the world? *Nat Clin Pract Cardiovasc Med.* 2005;2:60–61.
2. Brown JM, O'Brien SM, Wu C, et al. Isolated aortic valve replacement in North America comprising 108,687 patients in 10 years: changes in risks, valve types, and outcomes in the Society of Thoracic Surgeons National Database. *J Thorac Cardiovasc Surg.* 2009;137:82–90.
3. Kodali SK, Williams MR, Smith CR, et al. Two-year outcomes after transcatheter or surgical aortic-valve replacement. *N Engl J Med.* 2012;366:1686–1695.
4. Cesna S, De Backer O, Sondergaard L. Rapid adoption of transcatheter aortic valve replacement in intermediate- and high-risk patients to treat severe aortic valve stenosis. *J Thorac Dis.* 2017;9:1432–1436.
5. Yoganathan AP, Reamer HH, Corcoran WH, et al. The Starr-Edwards aortic ball valve: flow characteristics, thrombus formation, and tissue overgrowth. *Artif Organs.* 1981;5:6–17.
6. Pibarot P, Dumesnil JG, Briand M, et al. Hemodynamic performance during maximum exercise in adult patients with the ross operation and comparison with normal controls and patients with aortic bioprostheses. *Am J Cardiol.* 2000;86:982–988.
7. Nishimura RA, Otto CM, Bonow RO, et al. AHA/ACC focused update of the 2014 AHA/ACC guideline for the management of patients with valvular heart disease. *J Am Coll Cardiol 0.* 2017:252–289.
8. Mack MJ, Leon MB, Thourani VH, et al. Transcatheter aortic-valve replacement with a balloon-expandable valve in low-risk patients. *N Engl J Med.* 2019;380:1695–1705.
9. Popma JJ, Deeb GM, Yakubov SJ, et al. Transcatheter aortic-valve replacement with a self-expanding valve in low-risk patients. *N Engl J Med.* 2019;380:1706–1715.
10. Clavel MA, Webb JG, Pibarot P, et al. Comparison of the hemodynamic performance of percutaneous and surgical bioprostheses for the treatment of severe aortic stenosis. *J Am Coll Cardiol.* 2009;53:1883–1891.
11. Webb JG, Pasupati S, Humphries K, et al. Percutaneous transarterial aortic valve replacement in selected high-risk patients with aortic stenosis. *Circulation.* 2007;116:755–763.
12. Hahn RT, Pibarot P, Stewart WJ, et al. Comparison of transcatheter and surgical aortic valve replacement in severe aortic stenosis: a longitudinal study of echo parameters in cohort a of the PARTNER Trial. *J Am Coll Cardiol.* 2013;61:2514–2521.
13. Vahanian A, Alfieri O, Al-Attar N, et al. Transcatheter valve implantation for patients with aortic stenosis. *Eur Heart J.* 2008;29:1463–1470.
14. Leon MB, Smith CR, Mack M, et al. Transcatheter aortic-valve implantation for aortic stenosis in patients who cannot undergo surgery. *N Engl J Med.* 2010;363:1597–1607.
15. Athappan G, Patvardhan E, Tuzcu EM, et al. Incidence, predictors, and outcomes of aortic regurgitation after transcatheter aortic valve replacement: meta-analysis and systematic review of literature. *J Am Coll Cardiol.* 2013;61:1585–1595.
16. Grube E, Buellesfeld L, Mueller R, et al. Progress and current status of percutaneous aortic valve replacement: results of three device generations of the CoreValve Revalving system. *Circulation Cardiovasc Interv.* 2008;1:167–175.
17. Nombela-Franco L, Ruel M, Radhakrishnan S, et al. Comparison of hemodynamic performance of self-expanding CoreValve versus balloon-expandable Edwards SAPIEN aortic valves inserted by catheter for aortic stenosis. *Am J Cardiol.* 2013;111:1026–1033.
18. Bloomfield GS, Gillam LD, Hahn RT, et al. A practical guide to multimodality imaging of transcatheter aortic valve replacement. *JACC Cardiovasc Imag.* 2012;5:441–455.
19. Clavel MA, Rodes-Cabau J, Dumont E, et al. Validation and characterization of transcatheter aortic valve effective orifice area measured by Doppler echocardiography. *JACC Cardiovasc Imag.* 2011;4:1053–1062.
20. Baumgartner H, Schima H, Kuhn P. Discrepancies between Doppler and catheter gradients across bileaflet aortic valve prostheses. *Am J Cardiol.* 1993;71:1241–1243.
21. Aljassim O, Svensson G, Houltz E, Bech-Hanssen O. Doppler-catheter discrepancies in patients with bileaflet mechanical prostheses or bioprostheses in the aortic valve position. *Am J Cardiol.* 2008;102:1383–1389.
22. Garcia D, Pibarot P, Dumesnil JG, et al. Assessment of aortic valve stenosis severity: a new index based on the energy loss concept. *Circulation.* 2000;101:765–771.
23. Baumgartner H, Stefenelli T, Niederberger J, et al. "Overestimation" of catheter gradients by Doppler ultrasound in patients with aortic stenosis: a predictable manifestation of pressure recovery. *J Am Coll Cardiol.* 1999;33:1655–1661.
24. Garcia D, Dumesnil JG, Durand LG, et al. Discrepancies between catheter and Doppler estimates of valve effective orifice area can be predicted from the pressure recovery phenomenon: practical implications with regard to quantification of aortic stenosis severity. *J Am Coll Cardiol.* 2003;41:435–442.
25. Bech-Hanssen O, Caidahl K, Wallentin I, et al. Aortic prosthetic valve design and size: relation to Doppler echocardiographic findings and pressure recovery—an in vitro study. *J Am Soc Echocardiogr.* 2000;13:39–50.
26. Evin M, Pibarot P, Guivier-Curien C, et al. Localized transvalvular pressure gradients in mitral bileaflet mechanical heart valves and impact on gradient overestimation by Doppler. *J Am Soc Echocardiogr.* 2013;26:791–800.
27. Pibarot P, Dumesnil JG. Prosthetic heart valves: selection of the optimal prosthesis and long-term management. *Circulation.* 2009;119:1034–1048.
28. Dumesnil JG, Honos GN, Lemieux M, Beauchemin J. Validation and applications of indexed aortic prosthetic valve areas calculated by Doppler echocardiography. *J Am Coll Cardiol.* 1990;16:637–643.
29. Dumesnil JG, Honos GN, Lemieux M, Beauchemin J. Validation and applications of mitral prosthetic valvular areas calculated by Doppler echocardiography. *Am J Cardiol.* 1990;65:1443–1448.
30. Pibarot P, Dumesnil JG. Hemodynamic and clinical impact of prosthesis-patient mismatch in the aortic valve position and its prevention. *J Am Coll Cardiol.* 2000;36:1131–1141.
31. Pibarot P, Dumesnil JG. Prosthesis-patient mismatch: Definition, clinical impact, and prevention. *Heart.* 2006;92:1022–1029.
32. Rahimtoola SH. The problem of valve prosthesis-patient mismatch. *Circulation.* 1978;58:20–24.

110 Aortic Prosthetic Valves

Aaron C.W. Lin, Darryl J. Burstow

Transthoracic echocardiography (TTE) is established as the reference imaging modality for the routine evaluation of prosthetic valves because of the comprehensive anatomic, functional, and hemodynamic data obtained combined with its excellent safety profile. However, the unique acoustic properties of prosthetic valves can impair the echocardiographic examination, resulting in reduced diagnostic accuracy. To reduce errors in interpretation, an understanding of the distinctive structural and hemodynamic features of prosthetic valves is required combined with a standardized TTE examination protocol that includes integration of all data obtained from two-dimensional (2D), spectral, and color-flow Doppler modalities. In addition, knowledge of the limitations of TTE will enable the appropriate selection of cases in which additional imaging procedures, such as transesophageal echocardiography (TEE) and cine-fluoroscopy (CF), may be required.

STANDARD TRANSTHORACIC ECHOCARDIOGRAPHY ASSESSMENT OF AORTIC PROSTHETIC VALVE FUNCTION

Two-Dimensional Imaging

Before imaging, the type and size of the prosthetic valve should be established. The appearance and motion of the leaflets or occluder can then be assessed. Careful attention to specific imaging planes will reduce the problems caused by acoustic shadowing and improve diagnostic yield. If the ultrasound beam can be orientated parallel to the direction of occluder opening, acoustic shadowing across the plane of the valve is reduced with resultant improvement in visualization of occluder motion. This is particularly relevant in the assessment of aortic prostheses in which the apical five-chamber view can provide an improved view of the leaflets or occluder (Video 110.1).

Doppler Parameters Used to Assess Aortic Prosthetic Valve Function

All prosthetic valve designs cause variable degrees of obstruction to flow, resulting in measurable gradients. Doppler assessment allows the noninvasive measurement of flow velocities across prosthetic valves from which gradients are calculated. As with native aortic valve stenosis, Doppler interrogation of the aortic prosthesis should be performed from multiple acoustic windows to ensure the highest peak velocity and derived gradients have been obtained. Importantly, valve gradients are determined by both volumetric flow and the prosthetic valve area. Thus, in addition to valve gradients, the derivation of flow-independent parameters of prosthetic valve function such as effective orifice area (EOA) and dimensionless velocity index (DVI) is essential (Box 110.1).

Dimensionless Velocity Index

The DVI is a useful flow independent parameter of aortic prosthetic valve function that is easily derived (V_1/V_2) and does not require the measurement of a dimension such as the left ventricular outflow tract diameter (LVOTd), which can be technically difficult. In an individual patient, a baseline DVI value obtained in the early postoperative period can serve as the control value or "valve fingerprint" for future examinations. Providing prosthetic valve function remains normal, the DVI will remain constant even with changes in stroke volume.

Effective Orifice Area and Indexed Effective Orifice Area

The calculation of EOA using the continuity equation is shown in Box 110.1. It is important to follow correct methodology in measuring both LVOT parameters because inaccuracy in these measurements, particularly LVOTd, which is squared, will result in significant errors in the EOA calculation. The guiding principle is that both parameters are derived from the same anatomic location. As per American Society of Echocardiography (ASE) guidelines,[1] the cross-sectional area (CSA) is derived from the LVOTd measured just underneath the prosthesis from the parasternal long-axis view with care taken to measure to the outer margins of the valve sewing ring. The LVOT velocity time integral (VTI) is obtained by locating the pulsed-wave (PW) Doppler sample volume adjacent to the prosthesis while avoiding the region of subvalvular flow acceleration (this usually requires a position of 0.5–1 cm below the sewing ring). In a normally functioning prosthesis, the EOA obtained should fall in the normal reference range for that prosthetic valve subtype and size (Fig. 110.1 and Video 110.1D). The indexed EOA (IEOA) references the absolute EOA to patient body surface area (BSA) and is used to define and identify prosthesis–patient mismatch (PPM).

Measurement of Effective Orifice Area After Transcatheter Aortic Valve Replacement

Compared with surgically implanted prostheses, transcatheter aortic valve replacement (TAVR) valve designs have longer

---

BOX 110.1 Measured and Derived Parameters Used When Assessing Aortic Valve Replacement (AVR) Function

AVR VELOCITY (CW DOPPLER)

- Peak velocity (V_2) cm/s
- Maximum gradient ($4V_2^2$) mm Hg
- Mean gradient mm Hg
- AVR VTI cm
- AT/ET (AT ms, ET ms)

LVOT VELOCITY (PW DOPPLER)

- Peak velocity (V_1) cm/s
- LVOT VTI cm
- LVOTd cm

DVI = $V_1 \div V_2$

EOA (cm²) = (LVOT VTI × (LVOTd² × 0.785)/AVR VTI)

    = (LVOT VTI × LVOT CSA/AVR VTI)

AT, Acceleration time; *CSA*, cross-sectional area; *CW*, continuous-wave; *DVI*, Doppler velocity index; *EOA*, effective orifice area; *ET*, ejection time; *LVOT*, left ventricular outflow tract; *LVOTd*, left ventricular outflow tract diameter; *PW*, pulsed-wave; *VTI*, velocity time integral.

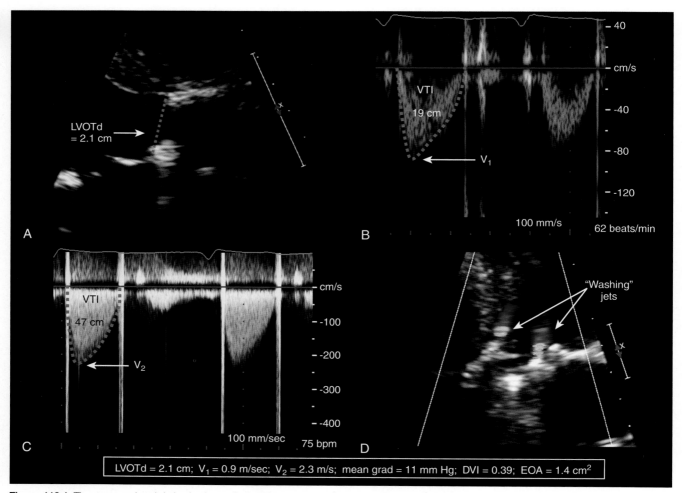

LVOTd = 2.1 cm; V_1 = 0.9 m/sec; V_2 = 2.3 m/s; mean grad = 11 mm Hg; DVI = 0.39; EOA = 1.4 cm²

Figure 110.1. The measured and derived echocardiographic parameters used to routinely assess aortic prosthetic valve function are illustrated in this case (21-mm St. Jude prosthesis). **A,** Left ventricular outflow tract diameter (LVOTd). **B,** LVOT peak velocity (V_1) and velocity time integral (VTI). **C,** Peak velocity (V_2) and VTI. **D,** Normal trivial transvalvular regurgitation ('washing jets'). All parameters (boxed area) are within the normal ranges for this valve and consistent with normal valvular function. (See accompanying Video 110.1D.) Doppler velocity index (DVI).

valve stents that project lower into the LVOT. This has resulted in revised recommendations for the measurement of LVOTd and LVOT VTI in these valves. Flow acceleration within the TAVR stent and proximal to the valve leaflets can cause erroneously elevated LVOT velocity and VTI measurements. Consequently, the derived valve area will be overestimated when using the continuity equation.[2] Thus, the European Association of Echocardiography (EAE)/ASE recommend that the LVOT velocity be measured prestent in the LVOT.[3] Consistent with the guiding principle that both parameters are derived from the same anatomic location, the LVOT diameter measurement should also be performed prestent.[4,5] The only exception to this is when the TAVR is implanted very low within the LVOT, preventing accurate measurement of the prestent diameter. In this case, the measurements should be made precusp within the stent.[6] It is important to apply this methodology consistently to obtain both accurate baseline valve hemodynamics and interpretable serial assessments. It is our practice to document the prestent LVOT methodology in the report and use the baseline prestent LVOTd in future studies. Also, if a prestent LVOTd has been obtained by TEE immediately after TAVR implantation, this value will be used as the default LVOTd value because of the superior resolution of TEE. It is also important to remember that TAVR implant

size correlates poorly with the LVOTd derived by 2D echocardiography and thus cannot be used as a substitute for the LVOTd.

Normal Doppler Values

After completion of the Doppler examination, reference should be made to the normal Doppler data available for the particular prosthetic valve subtype and size. A large amount of data[7] exist documenting the normal values for Doppler parameters of prosthetic valve function in surgically implanted prostheses. There are now more recent data available for balloon-expandable and self-expanding TAVR valves[8,9] documenting mean gradient, EOA, and DVI according to valve type and size.

DIAGNOSIS OF AORTIC PROSTHETIC VALVE DYSFUNCTION

Interpretation of Elevated Valve Gradients

The initial suspicion of prosthetic valve dysfunction is often raised by the detection of abnormally high prosthetic valve gradients during routine TTE assessment. The potential causes to be considered are (1) prosthetic valve obstruction, (2) PPM, (3) the phenomenon

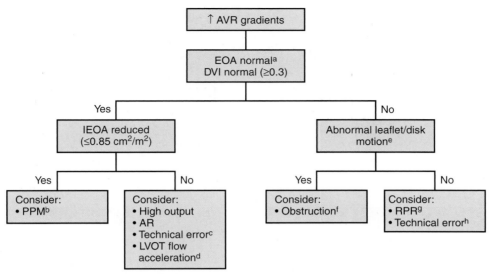

Figure 110.2. Algorithm for interpreting elevated prosthetic valve gradients after aortic valve replacement (AVR). [a]Normal values for valve subtype and size. [b]Indexed effective orifice area (IEOA) and Doppler velocity index (DVI) are typically unchanged compared with baseline study. [c]Consider overestimation of left ventricular outflow tract (LVOT) diameter, LVOT velocity time integral (VTI), or both. [d]Recalculate effective orifice area (EOA) using right ventricular outflow tract stroke volume. [e]If leaflet or disk motion is unclear by transthoracic echocardiography, consider cine fluoroscopy. [f]Consider significant prosthetic valve obstruction when aortic valve replacement (AVR) signal has a rounded velocity contour of AVR signal that peaks in midsystole, acceleration time (AT) is prolonged (>100 ms), and the ratio of AT to left ventricular ejection time is greater than 0.37. [g]Bileaflet valves only, small AVR size (19–21 mm). [h]Consider underestimation of LVOT diameter, LVOT VTI, or both. *AR,* Aortic regurgitation; *PPM,* prosthesis-patient mismatch; *RPR,* rapid pressure recovery. (Reproduced with permission from Anderson B: *A Sonographer's Guide to the Assessment of Heart Disease.* MGA Graphics Brisbane, Australia; 2014:311.)

of rapid pressure recovery (RPR), (4) significant aortic regurgitation (AR), and (5) high flow states (e.g., postsurgery, anemia, and sepsis). In PPM, AR, and high flow states, gradients are increased because of increased antegrade flow across the prosthesis. This emphasizes the value of the flow-independent parameters (EOA and DVI) for the interpretation of elevated gradients. By using these parameters in conjunction with an anatomical assessment of leaflet or occluder motion, an accurate diagnosis should be obtainable in most instances. A diagnostic algorithm for the interpretation of abnormally elevated gradients across aortic prostheses is presented in Fig. 110.2.

Prosthetic Valve Obstruction

In mechanical valves, the usual causes of valve obstruction are (1) thrombosis or (2) ingrowth of fibrous tissue called pannus below the inflow orifice of the valve restricting occluder motion. In bioprosthetic valves, structural valve degeneration is the usual cause. However, bioprosthetic valve thrombosis is an increasingly recognized complication in both surgically implanted valves[10–12] and TAVR valves.[13] Thus, cases of prosthetic valve obstruction will usually be associated with abnormal leaflet morphology or occluder mobility. TTE has major limitations in assessing the occluder and surrounding structures in mechanical valves because of a greater degree of reverberation artefact and acoustic shadowing caused by these devices. TAVR leaflets can also be more difficult to visualize than surgical bioprostheses because of the larger acoustic shadowing produced by the TAVR stents. This often necessitates supplementary imaging of the occluder or leaflets as will be discussed further later in this chapter. On Doppler examination, the hemodynamic diagnosis of aortic valve obstruction is suggested by (1) increased gradients for valve subtype and size, (2) decreased EOA and DVI below the normal reference range, and (3) significant deviation of EOA or DVI from the baseline study (Fig. 110.3 and Video 110.3C and F). Although individual EOA and DVI values

should always be referenced against normal values for the valve subtype and size, an EOA smaller than 0.8 cm^2 and a DVI less than 0.25[1,14] will almost always be abnormal and are useful numbers to memorize.

Prosthesis–Patient Mismatch

The most common cause of elevated aortic prosthetic valve gradients is said to be PPM.[15] These patients have a normal prosthetic valve, but the valve is too small for the patient. There are high absolute levels of flow across the valve generating high gradients. PPM is defined best by the IEOA, and this parameter has been shown to be predictive of abnormally elevated postoperative gradients and inferior clinical outcomes.[16] A value of 0.85 cm^2/m^2 or less is considered the threshold value for the presence of PPM with severe mismatch defined as an IEOA less than 0.65 cm^2/m^2. Therefore, PPM should be suspected if abnormally elevated Doppler gradients are obtained despite (1) no detectable structural abnormality of the prosthetic valve leaflets or occluders, (2) normal values for EOA and DVI for valve subtype and size, and (3) IEOA in the mismatch range. Typically, the prosthesis will be of small size and the patients of older age and with larger BSA.

Rapid Pressure Recovery

RPR is a phenomenon associated with bileaflet prosthetic valves, in which high Doppler gradients are recorded despite a normally functioning valve. The bileaflet design is characterized by localized high velocities within the divergent central orifice. In addition, there is RPR within the aorta immediately distal to the prosthetic valve, which may be further exaggerated if the aorta is of small diameter. This can result in high recorded Doppler gradients (typically in the small 19- and 21-mm sizes), which are significantly higher than those recorded by conventional cardiac

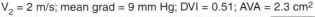

$V_2 = 2$ m/s; mean grad = 9 mm Hg; DVI = 0.51; AVA = 2.3 cm^2

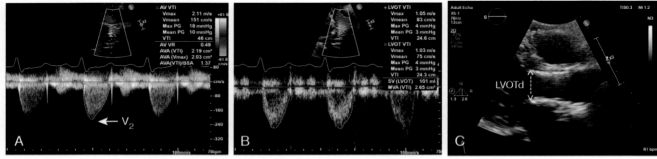

$V_2 = 3.2$ m/s; mean grad = 26 mm Hg; DVI = 0.22; AVA = 1.0 cm^2

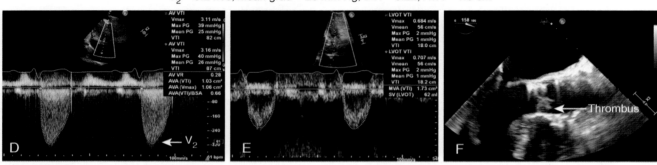

Figure 110.3. Measured and derived echocardiographic parameters in transcatheter aortic valve replacement (TAVR) are illustrated in this case (26-mm Edwards SAPIEN TAVR). **A** and **B,** Baseline TAVR and left ventricular outflow tract (LVOT) velocities with peak velocity (V$_2$), mean gradient (grad), dimensionless velocity index (DVI), and aortic valve area (AVA) within the normal range for this valve and consistent with normal valvular function. **C,** The recommended methodology for measurement of left ventricular outflow tract diameter (LVOTd) after TAVR; outer edge to outer edge prestent. **D** and **E,** TAVR and LVOT velocities 6 weeks after implant with elevated TAVR gradients associated with reduced DVI and AVA consistent with significant TAVR obstruction. **F,** Thrombus attached to the aortic aspect of the right coronary cusp on transesophageal echocardiogram confirming the cause of obstruction. (See accompanying Videos 110.3C and F.)

catheterization techniques. Therefore, RPR should be suspected in patients with small bileaflet prostheses who have (1) reduced EOA, IEOA, and DVI for valve subtype and size and (2) normal occluder motion.

Acceleration Time and Ejection Time

In patients with prosthetic valve obstruction, the acceleration time (AT, the time from the beginning of ejection to the prosthetic valve peak velocity) is prolonged and usually >100 ms with the ratio of AT to ejection time usually greater than 0.37.[17] This provides an additional assessment of prosthetic valve function in patients with elevated gradients and is particularly useful if flow independent parameters such as DVI have intermediate values between 0.25 and 0.29. Conversely, patients with high gradients and AT less than 100 ms are more likely to have high flow states or PPM.

AORTIC PROSTHETIC VALVE REGURGITATION
Physiologic or "Normal" Regurgitation

Most mechanical prostheses have mild valvular regurgitation that is "normal" and must be recognized and differentiated from pathological leaks. The commonest form is so called "leakage volume" in which regurgitation occurs through the gaps adjacent to the closed occluder. These jets are also termed "washing jets" because they are thought to prevent blood stasis and secondary thrombus formation and are typically transvalvular,

multiple, short in length, and of low turbulence (see Fig 110.1D). Mild central AR can also be seen in normally functioning bioprosthetic aortic valves.

Pathologic Regurgitation

Evaluation of aortic prosthetic valve regurgitation follows the general principles used for native valve regurgitation[1,18](i.e., an integrative approach using a number of semiquantitative and quantitative measurements). TTE usually provides adequate assessment of the severity of aortic prosthetic valve regurgitation using these standard parameters. The origin of regurgitation (valvular versus paravalvular) is routinely assessed in the parasternal short-axis view in which the full circumference of the annulus can be visualized. However, in an effort to avoid the acoustic shadow of the prosthesis, it is also important to interrogate the prosthesis from multiple acoustic windows, particularly the apical five-chamber and subcostal views in which the regurgitant jets may be more parallel to the ultrasound beam. The length of the jet is an unreliable indicator of severity and the proximal jet width or CSA of the jet beneath the prosthesis (within the LVOT) is preferred for assessing valvular jets. For regurgitation of valvular origin with central, noneccentric jets, the guidelines suggest using the following criteria for jet width based on the percentage LVOT diameter occupied: 25% or less suggests mild, 26% to 64% suggests moderate, and greater than 65% suggests severe.[19] The grading of paravalvular regurgitation (PVR) is technically more difficult because regurgitant jets are frequently multiple, eccentric, and irregular in shape. This

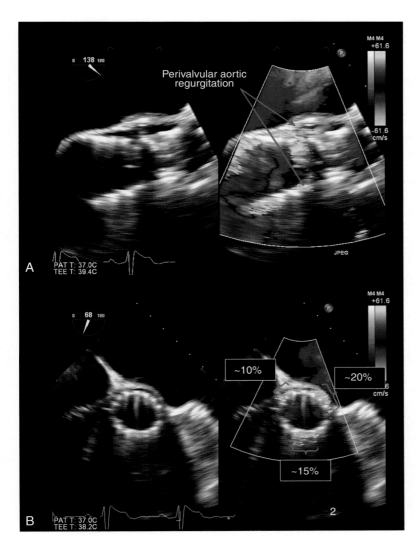

Figure 110.4. A, Transesophageal echocardiography long-axis view shows a CoreValve sitting low in the left ventricular outflow tract with significant paravalvular regurgitation. (See accompanying Video 110.4A.) **B,** The short-axis view is useful in quantifying the regurgitation severity by calculating its circumferential extent, which can then be expressed as a percentage of the total sewing ring circumference. In this case, approximately 45% of the circumference is involved, indicating severe paravalvular regurgitation.

is even more challenging in post-TAVR patients because the jets are affected by native calcium and leaflets as well as the discontinuous nature of the TAVR stent. Nonetheless, assessment of this complication is important because of the excess mortality and morbidity associated with post-TAVR moderate or severe AR.[20-22]

Technically, it is important to scan the full extent of the TAVR using color Doppler and identify the narrowest region of the vena contracta (VC) of each jet. In this context, a number of color Doppler measurements of the PVR jets appear most useful, including the VC width, the VC area, and the circumferential extent of PVR. A VC width of a single jet 0.6 cm or larger or total VC area 0.3 cm^2 or larger suggests severe PVR.[23] The circumferential extent of PVR is expressed as a percentage of the total sewing ring circumference to provide a semiquantitative guide to severity: (<10% = mild; 10%–29% = moderate; >30% = severe)[1,6,23] (Fig. 110.4 and Video 110.4A). Circumferential extent criteria appear the easiest approach to quantification of PVR; however, this method assumes an accurate measurement of the narrowest VC of all jets, and like all parameters, should not be used in isolation.[24] Because of the technical limitations of all semiquantitative parameters, it is important to grade the severity of regurgitation by reviewing the results of multiple Doppler parameters[1,6,23] and when feasible attempt the

quantitation of regurgitation by measurement of regurgitant volumes and regurgitant fractions (Fig. 110.5). 2D imaging may demonstrate the etiology of regurgitation by showing evidence of leaflet degeneration or thickening in bioprostheses or abnormal occluder motion in mechanical prostheses. In cases of infective endocarditis, vegetations and associated abnormalities of the valve annulus such as abscess cavities or valvular dehiscence may be seen. TEE further improves the detection of these anatomic abnormalities (see Video 110.3F), but as discussed later, may still miss abnormalities of occluder motion and anterior annular region.

Limitations of Transesophageal Echocardiography in Aortic Prostheses

Although TEE provides excellent imaging and a high diagnostic yield for mitral prostheses, the data are less convincing for mechanical valves in the aortic position. In one study,[25] the cause of mechanical AVR obstruction by TTE was correct in only 10% and increased to just 49% with TEE. Obstructing pannus in the presence of a coexistent mitral prosthesis was especially difficult to identify. This is because of the angle of the interrogating ultrasound beam, which with TEE is posterior and orthogonal to the prosthesis and LVOT, resulting in

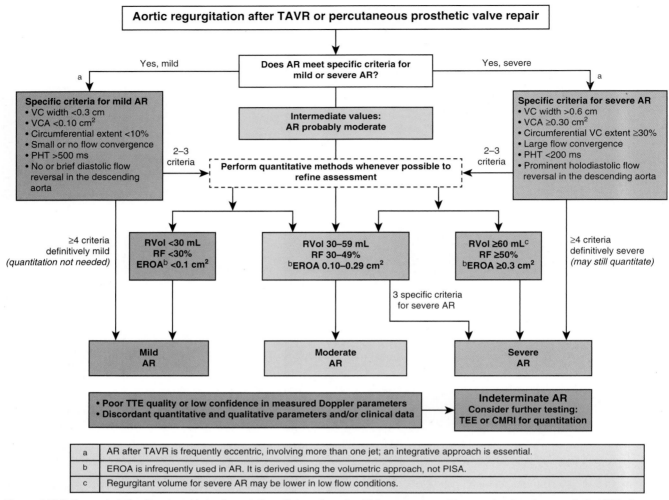

Figure 110.5. Suggested algorithm to guide implementation of integration of multiple parameters of the severity of aortic regurgitation (AR) after transcatheter aortic valve replacement (TAVR) or prosthetic aortic valve repair. Good-quality echocardiographic imaging and complete data acquisition are assumed. If imaging is technically difficult, consider transesophageal echocardiography (TEE) or cardiac magnetic resonance imaging (CMRI). The severity of AR may be indeterminate because of poor image quality, technical issues with data, internal inconsistency among echocardiography findings, or discordance with clinical findings. *EROA,* effective regurgitant orifice area; *PHT,* pressure half time; *PISA,* proximal isovelocity surface area; *RF,* regurgitant fraction; *RVol,* regurgitant volume; *TTE,* transthoracic echocardiography; *VC,* vena contracta; *VCA,* vena contracta area.

acoustic shadowing of the leaflets or occluder and anterior annulus (Fig. 110.6 and Video 110.6B–D). In these cases, CF is a safe and relatively rapid method of demonstrating occluder motion in mechanical prosthetic valves.[26] Despite this significant limitation of TEE, it is clearly superior to TTE for detection of prosthetic valve endocarditis and its complications and should be performed in all patients without a contraindication to esophageal intubation. In the assessment of aortic prosthetic valve regurgitation, TEE can provide additional data on both the mechanism and severity of prosthetic AR. Posterior paravalvular leaks are more visible on TEE and anterior jets on TTE. Using both techniques allows a full circumferential assessment of the annulus.

SUMMARY

This chapter has emphasized the central role of a standardized TTE protocol in the evaluation of prosthetic valves, a diagnostic framework for the interpretation of elevated prosthetic valve gradients, and the complementary role played by other imaging modalities in specific pathologies.

Please access ExpertConsult to view the corresponding videos for this chapter.

Acknowledgment

We thank Dr. Damian Roper for his contributions to the earlier edition of this chapter.

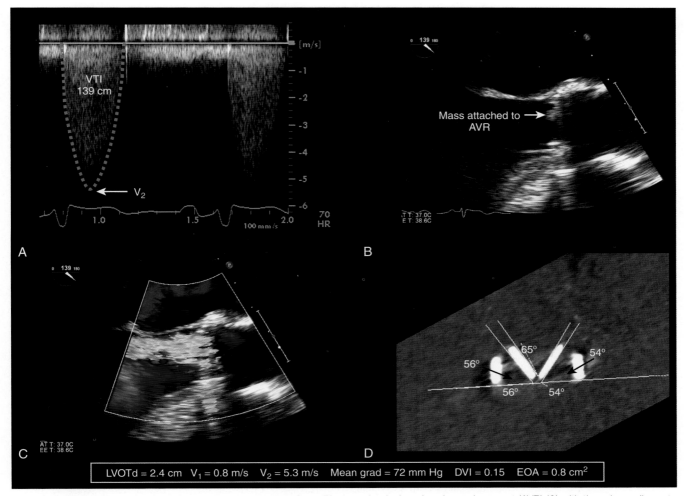

| LVOTd = 2.4 cm | V_1 = 0.8 m/s | V_2 = 5.3 m/s | Mean grad = 72 mm Hg | DVI = 0.15 | EOA = 0.8 cm² |

Figure 110.6. Elevated gradients across a 23-mm Medtronic Open Pivot mechanical aortic valve replacement (AVR) (**A**) with thrombus adherent to the left ventricular outflow tract (LVOT) aspect of the valve (**B**). Despite poor visualization of the AVR occluder motion, significant aortic regurgitation suggested that the thrombus was interfering with valvular function (**C**). Cardiac computed tomography (**D**) demonstrated reduced opening angles for both occluders (normal, 80%–85%). (See accompanying Video 110.6B–D.) *DVI*, Dimensionless velocity index; *EOA*, effective orifice area; *LVOTd*, left ventricular outflow tract diameter; *VTI*, velocity time integral.

REFERENCES

1. Zoghbi WA, Chambers JB, Dumesnil JG, et al. Recommendations for evaluation of prosthetic valves with echocardiography and Doppler ultrasound: a report from the American Society of Echocardiography's guidelines and standards Committee and the Task Force on prosthetic valves. *J Am Soc Echocardiogr.* 2009;22:975–1014. quiz 1082–1084.
2. Shames S, Koczo A, Hahn R, et al. Flow characteristics of the SAPIEN aortic valve: the importance of recognizing in-stent flow acceleration for the echocardiographic assessment of valve function. *J Am Soc Echocardiogr.* 2012;25:603–609.
3. Zamorano JL, Badano LP, Bruce C, et al. EAE/ASE recommendations for the use of echocardiography in new transcatheter interventions for valvular heart disease. *J Am Soc Echocardiogr.* 2011;24:937–965.
4. Clavel MA, Rodes-Cabau J, Dumont E, et al. Validation and characterization of transcatheter aortic valve effective orifice area measured by Doppler echocardiography. *JACC Cardiovasc Imag.* 2011;4:1053–1062.
5. Bloomfield GS, Gillam LD, Hahn RT, et al. A practical guide to multimodality imaging of transcatheter aortic valve replacement. *JACC Cardiovasc Imag.* 2012;5:441–455.
6. Pibarot P, Dumesnil JG. Doppler echocardiographic evaluation of prosthetic valve function. *Heart.* 2012;98:69–78.
7. Rosenhek R, Binder T, Maurer G, Baumgartner H. Normal values for Doppler echocardiographic assessment of heart valve prostheses. *J Am Soc Echocardiogr.* 2003;16:1116–1127.
8. Winter MP, Zbiral M, Kietaibl A, et al. Normal values for Doppler echocardiographic assessment of prosthetic valve function after transcatheter aortic valve replacement: a systematic review and meta-analysis. *Eur Heart J Cardiovasc Imag.* 2018;19:361–368.
9. Hahn RT, Leipsic J, Douglas PS, et al. Comprehensive echocardiographic assessment of normal transcatheter valve function. *JACC Cardiovasc Imaging.* 2019;12:25–34.
10. Pislaru SV, Hussain I, Pellikka PA, et al. Misconceptions, diagnostic challenges and treatment opportunities in bioprosthetic valve thrombosis: lessons from a case series. *Eur J Cardio Thorac Surg.* 2015;47:725–732.
11. Jander N, Sommer H, Pingpoh C, et al. The porcine valve type predicts obstructive thrombosis beyond the first three postoperative months in bioprostheses in the aortic position. *Int J Cardiol.* 2015;199:90–95.
12. Pislaru SV, Pellikka PA, Schaff HV, Connolly HM. Bioprosthetic valve thrombosis: the eyes will not see what the mind does not know. *J Thorac Cardiovasc Surg.* 2015;149. e86–8e7.
13. Latib A, Naganuma T, Abdel-Wahab M, et al. Treatment and clinical outcomes of transcatheter heart valve thrombosis. *Circ Cardiovasc Interv.* 2015;8. e001779.
14. Jamieson WR. Current and advanced prostheses for cardiac valvular replacement and reconstruction surgery. *Surg Technol Int.* 2002;10:121–149.
15. Pibarot P, Dumesnil JG. Hemodynamic and clinical impact of prosthesis-patient mismatch in the aortic valve position and its prevention. *J Am Coll Cardiol.* 2000;36:1131–1141.
16. Blais C, Dumesnil JG, Baillot R, et al. Impact of valve prosthesis-patient mismatch on short-term mortality after aortic valve replacement. *Circulation.* 2003;108:983–988.
17. Ben Zekry S, Saad RM, Ozkan M, et al. Flow acceleration time and ratio of acceleration time to ejection time for prosthetic aortic valve function. *JACC Cardiovasc Imag.* 2011;4:1161–1170.
18. Zoghbi WA, Enriquez-Sarano M, Foster E, et al. Recommendations for evaluation of the severity of native valvular regurgitation with two-dimensional and Doppler echocardiography. *J Am Soc Echocardiogr.* 2003;16:777–802.

19. Zoghbi WA, Adams D, Bonow RO, et al. Recommendations for noninvasive evaluation of native valvular regurgitation: a report from the American Society of Echocardiography developed in collaboration with the Society for Cardiovascular Magnetic Resonance. *J Am Soc Echocardiogr.* 2017;30:303–371.
20. Athappan G, Patvardhan E, Tuzcu EM, et al. Incidence, predictors, and outcomes of aortic regurgitation after transcatheter aortic valve replacement: meta-analysis and systematic review of literature. *J Am Coll Cardiol.* 2013;61:1585–1595.
21. Van Belle E, Juthier F, Susen S, et al. Postprocedural aortic regurgitation in balloon-expandable and self-expandable transcatheter aortic valve replacement procedures: analysis of predictors and impact on long-term mortality: Insights from the France2 registry. *Circulation.* 2014;129:1415–1427.
22. Kodali S, Pibarot P, Douglas PS, et al. Paravalvular regurgitation after transcatheter aortic valve replacement with the Edwards Sapien valve in the PARTNER trial: characterizing patients and impact on outcomes. *Eur Heart J.* 2015;36:449–456.
23. Zoghbi WA, Asch FM, Bruce C, et al. Guidelines for the evaluation of valvular regurgitation after percutaneous valve repair or replacement: a report from the American Society of Echocardiography. *J Am Soc Echocardiogr.* 2019;32:431–475.
24. Hahn RT, Pibarot P, Weissman NJ, et al. Assessment of paravalvular aortic regurgitation after transcatheter aortic valve replacement: intra-core laboratory variability. *J Am Soc Echocardiogr.* 2015;28:415–422.
25. Girard SE, Miller Jr FA, Orszulak TA, et al. Reoperation for prosthetic aortic valve obstruction in the era of echocardiography: trends in diagnostic testing and comparison with surgical findings. *J Am Coll Cardiol.* 2001;37:579–584.
26. Vogel W, Stoll HP, Bay W, et al. Cineradiography for determination of normal and abnormal function in mechanical heart valves. *Am J Cardiol.* 1993;71:225–232.

111 Mitral Prosthetic Valves

Katherine Lau, Darryl J. Burstow

Transthoracic echocardiography (TTE) is the essential imaging investigation for comprehensive baseline assessment and serial evaluation of mitral prosthetic valve function. It is important to understand the prosthetic valve design features to enhance interpretation of the anatomic and hemodynamic data. A standardized TTE protocol is essential in ensuring that all baseline parameters are assessed and documented during the initial postoperative assessment. Doppler examination at TTE provides accurate assessment of prosthetic valve hemodynamics but has limitations in detecting the cause of dysfunction and confirming the presence and mechanism of associated regurgitation. Because of the anatomical position of the prosthetic mitral valve, transesophageal echocardiography (TEE) provides an exceptional view of the mitral prosthesis and is essential in determining the mechanism and severity of prosthesis dysfunction in selected cases.

STANDARD TTE ASSESSMENT OF MITRAL PROSTHETIC VALVE FUNCTION
Two-Dimensional Imaging

The two-dimensional (2D) imaging component of the TTE examination provides anatomic information on prosthetic valve structure, sewing ring stability, and the surrounding structures. The prosthetic valve type (biologic or mechanical), valve size, and date of valve replacement must be established for accurate assessment of valve function. Basic clinical data, including body weight, height, blood pressure, and heart rate and rhythm, should be documented.

Assessment of the prosthetic leaflets or mechanical occluders can be assessed after orientation of the ultrasound beam to reduce acoustic shadowing and improve diagnostic yield. If the ultrasound beam is orientated parallel to the direction of occluder opening, acoustic shadowing across the plane of the valve is reduced with resultant improvement in visualization of occluder motion. For the mitral prosthesis, this is usually achieved from the apical two- or four-chamber window views depending on the implanted orientation of the prosthesis. Intermediate imaging planes scanning through the mitral annulus may also minimize acoustic shadowing and increase the detection of annular pathologies. In addition to assessing prosthetic valve structure, TTE also provides a complete assessment of concomitant native valvular disease, atrial dimensions, and ventricular size and function.

Doppler Parameters Used to Assess Mitral Prosthetic Valve Function

Doppler assessment allows the noninvasive measurement of flow velocities across prosthetic valves from which valve gradients can be calculated. However, as with all stenotic lesions, valve gradients are determined by both volumetric flow and the stenotic valve area. Thus, in addition to gradients, the derivation of flow-independent parameters of prosthetic valve function such as effective orifice area (EOA), pressure halftime (PHT), and dimensionless velocity index (DVI) are essential tools used to quantify mitral prosthetic valve function and are listed in Table 111.1.

Effective Orifice Area and Pressure Halftime

The EOA is calculated using the continuity equation, which requires stroke volumes at two chosen sites (see Table 111.1). It is important to note that significant aortic or mitral regurgitation (MR) >grade 1/4 invalidates this method. In the presence of aortic regurgitation, the right ventricular outflow tract is an alternative method for calculating the true systemic stroke volume. EOA should always be calculated using the continuity equation method, with normal values reported for different prosthesis types[1,2] and, as a general rule, is greater than 2.0 cm². Using the PHT method to derive EOA, as for native mitral stenosis, has not been validated for mitral prostheses and does not closely correlate with other measures of EOA.[1,2] However, PHT has been shown to lengthen with increasing obstruction across the prosthesis and remains a useful parameter for assessing valve function.[1] Therefore, it is important to record the PHT and compare it with available normal values documented for the particular valve subtype and size.

Dimensionless Velocity Index

The DVI is a useful flow-independent parameter of mitral prosthetic valve function. It is simple to derive requiring measurement of only two parameters (the velocity time integrals [VTIs] for the mitral prosthesis and the left ventricular outflow tract [LVOT]) and requires the absence of significant aortic regurgitation. At baseline analysis, it provides an assessment of the hemodynamic performance of a mitral prosthesis with the best performers, typically bileaflet mechanical prostheses, having lower DVI values than bioprostheses.[1] The baseline value can be used as the prosthetic valve "fingerprint" because this value should remain constant, regardless of changes in stroke volume, unless prosthetic valve dysfunction supervenes.[2] If prosthetic valve dysfunction develops (either obstruction or regurgitation), the DVI will increase as the mitral prosthesis VTI is elevated without a corresponding increase in LVOT VTI.[1] DVI has been shown to be one of the best predictors of prosthetic valve dysfunction (Fig. 111.1). The combination of DVI and early mitral diastolic velocity, E velocity, has been shown to improve the positive predictive value for prosthetic valve dysfunction[1] and aid in the selection of patients to undergo further assessment with TEE.

Normal Doppler Values

There is data documenting the normal values for Doppler parameters of various mitral prosthetic and bioprosthetic valve function.[2–5] After completion of the Doppler examination, reference should be made to the normal Doppler data available for that particular prosthetic valve subtype and size.

TABLE 111.1 Doppler Parameters Used to Quantify Mitral Prosthetic Valve Function[1]

Peak early mitral inflow velocity (E, m/s)	Refer to valve subtype; usually <2.2 m/s
Mean gradient (mm Hg)	Refer to valve subtype and size; usually <5 mm Hg
Pressure halftime (ms)	Refer to valve subtype and size; usually <100 ms
Effective orifice area (cm^2)	$(CSA_{LVOT} \times VTI_{LVOT}) \div VTI_{PMV}$ Refer to valve subtype and size
Dimensionless velocity index (unitless)	$PMV_{VTI}/LVOT_{VTI}$; usually <2.3 Refer to valve type and size

CSA, cross-sectional area; *LVOT*, left ventricular outflow; *PMV*, prosthetic mitral valve; *VTI*, velocity time interval.

DIAGNOSIS OF MITRAL PROSTHETIC VALVE DYSFUNCTION

Interpretation of Elevated Prosthetic Valve Gradients

Although a patient with prosthetic valve dysfunction may present with new symptoms or clinical signs, the initial suspicion of abnormality is often raised by the detection of elevated valve gradients, especially when there is a documented change in gradient greater than 50% from baseline during routine TTE assessment.[6] The potential causes to be considered include (1) prosthetic valve obstruction, (2) prosthesis–patient mismatch (PPM), (3) significant transvalvular regurgitation, and (4) high flow states (e.g., postsurgery, anemia, or sepsis). In PPM, MR, and high flow- states, valve gradients are increased because of increased antegrade flow across the prosthesis. This emphasizes the value of the flow-independent parameters (EOA, PHT, and DVI) for the interpretation of elevated gradients (see Fig. 111.1). By using these parameters in conjunction with an anatomical assessment of leaflet or occluder motion, an accurate diagnosis should be obtainable in most instances.

Prosthetic Valve Obstruction

In mechanical valves, the usual causes of valve obstruction are thrombosis or ingrowth of fibrous tissue called pannus below the inflow orifice of the valve, restricting occluder motion. In bioprosthetic valves, structural valve degeneration (SVD) was believed to the commonest cause of dysfunction (Figs. 111.2 and 111.3; Videos 111.3B and D). However, in recent times, it has been increasingly recognized that early bioprosthetic valve dysfunction from thrombosis can occur between 3 and 5 years after implantation, and the introduction of anticoagulation may help avoid the requirement for valve re-replacement.[7,8] 2D TTE imaging may be useful in assessing the cause of prosthetic valve obstruction by

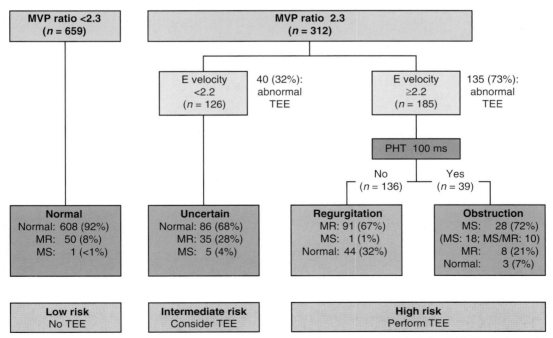

Figure 111.1. Clinical algorithm for the evaluation of mitral prostheses using the dimensionless velocity index (DVI), E velocity, and pressure halftime (PHT). In this study, DVI is referred to as the mitral valve prosthesis ratio (MVP ratio). A normal DVI is strongly predictive of normal mitral prosthetic valve function. Conversely, patients with an elevated DVI in combination with elevated E velocity have a high likelihood of dysfunction and in most cases should have further assessment with transesophageal echocardiography (TEE). PHT allows discrimination between stenosis and regurgitation. *MR*, Mitral regurgitation; *MS*, mitral stenosis. (Modified with permission from Usefulness of mitral valve prosthetic or bioprosthetic time velocity index ratio to detect prosthetic or bioprosthetic mitral valve dysfunction, *Am J Cardiol* 120:1373–1380, 2017)

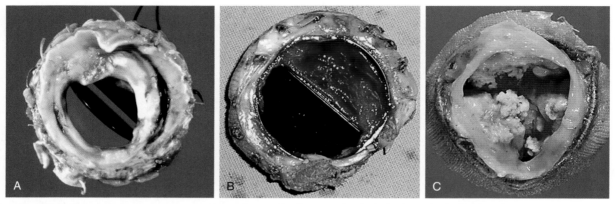

Figure 111.2. A, Pathological specimen of pannus ingrowth complicating a mechanical mitral prosthesis. **B,** Thrombosis of a mitral valve mechanical prosthesis. **C,** Structural valvular degeneration of a bioprosthetic mitral valve.

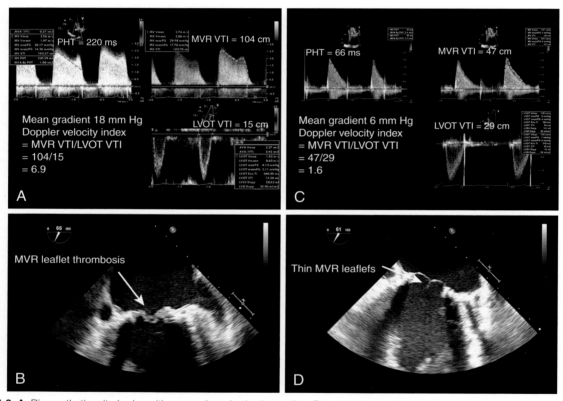

Figure 111.3. A, Bioprosthetic mitral valve with severe thrombotic obstruction. Doppler interrogation revealed markedly elevated mean gradient, prolonged pressure halftime (PHT), and elevated Doppler velocity index (DVI). **B,** Transesophageal echocardiographic (TEE) imaging revealed diffuse thickening and restriction of the prosthetic leaflets. **C,** After 3 months of warfarin therapy, repeat study revealed normalization of mean gradient, PHT, and DVI. **D,** Repeat TEE imaging demonstrating normal mitral leaflet thickness and motion. *LVOT,* Left ventricular outflow tract; *MVR,* mitral valve replacement (See accompanying Videos 111.3B and D.)

detecting leaflet thickening and reduced mobility in bioprosthetic valves but because of attenuation artefact has major limitations in assessing the occluder and surrounding structures in mechanical valves. Nevertheless, careful imaging from the apical window may demonstrate reduced occluder motion. Abnormalities may be subtle such as an absent occluder closing click and may vary with each cardiac cycle in cases of intermittent obstruction. Supplementary imaging of the occluder is usually required when prosthetic valve obstruction is suspected, and this is discussed later.

On Doppler examination, the hemodynamic diagnosis of mitral valve obstruction is suggested by (1) increased gradients for valve subtype and size, (2) decreased EOA below the normal reference range, (3) significant deviation of EOA from the baseline study, (4) increased PHT above the normal reference range, and (5) elevated DVI.[1] Although individual EOA, PHT, and DVI values should always be referenced against normal values for the valve subtype and size, an EOA smaller than 1.5 cm^2, PHT 100 ms or greater, and a DVI 2.3 or greater[1,2,5–9] are almost always abnormal and are useful numbers to remember (see Fig. 111.1).[1]

On rare occasions, usually associated with low flow states, mitral prosthetic valve dysfunction can occur without significant gradient elevation. DVI, being a flow-independent parameter, is also useful in this context. In a recent case, a small female patient with a large size bileaflet mechanical prosthesis (33 mm) presented with thrombotic obstruction with minimal elevation in mean gradient. DVI was abnormal emphasizing the value of flow-independent

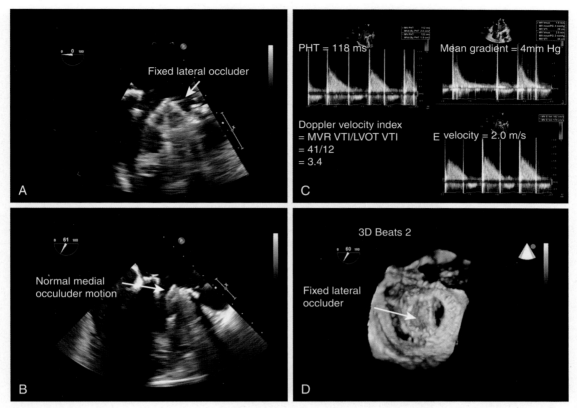

Figure 111.4. A and **B,** Mechanical mitral prosthetic valve with lateral occluder fixed in the closed position. **C,** Doppler interrogation revealed mitral valve obstruction suggested by elevated dimensionless velocity index (DVI) with pressure halftime greater than 100 ms despite a normal mean gradient. **D,** Transesophageal echocardiographic imaging showing a three-dimensional en face view of the fixed lateral occluder with normal medial occluder motion. *LVOT,* Left ventricular outflow tract; *MVR,* mitral valve replacement *VTI,* velocity time integral. (See accompanying Videos 111.4A, B and D.)

parameters of prosthetic valve function (Fig. 111.4; Videos 111.4A, B, and D).

Prosthesis–Patient Mismatch

Although a well-recognized cause of elevated gradients in aortic prostheses, PPM has also been described in mitral prosthetic valves.[10] It occurs when the prosthesis is inappropriately small for the size of the patient and, although uncommon in mitral prostheses because of their relatively large size, it may be seen in older teenagers or young adults when a small prosthesis was inserted in early childhood. Definitions for mitral PPM vary, but a value of less than 1.2 cm²/m² for the EOA indexed to body surface area (iEOA) has been proposed[10] and is predictive of early perioperative mortality and poorer late survival.[11] PPM should be suspected if abnormally elevated Doppler gradients are obtained despite (1) no detectable structural abnormality of the prosthetic valve leaflets or occluders, (2) normal values for EOA and DVI for valve subtype and size, and (3) iEOA in the mismatch range.

DOPPLER DETECTION AND QUANTITATION OF MITRAL PROSTHETIC VALVE REGURGITATION
"Normal" Regurgitation

Trivial to mild transvalvular MR is normal in mechanical mitral valve prostheses and is often present in a normal bioprosthetic valve. This normal regurgitation must be recognized and differentiated from pathological leaks. Two types of normal regurgitation occur with mechanical prostheses, "closing volume"

regurgitation, caused by transient displacement of blood by occluder closure, and so-called "leakage-volume" regurgitation, which occurs at occluder hinge points, resulting in multiple jets also referred to as "washing" jets. Typically, these jets are transvalvular, have a narrow vena contracta (VC) width, and do not project far back into the left atrium. Although it is possible to see a degree of "normal" regurgitation with TTE, it is seen more commonly with TEE.

Pathologic Regurgitation

Abnormal regurgitation of prosthetic valves may arise from valvular or perivalvular sites. Acoustic shadowing of the left atrium and surrounding structures by prosthetic valvular material reduces the detection, localization, and accurate quantitation of mitral prosthetic valve regurgitation by TTE. This is more pronounced with mechanical rather than bioprosthetic valves. Off-axis imaging to enable visualization of the left atrium free of acoustic shadow (e.g., from subcostal windows) may sometimes be helpful in detecting regurgitation. In view of these known difficulties, a number of indirect 2D and Doppler signs of significant regurgitation should be sought. These include (1) elevated DVI, (2) elevated mitral E velocity (≥2.2 m/s), (3) a dense continuous-wave regurgitant jet with early systolic peaking, (4) a large zone of systolic flow convergence on the left ventricular side of the prosthesis, and (5) elevated estimated pulmonary artery pressure. Elevated DVI cut-off values has been shown to vary with MVR subtypes[1] (≥2.2 for bileaflet mechanical valves and ≥2.6 for bioprostheses). As the DVI is elevated both by prosthetic valve obstruction (as discussed earlier) and by regurgitation, a PHT less than 100 ms in the presence of an

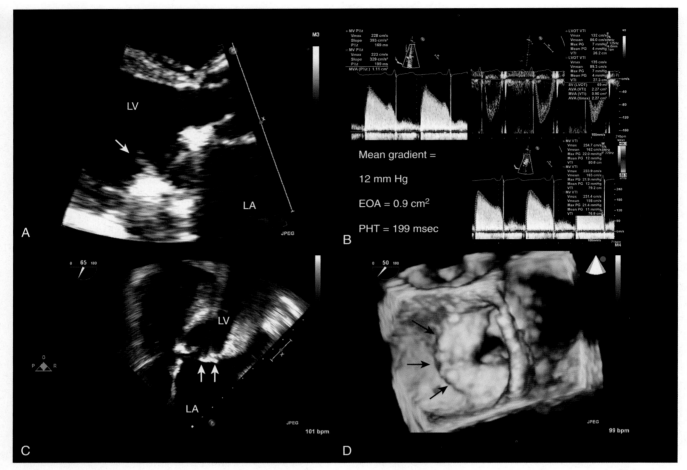

Figure 111.5. A, Mechanical prosthetic mitral valve with decreased occluder motion and associated thrombus on the left ventricular (LV) side of the prosthesis *(arrow)*. **B,** Doppler interrogation revealed an elevated E velocity and mean gradient, prolonged pressure halftime (PHT), and reduction in expected effective orifice area (EOA). **C,** In a separate case with elevated gradients across a bioprosthetic mitral valve, pannus is demonstrated by transesophageal echocardiographic imaging corresponding to the echogenic area on the atrial side of the prosthesis. **D,** Three-dimensional imaging more clearly demonstrates this on the lateral aspect of the valve and sewing ring. *LA,* Left atrium. (See accompanying Videos 111.5A, C, and D).

elevated DVI strongly suggests the presence of hemodynamically significant regurgitation, with a predictive accuracy of >greater than 80%[9], thus identifying patients in whom TEE should be performed to confirm the diagnosis[1] (see Fig. 111.1).

OPTIMAL USE OF TRANSESOPHAGEAL ECHOCARDIOGRAPHY

TEE provides excellent imaging of mitral prostheses and is recommended in the following scenarios: (1) Doppler hemodynamic evidence of prosthetic valve obstruction at TTE, (2) suspected prosthetic valve regurgitation, and (3) suspected or proven infective endocarditis.

Cause of Obstruction

TEE allows superior visualization of the prosthetic occluder or leaflets, resulting in improved detection of leaflet abnormalities and soft tissue masses, such as thrombus or chronic fibrosis tissue ingrowth (pannus), particularly when associated with mechanical valves.[12,13] The differentiation of thrombosis and pannus can often be difficult. Features favoring thrombus over pannus include "soft" echogenicity and large size, together with clinical factors such as short duration of symptoms and inadequate anticoagulation.[13,14] The advent of three-dimensional (3D) TEE, with its ability

to obtain en face views of the mitral prosthesis and annulus, and transgastric imaging of the ventricular aspect of the prosthesis, may further increase diagnostic accuracy (Figs. 111.4 and 111.5; Videos 111.4B and D and 111.5A, C, and D). Mitral prosthesis occluder motion is well seen on TEE; however, computed tomography or cine fluoroscopy can also used as supplementary information to assess prosthetic occluder motion.[15,16]

Confirmation of Regurgitation

TEE detection and semiquantitation of prosthetic mitral transvalvular and perivalvular regurgitation was one of the earliest applications of this technology, and the increased diagnostic yield compared with TTE is well established. The quantification of bioprosthetic transvalvular regurgitation is similar to the native valvular degeneration. In cases with perivalvular regurgitation, TEE provides additional data on the site of regurgitation with confirmation using color Doppler imaging to document the color jet passing outside of the sewing ring. 3D TEE imaging further enhances the visualization of the location and size of the ring dehiscence (Fig. 111.6; Videos 111.6A, C, and D). Identification of the VC and the jet's flow convergence is helpful to confirm the perivalvular leak. VC width correlates well with angiographic severity of MR; a width of 6 mm or larger correlates with severe MR.[17] As with native valves, an EROA can be calculated using the proximal isovelocity

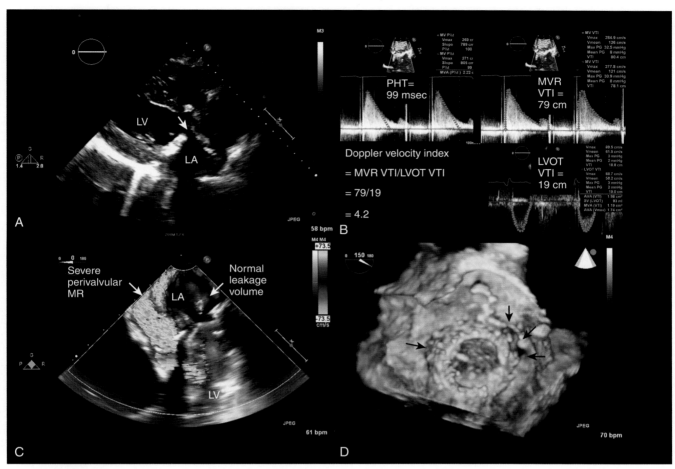

Figure 111.6. A, Dehiscence of a mechanical prosthetic valve. Readers should be alerted to the presence of mitral regurgitation (MR) by the elevated dimensionless velocity index (DVI) (≥2.2) in the presence of a normal pressure halftime (PHT) (**B**). **C,** Transesophageal echocardiographic imaging revealed a large perivalvular leak in addition to normal leakage volume regurgitation. **D,** Three-dimensional imaging confirmed the location of two areas of valvular dehiscence *(arrows)*. *LA,* Left atrium; *LV,* left ventricle; *LVOT,* left ventricular outflow tract; *MVR,* mitral valve replacement *VTI,* velocity time integral. (See accompanying Videos 111.6A, C, D.)

surface area method when a measurable flow convergence zone is visible. The regurgitation is often perivalvular and eccentric, which can lead to overestimated EROA, and hence the suggested cut-off for severe MR is higher at 50 mm² or greater.[17,18] It is essential to understand the limitations of 3D images caused by the "drop-out" artefact created by the prosthetic valves, sewing ring, and struts, which can be incorrectly identified as significant perivalvular dehiscence. Color Doppler is used to aid in the confirmation of a paravalvular regurgitant jet, assess the shape and extent of the perivalvular dehiscence, and generate multiplanar images to measure VC and 3D VC area for quantification of regurgitant orifice.[18,19] The 3D en face view is used in the identification of the locations, direction, and severity of the paravalvular jets, while real-time 3D is also used in the guidance of catheter-based closure devices.[19,20]

Infective Endocarditis

In cases of infective endocarditis, there may be vegetations, new bioprosthetic valvular regurgitation, or associated abnormalities of the valve annulus such as abscess cavities or prosthetic valve dehiscence. Because of the limitations from acoustic artefacts generated by prosthetic valves on TTE, early TEE is essential in all cases to further improve the detection of these anatomic abnormalities.[17,21–26] The sensitivity of TEE in detecting vegetations in prosthetic valve endocarditis verified at surgery or autopsy was 82%

compared with 36% for TTE.[12,27] It is also important to remember that developing perivalvular abscess may only be identified as nonspecific tissue thickening with serial TEE essential to confirm and assess the progression of disease.[24,26] TEE-generated 3D images have become a routine supplement in the accurate assessment of vegetation size, while color Doppler 3D is essential in determining the severity of perivalular regurgitation associated with dehiscence of the prosthetic valve and confirming the presence of bioprosthetic valve perforations[18] (Fig. 111.6 and Videos 111.6A, C, and D). Transgastric-acquired TEE images allow evaluation of the ventricular aspect of the mitral prosthesis, which is often hindered by acoustic artefact seen in esophageal views.

SUMMARY

This chapter has emphasized the central role of TTE in the evaluation of mitral prosthetic valves, its strengths and weaknesses, TTE clues to the presence of significant regurgitation, and the appropriate use of TEE in specific pathologies.

Please access ExpertConsult to view the corresponding videos for this chapter.

Acknowledgment

The authors acknowledge the contributions of Dr. Hillier, who was the author of this chapter in the previous edition.

REFERENCES

1. Luis SA, Blauwet LA, Samardhi H, et al. Usefulness of mitral valve prosthetic or bioprosthetic time velocity index ratio to detect prosthetic or bioprosthetic mitral valve dysfunction. *Am J Cardiol.* 2017;120:1373–1380.
2. Zoghbi WA, Chambers JB, Dumesnil JG, et al. Recommendations for evaluation of prosthetic valves with echocardiography and Doppler ultrasound. *J Am Soc Echocardiogr.* 2009;22:975–1014.
3. Blauwet LA, Malouf JF, Connolly HM, et al. Doppler echocardiography of 79 normal CarboMedics mitral prostheses: a comprehensive assessment including time-velocity integral ratio and prosthesis performance index. *J Am Soc Echocardiogr.* 2007;20:1125–1130.
4. Blauwet LA, Malouf JF, Connolly HM, et al. Doppler echocardiography of 240 normal Carpentier-Edwards Duraflex porcine mitral bioprostheses: a comprehensive assessment including time velocity integral ratio and prosthesis performance index. *J Am Soc Echocardiogr.* 2009;22:388–393.
5. Blauwet LA, Malouf JF, Connolly HM, et al. Comprehensive hemodynamic assessment of 368 normal St. Jude Medical mechanical mitral valve prostheses based on early postimplantation echocardiographic studies. *J Am Soc Echocardiogr.* 2013;26:381–389.
6. Egbe AC, Pislaru SV, Pellikka PA, et al. Bioprosthetic Valve thrombosis versus structural failure: clinical and echocardiographic predictors. *J Am Coll Cardiol.* 2015;66:2285–2294.
7. Egbe A, Pislaru SV, Ali MA, et al. Early prosthetic valve dysfunction due to bioprosthetic valve thrombosis: the role of echocardiography. *JACC Cardiovascular Imag.* 2018;11:951–958.
8. Butnaru A, Shaheen J, Tzivoni D, et al. Diagnosis and treatment of early bioprosthetic malfunction in the mitral valve position due to thrombus formation. *Am J Cardiol.* 2015;112:1439–1444.
9. Fernandes V, Olmos L, Nagueh SF, et al. Peak early diastolic velocity rather than pressure half-time is the best index of mechanical prosthetic mitral valve function. *Am J Cardiol.* 2002;89:704–710.
10. Magne J, Mathieu P, Dumesnil J, et al. Impact of prosthesis-patient mismatch on survival after mitral valve replacement. *Circulation.* 2007;115:1417–1425.
11. Sa M, Cavalcanti LRP, Rayol SDC, et al. Prosthesis-patient mismatch negatively affects outcomes after mitral valve replacement: meta-analysis of 10,239 patients. *Brazil J Cardiovasc Surg.* 2019;34:203–212.
12. Daniel WG, Mugge A, Grote J, et al. Comparison of transthoracic and transesophageal echocardiography for detection of abnormalities of prosthetic and bioprosthetic valves in the mitral and aortic positions. *Am J Cardiol.* 1993;71:210–215.
13. Saric M, Armour AC, Arnaout MS, et al. Guidelines for the use of echocardiography in the evaluation of a cardiac source of embolism. *J Am Soc Echocardiogr.* 2016;29:1–42.
14. Barbetseas J, Nagueh SF, Pitsavos C, et al. Differentiating thrombus from pannus formation in obstructed mechanical prosthetic valves: an evaluation of clinical, transthoracic and transesophageal echocardiographic parameters. *J Am Coll Cardiol.* 1998;32:1410–1417.
15. Nishimura RA, Otto CM, Bonow RO, et al. AHA/ACC guideline for the management of patients with valvular heart disease. *J Am Coll Cardiol.* 2014;63:e57–e185. 2014.
16. Nishimura RA, Otto CM, Bonow RO, et al. AHA/ACC focused update of the 2014 AHA/ACC guideline for the management of patients with valvular heart disease. *Circulation.* 2017;135:e1159–e1195. 2017.
17. Vitarelli A, Conde Y, Cimino E, et al. Assessment of severity of mechanical prosthetic mitral regurgitation by transoesophageal echocardiography. *Heart.* 2004;90:539–544.
18. Kinno M, Raissi SR, Olson KA, Rigolin VH. Three-dimensional echocardiography in the evaluation and management of paravalvular regurgitation. *Echocardiography.* 2018;35:2056–2070.
19. Zoghbi WA, Asch FM, Bruce C, et al. Guidelines for the evaluation of valvular regurgitation after percutaneous valve repair or replacement. *J Am Soc Echocardiogr.* 2019;32:431–475.
20. Franco E, Almeria C, de Agustin JA, et al. Three-dimensional color Doppler transesophageal echocardiography for mitral paravalvular leak quantification and evaluation of percutaneous closure success. *J Am Soc Echocardiogr.* 2014;27:1153–1163.
21. Lengyel M. The impact of transesophageal echocardiography on the management of prosthetic valve endocarditis: experience of 31 cases and review of the literature. *J Heart Valve Dis.* 1997;6:204–211.
22. Reynolds HRJM, Tunick PA, et al. Sensitivity of transthoracic versus transesophageal echocardiography for the detection of native valve vegetations in the modern era. *J Am Soc Echocardiogr.* 2003;16:67–70.
23. Tornos P, Iung B, Permanyer-Miralda G, et al. Infective endocarditis in Europe: lessons from the Euro heart survey. *Heart.* 2005;91:571–575.
24. Baddour LM, Wilson WR, Bayer AS, et al. Infective endocarditis in adults: diagnosis, antimicrobial therapy, and management of complications. *Circulation.* 2015;132:1435–1486.
25. Bai AD, Steinberg M, Showler A, et al. Diagnostic accuracy of transthoracic echocardiography for infective endocarditis findings using transesophageal echocardiography as the reference standard: a meta-analysis. *J Am Soc Echocardiogr.* 2017;30:639–646 e8.
26. Vilacosta I, Olmos C, de Agustin A, et al. The diagnostic ability of echocardiography for infective endocarditis and its associated complications. *Expert Rev Cardiovasc Ther.* 2015;13:1225–1236.
27. Daniel WG, Mugge A, Martin RP, et al. Improvement in the diagnosis of abscesses associated with endocarditis by transesophageal echocardiography. *N Engl J Med.* 1991;324:795–800.

112   Mitral Valve Repair

Stanton K. Shernan

Perioperative echocardiographers should approach patients scheduled for mitral valve (MV) surgery with several goals and the intention of using these data to facilitate clinical and surgical decision making. It is therefore important to (1) establish the cause, mechanism, and severity of MV dysfunction; (2) determine the presence of any echocardiographic predictors of a difficult MV repair; (3) obtain relevant measurements of the MV apparatus to assist in the development of a surgical treatment plan; and (4) diagnose postsurgical residual disease and complications.

PRE–CARDIOPULMONARY BYPASS TRANSESOPHAGEAL ECHOCARDIOGRAPHICEXAMINATION

Clinical studies have suggested that the pre–cardiopulmonary bypass (CPB) transesophageal echocardiographic (TEE) examination prompts changes in surgery in 9% to 13% of patients undergoing MV surgery.[1–3] During the pre-CPB TEE examination, the severity, mechanism, and location of MV disease, including subvalvular involvement, annular calcification, and dilatation, and leaflet motion abnormalities, as well as the status of left ventricular (LV)

function, should be identified to help determine whether an MV replacement, repair, or neither is indicated. It is particularly important to identify risk factors for difficult MV repair[4] (Box 112.1). In patients with functional mitral regurgitation (MR), approximately 30% of repairs may fail within the first 6 postoperative months.[5] Risk factors for limited durability include significant LV geometrical distortion, excessive apical tethering of the MV leaflets or annular dilatation, and severe MR.[6] Evidence in patients with ischemic functional MR undergoing coronary artery bypass grafting and randomized to either MV repair or MV replacement have demonstrated that although baseline echocardiographic measures of MV geometric leaflet tethering by themselves may not be associated with postoperative moderate or severe recurrent MR, the presence of LV basal aneurysm or dyskinesis is strongly associated with this outcome.[7] Others have shown that concurrent posteromedial MV leaflet tethering along with LV basal aneurysm or dyskinesis is most important for predicting MV repair failure associated with ischemic functional MR.[8] Difficult MV repair in patients with degenerative disease may be predicted by the presence of extensive anterior leaflet (AL) or multiple scallop involvement.[9] These patients may also be at risk for developing systolic anterior motion (SAM) with LV outflow tract obstruction, especially if they present

---

BOX 112.1 Feasibility of Mitral Valve Repair in Various Scenarios: Patient Selection

EASIEST TO REPAIR

- Pure mitral valve annular dilatation
- Ruptured chordate to posterior leaflet (especially the middle scallop [P2])
- Small perforation
- Pure rheumatic mitral stenosis without extensive subvalve involvement

HARDEST TO REPAIR

- Ruptured chordate to anterior leaflet
- Ruptured chordate to both leaflets
- Severe prolapsed of both leaflets
- Ruptured chordate near commissures
- Extensive leaflet fibrosis, retraction, or calcification
- Extensive calcification of mitral annulus

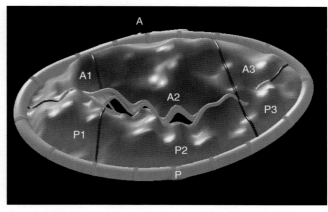

Figure 112.1. Parametric image (Q-labs; Philips Healthcare) of a complex mitral valve at risk for postrepair systolic anterior motion because of the presence of a long anterolateral (A1) and antero-middle (A2) segments. *A,* Anterior leaflet; *A3,* anteromedial segment; *P,* posterior leaflet; *P1,* posterolateral segment; *P2,* postero-middle segment; *P3,* posteromedial segment.

BOX 112.2 Use of Intraoperative Transesophageal Echocardiography to Predict Patients at Greatest Risk for Developing Systolic Anterior Motion[36]

- Coaptation–septum distance <25 mm
- Aortomitral angle <120 degrees
- Posterior leaflet height >15 mm
- Anteroposterior leaflet height ≤1.3
- Basal septal diameter >15 mm
- Left ventricular end-diastolic dimension <45 mm
- Hyperdynamic left ventricle

---

preoperatively with an excessively long or asymmetric AL; a redundant posterior leaflet (PL), especially when longer than the AL; a short coaptation–septal distance; a narrow mitral-aortic angle; or a nondilated LV[10–13] (Fig. 112.1 and Box 112.2). Finally, in patients with rheumatic heart disease, extensive mitral annular or subannular calcification, as well as a limited AL length, have been associated with an especially difficult MV repair.[14]

Determining the degree of MR intraoperatively can be particularly challenging because of the influence of changes in hemodynamic loading conditions on transmitral flow and pressure during general anesthesia, which may result in an underestimation of MR severity by TEE.[15] Furthermore, conventional two-dimensional echocardiographic techniques for estimating MR effective regurgitant orifice area, including vena contract width and proximal isovelocity surface area, may underestimate MR severity.[16] Thus, the American Society of Echocardiography guidelines recommend using both extensive qualitative and quantitative echocardiographic measures for assessing the severity of MR.[17,18]

POST–CARDIOPULMONARY BYPASS TRANSESOPHAGEAL ECHOCARDIOGRAPHIC EXAMINATION

Several studies have suggested that in approximately 5% to 10% of MV surgical procedures, the post-CPB TEE examination may identify persistent dysfunction that requires additional, immediate surgical intervention.[19–21] The initial post-CPB TEE examination is essential for determining the competency of the replaced or repaired MV. A full appreciation of the post-CPB TEE examination after MV repair requires a comprehensive understanding of the surgical procedure because numerous variations of both "resect" and "respect" techniques may be used along with a variety of partial band and full rings[22] (Fig. 112.2). Most small perivalvular jets are insignificant, although larger "leaks" may become associated with hemolysis, hemodynamic instability, or valvular dehiscence.[23] Loading conditions and LV function must also be taken into consideration in the assessment of residual MR (Fig. 122.3). After MV repair, SAM is more frequent in patients with persistent AL or PL redundancy, the use of an annuloplasty ring that is either too small or incorrectly oriented, and a hypertrophied or hyperdynamic left ventricle. Finally, iatrogenic MS, although rare, can occur in 2% of patients undergoing MV repair[24] but may be challenging to diagnose by conventional echocardiographic parameters in the hemodynamically volatile period because of the influence of cardiac output on measures of transvalvular pressure gradients.

THREE-DIMENSIONAL ECHOCARDIOGRAPHY FOR MITRAL VALVE SURGERY

Perioperative three-dimensional (3D) echocardiography may offer some advantages over two-dimensional (2D) echocardiography for patients undergoing MV repair. Preoperative 3D echocardiography has been very useful in delineating mechanisms of MV disease to potentially facilitate surgical planning.[25] In particular, identifying complex MV disease, including multisegment involvement,[26] commissural disease,[27] and clefts[28] (Figs. 112.1 and 112.4), is more accurately diagnosed with 3D TEE compared with 2D TEE. 3D intraoperative echocardiography can also provide a potentially more efficient process for acquiring a comprehensive echocardiographic examination of the MV, which may be particularly important in the volatile intraoperative environment where timely and effective clinically relevant decision making may be critical.[29–31]

A comprehensive intraoperative 3D TEE examination may also permit more accurate diagnoses and more effective communication with surgeons and interventionalists.[27,31,32] Novel imaging windows of the MV that are not readily obtainable with 2D TEE can be presented in en face perspectives to better appreciate anatomy, functional geometry, and pathophysiology, thereby attenuating the reliance on scanning and pattern recognition, as well as geometric assumptions[26,33] (see Fig. 122.4). Unique imaging planes also help to communicate relevant diagnostic information to those less familiar with conventional echocardiographic displays (see Fig. 122.4). Furthermore, accurately identifying the specific location and severity of MR jets, especially immediately after MV repair or replacement, can also facilitate decision making regarding the need for urgent further intervention[34] (Fig. 122.5). Finally,

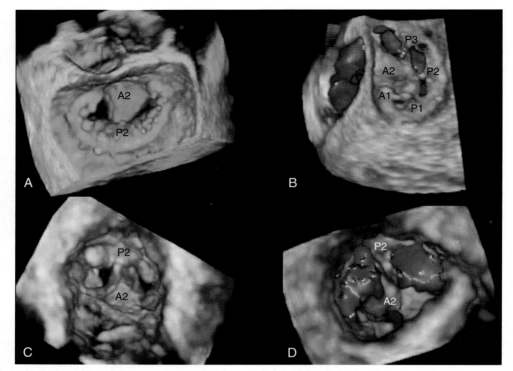

Figure 112.2. Mitral valve (MV) repair in a patient with myxomatous degeneration. **A,** Three-dimensional (3D) transesophageal echocardiography (TEE) en face view of the MV after a repair involving a posterolateral (P1) and middle segment of the posterior leaflet (P2) resection, along with a ring annuloplasty and an edge-to-edge repair between the middle scallops, A2 and P2. **B,** After the repair, color-flow Doppler demonstrated only trace residual mitral regurgitation. **C,** 3D TEE view of the postrepair MV from the left ventricular perspective showing the edge-to-edge repair between the middle scallops, A2 and P2. **D,** Color-flow Doppler 3D TEE view of the postrepair MV from the left ventricular perspective showing the edge-to-edge repair between the middle scallops, A2 and P2. *A1,* Anterolateral scallop; *A3,* anteromedial scallop; *P1,* posterolateral scallop; *P3,* posteromedial scallop.

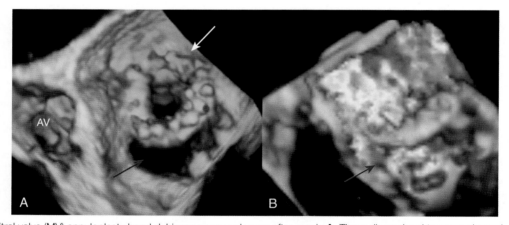

Figure 112.3. Mitral valve (MV) annuloplasty band dehiscence several years after repair. **A,** Three-dimensional transesophageal echocardiography image demonstrating an annuloplasty band *(white arrow)* that has dehisced *(blue arrow)* along the lateral aspect. **B,** Color flow Doppler demonstrating significant mitral regurgitation *(blue arrow)* at the site of dehiscence. *AV,* Aortic valve.

Figure 112.4. Three-dimensional transesophageal echocardiography full-volume data sets showing en face view of the mitral valve (MV) from the left atrial perspective with variations of degenerative disease. **A,** Posterior middle scallop (P2) cleft. **B,** P2 prolapse along with medial anterior (A3) and posterior (P3) leaflet scallop prolapse. *A1,* Anterolateral leaflet scallop; *A2,* antero-middle leaflet scallop; *P1,* posterolateral leaflet scallop.

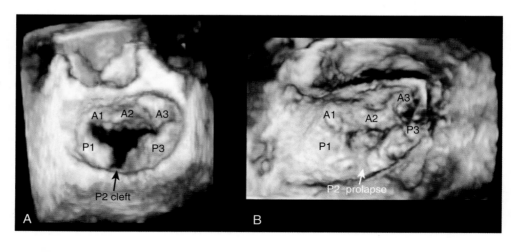

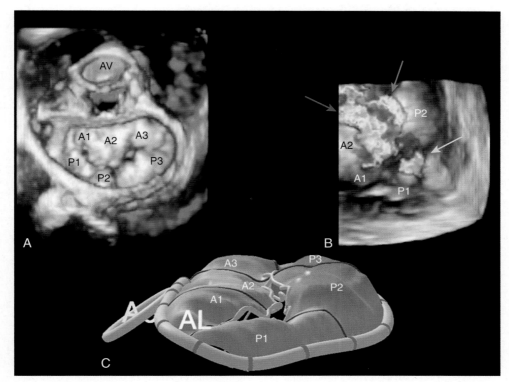

Figure 112.5. Myxomatous degeneration of the mitral valve (MV). **A,** Three-dimensional transesophageal echocardiographic image of an MV with myxomatous degeneration showing prolapse primarily of the antero-middle (A2) and anteromedial (A3) leaflet segments, as well as the postero-middle (P2) segment of the leaflet. **B,** Color-flow Doppler images show separate regurgitant jets associated with each prolapsing leaflet (anterior leaflet prolapse, *blue arrow,* and posterior leaflet prolapse, *red arrow*), as well as a jet associated with a functional, deep indentation or cleft between P2 and the lateral scallop (P1) of the posterior leaflet *(yellow arrow).* **C,** Parametric image (Q-labs; Philips Healthcare) of the same valve. *A1,* Anterolateral segment; *Ao,* aortic valve; *AL,* anterolateral commissure; *P3,* posteromedial segment.

3D echocardiography can assist in determining mechanisms and severity of dynamic pathophysiological states that often require surgical intervention, including MR associated with hypertrophic obstructive cardiomyopathy and SAM.[35]

REFERENCES

1. Stewart W, Currie P, Salcedo E, et al. Intraoperative Doppler color flow mapping for decision-making in valve repair for mitral regurgitation: technique and results in 100 patients. *Circulation.* 1990;81:556–566.
2. Sheikh K, deBruijn N, Rankin J, et al. The utility of transesophageal echocardiography and Doppler color flow imaging in patients undergoing cardiac valve surgery. *J Am Coll Cardiol.* 1990;15:363–372.
3. Eltzschig H, Rosenberger P, Löffler M, et al. Impact of intraoperative transesophageal echocardiography on surgical decision-making in 12,566 cardiac surgical patients. *Ann Thorac Surg.* 2008;85:845–852.
4. McGee E, Gillinov A, Blackstone E, et al. Recurrent mitral regurgitation after annuloplasty for functional ischemic mitral regurgitation. *J Thorac Cardiovasc Surg.* 2004;6:916–924.
5. Goldstein D, Moskowitz A, Gelijns A, et al. CTSN two-year outcomes of surgical treatment of severe ischemic mitral regurgitation. *N Engl J Med.* 2016;374:344–353.
6. Silbiger J. Mechanistic insights into ischemic mitral regurgitation: echocardiographic and surgical implications. *J Am Soc Echocardiogr.* 2011;24:707–719.
7. Kron I, Hung J, Overby J, et al. For the CTSN Investigators: predicting recurrent mitral regurgitation after mitral valve repair for severe ischemic mitral regurgitation. *J Thorac Cardiovasc Surg.* 2015;14:752–761.
8. Widjh-den Hamer I, Bouma W, Lai E, et al. The value of preoperative 3D over 2-dimensional valve analysis in predicting recurrent ischemic mitral regurgitation after mitral annuloplasty. *J Thorac Cardiovasc Surg.* 2016;152:847–859.
9. Shimokawa T, Kasegawa H, Katayama Y, et al. Mechanisms of recurrent regurgitation after valve repair for prolapsed mitral valve disease. *Ann Thorac Surg.* 2011;91:1433–1439.
10. Shah R, Raney A. Echocardiographic correlates of left ventricular outflow obstruction and systolic anterior motion following mitral valve repair. *J Heart Valve Disease.* 2011;10. 302–206.
11. Myers P, Khalpey Z, Maloney A, et al. Edge-to-edge repair for prevention and treatment of mitral valve systolic anterior motion. *J Thorac Cardiovasc Surg.* 2013;146:836–840.
12. Maslow A, Regan M, Haering M, et al. Echocardiographic predictors of left ventricular outflow tract obstruction and systolic anterior motion of the mitral valve after mitral valve reconstruction for myxomatous valve disease. *J Am Coll Cardiol.* 1999;34. 2096–104.
13. Varghese R, Itagaki S, Anyanwu A, et al. Predicting systolic anterior motion after mitral valve reconstruction: using intraoperative transoesophageal echocardiography to identify those at greatest risk. *Eur J Cardiothor Surg.* 2013;1–7.
14. Gupta A, Gharde M, Kumar A: Anterior mitral leaflet length: predictor for mitral valve repair in a rheumatic population, *Ann Thorac Surg.* 90:1930–3, 2010.
15. Aklog L, Filsoufi F, Flores KQ, et al. Does coronary artery bypass grafting alone correct moderate ischemic mitral regurgitation? *Circulation.* 2001;104. I-68–I-75.
16. Ashikmina E, Shook D, Cobey F, et al. Three-dimensional versus two-dimensional echocardiographic assessment of functional mitral regurgitation proximal isovelocity surface area. *Anesth Analg.* 2015;120:533–542.
17. Zogbhi W, Adams D, Bonow R, et al. Recommendations for noninvasive evaluation of native valvular regurgitation. *J Am Soc Echocardiogr.* 2017;30:303–371.
18. Nishimura R, Otto C, Bonow R, et al. Focused update of the 2014 AHA/ACC guideline for the management of patients with valvular heart disease. *J Am Coll Card.* 2017;7:252–289.
19. Click R, Martin A, Schaff H, Intraoperative TEE. 5-year prospective review of impact on surgical management. *Mayo Clin Proc.* 2000;75:241–247.
20. Stewart W, Thomas J, Klein A, et al. Ten-year trends in utilization of 6340 intraoperative echos. *Circulation.* 1995;92(Suppl I):2453.
21. Michel-Cherqui M, Ceddaha A, Liu N, et al. Assessment of systematic use of intraoperative transesophageal echocardiography during cardiac surgery in adults: a prospective study of 203 patients. *J Cardiothorac Vasc Anesth.* 2000;14:45–50.
22. Yacoub M, Cohn L. Novel approaches to cardiac valve repair: from structure to function: part II. *Circulation.* 2004;109:1064–1072.
23. Ruiz C, Hahn R, Berrebi A, et al. Clinical trial principles and endpoint definitions for paravalvular leaks in surgical prosthesis: an expert statement. *J Am Coll Cardiol.* 2017;69. 2067–87.
24. Riegel A, Busch R, Segal S, et al. Evaluation of transmitral pressure gradients in the intraoperative echocardiographic diagnosis of mitral stenosis after mitral valve repair. *PloS One.* 2011;6. e26559.

25. Chandra S, Salgo I, Sugeng L, et al. Characterization of degenerative mitral valve disease using morphologic analysis of real-time three-dimensional echocardiographic images: objective insight into complexity and planning of mitral valve repair. *Circ Cardiovasc Imag.* 2011;4:24–32.

26. Chikwe J, Adams D, Su K, et al. Can three-dimensional echocardiography accurately predict complexity of mitral valve repair? *Eur J Cardio Thorac Surg.* 2012;41:518–524.

27. Ben Zekry S, Nagueh S, Little S, et al. Comparative accuracy of two- and three-dimensional transthoracic and transesophageal echocardiography in identifying mitral valve pathology in patients undergoing mitral valve repair: initial observations. *J Am Soc Echocardiogr.* 2011;24:1079–1085.

28. Mantovani F, Clavel M, Vatury O, et al. Cleft-like indentations in myxomatous mitral valves by three-dimensional echocardiographic imaging. *Heart.* 2015;101:1111–1117.

29. Vegas A, Meineri M. Three-dimensional transesophageal echocardiography is a major advance for intraoperative clinical management of patients undergoing cardiac surgery: a core review. *Anesth Analg.* 2010;110:1548–1573.

30. Lang R, Badano L, Tsang W, et al. EAE/ASE Recommendations for image acquisition and display using three-dimensional echocardiography. *J Am Soc Echocardiogr.* 2012;25:3–46.

31. Skubas N, Shernan S. Intraoperative three-dimensional echocardiography for mitral valve surgery: just pretty pictures or ready for prime time? *Anesth Analg.* 2013;116:272–275.

32. Grewal J, Mankad S, Freeman W, et al. Real-time three-dimensional transesophageal echocardiography in the intraoperative assessment of mitral valve disease. *J Am Soc Echocardiogr.* 2009;22:34–41.

33. Salcedo E, Quaife R, Seres T, Carroll J. Framework for systematic characterization of the mitral valve by real-time three-dimensional transesophageal echocardiography. *J Am Soc Echocardiogr.* 2009;22. 1087–99.

34. Singh P, Manda J, Hsiung M. Live/real time three-dimensional transesophageal echocardiographic evaluation of mitral and aortic valve prosthetic paravalvular regurgitation. *Echocardiography.* 2009;26:980–987.

35. Jungwirth B, Adams D, Mathew J, et al. Mitral valve prolapse and systolic anterior motion illustrated by real time three-dimensional transesophageal echocardiography. *Anesth Analg.* 2008;107:1822–1824.

36. Varghese R, Hgaki S, Anyanwu AC, et al. Predicting systolic anterior motion after mitral valve reconstruction: using intraoperative transoesophageal echocardiography to identify those at greatest risk. *Eur J Cardio Thorac Surg.* 2014;45:132–137.

113 Tricuspid and Pulmonic Prosthetic Valves

Dimitrios Maragiannis, Sherif F. Nagueh

Various types of prosthetic heart valves (PHVs) have been available in clinical practice during the past five decades.[1] Tricuspid valve replacement (TVR) is now an uncommon procedure and has been described in fewer than 2% of all valve operations in one study.[2] Current guidelines recommend TVR is reasonable for severe tricuspid regurgitation (TR) secondary to diseased or abnormal tricuspid valve (TV) leaflets not amenable to annuloplasty or repair.[3] TVR is associated with high early 30-day mortality rate varying from 12% to 26% and a low 10-year survival rate among different studies.[4–8] A recent meta-analysis of 11 studies concluded that the surgeon's decision should depend on the individual patient's characteristics.[9]

TRICUSPID VALVE PROSTHESIS DYSFUNCTION

Prosthetic valve failure is usually caused by valve stenosis, regurgitation, or both. The most common causes of prosthetic valve stenosis are leaflet degeneration in bioprosthetic valves; endocarditis leading to leaflet destruction; and valve thrombosis and pannus formation in mechanical valves, which are associated with valve obstruction. Structural valve degeneration ranges from 0.4% to 2.2% patient-years in bioprosthetic valves.[4,7] The incidence of valve thrombosis has been reported at 0.5% to 3.3% patient-years in different studies.[7,10,11] Prosthetic transvalvular regurgitation can occur because of leaflet destruction from infective endocarditis, but paravalvular regurgitation can result from primary suture loosening or infective endocarditis.

Doppler echocardiography has been widely and accurately used to evaluate prosthetic valve function in the tricuspid position. Doppler measurements have been shown to correlate well with invasive hemodynamic data in cases of prosthetic valve stenosis.[12,13] However, diagnostic accuracy depends heavily on the quality of Doppler signals. Detailed assessment of TV prostheses is of crucial importance and requires imaging with two-dimensional (2D), continuous wave (CW) Doppler, and color-flow imaging.

ECHOCARDIOGRAPHIC ASSESSMENT OF PROSTHETIC TRICUSPID VALVE FUNCTION
Two-Dimensional Echocardiography

Prosthetic valves in the tricuspid position can be adequately imaged using standard echocardiographic views with transthoracic

echocardiography (TTE). Multiple views such as the right ventricular (RV) inflow view, four-chamber view, short-axis view (RV inflow and outflow), and subcostal view, are required for a comprehensive evaluation. 2D echocardiography confirms normal or abnormal leaflet motion and proper seating of the TV in the annulus. The type of each valve can be identified, and degenerative changes in bioprosthetic valves as thickening and calcification can be visualized. It is possible to diagnose the underlying causes of valve dysfunction such as thrombus, vegetations, or pannus by TTE or transesophageal echocardiography (TEE).

Color-Flow Imaging

Color-flow mapping describes the dynamic flow characteristics across the prosthesis. In normal prosthetic valves, the antegrade flow is central and consists usually of a wide jet (Figs. 113.1 and 113.2). The better views for assessing color flow through the prosthesis are the RV inflow and the subcostal views because in these views, acoustic shadowing interference is minimal in comparison with the apical four-chamber view. It is often possible to visualize aliasing as flow accelerates through a stenotic orifice. In cases with severe stenosis, the color jet has high velocities indicating turbulent flow (Fig. 113.3).

Doppler Echocardiography

Prosthetic TV evaluation is similar to that of native valves and is currently evaluated by Doppler echocardiography using peak velocity, mean gradient (MG), and effective orifice area (EOA) measured as proposed by American Society of Echocardiography (ASE) guidelines.[14] Past studies have included a small number of patients from the early postoperative period, as well as patients with older prostheses.[15–18] More recent studies have included larger patient populations and compared parameters from the early postoperative period (<30 days after surgery) with later measurements.[19,20] Patients with normally functioning valves have normal physical examinations, and the prostheses appears to have normal motion and flow pattern by TTE and TEE. Current guidelines recommend the early evaluation of tricuspid prosthesis postimplantation. It is important to average Doppler measurements from at least five cardiac cycles because measurements may vary significantly

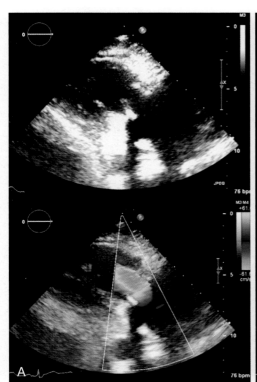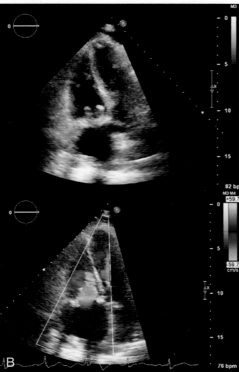

Figure 113.1. A, Two-dimensional (2D) and color-flow mapping of a normal tricuspid bioprosthesis in a 66-year-old woman from the right ventricular inflow view. **B,** 2D and color-flow mapping in the four-chamber view shows wide, smooth, unobstructed flow across the prosthesis. (See accompanying Video 113.1.)

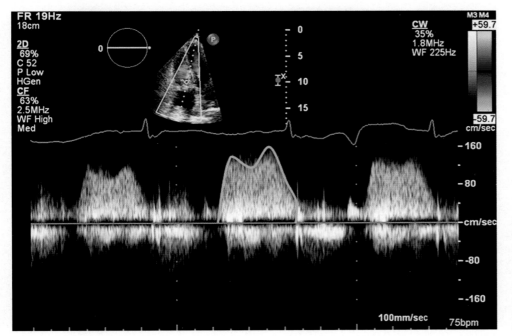

Figure 113.2. Continuous wave (CW) Doppler examination of a normal bioprosthetic tricuspid valve in the apical four-chamber view during the early postimplantation period by transthoracic echocardiography. The mean gradient was 4.8 mm Hg after averaging five cycles. (See accompanying Video 113.2.)

due to respiration.[14] Whereas Conolly and coworkers[16] averaged 10 cycles, recent studies from Blauwet and coworkers[19,20] have shown that averaging 5 cycles yields similar results to averaging 9 cycles. However, in cases of marked variation of velocities, more than 5 cycles should be measured, or signals should be obtained at end-expiratory apnea.

MG. The transvalvular gradient across the prosthesis is calculated using the modified Bernoulli equation $\Delta P = 4V^2$ in which ΔP is the transvalvular pressure gradient and V is the tricuspid inflow peak velocity by CW Doppler. The Doppler study should be performed from different transducer imaging positions to ensure acquisition of maximal velocity across the prosthesis. One should note the valve size and type when evaluating TV function. High flow states (anemia, hyperthyroidism, sepsis) should be taken into account when measuring transvalvular velocities because they can be associated with higher gradients in normal prosthetic valves. Other factors such as elevated RV diastolic pressures and constrictive pericarditis can affect these measurements. The peak gradient and MG across the prosthetic TV are measured with CW Doppler by tracing the tricuspid inflow velocities contour during diastole (see Fig. 113.2).

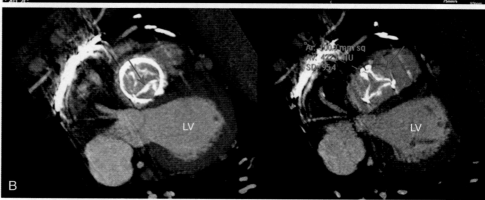

Figure 113.3. Transesophageal echocardiography images from a 40-year-old woman with severe prosthetic valve stenosis. **A,** The bioprosthetic tricuspid valve has severe calcification with stenosis, and color-flow mapping shows a prominent proximal isovelocity surface area (PISA) region *(yellow arrow)* caused by severe stenosis. **B,** The valve is imaged on multidetector computed tomography, which reveals the presence of degenerative and highly calcified leaflets in a short-axis view of the valve, with the anatomic area *(red arrow)* planimetered at 1.01 cm². *LV,* Left ventricle; *RA,* right atrium; *RV,* right ventricle. (See accompanying Video 113.3.)

ASE guidelines[14] recognize an MG less than 6 mm Hg as normal and values of 6 mm Hg or greater as suggesting prosthetic valve stenosis. A recent study[19] with a larger number of patients with bioprosthetic valves early after operation demonstrated that an MG greater than 9 mm Hg is highly suggestive of tricuspid bioprosthetic valve stenosis, and thus further imaging with TEE should be considered in these circumstances (Table 113.1). In the Blauwet and coworkers' study,[19] different prosthetic valves were evaluated, including the Carpentier-Edwards Duraflex, Medtronic Mosaic, St. Jude Medical Biocor, Carpentier-Edwards Perimount, and Medtronic Hancock II valves. In line with the guidelines, a large study[20] reported a normal MG at 5 mm Hg or less for bileaflet mechanical TV prosthesis, but values greater than 6 mm Hg were seen in patients with mechanical valve obstruction (Tables 113.2 to 113.4).

Pressure halftime (PHT). PHT is the time required for peak gradient across the prostheses to reach half of its initial value at valve opening. Earlier studies[16,18] have shown that a normal PHT ranges from 200 to 238 ms for bioprosthetic valves in tricuspid position and lies between 102 and 127 ms for St. Jude mechanical valves. Other studies[19,20] proposed a PHT of 200 ms or greater as indicating bioprosthetic valve stenosis, but a PHT of 130 ms or greater indicates bileaflet mechanical valve obstruction. According to the recent guidelines, the PHT for patients with normal xenograft prosthetic valves is 146 ± 39 ms; for normal caged ball valves, it is 144 ± 46 ms; and for normal St. Jude tricuspid prostheses, it is 108 ± 32 ms, with a PHT 230 ms or greater, highly suggestive of stenosis.[14]

TVI ratio for tricuspid valve prostheses. Blauwet and colleagues[19,20] proposed the use of the time velocity integral (TVI) ratio of the TV prosthesis (TVI_{TVP}) to the left ventricle outflow tract TVI (TVI_{LVOT}) as an index of prosthetic valve function. This ratio can be used to differentiate prosthetic valve stenosis from regurgitation because in both cases, the gradient is increased. For normal bioprosthetic TVs, the TVI ratio is less than 3.3. A peak tricuspid E velocity of 2.1 m/s or greater, TVI_{TVP}/TVI_{LVOT} 3.3 or greater, and PHT less than 200 ms are predictive of significant regurgitation in bioprosthetic valves, whereas a peak tricuspid E velocity of 1.9 m/s or greater, TVI_{TVP}/TVI_{LVOT} of 2.0 or greater, and PHT less than 130 ms occur in hemodynamically significant regurgitation in mechanical valves. Of note, these measurements appear useful even when color Doppler fails to show significant leaks.

EOA. EOA is a valuable parameter when evaluating tricuspid prosthetic valves and is calculated using the continuity equation dividing the LVOT stroke volume with the tricuspid prosthesis TVI. The LVOT stroke volume is calculated as $SV_{LVOT} = LVOT_{area} \times TVI_{LVOT}$. EOA can be of value in cases with suspected valve obstruction. In patients with significant aortic regurgitation, the right ventricular outflow tract (RVOT) stroke volume (SV_{RVOT}) can be used. However, with mixed lesions (regurgitation and stenosis), there are limitations for EOA calculation. Of note, EOA derived by PHT has not been validated in cases of prosthetic valves in tricuspid position.

PROSTHETIC VALVE REGURGITATION

Pathologic prosthetic valve regurgitation (PR) in the tricuspid position can be present either as paravalvular or transvalvular

TABLE 113.1 Normal Doppler Parameters in Bioprosthetic Tricuspid Valves

Parameter	ASE Guidelines[14] 2009	Blauwet et al[19] (threshold values)
Peak velocity (m/s)	≤1.7	<2.1
Mean pressure gradient (mm Hg)	<6	<8.8
Pressure halftime (ms)	<230	<193
Effective orifice area	No data available	No data available
TVI$_{TVR}$/TVI$_{LVOT}$	No data available	<3.3

ASE, American Society of Echocardiography; *LVOT,* left ventricular outflow tract; *TVI,* time velocity integral; *TVP,* tricuspid valve prosthesis.
Data from Zoghbi WA, et al: Recommendations for evaluation of prosthetic valves with echocardiography and Doppler ultrasound: A report From the American Society of Echocardiography's Guidelines and Standards Committee and the Task Force on Prosthetic Valves, *J Am Soc Echocardiogr* 22:975–1014, 2009; and Blauwet LA, et al: Comprehensive echocardiographic assessment of the hemodynamic parameters of 285 tricuspid valve bioprostheses early after implantation, *J Am Soc Echocardiogr* 23:1045–1059, 2010.

TABLE 113.2 Normal Doppler Parameters in Mechanical Tricuspid Valves and Normal Doppler Parameters in Bileaflet Mechanical Tricuspid Valves

Parameter	ASE Guideline[14] 2009	Blauwet et al[20]
Peak velocity (m/s)	≤1.7	<1.9
Mean pressure gradient (mm Hg)	<6	≤5
Pressure halftime (ms)	<230	<130
Effective orifice area	No data available	No data available
TVI$_{TVR}$/TVI$_{LVOT}$	No data available	<2

ASE, American Society of Echocardiography; *LVOT,* left ventricular outflow tract; *TVI,* time velocity integral; *TVP,* tricuspid valve prosthesis.
Data from Zoghbi WA, et al: Recommendations for evaluation of prosthetic valves with echocardiography and Doppler ultrasound: A report From the American Society of Echocardiography's Guidelines and Standards Committee and the Task Force on Prosthetic Valves, *J Am Soc Echocardiogr* 22:975–1014, 2009; and Blauwet LA, et al: Comprehensive echocardiographic assessment of mechanical tricuspid valve prostheses based on early post-implantation echocardiographic studies, *J Am Soc Echocardiogr* 24:414–424, 2011.

TABLE 113.3 Echocardiographic and Doppler Parameters in Grading Severity of Prosthetic Tricuspid Valve Regurgitation

Parameter	Mild	Moderate	Severe
Valve structure	Usually normal	Abnormal or valve dehiscence	Abnormal or valve dehiscence
Jet area by color Doppler, central jets only	<5 cm²	5–10 cm²	>10 cm²
Vena contracta width	Not defined	Not defined but <0.7 cm	>0.7 cm
Jet density and contour by CW Doppler	Incomplete or faint, parabolic	Dense, variable contour	Dense with early peaking
Doppler systolic hepatic flow	Normal or blunted	Blunted	Holosystolic reversal
Right atrium, right ventricle, inferior vena cava size	Normal	Dilated	Markedly dilated

CW, Continuous-wave.
From Zoghbi WA, et al: Recommendations for evaluation of prosthetic valves with echocardiography and Doppler ultrasound: A report From the American Society of Echocardiography's Guidelines and Standards Committee and the Task Force on Prosthetic Valves, *J Am Soc Echocardiogr* 22:975–1014, 2009.

TABLE 113.4 Doppler Parameters for Normal Bioprosthetic Valves in the Tricuspid Position[a]

Type of Prosthesis	Number of Patients (total, 285)	Mean Gradient (mm Hg)	Peak Velocity (m/s)	TVI$_{TVP}$/TVI$_{LVOT}$
Carpentier-Edwards Perimount	12	3.5 ± 1.31	1.3 ± 0.24	1.8 ± 0.29
Medtronic Mosaic	49	5.1 ± 1.52	1.5 ± 0.21	2.1 ± 0.53
Carpentier-Edwards Duraflex	177	5.5 ± 1.8	1.5 ± 0.26	2.3 ± 0.53
St. Jude Medical Biocor	36	4.3 ± 1.34	1.4 ± 0.28	2.0 ± 0.56
Medtronic Hancock II	11	5.6 ± 1.51	1.5 ± 0.25	2.3 ± 0.49

[a]Data are expressed as mean ± standard deviation.
LVOT, Left ventricular outflow tract; *TVI,* time velocity integral; *TVP,* tricuspid valve prosthesis.
From Blauwet LA, et al: Comprehensive echocardiographic assessment of the hemodynamic parameters of 285 tricuspid valve bioprostheses early after implantation, *J Am Soc Echocardiogr* 23:1045–1059, 2010.

TABLE 113.5 Doppler Parameters for Normal Mechanical Bileaflet Valves in the Tricuspid Position[a]

Type of Tricuspid Prosthesis	Number of Patients (total, 78)	Mean Gradient (mm Hg)	Peak Velocity (m/s)	TVI_{TVP}/TVI_{LVOT}
St. Jude Medical Standard	51	3.0 ± 1.22	1.3 ± 0.28	1.4 ± 0.29
CarboMedics Standard	17	3.5 ± 1.28	1.3 ± 0.17	1.7 ± 0.38
Starr-Edwards	10	5.1 ± 1.52	1.7 ± 0.33	1.9 ± 0.42

[a]Data are expressed as mean ± standard deviation.
LVOT, Left ventricular outflow tract; TVI, time velocity integral; TVP, tricuspid valve prosthesis.
From Blauwet LA, et al: Comprehensive echocardiographic assessment of mechanical tricuspid valve prostheses based on early post-implantation echocardiographic studies, J Am Soc Echocardiogr 24:414–424, 2011.

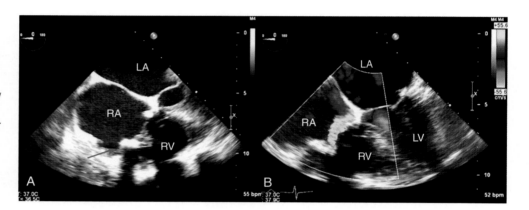

Figure 113.4. Transesophageal echocardiography (TEE) images from an 83-year-old woman with a bioprosthetic tricuspid valve. **A,** Midesophageal four-chamber view with rightward tilting showing the tricuspid bioprosthesis (red arrow). **B,** The same view with color-flow mapping revealing mild eccentric tricuspid regurgitation. LA, Left atrium; LV, left ventricle; RA, right atrium; RV, right ventricle. (See accompanying Video 113.4.)

regurgitation. Pathologic transvalvular regurgitation usually reflects degenerative mechanisms affecting valve leaflets, including calcification, thickening, and tears, but can also represent the results of leaflet destruction by infective endocarditis. In mechanical prostheses, transvalvular regurgitation is often combined with valve obstruction (thrombosis) where a stuck leaflet remains open throughout systole. Paravalvular regurgitation is a rare complication and is always pathologic. It is often caused by infective endocarditis or suture loosening. It is important to remember that mechanical prostheses normally have small regurgitant jets of a short duration and characteristic flow pattern. Normal bioprosthetic valves may have mild TR in the early postimplantation period. An integrated approach is recommend using 2D echocardiography, color-flow imaging, and spectral Doppler for assessment of valve regurgitation (Table 113.5).

Two-Dimensional Echocardiography

All echocardiographic standard views should be used for prosthetic valve evaluation using the transthoracic and, if needed, the transesophageal approach. RV and right atrial (RA) volumes are usually increased in patients with significant PR. A dilated inferior vena cava with minimal change on inspiration can be seen in the presence of elevated RA pressure, which is common with severe TR. Although the above findings can occur because of other reasons such as RV dysfunction, the presence of severe TR should be questioned in their absence. Furthermore, the rocking motion of a prosthetic valve is pathognomonic of dehiscence.

Color-Flow Imaging

Color-flow imaging in PR offers crucial information assessing the location of the jet, regurgitation severity, and the underlying mechanism (Fig. 113.4). It is possible to visualize and differentiate a paravalvular leak from a transvalvular jet. The severity of

TR can be assessed using the flow convergence area and vena contracta (VC) measurements. A VC[14] width greater than 0.7 cm is highly specific for severe TR. It is usually measured in the apical four-chamber view with TTE. However, reverberations by the prosthesis may conceal significant TR, and TEE may be needed in these cases.

Spectral Doppler

Both CW Doppler and pulsed-wave (PW) Doppler have been used for evaluation of prosthetic TR. A dense, early peaking jet by CW Doppler is seen in patients with severe TR. This characteristic contour reflects the markedly elevated systolic "V" wave in RA pressure tracing that is seen in severe TR. A holosystolic flow reversal in hepatic venous flow by PW Doppler is an additional finding in severe TR. However, it is not seen in all patients with severe lesions. An elevated tricuspid peak E velocity (≥1.9–2.1 m/s), although not specific, is a common finding in severe TR.

TRANSESOPHAGEAL ECHOCARDIOGRAPHY IN PATIENTS WITH PROSTHETIC TRICUSPID VALVES

TEE is an important modality for prosthetic valve function assessment, especially when combined with Doppler. Current guidelines recommend multiplane TEE in patients for the assessment of structure and function of PHVs, including the evaluation of paravalvular abscesses.[21] It is indicated for the evaluation of patients with the possible diagnosis of prosthetic valve endocarditis and valvular thrombosis, including reevaluation when a change in therapy is anticipated.[21] TEE is the modality of choice for guidance of transcatheter procedures and whenever TTE is nondiagnostic.[21] In cases of prosthetic valve thrombosis, TEE can be valuable in making decisions on the use of thrombolytic therapy because it allows measurement of thrombus size.[22] Standard

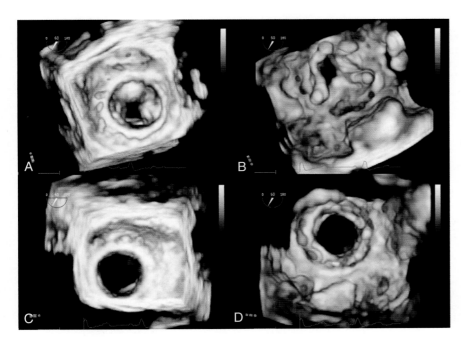

Figure 113.5. A–D, Three-dimensional images from a patient with a tricuspid valve-in-valve prosthesis. (Courtesy of Dr. Roberto Lang.)

views to image the tricuspid prosthesis are the midesophageal (ME) four-chamber view, the ME inflow–outflow view, the ME modified bicaval TV view, and the transgastric (TG) RV inflow–outflow view.[21] TEE can be used to examine leaflet motion and the seating of the valve and exclude the presence of vegetations or thrombi. Meanwhile, color Doppler may reveal abnormal blood flow patterns (flow convergence) and assess PR. Similar to TTE, CW Doppler can be used to measure transvalvular gradients and calculate EOA. However, it can be challenging to obtain good alignment of the Doppler beam.

THREE-DIMENSIONAL ECHOCARDIOGRAPHY

Current three-dimensional (3D) echocardiography technology is well validated in cases of native valve dysfunction. However, there are few data on prosthetic valve evaluation. 3D can complement traditional methods in investigating prosthetic valve dysfunction.[23,24] Current guidelines do not contain specific 3D protocols for imaging of prosthetic valves.[25] Recent TEE guidelines note that the native TV can be adequately assessed by 3D at the ME four-chamber-view from 0 to 30 degrees or at the 40-degree TG view with anteflexion.[21] A narrow-angle or a wide-angle acquisition mode using either single- or multiple-beat acquisition with adequate electrocardiographic gating can be used. Color-flow Doppler should be used in addition to multiple-beat acquisition in patients with prosthetic valves. Potential advantages include collection of the 3D data set, reconstruction and visualization of valve anatomy and its motion, and transvalvular flow with color Doppler in any plane. 3D TEE plays an important role not only in identifying multiple and complicated regurgitant jets, dehiscence sites, and paravalvular leaks but also in diagnosing the cause of valve stenosis as restricted leaflet motion and obstructing thrombi or vegetations.[26,27] Although promising, 3D has its limitations. These include a low frame rate and limited spatial resolution of the reconstructed image. Poor-quality images can result from stitching artifacts, which are more prominent in patients with arrhythmias, and tissue dropout with shadowing related to the highly reflective prosthesis.

TRANSCATHETER VALVE-IN-VALVE IMPLANTATION

Recent advances in novel percutaneous transcatheter valves have made it feasible to implant these valves as a treatment for bioprosthetic TV dysfunction in high-risk patients. To date, few reports have been reported to evaluate the feasibility of this technique.[28–35] Most of these reports used the transatrial, transjugular, or transfemoral approaches, implanting either the Melody valve (Medtronic) or Edwards SAPIEN transcatheter valve (Edwards Life Sciences). Although long-term follow-up and randomized trials are not available, this is a highly promising option for high-risk patients. 2D and 3D echocardiography have been successfully used to guide valve implantation and to evaluate the function of the percutaneously implanted valves (Fig. 113.5).

PROSTHETIC PULMONIC VALVES

Prosthetic pulmonic valves are often bioprosthetic, though at times mechanical valves are used. Because of coexisting subvalvular and supravalvular pathology in some patients, it is important to carefully visualize the RVOT and the valve itself so as to determine if there is subpulmonic stenosis that is the cause of increased velocities by CW Doppler. In younger individuals, it is usually possible to obtain satisfactory images of the valve and the RVOT by TTE in the parasternal short-axis view at the aortic valve level, as well as in the subcostal view. Importantly, both windows result in good alignment of the ultrasound beam with flow through the RVOT and through the pulmonic valve itself. Similar to other valves, it is important to use color Doppler. In the presence of significant stenosis, there is usually a zone of proximal flow acceleration that can be used to identify the site of stenosis. In addition, PW Doppler can be used to map the location of stenosis, which is recognized by aliasing. After the site the stenosis is identified, the severity is assessed by CW Doppler to measure the peak velocity and gradient. One should consider flow conditions before drawing conclusions based on the latter two measurements because increased transvalvular flow in the absence of stenosis leads to increased velocity and gradient across prosthetic valves. In addition, comparison with previous studies can be helpful because a serial increase in peak velocity and gradient occurs in the presence of stenosis. There are limited data on normal values, but in general, peak velocity increases from homografts (<2.5 m/s) to xenografts (<3.2 m/s).[14] In addition, RV systolic pressure increases with valve stenosis and can be estimated based on peak TR velocity. In addition, RV enlargement along with hypertrophy and systolic dysfunction can develop.

PROSTHETIC PULMONARY VALVE REGURGITATION

The general approach to grade PR is similar to that in patients with native valves. In patients with mild PR, the valve structure is usually normal, as are RV size and function unless the valve was implanted at a time when the RV was already dilated. In the latter situation, it is important to evaluate RV size and function in previous studies. PR jet occupies 25% or less of the pulmonary annulus, and the CW Doppler is faint with slow deceleration. RV is enlarged in patients with severe PR, and the jet occupies more than 50% of the pulmonary annulus.[14] CW Doppler signal is dense with steep deceleration and terminates before end-diastole because of the rapid rise in RV diastolic pressure as it approaches the PA diastolic pressure. Diastolic flow reversal can be recorded in the pulmonary artery. It is possible to quantify the PR volume as the difference between flow through the RVOT tract and left ventricular outflow tract. In severe PR, the regurgitant fraction is greater than 50%.

Please access ExpertConsult to view the corresponding videos for this chapter.

REFERENCES

1. Vongpatanasin W, Hillis LD, Lange RA. Prosthetic heart valves. *N Engl J Med.* 1996;335:407–416.
2. Committee for Scientific Affairs, Sakata R, Fujii Y, et al. Thoracic and cardiovascular surgery in Japan during 2009: annual report by the Japanese Association for Thoracic Surgery. *Gen Thorac Cardiovasc Surg.* 2011;59:636–667.
3. Bonow RO, Carabello BA, Chatterjee K, et al. American College of Cardiology/American Heart Association TaskForce on Practice Guidelines: 2008 focused update incorporated into the ACC/AHA2006 guidelines for the management of patients with valvular heart disease. *J Am Coll Cardiol.* 2008;52:e1–e142.
4. Ratnatunga CP, Edwards MB, Dore CJ, Taylor KM. Tricuspid valve replacement: UK Heart Valve Registry mid-term results comparing mechanical and biological prostheses. *Ann Thorac Surg.* 1998;66:1940–1947.
5. Filsoufi F, Anyanwu AC, Salzberg SP, et al. Long-term outcomes of tricuspid valve replacement in the current era. *Ann Thorac Surg.* 2005;80:845–850.
6. Guenther T, Noebauer C, Mazzitelli D, et al. Tricuspid valve surgery: a thirty-year assessment of early and late outcome. *Eur J Cardio Thorac Surg.* 2008;34:402–409.
7. Garatti A, Nano G, Bruschi G, et al. Twenty-five year outcomes of tricuspid valve replacement comparing mechanical and biologic prostheses. *Ann Thorac Surg.* 2012;93:1146–1153.
8. Marquis-Gravel G, Bouchard D, Perrault LP, et al. Retrospective cohort analysis of 926 tricuspid valve surgeries: clinical and hemodynamic outcomes with propensity score analysis. *Am Heart J.* 2012;163:851–858.
9. Rizzoli G, Vendramin I, Nesseris G, et al. Biological or mechanical prostheses in tricuspid position? A meta-analysis of intra-institutional results. *Ann Thorac Surg.* 2004;77:1607–1614.
10. Nakano K, Koyanagi H, Hashimoto A, et al. Tricuspid valve replacement with the bileaflet St. Jude Medical valve prosthesis. *J Thorac Cardiovasc Surg.* 1994;108:888–892.
11. Péterffy A, Szentkirályi I. Mechanical valves in tricuspid position: cause of thrombosis and prevention. *Eur J Cardio Thorac Surg.* 2001;19:735–736.
12. Wilkins GT, Gillam LD, Kritzer GL, et al. Validation of continuous-wave Doppler echocardiographic measurements of mitral and tricuspid prosthetic valve gradients: a simultaneous Doppler-catheter study. *Circulation.* 1986;74:786–795.
13. Burstow DJ, Nishimura RA, Bailey KR, et al. Continuous wave Doppler echocardiographic measurement of prosthetic valve gradients. A simultaneous Doppler-catheter correlative study. *Circulation.* 1989;80:504–514.
14. Zoghbi WA, Chambers JB, Dumesnil JG, et al. Recommendations for evaluation of prosthetic valves with echocardiography and Doppler ultrasound: a report from the American Society of Echocardiography's guidelines and standards Committee and the Task Force on prosthetic valves. *J Am Soc Echocardiogr.* 2009;22:975–1014.
15. Aoyagi S, Nishi Y, Kawara T, et al. Doppler echocardiographic evaluation of St. Jude Medical valves in the tricuspid position. *J Heart Valve Dis.* 1993;2:279–286.
16. Connolly HM, Miller Jr FA, Taylor CL, et al. Doppler hemodynamic profiles of 82 clinically and echocardiographically normal tricuspid valve prostheses. *Circulation.* 1993;88:2722–2727.
17. Sezai A, Shiono M, Akiyama K, et al. Doppler echocardiographic evaluation of St. Jude Medical valves in the tricuspid position: criteria for normal and abnormal valve function. *J Cardiovasc Surg.* 2001;42:303–309.
18. Aoyagi S, Tomoeda H, Kawano H, et al. Doppler echocardiographic evaluation of prosthetic valves in tricuspid position. *Asian Cardiovasc Thorac Ann.* 2003;11:193–197.
19. Blauwet LA, Danielson GK, Burkhart HM, et al. Comprehensive echocardiographic assessment of the hemodynamic parameters of 285 tricuspid valve bioprostheses early after implantation. *J Am Soc Echocardiogr.* 2010;23:1045–1059.
20. Blauwet LA, Burkhart HM, Dearani JA, et al. Comprehensive echocardiographic assessment of mechanical tricuspid valve prostheses based on early post-implantation echocardiographic studies. *J Am Soc Echocardiogr.* 2011;24:414–424.
21. Hahn RT, Abraham T, Adams MS, et al. Guidelines for performing a comprehensive transesophageal echocardiographic examination: recommendations from the American Society of Echocardiography and the Society of Cardiovascular Anesthesiologists. *J Am Soc Echocardiogr.* 2013;26:921–964.
22. Tong AT, Roudaut R, Ozkan M, et al. Prosthetic Valve Thrombolysis-Role of Transesophageal Echocardiography (PRO-TEE) Registry Investigators. Transesophageal echocardiography improves risk assessment of thrombolysis of prosthetic valve thrombosis: results of the international PRO-TEE registry. *J Am Coll Cardiol.* 2004;43:77–84.
23. Sugeng L, Shernan SK, Weinert L, et al. Real-time three-dimensional transesophageal echocardiography in valve disease: comparison with surgical findings and evaluation of prosthetic valves. *J Am Soc Echocardiogr.* 2008;21:1347–1354.
24. Krim SR, Vivo RP, Patel A, et al. Direct assessment of normal mechanical mitral valve orifice area by real-time 3D echocardiography. *JACC Cardiovasc Imag.* 2012;5:478–483.
25. Lang RM, Badano LP, Tsang W, et al. EAE/ASE recommendations for image acquisition and display using three-dimensional echocardiography. *Eur Heart J Cardiovasc Imag.* 2012;13:1–46.
26. Naqvi TZ, Rafie R, Ghalichi M. Real-time 3D TEE for the diagnosis of right-sided endocarditis in patients with prosthetic devices. *JACC Cardiovasc Imag.* 2010;3:325–327.
27. Cheng HL, Cheng YJ, Wang YC, Fan SZ. A stenotic bioprosthetic valve in the tricuspid position: real-time 3-dimensional transesophageal echocardiography as a useful supplement to conventional assessment. *Anesth Analg.* 2012;115:253–256.
28. Hon JK, Cheung A, Ye J, Carere RG, et al. Transatrial transcatheter tricuspid valve-in-valve implantation of balloon expandable bioprosthesis. *Ann Thorac Surg.* 2010;90:1696–1697.
29. Gurvitch R, Cheung A, Ye J, Wood DA, et al. Transcatheter valve-in-valve implantation for failed surgical bioprosthetic valves. *J Am Coll Cardiol.* 2011;58:2196–2209.
30. Hoendermis ES, Douglas YL, van den Heuvel AF. Percutaneous Edwards SAPIEN valve implantation in the tricuspid position: case report and review of literature. *Euro Intervention.* 2012;8:628–633.
31. Gaia DF, Palma JH, de Souza JA, Buffolo E. Tricuspid transcatheter valve-in-valve: an alternative for high-risk patients. *Eur J Cardio Thorac Surg.* 2012;41:696–698.
32. Petit CJ, Justino H, Ing FF. Melody valve implantation in the pulmonary and tricuspid position. *Catheter Cardiovasc Interv.* 2013;82:E944–E946.
33. Gerosa G, D'Onofrio A, Tessari C, et al. Open transcatheter tricuspid balloon expandable valve-in-valve implantation for failed bioprosthesis. *J Thorac Cardiovasc Surg.* 2013;146:e3–e5.
34. Ribichini F, Pesarini G, Feola M, et al. Transcatheter tricuspid valve implantation by femoral approach in trivalvular heart disease. *Am J Cardiol.* 2013;112:1051–1053.
35. Daneault B, Williams MR, Leon MB, et al. Transcatheter tricuspid valve-in-valve replacement resulting in 4 different prosthetic heart valves in a single patient. *J Am Coll Cardiol.* 2013;61:e3.

114 Infective Endocarditis: Role of Transthoracic Versus Transesophageal Echocardiography

Luca Longobardo, Bijoy K. Khandheria

Infective endocarditis (IE) is one of the most severe infectious diseases and is characterized by a poor prognosis and high mortality rates and associated with prolonged hospitalization and a high risk of need for surgery.[1] The incidence of IE ranges among countries from 3 to 10 episodes per 100,000 person years and increases dramatically with age, reaching a peak incidence of 14.5 episodes per 100,000 person years in patients aged 70 to 80 years.[2]

Since its first description in 1885, the epidemiology of the disease has greatly changed.[1] In the most developed countries, the increasing and widespread incidence of diabetes, chronic kidney failure requiring hemodialysis, and intravascular devices associated with progress in cardiac valve repair or replacement techniques have generated a new microbiological profile of IE, with a prevalence of infections caused by staphylococci, enterococci, fungi, and other resistant health care–related agents typically involving older patients with prosthetic valves or degenerative valve disease.[3] In contrast, developing countries are characterized by a prevalence of streptococcal infections and culture-negative IE affecting patients of younger age at presentation and higher incidence of structural cardiac predisposing risk factors such as rheumatic disease and untreated congenital heart disease.[2,4]

According to the site of infection and the presence of intracardiac materials, endocarditis can be classified as left-sided native valve IE, left-sided prosthetic valve IE, right-sided IE, or device-related IE (on pacemaker or defibrillator wires with or without associated valve involvement). This differentiation is important because the pathophysiology and diagnostic strategy of the different subtypes of endocarditis are different.

The diagnosis of IE is based on the clinical picture, echocardiographic findings, and microbiological diagnosis. The Duke criteria and the modified Duke criteria provide high sensitivity and specificity for diagnosis (Table 114.1).[2,5] IE can present acutely with septic changes and rapidly progressive infection but also as a subacute or chronic disease with a low-grade fever and nonspecific symptoms, which may delay the diagnosis, especially when occurring in patients with no previous history of valve disease. A range of other conditions, including rheumatic disease, chronic infection, malignancy, and autoimmune disease, can be suspected before the diagnosis of IE is established.

In IE caused by virulent organisms such as *Staphylococcus aureus*, the diagnosis can be missed when extracardiac signs of infection predominate and the clinical signs of valve disease are initially absent or difficult to evaluate (Videos 114.1 and 114.2). It is necessary to consider the diagnosis of IE in all cases of sepsis, particularly in all patients presenting with fever of unclear origin and an embolic episode even if there is no previous history of cardiac disease.[4]

ROLE OF ECHOCARDIOGRAPHY: TRANSTHORACIC VERSUS TRANSESOPHAGEAL ECHOCARDIOGRAPHY
Left-Sided Infective Endocarditis

Whenever IE is suspected, echocardiography is the first-line, gold-standard technique for the assessment of the diagnosis. The choice between transthoracic echocardiography (TTE) and transesophageal echocardiography (TEE) has been widely debated in the literature and often is not easy in clinical practice. Indeed, TTE is a fast, widely spread, noninvasive, and inexpensive technique, but it is affected by a low sensitivity, which ranges between 70% and 50% in patients with native and prosthetic valves, respectively. On the contrary, TEE is an invasive, more expensive, and less available technique that provides more reliable elements for the diagnosis of endocarditis, with a sensitivity that ranges between 96% and 92% in patients with native and prosthetic valves, respectively.[6] However, the wide availability of TTE and the need for a rapid diagnosis in patients with suspected endocarditis make TTE the first-line technique of choice in almost all patients. Indeed, Young and associates[7] reported that a fast diagnosis of IE impacts significantly on outcomes and complications; they compared the rate of complications in patients who underwent echocardiography late (≥4 days) and early (<4 days) and found that significantly more embolic events and severe valve destruction requiring valve surgery occurred when echocardiography was performed late. Moreover, it has been reported that clear leaflet visualization[8] and the use of strict criteria to exclude IE[9] significantly increase TTE sensitivity, particularly in patients with native valves without intracardiac devices. Furthermore, TTE is better than TEE for detecting anterior cardiac abscesses and for hemodynamic assessment of valvular dysfunction.[10] These data explain why the current guidelines[11,12] suggest the use of TTE in all patients as a first screening approach, although TTE may be negative or inconclusive in almost 30% of cases, especially in the presence of prosthetic valves or intracardiac electronic devices. It has been stated that when TTE findings are negative, image quality is optimal, and the risk profile of the patient is low, TEE can be safely delayed.[11,12] Thus, in this context, the pretest probability of the disease plays a central role in the diagnostic management of the patient. Several scores have been proposed for the assessment of risk of endocarditis to help the physician choose the most appropriate echocardiographic technique to avoid loss of time and money.[13–15] In particular, Palraj and coworkers[14] recently proposed a two-step scoring system for patients with *S. aureus* bacteremia that takes into account the mode of bacteremia acquisition, the presence of cardiac devices, and the duration of the bacteremia. This score, subsequently tested and modified by Longobardo and colleagues,[15] who included intravenous drug abuse as an element strongly correlated with endocarditis, identified patients at low risk for endocarditis, for whom a negative TTE safely excluded the diagnosis.

TABLE 114.1 Modified Duke Criteria for the Diagnosis of Infective Endocarditis

Major Criteria
BLOOD CULTURES POSITIVE FOR IE
Typical microorganisms consistent with IE from two separate blood cultures: • Viridans streptococci, *Streptococcus bovis*, HACEK group, *Staphylococcus aureus* or community-acquired enterococci in the absence of a primary focus • *Or* microorganisms consistent with IE from persistently positive blood cultures: at least two positive cultures of blood samples drawn >12 hours apart • *Or* All of three or a majority of four or more separate cultures of blood (with first and last sample drawn at least 1 hour apart) • *Or* single positive blood culture for *Coxiella burnetii* or phase I IgG antibody titer >1:800
EVIDENCE OF ENDOCARDIAL INVOLVEMENT
• Echocardiography positive for IE: vegetation, abscess, new partial dehiscence of prosthetic valve • New valvular regurgitation
MINOR CRITERIA
• Predisposition: predisposing heart condition, injection drug use • Fever: temperature >38°C • Vascular phenomena: major arterial emboli, septic pulmonary infarcts, mycotic aneurysm, intracranial hemorrhages, conjunctival hemorrhages, Janeway lesions • Immunologic phenomena: glomerulonephritis, Osler nodes, Roth spots, rheumatoid factor • Microbiological evidence: positive blood culture but does not meet a major criterion or serologic evidence of active infection with organism consistent with IE

Diagnosis of IE is definite in the presence of:	Diagnosis of IE is possible in the presence of:
• Two major criteria • *Or* one major and three minor criteria • *Or* five minor criteria	• One major and one minor criterion • *Or* three minor criteria

HACEK, Haemophilus spp., Aggregatibacter spp., Cardiobacterium hominis, Eikenella corrodens, and *Kingella spp.; IE,* infective endocarditis.
Adapted from Li JS, et al: Proposed modifications to the Duke criteria for the diagnosis of infective endocarditis, *Clin Infect Dis* 30:633–638, 2000.

Because of its better image quality and higher sensitivity, TEE should be considered the gold-standard echocardiographic technique for the detection of endocarditis. Indeed, the current guidelines suggest performing a TEE in case of negative TTE when there is a high index of suspicion for IE, when TTE is of suboptimal quality or in cases of positive TTE to rule out local complications.[11,12] Indeed, it has been widely demonstrated that TEE has significantly better accuracy in the detection of endocarditis, particularly in patients with prosthetic valves or intracardiac devices (Fig. 114.1).[16,17]

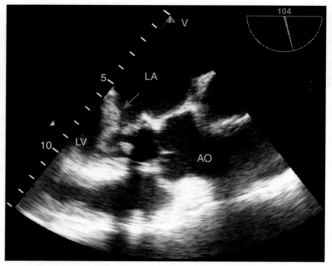

Figure 114.1. Transesophageal echocardiogram showing a big, mobile vegetation attached to the ventricular side of a biological mitral prosthesis *(red arrow)* and protruding into the left ventricular outflow tract. *AO,* Aorta; *LA,* left atrium; *LV,* left ventricle.

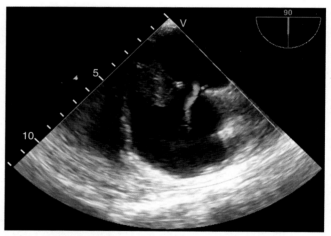

Figure 114.2. Transesophageal echocardiogram showing a big, round, mobile mass adherent to the right side of the interatrial septum near the junction of the inferior vena cava and right atrium. On color Doppler echocardiography, a left-to-right shunt at the level of the fossa ovalis also can be detected.

On the contrary, there are not clear results about the role of three-dimensional (3D) echocardiography in the diagnosis of endocarditis. It has been recently reported that 3D TEE showed greater accuracy in the detection of vegetations and in the quantification of vegetation size,[18,19] and particularly in patients with prosthetic valves, it improves the evaluation of periannular extensions of the disease, providing better delineation of the anatomical relationship of the proximal coronary arteries.[20] On the other hand, Pfister and coworkers[21] reported that in their cohort of patients, 3D TEE showed substantial lower sensitivity and negative predictive value for the diagnosis of IE compared with 2D TEE. Thus, further data about the effectiveness of 3D TEE are needed in this population of patients.

Right-Sided Infective Endocarditis

Right-sided IE shows different features compared with left-sided IE (Fig. 114.2). Patients with right-sided IE are usually younger, more frequently have antecedents of intravenous drug use or intracardiac

TABLE 114.2 Complications of Infective Endocarditis: Comparative Utility of Two-Dimensional Transthoracic Echocardiography Versus Two- or Three-Dimensional Transesophageal Echocardiography

Complication	2D TTE	2D TEE/3D TEE
Cardiac or paravalvular abscess	Echo-dense, thick-walled, or focal echolucency that commonly involves the aortic root Poor sensitivity; better visualization of anterior PV abscesses	Enhanced visualization of mitral annulus or valve, mitral–aortic intervalvular fibrosa; may detect septal abscess with more accuracy Better visualization of posterior PV aortic abscesses
Myocardial abscess	Single or multiple focal areas of myocardial depression; poor sensitivity	Will detect with much higher efficacy; 3D TEE has been shown to be effective on a case-by-case basis
Perforation or intracardiac fistulization or regurgitation	Result of abscess → pseudoaneurysm → rupture Regurgitant jet or turbulent flow will be visualized on color or Doppler flow; suboptimal for small perforation or intracardiac fistulization	Enhanced visualization of mitral–aortic leaflet perforation; 3D TEE can be helpful in diagnosing fistulas, abscesses, and small perforations missed on 2D TEE
Pseudoaneurysm	Presence of extraventricular cavity commonly involving the LV; bulging of aneurysm in systole; poor sensitivity	Enhanced detection of pseudoaneurysm; 3D TEE may provide additional anatomic information
Valve aneurysm	Focal saccular outpouching of valve; limited efficacy	Enhanced detection of aortic and mitral valve involvement

2D, Two-dimensional; *3D,* three-dimensional; *LV,* left ventricle; *PV,* prosthetic valve; *TEE,* transesophageal echocardiography; *TTE,* transthoracic echocardiography.
From Afonso L, et al: Echocardiography in infective endocarditis: State of the art, *Curr Cardiol Rep* 19):127, 2017.

devices, are more affected by *S. aureus*, have larger vegetations, have fewer periannular complications, and have better outcomes.[22] In this setting, San Roman and associates[23] reported that the effectiveness of TTE is quite similar to that of TEE in patients without intracardiac devices. The authors speculated that the good accuracy of TTE in the detection of right-sided endocarditis could be attributable to the younger age and the better acoustic window of typical drug abusers, the larger dimensions of vegetations, and the fact that right-sided vegetations are anterior structures that are closer to the transthoracic probe than to the transesophageal probe. However, these data are in contrast with data reported by other authors[24,25] who found a reduced effectiveness of TTE in the detection of endocarditis, especially of vegetations of the Eustachian valve, an uncommon entity that is often underdiagnosed. The accuracy of TTE is significantly lower in patients with intracardiac devices. In this subgroup of patients, the TTE sensitivity has been estimated to be 25%, whereas it is 84% for TEE.[23] These findings can be explained by the fact that intracardiac leads induce reverberations and artifacts that hinder the identification of a vegetation and that vegetations are frequently attached to the leads at the level of the superior vena cava or the upper part of the right atrium, areas that cannot be confidently seen by TTE.[23] Accordingly, TEE is mandatory in these patients when endocarditis is suspected.

COMPLICATIONS OF INFECTIVE ENDOCARDITIS

Although concordance between TTE and TEE is sufficient, immediate TEE should be performed in patients with a moderate or high likelihood of IE when at high risk for complications such as those with prolonged symptoms, hemodynamic instability, new onset of congestive heart failure, or new conduction abnormalities.[2,6]

A high incidence (30%–50%) of embolic events is reported in patients with IE, more so in cerebral circulation, and the role of echocardiography is pivotal for the evaluation of embolic risk through vegetation size and mobility.[26] In particular, vegetation length is a strong predictor of embolism, and the protective effect of surgical management within 48 hours is demonstrated in

patients with a vegetation larger than 10 mm associated with severe regurgitation.[27]

TEE is the echocardiographic technique of choice for the assessment of complications of endocarditis (Table 114.2).[28] Extravalvular extension of infection occurs most commonly in prosthetic valve–related IE in the form of periannular abscesses, often resulting in dehiscence of the prosthetic valve or paravalvular fistulae. Abscess formation in the context of native-valve IE is usually a complication of aortic valve infection, often involving the aortic annulus, mitral–aortic intervalvular fibrosa, the aortoseptal junction, or atrioventricular conduction pathways, and possibly leading to heart block.[3] The sensitivity and specificity for the diagnosis of a paravalvular abscess have been estimated at 28% and 98%, respectively, for TTE and 87% and 95%, respectively, for TEE[29]; for the diagnosis of fistulae, the sensitivity of TTE and TEE is estimated at 50% and 97%, respectively.[30]

Development of new or worsening congestive heart failure can be caused by acute valve regurgitation because of valve perforation. In this setting, TEE showed a sensitivity of 95% and a specificity of 98% compared with TTE, which had a sensitivity of 45% and specificity of 95% for the diagnosis.[31]

Finally, a rare but dangerous complication of endocarditis is the formation of a pseudoaneurysm, often placed in the region of the mitral–aortic intervalvular fibrosa and sometimes complicated by rupture into the left atrium, aorta, or pericardial space, leading to hemopericardium, tamponade, and death. TTE showed a sensitivity of 43% in the detection of pseudoaneurysm, whereas TEE had a sensitivity of nearly 100%.[32]

Please access ExpertConsult to view the corresponding videos for this chapter.

Acknowledgments

The authors gratefully acknowledge Susan Nord and Jennifer Pfaff for their editorial assistance and Brian Miller and Brian Schurrer for their help with the figures. We also thank Drs. Maria C. Todaro, Concetta Zito, and Scipione Carerj for their contributions to the previous edition of this chapter.

REFERENCES

1. Connolly K, Ong G, Kuhlmann M, et al. Use of the valve visualization on echocardiography grade tool improves sensitivity and negative predictive value of transthoracic echocardiogram for exclusion of native valvular vegetation. *J Am Soc Echocardiogr.* 2019;32:1551–1557.
2. Longobardo L, Zito C, Carerj S, et al. Role of echocardiography in assessment of cardioembolic sources: a strong diagnostic resource in patients with ischemic stroke. *Curr Cardiol Rep.* 2018;20:136.
3. Young WJ, Jeffery DA, Hua A, et al. Echocardiography in patients with infective endocarditis and the impact of diagnostic delays on clinical outcomes. *Am J Cardiol.* 2018;122:650–655.
4. Afonso L, Kottam A, Reddy V, et al. Echocardiography in infective endocarditis: State of the art. *Curr Cardiol Rep.* 2017;19:127.
5. Longobardo L, Klemm S, Cook M, et al. Risk assessment for infected endocarditis in Staphylococcus aureus bacteremia patients: when is transesophageal echocardiography needed? *Eur Heart J Acute Cardiovasc Care.* 2019;8:476–484.
6. Bai AD, Steinberg M, Showler A, et al. Diagnostic accuracy of transthoracic echocardiography for infective endocarditis findings using transesophageal echocardiography as the reference standard: a meta-analysis. *J Am Soc Echocardiogr.* 2017;30:639–646.
7. Pfister R, Betton Y, Freyhaus HT, et al. Three-dimensional compared to two-dimensional transesophageal echocardiography for diagnosis of infective endocarditis. *Infection.* 2016;44:725–731.
8. Sivak JA, Vora AN, Navar AM, et al. An approach to improve the negative predictive value and clinical utility of transthoracic echocardiography in suspected native valve infective endocarditis. *J Am Soc Echocardiogr.* 2016;29:315–322.
9. Baddour LM, Wilson WR, Bayer AS, et al. Infective endocarditis in adults: diagnosis, antimicrobial therapy, and management of complications. *Circulation.* 2015;132:1435–1486.
10. Lindner JR. Role of echocardiographic imaging in infective endocarditis. *ACC Curr J Rev.* 2002;11:40–43.
11. Cahill TJ, Prendergast BD. Infective endocarditis. *Lancet.* 2016;387:882–893.
12. Habib G, Lancellotti P, Antunes MJ, et al. ESC guidelines for the management of infective endocarditis. *Eur Heart J.* 2015;36:3075–3128. 2015.
13. Palraj BR, Baddour LM, Hess EP, et al. Predicting Risk of Endocarditis Using a Clinical Tool (PREDICT): scoring system to guide use of echocardiography in the management of staphylococcus aureus bacteremia. *Clin Infect Dis.* 2015;61:18–28.
14. Roldan CA, Tolstrup K, Macias L, et al. Libman-Sacks endocarditis: detection, characterization, and clinical correlates by three-dimensional transesophageal echocardiography. *J Am Soc Echocardiogr.* 2015;28:770–7799.
15. Tanis W, Teske AJ, van Herwerden LA, et al. The additional value of three-dimensional transesophageal echocardiography in complex aortic prosthetic heart valve endocarditis. *Echocardiography.* 2015;32:114–125.
16. Slipczuk L, Codolosa JN, Davila CD, et al. Infective endocarditis epidemiology over five decades: a systematic review. *PloS One.* 2013;8. e82665.
17. Thuny F, Gaubert JY, Jacquier A, et al. Imaging investigations in infective endocarditis: current approach and perspectives. *Arch Cardiovasc Dis.* 2013;106:52–62.
18. San Román JA, Vilacosta I, López J, et al. Role of transthoracic and transesophageal echocardiography in right-sided endocarditis: one echocardiographic modality does not fit all. *J Am Soc Echocardiogr.* 2012;25:807–814.
19. Thuny F, Grisoli D, Collart F, et al. Management of infective endocarditis: challenges and perspectives. *Lancet.* 2012;379:965–975.
20. Kaasch AJ, Fowler Jr VG, Rieg S, et al. Use of a simple criteria set for guiding echocardiography in nosocomial Staphylococcus aureus bacteremia. *Clin Infect Dis.* 2011;53:1–9.
21. Sudhakar S, Sewani A, Agrawal M, et al. Pseudoaneurysm of the mitral-aortic intervalvular fibrosa (MAIVF): a comprehensive review. *J Am Soc Echocardiogr.* 2010;23:1009–1018.
22. Habib G, Badano L, Tribouilloy C, et al. Recommendations for the practice of echocardiography in infective endocarditis. *Eur J Echocardiogr.* 2010;11:202–219.
23. Anguera I, Miro JM, San Roman JA, et al. Periannular complications in infective endocarditis involving prosthetic aortic valves. *Am J Cardiol.* 2006;98:1261–1268.
24. Bashore TM, Cabell C, Fowler Jr V. Update on infective endocarditis. *Curr Probl Cardiol.* 2006;31:274–352.
25. Thuny F, Di Salvo G, Belliard O, et al. Risk of embolism and death in infective endocarditis: prognostic value of echocardiography: a prospective multicenter study. *Circulation.* 2005;112:69–75.
26. Baddour LM, Wilson WR, Bayer AS, et al. Infective endocarditis: diagnosis, antimicrobial therapy, and management of complications. *Circulation.* 2005;111:e394–e434.
27. San Román JA, Vilacosta I, Sarriá C, et al. Eustachian valve endocarditis: is it worth searching for. *Am Heart J.* 2001;142:1037–1040.
28. Sawhney N, Palakodeti V, Raisinghani A, et al. Eustachian valve endocarditis: a case series and analysis of the literature. *J Am Soc Echocardiogr.* 2001;14:1139–1142.
29. De Castro S, Cartoni D, d'Amati G, et al. Diagnostic accuracy of transthoracic and multiplane transesophageal echocardiography for valvular perforation in acute infective endocarditis: correlation with anatomic findings. *Clin Infect Dis.* 2000;30:825–826.
30. De Castro S, Magni G, Beni S, et al. Role of transthoracic and transesophageal echocardiography in predicting embolic events in patients with active infective endocarditis involving native cardiac valves. *Am J Cardiol.* 1997;80:1030–1034.
31. San Román JA, Vilacosta I, Zamorano JL, et al. Transesophageal echocardiography in right-sided endocarditis. *J Am Coll Cardiol.* 1993;21:1226–1230.
32. Daniel WG, Mügge A, Martin RP, et al. Improvement in the diagnosis of abscesses associated with endocarditis by transesophageal echocardiography. *N Engl J Med.* 1991;324:795–800.

115 Echocardiography for Prediction of Cardioembolic Risk

Ferande Peters, Bijoy K. Khandheria, Muhamed Saric

SPECTRUM OF CARDIOEMBOLISM

The heart and the aorta are the sources of cardioembolism to any organ. Major clinical presentations involve either acute neurologic dysfunction—transient ischemic attack (TIA) or stroke—or peripheral vascular disease (e.g., acute limb ischemia, splenic or renal infarcts). All cardioembolic causes of TIA or stroke may also cause acute limb ischemia or organ infarcts, with additional thromboembolic sources being thrombus and atheroma in the descending thoracic and abdominal aorta. In 2016, the American Society of Echocardiography (ASE) issued comprehensive guidelines on the use of echocardiography for the evaluation of a cardiac source of emboli.[1]

Stroke

Stroke is the third leading cause of death in developed countries.[2,3] The most common type of stroke is ischemic, which accounts for approximately 85% of all strokes. The TOAST criteria are a useful epidemiologic tool to classify stroke.[4,5] Cardioembolic strokes by the TOAST criteria fall into either category 2 (proven cardioembolic strokes) or category 4 (cryptogenic strokes) (Table 115.1). ASGOD is an alternative stroke classification that expands on the TOAST concept by including the likelihood of a potential cardiac or aortic source to cause a stroke (Table 115.2). For instance, a patient with mitral valve endocarditis presenting with stroke would be classified as an ASCOD category C1 (probably cardioembolic cause).[6]

Cardioembolic strokes account for 15% to 30% of ischemic strokes.[7] The outcome of cardioembolic stroke is poor, with a 3-year mortality rate of almost 50% in some instances.[8–10] Cardiac and aortic sources have different embolic potential (Table 115.3). Intracardiac thrombi, vegetations, and tumors as well as aortic atheroma have high embolic potential. In contrast, some valvular pathologies (e.g., calcific aortic stenosis, mitral annular calcifications, and Lambl excrescences), abnormalities of the

TABLE 115.1 Classification of Ischemic Strokes by the TOAST Criteria

TOAST Subtype	Description	Relative Prevalence (%)
1. Large vessel stroke	Significant stenosis or occlusion of a large cervical or cerebral artery presumably caused by atherosclerosis	16
2. Cardioembolic stroke	Cerebral vessel occlusion caused by embolus arising in the heart (and thoracic aorta)	29
3. Small-vessel stroke	Lacunar brain infarcts	16
4. Cryptogenic stroke	Stroke of unknown cause	36
5. Stroke from other known causes	Vasculopathies, hypercoagulable states, and so on	3

Adapted from Adams HP Jr, et al: Classification of subtype of acute ischemic stroke. Definitions for use in a multicenter clinical trial. TOAST. Trial of Org 10172 in Acute Stroke Treatment, *Stroke* 24:35–41, 1993; and Petty GW, et al: Ischemic stroke subtypes: a population-based study of incidence and risk factors, *Stroke* 30:2513–2516, 1999.

TABLE 115.2 ASCOD Classification of Ischemic Strokes

	Stoke Type		Causality Likelihood Grade
A	Atherosclerosis	1	Potential
S	Small-vessel disease	2	Possible but uncertain
C	Cardioembolic	3	Unlikely
O	Other	0	Absent
D	Dissection	9	Nondiagnostic workup

Adapted from Amarenco P, et al: The ASCOD phenotyping of ischemic stroke (Updated ASCO Phenotyping), *Cerebrovasc Dis* 36:1–5, 2013.

TABLE 115.3 Cardiac Sources of Emboli and Their Embolic Potential[a]

High Risk Potential	Moderate Risk Potential

• **THROMBI**
  • Atrial fibrillation
  • Myocardial infarction
  • Cardiomyopathies
  • Mechanical prosthetic valves
• **VEGETATIONS**
  • Valvular and nonvalvular infective endocarditis
• **TUMORS**
  • Myxoma
  • Papillary fibroelastoma
• **AORTIC ATHEROMA**
	• **THROMBI AND SIMILAR PATHOLOGIES**
	  • "Smoke" and "sludge"
	  • Mitral stenosis with sinus rhythm
	  • Atrial flutter
	• **VALVULAR DISEASE**
	  • Bioprosthetic valves
	  • Giant Lambl excrescence
	  • Calcific aortic stenosis
	  • Mitral annular calcifications
	  • Mitral valve prolapse
	  • Nonbacterial thrombotic endocarditis
	• **ATRIAL SEPTUM**
	  • Atrial septal aneurysm
	  • Patent foramen ovale

[a]Cardiac sources differ in their embolic potential.

BOX 115.1 Brain Imaging Clues to Possible Cardioembolism

- Presence of older previous infarcts
- Multiple infarcts, especially in different arterial territories
- Hemorrhagic infarcts
- Infarct showing cortical extension
- Large lenticulostriate infarct
- Classic embolic sites
- Stem occlusion of the middle cerebral artery
- Bilateral sylvian fissure infarcts

The diagnostic yield of echocardiography in elucidating a cause of stroke depends on the clinical likelihood and findings on brain imaging (Box 115.1). Cardioembolism is a very likely cause of systemic embolism when one or more of the following is observed: (1) multiple organs are affected (e.g., brain, kidney, spleen), (2) multiple vascular territories are involved (infarcts in the territories of the right renal artery; left middle cerebral artery, right posterior cerebral artery), and (3) ischemic strokes and organ infarcts occurring at multiple time points (a combination of acute, subacute and chronic lesions).

Cardioembolic Stroke: Clinical and Neuroimaging Context

A complete medical history provides important clues to the possibility of cardioembolism. The abrupt onset of neurologic dysfunction with maximum deficit at the onset and absence of a stuttering course and a severe headache are important clues that suggest cardioembolism. Seizures that accompany such a presentation also may suggest cardioembolism. These clinical features are not always diagnostic because emboli fragment and reocclusion may present in a nonabrupt manner in some instances.[11]

Brain imaging, either computed tomography or magnetic resonance imaging, provides useful clues to the presence of a possible embolic presentation (see Box 115.1). Additional clues include a history of palpitations or documented atrial fibrillation (AF) or other signs of systemic embolism involving other organs. Some studies have suggested that the most specific features for cardioembolism are infarcts in multiple territories and concurrent systemic embolism.[12,13] In the absence of other competing mechanisms of stroke, clinical and brain imaging data must be combined to identify the potential cardioembolic pathology. Thus, finding concomitant low-risk pathology, such as fibrin strands or uncomplicated mitral valve prolapse, cannot be used to infer causality. An important part of the evaluation is to identify the presence of increased intracranial pressure because this may be a

interatrial septum (e.g., atrial septal aneurysm or patent foramen ovale [PFO]), and conditions of blood stasis (e.g., "smoke" and sludge) have a moderate embolic risk.

Echocardiography is essential for the evaluation, diagnosis, and management of stroke and systemic embolism. The 2016 guidelines on the use of echocardiography in the evaluation of a cardiac source of emboli provide comprehensive recommendations for both transthoracic echocardiography (TTE) and transesophageal echocardiography (TEE). They provide three levels of recommendations for each category of potential causes of cardioembolism: echocardiography recommended, echocardiography potentially useful, and echocardiography not recommended.

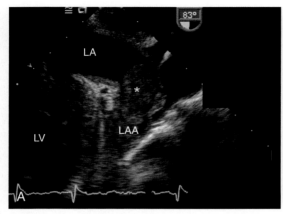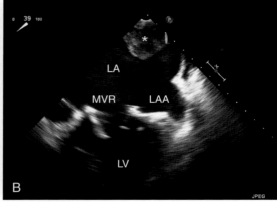

Figure 115.1. Cardioembolism: atrial fibrillation–related thrombi. **A,** Large mobile thrombus *(asterisk)* in the left atrial appendage in a patient with nonvalvular atrial fibrillation. **B,** Large sessile thrombus arising from the posterior left atrial wall in a patient with valvular atrial fibrillation with a history of rheumatic mitral stenosis and surgical mitral valve replacement. *LA,* Left atrium; *LAA,* left atrial appendage; *LV,* left ventricle; *MVR,* bioprosthetic mitral valve replacement. (See accompanying Video 115.1.)

relative contraindication against the use of early TEE in low-risk patients or patients with a normal TTE. Inappropriate agitation or straining during the procedure may worsen increased intracranial pressure.

Cryptogenic Stroke

Stroke presumed to be cryptogenic may have an embolic component that may not be considered based on clinical assessment but may become more obvious after TTE. The link with PFO is well established in this population, especially in those 55 years of age and younger. However, causality is more difficult to prove, and the outcome of intervention (closure of PFO) in the absence of recurrent neurologic events is questionable.

ECHOCARDIOGRAPHIC EVALUATION

TTE is the first-line imaging modality for evaluating cardioembolism because it is widely available, portable, cost effective, and, with the use of harmonic imaging and contrast, enables most predisposing factors to cardioembolism to be evaluated. TTE should be geared toward identifying three major pathophysiological predispositions. First, a careful, systematic, anatomical evaluation should occur to identify masses, such as thrombus, tumors, and vegetations within the heart, and atheroma and its complications within the aorta. Conditions that predispose to thrombus formation, such as old myocardial infarcts, severe left ventricular (LV) dysfunction, and valvular disease (e.g., mitral stenosis), should be explored. Last, a systematic evaluation to exclude conditions that serve as conduits for possible paradoxical embolism, such as PFO and atrial septal defect, should be performed.

TEE is superior to TTE in identifying thrombus within the left atrial appendage (LAA) and smaller vegetations and in the evaluation of prosthetic valves for thrombus or endocarditis. Contrast or agitated saline contrast to identify shunts may be used to enhance clinical decision making. TEE also may be required to evaluate patients for shunts that may predispose to paradoxical embolism, such as PFO and small atrial septal defects, and is useful in identifying thoracic aortic problems, such as thrombus, atherosclerotic plaques, and aortic dissection. A normal TTE may warrant further investigation by TEE if the suspicion or clinical presentation of cardioembolism is high because many of the aforementioned pathologies may be better identified using this latter technique.

SPECIFIC CARDIOEMBOLIC CLINICAL SITUATIONS
Atrial Fibrillation

AF is the most common predisposition to cardioembolism. Echocardiography is crucial in differentiating whether AF is valvular or nonvalvular. This distinction is important because the risk of stroke is much higher with valvular AF, and therapy may differ, such as in the use of novel anticoagulants, which currently are indicated only in nonvalvular AF. Valvular AF generally refers to AF in the setting of moderate to severe mitral stenosis (potentially requiring surgical intervention) or in the presence of an artificial (mechanical) heart valve. Nonvalvular AF does not imply absence of valvular heart disease; rather, it refers to AF in the absence of moderate to severe mitral stenosis or a mechanical heart valve.[14]

Furthermore, when assessing patients with nonvalvular AF for the use of anticoagulation using the CHA2DS2 VASc score, identifying LV hypertrophy and a low ejection fraction is important and may influence clinical decision making.[15] CHA2DS2-VASc is an acronym that refers to C: Congestive heart failure (or left ventricular systolic dysfunction); H: Hypertension: blood pressure consistently above 140/90 mmHg (or treated hypertension on medication); A2: Age ≥75 years; D: Diabetes Mellitus; S2: Prior Stroke or TIA or thromboembolism; V: Vascular disease (e.g., peripheral artery disease, myocardial infarction, aortic plaque); A: Age 65–74 years; Sc: Sex category (i.e., female sex); each parameter is worth 1 point except for A2 and S2 which are worth 2 points. The most common site of thrombus formation is the LAA (especially in nonvalvular AF), although thrombus may be found anywhere within the left atrium. Thrombi in the body of the left atrium is more likely to occur in valvular AF than nonvalvular AF (Fig. 115.1). Left atrial (LA) and LAA thrombi may occur in situations that may cause stasis within the LAA, such as mitral stenosis, even in the presence of sinus rhythm.

Left Heart Thrombus

Thrombus is a discrete echo-dense mass with defined margins that are distinct from the underlying wall. Ideally, thrombus should be seen in two different views. Thrombus causing systemic thromboembolism may be found in the left ventricle, left atrium, or LAA. TTE is best to visualize thrombus within the left ventricle because TEE is often inadequate to assess the LV apex, which is frequently foreshortened and in the far field.

LV thrombus usually occurs when the underlying walls are abnormal (i.e., either hypokinetic or akinetic) or in aneurysms (Fig. 115.2). In a postinfarction aneurysm, LV thrombus may be found

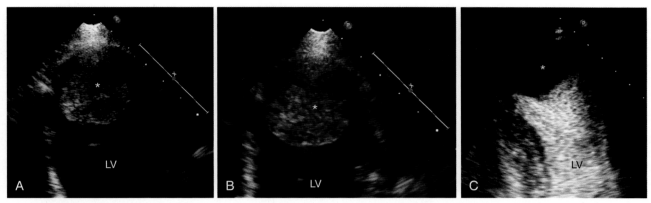

Figure 115.2. Cardioembolism: left ventricular (LV) thrombus. A large mobile thrombus *(asterisk)* arising from the akinetic LV apex in a patient with a history of myocardial infarction in the left anterior descending coronary artery presenting with stroke. The thrombus is visualized by noncontrast two-dimensional (2D) TTE (**A**), three-dimensional TTE (**B**), and (**C**) microbubble contrast-enhanced 2D TTE. (See accompanying Video 115.2.)

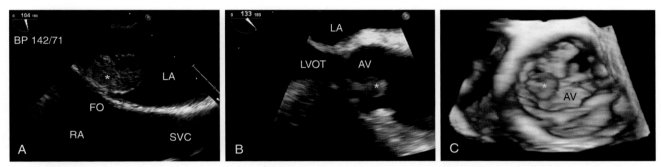

Figure 115.3. Cardioembolism: tumors. **A,** Two-dimensional (2D) transesophageal echocardiography (TEE) demonstrates a left atrial myxoma *(asterisk)* at its most common location attached to the fossa ovalis (FO). **B,** 2D TEE demonstrates a papillary fibroelastoma *(asterisk)* on the aortic side of the aortic valve (AV). **C,** Three-dimensional TEE demonstrates a highly mobile papillary fibroelastoma *(asterisk)* attached to the noncoronary cusp of the aortic valve. *LA,* Left atrium; *LVOT,* left ventricular outflow tract; *RA,* right atrium; *SVC,* superior vena cava. (See accompanying Video 115.3.)

in up to 50% of cases.[16] If the thrombus is found on an underlying normal wall, it may represent a manifestation of a hypercoagulable state or, far less commonly, thrombus in transit from another site. Attention to detailed global and regional wall assessment of the left ventricle are required to identify not only wall abnormalities but also the overlying thrombus. This may require off-axis two-dimensional (2D) TTE, biplane TTE imaging, or three-dimensional (3D) TTE. When the apex or walls cannot be adequately visualized, the use of contrast is mandatory to improve thrombus detection and function assessment.[17,18] LV thrombi must be distinguished from false tendons, trabeculae, and artifact. The exclusion of tumors can occasionally be challenging because a tumor may develop over the thrombus. Cardioembolism is a common complication in isolated LV noncompaction, but vigilance in identifying the thrombus and distinguishing it from trabeculation is required. After LV thrombus identification, evaluation of whether it is layered, calcified, pedunculated, or mobile or has central lucency will help determine the age of the thrombus. A central lucency may be associated with more recently formed thrombus and have greater potential for cardioembolism. It is also important to note that the mechanism of thrombus may not just relate to the underlying anatomical abnormality, but if there is concomitant stasis as in low ejection fraction or a possible accompanying hypercoagulable state (e.g., peripartum cardiomyopathy), LV thrombus is more likely to occur.

Masses

The most common masses encountered within the left heart are malignant metastatic tumors, including metastatic lung, breast, and prostate tumors; melanoma; and lymphoma. By the time cardiac involvement occurs, there usually is evidence of widespread tumor metastases. Metastatic tumors involving the heart may be associated with brain metastases, which may occasionally mimic the clinical presentation of a stroke. Primary tumors may rarely present as cardioembolic strokes and occur because of either detachment of tumor or emboli of superimposed thrombi.[19,20] The most common tumors are myxoma, which is commonly found attached via a pedicle to the interatrial septum, and, less commonly, papillary fibroelastoma, which is attached to valve leaflet (Fig. 115.3).

Resection of these tumors prevents stroke recurrence if successfully performed. It may be challenging to differentiate tumor from thrombus at times. The presence of a hemorrhagic pericardial effusion, mass extension into the underlying myocardium, and an irregular edge are clues that a tumor is more likely the culprit. However, if there is no widespread evidence of a tumor or classic features of certain benign tumors, cardiac magnetic resonance imaging may improve the ability to differentiate thrombus from tumor noninvasively.

Endocarditis

Echocardiography is important in diagnosing endocarditis as the source of cardioembolism. Vegetation, abscess, or new dehiscence of a prosthetic valve are major echocardiographic features that satisfy the Duke criteria for the diagnosis of infective endocarditis and point to the source of the cardioembolism within the right clinical context. To identify vegetations, TEE is superior to TTE in identifying smaller vegetations and those on prosthetic valves, which often are missed with TTE. Echocardiography also plays a role in

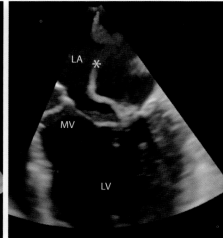

Figure 115.4. Cardioembolism: endocarditis. Hybrid two-dimensional–three-dimensional transesophageal echocardiography imaging (reference plane [RP] thickness imaging) demonstrates a massive vegetation on the atrial side of the mitral valve in a patient with *Streptococcus agalactiae* bacteremia presenting with stroke. (See accompanying Video 115.4.)

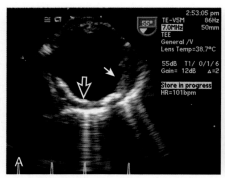
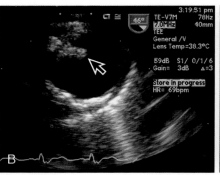
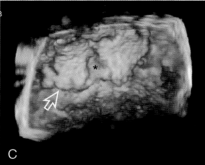

Figure 115.5. Embolism: aortic atheroma. **A,** Upper esophageal two-dimensional (2D) transesophageal echocardiography (TEE) view demonstrates severe nonmobile plaque *(thin arrow)* in the aortic arch that is partly calcified *(thick arrow)*. **B,** Upper esophageal 2D TEE view shows a mobile plaque in the aortic arch; the mobile component represents an overlying thrombus. **C,** Three-dimensional TEE reveals an en face view of a complex plaque *(arrow)* in the aortic arch with a larger central ulceration *(asterisk)*. (Reprinted with permission from Saric M, et al: Guidelines for the use of echocardiography in the evaluation of a cardiac source of embolism, *J Am Soc Echocardiogr* 29:1–42, 2016.) (See accompanying Video 115.5.)

providing information to predict cardioembolism. Vegetations typically larger than 10 mm located on the mitral valve may be useful in predicting cardioembolism (Fig. 115.4).[21] Recent data suggest that the use of 3D TEE is superior to that of 2D TEE in predicting vegetation size and the risk of cardioembolism.[22]

Aortic Pathology

The most important link to stroke involves the detection of complex aortic plaque. This may be defined as a plaque larger than 4 mm that may be protruding, mobile, or ulcerated. These plaques occur more commonly in the descending aorta and have been linked to cardioembolic stroke as well as peripheral vascular embolism. They are found more commonly among older patients and patients with traditional atherosclerotic risk factors such as diabetes and dyslipidemia and in up to 35% of patients with nonvalvular AF.[23] Thus, whether these plaques themselves cause cardioembolism or whether they are innocent bystanders in patients whose comorbid conditions may be causing the clinical scenario especially, for example, in stroke, has been debated. A more direct cause may occasionally be inferred when overlying mobile clot is noted overlying these complex aortic plaques (Fig. 115.5). A second scenario, though uncommon, is the syndrome of cholesterol emboli, which may occasionally develop after catheterization or after aortic manipulation.

Shunts

Any anatomic defect that allows left-to-right shunting can predispose to paradoxical embolism. Atrial septal defect or PFO in isolation or in combination with an atrial septal aneurysm is considered a conduit for paradoxical embolism (Fig. 115.6). One of the major problems with this postulate for cardioembolism is that often there is no accompanying evidence of concurrent venous thrombosis in these patients. Thus, with regard to the clinical presentation of stroke, careful cardiac and neurologic evaluations of the patient are required to reach a feasible consensus on whether a conduit is the likely cause of stroke. The technical diagnostic issues and clinical relevance of PFO in cardioembolism are discussed elsewhere in this text.

Prosthetic Valves

Prosthetic valves may predispose to cardioembolism either as a result of thromboemboli from thrombus formation on the valve or as a consequence of prosthetic valve endocarditis. In both instances, TEE is the diagnostic modality of choice, and data obtained must be integrated within the clinical context to make the right diagnosis because differentiating endocarditis from thrombus can occasionally be challenging. Fibrin strands on prosthetic valves in patients with stroke or cardioembolism may be a mechanism for cardioembolism, especially in patients with recurrent cardioembolic events associated with

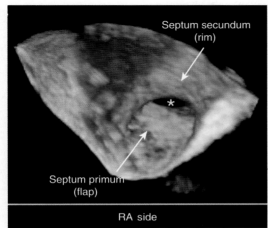
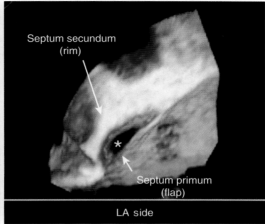

Figure 115.6. Cardioembolism: patent foramen ovale (PFO). Three-dimensional transesophageal echocardiography imaging demonstrates a PFO from the right atrial (RA) and left atrial (LA) side. (See accompanying Video 115.6.)

persistence of these findings. A final but common association is that of paroxysmal AF, which may be the mechanism for cardioembolism and not the valve itself. This may occur in normally functioning prosthetic valves or in a dysfunctional prosthetic valve (e.g., prosthetic valve stenosis caused by pannus or because of severe LV dysfunction that may be unrelated to the current normally functioning prosthetic valve). Thus, echocardiographers need to judiciously evaluate LV and LA anatomy and function in addition to prostheses to carefully unravel any potential mechanism for cardioembolism.

CONDITIONS THAT ARE LOW OR UNCERTAIN RISK FOR CARDIOEMBOLISM

Conditions that are low or uncertain risk for cardioembolism include mitral valve prolapse, mitral annular calcification, aortic sclerosis or stenosis, and prominent Lambl excrescences. No certain causal relationship has been established between these pathologies and cardioembolism because some of these findings may constitute chance findings in normal individuals and be more common in older individuals. In particular, mitral valve prolapse in the absence of significant mitral regurgitation, AF, or associated endocarditis is currently thought not to be associated with an increased risk of stroke.[24,25]

CONCLUSION

Echocardiography is an essential tool in the investigation of patients who may have a clinical presentation that may be related to cardioembolism. The systematic use of various echocardiography techniques allow for a thorough evaluation, and these findings are judiciously integrated into clinical decision making with regard to causation. By using the appropriate clinical decision pathways, the addition of echocardiography offers insight into the pathogenesis, guides therapeutic selection, and may prevent future events and potentially alter the prognosis in certain conditions.

Please access ExpertConsult to view the corresponding videos for this chapter.

REFERENCES

1. Saric M, Armour AA, Arnaout S, et al. Guidelines for the use of echocardiography in the evaluation of a cardiac source of embolism. *J Am Soc Echocardiogr.* 2016;29:1–42.
2. Goldstein LB, Adams R, Alberts MJ, et al. Primary prevention of ischemic stroke. *Stroke.* 2006;37:1583–1633. Erratum in Stroke 38:207, 2007.
3. Sacco RL, Adams R, Albers G, et al. Guidelines for prevention of stroke in patients with ischemic stroke or transient ischemic attack. *Stroke.* 2006;37:577–617.
4. Adams Jr HP, Bendixen BH, Kappelle LJ, et al. Classification of subtype of acute ischemic stroke. Definitions for use in a multicenter clinical trial. TOAST. *Trial of Org 10172 in Acute Stroke Treatment, Stroke.* 1993;24:35–41.
5. GW1 P, Brown Jr RD, Whisnant JP, et al. Ischemic stroke subtypes: a population-based study of incidence and risk factors. *Stroke.* 1999;30:2513–2516.
6. Amarenco P, Bogousslavsky J, Caplan LR, et al. The ASCOD phenotyping of ischemic stroke (Updated ASCO Phenotyping). *Cerebrovasc Dis.* 2013; 36:1–5.
7. Ferro JM. Cardioembolic stroke: an update. *Lancet Neurol.* 2003;2:177–188.
8. Kolominsky-Rabas PL, Weber M, Gefeller O, et al. Epidemiology of ischemic stroke subtypes according to TOAST criteria. *Stroke.* 2001;32:2735–2740.
9. Lip GY, Lim HS. Atrial fibrillation and stroke prevention. *Lancet Neurol.* 2007;6:981–993.
10. de Jong G, van Raak L, Kessels F, et al. Stroke subtype and mortality: a follow-up study in 998 patients with a first cerebral infarct. *J Clin Epidemiol.* 2003;56:262–268.
11. Arboix A, Oliveres M, Massons J, et al. Early differentiation of cardioembolic from atherothrombotic cerebral infarction: a multivariate analysis. *Eur J Neurol.* 1999;6:677–683.
12. Kittner SJ, Sharkness CM, Price TR, et al. Infarcts with a cardiac source of embolism in the NINCDS stroke data bank: historical features. *Neurology.* 1990;40:281–284.
13. Bogousslavsky J, Cachin C, Regli F, et al. Cardiac sources of embolism and cerebral infarction—clinical consequences and vascular concomitants. *Neurology.* 1991;41:855–859.
14. January CT, Wann LS, Calkins H, et al. AHA/ACC/HRS focused update of the 2014 AHA/ACC/HRS guideline for the management of patients with atrial fibrillation. *Heart Rhythm.* 2019;16:e66–e93. 2019.
15. Mason PK, Lake DE, DiMarco JP, et al. Impact of the CHA2DS2-VASc score on anticoagulation recommendations for atrial fibrillation. *Am J Med.* 2012;125:e1–e6.
16. Nihoyannopoulos P, Smith GC, Maseri A, et al. The natural history of left ventricular thrombus in myocardial infarction. *J Am Coll Cardiol.* 1989;14:903–911.
17. Kurt M, Shaikh KA, Peterson L, et al. Impact of contrast echocardiography on evaluation of ventricular function and clinical management in a large prospective cohort. *J Am Coll Cardiol.* 2009;53:802–810.
18. Senior R, Becher H, Monaghan M, et al. Contrast echocardiography: evidence-based recommendations by European Association of Echocardiography. *Eur J Echocardiogr.* 2009;10:194–212.
19. Rahmatullah AF, Rahko PS, Stein JH. Transesophageal echocardiography for the evaluation and management of patients with cerebral ischemia. *Clin Cardiol.* 1999;22:391–396.
20. Reynen K. Cardiac myxomas. *N Engl J Med.* 1995;333:1610–1617.
21. Okonta KE, Adamu YB. What size of vegetation is an indication for surgery in endocarditis. *Interact Cardiovasc Thorac Surg.* 2012;15:1052–1056.
22. Berdejo J, Shibayama K, Harada K, et al. Evaluation of vegetation size and its relationship with embolism in infective endocarditis. *Circ Cardiovasc Imag.* 2014;7:149–154.
23. Transesophageal echocardiographic correlates of thromboembolism in high-risk patients with nonvalvular atrial fibrillation. *Ann Intern Med.* 1998;128:639–647.
24. Nishimura RA, McGoon MD. Perspectives on mitral-valve prolapse. *N Engl J Med.* 1999;341:48–50.
25. Cardiogenic brain embolism. The second report of the cerebral embolism Task Force. *Arch Neurol.* 1989;46:727–743. Erratum in *Arch Neurol* 46:1079, 1989.

116 Limitations and Technical Considerations in Infective Endocarditis

Kate Rankin, Paaladinesh Thavendiranathan

Guidelines recommend echocardiography as the imaging modality of choice in the diagnosis and management guidance in patients with suspected infective endocarditis (IE).[1,2] Although echocardiographic findings lead to definitive diagnosis in the majority of patients, atypical results or results of uncertain clinical significance are not rare. The diagnostic yield and limitations of transthoracic echocardiography (TTE) and transesophageal echocardiography (TEE) depend on several factors, including (1) image quality, (2) the specific pathology associated with endocarditis (i.e., vegetations, valvular dysfunction or perivalvular extension), (3) the presence of prosthetic valve or device involvement, and (4) the index of clinical suspicion in the patient being investigated.

ECHOCARDIOGRAPHY IN DIAGNOSIS OF NATIVE VALVE INFECTIVE ENDOCARDITIS

Early studies demonstrated that M-mode echocardiography was able to detect approximately one-third of native valve vegetations.[3] With the advent of real-time two-dimensional and more recently three-dimensional (3D) echocardiography along with color and spectral Doppler capabilities, echocardiography is now well established as the gold standard for imaging diagnosis of IE and is incorporated into the modified Duke criteria as a major criterion.[2] Echocardiography is capable of detecting the three major findings involving endocarditis: vegetations, valvular dysfunction and perivalvular extension, with varying accuracy, depending on both patient and imaging factors.

The clinical index of suspicion of endocarditis in a particular patient influences the specificity of TTE and TEE. Clinical index of suspicion is assessed via the Duke criteria, incorporating major (microbiological and echocardiographic) and minor (clinical and microbiological) criteria to categorize presentations into definite, possible or rejected IE.[2,4,5] Current Appropriate Use Criteria guidelines for echocardiography that incorporate clinical suspicion of disease are summarized in Table 116.1. It is recommended that any patient suspected of having IE by appropriate clinical criteria (positive blood cultures or new murmur) should be screened with TTE. If the images are of good quality and the study result is negative in a patient with a low index of clinical suspicion, an alternative diagnosis should be sought. TEE should be performed when clinical suspicion is high (staphylococcal bacteremia, fungemia, prosthetic heart valve or intracardiac device).[6] Additionally, a repeat TEE should be performed 7 to 10 days after the initial study in cases of persisting high index of clinical suspicion and even earlier when indicated by the clinical situation such as suspected postoperative staphylococcal prosthetic valve endocarditis.[7] The importance of applying clinical criteria to determine investigation approach cannot be overstated. Greaves and colleagues demonstrated that the absence of five clinical characteristics (embolic phenomena, central venous access, intravenous drug use, prosthetic valve, and positive blood culture) virtually ruled out that a TTE would demonstrate evidence of endocarditis.[8]

It is essential that the clinician is aware that both TTE and TEE are not 100% sensitive and specific.[9] Depending on the patient population studied, the sensitivity of TTE for detection of native valvular vegetations has been reported to be between 21% and 87%[10–21] (Table 116.2). Echocardiographic diagnosis of IE on TTE is limited by generally accepted limitations of image quality, including patient body habitus, mechanical ventilation, presence of chest wall deformities, and interposing lung tissue.[10] In contrast, TEE is not limited by the aforementioned issues. TEE's superior image quality is the main reason it demonstrates greater diagnostic accuracy compared with TTE, with studies reporting sensitivity ranges between 86% and 100%[10–16,21] for native valvular vegetations (Fig. 116.1).

The use of harmonic imaging improves image quality of TTE compared with fundamental imaging, leading to improved sensitivity; however, it is suboptimal for the assessment of certain complications such as annular abscesses, which are superiorly defined with TEE,[22] particularly in this era of high-frequency, multiplanar probes. The use of 3D echocardiography may further improve the detection of vegetations on transthoracic studies (see Fig. 116.1).[23]

Near-field windows provided by TEE for left-sided aortic and semilunar valves ensure diagnostic superiority of TEE for the assessment of left-sided structures; however, comparatively, the

TABLE 116.1 Appropriate Use Criteria for Transthoracic and Transesophageal Echocardiography According to the 2011 ACCF/ASE/AHA/ASNC/HFSA/HRS/SCAI/SCCM/SCCT/SCMR 2011 Appropriate Use Criteria for Echocardiography

Transthoracic Echocardiography	Appropriate	Score
Initial evaluation of suspected IE with positive blood cultures or new murmur	Yes	9
Transient fever without evidence of bacteremia or a new murmur	No	2
Transient bacteremia with a pathogen not typically associated with IE and/or a documented nonendovascular source of infection	No	3
Reevaluation of IE at high risk for progression or complication or with a change in clinical status or cardiac examination	Yes	9
Routine surveillance of uncomplicated IE when no change in management is contemplated	No	2

Transesophageal Echocardiography	Appropriate	Score
To diagnose IE with a low pretest probability (e.g., transient fever, known alternative source of infection, or negative blood cultures or atypical pathogen for IE)	No	3
To diagnose IE with moderate or high pretest probability (e.g., staphylococcal bacteremia, fungemia, prosthetic heart valve or intracardiac device)	Yes	9

ACCF, American College of Cardiology Foundation; *AHA*, American Heart Association; *ASE*, American Society of Echocardiography; *ASNC*, American Society of Nuclear Cardiology; *HFSA*, Heart Failure Society of America; *HRS*, Heart Rhythm Society; *IE*, infective endocarditis; *SCAI*, Society for Cardiovascular Angiography and Interventions; *SCCT*, Society of Cardiovascular Computed Tomography; *SCCM*, Society of Critical Care Medicine; *SCMR*, Society for Cardiovascular Magnetic Resonance.

TABLE 116.2 Sensitivity and Specificity of Transthoracic and Transesophageal Echocardiography in the Diagnosis of Valvular Vegetations in Native Valve Endocarditis

Study	Patients (n)	Valve	TTE		TEE	
			Sensitivity (%)	Specificity (%)	Sensitivity (%)	Specificity (%)
Erbel et al[10] (1988)	96		63	98	100	98
Shively et al[11] (1991)	62		44	98	94	100
Pedersen et al[12] (1991)	24		50		100	
Birmingham et al[14] (1992)	61	Aortic	25		88	
		Mitral	50		100	
Sochowski et al[13] (1993)	105				91	
Shapiro et al[15] (1994)	64		60	91	87	91
De Castro et al[16] (1997)	57		80		95	
Reynolds et al[17] (2003)	50	All	55		N/A (TEE as standard)	
		Aortic	50			
		Mitral	62			
Jassal et al[18] (2007)	36		84	88	N/A (TEE as standard)	
Casella et al[19] (2009)	75	All	87	86	N/A (TEE as standard)	
		Aortic		71		
		Mitral		87		
Kini et al[20] (2010)	511		45	79	N/A (TEE as standard)	
Sekar et al[21] (2017)	119		21	100	86	97
Range			**21–87**	**79–100**	**86–100**	**91–100**

N/A, Not applicable; *TEE,* transesophageal echocardiography; *TTE,* transthoracic echocardiography.

anterior positioning of right-sided aortic and semilunar valves often lends itself to better visualization with TTE.[9]

Echocardiographic studies are more likely to be falsely negative in the setting of small vegetations.[24] The limits of image resolution allow for the detection of vegetations as small as 3 to 4 mm for TTE; however, only 25% of vegetations smaller than 5 mm and 70% between 6 and 10 mm are identified.[10] Although the higher resolution of TEE detects smaller vegetations, Sochowski and colleagues reported that 5 of 65 (7.6%) patients with an initially negative TEE result were eventually diagnosed with IE on a repeat TEE study 1 to 2 weeks later.[13] This reiterates the importance of repeating TEE at 7 to 10 days when clinical index of suspicion remains high because early on, vegetations may be too small to be detected. Atypically located or nonoscillating vegetations are also more likely to be missed because vegetations have a similar echogenicity to normal myocardium.[9]

The presence of preexisting significant valvular lesions such as mitral valve prolapse or valvular degenerative disease makes identification of vegetations challenging and can lead to false-negative results[24] (Fig. 116.2). Acoustic shadowing from prosthetic material or valvular calcification, leading to incomplete visualization of the entire valve apparatus, affects the diagnostic accuracy of TTE.[19]

False-positive echocardiographic results[24] leading to an incorrect diagnosis of IE can also occur. Vegetations can be difficult to differentiate from thrombi, cusp prolapse, flail chords, cardiac tumors, myxomatous changes, Lambl excrescences, and prominent Eustachian valves (see Fig. 116.2).[24] Thin linear strands can be seen commonly on native valves along the leaflet coaptation zone and may be misidentified as vegetation. Noninfective vegetations (marantic endocarditis) are impossible to differentiate from infective vegetations (Fig. 116.3) but can be suspected in the setting of multiple small vegetations without associated valvular destruction or perivalvular abscess.[9]

Owing to the possibility of both false-positive and false-negative echocardiographic study results, an individualized approach to each case is essential, incorporating echocardiographic data in combination with supportive clinical and microbiological evidence in making a definitive diagnosis of IE.

ECHOCARDIOGRAPHY IN THE DIAGNOSIS OF PROSTHETIC VALVE ENDOCARDITIS

TEE is strongly favored in the diagnosis of prosthetic valve endocarditis, with far superior sensitivity compared with TTE, providing

real-time assessment of prosthetic valvular function and concurrently assessing for the presence of vegetations or perivalvular extension.[9] TEE has demonstrated a sensitivity of 83% to 94% and specificity of 87% to 100% for prosthetic valve vegetation detection (Table 116.3).[11,20,25] This is compared with TTE, which has been shown to have a sensitivity of 22% to 65%.[11,20,25] Considering this, TEE is recommended for all patients with prosthetic valves who are considered at least "possible IE" according to the Duke criteria.[26]

Prosthetic valves present particular challenges for sonographers and reporting echocardiographers. Prosthetic material is strongly echogenic and causes numerous artifacts that can obscure visualization and impair assessment. The mitral prosthesis, when assessed on TTE, shadows the left atrium in the far field, and therefore color Doppler assessment of mitral prosthetic regurgitation is challenging. The left atrial side of a mitral prosthesis and therefore mitral regurgitation is more thoroughly assessed on TEE, whereas the subvalvular apparatus and LV systolic function are better assessed with TTE. The anterior portions of the aortic prosthesis are optimally visualized by TTE compared with TEE. Conversely, the posterior portion of the aortic prosthesis is superiorly assessed on TEE rather than TTE. Owing to the echogenicity of the sewing ring and support structures of prosthetic valves and the potential for artifacts to prevent detection of vegetation within the valve apparatus or its shadow (Fig. 116.4), both TTE and TEE may be required for complete visualization of the prosthetic valve apparatus when IE is suspected.

Small sterile strands can be frequently seen on prosthetic valves and are of uncertain significance. Prosthesis-associated thrombus, pannus, fibrin strands, and suture material are also commonly mistaken for an infectious process, leading to false-positive study results.[27]

ECHOCARDIOGRAPHY IN DIAGNOSIS OF INFECTIVE ENDOCARDITIS COMPLICATIONS OR PERIVALVULAR EXTENSION

Periannular extension of infection is a feared complication of IE and is associated with significantly higher morbidity and mortality.[28] Aortic infection, prosthetic endocarditis, new atrioventricular block, and coagulase-negative staphylococci are considered independent risk factors for periannular complications.[29] Complications of IE are best diagnosed on echocardiography and are essential to

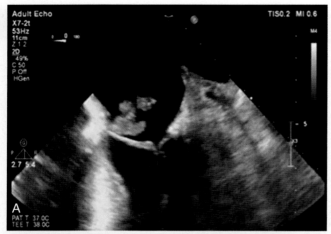

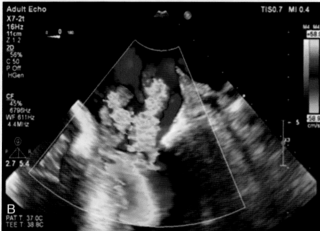

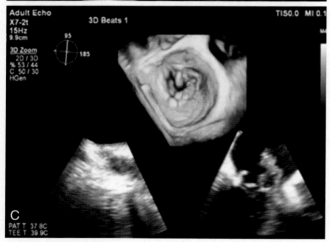

Figure 116.1. Native mitral valve infective endocarditis with large vegetation. Transesophageal echocardiography (TEE) 0-degree midesophageal view (**A**) with large, multilobed vegetation seen attached to the anterior mitral valve leaflet and severe mitral regurgitation seen on color Doppler (**B**). **C,** Three-dimensional TEE image of the same vegetation seen attached to the A3 segment of the anterior mitral valve leaflet.

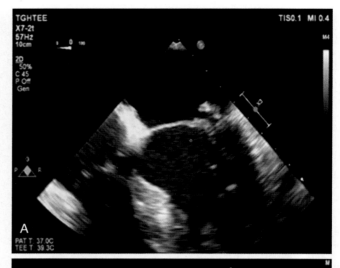

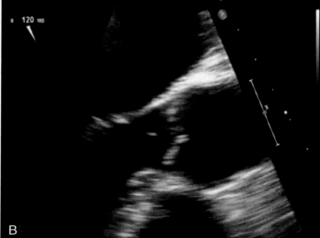

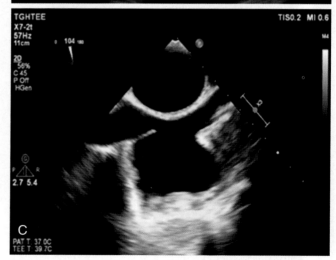

Figure 116.2. Examples of structures commonly leading to a false-positive diagnosis of infective endocarditis on echocardiography. **A,** Myxomatous, thickened posterior mitral valve leaflet with posterior leaflet prolapse/flail *(arrow)*. **B,** Lambl excrescence of the aortic valve *(arrow)*. **C,** Prominent Eustachian valve in the right atrium *(arrow)*.

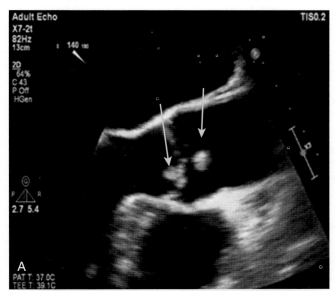

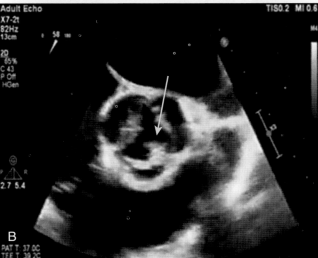

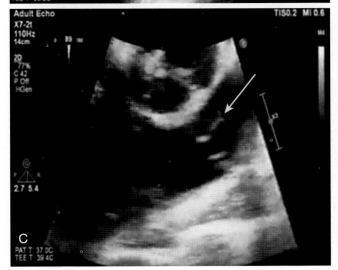

Figure 116.3. Marantic (noninfective) endocarditis involving both the aortic valve and pulmonic valve with multiple small vegetations seen without associated valvular destruction or perivalvular abscess. **A,** Transesophageal echocardiography (TEE) 120-degree (long-axis) view of the aortic valve with several small vegetations seen *(arrows).* **B,** TEE 60-degree (short-axis) view of the aortic valve with the same vegetations seen. **C,** TEE 60-degree view of the pulmonic valve with linear echodensity seen in the same patient.

evaluate thoroughly, as the presence of such dictates urgency of surgical intervention.

The diagnosis of perivalvular abscesses can be challenging. Valvular abscesses are rarely detected by TTE. Conversely, the specificity of TEE in the diagnosis of perivalvular extension including abscess, aneurysm, or fistula formation is high (Tables 116.4 and 116.5).[30] False-negative results can occur, particularly with small abscesses, early in the course of the disease or in the presence of prosthetic material or annular calcifications obscuring visualization of the perivalvular apparatus. Hill and colleagues demonstrated that the most commonly missed abscesses were localized around areas of calcification in the posterior mitral annulus and that such missed abscess cases had a resultant delay in surgical intervention but no significant effect on mortality rate[30].

Special Considerations

Catheter-related infections are common in patients with long-standing indwelling vascular access.[31] Infections of cardiac devices (pacemaker or implantable cardioverter-defibrillator leads) are also common and are associated with significant morbidity and mortality.[9] Vegetations attached to indwelling devices can be difficult to diagnose with TTE because of reverberation artefacts.[9] Often, vegetations may not involve valves or endocardial surfaces but may be attached to the line or pacing lead more proximally within the superior vena cava; therefore, it is essential to evaluate the whole lead course.[9] TTE is not sensitive enough to detect such vegetations; therefore, TEE is indicated in patients in whom line infection is suspected, particularly with persistent fever or positive blood culture results.[32] In most patients, vegetations attached to a central venous catheter or pacemaker lead present with typical motion and morphology; however, some may have a "sleeve-like" appearance and can be difficult to distinguish from thrombi.[9] When clinical suspicion of device-related infection is high and results from a TEE are negative, repeat TEE is warranted within 7 days.[9]

The pulmonic valve poses a particular challenge because it is often challenging to optimally visualize with either echocardiographic approach because of its anatomic position. Pulmonic valve IE is a rare clinical entity (<2% of IE cases). TTE has an estimated sensitivity for pulmonic valve vegetations of 70%, and owing to its anterior position, visualization of the pulmonic valve with TEE is often suboptimal.[33] Thus, alternative imaging techniques may need to be considered in cases of high clinical suspicion but equivocal echocardiographic findings to allow for more rapid diagnosis.

Recent advances in multimodality imaging techniques, including computed tomography (CT) and magnetic resonance imaging (MRI), are important to note. CT provides superior assessment of the aortic root and ascending aorta and higher sensitivity for the diagnosis of aortic annular involvement and aortic root abscess or pseudoaneurysm.[34] Although vegetations can also be diagnosed by MRI, diagnosis can often be limited by lower temporal resolution especially in the context of small highly mobile vegetations. Delayed enhancement depicting endothelial inflammation has been suggested as an adjunctive technique for vegetations[35]; however, further validation is needed. Positron emission tomography/CT is a useful adjunctive test in the evaluation of diagnostically challenging cases of IE, particularly involving prosthetic valves, having the potential to also detect extracardiac foci of infection.[36]

In summary, TTE and TEE both play a vital role in the diagnosis of IE. The diagnostic utility of these imaging modalities is influenced by a number of factors, including patient factors, index of clinical suspicion, the valve or anatomic structure in question, the presence of prosthetic valves, and the specific abnormality associated with endocarditis (e.g., vegetation, valvular dysfunction, perivalvular extension).

TABLE 116.3 Sensitivity and Specificity of Transthoracic and Transesophageal Echocardiography in the Diagnosis of Prosthetic Valve Endocarditis

Study	Patients (n)	PVE (n)	TTE		TEE	
			Sensitivity (%)	Specificity (%)	Sensitivity (%)	Specificity (%)
Shively et al[11] (1991)	61	3	44	98%	94%	100%
Daniel et al[25] (1993)	126	101 (bioprosthetic)	65	78%	87%	91%
		23 (mechanical)	22	48%	83%	87%
		Total	57	63%	86%	88%
Kini et al[20] (2010)	114 of 511		64		N/A	N/A
Range			**22–65**	**48–98**	**83–94**	**87–100**

N/A, Not applicable; *PVE,* prosthetic valve endocarditis; *TEE,* transesophageal echocardiography; *TTE,* transthoracic echocardiography.

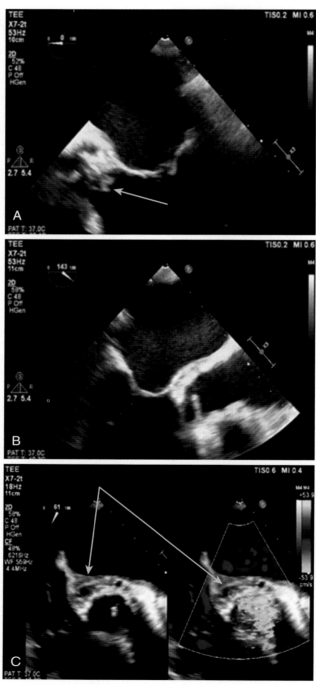

Figure 116.4. An example of the importance of acquiring multiple, off-axis images to rule out infective endocarditis in the presence of a prosthetic valve. Prosthetic valve endocarditis involving an aortic valve prosthesis where in an off-axis view, a vegetation is clearly seen (**A**), whereas in the on-axis (120-degree) view (**B**), the vegetation is not appreciated because of shadowing or artifact from the valve prosthesis. **C,** On further assessment, there is clearly an abscess involving the posterior aortic root (*arrow*) with color flow within the abscess seen on color Doppler (*arrow*).

TABLE 116.4 Sensitivity and Specificity of Transthoracic and Transesophageal Echocardiography in the Diagnosis of Native Valve Perivalvular Extension (i.e., abscess)

Study	Patients (n)	Valve	TTE		TEE	
			Sensitivity (%)	Specificity (%)	Sensitivity (%)	Specificity (%)
Daniel et al[37] (1991)	118		28	99	87	95
Leung et al[38] (1994)	34	Aortic	36		100	
Choussat et al[39] (1999)	233		36		80	
Graupner et al[29] (2002)	211				80	92
Hill et al[30] (2007)	115	Surgery				48
Range			28–36	99	80–100	48–95

TEE, Transesophageal echocardiography; *TTE,* transthoracic echocardiography.

TABLE 116.5 Sensitivity and Specificity of Transthoracic and Transesophageal Echocardiography in the Diagnosis of Periannular Complications of Prosthetic Valve Endocarditis

Study	Patients (n)	PVE Periannular Extension (n)	TTE		TEE	
			Sensitivity (%)	Specificity (%)	Sensitivity (%)	Specificity (%)
Daniel et al[37] (1991)	46 of 118	12	28	99	87	95
Zabalgoitia et al[40] (1993)	44	Bioprosthetic	25		100	
Choussat et al[38] (1999)	233	77	36	N/A	80	N/A
Hill et al[30] (2007)	44 of 115	26	N/A	N/A	48	99
Range			28–36	99	48–87	95–99

N/A, Not applicable; *PVE,* prosthetic valve endocarditis; *TEE,* transesophageal echocardiography; *TTE,* transthoracic echocardiography.

REFERENCES

1. American College of Cardiology/American Heart Association Task Force on Practice Guidelines, Society of Cardiovascular Anesthesiologists, Society for Cardiovascular Angiography and Interventions, et al: ACC/AHA 2006 guidelines for the management of patients with valvular heart disease: a report of the American College of Cardiology/American Heart Association Task Force on Practice Guidelines (writing Committee to Revise the 1998 guidelines for the management of patients with valvular heart disease) developed in collaboration with the Society of Cardiovascular Anesthesiologists endorsed by the Society for Cardiovascular Angiography and Interventions and the Society of Thoracic Surgeons. *J Am Coll Cardiol.* 2006;48:e1–e148.
2. Habib G, Hoen B, Tornos P, et al. Guidelines on the prevention, diagnosis, and treatment of infective endocarditis (new version 2009): The Task Force on the prevention, diagnosis, and Treatment of infective endocarditis of the European Society of Cardiology (ESC). Endorsed by the European Society of clinical Microbiology and infectious diseases (ESCMID) and the International Society of Chemotherapy (ISC) for infection and Cancer. *Eur Heart J.* 2009;30:2369–2413.
3. Wann LS, Dillon JC, Weyman AE, Feigenbaum H. Echocardiography in bacterial endocarditis. *N Engl J Med.* 1976;295:135–139.
4. Durack DT, Lukes AS, Bright DK. New criteria for diagnosis of infective endocarditis: Utilization of specific echocardiographic findings. *Duke Endocarditis Service, Am J Med.* 1994;96:200–209.
5. Lindner JR, Case RA, Dent JM, et al. Diagnostic value of echocardiography in suspected endocarditis. An evaluation based on the pretest probability of disease. *Circulation.* 1996;93:730–736.
6. American College of Cardiology Foundation Appropriate Use Criteria Task Force, American Society of Echocardiography, American Heart Association, et al: ACCF/ASE/AHA/ASNC/HFSA/HRS/SCAI/SCCM/SCCT/SCMR 2011 Appropriate Use Criteria for Echocardiography. A Report of the American College of Cardiology Foundation Appropriate Use Criteria Task Force, American Society of Echocardiography, American Heart Association, American Society of Nuclear Cardiology, Heart Failure Society of America, Heart Rhythm Society, Society for Cardiovascular Angiography and Interventions, Society of Critical Care Medicine, Society of Cardiovascular Computed Tomography, and Society for Cardiovascular Magnetic Resonance Endorsed by the American College of Chest Physicians. *J Am Coll Cardiol.* 2011;57:1126–1166.
7. Evangelista A, Gonzalez-Alujas MT. Echocardiography in infective endocarditis. *Heart.* 2004;90:614–617.
8. Greaves K, Mou D, Patel A, Celermajer DS. Clinical criteria and the appropriate use of transthoracic echocardiography for the exclusion of infective endocarditis. *Heart.* 2003;89:273–275.
9. Habib G, Badano L, Tribouilloy C, et al. Recommendations for the practice of echocardiography in infective endocarditis. *Eur J Echocardiogr.* 2010;11:202–219.
10. Erbel R, Rohmann S, Drexler M, et al. Improved diagnostic value of echocardiography in patients with infective endocarditis by transoesophageal approach. A prospective study. *Eur Heart J.* 1988;9:43–53.
11. Shively BK, Gurule FT, Roldan CA, et al. Diagnostic value of transesophageal compared with transthoracic echocardiography in infective endocarditis. *J Am Coll Cardiol.* 1991;18:391–397.
12. Pedersen WR, Walker M, Olson JD, et al. Value of transesophageal echocardiography as an adjunct to transthoracic echocardiography in evaluation of native and prosthetic valve endocarditis. *Chest.* 1991;100:351–356.
13. Sochowski RA, Chan KL. Implication of negative results on a monoplane transesophageal echocardiographic study in patients with suspected infective endocarditis. *J Am Coll Cardiol.* 1993;21:216–221.
14. Birmingham GD, Rahko PS, Ballantyne 3rd F. Improved detection of infective endocarditis with transesophageal echocardiography. *Am Heart J.* 1992;123:774–781.
15. Shapiro SM, Young E, De Guzman S, et al. Transesophageal echocardiography in diagnosis of infective endocarditis. *Chest.* 1994;105:377–382.
16. De Castro S, Magni G, Beni S, et al. Role of transthoracic and transesophageal echocardiography in predicting embolic events in patients with active infective endocarditis involving native cardiac valves. *Am J Cardiol.* 1997;80:1030–1034.
17. Reynolds HR, Jagen MA, Tunick PA, Kronzon I. Sensitivity of transthoracic versus transesophageal echocardiography for the detection of native valve vegetations in the modern era. *J Am Soc Echocardiogr.* 2003;16:67–70.
18. Jassal DS, Aminbakhsh A, Fang T, et al. Diagnostic value of harmonic transthoracic echocardiography in native valve infective endocarditis: comparison with transesophageal echocardiography. *Cardiovasc Ultrasound.* 2007;5:20.
19. Casella F, Rana B, Casazza G, et al. The potential impact of contemporary transthoracic echocardiography on the management of patients with native valve endocarditis: a comparison with transesophageal echocardiography. *Echocardiography.* 2009;26:900–906.
20. Kini V, Logani S, Ky B, et al. Transthoracic and transesophageal echocardiography for the indication of suspected infective endocarditis: vegetations, blood cultures and imaging. *J Am Soc Echocardiogr.* 2010;23:396–402.
21. Sekar P, Johnson JR, Thurn JR, et al. Comparative sensitivity of transthoracic and transesophageal echocardiography in diagnosis of infective endocarditis among veterans with staphylococcus aureus bacteremia. *Open Forum Infect Dis.* 2017;4(2): ofx035.
22. Chirillo F, Pedrocco A, De Leo A, et al. Impact of harmonic imaging on transthoracic echocardiographic identification of infective endocarditis and its complications. *Heart.* 2005;91:329–333.
23. Berdejo J, Shibayama K, Harada K, et al. Evaluation of vegetation size and its relationship with embolism in infective endocarditis: a real-time 3-dimensional transesophageal echocardiography study. *Circ Cardiovasc Imag.* 2014;7:149–154.
24. Habib G. Management of infective endocarditis. *Heart.* 2006;92:124–130.
25. Daniel WG, Mugge A, Grote J, et al. Comparison of transthoracic and transesophageal echocardiography for detection of abnormalities of prosthetic and bioprosthetic valves in the mitral and aortic positions. *Am J Cardiol.* 1993;71:210–215.

26. Baddour LM, Wilson WR, Bayer AS, et al. Infective endocarditis: diagnosis, antimicrobial therapy, and management of complications: a statement for healthcare professionals from the Committee on Rheumatic fever, endocarditis, and Kawasaki disease, Council on Cardiovascular disease in the Young, and the Councils on clinical Cardiology, Stroke, and Cardiovascular Surgery and Anesthesia, American heart association: endorsed by the infectious diseases Society of America. *Circulation*. 2005;111:e394–e434.

27. Rozich JD, Edwards WD, Hanna RD, et al. Mechanical prosthetic valve-associated strands: pathologic correlates to transesophageal echocardiography. *J Am Soc Echocardiogr*. 2003;16:97–100.

28. Anguera I, Miro JM, Cabell CH, et al. Clinical characteristics and outcome of aortic endocarditis with periannular abscess in the International Collaboration on Endocarditis Merged Database. *Am J Cardiol*. 2005;96:976–981.

29. Graupner C, Vilacosta I, SanRoman J, et al. Periannular extension of infective endocarditis. *J Am Coll Cardiol*. 2002;39:1204–1211.

30. Hill EE, Herijgers P, Claus P, et al. Abscess in infective endocarditis: the value of transesophageal echocardiography and outcome: a 5-year study. *Am Heart J*. 2007;154:923–928.

31. Shah H, Bosch W, Thompson KM, Hellinger WC. Intravascular catheter-related bloodstream infection. *Neurohospitalist*. 2013;3:144–151.

32. Chao TF, Chen SJ, Ho SJ, et al. Vegetation in the superior vena cava: a complication of tunneled dialysis catheters. *Kidney Int*. 2010;77:836.

33. Abdelbar A, Azzam R, Yap KH, Abousteit A. Isolated pulmonary infective endocarditis with septic pulmonary embolism complicating a right ventricular outflow tract obstruction: Scarce and devious presentation. *Case Rep Surg*. 2013:746589. 2013.

34. Feuchtner GM, Stolzmann P, Dichtl W, et al. Multislice computed tomography in infective endocarditis: comparison with transesophageal echocardiography and intraoperative findings. *J Am Coll Cardiol*. 2009;53:436–444.

35. Dursun M, Yilmaz S, Yilmaz E, et al. The utility of cardiac MRI in diagnosis of infective endocarditis: Preliminary results. *Diagn Interv Radiol*. 2015;21:28–33.

36. Mahmood M, Kendi AT, Ajmal S, et al. Meta-analysis of 18F-FDG PET/CT in the diagnosis of infective endocarditis. *J Nucl Cardiol*. 2019;26:922–935.

37. Daniel WG, Mugge A, Martin RP, et al. Improvement in the diagnosis of abscesses associated with endocarditis by transesophageal echocardiography. *N Engl J Med*. 1991;324:795–800.

38. Leung DY, Cranney GB, Hopkins AP, et al. Role of transoesophageal echocardiography in the diagnosis and management of aortic root abscess. *Br Heart J*. 1994;72:175–181.

39. Choussat R, Thomas D, Isnard R, et al. Perivalvular abscesses associated with endocarditis: clinical features and prognostic factors of overall survival in a series of 233 cases. Perivalvular Abscesses French Multicentre, *Study Eur Heart J*. 1999;20:232–241.

40. Zabalgoitia M, Herrera CJ, Chaudhry FA, et al. Improvement in the diagnosis of bioprosthetic valve dysfunction by transesophageal echocardiography. *J Heart Valve Dis*. 1993;2(5):595–603.

117 Echocardiography and Decision Making for Surgery

Andrew C. Peters, Vera H. Rigolin

The diagnosis and management of patients with infective endocarditis (IE) can be a challenging. Because of the wide spectrum of presentations seen in IE, the current diagnostic approach incorporates clinical, pathological, serologic, and echocardiographic criteria into a strategy that maintains both sensitivity and specificity for this disease entity. This multimodality approach, in turn, leads to earlier diagnosis and therefore prompt implementation of appropriate therapies. Echocardiography remains the key imaging modality in diagnosing IE and its local complications. Knowing when to implement transthoracic echocardiography (TTE) versus transesophageal echocardiography (TEE) and recognizing key cardiac complications on echocardiography that warrant surgery is paramount to the successful management of patients with IE.

TRANSTHORACIC ECHOCARDIOGRAPHY VERSUS TRANSESOPHAGEAL ECHOCARDIOGRAPHY IN INFECTIVE ENDOCARDITIS

Choosing the correct echocardiographic modality in patients with suspected IE allows for earlier diagnosis and therefore a greater opportunity to initiate antimicrobial therapy and identify patients who are at high risk for complications requiring surgery. Echocardiographic features consistent with IE form part of the major modified Duke criteria, further underscoring the critical role of echocardiography in this context. TTE is the initial imaging modality of choice for both suspected native and prosthetic heart valve endocarditis.[1–3] The specificity of TTE is greater than 90%, but sensitivity is less (62%–79%) because of insufficient spatial resolution to detect vegetations smaller than 2 to 3 mm in size.[4] Clinicians are recommended to proceed to TEE when a TTE is nondiagnostic, if complications develop, if a prosthetic valve is present, or if an intracardiac device or leads are present.[1–3] TEE is superior to TTE in identifying valvular complications such as leaflet perforation or annular abscess formation.[4] For example, if an initially low-risk patient should develop unexplained persistent fevers, atrioventricular (AV) block, or heart failure, TEE should be pursued to evaluate for IE findings that were not appreciated on the initial TTE. Clinicians should have a lower threshold to proceed to TEE in the setting of a nondiagnostic TTE for prosthetic valve endocarditis because

the sensitivity of TTE declines to 20% to 40% for aortic or mitral prostheses compared with a sensitivity of 80% to 90% for TEE.[4] Further investigation with TEE may also be warranted in patients with clinical features that confer a higher risk of IE such as prior history of IE, congenital heart disease, new murmur, and stigmata of embolic and vascular phenomena.[5] Additionally, it is a class IIa indication to perform a TEE in patients with persistent staphylococcal bacteremia when a source cannot be identified and in a patient with a prosthetic valve with recurrent fevers despite negative blood cultures.[1,2]

By following this imaging strategy, IE may be detected and treated earlier, which translates into improved patient outcomes. In addition, local complications requiring surgery may be recognized and addressed before clinical deterioration takes place and operative risks become prohibitive.

ECHOCARDIOGRAPHY AND SURGICAL DECISION MAKING IN INFECTIVE ENDOCARDITIS

Criteria have been published to guide clinicians on when to pursue valve surgery in IE. Whereas some of these criteria relate to extracardiac complications of IE, many are rooted in local, cardiac complications of IE that are typically diagnosed and monitored by echocardiography. Although some differences exist in the surgical guidelines for native valve versus prosthetic valve IE, the indications and their respective themes are generally similar and focus on shared decision making by a multispecialty heart valve team consisting of a cardiologist, cardiothoracic surgeon, and infectious disease specialist.[1,2]

First, both the American Heart Association (AHA)/American College of Cardiology (ACC) and European Society of Cardiology (ESC) guidelines recommend early surgery for native and prosthetic heart valve dysfunction resulting in signs or symptoms of heart failure.[1–3] Heart failure in this context may be diagnosed based on clinical grounds alone; however, certain echocardiography findings lend support to the diagnosis. Elevated left ventricular and left atrial pressures are suggested by premature closure of the mitral valve with acute aortic regurgitation (Figs. 117.1 to 117.3; Videos 117.2 and 117.3), rapid deceleration of the mitral regurgitation signal by continuous-wave Doppler, and moderate or severe

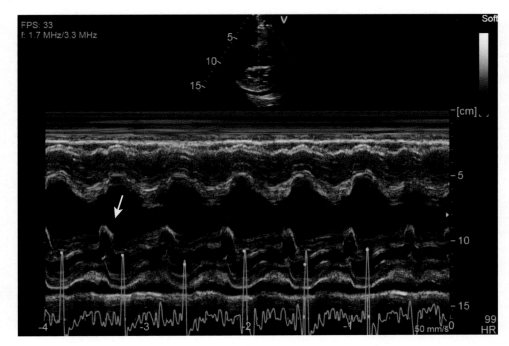

Figure 117.1. M-mode tracing on transthoracic echocardiography of the mitral valve in short-axis view in a patient with acute severe aortic regurgitation caused by endocarditis. Early closure of the mitral valve is demonstrated *(arrow)*.

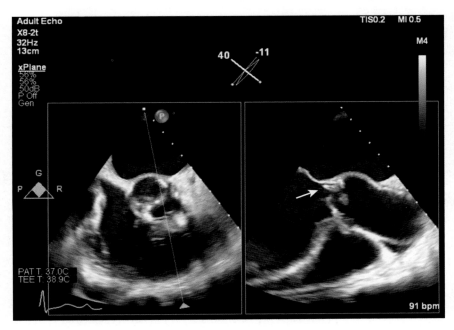

Figure 117.2. Transesophageal echocardiogram performed in a 74-year-old man who presented with fevers and was found to have enterococcus bacteremia. Biplane imaging through the aortic valve shows a bicuspid aortic valve with a mobile vegetation on the ventricular aspect of the noncoronary cusp *(arrow)* and a flail coronary cusp. (See accompanying Video 117.2).

pulmonary hypertension.[6] Rapid recognition of heart failure in this context is critical because surgical risks may become prohibitive after advanced-stage heart failure and renal insufficiency develop, particularly in older adults.[5]

Second, surgery is indicated for uncontrolled infection. In particular, IE caused by fungal organisms are commonly resistant to antimicrobial therapy. Fungal IE, although relatively uncommon, causes large vegetations, and *Candida* spp., in particular, should be considered in patients with prosthetic valves, an immunocompromised state, or a history of intravenous drug abuse.[1–3] Fungal endocarditis can be especially destructive because antifungal medications penetrate the vegetations poorly.[7] In general, a large vegetation (>1 cm) seen on echocardiography should raise the concern for fungal or HACEK group organisms (*Haemophilus, Actinobacillus, Cardiobacterium, Eikenella*, and *Kingella* spp.), noting that large vegetations are

associated with a higher embolic potential, particularly when present on the anterior mitral valve leaflet.[5]

Third, surgery is indicated in IE when local extension and complications occur. These complications, which can be devastating, are often suspected based on clinical and microbial grounds and subsequently confirmed by echocardiography. Examples include perivalvular abscess; penetrating lesion formation, such as a sinus of Valsalva fistula; extension onto the anterior mitral valve leaflet in aortic valve endocarditis; and AV block.[1–3] In addition, surgery is indicated for prosthetic valve dehiscence, as appreciated by either cine fluoroscopy or echocardiography.[1–3]

Perivalvular abscess, in particular, is associated with increased morbidity and mortality.[8] Early recognition and surgical intervention are critical to patient outcomes. A perivalvular abscess may be missed by TTE because of its low sensitivity for this finding.[6]

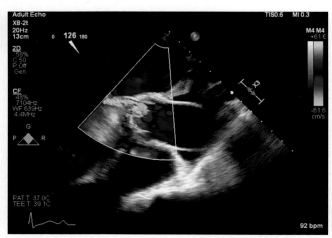

Figure 117.3. Transesophageal echocardiographic image of the left ventricular outflow tract with color Doppler demonstrates severe aortic regurgitation with a posteriorly directed jet caused by valve destruction from endocarditis, resulting in a flail coronary cusp. (See accompanying Video 117.3).

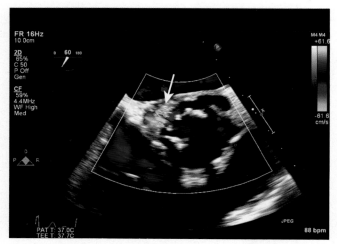

Figure 117.4. A complex circumferential perivalvular abscess with moderate perivalvular regurgitation (arrow) and partial valve dehiscence confirmed by transesophageal echocardiography. (See accompanying Video 117.4).

The estimated sensitivities of TTE and TEE for the diagnosis of a perivalvular abscess are 28% and 87%, respectively.[9] Therefore, TEE should be performed when a perivalvular abscess is suspected, particularly in the setting of prosthetic valve endocarditis.

On echocardiography, a perivalvular abscess appears as an echo-dense or echolucent mass within the annular tissue[6,9] (Figs. 117.4 to 117.6). Perivalvular abscesses are frequently seen in prosthetic valve endocarditis because the valve annulus, not the leaflets, is the primary site of infection. Abscess formation can also occur in native valve endocarditis; it is most common in aortic valve endocarditis near the membranous septum and the AV node, which is the weakest portion of the aortic annulus.[5] Annular weakness at this location also explains why AV conduction abnormalities are known complications of both prosthetic and native aortic valve endocarditis.

In the face of systemic intravascular pressures, perivalvular abscesses may lead to the formation of cardiac fistulae. These fistulae, which communicate with either an intracardiac chamber or the pericardial space, are associated with devastating hemodynamic consequences and require urgent surgical intervention.[5] This

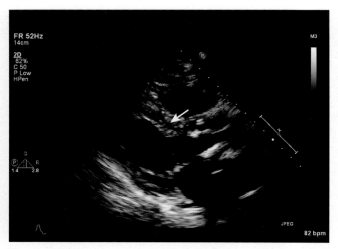

Figure 117.5. Follow-up transthoracic echocardiography obtained for a new left bundle branch block reveals a new linear echolucent space (arrow) in the basal interventricular septum, consistent with perivalvular abscess extension. (See accompanying Video 117.5).

complication, which is detected by color Doppler imaging, is also best appreciated by TEE.

Fourth, surgery may be indicated to prevent embolic phenomenon. The ESC gives a class I indication for surgery with aortic or mitral native/prosthetic valve endocarditis with a vegetation larger than 10 mm after more than one embolic episode despite antimicrobial therapy.[3] The AHA/ACC guidelines confer a class IIa recommendation on early surgery in patients with recurrent emboli and an enlarging vegetation despite antimicrobial therapy or in patients with severe valvular regurgitation and mobile vegetations larger than 10 mm.[1,2]

Fifth, surgery is a class IIa indication for native and prosthetic valve IE in the setting of persistent bacteremia, persistent vegetation, or recurrent emboli despite appropriate antibiotic therapy.[1,2] Figs. 117.4 to 117.6 and Videos 117.4 and 117.5 illustrate a case of culture-negative bioprosthetic aortic valve endocarditis in a patient with new-onset heart failure and echocardiographic features requiring urgent surgical intervention. The initial TTE demonstrated filamentous strands on the ventricular surface of the valve, concerning for IE, as well as "rocking" motion of the prosthesis and multiple jets of regurgitation, both concerning for valve dehiscence. TEE was appropriately performed later that same day. This study demonstrated no obvious vegetation, which is common in prosthetic valve endocarditis for reasons outlined earlier; however, a complex circumferential perivalvular abscess with moderate perivalvular regurgitation and partial valve dehiscence were confirmed (see Fig. 117.4 and Video 117.4). An electrocardiogram the following day showed a new left bundle branch block, for which an urgent TTE was obtained. This study revealed a new linear echolucent space in the basal interventricular septum, consistent with extension of the perivalvular abscess (see Fig. 117.5 and Video 117.5). The patient underwent urgent surgery for removal of the infected bioprosthesis, annular debridement, and placement of an aortic valve homograft. Intraoperative TEE also revealed abscess extension onto the anterior mitral valve leaflet, causing destabilization of the aortomitral curtain and moderate to severe mitral regurgitation (Fig. 117.6 and Video 117.6).

Sixth, in patients with implanted pacemakers or defibrillators and evidence of device or lead infection, complete extraction of the device is recommended. Patients with a pacemaker or defibrillator and *Staphylococcus aureus* or fungal endocarditis without evidence of device infection or those undergoing valve surgery have a class IIa

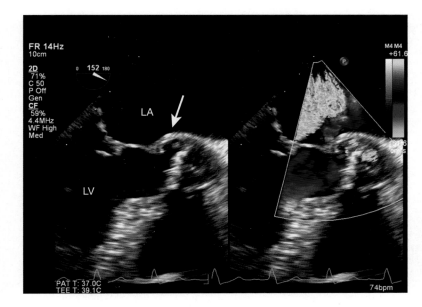

Figure 117.6. Intraoperative transesophageal echocardiogram demonstrates further abscess extension onto the anterior mitral valve leaflet causing destabilization of the aortomitral curtain *(arrow)* and moderate to severe mitral regurgitation. *LA*, Left atrium; *LV*, left ventricle. (See accompanying Video 117.6).

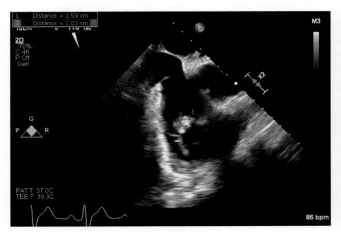

Figure 117.7. A 42-year-old man with prior dual-chamber implantable cardiac defibrillator for Brugada syndrome presented with fevers and malaise and was found to have methicillin-sensitive *Staphylococcus aureus* bacteremia. Transesophageal echocardiography demonstrates a 1.6- × 1-cm vegetation on the atrial aspect of the defibrillator lead. (See accompanying Video 117.7).

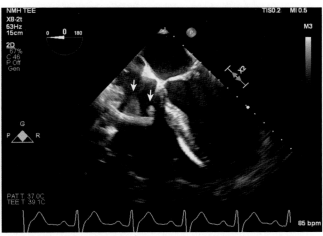

Figure 117.8. Four-chamber transesophageal view shows two separate vegetations *(arrows)* on the atrial aspect of the implantable cardiac defibrillator lead. (See accompanying Video 117.8).

recommendation for percutaneous or surgical device extraction.[1,2] Cardiac device infection has been increasing out of proportion to device implants with an incidence of 1 to 10 per 1000 device years for first implant.[10] TEE has better sensitivity for evaluating lead endocarditis, but it may be difficult to distinguish a vegetation from a sterile thrombus which is commonly seen.[10] When IE of a cardiac device is identified (Figs. 117.7 and 117.8; Videos 117.7 and 117.8), removal of the system is essential to management because antibiotics alone are associated with an increased risk of recurrence and death.[10]

CONCLUSION

In summary, IE is a complex disease process that requires a multimodality approach to diagnosis and management. Echocardiography plays an integral in role in this approach, particularly in regard to surgical decision making. Knowing when to select TTE or TEE as the initial study of choice allows patients who require surgery to be identified early and managed accordingly. In addition, clinicians must understand the indications for surgery in native and prosthetic valve IE and recognize the vital role of echocardiography in bringing these surgical indications to light.

Please access ExpertConsult to view the corresponding videos for this chapter.

Acknowledgment

The authors acknowledge the contributions of Dr. Laila A. Payvandi, who was the author of this chapter in the previous edition.

REFERENCES

1. Nishimura RA, Otto CM, Bonow RO, et al. AHA/ACC guideline for the management of patients with valvular heart disease: Executive summary: a report of the American College of Cardiology/American Heart Association Task Force on Practice guidelines. *J Am Coll Cardiol.* 2014;63:2438–2488. 2014.

2. Nishimura RA, Otto CM, Bonow RO, et al. AHA/ACC focused update of the 2014 AHA/ACC guideline for the management of patients with valvular heart disease: a report of the American College of Cardiology/American Heart Association Task Force on Clinical Practice Guidelines. *J Am Coll Cardiol.* 2017;70:252–289. 2017.
3. Habib G, Lancellotti P, Antunes MJ, et al. ESC guidelines for the management of infective endocarditis: the Task Force for the management of infective endocarditis of the European Society of Cardiology (ESC). Endorsed by: European association for Cardio-Thoracic surgery (EACTS), the European association of Nuclear medicine (EANM). *Eur Heart J.* 2015;36:3075–3128. 2015.
4. Saric M, Armour AC, Arnaout MS, et al. Guidelines for the use of echocardiography in the evaluation of a cardiac source of embolism. *J Am Soc Echocardiogr.* 2016;29:1–42.
5. Baddour LM, Wilson WR, Bayer AS, et al. Infective endocarditis: diagnosis, antimicrobial therapy, and management of complications. *Circulation.* 2005;111:e394–e434.
6. Armstrong WF, Ryan T. Infective endocarditis. In: Armstrong WF, Ryan T, eds. *Feigenbaum's Echocardiography.* 7th ed. Philadelphia: Lippincott Williams & Wilkins; 2010:361–383.
7. Delahaye F, Célard M, Roth O, et al. Indications and optimal timing for surgery in infective endocarditis. *Heart.* 2004;90:618–620.
8. Blumberg EA, Karalis DA, Chandrasekaran K, et al. Endocarditis-associated paravalvular abscesses. Do clinical parameters predict the presence of abscess? *Chest.* 1995;107:898–903.
9. Zoghbi WA, Chambers JB, Dumesnil JG, et al. Recommendations for evaluation of prosthetic valves with echocardiography and Doppler ultrasound. *J Am Soc Echocardiogr.* 2009;22:975–1014.
10. Cahill TJ, Baddour LM, Habib G, et al. Challenges in infective endocarditis. *J Am Coll Cardiol.* 2017;69:325–344.

118 Intraoperative Echocardiography in Infective Endocarditis

Kamari C. Jackson, Duc Thinh Pham, Vera H. Rigolin

Infective endocarditis (IE) is a serious condition associated with a 30% to 40% mortality rate.[1-3] The prevalence of IE has continued to increase likely because of an aging population and increasing use of prosthetic valves and indwelling cardiac devices.[2-3] IE can lead to complications such as embolic phenomenon, valvular destruction, perivalvular extension, and heart failure.[4] Echocardiography remains the cornerstone for the diagnosis and prognostication of IE. Transthoracic echocardiography (TTE) has a 70% to 75% sensitivity in detecting native valve endocarditis and is considered the first-line imaging modality in suspected IE.[3,5] Transesophageal echocardiography (TEE) has a greater sensitivity in detecting IE and plays a critical role in the management of this disorder.

Intraoperative TEE is especially beneficial given the dynamic nature of IE over time. From the time of the preoperative echocardiogram, vegetations may change in size, lead to abscess formation, extend beyond the valve tissue, and extend onto other valves.[6] Intraoperative TEE is therefore useful at the time of surgery to confirm the vegetation size and location, evaluate for preexisting valvular disease that may have predisposed to endocarditis, and assess for the mechanism and severity of valvular regurgitation (Figs. 118.1 and 118.2; Videos 118.1 to 118.5). It is also important to detect rupture of chordae, leaflet perforation, and presence of leaflet or annular abscess (see Fig. 118.1). Intraoperative TEE has also been shown to influence the operative plan. In one study, intraoperative TEE altered the initial operative plan in 11.5% of patients undergoing surgery.[7] An earlier study showed that intraoperative TEE affected the therapeutic decision making in nearly 30% of patients.[7,8] Intraoperative TEE can also be used to identify issues causing prolonged cardiopulmonary bypass wean and monitor for operative complications such as air emboli.[1,7] Finally, TEE immediately after cardiopulmonary bypass can assess for any residual or new valvular or perivalvular regurgitation. The American Heart Association/American College of Cardiology and the European Society of Cardiology confirm the importance of intraoperative TEE and recommend it in patients undergoing surgery for IE as a class IB indication.[1,5]

To provide the most accurate information for surgical planning in patients with IE, echocardiographers must remain up to date in all new devices and treatments. Transcatheter aortic valve replacement (TAVR) endocarditis is of particular interest given the rise in the number of TAVRs performed in the last decade. Recently, the Placement of Aortic Transcatheter Valves 3 (PARTNER) trial showed that patients with severe aortic stenosis and a low risk for surgery had a lower 1-year rate of death with TAVR compared with surgical valve replacement.[9] With the findings from all of the PARTNER trials, TAVR may soon be considered as an option for nearly all patients with severe, symptomatic aortic stenosis.

In TAVR endocarditis, vegetations are often seen by echocardiography on the prosthetic leaflet or stent frame and can extend to the mitral valve.[10] Echocardiographic imaging can be difficult because of shadow artifact from the metallic stent frame. A new elevation in transvalvular gradient suggesting obstruction may be seen in TAVR IE and may be the first hint of the presence of a vegetation.[11,12]

Although echocardiography remains the study of choice in patients with IE, there has been increasing interest in a multimodality imaging approach in the preoperative evaluation, particularly regarding the use of multislice computed tomography (CT). One study showed that TEE was superior in detecting small vegetations (<10 mm), valve perforation, and intracardiac fistula compared with cardiac CT.[10] Cardiac CT, on the other hand, was superior in detecting perivalvular abscess[13] (Fig. 118.3). These findings suggest that cardiac CT is a reasonable tool to evaluate suspected perivalvular disease when it is not clearly demonstrated on TEE and thus may help with preoperative planning. Cardiac CT is also useful to identify vegetations on TAVR valves (Fig. 118.4).

In summary, intraoperative TEE plays a crucial role in the management of patients with IE and is warranted in patients undergoing surgery. Echocardiography remains the imaging study of choice for the evaluation of IE before, during, and after surgery. It is imperative that echocardiographers be familiar with the complications associated with IE in native and prosthetic valves. In addition, familiarity with newer devices such as TAVR valves and the unique ways that IE presents on these structures is critical to provide optimal care to patients. Finally, additional imaging modalities such as multislice CT may aid in preoperative planning when the information demonstrated on echocardiography is insufficient.

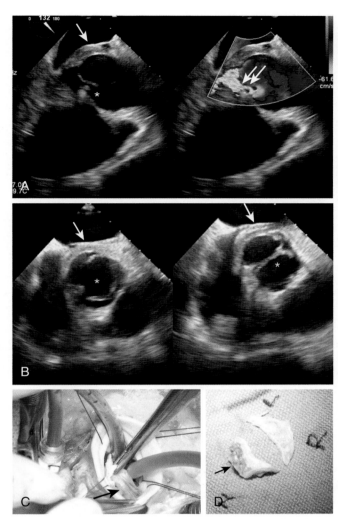

Figure 118.1. A, Transesophageal echocardiography image of an aortic root abscess *(single arrow)* in a patient with a bicuspid aortic valve *(asterisk)* and severe aortic regurgitation *(double arrow)*. **B,** Bicuspid valve in diastole on the *left* and systole on the *right*. The abscess is again shown by the *arrow*. (See accompanying Videos 118.1 and 118.2.) **C,** Intraoperative view of the aortic valve. The abscess was noted to be adjacent to the noncoronary cusp *(arrow)*. **D,** Explanted valve leaflets. Note the fusion of the left and right cusps and the residual abscess material on the noncoronary leaflet *(arrow)*.

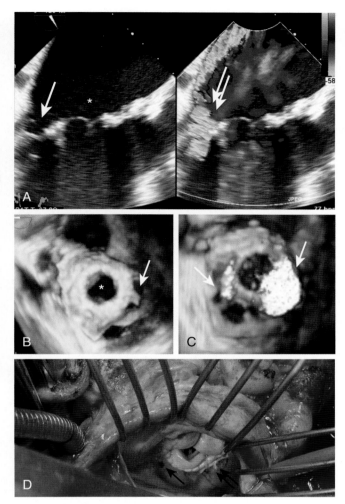

Figure 118.2. Transesophageal echocardiographic images demonstrating a bioprosthetic mitral valve *(asterisk)* in a patient with endocarditis. Long-axis view showing the valve dehiscence *(arrow)*, resulting in severe paravalvular regurgitation (**A**, *double arrows*). The area of dehiscence *(arrow)* is well demonstrated on the three-dimensional (3D) image of the prosthesis (**B**). The corresponding 3D color image (**C**) shows two area of paravalvular regurgitation *(arrows)*. (See accompanying Videos 118.3 to 118.5.) Intraoperative view of the mitral prosthesis (**D**). Note the large area of dehiscence of the mitral prosthesis *(double arrows)* and an abscess cavity with associated perforation *(single arrow)*.

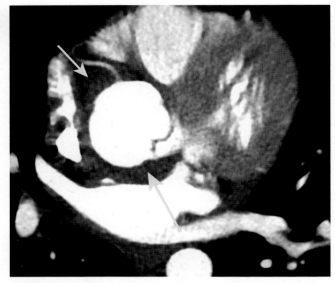

Figure 118.3. Computed tomography image taken from the patient with a bicuspid aortic valve and endocarditis shown in Fig.118.1. The gray soft tissue densities (*yellow arrows*) surrounding the aortic root are consistent with abscess.

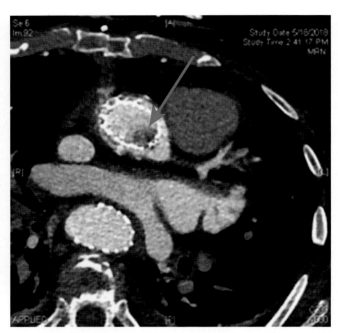

Figure 118.4. Computed tomography image in a patient with positive blood cultures. Note the vegetation on the transcatheter aortic valve replacement aortic prosthesis (*arrow*).

Please access ExpertConsult to view the corresponding videos for this chapter.

REFERENCES

1. Nishimura RA, Otto CM, Bonow RO, et al. AHA/ACC guideline for the management of patients with valvular heart disease. *J Am Coll Cardiol.* 2014;63. e57–185, 2014.
2. Feuchtner GM, Stolzmann P, Dichtl W, et al. Multislice computed tomography in infective endocarditis. *J Am Coll Cardiol.* 2009;53:436–444.
3. Cahill TJ, Prendergast BD. Infective endocarditis. *Lancet.* 2016;387:882–893.
4. Hasbun R, Vikram HR, Barakat LA, et al. Complicated left sided native valve endocarditis in adults: risk classification for mortality. *J Am Med Assoc.* 2003;289:1933–1940.
5. Habib G, Lancellotti P, Antunes MJ, et al. ESC Guidelines for the management of infective endocarditis. *Eur Heart J.* 2015;36:3075–3123. 2015.
6. Piper C, Hetzer R, Korfer R, et al. The importance of secondary mitral valve involvement in primary aortic valve endocarditis: the mitral kissing vegetation. *Eur Heart J.* 2002;23:79–86.
7. Shapira Y, Weisenberg DE, Vaturi M, et al. The impact of intraoperative transesophageal echocardiography in infective endocarditis. *Isr Med Assoc J.* 2007;9:299–302.
8. Shapira Y, Vaturi M, Weisenberg DE, et al. The impact of intraoperative transesophageal echocardiography in patients undergoing valve replacement. *Ann Thorac Surg.* 2004;78:579–583.
9. Mack MJ, Leon MB, Makkar R, et al. Transcatheter aortic-valve replacement with a balloon-expandable valve in low risk patients. *N Engl J Med.* 2019;380:1695–1705.
10. Kuttamperoor F, Yandrapalli S, Siddhamsetti S, et al. Infectious endocarditis after transcatheter aortic valve replacement: epidemiology and outcomes. *Cardiol Rev.* 2019;27:236–241.
11. Miranda WR, Connolly HM, Baddour LM, et al. Infective endocarditis following transcatheter aortic valve replacement: diagnostic yield of echocardiography and associated echo-Doppler findings. *Int J Cardiol.* 2018;271:392–395.
12. Salaun E, Sportouch L, Barral PA, et al. Diagnosis of infective endocarditis after TAVR: valve of a multimodality imaging approach. *JACC Cardiovasc Imag.* 2018;11:143–146.
13. Kim IC, Chang S, Hong GR, et al. Comparison of cardiac computed tomography with transesophageal echocardiography for identifying vegetation and intracardiac complications in patients with infective endocarditis in the era of 3-dimensional images. *Circ Cardiovasc Imag.* 2018;11:e006986.

119 Normal Pericardial Anatomy

Steven Giovannone, Robert Donnino, Muhamed Saric

The pericardium is a membranous sac that envelops almost the entire heart (with the exception of the region of the left atrium around the pulmonary venous ostia) as well as the origins of the great cardiac vessels (the ascending aorta, the main pulmonary artery, and the venae cavae). The term "pericardium" is a Latinized version of the Greek word περικάρδιον, which literally means "that which is around the heart." As an anatomic term, the word has been used at least since the time of the Greco-Roman physician Galen around AD 160, when he used it to describe stab wounds of gladiators resulting in pericardial effusions.[1] In English, the word "pericardium" first appears in print around 1425 in a Middle English translation of *Chirurgia Magna*, a surgical treatise written in Latin by the French physician Guy de Chauliac (c. 1300–1368).[2]

PHYLOGENY AND EMBRYOLOGY

The pericardium envelops the heart of all vertebrates, including fishes, amphibians, reptiles, birds, and mammals. As such a phylogenetically ancient structure, it forms very early during embryologic development in humans (starting at around 5 weeks' gestation) by the division of the coelom—the original visceral cavity—into pericardial, pleural, and peritoneal spaces. Through incompletely understood mechanisms, embryologic mishaps may result in a congenitally absent pericardium or pericardial cysts.

BASIC ANATOMY

The normal pericardium (Fig. 119.1) consists of a double-layered sac: an outer fibrous envelope (fibrous pericardium) and an inner serous sac (serous pericardium). The serous pericardium can be divided into an outer (parietal) and an inner (visceral) layer. The parietal layer normally fuses with the fibrous pericardium to create an inseparable outer layer of the pericardium. The fibrous pericardium is contiguous with the adventitia of the great arteries. The visceral layer of the serious pericardium is synonymous with the epicardium.[3] Between these two layers there is a virtual space that contains a very small amount of clear serous fluid, as discussed later.[4]

The pericardium spans the space between the third and the seventh rib. Strong superior and inferior sternopericardial ligaments anchor the pericardial sac to the posterior aspect of the sternum. In addition, loose fibrous tissue binds the pericardium to the diaphragm and surrounding thoracic structures, including pleurae. The right and left phrenic nerves travel in this loose tissue between the fibrous pericardium and the pleurae. The arterial supply to the pericardium is provided by the branches of the internal mammary arteries (especially the pericardiophrenic artery) and the descending thoracic aorta. The pericardiophrenic vein, ultimately draining into the brachiocephalic vein, provides the principal venous drainage of the pericardium. The nerves of the pericardium are derived from the sympathetic trunks as well as the vagus and phrenic nerves.

PERICARDIAL THICKNESS

Normal pericardial wall thickness is approximately 1 to 2 mm. Transthoracic echocardiography (TTE) does not delineate the pericardial wall boundaries well enough; therefore, TTE is not recommended for measurements of pericardial thickness by either the American Society of Echocardiography[5] or the European Society of Cardiology[6] guidelines on proper use of echocardiography in pericardial disorders. In contrast, pericardial thickness can be obtained by transesophageal echocardiography (TEE)[7] but is less reliable compared to the gold standard of computed tomography (CT) and cardiac magnetic resonance imaging (CMRI) (Fig. 119.2). Increased pericardial thickness caused by fibrosis and calcification is the hallmark of constrictive pericarditis.

PERICARDIAL FLUID

Under physiologic conditions, there is only a very small amount of clear straw-colored pericardial fluid (typically <50 mL) representing an ultrafiltrate of plasma. On echocardiography, the separation between parietal and visceral layers of the serous pericardium either is imperceptible or is seen only during ventricular systole as a slitlike echolucent area between the two pericardial layers. This small amount of fluid has multiple physiologic roles: it diminishes friction between the two pericardial layers; by being an incompressible fluid, it protects the heart from minor injuries; and it provides a source of vasoactive substances that may regulate the function of the heart and the coronary arteries.[8]

INTRAPERICARDIAL PRESSURE

The intrapericardial pressure (P) is a product of the intrapericardial fluid volume (V) and the pericardial stiffness ($\Delta P/\Delta V$):

$$P = V \times \frac{\Delta P}{\Delta V}$$

Pericardial stiffness, an inverse of pericardial compliance, is the slope of the intrapericardial pressure–volume curve. Because a normal pericardium is not an impediment for transmission of intrathoracic pressure changes into the pericardial space during physiologic respiration and because the physiologic amount of pericardial fluid is small, a normal intrapericardial pressure is close to 0 mm Hg or even negative (subatmospheric).

Under pathologic conditions, the intrapericardial pressure may rise either because of an increase in the amount of pericardial fluid (as with pericardial effusion) or because of pronounced pericardial stiffness (as in rapidly accumulating pericardial effusion or with effusive-constrictive pericarditis). The pericardial pressure–volume relationship is nonlinear; initially, the slope is flat but subsequently becomes very steep. This nonlinear relationship explains why

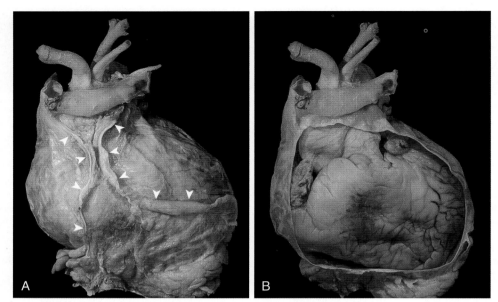

Figure 119.1. Gross anatomy of normal human pericardium. **A,** Anterior view of the intact parietal pericardial sac. The attachment of the fibrous sac to the diaphragm is seen at the base. Abundant epipericardial fat is conspicuously present at the pericardium–diaphragm junction. The mediastinal pleura invests the lateral portion of fibrous pericardium. The anterior reflections of the mediastinal pleura are indicated by the *white arrowheads*. The space between the *arrowheads* corresponds to the attachment of the pericardium to the posterior surface of the sternum. Superiorly, the left innominate vein is seen merging with the superior vena cava. The arterial branches of the aortic arch are just dorsal to the innominate vein. **B,** The anterior portion of the pericardial sac has been removed to show the heart and great vessels in anatomic position. It distinctly shows how the proximal segments of the great arteries are intrapericardial. At that point, there is fusion of the adventitia of the great vessels with the fibrous pericardium. (Reproduced with permission from Klein AL, et al: American Society of Echocardiography clinical recommendations for multimodality cardiovascular imaging of patients with pericardial disease, *J Am Soc Echocardiogr* 26:965–1012, e15, 2013.)

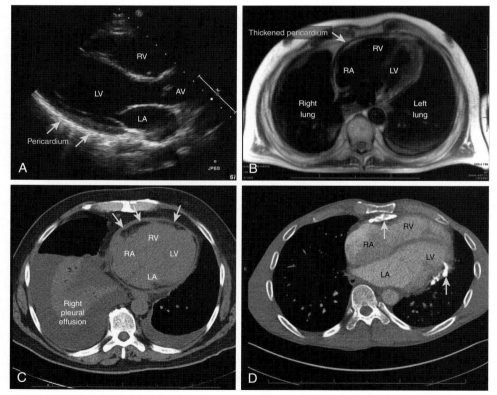

Figure 119.2. Imaging of pericardial thickness and calcifications. **A,** Transthoracic echocardiography (TTE). Although the pericardium can be visualized by TTE *(arrows)*, the exact thickness of the pericardium cannot be accurately measured by this means. **B,** Cardiac magnetic resonance demonstrates thickened pericardium *(arrow)* adjacent to the right heart on a T2-weighted spin echo axial image; this is the sequence that often shows the thickening the best. **C,** Chest computed tomography (CT) without contrast enhancement. Axial slice demonstrates a thickened pericardium, most prominent anteriorly *(arrows)*. **D,** Intravenous contrast–enhanced CT of the chest. Axial image shows areas of focal thickening with calcification in the pericardium *(arrows)*. *AV,* Aortic valve; *LA,* left atrium; *LV,* left ventricle; *RA,* right atrium; *RV,* right ventricle.

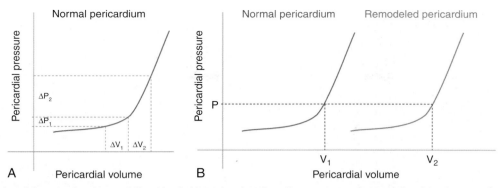

Figure 119.3. Pericardial pressure–volume relationship. **A**, Normal pericardium: the pressure–volume relationship of a normal pericardium is nonlinear. Note that the same unit increase in the volume of pericardial effusion ($\Delta V_1 = \Delta V_2$) produces markedly different intrapericardial pressure changes ($\Delta P_2 \gg \Delta P_1$) depending on the slope of the pressure–volume relationship. The steeper the slope, the greater the increase in intrapericardial pressure relative to increases in intrapericardial volume. **B**, Normal versus remodeled pericardium: the *left curve* demonstrates pressure–volume relationship with acute pericardial effusion in the setting of normal pericardial stiffness. The *right curve* demonstrates pressure relationship with chronic pericardial effusion; the pericardium remodels to accommodate the slowly accumulating fluid. Note that much greater amounts of pericardial fluid (V_2 vs V_1) are needed to produce the same pericardial pressure (P).

increases in the size of pericardial effusion initially may only modestly elevate intrapericardial pressures when the slope is flat. However, when the steep portion of the curve is reached, even a small additional increase in the size of pericardial effusion leads to marked increases in intrapericardial pressure (Fig. 119.3A).

When the intrapericardial pressure exceeds the pressure in any of the cardiac chambers during at least part of the cardiac cycle, tamponade physiology develops. Conversely, even removal of a relatively small amount of pericardial effusion may rapidly relieve signs and symptoms of tamponade. With slowly accumulating pericardial effusions, pericardial stiffness gradually falls, and thus the intrapericardial pressure remains near normal for longer periods of time compared with acute pericardial effusions. Mathematically, this corresponds to a shift of the pressure–volume relationship to the right (Fig. 119.3B).

INTRAPERICARDIAL VERSUS EXTRAPERICARDIAL HEART STRUCTURES

To fully understand pericardial physiology and pathology, it is important to recognize which heart structures lie within and which lie outside the pericardial sac. The proximal portions of the great arteries (the ascending aorta and the main pulmonary artery) are located within the pericardial sac, whereas the superior portion of the left atrium and the ostia of the pulmonary veins are outside of the pericardial sac. Dissections or other injuries of proximal portions of the great arteries may result in the development of a pericardial effusion.

In contrast, the extrapericardial location of the pulmonary veins contributes to exaggerated respiratory variations in tamponade and constrictive pericarditis. Briefly, under physiologic conditions during inspiration, the intrathoracic pressure drops, which leads to a drop in both pulmonary vein and intracardiac pressures. The opposite occurs during expiration. Because intrathoracic pressures changes affect the pulmonary veins and the left heart almost equally, the pressure gradient between the pulmonary vein and the left atrium does not change substantially. Therefore, under physiologic conditions, there is only a minor decrease of left heart filling during inspiration.

Significant pericardial effusions and constrictive pericarditis insulate intracardiac chambers from changes in intrathoracic pressures during respiration. Thus, in such pathologic conditions,

the normal inspiratory drop in intrathoracic pressures leads to a drop in the pulmonary vein pressure without a concomitant drop in the left atrial pressure. The resulting decrease in the pressure gradient between the pulmonary vein and the left atrium leads to a marked drop in the filling of the left heart during inspiration. The concept of these exaggerated respiratory variations in tamponade and constrictive pericarditis is further discussed in other chapters of this book.

PERICARDIAL FAT

A variable amount of fat may be present in and around the pericardial sac; collectively, this adipose tissue is referred to as the pericardial fat pad. Intrapericardial fat accumulates preferentially along the coronary arteries and in the atrioventricular groove; this is referred to as epicardial fat. Additional fat tissue may also accumulate outside the pericardium in the nearby mediastinum, particularly anterior to the right heart; this is referred to as mediastinal fat. On imaging, the epicardial and mediastinal fat layers should not be mistaken for a loculated pericardial effusion. Echocardiographically, pericardial fat is a noncircumferential accumulation of ultrasonographically heterogeneous material that moves in concert with the heart. In contrast, pericardial effusions are typically stationary, echolucent, and circumferential rather than restricted to the region around the right heart. Pericardial fat can also be well visualized by cardiac CT or CMRI (Fig. 119.4 and Video 119.4A).

PERICARDIAL EXTENSIONS

The main pericardial sac communicates with several extensions that are referred to as sinuses and recesses.[9] There are two sinuses (oblique sinus and transverse sinus) and multiple recesses. The two sinuses do not communicate directly. Occasionally, pericardial effusion may only be present in one or more of these sinuses and recesses and absent from the main pericardial cavity (Fig. 119.5 and Video 119.5). The oblique sinus is a blind pouch or cul-de-sac that overlies the posterior aspect of left atrium, normally between all four pulmonary veins, as well as a portion of the right atrium. The transverse sinus is bounded anteriorly by the origins of the great arteries; inferiorly by the roof of the left atrium; and posteriorly by the superior vena cava, the atria, and the left atrial appendage.

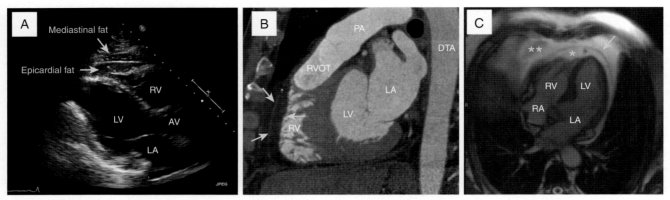

Figure 119.4. Imaging of pericardial fat. **A,** Transthoracic echocardiogram (TTE): pericardial fat pad consists of epicardial fat inside the pericardium and mediastinal fat just outside the pericardial sac. On TTE, pericardial fat *(arrows)* appears as noncircumferential accumulation of ultrasonographically heterogeneous material that moves in concert with the heart. In contrast, pericardial effusions are typically stationary, echolucent, and circumferential rather than restricted to the region around the right heart. (See accompanying Video 119.4A.) **B,** Computed tomography (CT): intravenous contrast CT image in the sagittal projection demonstrates a pericardial fat pad *(thick arrow)* area between the right ventricle (RV) and the fibrous pericardium *(thin arrow)*. **C,** Cardiac magnetic resonance: steady-state free precession image in axial projection demonstrates fat surrounding the pericardium *(arrow)*. Epicardial fat *(asterisk)* is inside the pericardium, and mediastinal fat *(double asterisk)* is just outside the pericardium. *AV,* Aortic valve; *DTA,* descending thoracic aorta; *LA,* left atrium; *LV,* left ventricle; *PA,* pulmonary artery; *RA,* right atrium; *RV,* right ventricle; *RVOT,* right ventricular outflow tract.

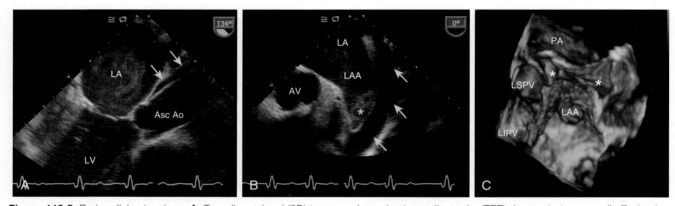

Figure 119.5. Pericardial extensions. **A,** Two-dimensional (2D) transesophageal echocardiography (TEE) demonstrates a small effusion in the aortic recess of the transverse sinus of the pericardium *(arrows)*. **B** and **C,** A small effusion in the pulmonic recess of the pericardium around the left atrial appendage (LAA) is seen on 2D TEE *(arrows in **B**)* and 3D TEE *(asterisks in **C**)*. *Asc Ao,* Ascending aorta; *LA,* left atrium; *LIPV,* left inferior pulmonary vein; *LSPV,* left superior pulmonary vein; *LV,* left ventricle; *PA,* pulmonary artery. (See accompanying Video 119.5.)

Extensions of the transverse sinus include the superior aortic recess (between the ascending aorta and the superior vena cava), the inferior aortic recess (between the ascending aorta and the right atrium), and the right and left pulmonic recesses (around the right and left pulmonary arteries). Pericardial effusions localized in the transverse sinus and its recesses should not be mistaken for other pathologies such as type A aortic dissection. The postcaval recess is an extension of the main pericardial cavity; it lies posterior and to the right of the superior vena cava.[10,11]

Please access ExpertConsult to view the corresponding videos for this chapter.

REFERENCES

1. Beck CS. Wounds of the heart. *Arch Surg.* 1926;13:205–227.
2. Oxford English Dictionary. http://www.oed.com/view/Entry/140863#eid3126185. Accessed on March 2, 2014.
3. Willians PL, Warmick R, eds. *Gray's Anatomy.* 36th ed. Philadelphia: WB Saunders; 1980.
4. Spodick DH, ed. *The Pericardium: A Comprehensive Textbook.* New York: Marcel Dekker; 1997.
5. Klein AL, Abbara S, Agler DA, et al. American Society of Echocardiography clinical recommendations for multimodality cardiovascular imaging of patients with pericardial disease. *J Am Soc Echocardiogr.* 2013;26:965–1012. e15, 2013.
6. Adler Y, Charron P, Imazio M, et al. ESC guidelines for the diagnosis and management of pericardial diseases. *Eur Heart J.* 2015;36:2921–2964. 2015.
7. Ling LH, Oh JK, Tei C, et al. Pericardial thickness measured with transesophageal echocardiography. *J Am Coll Cardiol.* 1997;29:1317–1323.
8. Mebazaa A, Wetzel RC, Dodd-o JM, et al. Potential paracrine role of the pericardium in the regulation of cardiac function. *Cardiovasc Res.* 1998;40:332–342.
9. Choe YH, Im JG, Park JH, et al. The anatomy of the pericardial space: a study in cadavers and patients. *AJR Am J Roentgenol.* 1987;149:693–697.
10. Vesely TM, Cahill DR. Cross-sectional anatomy of the pericardial sinuses, recesses and adjacent structures. *Surg Radiol Anat.* 1986;8:221–227.
11. Chaffanjon P, Brichon PY, Faure C, et al. Pericardial reflection around the venous aspect of the heart. *Surg Radiol Anat.* 1997;19:17–21.

120 Pericarditis

Sushil Allen Luis, Sunil V. Mankad

DEFINITION

Pericarditis refers to a symptomatic inflammation of the pericardium and can be categorized as acute, incessant (episode lasting 4–12 weeks without remission), recurrent, or chronic (episodes lasting >3 months).[1] Myopericarditis implies associated inflammation, often with coinciding tissue necrosis of the myocardium.[2] Acute pericarditis is the most common manifestation of pericardial disease.

EPIDEMIOLOGY

The incidence and prevalence of acute pericarditis are difficult to determine because of the presence of subclinical disease, the variability of the clinical presentation, and referral bias. Observational national registry data suggests a standardized incidence rate of 3.32 cases per 100,000 person years among patients requiring hospitalization, accounting for 0.2% of all cardiology admissions.[3]

ETIOLOGY

Acute, recurrent, or chronic pericarditis can be encountered in a myriad of clinical settings. An elegant yet simple etiologic classification has been described and includes (1) infectious, (2) autoimmune, (3) reactive, (4) metabolic, (5) traumatic or iatrogenic, and (6) neoplastic.[1] The vast majority of cases in Western Europe and North America are of viral or idiopathic etiology. Pericardial irritation secondary to cardiothoracic surgery, percutaneous device implantations, and endocardial and epicardial catheter-based ablation procedures are also increasing in frequency. There is a global geographical variation in infectious agents, with tuberculous and human immunodeficiency virus (HIV) pericarditis being more common in low- and middle-income countries.

DIAGNOSTIC EVALUATION

Acute pericarditis is diagnosed in the presence of at least two of the following four criteria: (1) pericarditic chest pain, (2) pericardial friction rub, (3) electrocardiographic (ECG) features, and (4) new or worsening pericardial effusion.[1] The most important aspect of the diagnostic evaluation is to distinguish pericarditis from other potentially fatal causes such as acute coronary syndromes, pulmonary thromboembolic disease, and aortic dissection. Published guidelines outline a useful diagnostic pathway.[1,4]

CLINICAL FEATURES
Symptoms

Chest pain is the most common presenting symptom. It may be sudden or gradual in onset, sharp and akin to pleurisy, and, in many, agonizingly limiting. The pain characteristically radiates to the trapezius ridge, is aggravated by lying down, and is ameliorated by sitting and leaning forward. A preceding flu-like illness may be present in viral pericarditis. The development of pericarditic pain in a post–acute myocardial infarction (MI) patient should flag concern for pericardial irritation from a pseudoaneurysm or contained myocardial rupture but can also be seen with transmural myocardial injury.

Signs

A pericardial friction rub is the pathognomonic auscultatory finding. It is described as a harsh, "scratchy" sound that can vary in intensity and can be heard in up to three phases including atrial systole, ventricular systole, and ventricular diastole.[5]

ELECTROCARDIOGRAPHY

Pericarditis is associated with diagnostic ECG changes secondary to epicardial inflammatory injury.[6] These changes have been observed to evolve through four stages[7,8]: (1) widespread, saddle-shaped ST-segment elevation in most leads (except in aVR) with upright T waves, (2) diffuse PR segment depression in all leads except in lead aVR (where the PR segment is elevated), (3) diffuse T-wave inversion, and (4) normalization of changes with return to baseline ECG. The diffuse, concave ST-segment elevation is easily distinguishable from the regional, convex ST-segment elevation in acute MI. Sinus tachycardia is common. Low voltage should arouse suspicion for pericardial effusion, and electrical alternans is highly specific for cardiac tamponade.[9] An example of the cardinal ECG features of acute pericarditis is shown in Fig. 120.1. The ECG changes can be subtle or localized in post-MI, postsurgical, or postprocedural pericarditis.

CHEST RADIOGRAPHY

The chest radiograph is typically unrevealing. Occasionally, a large pericardial effusion can result in an enlarged cardiac silhouette. A small, left-sided pleural effusion may also be seen in the presence of coexistent pleuritis.

LABORATORY STUDIES

Inflammatory markers such as an elevated erythrocyte sedimentation rate (ESR), serum C-reactive protein (CRP), or both are frequently, but not always, present. Persistently elevated CRP can identify patients at higher risk of recurrence and help guide duration of therapy.[10] Elevation of cardiac biomarkers such as creatine kinase MB (CK-MB) fraction and troponins suggests associated myopericarditis.[11,12]

ECHOCARDIOGRAPHY

Transthoracic echocardiography is recommended as the initial imaging modality of choice amongst patients with suspected pericarditis.[1,13] Although the majority of patients with suspected pericarditis have normal echocardiograms, current American Society of Echocardiography guidelines recommend that all patients with acute pericarditis should undergo transthoracic echocardiography to assess for a pericardial effusion and its hemodynamic impact (Figs. 120.2 to 120.4).[4] The prevalence of pericardial effusions among patients with acute pericarditis has been estimated at 60% in one series, of which most effusions are small (79%) and cardiac tamponade infrequent (5%).[14] Pericardial stranding may be seen in hemorrhagic or purulent effusions. It should be remembered that pericardial effusion size cannot be used as an independent marker of tamponade physiology, and even small effusions can accumulate rapidly, resulting in cardiac tamponade. Loculated or

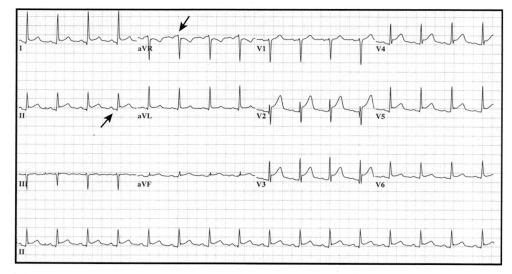

Figure 120.1. The classic features of acute pericarditis: diffuse concave upward S-T (J-point) elevation with S-T depression in lead aVR consistent with epicardial inflammation. The PR segment elevation in aVR and depression in lead II may be present in stage 1 or 2 of acute pericarditis *(arrows)*.

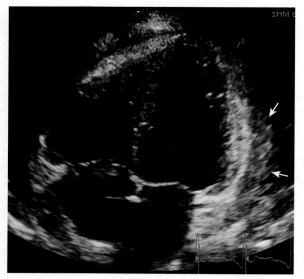

Figure 120.2. Apical four-chamber view demonstrating a pericardial "rind" or thickening of the visceral pericardial surface secondary to inflammation related to acute pericarditis. This is best seen adjacent to the lateral wall of the left ventricle *(arrows)*. (See accompanying Video 120.2.)

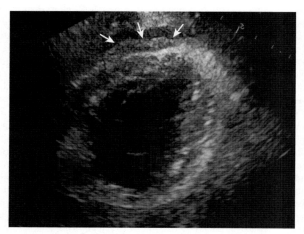

Figure 120.3. Modified apical two-chamber view again demonstrates a pericardial "rind" or thickening of the visceral pericardial surface secondary to inflammation related to acute pericarditis. This is best seen adjacent to the lateral wall of the left ventricle *(arrows)*. (See accompanying Video 120.3.)

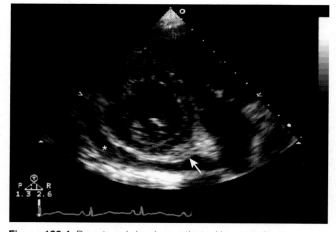

Figure 120.4. Parasternal view in a patient with acute chest pain secondary to acute pericarditis demonstrating a small to moderate pericardial effusion *(asterisk)*. Note the thickening on the visceral pericardial surface *(arrow)* and lack of regional wall motion abnormalities in the short-axis view of the left ventricle. (See accompanying Video 120.4.)

posterior effusions are encountered in the setting of cardiac surgery or catheter-based procedures and must be carefully sought in multiple and modified imaging windows. Large pericardial effusion and cardiac tamponade are potential risk factors for development of constriction.[15]

Acute pericarditis may be associated with significant pericardial inflammation and edema, resulting in constrictive pericardial physiology, a phenomenon known as "transient constrictive pericarditis." Careful and detailed echocardiographic assessment should be performed in patients with suspected pericarditis to exclude constrictive pericardial physiology because this would provide supportive diagnostic evidence among patients with pericardial chest pain. Evaluation should include assessment for the presence of ventricular interdependence by two-dimensional (2D) and M-mode imaging, respirophasic mitral and tricuspid pulsed-wave Doppler inflow variation, annulus reversus (medial > lateral mitral annular tissue Doppler velocities), and expiratory hepatic venous diastolic flow reversals. Transient constrictive pericarditis is a reversible phenomenon warranting aggressive antiinflammatory therapy.

Additional findings supporting the diagnosis of pericarditis include pericardial thickening. The normal pericardium is a thin echogenic layer that cannot be easily distinguished from the epicardium. When the pericardium is inflamed and thickened more than 5 mm, it can appear as a bright echogenic layer on 2D and M-mode echocardiography. This is best appreciated in the presence of a pericardial effusion. A thickened pericardium should increase the suspicion for coexistent constrictive physiology. Regional wall motion abnormalities, cardiac chamber dilatation with increase in sphericity,[16] diffuse or patchy left ventricular dysfunction, decrease in ejection fraction, and right ventricular involvement should raise suspicion for associated myocarditis.

The main advantages of echocardiography are quick bedside accessibility and its ability to provide both anatomic and physiologic details and guide therapeutic interventions such as pericardiocentesis. In addition, important differential diagnoses such as coronary ischemia and aortic pathology can be evaluated.

MAGNETIC RESONANCE IMAGING

Cardiac magnetic resonance imaging (CMRI) is a valuable diagnostic testing in the assessment of acute pericarditis. In addition to assessing the presence of pericardial effusions and pericardial thickness, CMRI also offers the opportunity to determine the presence of pericardial inflammation (as defined by the presence of pericardial delayed gadolinium enhancement) and edema (as assessed by T2-weighted imaging). Delayed gadolinium enhancement has been reported to have a 94% sensitivity for the diagnosis of inflammatory pericarditis in one series. Additionally, pericardial edema was present in 63% of such patients with each of these patients having significant pericardial edema proven on pathological examination.[4] Disadvantages of CMRI include high cost, limited availability, and technical contraindications, including the inability to administer gadolinium contrast among patients with advanced (stage IV or V) kidney disease. Hence, current guidelines recommend use of CMRI as a second-line imaging technique among patients with atypical clinical presentations or inconclusive echocardiographic findings.

COMPUTED TOMOGRAPHIC IMAGING

Pericardial effusion and thickened noncalcified pericardium support the diagnosis.[4,17]

TREATMENT

A combination of nonsteroidal antiinflammatory drugs (NSAIDs) with colchicine is the recommended first-line therapy for uncomplicated idiopathic pericarditis.[1,9–22] In patients with renal dysfunction in whom NSAIDs are contraindicated, colchicine may be used in combination with corticosteroid therapy. Corticosteroid therapy may also be associated with an increased risk of recurrent pericarditis,[20] and its use should be restricted to patients who are intolerant or unresponsive to the foregoing therapy and in the setting of autoimmune disease or uremia. Aspirin is the drug of choice in patients with post-MI pericarditis because of the increased risk of myocardial thinning and rupture with NSAIDs and corticosteroids. In cases with a known cause, treatment of the primary inciting cause should be addressed.

Please access ExpertConsult to view the corresponding videos for this chapter.

Acknowledgment

The authors thank Dr. Sonia Jain for her contribution to this chapter in the previous edition.

REFERENCES

1. Adler Y, Charron P, Imazio M, et al. 2015 ESC guidelines for the diagnosis and management of pericardial diseases. *Eur Heart J.* 2015;36:2921–2964.
2. Imazio M, Cecchi E, Demichelis B, et al. Myopericarditis versus viral or idiopathic acute pericarditis. *Heart.* 2008;94:498–501.
3. Kyto V, Sipila J, Rautava P. Clinical profile and influences on outcomes in patients hospitalized for acute pericarditis. *Circulation.* 2014;130:1601–1606.
4. Klein AL, Abbara S, Agler DA, et al. American Society of Echocardiography clinical recommendations for multimodality cardiovascular imaging of patients with pericardial disease. *J Am Soc Echocardiogr.* 2013;26:965–1012. e15.
5. Spodick DH. Pericardial rub. Prospective, multiple observer investigation of pericardial friction in 100 patients. *Am J Cardiol.* 1975;35:357–362.
6. Alraies MC, Klein AL. Q: should we still use electrocardiography to diagnose pericardial disease? *Cleve Clin J Med.* 2013;80:97–100.
7. Spodick DH. Diagnostic electrocardiographic sequences in acute pericarditis. Significance of PR segment and PR vector changes. *Circulation.* 1973;48:575–580.
8. Spodick DH. Electrocardiogram in acute pericarditis. Distributions of morphologic and axial changes by stages. *Am J Cardiol.* 1974;33:470–474.
9. Eisenberg MJ, de Romeral LM, Heidenreich PA, et al. The diagnosis of pericardial effusion and cardiac tamponade by 12- lead ECG. A technology assessment. *Chest.* 1996;110:318–324.
10. Imazio M, Brucato A, Maestroni S, et al. Prevalence of C-reactive protein elevation and time course of normalization in acute pericarditis. *Circulation.* 2011;123:1092–1097.
11. Smith SC, Ladenson JH, Mason JW, et al. Elevations of cardiac troponin I associated with myocarditis. Experimental and clinical correlates. *Circulation.* 1997;95:163–168.
12. Bonnefoy E, Godon P, Kirkorian G, et al. Serum cardiac troponin I and ST-segment elevation in patients with acute pericarditis. *Eur Heart J.* 2000;21:832–836.
13. Yared K, Baggish AL, Picard MH, et al. Multimodality imaging of pericardial diseases. *JACC Cardiovasc Imag.* 2010;3:650–660.
14. Imazio M, Demichelis B, Parrini I, et al. Day-hospital treatment of acute pericarditis: a management program for outpatient therapy. *J Am Coll Cardiol.* 2004;43:1042–1046.
15. Imazio M, Brucato A, Maestroni S, et al. Risk of constrictive pericarditis after acute pericarditis. *Circulation.* 2011;124:1270–1275.
16. Mendes LA, Picard MH, Dec GW, et al. Ventricular remodeling in active myocarditis. Myocarditis Treatment Trial. *Am Heart J.* 1999;138(2 Pt 1):303–308.
17. Sa MI, Kiesewetter CH, Jagathesan R, et al. Images in cardiovascular medicine. Acute pericarditis assessed with magnetic resonance imaging. *Circulation.* 2009;119:e183–e186.
18. Khandaker MH, Espinosa RE, Nishimura RA, et al. Pericardial disease: diagnosis and management. *Mayo Clin Proc.* 2010;85:572–593.
19. Young PM, Glockner JF, Williamson EE, et al. MR imaging findings in 76 consecutive surgically proven cases of pericardial disease with CT and pathologic correlation. *Int J Cardiovasc Imag.* 2012;28:1099–1109.
20. Imazio M, Bobbio M, Cecchi E, et al. Colchicine in addition to conventional therapy for acute pericarditis: results of the COlchicine for acute PEricarditis (COPE) trial. *Circulation.* 2005;112:2012–2016.
21. Imazio M, Bobbio M, Cecchi E, et al. Colchicine as first-choice therapy for recurrent pericarditis: results of the CORE (COlchicine for REcurrent pericarditis) trial. *Arch Intern Med.* 2005;165:1987–1991.
22. Imazio M, Brucato A, Cemin R, et al. Colchicine for recurrent pericarditis (CORP): a randomized trial. *Ann Intern Med.* 2011;155:409–414.

121 Pericardial Effusion and Cardiac Tamponade

Bryan Doherty, Itzhak Kronzon

NORMAL ANATOMY OF THE PERICARDIUM

The pericardium is a two-layered fibroelastic membrane or sac that surrounds the heart and proximal segments of the aorta, pulmonary artery, pulmonary veins, and vena cava. A small physiologic amount of fluid is present between the fibrous parietal layer and the single-cell-thickness visceral layer. The small volume of normal pericardial fluid plasma ultrafiltrate is usually less than 50 mL[1,2] and is believed to come from the visceral pericardium. Normal pericardial pressure is 0 to 3 mm Hg, varying with respiration. The pericardial space drains via lymphatics through both the thoracic duct and the right lymphatic duct. The pericardial space in normal health is more potential than actual, containing only enough fluid to allow for smooth sliding of the serosal layers over one another during cardiac motion. However, a wide variety of diseases affecting the pericardium can lead to an abnormal increase in pericardial fluid.

PERICARDIAL EFFUSION

Accumulations of fluid within the pericardial space may be caused by transudate, exudate, hemopericardium, and pyopericardium.[3] Table 121.1 describes some of the most common causes of pericardial effusions.[4] The presence or absence of symptoms or signs of pericardial effusion depend on many factors, including the cause of the fluid, the size of the effusion, and most important from a hemodynamic standpoint, the rate of fluid accumulation. Typically, a small noninflammatory pericardial effusion is asymptomatic and may be discovered only incidentally when an imaging study (usually either echocardiography or chest computed tomography [CT]) is ordered for other reasons. Large pericardial effusions may also be asymptomatic if they develop slowly; however, large effusions can cause symptoms if associated with increased intrapericardial pressure (discussed later under Cardiac Tamponade) or if they cause mechanical compression of structures adjacent to the heart. Specifically, esophageal compression can cause dysphagia, bronchial or tracheal compression can cause cough, phrenic nerve compression can cause hiccups, recurrent laryngeal nerve compression can result in hoarseness, and lung compression or atelectasis can cause dyspnea. Various arbitrary definitions have been promulgated[5] to define pericardial effusion size into small, moderate, and large categories. Small effusions are usually defined as 50 to 100 mL,

moderate as 100 to 500 mL, and large as greater than 500 mL. It is important to note that there is often a poor correlation between the volume of pericardial fluid and hemodynamic effects.

Echocardiography in Pericardial Effusion

Echocardiography has long been considered the first-line imaging test to diagnose pericardial effusion. Echocardiography takes advantage of the different acoustic properties of pericardial fluid as compared with the myocardium and parietal pericardium because pericardial fluid is typically echolucent, and the myocardium and pericardial membrane are echo dense. The detection of pericardial effusion was one of the first clinically useful applications of echocardiography,[6] which continues being the most practical way to diagnose, assess the severity of, and follow pericardial effusions.

Pericardial fluid, when trivial or small, tends to first accumulate posteriorly behind the left ventricle in the oblique sinus and is best imaged in the parasternal long-axis view. It is seen (when trivial) as an echolucent space between the posterior left ventricular (LV) myocardium and pericardial reflection only in systole. As the fluid volume increases, the echolucent posterior separation occurs in both systole and diastole. As the fluid accumulates to greater than 100 mL, it tends to become circumferential, and an echolucent space appears both anteriorly and posteriorly. Measuring the depth in millimeters of the echolucent separation of pericardial reflection from the myocardium or epicardium on two-dimensional (2D) echocardiography is an accepted semiquantitative way to size pericardial effusion (Table 121.2).

There are both normal anatomic variants (epicardial fat) and nonpericardial processes that can sometimes confuse and potentially mimic the echocardiographic appearance of pericardial effusion (Table 121.3). As noted in Table 121.3, left pleural effusion may also appear as an echolucent space posterior to the heart. However, the 2D parasternal long-axis view shows this fluid as posterior to the descending thoracic aorta, whereas pericardial fluid tracks anterior to the descending aorta (Fig. 121.1). Pericardial cysts and LV pseudoaneurysms can also occasionally be mistaken for loculated pericardial effusions. Epicardial fat can appear as a relatively echolucent space most often anteriorly within the pericardial reflection. The stippled appearance of epicardial fat is often seen to move in unison with cardiac motion (Fig. 121.2). Increased epicardial fat is typically seen in older adults, particularly in obese women.[6]

TABLE 121.1 Causes of Pericardial Effusion

Inflammatory
- Infectious
- Autoimmune

NEOPLASTIC

Endocrine or Metabolic
- Myxedema
- Uremia

Trauma, Iatrogenic, or Surgery

Radiation Treatment

Volume Overload States
- Congestive heart failure
- Cirrhosis

Myocardial Infarction

Idiopathic

TABLE 121.2 Echocardiographic Quantification of Pericardial Effusion

Trivial	Echolucent space <10 mm Seen only in systole
Small	Echolucent space <10 mm Seen in systole and diastole
Moderate	Echolucent space 10–20 mm
Large	Echolucent space >20 mm

TABLE 121.3 Mimics of Pericardial Effusion

Pleural effusion
Epicardial fat
Left ventricular pseudoaneurysm
Pericardial cyst

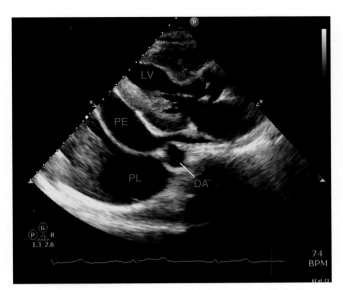

Figure 121.1. Parasternal long-axis image in a patient with both pericardial (PE) and pleural (PL) effusions. Note that the pericardial fluid lies anterior to the descending thoracic aorta (DA). The left ventricle (LV) is marked for reference.

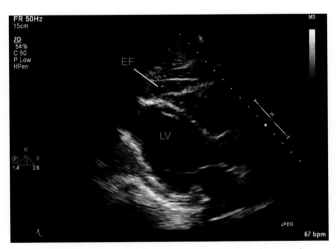

Figure 121.2. Parasternal long-axis image demonstrating anterior epicardial fat (EF). Note the typical stippled appearance of the tissue. The left ventricle (LV) is marked for reference. (See accompanying Video 121.2.)

Pericardial effusions are not always completely echolucent on echocardiography and may have varying degrees of echogenicity related to the presence of fibrin or clot, protein content, chyle, tumor cells, bacteria, and so on. The specific fluid density can be better defined sometimes with other imaging modalities such as CT and magnetic resonance imaging (MRI). However, the relative echogenicity on echocardiography should always be noted and characterized in the report because the fluid appearance (echolucent vs fibrin stranding and organization) can sometimes provide clues to the cause of the pericardial effusion and can also help decide whether drainage (if indicated) would be better accomplished with needle pericardiocentesis or surgically, with highly organized effusions most often requiring operative intervention because of loculation.

CARDIAC TAMPONADE

Cardiac tamponade is an abnormal accumulation of fluid or blood (or both) in the pericardial space that both compresses the cardiac

TABLE 121.4 Clinical and Echocardiographic Findings in Cardiac Tamponade

Clinical Findings	Echocardiographic Findings
Hypotension	Pericardial effusion
Elevated JVP	Chamber collapse
Pulsus paradoxus	IVC plethora
Tachycardia or tachypnea	Hepatic venous flow pattern change
Diminished heart sounds	Exaggerated respiratory-related changes in RV and LV size and Doppler inflow velocities
	Swinging heart

IVC, Inferior vena cava; *JVP,* jugular venous pressure; *LV,* left ventricular; *RV,* right ventricular.

chambers and inhibits chamber filling, leading to varying degrees of decreased cardiac output. When severe, it is characterized by elevated and equalized diastolic chamber and pericardial pressures, an exaggerated drop in blood pressure during inspiration (pulsus paradoxus: a >10-mm drop in systolic blood pressure with inspiration), and a reduced blood pressure (Table 121.4). It is important to remember that cardiac tamponade occurs along a continuum ranging from mild (in which clinical or bedside signs may be absent) to severe (cardiogenic shock and ultimately death). The amount of fluid or blood needed to cause cardiac tamponade is determined primarily by two interacting factors: rate of fluid accumulation (ranging from slow to very fast) and pericardial compliance or elasticity.[7]

Acute Tamponade

Rapid accumulation of as little as 150 mL of fluid or blood can cause profound tamponade physiology. This situation, known as acute tamponade, involves abrupt bleeding into a relatively stiff pericardial space, resulting in rapidly rising intrapericardial pressure (>15 mm Hg), chamber compression, and hypotension, leading to cardiogenic shock. Acute tamponade can occur with penetrating chest wounds, cardiac contusion, complication of diagnostic or therapeutic invasive cardiac procedures (coronary angiography, pacemaker implantation, cardiac ablation, and so on), free wall LV rupture as a late complication of acute myocardial infarction, and proximal aortic dissection rupturing into the pericardial space.

Subacute Tamponade

When pericardial effusion develops gradually, the pericardium stretches and can allow for the accumulation of large amounts of pericardial fluid (>1000 mL) without any significant increase in intrapericardial pressure (<10 mm Hg). Eventually, increasing pericardial fluid volume reaches a critical point at which the pericardium can no longer stretch, and even small additional pericardial fluid may cause a marked increase in intrapericardial and intracardiac pressures, leading to cardiac tamponade. Importantly, these more chronic effusions can result in tamponade if there is a decrease in intracardiac pressure (e.g., with diuresis, acute blood loss, and hemodialysis), resulting in so-called "low-pressure tamponade."[8,9]

Echocardiography in Cardiac Tamponade

As noted earlier, cardiac tamponade can occur with relatively small pericardial collections, whereas large pericardial effusions sometimes do not have hemodynamic import. Thus, the echocardiography and Doppler examination needs to assess the hemodynamic significance of the pericardial effusion. Many echocardiographic and Doppler signs of cardiac tamponade have been described; these are described in the following paragraphs. In any individual patient case, the number of abnormal echocardiography and Doppler signs

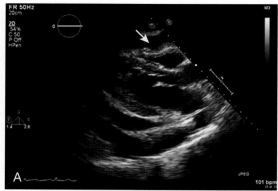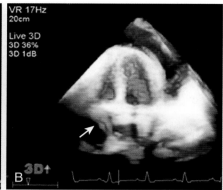

Figure 121.3. Chamber collapse. **A,** Parasternal long-axis view shows right ventricle (RV) collapse *(arrow)* in end-diastole. **B,** Three-dimensional apical four-chamber view demonstrating right atrial collapse. **C,** Note the open mitral valve and indented RV cavity during diastole. RV collapse may also be seen on parasternal short-axis views. (See accompanying Video 121.3.)

of cardiac tamponade present increases as the hemodynamic or clinical severity of the pericardial effusion progresses.

The reported echocardiography and Doppler signs of cardiac tamponade are given in Table 121.4.

Chamber Collapse

As intrapericardial pressure rises with increasing pericardial fluid, intrapericardial pressure begins to exceed diastolic intracardiac pressure and cause partial chamber wall collapse. This usually occurs with the right heart chambers because they operate at lower diastolic pressure and have thin or compliant walls (Fig. 121.3).

1. *Right atrial (RA) chamber collapse (inversion).*[10] As the intrapericardial pressure rises, it will exceed RA intracardiac pressure first in late diastole, when RA pressure is lowest, at the onset of atrial relaxation. RA chamber collapse is often seen early in the course of tamponade physiology, commonly preceding typical clinical or bedside signs of tamponade, such as hypotension or pulsus paradoxus. Thus, RA collapse is sensitive but not a specific sign of cardiac tamponade. However, the specificity of this sign improves if the duration of RA collapse exceeds 30% of the cardiac cycle.[11] RA collapse is often best imaged either in the apical or subcostal four-chamber 2D views.

2. *Right ventricular (RV) chamber collapse (inversion).*[12] RV wall inversion occurs typically in early diastole, when intracavitary RV pressure and volume is at its nadir. Again, as in RA wall collapse, the RV wall inversion extends further into diastole (longer duration) as the hemodynamics of tamponade worsen. This echocardiography finding is often best seen in the parasternal long-axis view, with transient "dimpling" of the RV outflow tract anterior wall noted when the mitral valve opens. If the patient is tachycardic, the timing of this early diastolic inward motion of the RV wall can sometimes be better appreciated using M-mode recording.

Both of these right heart chamber signs of compression depend on the intrapericardial pressure rising above the intracardiac chamber pressure. Thus, any preexisting condition associated with elevated right heart pressure may potentially mask these signs.[12] Conditions including RV hypertrophy and significant pulmonary hypertension are examples. In addition, cardiac tamponade physiology without right heart collapse has also been described[13] in the setting of infected or organized pericardial collections (tuberculosis and pyogenic), in which it is hypothesized that intrapericardial adhesions prevent the development of collapse.

3. *Left-sided chamber collapse.* Left atrial (LA) and LV chamber compression has almost exclusively been described[14–16] as related to loculated or regional collections occurring postoperatively in the cardiac or thoracic surgical patients and is discussed further later. However, circumferential pericardial effusion leading to cardiac tamponade from LV diastolic compression has rarely been reported in the setting of severe pulmonary hypertension.[7]

Inferior Vena Cava Plethora

A dilated (≥2.1 cm) inferior vena cava (IVC) with associated minimal (<50%) respiratory change in size is considered a sensitive sign of cardiac tamponade physiology, reflecting the elevated intrapericardial pressure transmitted to the right heart chambers. Studies have found a sensitivity of greater than 90% for cardiac tamponade in patients with both pulsus paradoxus and dilated IVC, with improvement after pericardial drainage.[18] Because a dilated IVC is seen in many other conditions, IVC plethora is considered a nonspecific sign of cardiac tamponade. However, its presence in the setting of a patient with a moderate or large pericardial effusion is helpful in implying that the pericardial fluid has a hemodynamic burden. This echocardiographic sign, often obvious to experienced readers with 2D imaging subcostally, can be better visualized with M-mode recording of the IVC, allowing measurement of size and greater than 50% variation in size with respiration or sniff (Fig. 121.4). Of note, IVC plethora is typically absent with low-pressure tamponade because patients have decreased right heart filling pressure.

Echocardiography and Doppler Signs of Increased Ventricular Interdependence

As increasing pericardial fluid leads to increasing intrapericardial pressure, the cardiac chambers "compete" for increasingly more limited space. Thus, an increase in filling of one ventricle causes a decrease in filling of the other. This is a respiration-related finding, which occurs for two reasons:

- Inspiration-related drop in intrathoracic pressure (and pulmonary venous pressure) is not transmitted to the heart and left heart chambers (shielded by high intrapericardial pressure or volume); thus, the pulmonary venous to LA pressure gradient is reduced in inspiration, lessening flow during inspiration into the left heart.[19]
- The systemic venous to RA pressure gradient is less affected with inspiration, favoring flow into the right heart during inspiration. The only RV wall with any "give" is the interventricular septum, which shifts leftward during inspiration. This septal shift increases RV size and reduces LV size and filling.

Doppler mitral and tricuspid diastolic inflow velocities are the most useful and practical way to quantify the exaggerated changes

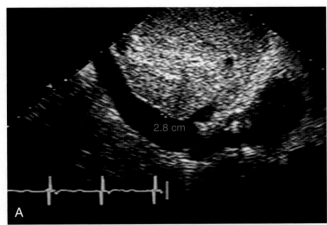

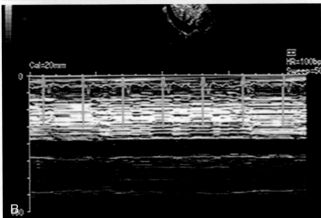

Figure 121.4. A, Subcostal view shows engorgement of the inferior vena cava. **B,** M-mode echocardiography shows an absence of inspiratory collapse.

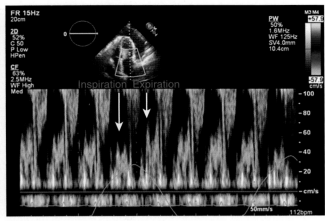

Figure 121.5. Respiratory variation in flow across the mitral valve as measured by Doppler echocardiography. Note the inspiratory decrease in left ventricular inflow.

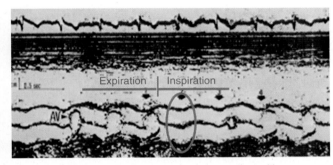

Figure 121.6. Absolute pulsus paradoxus in a patient with pericardial tamponade. Note that the aortic valve fails to open during inspiration—a dramatic M-mode representation of decreased left ventricular stroke volume.

in right and LV filling related to breathing.[20] Specifically, mitral inflow E-velocity decreases with inspiration: a drop of greater than 30% compared with expiration during regular breathing is considered consistent with significant tamponade physiology. Conversely, tricuspid inflow E velocities are significantly increased with inspiration, and a greater than 60% increase is seen compared with expiration. These changes are usually best demonstrated with pulsed-wave Doppler recording (and superimposed respirometer) from the apical four-chamber view at a slow sweep speed (Fig. 121.5). Prolongation of the isovolumetric relaxation time, measured at the mitral valve annulus on tissue Doppler images, is also increased with inspiration, reflecting increased LV filling pressure.[21] The 2D echo correlate to these Doppler findings is the presence of a noticeable sudden leftward shift of the interventricular septum toward the left ventricle with inspiration. This finding is best appreciated in the apical four-chamber view.

These echocardiography and Doppler signs of increased ventricular interdependence, along with their clinical correlate of pulsus paradoxus (Fig. 121.6), are not specific for cardiac tamponade[22] (Table 121.5). Marked dyspnea, severe chronic obstructive pulmonary disease, and pulmonary embolism have all been associated with both pulsus paradoxus and the above-described echocardiography and Doppler findings. Thus, clinical history together with presence or absence of pericardial effusion is often required to clarify the cause.

Certain conditions, when present in a patient with other signs of cardiac tamponade, may prevent or lessen this enhanced interventricular interaction (see Table 121.5). Pulsus paradoxus and the echocardiography and Doppler signs of exaggerated ventricular

TABLE 121.5 Presence of Pulsus Paradoxus in the Presence of Tamponade

Pulsus Paradoxus+, Tamponade-	Pulsus Paradoxus+, Tamponade-
Constrictive pericarditis	Positive-pressure ventilation
Pulmonary embolus	Atrial septal defect
COPD	Aortic insufficiency
Rapid, deep breathing	High LV filling pressure

COPD, Chronic obstructive pulmonary disease; *LV,* left ventricular.

interaction may not occur if the LV diastolic pressure is markedly elevated. Also, atrial septal defect, in which the increased inspiratory systemic venous return is shared between both sides of the heart, may prevent these findings. Significant aortic regurgitation and positive-pressure ventilation are two additional conditions in which pulsus paradoxus may be absent in cardiac tamponade.[23,24]

Caveats

- Loculated pericardial collections causing "regional" cardiac tamponade. This scenario is most commonly seen in early postoperative cardiac surgery patients[14,25] and often is related to a collection of blood clot compressing an individual chamber, most commonly the atria. Given the often limited transthoracic windows available in these patients, together with the localized or loculated nature of these collections, both a high index of suspicion together with other imaging modalities (transesophageal echocardiography, CT, cardiac MRI [CMRI]) are often necessary to diagnose these situations of regional cardiac tamponade, particularly as typical compressive right heart findings may be absent.

- Large left pleural effusions[26] have occasionally been described as causing tamponade physiology, sometimes with echocardiography signs such as RV diastolic collapse. In these situations, there is often pericardial effusion present, and it can be difficult to decide which collection is more significant. Clinical experience usually favors first draining the more accessible pleural fluid and then reassessing both clinically and by echocardiography.
- Hepatic venous Doppler recording,[4,13] although not always easy to obtain, can show characteristic findings in cardiac tamponade. Specifically, reduced velocities (decrease from the normal 50-cm/s range to 20 to 40 cm/s in tamponade) and a marked predominance of flow in systole is seen. In addition, the most characteristic sign of tamponade is noted on the first beat of expiration, showing absent or reversed diastolic flow. When these findings can be obtained, they are believed to be highly specific for cardiac tamponade. However, in addition to the technical difficulties in obtaining these recordings, the presence of either atrial fibrillation or significant tricuspid regurgitation may confound these hepatic venous changes.
- Swinging of the heart sometimes occurs with large pericardial effusions and cardiac tamponade as the heart swings toward and away from the chest wall and is easily appreciated with 2D echocardiographic imaging. This excessive cardiac motion is the basis for the classic ECG finding of electrical alternans (Fig. 121.7). This phenomenon is caused by beat-to-beat reciprocal variation in ventricular size. Removal of even small amounts of fluid may relieve the tamponade and this excess cardiac motion.

ECHOCARDIOGRAPHY-GUIDED PERICARDIOCENTESIS

Most hospitals now perform pericardiocentesis under echocardiographic guidance. This technique, championed by the Mayo Clinic,[27] involves transthoracic preprocedural imaging to select the optimal location on the chest with the most direct route to the largest collection of pericardial fluid, preferably at a minimal distance from the skin to fluid, and avoiding unintended structures such as the left lung or internal thoracic arteries. The most common approach with echo guidance is from the paraapical cardiac region[28] and has been performed in experienced hands with more than 99% success, no deaths, and a low complication rate. Imaging during the procedure, sometimes with injection of agitated saline to document proper needle and catheter position in the pericardial space, allows for assessment of success in eliminating the fluid.

SUMMARY

Echocardiography is particularly well-suited for the assessment of pericardial effusion presence, size, and hemodynamic significance. Coupled with careful clinical assessment, echocardiography and Doppler are often essential in helping to decide when and whether pericardial effusion should be drained and even how (surgical or pericardiocentesis) to treat it. When a pericardial effusion is large, circumferential, and not organized, most centers now favor needle pericardiocentesis as the procedure of choice. Other imaging modalities (CT and CMRI) are of significant value in complex pericardial effusions (but not life-threatening tamponade) for both tissue characterization of fluid and to define the feasibility of percutaneous versus surgical intervention.

Please access ExpertConsult to view the corresponding videos for this chapter.

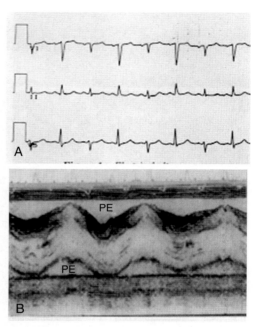

Figure 121.7. Electrical alternans on electrocardiography (**A**) and M-mode echocardiography (**B**). Swinging of the heart in the pericardial fluid (PE) alters the vectors on electrocardiography in every other beat.

Acknowledgments

The authors acknowledge the coauthors of the preceding editions of the chapter on pericardial tamponade—Drs. Richard Kutnick, R. Parker Ward, and Roberto M. Lang—for providing the structure for the current update and the included echocardiography and Doppler illustrations.

REFERENCES

1. Spodick DH. *The Pericardium: A Comprehensive Textbook.* New York: Marcel Dekker; 1997.
2. Otto CM. *The Practice of Clinical Echocardiography.* 2nd ed. Philadelphia: WB Saunders; 2002.
3. Maisch B, Seferovic PM, Ristic AD, et al. Guidelines on the diagnosis and management of pericardial diseases executive summary: the Task Force on the Diagnosis and Management of Pericardial Diseases of the European Society of Cardiology. *Eur Heart J.* 2004;25:587–610.
4. Klein AL, Abbara S, Agler DA, et al. American Society of Echocardiography clinical recommendations for multimodality cardiovascular imaging of patients with pericardial disease. *J Am Soc Echocardiogr.* 2013;26:965–1012.
5. Feigenbaum H, Waldhausen JA, Hyde LP. Ultrasound diagnosis of pericardial effusion. *J Am Med Assoc.* 1965;191:107.
6. Savage D, Garrison R, Brand F, et al. Prevalence and correlates of posterior extra echocardiographic spaces in a free-living population based on Framingham study. *Am J Cardiol.* 1983;51:1207–1212.
7. Spodick DH. Acute cardiac tamponade. *N Engl J Med.* 2003;349:684–690.
8. Antman EM, Cargill V, Grossman W. Low-pressure cardiac tamponade. *Ann Intern Med.* 1979;91:403–406.
9. Sagrista-Sauleda J, Angel J, Sambola A, et al. Low-pressure cardiac tamponade: clinical and hemodynamic profile. *Circulation.* 2006;114:945–952.
10. Kronzon I, Cohen ML, Winer HE. Diastolic atrial compression: a sensitive echo sign of cardiac tamponade. *J Am Coll Cardiol.* 1983;2:770–775.
11. Gillam LD, Guyer DE, Gibson TC, et al. Hydrodynamic compression of the right atrium: a new echo sign of cardiac tamponade. *Circulation.* 1983;68:294–301.
12. Leimgruber PP, Klopfenstein HS, Wann LS, et al. The hemodynamic derangement associated with right ventricular diastolic collapse in cardiac tamponade: an experimental echo study. *Circulation.* 1983;68:612–620.
13. Merce J, Sagrista-Sauleda J, Permanyer-Miralda G, et al. Correlation between clinical and Doppler echo findings in patients with moderate and large pericardial effusion: Implications for the diagnosis of cardiac tamponade. *Am Heart J.* 1999;138:759–764.
14. Brooker R, Farah M. Postoperative left atrial compression diagnosed by transesophageal echocardiography. *J Cardiothorac Vasc Anesth.* 1995;9:304–307.
15. Torelli J, Marwick T, Salcedo E. Left atrial tamponade: diagnosis by transesophageal echocardiography. *J Am Soc Echocardiogr.* 1991;4:413–414.

16. Fusman B, Schwinger M, Charney R, et al. Isolated collapse of left-sided heart chambers in cardiac tamponade: demonstration by two-dimensional echocardiography. *Am Heart J.* 1991;121:613–616.

17. Frey MJ, Berko B, Palevsky H, et al. Recognition of cardiac tamponade in the presence of severe pulmonary hypertension. *Ann Intern Med.* 1989;111:615–617.

18. Himelman RB, Kircher B, Rockey DC, et al. Inferior vena cava plethora with blunted respiratory response: a sensitive echo sign of cardiac tamponade. *J Am Coll Cardiol.* 1988;12:1470–1477.

19. Reddy P, Curtiss E, O'Toole J, et al. Cardiac tamponade: hemodynamic observations in man. *Circulation.* 1978;58:265–272.

20. Leeman DE, Levine MJ, Come PC. Doppler echocardiography in cardiac tamponade: exaggerated respiratory variation in transvalvular blood flow velocity integrals. *J Am Coll Cardiol.* 1988;11:572–578.

21. Appleton CP, Hatle LK, Popp RL. Cardiac tamponade and pericardial effusion: respiratory variation in transvalvular flow velocities studied by Doppler echocardiography. *J Am Coll Cardiol.* 1988;11:1020–1030.

22. Hoit BD, Shaw D. The paradoxical pulse in tamponade: mechanisms and echocardiographic correlates. *Echocardiography.* 1994;11:477–487.

23. Faehnrich JA, Noone Jr RB, White WD, et al. Effects of positive-pressure ventilation, pericardial effusion, and cardiac tamponade on respiratory variation in transmitral flow velocities. *J Cardiothorac Vasc Anesth.* 2003;17:45–50.

24. Braunwald E. *Heart Disease.* 5th ed. Philadelphia: WB Saunders; 1997:1485–1495.

25. Kochar G, Jacobs L, Kotler M. Right atrial compression in postoperative cardiac patients: detection by transesophageal echocardiography. *J Am Coll Cardiol.* 1990;16:511–516.

26. Kaplan L, Epstein S, Schwartz S, et al. Clinical, echocardiographic, and hemodynamic evidence of cardiac tamponade caused by large pleural effusions. *Am J Respir Crit Care Med.* 1995;151:904–908.

27. Callahan J, Seward J, Nishimura R, et al. Two-dimensional echocardiographically guided pericardiocentesis: experience in 117 consecutive patients. *Am J Cardiol.* 1985;55:476–479.

28. Tsang T, Freeman W, Sinak L, et al. Echocardiographically guided pericardiocentesis: evolution and state of the art technique. *Mayo Clinic Proc.* 1998;73:647–652.

122 Constrictive Pericarditis

Itzhak Kronzon, Arber Kodra

Constrictive pericarditis (CP) is a relatively rare disorder in which the stiff, poorly compliant pericardium interferes with ventricular filling, causing elevation of ventricular diastolic pressure and, as a result, increased atrial pressures. This condition is responsible for a unique form of diastolic dysfunction and diastolic heart failure characterized by abnormal passive compliance, without myocardial involvement or systolic dysfunction and without active diastolic relaxation abnormalities. CP may be acute and transient or chronic and progressive.[1] Recognition of this disorder is extremely important because pericardiectomy may offer a complete cure. The differential diagnosis includes restrictive cardiomyopathy (RCM), another form of ventricular compliance abnormality in which the culprit is the poorly compliant ventricular myocardium.

CP and RCM may imitate one another, and the differential diagnosis may be extremely difficult. The symptoms, physical findings, and many commonly used diagnostic techniques frequently fail to make the correct diagnosis. Sometimes the diagnosis can be established only after exploratory thoracotomy.

During the past two decades, echocardiography has been proven to be the technique of choice for the diagnosis of CP.[2–4] Echocardiographic diagnosis requires state-of-the-art equipment, understanding of the underlying pathophysiology, and attention to details that can be easily missed on a routine examination. Clinical and echocardiographic findings in CP and RCM are summarized in Tables 122.1 and 122.2.

DEMOGRAPHICS AND PRESENTING SYMPTOMS

The causes of CP include pericardial inflammation, infection, blunt trauma, radiation, and complications of cardiac surgery. In 30% to 70% of patients, the cause cannot be established (idiopathic CP).[5] The distribution of the causes varies geographically. In the United States and other Western countries, iatrogenic CP (as a result of cardiac surgery and radiation therapy) is more common. It is estimated that 0.3% of all patients who undergo cardiac surgery will develop CP. Longer survival in patients with Hodgkin lymphoma also leads to increasing numbers of patients who develop CP 10 to 20 years after mantle radiation. In developing countries, infection is a more common cause, with tuberculous, bacterial, fungal, and parasitic CP being more prevalent.[5]

Symptoms include those of elevated atrial pressure and low cardiac output. Characteristically, diastolic left and right heart pressures are elevated and equal; however, elevated right atrial (RA) pressure produces symptoms at a lower pressure. Symptoms include general malaise, weakness, leg edema, ascites, and shortness of breath.

PATHOPHYSIOLOGY

With the entire heart encased by a stiff, poorly compliant pericardium, diastolic filling is impaired. The end-diastolic pressure volume relation curve shifts upward and to the left, and all diastolic pressures are elevated and equal. Because the intrapericardial space is limited and fixed, an increase in the volume of one ventricle may necessitate a decrease in the other's ventricular volume. During inspiration, intrathoracic pressure decreases. The pressure in the pulmonary veins, which are intrathoracic structures, also declines accordingly. In contrast, the decline in intrathoracic pressure is not transmitted to the heart, which is isolated by the thick, rigid pericardium. As a result, the pressure gradient between the pulmonary veins and the left atrium declines, and therefore the flow into the left atrium decreases. This leads to a decline in transmitral flow and left ventricular (LV) filling during inspiration. With a smaller inspiratory LV volume, more intrapericardial space becomes available for the right ventricle, which is now able to expand and accommodate increased systemic venous return. As the result of these events, the interventricular septum shifts toward the left. With expiration, the intrathoracic pressure increases, the gradient between the pulmonary veins and the left atrium increases, and as a result transmitral blood flow and LV volume during expiration increase. The larger LV volume permits less expiratory intrapericardial space for the right ventricle, which is now unable to expand appropriately during expiration. This leads to expiratory reversal of flow in the systemic veins even before atrial contraction. This abnormal finding is best demonstrated in the hepatic veins using Doppler echocardiography.

DIAGNOSTICS

The physical examination shows signs of right heart failure. A rapid Y descent can be seen in the engorged jugular veins. Cardiac auscultation is remarkable for a lack of murmurs. A pericardial knock is occasionally heard in early diastole. The electrocardiogram is not diagnostic. It may show nonspecific ST-T changes. Low voltage may be seen (<50%). Chest radiography and fluoroscopy show

TABLE 122.1 Clinical Data in Constrictive Pericarditis Versus Restrictive Cardiomyopathy

	Constriction	Restriction
HISTORY		
Right heart failure	Present	Present
Left heart failure (pulmonary congestion)	Uncommon	More common
Low cardiac output	Present	Present
Palpitations, arrhythmia	Present	Present
PHYSICAL EXAMINATION		
Pericardial knock	Present	Absent
S2, S4	Absent	Present
Apical impulse	Decreased	Present
Pericardial knuckle	Present	Absent
CARDIAC CATHETERIZATION		
High diastolic pressure	Present	Present
Square root sign	Present	Present
LV vs RV diastolic pressure	Equal	Unequal (left > right)
OTHER DIAGNOSTIC TESTS		
Pericardial calcification	May be present	Absent
Pericardial thickening	Present	Absent
Low-voltage ECG	May be present	May be present (amyloid)
Myocardial biopsy	Normal	Abnormal

ECG, Electrocardiogram; *LV,* left ventricular; *RV,* right ventricular.

TABLE 122.2 Echocardiography in Constrictive Pericarditis Versus Restrictive Cardiomyopathy

	Constriction	Restriction
M-MODE AND TWO-DIMENSIONAL ECHOCARDIOGRAPHY		
IVC plethora	Present	Present
Premature pulmonic valve opening	Present	Absent
Septal bounce	Present	Absent
DOPPLER ECHOCARDIOGRAPHY		
Mitral E-wave velocity	Increased	Increased
Mitral E/A ratio	Increased	Increased
Mitral deceleration time (ms)	<160	<160
E-wave respiratory variations	>25%	Absent
Hepatic vein expiratory flow reversal	Present	Absent
Increased expiratory pulmonary venous flow velocity	Present	Absent
M-mode color-flow propagation velocity	Normal or increased	Decreased
MITRAL RING TISSUE DOPPLER		
e′ velocity	Normal or increased	Decreased
E/e′ ratio	Normal or decreased	Increased
Lateral e′ < medial e′ (annulus reversus)	Present	Absent
Longitudinal strain	Preserved	Diminished

IVC, Inferior vena cava.

clear lungs and a normal or smaller than normal cardiac silhouette. Pericardial calcification may be seen.

Cardiac catheterization, once the gold standard for presurgical diagnosis, demonstrates elevation and equalization of all intracardiac diastolic pressures, with a characteristic dip and plateau appearance of the right ventricular (RV) and LV diastolic pressures ("square root sign"). The pulmonary artery pressure is not markedly elevated, and the RV diastolic pressure reaches one-third or more of the systolic pressure. In contrast, systolic RV pressure in RCM may be higher, but LV diastolic pressure is higher than the right. Occasionally, when diastolic pressures are equal, a change in loading conditions (e.g., intravenous administration of 500 mL of saline) is required for the differential diagnosis between CP and RCM. In CP, diastolic pressures maintain their equalization, whereas in RCM, they separate as the LV diastolic pressure exceeds the RV diastolic pressure.[6]

The use of transthoracic Doppler echocardiography has now replaced cardiac catheterization as the initial test for CP. Cardiac magnetic resonance (CMRI) and computed tomography (CT) are considered complementary techniques to confirm CP and can be important tools in selected patients with poor echocardiographic windows or unclear findings. A CT scan can reveal pericardial thickening (>4 mm) and occasionally calcification (Fig. 122.1). Indirect findings may include tubular deformity of the ventricles, a dilated inferior vena cava (IVC) or hepatic vein (HV), ascites, or pleural effusions. CMRI can also demonstrate pericardial thickening (Fig. 122.2). However, a lack of calcification or thickening does not rule out CP, but their presence does not always determine the diagnosis.[7] Cine CMRI can also demonstrate diastolic septal bounce, abrupt cessation of diastolic filling, ventricular interdependence, and tethering of the thickened pericardium caused by adhesions between the pericardium and myocardium.

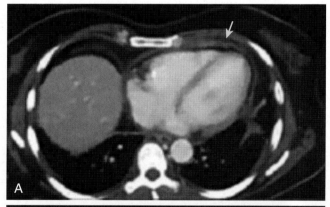
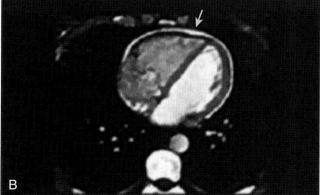

Figure 122.1. Computed tomography scan of the chest. **A,** Increased pericardial thickness *(arrow)*. **B,** Calcification of the pericardium *(arrow)*.

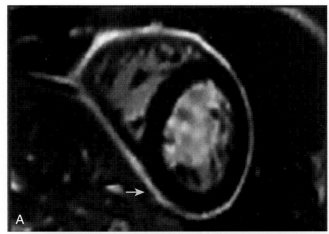

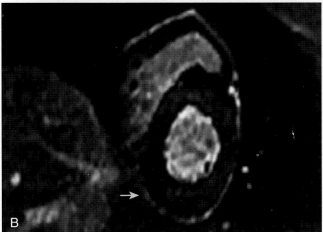

Figure 122.2. Cardiac magnetic resonance imaging of the heart. **A,** Severe late gadolinium enhancement before treatment with prednisone *(arrow)*. **B,** Minimal late gadolinium enhancement after treatment with prednisone *(arrow)*.

ECHOCARDIOGRAPHY

Echocardiographic findings are summarized in Figs. 122.3 and 122.4. M-mode and two-dimensional echocardiography can show the characteristic diastolic septal bounce (see Fig. 122.3A). There are respiratory variations in ventricular volumes. The dilated IVC with a lack of respiratory variation in diameter is highly suggestive of markedly elevated RA pressures (see Fig. 122.3B). An elevated RV diastolic pressure with a normal or near-normal pulmonary artery pressure may result in premature pulmonic valve opening at end-diastole because the pressure in the right ventricle equals or exceeds pulmonary artery diastolic pressure. Pericardial thickening and a small pericardial effusion (in the constrictive-effusive variant) are occasionally demonstrated.

PULSED DOPPLER STUDIES

The transmitral flow velocity pattern is characteristic of markedly elevated LV filling pressure (restrictive pattern). The high left atrial (LA) pressure is associated with high LA–LV pressure gradient at the time of mitral valve opening and therefore high E-wave velocity, low A velocity, and higher than normal E/A ratio (Fig. 122.4A). Poor LV compliance results in a rapid rise of LV early diastolic pressure, which leads to a rapid decline of

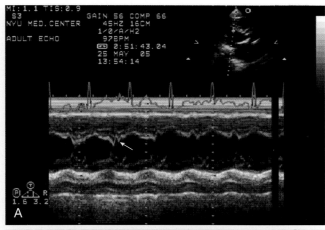

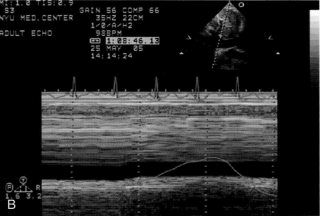

Figure 122.3. M-mode echocardiography in constrictive pericarditis. **A,** Diastolic septal bounce. **B,** The inferior vena cava is dilated without respiratory variations in diameter.

LV–LA pressure gradient. As a result, there is a rapid, early diastolic deceleration of transmitral flow, with shorter than normal deceleration times (<160 ms) (see Fig. 122.4A). These findings are seen in both CP and RCM.

Exaggerated respiratory variation in transmitral flow is frequently seen in CP (and not in RCM). With inspiration, the early diastolic (E wave) velocity decreases. An inspiratory decline of 25% or more is considered significant (see Fig. 122.4A). In CP, there is also an exaggerated inspiratory decrease in transaortic valve flow velocity, whereas the flow velocity across the right heart valves increases with inspiration.[2] In patients with CP, the early diastolic flow velocity across the tricuspid valve (E wave) increases by 40% or more with inspiration (Fig. 122.4B).

The pulmonary venous flow can be evaluated during a transthoracic and, even better, during a transesophageal study. In both CP and RCM, the antegrade diastolic velocity wave is higher than the systolic, and the retrograde flow velocity wave during atrial contraction is higher than normal. However, only in CP does the diastolic wave velocity increase with expiration.

Pulsed Doppler studies of hepatic vein flow can be obtained from the subxiphoid window. In both CP and RCM, the antegrade flow velocity is higher in diastole than in systole. In patients with CP (but not with RCM), there is frequently an expiratory reversal of diastolic hepatic venous flow[3] (Fig. 122.4C). This is in contrast to the pulsed Doppler of the superior vena cava, which shows little respiratory changes in systolic forward flow velocity from inspiration to expiration (Fig. 122.4D).

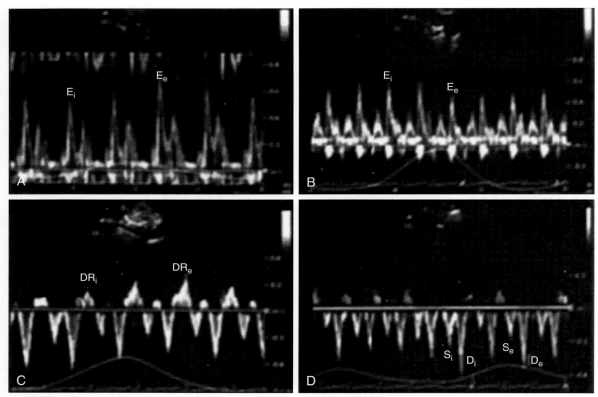

Figure 122.4. Doppler echocardiography in constrictive pericarditis. **A,** Transmitral flow velocity tracing (pulsed Doppler) demonstrates high E wave, low A wave, and short deceleration time (restrictive pattern). **B,** Pulsed Doppler tracing shows inspiratory increase of in tricuspid velocity with inspiration and opposite changes in expiration. **C,** Pulsed Doppler tracing demonstrates expiratory diastolic flow reversal in the hepatic vein. **D,** Pulse Doppler tracing demonstrating flow through the superior vena cava with respiration.

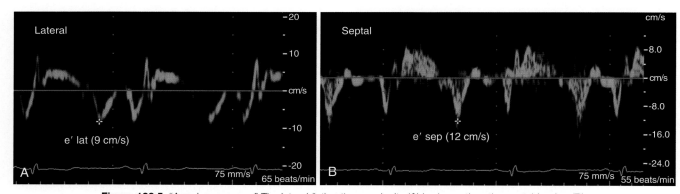

Figure 122.5. "Annulus reversus." The lateral (lat) e' tissue velocity (**A**) is slower than the septal (sep) e' (**B**).

TISSUE DOPPLER

In CP, the myocardium is normal. Therefore, early diastolic LV active relaxation is normal. The longitudinal early diastolic tissue velocity measured with the sample volume at the mitral ring (e' wave) is normal or even increased (Fig. 122.5). Thus, although the transmitral E-wave velocity is higher than normal, the E/e' ratio is within normal limits or decreased (≤ 8). This unusual combination of high filling pressure and normal E/e' ratio is pathognomonic of CP. In these patients, the E/e' ratio is inversely related to the LV filling (wedge) pressure (annulus paradoxus). In contrast, the myocardium, the active early diastolic relaxation, and therefore the early diastolic tissue velocity are abnormal in RCM. In RCM, the e'-wave peak velocity is smaller than normal, and the E/e' ratio is high, usually 15 or more.[4]

Color M-mode flow propagation in the left ventricle is yet another method to demonstrate normal active relaxation and normal LV myocardium in CP. The flow propagation velocity is normal in CP (usually ≥ 45 cm/s) and slower than normal in RCM.[8]

In patients with CP, the lateral mitral ring motion at early diastole (e') is limited because of tethering of the lateral part of the mitral ring to the thickened pericardium. Thus, the septal part of the mitral ring tissue e' velocity is higher than the lateral velocity. This finding (known as "annulus reversus") (see Fig. 122.5) is not observed in patients with RCM and in normal individuals.[9] The RV wall motion may also be restricted and slower than normal in patients with CP.

Strain imaging is also useful in the differentiation between CP and RCM. In CP, whereas the circumferential, torsion, and early diastolic untwisting are reduced, global longitudinal strain, displacement, and early diastolic tissue velocity are unchanged. In RCM, the longitudinal strain is decreased, but the circumferential strain and early diastolic twisting are unchanged.[10]

Doppler echocardiography is superior to all other invasive and noninvasive techniques in the diagnosis of CP in symptomatic patients with apparent right heart failure. The combination of characteristic respiratory variation in transmitral flow, hepatic vein flow, and normal tissue Doppler e′ wave velocity and E/e′ ratio correctly predicted CP in more than 90% of patients in whom the diagnosis was confirmed by surgery.

A recent American Society of Echocardiography expert consensus document describes in details the role of echocardiography and other imaging modalities in patients with pericardial disease.[11]

TREATMENT

Recent-onset, symptomatic CP of various etiologies may be transient, with remarkable recovery within an average time of 2 months.[1] In the absence of a medical emergency, CP should be observed and treated medically. Pericardiectomy should be considered in chronic, symptomatic CP. The perioperative mortality rate is 5% to 8%. Survivors have fewer or no symptoms, with marked improvement of the New York Heart Association (NYHA) class. The late survival of those operated is still inferior to age- and sex-matched control participants. Predictors of long-term mortality include age older than 55 years, previous history of radiation, preoperative NYHA class IV, and incomplete pericardiectomy.[5,12]

Acknowledgment

The authors acknowledge the American Society of Echocardiography for allowing us to reproduce Figs. 122.1 to 122.3.

REFERENCES

1. Haley JH, Tajik AJ, Danielson GK, et al. Transient constrictive pericarditis: causes and natural history. *J Am Coll Cardiol.* 2004;43:271–275.
2. Oh JK, Hatle JK, Seward JB, et al. Diagnostic role of echocardiography in constrictive pericarditis. *Am J Cardiol.* 1994;23:154–162.
3. Von Bibra H, Schober K, Jenni R, et al. Diagnosis of constrictive pericarditis by pulsed Doppler echocardiography. *Am J Cardiol.* 1989;63:483–488.
4. Ha J, Ommen SR, Tajik AJ, et al. Differentiation of constrictive pericarditis from restrictive cardiomyopathy using mitral annular velocity by tissue Doppler echocardiography. *Am J Cardiol.* 2004;94:316–319.
5. Ling LH, Oh JK, Schaff HV, et al. Constrictive pericarditis in the modern era: evolving clinical spectrum and impact on outcome after pericardiectomy. *Circulation.* 1999;100:1380–1386.
6. Nishimura RA, Connolly DC, Parkin TW, Stanson AW. Constrictive pericarditis: assessment of current diagnostic procedures. *Mayo Clin Proc.* 1985;60:397.
7. Talreja DR, Edwards WD, Danielson WD, et al. Constrictive pericarditis in 26 patients with histologically normal pericardial thickness. *Circulation.* 2003;108:1852–1857.
8. Rajagopalan N, Garcia MJ, Rodriguez L, et al. Comparison of new Doppler echocardiography methods to differentiate constrictive pericardial heart disease and restrictive cardiomyopathy. *Am J Cardiol.* 2001;87:86–94.
9. Reus CS, Wilansky SM, Lester SJ, et al. Mitral "annulus reversus" to diagnose constrictive pericarditis. *Eur J Echocardiogr.* 2009;10:372–375.
10. Sengupta PP, Krishnamurty VK, Abbayaratna WP, et al. Disparate patterns of left ventricular mechanics differentiate constrictive pericarditis from restrictive cardiomyopathy. *JACC Cardiovasc Imag.* 2008;1:29–38.
11. Klein AL, Abhara S, Agler DA, et al. American Society of Echocardiography clinical recommendation for multimodality cardiovascular imaging of patients with pericardial disease. *J Am Soc Echocardiogr.* 2013;26:965–1012.
12. Moosdorf R. Indications, results and pitfalls in the surgery of constrictive pericarditis. *Herz.* 2000;25:794–798.

123 Effusive Constrictive Pericarditis

Eric Berkowitz, Itzhak Kronzon

Effusive constrictive pericarditis is the least common of the pericardial constraint syndromes. It is defined as the persistence of elevated intracardiac pressure after pericardiocentesis for pericardial tamponade. It was first recognized in the 1920s and 1930s when surgical pericardiectomy became an established therapy for constrictive pericarditis. The syndrome combines elements of pericardial effusion or tamponade with a visceral constrictive pericarditis.[1,2]

EPIDEMIOLOGY

The prevalence of effusive constrictive pericarditis differs based on presentation. It has been reported to be present in 1.3% of patients with pericarditis.[2] In those presenting with pericardial effusions, the prevalence was 1.4% to 3.6%,[3,4] and for those who present with tamponade, it was as high as 6.9% to 7.9%.[1,2] In one surgical series, 24% of patients requiring pericardiectomy for constrictive pericarditis had effusive constrictive pericarditis.[5] Given that many of these numbers come from patients who underwent left and right heart catheterizations, they may underestimate the true prevalence of effusive constrictive pericarditis. In a recent study, the incidence of constrictive physiology on postpericardiocentesis echocardiography Doppler examination was 16.1%. This suggests that the actual incidence may be considerably higher than previously thought.[6]

CAUSE

The cause of effusive constrictive pericarditis greatly depends on the geographic location. In areas where tuberculosis is endemic, it is responsible for the vast majority of pericardial disease, such as in South Africa, where 70% of pericardial effusions are tuberculous.[7] The incidence of effusive constrictive pericarditis in patients with tuberculous pericarditis in endemic areas was found to be 2.6% to 15%.[8–10] In one study, in which invasive measurements were used during the drainage of tuberculous pericardial effusions, 38% met the hemodynamic criteria for effusive constrictive pericarditis.[11] This is in contrast to the findings in Western countries, where tuberculosis is far less prevalent. In these geographic regions, findings mirror other pericardial diseases in which a broad spectrum of causes are reported, with idiopathic being the most common. However, in contrast to chronic noneffusive constrictive pericarditis, radiation-related and malignancy-related causes occur more frequently than after pericardiotomy.[1,2]

PATHOPHYSIOLOGY

The pericardium consists of two layers forming a sac around the heart. These layers are the visceral and parietal pericardium. The visceral pericardium, which is a cellular monolayer adherent to the myocardium, and the fibrous parietal pericardium are separated by a space that usually contains 10 to 50 mL of lubricating fluid. The relatively inelastic pericardium exerts pressure on the underlying myocardial chambers. The greatest of these mechanical effects is on the thinner-walled right atrium and right ventricle, in which at least 50% of normal diastolic pressure is caused by pericardial influence.[1]

Although features can overlap with both constrictive pericarditis and pericardial effusion, there are findings unique to effusive constrictive pericarditis. These characteristic findings are found at pericardiectomy and include thickening of both parietal and visceral pericardium with fibrosis and nonspecific inflammation with interspersed adhesions and fluid.

Despite findings of thickened parietal and visceral pericardium, the unique pathophysiological feature of this form of cardiac compression is the constricted visceral pericardium, which is associated with concomitant pericardial effusion. These two disease processes have combined, thereby reducing myocardial transmural pressure and restricting chamber filling. The compression from the affected visceral membrane will ultimately lead to underlying myocardial fiber atrophy. In contrast to chronic constrictive pericarditis, pericardial calcification is rarely seen, and when it does occur, it does so in unusual locations.[1,2,12]

Although presentation can vary, patients tend to present with three clinical scenarios:

1. The first occurs in patients presenting with initial hemodynamics resembling tamponade. The hallmark of effusive constrictive pericarditis is seen with removal of pericardial fluid and reduction in intrapericardial pressure. When intrapericardial pressure is normalized, there is persistence of diastolic filling abnormalities within the cardiac chambers, although generally less pronounced. At this point, there is a transition from tamponade physiology to that of constrictive pericarditis in which the compressive effects are generally seen when the heart exceeds a critical size during diastolic filling. The continued hemodynamic abnormality is reflected by persistent elevation of right and left heart filling pressures. This is also expressed clinically with symptoms of right heart failure.[2,13]
2. Chronic or subacute constrictive pericarditis with associated pericardial effusion, which is generally partially organized and composed of echogenic material[13]
3. Chronic pericardial effusion with signs and symptoms of right heart failure

In the latter two scenarios, both invasive and noninvasive evaluations resemble those of constrictive pericarditis on initial presentation.[13]

DIAGNOSTIC TESTS

Invasive hemodynamic measurements have historically been the gold standard by which effusive constrictive pericarditis has been diagnosed. This generally is done on patients presenting with either tamponade or large pericardial effusions requiring pericardiocentesis. If at the time of pericardiocentesis, intracardiac and intrapericardial pressure monitoring is performed, one would see a failure of right atrial pressure to fall by 50% or to a new level of 10 mmHg or less after the intrapericardial pressure is normalized. In addition, on the ventricular pressure waveform, there may be a transition to a dip-plateau morphology without significant drop in end-diastolic pressures.[2]

Pericardial fluid analysis should be undertaken whenever a pericardiocentesis is performed. Patients with constrictive physiology after pericardiocentesis are more likely to have a higher percentage of neutrophils and a lower percentage of monocytes compared with the fluid of patients without constrictive physiology.[6] When this pattern is found on fluid analysis, one should have a higher suspicion for effusive constrictive pericarditis.

Any patient presenting with right heart failure with a pericardial effusion or recent pericardiocentesis must have effusive constrictive pericarditis in the differential diagnosis. In addition, patients with recent acute pericarditis, especially those with associated pericardial effusions, in whom signs and symptoms of right heart failure occur within weeks of the inciting injury, should undergo further workup for effusive constrictive pericarditis.

Echocardiography

Echocardiography should be performed in all patients with suspected effusive constrictive pericarditis. Special attention should be given to pericardial thickening and the presence of a pericardial effusion. In addition, a full, comprehensive evaluation of diastolic function is in order.

The interpretation of the echocardiographic features of effusive constrictive pericarditis depends on the clinical presentation. In patients presenting with large pericardial effusions, the initial M-mode, two-dimensional, (2D) and Doppler features will be most consistent with a sizable pericardial effusion and cardiac tamponade (Fig. 123.1). Some findings include plethoric inferior vena cava and hepatic veins, cardiac chamber collapse, respiratory variation in chamber size, respiratory variation in transvalvular velocities, an increased isovolumic relaxation time with inspiration, and low hepatic vein velocities with diastolic expiratory reversals. On drainage of the pericardial effusion, there should be a transition from tamponade features to constrictive features on echocardiography. These findings may include diastolic flattening of the left ventricular (LV) posterior wall endocardium with little or absent respiratory movement, decreased LV posterior wall movement in early diastole, septal bounce, marked dilatation and absent or diminished collapse of the inferior vena cava and hepatic veins, more than a 25% fall in mitral inflow velocity, and an increase of greater than 40% in tricuspid velocity in the first beat after inspiration, with opposite changes occurring during expiration and with low hepatic vein velocities with decreased expiratory diastolic hepatic vein velocities and large diastolic flow reversal.[13] The specific echocardiographic features of both tamponade and constrictive pericarditis are covered in their respective chapters. Although not validated, an early feature that may be present immediately after drainage is M-mode and 2D imaging depicting a persistence of a plethoric and noncollapsible inferior vena cava (see Fig. 123.1 B and D). This represents a persistent elevation in right atrial pressure.

For patients presenting with either chronic effusion or chronic constrictive pericarditis, there is generally a transition to or the presence of organized intrapericardial material evidenced by an echogenic pericardial effusion (see Fig. 123.1C).[10,13–15] Imaging of the pericardial effusion may reveal bandlike fibrinous strands that traverse the pericardial cavity from visceral to parietal surfaces, resulting in loculation of the effusion. With loculated and organized effusions, there may not be alterations in the location of pericardial fluid with position change. Visceral pericardial thickening and irregularities are sometimes appreciated.[13,15]

OTHER TECHNIQUES

Computed tomography (CT) and cardiac magnetic resonance imaging (CMRI) are complementary to echocardiography in the workup of suspected effusive constrictive pericarditis. CT may help in the evaluation of the pericardium by measuring the degree of pericardial thickening. A thickness greater than 3 mm is considered abnormal. Other findings on CT may include high-attenuation material in the effusion, enhancing pericardial layers with or without bandlike strands, nodular thickening of the pericardial surface, pericardial calcification, and loculations.[13]

CMRI can also evaluate the degree of pericardial thickening. Slow phase-contrast flow MRI has the ability to distinguish pericardial fluid from the pericardium and to detect inflammation (Fig. 123.2 and Video 123.2). Tagged cine CMRI may demonstrate adhesions in areas without pericardial fluid, as is the case with loculations. Functional studies looking at chamber morphology and volumes may reveal increased ventricular interdependence, resulting in flattening or inversion of the septum.[13,16]

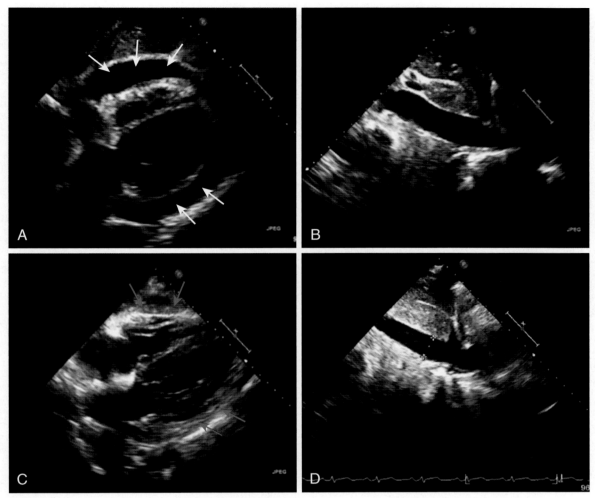

Figure 123.1. A patient with uremic effusive constrictive pericarditis initially presented with a large pericardial effusion *(white arrows)* and tamponade features on echocardiography (**A**), including a plethoric, noncollapsing inferior vena cava (**B**). After pericardiocentesis, the patient continued to have right heart failure, and on repeat echocardiography, there was transition to an organized, echogenic effusion (**C;** *red arrows*) with persistence of the plethoric, noncollapsing inferior vena cava (**D**), indicating failure of right atrial pressure to fall by 50%.

TREATMENT

Therapy should aim to relieve any hemodynamic compromise. If tamponade is present or suspected, timely drainage of the pericardial effusion should be performed. In addition, if a patient has refractory heart failure with end-organ hypoperfusion, an early surgical approach may be considered. Many patients may eventually require surgical intervention. One study suggested that as many as 65% will require intervention within the first year of diagnosis.[11] Epicardiectomy (i.e., removal of the visceral pericardium), and not just pericardiectomy, is considered the procedure of choice.

Although many patients will require surgery, there is a group of patients in whom surgery may be avoided. Nearly half of individuals with effusive constrictive pericarditis may have a transient form of the disease with three distinct phases. Phase I is an acute presentation of pericarditis with pericardial effusion of any cause. During phase II, there are resolution and marked improvement of the pericardial effusion with constrictive physiology and heart failure symptoms persisting. In phase III, there is resolution of constrictive physiology and heart failure symptoms. The mean time to phase III is 2.7 months (12 days to 10 months).[17] Patients with transient constriction are more likely to have an idiopathic or noncalcific tuberculous effusive constrictive pericarditis.[1,2]

In these patients, a conservative approach with medical therapy may lead to complete or partial resolution. The mainstay of a medical strategy should be therapy targeting the underlying cause of the pericardial disease.[1] The clinical picture should be a factor when deciding on an antiinflammatory agent. For patients with severely compromised hemodynamics, high-dose steroids may be used. In patients with less compromised hemodynamics, a less potent antiinflammatory agent may be considered. It is important to allow adequate time to assess for response to medical therapy, given the high morbidity and mortality associated with surgery. Some studies have reported an early surgical mortality rate as high as 15% to 30%.[1,2,12] Despite these findings, good long-term outcomes can be seen in patients who respond to medical therapy or survive pericardiectomy.

Please access ExpertConsult to view the corresponding video for this chapter.

REFERENCES

1. Syed F, Ntsekhe M, Mayosi B, et al. Effusive-constrictive pericarditis. *Heart Fail Rev.* 2013;18:277–287.
2. Sagrista-Sauleda J, Angel J, Sanchez A, et al. Effusive-constrictive pericarditis. *N Engl J Med.* 2004;350:469–475.
3. Nugue O, Millaire A, Porte H, et al. Pericardioscopy in the etiologic diagnosis of pericardial effusion in 141 consecutive patients. *Circulation.* 1996;94:1635–1641.
4. Tsang T, Barnes M, Gersh B, et al. Outcomes of clinically significant idiopathic pericardial effusion requiring intervention. *Am J Cardiol.* 2003;91:704–707.

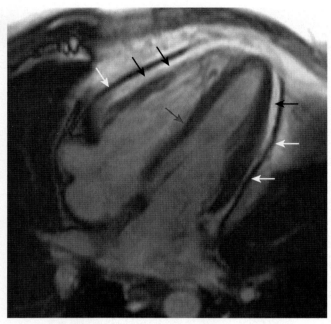

Figure 123.2. Cine cardiovascular magnetic resonance (CMRI) imaging of effusive constrictive pericarditis. Dynamic cine CMRI images in long axis demonstrate a dark and thickened pericardium *(white arrows)* along with a bright pericardial effusion *(black arrows)*. In addition, a septal bounce *(red arrow)* can be seen with pericardial tethering by the right ventricular free wall (Courtesy of Dr. Monvadi B. Srichai, NYU Langone Medical Center. (See accompanying Video 123.2.))

5. Cameron J, Oesterle SN, Baldwin JC, Hancock EW. The etiologic spectrum of constrictive pericarditis. *Am Heart J.* 1987;113:354–360.
6. Kim K, Miranda W, Sinak L, et al. Effusive-constrictive pericarditis after pericardiocentesis: incidence, associated findings, and natural history. *JACC Cardiovasc Imaging.* 2018;11(4):534–541.
7. Reuter H, Oesterle S, Baldwin J, et al. Epidemiology of pericardial effusions at a large academic hospital in South Africa. *Epidemiol Infect.* 2005;133:393–399.
8. Reuter H, Burgess L, Louw V, et al. The management of tuberculous pericardial effusion: experience in 233 consecutive patients. *Cardiovasc J S Afr.* 2007;18:20–25.
9. Sagrista-Sauleda J, Permanyer-Miralda G, Soler-Soler J. Tuberculous pericarditis: ten year experience with a prospective protocol for diagnosis and treatment. *J Am Coll Cardiol.* 1988;11:724–728.
10. Choi H, Song J, Shim T, et al. Prognostic value of initial echocardiographic features in patients with tuberculous pericarditis. *Korean Circ J.* 2010;40:377–386.
11. Ntsekhe M, Syed F, Russell J, et al. The prevalence of effusive constrictive pericarditis in patients with confirmed tuberculous pericarditis. *J Am Coll Cardiol.* 2009;53:A169.
12. Hancock E. Subacute effusive-constrictive pericarditis. *Circulation.* 1971;43:183–192.
13. Klein A, Abbara S, Agler D, et al. American Society of Echocardiography clinical recommendations for multimodality cardiovascular imaging of patients with pericardial disease. *J Am Soc Echocardiogr.* 2013;26:965–1012.
14. Martin R, Bowden R, Filly K, et al. Intrapericardial abnormalities in patients with pericardial effusion. Findings by two- dimensional echocardiography. *Circulation.* 1980;61:568–572.
15. Baker C, Orsinelli D. Subacute effusive-constrictive pericarditis: diagnosis by serial echocardiography. *J Am Soc Echocardiogr.* 2004;17:1204–1206.
16. Bogaert J, Francone M. Cardiovascular magnetic resonance in pericardial diseases. *J Cardiovasc Magn Reson.* 2009;11(1–14).
17. Haley J, Tajik A, Danielson G, et al. Transient constrictive pericarditis: causes and natural history. *J Am Coll Cardiol.* 2004;43:271–275.

124 Pericardial Cysts and Congenital Absence of the Pericardium

Sushil Allen Luis, John Gorcsan III, Sunil V. Mankad

PERICARDIAL CYSTS

Pericardial cysts are benign intrathoracic lesions accounting for 6% of all mediastinal masses.[1] They are typically unilocular, contain serous fluid, and range from 1 to 5 cm in diameter, although giant cysts have been reported.[2] Inflammatory cysts and pseudocysts are caused by pericardial inflammation or loculated effusion from surgery, trauma, pericarditis, or chronic bacterial or tuberculous infection. A parasitic or hydatid cyst is typically multilocular.

Clinical Presentation

Most cysts are found by incidental imaging studies performed for other indications. Although many are asymptomatic and have a benign course, up to one-third of patients report atypical chest pain, dyspnea, or persistent cough.[3] Potential complications include cyst infection, hemorrhage or rupture, erosion into adjacent structures such as the superior vena cava (SVC) or right ventricular (RV) free wall, cardiac tamponade, RV outflow tract obstruction, atrial fibrillation, obstruction of the right main bronchus, or sudden death.[4]

Imaging Modalities

The characteristic chest radiography finding is a rounded, well-circumscribed radiodense mass at the right cardiophrenic angle, abutting the diaphragm. Other locations such as the left cardiophrenic angle, hila, or elsewhere in the superior mediastinum have been reported.[3]

On echocardiography, the cyst appears as a rounded, echolucent cystic structure adjacent to the right atrium, which do not communicate with the pericardial space. Transesophageal echocardiography may offer better delineation.[4] Large pericardial cysts may result in right-sided cardiac chamber compression, resulting in symptoms. The differential diagnosis for a pericardial cyst, include a pericardial diverticulum. Pericardial diverticula are extremely rare outpouchings through a defect in the parietal pericardium. Pericardial diverticula communicate with the pericardial space and defect in the pericardial lining and may be noted on echocardiography. Additionally, given their communication with the pericardial space, pericardial diverticula may change in size and shape with repositioning and respiration.[5]

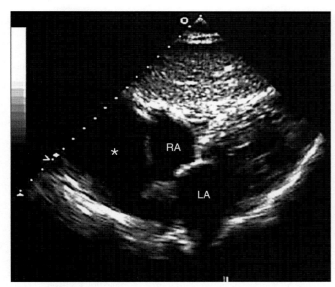

Figure 124.1. Subcostal view of a pericardial cyst *(asterisk)* adjacent to the right atrium (RA). Note the smooth border and that there is no compression of the RA. *LA,* Left atrium. (See accompanying Video 124.1.)

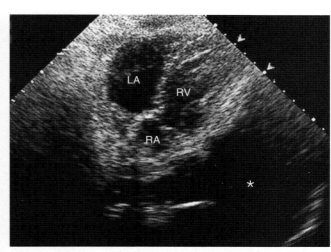

Figure 124.3. Subcostal view of the same giant pericardial cyst as in Fig. 124.2. The true enormity of the size of the cyst *(asterisk)* is better revealed from the subcostal view, and the decision was made to percutaneously drain the cyst. A total of 1100 mL of fluid was removed. *LA,* Left atrium; *RA,* right atrium; *RV,* right ventricle. (See accompanying Video 124.3.)

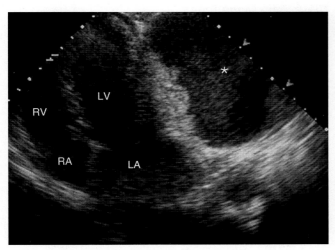

Figure 124.2. Apical four-chamber view demonstrating a giant pericardial cyst *(asterisk)* adjacent to the left ventricle (LV) and left atrium (LA). *RA,* Right atrium; *RV,* right ventricle. (See accompanying Video 124.2.)

Cardiac magnetic resonance imaging (CMRI) or computed tomography (CT) is usually pursued to confirm the diagnosis, ascertain other anatomic details, and distinguish from neoplasms and aneurysms.[5]

An example of a typical pericardial cyst adjacent to the right atrium is shown in Fig. 124.1 and Video 124.1. A giant pericardial cyst adjacent to the left ventricle is shown in Figs. 124.2 and 124.3 and Videos 124.2 and 124.3. The impressive chest radiograph that led to the echocardiographic study demonstrating the giant pericardial cyst is also shown (Fig. 124.4).

Differential Diagnosis

The main differential diagnoses are cardiac and mediastinal tumors, noncardiac cysts, abscesses, and visceral hernias.

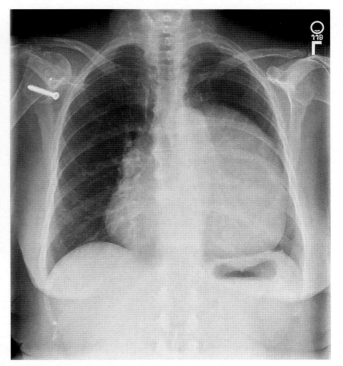

Figure 124.4. Associated chest radiography (same patient as in Fig. 124.2) demonstrating a markedly enlarged cardiac silhouette caused by the giant pericardial cyst.

Treatment

Asymptomatic patients require periodic follow-up, typically with serial CT or CMRI evaluations every 1 to 2 years.[5] In the setting of symptoms or diagnostic ambiguity, percutaneous aspiration with possible ethanol sclerosis is recommended. Thoracoscopic or open surgical resection may be warranted when there is diagnostic uncertainty or for recurrent cysts despite percutaneous aspiration. Surgical excision of echinococcal cysts should be avoided. Instead, albendazole pretreatment followed by ethanol or silver nitrate instillation is advised.[1]

ABSENCE OF THE PERICARDIUM

Absence of the pericardium is rare and either acquired or congenital.

Epidemiology

Congenital absence is an uncommon entity (<1:100,000)[1] with a 3:1 or 4:1 male preponderance.[6] Absence of the left side is the most common, seen in 67% of cases.[6,7] Rarer subtypes are total absence, right-sided, and diaphragmatic defects. The more common acquired variant is nearly always consequent to surgical pericardiectomy.

Pathogenesis

Absence of the pericardium occurs as a result of premature atrophy of the left common cardiac vein (duct of Cuvier) during fetal development, leading to pericardial hypoperfusion and agenesis.

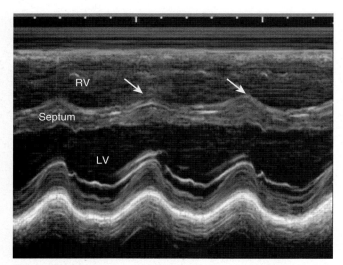

Figure 124.5. M-mode echocardiography from the parasternal long-axis view demonstrating abnormal septal motion in a patient with complete absence of the pericardium. Note the movement of the septum anteriorly in systole *(white arrows)* and posteriorly in diastole. *LV,* Left ventricle; *RV,* right ventricle.

Associated Anomalies

Thirty percent of patients with congenital absence of the pericardium have coexisting anomalies.[8] Cardiac associations include atrial septal defect, bicuspid aortic valve, patent ductus arteriosus, and tetralogy of Fallot. Extracardiac pulmonary sequestration, bronchogenic cysts, and congenital diaphragmatic hernia have also been noted.[8] Reported syndromic associations are VATER syndrome (vertebral defects, anal atresia, tracheoesophageal fistula, radial and renal dysplasia), Marfan syndrome, and Pallister–Killian syndrome.[8]

Clinical Presentation

Most patients are asymptomatic. Often the diagnosis comes to light by incidental discovery on imaging studies, cardiac surgery, or autopsy. Both clinical and imaging manifestations are caused by loss of pericardial restraint and the ensuing exaggerated leftward and posterior swing of the heart. A typical symptomatic patient is a young male presenting with intermittent nonexertional, stabbing chest pain; dyspnea; or subjective palpitations in the left lateral position.[9] Rarely, sequelae such as tricuspid regurgitation caused by chordal rupture or annular dilatation and cardiac herniation may be encountered.[10] Physical examination findings may be limited to a laterally displaced apical impulse or nonspecific systolic murmurs.[9] Complete pericardial absence is usually benign, whereas partial pericardial absence may cause cardiac entrapment.

Diagnostic Modalities

Right axis deviation, incomplete right bundle branch block, and poor R-wave progression in precordial leads maybe seen on electrocardiography (ECG). The ECG axis as well as morphology of ST-T waves may also change with varying body positions and may be an important clue to the diagnosis. Chest radiography abnormalities include levoposition of the heart, elongated left ventricular silhouette, and interposed lung tissue appearing as a radiolucent area between the heart and diaphragm or aorta and pulmonary arteries.[6]

Echocardiography

Typical echocardiography features have been reported.[6,9,11] The transducer position is unusually lateral for both parasternal and apical imaging. The levoposition and exaggerated left posterior mobility of the heart cause the appearance of abnormal paradoxical septal motion and right-sided chamber enlargement. The term "teardrop shape" has been used to describe the elongated atria and rounded ventricle.[8] The enlarged right ventricle and paradoxical movement of the septum anteriorly in systole and posteriorly in diastole can be well appreciated on M-mode echocardiography. The classic features of complete absence of the pericardium are shown in

Figure 124.6. Parasternal long-axis views in a patient with complete congenital absence of the pericardium. **A,** End-diastolic frame. **B,** End-systolic frame. The swinging nature of the heart and abnormal septal motion are demonstrated in the accompanying Video 124.6. *LV,* Left ventricle; *RV,* right ventricle.

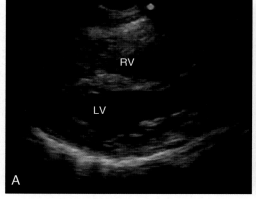

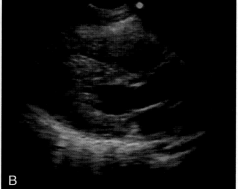

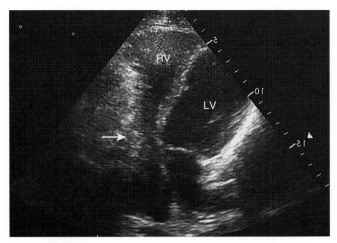

Figure 124.7. Apical four-chamber view in a patient with partial absence of the pericardium. The "teardrop shape" of the right ventricle (RV) caused by herniation is well demonstrated with focal constriction or entrapment noted *(white arrow)*. Also demonstrated are an elongated atria and a rounded left ventricle (LV). (See accompanying Video 124.7.)

Figs. 124.5 and 124.6 and Video 124.6. An example of partial absence of the pericardium with herniation and cardiac entrapment is shown in Fig. 124.7 and Video 124.7. Absence of intrapericardial pressure attenuates atrial filling in systole reflected in characteristic pulsed Doppler flow patterns. There is also a decrease in systolic flow in the SVC and pulmonary veins and reduced pulmonary venous systolic-to-diastolic flow ratio.[12,13]

Cardiac Magnetic Resonance Imaging and Cardiac Computed Tomography

Additional imaging should be reserved for select patients with significant symptoms or associated anomalies and in those undergoing surgical evaluation. CMRI or CT is recommended to confirm the diagnosis and delineate other structural defects.[5]

Treatment

Treatment is not indicated in most patients. Patients with partial left-sided defects who are at risk of herniation of cardiac tissue, especially the left atrium, may require pericardioplasty.[9,10]

Please access ExpertConsult to view the corresponding videos for this chapter.

Acknowledgement

The authors thank Dr. Sonia Jain for her contribution to this chapter in the previous edition.

REFERENCES

1. Maisch B, Seferovic PM, Ristic AD, et al. Guidelines on the diagnosis and management of pericardial diseases executive summary. *Eur Heart J*. 2004;25(7):587–610.
2. Satur CM, Hsin MK, Dussek JE. Giant pericardial cysts. *Ann Thorac Surg*. 1996;61:208–210.
3. Feigin DS, Fenoglio JJ, McAllister HA, et al. Pericardial cysts: a radiologic-pathologic correlation and review. *Radiology*. 1977;125:15–20.
4. Patel J, Park C, Michaels J, et al. Pericardial cyst: case reports and a literature review. *Echocardiography*. 2004;21:269–272.
5. Klein AL, Abbara S, Agler DA, et al. American Society of Echocardiography clinical recommendations for multimodality cardiovascular imaging of patients with pericardial disease. *J Am Soc Echocardiogr*. 2013;26:965–1012.
6. Connolly HM, Click RL, Schattenberg TT, et al. Congenital absence of the pericardium: echocardiography as a diagnostic tool. *J Am Soc Echocardiogr*. 1995;8:87–92.
7. Abbas AE, Appleton CP, Liu PT, et al. Congenital absence of the pericardium: case presentation and review of literature. *Int J Cardiol*. 2005;98:21–25.
8. Alizad A, Seward JB. Echocardiographic features of genetic diseases: part 8. Organ system. *J Am Soc Echocardiogr*. 2000;13:796–800.
9. Gatzoulis MA, Munk MD, Merchant N, et al. Isolated congenital absence of the pericardium: clinical presentation, diagnosis, and management. *Ann Thorac Surg*. 2000;69:1209–1215.
10. Van Son JA, Danielson GK, Schaff HV, et al. Congenital partial and complete absence of the pericardium. *Mayo Clin Proc*. 1993;68:743–747.
11. Payvandi MN, Kerber RE. Echocardiography in congenital and acquired absence of the pericardium: an echocardiographic mimic of right ventricular volume overload. *Circulation*. 1976;53:86–92.
12. Fukuda N, Oki T, Iuchi A, et al. Pulmonary and systemic venous flow patterns assessed by transesophageal Doppler echocardiography in congenital absence of the pericardium. *Am J Cardiol*. 1995;75:1286–1288.
13. Topilsky Y, Tabatabaei N, Freeman WK, et al. Images in cardiovascular medicine. Pendulum heart in congenital absence of the pericardium. *Circulation*. 2010;121:1272–1274.

125 Primary Benign, Malignant, and Metastatic Tumors of the Heart

Jeanne M. DeCara, Corey Rearick

Cardiac masses are often the subject of case reports because of their rarity. However, because they are so infrequent, they often challenge the diagnostic skills of even the most experienced physician. Improvements in echocardiography, including real-time three-dimensional (3D) echocardiography, as well as cardiac computed tomography (CT) and cardiac magnetic resonance imaging (CMRI), have enabled cardiologists to better refine the differential diagnosis of cardiac masses.

Cardiac masses are generally first noted antemortem with echocardiography. The sensitivity and specificity of echocardiography for the detection of cardiac masses is difficult to precisely discern because the incidence of cardiac tumors is low, especially for primary tumors. Data from several small case series, however, offer some insight about the diagnostic yield from two-dimensional (2D) echocardiography. For instance, the sensitivity of 2D transthoracic echocardiography for the detection of a pathologically confirmed tumor was 93.3% with a minimal detectable tumor size of 0.5 to 1.0 cm^2 in one series of 149 patients. In the same series, 2D transesophageal echocardiography (TEE) had a sensitivity of 96.8%.[1]

Three-dimensional echocardiography appears to have incremental yield when used as an adjunct to 2D echocardiography. Its value lies in its ability to provide additional information about the location of a mass, its size, site of attachment, and potential approach for surgical resection. In one series, 3D TEE provided incremental information over 2D echocardiography for the preoperative assessment of 37% of the patients studied and was estimated to be able to do so in approximately 18% of all intracardiac masses.[2] Another way in which 3D echocardiography may be helpful is in determining the size of a cardiac mass. Compared with real-time 3D echocardiography, 2D transthoracic echocardiography has been shown to underestimate the diameter of cardiac masses by as much as 24.6%. Similarly, 2D TEE can underestimate mass diameter by 19.8% compared with real-time 3D echocardiography.[3] This has clinical importance because the diameter of a mass, whether it is a vegetation, thrombus, or tumor, has important implications for patient prognosis and embolic potential. Advanced cardiac imaging is now more readily available for diagnostic evaluation of cardiac masses. CMRI is the most commonly used imaging modality after echocardiography; at present, cardiac CT has a more limited role.

TUMOR CLASSIFICATION AND FREQUENCY

Cardiac masses can be classified as primary or secondary, benign or malignant, or by their location: atrial, ventricular, or valvular. Tables 125.1 and 125.2 show the relative frequencies of primary benign, primary malignant, and metastatic neoplasms.[4] Fig. 125.1 illustrates how the location of a mass may provide a helpful clue to its cause.

PRIMARY BENIGN TUMORS

Myxomas are the most common adult primary cardiac benign tumors.[5] Symptom presentation can be variable and ranges from subtle to overt. For instance, some patients present only with vague constitutional symptoms, whereas others may experience overt heart failure or syncope secondary to obstruction to ventricular filling in cases in which the tumor is sufficiently large (Fig. 125.2 and Video 125.2A). Patients may also present with embolic events, including stroke, thought to arise from the friable surface of the tumor and possibly adherent thrombus. Myxomas are classically described as mobile lobular masses located in the left atrium attached via a pedicle to the interatrial septum, often in the region of the fossa ovalis. Less frequently, they can be located in the right atrium or in the ventricles.[6] These masses may appear heterogeneous because of areas of necrosis and hemorrhage (Video 125.2B). Differentiating this tumor from thrombus becomes challenging when the myxoma is sessile and in an atypical location within the atrium. In such cases, it is important to elicit clinical context favoring thrombus formation, such as the presence of atrial dysrhythmias, recent ablation for atrial dysrhythmias, or mitral stenosis. Myxomas are mainly solitary masses, although familial syndromes may be diagnosed by the presence of multiple lesions.[5] After the diagnosis of myxoma is confirmed, prompt surgical resection yields good results, although there is a 2% to 5% recurrence rate.[7,8] Recurrence is often either at the site of the initial myxoma, indicating incomplete resection, or from an additional undiscovered focus.[9,10] This underscores the importance of a thorough intraoperative transesophageal echocardiographic examination.

Papillary fibroelastomas are the second most common primary benign neoplasm of the heart. These round and solitary lesions are most commonly located on the aortic valve (44%) followed closely by the mitral valve (35%) and less commonly on the tricuspid valve (15%) and pulmonic valves (8%). The valvular location of papillary fibroelastomas—along with their frondlike surface, the latter giving them a shimmering appearance on echocardiography—distinguishes these tumors from myxomas[11] (Fig. 125.3). Although these masses may be discovered incidentally on echocardiography, embolic events associated with these lesions are known to occur and are more common when the fibroelastoma is mobile and attached to a stalk.[12] Cropping and manipulation of 3D echocardiographic images may aid in the detection of a discrete stalk if not readily apparent on 2D images. The identification of a stalk can be the first clue to help distinguish a fibroelastoma from other entities such as Libman-Sacks endocarditis, in which the lesion is sessile and along the coaptation point of the valve leaflets. Because of its valvular location, a papillary fibroelastoma may initially be mistaken for vegetation until conditions predisposing to endovascular infection have been excluded. Unlike vegetations, which may be irregularly

TABLE 125.1 Armed Forces Institute of Pathology 1976 to 1993 Report on the Most Common Primary Benign and Malignant Tumors of the Heart

Tumor	Total	Surgical	Autopsy	Age 15 Years or Younger at Diagnosis
Primary *Benign* Neoplasms of the Heart				
Myxoma	114	102	12	4
Rhabdomyoma	20	6	14	20
Fibroma	20	18	2	13
Hemangioma	17	10	7	2
Atrioventricular nodal	10	0	10	2
Granular cell	4	0	4	0
Lipoma	2	2	0	0
Paraganglioma	2	2	0	0
Myocytic hamartoma	2	2	0	0
Histiocytoid cardiomyopathy	2	0	2	2
Inflammatory pseudotumor	2	2	0	1
Fibrous histiocytoma	1	0	1	0
Epithelioid hemangioendothelioma	1	1	0	0
Bronchogenic cyst	1	1	0	0
Teratoma	1	0	1	1
Totals	**199**	**146 (73%)**	**53 (27%)**	**45 (23%)**
Primary *Malignant* Tumors of the Heart				
Sarcoma	137 (95%)	116	21	11 (8%)
Angioma	33	22	11	1
Unclassified	33	30	3	3
Fibrous histiocytoma	16	16	0	1
Osteoma	13	13	0	0
Leiomyoma	12	11	1	1
Fibroma	9	9	0	1
Myxoma	8	8	0	1
Rhabdomyoma	6	2	4	3
Synovial	4	4	0	0
Lipoma	2	0	2	0
Schwannoma	1	1	0	0
Lymphoma	7 (5%)	1	6	0
Totals	**144**	**117 (81%)**	**27 (19%)**	**11 (8%)**

Modified from Burke A, Virmani R: *Atlas of Tumor Pathology. Tumors of the Heart and Great Vessels*. Washington, DC: Armed Forces Institute of Pathology 1996:231.

TABLE 125.2 Metastatic Neoplasms of the Heart at Necropsy: Order of Frequency of Cancers Encountered[a]

Primary Tumor	Total Autopsies	Metastases to the Heart
Lung	1037	180 (17%)
Breast	685	70 (10%)
Lymphoma	392	67 (17%)
Leukemia	202	66 (33%)
Esophagus	294	37 (13%)
Uterus	451	36 (8%)
Melanoma	69	32 (46%)
Stomach	603	28 (5%)
Sarcoma	159	24 (15%)
Oral cavity and tongue	235	22 (9%)
Colon and rectum	440	22 (5%)
Kidney	114	12 (11%)
Thyroid gland	97	9 (9%)
Larynx	100	9 (9%)
Germ cell	21	8 (38%)
Urinary bladder	128	8 (6%)
Liver and biliary tract	325	7 (2%)
Prostate gland	171	6 (4%)
Pancreas	185	6 (3%)
Ovary	188	2 (1%)
Nose (interior)	32	1 (3%)
Pharynx	67	1 (1%)
Miscellaneous	245	0
Total	6240	653 (10%)

[a]In this series including some of the more commonly encountered malignancies, melanoma is the primary tumor for which metastatic tumors were most commonly found in the heart on autopsy.

Modified from Burke A, Virmani R: *Tumors of the Cardiovascular System. Atlas of Tumor Pathology*. Washington, DC: Armed Forces Institute of Pathology 1996:231; and Mukai K, et al: The incidence of secondary tumors of the heart and pericardium: a 10-year study, *Jpn N Clin Oncol* 18:195-201, 1988.

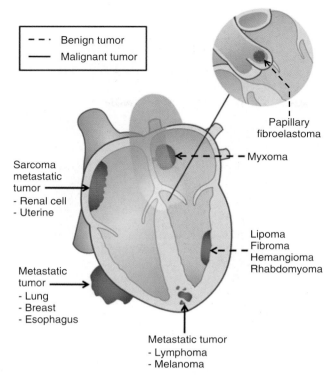

Figure 125.1. Schematic of the typical locations for common benign, malignant, and metastatic tumors in the heart. (Courtesy of Jason Kim.)

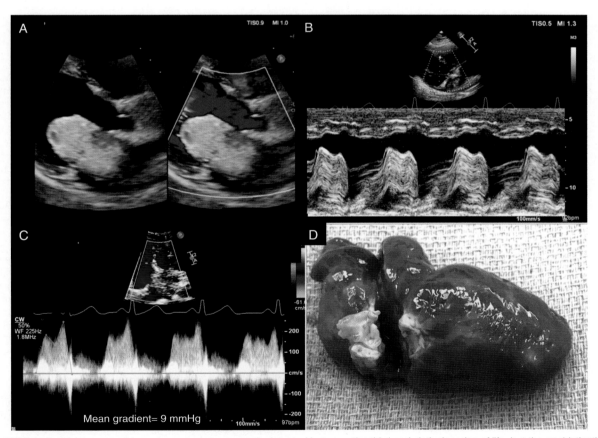

Figure 125.2. Left atrial myxoma. Myxomas are most commonly detected between the third and sixth decades of life, but the sophistication of echocardiography has led to more frequent diagnoses among older patients. Myxomas are grossly round but on closer inspection may have a villous surface, consistent with their gross pathologic description as gelatinous tumors because of their large collagenous content. They may become quite large and cause hemodynamic obstruction. **A,** A large left atrial myxoma enters the mitral valve inflow as seen on both transthoracic and transesophageal echocardiogram. (See accompanying Video 125.2A.) **B,** M-mode echocardiography of the mitral valve shows the prolapsing mass. **C,** The myxoma causes a pseudo mitral stenosis with an elevated mean mitral valve gradient of 8 mm Hg. **D,** The excised mass appears relatively smooth, somewhat uncharacteristic of the friable and multilobular nature of many myxomas, many of which have areas of hemorrhage or necrosis. (See accompanying Video 125.2B.)

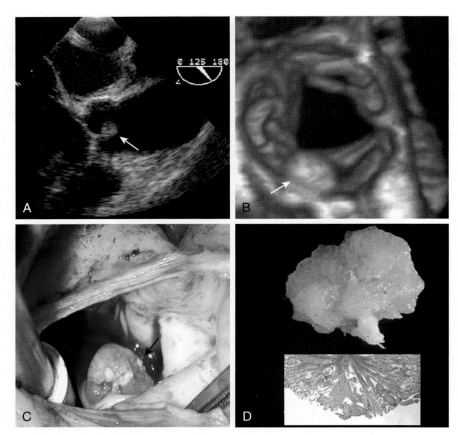

Figure 125.3. Papillary fibroelastoma of the aortic valve (arrows). Ninety-five percent of fibroelastomas are found in the left heart, most frequently seen on the midportion of the valve leaflets. The characteristic features of this tumor include frondlike extensions, a high degree of mobility, and a stalklike attachment to the valve leaflet. Like myxomas, these tumors are associated with peripheral and systemic emboli. However, unlike myxomas, they are infrequently attached to nonvalvular sites and are not associated with constitutional symptoms. Although many fibroelastomas are incidental findings, this patient presented with a stroke. Transesophageal echocardiogram revealed a gelatinous-appearing, mobile echodensity attached to the aortic valve. **A,** Three-dimensional echocardiography localized this mass to the midportion of the noncoronary cusp of the aortic valve (**B** and **C**). Surgical pathology (**D**) confirmed the diagnosis of papillary fibroelastoma.

shaped and disrupt valve function, papillary fibroelastomas appear more discrete and do not tend to cause valve regurgitation or stenosis. A Lambl excrescence may also be in the differential diagnosis of a papillary fibroelastoma; however, whereas the former have a wispy, fibrolinear nature, the latter are round and well formed.

In children, **rhabdomyomas** and **fibromas** are the most common benign tumors, yet despite their benign nature, they can be associated with conduction abnormalities, arrhythmias, and even sudden death. Unlike myxomas, these neoplasms are commonly located in the ventricular myocardium. Rhabdomyomas tend to be small and may be multiple or solitary in nature. Fibromas are larger tumors, and as a result, they are symptomatic in many patients. Fibromas (Fig. 125.4)[13] tend to be hyperreflective on echocardiography, whereas other rare benign masses such as hemangiomas (Fig. 125.5) are highly vascular tumors that show evidence of perfusion on contrast echocardiography.[14]

PRIMARY MALIGNANT TUMORS

Cardiac sarcomas are the most common primary malignancies of the heart. These include (in order of frequency) angiosarcoma, rhabdomyosarcoma, fibrosarcoma, and leiomyosarcoma. Their large size and predilection for the right atrium point toward this diagnosis[15–18] (Fig. 125.6). These tumors often take the form of broad-based, lobular masses; however, they may alternatively be polypoid or intramyocardial and can extend into the inferior vena cava. Calcification may be noted in the case of osteosarcomas. Cardiac sarcomas are aggressive tumors that spread rapidly from an intramural location into the cardiac chambers, pericardium, or both. They tend to manifest with obstructive symptoms associated with impaired right heart filling, pericardial effusion, or tamponade. Arrhythmias or embolization may also occur. By the time of diagnosis, metastases are often present.[16] Rhabdomyosarcomas are more common in children and

are found in both ventricular and atrial locations.[17] Although optimal management of sarcomas includes chemotherapy and radiotherapy and complete surgical resection, this is frequently not possible owing to their dimensions and intramyocardial location.[15] Overall, the prognosis remains very poor; the median survival time is 6 to 12 months.[18]

Sarcomas must be differentiated from **primary cardiac lymphomas.** Although metastatic lymphoma is much more common than primary cardiac lymphoma, the latter, like sarcomas, has a predilection for the right heart, particularly the right atrium. Morphologically, they do not have a classic pattern. However, an associated pericardial effusion is common. Surprisingly, constitutional symptoms typical of lymphoma are not usually present. Patients instead may complain of precordial pain or dyspnea. The majority of reported primary cardiac lymphomas have been of the diffuse large B cell variety.[19,20] In contrast to sarcomas, a favorable response to surgery or anthracycline-based therapy (or both) has been reported for primary cardiac lymphomas when detected early with cardiac imaging. Therefore, obtaining a definitive pathologic diagnosis can be important in determining prognosis and treatment options when a primary malignant cardiac tumor is suspected.

METASTATIC TUMORS

Metastatic disease has been found in 10% to 25% of patients in autopsy series of patients with cancer.[21,22] In the majority of clinical cases, metastatic disease is known before cardiac involvement is discovered on echocardiogram. Symptoms may include embolic events, congestive heart failure in cases in which intramyocardial extension has compromised systolic function, pericardial tamponade, intracavitary obstruction, or arrhythmia. Cardiac metastatic foci may present as multiple or solitary lesions. There are a variety of mechanisms for cardiac metastasis, including direct invasion

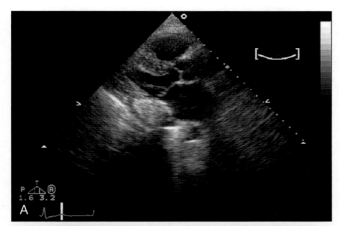

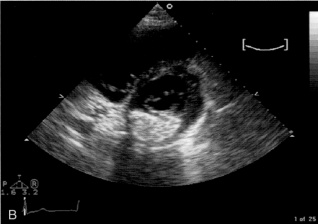

Figure 125.4. Fibroma. Of fibroblast origin, these benign tumors are more often located in the ventricles rather than the atria. Echocardiographically, they are echodense round masses embedded within the myocardium (**A**) and often speckled with calcium (**B**). Ventricular arrhythmias and sudden death have been reported in patients with fibromas. Echocardiography is pivotal in determining the precise location and extent of these tumors before resection because they may course close to the coronary arteries. (From Cho J, et al: Surgical resection of ventricular cardiac fibromas: early and late results, *Ann Thorac Surg* 76:1929–1934, 2003.)

from the mediastinum, hematologic spread, lymphatic spread, or venous extension into the heart. Metastatic foci in the right heart commonly originate from extension of the tumor from the inferior vena cava. This can be observed with **renal cell carcinoma, leiomyosarcoma,** and **some gynecologic malignancies.** In the left heart, the pulmonary veins may serve as a conduit for lung cancer extension into the heart. Not only do solid tumors metastasize to the heart, but hematologic malignancies may also become manifest in the heart, particularly in the pericardium or myocardium. For lymphoma, this may involve actual tumor foci on the pericardium or myocardium with clinical manifestations, whereas leukemic infiltration of the heart may be subtler, even though cardiac metastasis is reported to be more common.[23] Generally, metastatic disease involving the heart, regardless of the primary malignancy, is a sign of widely disseminated disease and associated with a poor prognosis. In most cases, treatment is largely palliative.

Complementary Role of Advanced Cardiac Imaging

Echocardiography is a key first-line imaging modality to diagnose a mass and generate a differential diagnosis for its cause. Its strength is its ability to determine the location, size, site of attachment, and hemodynamic importance. Advanced cardiac imaging plays a complementary role in refining the differential diagnosis by offering tissue characterization and multiplanar assessment of a mass's location relative to other structures important in anticipating adverse sequelae and for surgical planning (Table 125.3, Fig. 125.7, and Video 125.7). CMRI has the advantage of offering soft tissue characterization of masses and evaluation of perfusion within a mass, which is useful to differentiate tumor from thrombus. In a 10-year retrospective review of CMRI performed to further characterize cardiac masses found on echocardiography, CMRI was able to identify a mass in 82% of cases and categorize masses in three categories: tumor (76%), thrombi (20%), and inconclusive (4%). CMRI was found to be very accurate in its distinction of tumor from thrombus (diagnostic accuracy 97% and 94%, respectively). Lack of postcontrast enhancement was a useful determinant of thrombus.[24] CMRI findings correlated well clinically with mass or tissue histopathology or thrombus size reduction with therapeutic anticoagulation.

CMRI has been studied not only in its ability to distinguish thrombus from tumor but also in its capacity to delineate morphologic features of tumors that help differentiate them as

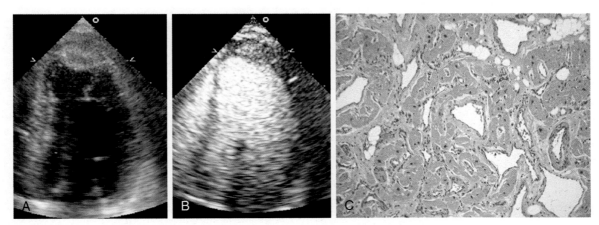

Figure 125.5. Hemangioma of the left ventricular apex. As shown here, these benign tumors are often not initially appreciated as vascular entities on a standard echocardiogram (**A**) without the use of echocardiographic contrast. **B** clearly demonstrates the uptake of echocardiographic contrast in the vasculature of this tumor that is also evident on pathology (**C**). Hemangiomas are typically intramyocardial, although most often involve the base of the heart and are known to be associated with pericardial effusions. These benign tumors can have serious sequelae such as arrhythmias and sudden death.

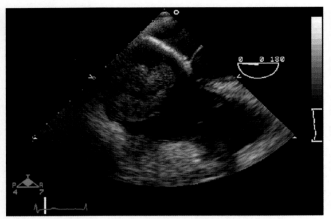

Figure 125.6. Angiosarcoma. In this example, the angiosarcoma was found in the right atrium, but these tumors have been reported in all four chambers. The large size of the mass seen in this patient is not unusual for this tumor type given its rapid and aggressive growth pattern. In this case, the tumor had invaded beyond the margins of the right atrial free wall. In addition, the tumor intermittently occluded the tricuspid valve, causing right heart failure symptoms. In such situations, hemorrhagic pericardial effusions are common.

malignant or benign. In one study of evaluating CMRI in the evaluation of 66 cardiac and paracardiac masses, CMRI defined the characteristic features that were suggestive of malignant tumors, which included infiltration into the free wall (54% of malignant tumors vs 0% of benign), infiltration into adjacent structures (49% vs 0%), and concurrent pericardial effusion (41%, vs 7%).[25] Two capabilities of CMRI that uniquely distinguish its role as complementary imaging in the evaluation of cardiac masses characterization of the vascular components of masses with first-pass perfusion (FPP) as well as tissue fibrosis characterization with late gadolinium enhancement (LGE). Both FPP and LGE were found to occur more frequently in malignant tumors than in benign tumors. Enhancement on FPP was evident in all malignant tumors (100% sensitive). FPP was also seen on about 30% of benign tumors but tended to be less homogenous compared with the pattern seen with malignant tumors. LGE was also present in all malignant tumors (100% sensitive) but was also seen in 59% of benign tumors. Large tumor size (5 cm vs 3 cm) and concurrent pericardial effusion were also markers of malignant tumors. T1- and T2-weighted imaging in this particular series was not a good differentiator between malignant and benign tumors. This is in contrast to other reports suggesting it may be useful.[26]

Although CMRI has high temporal resolution, its diagnostic capacity for cardiac masses has some limitations because of its limits in spatial resolution, particularly when the mass size is smaller

TABLE 125.3 Imaging Features of Common Cardiac Masses: Comparing Echo With Cardiac Magnetic Resonance Imaging

Classification	Mass Type	TTE or TEE	CMRI
Non-neoplastic	Thrombus	Any chamber, mobile or mural associated with wall motion abnormalities or attached to a catheter or device; spontaneous echocardiography contrast may be associated	Acute: hyperintense T1W imaging, hyperintense T2W imaging, no enhancement Chronic: hypointense T1W imaging, hypointense T2W imaging, rarely have rim of enhancement after contrast
Primary benign	Lipoma	Mainly in the subendocardium but pericardial and valve locations possible, broad based, well circumscribed	Well-encapsulated; hyperintense T1W imaging, hyperintense T2W imaging; hypointense on fat suppression; no enhancement with contrast
Primary benign	Myxoma	Round, more often left sided, sessile or pedunculated, typically attached near the foramen ovale but other locations possible; may be helpful to identify a stalk and site of attachment	Isointense or hypointense T1W imaging, hyperintense T2W imaging, minimal enhancement (may be heterogeneous) on early or delayed postcontrast imaging
Primary benign	Papillary fibroelastoma	Small, round, pedunculated, attached to valves (most commonly the aortic valve), shimmering surface; TEE and 3D echocardiography may be helpful in determining the presence of a stalk and point of attachment	Size and mobility limit CMRI evaluation; isointense T1W imaging, isointense T2W imaging; minimal or pronounced enhancement, the later the imaging after contrast injection, the more pronounced the enhancement
Primary benign	Rhabdomyoma	More common in children, multiple lesions, intramyocardial ventricular or AV valvular locations predominate, nodular or pedunculated, variable size; hyperechoic; may regress	Intramural, isointense T1W imaging, hyperintense T2W imaging, variable contrast enhancement
Primary benign	Fibroma	More common in children, large, hyperechoic and can have calcification, left ventricular intramyocardial location, can cause cavity obstruction	Well-circumscribed, isointense or hypointense T1W imaging, hypointense T2W imaging, little to no enhancement on first-pass or delayed imaging postcontrast because of nonenhancing fibrous core
Primary malignant	Sarcoma	Angiosarcomas most common in right atrium; bulky, irregular, heterogenous-appearing mass, more often right sided, invasive, may cause hemodynamic obstruction of tricuspid valve; other sarcoma types, including rhabdomyosarcoma, leiomyosarcoma, and osteosarcoma, may have a variety of other locations; left atrial location predominates for sarcomas as a group	Angiosarcomas: isointense T1W imaging, hyperintense T2W imaging, heterogeneous contrast enhancement
Primary malignant	Lymphoma	Right-sided predilection, nodular or infiltrating, homogeneous, may be associated with pericardial disease, may cause mechanical obstruction or constrictive physiology (if associated with pericardial infiltration)	Hypointense T1W imaging, hyperintense T2W imaging, heterogenous contrast enhancement

AV, Atrioventricular; *CMRI,* cardiac magnetic resonance imaging; *TEE,* transesophageal echocardiography; *TTE,* transthoracic echocardiography.

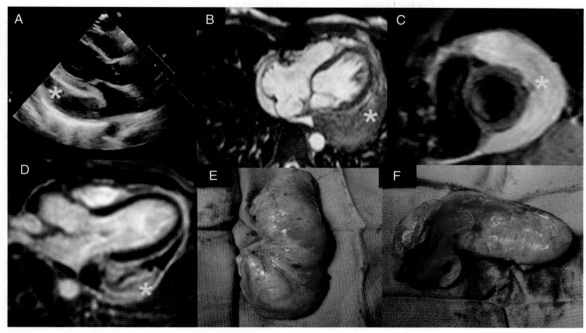

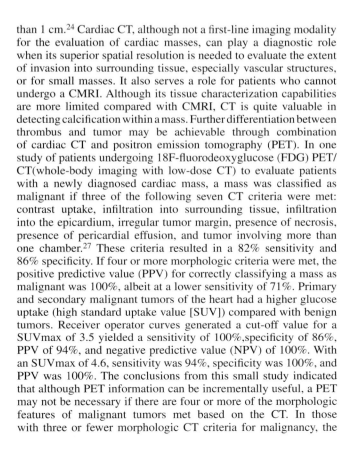

Figure 125.7. Synovial sarcoma. This is an example of the complementary role that cardiac magnetic resonance imaging (CMRI) played in a patient with equivocal echocardiographic findings. **A,** Transthoracic echocardiogram demonstrated an echodensity in the pericardial sac adjacent to left ventricular inferolateral wall *(asterisk)*. This was thought to be either a loculated pericardial effusion or a heterogeneous mass. **B,** CMRI demonstrated a solid-appearing mass, not a pericardial effusion *(asterisk)*. **C,** T2-weighted imaging showed a hyperintense signal *(asterisk)*. **D,** Whereas first-pass perfusion revealed a perfused mass (see accompanying Video 125.7), the late gadolinium images showed contrast uptake in the mass consistent with tumor *(asterisk)*. **E** and **F,** Using the multiplanar data from CMRI to plan the resection, the mass was carefully excised. Pathology was consistent with a synovial sarcoma.

than 1 cm.[24] Cardiac CT, although not a first-line imaging modality for the evaluation of cardiac masses, can play a diagnostic role when its superior spatial resolution is needed to evaluate the extent of invasion into surrounding tissue, especially vascular structures, or for small masses. It also serves a role for patients who cannot undergo a CMRI. Although its tissue characterization capabilities are more limited compared with CMRI, CT is quite valuable in detecting calcification within a mass. Further differentiation between thrombus and tumor may be achievable through combination of cardiac CT and positron emission tomography (PET). In one study of patients undergoing 18F-fluorodeoxyglucose (FDG) PET/CT(whole-body imaging with low-dose CT) to evaluate patients with a newly diagnosed cardiac mass, a mass was classified as malignant if three of the following seven CT criteria were met: contrast uptake, infiltration into surrounding tissue, infiltration into the epicardium, irregular tumor margin, presence of necrosis, presence of pericardial effusion, and tumor involving more than one chamber.[27] These criteria resulted in a 82% sensitivity and 86% specificity. If four or more morphologic criteria were met, the positive predictive value (PPV) for correctly classifying a mass as malignant was 100%, albeit at a lower sensitivity of 71%. Primary and secondary malignant tumors of the heart had a higher glucose uptake (high standard uptake value [SUV]) compared with benign tumors. Receiver operator curves generated a cut-off value for a SUVmax of 3.5 yielded a sensitivity of 100%,specificity of 86%, PPV of 94%, and negative predictive value (NPV) of 100%. With an SUVmax of 4.6, sensitivity was 94%, specificity was 100%, and PPV was 100%. The conclusions from this small study indicated that although PET information can be incrementally useful, a PET may not be necessary if there are four or more of the morphologic features of malignant tumors met based on the CT. In those with three or fewer morphologic CT criteria for malignancy, the

additional metabolic information obtained from PET resulted in a NPV of 100%. Larger studies are needed to validate this or the use of alternative diagnostic algorithms involving 18F-FDG PET/CT or CMRI.

SUMMARY

Cardiac tumors are rare clinical entities that challenge our diagnostic acumen. Tumor features such as location, size, and means of attachment as well as clinical context are important clues to refining the differential diagnosis. Although most masses are first discovered with 2D echocardiography, real-time 3D echocardiography may have an additive role in determining the potential cause of a cardiac mass. By nature of its volumetric data acquisition, 3D echocardiography can yield potential prognostic information by providing information on the size of a mass as it relates to its embolic potential. In addition, 2D and 3D TEE is of value in defining potential surgical approaches whenever resection is planned. MRI and cardiac CT complement the role of echocardiography in refining the differential diagnosis through tissue characterization and localization of the mass relative to other structures relevant to surgical planning.

Please access ExpertConsult to view the corresponding videos for this chapter.

Acknowledgments

The authors acknowledge the contribution of Jason Kim, who provided Fig. 125.1, and the contributions of Drs. Zoe Yu and Gillian Murtagh, who were authors of this chapter in the previous edition.

REFERENCES

1. Meng Q, Lai H, Lima J, et al. Echocardiographic and pathologic characteristics of primary cardiac tumors: a study of 149 cases. *Int J Cardiol.* 2002;84:69–75.

2. Muller S, Feuchtner G, Bonatti J, et al. Value of transesophageal 3D echocardiography as an adjunct to conventional 2D imaging in preoperative evaluation of cardiac masses. *Echocardiography.* 2008;25:624–631.

3. Asch F, Bieganski S, Panza J, et al. Real-time 3-dimensional echocardiography evaluation of intracardiac masses. *Echocardiography.* 2006;23:218–224.

4. Roberts W. Primary and secondary neoplasms of the heart. *Am J Cardiol.* 1997;80:671–682.

5. Reynen K. Cardiac myxomas. *N Engl J Med.* 1995;333:1610–1617.

6. Sarjeant J, Butany J, Cusimano R. Cancer of the heart: epidemiology and management of primary tumors and metastases. *Am J Cardiovasc Drugs.* 2003;3:407–421.

7. D'Alfonso A, Catania S, Pierri M, et al. Atrial myxoma: a 25-year single-institutional follow-up study. *J Cardiovasc Med.* 2008;9:178–181.

8. Pinede L, Duhaut P, Loire R. Clinical presentation of left atrial cardiac myxoma. A series of 112 consecutive cases. *Medicine.* 2001;80:159–172.

9. McCarthy P, Piehler J, Schaff H, et al. The significance of multiple, recurrent, and "complex" cardiac myxomas. *J Thorac Cardiovasc Surg.* 1986;91:389–396.

10. Waller D, Ettles D, Saunders N, et al. Recurrent cardiac myxoma: the surgical implications of two distinct groups of patients. *Thorac Cardiovasc Surg.* 1989;37:226–230.

11. Gowda R, Khan I, Nair C, et al. Cardiac papillary fibroelastoma: a comprehensive analysis of 725 cases. *Am Heart J.* 2003;146:404–410.

12. Sun J, Asher C, Yang X, et al. Clinical and echocardiographic characteristics of papillary fibroelastomas: a retrospective and prospective study in 162 patients. *Circulation.* 2001;103:2687–2693.

13. Cho J, Danielson G, Puga F, et al. Surgical resection of ventricular cardiac fibromas: early and late results. *Ann Thorac Surg.* 2003;76:1929–1934.

14. Kirkpatrick J, Wong T, Bednarz J, et al. Differential diagnosis of cardiac masses using contrast echocardiographic perfusion imaging. *J Am Coll Cardiol.* 2004;43:1412–1419.

15. Fatima J, Duncan A, Maleszewski J, et al. Primary angiosarcoma of the aorta, great vessels, and the heart. *J Vasc Surg.* 2013;57:756–764.

16. Look Hong N, Pandalai P, Hornick J, et al. Cardiac angiosarcoma management and outcomes: 20-year single-institution experience. *Ann Surg Oncol.* 2012;19:2707–2715.

17. Ragland M, Tak T. The role of echocardiography in diagnosing space-occupying lesions of the heart. *Clin Med Res.* 2006;4:22–32.

18. Simpson L, Kumar S, Okuno S, et al. Malignant primary cardiac tumors: review of a single institution experience. *Cancer.* 2008;112:2440–2446.

19. Gowda R, Khan I. Clinical perspectives of primary cardiac lymphoma. *Angiology.* 2003;54:599–604.

20. Nascimento A, Winters G, Pinkus G. Primary cardiac lymphoma: clinical, histologic, immunophenotypic, and genotypic features of 5 cases of a rare disorder. *Am J Surg Pathol.* 2007;31:1344–1350.

21. Goudie R. Secondary tumours of the heart and pericardium. *Br Heart J.* 1955;17:183–188.

22. Reynen K, Köockeritz U, Strasser R. Metastases to the heart. *Ann Oncol.* 2004;15:375–381.

23. Javier B, Yount W, Crosby D, et al. Cardiac metastasis in lymphoma and leukemia. *Dis Chest.* 1967;52:481–484.

24. Sloninsky E, Konen O, Segni ED, et al. Cardiac MRI: a useful too for differentiating cardiac thrombi from tumors. *Isr Med Assoc J.* 2018;20:472–475.

25. Kassi M, Polsani V, Schutt RC, et al. Differentiating benign from malignant cardiac tumors with cardiac magnetic resonance imaging. *J Thorac Cardiovasc Surg.* 2019;157:1912–1922. e2.

26. Caspar T, El Ghannudi S, Ohana M. Magnetic resonance evaluation of cardiac thrombi and masses by T1 and T2 mapping: an observational study. *Int J Cardiovasc Imag.* 2017;33:551–559.

27. Rhabar K, Seifarth H, Schafers M, et al. Differentiation of malignant and benign cardiac tumors using 18F-FDG PET/CT. *J Nucl Med.* 2012;53:856063.

126 Left Ventricular Thrombus

Biana Trost, Itzhak Kronzon

LEFT VENTRICULAR THROMBUS WITH IMPAIRED LEFT VENTRICULAR FUNCTION

Thrombus formation within the left ventricle can be noted 24 hours after an acute myocardial infarction (AMI); 90% of the time they are formed within 2 weeks following the event, but they can form within the first 3 months (Fig. 126.1). The incidence of LV thrombus after an AMI has been reported to be between 7% and 46%, depending on the diagnostic modality used for detection. However, contemporary literature reports a declining incidence of left ventricular (LV) thrombus after AMI, mainly attributed to the growing use of primary percutaneous coronary intervention (PCI), which varies between 5% and 15% in patients receiving percutaneous treatment. LV thrombus usually occurs after AMI in the left anterior descending artery (LAD) territory being less common after infarction in non-LAD territories. About 11% of clots may occur in the septal wall, and 3% occur in the inferior wall (Fig. 126.2 and Video 126.2), particularly when the infarct extends to the lateral wall.[1]

Aside from patients with apical aneurysm, the prevalence of LV thrombus is more likely to be present in patients with systolic dysfunction (ejection fraction [EF] <40%), previous myocardial infarction, multivessel coronary artery disease, high creatinine kinase levels, and large scar burdens identified by delayed enhanced magnetic resonance imaging (MRI).[1–3] In addition, Doppler analysis of apical flow patterns has been suggested to help identify which of these patients are at highest risk of thrombus formation. Evidence of apical flow stasis or of continuous flow swirling around the apex is thought to identify patients at particular risk for apical thrombus.[4] In the presence of a pseudoaneurysm, the clot occurs lining the LV wall at the site of rupture contained by the pericardium.[4]

The use of angiotensin-converting enzyme inhibitors after AMI has not been associated with a decreased incidence of thrombus despite improved remodeling, and the effect of β-blockers is also controversial. LV thrombus formation is more likely to occur before the full effect of remodeling takes place. It has been demonstrated that levels of soluble tissue factor, D-dimer, and anticardiolipin are increased in patients with LV clot after AMI. However, the clinical value of following these levels is unknown.[1]

On the other hand, in patients with cardiomyopathy (Fig. 126.3), an EF less than 20% provides the highest risk with a reported incidence of thrombus formation of almost 50%.[5] The presence of mitral regurgitation appears to be protective in these patients against developing clot. However, a similar association has not been demonstrated after AMI.[1]

LEFT VENTRICULAR THROMBUS WITH PRESERVED LEFT VENTRICULAR FUNCTION

Thrombus within the LV cavity has been reported in patients with preserved LV function. This occurs rarely in the setting of endothelial damage as with trauma, eosinophilic endocarditis (Fig. 126.4), tumors, or device leads (Fig. 126.5) or in the setting of hypercoagulable states. In eosinophilic endocarditis, thrombus can occur in the left or the right ventricle in the presence of normally contracting heart regions. The treatment is targeted to the underlying pathology, along with the use of anticoagulation.[6]

LV THROMBUS WITH IMPAIRED LV FUNCTION (MORE COMMON)

- LV apical aneurysm
- After MI with apical akinesis
- After MI in segments other than LAD territory
- LV pseudoaneurysm
- Dilated cardiomyopathy
- Apical ballooning (takotsubo) syndrome

LV THROMBUS WITH PRESERVED LV FUNCTION (EXTREMELY RARE)

- Eosinophilic endocarditis
- Hypercoagulable states
  - Antiphospholipid antibody
  - Protein C deficiency
- Myeloproliferative disorders
- Essential thrombocythemia
- Myelofibrosis
- Salmonella septicemia
- Cardiac trauma
- Connective tissue disease
  - Systemic lupus erythematosus
  - Behçet disease
- On the surface of LV tumors
- On device leads that inadvertently migrate to the left ventricle
- Administration of large doses of erythropoietin

LAD, Left anterior descending coronary artery; *LV,* left ventricular; *MI,* myocardial infarction.

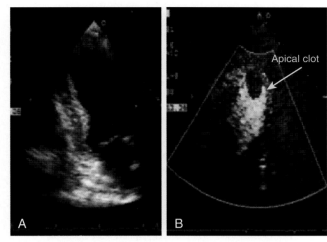

Figure 126.1. A, A patient with anterior myocardial infarction and no clot evident on noncontrast image. Note the poor apical endocardial border delineation. **B,** After contrast administration, an apical clot is visualized. Note that the mass is avascular with no contrast uptake.

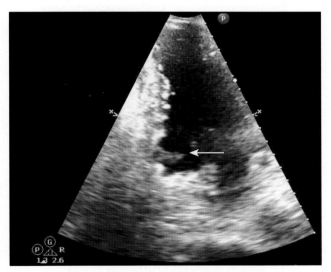

Figure 126.2. Transthoracic echocardiography of an apical two-chamber view revealing a basal inferior aneurysm with a mobile thrombus inside the aneurysm *(arrow).* (See accompanying Video 126.2.)

DIAGNOSTIC TESTS AND THE ROLE OF ECHOCARDIOGRAPHY

A space-occupying mass in the LV can be classified as either neoplastic or non-neoplastic. An LV thrombus is an example of a non-neoplastic mass, and although echocardiography does not provide histologic diagnosis, certain features, when present, suggest that the mass is indeed a thrombus. A mass noted in a segment of the LV where there is a wall motion abnormality that is avascular (based on either color Doppler or use of contrast) and in an apical location suggests thrombus as its cause.

There are three types of thrombi that can be identified within the left ventricle:

1. Mural thrombus (only one surface exposed to the blood pool; flat and parallel to the endocardial surface) (Figs. 126.6 and 126.7)
2. Protruding thrombus (more than one surface exposed to the blood pool and protruding into the LV cavity)
3. Mobile thrombus with independent motion (either in parts of the thrombus or its entirety)

A fresh thrombus often protrudes into the LV cavity and is highly mobile, whereas more chronic thrombi are often sessile in appearance. However, studies have shown that thrombi can change in shape and mobility in the first several months after AMI.[7] The predictive accuracy of transthoracic echocardiography (TTE) for the detection of LV thrombus is dependent on clear delineation of all endocardial borders. Therefore, meticulous imaging is imperative, and one should have a low threshold for the use of echocardiographic contrast if endocardial border delineation is suboptimal.[8] The sensitivity and specificity to detect an LV thrombus have been reported to be 92% to 95% and 86% to 88%, respectively.[9] The diagnostic ability of echocardiography is increased in the presence of large protuberant clots. False tendons, trabeculations, near-field clutter artifact, and misplaced papillary muscles can all cause false-positive results.[1] Conversely, poor endocardial border delineation, small clot size, mural thrombus, and image foreshortening may yield false-negative results.

Cardiac MRI has an increased sensitivity to detect LV thrombus and should be considered when the TTE evaluation is equivocal or suboptimal.[1,10] Transesophageal echocardiography (TEE) has a much lower sensitivity in the detection of LV thrombus because the apex is farthest from the transducer and frequently is foreshortened or not well seen. Although three-dimensional echocardiography has lower frame rates and inferior resolution to two-dimensional imaging, it may still enhance identification of LV thrombus with a more detailed depiction of the LV apex (Fig. 126.8 and Video 126.8).

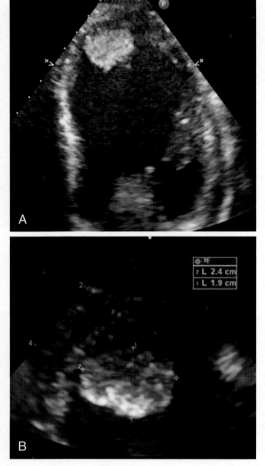

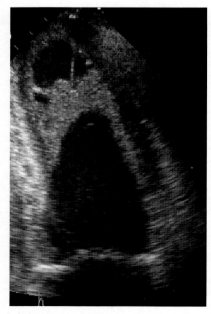

Figure 126.3. Apical four-chamber view demonstrating a protruding apical left ventricular thrombus with mobile elements in a patient with dilated cardiomyopathy (**A**). A zoomed-in view of the thrombus showing the measurements of 2.4 × 1.9 cm (**B**).

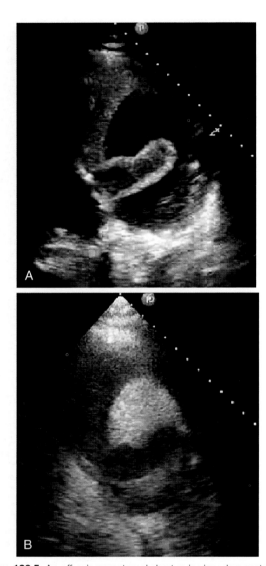

Figure 126.5. An off-axis parasternal short-axis view demonstrating a left ventricular (LV) clot formed on a migrated automatic implantable cardioverter-defibrillator lead in a patient with dilated cardiomyopathy and severely reduced LV systolic function without (**A**) and with (**B**) contrast enhancement.

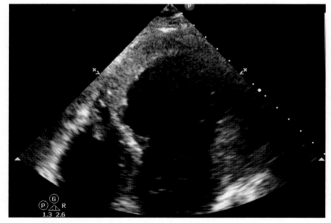

Figure 126.4. Apical two-chamber view demonstrating a left ventricular thrombus in a patient with hypereosinophilic syndrome.

Figure 126.6. Four-chamber view showing aneurysmal apical segments with a mural thrombus along the apical septum and apex proper.

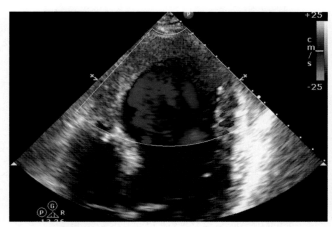

Figure 126.7. Same patient as in Fig. 126.6. Low-velocity color Doppler signal demonstrating no flow entering the mural thrombus.

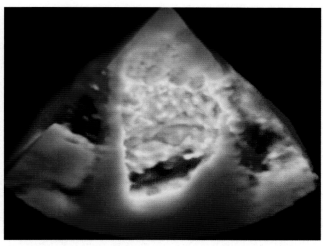

Figure 126.8. Transillumination view of an apical thrombus. (See accompanying Video 126.8.)

PROGNOSIS AND TREATMENT

When present, LV thrombus poses risk for thromboembolic complications, with stroke being the most feared. Risk factors that predispose patients with cardiomyopathies to have thromboembolic events include extensive regional wall motion abnormalities, severely dilated left ventricles, low cardiac output with slow flow (stasis) of blood, and hypertrophic cardiomyopathy with apical aneurysms, particularly if there is concomitant atrial fibrillation.

Clot protrusion and mobility have been associated with risk of embolization.[1] Other findings associated with increased risk for embolization include heart failure, advanced age, previous emboli, and hyperdynamic adjacent segment. Apical aneurysm may be protective against embolization because the lack of adjacent contractility results in less chance of dislodgement.[1] The incidence of embolization is lowest for a mural thrombus and highest for a mobile thrombus.[11,12]

After a thrombus is identified, anticoagulation is the mainstay of therapy, with serial imaging to evaluate for thrombus regression or organization. The duration of anticoagulation is a minimum of 3 months according to the 2013 American College of Cardiology Foundation/American Heart Association guidelines[13]; however, duration is influenced by the underlying condition and depends on whether serial imaging shows thrombus resolution or organization.[1] In addition, management of the underlying predisposing condition, as with immunosuppressive therapy in patients with connective tissue disease or eosinophilic endocarditis, is essential.

The prognosis of patients with LV thrombus is highly dependent on the causing factors and the extent and severity of LV dysfunction.

SUMMARY

LV thrombus occurs most commonly in the presence of decreased LV systolic function but in certain conditions may occur in those with preserved LVEF. TTE is the principal noninvasive diagnostic tool used for detection, with contrast echocardiography increasing both its sensitivity and specificity. Thrombi that protrude into the lumen of the LV and are highly mobile have the highest thromboembolic potential. Current treatment is primarily focused on management of the underlying predisposing condition along with anticoagulation.

Please access ExpertConsult to view the corresponding videos for this chapter.

Acknowledgments

The authors acknowledge the contributions of Drs. Amr E. Abbas, MD, and Steven J. Lester, MD, who were the authors of this chapter in the previous edition.

REFERENCES

1. Delewi R, Zijlstra F, Piek J, et al. Left ventricular thrombus formation after acute myocardial infarction. *Heart.* 2012;98:1743–1749.
2. Okuyan E, Okcun B, Dinckal M, Mutlu H. Risk factors for development of left ventricular thrombus after first acute myocardial infarction—association with anticardiolipin antibodies. *Thromb J.* 2010;8(15).
3. Weinsaft JW, Kim HW, Shah DJ, et al. Detection of left ventricular thrombus by delayed-enhancement cardiovascular magnetic resonance. *J Am Coll Cardiol.* 2008;52:148–157.
4. Otto CM. Cardiac masses and potential cardiac "source of embolus." In: *Textbook of Clinical Echocardiography.* 4th ed. Philadelphia: Saunders; 2009.
5. Mazzone M, La Sala M, Portale G, et al. Review of dilated cardiomyopathies. Dilated cardiomyopathies and altered prothrombotic state. *Panminerva Med.* 2005;47:157–167.
6. Alzand M, Meeder JG. Thrombus in a normal ventricle. *Neth Heart J.* 2008;16:24–25.
7. Haugland JM, Asinger RW, Mikell FL, et al. Embolic potential of left ventricular thrombi detected by two-dimensional echocardiography. *Circulation.* 1984;70:588–598.
8. Kurt M, Shaikh KA, Peterson L, et al. Impact of contrast echocardiography on evaluation of ventricular function and clinical management in a large prospective cohort. *J Am Coll Cardiol.* 2009;53:802–810.
9. Visser CA, Kan G, Lie KI, et al. Left ventricular thrombus following acute myocardial infarction: a prospective serial echocardiographic study of 96 patients. *Eur Heart J.* 1983;4:333–337.
10. Srichai MB, Junor C, Rodriguez LL, et al. Clinical, imaging, and pathological characteristics of left ventricular thrombus. *Am Heart J.* 2006;152:75–84.
11. Meltzer RS, Visser CA, Fuster V. Intracardiac thrombi and systemic embolization. *Ann Intern Med.* 1986;104:689–698.
12. Johannessen KA, Nordrehaug JE, von der Lippe G, Vollset SE. Risk factors for embolisation in patients with left ventricular thrombi and acute myocardial infarction. *Br Heart J.* 1988;60:104–110.
13. O'Gara PT, Kushner FG, Ascheim DD, et al. 2013 ACCF/AHA guidelines for the management of ST elevation myocardial infarction. *J Am Coll Cardiol.* 2013;61:e78–e140.

127 Left Atrial Appendage Thrombus

Michael Morcos, James N. Kirkpatrick

PATHOGENESIS OF LEFT ATRIAL APPENDAGE THROMBUS FORMATION

The left atrial appendage (LAA) is by far the most common location for an atrial thrombus with extra-appendage thrombi being very rare in nonvalvular atrial fibrillation (AF).[1] Thrombus forms within the LAA primarily as a result of stasis within the cavity, although additional components of the Virchow triad, such as hypercoagulable state and endothelial dysfunction, likely also contribute.[2] The cul-de-sac morphology of the LAA may also predispose to variable contractile dysfunction and stasis. Atrial arrhythmias such as AF and atrial flutter (AFL) are associated with left atrial (LA) contractile dysfunction; however, there is a significant heterogeneity in the degree of LA dysfunction depending on the arrhythmia (in general, more contractility from AFL than AF) and duration of arrhythmia (long-standing arrhythmias associated with worse contraction).[3] Additionally, elevated LA or left ventricular (LV) filling pressures and mitral valve disease (mitral stenosis in particular) also lead to decreased LA contractile function, which can promote stasis. This may also be seen in surgical or catheter-based procedures that cause endocardial damage within the left atrium (fibrosis after catheter-based ablation, interatrial septal or LAA occluder devices, or surgical incisions for cardiac surgery).

LA thrombus is infrequently demonstrated on transesophageal echocardiography (TEE) performed in patients with sinus rhythm (SR)[4]; nonetheless, it may be seen in patients without atrial arrhythmias in the setting of severe LA stasis or cardiac dysfunction (particularly with infiltrative process such as cardiac amyloidosis) or in those with transient episodes of AF that are clinically undetected. Transient LA dysfunction ("stunning") occurring after conversion from AF or AFL into SR caused by pharmacologic or electric cardioversion is well described[3] and one of the primary reasons that uninterrupted anticoagulation is recommended for at least 4 weeks after cardioversions.[5]

TRANSESOPHAGEAL ECHOCARDIOGRAPHIC DIAGNOSIS OF LEFT ATRIAL THROMBUS

TEE is an ideal imaging modality for the left atrium because of its anatomic position and proximity to the esophagus.[6,7] In the evaluation for intracardiac thrombus, the LAA and LA should be scanned separately and meticulously for the presence of thrombus. Because of the highly variable morphology and potential for multiple lobes, the LAA should be systematically scanned in multiple omniplane angles.[8] Scanning should be performed from the mid-esophageal position with mild probe anteflexion. To fully delineate the LAA cavity and its multiple lobes, the scanning omniplane angle should be gradually changed from 0 degrees to 150 degrees (the latter allowing for visualization of the LAA in its widest dimension). Effort should be made to isolate the LAA to the middle of the imaging window and limit any superficial structures that may contribute to shadowing or imaging artifact. Three-dimensional (3D) echocardiography may also aid in the detection of LAA thrombus.[9] The main LA cavity, a much less common location of intracardiac thrombi, should be scanned in a vertical (90-degree) scanning plane with gradual clockwise rotation of the TEE probe from the left pulmonary veins (adjacent to the LAA) to the right pulmonary veins. When indicated, vertical scanning may be supplemented by horizontal (0-degree) scanning, with a gradual inferior-to-superior outward motion of the TEE probe, from the inferior to the superior aspect of the LA body.

Acute LA mural thrombi may have variable size, morphology, and locations; however, it usually appears as a heterogenous mass with lower echogenicity than the surrounding LA walls and can be associated with LAA thrombus (Fig. 127.1 and Video 127.1). A chronic LA thrombus may appear more echogenic than the surrounding walls and may occasionally have calcifications. After diagnosis, it is important to characterize the embolic potential of the thrombus based on its size, morphology, attachment points (if there is an associated narrow stalk), and mobility. Echodensities in the LAA often represent normal variants (pectinate muscles) or artifacts, and additional imaging modalities may be necessary for further characterization.

Comprehensive scanning of the LA and LAA will help overcome several diagnostic pitfalls, including incorrectly diagnosing prominent pectinate muscles as LAA thrombi (Fig.127.2 and Video 127.2), overlooking the presence of a thrombus in a multilobed LAA, and incorrectly interpreting various artifacts as thrombi. Limited quality near-field imaging of the LA body adjacent to the TEE probe can also be overcome with comprehensive scanning.

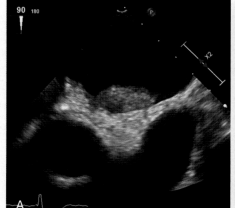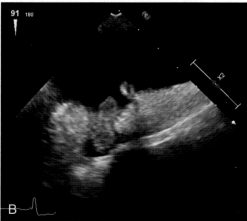

Figure 127.1. A, Large left atrial appendage thrombus. **B,** Layered left atrial mural thrombus associated with the left atrial appendage thrombus. (Also see Video 127.1.)

If LAA thrombus is confirmed, the right atrial appendage (RAA) should also be evaluated. Spontaneous RAA thrombus is rare, but the presence of LAA thrombus makes it significantly more likely (Fig. 127.3 and Video 127.3).[10]

In addition to the confirmation or exclusion of LA and LAA thrombus, additional imaging findings can assist in assessing thromboembolic risk, including the presence of spontaneous echocardiographic contrast (SEC) or "smoke" within the LA or LAA, and in selected cases, assessment of LAA contractile function. Although attempts to semiquantify the degree of LAA SEC have been previously reported,[11] it is practical and clinically sufficient to categorize SEC as either mild or severe ("dense") (Fig. 127.4 and Video 127.4). If dense LAA SEC is appreciated, special attention and a systematic approach should be pursued to exclude the presence of LAA thrombus because dense SEC is almost uniformly associated with the presence of thrombus. Because the appearance of the SEC may be significantly affected by various echocardiographic machine settings, mainly gain, the image quality of the surrounding LA walls and the adjacent cardiac structures should be optimized to avoid overestimation or underestimation of SEC severity. Additionally, dense SEC may appear as "sludge," which may be difficult to differentiate from a "soft" thrombus (Fig. 127.5 and Video 127.5), and clinical considerations to treat these patients as if a LAA thrombus exists are recommended.

LAA contractile function can be challenging to assess but may play an important role in cardioembolic risk assessment in patients undergoing TEE. Visual function assessment, pulsed-wave (PW) Doppler measurements of flow at the proximal LAA cavity (adjacent to the LAA orifice), measurements of LAA wall motion velocities by tissue Doppler, and LAA wall speckle

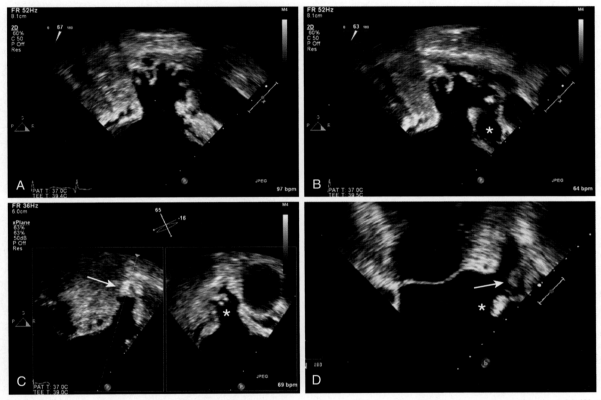

Figure 127.2. Potential diagnostic caveats in imaging of the left atrial appendage (LAA). Prominent pectinate muscles within the LAA (**A**) and a multilobed LAA (**B;** additional lobe marked with an *asterisk*). **C,** An apparent "mass" at the tip of the LAA (*left; arrow*), which may be mistaken for a thrombus. Imaging at an orthogonal plane (*right*), using the transesophageal echocardiography matrix probe with biplane imaging, clearly shows that this mass is caused by normal pectinate muscles *(asterisk)*. **D,** Shadowing of the LAA *(arrow)* by a thickened septum *(asterisk)* between the LAA and the adjacent left upper pulmonary vein ("Q-tip"; ligament of Marshall), which may appear like a thrombus or obscure a thrombus, causing both false-positive and false-negative diagnoses of an LAA thrombus. (Also see Video 127.2.)

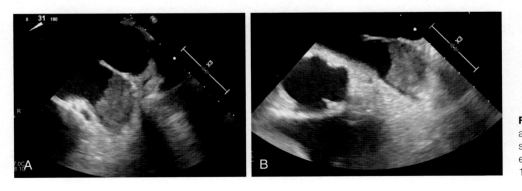

Figure 127.3. A and **B,** Left atrial and right atrial appendage thrombi seen in the same transesophageal echocardiogram. (Also see Video 127.3.)

tracking to measure strain, as well as the presence of atrial wave forms on PW Doppler have all been described as quantitative and qualitative parameters of LAA contractility.[3,12,13] Although the hypothesis that preserved LAA contractile function decreases the likelihood of LAA thrombus formation, the clinical implications of LAA contractility are less established. Additionally, there may be cause other than atrial arrhythmias for profound LAA contractile dysfunction such as severe LV dysfunction or mitral stenosis.

In addition to two-dimensional (2D) echocardiography, 3D echocardiography can be helpful in defining the presence of LA thrombi, particularly when there are multiple lobes of the LAA and can be used to help differentiate pectinate muscles from thrombi. The use of 3D was evaluated in a small, single-center trial wherein TEEs were reviewed with both 2D and 3D imaging. Of the studies, a total of 12 were equivocal on 2D imaging for the presence or exclusion of a LAA thrombus. 3D TEE was able to further characterize 11 of the 12 equivocal studies (1 thrombus, 10 without thrombus) and otherwise had excellent agreement with 2D.[14] When there remains uncertainty regarding the presence of LAA thrombus, the use of ultrasound-enhancing agents (UAEs; microbubble contrast) during TEE has been demonstrated to increase the accuracy of detecting LAA thrombus.[15]

ADDITIONAL DIAGNOSTIC TECHNIQUES

At times, large LA or LAA thrombi may be visualized using trans-thoracic echocardiography (TTE) (Fig. 127.6 and Video 127.6). In a small pilot multicenter trial of 118 patients with AF for more than 48 hours' duration, TTE with UAEs (microbubble contrast) administration and measurement of LAA wall velocities by tissue Doppler were compared with TEE images as the diagnostic gold standard. TTE correctly identified the two patients with thrombi, whereas low tissue Doppler velocities of the LAA wall were associated with the presence of severe LAA SEC, sludge, or thrombus on TEE.[16] Although these results are encouraging, overall, TTE is not yet sensitive enough to rule out the presence of LA or LAA thrombus and should not be relied on clinically before cardioversions or in the workup of cerebral or systemic emboli.

CARDIAC COMPUTED TOMOGRAPHY AND MAGNETIC RESONANCE IMAGING

Cardiac computed tomography angiography (CTA) may detect LA and LAA thrombi (Fig. 127.7), particularly when TEE is contra-indicated or nondiagnostic. The detection of LAA thrombi with CTA is highly sensitive (~100%); however, the specificity of the test ranges widely depending on the technique and patient population (positive predictive value has ranged between 25% and 100%

in various studies).[17] Although the examination may be performed using nongated imaging acquisition, the standard cardiac CTA procedure is electrocardiography gated. Additionally, the ideal imaging acquisition time occurs during or immediately after contrast bolus reaching the LA or thoracic aorta. This usually results in excellent contrast between the intracardiac blood and the cardiac tissues, assuming rapid mixing of blood within each cavity. In the presence of sluggish flow with the LAA, such as that occurring in the context of poor LAA contractility or SEC by TEE, this mixing may not be complete and may result in false-positive diagnosis. Several solutions to improve the accuracy of the cardiac CTA have been proposed such as scanning at a later phase (to test whether

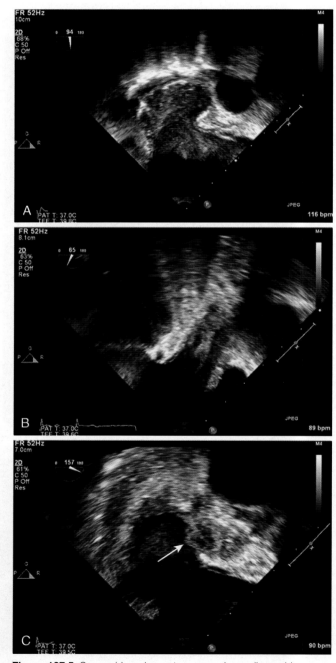

Figure 127.5. Severe (dense) spontaneous echocardiographic contrast (**A**) and left atrial appendage "sludge" or soft thrombus (**B** and **C**). (Also see Video 127.5.)

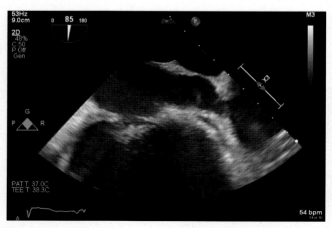

Figure 127.4. Spontaneous echocardiographic contrast seen within the left atrial appendage. (Also see Video 127.4.)

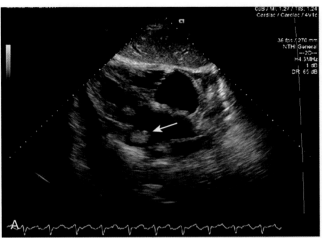

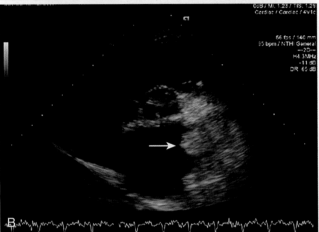

Figure 127.6. Left atrial appendage thrombus visualized via transthoracic echocardiography in subcostal (**A**, *arrow*) and parasternal short-axis (**B**, *arrow*) view in a patient with severe mitral stenosis and atrial flutter. (Also see Video 127.6.)

any filling defect is persistent or transient) and measuring the CT enhancement in the suspected area within the LAA.

Magnetic resonance imaging (MRI) is also highly sensitive for the detection of intracardiac thrombus using both gadolinium and nongadolinium approaches. MRI has been less widely used for the purpose of excluding LAA thrombi, and to date, there are limited data on the use of cardiac MRI specifically for this purpose.

CLINICAL IMPLICATIONS OF THE DIAGNOSIS OF LEFT ATRIAL THROMBUS BY TRANSESOPHAGEAL ECHOCARDIOGRAPHY

The appropriate use criteria for TEE in diagnosing LA thrombus, adopted by multiple cardiac imaging societies (including the American Society of Echocardiography), are presented in Table 127.1.[18]

Cardiac Source of Embolism

TEE is commonly used to identify a potential cardiac source of embolism in patients with a cerebrovascular accident (CVA) or systemic embolic event.[19] The appropriate use criteria support the use of TEE in the evaluation of CVA when an alternative, noncardiac source is not identified or if confirmation of a cardiac source of embolism will affect management. LA thrombus is most frequently detected in patients with ischemic events in association with AF (paroxysmal, persistent, or permanent). In this setting, lifelong anticoagulation is strongly recommended, even without the demonstration of LAA thrombus. In this scenario, because the treatment strategy will be unchanged with confirmation or exclusion of LAA thrombus, TEE would not be clinically indicated.

LA thrombus may infrequently form in the absence of atrial arrhythmias, but as previously mentioned, additional physiologic features may predispose to LAA stasis and subsequent thrombus formation. Additionally, given the paroxysmal nature of many atrial arrhythmias, the absence of documented AF, for example, on telemetry monitoring does not rule out the presence of paroxysmal AF. The frequency of LA

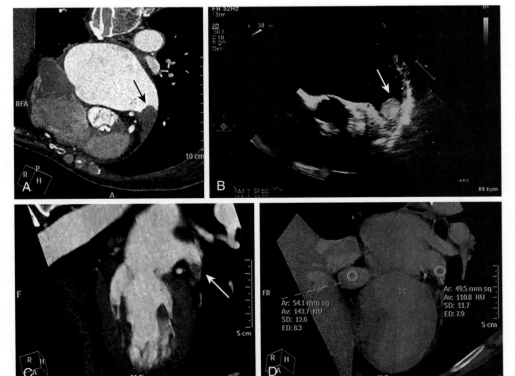

Figure 127.7. Left atrial appendage (LAA) thrombus *(arrows)* detected by computed tomography (**A**) and the corresponding image by transesophageal echocardiography (TEE) (**B**). In a different patient, a filling defect detected in an early scan (**C**) disappears in a late scan 1 minute later (**D**). The ratio of enhancement in the LAA versus the aorta is greater than 0.5 (**D**), indicating that the defect represents slow flow and not a thrombus. TEE (not shown) did not show a thrombus in the LAA.

TABLE 127.1 Appropriate Criteria[a] for the Use of Transesophageal Echocardiography for Diagnosis of Left Atrial Thrombus

1. TEE as initial test: AF or AFL
   a. Evaluation to facilitate clinical decision making with regard to anticoagulation, cardioversion, or radiofrequency ablation (**Appropriate: 9**)
   b. Evaluation when a decision has been made to anticoagulate and not to perform cardioversion (**Inappropriate: 2**)
2. TEE as initial or supplemental test—embolic event[b]
   a. Evaluation for cardiovascular source of embolus with no identified noncardiac source (**Appropriate: 7**)
   b. Evaluation for cardiovascular source of embolus with a previously identified noncardiac source (**Uncertain: 5**)
   c. Evaluation for cardiovascular source of embolus with a known cardiac source in which a TEE would not change management (**Inappropriate: 1**)
3. TEE as initial or supplemental test: general uses a. Reevaluation of prior TEE finding for interval change (e.g., resolution of thrombus after anticoagulation) when a change in therapy is anticipated (**Appropriate: 8**)

[a]Appropriateness scores in parentheses (7–9 = appropriate; 4–6 = uncertain; 1–3 = inappropriate).
[b]Evaluation for various cardiovascular sources of embolism, including a left atrial thrombus.
AF, Atrial fibrillation; *AFL,* atrial flutter; *TEE,* transesophageal echocardiography.
From American College of Cardiology Foundation Appropriate Use Criteria Task Force; American Society of Echocardiography; American Heart Association; et al: A Report of the American College of Cardiology Foundation Appropriate Use Criteria Task Force, American Society of Echocardiography, American Heart Association, American Society of Nuclear Cardiology, Heart Failure Society of America, Heart Rhythm Society, Society for Cardiovascular Angiography and Interventions, Society of Critical Care Medicine, Society of Cardiovascular Computed Tomography, Society for Cardiovascular Magnetic Resonance American College of Chest Physicians, *J Am Soc Echocardiogr* 24:229–267, 2011.

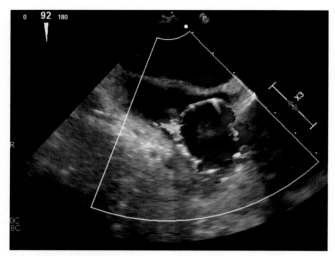

Figure 127.8. Left atrial appendage occlusion device with peridevice leak noted with color Doppler. (Also see Video 127.8.)

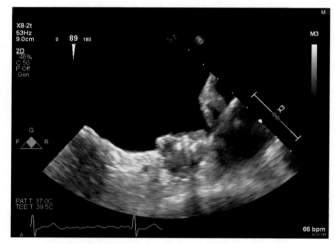

Figure 127.9. Left atrial appendage occlusion device with associated thrombus on two- and three-dimensional imaging. (Also see Video 127.9.)

thrombi in patients with SR at the time of the echocardiographic examination has been examined in a large series of more than 20,000 consecutive TEE examinations performed for various indications in which 380 LA thrombi were detected, mostly in patients with AF.[4] LA thrombi were evident in only 20 patients who had SR during TEE (0.1% of all TEE examinations), and of these, 19 patients were clearly at risk for LA dysfunction and thrombus formation because of high-risk hemodynamic features or previously documented AF. Thus, it appears that LA thrombus formation caused by occult AF is an extremely rare phenomenon. Nevertheless, because TEE may detect other potential cardiovascular sources of embolism, including the presence of a large patent foramen ovale and mobile plaque in the aorta, it is commonly performed in patients with CVA, especially in those who are relatively young, without an obvious cause of the event.

Cardioversion of Atrial Fibrillation

TEE has remained the standard imaging modality of choice before cardioversion or planned AF or AFL ablations in patients who are not sufficiently anticoagulated before procedure (at least 3 weeks of uninterrupted, therapeutic anticoagulation).[20] In addition, TEE can be useful to follow up on previously noted LAA thrombus after initiation of anticoagulation. TEE-guided cardioversion is very safe, feasible procedure associated with high success rates of cardioversion with low risk of thromboembolism.[21] Therapeutic anticoagulation should be confirmed at the time of the TEE cardioversion, and it remains extremely important to instruct patients, even if TEE excludes the presence

of LAA thrombus, to remain on uninterrupted, therapeutic anticoagulation for at east 4 weeks after cardioversion because of the risk of thrombus formation secondary to myocardial and LA "stunning."[5]

Left Atrial Appendage Occlusion Devices

TEE has become the imaging modality of choice to assist with implantation of left atrial appendage occlusion (LAAO) devices as well as the routine monitoring for successful implantation in the postprocedure period. It is currently recommended to obtain a TEE 45 days after device implantation to evaluate for the presence of peridevice leak and device-associated thrombus.[22] Cautious and systemic approach should be taken to evaluate LAAO devices using multibeat acquisitions of the LAA at several different omniplane angles. The presence of a large leak (>5 mm) (Fig. 127.8 and Video 127.8) or device-associated thrombus (Fig. 127.9 and Video 127.9) should prompt consideration for continuing anticoagulation past the 45 day postprocedure period and, in the latter case, considering repeat TEE.

Please access ExpertConsult to view the corresponding videos for this chapter.

REFERENCES

1. Cresti A, García-Fernández MA, Sievert H, et al. Prevalence of extra-appendage thrombosis in non-valvular atrial fibrillation and atrial flutter in patients undergoing cardioversion: a large transesophageal echo study. *EuroIntervention.* 2019;15:e225–e230.
2. Watson T, Shantsila E, Lip GY. Mechanisms of thrombogenesis in atrial fibrillation: Virchow's triad revisited. *Lancet.* 2009;373:155–166.
3. Agmon Y, Khandheria BK, Gentile F, Seward JB. Echocardiographic assessment of the left atrial appendage. *J Am Coll Cardiol.* 1999;34:1867–1877.
4. Agmon Y. Clinical and echocardiographic characteristics of patients with left atrial thrombus and sinus rhythm. *Circulation.* 2002;105:27–31.
5. January C, Wann LS, Alpert JS, et al. AHA/ACC/HRS Guideline for the management of patients with atrial fibrillation; executive summary. *Circulation.* 2014;130(23). 2014.
6. Flachskampf F, Badano L, Daniel WG, et al. Recommendations for transesophageal echocardiography: Update. *Eur J Echocardiogr.* 2010;11:557–576. 2010.
7. Hahn R, Abraham T, Adams MS, et al. Guidelines for performing a comprehensive transesophageal echocardiographic examination. *J Am Soc Echocardiogr.* 2013;26:921–964.
8. Veino J, Harrity PJ, Gentile F, et al. Anatomy of the normal left atrial appendage: a quantitative study of age-related changes in 500 autopsy hearts: implications for echocardiographic examination. *Circulation.* 1997;96:3112–3115.
9. Melillo E, Palmiero G, Ferro A, et al. Diagnosis and management of left atrium appendage thrombosis in atrial fibrillation patients undergoing cardioversion. *Medicina.* 2019;55(51).
10. Cresti A, García-Fernández MA, Miracapillo G, et al. Frequency and significance of right atrial appendage thrombi in patients with persistent atrial fibrillation or atrial flutter. *J Am Soc Echocardiogr.* 2014;11:1200–1207.
11. Donal E, Sallach JA, Murray RD, et al. Contrast-enhanced tissue Doppler imaging of the left atrial appendage is a new quantitative measure of spontaneous echocardiographic contrast in atrial fibrillation. *Eur J Echocardiogr.* 2008;9:5–11.
12. Biase L, Mohanty S, Trivedi C, et al. Stroke risk in patients with atrial fibrillation undergoing electric isolation of the left atrial appendage. *J Am Coll Cardiol.* 2019;74:1019–1029.
13. Saracoglu E, Ural D, Sahin T, et al. Assessment of left atrial appendage function by 2-dimensional speckle-tracking imaging in transesophageal echocardiography. *JACC.* 2013;62(Suppl. 2):18.
14. Squara F, Bres M, Baudouy D, et al. Transesophageal echocardiography for the assessment of left atrial appendage thrombus: study of the additional value of systematic real time 3D imaging after regular 2D evaluation. *Echocardiography.* 2018;35:474–480.
15. Koukky R, Donenberg MJ, Parker J, et al. Use of ultrasound enhancing agents in transesophageal echocardiography to improve interpretive confidence of left atrial appendage thrombus. *Echocardiography.* 2019;2:362–369.
16. Sallach J, Puwanant S, Drinko JK, et al. Comprehensive left atrial appendage optimization of thrombus using surface echocardiography: the CLOTS multicenter pilot trial. *J Am Soc Echocardiogr.* 2009;22:1165–1172.
17. Romero J, Husain SA, Kelesidis I, et al. Detection of left atrial appendage thrombus by cardiac computed tomography in patients with atrial fibrillation: a meta-analysis. *Circ Cardiovasc Imag.* 2013;6:185–194.
18. American College of Cardiology Foundation Appropriate Use Criteria Task Force; American Society of Echocardiography; American Heart Association; et al: a Report of the American College of Cardiology Foundation Appropriate Use Criteria Task Force, American Society of Echocardiography, American Heart Association, American Society of Nuclear Cardiology, Heart Failure Society of America, Heart Rhythm Society, Society for Cardiovascular Angiography and Interventions, Society of Critical Care Medicine, Society of Cardiovascular Computed Tomography, Society for Cardiovascular Magnetic Resonance American College of Chest Physicians. *J Am Soc Echocardiogr.* 2011;24:229–267.
19. Pepi M, Evangelista A, Nihoyannopoulos P, et al. Recommendations for echocardiography use in the diagnosis and management of cardiac sources of embolism. *Eur J Echocardiogr.* 2010;11:461–476.
20. Yarmohammadi H, Klosterman T, Grewal G, et al. Transesophageal echocardiography and cardioversion trends in patients with atrial fibrillation: a 10 year survey. *J Am Soc Echocardiogr.* 2012;25:962–968.
21. Klein A, Grimm RA, Murray RD, et al. Use of transesophageal echocardiography to guide cardioversion in patients with atrial fibrillation. *N Engl J Med.* 2001;344:1411–1420.
22. Holmes RVY, Turi ZG, et al. Percutaneous closure of the left atrial appendage versus warfarin therapy for prevention of stroke in patients with atrial fibrillation: a randomised non-inferiority trial. *Lancet.* 2009;374:534.

128 Right Heart Thrombi

Gregory J. Sinner, Steve W. Leung, Vincent L. Sorrell

Right heart thrombi (RHT) are relatively common but can often be missed on routine echocardiography without careful image acquisition and high suspicion. Because of increased use of right heart catheters, pacemakers, and other devices coupled with a growing population of adults with congenital heart diseases and end-stage heart failure, the incidence of RHT is expected to climb. Despite an association with symptomatic pulmonary embolism (PE), RHT often remain asymptomatic and are incidentally identified during contrast-enhanced echocardiography, cardiovascular magnetic resonance imaging (CMRI), or cardiac computed tomography (CT). Documented reports of detectable RHT in the general population likely underestimate the true frequency of occurrence based on conventional two-dimensional (2D) echocardiography. This chapter reviews risk factors, at-risk patient populations, and characteristics of RHT and offers suggestions on echocardiographic image acquisition, optimization, and interpretation. It concludes with a brief overview on both traditional and novel, innovative treatment approaches.

INCIDENCE

The true incidence of RHT is difficult to determine because of inconsistent definitions, the clinically silent nature of many of these thrombi, and variations in diagnostic techniques employed. In a large, Swedish, population-based autopsy study that included both in- and out-of-hospital deaths, the reported incidence of RHT was 3.4%. PE was identified in 22.8% of all cases and in 43.4% of patients with RHT.[1] In hemodynamically stable patients with PE assessed by echocardiography, 2% to 3% have RHT. Among unstable patients with acute massive PE, the incidence of RHT is as high as 18%.[2] In the Italian PE registry, echocardiography within 48 hours of admission identified RHT in 4.5% of all patients. When risk stratified, incidences were 0.3%, 3.8%, and 16% in low-, intermediate-, and high-risk patients, respectively.[3] Variable terminology, such as thrombi-in-transit, free-floating thrombi in the right heart (FFTRH), right-sided intracardiac thrombus, and RHT may be the largest contributor to ambiguity in incidence reporting. When associated with PE, RHT are thought to be residual thrombi in transit from the deep venous system to the pulmonary vasculature. However, it is likely that some thrombi form in situ within the right atrium (RA) or right ventricle (RV), as may be the case with catheter- and cardiomyopathy-associated intracardiac thromboses, respectively.

RISK FACTORS

A myriad of modifiable and nonmodifiable risk factors predispose patients to the development of RHT. Knowledge of these risk factors is important to ensure image acquisition and interpretation is performed with a higher degree of scrutiny, allowing for earlier detection of RHT in at-risk patients (Table 128.1).

TABLE 128.1 Risk Factors for Right Heart Thrombi

Patient Characteristics	Disease State	Catheter or Device	Drug or Substance Intake
Male	Malignancy	CVC (size, type)	Amphotericin B
Age (65 years or older)	COPD	Pacemaker (especially temporary)	Parenteral nutrition
Hypercoagulable	Chronic hemodialysis	Multiple	No prophylaxis
Obesity	Congestive heart failure	PICC size	Cigarettes
Immobility	Atrial fibrillation or flutter	Internal jugular location	Contraceptives
Pregnancy	Cardiomyopathy	Subclavian vein location	
Trauma or surgery	Cor pulmonale	Distal position	
Protein C/S deficiency	RV contusion	Duration (>6 days)	
Thrombophilia	RV infarct		
APLS	ARVD/C		
	IBD		
	Behçet disease		

APLS, Antiphospholipid syndrome; *ARVC/D,* arrhythmogenic right ventricular cardiomyopathy/dysplasia; *COPD,* chronic obstructive pulmonary disease; *CVC,* central venous catheter; *IBD,* inflammatory bowel disease; *PICC,* peripherally inserted central catheter; *RV,* right ventricular.

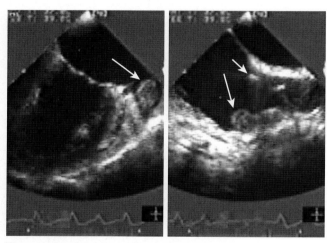

Figure 128.1. An early multiplane transesophageal echocardiographic examination (circa 1994), 90-degree orientation, performed for atrial fibrillation. Leftward rotation revealed a large thrombus *(arrow)* in the right atrial appendage. A linear echodense line seen entering the superior vena cava is a pacemaker wire *(arrow).* (See accompanying Video 128.1.)

Central Venous Catheters

Central venous catheters (CVCs) are used in up to 8% of hospitalized patients and can lead to thrombotic complications in up to 66% of those individuals. CVC tip-associated thrombi at the cavoatrial junction or within the RA, RV, or pulmonary artery (PA) are often detected by echocardiography. Catheter-related RHT are identified on autopsy in up to 29% of cases when CVCs are present at the time of death; however, frequency varies among reports of live patient populations. Their presence is likely related to tip position, catheter type, concomitant infection, and patient comorbidities.[4]

Catheter-related right atrial thrombi identified by transthoracic echocardiography (TTE) have been reported in up to 9% of children with malignancy and up to18% of patients with hemodialysis catheters.[5] Yet no guidelines for management of these thrombi currently exist. Among several proposed treatment algorithms, catheter removal and 3 to 6 months of anticoagulation is the most commonly recommended strategy, likely derived from published guidelines on treatment of catheter-related upper extremity venous thrombosis and intracardiac thrombi.

Atrial Fibrillation and Flutter

The incidence of atrial fibrillation (AF) and flutter (AFL) is high, especially in older adults. It is well-appreciated that thrombi form in the left atrial appendage (LAA), increasing the likelihood for systemic embolization and stroke. Therefore, transesophageal echocardiography (TEE) before elective electrical cardioversion is standard clinical practice.

The RAA, despite having a wider mouth and less deep recesses, is also subject to low flow, spontaneous echocardiographic contrast (SEC), and thrombus development in AF and AFL (Fig. 128.1 and Video 128.1). The incidence of RAA thrombi in AF varies from 0.4% to 7.5%. In the Assessment of Cardioversion Using Transesophageal Echocardiography (ACUTE) trial, 9 of 549 patients (1.6%) with AF had a right heart thrombus, without specifying the number of RAA thrombi. Similarly, in another large investigation of 983 patients with AF and AFL presenting to the emergency department, 0.73% had RAA thrombi. RAA peak emptying velocities were lower, similar to velocities in the LAA. Four of 7 patients with RAA thrombi had isolated right-sided clots, and all patients had decompensated congestive heart failure.[6] As in the LAA, SEC in the RA is a marker for organized embolic potential. Compared with patients with nonvalvular AF without RA SEC, the incidence of pulmonary defects on pulmonary scintigraphy in patients with RA SEC was 40% versus 7% (*P* = .006) despite similar D-dimer and fibrinogen serum thrombotic markers.[7]

Indwelling Cardiac Devices

Intracardiac devices, including implantable electronic device leads, occlude devices, ventricular assist devices (VADs), and extracorporeal membrane oxygenation (ECMO) circuits, have become common in cardiology practice. These devices are inherently prothrombotic because of the foreign materials they are made of (Fig. 128.2 and Video 128.2).

Patients with VADs are prone to complications of low-flow conditions and artificial cannulas. Pump thrombosis, a devasting complication often requiring pump exchange, is more common with RVADs than LVADs. Among patients with severe right ventricular failure necessitating RVAD, more than 30% experience right-sided pump thrombosis.[8] Although left-sided intracardiac thrombosis is a known complication of ECMO, RHT are much less common, with reported incidences limited to case reports only.[9] Low-flow states, right ventricular infarction, and right-sided valvular stenosis are likely contributing factors in these patients.

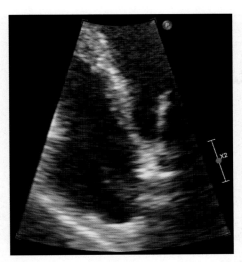

Figure 128.2. Transthoracic echocardiogram: right ventricle focused apical four-chamber zoom view. A mobile thrombus is attached to the right atrial surface of a recently placed atrial septal defect occluder device. (See accompanying Video 128.2.)

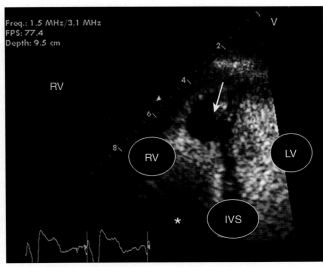

Figure 128.3. Transthoracic echocardiogram: right ventricle focused apical four-chamber zoom view. During maximal contrast enhancement of the right ventricle (RV), a large (>1.0 cm) filling defect is seen in the apex *(arrow)*. An attenuation artifact from the contrast (activated perflutren) is seen *(asterisk)*. *IVS*, Interventricular septum; *LV*, left ventricle. (See accompanying Video 128.3.)

Adult Congenital Heart Disease

The incidence of intracardiac thrombus in Fontan patients is 8% to 13%, likely related to postsurgical hypercoagulability, the presence of thrombogenic graft material, and sluggish flow inherent to bidirectional shunts, blind pulmonary stumps, and ventricular dysfunction. The 1-year mortality rate approaches 20% in these patients, with nearly 40% having residual clot on repeat imaging regardless of treatment strategy (anticoagulation, fibrinolysis, or surgery).[10]

In Eisenmenger syndrome, pulmonary arterial thrombosis is equally prevalent, observed in 20% of in vivo patients and 25% of necropsy studies. Local vascular injury, hypercoagulability, hypoxemia, and sluggish pulmonary flow are contributing factors. Thrombosis necessitates anticoagulation, but because these patients are innately at risk for hemoptysis, the safety of empiric treatment remains controversial and used on a per-patient basis.[10]

Children

The incidence of RHT in children is still uncertain. A meta-analysis of 27 publications identified 122 cases of RA thrombi in children, 91% of which were associated with CVCs. Coexisting hypercoagulable conditions such as malignancy or postoperative state were present in 20% and 25% of these cases, respectively. The majority of identified thrombi were clinically asymptomatic and associated with favorable patient outcomes. Fifty of the 122 cases included a detailed echocardiographic description of the RA thrombus, and high-risk features included a snakelike shape, pedunculated attachment, excessive mobility, and size greater than 2 cm. Children with high-risk thrombi had an increased mortality rate compared with those with low-risk thrombi (17% [3 of 18] vs 0% [0 of 32]).[11]

Systemic Inflammatory Disease

Thromboembolism in patients with systemic inflammatory conditions is common, and active inflammation, prothrombotic state, and dysfunctional endothelium are likely contributing factors. Intracardiac thrombi in these disease states is much less common but have been reported in systemic lupus erythematosus, Takayasu arteritis, and inflammatory bowel disease. Behçet disease, in which up to 1% of affected patients are thought to have cardiac mass lesions, is the only inflammatory disease consistently linked to RHT.[12]

ECHOCARDIOGRAPHIC IMAGING OF RIGHT HEART THROMBI

2D TTE is a portable, noninvasive, nonirradiating, and comprehensive tool regarded as the primary diagnostic imaging modality used in the evaluation of cardiac mass lesions.[13] It provides immediate, real-time, cross-sectional details on the size, shape, mobility, location, and attachment site of intracardiac masses and can be invaluable in the detection of thrombi. Serial echocardiographic examinations performed during moments of rapid clinical deterioration can identify a thrombus not detected on initial examination.

TEE is more sensitive than TTE to detect small thrombi and may be more useful to visualize the superior and inferior vena cava as they enter the RA. With respect to RA thrombi, TEE and TTE have reported sensitivities of 97% and 60%, respectively. TEE's superiority in visualizing the right heart is most evident in congenital heart disease, after cardiac surgery, and evaluation of indwelling catheters and devices. Intracardiac echocardiography (ICE), commonly used during catheter-based cardiac interventions, is considered to be 100% sensitive for RA masses, but its diagnostic role remains limited because of its invasive nature.[14]

Expanded capabilities of CMRI and cardiac CT allow for enhanced detection of RHT. CMRI is the reference standard for classifying cardiac masses, and CT is an acceptable alternative. TTE will likely remain the initial diagnostic tool for evaluating known or suspected intracardiac thrombi. Its contribution to the success of CMRI should not be underestimated because most CMRI examinations are performed with echocardiography interrogation a priori.[15] Advancements in modern ultrasound transducers provide improved RHT detection, and manufactured ultrasound contrast agents (ultrasound-enhancing agents [UEAs]) are available to further enhance diagnostic acumen (Fig. 128.3 and Video 128.3).[16]

Optimal imaging of the right heart is key to diagnosis and necessitates adjunctive echocardiographic views relative to the standard TTE examination. M-mode, 2D, and three-dimensional (3D) acquisitions from parasternal, apical, and subcostal views aligned toward the right side along with physiologic data obtained from pulsed-wave, continuous-wave, and tissue Doppler permit comprehensive right heart evaluation. Because right ventricular

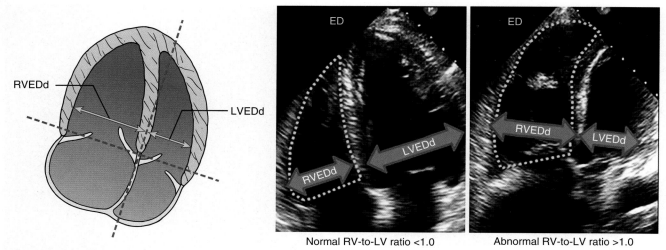

Figure 128.4. Schematic of an apical four-chamber view demonstrating the method of measuring the subannular interventricular right ventricular (RV) to left ventricular (LV) ratio (see text for details). A *dotted blue line* along the interventricular groove at the cardiac crux provides an alignment to draw a perpendicular intersecting line along the atrial–ventricular plane. The right and left ventricular end-diastolic diameters (RVEDd and LVEDd, respectively) are measured parallel to this plane. An example from a normal and abnormal RV-to-LV ratio are shown. Note how these measures are varied based on patient disease. *ED*, End-diastole. (Adapted from Rudski LG, et al: Guidelines for the echocardiographic assessment of the right heart in adults: a report from the American Society of Echocardiography endorsed by the European Association of Echocardiography, a registered branch of the European Society of Cardiology, and the Canadian Society of Echocardiography. *J Am Soc Echocardiogr* 23:685–713, 2013.)

TABLE 128.2 Right Heart Thrombus Morphology

Characteristic	Type A	Neither (AB)	Type B
Shape	Wormlike	Mixed	Round
Mobility	+++	+/++	–/+
DVT	Likely	Unknown	Rare
RH pathology	Absent	Unknown	Present
PE (any)	100%	Unknown	40%
PE (fatal)	27%		0%

DVT, Deep vein thrombosis; *PE*, pulmonary thromboembolism; *RH*, right heart.

Reproduced with permission from Kronik G: The European cooperative study on the clinical significance of right heart thrombi. European Working Group on Echocardiography, *Eur Heart J* 10(12):1046–1059, 1989.

dilatation and dysfunction have grave prognostic implications, a thorough understanding of right ventricular anatomy is vital.[17]

In contrast to RA thrombi, clots within the RV, right ventricular outflow tract, or PA are often symptomatic with echocardiographic signs of cor pulmonale (subannular interventricular RV-to-LV ratio >1.0, right ventricular dysfunction, tricuspid regurgitation maximum velocity ≥2.8 m/s). The interventricular RV-to-LV ratio is often used for risk stratification and management guidance in patients with documented PE, and a ratio greater than 1.0 by echocardiography (Ultrasound Accelerated Thrombolysis of Pulmonary Embolism [ULTIMA]) or CT angiography (Submassive and Massive Pulmonary Embolism Treatment with Ultrasound Accelerated Thrombolysis Therapy (SEATTLE II) Trial and Optimum Duration of Acoustic Pulse Thrombolysis Procedure in Acute Intermediate-Risk Pulmonary Embolism (OPTALYSE-PE) Trial) were the inclusion criteria in all of the major catheter-based thrombolysis trials published this decade.[18] Therefore, the RV-to-LV ratio measurement should be accurately obtained, highly scrutinized, and carefully reported because major management decisions are commonly determined by this value (Fig. 128.4).

The tricuspid valve (TV) apparatus seemingly acts to prevent or delay the advancement of thrombi into the RV or PA. FFTRH are often identified within multiple chambers simultaneously and are commonly associated with massive PE.[3] Because of the increased mortality rate in these patients, echocardiographic detection of this RHT subtype is of absolute importance.[3]

Last, TTE may prove useful in detecting a patent foramen ovale (PFO), an embryonic remnant present in up to 34% of normal adults. The combination of RHT, PE, and PFO lends itself to greater risk of systemic embolism, specifically when RV and PA pressures are high. Congenital heart disease can also create an environment susceptible to this devastating occurrence.[19]

RIGHT HEART THROMBI MORPHOLOGY

In 1989, an RHT-specific classification scheme was developed, categorizing thrombi by morphology and linking shape to prognosis (Table 128.2).[20] Thirty years later, the echocardiographic appearance of RHT is suggestive of embolic potential, morbidity, and mortality.

RHT contour often mimics the chamber in which they form. Thrombi originating in the RV, whether on a foreign body or as a result of myocardial dysfunction or endothelial injury, are often asymptomatic. RHT from the lower extremity venous system are often lengthy and serpiginous. In situ formation in the RA often cultivates a round, ball-like shape.[20,21]

The highest-risk RHT (FFTRH) are mobile, vessel-shaped masses that may extend from the RA across the TV orifice and into the RV or PA (type A). These thrombi can be exceedingly long and extend from the cavoatrial junction into the main or branch PAs (Figs. 128.5 and 128.6; Videos 128.5 and 128.6). Type A RHT coincides with a high incidence of deep venous thrombosis and a strong association with PE.[21] Of patients with PE, 3.5% have FFTRH, and these patients present more often with dyspnea, tachycardia, cardiogenic shock, and cardiac arrest. Not surprisingly, the mortality rate is reported to be as high as 50% in these patients.[20]

Type A RHT have a propensity for transit through a PFO because of the association with massive PE and concomitant pulmonary arterial hypertension (Fig. 128.7 and Video 128.7). Formerly thought to be a rare occurrence, multiple case reports have

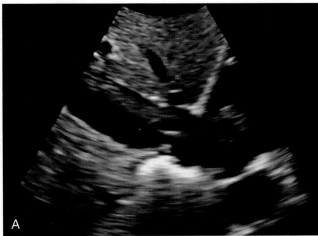

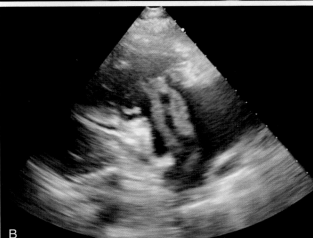

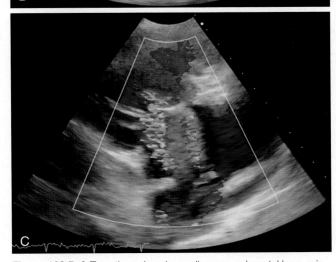

Figure 128.5. A, Transthoracic echocardiogram: subcostal long-axis view of the inferior vena cava (IVC). A large, echodense, highly mobile mass (embolized deep venous thrombosis) is seen in the IVC and right atrium (RA). **B,** Parasternal long-axis view of right ventricle (RV) inflow. The thrombus straddles the tricuspid valve, resting in both the RA and RV. **C,** Color Doppler of right ventricular inflow showing severe tricuspid regurgitant jet. (See accompanying Video 128.5.)

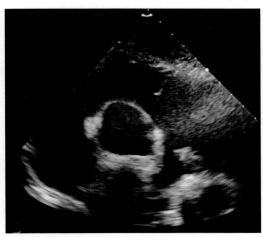

Figure 128.6. Transthoracic echocardiogram: parasternal long-axis view with focus on the pulmonary artery (PA) and branches. A mobile mass is seen at the main PA bifurcation. (See accompanying Video 128.6.)

described RHT that have become lodged or "trapped" within a PFO. A meta-analysis of observational studies and case reports by Myers and coworkers identified 174 patients with impending paradoxical embolism, defined as a biatrial thromboembolism caught in transit across a PFO. PE was present in 91% of these patients, and the 24-hour and 30-day mortality rates in this review were 11.5% and 18.4%, respectively. A total of 55% had evidence of systemic embolism (cerebral, peripheral vascular, or abdominal ischemia), underscoring the heightened morbidity associated with IPDE.[22]

Lower risk RHT are typically immobile and laminated (attached to the chamber wall) and have an amorphous shape (type B). These thrombi are morphologically similar to left-sided intracardiac thrombi. Because they often develop within the right heart chambers, they are commonly associated with underlying cardiac pathology. Unlike type A RHT, type B RHT typically run a more benign course despite a relatively common, nonfatal PE event rate of 40%.[20]

A third morphologic description of RHT has echocardiographic features of both type A and B clots and is labeled type AB or type C RHT, depending on the source. These intermediate RHT are described as highly mobile but not "vessel shaped" (Fig. 128.8 and Video 128.8).[20]

SPECIFIC ECHOCARDIOGRAPHY IMAGING STRATEGIES FOR RIGHT HEART THROMBI

Echocardiographic evaluation of RHT should begin with a thorough assessment of the right heart per established guidelines.[17] Because type A RHT are often identified spanning one or more cardiac chambers and type B thrombi can form in the ventricular apex, the apical and subcostal views may be most valuable. Images from multiple, off-axis, nonstandard views, including image sweeps, should be obtained to better define complete location, size, and shape.[13]

Techniques for better visualization include reducing depth (or zoom) and narrowing sector width. A high-frequency (pediatric transducer) probe or manipulation of the adult multifrequency (emphasizing resolution more than penetration) imaging probe should be used. For the latter, adjustments should be made to maximize temporal and spatial resolution. Sweeps from multiple perspectives with and without harmonics are recommended, as is the use of 3D and simultaneous multiplane imaging. Real-time 3D TTE may further clarify the size, shape, consistency, mobility, and location to help differentiate thrombus from other cardiac masses (Fig. 128.9 and Video 128.9).[13]

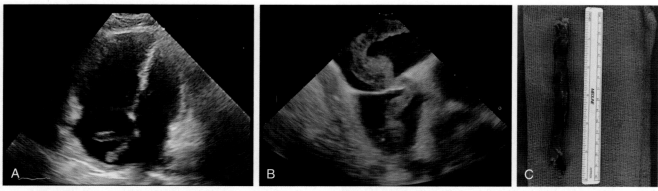

Figure 128.7. Transthoracic echocardiogram: right ventricle–focused apical four-chamber view. **A,** A large, snakelike mass is seen in the right atrium and is noted to cross through the patent foramen ovale (PFO). **B,** Intracardiac echocardiogram. Interatrial septal view showing the mass (embolized deep venous thrombosis) "trapped" in the PFO. **C,** The extracted thrombus measured nearly 6 inches after successful percutaneous retrieval. (See accompanying Video 128.7.)

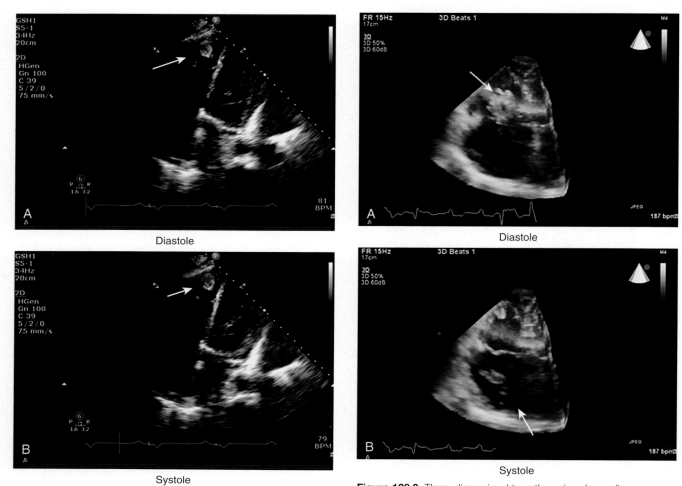

Figure 128.8. Transthoracic echocardiogram: right ventricle (RV)–modified apical four-chamber view. Patient had severe RV systolic dysfunction and type AB (round and mobile) right heart thrombus in the RV apex *(arrow).* Note subtle position change in A, diastole and B, systole due to thrombus mobility. (See accompanying Video 128.8.)

Figure 128.9. Three-dimensional transthoracic echocardiogram: right ventricular (RV)–aligned view, apical four-chamber view. **A,** Type A right heart thrombus protrudes across the tricuspid valve *(arrow)* in diastole. **B,** In systole, the thrombus is seen anchored in the right atrium and entering via the superior vena cava *(arrow).* (See accompanying Video 128.9.)

Normal cardiac structures and intracardiac devices and catheters should not be confused with RHT. The septomarginal muscle bundle and moderator band are present in the distal third of the RV, and although they can be indiscriminate, they are commonly hypertrophied in patients with pulmonary hypertension.[17]

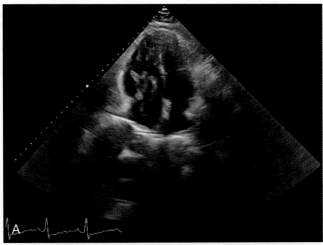

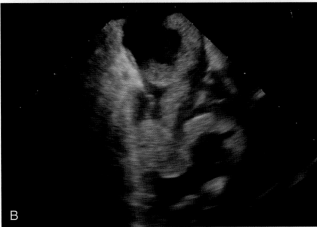

Figure 128.10. Transthoracic echocardiogram: apical four-chamber view. **A,** A large, snakelike mass is seen in the right atrium and right ventricle. **B,** Intracardiac echocardiogram. RV inflow "home view." The embolized deep venous thrombosis passes through the tricuspid valve during ventricular diastole. The patient underwent successful, urgent percutaneous retrieval of the thrombus-in-transit. (See accompanying Video 128.10.)

UEAs can be useful to improve endocardial definition and identify structures within the RV, specifically when images are suboptimal (see Fig. 128.3 and Video 128.3). Although agitated saline is a simple, low-cost contrast agent that can routinely visualize the right ventricular cavity and apex, saline microbubbles are unstable and less homogenous compared with UEA. Despite these obvious limitations, agitated saline contrast provides a quick and simple method for visualization during maximal, albeit transient, opacification.[13,16]

When it comes to echocardiographic imaging of the right heart, ICE may be the best modality. It is commonly used by some centers during interventional catheterization and electrophysiologic procedures to improve the efficacy and safety of complex procedures. ICE transducers transmit with higher frequency (9–12 MHz) with accompanying greater spatial resolution and lower penetration than those used in TEE. Therefore, imaging with these catheters requires close proximity of the probe to the structure of interest (Fig. 128.10 and Video 128.10). ICE imaging detects intracardiac thrombus formation on sheaths, catheters, and device leads in the RA, a finding that occurs with an incidence of 30% of patients undergoing ablation.[23]

TISSUE CHARACTERIZATION AND CONTRAST PERFUSION

The acuity of intracardiac thrombi can have important embolic and treatment implications, necessitating enhanced tissue characterization. Chronic thrombi often have an organized, laminated appearance and are thought to have a lower incidence of embolization. Echo density is greater compared with myocardial boundaries, and there is an absence of tumor stalk or invasion of surrounding myocardium. Acute thrombi are often freely mobile and less echo dense and may have an associated, stringlike attachment, features that contribute to diagnostic complexity in differentiating thrombi from cardiac tumors.[24]

UEAs may help to discriminate thrombi from tumors. Contrast perfusion sequences applying a high-mechanical index impulse (flash) after contrast opacification result in immediate or transient microbubble destruction. The rate of UEA replenishment can delineate blood flow within cardiac masses (i.e., whereas rapid replenishment identifies vascular, malignant tumors, slow or nonexistent replenishment is representative of avascular masses such as thrombi) (Fig. 128.11). Thrombi can be further distinguished from low-vascularized masses by using low-mechanical index ultrasonography.[16] Desire to further characterize the histopathology of intracardiac masses has prompted molecular imaging research and development of novel, designer UEAs that are targeted toward or activated by a specific disease state (i.e., thrombus imaging). Targeted UEAs use microbubbles that recognize platelet glycoprotein IIb/IIIa receptors, aiding in the ultrasonic visualization of acute arterial thrombotic occlusion in in vitro and in vivo models. These agents have not yet been adapted into clinical use.[25]

UEAs can miss thrombi that are mural in shape, apically oriented, or small in size. Laminated mural thrombi may masquerade as regional

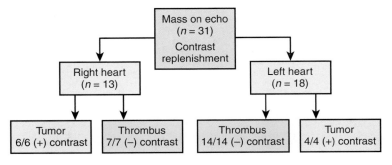

Figure 128.11. Myocardial contrast echocardiography using a replenishment imaging technique. This technique was able to accurately distinguish an intracardiac tumor (+ contrast enhancement) from thrombus (– contrast enhancement) in both the left and right heart chambers (see text for details).

myocardial thickening, and small apical thrombi may be difficult to discern from the heavily trabeculated, corrugated appearance of the normal right ventricular myocardium. CMRI is a noninvasive, nonirradiating modality that offers enhanced tissue characterization and is considered to be the reference standard for assessment of intracardiac masses when clinical indecision remains after echocardiography has been obtained.[26] Cardiac CT, although not routinely used for the workup of cardiac masses, can also provide complementary information in the form of tissue characterization. Because of mixing of peripherally injected contrast and noncontrast blood, the accuracy of identifying right atrial thrombus is lower with cardiac CT.

CONVENTIONAL MANAGEMENT STRATEGIES

The echocardiographic appearance and coexisting cardiac pathology help determine the optimal treatment strategy. Type A RHT warrant care in an intensive care unit setting because of a high risk of migration and catastrophic cardiovascular collapse. Regardless of treatment approach (anticoagulation, fibrinolysis, or embolectomy), the mortality rate in untreated patients with RHT and PE approaches 100%, and most deaths occur within the first 24 hours of hospitalization. In a retrospective analysis of 177 cases of RHT, mortality rates were 100%, 29%, 24%, and 11% for patients who received no treatment, anticoagulation only, surgical embolectomy, or fibrinolysis, respectively.[27] Therefore, individualized treatment options need to be considered and carried out expeditiously. Any further diagnostic investigations (CT angiography, lung perfusion scintigraphy, or invasive pulmonary angiography) can be performed after treatment has been initiated.

Surgical embolectomy and fibrinolysis enhance survival in selected patients with RHT and PE, but the best treatment approach remains controversial. A surgical approach is preferred for very large RHT, obstruction of right ventricular inflow, entrapment within a PFO, fibrinolytic failure, or contraindications to fibrinolysis, requiring cardiopulmonary bypass and an experienced surgeon for open inspection and thrombus extraction. Fibrinolytics represent a convenient treatment option for patients with PE and concomitant hemodynamic compromise or right ventricular failure, providing the added benefit of simultaneously treating the PE, RHT, and any residual DVT. Nonrandomized, prospective clinical trials suggest systemic lysis is safe, efficient, and effective, with complete resolution of thrombi within 24 hours and often as soon as 2 hours after fibrinolytic treatment.

The Registro Informatizado de Enfermedad TromboEmbolica (Computerized Registry of Patients with Venous Thromboembolism) registry data did not detect a difference in mortality rate between fibrinolytic therapy and routine anticoagulation (4.7% vs 7.8%; $P = .47$). These findings coincide with older data suggestive of similar survival curves in patients receiving heparin, fibrinolytics, or embolectomy. Thus, RHT in isolation (without hemodynamic instability or entrapment within a PFO) do not warrant riskier interventions other than standard anticoagulation. Thus, the 2019 European guidelines for the diagnosis and management of acute PE recommend fibrinolysis for patients with circulatory collapse without contraindications (class I; level of evidence: B) and embolectomy for those in whom fibrinolysis is contraindicated or has failed (class I; level of evidence: C).[28] The same document does provide guidance for impending paradoxical embolism, but the 2011 American Heart Association scientific statement recommends considering embolectomy for this scenario (class IIb; level of evidence: C).[29]

CONTEMPORARY MANAGEMENT STRATEGIES

Given the propensity for PE and associated mortality of type A RHT, a basic understanding of contemporary treatment strategies is necessary. Novel catheter-based interventions such as ultrasound-facilitated catheter-directed thrombolysis (USCDT) and AngioVac (AngioDynamics) are interventions with therapeutic potential. USCDT uses the EkoSonic

Endovascular System (EKOS Corporation) and combines catheter-directed thrombolysis with pulsed, high-frequency ultrasound waves to enhance PTE lysis efficiency.[18] AngioVac, approved in 2014 for the filtration of intravascular thrombi and emboli, is a venovenous filtration apparatus that uses extracorporeal drainage and reinfusion cannulas to aspirate and debulk RHT and PE.[30]

The aim of USCDT is to deliver the reperfusion capabilities of fibrinolytics with a reduced risk of adverse effects such as major bleeding including intracranial hemorrhage (ICH). The ULTIMA and SEATTLE II trials were prospective, multicenter studies of patients with acute massive or submassive PTE demonstrating a reduced RV-to-LV diameter ratio at 24- and 48-hours post-USCDT, respectively. The Optimum Duration of Acoustic Pulse Thrombolysis Procedure in Acute Intermediate-Risk Pulmonary Embolism (OPTALYSE-PE) trial examined fibrinolytic dosing, reporting efficacy at reducing thrombus burden with shorter delivery time and lower dose tissue plasminogen activator (4 mg/lung/2 hours). In general, major bleeding (4.65%) and ICH (0.35%) remain significant detriments to widespread use. In the absence of randomized clinical trials comparing USCDT with anticoagulation alone, conclusions regarding safety and efficacy cannot be made.[18]

AngioVac is an option for extraction of RHT in a select patient population, particularly in sicker patients considered to be at prohibitive risk for open surgery. Thus far, safety and efficacy data on AngioVac are limited. A meta-analysis of 42 published reports (182 total patients; 101 thrombus and 81 vegetation) on AngioVac found a success rate of 80.5% for removal of right atrial or caval thrombi with a mortality rate of 14.8%. For PTE, success and mortality rates were 32.4% and 32.3%, respectively.[30] It should be noted that studies in this review were those of single-center experiences, and randomized, controlled trials have yet to validate the results of this novel technology.

CONCLUSION

RHT are not uncommon, possibly increasing in incidence, potentially underreported, and associated with poorly appreciated risk factors such as AF. Echocardiography accurately discriminates high-risk (type A) from low-risk (type B) morphologic features and helps dictate who needs critical monitoring and urgent treatment. UEA can be used to evaluate perfusion of masses and helps TTE in distinguishing tumors from thrombi. 3D echocardiography is an important complementary tool for complete mass assessment. TEE, CMRI, cardiac CT, and ICE remain important additional diagnostic tools with unique strengths and weaknesses. USCDT and AngioVac offer alternative treatment options to conventional methods, and each relies heavily on accurate echocardiographic evaluation of the right heart.

Please access ExpertConsult to view the corresponding videos for this chapter.

Acknowledgment

The authors acknowledge the contributions of Dr. Vrinda Sardana, who was the author of this chapter in the previous edition.

REFERENCES

1. Ogren M, Bergqvist D, Eriksson H, et al. Prevalence and risk of pulmonary embolism in patients with intracardiac thrombosis: a population-based study of 23 796 consecutive autopsies. *Eur Heart J*. 2005;26(11):1108–1114.
2. Barrios D, Rosa-Salazar V, Jimenez D, et al. Right heart thrombi in pulmonary embolism. *Eur Respir J*. 2016;48(5):1377–1385.
3. Casazza F, Becattini C, Guglielmelli E, et al. Prognostic significance of free-floating right heart thromboemboli in acute pulmonary embolism: results from the Italian Pulmonary Embolism Registry. *Thromb Haemost*. 2014;111(1):53–57.
4. Rossi L, Libutti P, Casucci F, et al. Is the removal of a central venous catheter always necessary in the context of catheter-related right atrial thrombosis? *J Vasc Access*. 2019;20(1):98–101.
5. Jeung S, Kang SM, Seo Y, et al. A case series of asymptomatic hemodialysis catheter-related right atrial thrombi that are incidentally detected prior to kidney transplantation. *Transplant Proc*. 2018;50(10):3172–3180.

6. Cresti A, Garcia-Fernandez MA, Miracapillo G, et al. Frequency and significance of right atrial appendage thrombi in patients with persistent atrial fibrillation or atrial flutter. *J Am Soc Echocardiogr.* 2014;27(11):1200–1207.

7. Yasuoka Y, Naito J, Hirooka K, et al. Right atrial spontaneous echo contrast indicates a high incidence of perfusion defects in pulmonary scintigraphy in patients with atrial fibrillation. *Heart Ves.* 2009;24(1):32–36.

8. Shah P, Ha R, Singh R, et al. Multicenter experience with durable biventricular assist devices. *J Heart Lung Transplant.* 2018;37(9):1093–1101.

9. Bhat AG, Golchin A, Pasupula DK, et al. Right sided intracardiac thrombosis during veno-arterial extracorporeal membrane oxygenation: a case report and literature review. *Case Rep Crit Care.* 2019;8594681.

10. Ohuchi H. Adult patients with Fontan circulation: what we know and how to manage adults with Fontan circulation. *J Cardiol.* 2016;68(3):181–189.

11. Yang JY, Williams S, Brandao LR, Chan AK. Neonatal and childhood right atrial thrombosis: recognition and a risk-stratified treatment approach. *Blood Coagul Fibrinolysis.* 2010;21(4):301–307.

12. Misra DP, Shenoy SN. Cardiac involvement in primary systemic vasculitis and potential drug therapies to reduce cardiovascular risk. *Rheumatol Int.* 2017;37(1):151–167.

13. Saric M, Armour AC, Arnaout MS, et al. Guidelines for the use of echocardiography in the evaluation of a cardiac Source of embolism. *J Am Soc Echocardiogr.* 2016;29(1):1–42.

14. Obeid AI, al Mudamgha A, Smulyan H. Diagnosis of right atrial mass lesions by transesophageal and transthoracic echocardiography. *Chest.* 1993;103(5):1447–1451.

15. Rathi VK, Czajka AT, Thompson DV, et al. Can cardiovascular MRI be used to more definitively characterize cardiac masses initially identified using echocardiography. *Echocardiography.* 2018;35(5):735–742.

16. Porter TR, Mulvagh SL, Abdelmoneim SS, et al. Clinical applications of ultrasonic enhancing agents in echocardiography: 2018 American Society of Echocardiography Guidelines Update. *J Am Soc Echocardiogr.* 2018;31(3):241–274.

17. Lang RM, Badano LP, Mor-Avi V, et al. Recommendations for cardiac chamber quantification by echocardiography in adults: an update from the American Society of Echocardiography and the European Association of Cardiovascular Imaging. *J Am Soc Echocardiogr.* 2015;28(1):1–39. e14.

18. Rali PM, Criner GJ. Submassive pulmonary embolism. *Am J Respir Crit Care Med.* 2018;198(5):588–598.

19. Lu C, Li J, Wang W, et al. Large thrombus-in-transit within a patent foramen ovale in a patient with pulmonary embolism: a case report. *J Int Med Res.* 2018;46(10):4332–4337.

20. Kronik G. The European cooperative study on the clinical significance of right heart thrombi. European Working Group on Echocardiography. *Eur Heart J.* 1989;10(12):1046–1059.

21. Charif F, Mansour MJ, Hamdan R, et al. Free-floating right heart thrombus with acute massive pulmonary embolism: a case report and review of the literature. *J Cardiovasc Echogr.* 2018;28(2):146–149.

22. Myers PO, Bounameaux H, Panos A, et al. Impending paradoxical embolism: Systematic review of prognostic factors and treatment. *Chest.* 2010;137(1):164–170.

23. Enriquez A, Saenz LC, Rosso R, et al. Use of intracardiac echocardiography in interventional cardiology: working with the anatomy rather than fighting it. *Circulation.* 2018;137(21):2278–2294.

24. Basso C, Rizzo S, Valente M, Thiene G. Cardiac masses and tumours. *Heart.* 2016;102(15):1230–1245.

25. Brown E, Lindner JR. Ultrasound molecular imaging: principles and applications in cardiovascular medicine. *Curr Cardiol Rep.* 2019;21(5):30.

26. Weinsaft JW, Kim J, Medicherla CB, et al. Echocardiographic algorithm for post-myocardial infarction lv thrombus: a gatekeeper for thrombus evaluation by delayed enhancement CMRI. *JACC Cardiovasc Imag.* 2016;9(5):505–515.

27. Chartier L, Bera J, Delomez M, et al. Free-floating thrombi in the right heart: diagnosis, management, and prognostic indexes in 38 consecutive patients. *Circulation.* 1999;99(21):2779–2783.

28. Konstantinides SV, Meyer G, Becattini C, et al. ESC guidelines for the diagnosis and management of acute pulmonary embolism developed in collaboration with the European Respiratory Society (ERS). *Eur Heart J.* 2019;54:1901647. 2019.

29. Jaff MR, McMurtry MS, Archer SL, et al. Management of massive and submassive pulmonary embolism, iliofemoral deep vein thrombosis, and chronic thromboembolic pulmonary hypertension: a scientific statement from the American Heart Association. *Circulation.* 2011;123(16):1788–1830.

30. Hameed I, Lau C, Khan FM, et al. AngioVac for extraction of venous thromboses and endocardial vegetations: a meta-analysis. *J Card Surg.* 2019;34(4):170–180.

129 Normal Anatomic Variants and Artifacts

Steven A. Goldstein

Echocardiography has greatly enhanced the field of cardiology. However, optimal use of echocardiography requires the ability to recognize and differentiate pathological conditions from normal cardiac structures and their variants that may simulate serious pathology. Although errors can occur with both transthoracic echocardiography (TTE) and transesophageal echocardiography (TEE), they are especially common with TEE. Despite its superior image resolution—in fact, partly because of it—TEE is particularly prone to a variety of pitfalls. Several of these pitfalls are related to embryologic remnants, other to oblique views, and yet others to variants of normal structures. Categories of echocardiographic pitfalls are shown in Box 129.1. A list of pitfalls that are discussed and illustrated in this subsection is shown in Box 129.2.

CRISTA TERMINALIS

The crista terminalis (CT), or terminal ridge, is a crescent-shaped (or C-shaped) muscular ridge that spans from the anteromedial wall of the right atrium (just to the left of the orifice of the superior vena cava [SVC]) near the right atrial (RA) appendage toward the vicinity of the inferior vena cava (IVC).[1–4] In some instances the crista terminalis merges with the valve of the IVC (eustachian valve [EV]). Its length is up to 4 to 5 cm, which decreases with age.[4] The CT is derived from the regression of the embryologic septum spurium as the sinus venosus is incorporated into the RA wall.[5] This process of regression varies widely, resulting in considerable variability in appearance in imaging modalities.[6,7] When it is prominent, this

fibromuscular ridge can protrude into the RA cavity and resemble a mass, such as a neoplasm or thrombus.[6–9] Thus, awareness of the variable and often prominent echocardiographic features of this structure can prevent the misdiagnosis of a "tumor." In at least one case, the significance of this structure was not appreciated, resulting in unnecessary open heart surgery for removal of a presumed intracardiac tumor.[6] Using the transesophageal echocardiographic bicaval view, the CT will appear as a protuberance originating from the SVC extending for a variable distance along the lateral RA wall (Fig. 129.1). This anatomic structure has gained increased attention recently because the sinoatrial node lies in its superior aspect and its location is important for electrophysiologic studies.[2] In addition, some authors have described the CT to be larger (greater in height, width, and area) in patients with atrial flutter (AFL) than in those without AFL.[3,4,10,11] Moreover, AFL and other reentry arrhythmias can be eliminated by ablation of the region of the CT.[12–15]

EUSTACHIAN VALVE

The EV, or valve of the inferior cava, is a remnant of the embryonic right valve of the sinus venosus. In the fetal circulation, the EV performs the important function of directing oxygenated blood from the IVC toward the foramen ovale and into the left atrium. The EV generally regresses during childhood but can persist into adulthood. Although usually vestigial or small, its size and shape in adults can vary considerably. In fact, Eustachius, writing in 1563, was the first to describe and classify its variations.[16] There is also wide

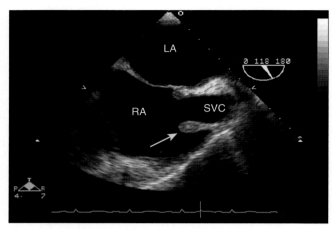

Figure 129.1. Transesophageal echocardiographic bicaval view illustrates a prominent crista terminalis *(yellow arrow)*. *LA,* Left atrium; *RA,* right atrium; *SVC,* superior vena cava.

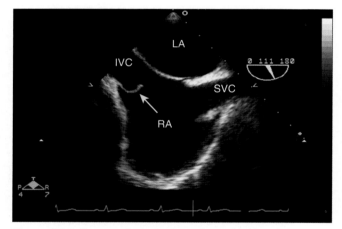

Figure 129.2. Transesophageal echocardiographic bicaval view illustrates a prominent eustachian valve *(yellow arrow)* in the right atrium (RA) at the inlet of the inferior vena cava (IVC). *LA,* Left atrium; *SVC,* superior vena cava.

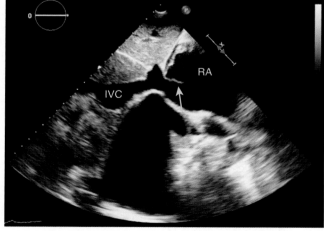

Figure 129.3. Transthoracic echocardiographic (TTE) subxiphoid view that illustrates the entrance of the inferior vena cava (IVC) into the right atrium (RA). A Eustachian valve is indicated by the *yellow arrow*.

echocardiographic variability.[17–19] At one end of the spectrum, the EV may be totally absent or present only as a thin ridge. Most commonly, it appears as a crescent fold of tissue arising from the anterior rim of the IVC and may be rigid or slightly mobile (Figs. 129.2 and 129.3). At the other end of the spectrum, it appears as an elongated, mobile structure projecting several centimeters into the RA cavity, demonstrating an undulating motion. The average length of the EV has been reported to be 3.6 mm with a range of 1.5 to 22 mm.[17,20] On TEE, the EV is best visualized in the midesophageal four-chamber view or the midesophageal bicaval view, where it usually appears as an undulating flap of tissue where the IVC enters the right atrium. When prominent, it may be confused with an RA tumor, thrombus, or vegetation.[21–23]

The EV, even when prominent, is a benign and incidental finding. However, complications have been reported. Endocarditis and thrombus formation are extremely rare complications.[24–29] Even more rare, cases of RA myxoma or papillary fibroelastoma originating from the EV have been reported.[30] Last, there have been reports of a prominent EV causing problems during catheter-based interventional procedures and even surgery, in which a prominent EV was mistaken for an atrial septal defect and inadvertently closed[31] (Fig. 129.4).

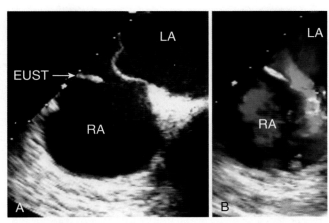

Figure 129.4. Transesophageal echocardiogram illustrating how the presence of a prominent eustachian valve (EUST, **A**) can be mistaken for the atrial septum, and therefore normal flow entering from the inferior vena cava (IVC) can mimic an atrial septal defect (ASD). **B,** The blue jet is caused by blood entering the right atrium (RA) from the IVC; this jet can be misdiagnosed as flow across an ASD. *LA,* Left atrium.

CHIARI NETWORK

The Chiari network is an embryologic remnant resulting from incomplete resorption of the right sinus venosus valve that persists as a reticular network of fine or lacelike strands or a fenestrated membrane with variable attachments to the crista terminalis, Thebesian valve, upper region of the RA wall, or interatrial septum or to the "floor" of the right atrium in the region of the opening of the coronary sinus (CS).[32,33] Because of its fenestrations, the Chiari network does not cause obstruction to flow. In 1897, the Austrian anatomist Hans Chiari described 11 cases in which the valve of the IVC (the EV) was represented by networks with widespread attachments that differed from the EV, which was derived only from the valve of the IVC.[34] Although not all studies make a clear morphologic distinction between these two entities and a precise definition and classification of the EV versus a Chiari network differs among manuscripts, most authors, like Chiari himself,[34] stress the importance of differentiating these entities. A Chiari network is generally more extensive, attaches to two or more regions, and is typically fenestrated or netlike.[33] The EV, even though it may also be mobile and even fenestrated, does not have additional attachments.

Echocardiographically, a Chiari network is seen as a long, thin, sometimes curvilinear, highly mobile structure with variable insertion sites from the valve of the IVC to the additional sites previously mentioned. Because of its rapid mobility and whiplike motion, this structure tends to move into and out of the scan plane. Moreover, because of its fenestrated or weblike nature, echocardiographic "dropout" of parts of this highly mobile structure is found in about 2% to 3% of hearts at autopsy.[35,36] The incidence detected by TTE is very low (<0.6%), but by TEE, it is comparable to that at autopsy.[33,37–40] The role of the echocardiographer is to recognize this structure as a Chiari network and to differentiate it from pathologic RA abnormalities such as a thrombus, vegetation, pedunculated tumor, or tricuspid chordal rupture. Congenital remnants such as Chiari networks generally have no clinical significance.[33,39] Rarely, however, Chiari networks may be associated with complications such as thrombus formation,[41] embolus entrapment,[42] arrhythmias,[43] tumor development,[44] catheter entrapment,[45] infection,[46] and entanglement of a atrial septal occluder device[37] (Box 129.3).

The presence of the Chiari network may be confused with the diagnosis of cor triatriatum dexter.[47–49] Cor triatriatum dexter also results from incomplete resorption of the right sinus venosus valve, but the dividing septum of cor triatriatum dexter is much thicker

BOX 129.3 Clinical Relevance of Chiari Networks: Rare Associations

- Site of thrombus formation
- Site of infectious endocarditis
- Ensnarement of thrombus-in-transit (prevention of pulmonary emboli)
- Entrapment of pacemaker electrodes, Swan-Ganz catheters, and so forth
- Arrhythmias
- Site of tumor development
- Entanglement of atrial septal occluder device

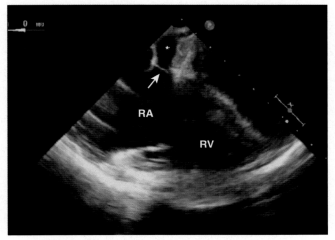

Figure 129.5. Transesophageal echocardiogram lower esophageal view illustrates the Thebesian valve *(arrow)* "guarding" the orifice of the coronary sinus *(asterisk)*. *RA,* Right atrium; *RV,* right ventricle.

with few or no fenestrations. Unlike the Chiari network, it may cause obstruction to blood flow and is usually associated with other congenital abnormalities such as atrial septal defect and tricuspid atresia.[47,48,50]

THEBESIAN VALVE

The CS receives the majority of cardiac venous blood and opens directly into the right atrium. Embryologically, it is a caudal remnant of the sinoatrial valves. The CS ostium is situated in the posteroinferior surface of the heart between the IVC opening and the inferior tricuspid orifice.[51] It serves as an anatomic landmark as well as a conduit for diagnostic and therapeutic procedures.

The ostium of the CS is "guarded" by a fold of endocardial tissue called the Thebesian valve. The Thebesian valve was first described by Adam Christain Thebesius in 1708.[51,52] The Thebesian valve morphology is variable in size, shape (semilunar, linear, circular), composition (membranous, fibrous, fibromuscular), presence or absence of fenestrations, and extent of coverage (occlusion) of the CS ostium.

The CS is a frequently cannulated structure in patients undergoing cardiac resynchronization therapy, catheter ablation of arrhythmias, perfusion therapy, mitral valve annuloplasty, and targeted drug delivery. A typical Thebesian valve leaves enough space for the passage of a standard catheter, but when it covers all or most of the CS orifice, the Thebesian valve can pose difficulties for such procedures.[51,53–55] Therefore, procedural and perioperative echocardiographers must be aware of the Thebesian valve and predictive factors for difficult CS cannulation. Lower esophageal four-chamber view (Fig. 129.5) and modified midesophageal bicaval views are useful in evaluating Thebesian valve anatomy.

TABLE 129.1 Incidence of Lipomatous Hypertrophy of the Atrial Septum

Author	Year	Diagnostic Modality	Patients (*n*)	Patients (%)
Reyes and Jablokow[59]	1979	Necropsy	38 of 4591	0.8
Pochis et al[60]	1992	TEE	8 of 107	7.6
Heyer et al[61]	2003	Multislice CT	28 of 1292	2.2
Kuester et al[62]	2005	PET–CT fusion	23 of 802	2.8
Czekajska-Chehab et al[63]	2012	Multislice CT	56 of 5786	0.96

CT, Computed tomography; *PET,* positron emission tomography; *TEE,* transesophageal echocardiography.

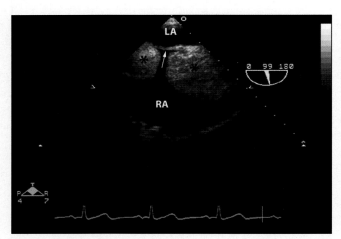

Figure 129.6. Transesophageal echocardiogram of a patient with lipomatous hypertrophy of the atrial septum (LHAS) illustrating the typical "dumbbell" shape created by sparing of the fossa ovalis *(arrow)* region. The hypertrophied portions of the atrial septum are indicated by *asterisks*. *LA,* Left atrium; *RA,* right atrium.

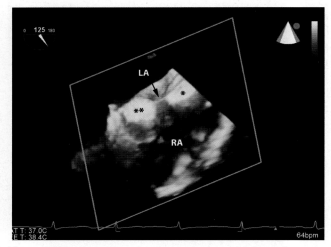

Figure 129.7. Three-dimensional transesophageal echocardiogram illustrating lipomatous hypertrophy of the atrial septum (LHAS). Note the thicker cephalad portion *(two asterisks)* and the thinner caudal portion *(one asterisk),* the usual distribution of LHAS. The *arrow* points to the thin septum primum. The fossa ovalis region is spared from fat deposition, leading to the typical "dumbbell" appearance of the atrial septum. *LA,* Left atrium; *RA,* right atrium.

LIPOMATOUS HYPERTROPHY OF THE ATRIAL SEPTUM

Lipomatous hypertrophy of the atrial septum (LHAS) is a condition characterized by an unencapsulated but circumscribed accumulation of excessive adipose tissue in the atrial septum, resulting in a globular thickening of the atrial septum.[56] This thickening is caused by a proliferation of mature fat cells rather than hypertrophy of the cells.[56] Nevertheless, the designation "lipomatous hypertrophy of the interatrial (or atrial) septum" persists.

LHAS is an uncommon but increasingly recognized benign mass lesion. This entity was first described in 1964 at autopsy[57] and was first diagnosed in a living patient in 1982 by computed tomography.[58] Since then this condition has been reported widely, with an incidence between 1% and 8% depending on the series and methods used for detection[59–63] (Table 129.1). No absolute diagnostic criteria have been established, but a septal thickness of 15 to 20 mm is often quoted.[64–66] In a series of 32 autopsy specimens reported by McAllister and Fenoglio,[65] the maximal diameter ranged from 1 to 8 cm. The defining characteristic feature is the septal location of the atrial thickening, which typically spares the fossa ovalis, leading to a classic "dumbbell" or "hourglass" shape[67] (Figs. 129.6 and 129.7). The cephalad portion of the mass is often thicker than the caudal portion.[57] The fat accumulation often extends to the atrial wall and on occasion to the ventricular septum. These features are typical, and the diagnosis is easily made by TTE or TEE.[56,68–72] Additional imaging is not usually required, but the diagnosis can also be made by magnetic resonance imaging and computed tomography.

LHAS is associated with increasing age and obesity.[59,61,66,73] LHAS is generally a benign abnormality and is most often detected as an incidental finding on cardiac imaging, surgery, or autopsy.[71,72,74] Although the vast majority of patients with LHAS are asymptomatic, LHAS may be associated with supraventricular arrhythmias.[56,61,71,73] In extreme cases, it can cause SVC obstruction.[56,74–76] Surgical resection of LHAS should be reserved for patients with SVC obstruction because important morbidity exists when large portions of the atrial septum are excised, requiring reconstruction with pericardium or Dacron.[75–77]

With the increasing use of transseptal puncture for a variety of "structural heart disease" interventions, knowledge of the anatomy of the atrial septum, including LHAS, is crucial for echocardiographers. First, LHAS can interfere with the transseptal puncture itself. Second, puncturing of the hypertrophied area may reduce the maneuverability of catheters, wires, and devices.[78,79]

FAT INFILTRATION OF THE TRICUSPID ANNULUS

As previously described, LHAS is characterized by deposition of adipose tissue in the atrial septum. Although less well reported, fatty accumulation can occur in the tricuspid annulus and also, rarely, in the atrial wall.[80] Because of the normal motion of the tricuspid annulus throughout the cardiac cycle, a prominent fatty tricuspid annulus can simulate a mobile mass such as a neoplasm. Clues to avoid this mistaken diagnosis include (1) a fatty tricuspid annulus tends to be triangular, and (2) the base of the anterior tricuspid leaflet comes off the apex of this triangular "mass" as in Fig. 129.8.

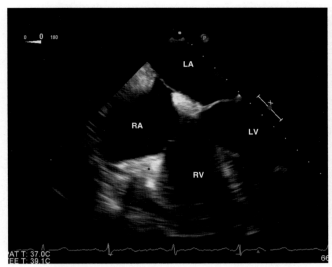

Figure 129.8. Transesophageal midesophageal four-chamber view illustrates prominent triangular-shaped fatty infiltration in the tricuspid annulus *(asterisk)* in a patient who also has lipomatous hypertrophy of the atrial septum. *LA,* Left atrium; *LV,* left ventricle; *RA,* right atrium; *RV,* right ventricle.

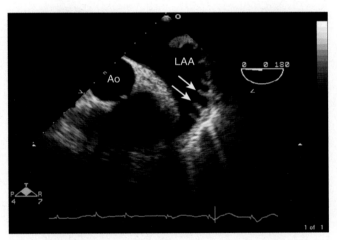

Figure 129.9. Transesophageal echocardiographic image of the left atrial appendage (LAA) illustrates the typical appearance of prominent pectinate muscles *(arrows)* that appear as parallel ridges appearing to protrude into the lumen of the LAA. *Ao,* Aorta.

PECTINATE MUSCLES IN THE LEFT ATRIAL APPENDAGE

A series of parallel ridges known as pectinate muscles course along the endocardial surfaces of both the left and right atria, including the appendages. Generally, they are only imaged with TEE. When prominent, they can appear to protrude into the lumen of the left atrial appendage (LAA) and may mimic thrombi (Fig. 129.9). The following features help differentiate pectinate muscles from thrombi:

1. Lack of independent mobility of the atrial wall but move in concert with it
2. Relatively small and linear
3. Typically, they have a multiple, parallel ridgelike appearance, like the teeth of a comb.

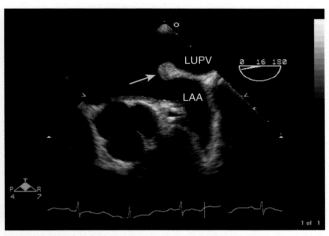

Figure 129.10. Transesophageal echocardiogram illustrates a prominent "Q-tip"–shaped muscular ridge *(yellow arrow)* between the left atrial appendage (LAA) and the left upper pulmonary vein (LUPV).

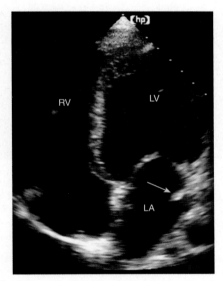

Figure 129.11. Transthoracic echocardiographic apical four-chamber view that illustrates the muscular ridge *(yellow arrow)* that separates the left atrial appendage (not imaged) from the left superior pulmonary vein. *LA,* Left atrium; *LV,* left ventricle; *RV,* right ventricle.

PROMINENT RIDGE OF TISSUE BETWEEN THE LEFT ATRIAL APPENDAGE AND THE LEFT UPPER PULMONARY VEIN

Within the left atrium, there is a ridge, or diaphragm, that separates the LAA and the left upper pulmonary vein. This dividing membrane is composed of cardiac muscle covered by endocardial tissue.[81] When prominent, this structure can resemble a mass and can be misdiagnosed as an atrial tumor or thrombus[82] (Figs. 129.10 and 129.11). Experienced echocardiographers recognize this as a normal anatomic structure and avoid such misdiagnosis. It often has the appearance of a "matchstick" or "Q-tip."

FLUID IN THE TRANSVERSE SINUS

The transverse sinus is the potential space between the ascending aorta and the left atrium. It is visualized only when fluid is present and almost exclusively by TEE, often surrounding the LAA

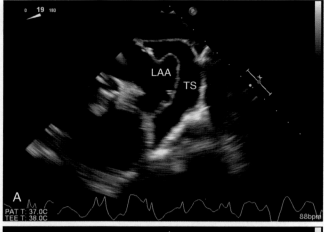

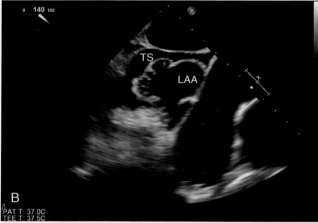

Figure 129.12. A, Transesophageal echocardiogram (TEE) at 19 degrees showing the left atrial appendage (LAA) surrounded by fluid in the transverse sinus (TS). **B,** TEE at 140 degrees showing the LAA identified by multiple "comblike" pectinate muscles surrounded by fluid in the transverse sinus (TS).

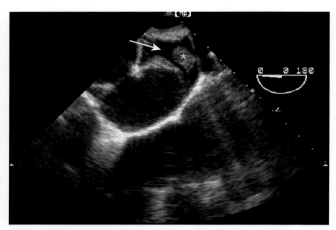

Figure 129.13. Transesophageal echocardiogram of a patient in whom the tip of the atrial appendage appears like a solid mass *(yellow asterisk)* within the transverse sinus *(arrow)*.

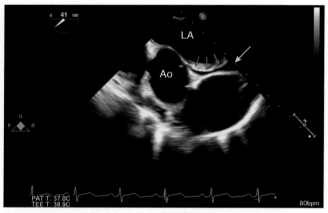

Figure 129.14. Transesophageal echocardiogram illustrates fluid in the transverse sinus *(red arrows)* that can mimic a coronary artery. Note that the walls of this structure are not parallel as they would be for a tubular structure such as a coronary artery but diverge *(yellow arrow)*. *Ao,* Aorta; *LA,* left atrium.

as shown in Fig. 129.12. In the presence of pericardial effusion, the apex of the LAA can appear as a mobile mass "inside" this fluid-filled space, mimicking a mass lesion (Fig. 129.13). Careful imaging, including electronic rotation of the imaging plane, can correctly identify this pseudomass as part of the LAA. In addition, pericardial effusion within the transverse sinus may harbor fibrinous material, which can also be erroneously interpreted as a mass. Another pitfall of the transverse sinus is its potential to be confused for the left coronary artery. With careful scanning and probe manipulation, the transverse sinus, unlike coronary arteries, can be demonstrated to have a nontubular shape (Fig. 129.14). Color and pulsed-wave Doppler can also document flow in the true coronary artery.

The oblique sinus (OS) is a cul-de-sac located behind the posterior wall of the left atrium.[83] The OS is not visible unless there is an abnormal collection of fluid within the pericardial space.[84] Effusions filling the OS appear as an echo-free space posterior to the left atrium as in Fig. 129.15.

False Tendons

Left ventricular false tendons (LVFTs) are discrete, linear, fibrous (majority) or fibromuscular bands of varying lengths and thickness that traverse the left ventricular (LV) cavity. They usually extend between the ventricular septum and LV free wall, papillary muscle, or LV apex but do not connect, like chordate tendinae, to the mitral

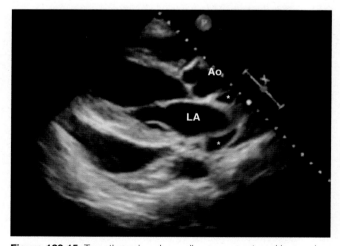

Figure 129.15. Transthoracic echocardiogram parasternal long-axis view illustrates the transverse sinus *(white asterisk)*, which is the echo-free space posterior to the posterior aspect of the ascending aorta (Ao) and the oblique sinus *(yellow asterisk)*, which is the echo-free space posterior to the left atrium (LA).

TABLE 129.2 Various Terms Used for Left Ventricular False Tendons in the Literature

Authors	Year	Terms Used
Turner[82]	1893	Moderator band in the left ventricle
Roberts[105]	1969	Anomalous LV strands
Gueron and Cohen[106]	1972	Anomalous LV chordae tendinae
Pomerance[107]	1975	False tendons
Gerlis et al[88]	1984	LV bands
Gryzbiak et al[108]	1996	Fibromuscular ribbons
Bhatt et al[109]	2009	LV false tendons

LV, Left ventricular.

leaflets.[85,86] Histologic analysis of LVFTs show that they contain fibrous tissue, myocardial fibers, elastic fibers, blood vessels, and conduction tissue.[87–89] Various names have been ascribed to false tendons (Table 129.2).

LVFTs are commonly visualized on echocardiography and at autopsy. They are readily detected by routine transthoracic two-dimensional echocardiographic apical views. They appear as distinctive linear echogenic strands traversing the LV cavity, connecting the free wall or papillary muscle to the ventricular septum (Fig. 129.16). Typically, they are stretched (taut) in diastole and flaccid (lax) in systole (Video 129.1). Special care is required to differentiate LVFTs from other entities such as ventricular trabeculations, masses or tumors, discrete subaortic membrane, accessory mitral valve leaflet tissue, and flail mitral chordae tendinae.

Although LVFTs are generally considered benign anatomic variants, there is no consensus on their clinical significance. Some authors have suggested that they may be associated with repolarization abnormalities on resting electrocardiography preexcitation, ventricular arrhythmias, dilated left ventricles, and heart murmurs. Others have touted a protective effect by preventing adverse remodeling of the LV because they tether opposing LV wall or by reducing the severity of mitral regurgitation by stabilizing the position of papillary muscle(s) as the left ventricle enlarges.[86]

CASEOUS CALCIFICATION OF THE MITRAL ANNULUS

Mitral annular calcification (MAC) is a common degenerative abnormality of the cardiac fibrous skeleton that occurs mostly in older adults and in patients with end-stage renal failure. Caseous calcification of the mitral annulus is a relatively rare and underappreciated variant of MAC. There are several published reports and several names applied to this unusual entity (Box 129.4) in which there is central liquefaction necrosis composed of a mixture of calcium, fatty acids, and cholesterol with a "toothpaste-like" or "putty-like" texture[90–100] The incidence reported by Pomerance in a necropsy study was 2.7% of all autopsies with MAC in patients older than 50 years.[90] Harpaz and colleagues[97] reported an echocardiographic prevalence of 0.63% (19 of 3007) in patients with MAC and 0.067% (19 of 28,364) in a general adult population referred for echocardiography. This is similar to the 0.055% prevalence suggested by Kronzon and associates[91] (5 of 9000 echocardiograms). Caseous calcification of the mitral annulus is usually detected as an incidental finding by TTE or TEE. The characteristic echocardiographic appearance is a large, round echodense mass in the mitral periannular region with a clear central echolucent zone[92,94–100] (Fig. 129.17). An absence of acoustic shadowing behind the mass suggests the absence of a more typical solid, dense calcium deposition of MAC. As previously stated, this entity is underrecognized

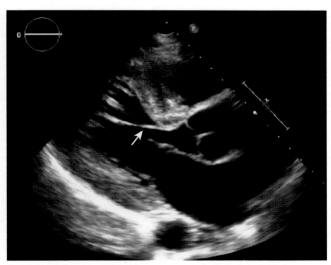

Figure 129.16. Transthoracic echocardiogram parasternal long-axis view illustrates a left ventricular false tendon *(arrow)* traversing from the apex to the basal septum.

BOX 129.4 Caseous Calcification of the Mitral Annulus: Other Terms in Various Publications

- Caseous "tumor" of the mitral annulus
- Mitral annular calcification with central caseation
- Sterile, caseous mitral valve annular abscess
- Tumorlike mild annular calcification with central liquefaction
- Sterile caseous mass of the mitral valve
- Liquefaction necrosis of mitral annular calcification

---

but is important because it can be misdiagnosed as a myocardial abscess[90,92–94,96] or tumor,[92–94] leading in some cases to unnecessary explorative cardiotomy.[92,93]

ARTIFACTS OF THE THORACIC AORTA

The proximal ascending aorta frequently displays artifacts that can simulate an aortic dissection flap, especially when the ascending aorta is dilated.[101–104] These artifacts include ultrasound "ghosts," reverberations from calcified atherosclerotic plaques, calcium deposition in the sinotubular junction (Fig. 129.18), and reverberations from catheters and pacemakers in the right heart. These artifacts, unlike dissection flaps, often appear to move outside the confines of the aorta itself. Color Doppler can be useful in differentiating these artifacts from a true dissection by the absence of turbulent flow or flow differential (i.e., different flow velocities in true and false lumens). Occasionally with TEE, there is a mirror image of the descending thoracic aorta because of an artifact related to reverberations. Sound bounces (reflects) from an object to the transducer, and some sounds make the round trip again; thus, the echocardiography machine "sees" a similar object twice as far away as the actual one. This artifact is most commonly encountered in longitudinal views of the descending thoracic aorta (Fig. 129.19). These "two" aortas should not be confused with true and false lumens of an aortic dissection. On occasion, normal flow, because it spirals down the descending thoracic aorta, will appear to be bidirectional by color Doppler in a cross-sectional view and may mimic the true and false lumen of an aortic dissection as seen in Fig. 129.20.

Please access ExpertConsult to view the corresponding video for this chapter.

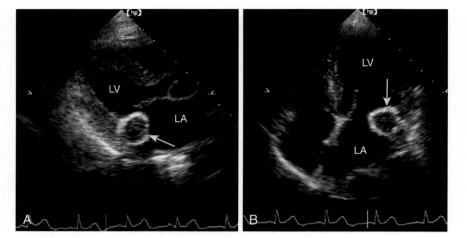

Figure 129.17. Parasternal long-axis (**A**) and apical four-chamber (**B**) views of the same patient illustrating a relatively large, round, echodense mass in the mitral periannular region, with a relatively echolucent center typical of caseous mitral annular calcification. *LA,* Left atrium; *LV,* left ventricle.

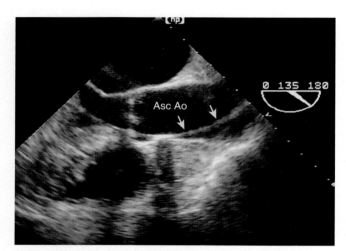

Figure 129.18. Longitudinal views of the aortic root in two patients illustrating an arclike reverberation *(yellow arrows)* from calcium in the sinotubular junction, which could be misinterpreted as an aortic dissection flap. *Asc Ao,* Ascending aorta.

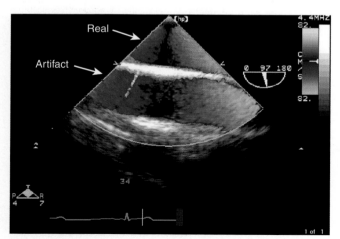

Figure 129.19. Transesophageal echocardiographic longitudinal view of the mid–descending thoracic aorta, which shows the true (Real) and pseudo (Artifact) aortas.

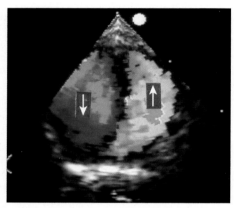

Figure 129.20. Transesophageal echocardiographic cross-section view of descending thoracic aorta that illustrates yellow and blue flow on color Doppler (caused by normal unidirectional flow that spirals down the descending thoracic aorta) that mimics bidirectional flow (which could be misinterpreted as flow in true and false lumens and thus potentially leading to a false-positive diagnosis of aortic dissection).

REFERENCES

1. Matsuyama TA, Inoue S, Kobayashi Y, et al. Anatomical diversity and age-related histological changes in the human right atrial posterolateral wall. *Europace.* 2004;6:307–315.
2. Loukas M, Tubbs RS, Tongson JM, et al. The clinical anatomy of the crista terminalis, pectinate muscles, and teniae sagittalis. *Ann Anat.* 2008;190:81–87.
3. Morita N, Kobayashi Y, Iwasaki YK, et al. Characterization of transient atrial rhythm occurring between typical atrial flutter and its termination with class III drugs. *Pacing Clin Electrophysiol.* 2008;31:943–954.
4. Saoudi N, Ercyies D, Anselme F. Why do patients develop atrial flutter? Is this crista terminalis geometry? *Pacing Clin Electrophysiol.* 2009;32:866–867.
5. Edwards JE. Congenital malformation of the heart and great vessels—a. Malformations of the atrial septal complex. In: Gould SE, ed. *Pathology of the Heart.* Springfield, IL: Bannerstone House; 1960:287–289. 61–63.
6. Mirowitz SA, Gutiernez FR. Fibromuscular elements of the right atrium; pseudomass at MR imaging. *Radiology.* 1992;182:231–233.
7. Meier RA, Hartnell GG. MRI of right atrial pseudomass: is it really a diagnostic problem? *J Comput Assist Tomogr.* 1994;18:398–401.
8. Pharr JR, West MB, Kusumoto FM, Figueredo VM. Prominent crista terminalis appearing as a right atrial mass on transthoracic echocardiogram. *J Am Soc Echocardiogr.* 2002;15:753–755.

9. Ackay M, Bilen ES, Bilge M, et al. Prominent crista terminalis: as an anatomic structure leading to atrial arrhythmias and mimicking right atrial mass. *J Am Soc Echocardiogr.* 2007;20:e9–e10.

10. Mizumaki K, Fujiki A, Nagasawa H, et al. Relation between transverse conduction capability and the anatomy of the crista terminalis in patients with atrial flutter and atrial fibrillation. *Circ J.* 2002;66:1113–1118.

11. Okumura Y, Watanabe I, Ashino S, et al. Electrophysiologic and anatomical characteristics of the right atrial posterior wall in patients with and without atrial flutter. *Circ J.* 2007;71:636–642.

12. Marchlinski FE, Ren JF, Schwartzman D, et al. Accuracy of fluoroscopic localization of the crista terminalis documented by intracardiac echocardiography. *J Interv Card Electrophysiol.* 2000;4:415–421.

13. Sanchez-Quintana D, Anderson RH, Cabrera JA, et al. The terminal crest: morphological features relevant to electrophysiology. *Heart.* 2002;88:406–411.

14. Tai CT, Huang JL, Lee PC, et al. High-resolution mapping around the crista terminalis during typical atrial flutter. *J Cardiovasc Electrophysiol.* 2004;15:406–414.

15. Zhao Q-Y, Huang H, Tang Y-H, et al. Relationship between the automatic innervations in crista terminalis and atrial arrhythmia. *J Cardiovasc Electrophysiol.* 2009;20:551–557.

16. Powell EDU, Mullaney JM. The Chiari network and the valve of the inferior vena cava. *Br Heart J.* 1960;22:579–584.

17. Limacher MC, Gutgesell HP, Vick GW, et al. Echocardiographic anatomy of the Eustachian valve. *Am J Cardiol.* 1986;57:363–365.

18. Yavuz T, Nazli C, Kinay O, Kutsal A. Giant Eustachian valve with echocardiographic appearance of divided right atrium. *Tex Heart Inst J.* 2002;129:336–338.

19. Okamoto M, Beppu S, Nagata S. Echocardiographic features of the Eustachian valve and its clinical significance. *J Cardiogr.* 1981;11:271–276.

20. Asirdizer M, Tatlisumak E. The role of the Eustachian valve and patent foramen ovale in sudden death. *J Clin Forensic Med.* 2006;13:262–267.

21. Ducharme A, Tardif JC, Mercier LA, et al. Remnants of the right valve of the sinus venous presenting as a right atrial mass on transthoracic echocardiography. *Can J Cardiol.* 1997;13:573–576.

22. Carson W, Chiu SS. Eustachian valve mimicking intracardiac mass. *Circulation.* 1998;97:2188.

23. Malaterre HR, Kallee K, Perier Y. Eustachian valve mimicking a right atrial cystic tumor. *Int J Card Imag.* 2000;16(4):305–307.

24. Palakodeti V, Keen Jr WD, Rickman LS, Blanchard DG. Eustachian valve endocarditis: detection with multiplane transesophageal echocardiography. *Clin Cardiol.* 1997;20:579–580.

25. Bowers J, Krimsky W, Graden JD. The pitfalls of transthoracic echocardiography. A case of Eustachian valve endocarditis. *Tex Heart Inst J.* 2001;28:57–59.

26. Ponzo F, Guarini P, De Michele M, et al. Eustachian valve endocarditis in an elderly woman. *Echocardiography.* 1999;16:259–261.

27. Pellicelli AM, Pino P, Terranova A, et al. Eustachian valve endocarditis: a rare localization of right side endocarditis. *Cardiovasc Ultrasound.* 2005;3(30).

28. Gill DS, Birchley S. Eustachian valve endocarditis. *Echocardiography.* 2006;23:256–257.

29. Jolly N, Kaul UA, Khalilullah M. Right atrial thrombus over eustachian valve—Successful lysis with streptokinase. *Int J Cardiol.* 1991;30:354–356.

30. Teoh KH, Mulji A, Tomlinson CW, Lobo FV. Right atrial myxoma originating from the eustachian valve. *Can J Cardiol.* 1993;9:441–443.

31. Becker A, Buss M, Sebening W, et al. Acute inferior cardiac inflow obstruction resulting from inadvertent surgical closure of a prominent Eustachian valve mistaken for an atrial septal defect. *Pediatr Cardiol.* 1999;20:155–157.

32. Powell EDU, Mullaney JM. The Chiari network and the valve of the inferior vena cava. *Br Heart J.* 1960;22:579–584.

33. Schneider B, Hofmann T, Justen M, et al. Chiari's network: normal anatomic variant or risk factor for arterial embolic events? *J Am Coll Cardiol.* 1995;26:203–210.

34. Chiari H. Ueber Netzbildungen in rechten Vorhofe des Herzens. *Beitr Path Anat.* 1897;22:1–10.

35. Yater WM. The paradox of Chiari's network. Review and report of a case of Chiari's network ensnaring a large embolus. *Am Heart J.* 1936;11:541–553.

36. Ralston L, Wasdahl W. Chiari's network. *Am J Med.* 1958;25:810–813.

37. Pellett AA, Kerut EK. The Chiari network in an echocardiography student. *Echocardiography.* 2004;21:91–93.

38. Cooke JC, Gelman JS, Harper RW. Chiari network entanglement and herniation into the left atrium by an atrial septal defect occluder device. *J Am Soc Echocardiogr.* 1999;12:601–603.

39. Werner IA, Cheitlin MD, Gross BW, et al. Echocardiographic appearance of the Chiari network: differentiation from right-heart pathology. *Circulation.* 1981;63:1104–1109.

40. Cujec B, Mycyk T, Khouri M. Identification of Chiari's network with transesophageal echocardiography. *J Am Soc Echocardiogr.* 1992;5:96–99.

41. Benbow EW, Lone EM, Love HG, et al. Massive right atrial thrombus associated with a Chiari network and a Hickman catheter. *Am J Clin Pathol.* 1987;88:243–248.

42. Goedde TA, Conetta D, Rumisek JD. Chiari network entrapment of thromboemboli: congenital inferior vena cava filler. *Ann Thorac Surg.* 1990;49:317–318.

43. Clements J, Sobotka-Plojhar M, Exlato N, et al. A connective tissue membrane in the right atrium (Chiari network) as a cause of fetal cardiac arrhythmia. *J Obstet Gynecol.* 1982;142:709–712.

44. Wasdahl DA, Wasdahl WA, Edwards WD. Fibroelastic papilloma arising in a Chiari network. *Clin Cardiol.* 1992;15:45–47.

45. Goldschlager A, Goldschlager N, Brewster H, et al. Catheter entrapment in a Chiari network involving an atrial septal defect. *Chest.* 1972;61:345–346.

46. Payne DM, Basket RIF, Hirsch GM. Infectious endocarditis of a Chiari network. *Ann Thorac Surg.* 2003;76:1303–1305.

47. Hansing CE, Young WP, Rowe GG. Cor triatriatum dexter. *Am J Cardiol.* 1972;30:559–564.

48. Lanzarini L, Lucca E. Persistence of the right valve of the sinus venosus resulting in an unusually prominent Chiari network remnant mimicking cor triatriatum dexter. *Pediatr Cardiol.* 2001;23:103–105.

49. Loukas M, Sullivan A, Tubbs RS, et al. Chiari's network: review of the literature. *Surg Radiol Anat.* 2010;32(10):895–901.

50. Islam AKMM, Sayami LA, Zaman S. Chiari network: a case report and brief overview. *J Saudi Heart Assoc.* 2013;25:225–229.

51. Mak GS, Hill AJ, Moisiuc F, Krishnan SC. Variations in Thebesian valve anatomy and coronary sinus ostium: implications for invasive electrophysiology procedures. *Europace.* 2009;11(9):1188–1192.

52. Loukas M, Clarke P, Tubbs RS, et al. Adam Christian Thebesius, a historical perspective. *Int J Cardiol.* 2008;129(1):138–140.

53. Kulkarni V, Kulkarni V, Vagdevi HS, Kumar V. Morphological and clinical significance of Thebesian valve guarding ostium of coronary sinus. *Natl J Clin Anat.* 2019;8:62–65.

54. Kautzner J. Thebesian valve: the guard dog of the coronary sinus? *Europace.* 2009;11(9):1136–1137.

55. Ghosh SK, Raheja S, Tuli A. Obstructive Thebesian valve: anatomical study and implications for invasive cardiologic procedures. *Anat Sci Int.* 2014;89(2):85–94.

56. O'Connor S, Recvarren R, Nichols LC, et al. Lipomatous hypertrophy of the interatrial septum. An overview. *Arch Pathol Lab Med.* 2006;130:397–399.

57. Prior JT. Lipomatous hypertrophy of the cardiac interatrial septum. *Arch Pathol.* 1964;78:11–15.

58. Isner JM, Swan CS, Mikus P, et al. Lipomatous hypertrophy of the interatrial septum: in vivo diagnosis. *Circulation.* 1982;66:470–473.

59. Reyes CV, Jablokow VR. Lipomatous hypertrophy of the cardiac interatrial septum: a report of 38 cases and review of the literature. *Am J Clin Pathol.* 1979;72:785–788.

60. Pochis WT, Saeian K, Sagar KB. Usefulness of transesophageal echocardiography in diagnosing lipomatous hypertrophy of the atrial septum with comparison to transthoracic echocardiography. *Am J Cardiol.* 1992;70:396–398.

61. Heyer CM, Kagel T, Lemburg SP, et al. Lipomatous hypertrophy of the interatrial septum: a prospective study of incidence, imaging findings, and clinical symptoms. *Chest.* 2003;124:2068–2073.

62. Kuester LB, Fischman AJ, Fan CM, et al. Lipomatous hypertrophy of the interatrial septum: prevalence and features on fusion ^{18}F-fluorodeoxyglucose positron emission tomography/CT. *Chest.* 2005;128:3888–3893.

63. Czekajska-Chehab E, Tomaszewska M, Olchowik G, et al. Lipomatous hypertrophy of the interatrial septum in ECG-gated multislice computed tomography of the heart. *Med Sci Monit.* 2012;18:MT54–MT59.

64. Hutter Jr PM, Page DL. Atrial arrhythmias and lipomatous hypertrophy of the cardiac interatrial septum. *Am Heart J.* 1971;82:16–21.

65. McAllister HA, Fenoglio Jr JR. Tumors of the cardiovascular system. In: *Atlas of Tumor Pathology, Ser 2, Fascicle 27*. Washington, DC: Armed Forces Institute of Pathology; 1978:40–46.

66. Burke AP, Litovsky S, Virmani R. Lipomatous hypertrophy of the atrial septum presenting as a right atrial mass. *Am J Surg Pathol.* 1996;20:678–685.

67. Fyke III FE, Tajik AJ, Edwards WD, et al. Diagnosis of lipomatous hypertrophy of the atrial septum by two-dimensional echocardiography. *J Am Coll Cardiol.* 1983;1:1352–1357.

68. Kindman LA, Wright A, Tye T, et al. Lipomatous hypertrophy of the interatrial septum: characterization by transesophageal and transthoracic echocardiography, magnetic resonance imaging, and computed tomography. *J Am Soc Echocardiogr.* 1988;1:450–454.

69. Journet A, Batalla J, Uson M, et al. Lipomatous hypertrophy of the interatrial septum. *Echocardiography.* 1992;9:501–503.

70. Munoz J, Losada A, Ibanez M, et al. Lipomatous hypertrophy of the atrial septum: Complementary diagnosis by transesophageal echocardiography and nuclear magnetic resonance imaging. *Eur Heart J.* 1996;17:1290–1291.

71. Nadra I, Dawson D, Schmitz SA, et al. Lipomatous hypertrophy of the interatrial septum: a commonly misdiagnosed mass often leading to unnecessary cardiac surgery. *Heart.* 2004;90:e66.

72. Bhattacharjee M, Netigan MC, Dervan P. Lipomatous hypertrophy of the interatrial septum: an unusual intraoperative finding. *Br Heart J.* 1991;65:49–50.

73. Gay JD, Guileyardo JM, Townsend-Parchman JK, et al. Clinical and morphological features of lipomatous hypertrophy ("massive fatty deposits") of the interatrial septum. *Am J Forensic Med Pathol.* 1996;17:43–48.

74. Shirani J, Roberts WC. Clinical electrocardiographic and morphologic features of massive fatty deposits ("lipomatous hypertrophy") in the atrial septum. *J Am Coll Cardiol.* 1993;22:226–238.

75. McNamara RF, Taylor AE, Panner BJ. Superior vena caval obstruction by lipomatous hypertrophy of the right atrium. *Clin Cardiol.* 1987;10:609–610.

76. Zeebregts CJAM, Hensens AG, Timmermans J, et al. Lipomatous hypertrophy of the interatrial septum: indication for surgery? *Eur J Cardio Thorac Surg.* 1997;11:785–787.

77. Oxorn DC, Edelist G, Goldman BS, et al. Echocardiography and excision of lipomatous hypertrophy of the interatrial septum. *Ann Thorac Surg.* 1999;67:852–854.

78. Ho SY, McCarthy KP, Faletra FF. Anatomy of the left atrium for interventional echocardiography. *Eur J Echocardiogr.* 2011;12. i11–15.

79. Laura DM, Donnino R, Kim EE, et al. Lipomatous atrial septal hypertrophy: a review of its anatomy, pathophysiology, multimodality imaging, and relevance to percutaneous interventions. *J Am Soc Echocardiogr.* 2016;29(8):717–723.

80. Cohen IS, Raiker K. Atrial lipomatous hypertrophy: lipomatous atrial hypertrophy with significant involvement of the right atrial wall. *J Am Soc Echocardiogr.* 1993;6:30–34.

81. Van Pragh R, Corsini I. Postmortem cases and a study of normal development of the pulmonary vein and atrial septum in 83 human embryos. *Am Heart J.* 1969;78:379–405.

82. Turner W. Another heart with moderator band in the left ventricle. *J Anat Physiol.* 1896;30:568–569.

83. Rodriquez ER, Tan CD. Structure and anatomy of the human pericardium. *Prog Cardiovasc Dis.* 2017;59:327–340.

84. Penmasta S, Silbiger JJ. The transverse and oblique sinuses of the pericardium: anatomic and echocardiographic insights. *Echocardiography.* 2019;36:170–176.

85. Kenchaiah S, Benjamin EJ, Evans JC, et al. Epidemiology of left ventricular false tendons: clinical correlates in the Framingham study. *J Am Soc Echocardiogr.* 2009;22:739–745.

86. Silbiger JJ. Left ventricular false tendons: anatomic echocardiographic, and pathophysiologic insights. *J Am Soc Echocardiogr.* 2013;26:582–588.

87. Philip S, Cherian KM, Wu M, Lue H. Left ventricular false tendons: echocardiographic, morphologic, and histopathologic studies and review of the literature. *Pediatr Neonatal.* 2001;52:279–286.

88. Gerlis LM, Wright HM, Wilson N, et al. Left ventricular bands: a normal anatomical feature. *Br Heart J.* 1984;52:641–647.

89. Kervancioglu M, Ozbaf D, Kervancioglu P, et al. Echocardiographic and morphologic examination of left ventricular false tendons in human and animal hearts. *Clin Anat.* 2003;16:389–395.

90. Pomerance A. Pathological and clinical study of the calcification of the mitral valve ring. *J Clin Pathol.* 1970;23:354–361.

91. Kronzon I, Winer HE, Cohen ML. Sterile, caseous mitral annular abscess. *J Am Coll Cardiol.* 1983;2:186–190.

92. Teja K, Gibson RS, Nolan SP. Atrial extension of mitral annular calcification mimicking intracardiac tumor. *Clin Cardiol.* 1987;10:546–548.

93. Borowski A, Korb H, Voth E, et al. Asymptomatic myocardial disease. *Thorac Cardiovasc Surg.* 1988;36:338–340.

94. Kautzner J, Vondracek V, Jirasek A, Belohlavek M. Tumor-like mitral annular calcification with central liquefaction. *Echocardiography.* 1993;10:459–463.

95. Prasad NK, Alam M, Rosman HS. Mitral annular calcification mimicking an intracardiac mass. *Echocardiography.* 1995;12:609–612.

96. Gilbert HM, Grodman R, Chung MH, et al. Sterile, caseous mitral valve "abscess" mimicking infective endocarditis. *Clin Infect Dis.* 1997;24:1015–1076.

97. Harpaz D, Auerbach I, Vered Z, et al. Caseous calcification of the mitral annulus: a neglected, unrecognized diagnosis. *J Am Soc Echocardiogr.* 2001;14:825–831.

98. Morgan-Hughes G, Zacharkiw L, Roobottom C, et al. Images in cardiovascular medicine. Tumor-like calcification of the mitral annulus: diagnosis with multislice computed tomography. *Circulation.* 2003;107:355–356.

99. Novaro GM, Griffin BP, Hammer DF. Caseous calcification of the atrial annulus: an underappreciated variant. *Heart.* 2004;90:388.

100. Alkadhi H, Leschka S, Pretre R, et al. Caseous calcification of the mitral annulus. *J Thorac Cardiovasc Surg.* 2005;129:1438–1440.

101. Kronzon J, Demopoulos L, Schrem SS, et al. Pitfalls in the diagnosis of thoracic aortic aneurysm by transesophageal echocardiography. *J Am Soc Echocardiogr.* 1990;3:145–148.

102. Applebe AF, Walker PG, Yeoh JK, et al. Clinical significance and origin of artifacts in transesophageal echocardiography of the thoracic aorta. *J Am Coll Cardiol.* 1993;21:754–760.

103. Losi MA, Betocchi S, Briguori C, et al. Determinants of aortic artifacts during transesophageal echocardiography of the ascending aorta. *Am Heart J.* 1999;137:967–972.

104. Vignon P, Spencer KT, Rambaud G, et al. Differential transesophageal echocardiographic diagnosis between linear artifacts and intramural flap of aortic dissection or disruption. *Chest.* 2001;119:1778–1790.

105. Roberts WC. Anomalous left ventricular band: an unemphasized cause of a precordial musical murmur. *Am J Cardiol.* 1969;23:736–768.

106. Gueron M, Cohen W. Anomalous left ventricular chordate tendinae and pre-excitation, unusual cause of precordial systolic murmur in a baby with fibroelastosis. *Br Heart J.* 1972;34:966–968.

107. Pomerance A. Rarities and miscellaneous endocardial abnormalities. In: Pomerance A, Davies MJ, eds. *The Pathology of the Heart.* Oxford: Blackwell Scientific Publications; 1975:483.

108. Gryzbiak M, Lotkowski D, Kozlowski D. False tendons in the left ventricle of the heart in humans during pre and postnatal periods. *Folia Morphol (Warsz).* 1996;55:89–99.

109. Bhatt MR, Alfonso CE, Bhatt EM, et al. Effects and mechanisms of left ventricular false tendons on functional mitral regurgitation in patients with severe cardiomyopathy. *J Thorac Cardiovasc Surg.* 2009;138:1123–1128.

130 Aortic Atherosclerosis and Embolic Events

Astha Tejpal, Itzhak Kronzon

Nearly 150 years ago, P.L. Panum suggested that atherosclerotic material within the aorta can embolize to peripheral arteries.[1] In a 1945 paper based on an autopsy, Flory showed that arterial occlusion was the result of aortic atherosclerotic plaque.[2] However, modern imaging technologies, which include contrast angiography, computed tomography (CT), magnetic resonance imaging (MRI), transthoracic echocardiography (TTE), and transesophageal echocardiography (TEE), are required to evaluate aortic atherosclerosis in vivo. At present, two- and three-dimensional (3D) TEE provides accurate, high-resolution images of the thoracic aortic wall. This technique has also established the correlation among severe aortic plaque, stroke, and peripheral aortogenic embolism.[3] Box 130.1 shows various names used in the medical literature to define this aortic pathology. For the sake of simplicity, we will use the term *aortic plaque*.

TRANSESOPHAGEAL ECHOCARDIOGRAPHY AND AORTIC PLAQUE

Almost the entire thoracic aorta can be visualized during a transesophageal examination. Multiplane views permit the visualization of each aortic segment except for a short segment at the junction of the aortic arch and the ascending aorta, which is masked by the air column inside the trachea. Normally, the aortic intima is smooth and thin (Fig. 130.1A). There is no evidence of irregularity, protrusion, calcification, or ulceration. Aortic plaque is considered mild when intimal thickness is 3 mm or less (Fig. 130.1B). Severe plaque is determined by intimal thickness of equal or more than 4 mm (Fig. 130.1C). If the plaque is unstable, there may be rupture and thrombus formation, which may be seen as a mobile mass (Fig. 130.1D and Videos 130.1 to 130.3). Plaques can also show calcification (Fig. 130.1E) or ulcerations (Fig. 130.1F). 3D echocardiography may provide a more detailed and accurate topographic representation of aortic plaque, including exact location, shape, and thickness (Fig. 130.1G and Video 130.4) but can be a time-consuming process.[4] Semiautomated plaque analysis systems are being studied for their role in plaque detection using 3D echocardiography and quantification of plaque size, thickness, and volume (Fig. 130.2).[5]

BOX 130.1 Names Used in the Medical Literature to Describe Aortic Plaque

- Aortic plaque
- Complex aortic plaque
- Eroded atheromatous plaque
- Arteriosclerotic plaque
- Aortic atheroma
- Atheromatous aorta
- Protruding atheroma
- Aortic atherosclerosis
- Atherosclerotic atheromatosis
- Atherosclerotic debris

This technology may provide a useful and more efficient way to determine disease severity and plaque burden in the future.

Plaques with thickness of 4 mm or more and those that contain ulceration or thrombus are defined as *complex plaques*. Many investigators have shown that complex plaques are associated with stroke and embolic events. Noncomplex plaques (i.e., <4 mm with no evidence of ulceration or clot) are significantly less dangerous.[6] The amount of aortic plaque (also known as atherosclerotic burden) increases from the ascending aorta distally. It is also obvious that aortic plaques are only one manifestation of atherosclerosis and therefore are associated with a higher prevalence of coronary artery disease, carotid artery disease, renal artery stenosis, abdominal aortic aneurysms, and all the atherosclerotic risk factors.[7]

OTHER IMAGING MODALITIES

TTE occasionally demonstrates ascending aortic plaques. The aortic arch can be evaluated for plaques using the suprasternal window. The descending aorta may be visualized from the apical window. The quality of these images is frequently suboptimal. CT with contrast and MRI have been used to evaluate aortic plaques when TEE was not available or possible.[8-10] Both technologies can visualize the entire aorta, including the proximal arch (which may not be seen on TEE), the abdominal aorta, and the aortic branches. CT can assess aortic wall calcification (Fig. 130.1H) whereas MRI can provide information about the composition of the plaque (e.g., fibrous vs fatty) (Fig. 130.1I).

CLOT EMBOLIZATION VERSUS CHOLESTEROL EMBOLIZATION

Aortic atherosclerosis is associated with two different embolic syndromes. The first is clot embolization. It is estimated that 99% of all embolization cases associated with aortic plaque are embolization of clot that was superimposed on the plaque. The embolus occludes large to midsized arteries and causes stroke because of significant brain infarct and infarct in other organs such as the spleen, kidney, or limb.

The second embolic syndrome, cholesterol crystal embolization, is much less common. It is estimated that only 1% of all aortic plaque–related embolic events are associated with cholesterol embolization. The most frequent cause of cholesterol embolization is iatrogenic rupture of a plaque during invasive aortic instrumentation; however, spontaneous rupture may occur as well.[11] Showering of cholesterol crystals may lead to bilateral "blue toe syndrome," livedo reticularis, Hollenhorst plaques from retinal artery embolization, renal failure, gastrointestinal infarction, and diffuse cerebral dysfunction.[12,13]

HIGH-RISK PLAQUE

The risk of embolization is directly related to plaque thickness. The odds ratio for embolization of plaque less than 4 mm in thickness was found in one study to be 4, whereas the odds ratio for plaques with a thickness of 4 mm or more was 13.8.[14] Naturally, the distribution of

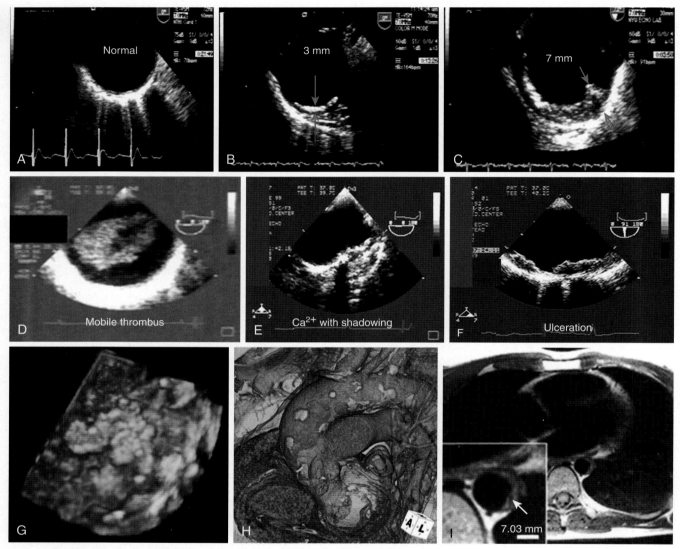

Figure 130.1. Transesophageal echocardiography shows a normal aortic intima (**A**), mild plaque (**B,** *red arrows*), severe plaque (**C,** *red arrows*), large superimposed thrombus (**D**), calcification (**E**), and ulceration (**F**). **G,** Three-dimensional transesophageal echocardiographic image shows the distribution, shape, and size of aortic arch plaques. **H,** Cardiac computed tomography demonstrates the distribution of aortic calcified plaques. **I,** Magnetic resonance imaging shows severe descending aortic plaque. Note the relatively lucent lipid core *(arrow)*. (Reproduced with permission from Tunick PA, et al: Diagnostic imaging of thoracic aortic atherosclerosis, *Am J Roentgenol* 174:1119–1125, 2000.)

the emboli is directly related to the plaque location within the thoracic aorta, and thus strokes are likely to occur in patients with plaques in the ascending aorta and the aortic arch and not in patients with isolated descending aortic plaques. The incidence of embolic stroke in patients with aortic arch complex plaques was found by three different studies to be 12% in the first year.[6] Plaque morphology may contribute to the embolization risk. Noncalcified plaques have the highest stroke risk. Also, when a higher proportion of plaque is occupied by lipid (which appears hypoechoic by echocardiography) or when a plaque is thrombosed, embolic risk is higher as well.[15]

AORTIC PLAQUE AND EMBOLIC EVENTS IN HEART SURGERY AND INVASIVE INTRAVASCULAR PROCEDURES

Cardiac catheterization carries a low but definite risk for embolic stroke (<1:1,000). During percutaneous transcatheter coronary angioplasty, the rate of stroke is 0.2%.[16] Most of these strokes occur in patients who have aortic plaque.[17] Patients at a higher risk for stroke during cardiac catheterization or intervention are those with previously known severe ascending aorta and aortic arch plaque or those who have a previous history of embolic stroke. The right brachial artery approach in those patients may decrease the risk of embolic stroke by avoiding negotiation of the more distal arch (and avoid other embolic events related to plaque in the abdominal and thoracic aorta). However, to date, there are no data showing that this approach can indeed prevent stroke.

Stroke is common in patients who undergo cardiac surgery. The risk of stroke in these patients may reach 7%.[18] Of patients who undergo coronary artery bypass grafting, 25% have complex aortic arch plaque, and it has been demonstrated that cannulation of the arch in those patients may be the culprit for this devastating outcome.[19] The risk of embolic complication and death in a patient undergoing open-heart surgery is sixfold higher in patients with

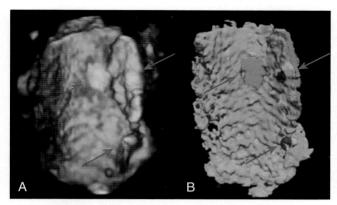

Figure 130.2. A, Three-dimensional transesophageal echocardiographic image of a diseased aorta. **B,** Processed image of the diseased aorta using an automated analysis software to analyze the characteristics of the plaque. *Red arrows* indicate atherosclerotic plaques (Reproduced with permission from Piazzese C, et al: Semiautomated detection and quantification of aortic plaques from three-dimensional transesophageal echocardiography, *J Am Soc Echocardiogr* 27:758–766, 2014.)

complex aortic arch plaque.[20] It appears that off-pump coronary artery bypass done with full sternotomy or minimally invasive surgery (mini-thoracotomy), which prevents any manipulation of the aorta (no aortic cannulation or cross-clamping), is associated with a lower incidence of intraoperative stroke.[21]

MANAGEMENT OPTIONS

The optimal treatment of aortic plaque is not known. However, statins appear to be of value in long-term prevention of recurrent embolic events in these patients.[22] No prospective, randomized study has yet established the value of anticoagulants and antiplatelet agents. Small studies have shown that, in addition to antiplatelet therapy, anticoagulation therapy may have a role in treating large aortic plaques, especially if mobile thrombus is present; however, the data are limited.[23] A study by Di Tullio and coworkers showed that patients with prior strokes, especially cryptogenic strokes, with severe aortic plaques had similar rates of recurrent stroke and death at 2 years whether they were treated with aspirin or warfarin (mean international normalized ratio, 2.03 for patients with large plaques).[24] The safety and efficacy of direct oral anticoagulants for aortic plaque have not been adequately studied. Avoiding the aorta during coronary bypass decreases the rate of complications and the number of strokes. Endovascular stenting with possible grafting may have a role for treating thoracic or abdominal aortic atheroembolic disease.[6]

Please access ExpertConsult to view the corresponding videos for this chapter.

Acknowledgment

The authors would like to acknowledge the contribution of Dr. Paul A. Tunick, who was one of the authors for this chapter in the previous edition.

REFERENCES

1. Panum PL. Experimentelle Beitrage zur Lehre von der Embolie. *Virchows Arch Pathol Anat Physiol.* 1862;25:308–310.
2. Flory CM. Arterial occlusions produced by eroded aortic atheromatous plaques. *Am J Pathol.* 1945;21:549–558.
3. Tunick PA, Kronzon I. Atheromas of the thoracic aorta: clinical and therapeutic update. *J Am Coll Cardiol.* 2000;35:545–554.
4. Weissler-Snir A, Greenberg G, Shapira Y, et al. Transesophageal echocardiography of aortic atherosclerosis: the additive value of three-dimensional over two-dimensional imaging. *Eur Heart J Cardiovasc Imag.* 2015;16:389–394.
5. Piazzese C, Tsang W, Sotaquira M, et al. Semiautomated detection and quantification of aortic plaques from three-dimensional transesophageal echocardiography. *J Am Soc Echocardiogr.* 2014;27:758–766.
6. Kronzon I, Tunick PA. Aortic atherosclerotic disease and stroke. *Circulation.* 2006;114:63–75.
7. Kronzon I, Tunick PA. Atheromatous disease of the thoracic aorta: pathologic and clinical implications. *Ann Intern Med.* 1997;126:629–637.
8. Schwammenthal E, Schwammenthal Y, Tanne D, et al. Transcutaneous detection of aortic arch atheromas by suprasternal harmonic imaging. *J Am Coll Cardiol.* 2002;39:1127–1132.
9. Tenenbaum A, Garniek A, Shemesh J, et al. Dual-helical CT for detecting aortic atheromas as a source of stroke: comparison with transesophageal echocardiography. *Radiology.* 1998;208:153–158.
10. Tunick PA, Krinsky GA, Lee VS, Kronzon I. Diagnostic imaging of thoracic aortic atherosclerosis. *Am J Roentgenol.* 2000;174:1119–1125.
11. Caron F, Anand SS. Antithrombotic therapy in aortic diseases: a narrative review. *Vasc Med.* 2017;22(1):57–65.
12. Applebaum RM, Kronzon I. Evaluation and management of cholesterol embolization and the blue toe syndrome. *Curr Opin Cardiol.* 1996;11:533–542.
13. Kronzon I, Saric M. Cholesterol embolization syndrome. *Circulation.* 2010;122:631–641.
14. Amarenco P, Cohen A, Hommel M, et al. The French study of aortic plaques in stroke group: atherosclerotic disease of the aortic arch as a risk factor for recurrent ischemic stroke. *N Engl J Med.* 1996;334:1216–1221.
15. Davies MJ, Richardson PD, Woolf N, et al. Risk of thrombosis in human atherosclerotic plaques: role of extracellular lipid, macrophage, and smooth muscle cell content. *Br Heart J.* 1993;69:377–381.
16. Wong SC, Minutello R, Hong MK. Neurologic complications following percutaneous coronary interventions. *Am J Cardiol.* 2005;96:1248–1250.
17. Karalis DG, Quinn V, Victor MF, et al. Risk of catheter-related emboli in patients with atherosclerotic debris in the thoracic aorta. *Am Heart J.* 1996;131:1149–1155.
18. Gardner TJ, Korneffer P, Manolio TA, et al. Stroke following coronary artery bypass grafting: a ten year study. *Ann Thorac Surg.* 1985;40:574–581.
19. Katz ES, Tunick PA, Rusinek H, et al. Protruding aortic atheromas predict stroke in elderly patients undergoing cardiopulmonary bypass: a review of our experience with intraoperative transesophageal echocardiography. *J Am Coll Cardiol.* 1992;20:70–77.
20. Stern A, Tunick PA, Culliford AT, et al. Protruding aortic arch atheromas: risk of stroke during heart surgery with and without aortic arch endarterectomy. *Am Heart J.* 1999;138:746–752.
21. Sharony R, Bizekis CS, Kanchuger M, et al. Off-pump coronary artery bypass grafting reduces mortality and stroke in patients with atheromatous aortas. *Circulation.* 2003;(suppl 1):II15–II20.
22. Tunick PA, Nayar AC, Goodkin GM, et al. Effect of treatment on the incidence of stroke and other emboli in 519 patients with severe thoracic aortic plaque. *Am J Cardiol.* 2002;90:1320–1325.
23. Dressler FA, Craig WR, Castello R, et al. Mobile aortic atheroma and systemic emboli: efficacy of anticoagulation and influence of plaque morphology on recurrent stroke. *J Am Coll Cardiol.* 1998;31:134–138.
24. Di Tullio MR, Russo C, Jin Z, et al. Aortic arch plaques and risk of recurrent stroke and death. *Circulation.* 2009;119:2376–2382.

131 Aortic Aneurysm

Arturo Evangelista, Ángela López-Sainz, José F. Rodríguez Palomares

Imaging techniques play a pivotal role in the diagnosis, follow-up and management of aortic aneurysms. Ultrasonography, computed tomography (CT) and magnetic resonance imaging (MRI) have strengths and limitations in the assessment of this disease depending on the aortic segment involved and reasons for the study. Ultrasonography is useful in the diagnosis and follow-up of proximal ascending aorta and abdominal aorta aneurysms, respectively. However, other imaging modalities are required to confirm measurements and add information on adjacent structures or aortic branches. Transesophageal echocardiography (TEE) is frequently limited to perioperative indications. CT plays a central role in the diagnosis, risk stratification, and management of most aneurysms. Advantages of CT over other imaging modalities include rapid image acquisition, multiplanar capacity with submillimeter spatial resolution, and wide field of view. MRI is less readily available but adds functional and biomechanical information. Aortic diameters are the cornerstone of current clinical practice in aortic aneurysms. However, new biomechanical information could potentially provide reliable prediction of aneurysm dilatation and rupture.

Aortic dilatation is defined by a size measurement of the aorta that exceeds normal range for a given age and body size and an aneurysm by an increase of more than 50% above the normal diameter range. From a practical point of view, an aortic aneurysm is diagnosed when diameters exceed 50 mm in the ascending and 40 mm in the descending aorta. The estimated incidence of thoracic aortic aneurysm is 5.6 to 10.4 cases per 100,000 patient-years.[1] Sixty percent involve the aortic root, ascending aorta, or both; 40% involve the descending aorta; 10% involve the arch; and 10% involve the thoracic abdominal aorta, with some involving more than one segment.[2] Abdominal aortic aneurysms (AAAs) are much more common than thoracic aortic aneurysms. Screening of subgroups at risk (i.e., male sex, older than 65 years of age, smokers, and those with a family history) shows the prevalence to be on average 5.5%.[2] The cause, natural history, and treatment of thoracic aneurysms differ for each segment.

CAUSE

The formation and expansion of thoracic aneurysms are multifactorial and involve the interplay of genetic predisposition, cellular imbalances, and hemodynamic factors.[3] Causes of thoracic aneurysms are listed in Table 131.1. In older patients, the most common cause is a degenerative process associated with hypertension, hyperlipidemia, or smoking. However, a genetic cause should be suspected[2,4,5] in young patients and in those without cardiovascular risk factors.

MORPHOLOGY

Aneurysms of the aorta can be classified in two morphologic types: fusiform and saccular. Morphologic shapes of the aortic root and ascending aorta are (1) annuloaortic ectasia, characterized by a "pear-shaped" aortic root with dilatation localized to the annulus and sinuses of Valsalva; (2) dilatation involving the annulus, sinuses of Valsalva and the tubular part of the ascending aorta; and (3) dilatation beginning at the sinotubular junction but sparing the aortic annulus and sinuses of Valsalva (Fig. 131.1 and Video 131.1).

Annuloaortic ectasia is common in patients with Marfan syndrome (MFS).[6] However, it may also be present in patients with no other conditions. Other cases of ascending aortic aneurysm are associated with an underlying bicuspid aortic valve (BAV), with dilatation localized most frequently to the level of the tubular portion of the ascending aorta in 44% and 20% at the sinus level. Proximal atherosclerotic aneurysms are typically fusiform and may extend into the arch and constitute the predominant etiology of aneurysms of the descending thoracic and abdominal aorta.[7]

DIAGNOSIS

Thoracic aortic enlargement is often diagnosed on imaging studies performed for unrelated indications. An abnormal contour of the superior mediastinum on chest radiography may raise the suspicion. Transthoracic echocardiography (TTE) is very useful for the diagnosis and follow-up of aortic root aneurysms, which is crucial for patients with annuloaortic ectasia or Marfan syndrome (see Fig. 131.1A). Because the predominant area of dilatation is in the proximal aorta, TTE often suffices for screening. This is the technique of choice in the serial measurement of maximum aortic root diameters, evaluation of aortic regurgitation (see Video 131.1), and timing of elective surgery. TTE is relatively accurate, inexpensive, and noninvasive. The suprasternal view primarily shows the aortic arch and the three major supra-aortic vessels, with variable lengths of the ascending and descending aorta. The entire thoracic descending aorta is not well visualized by TTE. In contrast, the abdominal aorta is relatively easily visualized in sagittal subcostal views. Abdominal ultrasonography by curvilinear array transducers provides good visualization of the abdominal aorta; however, the phased-array probes used for echocardiography may also suffice. Scanning the abdominal aorta consists of obtaining longitudinal and transverse images from the diaphragm to the bifurcation of the aorta (Fig. 131.2). The maximum diameter is obtained in the longitudinal and transverse views, with the diameter perpendicular to the longitudinal axis of the aorta.

TEE provides high-quality imaging of nearly all the thoracic aorta owing to the close proximity of the esophagus to the aorta and the use of high-frequency transducers. A portion of the distal ascending aorta and proximal aortic arch may not be visible because of interposition of the trachea. TEE is highly useful in the assessment of aortic regurgitation mechanisms and may be warranted when the type of surgical treatment (repair or valve replacement) is being considered (Fig. 131.3; Videos 131.3A and 131.3D). The main limitation of this test is that it is semi-invasive and not accurate in the measurement and location of arch or descending aorta aneurysms. Although three-dimensional (3D) TTE and 3D TEE enable short-axis views of the aortic root, the spatial resolution of 3D limits its use for aortic measurements in the majority of cases. TTE and TEE cannot correctly visualize the distal ascending aorta. For measuring the upper part of the ascending aorta by TTE, it is recommended to move the transducer to one upper intercostal space (see Fig. 131.1D) or in some cases to use the right parasternal window.

Contrast-enhanced CT and MRI may visualize the entire aorta and its major branches and accurately detect the size of thoracic aortic aneurysms. The multiplanar capacity of multidetector CT, together with its submillimeter spatial resolution, offers the best visualization of thoracic aortic aneurysms. This technique permits easy identification of the maximum aortic diameter plane, which must be doubly orthogonal to the longitudinal plane of the aortic segment. Using the parasagittal plane, the oblique maximum intensity projection plane is reproducible and comparable in follow-up studies.[8]

AORTIC SIZE

Aortic root dimensions are assessed by TTE at end-diastole in the parasternal long-axis view at four levels: annulus, sinuses of

TABLE 131.1 Causes of Thoracic Aortic Aneurysm

Degenerative	
	• Associated with age, hypertension
	• With atherosclerotic risk factors, frequently involves descending aorta
	• With aortic valve disease, involves ascending aorta
Genetically Triggered Diseases	
Marfan syndrome	Aortic root dilatation in >75% of cases
	Annuloaortic ectasia
	Descending aorta dilatation is infrequent
Loeys-Dietz syndrome	Aggressive vasculopathy
	Arterial tortuosities
	Higher risk of dissection than Marfan syndrome
Bicuspid aortic valve	Ascending aorta dilatation in >50% of cases
	Valsalva sinus involvement in >20% of cases
	Faster growth rate than tricuspid valves
Turner syndrome, Ehlers-Danlos syndrome	More common in the ascending aorta
Familial nonsyndromic aneurysms	New mutations: ACTA-II and so on; may involve various aortic segments
Aortitis	
Infectious	Syphilis, *Salmonella* spp., *Mycobacterium* spp., others
Inflammatory	Giant cell and Takayasu arteritis, others
Trauma	
	Typical location at the aortic isthmus

Valsalva, supra-aortic ridge and proximal ascending aorta (AA). Measurements should be made perpendicular to the long axis of the aorta with the use of the leading-edge method.[9] Some experts[10] favor inner edge to inner edge to match the method used by MRI and CT scanning. However, the 3 to 4 mm of underestimation of aortic diameter size using this method owing to false oversizing of the aorta wall thickness may mislead the management of these diseases.[9] TTE is not useful for evaluating descending thoracic aorta aneurysm. Although TEE can visualize the entire descending thoracic aorta, it is limited for identifying the precise aorta level where the measurement is taken and for obtaining an axial plane perpendicular to the aortic lumen, mainly in the presence of tortuosity. Distal to the aorta root, CT or MRI is indicated to assess aortic size. Because the ascending aorta is not totally vertical and may be asymmetrical, aortic size may be overestimated using axial planes. Thus, double-oblique planes by CT or MRI should be used to measure the aorta lumen perpendicularly and avoid axial obliquities. In the descending thoracic aorta, multidetector CT with multiplanar reformation offers accurate measurement of aortic aneurysm size, and 3D volume-rendering reconstruction is useful for depicting the spatial relationship of aneurysms with adjacent structures. Similarly, magnetic resonance angiography (MRA)–acquired data can be reformatted to yield two-dimensional images along any plane and 3D images. The information provided by MRA in aortic aneurysm assessment is similar to that offered by CT. It is recommended to conduct a functional study through the aortic valve using cine MR sequences to rule out associated valvular disease that may be related to aortic dilatation.[11]

AAAs, mostly infrarenal, are usually defined as a diameter of 30 mm or greater. Ultrasonography is an excellent tool for their screening and surveillance, without risk and at low cost. Screening is recommended in all men older than 65 years of age and may be considered in women older than 65 years of age with a history of smoking. Opportunistic screening during TTE should be considered in the same population and in all patients with a thoracic aortic aneurysm. CTA and MRA have emerged as the current gold standards in the evaluation of AAA. CTA is a rapid and reproducible modality and provides all necessary detailed anatomic information of the aorta and surrounding structures. CTA can accurately visualize aortoiliac lesions, including calcifications, and contrast-enhanced MRA allows ready acquisition of images in any plane.

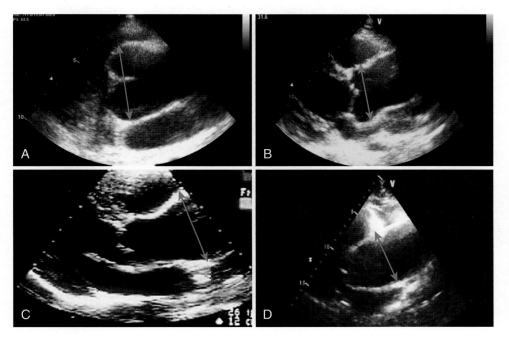

Figure 131.1. Parasternal long-axis view by transthoracic echocardiography. **A,** Annuloaortic ectasia *(arrow)* with pyriform. **B,** Mild aortic root *(arrow)* and ascending aorta dilatation. **C,** Ascending aorta dilatation located in the upper part of the sinotubular junction *(arrow).* **D,** Ascending aorta dilatation at the tubular level *(arrow)* visualized by moving the transducer one upper intercostal space. (See accompanying Video 131.1)

BIOMECHANICAL INFORMATION

MRI has been established as an accurate noninvasive tool for the assessment of aortic distensibility and pulse wave velocity with acceptable reproducibility.[12] These methods have been used to assess aortic elasticity in patients with MFS,[13,14] BAV, and aortic aneurysms.[15]

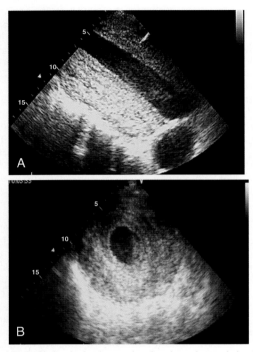

Figure 131.2. Abdominal echography showing a large abdominal aneurysm partially thrombosed in longitudinal view (**A**) and transversal view (**B**).

Some authors recently showed that ascending aorta flow patterns as assessed by four-dimensional (4D) MRI are a major contributor to aortic dilatation in BAV disease.[16] A short series found that almost 50% of first-degree relatives with BAV with ascending aorta dilatation but tricuspid aortic valve (TAV) defined by TTE presented a mini-raphe by CT and similar ascending aorta flow abnormalities by 4D MRI to patients with BAV, suggesting that this disturbed flow secondary to the mini-raphe may be related to their ascending aorta dilatation.[17] Although aorta distensibility and stiffness may be assessed by TTE, MRI, particularly 4D MRI, has significantly improved this evaluation.[18] A recent analysis showed the mechanical properties of AAAs to be similar in patients with BAV and TAV, whereas patients with MFS have stiffer aortas. Aortic stiffness strongly depends on dilatation severity. Ascending aorta pulse wave velocity resulted in a potentially clinically useful biphasic trend with respect to aneurysm diameter, whereas distensibility did not discern mildly dilated aorta. Beyond clinical risk factors, PWV but not AD was independently related to AAo dilatation in patients with BAV.[18] A new parameter, the proximal aorta longitudinal strain determined by MRI, has been reported to be independently related to the aortic root dilatation rate and aortic events in addition to aortic root diameter, clinical risk factors, and demographic characteristics in patients with MFS.[19]

NATURAL HISTORY AND COMPLICATIONS

Aortic size is the principal predictor of aortic rupture or dissection, the risk of which is almost 7% per year for a diameter larger than 60 mm. The odds ratio for rupture increased 27-fold compared with lower values.[20] Davies and associates showed aortic size index to be a significant predictor of aortic rupture with a moderate risk when the aortic size index is larger than 2.75 cm/m^2.[21] A recent study from the same center showed that compared with indices including weight, the simpler height-based ratio (excluding weight and body surface area calculations) yielded satisfactory results for evaluating the risk of natural complications in patients with ascending thoracic aneurysms.[22] The rate of aneurysmal expansion is not constant, however, because growth rates accelerate as the aneurysm enlarges. Risk

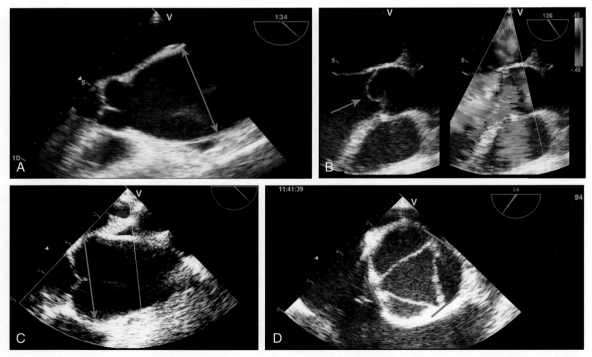

Figure 131.3. Transesophageal echocardiography. **A,** Ascending aorta aneurysms *(arrow)* with normal aortic root, **B,** Valvular abnormality with aortic leaflet prolapse *(arrows, left)*, which leads to significant aortic regurgitation *(right)*. **C,** Aortic root dilatation *(arrow)* in a patient with Marfan syndrome. **D,** Measurement of the three intercommisural length *(red lines)* before David surgery. (See accompanying Videos 131.3A and 131.3D.)

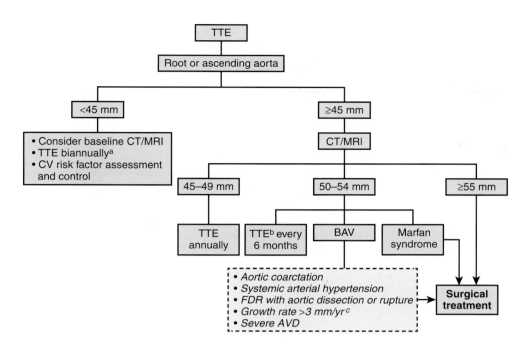

Figure 131.4. Proposed algorithm for the surveillance and surgical indication workup of ascending aorta dilatation. Notes: [a]When aortic valve disease does not require more frequent study. [b]When transthoracic echocardiography (TTE) has similar maximum aortic diameter, use computed tomography (CT)/magnetic resonance imaging (MRI); if not, use CT/MRI. [c]On repeated measurements using the same electrocardiography-gated imaging technique, measured at the same aorta level with side-by-side comparison. *AVD,* Aortic valve disease; *BAV,* bicuspid aortic valve; *CV,* cardiovascular; *FDR,* first-degree relative.

factors for increased growth of thoracic aortic aneurysms include older age, female sex, chronic obstructive pulmonary disease, hypertension, and a positive family history. A growth rate greater than 5 mm/yr is associated with an increased risk of rupture.[23]

Serial Imaging

Careful follow-up of maximum aortic diameter is paramount for correct therapeutic management. Aneurysms affecting the aortic root can be correctly followed by TTE if the echocardiographic window is adequate. The excellent reproducibility of measurements at this level and information from other parameters such as aortic regurgitation severity and ventricular function facilitate appropriate follow-up. Serial follow-up evaluation of proximal ascending aorta diameters should be made by echocardiography every 6 to 12 months depending on aortic dimensions, rate of expansion, and aortic valve dysfunction. However, it is advisable to perform a CT/MRI study when aortic root or ascending aortic diameter is 45 mm by TTE to confirm measurement agreement, rule out aortic section asymmetry,[24] and obtain a basal measurement to compare when enlargement nears surgical indication (Fig. 131.4). CT and MRI are the techniques of choice in the follow-up of aortic aneurysms located in the upper part of the ascending aorta or more distal segments. Use of the same modality at the same institution should be considered so that similar images of matching anatomic segments can be compared side by side. In patients with nephropathy or in young patients, MRI without gadolinium is a reasonable alternative to CT. For correct monitoring, it is necessary to measure aortic diameter in the same location and the same spatial plane. We believe that only a growth rate greater than 3 mm/yr with and greater than 5 mm/yr without electrocardiographic gating may represent reasonable benchmarks of a clinically meaningful change.[25]

If the only indication for surgery is a growth rate of 2 to 3 m/yr, it would be advisable to confirm this tendency in a new control performed at 6 months with the same imaging technique. In asymptomatic patients with aortic aneurysm, imaging controls should be annual. However, when aortic size is near to indicating surgery, it is advisable to repeat the test every 6 months.

Surgical Indication

The clinical significance of maximum aortic diameter in the indication of prophylactic surgical treatment implies taking measurements as accurately as possible (see Fig. 131.4).[4] Indications for surgery are based mainly on aortic diameter and derived from findings on natural history regarding the risk of complications versus the risk of elective surgery. Although several modalities serve for this purpose, CT is frequently used because it offers comprehensive imaging of the entire aorta, provides high spatial resolution data, and permits assessment of coronary abnormalities, which reduces the need for invasive coronary angiography.[26] The surgical options for repair of ascending aortic aneurysms depend on the presence of aortic valve disease, dilatation of the sinuses of Valsalva, and distal extension of the aneurysm into the aortic arch.[27] Intraoperative TEE is useful for evaluating the aortic valve to determine whether valve-sparing surgery is feasible, define the aortic valve annular diameter in relation to the diameter of the sinotubular junction to establish the need for aortic root replacement, and detect and quantify the presence of aortic regurgitation after valve repair.

Please access ExpertConsult to view the corresponding videos for this chapter.

REFERENCES

1. Clouse WD, Hallett JWJ, Schaff HV, et al. Improved prognosis of thoracic aortic aneurysms: a population-based study. *J Am Med Assoc.* 1998;280:1926–1929.
2. Isselbacher EM. Thoracic and abdominal aortic aneurysms. *Circulation.* 2005;111:816–828.
3. Kuivaniemi H, Platsoucas CD, Tilson MD 3rd. Aortic aneurysms: an immune disease with a strong genetic component. *Circulation.* 2008;117:242–252.
4. Loeys BL, Schwarze U, Holm T, et al. Aneurysm syndromes caused by mutations in the TGF-beta receptor. *N Engl J Med.* 2006;355:788–798.
5. Fedak PWM, Verma S, David TE, et al. Clinical and pathophysiological implications of a bicuspid aortic valve. *Circulation.* 2002;106:900–904.
6. Ha H Il, Seo JB, Lee SH, et al. Imaging of Marfan syndrome: multisystemic manifestations. *Radiographics.* 2007;27:989–1004.
7. Evangelista A, Gallego P, Calvo-Iglesias F, et al. Anatomical and clinical predictors of valve dysfunction and aortic dilation in bicuspid aortic valve disease. *Heart.* 2018;104:566–573.
8. Goldstein SA, Evangelista A, Abbara S, et al. Multimodality imaging of diseases of the thoracic aorta in adults. *J Am Soc Echocardiogr.* 2015;28:119–182.
9. Rodriguez-Palomares JF, Teixido-Tura G, Galuppo V, et al. Multimodality assessment of ascending aortic diameters: comparison of different measurement methods. *J Am Soc Echocardiogr.* 2016;29:819–826. e4.
10. Mirea O, Maffessanti F, Gripari P, et al. Effects of aging and body size on proximal and ascending aorta and aortic arch: inner edge-to-inner edge reference values in a large adult population by two-dimensional transthoracic echocardiography. *J Am Soc Echocardiogr.* 2013;26:419–427.
11. Bolen MA, Popovic ZB, Rajiah P, et al. Cardiac MR assessment of aortic regurgitation: holodiastolic flow reversal in the descending aorta helps stratify severity. *Radiology.* 2011;260:98–104.

12. Grotenhuis HB, Westenberg JJM, Steendijk P, et al. Validation and reproducibility of aortic pulse wave velocity as assessed with velocity-encoded MRI. *J Magn Reson Imag*. 2009;30:521–526.
13. Teixido-Tura G, Redheuil A, Rodriguez-Palomares J, et al. Aortic biomechanics by magnetic resonance: early markers of aortic disease in Marfan syndrome regardless of aortic dilatation. *Int J Cardiol*. 2014;171:56–61.
14. Redheuil A, Wu CO, Kachenoura N, et al. Proximal aortic distensibility is an independent predictor of all-cause mortality and incident CV events: the MESA study. *J Am Coll Cardiol*. 2014;64:2619–2629.
15. Bissell MM, Hess AT, Biasiolli L, et al. Aortic dilation in bicuspid aortic valve disease: flow pattern is a major contributor and differs with valve fusion type. *Circ Cardiovasc Imag*. 2013;6:499–507.
16. Rodriguez-Palomares JF, Dux-Santoy L, Guala A, et al. Aortic flow patterns and wall shear stress maps by 4D-flow cardiovascular magnetic resonance in the assessment of aortic dilatation in bicuspid aortic valve disease. *J Cardiovasc Magn Reson*. 2018;20:28.
17. Guala A, Rodriguez-Palomares J, Galian-Gay L, et al. Partial aortic valve leaflet fusion is related to deleterious alteration of proximal aorta hemodynamics. *Circulation*. 2019;23:2707–2709.
18. Guala A, Rodriguez-Palomares J, Dux-Santoy L, et al. Influence of aortic dilation on the regional aortic stiffness of bicuspid aortic valve assessed by 4-dimensional flow cardiac magnetic resonance: comparison with Marfan syndrome and degenerative aortic aneurysm. *JACC Cardiovasc Imag*. 2019;12:1020–1029.
19. Guala A, Teixido-Tura G, Rodriguez-Palomares J, et al. Proximal aorta longitudinal strain predicts aortic root dilation rate and aortic events in Marfan syndrome. *Eur Heart J*. 2019;40:2047–2055.
20. Coady MA, Rizzo JA, Hammond GL, et al. What is the appropriate size criterion for resection of thoracic aortic aneurysms. *J Thorac Cardiovasc Surg*. 1997;113:476–491.
21. Davies RR, Gallo A, Coady MA, et al. Novel measurement of relative aortic size predicts rupture of thoracic aortic aneurysms. *Ann Thorac Surg*. 2006;81:169–177.
22. Zafar MA, Li Y, Rizzo JA, et al. Height alone, rather than body surface area, suffices for risk estimation in ascending aortic aneurysm. *J Thorac Cardiovasc Surg*. 2018;155:1938–1950.
23. Hiratzka LF, Bakris GL, Beckman JA, et al. 2010 ACCF/AHA/AATS/ACR/ASA/SCA/SCAI/SIR/STS/SVM guidelines for the diagnosis and management of patients with thoracic aortic disease: executive summary. *Catheter Cardiovasc Interv*. 2010;76:E43–F86.
24. Vis JC, Rodriguez-Palomares JF, Teixido-Tura G, et al. Implications of asymmetry and valvular morphotype on echocardiographic measurements of the aortic root in bicuspid aortic valve. *J Am Soc Echocardiogr*. 2019;32:105–112.
25. Evangelista A. Imaging aortic aneurysmal disease. *Heart*. 2014;100:909–915.
26. Erbel R, Aboyans V, Boileau C, et al. [2014 ESC guidelines on the diagnosis and treatment of aortic diseases]. *Kardiol Pol*. 2014;72:1169–11252.
27. Borger MA, Fedak PWM, Stephens EH, et al. The American Association for Thoracic Surgery consensus guidelines on bicuspid aortic valve-related aortopathy: executive summary. *J Thorac Cardiovasc Surg*. 2018;156:473–480.

132 Sinus of Valsalva Aneurysm

Reza Arsanjani, Farouk Mookadam

The sinuses of Valsalva are cuplike dilatations in the aortic wall just above the three cusps of the aortic valve (AV). These sinuses function in part to suspend the AV between the valve annulus and the sinotubular ridge. In addition, the left and right sinuses house the ostia of the left and right coronary arteries (Fig. 132.1). Aneurysm of the sinus of Valsalva was first described by Hope in 1839.[1] In 1840, the first six cases were described by Thurnam[2,3] with a description that aneurysms of the sinuses of Valsalva usually protrude into one of the cardiac chambers. Subsequently, Smith and coworkers[4] described sinus of Valsalva aneurysms (SOVAs) found during postmortem examination. Aneurysms of the sinus of Valsalva are thought to result from incomplete fusion of the medial layer of the aorta with the annulus fibrosis of the AV. The medial layer lacks an elastic lamellae, which creates a weakness in the aortic wall, making it susceptible to dilatation and aneurysm formation, especially in the presence of hypertension.

CLINICAL SIGNIFICANCE

In general, sinuses of Valsalva aneurysms are rare, and they may be caused by acquired conditions or congenital conditions (Table 132.1). SOVAs are frequently associated with other cardiac congenital abnormalities such as ventricular septal defect (VSD), anomalous coronary arteries, or abnormal AV cusps (bicuspid and quadricuspid). In instances of bicuspid AV, not only does the congenitally abnormal valve result in complications, such as regurgitation or stenosis, but a concomitant aortopathy may coexist. The aortopathy most commonly affects the ascending aorta; however, SOVA may also be an accompaniment of bicuspid or quadricuspid AV (Fig. 132.2).[5]

The clinical presentation varies depending on the site and size and whether compressive symptoms or rupture into a cardiac chamber or extracardiac site occurs. Hence, with sinus of Valsalva

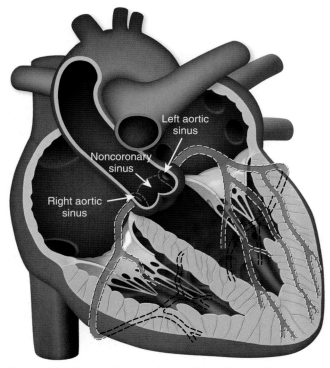

Figure 132.1. Schematic of heart in sagittal section showing sinuses of Valsalva and their relationship to the aortic valve leaflets, sinotubular junction, and coronary ostia. (By permission of Mayo Foundation for Medical Education and Research. All rights reserved.)

causing right ventricular inflow or outflow tract obstruction, right-sided heart failure symptoms will predominate. A fistula into the right atrium (RA) or right ventricle (RV) will present the same, but fistula into the left atrium may present with predominantly left-sided heart failure (Fig. 132.3).

The sinuses of Valsalva characteristically rupture into an adjacent chamber (Table 132.2 and Fig. 132.3). The cause is generally thought to be congenital because of abnormal ultrastructural changes in the medial layer (cystic medial necrosis) of the sinus

wall. This may be congenital or acquired as in endocarditis or rarely may be iatrogenic after coronary angiography or after AV surgery. In known connective tissue disease abnormalities (Marfan, Treacher-Collins, or Ehlers-Danlos syndromes) or in patients with a unicuspid, bicuspid, or quadricuspid AV or coarctation of the aorta, abnormal elastic tissue may be seen.[6]

In the presence of a membranous VSD, prolapse of the noncoronary cusp or the right coronary cusp into the VSD by a windsock mechanism may occur.[7] In one large study of SOVAs spanning almost half a century,[8] 63% of participants were male; asymptomatic incidental murmur was noted in 20%; fatigue was noted in 45%; and dyspnea and chest pain were noted in 36% and 19%, respectively; and palpitations were noted in 5%.[8] Symptoms in SOVA are largely dependent on which sinus dilates and the size and the relationship with adjacent structures. Symptoms may be caused by compressive aneurysms on the coronary arteries or obstructive to right ventricular inflow or right ventricular outflow tract (RVOT) outflow or left-to-right or left-to-left shunting or less commonly may cause conduction system abnormalities by

TABLE 132.1 Causes of Sinus of Valsalva Aneurysms

Congenital	Acquired
Bicuspid aortic valve	Endocarditis
Connective tissue disease	Iatrogenic postaortic valve surgery
• Marfan disease	or cardiac catheterization
• Ehlers-Danlos syndrome	
	Atherosclerotic degeneration

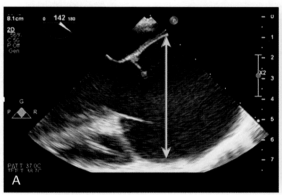
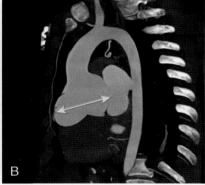

Figure 132.2. Long-axis view of the aortic valve on transesophageal echocardiogram (**A**) in a patient with bicuspid aortic valve and aortic root aneurysm *(yellow arrow)*. Sagittal view on computed tomography (**B**) of the same patient demonstrating a significantly dilated aortic root *(yellow arrow)*.

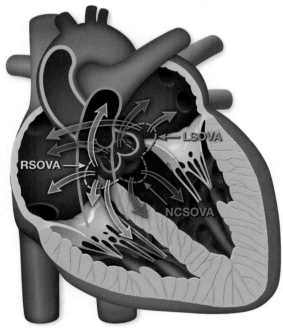

LSOVA
- May rupture into the LA or RA
- Can cause LA compression

NCSOVA
- May rupture into the LA, RA, LV, or ventricular septum

RSOVA
- May rupture into the RA, RV, or adjacent main pulmonary artery
- Can cause RVOT obstruction
- May result in RCA dissection or compression and acute MI
- May compress the conduction system and cause heart block
- May rupture into the pericardium and cause tamponade

Figure 132.3. Sinuses of Valsalva with likely chambers into which aneurysm may protrude or rupture. Colors of *arrows* show each of the sinuses and direction of enlargement or rupture: *green* indicates left sinus of Valsalva aneurysm (LSOVA), *purple* indicates noncoronary sinus of Valsalva aneurysm (NCSOVA), and *yellow* indicates right sinus of Valsalva aneurysm (RSOVA). *LA,* Left atrium; *LV,* left ventricle; *MI,* myocardial infarction; *RA,* right atrium; *RCA,* right coronary artery; *RV,* right ventricle; *RVOT,* right ventricular outflow tract. (By permission of Mayo Foundation for Medical Education and Research. All rights reserved.)

TABLE 132.2 Sinus of Valsalva Aneurysms and Likely Chamber Into Which It May Rupture and Cause a Fistulous Communication

Ruptured Sinuses	Unruptured Sinuses
RSOVA may rupture into RA, RV, or adjacent main pulmonary artery	RSOVA can cause RVOT obstruction
LSOVA will rupture into the LA or RA	LSOVA can cause LA compression
RSOFA may result in right coronary artery dissection or compression and acute MI	RSOVA may compress the conduction system and cause heart block
RSOVA may rupture into the pericardium with tamponade	

LA, Left atrium; *LSOVA,* left sinus of Valsalva aneurysm; *MI,* myocardial infarction; *MPA,* main pulmonary artery; *RA,* right atrium; *RSOVA,* right sinus of Valsalva aneurysm; *RV,* right ventricle; *RVOT,* right ventricular outflow tract obstruction.

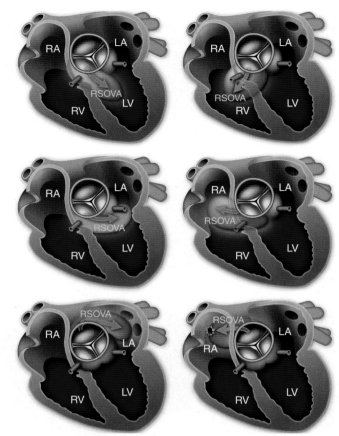

Figure 132.4. Outlines some examples of a right sinus of Valsalva aneurysm (RSOVA) and noncoronary sinus of Valsalva aneurysm (NCSOVA) and putative cardiac chamber into which it may enlarge. Note that the relationship of the SOVA and coronary arteries displays the mechanism for coronary artery compression and angina-type pain or acute coronary syndrome that may result. *LA,* Left atrium; *LV,* left ventricle; *RA,* right atrium; *RV,* right ventricle. (By permission of Mayo Foundation for Medical Education and Research. All rights reserved.)

impinging on conduction fibers in the interventricular septum or atrial ventricular node. Extracardiac rupture within the pericardium or mediastinum is extremely uncommon. Aneurysms arose from the right coronary sinus in 70%, the noncoronary sinus in 25%, and the left coronary sinus in 5% of patients.[8] The aneurysms had ruptured in 29 of the patients (34%). Twenty percent ruptured into the RV and 13% into the RA.[8] All the ruptured aneurysms arose from the right coronary sinus (76%) or the noncoronary sinus (24%).[8] Aneurysms originating in the noncoronary sinus tended to rupture into the RA (86%), and those originating in the right coronary sinus tended to rupture into the RV (73%).[8] Most right coronary sinus aneurysms rupture into the RV, either into the body or into the outflow tract.[9] In the Mayo series, 20% of all SOVAs opened into the RV and 13% into the RA. Of the right coronary sinus aneurysms, most (73%) opened into the RV. Aneurysms of the noncoronary sinus ruptured into the RA in 86% of patients. Rarely, rupture may occur into the left ventricle, left atrium, pulmonary artery, pericardium, interventricular septum, or superior vena cava.[10–12] It is safe to say that approximately two-thirds of SOVAs arise from the right sinus of Valsalva; two-thirds will rupture into the RV, two-thirds are male, one-third arise from the noncoronary sinus of Valsalva, one-third rupture into the RA, one-third present with rupture, and 20% to 25% are asymptomatic and discovered incidentally. Approximately 6% have endocarditis. Frequently, the presentation may be insidious with gradual symptom presentation over several years. It may be discovered incidentally on imaging or clinically through a continuous murmur.[13] The subacute or insidious presentation is that of congestive heart failure from volume overload or RVOT obstruction.

With regard to clinical presentation, it generally may be acute with chest pain or more commonly with heart failure. Symptoms of acute or subacute dyspnea on exertion or right-sided heart failure symptoms if the aneurysm results in right-sided volume overload by rupture into the RA or RV or if RVOT obstruction or tricuspid valve inflow obstruction occurs. Fig. 132.4 outlines examples of a right and noncoronary SOVA and putative chamber into which it may enlarge. These account for greater than 90% of all SOVAs. Of note, the relationship of the SOVA and coronary arteries reflects the mechanism for coronary artery compression and angina type pain or acute coronary syndrome that may result.

DIAGNOSIS

The physical examination may reveal a wide pulse pressure, especially if significant aortic regurgitation is present, and a long diastolic murmur from aortic regurgitation or a continuous murmur if a sinus to cameral (aortocameral shunt) is present. The 12-lead electrocardiogram shows no pathognomonic findings, but LV hypertrophy is a common finding. The chest radiograph may show

unfolding of the aorta or, more commonly, cardiomegaly and features of congestive heart failure.[14] Transthoracic echocardiography (TTE) allows views of the proximal ascending aorta, including the sinuses of Valsalva, the sinotubular junction, the proximal mid-distal ascending aorta, and the aortic arch from suprasternal or high parasternal views. Transesophageal echocardiography (TEE) provides a more comprehensive view of the anatomy of the aorta in its entirety.

TTE using the left parasternal long-axis view allows visualization of the cardiac chambers and ascending aorta, sinotubular junction, sinuses of Valsalva (right and noncoronary), and associated AV. In older patients or those with chronic hypertension, the aortas is unfolded, therefore moving up an interspace will allow better visualization of the aortic anatomy. Color Doppler to assess flow acceleration or AV regurgitation can be assessed. The apical long-axis views are used to corroborate any findings from the parasternal views. In addition, the AV itself can be better assessed for regurgitation or stenosis. Coupled with a basal short-axis view of the AV and sinuses, a significant amount of information is gleaned.

TEE provides greater resolution because of proximity of the esophagus to the cardiac structures. The entire ascending aorta, arch, and descending thoracic aorta, including the abdominal aorta, can be clearly visualized. Because of the location of the left main bronchus, a segment of the proximal arch is incompletely visualized. However, sufficient detail of the remaining segments of

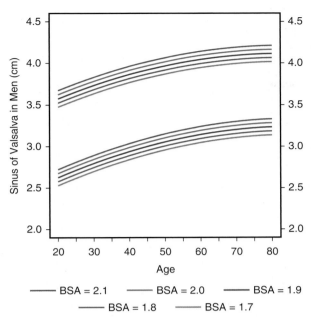

Figure 132.5. Fifth and 95th percentiles based on echocardiographic leading-edge-to-leading-edge diameters of the sinus of Valsalva and ascending aorta in 815 men with normal cardiac findings on transthoracic echocardiogram. *BSA,* Body surface area. (Reproduced from Biaggi P, et al: Gender, age, and body surface area are the major determinants of ascending aorta dimensions in subjects with apparently normal echocardiograms, *J Am Soc Echocardiogr* 22:720, 2009. Illustration used with permission of Elsevier.)

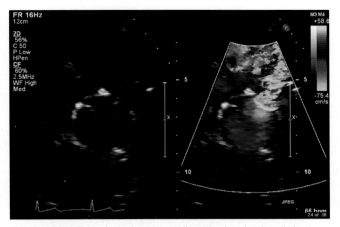

Figure 132.6. Transthoracic echocardiogram showing basal short-axis view at the level of the sinuses of Valsalva (*left*) and with color Doppler (*right*). A rupture into the right ventricular outflow tract (RVOT) (*arrows*) is noted. Systolic flow from the sinus of Valsalva aneurysm (SOVA) into right ventricular outflow tract (RVOT) is shown. Color Doppler imaging shows a prominent jet into the RVOT.

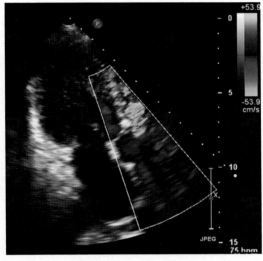

Figure 132.7. Transthoracic echocardiogram showing three-chamber long-axis view with color Doppler imaging showing a prominent jet from the sinus of Valsalva into the right ventricular outflow tract.

aorta allows for accurate measurement of the sinuses of Valsalva, sinotubular junction, and all components of the aorta. Atheroma, intramural hematoma, penetrating aortic ulcer, dissection, and aortic calcification can be well visualized with TEE. Proximal coronary arteries can be also visualized as well.

Color-flow Doppler imaging by TTE and TEE is necessary to identify associated conditions with a SOVA. These include aortic regurgitation or rupture of the sinus of Valsalva into the RV, right atrium, or left ventricle. An accepted definition for what constitutes a SOVA has not been well established. However, using the proximal ascending aorta as a guide for normative values in adults individualized by gender, sinuses should measure 3.7 cm or less (Fig. 132.5).[15] In a retrospective study of patients undergoing surgery for SOVA sac, the median age is 45 years (range, 5–80 years).[8] Rupture occurred in about 34% of patients. The predominant fistula was from the right sinus of Valsalva to the RV.[8] Echocardiographic diagnosis occurred in 65% of patients with the remaining third diagnosed at cardiac catheterization. Aortic regurgitation occurred in 44% of patients.[8] The most likely location of the aneurysm of the sinus of Valsalva is the right coronary sinus followed by the noncoronary sinus, with the left coronary sinus being least common. Infrequently, the aneurysm ruptures into the left ventricle or into the left atrium, and associated atrial septal defect or VSD may also be present.[8]

Routine TTE can make the diagnosis. Two-dimensional (2D) or three-dimensional (3D) TEE can increasingly make the diagnosis, including size and site of rupture, more easily and with better information regarding the site, size, and receiving chamber into which the sinus protrudes or communicates. Echocardiography plays an important role in diagnosing SOVAs and rupture. Based on published case reports, more than 90% cases can be diagnosed by color Doppler echocardiography. 2D echocardiography identifies the site and size of aneurysm and its relationship to adjacent structures such as coronary arteries, RVOT, or RV inflow (Figs. 132.6 and 132.7). The *right panel* of

Fig. 132.8 shows a parasternal long-axis view with a right SOVA that ruptures into the RV, and the *left panel* shows color Doppler of a high-velocity jet into the RV. Color Doppler shows turbulent flow across the site of rupture and spectral Doppler confirms a high-velocity continuous shunt throughout the cardiac cycle.

The high-velocity continuous nature, with prolonged diastolic phase of the jet spanning the entire cardiac cycle or predominantly diastolic phase (Fig. 132.9), helps distinguish aneurysm rupture into the RV from a VSD, where the flow is restricted mainly to the systolic phase Although in some adult patients with VSD and increased left ventricular end-diastolic pressure, diastolic left-to-right shunt can be present, the diastolic flow velocity is usually low (<2 m/s) because left ventricular diastolic pressure is much lower than diastolic pressure in the ascending aorta. With large ruptures, Doppler interrogation in the descending aorta can also demonstrate diastolic flow reversal. Echocardiography can also be used for serial follow-up of smaller asymptomatic SOVAs as well as those who underwent repair. This strategy again is akin to following ascending aorta aneurysms serially. Serial follow-up should be directed at interrogation of the aneurysm,

AV regurgitation, or the known complications that may occur in these patients. Further delineation of the anatomy of aneurysms can be obtained by cardiac magnetic resonance (CMRI) and electrocardiogram-gated contrast-enhanced computed tomography

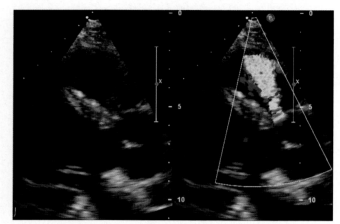

Figure 132.8. Transthoracic echocardiography parasternal long-axis view (left) and with color Doppler (right) in a 33-year-old patient with known ventricular septal defect presenting with acute chest pain and shortness of breath.

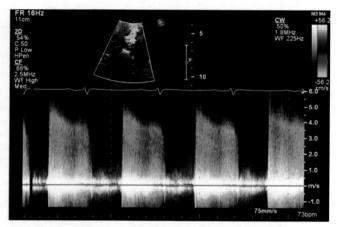

Figure 132.9. Doppler imaging demonstrating a prominent jet gradient into the right ventricular outflow tract (flow velocity, 5 m/s).

(CT) (Fig. 132.10). These imaging modalities provide better spatial resolution of cardiac structures and greater anatomic delineation of the Valsalva aneurysms and surrounding structures.

Heretofore, it was thought that angiography was the gold standard; however, cardiac CT angiography and CMRI have been increasingly described as adjunctive tools in confirming the diagnosis and aiding surgical management. Cardiac CT is also helpful in identifying coronary anomalies that may accompany abnormal AV morphology or abnormalities of the aorta such as coarctation of the aorta.

TREATMENT

In general, treatment for both ruptured and unruptured SOVAs if associated with symptoms is surgical. Asymptomatic SOVAs, depending on the size, may also require surgery to avoid complications such as acute rupture, which can be devastating when accompanied by hemodynamic compromise and may even result in death. The SOVA also can be complicated by endocarditis or thrombus formation with central or peripheral embolization. More recently, and increasingly, transcatheter repair is being used with increasing success.[16] 3D live imaging is an emergent and important tool that is readily available to delineate the features of SOVA.[17,18] Cardiac CT angiography can be beneficial in both diagnosis as well as surgical planning. More important, percutaneous closure (PC) may benefit from a combined echocardiography and thoracic aortogram information.[19] Similarly, CMRI may be used with appropriate protocols in the assessment of SOVA.[20,21]

Although historically SOVAs have been repaired surgically, PC is an emerging therapeutic intervention that is being used with increasing frequency.[22–24] Recent information supports PC with good safety and efficacy in a total of 877 infants treated for ruptured SOVA,[25] with similar demographics, anatomic pathology, and sites of rupture. Selection of patients in skilled hands makes this an attractive alternative to surgery with very good short- and midterm outcomes in experienced hands. Surgical closure is still reserved for patients that are more complicated, those who have associated significant aortic regurgitation, presence of endocarditis, bicuspid AV, or a tunnel type fistulous connection, larger defects or multiple sites of rupture. Percutaneous sinus of Valsalva closure may be reasonable in patients who may have prohibitive surgical risk for cardiopulmonary bypass or have significant medical comorbidities.

INDICATIONS FOR SURGERY

When left untreated, ruptured SOVAs have a high 1-year mortality rate, with an estimated mean survival time after diagnosis of 3.9 years.[26] Hence, a ruptured SOVA almost always mandates surgical intervention. An unruptured SOVA, when symptomatic with heart

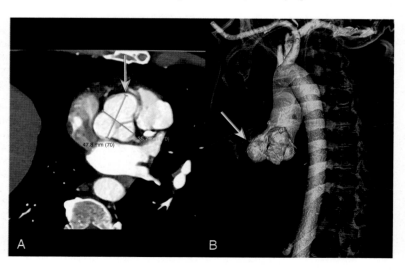

Figure 132.10. Short-axis view of the aortic valve on computed tomography demonstrating right sinus of Valsalva aneurysm (SOVA; **A,** *yellow arrow*). Volume-rendered view on computed tomography (**B**) of the same patient again demonstrating SOVA *(yellow arrow).*

failure, conduction system aberrations, arrhythmia or compressive symptoms on the coronary arteries RV inflow, RV outflow tract, or suspicion for endocarditis are also reasons for surgical intervention. Patients with asymptomatic unruptured SOVA may be monitored closely. In the event of symptoms or significant aortic valvular regurgitation or evidence if rapid growth ensues or attainment of severe enlargement with or without fistulous communication, surgery may be indicated with similar criteria used for ascending aortic aneurysms. There are few data to support this approach, but it provides a framework for clinical decision making. In the event that during follow-up of these patients, rupture or compressive symptoms or infections supervene, surgical intervention is again recommended. The operative mortality rate is low at less than 1% in uncomplicated SOVA; however, in the presence of endocarditis or acute hemodynamic collapse, the mortality rate may be higher. Long-term survival is excellent with surgery for SOVA repair, with 5- to 10-year survival rates between 82% and 97%.[8,27]

REFERENCES

1. Hope J. *A Treatise on the Diseases of the Heart and Great Vessels, and on the Affections Which May Be Mistaken for Them*. 3rd ed. Vol. 8. London: Churchill; 1839:639.
2. Boutefeu JM, Moret PR, Hahn C, Hauf E. Aneurysms of the sinus of Valsalva. Report of seven cases and review of the literature. *Am J Med*. 1978;65:18–24.
3. Thurnam J. On aneurisms, and especially spontaneous varicose aneurisms of the ascending aorta, and sinuses of Valsalva, with cases. *Med Chir Trans*. 1840;23:323–384.
4. Smith W. Aneurysm of the sinus of Valsalva with report of two cases. *J Am Med Assoc*. 1914;LXII:1878–1880.
5. Cedars A, Braverman A. The many faces of bicuspid aortic valve disease. *Prog Pediatr Cardiol*. 2012;34:91–96.
6. Yang EH, Rawal M, Pillutla P, Criley JM. Quadricuspid aortic valve with sinus of Valsalva rupture. *Congenit Heart Dis*. 2011;6:170–174.
7. Mariucci EM, Donti A, Picchio FM, Gargiulo GD. Noncoronary aortic cusp rupture in an adult patient with ventricular septal defect: echocardiographic diagnosis. *Pediatr Cardiol*. 2011;32:527–529.
8. Moustafa S, Mookadam F, Cooper L, et al. Sinus of Valsalva aneurysms: 47 years of a single center experience and systematic overview of published reports. *Am J Cardiol*. 2007;99:1159–1164.
9. Chu SH, Hung CR, How SS, et al. Ruptured aneurysms of the sinus of Valsalva in Oriental patients. *J Thorac Cardiovasc Surg*. 1990;99:288–298.
10. Kaye GC, Edmonson SJ, Caplin JL, Tunstall-Pedoe DS. Rupture of an aneurysm of the sinus of Valsalva into the superior vena cava. *Thorax*. 1984;39:475–476.
11. Killen DA, Wathanacharoen S, Pogson GW. Repair of intrapericardial rupture of left sinus of Valsalva aneurysm. *Ann Thorac Surg*. 1987;44:310–311.
12. Scagliotti D, Fisher EA, Deal BJ, et al. Congenital aneurysm of the left sinus of Valsalva with an aortopulmonary tunnel. *J Am Coll Cardiol*. 1986;7:443–445.
13. Moustafa S, Mookadam F, Connelly MS. Reticent uneventful rupture of right coronary sinus of Valsalva aneurysm into right ventricle. *Heart Lung Circ*. 2013;22:390–391.
14. Feldman DN, Roman MJ. Aneurysms of the sinuses of Valsalva. *Cardiology*. 2006;106:73–81.
15. Biaggi P, Matthews F, Braun J, et al. Gender, age, and body surface area are the major determinants of ascending aorta dimensions in subjects with apparently normal echocardiograms. *J Am Soc Echocardiogr*. 2009;22:720–725.
16. Sinha SC, Sujatha V, Mahapatro AK. Percutaneous transcatheter closure of ruptured sinus of Valsalva aneurysm: immediate result and long-term follow-up. *Int J Angiol*. 2015;24:99–104.
17. Chandra S, Vijay SK, Dwivedi SK, Saran RK. Delineation of anatomy of the ruptured sinus of Valsalva with three-dimensional echocardiography: the advantage of the added dimension. *Echocardiography*. 2012;29:E148–E151.
18. Raslan S, Nanda NC, Lloyd L, et al. Incremental value of live/real time 3D transesophageal echocardiography over the two-dimensional technique in the assessment of sinus of Valsalva aneurysm rupture. *Echocardiography*. 2011;28:918–920.
19. Mandel L, Gakhal M, Hopkins J. Percutaneous closure of recurrent noncoronary sinus of Valsalva aneurysm rupture: utility of computed tomography in procedural planning. *J Invasive Cardiol*. 2010;22:336–338.
20. Hoey ETD, Kanagasingam A, Sivananthan MU. Sinus of Valsalva aneurysms: assessment with cardiovascular MRI. *AJR Am J Roentgenol*. 2010;194:W495–W504.
21. Ro TK, Cotter BR, Simsir SA, Karlsberg RP. Complicated ruptured sinus of Valsalva: cardiac computed tomographic angiography (64 slice) predicts surgical appearance and obviates need for invasive cardiac catheterization. *Interact Cardiovasc Thorac Surg*. 2009;9:888–890.
22. Karlekar SM, Bhalghat P, Kerkar PG. Complete heart block following transcatheter closure of ruptured sinus of Valsalva aneurysm. *J Invasive Cardiol*. 2012;24:E314–E317.
23. Kenny D, Hijazi ZM. Transcatheter approaches to non-valvar structural heart disease. *Int J Cardiovasc Imag*. 2011;27:1133–1141.
24. Kerkar PG, Lanjewar CP, Mishra N, et al. Transcatheter closure of ruptured sinus of Valsalva aneurysm using the Amplatzer duct occluder: immediate results and mid-term follow-up. *Eur Heart J*. 2010;31:2881–2887.
25. Kuriakose EM, Bhatla P, McElhinney DB. Comparison of reported outcomes with percutaneous versus surgical closure of ruptured sinus of Valsalva aneurysm. *Am J Cardiol*. 2015;115:392–398.
26. Sawyers JL, Adams JE, Scott HW. A method of surgical repair for ruptured aortic sinus aneurysms with aorticoatrial fistula. *South Med J*. 1957;50:1075–1078.
27. Vural KM, Sener E, Taşdemir O, Bayazit K. Approach to sinus of Valsalva aneurysms: a review of 53 cases. *Eur J Cardio Thorac Surg*. 2001;20:71–76.

133 Aortic Dissection

Muhamed Saric, Itzhak Kronzon

Aortic dissection (AD) is a form of acute aortic syndrome (AAS). This syndrome encompasses several life-threatening clinical entities with overlapping features, including acute onset of chest pain, disruption of the aortic wall media, and a need for urgent medical care (Fig. 133.1). The term *acute aortic syndrome* was first proposed in 2001 by the Spanish physicians Vilacosta and San Román.[1] Originally, the spectrum of AAS included AD, intramural hematoma (IMH), and penetrating atherosclerotic ulcer (PAU). AAS now also included traumatic aortic rupture (TAR; transection) caused by blunt deceleration trauma as well as aortic aneurysm leak and rupture.[2] AD, the most common clinical presentation of AAS, is discussed in this chapter; the other forms of AAS are described elsewhere in this book. The cardinal features of an AD are (1) intimal tear (which may be primary or secondary); (2) abnormal blood flow from the aortic lumen into the media, which is typically already weakened by chronic hypertension, connective tissue disorders, or trauma (medial degeneration); (3) longitudinal cleavage of aortic wall by blood flow, leading to creation of a false lumen separated from the true lumen by an intimomedial dissection flap;

(4) development of complications such as tamponade, aortic regurgitation, and malperfusion in the territories of aortic branch vessels; and (5) long-term changes in the aortic anatomy (e.g., false-lumen thrombosis and aneurysm formation).

HISTORY

The British royal physician Frank Nichols provided the first unequivocal description of AD on the autopsy of the English king George II, who had died in 1760 of an ascending AD after straining on a commode.[3] The term "dissection" appears to have been first applied to blood vessels and the aorta in 1802 by the Swiss surgeon Jean Pierre Maunoir.[4,5] In 1826, the French physician René Laënnec introduced the term *dissecting aneurysm* (*anévrysme disséquant*).[6] Until the introduction of aortography in 1929 by the Portuguese physician Reynaldo dos Santos,[7] AD was exclusively a postmortem diagnosis. Aortography remained the primary means of diagnosing AD until the introduction of echocardiography, computed tomography (CT), and magnetic resonance imaging (MRI).

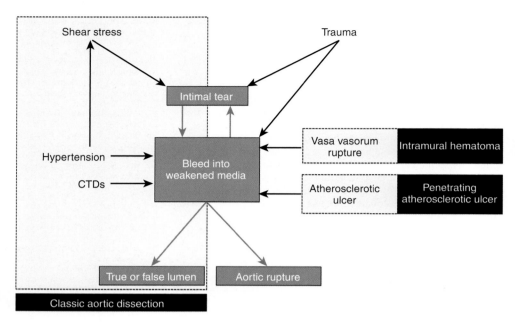

Figure 133.1. The spectrum of acute aortic syndrome. Note that although a primary intimal tear, a rupture of vasa vasorum or an ulceration of an atherosclerotic plaque may initiate the cascade, preexisting abnormalities in the aortic wall in the setting of hypertension, connective tissue disorders (CTDs; e.g., Marfan syndrome, Loeys-Dietz syndrome, Ehlers-Danlos syndrome type 4, Turner syndrome, bicuspid valve aortopathy), or trauma facilitate the development of an acute aortic syndrome.

The first successful surgical repair of a descending AD was reported in 1955 by Michael DeBakey, an American surgeon of Lebanese origin.[8] The first successful surgical repair of an ascending AD was reported in 1962 by the American surgeons Frank Spencer and Hu Blake.[9]

DeBakey[10] and Stanford University[11] are the two major classifications of AD. Because AD is a rare diagnosis, the International Registry of Acute Aortic Dissection (IRAD) was established in 1996 to pool data from leading centers in North America, Europe, and Asia.[12] Methods for percutaneous endovascular repair of AD are replacing surgical repair of AD in some patients.[13]

CLASSIFICATIONS OF AORTIC DISSECTION
Temporal

Dissections that are diagnosed within the first 2 weeks of presentation are termed acute; after the 2-week mark is passed, they are referred to as chronic dissections.

Spatial

Stanford classification. All dissections are either type A or type B. Any involvement of the ascending aorta classifies the dissection as type A irrespective of whether the dissection is contained within the ascending aorta or extends farther distally into the aortic arch, descending thoracic aorta, abdominal aorta, and beyond. Type B dissections are confined to the descending aorta.

DeBakey classification. Dissections contained within the ascending aorta are termed DeBakey II, whereas those extending any length distally from the ascending aorta are classified as DeBakey I. Thus, DeBakey types I and II correspond to Stanford type A. Dissections limited to the descending aorta are labeled DeBakey III and are equivalent to Stanford type B. DeBakey III dissections that are confined to the descending thoracic aorta are labeled as IIIa; those extending into the abdominal aorta are called IIIb (Fig. 133.2).

Epidemiology

AD is the most common form of catastrophic aortic disease and comprises the majority of all AAS cases.[14] The overall incidence of AD is low and is estimated at 0.5 to 4.0 annual cases per 100,000

individuals; only a few thousand new AD cases are diagnosed worldwide each year. Men are approximately twice as likely as women to develop AD. In the initial IRAD database, Stanford type A comprised approximately two-thirds and Stanford type B approximately one-third of all ADs.[15]

The prevalence of AD has a bimodal distribution with one cluster in younger patients (around 40 years of age) and the other in older patients (around 60 years of age). Risk factors mediate the pathogenesis of AD either by triggering initial events (intimal tear or vasa vasorum rupture) or by promoting chronic medial degeneration that facilitates subsequent dissection.

In younger patients, connective tissue disorders are the predominant risk factor, whereas hypertension is particularly prevalent among older patients with AD. Systemic hypertension is present in about three-fourths of cases and promotes both intimal tear formation and chronic medial denegation.[16] Cocaine use preferentially leads to type B dissections.[17]

Certain inherited connective tissue disorders are the strongest risk factor for the development of ADs, especially type A. Except for Turner syndrome, these disorders tend to have an autosomal-dominant pattern of inheritance. They include Marfan syndrome (caused by mutations in the fibrillin gene), Loeys-Dietz syndrome (mutation in the genes encoding transforming growth factor β receptor 1 and 2), Ehlers-Danlos syndrome type 4 (mutations in the collagen gene), bicuspid aortic valve (mutations in, e.g., the *NOTCH1* gene), and aortic coarctation (e.g., chromosome X monosomy in Turner syndrome). Although these disorders are rare, they account for a high percentage of ADs, especially before the age of 40 years. For instance, the prevalence of Marfan syndrome in the general population is about 0.02% (1 in 5000), yet Marfan syndrome accounts for about 5% of all ADs.[15]

Pregnancy is a risk factor for AD, particularly in Marfan syndrome and bicuspid aortic valve aortopathy. About half of all ADs in women younger than 40 years occur during pregnancy, especially in the last trimester or early postpartum period.[18] Occasionally, AD is iatrogenic as a complication of aortic cannulation or surgery. Atherosclerosis is not considered a direct risk factor for AD unless associated with PAUs.

Pathophysiology

The aortic wall consists of three layers. The media, a thick middle layer filled with strong elastic fibers, is bounded by the thin intima,

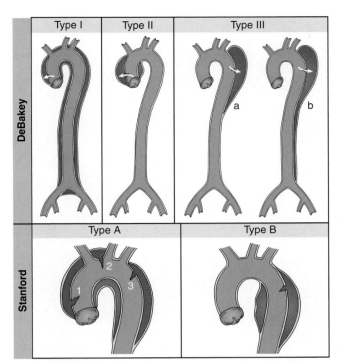

Figure 133.2. Classifications of aortic dissection. DeBakey *(top)* and Stanford *(bottom)* are the most common classifications of aortic dissections. Note that DeBakey I and II correspond to Stanford type A, whereas DeBakey III corresponds to Stanford type B. The figure is based on drawings from original publications (DeBakey in 1966 and Stanford in 1970).

which lines the aortic lumen, and the adventitia, which covers the outer wall of the aorta and provides most of the wall's tensile strength. The wall is nourished through vasa vasorum, small arteries that penetrate the wall from the adventitial side.

Basic Features

AD occurs when the normal intraluminal blood flow gains access to the aortic media and cleaves it longitudinally in either antegrade or retrograde direction. The cleavage creates an intimomedial flap (often incorrectly referred to as an "intimal flap") that separates the false lumen in the media from the aortic lumen (true lumen). Disruption of the media may lead to a variety of complications whose clinical presentation depends on the location of AD. Type A dissection may lead to tamponade, aortic regurgitation, and malperfusion of coronary or cerebral circulation. Type B dissection may lead to malperfusion in the spinal and visceral arterial circulation.

In the classic form of AD, an intimal tear starting at the luminal side is the primary event, triggering a cascade of subsequent blood flow–driven longitudinal cleavage of the aortic wall. The higher the amplitude and the rate of rise in systolic blood pressure, the stronger the cleavage force within the aortic media. Preexisting structural abnormalities of the media (e.g., connective tissue disorders or chronic hypertension) greatly enhance the propagation of cleavage. Historically, the histologic substrate underlying AD was described as cystic medial necrosis,[19] but this is inaccurate because the change is neither cystic nor necrotic; medial degeneration is probably a better term.

Although an intimal tear may affect any portion of the aorta, it typically occurs at one of the two sites with highest shear stress: (1) the right side of the ascending aorta just distal to the ostium of the right coronary artery in type A dissection and (2) just distal

to the ostium of the subclavian artery and close to the attachment of the ligamentum arteriosum in type B dissection. IMH may be considered a variant of AD in which the initial event is rupture of the vasa vasorum, leading to wall hematoma that erodes into the lumen, creating an intimal tear from the medial site into the aortic lumen.[20] With IMH, an intimal tear is not a primary event (as in classic dissection) but rather a secondary phenomenon. PAUs, first described in 1934, may also lead to AD, although contained rupture is a more common presentation of an ulcer.[21] Irrespective of how an AD starts, the intimomedial flap may have additional entry and exit points along the dissection path.

COMPLICATIONS

AD may be complicated by malperfusion syndromes, aortic regurgitation, and rupture into an adjacent cavity. Malperfusion syndromes in the territories of aortic side branches may lead to coronary and cerebral ischemia in type A dissection, or spinal, limb, and/or abdominal ischemia in type A or B dissections. The mechanism of aortic valvular regurgitation in AD may be caused by effacement of the sinotubular junction loss of leaflet support, prolapse of the intimal flap through the aortic valve into the left ventricle. AD may rupture into the pericardial, pleural, and/or peritoneal space, leading to hemorrhagic effusions. Pericardial tamponade is likely the most common cause of death in type A dissection; urgent surgical repair of the AD rather than pericardiocentesis is the treatment of choice.

LONG-TERM CHANGES

If the patient survives and no surgical intervention is performed within 2 weeks of dissection onset, AD enters a chronic phase in which the false lumen either undergoes thrombosis or remains permanently patent. Thrombosis obliterates the true lumen and allows for reestablishment of physiologic flow confined to the true lumen. False-lumen thrombosis is preceded by blood stasis, seen on echocardiography as spontaneous echocardiographic contrast ("smoke") in the false lumen. Permanent patency of the false lumen is enhanced by the presence of reentry fenestrations. The cleaved media of the chronically patent false lumen may endothelialize to give rise to the so-called double-barrel aorta. In addition, progressive weakening of the false lumen's adventitial wall may give rise to secondary aortic aneurysms.

DIAGNOSIS OF AORTIC DISSECTION

The diagnosis of AD requires a high index of suspicion because AD is rare disorder. Classically, AD presents with severe tearing and often migratory chest pain. Physical diagnosis is notoriously unreliable; pathognomonic physical findings (e.g., pulse deficits or focal neurological signs) only occur in one-third of the cases or fewer.[15] Four imaging techniques are used to diagnose AD: echocardiography, CT (Fig. 133.3A and B), MRI (Fig. 133.3C and D), and aortography. Either transesophageal echocardiography (TEE) or CT is the initial diagnostic test of choice for acute dissections. Only occasionally can transthoracic echocardiography (TTE) establish the diagnosis of AD (Fig. 133.4 and Video 133.4). MRI is best suited for chronic dissections. Invasive aortography typically adds no incremental diagnostic value but is still useful intraprocedurally during stent placement or palliative creation of iatrogenic fenestrations in the intimomedial tear.

ECHOCARDIOGRAPHY IN AORTIC DISSECTION

The principal goal of any imaging is to identify the three fundamental features of AD: basic findings, complications, and long-term changes. TEE (Figs. 133.5 and 133.6 and Videos 133.5 and 133.6) is the echocardiographic test of choice for the diagnosis of

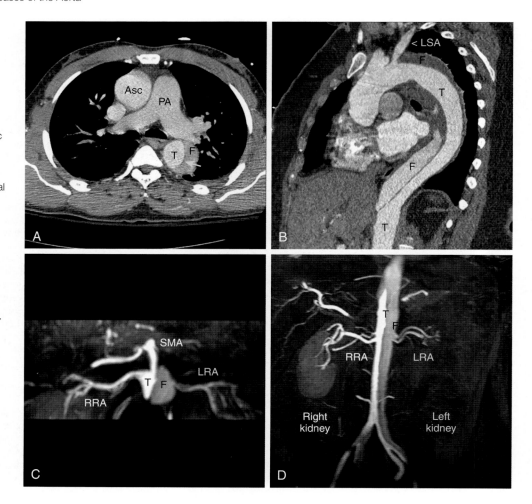

Figure 133.3. Computed tomography (CT) and magnetic resonance imaging (MRI) in aortic dissection. **A** and **B,** Contrast-enhanced CT demonstrates an acute type B aortic dissection. Axial images in **A** show the typical appearance of a dissection flap in the descending thoracic aorta *(arrow)* separating the true (T) from the false (F) lumen. Note the absence of dissection in the ascending (Asc) aorta. Sagittal images in **B** demonstrate the typical origin *(arrow)* of type B dissection just distal to the origin of the left subclavian artery *(LSA).* **C** and **D,** MRI demonstrates a chronic type B aortic dissection extending from the thoracic aorta into the abdominal aorta. Axial (**C**) and coronal (**D**) images demonstrate that the right renal artery (RRA) originates from the true (T) lumen, and the left renal artery (LRA) originates from the false lumen, leading to hypoperfusion of the left kidney. *PA,* Pulmonary artery; *SMA,* superior mesenteric artery.

AD because TTE lacks sensitivity and specificity in diagnosing AD. Nonetheless, TTE may be invaluable in visualizing complications of AD.

On echocardiography, the dissection flap separating the true lumen from the false lumen appears as an undulating membrane parallel to the long axis of the aorta. The intimomedial flap is often easier to visualize in the short rather than the long axis of the aorta. A linear reverberation artifact in the ascending aorta should not be mistaken for type A dissection. Similarly, the band of tissue separating a prominent azygos vein from the descending thoracic aorta should not be misinterpreted as a dissection flap (Fig. 133.7 and Video 133.7).

The true lumen is often smaller than the false lumen, expands in systole, and shrinks in diastole. Because the true lumen is lined by the intima and the false lumen by the cleaved media, the presence of intimal atherosclerotic changes helps identify the true lumen. The false lumen more often features blood stasis, leading to spontaneous echo contrast ("smoke") and thrombus formation. Microbubble contrast may help distinguish the true from the false lumen because the contrast typically fills the true lumen before the false lumen (Fig. 133.8 and Video 133.8).

Entry sites from the true lumen into the false lumen are visualized as color Doppler jets extending from the true lumen into the false lumen, often at predilection sites (a few centimeters distal to the right coronary cusp in type A dissections or in the descending thoracic aorta just distal to the origin of the left subclavian artery in type B dissections). Similarly, exit holes may be seen on the distal portions of the dissection flap, with color jets exiting the false lumen into the true lumen.

Complications of AD are easily visualized by TEE or TTE such as aortic regurgitation, segmental left ventricular wall motion caused by a coronary artery dissection, pericardial effusion, or dissection flap extensions into aortic branch vessels. Long-term changes in the false lumen start with development of spontaneous echocardiographic contrast in the false lumen, leading to clot formation and obliteration of the false lumen (Fig. 133.9 and Video 133.9). TEE may also be used for serial monitoring of aortic aneurysm formation after AD.

The major drawback of TEE is its inability to visualize the portion of the thoracic aorta around the brachiocephalic trunk ostium because of interposition of the trachea and the left main bronchus between the aorta and the esophagus. This region, however, can often be well visualized on suprasternal TTE imaging.

THERAPY AND PROGNOSIS

Type A AD is an absolute medical emergency requiring prompt surgical repair because the likelihood of survival decreases with each passing hour. Up to 90% of unoperated patients with type A dissection die within 3 months of presentation. For type B dissections, patients who undergo medical therapy have on average a lower mortality rate than those who undergo surgical repair. Percutaneous endovascular stent graft placement is becoming an alternative to surgical repair of AD. Medical therapy is used in all patients irrespective of whether they are operated or not. A multidrug regimen including a β-blocker is recommended to control the systemic blood pressure and to decrease the rate of rise of systemic blood pressure.

Please access ExpertConsult to view the corresponding videos for this chapter.

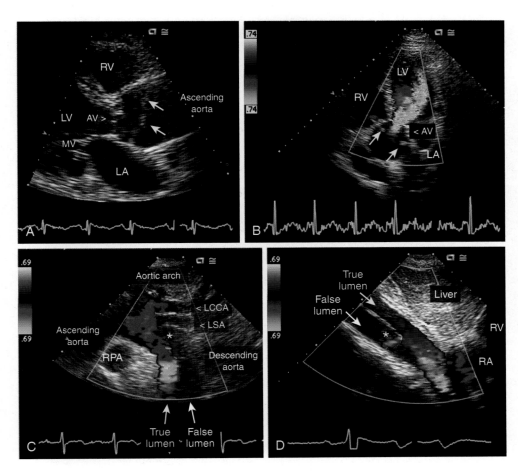

Figure 133.4. Transthoracic echocardiography in aortic dissection. **A,** Dissection flap *(arrows)* in the aortic root of a patient with acute type A dissection on the parasternal long-axis view. **B,** Severe aortic regurgitation caused by type A aortic dissection *(arrows)* on the apical five-chamber view. **C,** Type B aortic dissection seen on the suprasternal view. Note the typical origin *(asterisk)* of the dissection flap just distal to the ostium of the left subclavian artery (LSA). **D,** Subcostal imaging demonstrates dissection flap extending from the distal thoracic aorta into the abdominal aorta. The *asterisk* denotes a secondary communication between the true and false lumen with a to-and-fro flow. *AV,* Aortic valve; *LA,* left atrium; *LCCA,* left common carotid artery; *LV,* left ventricle; *MV,* mitral valve; *RA,* right atrium; *RPA,* right pulmonary artery; *RV,* right ventricle. (See accompanying Video 133.4.)

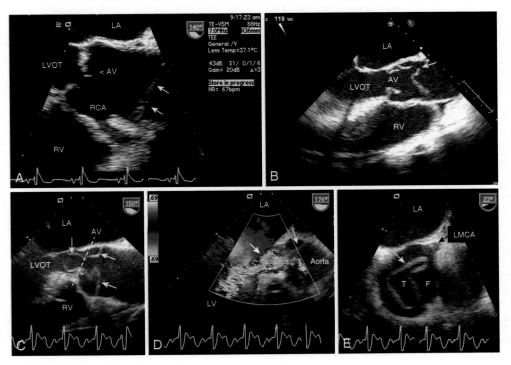

Figure 133.5. Type A dissection on transesophageal echocardiography. **A,** Typical origin of the type A aortic dissection flap *(arrows)* just distal to the ostium of the right coronary artery (RCA). **B,** The dissection flap *(arrow)* remains in the ascending aorta during diastole and does not prolapse through the aortic valve in this patient. In contrast, **C** and **D** demonstrate dissection flaps *(yellow arrows)* through the aortic valve (AV) during diastole. Dissection flap prolapse is one of several mechanisms that lead to aortic regurgitation *(white arrow)* in type A dissection. **E,** Circumferential dissection flap in the ascending aorta seen in a short-axis view separating the true (T) from the false (F) lumen. *LA,* Left atrium; *LMCA,* left main coronary artery; *LV,* left ventricle; *LVOT,* left ventricular outflow tract; *RV,* right ventricle. (See accompanying Video 133.5.)

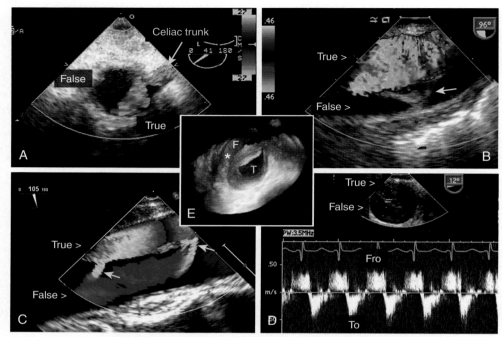

Figure 133.6. Type B dissection on transesophageal echocardiography (TEE). **A,** The color-filled true lumen gives rise to the celiac trunk. The false lumen is to the left of the true lumen and shows little flow on color Doppler. **B,** Type B dissection in the descending thoracic aorta. The *arrow* points to incomplete dissection of the media at this level. Findings of strands of media tissues still intact help identify the false lumen. **C,** Two secondary communications *(arrows)* between the true and the false lumen. **D,** Flow in these secondary communications frequently demonstrates a to-and-fro pattern on spectral Doppler. **E,** Three-dimensional TEE image demonstrate a dissection flap separating the true (T) from the false (F) lumen. Note the acute angle *(asterisk)* between the false lumen and the dissection flap. This acute angle helps identify the false lumen. (See accompanying Video 133.6.)

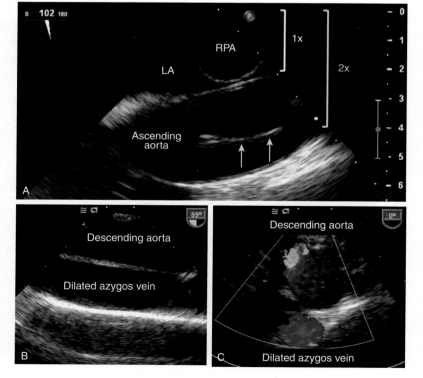

Figure 133.7. Masqueraders of aortic dissection flap. **A,** A true type A aortic dissection flap should not be confused with the reverberation artifact in the ascending aorta. Note that the reverberation artifact is located twice as deep (2×) as the anterior aortic wall (1×) that gives rise to the reverberation artifact *(arrows)*. **B** and **C,** The wall separating the descending aorta from a prominent azygos vein should not be mistaken for a type B aortic dissection flap. In this patient, the azygos vein is unusually larger because of azygos continuation of the inferior vena cava (IVC) in the setting of congenital absence of the intrahepatic portion of the IVC. *LA,* Left atrium; *RPA,* right pulmonary artery. (See accompanying Video 133.7.)

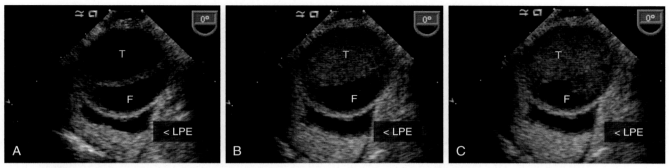

Figure 133.8. Use of microbubble contrast in diagnosis of aortic dissection. Intravenously given microbubble echo contrast helps distinguish the true (T) from the false (F) lumen. In this patient with a dissection flap in the descending thoracic aorta (**A**), the contrast agent fills the true lumen first (**B**) and then enters the false lumen (**C**). Images also show a left pleural effusion (LPE), which is often a complication of aortic dissection. (See accompanying Video 133.8.)

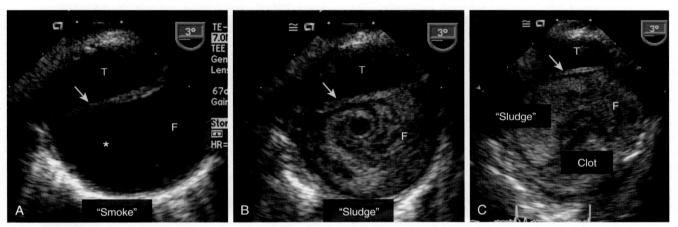

Figure 133.9. Long-term changes in the false lumen. **A,** Only a small amount of spontaneous echo contrast or "smoke" *(asterisk)* is seen in the false lumen (F) in the proximal descending thoracic aorta. This indicates the presence of stasis in the false lumen. Note the absence of "smoke" in the true (T) lumen. The *arrow* points to the dissection flap. **B,** The "smoke" turns into even denser "sludge" indicative of a higher degree of stasis in the false lumen in the midportion of the descending thoracic aorta. The *arrow* points to the dissection flap. **C,** In the distal descending thoracic aorta, a clot has started to form within the "sludge." The *arrow* points to the dissection flap. (See accompanying Video 133.9.)

REFERENCES

1. Vilacosta I, San Román JA. Acute aortic syndrome. *Heart*. 2001;85:365–368.
2. Nienaber CA, Powell JT. Management of acute aortic syndromes. *Eur Heart J*. 2012;33(1):26–35.
3. Nichols F. Observations concerning the body of his late majesty. *Phil Trans Lond*. 1761;52:265–274.
4. Maunoir JP. *Mémoires physiologiques et pratiques sur l'anévrisme et la ligature des artères*. Geneva: JJ Paschoud; 1802.
5. Cumston CG. A contribution to the history of the surgical treatment of aneurysm, from the notes of Dr. Charles T. Maunoir, of Geneva, made during the year 1802. *Proc R Soc Med*. 1919;12(Suppl):63–69.
6. Laennec RTH. Anévrysme disséquant de l'aorte, chez un sujet attaqué d'hypertrophie simple du ventricule droit. In: *I, De l'auscultation médiate ou traité du diagnostic des maladies des poumons et du cœur*. 2nd ed. Paris: J. S. Chaudé; 1826:696.
7. Dos Santos R, Lamas A, Pereirgi CJ. L'artériographie des members de l'aorte et ses branches abdominals. *Bull Soc Nat Chir*. 1929;55:587.
8. DeBakey ME, Cooley DA, Creech O Jr. Surgical considerations of dissecting aneurysm of the aorta. *Ann Surg*. 1955;142:586–612.
9. Spencer FC, Blake H. A report of the successful surgical treatment of aortic regurgitation from a dissecting aortic aneurysm in a patient with the Marfan syndrome. *J Thorac Cardiovasc Surg*. 1962;44:238.
10. Debakey ME, Henly WS, Cooley DA, et al. Surgical management of dissecting aneurysms of the aorta. *J Thorac Cardiovasc Surg*. 1965;49:130–149.
11. Daily PO, Trueblood HW, Stinson EB, et al. Management of acute aortic dissections. *Ann Thorac Surg*. 1970;10(3):237–247.
12. International Registry of Acute Aortic Dissections. http://www.iradonline.org/irad.html. Accessed on January 20, 2014.
13. Svensson LG, Kouchoukos NT, Miller DC, et al. Society of Thoracic Surgeons Endovascular Surgery Task Force: Expert consensus document on the treatment of descending thoracic aortic disease using endovascular stent-grafts. *Ann Thorac Surg*. 2008;85(1 Suppl):S1–S41.
14. Lansman SL, Saunders PC, Malekan R, Spielvogel D. Acute aortic syndrome. *J Thorac Cardiovasc Surg*. 2010;140(6 Suppl):S92–S97.
15. Hagan PG, Nienaber CA, Isselbacher EM, et al. The International Registry of acute aortic dissection (IRAD): new insights into an old disease. *J Am Med Assoc*. 2000;283(7):897–903.
16. Braverman AC. Acute aortic dissection: Clinician update. *Circulation*. 2010;122:184–188.
17. Tsai TT, Nienaber CA, Eagle KA. Acute aortic syndromes. *Circulation*. 2005;112:3802–3813.
18. Immer FF, Bansi AG, Immer-Bansi AS, et al. Aortic dissection in pregnancy: Analysis of risk factors and outcome. *Ann Thorac Surg*. 2003;76(1):309–314.
19. Larson EW, Edwards WD. Risk factors for aortic dissection: a necropsy study of 161 cases. *Am J Cardiol*. 1984;53(6):849–855.
20. Krukenberg E. Beiträge zur Frage des Aneurysma dissecans. *Beitr Pathol Anat Allg Pathol*. 1920;67:329–351.
21. Shennan T: Dissecting Aneurysms. Medical Research Council, Special Report Series, No Vol. 193; 1934, London, His Majesty's Stationary Office.

134 Penetrating Atherosclerotic Ulcer and Intramural Hematoma

Philippe B. Bertrand, Eric M. Isselbacher

Intramural hematoma (IMH) and penetrating atherosclerotic ulcers (PAU), along with acute aortic dissection (AD), are part of the spectrum of acute aortic syndromes, which involve disruption of the medial layer of the aortic wall (Fig. 134.1). Of these, AD is the most common (62%–88%), followed by IMH (10%–30%) and PAU (2%–8%).[1] Noninvasive imaging techniques—including echocardiography, computed tomography (CT), and magnetic resonance imaging (MRI)—play a crucial role in ensuring early and accurate diagnosis of these potentially life-threatening conditions.[2,3] This chapter focuses on the clinical presentation, etiology, and noninvasive imaging findings in IMH and PAU, along with guidance for diagnosis and management.

INTRAMURAL HEMATOMA

IMH is defined as the presence of blood or thrombus within the medial layer of the aortic wall but without evidence of overt communication with the aortic lumen or flow within the wall. Historically, IMH has been believed to result from rupture of the vasa vasorum, the small blood vessels that nourish the aortic media, leading to bleeding directly within the aortic media. However, more recent evidence suggests that many IMHs are caused by very small intimal tears that allow blood to seep into the medial layer and thrombose, preventing ongoing or visible flow within the media.[4] IMHs are considered a variant of classic AD, accounting for approximately 10% to 25% of patients with acute aortic syndrome. In contrast to a classic AD, IMHs do not have a dissection flap, a reentry site, or the presence of a double-channel aorta. Importantly, the prognosis of IMH appears to be similar to that of classic acute dissection.[5,6]

CLINICAL PRESENTATION

Abrupt onset of severe pain in the chest or back is the typical presenting symptom of IMH, making it indistinguishable from classic AD on clinical grounds alone. Migration of the pain can be similar to AD but rarely reaches the legs. IMH tends to occur more frequently in the descending (Stanford type B) than the ascending thoracic aorta (Stanford type A).[5,7] Patients with IMH are less likely to develop aortic regurgitation or pulse deficits than patients with AD but are more likely to develop periaortic hematoma and pericardial effusion and are still prone to rupture.[8] The most common risk factors include arterial hypertension, hypercholesterolemia, and a history of smoking; conversely, IMH is not commonly associated with Marfan syndrome or bicuspid aortic valves. Of note, IMH can also be caused by blunt trauma to the thorax or can be iatrogenic after catheter manipulations.[9]

NONINVASIVE IMAGING FEATURES

The diagnosis of IMH is more challenging than that of classic AD. IMH typically presents as a crescentic or circumferential thickening of the aortic wall, with a thickness typically greater than 5 mm and without a gross entry tear or mobile dissection flap (Fig. 134.2). The hematoma typically bulges outward, so the shape of the aortic lumen is preserved, whereas in classic AD, the false lumen usually pushes the dissection flap inward, distorting the shape of the true lumen. In IMH, the luminal surface is usually curvilinear and

smooth (Fig. 134.3), as opposed to the rough, irregular border seen with aortic atherosclerosis and PAUs (Fig. 134.4). However, these conditions may coexist.

IMHs can be difficult to distinguish from a thrombosed false lumen of classic AD because sometimes the latter can also appear as a crescent-shaped thickening of the aortic wall. In addition, IMH is often confused with intraluminal mural thrombus; however, IMH can usually be distinguished by the smoothness of its inner surface, whereas mural thrombus tends to have an irregular surface and inward displacement of intimal calcium, whereas intimal calcium is located outside of mural thrombus (Fig. 134.5). An overview of the characteristics that are key for differentiation between intraluminal thrombus and IMH is presented in Table 134.1.

Transesophageal echocardiography (TEE) is superior to transthoracic echocardiography (TTE) in the diagnosis of IMH. The characteristic finding of crescentic or circumferential aortic

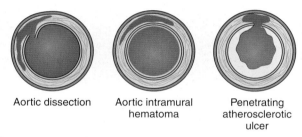

Figure 134.1. Acute aortic syndromes. (Adapted with permission, from Baliga RR, et al. The role of imaging in aortic dissection and related syndromes, *JACC Cardiovasc Imag* 7:406–424, 2014.)

Aortic dissection   Aortic intramural hematoma   Penetrating atherosclerotic ulcer

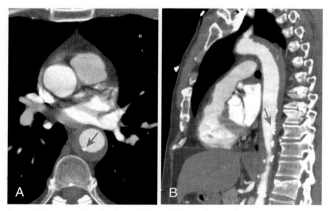

Figure 134.2. Type B intramural hematoma (IMH). Computed tomography angiography in a patient with type B IMH as shown by the abnormal thickening of the descending aortic wall on both axial (**A**) and sagittal (**B**) imaging. Note the inward displacement of inward calcium *(arrow)* and the curvilinear smooth luminal surface in axial imaging. (© Massachusetts General Hospital Thoracic Aortic Center, used with permission.)

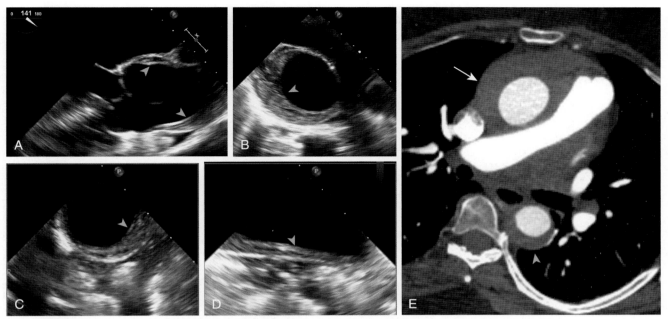

Figure 134.3. Type A intramural hematoma (IMH). Transesophageal echocardiographic images (**A–D**) obtained in a patient with type A IMH extending from the aortic root and ascending aorta (*hollow arrowheads*, A and B, Videos 134.3A and B) to the descending thoracic aorta (*full arrowheads*, C and D, Video 134.3C). Axial computed tomography angiography image (**E**) shows both the IMH in both the ascending (*hollow arrowhead*) and descending thoracic aorta (*full arrowhead*). (© Massachusetts General Hospital Thoracic Aortic Center, used with permission.)

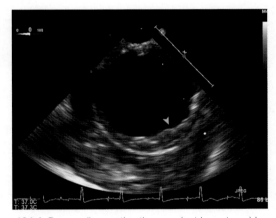

Figure 134.4. Descending aortic atheroma (not hematoma) by transesophageal echocardiography, with irregular intraluminal borders (*arrowhead*). (© Massachusetts General Hospital Thoracic Aortic Center, used with permission.)

wall thickening requires further attention, and differentiation from mural thrombus or extensive atheroma can be made based on above features. There may be areas of echolucency within the aortic wall hematoma but no communication of flow to the aortic lumen (see Fig. 134.3). TEE is helpful in assessing IMHs in the ascending aorta, aortic arch, and descending aorta and is useful in assessing for associated pericardial effusion and aortic regurgitation. However, IMH in the distal ascending aorta or proximal aortic arch can be missed if in the TEE blind spot.

CT is the preferred imaging modality for diagnosis and follow-up of IMH (and other acute aortic syndromes). On noncontrast CT, IMH is diagnosed when thickening of the aortic wall is observed with higher attenuation than intraluminal blood. Noncontrast CT is helpful in distinguishing IMH from atheroma, mural thrombus, motion artifacts, and other aortic wall thickening (see Fig. 134.5).[10]

Alternatively, contrast-enhanced CT is useful to assess for the presence of focal contrast enhancement within the IMH. This comprises small contrast-enhanced islandlike lesions within the hematoma without direct communication with the true lumen or a localized blood-filled pouch protruding into the thrombosed lumen of the aorta, resulting in an ulcerlike projection into the hematoma (Fig. 134.6). Ulcerlike projections have prognostic impact in IMH because they are associated with increased progression to dissection or rupture.[11,12]

MRI, with its superior tissue characterization and contrast, might have a role in the diagnosis of IMH, particularly in small IMHs or when differential diagnosis is unclear. Differences in imaging modalities for IMHs and PAUs are listed in Table 134.2.

The main limitation for all the imaging modalities is the aspect of time. IMH can be progressive over the course of hours or days, and imaging the aortic wall at the time of presentation can miss an IMH in formation (or complication of IMH) that will only be evident on subsequent imaging.

MANAGEMENT AND PROGNOSIS

Predictors of progression of IMH to classic AD or rupture are shown in Box 134.1.[13] The natural evolution in IMH is variable: regression of the hematoma was observed in 40%, but in 60%, progression occurred to either aneurysm, localized AD (or ulcerlike projection), classical AD with longitudinal propagation, or aortic rupture.[14] Accordingly, serial imaging is required to rule out progression in patients managed medically because clinical signs and symptoms cannot predict progression (Fig. 134.7). Current international guidelines recommend treating IMHs as classic AD.[15] Type A IMHs are usually managed with urgent surgery to repair the ascending aorta. Type B IMHs are usually managed with medical therapy and careful surveillance imaging with the option of thoracic endovascular aortic repair (TEVAR) or, rarely, surgery in the setting of complications. However, there has been an increasing interest in considering early TEVAR if there are indications that the patient is at increased risk of complications.[16,17]

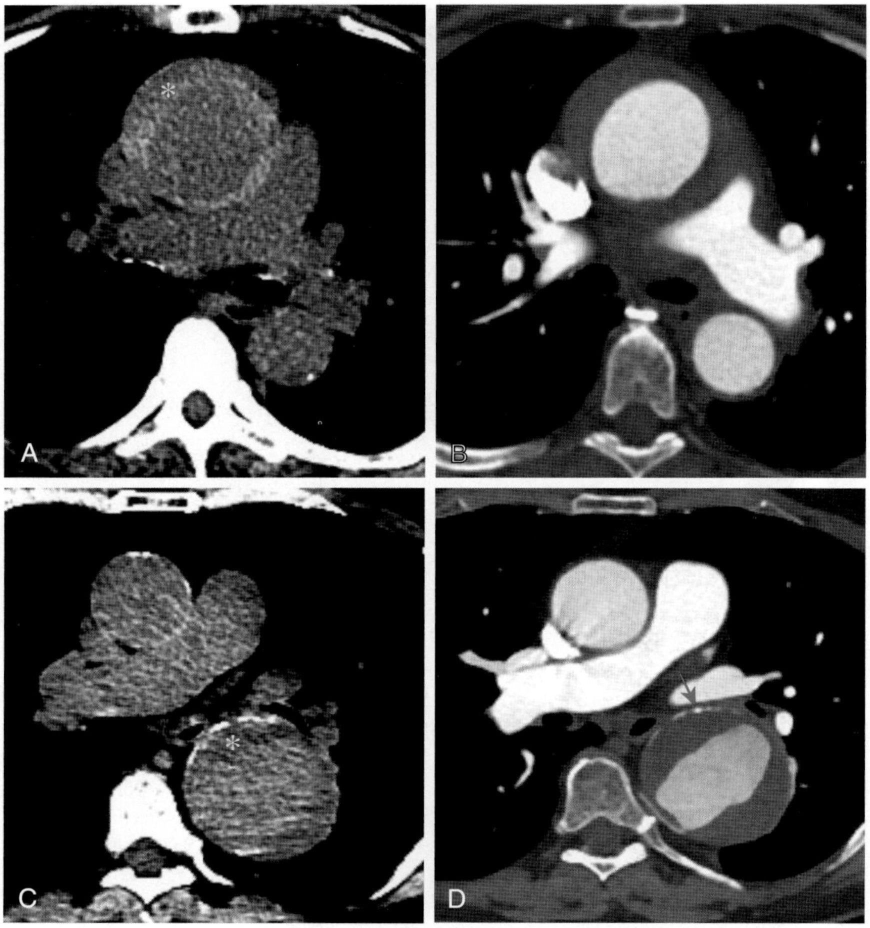

Figure 134.5. Intramural hematoma (IMH) versus mural thrombus. Noncontrast computed tomography (CT) of the aorta shows hyperattenuation *(asterisk)* in case of intramural hematoma (IMH) (**A**) as opposed to hypoattenuation in case of mural thrombus (**C**). By contrast-enhanced CT, IMH has a smooth, curvilinear luminal border (**B**) as opposed to the irregular border in case of mural thrombus (**D**). Also note the intimal calcium on the outside of the mural thrombus (**D**, *arrow*). (© Massachusetts General Hospital Thoracic Aortic Center, used with permission.)

TABLE 134.1 Characteristics of Intramural Hematoma Versus Mural Thrombus

	Intramural hematoma	Mural thrombus
Aortic diameter	Often normal	Aneurysmal
Spontaneous echocontrast along lumen wall	Absent	Often present
Shape of thickened wall	Crescentic	Irregular
Inner surface of wall	Smooth	Irregular/rough
Intimal calcium	Next to the lumen	Under the thrombus
Echolucent areas within thickened wall	May be present	Absent

PENETRATING ATHEROSCLEROTIC ULCER

The term *penetrating atherosclerotic ulcer*, also called penetrating aortic ulcer (PAU), describes a condition in which ulceration of an atherosclerotic lesion penetrates the aortic internal elastic lamina and into the aortic media (see Fig. 134.1). Although the clinical presentation of PAU can be similar to that of classic AD, PAU is primarily a disease of the intima (aortic atherosclerosis), whereas AD and IMH are diseases of the media (degeneration of the elastic fibers and smooth muscle cells).

Pathophysiology

In its most common form, a PAU is caused by erosion or rupture of an atherosclerotic plaque, in which the disruption of the fibrous cap leads to ulceration. This ulceration may be restricted to the intima but can progress to penetrate the media or even the adventitia. Penetration of the medial layer can lead to a hematoma, which may be localized or extend proximally or distally within the outer third of the aortic media for a varying length. On occasion, the hematoma may break through the outer medial wall, cleaving the media from the adventitia.[18] After they have formed, PAUs may remain quiescent, but the weakened aortic wall may allow progression to saccular, fusiform, or false aneurysms (pseudoaneurysms).[19] External rupture into the mediastinum or the right or left pleural space may occur, but this is uncommon. Embolization of thrombus or atherosclerotic debris from the ulcer to the distal arterial circulation may also occur. Rarely, the medial hematoma ruptures back into the aortic lumen, resulting in an appearance similar to AD, with flow in both lumens.

Clinical Presentation

Risk factors for the development of PAU include age, hypertension, atherosclerosis, and smoking. PAUs can occur anywhere along the length of the aorta but appear most often in the mid and distal portions of the descending thoracic aorta (~90%). They may also present in the abdominal aorta or the aortic arch but are rarely seen in the ascending aorta.[19] Although PAUs can present with severe chest or back pain of acute onset, most often they are discovered as an

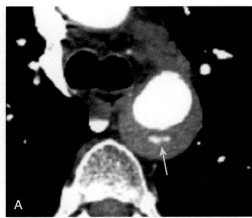

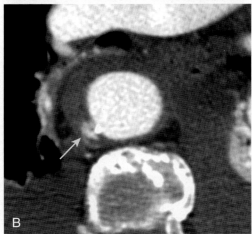

Figure 134.6. A and **B,** Ulcerlike projections in intramural hematoma (IMH). Ulcerlike projections *(arrows)* are small, localized, contrast-filled outpouchings the protrude from the aortic lumen into the thrombus of an IMH. (© Massachusetts General Hospital Thoracic Aortic Center, used with permission.)

TABLE 134.2 Differences Between Imaging Modalities to Diagnose Intramural Hematoma and Penetrating Aortic Ulcer

Modality	Advantages	Disadvantages
TEE	No radiation exposure Assessment of aortic regurgitation Assessment of pericardial fluid Differential diagnosis of IMH, dissection, mural thrombus, or atheroma; differentiating PAU from ULP	TEE blind spot Operator and patient dependent Less well studied than CT or MRI Semi-invasive
CT	Permits assessment of entire aorta and other thoracic structures Superior to TEE for detecting IMH and PAU, especially when small or localized Detects extraluminal and extracardiac abnormalities better than TEE (e.g., pseudoaneurysm, mediastinal fluid) Ideal for serial imaging or comparison; follow-up by CT scan recommended	Ionizing radiation exposure Iodinated contrast material
MRI	Provides multiple images without contrast Detecting associated IMH complicating PAU Differentiating primary IMH from atherosclerotic plaque and intraluminal thrombus	Availability Operator dependent

CT, Computed tomography; *IMH,* intramural hematoma; *MRI,* magnetic resonance imaging; *PAU,* penetrating atherosclerotic ulcer; *TEE,* transesophageal echocardiography; *ULP,* ulcerlike projections.

BOX 134.1 Adverse Predictors of Progression to Dissection or Rupture of Type A and Type B Intramural Hematoma

- Younger age
- Persistent pain
- Aortic diameter ≥50–53 mm
- Aortic wall thickness ≥11–16 mm
- Intramural hematoma expansion
- Compression of the aortic lumen
- Associated penetrating ulcer
- Periaortic bleeding
- Pericardial effusion
- Increasing pleural effusion
- Absence of long-term β-blocker use
- Marfan syndrome

Reproduced from Pelzel JM, et al: International heterogeneity in diagnostic frequency and clinical outcomes of ascending aortic intramural hematoma, *J Am Soc Echocardiogr* 20:1260–1268, 2007.

incidental finding on an imaging study in asymptomatic patients.[19] Although they are more commonly found in the setting of aortic dilatation, PAUs can occur in normal caliber aortas as well.

Noninvasive Imaging Features

The diagnosis of PAU requires demonstration of an ulcer or a craterlike outpouching in the aortic wall (Fig. 134.8). Because protrusion through the internal elastic lamina cannot be identified, PAUs can only be detected when they permit blood to protrude outside the normal contour of the aortic lumen. Another entity that may be mistaken for a PAU is an ulcerlike projection that may arise in an IMH.[20] These are localized, blood-filled pouches that protrude from the lumen into the hematoma, typically with a communicating orifice 3 mm or more. Ulcerlike projections are believed to be the consequence of a focal tear of the intimal layer in the absence of an atherosclerotic plaque. Differentiation from a PAU may be difficult, but ulcerlike projections are associated with a smooth intima, whereas PAUs typically have jagged edges and are associated with irregularities of the intimal layer.

Echocardiography, CT, and MRI are all useful in detecting the presence of a PAU and its complications. After it has been identified, attention should be directed to assessing (1) the maximum depth of penetration of the ulcer, measured from the aortic lumen; (2) the maximum width at the entry site; and (3) the axial length of the associated medial hematoma.

TTE can sometimes identify the presence of a PAU (Fig. 134.9), but it usually cannot provide sufficient anatomic information for clinical decision making, so additional imaging is typically necessary. TEE is helpful in visualizing PAUs in the ascending aorta, aortic arch, and descending aorta (Fig. 134.10) but is not well suited to image the abdominal aorta.[21] Ulcers located in the distal ascending aorta or proximal aortic arch may be in the TEE blind spot and therefore missed. The characteristic finding, similar to what is seen with CT and MRI, is a craterlike outpouching of the aortic wall, often with jagged edges, which is usually associated with extensive aortic atheroma. Although uncommon, a localized aortic dissection may also be present, but the dissection flap, if present, tends to be thick, irregular, nonoscillating, and typically of limited length.[22]

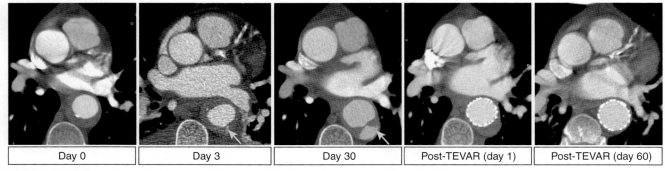

Figure 134.7. Progression of type B intramural hematoma (IMH). Axial computed tomography images of a patient presenting with an initially uncomplicated type B IMH. After 3 days, a small ulcerlike projection is noted (*arrow,* day 3), progressing to a localized dissection at 30 days (*arrow,* day 30). After treatment with thoracic endovascular aortic repair (TEVAR), the false lumen of the dissection thromboses (post-TEVAR day 1) and the hematoma is then gradually resorbed (post-TEVAR day 60). (© Massachusetts General Hospital Thoracic Aortic Center, used with permission.)

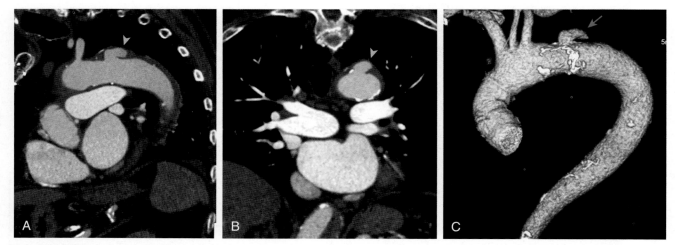

Figure 134.8. Penetrating atherosclerotic ulcer in the descending thoracic aorta, as visualized by computed tomography (CT) imaging. A large penetrating atherosclerotic ulcer *(arrow)* of the proximal descending thoracic aorta is demonstrated on a contrast-enhanced CT angiography in the sagittal projection (**A**), coronal projection (**B**), and a three-dimensional surface-shaded display (**C**). Notice the burden of atherosclerosis in the descending thoracic aorta adjacent to the ulcer (*white* on the display in **C**). (© Massachusetts General Hospital Thoracic Aortic Center, used with permission.)

CT is considered the first-line diagnostic imaging modality for PAU. It is widely available, permits assessment of other thoracic structures, and provides three-dimensional reconstructed images that are essential in planning open surgery or TEVAR. The typical CT finding of a PAU is a localized, contrast-filled outpouching of the aortic wall communicating with the lumen. Thickening (enhancement) of the aortic wall external to sites of intimal calcification suggests the presence of a localized IMH. These findings are usually seen in conjunction with severe atherosclerosis. CT is preferred to TEE because it can examine the aortic segments not visualized by TEE, allowing for a more thorough evaluation, and CT angiography (CTA) is also more likely than TEE to demonstrate extraluminal abnormalities, including pseudoaneurysm or blood extravasation in the mediastinum or pleural space.

MRI can visualize the entire aorta in multiple planes even without the use of intravascular contrast. MRI is excellent for detecting focal or extensive IMHs, which appear as areas of high-signal intensity within the aortic wall on T1-weighted images. MRI is excellent for differentiating PAUs from IMH, atherosclerotic plaque, and intraluminal chronic mural thrombus.[23]

PROGNOSIS AND MANAGEMENT

Despite differences in opinion regarding the natural history and management of PAUs, there is agreement that all PAUs, even those found incidentally, warrant close clinical and imaging follow-up, usually by CTA.[24] Surveillance imaging should be performed at intervals similar to those recommended for AD. Box 134.2 summarizes the clinical characteristics and imaging features of PAUs that mark a higher risk of progression or rupture and therefore might warrant closer follow-up or consideration for intervention.[25]

The excellent visualization of PAU by CTA has facilitated the treatment of symptomatic or high-risk PAU cases with TEVAR (Fig. 134.11), which has a significantly lower morbidity and mortality than does open surgical repair.[26] However, because this particular population tends to be older adults with extensive aortic atherosclerosis and high likelihood of concomitant coronary or cardiovascular disease, any intervention comes at increased periprocedural risk.

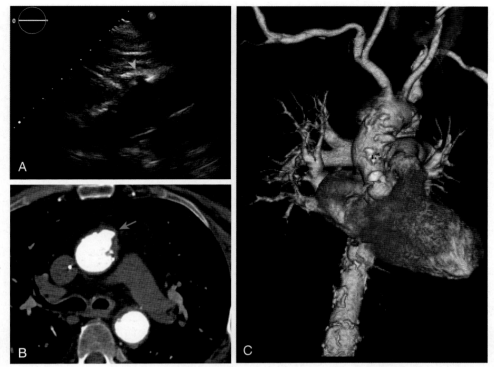

Figure 134.9. Penetrating aortic ulcer in the ascending aorta as initially detected on a transthoracic echocardiogram (**A**, *arrowhead*, Video 134.9). Subsequent axial contrast-enhanced computed tomography (CT) image confirms the presence of the penetrating atherosclerotic ulcer in the anterior wall of the ascending thoracic aorta (**B**, *arrow*). A surface-shaded display of CT angiography reveals multiple ulcers and a significant burden of aortic atherosclerosis in multiple segments of the aorta (**C**). (© Massachusetts General Hospital Thoracic Aortic Center, used with permission.)

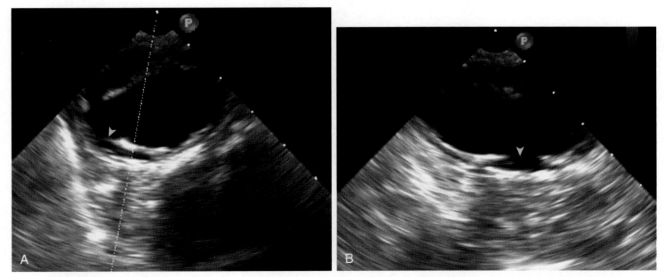

Figure 134.10. Penetrating aortic ulcer *(arrows)* in the descending aorta as visualized on biplane transesophageal echocardiography in the short-axis view (**A**) and the long-axis view (**B**). (© Massachusetts General Hospital Thoracic Aortic Center, used with permission.) (See accompanying Video 134.10.)

Please access ExpertConsult to view the corresponding videos for this chapter.

Acknowledgment

The authors acknowledge the contributions of Dr. Raimund Erbel, Dr. Sofia Churzidse, Dr. Riccardo Gorla, and Dr. Alexander Janosi, who were the authors of this chapter in the previous edition.

BOX 134.2 Adverse Predictors of Progression to Dissection or Rupture of Penetrating Aortic Ulcer

- Persistent symptoms despite medical treatment
- Enlarging pleural effusion
- Presence of intramural hematoma
- Maximal aortic diameter at ulcer site >55 mm
- Large size of initial penetrating aortic ulcer
  - Depth >10 mm
  - Width >20 mm
- Rapid rate of growth

Adapted with permission from Evangelista A, et al: Interdisciplinary expert consensus on management of type B intramural haematoma and penetrating aortic ulcer, Eur J Cardiothorac Surg 47:209–217, 2015.

REFERENCES

1. Clough RE, Nienaber CA. Management of acute aortic syndrome. *Nat Rev Cardiol*. 2015;12:103–114.
2. Evangelista A, Carro A, Moral S, et al. Imaging modalities for the early diagnosis of acute aortic syndrome. *Nat Rev Cardiol*. 2013;10:477–486.
3. Baliga RR, Nienaber CA, Bossone E, et al. The role of imaging in aortic dissection and related syndromes. *JACC Cardiovasc Imag*. 2014;7:406–424.
4. Kitai T, Kaji S, Yamamuro A, et al. Detection of intimal defect by 64-row multidetector computed tomography in patients with acute aortic intramural hematoma. *Circulation*. 2011;124(Suppl):S174–S178.
5. Evangelista A, Isselbacher EM, Bossone E, et al. Insights from the international Registry of acute aortic dissection: a 20-year experience of collaborative clinical research. *Circulation*. 2018;137:1846–1860.
6. Mussa FF, Horton JD, Moridzadeh R, et al. Acute aortic dissection and intramural hematoma: a systematic review. *J Am Med Assoc*. 2016;316:754–763.
7. Harris KM, Braverman AC, Eagle KA, et al. Acute aortic intramural hematoma: an analysis from the International Registry of Acute Aortic Dissection. *Circulation*. 2012;126(Suppl):S91–S96.
8. Alomari IB, Hamirani YS, Madera G, et al. Aortic intramural hematoma and its complications. *Circulation*. 2014;129:711–716.
9. Evangelista A, Maldonado G, Moral S, et al. Intramural hematoma and penetrating ulcer in the descending aorta: differences and similarities. *Ann Cardiothorac Surg*. 2019;8:456–470.
10. Gutschow SE, Walker CM, Martinez-Jimenez S, et al. Emerging concepts in intramural hematoma imaging. *Radiographics*. 2016;36:660–674.
11. Kitai T, Kaji S, Yamamuro A, et al. Impact of new development of ulcer-like projection on clinical outcomes in patients with type B aortic dissection with closed and thrombosed false lumen. *Circulation*. 2010;122:S74–S780.

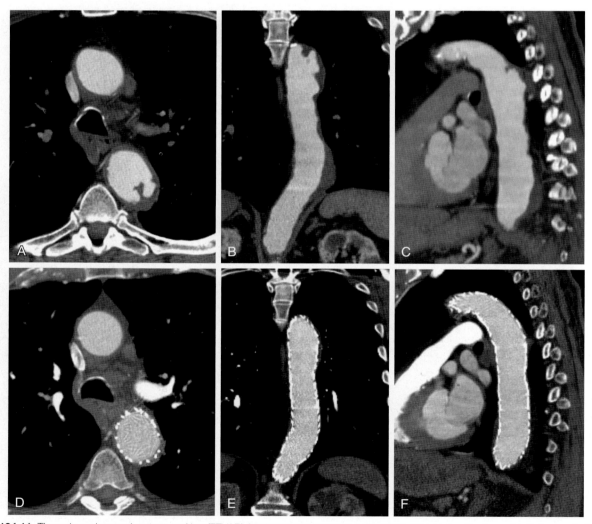

Figure 134.11. Thoracic endovascular stent grafting (TEVAR) for the management of penetrating atherosclerotic ulcers. Multiple penetrating aortic ulcers are present in the descending thoracic aorta as visualized on axial (**A**), coronal (**B**), and sagittal computed tomography angiography (**C**) images. After placement of an endovascular stent graft, marked regression of the ulcers is observed in the axial (**D**), coronal (**E**), and sagittal (**F**) images. (© Massachusetts General Hospital Thoracic Aortic Center, used with permission.)

12. Moral S, Cuellar H, Avegliano G, et al. Clinical implications of focal intimal disruption in patients with type B intramural hematoma. *J Am Coll Cardiol.* 2017;69:28–39.
13. Pelzel JM, Braverman AC, Hirsch AT, Harris KM. International heterogeneity in diagnostic frequency and clinical outcomes of ascending aortic intramural hematoma. *J Am Soc Echocardiogr.* 2007;20:1260–1268.
14. Evangelista A, Mukherjee D, Mehta RH, et al. Acute intramural hematoma of the aorta: a mystery in evolution. *Circulation.* 2005;111:1063–1070.
15. Hiratzka LF, Bakris GL, Beckman JA, et al. 2010 ACCF/AHA/AATS/ACR/ASA/SCA/SCAI/SIR/STS/SVM guidelines for the diagnosis and management of patients with thoracic aortic disease. *Circulation.* 2010;121:e266–e369.
16. Piffaretti G, Lomazzi C, Benedetto F, et al. Best medical treatment and selective stent-graft repair for acute type B aortic intramural hematoma. *Semin Thorac Cardiovasc Surg.* 2018;30:279–287.
17. Eggebrecht H, Plicht B, Kahlert P, Erbel R. Intramural hematoma and penetrating ulcers: indications to endovascular treatment. *Eur J Vasc Endovasc Surg.* 2009;38:659–665.
18. Stanson AW, Kazmier FJ, Hollier LH, et al. Penetrating atherosclerotic ulcers of the thoracic aorta: natural history and clinicopathologic correlations. *Ann Vasc Surg.* 1986;1:15–23.
19. Nathan DP, Boonn W, Lai E, et al. Presentation, complications, and natural history of penetrating atherosclerotic ulcer disease. *J Vasc Surg.* 2012;55:10–15.
20. Sebastia C, Evangelista A, Quiroga S, et al. Predictive value of small ulcers in the evolution of acute type B intramural hematoma. *Eur J Radiol.* 2012;81:1569–1574.
21. Vilacosta I, San Roman JA, Aragoncillo P, et al. Penetrating atherosclerotic aortic ulcer: Documentation by transesophageal echocardiography. *J Am Coll Cardiol.* 1998;32:83–89.
22. Welch TJ, Stanson AW, Sheedy PF 2nd, et al. Radiologic evaluation of penetrating aortic atherosclerotic ulcer. *Radiographics.* 1990;10:675–685.
23. Yucel EK, Steinberg FL, Egglin TK, et al. Penetrating aortic ulcers: diagnosis with MR imaging. *Radiology.* 1990;177:779–781.
24. Gifford SM, Duncan AA, Greiten LE, et al. The natural history and outcomes for thoracic and abdominal penetrating aortic ulcers. *J Vasc Surg.* 2016;63:1182–1188.
25. Evangelista A, Czerny M, Nienaber C, et al. Interdisciplinary expert consensus on management of type B intramural haematoma and penetrating aortic ulcer. *Eur J Cardio Thorac Surg.* 2015;47:209–217.
26. Eggebrecht H, Herold U, Schmermund A, et al. Endovascular stent-graft treatment of penetrating aortic ulcer: results over a median follow-up of 27 months. *Am Heart J.* 2006;151:530–536.

135 Blunt Aortic Trauma

Philippe Vignon, Roberto M. Lang

Blunt aortic trauma (BAT) is a life-threatening injury because most patients die at the scene, and delayed adventitial rupture may occur during hospitalization.[1] Multiplane transesophageal echocardiography (TEE) and contrast-enhanced helical computed tomography (CT) have similar diagnostic accuracy for the identification of BAT that requires repair.[2,3] Historically, BAT constituted a surgical emergency to avoid lethal adventitial rupture. Progressively, delayed repair was proposed in specific patients, and aortic stent grafting has supplanted conventional surgery.[1] Subtle aortic injuries with spontaneous favorable outcome may also be encountered.[3,4]

PATHOPHYSIOLOGY AND CLASSIFICATION

BAT involves the aortic isthmus in about 90% of the cases.[1] This aortic segment is located between the origin of the left subclavian artery and the first intercostal arteries, where the mobile aortic arch becomes relatively fixed to the thoracic cage. During an abrupt deceleration (e.g., head-on collision, lateral impact, vertical deceleration), generated traction, rotation, and shearing forces act maximally in this region.[5] BAT rarely involves other anatomic segments of the aorta in patients who reach the hospital alive. Direct aortic injury is uncommon. Because blunt cardiac injuries share the same pathophysiology,[5] they may be associated with BAT.[6]

The most common BAT type is contained disruptions involving the entire depth of intimal and medial layers. In this case, adventitia and surrounding tissues allow a temporary hemostasis. Because of the risk of lethal free rupture, timely diagnosis, rigorous blood pressure control, and rapid repair of contained BAT are widely advocated.[1,5] Traumatic aortic dissection and intramural hematoma are less frequent. Superficial aortic injuries solely involve the intimal layer. They are too small and superficial to exert an excess of pressure on the adventitial layer and therefore have a benign natural history.[3,4]

A classification of BAT has been proposed[4]: type I, intimal tear; type II, intramural hematoma; type III, pseudoaneurysm; and type IV, rupture. Type I injuries usually heal spontaneously,[3,4] whereas other types require correction. Exposed collagenous fibers by an intimal tear may constitute a nidus on which acute thrombus formation and related arterial embolism may occur (Fig. 135.1). False aneurysm formation associated with types III and IV may be asymmetrical. Type IV injuries may lead to abrupt death if blood extravasation is not temporarily contained by adjacent anatomical structures.

DEMOGRAPHICS AND PRESENTING SYMPTOMS

BAT is usually diagnosed in individuals involved in high-velocity motor vehicle crashes or falls from heights or in pedestrians hit by motor vehicles.[1] Patients sustaining a BAT frequently fail to exhibit external signs of direct chest wall injury[2] but commonly present with severe multisystem trauma.[1,7] Among described radiographic findings,[2] the presence of a widened mediastinum is most frequently sought on clinical grounds to suspect BAT.[7] Nevertheless, an apparently unremarkable mediastinal contour does not exclude the presence of an underlying BAT.[1,8] Accordingly, no clinical or radiographic sign is accurate enough to efficiently identify patients presenting with a BAT. Indicators suggestive of high-energy impact to the body can be used to select high-risk patients who should undergo additional work-up to confidently exclude a BAT[7] (Table 135.1).

TRANSESOPHAGEAL ECHOCARDIOGRAPHIC FINDINGS

Because BAT involves almost exclusively the anatomic region corresponding to the aortic isthmus,[1] transthoracic echocardiography (TTE) is *not* indicated because of poor diagnostic capability.[9] In contrast, TEE allows precise assessment of this aortic segment and provides valuable information on both the depth and extension of BAT at the bedside.[3,10] This allows best guiding initial management of these frequently unstable patients because BAT at risk of blood extravasation require prompt correction, as opposed to type I injuries[11] (see Fig. 135.1).

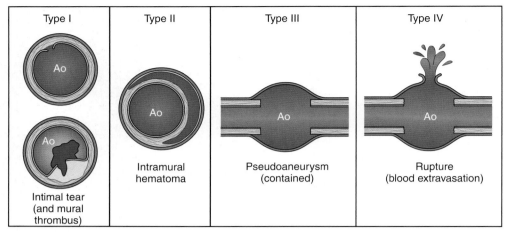

Figure 135.1. Schematic representation of proposed classification for blunt aortic trauma. Type I injuries may be managed conservatively because they usually heal spontaneously, whereas other types require correction (see text for details). *Ao,* Aorta. (Adapted from Azizzadeh A, et al: Blunt traumatic aortic injury: initial experience with endovascular repair, *J Vasc Surg* 49:1403–1408, 2009.)

TABLE 135.1 Indicators Used to Identify Patients at High Risk of Sustaining Blunt Aortic Trauma

- Violent deceleration (head-on collision, lateral impact, fall from a height >4 m), unrestrained patient ejected from vehicle, pedestrian or bicyclist struck by a motor vehicle, death(s) in accident
- Chest trauma requiring mechanical ventilation, associated traumatic injury reflecting marked shearing forces transmitted to deep organs at the time of impact (e.g., diaphragmatic rupture, mesenteric tear)
- Pseudocoarctation syndrome, large left hemothorax, unexplained hypotension or shock
- Radiographic findings consistent with mediastinal hematoma or false aneurysm formation: widened mediastinum, abnormal mediastinal contour

TABLE 135.2 Differential Diagnostic Criteria Using Transesophageal Echocardiography to Distinguish Subadventitial Blunt Aortic Trauma and Aortic Dissection

Subadventitial Blunt Aortic Trauma	Aortic Dissection
TWO-DIMENSIONAL IMAGING	**TWO-DIMENSIONAL IMAGING**
• Medial flap reflecting disrupted aortic wall (entire depth of intimal and medial layers): thick, near perpendicular to aortic walls (90 degrees), reduced mobility	• Intimal flap reflecting dissected aortic wall (delimits two distinct channels): thin, near parallel to aortic walls (90 degrees), variable mobility within cardiac cycle
• False aneurysm formation: abnormal aortic contour (because frequently asymmetrical), variable enlargement	• No false aneurysm: normal aortic contour, consistent symmetrical enlargement
• Mediastinal hematoma: frequent (large)[a]	• Mediastinal hematoma: not frequent
• Left hemothorax: frequent (large)[b]	• Left hemothorax: not frequent
COLOR DOPPLER MAPPING	**COLOR DOPPLER MAPPING**
• Similar blood flow velocities on both sides of the medial flap	• Slower blood flow velocities in the false lumen ± thrombus formation
• Mosaic of colors surrounding the disrupted wall (blood flow turbulence)	• Near laminar flow (except in the vicinity of an entry or reentry tear)
• No entry or reentry tear	• Presence of entry or reentry tears
LOCATION OF ECHOCARDIOGRAPHIC FINDINGS	**LOCATION OF ECHOCARDIOGRAPHIC FINDINGS**
• Confined to the aortic isthmus (25–35 cm from incisors)	• Variable spatial extension on the thoracic aorta, according to anatomic type

[a]Consistent with type IV blunt aortic trauma when large and not associated with other sources of posterior hemomediastinum (e.g., vertebral fractures).[12]

[b]Consistent with type IV blunt aortic trauma when large and no other explanation.

Adapted from Vignon P, et al: Role of transesophageal echocardiography in the diagnosis and management of traumatic aortic disruption, *Circulation* 92:2959–2968, 1995.

TEE findings associated with subadventitial (i.e., contained) BAT (type III injury) are usually confined to the aortic isthmus and must be differentiated from those encountered in spontaneous aortic dissection (Table 135.2).[10] The presence of a thick and irregular medial flap or torn aortic wall appendages within the aortic lumen reflects the injury to both the intimal and medial layers.[10] In the longitudinal view (90 degrees), the medial flap typically crosses the entire vascular lumen almost perpendicularly to the aortic wall because the disruption is confined to the aortic isthmus (Fig. 135.2). It usually fails to oscillate during the cardiac cycle and to delimit two distinct aortic channels, as opposed to the intimal flap of aortic dissection. Accordingly, blood flow velocities evaluated by color Doppler are usually similar on both sides of the medial flap.[10] A mosaic of colors is frequently observed at the site and vicinity of the aortic wall disruption because of the presence of local blood flow turbulence (see Fig. 135.2). A pseudocoarctation syndrome may be identified in the presence of a vascular obstruction by the disrupted aortic wall (Fig. 135.3). Acute false aneurysm formation resulting from excess of pressure on adventitial layer usually appears as a localized deformity of the vascular lumen, which may increase aortic size or not.[10] Concomitant hemomediastinum and left hemothorax are frequently observed (see Table 135.2). Although nonspecific, large hemomediastinum and major left hemothorax more likely reflect BTA with associated blood extravasation, consistent with a type IV injury.[12] The size of aortic false aneurysm and hemomediastinum indirectly reflects the risk of free adventitial rupture (type IV injury) (Fig. 135.4).[13]

Traumatic aortic dissection may occur at any age secondary to severe blunt chest trauma.[1,14] TEE findings are similar to those associated with spontaneous aortic dissection (see Table 135.2 and Fig. 135.2). It usually involves the descending thoracic aorta (Fig. 135.5). Traumatic intramural hematoma

Aortic disruption

Aortic dissection

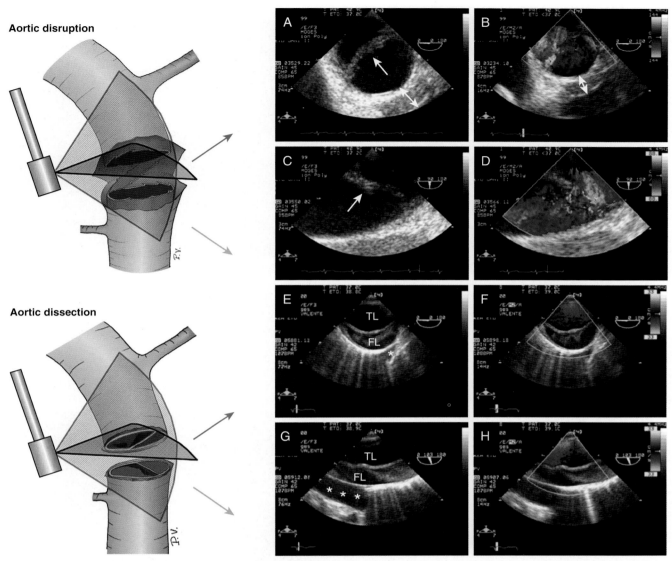

Figure 135.2. Schematic representation and comparative transesophageal echocardiography findings associated with subadventitial disruption (type III injury) of the aortic isthmus *(upper panels)* and spontaneous aortic dissection *(lower panels)* in both the transversal (0 degrees, **A, B, E,** and **F**) and longitudinal (90 degrees, **C, D, G,** and **H**) views. The thick medial flap associated with aortic disruption (**A,** *arrow*) is associated with a mild hemomediastinum (**A** and **B,** *double-headed arrows*). It fails to delimit two aortic channels as depicted by color Doppler (**B**) and is confined to the aortic isthmus because it appears almost perpendicular to aortic walls in the longitudinal view (**C,** *arrow*). Blood turbulences are depicted by color Doppler in the vicinity or disrupted aortic wall (**D**). In contrast, the intimal flap of aortic dissection is thinner and delimits a true lumen (TL) and a false lumen (FL; **E** and **G**). It is almost parallel to aortic walls in the longitudinal view because the process is more extended anatomically (**G** and **H**). Blood flow velocity is lower in the false lumen, as reflected by color Doppler (**F** and **H**) and a thrombus formation (**E–H**). Note the presence of a small left pleural effusion (**E** and **G,** *asterisks*).

(type II injury) also commonly involves the descending thoracic aorta. Similar to spontaneous intramural hematoma,[15] it appears as a circular or crescentic thickening of the aortic wall with no flap (see Fig. 135.4).

Superficial BAT (type I injuries) include intimal tears and potentially associated mobile thrombi (see Fig. 135.1). They are also commonly located at or in the vicinity of the aortic isthmus.[3,10] Both the aortic size and contour are unchanged, and blood flow assessed by color Doppler remains laminar. Associated hemomediastinum is uncommon. Intimal tears appear as thin and mobile intraluminal appendages of the aortic wall[10] (see Fig. 135.4). Wall thrombi may be voluminous and may result in peripheral arterial emboli when highly mobile (see Fig. 135.4). The

frequency of these aortic injuries is presumably underrated because they usually remain underestimated by CT.[3,10]

DIAGNOSIS

TTE is not adequately suited for the accurate identification of BAT and should therefore not be used in this specific clinical setting.[9] TEE and CT have a similar diagnostic accuracy for the identification of type III and type IV BAT, whereas TEE appears more sensitive for the diagnosis of type I injuries and of blunt cardiac injuries.[3,10] CT is advantageously used in hemodynamically stable patients with multisystem trauma because it allows a precise identification of frequently associated traumatic injuries.[3] Alternatively,

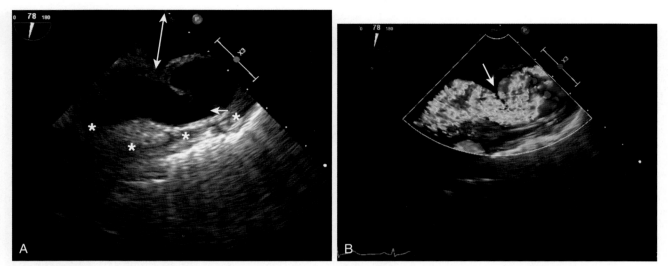

Figure 135.3. Subadventitial aortic disruption (type III injury) with associated pseudocoarctation syndrome. In the longitudinal transesophageal echocardiography view, the torn aortic walls result in a pseudocoarctation syndrome (**A**, *arrow*), as reflected by a highly turbulent and narrowed descending aortic blood flow depicted by color Doppler (**B**). Note the presence of a large hemomediastinum (**A**, *double-headed arrow* and *asterisks*).

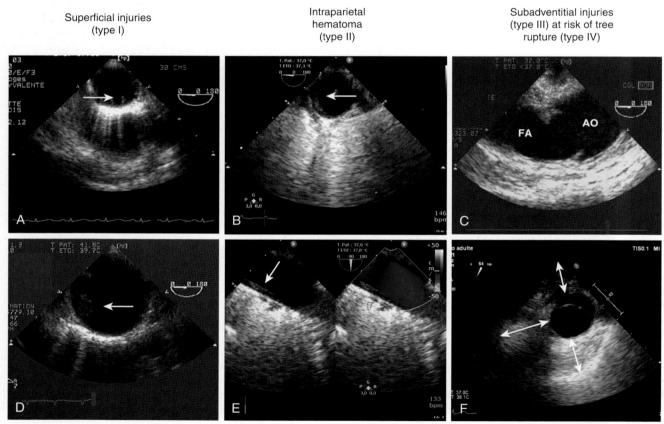

Figure 135.4. Examples of blunt aortic injuries depicted by transesophageal echocardiography. Superficial blunt injuries (type I) to the aortic isthmus (AO) include intimal tears (**A**, *arrow*) and mural thrombus (**D**, *arrow*). They are not associated with abnormal aortic contour or size or with associated hemomediastinum. These superficial lesions usually regress spontaneously with conservative management. Intramural hematoma (type II injury) also predominantly involves the descending thoracic *aorta*. It appears as a crescentic thickening of the aortic wall with no flap in the transversal view (**B**, *arrow*), and as a linear thickening of the injured aortic wall with normal laminar blood flow in the longitudinal view (**D**, *arrow*). Subadventitial aortic disruption (type III injury) may be associated with a large false aneurysm (FA) formation (**C**) or large posterior hemomediastinum surrounding the disrupted descending thoracic aorta (**F**, *double-headed arrows*). These findings should be interpreted as severity signs indirectly reflecting the threat of imminent free adventitial rupture (type IV injury). These aortic injuries must be repaired immediately (see text for details).

TEE is ideally suited for the assessment of ventilated, hemodynamically unstable patients at the bedside.[3] Its diagnostic accuracy for the identification of BAT has been reviewed elsewhere.[16] Traumatic injuries to aortic branches lead to false-negative TEE findings.[3] False-positive TEE findings may be related to ultrasound artifacts or atherosclerotic change.[17,18] Simple TEE differential diagnostic criteria allow accurate distinction between linear intraluminal artifacts and aortic flaps.[19] European Society of Cardiology guidelines recommend performing CT when BAT is suspected (class I, level C) and to consider using TEE if CT is not available (class II, level C).[20] Eastern Association for the Surgery of Trauma (EAST) guidelines strongly recommend the use of CT in patients with suspected BAT.[21]

Intravascular ultrasonography has been proposed as an alternative imaging modality in the presence of equivocal CT but also to help determining the optimal size and point of implantation of aortic stent graft in patients with BAT who are eligible for endovascular repair.[22] Magnetic resonance imaging has been proposed to serially assess stabilized patients with BAT,[23] but imaging time and inaccessibility of the patient during the procedure preclude its routine use in unstable trauma patients. Angiography has virtually no indication other than suspected disruption of aortic branches.

INITIAL MANAGEMENT

Rigorous blood pressure control and timely correction of BAT remain widely advocated to prevent lethal adventitial rupture.[1] To reduce the risk of aortic rupture, mean blood pressure should not exceed 80 mm Hg.[4,24] Historically, immediate surgical repair was the reference treatment of BAT because more than 90% of lethal adventitial rupture occur within the first 24 hours after hospital admission.[24] To reduce the risk of worsening associated injuries by surgery and circulatory assistance techniques, delayed BAT repair was then proposed, with improved survival.[25] During the past decade, endovascular repair of BAT has progressively supplanted conventional surgery[1,26] because it minimizes the risk of paraplegia and reduces mortality rates.[26,27] Nevertheless, the high incidence of device-related serious complications remains a concern, the most common being the presence of endoleak.[1] In addition, the long-term mechanical properties of stent grafts are yet unknown.[1] Current recommendations, which are weak with a very low quality of evidence (grade 2, level C), suggest early (<24-hour) endovascular repair of types II to IV BAT with suitable anatomy rather than surgery,[11,20] barring associated severe injuries, or immediately after other injuries have been treated.[11] EAST strongly recommend the use of endovascular repair in patients diagnosed with BAT who do not have contraindications for aortic stent grafting.[21] The early (<24-hour)[11] versus delayed (>24-hour)[21] timing of BAT correction remains debated. Immediate endovascular repair is indicated in patients with complete aortic rupture and free bleeding into the mediastinum (type IV injury)[20,28] or pseudocoarctation syndrome.[28] In other cases, BAT repair may be delayed to allow for patient stabilization before performing the procedure in the best possible conditions.[20,28]

In addition to its diagnostic capacity, TEE provides valuable information that helps guide early management of patients with BAT.[13] The severity TEE findings, which include the presence of a large posterior hemomediastinum (blood extravasation), deep false aneurysm formation (imminent risk of free adventitial rupture), or pseudocoarctation syndrome (risk of organ hypoperfusion), should prompt BAT repair[13] (see Fig. 135.4). When endovascular repair is indicated, TEE allows real-time guidance of endovascular stent-graft implantation and early diagnosis of related complications[29]

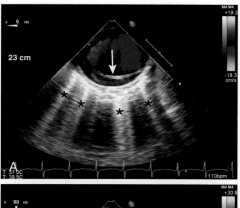

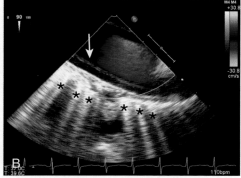

Figure 135.5. Traumatic dissection of the descending thoracic aorta depicted by color Doppler transesophageal echocardiography. In the transverse view, a thin intimal flap (**A**, *arrow*) separates the true circulating lumen from the noncirculating and partially thrombosed false lumen. In the longitudinal view, the intimal flap is parallel to aortic walls because the dissection extends to the entire descending thoracic aorta (**B**, *arrow*). Note the moderate and regular (symmetrical) enlargement of the aorta without associated hemomediastinum or left hemothorax, as reflected by the presence of B lines *(asterisks)*.

(Fig. 135.6 and Video 135.6). Type I BAT can be managed conservatively with serial imaging follow-up[11,20] because they typically regress spontaneously.[3,10] The decision to intervene and its timing should be guided by potential symptoms and progression of BAT.[11] Although safe conservative management of Type II injuries has recently been reported,[30] further prospective confirmation is required.

CONCLUSION

In the setting of ventilated unstable patients sustaining severe multisystem trauma who are at risk of BAT, TEE allows an alternative, safe, rapid, and accurate identification of cardiovascular injuries at the bedside. TEE also helps guiding initial therapeutic management of patients with BAT in precisely characterizing the depth and extension of vessel injury, monitoring endovascular stent-graft implantation, and diagnosing potential early related complications. CT is recommended as the first-line imaging modality for the evaluation of patients at high risk of BAT and for follow-up after aortic repair but appears less sensitive than TEE for the diagnosis of superficial aortic injuries and potentially associated cardiac trauma.

Please access ExpertConsult to view the corresponding videos for this chapter.

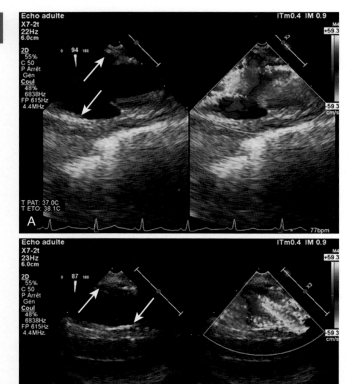

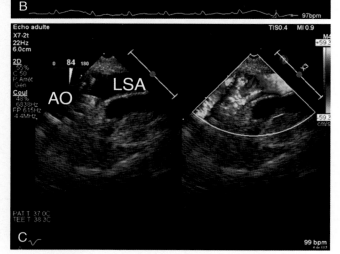

Figure 135.6. Transesophageal echocardiography (TEE)–guided thoracic endovascular repair of a traumatic false aneurysm formation. In the longitudinal view of the proximal descending aorta, TEE depicts a false aneurysm formation (**A,** *arrows*) associated with a mild hemomediastinum and limited blood flow turbulences using color Doppler mapping. TEE confirms the adequate deployment and location of aortic stent graft in the proximal descending aorta that fully covers the false aneurysm formation (**B,** *arrows*). TEE also allows visualizing the take-off and initial anatomic portion of the left subclavian artery to ensure adequate perfusion after the deployment of covered endovascular stent with color Doppler mapping (**C,** *arrow*). *AO,* Distal aortic arch; *LSA,* take-off of the left subclavian artery. (Also see Video 135.6.)

REFERENCES

1. Demetriades D. Blunt thoracic aortic injuries: crossing the Rubicon. *J Am Coll Surg.* 2012;214:247–259.
2. Patel NH, Stephens KE, Mirvis SE, et al. Imaging of acute thoracic aortic injury due to blunt trauma: a review. *Radiology.* 1998;209:335–348.
3. Vignon P, Boncoeur MP, François B, et al. Comparison of multiplane transesophageal echocardiography and contrast-enhanced helical CT in the diagnosis of blunt traumatic cardiovascular injuries. *Anesthesiology.* 2001;94:615–622.
4. Azizzadeh A, Keyhani K, Miller CC, et al. Blunt traumatic aortic injury: initial experience with endovascular repair. *J Vasc Surg.* 2009;49:1403–1408.
5. Prêtre R, Chilcott M. Blunt trauma to the heart and great vessels. *New Engl J Med.* 1997;336:626–632.
6. Rambaud G, François B, Cornu E, et al. Diagnosis and management of traumatic aortic regurgitation associated with laceration of the aortic isthmus. *J Trauma.* 1999;46:717–720.
7. Mosquera VX, Marini M, Muniz J, et al. Traumatic aortic injury score (TRAINS): an easy and simple score for early detection of traumatic aortic injuries in major trauma patients with associated blunt chest trauma. *Intensive Care Med.* 2012;38:1487–1496.
8. Vignon P, Lagrange P, Boncoeur MP, et al. Routine transesophageal echocardiography for the diagnosis of aortic disruption in trauma patients without enlarged mediastinum. *J Trauma.* 1996;40:422–427.
9. Chirillo F, Totis O, Cavarzerani A, et al. Usefulness of transthoracic and transesophageal echocardiography in recognition and management of cardiovascular injuries after blunt chest trauma. *Heart.* 1996;75:301–306.
10. Vignon P, Guéret P, Vedrinne JM, et al. Role of transesophageal echocardiography in the diagnosis and management of traumatic aortic disruption. *Circulation.* 1995;92:2959–2968.
11. Lee WA, Matsumura JS, Mitchell RS, et al. Endovascular repair of traumatic thoracic aortic injury: clinical practice guidelines of the Society for Vascular Surgery. *J Vasc Surg.* 2011;53:187–192.
12. Vignon P, Rambaud G, François B, et al. Quantification of traumatic hemomediastinum using transesophageal echocardiography: impact on patient management. *Chest.* 1998;113:1475–1480.
13. Vignon P, Martaillé JF, François B, et al. Transesophageal echocardiography and therapeutic management of patients sustaining blunt aortic injuries. *J Trauma.* 2005;58:1150–1158.
14. Rogers FB, Osler TM, Shackford SR. Aortic dissection after trauma: case report and review of the literature. *J Trauma.* 1996;41:906–908.
15. Vilacosta I, San Roman JA, Ferreiros J, et al. Natural history and serial morphology of aortic intramural hematoma: a novel variant of aortic dissection. *Am Heart J.* 1997;134:495–507.
16. Cinnella G, Dambrosio M, Brienza N, et al. Transesophageal echocardiography for diagnosis of traumatic aortic injury: an appraisal of the evidence. *J Trauma.* 2004;57:1246–1255.
17. Oxorn D, Towers M. Traumatic aortic disruption: false positive diagnosis on transesophageal echocardiography. *J Trauma.* 1995;39:386–387.
18. Minard G, Schurr MJ, Croce MA, et al. A prospective analysis of transesophageal echocardiography in the diagnosis of traumatic disruption of the aorta. *J Trauma.* 1996;40:225–230.
19. Vignon P, Spencer KT, Rambaud G, et al. Differential transesophageal echocardiographic diagnosis between linear artifacts and intraluminal flap of aortic dissection or disruption. *Chest.* 2001;119:1778–1790.
20. Erbel R, Aboyans V, Boileau C, et al. ESC guidelines on the diagnosis and treatment of aortic diseases. *Eur Heart J.* 2014;35:2873–2926. 2014.
21. Fox N, Schwartz D, Salazar JH, et al. Evaluation and management of blunt traumatic aortic injury: a practice guideline from the Eastern Association for the Surgery of Trauma. *J Trauma Acute Care Surg.* 2015;78:136–146.
22. Shi Y, Tsai PI, Wall MJ, et al. Intravascular ultrasound enhanced aortic sizing for endovascular treatment of blunt aortic injury: results of an American Association for the Surgery of Trauma multicenter study. *J Trauma Acute Care Surg.* 2015;79:817–821.
23. Fattori R, Celletti F, Bertaccini P, et al. Delayed surgery of traumatic aortic rupture. Role of magnetic resonance imaging. *Circulation.* 1996;94:2865–2870.
24. Fabian TC, Richardson D, Croce MA, et al. Prospective study of blunt aortic injury: multicentre trial of the American Association for the Surgery of Trauma. *J Trauma.* 1997;42:374–380.
25. Demetriades D, Velmahos GC, Scalea TM, et al. Blunt traumatic thoracic aortic injuries: early or delayed repair—results of an American Association for the Surgery of Trauma prospective study. *J Trauma.* 2009;66:967–973.
26. Scalea TM, Feliciano DV, DuBose JJ, et al. Blunt thoracic aortic injury: endovascular repair is now the standard. *J Am Coll Surg.* 2019;228:605–612.
27. Demetriades D, Velmahos GC, Scalea TM, et al. Operative repair or endovascular stent graft in blunt traumatic thoracic aortic injuries: results of an American Association for the Surgery of Trauma multicenter study. *J Trauma.* 2008;64:561–570.
28. Grabenwoger M, Alfonso F, Bachet J, et al. Thoracic endovascular aortic repair (TEVAR) for the treatment of aortic diseases: a position statement from the European association for Cardio-thoracic surgery (EACTS) and the European Society of Cardiology (ESC), in collaboration with the European association of Percutaneous cardiovascular Interventions (EAPCI). *Eur Heart J.* 2012;33:1558–1563.
29. Metaxa V, Tsagourias M, Matamis D. The role of echocardiography in the early diagnosis of the complications of endovascular repair of blunt aortic injury. *J Crit Care.* 2011;26. 434.e7–434.e12.
30. Spencer SM, Safcsak K, Smith CP, et al. Nonoperative management rather than endovascular repair may be safe for grade II blunt traumatic injuries: an 11-year retrospective analysis. *J Trauma Acute Care Surg.* 2018;84:133–138.

136 Intraoperative Echocardiography

Erin S. Grawe, Jack S. Shanewise

Transesophageal echocardiography (TEE) was used as a monitoring and diagnostic tool during cardiac surgery in the operating room (OR) as soon as TEE probes became available in the 1980s. The first report of use in the OR came in 1980 from New York City, where transesophageal M-mode echocardiography was used to monitor left ventricular dimensions during various stages of cardiac surgery. Not only were the TEE images found to correlate well with the standard parasternal transthoracic echocardiography (TTE) images, but the findings were also consistent with changes seen in cardiac output and atrial pressures measured by pulmonary artery catheter.[1] In 1982, a 3.5-MHz phased-array TEE probe was introduced that could create two-dimensional (2D) images of the heart as well as Doppler measurements of the mitral valve flow.[2] Due to its ability to acquire high-quality images of the heart in real time without interfering in the surgical field, TEE quickly became a widely used imaging modality during cardiac surgery. In 1985, Smith and colleagues reported that new segmental wall motion abnormalities detected using TEE 2D images were a more sensitive indicator of myocardial ischemia than electrocardiography in high-risk patients undergoing coronary bypass grafting (CABG) or vascular surgery.[3]

Since then, TEE has become a common monitor for the diagnosis and management of patients undergoing cardiac surgery. Its advantages are that it is minimally invasive, easy to introduce, does not interfere with the surgical field, and provides real-time information on cardiac performance during surgery in which hemodynamic conditions change very rapidly. It allows for the evaluation of structural and functional aspects of the heart, and it serves as a useful hemodynamic monitoring tool, providing information regarding cardiac output and fluid responsiveness during changing intraoperative conditions. Finally, TEE can also identify residual defects after surgical intervention to enable an immediate correction if necessary.

Intraoperative TEE findings influence surgical decision making in 7% to 25% of CABG and valve cases.[4–6] TEE has also been shown to provide useful information during congenital cardiac surgery[7] and the growing field of ventricular assist device implantation and management.[8] TEE findings can contribute to anesthetic management during cardiac surgery, including decisions regarding fluid administration, initiation of anti-ischemic therapy, vasopressor or inotropic support, vasodilator therapy, and adjusting the depth of anesthesia.[9,10] These studies provide support that TEE monitoring is a safe and viable tool that significantly affects the decision-making process in the intraoperative care of cardiac surgery patients and may contribute to optimal care.

Intraoperative TEE differs from standard diagnostic TEE is several critical ways: time constraints may require a more focused examination; altered loading conditions of general anesthesia may affect the evaluation of valve and ventricular dysfunction' baseline and postintervention evaluations should have matched loading conditions for valid comparisons; and urgent decision making based on imaging information may be necessary.[11] The American Society of Echocardiography (ASE) and the Society of Cardiovascular Anesthesiologists (SCA) have issued guidelines for performing an intraoperative TEE[12] and for training in perioperative echocardiography.[13] In 1996, the American Society of Anesthesiologists and SCA published practice guidelines for perioperative TEE,[14] which were updated in 2010.[15]

INTRAOPERATIVE TRANSESOPHAGEAL ECHOCARDIOGRAPHY: THE THORACIC AORTA

The ASE/SCA guidelines on performing an intraoperative TEE describe six views of the thoracic aorta[12]; these are the short- and long-axis views of (1) the proximal and mid ascending aorta, (2) the thoracic descending aorta, and (3) the distal and mid aortic arch. The proximal and mid ascending aorta are seen through a midesophageal window with the probe advanced about 30 cm from the incisors. This places the transducer at the level of the right pulmonary artery. The ascending aorta short-axis view is developed by placing the ascending aorta in the center of the screen and adjusting the multiplane angle between 0 and 60 degrees until it appears as a circular structure. The multiplane angle is then advanced between 100 and 150 degrees to develop the ascending aorta long-axis view, in which it appears as a tubular structure (Fig. 136.1A and B). Evaluation of the descending thoracic aorta is accomplished by rotating the probe counterclockwise to the patient's left from the midesophageal four-chamber view until the descending thoracic aorta is seen in short axis. The image depth is decreased to 6 or 8 cm, and the focus field is adjusted to the near field to optimize image quality. The entire descending thoracic aorta and upper abdominal aorta is imaged by advancing and withdrawing the probe along the esophagus and into the stomach. The long-axis view of the descending aorta is achieved by adjusting the multiplane angle from 0 to between 90 and 110 degrees until the structure appears in long axis (Fig. 136.1C and D). Modern echocardiographic systems with three-dimensional capability allow simultaneous viewing of the short and long-axis views. Finally, the aortic arch is visualized with the multiplane angle at 0 degrees. This is usually achieved by first finding the descending thoracic aorta in short axis, then withdrawing the probe, while maintaining the image in the center of the screen, until the upper esophagus is reached, approximately 20 to 25 cm from the incisors. This will develop the distal aortic arch in long axis. To visualize the mid aortic arch, the probe is withdrawn farther and turned to the right to keep the vessel in view. The multiplane angle is then advanced to 90 degrees to develop the aortic arch in short axis (Fig. 136.1E and F). The probe is rotated to the patient's right to visualize the arch proximally and to the left to visualize the arch more distally. The thoracic aorta should be examined carefully with TEE from the diaphragm to the aortic valve looking for abnormalities such as atherosclerosis, aneurysm, and dissection.

One of the main goals of the evaluation of the thoracic aorta by TEE during cardiac surgery in adults is to assess the atherosclerotic burden. Cardiac surgery typically involves cannulating and clamping of the ascending aorta. It is well known that atherosclerosis of the ascending aorta and the aortic arch are important risk factors for perioperative stroke secondary to a cerebral embolism during aortic cannulation and cardiopulmonary bypass (CPB).[16–21] In an attempt to define the risk of atheromatous embolization during surgical manipulation, several grading systems have been developed using TEE imaging to quantify the severity of plaque burden.[22] Most of these grading systems take into account the degree of intimal thickness, the distance the atheroma protrudes into the aortic lumen, and the presence of mobile components.[16–18,20] There have been no studies to date validating one grading system over another. However, there have been several studies that demonstrate an association between the severity of atheromatous plaque and adverse

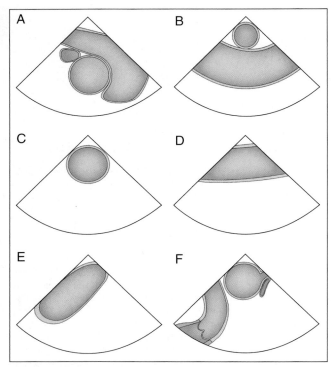

Figure 136.1. Cross-sectional transesophageal echocardiography views of the ascending aorta short axis (**A**), ascending aorta long axis (**B**), descending thoracic aorta short axis (**C**), descending thoracic aorta long axis (**D**), aortic arch long axis (**E**), and aortic arch short axis (**F**). (Adapted with permission from Shanewise JS, et al: ASE/SCA guidelines for performing a comprehensive intraoperative multiplane transesophageal echocardiography examination, *J Am Soc Echocardiogr* 12:884–900, 1999.)

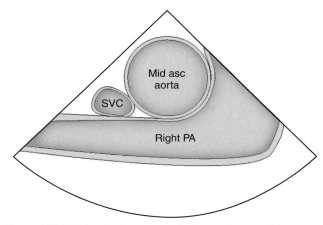

Figure 136.2. Epiaortic ultrasonography image diagram of the short-axis view. *Mid asc,* Mid ascending; *PA,* pulmonary artery; *SVC,* superior vena cava.

neurologic injury form embolization.[19–21] Literature does agree that certain plaque characteristics are associated with a higher risk of neurologic injury; these include a height or thickness greater than 3 mm, location in the ascending aorta, or any mobile component to the plaque.[22] Thus, it is imperative that when performing a TEE examination of the thoracic aorta, these characteristics are identified and discussed with the surgical team before aortic manipulation.

Although most of the thoracic aorta can be imaged with a multiplane TEE, there is a variably sized "blind spot" in the distal ascending aorta and proximal aortic arch that cannot be seen because the air-filled trachea is interposed between the esophagus and this area of the aorta. This, unfortunately, is typically the site of aortic manipulation during cardiac surgery (aortic cannulation for CPB, aortic cross-clamping, and proximal bypass anastomosis). Konstadt and colleagues found that the "blind spot" that cannot be assessed by TEE is anywhere between 0.2 and 4.5 cm of the distal ascending aorta.[23] Epiaortic ultrasonography (EAU) in the surgical field after sternotomy can be used to examine this area by covering a high-frequency transducer with a sterile sheath and placing it directly on the ascending aorta.

EPIAORTIC SCANNING: A SOLUTION TO THE "BLIND SPOT"

Intraoperative epicardial echocardiography has been used as an adjunct to TEE in cardiac surgery for many years. Its earliest application included the diagnosis of intracardiac pathology, specifically valvular disease. However, more recently, EAU imaging of the ascending aorta has been advocated as part of a multifaceted approach to reduce intraoperative atherosclerotic embolism.[22] Wareing and colleagues reported that EAU is more effective at

determining the size and extent of atherosclerotic plaque in the ascending aorta compared with surgical palpation alone.[24]

In 2008, the ASE and SCA published guidelines for the performance of a comprehensive intraoperative EAU examination.[22] Based on available evidence, the writing committee recommends that EAU be performed on all cardiac patients at risk for embolic stroke; this includes patients with a history of cerebrovascular or peripheral vascular disease and patients with evidence of atherosclerotic disease diagnosed by other imaging techniques including intraoperative TEE, preoperative TTE, chest magnetic resonance imaging, computed tomography, or radiography.

The guidelines recommend that EAU be performed using a high-frequency (>7-MHz) linear- or phased-array transducer. The transducer needs to be inserted into a sterile sheath filled with either sterile water or ultrasound transmission gel before being brought into the surgical field and placed on the aorta. Warm sterile saline can be used to fill the pericardial cavity to enhance ultrasound transmission. A complete EAU examination includes multiple views of the ascending aorta in both short and long axes from the sinotubular junction to the origin of the innominate artery as well as the aortic arch in long axis. The proximal ascending aorta is defined as the region from the sinotubular junction to the proximal intersection of the right pulmonary artery. The mid ascending aorta is defined as the region of the aorta anterior to the right pulmonary artery. The distal ascending aorta extends from the intersection of the right pulmonary artery to the origin of the innominate artery. To obtain these images, start with a short-axis view of the proximal ascending aorta. The ultrasound probe should be placed as proximal as possible with the orientation marker directed toward the patient's left shoulder. Minor manipulations in the angulation of the probe are necessary to center the aorta in the imaging plane and create a circular structure. Next, slowly move the probe in a cephalad direction along the aorta to obtain images of the mid ascending aorta (Fig. 136.2 and Videos 136.1 to 136.3). Further advancement along the aorta brings into view the distal ascending aorta. It is often necessary to rotate the probe in a clockwise fashion to maintain the short-axis orientation as the probe gets closer to the innominate artery. The long-axis images are achieved by rotating the probe 90 degrees from the short-axis orientation. Again, start as proximally as possible and advance the probe in a cephalad direction along the ascending aorta, changing the rotation and angulation as necessary to keep the aorta as a tubular structure (Fig. 136.3). Imaging of the ascending aorta should include the origin of the innominate artery. The probe can be advanced slightly farther to visualize the aortic arch and the origins of the other great vessels.

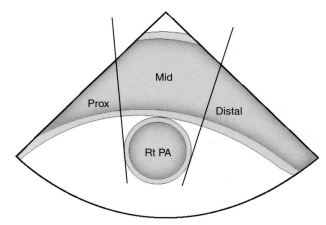

Figure 136.3. Epiaortic ultrasonography image diagram of the long-axis view. *Distal,* Distal third of the ascending aorta; *Mid,* middle third of the ascending aorta; *proximal,* proximal third of the ascending aorta; *Rt PA,* right pulmonary artery.

For each of the three segments of the ascending aorta, four measurements should be recorded and reported: maximal aortic diameter, maximal plaque height or thickness, location of the maximal plaque within the ascending aorta, and the presence of any mobile components. Because of the increased risk of embolic stroke in patients with plaque larger than 3 mm or mobile components, the presence and location of these plaques should be discussed with the surgeon before aortic manipulation.[22]

Several studies have sought to evaluate the impact of EAU on surgical decision making and outcome in cardiac surgery patients. Wareing and colleagues were the first to report that using EAU to evaluate for ascending aortic atheroma and modifying surgical technique in patients found to have moderate to severe aortic atherosclerotic disease may reduce the incidence of postoperative stroke.[25] Subsequent studies have shown similar results.[26–29] Although EAU is a very sensitive technique for identifying and delineating atherosclerosis in the ascending aorta during cardiac surgery, the modifications of surgical technique based on this information that can actually improve clinical outcomes have yet to be clearly defined and validated.

Please access ExpertConsult to view the corresponding videos for this chapter.

REFERENCES

1. Matsumoto M, Oka Y, Strom J, et al. Application of transesophageal echocardiography to continuous intraoperative monitoring of left ventricular performance. *Am J Cardiol.* 1980;46:95–105.
2. Souquet J, Hanrath P, Zitelli L, et al. Transesophageal phased array for imaging the heart. *IEEE Trans Biomed Eng.* 1982;29:707–712.
3. Smith JS, Cahalan MK, Benefiel DJ, et al. Intraoperative detection of myocardial ischemia in high-risk patients: electrocardiography versus two-dimensional transesophageal echocardiography. *Circulation.* 1985;72:1015–1021.
4. Eltzschig HK, Rosenberger P, Löffler M, et al. Impact of intraoperative transesophageal echocardiography on surgical decisions in 12,566 patients undergoing cardiac surgery. *Ann Thorac Surg.* 2008;85:845–852.
5. Minhaj M, Patel K, Muzic D, et al. The effect of routine intraoperative transesophageal echocardiography on surgical management. *J Cardiothorac Vasc Anesth.* 2007;21:800–804.
6. Kato M, Nakashima Y, Levine J, et al. Does transesophageal echocardiography improve postoperative outcome in patients undergoing coronary artery bypass surgery. *J Cardiothorac Vasc Anesth.* 1993;7:285–289.
7. Kamra K, Russell I, Miller-Hance WC. Role of transesophageal echocardiography in the management of pediatric patients with congenital heart disease. *Paediatr Anaesth.* 2011;21:479–493.
8. Sheinberg R, Brady MB, Mitter N. Intraoperative transesophageal echocardiography and ventricular assist device insertion. *Semin CardioThorac Vasc Anesth.* 2011;15:14–24.
9. Bergquist BD, Bellows WH, Leung JM. Transesophageal echocardiography in myocardial revascularization: II. Influence on intraoperative decision making. *Anesth Analg.* 1996;82:1139–1145.
10. Savage RM, Lytle BW, Aronson S, et al. Intraoperative echocardiography is indicated in high-risk coronary artery bypass grafting. *Ann Thorac Surg.* 1997;64:368–374.
11. Otto C. Intraoperative and interventional echocardiography. In: *Textbook of Clinical Echocardiography.* 5th ed. Philadelphia: Elsevier Saunders; 2013:475–476.
12. Shanewise JS, Cheung AT, Aronson S, et al. ASE/SCA guidelines for performing a comprehensive intraoperative multiplane transesophageal echocardiography examination. *J Am Soc Echocardiogr.* 1999;12:884–900.
13. Cahalan MK, Stewart W, Pearlman A, et al. American Society of Echocardiography and Society of Cardiovascular Anesthesiologists task force guidelines for training in perioperative echocardiography. *J Am Soc Echocardiogr.* 2002;15:647–652.
14. Cahalan MK, Stewart W, Pearlman A. Practice guidelines for perioperative transesophageal echocardiography. *J Am Soc Echocardiogr.* 1996;84:986–1006.
15. Practice guidelines for perioperative transesophageal echocardiography. An updated report by the American Society of Anesthesiologists and the Society of Cardiovascular Anesthesiologists task force on transesophageal echocardiography. *Anesthesiology.* 2010;112:1084–1096.
16. Katz ES, Tunick PA, Rusinek H, et al. Protruding aortic atheromas predict stroke in elderly patients undergoing cardiopulmonary bypass: experience with intraoperative transesophageal echocardiography. *J Am Coll Cardiol.* 1992;20. 70–7.
17. Amarenco P, Cohen A, Tzourio C, et al. Atherosclerotic disease of the aortic arch and the risk of ischemic stroke. *N Engl J Med.* 1994;331:1474–1479.
18. Dávila-Román VG, Barzilai B, Wareing TH, et al. Atherosclerosis of the ascending aorta: prevalence and role as an independent predictor of cerebrovascular events in cardiac patients. *Stroke.* 1994;25:2010–2016.
19. Ferrari E, Vidal R, Chevallier T, et al. Atherosclerosis of the thoracic aorta and aortic debris as a marker of poor prognosis: benefit of oral anticoagulants. *J Am Coll Cardiol.* 1999;33:1317–1322.
20. Trehan N, Mishra M, Kasliwal RR, et al. Reduced neurological injury during CABG in patients with mobile aortic atheromas: a five-year follow-up study. *Ann Thorac Surg.* 2000;70:1558–1564.
21. van der Linden J, Hadjinikolaou L, Bergman P, et al. Postoperative stroke in cardiac surgery is related to the location and extent of atherosclerotic disease in the ascending aorta. *J Am Coll Cardiol.* 2001;38:131–135.
22. Glas KE, Swaminathan M, Reeves ST, et al. Guidelines for the performance of a comprehensive intraoperative epiaortic ultrasonographic examination. *J Am Soc Echocardiogr.* 2007;20:1227–1235.
23. Konstadt SN, Reich DL, Quintana C, et al. The ascending aorta: how much does transesophageal echocardiography see. *Anesth Analg.* 1994;78:240–244.
24. Wareing TH, Davila-Roman VG, Barzilai B, et al. Management of the severely atherosclerotic ascending aorta during cardiac operations: a strategy for detection and treatment. *J Thorac Cardiovasc Surg.* 1992;103:453–462.
25. Wareing TH, Davila-Roman VG, Daily BB, et al. Strategy for the reduction of stroke incidence in cardiac surgical patients. *Ann Thorac Surg.* 1993;55:1400–1408.
26. Hangler HB, Nagele G, Danzmayr M, et al. Modification of surgical technique for ascending aortic atherosclerosis: impact on stroke reduction in coronary artery bypass grafting. *J Thorac Cardiovasc Surg.* 2003;126:391–400.
27. Zingone B, Rauber E, Gatti G, et al. The impact of epiaortic ultrasonographic scanning on the risk of perioperative stroke. *Eur J Cardio Thorac Surg.* 2006;29:720–728.
28. Rosenberger P, Shernan SK, Löffler M, et al. The influence of epiaortic ultrasonography on intraoperative surgical management in 6051 cardiac surgical patients. *Ann Thorac Surg.* 2008;85:548–553.
29. Joo HC, Youn YN, Kwak YL, et al. Intraoperative epiaortic scanning for preventing early stroke after off-pump coronary artery bypass. *Br J Anaesth.* 2013;111:374–381.

137 Postoperative Echocardiography of the Aorta

Steven A. Goldstein

POSTSURGICAL IMAGING OF THE AORTIC ROOT AND AORTA

Advances in imaging have raised expectations of improved outcomes for both emergency and elective surgery of the aorta. These advances have allowed early diagnosis and more prompt surgical intervention. Simultaneous with improvements in imaging, improved surgical techniques and postoperative care have enhanced outcomes. As a consequence, more patients are presenting for follow-up care.

For both aortic aneurysms and aortic dissections involving the ascending aorta, the surgeon usually resects the diseased segment and interposes a Dacron graft. Importantly, this approach occasionally does not address diseased segments of the proximal aortic root, arch, or descending aortic segments, which leaves behind a weakened aortic wall because of the effects of the primary disease process. Thus, survivors of the initial repair may remain at considerable risk of future complications, including aneurysmal dilatation and eventual rupture. Consequently, appropriate follow-up requires long-term clinical monitoring and follow-up imaging designed to detect such complications and to allow for timely surgical or percutaneous reintervention. The foundation for such follow-up imaging is adequate baseline imaging that provides a reference for future comparisons of aortic size and appearance. Moreover, baseline imaging will detect technical failures and improper or incomplete repairs that have the potential for subsequent complications.

What the Imager Needs to Know

To evaluate postoperative findings accurately, the imaging physician must possess a general understanding of the surgical technique available for aortic diseases and a full knowledge of the details of the surgical procedure that has been used in the individual patient. In most instances, the postoperative image may differ in important ways from the image seen before the surgical intervention. The expected postoperative image and any possible variations as presented by the relevant imaging modality must be understood. Only then can the spectrum of potential postsurgical complications be accurately recognized and distinguished from the expected postoperative appearance.

COMMON AORTIC SURGICAL TECHNIQUES

Boxes 137.1 and 137.2 list some of the more common aortic procedures and some of the alternative or less common procedures. A brief discussion of some of the more common procedures follows. The scope of this chapter does not permit detailed discussion of modifications of standard procedures or of less commonly used techniques.

Interposition Technique

This currently standard technique includes excision of the diseased segment of the native ascending aorta and its replacement with a polyester (Dacron) graft (Fig. 137.1). The proximal anastomotic site is often supracoronary, typically at the sinotubular junction, and the distal anastomotic site is immediately proximal to the brachiocephalic artery. The anastomotic sites are often reinforced with externally placed circumferential strips of Teflon felt (DuPont).

Inclusion Technique

The inclusion technique consists of an aortotomy, placement of an artificial graft within the diseased native aorta, and enclosing or wrapping the graft with the native aorta, which is sutured around the graft. This procedure creates a potential space between the graft and the native aortic wall, which has important imaging implications. The use of this technique has diminished significantly (and is largely of historical significance) because of improved graft materials and techniques that have led to decreased bleeding. (This technique was used to provide a space into which leakage through relatively porous grafts could occur to minimize extensive bleeding into the mediastinum.)

Composite Grafts

The standard approach for repair of acute type A aortic dissection and aneurysms that involve the aortic root is replacement of the aortic valve, root, and ascending aorta with a composite graft. A composite graft, or conduit, is a synthetic (commonly Dacron) aortic graft that includes a directly attached mechanical valve (less

---

BOX 137.1 Common Aortic Surgical Procedures

1. Valveless ascending grafts
   a. Interposition technique
   b. Inclusion technique
2. Composite grafts
3. Aortic arch grafts
4. Descending grafts
5. Endovascular stent grafts
6. Resuspension of the aortic valve
7. Valve-sparing root replacement
8. Use of biologic adhesives and sealants
9. Coronary artery reimplantation

BOX 137.2 Less Common Aortic Surgical Procedures

1. Elephant trunk procedure
2. Cabrol shunt procedure
3. Cabrol coronary graft procedure
4. Aortic tailoring (aortoplasty)
5. Fenestration
6. Obliteration of false lumen (primary repair)
   a. Glue aortoplasty
   b. Insertion of foreign material
   c. Thromboexclusion
7. Aortic girdling (wrapping the aorta with Dacron mesh)

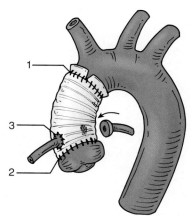

Figure 137.1. The Bentall procedure. The dilated portion of the ascending aorta has been resected and replaced with a Dacron graft. A coronary "button" *(curved arrow)* was removed from the resected native aorta and is ready to be sutured to the graft. The numbers *1, 2,* and *3* represent potential sites of pseudoaneurysm formation: *1* and *2* indicate the proximal and distal anastomotic sites of the graft, and *3* indicates the anastomotic site of the reimplanted coronary artery.

commonly a bioprosthetic valve because currently there is no pre-fabricated composite with a bioprosthetic valve). With composite graft replacement, the coronary ostia are dissected from the native aorta with a rim of the surrounding aorta (button technique) and reanastomosed individually to the composite graft. In select cases of nonpathologic aortic valves, reimplantation or remodeling procedures have become valve-sparing alternatives. Newer graft designs, such as the Valsalva-design graft, recreate the sinuses of Valsalva and more closely resemble the shape and dimensions of the normal aortic root.[1,2] This type of graft (Fig. 137.2) theoretically promotes sinus expansion, improves coronary blood flow, and decreases mechanical leaflet stress.

Reduction Aortic Aortoplasty

Reduction ascending aortoplasty (RAA) is an alternative to ascending aortic replacement with synthetic grafts, especially in patients with only a moderately dilated aorta without aortic root involvement and when a decreased aortic cross-clamp time is desirable.[3,4] Advantages of RAA include its being a simpler procedure than Dacron graft replacement and having a shorter cross-clamp time, less bleeding, and lower rates of mortality and morbidity.[3–7] A major concern about RAA is that it exposes the patient to the risk of redilatation, rupture, or dissection because it may leave intrinsically diseased native aortic wall tissue in place.[8,9] Several variations of reduction aortoplasty of the ascending aorta, with or without external wrapping, exist.[7,10–13] The details of the diverse number of technical variants of this procedure are beyond the scope of this chapter. All of these variants reduce the diameter of the aorta, which theoretically restores normal wall tension according to the law of Laplace.

Aortoplasty is performed by resecting an elliptical portion of the dilated aortic wall along a longitudinal aortotomy. The aortotomy is then closed using two layers of sutures, which are often reinforced with Teflon strips to tailor the aortic shape and to obtain a normal diameter (Fig. 137.3). Some authors advise wrapping of this segment after completion of the suture line to provide reinforcement of the vessel wall and prevent further dilatation (see next section).

External Reinforcement (Wrapping)

Aortic wrapping (or girdling) is a relatively simple alternative to conventional graft replacement for mild to moderately dilated

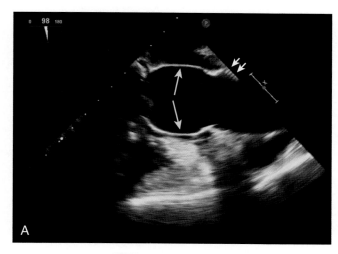

A

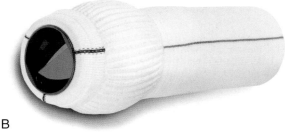

B

Figure 137.2. A, Transesophageal echocardiogram (longitudinal view of the aorta) illustrates a Valsalva graft. The *large yellow arrows* indicate the portion of the graft that recreates the sinuses of Valsalva. The *small white arrows* indicate the "corrugated" appearance of grafts seen on echo. **B,** An actual composite Vascutek Gelweave Valsalva graft with a mechanical bileaflet tilting disc prosthetic valve. (Courtesy of Sorin Group, Arveda, CO, and Vascutek Ltd., Inchinnan, Scotland. Vascutek and Gelweave are trademarks of Vascutek Ltd.)

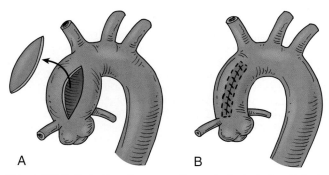

A   B

Figure 137.3. Reduction of an ascending aortoplasty. **A,** An elliptical segment *(arrow)* is excised from the maximally convex portion of the ascending aorta. **B,** The aortic diameter is reduced to normal as the aortotomy is closed with a running mattress suture in an over-and-over nonabsorbable suture.

ascending aortas. Wrapping is most appropriate for older adults and high-risk patients who have multiple comorbidities and for whom a prolonged operative time would significantly increase the mortality rate.[3,14,15] Wrapping theoretically prevents further dilatation by reinforcing the aorta.[16,17] Although usually performed in combination with reduction aortoplasty, as described previously, wrapping can also be performed as a definitive procedure (Fig. 137.4), especially when performed concomitantly with coronary artery bypass surgery or aortic valve replacement.[18–20] Materials used for

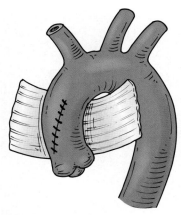

Figure 137.4. The external wrapping technique. The aortic diameter that was reduced by the aortoplasty is now closed by the suture line. The Dacron wrap will be closed with sutures and fixed to the aorta by proximal and distal sutures (not shown).

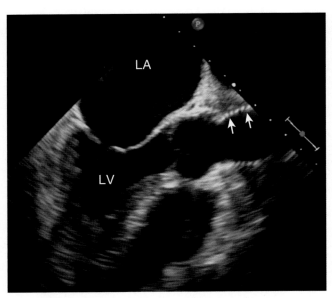

Figure 137.5. Transesophageal echocardiogram (longitudinal view of the aorta) illustrates the proximal portion of an interposition graft that begins at the sinotubular junction. The *small arrows* illustrate the typical "corrugations" of Dacron grafts as seen by echocardiography. *LA*, Left atrium; *LV*, left ventricle.

wrapping include Dacron, bovine pericardium, CorMartix ECM (extracellular matrix), and felt. Potential disadvantages of wrapping include a risk of hematoma formation underneath the wrap, which can cause external compression and narrowing of the aorta or degeneration and erosion of the underlying aortic wall.[21,22]

Aortic Arch Grafts

For select patients with aortic arch involvement, open surgery may range from partial to complete arch replacement with or without debranching and reattachment of one or more of the arch vessels.

Elephant Trunk Procedure

Surgery for treatment of diffuse or extensive thoracic aortic disease (e.g., aneurysms involving both the ascending and descending thoracic aorta or the mega aorta) is commonly performed via a two-stage operation known as the *elephant trunk* (ET) procedure.[23,24] Staged repair, introduced by Borst and coworkers in 1983, is required because it is not feasible to expose both the ascending and descending thoracic aortas with a single incision.[25] The first stage, performed via a sternotomy, consists of repair of the ascending aorta, aortic arch, and reconstruction of the great vessels (if needed); the ET is the distal segment of the aortic graft material that floats freely within the descending thoracic aorta (like an elephant's trunk dangles freely from its face). The second stage, repair of the descending or thoracoabdominal aorta, is performed via a left thoracotomy using the ET, which is suspended freely in the descending thoracic aorta. Alternatively, the second stage can be performed transarterially with an endovascular stent graft. An important advantage of the ET technique is that the second stage avoids a difficult dissection at the initial anastomotic region where firm and hazardous adhesions are present.

The ET technique has undergone a number of modifications, and the technical details vary among surgeons and are also tailored to individual situations. The imager must be aware of the specific details of the surgical technique in a given patient, as well as the potential complications related to this procedure, which include kinking, obstruction, and graft entrapment in the false lumen.[23,24,26]

Cabrol Shunt Procedure

The Cabrol shunt procedure is an uncommon adjunct to the inclusion graft technique, and it is performed to prevent progressive bleeding into the potential space between the graft and the native aortic wall, as described earlier. This procedure consists of a surgically created shunt between this space and the right atrium to alleviate pressure in the perigraft space. Because the inclusion technique has fallen out of favor, the Cabrol shunt is rarely performed today.

Technical Adjuncts

For all types of grafts, circumferential felt or pericardial strips are often used to buttress anastomoses. Felt pledgets are also used to reinforce the graft or the native aortic wall at sites of intraoperative cannula placement. These strips and pledgets have imaging implications for each of the imaging modalities, such as otherwise unexplained thickenings, reverberations, and acoustic shadowing. A variety of adhesives, or biologic glues, have been used as an adjunct to standard methods of achieving anastomotic hemostasis (e.g., sutures and clips). These bioglues have also been used for reapproximating layers of the dissected aorta and for strengthening weakened aortic tissues by a tanning process. Although the value of these tissue adhesives has been recognized, there are reports of tissue necrosis leading to false aneurysms.[27] Moreover, these substances may produce edema inflammation and fibrosis that leads to thickening of the aortic wall or adjacent tissues. Such thickening can be confused with leakage and hematomas in imaging techniques.

NORMAL POSTOPERATIVE FEATURES

The details of the surgery that has been performed will determine the appearance of the ascending aorta on prospective imaging studies. There are only a few descriptions of the echocardiographic appearance of the ascending aorta after reconstruction. More information is available on computed tomography (CT) scans and magnetic resonance imaging (MRI) findings. An aortic interposition graft is visualized as a thin, corrugated echo-dense tube (Fig. 137.5). There is usually a noticeable change between the graft and the native aorta. The felt strips that are used to reinforce the anastomoses provide visual markers of the anastomoses. Occasionally, there is angulation of the aortic graft, especially near the anastomoses. These points of angulation are not clinically significant, but they can simulate a dissection flap, especially on axial CT images.

BOX 137.3 Potential Postoperative Complications of Aortic Surgery

1. Anastomotic leakage or disruption dehiscence
2. Pseudoaneurysm (at proximal, distal, or coronary anastomotic site)
3. Progressive aortic regurgitation
4. Involvement of aortic branches
5. Perigraft infection
6. Compression of graft by hematoma (inclusion technique)
7. Aneurysmal dilatation of false lumen (after dissection repair)
8. Compression or collapse of true lumen (by expanding false lumen)
9. Frank rupture
10. Anastomotic stenosis
11. Development of recurrent dissection or aneurysm proximal to a graft in patients in whom a supracoronary procedure has been performed
12. Aortoesophageal or aortopulmonary fistula
13. Graft herniation into thoracotomy defect

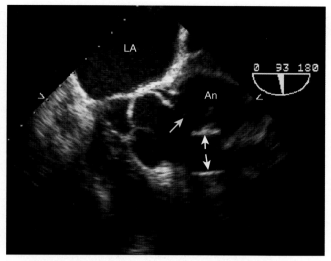

Figure 137.6. Transesophageal echocardiogram (longitudinal view of the aorta) that illustrates a pseudoaneurysm (An) that occurred at the proximal anastomotic site of a Dacron graft *(small white arrows)*, which originally began at the sinotubular junction but is now partially dehisced. The *yellow arrow* designates entrance into the pseudoaneurysm. *LA,* Left atrium.

A small amount of perigraft thickening (<10 mm thick) is a common postoperative finding. This presumably results from minor leakage at the anastomotic suture lines created by needle holes, edema, or inflammation. The uniform and concentric distribution of this thickening helps to differentiate it from more serious leakage. Another mimicker of pathology can be seen at the site of coronary anastomoses. When the coronary arteries are resected with a rim of native aortic tissue (button technique), a focal bulge at this site can be misinterpreted as an incipient pseudoaneurysm. Importantly, the inclusion graft technique creates a potential space between the graft and its wrap, which is the native aorta. This space often contains fluid or hematomas, which can be a normal finding with no clinical significance, especially when the space is smaller than 10 mm.

After repair of a type A dissection, a persistent dissection flap is seen distal to the graft in 80% of cases.[28] This persistence of a double-channel aorta after surgery is not considered a complication, provided it does not increase in size. In chronic dissections, the residual dissection flap becomes thickened because of collagen deposition and becomes less oscillatory or even immobile.

Many early postoperative CT studies show pleural or pericardial effusion, mediastinal lymph node enlargement, or left lobe atelectasis. These findings diminish in frequency over time and presumably represent normal postoperative findings without adverse clinical consequences.

COMPLICATIONS AFTER AORTIC REPAIR

Total removal of the diseased aortic segment is often not possible with surgical repair of aortic lesions (e.g., aneurysm and dissection), and the anastomoses between the graft and the native aorta are potential sites for problems. Therefore, periodic postoperative surveillance by cardiovascular imaging specialists who are familiar with aortic diseases and surgical procedures cannot be overemphasized. Early detection of complications can facilitate optimal management, including reoperation. Potential postoperative complications are listed in Box 137.3. Awareness of these complications and differentiation of these from the spectrum of normal postoperative findings is obviously important. Some of the more common complications are discussed.

Pseudoaneurysm

Pseudoaneurysm is an important early or late complication that can occur after elective surgery for aneurysm or emergency surgery for acute dissection. In the majority of patients, pseudoaneurysm

is not associated with any clinical symptoms.[29] The silent nature of these potentially life-threatening complications emphasizes the need for imaging surveillance. Pseudoaneurysms usually occur at anastomoses (Fig. 137.6). They may form at the site of needle holes even when the suture lines are intact. More commonly, they originate from partial dehiscence of the proximal or distal suture lines or at the site of coronary reimplantation. The size of the pseudoaneurysm, its change over time, and the patient's clinical symptoms determine management. Small, sterile pseudoaneurysms can remain stable for years without intervention. Pseudoaneurysms are readily detectable by both CT scan and MRI. Transesophageal echocardiography (TEE) is also reliable for detecting pseudoaneurysms of the aortic root and proximal ascending aorta. However, TEE may miss this lesion in the distal ascending aorta because of interposition of the trachea.

False Lumen Dilatation

Surgery for type A aortic dissection is usually limited to the ascending aorta. Distal to the ascending aortic graft, a dissection flap and a false lumen with demonstrable blood flow are present in approximately 80% of patients.[28] Strictly speaking, this is not a complication, but there is a potential for false lumen expansion. Typically, the median diameter of the aortic arch, descending thoracic aorta, and abdominal aorta are all mildly enlarged after type A aortic dissection repair.[30] Although expansion rates are low, progressive dilatation of the patent false lumen, which is facilitated by the poor condition of the weakened and thinned wall, often occurs. This may result in late aortic rupture or compression of the true lumen. In the minority of patients, the false lumen can become thrombosed. Although the influence of thrombosis of the false lumen on long-term survival remains speculative, it may be associated with better survival.

Involvement of Aortic Branches

Extension of a dissection flap or intramural hematoma into an aortic branch may result in luminal narrowing or total obstruction. In addition, dilatation of a patent false lumen and associated collapse of the true lumen may also affect the branch vessels. These complications may occur in the coronary arteries, supraaortic vessels, or visceral vessels.

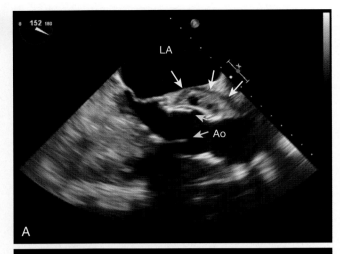

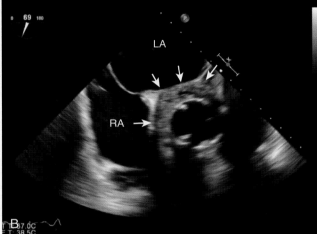

Figure 137.7. Transesophageal echocardiogram of a patient with an infected composite Valsalva graft. **A,** The longitudinal view illustrates a perigraft abscess indicated by the *three small white arrows*. The composite graft contained a bioprosthetic valve. Two of the three stents are shown *(small white arrows)*. **B,** Short-axis view illustrates the extensive degree of the abscess *(four small white arrows)*. *Ao,* Ascending aortic portion of the graft; *LA,* left atrium; *RA,* right atrium.

Infection

Early or late-onset infection complicates prosthetic aortic graft insertion in 0.5% to 5% of cases.[31] CT is considered to be the standard imaging method for aortic graft infection.[31] The role of TEE for detection for graft infection has not been thoroughly investigated. Fig. 137.7 illustrates an infected graft detected by TEE. Fig. 137.1 illustrates the typical sites of pseudoaneurysm formation. The diagnosis of infection is suspected with fever, elevated serum C-reactive protein and leukocytes, and fluid collection around a graft on CT scan, in the absence of other possible causes of fever. In unclear cases, fluorodeoxyglucose positron emission tomography CT has proven to be a useful tool in the workup for diagnosis of aortic graft infection.[32,33]

COMPOSITE GRAFT DEHISCENCE

Dehiscence of a composite aortic graft is a very rare postoperative complication after aortic root replacement[34] (Video 137.1). Graft dehiscence can occur in both infectious and noninfectious settings.[35] The time interval between the initial surgical procedure

TABLE 137.1   Follow-Up: Investigational Methods, Indications, and Time Frame

Time	Method	Indication
Before hospital discharge	CT scan	Every patient
	TTE	Every patient
	TEE	Valve reconstruction
	MRI	Young patients (instead of CT scan, where available)
INITIAL EXAMINATIONS AFTER DISCHARGE		
3 months after discharge	CT scan (MRI)	Dilated residual aorta
	TTE or TEE	Valve reconstruction
6 months after discharge	CT scan (MRI)	Normal aortic diameter
	TTE or TEE	Valve reconstruction
SUBSEQUENT EXAMINATIONS		
Every 6 months	CT scan (MRI)	Progression of aortic disease
Every 12 months	CT scan (MRI)	Aortic diameter ≥4.5 cm
Every 24 months	CT scan (MRI)	Aortic diameter <4.0 cm

CT, Computed tomography; *MRI,* magnetic resonance imaging; *TEE,* transesophageal echocardiography; *TTE,* transthoracic echocardiography.

and discovery of this complication is variable but has been reported up to 17 years after the initial operation.[34]

RECOMMENDATIONS FOR SERIAL IMAGING TECHNIQUES AND SCHEDULES

The imaging modality of choice for evaluating the postoperative aorta has not been clearly determined. Both CT scan and MRI are reasonable choices. These techniques provide precise and reproducible measurements of the native aorta diameter at any level and have the advantage, compared with TEE, of including the supraaortic and visceral vessels in a single examination.

Transthoracic echocardiography (TTE), although a routine study for many cardiology patients, is limited for follow-up after surgery. TTE provides assessment of the aortic valve, aortic root, and proximal ascending aorta, but it is limited for the remainder of the aorta.

Contrast CT scan is the preferred diagnostic tool for follow-up of patients after surgery for aortic disease. MRI is also valuable for serial follow-up. Image resolution is comparable to that of CT scanning. In some patients, MRI may be preferable because neither radiation nor contrast media is required. However, MRI is less practical as the primary investigation for follow-up because it is still more expensive and less available than CT scanning.

TEE has some advantages over CT scan and MRI. It is portable, provides excellent images of the aortic root, can precisely assess the morphology and function of the aortic valve, and provides information on left ventricular function. However, it may not image the distal ascending aorta (site of the distal anastomoses), the aortic arch, the abdominal aorta, and the aortic branch vessels. Moreover, it does not assess the relationship of pseudoaneurysms to other structures (e.g., the lung or mediastinum). Last, its semi-invasive nature is a drawback for serial, repeated evaluations.

The organization of the follow-up should not be left to practitioners or cardiologists alone. Primary responsibility should be clarified and should include the surgeon. Ideally, there should be a computer database into which every patient with aortic disease is entered. Details of the intraoperative and postoperative findings should be recorded. Interval and the follow-up imaging modality should be based on progression of the disease and the expertise available, according to the preceding comments and to the factors outlined in Table 137.1. The examination can be performed near the patient's home, but the patient should be sent to a site with aortic experience for comparison and reevaluation. The guidelines mentioned in Table 137.1 should be modified depending on aortic size. Patients with small aortas can be followed at less frequent intervals than those with larger aortas.

The importance of indefinite surveillance after surgery of the aorta cannot be overemphasized. The imager must understand thoracic aortic surgical techniques and must be aware of the spectrum of normal and pathologic findings after surgery to detect or exclude clinically significant abnormalities. Thus, ideally, cardiovascular or radiology specialists familiar with aortic diseases and surgical procedures should perform and interpret these examinations.

Please access ExpertConsult to view the corresponding video for this chapter.

REFERENCES

1. De Paulis R, DeMatteis GM, Nardi P, et al. One-year appraisal of a new aortic root conduit with sinuses of Valsalva. *J Thorac Cardiovasc Surg.* 2002;123:33–39.
2. DePaulis R, Scaffa R, Nardella S, et al. Use of the Valsalva graft and long-term follow-up. *J Thorac Cardiovasc Surg.* 2010;140:523–527.
3. Robicsek F. A new method to treat fusiform aneurysms of the ascending aorta associated with aortic valve disease: an alternative to radical resection. *Ann Thorac Surg.* 1982;34:92–94.
4. Carrrel T, von Segesser L, Jenni R, et al. Dealing with dilated ascending aorta during aortic valve replacement: advantages of conservative surgical approach. *Eur J Cardio Thorac Surg.* 1991;5:137–143.
5. Arsan S, Akgun S, Kurtoglu N, et al. Reduction aortoplasty and external wrapping for moderately sized tubular ascending aortic aneurysm with concomitant operations. *Ann Thorac Surg.* 2004;78:858–861.
6. Zhang H, Lu F, Qu D, et al. Treatment of fusiform ascending aortic aneurysms: a comparative study with 2 options. *J Thorac Cardiovasc Surg.* 2011;141:738–743.
7. Della Corte A, De Feo M, Bancone C, et al. Long-term follow-up of reduction ascending aortoplasty with autologous partial wrapping: for which patient is waistcoat aortoplasty best suited. *Interact Cardiovasc Thorac Surg.* 2012;14:56–63.
8. Sievers HH. Reflections on reduction ascending aortoplasty's liveliness. *J Thorac Cardiovasc Surg.* 2004;128:499–501.
9. Sundt 3rd T. Unsupported reduction ascending aortoplasty: fate of diameter and Windkessel function. *Ann Thorac Surg.* 2007;83:1053–1054.
10. Robicsek F, Thubrikar MJ. Conservative operation in the management of annular dilatation and ascending aortic aneurysm. *Ann Thorac Surg.* 1994;57:1672–1674.
11. Harrison Jr LH, Heck Jr HA. Shawl lapel aortoplasty. *Ann Thorac Surg.* 1996;62:1867.
12. Walker T, Bail DH, Gruler M, et al. Unsupported reduction ascending aortoplasty: fate of diameter and of Windkessel function. *Ann Thorac Surg.* 2007;83:1047–1053.
13. Ozcan AV, Alsalaldeh M, Boysan E, Goksin I. Ascending aortic aneurysm treatment with linear plication and external wrapping technique: mid-term results. *J Card Surg.* 2013;28:421–426.
14. Feindt P, Litmathe J, Borgens A, et al. Is size-reducing ascending aortoplasty with external reinforcement an option in modern aortic surgery? *Eur J Cardio Thorac Surg.* 2007;31:614–617.
15. Belov IV, Stepanenko AB, Gens AP, et al. Reduction aortoplasty for ascending aortic aneurysm: a 14-year experience. *Asian Cardiovasc Thorac Ann.* 2009;17:162–166.
16. Hess Jr PJ, Harman PK, Klodell CT, et al. Early outcomes using the Florida repair for correction of aortic insufficiency due to root aneurysm. *Ann Thorac Surg.* 2009;87:1161–1169.
17. Hetzer R, Komoda T, Komoda S, et al. New aortic root remodeling surgery in aortic root aneurysm. *Ann Thorac Surg.* 2010;89:1260–1264.
18. Cohen O, Odim J, De La Zerda D, et al. Long-term experience of girdling the ascending aorta with Dacron mesh as definitive treatment for aneurysmal dilatation. *Ann Thorac Surg.* 2007;83:S780–S784.
19. Ang K-L, Raheel F, Bajaj A, et al. Early impact of aortic wrapping on patients undergoing aortic valve replacement with mild to moderate ascending aorta dilatation. *J Cardiothorac Surg.* 2010;5:58–61.
20. Park JY, Shin J-K, Chung JW, et al. Short-time outcomes of aortic wrapping for mild to moderate ascending aorta dilatation in patients undergoing cardiac surgery. *Korean J Thorac Cardiovasc Surg.* 2012;45:148–154.
21. Neri E, Massetti M, Tanganelli P, et al. Is it only a mechanical matter? Histologic modifications of the aorta underlying external banding. *J Thorac Cardiovasc Surg.* 1999;118:1116–1118.
22. Bauer M, Grauhan O, Hetzer R. Dislocated wrap after previous aortoplasty causes erosion of the ascending aorta. *Ann Thorac Surg.* 2003;75:583–584.
23. Schepens MA, Dossche KM, Morshuis WJ, et al. The elephant trunk technique: operative results in 100 consecutive patient. *Eur J Cardio Thorac Surg.* 2002;21:276–281.
24. Safi HJ, Miller 3rd CC, Estera AL, et al. Staged repair of extensive aortic aneurysms: long-term experience with the elephant trunk technique. *Ann Surg.* 2004;240:677–685.
25. Borst HG, Walterbusch G, Schaps D. Extensive aortic replacement using "elephant trunk" prosthesis. *Thorac Cardiovasc Surg.* 1983;31:37–40.
26. Ius F, Hagl C, Haverich A, Pichlmaier M. Elephant trunk procedure 27 years after Borst: what remains and what is new. *Eur J Cardio Thorac Surg.* 2011;40:1–11.
27. Furst W, Banerjee A. Release of glutaraldehyde from an albumin-glutaraldehyde tissue adhesive causes significant in vitro and in vivo toxicity. *Ann Thorac Surg.* 2005;79:1522–1528.
28. Goldstein SA, Mintz GS, Lindsay JJ. Aorta: comprehensive evaluation by echocardiography and transesophageal echocardiography. *J Am Soc Echocardiogr.* 1993;6:634–659.
29. Mesana TG, Caus T, Gaubert J, et al. Late complications after prosthetic replacement of the ascending aorta: what did we learn from routine magnetic resonance imaging follow-up? *Eur J Cardio Thorac Surg.* 2000;18:313–320.
30. Halstead JC, Meier M, Etz C, et al. The fate of the distal aorta after repair of acute type A aortic dissection. *J Thorac Cardiovasc Surg.* 2007;113:127–135.
31. Orton DF, LeVeen RF, Saigh JA, et al. Aortic prosthetic graft infections: Radiologic manifestations and implications for management. *Radiographics.* 2000;20:977–993.
32. Bruggink J, Glaudemans A, Saleem B. Accuracy of FDG-PET-CT in the diagnostic work-up of vascular prosthetic graft infection. *Eur J Vasc Endovasc Surg.* 2010;40:348–354.
33. Rojoa D, Kontopodis N, Antoniou SA, et al. 18F-FDG-PET in the diagnosis of vascular prosthetic graft infection: a diagnostic test accuracy meta-analysis. *Eur J Vasc Endovasc Surg.* 2019;57:292–301.
34. Mohammadi S, Bonnet N, Leprince P, et al. Reoperation for false aneurysm of the ascending aorta after its prosthetic replacement: surgical strategy. *Ann Thorac Surg.* 2005;79:147–152.
35. Stiver K, Bayram M, Orsinelli D. Aortic root Bentall graft disarticulation following repair of type A aortic dissection. *Echocardiography.* 2010;27:E27–E2-E9.

138 Aortitis

Steven A. Goldstein

Aortitis is a general and nonspecific term that refers to a broad group of infectious and noninfectious conditions in which there is abnormal inflammation of the aortic wall. These inflammatory conditions have different clinical and morphologic features and variable prognoses. Some conditions exclusively affect the aorta, whereas others may also extend to its major branches. The clinical manifestations are often vague and nonspecific, including nonspecific pain, fever, malaise, elevated levels of acute phase reactants (e.g., serum C-reactive protein and erythrocyte sedimentation rate), and other systemic manifestations. As a result, aortitis is often overlooked during the initial workup of patients with constitutional symptoms and systemic disorders. In addition, organ ischemia and acute life-threatening aortic syndromes, such as aortic dissection or rupture, can complicate the course in some patients.

A multimodality imaging approach is often required for assessment of both the aortic wall and aortic lumen. Imaging techniques include ultrasonography, echocardiography, multidetector computed tomography (CT), magnetic resonance imaging (MRI), nuclear medicine imaging with fluorine 18-fluorodeoxyglucose

---

BOX 138.1 Classification of Aortitis

NONINFECTIOUS AORTITIS

Large-Vessel Vasculitides

- Giant cell arteritis (especially in older patients)
- Takayasu arteritis (especially in younger patients)
- Immunoglobulin G4–related aortitis
- Rheumatoid arthritis
- Systemic lupus erythematosus
- Ankylosing spondylitis
- Reiter syndrome
- Cogan syndrome

Medium- and Small-Vessel Vasculitides

- Wegener's arteritis
- Polyarteritis nodosa
- Behcet disease
- Relapsing polychondritis
- Sarcoid

Idiopathic Conditions

- Idiopathic aortitis
- Inflammatory aortic aneurysm
- Idiopathic retroperitoneal fibrosis (periaortitis)

Radiation-Induced Aortitis

INFECTIOUS AORTITIS

- Bacterial (e.g., caused by Salmonella, Staphylococcus, or Pseudomonas)
- Luetic (syphilis)
- Mycobacterial
- Viral (HIV)
- Fungal

BOX 138.2 American College of Rheumatology Criteria for Giant Cell Arteritis[a]

- Age older than 50 years
- Recent-onset localized headache
- Temporal artery pulse attenuation or tenderness
- Erythrocyte sedimentation rate >50 mm/hr
- Arterial biopsy: necrotizing vasculitis
- No imaging findings are required for diagnosis

[a]Three of five criteria are required for diagnosis.
Data from Gornik HL, Creager MA: Aortitis, *Circulation* 117:3039–3051, 2008.

(18F-FDG) positron emission tomography/CT fusion (PET/CT) or gallium 67 (67GA), and conventional angiography. Each of these modalities has strengths and limitations. Regardless of the imaging modality used, changes in the aortic wall and aortic lumen must be evaluated. Imaging is also required for surveillance of disease activity and treatment planning.

CLASSIFICATION

There are various classifications, but a simple classification of aortic inflammation into two broad categories (noninfectious and infectious) is practical and clinically useful (Box 138.1). Noninfectious aortitis can be subdivided into large-, medium-, and small vessel vasculitis because diseases in this category commonly affect other vessels and may be part of a systemic disorder.[1] It is essential to differentiate between noninfectious causes of aortitis and the much rarer infectious causes because the treatment differs greatly.

Takayasu arteritis (TA) and giant cell arteritis (GCA) are the most common causes of noninfectious aortitis.[1] Immunoglobulin (Ig) G4–related aortitis has recently emerged as a new subtype.[2–4] This chapter focuses largely on TA, GCA, and IgG4-related aortitis.

GIANT CELL ARTERITIS

GCA, also known as temporal arteritis, classically involves cranial arteries such as the temporal and ophthalmic artery. However, it may also involve the aorta. In fact, patients with clinically apparent cranial GCA will have aortic involvement in 15%[5] to 50%[6] or higher.[7] In fact, GCA is the most common form of aortitis in North America, accounting for more than 75% of cases.[5] As opposed to predominantly young patients affected by TA, GCA is usually seen almost exclusively in persons older than age 50 years old with an incidence peaking in the 80th decade of life.[8] Two-thirds of those affected are women.[9] Box 138.2 lists the American College of Rheumatology diagnostic criteria.[1]

GCA typically causes vasculitis of the extracranial branches of the aorta and spares the intracranial vessels. Branches of the external and internal carotid arteries are particularly susceptible. Their involvement leads to classic manifestations of blindness, headache, scalp tenderness, and jaw claudication. Involvement of the subclavian, axillary, and proximal brachial arteries leads to the aortic arch syndrome of claudication of the arms or asymmetrical pulses.[9]

Whereas GCA of the medium-sized arteries results almost exclusively in narrowing and obstruction of vessels, the complications of aortitis, which most often occur in the ascending aorta, are aneurysm formation, dissection, and rupture.[6,10] Importantly, aortic involvement in GCA may be associated with an aggressive disease course with increased risk of death from complications, such as aneurysm, aneurysmal rupture, and aortic dissection.[6] These occur predominantly in the ascending aorta (Fig. 138.1). Aortic stenosis is less common than with TA, but annuloaortic ectasia and ascending thoracic aneurysms that can extend into the aortic arch are more common than in TA.[11]

IMAGING IN GCA

Ultrasonography is the primary imaging test in patients with cranial GCA and cranial symptoms. The "halo" sign of temporal arteritis has been defined as a "homogeneous, hypoechoic wall thickening that is well-delineated toward the luminal side that is visible in both longitudinal and transverse planes"[12] (Fig. 138.2 and Video 138.2). The "halo sign" typically resolves within 2 to 4 weeks of steroid therapy.[13–15] Aortitis in the setting of GCA may reveal thickening of the ascending aorta or dilatation. According to one study, 18F-FDG uptake of the aorta predicts progression and aortic dilatation.[16] Fig. 138.3 illustrates a PET/CT image of a patient with aortitis.

Takayasu Arteritis

TA is the prototypical inflammatory aortic disease of the young. It typically presents in individuals younger than 50 years, especially in young women (female-to-male ratio of 8–9 to 1) of Asian descent. Because of its predilection for the arch vessels, which may result in loss of circulation to the upper extremities, this arteritis has been labeled *pulseless disease* and *aortic arch syndrome*.[17] As with other forms of aortitis, this disease may be asymptomatic or may present with a spectrum of symptoms and clinical signs. The initial presentation is usually nonspecific and consists of systemic symptoms, including fever, fatigue, arthralgias, and night sweats. Because of the nonspecific presentation, the diagnosis of TA is often missed

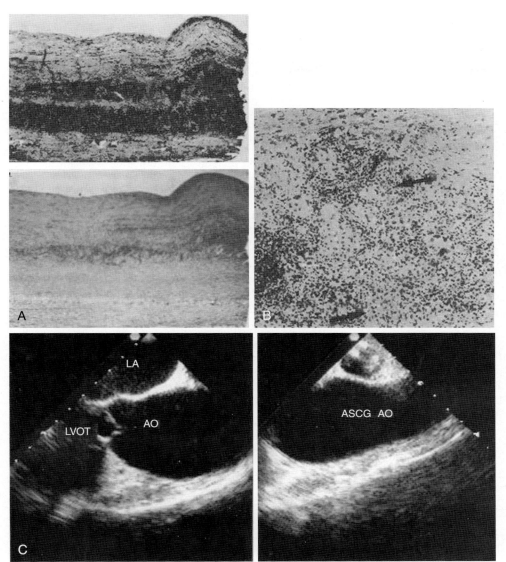

Figure 138.1. A, Low-power photomicrographs of the aortic wall obtained at aortic valve replacement in a 67-year-old woman who presented with severe aortic regurgitation. Movat *(top)* and hematoxylin-and-eosin *(bottom)* staining demonstrate replacement of the normal aortic media by granulomatous inflammation. Preserved elastic fibers (stained *black* by the Movat stain) are seen nearest the intimal surface. **B,** High-power photomicrograph of the granulation tissue. Lymphocytes and giant cells *(arrows)* are prominent. (**C,** Views from the transesophageal echocardiogram of the same patient. Dilatation of the proximal aorta (AO) is demonstrated. At operation, the aorta was thick and "leathery," not thinned as is the case in typical annuloaortic ectasia. *ASCG AO,* Ascending aorta; *LA,* left atrium; *LVOT,* left ventricular outflow tract. (Part B courtesy of Dr. Lucy Nam, Department of Pathology, Washington Hospital Center.)

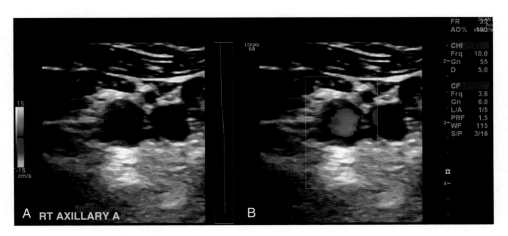

Figure 138.2. A and **B,** Color duplex ultrasonography demonstrates hypoechoic circumferential wall thickening (halo sign) and normal luminal flow in a right axillary artery in a 59-year-old woman with temporal artery biopsy-proven giant cell arteritis. (Courtesy of Dr. Ayaz Aghayev and Dr. Umberto Campia.) (Also see accompanying Video 138.2.)

or misdiagnosed. Unfortunately, there is no diagnostic test for TA. Therefore, to suspect TA, consider the findings listed in Box 138.3. Cardiac manifestations may result from dilatation of the aortic root (with or without aortic regurgitation) or coronary ostial stenosis as a result of the aortitis. Box 138.4 lists the American College of Rheumatology diagnostic criteria.

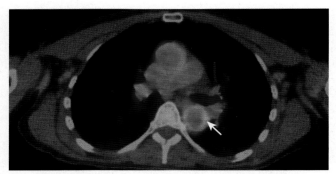

Figure 138.3. Positron emission tomography/computed tomography scan of the descending thoracic aorta shows "intense" yellow wall thickening (arrow) indicating active inflammation (aortitis) in the same 59-year-old woman as in Fig. 138.2. (Courtesy of Dr. Ayaz Aghayev and Dr. Umberto Campia.)

BOX 138.3 When to Suspect Takayasu Arteritis

- Young women with nonspecific systemic symptoms
- Reduced or absent peripheral pulses
- Carotid or subclavian bruits
- Circumferential thickening of the aortic wall (TEE, CT, MRI)
- Co-occurrence of occlusive and dilated lesions

CT, Computed tomography; *MRI,* magnetic resonance imaging; *TEE,* transesophageal echocardiography.

BOX 138.4 American College of Rheumatology Criteria for Takayasu Arteritis[a]

- Age at onset younger than 40 years
- Intermittent claudication of extremities
- Diminished brachial artery pulse
- Subclavian artery or abdominal aortic bruit
- Blood pressure difference >10 mm Hg between arms
- Angiographic (CT, MRI) evidence of stenosis

[a]Highly probable in the presence of three or more criteria; sensitivity is 91%, and specificity is 98%.
CT, Computed tomography; *MRI,* magnetic resonance imaging.
Data from Gornik HL, Creager MA: Aortitis, *Circulation* 117:3039–3051, 2008.

Imaging studies are essential for establishing the diagnosis of TA and determining the extent of involvement. Typical ultrasound finding of the aortic arch branches is circumferential thickening of the wall of the coronary arteries (so-called "macaroni sign").[18] The thoracic aorta is nearly always affected by TA. Echocardiography plays an important role in the assessment of the aortic root and aortic valve in the setting of aortitis of the ascending aorta associated with aortic regurgitation. In some patients, the typical concentric wall thickening of the aortic arch can be visualized from the suprasternal approach.[19] Transesophageal echocardiography (TEE) or CT may also provide evaluation of the thickness of the aortic wall and the exclusion of other pathologies that may resemble aortitis, including intramural hematoma and aortic dissection. The character of the aortic wall depends on the phase of the disease at the time of imaging or resection. In the acute phase, the aortic wall may be thinned. Chronic or late-phase disease may manifest as wall thickening, sometimes striking. The thickening is often circumferential producing regions of stenosis in the aortic branches.

Based on expert consensus, patients with suspected TA should be evaluated with MRI, assuming prompt availability and expertise.[20] MRI avoids radiation in these younger patients. It is not clear whether MRI can discriminate between active disease and remission. MRI may also have a prognostic role.[21] The role of 18F-FDG/PET is increasing, and FDG uptake can facilitate recognition of extension and intensity of inflammatory changes of the aorta and its branches. Moreover, the maximum FDG on serial PET scans can be used to monitor the response of TA to therapy.[22]

Immunoglobulin G4–Related Aortitis

IgG4-related disease is a recently recognized immune-mediated inflammatory condition characterized by elevated IgG4 levels. It involves multiple organs, including the aorta. The increasing interest in IgG4-related disease and the improvement of available histologic techniques have led to more frequent diagnosis of this relatively "young" entity.[3,23–26] In fact, IgG4-related aortitis has emerged as a new subtype of noninfectious aortitis with a frequency approaching that of GCA and TA. In IgG4-related aortitis, there is a male predominance in most series, whereas GCA and TA are more common in female patients (Table 138.1).

The most common pattern of involvement is the abdominal aorta, ascending aorta, arch, and descending aorta in that order.[3] Clinical manifestations are nonspecific, making presurgical diagnosis difficult. Although echocardiography may accidentally detect IgG4-related aortitis, this inflammatory aortic disease is rarely detected by echocardiography until complications such as aneurysm formation or aortic dissection occurs. In the experience of one group, in a cohort of 160 IgG4-related diseases, PET/CT with angiography, including noncontrast, postcontrast, and delayed phases, is the most appropriate imaging study to evaluate vessel walls for evidence of enhancement, thickening, and aneurysm formation.[2] FDG PET/CT can also provide information about the extent of disease, the presence of active inflammation, and the optimum site for biopsy.[27] Measurement of IgG4 levels and tissue biopsy are necessary for definitive diagnosis.

TABLE 138.1 Characteristic Features of Takayasu Arteritis, Giant Cell Arteritis, and Immunoglobulin G4–Related Cardiovascular Disease

Feature	Takayasu Arteritis	Giant Cell Arteritis	Immunoglobulin G4–Related Cardiovascular Disease
Sex	Females > males	Females > males	Males > females
Age	Typically 20–30 years	Typically older than 50 years	Typically older than 60 years
Most common site	Thoracic aorta	Temporal artery Thoracic aorta	Abdominal aorta
Involved region of aortic wall	Media, adventitia	Media	Adventitia
Associated coronary aneurysm	Yes	No	Yes

BOX 138.5 Risk Factors for Infectious Aortitis

- Atherosclerosis
- Infective endocarditis
- Aortic trauma (including complications of aortic angiography)
- Congenital aortic anomalies (e.g., patent ductus arteriosus, coarctation)
- Conditions causing impaired immunity

Histopathologic analysis shows inflammation mostly in the adventitia in IgG4-related aortitis, whereas inflammation is seen in the medial layer in GCA and in the medial layer and adventitia in TA.[5] Because IgG4-related aortitis predominantly involves the adventitia, it is often referred to as periaortitis or periarteritis, depending on the vessel involved.[4]

Infectious Aortitis

With the advent of antibiotics, infectious aortitis has become an uncommon occurrence. The historical term "mycotic aneurysm," coined by Osler, is confusing because it does not refer to a fungal infection but rather infection of the aorta by any microorganism. The aorta is normally very resistant to infection; however, infection of the aorta can arise by several mechanisms: (1) bacteremic seeding of an existing intimal injury or atherosclerotic plaque (the most common mechanism), (2) septic emboli of the vasa vasorum (typically in infective endocarditis), (3) contiguous infective focus extending to the aortic wall (rare), (4) direct bacterial invasion at the time of trauma (e.g., penetrating trauma), and (5) iatrogenic vascular manipulation.[28–30] Risk factors for aortic infections are listed in Box 138.5. Although any microorganism can cause infectious aortitis, some bacteria have a propensity for this location, including *Staphylococcus* spp., *Enterococcus* spp., *Streptococcus pneumoniae,* and *Salmonella* spp. Aortic infection by *Mycobacterium tuberculosis* may occur as a result of extension to the aortic wall from a contiguous infected focus (lymph nodes, lung). *Treponema pallidum* is currently exceedingly rare. Fungal aortitis (e.g., Candida and Aspergillus spp.) represents other rare pathogens.

It is extremely important to establish an early diagnosis of infectious aortitis because this condition is associated with a high rate of aortic rupture and mortality if left untreated.[1] However, the diagnosis is frequently delayed because the clinical manifestations are usually nonspecific, and the first symptoms may result from expansion or rupture of an aneurysm. Infective aortitis should always be considered in patients with endocarditis and if a TEE is a part of the workup, careful assessment of the aorta should always be performed. TEE can usually distinguish intramural hematoma, noninfected aneurysm, and aortic dissection. The TEE shown in Fig. 138.4 illustrates how rapidly an infectious aneurysm can progress.

CT with contrast enhancement is also an excellent imaging modality. CT also provides exclusion of other pathologies that may resemble acute aortitis, such as intramural hematoma, aortic dissection, and penetrating ulcer.[1] Diagnostic CT findings of aortic inflammation include mural thickening, periaortic soft tissue density, rim enhancement, air in the aortic wall, periaortic stranding or fluid retention, saccular or fusiform aneurysm.[31,32]

MRI with gadolinium enhancement is emerging as an excellent imaging modality for aortitis. It provides an entire aorta image with excellent resolution and without radiation exposure. Areas of aortitis may appear as vessel wall edema, enhancement, or wall thickening.

The use of FDG PET/CT may be helpful in cases when the previously mentioned imaging methods fail to yield unequivocal findings or when differentiation from other possible infectious foci is necessary.[30,33,34]

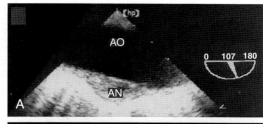
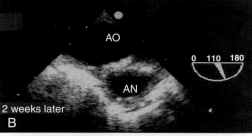
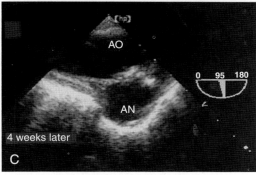

Figure 138.4. A–C, Serial transesophageal echocardiograms performed at 2-week intervals in a 32-year-old man with aortic valve endocarditis illustrating rapid progression in size of a mycotic aneurysm (AN) of the proximal descending thoracic aorta (AO).

Echocardiography for Aortitis

As noted, the clinical features of both noninfectious and infectious aortitis are protean. Therefore, imaging plays a key role for the initial diagnosis, assessment of disease activity, and follow-up. Noninvasive cross-sectional imaging modalities such as contrast-enhanced CT, MRI, and PET are considered the first-line modalities.

SUMMARY

Echocardiography and vascular ultrasonography are seldom first-line methods for the diagnosis of aortitis. However, transthoracic echocardiography, TEE, abdominal ultrasonography, and peripheral vascular ultrasonography may provide useful information. These techniques may demonstrate thickening of the aortic wall, an echolucent "halo" caused by mural edema, and aortic aneurysm.[1] In addition, Doppler provides functional assessment of stenotic segments. Echocardiography is primarily used for identifying complications of aortitis, such as aortic root dilatation, aortic regurgitation, aortic dissection, intramural hematoma, penetrating ulcer, and left ventricular dysfunction.[35]

Please access ExpertConsult to view the corresponding video for this chapter.

REFERENCES

1. Gornik HL, Creager MA. Aortitis, *Circulation.* 2008;117:3039–3051.
2. Perugino CA, Wallace ZS, Meyersohn N, et al. Large vessel involvement by IgG4-related disease. *Medicine.* 2016;95:e3344–e3356.

3. Perez-Garcia CN, Olmos C, Vivas D, et al. IgG4-aortitis among thoracic aneurysms. *Heart*. 2019;105:1583–1589.
4. Mizushima I, Kasashima S, Fujinaga Y, et al. IgG4-related periaortitis/periarteritis: an under-recognized condition that is potentially life-threatening. *Modern Rheum*. 2019;29:240–250.
5. Pacini D, Leone O, Turci S, et al. Incidence, etiology, histologic findings, and course of thoracic inflammatory aortopathies. *Ann Thorac Surg*. 2008;86:1518–1523.
6. Martinez-Valle F, Solans-Laque R, Bosch-Gil J, et al. Aortic involvement in giant cell arteritis. *Autoimmun Rev*. 2010;9:521–524.
7. Prieto-Gonzalez S, Arguis P, Garcia-Martinez A, et al. Large vessel involvement in biopsy-proven giant cell arteritis: prospective study in 40 newly diagnosed patients using CT angiography. *Ann Rheum Dis*. 2012;71: 1170–116.
8. Hunder GG, Bloch DA, Michel BA, et al. The American College of Rheumatology 1990 criteria for the classification of giant cell arteritis. *Arthritis Rheum*. 1990;33:1122–1128.
9. Weyand CM, Goronzy JJ. Medium- and large-vessel vasculitis. *N Engl J Med*. 2003;349:160–169.
10. Gravanis MB. Giant cell arteritis and Takayasu arteritis: morphologic, pathologic, and etiologic factors. *Int J Cardiol*. 2000;75(suppl 1):S21–S33.
11. Zehr KJ, Mathur A, Orszulak TA, et al. Surgical treatment of ascending aortic aneurysms in patients with giant cell aortitis. *Ann Thorac Surg*. 2005;79:1512–1517.
12. Chrysidis S, Duftner C, Dejaco C, et al. Definitions and reliability assessment of elementary ultrasound lesions in giant cell arteritis: a study from the OMERACT Large Vessel Vasculitis Ultrasound Working Group. *Rheumatology*. 2018;57:227–235.
13. De Miguel E, Roxo A, Castillo C, et al. The utility and sensitivity of colour Doppler ultrasound in monitoring changes in giant cell arteritis. *Clin Exp Rheumatol*. 2012;30(1 suppl 70):S34–S38.
14. Habib HM, Essa AA, Hassan AA. Color duplex ultrasonography of temporal arteries: role in diagnosis and follow-up of suspected cases of temporal arteritis. *Clin Rheumatol*. 2012;31:231–237.
15. Schmidt WA, Blockmans D. Use of ultrasonography and positron emission tomography in the diagnosis and assessment of large-vessel vasculitis. *Curr Opin Rheumatol*. 2005;17:9–15.
16. Blockmans D, Coudyzer W, Vanderschueren S, et al. Relationship between fluorodeoxyglucose uptake in the large vessels and late aortic diameter in giant cell arteritis. *Rheumatology*. 2008;47:1179–1184.
17. Restropo CS, Ocazionez D, Suri R, Vargas D. Aortitis: imaging spectrum of the infectious and inflammatory conditions of the aorta. *Radiographics*. 2011;31:435–451.
18. Maeda H, Handa N, Matsumoto M, et al. Carotid lesions detected by B-mode ultrasonography in Takayasu's arteritis: "Macaroni sign" as an indicator of the disease. *Ultrasound Med Biol*. 1991;17:695–701.
19. Bezerra Lira-Filho E, Campos O, et al. Thoracic aorta evaluation in patients with Takayasu's arteritis by transesophageal echocardiography. *J Am Soc Echocardiogr*. 2006;19:829–834.
20. Dejaco C, Ramiro S, Duftner C, et al. EULAR recommendations for the use of imaging in large vessel vasculitis in clinical practice. *Ann Rheum Dis*. 2018;77:636–643.
21. Dellavedova L, Carletto M, Faggioli P, et al. The prognostic value of baseline (18)F-FDG PET/CT in steroid-naïve large-vessel vasculitis: introduction of volume-based parameters. *Eur J Nucl Med Mol Imag*. 2016;43:340–348.
22. Caubert O, Meunier V, Marthan R, Laffon E. Early assessment of treatment response in Takayasu arteritis: an 18FDG PET procedure. *Clin Nucl Med*. 2016;41:743–745.
23. Hiratzka LF, Bakris GL, Beckman JA, et al. 2010ACCF/AHA/AATS/ACR/ASA/SCA/SCAI/SIR/STS/SVM guidelines for the diagnosis and management of patients with thoracic aortic disease. *Circulation*. 2010;121:e266–e369.
24. Settepani F, Monti L, Antunovic L, et al. IgG4-related aortitis: multimodality imaging approach. *Ann Thorac Surg*. 2017;103:e289.
25. Mavrogeni S, Markousis-Mavrogenis G, Kolovou G. IgG4-related cardiovascular disease. The emerging role of cardiovascular imaging. *Eur J Radiol*. 2017;86:169–175.
26. Aguirre V, Connolly C, Stuklis R. IgG4-aortopathy: an underappreciated cause of non-infectious thoracic aortitis. *Heart Lung Circ*. 2017;26:e79–e81.
27. Takahashi M, Shimizu T, Inajima T, et al. A case of localized IgG4-related thoracic periarteritis and recurrent nerve palsy. *Am J Med Sci*. 2011;341:166–169.
28. Foote EA, Postier RG, Greenfield RA, et al. Infectious aortitis. *Curr Treat Options Cardiovasc Med*. 2005;7:89–97.
29. Revest M, Decaux O, Cazalets C, et al. Thoracic infectious aortitis: microbiology, pathophysiology, and treatment. *Rev Med Interne*. 2007;28:108–115.
30. Topel I, Zorger N, Steinbauer M. Inflammatory diseases of the aorta. Part 2: infectious aortitis. *Gefässchirurgie*. 2016;21(suppl 2):S87–S93.
31. Lin MP, Chang SC, Wu RH, et al. A comparison of computed tomography, magnetic resonance imaging, and digital subtraction angiography findings in the diagnosis of infected aortic aneurysm. *J Comput Assist Tomogr*. 2008;32(4):616–620.
32. Macedo TA, Stanson AW, Oderich GS, et al. Infected aortic aneurysms: imaging findings. *Radiology*. 2004;231:250–257.
33. Blockmans D. PET in vasculitis. *Ann NY Acad Sci*. 2011;1228:64–70.
34. Einspieler I, Thurmel K, Eiber M, et al. First experience of imaging large vessel vasculitis with fully integrated positron emission tomography/MRI. *Circ Cardiovasc Imag*. 2013;6:1117–1119.
35. Evangelista A, Mukherjee D, Mehta RH, et al. Acute intramural hematoma of the aortic: a mystery in evolution. *Circulation*. 2005;111:1063–1070.

139 Congenital Heart Disease: Basic Principles

Talha Niaz, Benjamin W. Eidem

Over the past few decades, there has been a tremendous advancement in the medical and surgical management of patients with congenital heart disease (CHD), leading to an improved survival into adulthood. It has been estimated in various population-based studies worldwide that the prevalence of patients with adult congenital heart disease (ACHD) ranges between 2.17 and 6.12 per 1000 adults (Fig. 139.1).[1–4] The most striking improvement in survival is among the patients with complex CHD (Fig. 139.2). Approximately 90% children with complex CHD are now expected to survive to 18 years of age in the current era.[5] The majority of patients with simple CHD and almost all patients with complex CHD require specialized care throughout their lives for long-term sequelae and complications resulting from the surgical repair or palliation. Moreover, women with CHD not only require prepregnancy counseling for an individualized risk assessment but also monitoring during pregnancy and delivery as well as the peripartum period.[6] To ensure high-quality care for the ongoing increasing demands of this population, adult cardiology practice will need the knowledge and skills to provide optimum care to these patients.

ACHD comprises a heterogeneous group of patients with enormous variations in the underlying anatomy, physiology and surgical repair or palliative techniques. Recently, 2018 American Heart Association/American College of Cardiology guidelines for ACHD patients have classified these cardiac lesions on the basis of anatomic and physiologic complexity (Boxes 139.1 and 139.2).[7] The complexity of these lesions range from an isolated atrial or ventricular septal defect to those with complex atrioventricular and ventriculoarterial connections in heterotaxy. The assessment of the severity of CHD should also include physiological factors, including hemodynamically significant intracardiac shunts, hypoxemia, pulmonary hypertension, end-organ dysfunction, exercise limitation, and associated arrhythmias.[7] It is also critical to have knowledge of the original anatomic diagnosis, type of surgical repair or palliation, and the expected complications that may arise over time. Therefore, a comprehensive echocardiographic evaluation of a patient with ACHD should take into account the interplay of these physiologic factors with the underlying anatomy while paying special attention to the expected complications in different lesions (Fig. 139.3).

Advancement in many cardiac imaging modalities has greatly facilitated improved precision in the diagnosis and quantitative assessment of the functional status of patients with CHD. Transthoracic echocardiography (TTE), however, remains the mainstay because of its wide availability, portability, lack of radiation, and cost effectiveness. Over the past two decades, technological advancements have led to improved image quality and the development of new techniques, including three-dimensional (3D) echocardiography and speckle tracking. 3D echocardiography has shown promise in evaluating complex 3D structures and valvular heart disease, especially mitral valve anatomy and the mechanisms of valvular regurgitation via real time en face imaging (Fig. 139.4).[8]

In addition, reproducible 3D quantitative volumetric and functional assessment have greatly enhanced its value in the serial assessment of patients with ACHD.[9] Quantification of right ventricular (RV) size and systolic function also hold a crucial importance in patients with CHD, especially in patients with congenitally corrected transposition and d-transposition of great arteries after atrial switch, in which the right ventricle serves as the systemic ventricle. RV size and function are also key determinants in the timing of pulmonary valve replacement in patients with tetralogy of Fallot and other similar lesions.[7] In patients with functional single-ventricle anatomy, quantitative assessment of ventricular function can be challenging, and in most cases, a visual estimate of systolic function is used. Transesophageal echocardiography (TEE) can contribute valuable data in patients with limited acoustic windows. Intraoperative TEE has become the preferred modality during surgical repair of CHD for intraoperative monitoring, assessment of postbypass cardiac function, and determination of hemodynamically significant residual lesions.[10,11] Similarly, TEE and intracardiac echocardiography have also become necessity for procedural guidance during transcatheter interventions such as device closure of septal defects, intravascular stent placement, and percutaneous valve replacement (Fig. 139.5).[12,13] Other echocardiographic techniques that are currently used in the field of ACHD include stress echocardiography, contrast echocardiography, and echocardiographically guided cardiac resynchronization therapy.[14]

The chapters that follow provide a systemic approach to the echocardiographic assessment of adults with CHD.

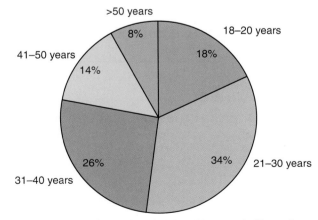

Figure 139.1. Age distribution of adults with congenital heart disease (CHD) in the United States as derived from the Adult Congenital Heart Association's clinic directory. More than half of the adult population with CHD seen in adult CHD clinics is between 18 and 30 years of age. (Adapted with permission from Patel MS, Kogon BE: Care of the adult congenital heart disease patient in the United States: A summary of the current system. *Pediatr Cardiol* 31:511–514, 2010.)

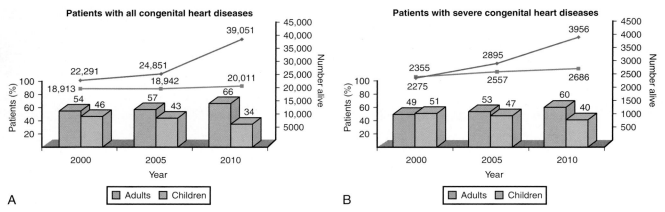

A **B**

Figure 139.2. The numbers and proportions of adults and children with congenital heart disease (CHD) over time in 2000, 2005, and 2010 in Quebec, Canada. **A,** Patients with all forms of CHD. **B,** Patients with severe CHD. (Adapted with permission from Marelli AJ, et al: Lifetime prevalence of congenital heart disease in the general population from 2000 to 2010, *Circulation* 130:749–756, 2014.)

BOX 139.1 Simple and Moderately Complex Congenital Heart Diseases

SIMPLE CONGENITAL HEART DISEASES
- Isolated small ASD or VSD
- Mild isolated pulmonic stenosis
- Repaired ASD, VSD, or PDA

MODERATELY COMPLEX CONGENITAL HEART DISEASES
- Moderate or large unrepaired ASD, PDA, or VSD
- Ostium primum or sinus venosus ASD
- Moderate or greater pulmonary stenosis
- Congenital aortic valve disease
- Subvalvar or supravalvar aortic stenosis
- Congenital mitral valve disease
- Coarctation of the aorta
- Ebstein anomaly
- Tetralogy of Fallot
- Anomalous pulmonary venous connection, partial or total
- Anomalous coronary artery arising from the pulmonary artery or from opposite sinus
- Aorto-left ventricular fistula

ASD, Atrial septal defect; *PDA,* patent ductus arteriosus; *VSD,* ventricular septal defect.
Modified with permission from Stout KK, et al: 2018 AHA/ACC guideline for the management of adults with congenital heart disease, *J Am Coll Cardiol* 73:e81–e192, 2019.

BOX 139.2 Severe and Complex Congenital Heart Diseases

SEVERELY COMPLEX CONGENITAL HEART DISEASE
- Cyanotic congenital heart defect (unrepaired or palliated)
- Double-outlet ventricle
- Fontan procedure
- Interrupted aortic arch
- Mitral atresia
- Single ventricle (including double inlet left ventricle, tricuspid atresia, hypoplastic left heart, any other anatomic abnormality with a functionally single ventricle)
- Pulmonary atresia (all forms)
- Transposition of great arteries (all forms)
- Truncus arteriosus

Modified with permission from Stout KK, et al: 2018 AHA/ACC guideline for the management of adults with congenital heart disease, *J Am Coll Cardiol* 73:e81–e192, 2019.

Complications of surgical repairs

Tetralogy of fallot: pulmonary valve regurgitation requiring valve replacement

d-TGA after atrial switch: systemic and pulmonary venous baffle obstruction or leak

Atrioventricular (AV) septal defects: progressive AV valve regurgitation and left ventricular outflow tract obstruction

Coarctation of the aorta: recoarctation

Fontan: narrowing of superior or inferior vena cava pathways; progressive systemic ventricle dysfunction

Truncus arteriosus: truncal valve dysfunction

Aortic aneurysm and dissection: Turner syndrome, patients with connective tissue disorders or genetically triggered aorotopathy

Patients with ACHD

- NYHA classification
- Arrhythmias and sudden death
- Residual shunts
- Valvular dysfunction
- Pulmonary hypertension
- Recurrent lesions

Figure 139.3. Long-term complications and residual lesions in adult patients with congenital heart disease. *ACHD,* Adult congenital heart disease; *AV,* atrioventricular; *d-TGA,* dextrotransposition of the great arteries; *NYHA,* New York heart classification.

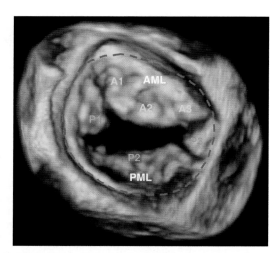

Figure 139.4. Three-dimensional en face transesophageal echocardiogram image demonstrating mitral valve anatomy. Anterior and posterior mitral valve leaflets (AML and PML, respectively) are divided into scallops designated as A1 to A3 and P1 to P3, respectively.

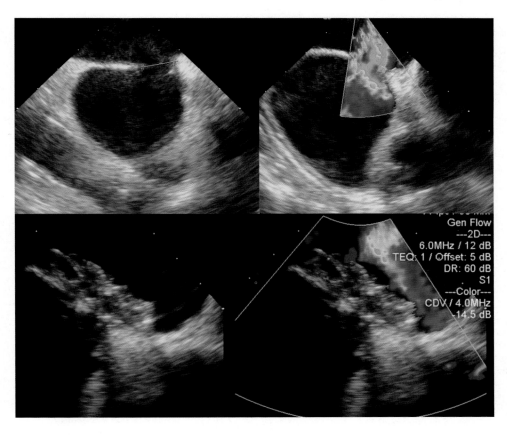

Figure 139.5. Intracardiac echocardiography demonstrating atrial septal defect closure with Gore Cardioform septal occluder device in a 55-year-old patient.

REFERENCES

1. Marelli AJ, Ionescu-Ittu R, Mackie AS, et al. Lifetime prevalence of congenital heart disease in the general population from 2000 to 2010. *Circulation.* 2014;130:749–756.
2. van der Bom T, Bouma BJ, Meijboom FJ, et al. The prevalence of adult congenital heart disease, results from a systematic review and evidence based calculation. *Am Heart J.* 2012;164:568–575.
3. Warnes CA, Liberthson R, Danielson GK, et al. Task force 1: the changing profile of congenital heart disease in adult life. *J Am Coll Cardiol.* 2001;37:1170–1175.
4. Wu MH, Lu CW, Chen HC, et al. Adult congenital heart disease in a nationwide population 2000-2014: epidemiological trends, arrhythmia, and standardized mortality ratio. *J Am Heart Assoc.* 2018;7(4):e007907.
5. Gilboa SM, Salemi JL, Nembhard WN, et al. Mortality resulting from congenital heart disease among children and adults in the United States, 1999 to 2006. *Circulation.* 2010;122:2254–2263.
6. Balint OH, Siu SC, Mason J, et al. Cardiac outcomes after pregnancy in women with congenital heart disease. *Heart.* 2010;96:1656–1661.
7. Stout KK, Daniels CJ, Aboulhosn JA, et al: 2018 AHA/ACC guideline for the management of adults with congenital heart disease, *Circulation.* 2019;139:e698–e800.
8. Tsang W, Lang RM. Three-dimensional echocardiography is essential for intraoperative assessment of mitral regurgitation. *Circulation.* 2013;128:643–652.
9. Lang RM, Addetia K, Narang A, et al. 3-dimensional echocardiography: latest developments and future directions. *JACC Cardiovasc Imag.* 2018;11:1854–1878.
10. Ungerleider RM, Greeley WJ, Sheikh KH, et al. The use of intraoperative echo with Doppler color flow imaging to predict outcome after repair of congenital cardiac defects. *Ann Surg.* 1989;210:526–534.
11. O'Leary PW, Hagler DJ, Seward JB, et al. Biplane intraoperative transesophageal echocardiography in congenital heart disease. *Mayo Clinic Proc.* 1995;70:317–326.
12. Inglessis I, Landzberg MJ. Interventional catheterization in adult congenital heart disease. *Circulation.* 2007;115:1622–1633.
13. Enriquez A, Saenz LC, Rosso R, et al. Use of intracardiac echocardiography in interventional cardiology. *Circulation.* 2018;137:2278–2294.
14. Patel MS, Kogon BE. Care of the adult congenital heart disease patient in the United States: a summary of the current system. *Pediatr Cardiol.* 2010;31:511–514.

140 Systematic Approach to Adult Congenital Heart Disease

Pooja Gupta, Yamuna Sanil, Richard Humes

To efficiently perform an echocardiographic study on an adult with congenital heart disease (CHD), it is extremely important to understand the following: (1) the role of history and natural history, (2) location of the surgical scar(s) and probable surgical repair, (3) knowledge of segmental analysis, (4) special pediatric views and their significance, and (5) the role of transesophageal echocardiography (TEE), particularly with certain CHDs and those with poor acoustic windows.

HISTORY AND NATURAL HISTORY

Lack of awareness of their CHD and the anatomic diagnosis is common among adult patients for whom diagnosis and possible intervention occurred early in life.[1–4] Information about procedures was provided to the parents, not to the current adult patient, whose understanding will be modified by time and the second telling. If the patient knows the diagnosis, this provides important information to

TABLE 140.1 Incidence and Sex Predilection of Congenital Heart Disease: Frequency of Individual Defects

Cardiac Malformation[a]	CHD (%)	Male-to-Female Ratio
Ventricular septal defect	18–28	1:1
Patent ductus arteriosus	10–18	1:2–3
Tetralogy of Fallot	10–13	1:1
Atrial septal defect	7–8	1:2–4
Pulmonary stenosis	7–8	1:1
Transposition of the great arteries	4–8	2–4:1
Coarctation of the aorta	5–7	2–5:1
Atrioventricular canal defect	2–7	1:1
Aortic stenosis	2–5	4:1
Truncus arteriosus	1–2	1:1
Tricuspid atresia	1–2	1:1
Total anomalous pulmonary venous connection	1–2	1:1

[a]Excludes mitral valve prolapse and bicuspid aortic valve
Data reproduced with permission from Hoffman JI, Kaplan S: The incidence of congenital heart disease, *J Am Coll Cardiol* 39:1890–1900, 2002.

TABLE 140.2 Examples of Closed and Open-Heart Operations[a]

Closed Heart Operations	Open Heart Operations
Ligation of patent ductus arteriosus	Closure of atrial septal defect
Repair of coarctation of the aorta	Closure of ventricular septal defect
Pulmonary artery banding	Repair of tetralogy of Fallot
Division of vascular ring or double aortic arch	Arterial or atrial switch operation (for d-TGA)
Blalock-Taussig shunt	Fontan procedure
Transventricular aortic or pulmonary valvotomy	Repair of complete atrioventricular canal defect

[a]Operations done via a "closed" heart technique implies no use of cardiopulmonary bypass. "Open" heart surgery generally is done using bypass and generally through a median sternotomy.
d-TGA, D-transposition of great arteries.

the sonographer that can be beneficial while performing an echocardiogram. Patients without the particulars of diagnosis might use statements such as, "My arteries were backwards," which might mean transposition of great arteries, or "I was born with half a heart," which might mean a single ventricle of some sort. The statement "I had a hole in my heart" can have many meanings ranging from simple to complex problems.[5] Patients may refer to their defect as a "heart murmur," with no understanding of the implications.

If medical records are available, it is worth spending time reviewing this information before initiating an echocardiographic study. If records are not available, clinicians should make every attempt to procure them from the treatment facility (an important historical question), which is often known. Specific knowledge of surgical procedures is vital to understanding the patient and interpreting the echocardiogram. Subtle, but important, details such as an absent pulmonary artery or a right-sided aortic arch will make the echocardiographic examination much smoother and less time consuming.

The natural history of CHD varies tremendously depending on the defect. Not all CHD is lethal. CHD occurs in about 0.8% of live births.[6] In the current era of significantly improved survival,[7,8] adults with complex CHDs have outnumbered children.[9,10] The total number of adults with CHD is estimated to be more than 1 million.[11] Patients who claim to have CHD will be more likely to have a defect that is more prevalent. The actual prevalence of various forms of CHD varies depending on the study cited or methodology used for diagnosis. Bicuspid aortic valve is likely the most common "defect" but is often left out of many lists of CHD as a normal variation. Ventricular septal defect is the next most common CHD, comprising 18% to 28% of the total. A list of the rough incidence percentages of CHD is shown in Table 140.1.[6,12] When performing an echocardiogram on an uninformed adult with CHD, knowledge of commonly found CHD and its natural history is helpful.

Details such as the year of surgery and the total number of surgeries a patient has gone through may help to define the type of surgical repair the patient might have had. A detailed listing of timeline for various surgical procedures is provided in another chapter. Gathering all of this information may take some detective work on the part of the sonographer or cardiologist. A good example is the case of d-transposition of great arteries, which was repaired by performing an atrial switch operation (also referred to as Mustard/Senning procedure) for the first time in 1954. With advancement in surgical techniques, the approach of switching the atria was changed to performing the arterial switch operation (also referred to as Jatene procedure) for the first time in 1976. However, acceptance of this newer procedure was not immediate

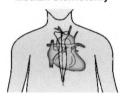

Median sternotomy

Lateral thoracotomy

4th
5th

Median sternotomy
- Most open heart procedures using cardiopulmonary bypass (VSD, ASD, tetralogy of Fallot, Fontan, Mustard, etc.)

Right lateral thoracotomy
- Right Blalock-Taussig shunt
- Waterston shunt

Left lateral thoracotomy
- Left Blalock-Taussig shunt
- Pulmonary artery band
- Coarctation repair
- PDA ligation
- Potts shunt

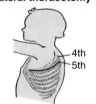

Figure 140.1. Schematic representation of the chest incisions and the likely congenital heart operations that may be performed through this approach. This information can be very helpful when the patient is unaware of the procedure or procedures that were performed. *ASD,* Atrial septal defect; *PDA,* patent ductus arteriosus; *VSD,* ventricular septal defect.

everywhere, implying that patients born before 1976 most likely had atrial switch operations, and those born after early 1980s very likely had arterial switch operations. It is also important to know if the patient had any form of catheter-based intervention such as a device or a stent, which were not common before the mid-1990s. Many patients may also confuse a catheter-based intervention or even a diagnostic catheterization with a "surgery."

LOCATION OF THE SCAR: "THE SCAR IS THE CLUE"

Optimal timing for repairing a particular CHD has evolved with time and advancement in surgical technique. We are now increasingly performing complete repairs for several CHDs in the neonatal period and fewer palliative operations (Table 140.2). Primary open-heart repair using cardiopulmonary bypass is most frequently performed through a median sternotomy and a midline chest incision. By contrast, in earlier years, palliative operations were frequently performed using lateral or posterolateral thoracotomies. A midline sternotomy scar versus a right or left lateral thoracotomy scar can help discern the probable surgical repair and, in some cases, the possible diagnosis. Some of the operations that could be performed without opening the heart were performed via a lateral thoracotomy (Fig. 140.1).

SEGMENTAL ANALYSIS

An echocardiographic strategy, which encompasses identification of the blood flow in and out of the heart and the connection of the various segments of the heart, is called *segmental analysis*. This includes systematic determination of the position of the cardiac apex, situs of the atrium, the atrioventricular (AV) relationship, and the ventriculoarterial relationship.[13–15] In CHD, the pathway that the blood takes and the connections between the cardiac segments are the focus, particularly in those with complex CHD. Standard American Society of Echocardiography (ASE) imaging protocols[16,17] allow the examiner to identify these points of anatomic interest and recognize the deviation from normal. It is the thinking, not just the protocol, that needs emphasis in terms of segmental analysis. Segmental thinking includes:

1. Cardiac position and position of the visceral organs (visceral situs)
   a. Position of the heart in the chest and the visceral organs in the abdomen
   b. Relative position of the atria, identified morphologically
   c. Relative position of the ventricles, identified morphologically
2. Blood flow into the heart
   a. Identification of systemic veins and its drainage
   b. Identification of pulmonary veins and its drainage
   c. Identification of additional venous anomalies
3. Blood flow through the heart
   a. Atrioventricular connections, identified morphologically
   b. Ventriculoarterial connections, identified morphologically
   c. Shunts
   d. Obstructions
4. Blood flow out of the heart
   a. Aortic arch patency and branching pattern
   b. Pulmonary artery patency, bifurcation, and size
   c. Presence and size of the ductus arteriosus
5. Coronary artery anatomy

Cardiac Position and Visceral Situs

Abnormalities of cardiac position and visceral situs may be associated with complex CHDs. Imaging difficulties or confusion about complex anatomy can be made clearer after defining these points. An unusual or confusing appearance of the heart from standard left parasternal imaging planes may imply abnormal cardiac position such as dextrocardia or mesocardia.

Cardiac position and identification of visceral situs are best performed in a transverse plane from the subcostal or subxiphoid location. The transducer positioned with the notch at 3 o'clock position will demonstrate the relative position of the abdominal viscera such as liver and stomach.

Visceral Situs

- Situs solitus (normal): The stomach, spleen, pancreas, and sigmoid colon are left-sided structures, and the liver, cecum, and appendix are right-sided organs. On echocardiogram, we only show the liver and the air in the stomach along with portions of inferior vena cava (IVC) and descending aorta (Ao) (Fig. 140.2A, and Video 140.2A).
- Situs inversus: mirror image of normal (Fig. 140.2B and Video 140.2B)
- Situs ambiguous: does not fit into normal or inversus pattern. The abdominal or thoracic organ arrangements are inconsistent and or abnormally symmetric with duplication or absence of organs. The liver is often midline, and there could be either multiple or absent spleen (Fig. 140.2C and Video 140.2C).

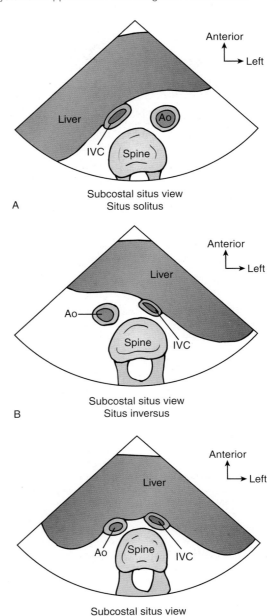

Figure 140.2. A, Normal visceral situs is described as situs solitus with the liver mainly on the right, the stomach on the left, and the aorta (Ao) to the left of the spine. Abnormalities of situs are frequently associated with cardiac anomalies that are often complex. This is particularly true when the visceral situs and cardiac position are discordant. For example, visceral situs solitus and dextrocardia has a high incidence of congenital heart disease, as does situs inversus and levocardia. **B,** Visceral situs is referred to as inversus when liver is mainly on the left and stomach and aorta on the right of the spine. **C,** When the position of the vessels and the liver cannot be reliably determined, it is referred to as situs ambiguous. This finding has a higher incidence of associated congenital cardiac defects. *IVC*, Inferior vena cava. (See accompanying Video 140.2.)

- Tilting the probe toward the patient's left shoulder will bring in the four-chamber view, and the direction of the cardiac apex will determine the cardiac position (Fig. 140.3 and Video 140.3).
  - Apex pointing to the left: levocardia (normal)
  - Apex pointing to the right: dextrocardia
  - Apex pointing to the midline: mesocardia

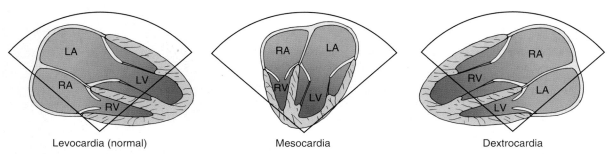

Levocardia (normal)   Mesocardia   Dextrocardia

Figure 140.3. Cardiac position is best determined from subcostal imaging. This view is obtained by placing the transducer in the subcostal space in a transverse orientation with the indicator notch pointed to the patient's left. An "apex-down" view is the most anatomically correct and is a less confusing view to determine the direction of the apex. Apex pointing to the patient's left is referred to as levocardia, to the middle is mesocardia, and to the right is dextrocardia. Although dextrocardia in this example is shown with the left atrium (LA) and left ventricle (LV) as a mirror image, this is not always the case. Dextrocardia may also present with the LV and LA being leftward of the right-sided chamber in the right chest. True mesocardia is quite rare. The apex almost always favors one side or the other. The sonographer must take care to display the image exactly as it appears. The orientation of patient right and left should remain constant, and no attempt should be made to make the image appear "normal" by changing right–left orientation. *RA,* Right atrium; *RV,* right ventricle. (See accompanying Video 140.3.)

Atrial Situs

Distinctive morphologic features determine atrial sidedness and not their relative position in the chest. The atria can sometimes be recognized based on the appearance of their appendage. A *morphologic right atrium (RA)* has a broad-based, triangular appendage, whereas a *morphologic left atrium (LA)* has a narrow, elongated, fingerlike appendage. Interestingly, in certain complex CHDs, the *morphologic RA* can be positioned on the left side of the heart and chest, and the *morphologic LA* can be on the right side of the heart and chest. Practically speaking, it is challenging to image the atrial appendage, and in most cases, atrial situs follows abdominal visceral situs as determined from the subcostal view. It is also a reasonable assumption that the morphologic RA receives the systemic veins and the morphologic LA the pulmonary veins.

Atrial position is described as atrial situs solitus, which is a normal morphologic RA on the right side and a morphologic LA on the left side), atrial situs inversus (morphologic atria on the opposite sides), or atrial situs ambiguous (also referred to as *atrial isomerism*; the atria duplicated or atrial sidedness cannot be determined).

Ventricular Position and Morphologic Identification

Right or left ventricular identification is more properly based on their specific morphologic characteristics and not on their relative position in the chest. The right ventricle (RV) has a triangular shape with coarse trabeculations and the presence of a prominent muscle bundle called a moderator band with a septal band along the septal surface. Compared with the RV, the left ventricle (LV) is cone shaped and finely trabeculated and has a smooth septal surface with no moderator band and a more superior level of insertion of the mitral valve to the ventricular septum. Two papillary muscles that attach to the left ventricular free wall with no attachment to the interventricular septum are usually present. It is also important to remember that embryologically, the AV valves arise from their respective ventricles and are inseparable. Thus, the tricuspid valve always accompanies the morphologic RV irrespective of its position or attachment to the atria or the great vessel, and the same rule applies to the LV and mitral valve. While imaging patients with CHD, it is also useful to remember that the tricuspid valve is inserted more apically along the ventricular septum compared with the mitral valve, and this may further facilitate identification of the ventricles.

Blood Flow Into the Heart

Echocardiographic imaging of the systemic and pulmonary veins requires skill and training to identify any deviation from normal. It is important to know and understand the anomalies of systemic and pulmonary venous return and their echocardiographic appearance. A combination of suprasternal and subcostal or subxiphoid views is helpful in defining the venous anatomy. Morphologic identification of the individual cardiac segments is followed by tracing the course of blood flow through the heart.

Blood Flow Through the Heart

Blood in the RA may enter the right or the LV depending on the AV relationship, which can be described as AV concordance or discordance. When the morphologic RA drains into the morphologic RV, it is referred to as *AV concordance* (normal), and when the morphologic RA drains into the morphologic LV, it is referred to as *AV discordance*. In addition, blood flow through the heart requires a systematic assessment for shunts, which may occur at atrial, ventricular, or great artery levels. Evaluation of flow across the valves will determine the presence of obstruction, stenosis, or regurgitation.

Blood Flow Out of the Heart

Identifying flow out of the heart begins by defining the ventriculoarterial relationship, which can, again, be described as ventriculoarterial concordance (normal), ventriculoarterial discordance, or double-outlet right or LV. Knowledge of the echocardiographic appearance of abnormal great artery relationships is crucial for imaging patients with CHDs. The pulmonary artery and pulmonary valve can be identified by visualizing the bifurcation into the left and right branch pulmonary artery. The aorta and aortic valve will demonstrate the origin of coronary arteries and the head and neck vessels. Arch sidedness and its patency should be established as part of a systematic segmental approach. The connection of the morphologic RV to the pulmonary artery is referred to as *ventriculoarterial concordance*, and connection of the morphologic LV to the pulmonary artery is *ventriculoarterial discordance*. When more than 50% of both arteries arise from a particular ventricle, it is referred to as double-outlet right or LV based on the ventricle of origin.

Coronary Artery Anatomy

In a pediatric echocardiographic laboratory, it is routine practice to image the origin and proximal course of the coronary arteries.[17] The coronary artery anatomy may be difficult to image in larger adult patients with difficult echocardiographic windows. However, it should be attempted to develop the skill and particularly in certain CHDs that are known to be associated with a coronary artery

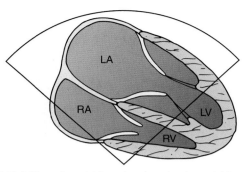

Figure 140.4. The subcostal four-chamber view is useful for evaluating atrial chamber size and particularly for looking at the atrial septum. It is obtained from the subxiphoid space with the transducer pointed at the left shoulder and the indicator notch to the patient's left. *LA,* Left atrium; *LV,* left ventricle; *RA,* right atrium; *RV,* right ventricle. (See accompanying Video 140.4.)

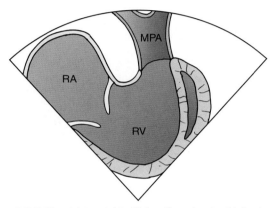

Figure 140.5. The right ventricle (RV) outflow view is obtained by rotating the transducer 45 degrees counterclockwise from the subcostal four-chamber view. This is an excellent view for evaluating the entire RV outflow tract, particularly when there is stenosis or hypoplasia at one or more levels along the tract. This view offers good alignment for Doppler assessment. *MPA,* Main pulmonary artery; *RA,* right atrium. (See accompanying Video 140.5.)

anomaly. In some cases, the coronary artery anatomy might even have implications during surgical intervention or reintervention.

SPECIAL PEDIATRIC VIEWS AND THEIR SIGNIFICANCE

As described by the ASE, five different locations, including subcostal or subxiphoid, apical, left parasternal, right parasternal, and suprasternal views, are used for performing a detailed pediatric echocardiogram.[17] In this chapter, we describe some of the special pediatric views and their role in defining CHD.

The subcostal or subxiphoid long-axis view (four-chamber view) is useful for evaluating atrial chamber size and particularly for visualization of the atrial septum. The transducer is pointed at the left shoulder, and the indicator notch is to the patient's left (3 or 4 o'clock position). Color-flow mapping from this view is very helpful in identifying the presence of atrial level shunting, as well as its magnitude and direction (Fig. 140.4 and Video 140.4). The right ventricular outflow view is obtained by rotating the transducer 45 degrees counterclockwise from the subcostal or subxiphoid long-axis view and angulating anteriorly (Fig. 140.5 and Video 140.5). This is an excellent view for evaluating the right ventricular outflow tract, particularly when there is suspected stenosis or hypoplasia.

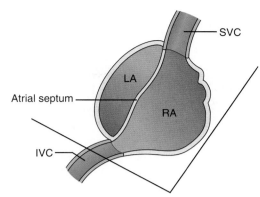

Figure 140.6. The subcostal or subxiphoid bicaval view is obtained by rotating the transducer 45 degrees farther counterclockwise from the subcostal right ventricular outflow tract view (indicator notch at 12 o'clock position) and angulating it anterosuperiorly. The superior vena cavae (SVCs), atrial septum (AS), and right upper pulmonary vein are well visualized in this view. *IVC,* Inferior vena cava; *RA,* right atrium. (See accompanying Video 140.6.)

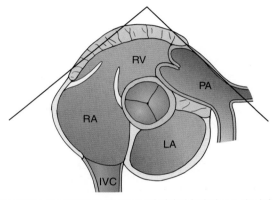

Figure 140.7. In patients with poor subxiphoid windows, the left parasternal short-axis view may be used to visualize the atrial septum (transducer in left parasternal location and notch directed at the 3 o'clock position). *IVC,* Inferior vena cava; *LA,* left atrium; *PA,* pulmonary artery; *RA,* right atrium; *RV,* right ventricle. (See accompanying Video 140.7.)

The subcostal or subxiphoid bicaval view is obtained by rotating the transducer 45 degrees farther anticlockwise from the subcostal right ventricular outflow tract view (indicator notch at 12 o'clock position) and angulating it anterosuperiorly (Fig. 140.6 and Video 140.6). The superior and inferior vena cavae, atrial septum, and the right upper pulmonary vein are well visualized in this view. This is particularly beneficial for identifying sinus venosus atrial septal defects. Color-flow mapping demonstrates the direction and magnitude of the atrial-level shunt.

In patients with poor subxiphoid windows, the left parasternal short-axis view (Fig. 140.7 and Video 140.7) may be used to visualize the atrial septum (transducer in the left parasternal location and notch directed at 3 o'clock position). Sweeping the transducer is important to establish relationships between contiguous structures. The left parasternal short-axis sweep (transducer in left parasternal position, notch pointing toward the 2 o'clock position) begins with the transducer tilted toward the right shoulder and progresses from the base of the heart to the apex. This sweep is particularly important for evaluating the ventricular septum. This is useful in the two-dimensional examination as well as in color-flow mapping. While sweeping toward the apex, it may be necessary to slide the transducer inferiorly between rib interspaces toward the cardiac apex in an attempt to cover the

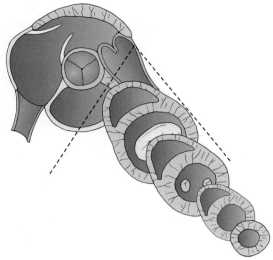

Figure 140.8. Sweeps are important to establish relationships between contiguous structures. The parasternal short-axis sweep is performed from a parasternal location with the transducer in a short-axis plane. This view is particularly important for evaluating the entire ventricular septum from the base to the apex as well as the mitral valve apparatus. Color-flow mapping aids the diagnosis of shunts across the ventricular septum as well as valvular regurgitation. (See accompanying Video 140.8.)

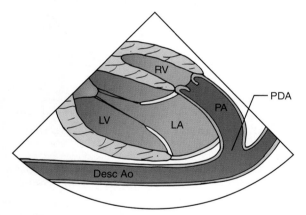

Figure 140.9. The "ductal view" is obtained by placing the transducer in a sagittal orientation from a high left parasternal location with the indicator notch directly superior. The main pulmonary artery (PA), patent ductus arteriosus (PDA), and descending aorta (Desc Ao) are all seen in a continuation. Color-flow mapping is an essential part of imaging. However, recognition of blue flow (representing right-to-left ductus) requires caution. *LA,* Left atrium; *LV,* left ventricle; *RA,* right atrium; *RV,* right ventricle. (See accompanying Video 140.9.)

entire ventricular septum, particularly the apical muscular septum (Fig. 140.8 and Video 140.8). In addition to the ventricular septum and the details of the aortic and pulmonary valve, this view is excellent for visualization of the mitral valve and papillary muscles.

The *ductal view* is obtained by aligning the transducer in a sagittal plane from a high left parasternal location (notch positioned between the 12 and 1 o'clock positions) (Fig. 140.9 and Video 140.9). This view aligns the main pulmonary artery, the ductus arteriosus, and the descending aorta in a single plane. Color-flow mapping helps confirm the absence or presence of a ductus and the direction of blood flow in this vessel. This view also allows a better visualization of ductal size. In cases with a good echocardiographic window, this view is also excellent for visualization of the isthmus

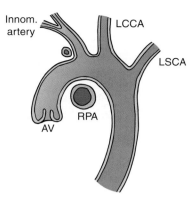

Figure 140.10. Arch configuration and patency may be obtained from the suprasternal long-axis view, with the transducer in the suprasternal notch and the transducer parallel to a plane between the left shoulder and right hip. Specific attention to the distance between head and neck vessels and color-flow mapping may be necessary to assess for coarctation. *AV,* Aortic valve; *Innom. artery.* innominate artery; *LCCA,* left common carotid artery; *LSCA,* left subclavian artery; *RPA,* right pulmonary artery. (See accompanying Video 140.10.)

(narrowest portion of the arch) and the upper descending aorta. Hence, this view is of particular significance in recognizing the presence and severity of coarctation of the aorta.

Aortic arch pathology may exist independently or coexist with a CHD, making imaging of this structure an important part of the examination. The aortic arch is best visualized from a *suprasternal long-axis view* (transducer in the suprasternal notch and parallel to a plane between the left shoulder and right hip). The transducer indicator notch is approximately at the 1 o'clock position with the patient positioned supine with head and neck extended with the help of a wedge under the shoulder (Fig. 140.10 and Video 140.10). If the arch is difficult to visualize from a standard suprasternal long-axis view, a right aortic arch may be suspected, which requires an opposite tilt and counterclockwise transducer rotation of about 30 degrees to demonstrate it.

The *suprasternal short-axis* view is obtained by rotating the transducer about 60 degrees clockwise from the long-axis view (indicator notch at the 3 o'clock position) and is useful for evaluating pulmonary veins as well as the superior vena cava (Fig. 140.11 and Video 140.11). This is also an excellent view for visualization of the right pulmonary artery, which is used as a landmark. While in the suprasternal short-axis view, with some further clockwise rotation and superior tilt toward the contralateral shoulder, the branching pattern of the innominate artery may be visualized to aid in identification of arch-sidedness (Fig. 140.12 and Video 140.12).

THE ROLE OF TRANSESOPHAGEAL ECHOCARDIOGRAPHY IN AN ADULT PATIENT WITH CONGENITAL HEART DISEASE

The indications for TEE in an adult patient with CHD include diagnosis and guidance during percutaneous interventions or surgical repairs (intraoperative). In the presence of poor acoustic transthoracic windows, TEE can be extremely helpful for establishing a diagnosis and guiding their management. TEE offers better visualization of interatrial shunts, pulmonary venous drainage, aortic dissection, abscesses or vegetations, intracardiac thrombus, intracardiac baffles, and prosthetic valves compared with transthoracic echocardiography (TTE).[18–24] Surgical baffles and conduits may be better visualized by TEE than TTE.[23,24] In the interventional cardiac laboratory and operating room, TEE is an extremely helpful

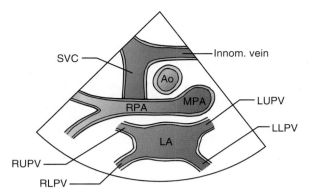

Figure 140.11. Suprasternal short-axis views are obtained by rotating the transducer about 60 degrees in clockwise direction from the suprasternal long-axis view. This view is very useful for evaluating pulmonary veins as well as the superior vena cava (SVC). This is also an excellent view for assessment of the right pulmonary artery (RPA), which is used as a landmark for obtaining the view. *Ao,* Aorta; *Innom. vein,* innominate vein; *LA,* left atrium; *LLPV,* left lower pulmonary vein; *LUPV,* left upper pulmonary vein; *MPA,* main pulmonary artery; *RLPV,* right lower pulmonary vein; *RUPV,* right upper pulmonary vein. (See accompanying Video 140.11.)

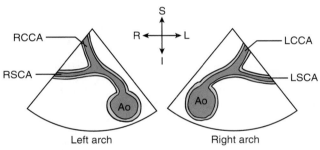

Figure 140.12. From the suprasternal short-axis view, farther clockwise rotation and slight angulation of the transducer toward the contralateral shoulder demonstrate the branching pattern of the innominate artery as an aid in identification of arch sidedness. The first branch going to the right side and bifurcating suggests a left arch, and the first branch going to the left and bifurcating suggests a mirror-image right arch. *Ao,* Aorta; *I,* inferior; *L,* left; *LCCA,* left common carotid artery; *LSCA,* left subclavian artery; *R,* right; *RCCA,* right common carotid artery; *RSCA,* right subclavian artery; *S,* superior. (See accompanying Video 140.12.)

modality for cardiac imaging and a standard of care.[25,26] Recent advances in high-resolution real-time image acquisition, cropping tools, and quantification software have made three-dimensional (3D) TEE an important adjunct for imaging adults with CHD. 3D TEE is especially useful in providing guidance during cardiac interventions and for preoperative assessment of CHD.[18,27,28] Real-time, 3D zoom or full-volume modalities can be used depending on the structure of interest. Puchalski and colleagues describe specific TEE views recommended in specific diagnostic scenarios for adult patients with CHD.[18] They also alert clinicians to the sedation requirements of this group of patients during TEE and the need for closer monitoring.[18] The utility of TEE may be regarded as an alternative to cardiac magnetic resonance (CMRI) imaging in certain cases or as an adjunct to it in other cases. Depending on the questions being asked and the setting, one may be preferred over the other. CMRI may provide additional information in cases of intracardiac baffles, extracardiac baffles, and conduits.[2,23,29] CMRI is now the imaging test of choice in adult patients with tetralogy of Fallot for quantification of right ventricular volumes, estimation of pulmonary regurgitation

fraction, and quantification of other shunt flows and collateral flow. It is also the recommended imaging test for measurement of aortic root size in patients with bicuspid aortic valve or Marfan syndrome. Intracardiac echocardiography (ICE) is now being increasingly used for interventional procedures in some centers.[30]

SUMMARY

- Historical details are the key (including the surgical details).
- If the history is incomplete, be a detective—find out when the repair was done, where the scar is, and so on.
- Know which operations are done through the side versus midline incision.
- Know the timeline of the various surgical repairs and which procedure is currently being done for a particular CHD and those that are now abandoned.
- Understand the segmental approach to the identification of cardiac anatomy.
- Know the specific morphologic characteristics of all the cardiac structures and chambers.
- Know and practice the special pediatric views.
- Know the commonly occurring complications and consequences of various forms of CHD.
- Understand the role of TTE, TEE, ICE, and CMRI in these patients.

  Please access ExpertConsult to view the corresponding videos for this chapter.

REFERENCES

1. Valente AM, Landzberg MJ, Gianola A, et al. Improving heart disease knowledge and research participation in adults with congenital heart disease. *Int J Cardiol.* 2013;168:3236–3240.
2. Moons P, De Volder E, Budts W, et al. What do adult patients with congenital heart disease know about their disease, treatment, and prevention of complications? *Heart.* 2001;86:74–80.
3. Fernandes SM, Verstappen A, Ackerman K, et al. Parental knowledge regarding lifelong congenital cardiac care. *Pediatrics.* 2011;128:e1489–e1495.
4. Chessa M, De Rosa G, Pardeo M, et al. Illness understanding in adults with congenital heart disease. *Ital Heart J.* 2005;6:895–899.
5. Verstappen A, Pearson D, Kovacs AH. Adult congenital heart disease: the patient's perspective. *Cardiol Clin.* 2006;24:515–529.
6. Hoffman JI, Kaplan S. The incidence of congenital heart disease. *J Am Coll Cardiol.* 2002;39:1890–1900.
7. Mahle WT, Spray TL, Wernovsky G, et al. Survival after reconstructive surgery for hypoplastic left heart syndrome. *Circulation.* 2000;102:III136–III141.
8. Warnes CA, Liberthson R, Danielson GK, et al. Task force 1: the changing profile of congenital heart disease in adult life. *J Am Coll Cardiol.* 2001;37:1170–1175.
9. Brickner ME, Hillis LD, Lange RA. Congenital heart disease in adults. *N Engl J Med.* 2000;342:256–263.
10. Williams RG, Pearson GD, Barst RJ, et al. Report of the National heart, Lung, and Blood Institute working group on research in adult congenital heart disease. *J Am Coll Cardiol.* 2006;47:701–707.
11. Gilboa SM, Devine OJ, Kucik JE, et al. Congenital heart defects in the United States. *Circulation.* 2016;134:101–109.
12. Ferencz C, Rubin JD, McCarter RJ, et al. Congenital heart disease: prevalence at livebirth. *Am J Epidemiol.* 1985;121:31–36.
13. Lev M. Pathologic diagnosis of positional variations in cardiac chambers in congenital heart disease. *Lab Invest.* 1954;3:71–82.
14. Van Praagh R. Diagnosis of complex congenital heart disease: morphologic-anatomic method and terminology. *Cardiovasc Intervent Radiol.* 1984;7:115–120.
15. Anderson RH, Becker AE, Freedom RM, et al. Sequential segmental analysis of congenital heart disease. *Pediatr Cardiol.* 1984;5:281–287.
16. Lopez L, Colan SD, Frommelt PC, et al. Recommendations for quantification methods during the performance of a pediatric echocardiogram. *J Am Soc Echocardiogr.* 2010;23:465–495.
17. Lai WW, Geva T, Shirali GS, et al. Guidelines and standards for performance of a pediatric echocardiogram. *J Am Soc Echocardiogr.* 2006;19:1413–1430.
18. Puchalski MD, Lui GK, Miller-Hance WC, et al. Guidelines for performing a comprehensive transesophageal echocardiographic: examination in children and all patients with congenital heart disease. *J Am Soc Echocardiogr.* 2019;32:173–215.
19. Sreeram N, Stumper OF, Kaulitz R, et al. Comparative value of transthoracic and transesophageal echocardiography in the assessment of congenital abnormalities of the atrioventricular junction. *J Am Coll Cardiol.* 1990;16:1205–1214.
20. Hausmann D, Daniel WG, Mugge A, et al. Value of transesophageal color Doppler echocardiography for detection of different types of atrial septal defect in adults. *J Am Soc Echocardiogr.* 1992;5:481–488.

21. Feltes TF, Friedman RA. Transesophageal echocardiographic detection of atrial thrombi in patients with nonfibrillation atrial tachyarrhythmias and congenital heart disease. *J Am Coll Cardiol.* 1994;24:1365–1370.

22. Fyfe DA, Kline CH, Sade RM, et al. Transesophageal echocardiography detects thrombus formation not identified by transthoracic echocardiography after the Fontan operation. *J Am Coll Cardiol.* 1991;18:1733–1737.

23. Hirsch R, Kilner PJ, Connelly MS, et al. Diagnosis in adolescents and adults with congenital heart disease. Prospective assessment of individual and combined roles of magnetic resonance imaging and transesophageal echocardiography. *Circulation.* 1994;90:2937–2951.

24. Ayres NA, Miller-Hance W, Fyfe DA, et al. Indications and guidelines for performance of transesophageal echocardiography in the patient with pediatric acquired or congenital heart disease. *J Am Soc Echocardiogr.* 2005;18:91–98.

25. Stevenson JG. Utilization of intraoperative transesophageal echocardiography during repair of congenital cardiac defects: a survey of North American centers. *Clin Cardiol.* 2003;26:132–134.

26. Stevenson JG, Sorensen GK, Gartman DM, et al. Transesophageal echocardiography during repair of congenital cardiac defects: identification of residual problems necessitating reoperation. *J Am Soc Echocardiogr.* 1993;6:356–365.

27. Simpson J, Lopez L, Acar P, et al. Three-dimensional echocardiography in congenital heart disease. *J Am Soc Echocardiogr.* 2017;30:1–28.

28. Cossor W, Cui VW, Roberson DA. Three-dimensional echocardiographic en face views of ventricular septal defects: Feasibility, accuracy, imaging protocols and reference image collection. *J Am Soc Echocardiogr.* 2015;28:1020–1029.

29. Hoppe UC, Dederichs B, Deutsch HJ, et al. Congenital heart disease in adults and adolescents: comparative value of transthoracic and transesophageal echocardiography and MR imaging. *Radiology.* 1996;199:669–677.

30. Mullen MJ, Dias BF, Walker F, et al. Intracardiac echocardiography guided device closure of atrial septal defects. *J Am Coll Cardiol.* 2003;41:285–292.

141 Common Congenital Heart Defects Associated With Left-to-Right Shunts

David A. Roberson, Eleanor Ross, Vivian W. Cui

Congenital heart defects (CHDs) associated with left-to-right shunts are among the most common anomalies.[1] The most common types of left-to-right shunt lesions include atrial septal defect (ASD), ventricular septal defect (VSD), atrioventricular septal defect (AVSD), and patent ductus arteriosus (PDA) (Table 141.1). Their clinical significance is based on volume overload, congestive heart failure, pulmonary hypertension, and endocarditis. Some defects may close spontaneously, such as PDA, secundum ASD, muscular VSD, and less commonly perimembranous VSD.[2,3] Some are amenable to device closure, including secundum ASD, muscular VSD, some perimembranous VSD, and PDA.[4–7] The remaining types of defects require surgical closure when they are clinically significant. In this chapter, we focus on these more common defects in the absence of additional cardiac defects. The less common left-to-right shunt anomalies such as fistulas, arteriovenous malformations, and aortopulmonary window, are excluded from this discussion. The goal of echocardiography is to define the type, size, number, location, chamber dimensions, shunt size, and pulmonary artery pressures.

ATRIAL SEPTAL DEFECT

ASD is associated with increased pulmonary blood flow, right heart chamber enlargement caused by volume overload, exercise intolerance, and pulmonary hypertension if left untreated for an extensive period.[8–10] The most common type is the ostium secundum ASD, which is located within the oval fossa (Fig. 141.1). Many of these are amenable to device closure.[4,11] The second most common type is ostium primum ASD, which is located at the apical aspect of the atrial septum adjacent to the atrioventricular (AV) valves.[12] This defect is typically associated with a cleft in the mitral valve and is within the AVSD spectrum (Fig. 141.2 and Video 141.2). Sinus venosus ASDs are located at the cavoatrial junction and typically are associated with partial anomalous pulmonary venous connections of the right pulmonary veins.[13] The superior type, which is adjacent to the superior vena cava (SVC), is more common than the inferior type adjacent to the inferior vena cava (Fig. 141.3 and Video 141.3). The coronary sinus type ASD is caused by unroofing of the coronary sinus, resulting in a communication with the floor of the left atrium. It is very rare and usually associated with

a connection of the left SVC to the coronary sinus (Fig. 141.4 and Video 141.4).[14]

VENTRICULAR SEPTAL DEFECT

VSD is a very common CHD, either as an isolated anomaly or in combination with a large variety of other defects.[1] In this chapter, we focus on VSD as an isolated anomaly. VSD may be associated with increased pulmonary blood flow, left heart chamber enlargement, congestive heart failure, exercise intolerance, endocarditis, and pulmonary hypertension if left untreated for an extensive period.[3,15,16]

Muscular VSDs are completely surrounded by septal myocardium.[17,18] They may be single or multiple, vary widely in size, and are most commonly located in the region of the moderator band or apex (Figs. 141.5 and 141.6; Video 141.6). Many of these presenting in the newborn period will close spontaneously.[19] Large or persistent multiple muscular VSD may require treatment with device closure or surgery.[6,20]

Perimembranous VSD involves the membranous portion of the ventricular septum and surrounding tissue (Fig. 141.7 and Video 141.7).[17,18] There is contact between the tricuspid, mitral, and aortic valves. There is often a pouch of tissue related to the tricuspid valve that partially occludes the defect. Some are amenable to device closure, and others require surgery to close.[7,20]

Malaligned VSD is caused by malalignment and deficiency of ventricular septal myocardial components.[18] Most malalignment defects are associated with other anomalies such as anterior malalignment present in tetralogy of Fallot and double-outlet right ventricle[21] (Fig. 141.8 and Video 141.8). Anterior deviation of the conal septum without outflow tract obstruction, the so-called Eisenmenger type, is one of the least common types of malaligned VSD. Posterior malalignment VSD is associated with coarctation and interrupted aortic arch complex (Fig. 141.9). Surgical repair is needed for malalignment type VSD.

Outlet VSD is located in the ventricular outflow tract beneath the semilunar valves and requires surgical closure.[18] These defects are sometimes referred to as supracristal or doubly committed subarterial VSD (Fig. 141.10 and Video 141.10).[17] They may be associated with prolapse of the aortic valve into the defect, causing

TABLE 141.1 Congenital Heart Disease with Left-to-Right Shunt

Atrial Septal Defect (ASD)	
Type	**Description**
Secundum	In the region of the oval fossa; may have multiple orifices; often amenable to device closure
Primum	In the apical region of the atrial septum; associated with cleft mitral valve; within the spectrum of AVSDs
Sinus venosus	Superior type with SVC override is more common than the inferior type with IVC override; associated with anomalous right pulmonary vein connections
Coronary sinus	Shunt through the coronary sinus is associated with partial or complete unroofing of the coronary sinus and persistent left superior vena cava

Ventricular Septal Defect (VSD)	
Type	**Description**
Muscular	Completely surrounded by septal myocardium; various locations and multiple defects possible
Perimembranous	Deficiency of membranous septum and surrounding region; fibrous continuity of tricuspid, mitral, and aortic valves
Malaligned	Deviated conal septum; seen in tetralogy of Fallot, double-outlet RV, interrupted aortic arch complex
Outlet VSD	Deficient or absent outlet portion of ventricular septum; seen in doubly committed subarterial VSD and truncus arteriosus
Inlet VSD	Caused by absent or deficient AV septum; has coplanar AV valves

Atrioventricular Septal Defect (AVSD)	
Type	**Description**
Primum ASD	Located in the apical region of the atrial septum; associated with cleft mitral valve
Intermediate	Includes primum ASD, common AV valve with divided orifice and inlet VSD with pouch
Complete	Includes primum ASD, common AV valve with common orifice and inlet VSD

Patent Ductus Arteriosus (PDA)	
Type	**Description**
Premature	May cause high pulmonary blood flow and CHF; can be closed with indomethacin, percutaneous device, or surgery
Older patients	Rarely causes CHF; typically closed with a percutaneous device

CHF, Congestive heart failure; *IVC,* inferior vena cava; *RV,* right ventricle; *SVC,* superior vena cava.

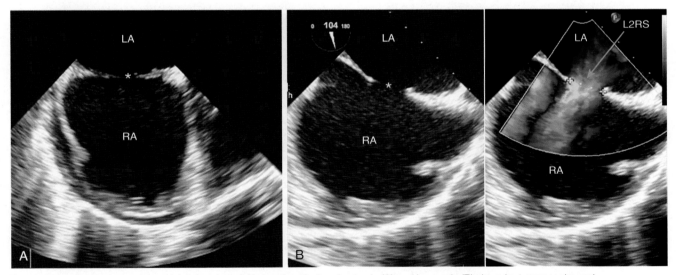

Figure 141.1. Secundum atrial septal defect *(asterisk)* visualized in the short-axis (**A**) and long-axis (**B**) views by transesophageal echocardiography. Color Doppler imaging shows the left-to-right shunt (L2RS). *LA,* Left atrium; *RA,* right atrium.

aortic valve insufficiency.[22] This type of VSD is also present in truncus arteriosus (Fig. 141.11 and Video 141.11B).[23] Surgical repair is needed for outlet-type VSD.

Inlet VSD is located in the inlet portions of the ventricular septum, within the confines of the attachments of the tricuspid valve apparatus (Fig. 141.12).[18] It is characterized by coplanar AV valves and is often associated with a cleft in the anterior leaflet of the mitral valve. Inlet VSD is present in AVSD and is treated with surgery.[24]

ATRIOVENTRICULAR SEPTAL DEFECT

AVSD, also called AV canal defect, is caused by a defect in AV septation that results in abnormalities of the atrial septum, ventricular septum, and AV valves (Fig. 141.13).[12,24] Partial AVSD, with primum ASD and cleft mitral valve, was discussed earlier. Intermediate AVSD consists of a primum ASD, common AV valve with separate right and left orifice, and an inlet VSD completely or partially closed by pouchlike tissue related to the AV valves

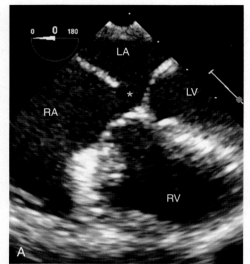

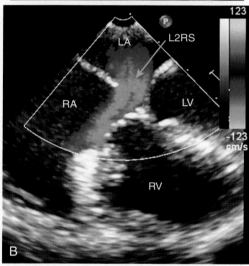

Figure 141.2. A, Primum atrial septal defect *(asterisk)* visualized in the midesophageal four-chamber view by transesophageal echocardiography. **B,** Color Doppler imaging shows the left-to-right shunt (L2RS). *LA,* Left atrium; *LV,* left ventricle; *RA,* right atrium; *RV,* right ventricle. (See accompanying Video 141.2)

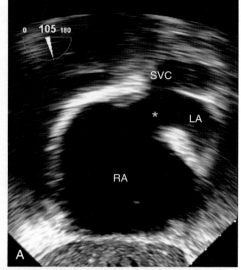

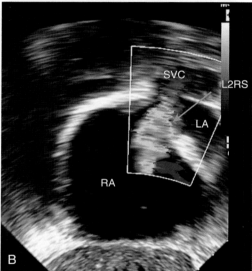

Figure 141.3. A, Superior sinus venosus atrial septal defect *(asterisk)* visualized in the transgastric view by transesophageal echocardiography. **B,** Color Doppler imaging shows the left-to-right shunt (L2RS). *LA,* Left atrium; *RA,* right atrium; *SVC,* superior vena cava. (See accompanying Video 141.3)

(Fig. 141.14 and Video 141.14). Complete AVSD has a primum ASD, common AV valve with common orifice, and inlet VSD (Fig. 141.15 and Video 141.15). These defects require surgical closure.

PATENT DUCTUS ARTERIOSUS

PDA is caused by the persistent patency of the fetal artery that connects the main pulmonary artery and the descending aorta (Fig.

141.16 and Video 141.16). Failure of spontaneous PDA closure in preterm infants is associated with pulmonary overcirculation.[15] In this setting, the PDA may be closed with indomethacin, a percutaneous device, or surgically if medical treatment fails.[15,25] Older patients with PDA are often asymptomatic and are treated most commonly with device closure, which has largely replaced surgical treatment.[5]

Please access ExpertConsult to view the corresponding videos for this chapter.

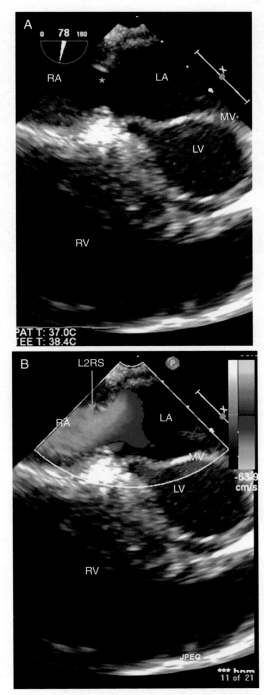

Figure 141.4. A, Coronary sinus atrial septal defect *(asterisk)* visualized by transesophageal echocardiography. **B,** Color Doppler imaging shows the left-to-right shunt (L2RS). *LA,* Left atrium; *LV,* left ventricle; *MV,* mitral valve; *RA,* right atrium; *RV,* right ventricle. (See accompanying Video 141.4)

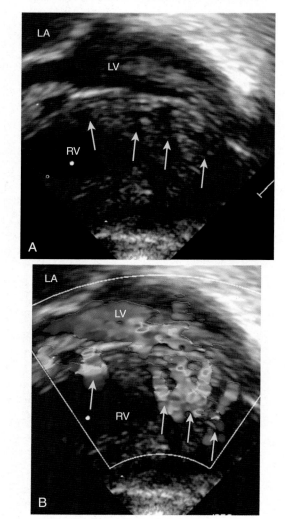

Figure 141.5. A, Apical muscular ventricular septal defect (VSD; *arrow*) visualized by transthoracic echocardiography in the parasternal long-axis view with color Doppler imaging. **B,** Spectral Doppler interrogation shows that VSD is restrictive, with peak gradient greater than 90 mm Hg. *LA,* Left atrium; *LV,* left ventricle; *RV,* right ventricle.

Figure 141.6. A, Multiple small muscular ventricular septal defects (VSDs; *arrows*) visualized by transthoracic echocardiography in the subcostal view. **B,** Color Doppler imaging shows the multiple left-to-right shunts, so-called Swiss cheese VSD. *LA,* Left atrium; *LV,* left ventricle; *RV,* right ventricle. (See accompanying Video 141.6)

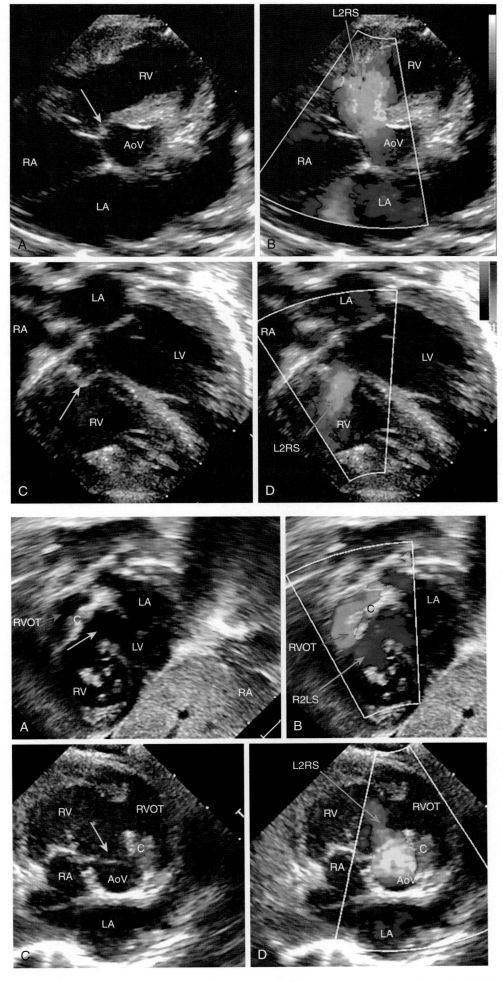

Figure 141.7. *Top*, Perimembranous ventricular septal defect (VSD; *yellow arrow*) visualized by transthoracic echocardiogram in the parasternal short-axis view by two-dimensional (**A**) and color Doppler imaging (**B**). *Bottom*, Subcostal views of the same perimembranous VSD *(yellow arrow)*, showing the defect with tricuspid valve pouch tissue by two-dimensional (**C**) and the left-to-right shunt (L2RS) by color Doppler imaging (**D**). *AoV,* Aortic valve; *LA,* left atrium; *LV,* left ventricle; *RA,* right atrium; *RV,* right ventricle. (See accompanying Video 141.7, *A-D*)

Figure 141.8. Malaligned ventricular septal defect (VSD; *yellow arrow*) in tetralogy of Fallot with anterior deviation of the conal septum *(C)* and resultant narrowing of the right ventricular outflow tract (RVOT). *Top*, VSD visualized by transthoracic echocardiography in the subcostal view by two-dimensional (**A**) and color Doppler imaging (**B**) right-to-left shunt (R2LS). *Bottom*, Subcostal views of the same malaligned VSD *(yellow arrow)*, showing the defect with tricuspid valve pouch tissue by two-dimensional (**C**) and the left-to-right shunt (L2RS) by color Doppler imaging (**D**). *AoV,* Aortic valve; *LA,* left atrium; *LV,* left ventricle; *RA,* right atrium; *RV,* right ventricle. (See accompanying Video 141.8, *A-D*)

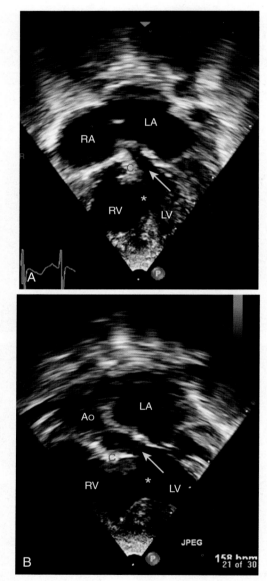

Figure 141.9. Malaligned ventricular septal defect (VSD; *asterisk*) in patient with interrupted aortic arch, shown by transthoracic echocardiogram in the apical view. There is subaortic narrowing *(arrow)*. **A,** Posterior deviation of the conal septum *(C)*. **B,** Orthogonal view with the same findings. *Ao,* Ascending aorta; *LA,* left atrium; *LV,* left ventricle; *RA,* right atrium; *RV,* right ventricle.

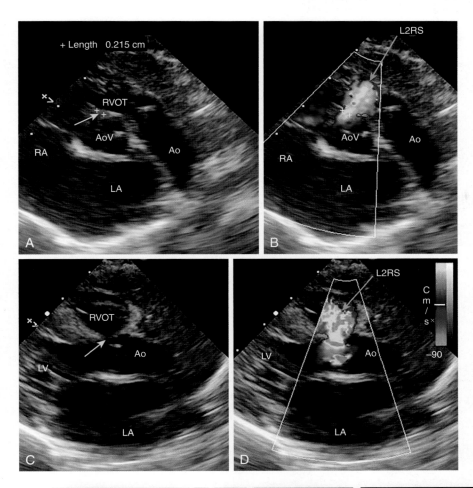

Figure 141.10. *Top,* Supracristal type outlet ventricular septal defect (VSD; *yellow arrow*) visualized by transthoracic echocardiography in the parasternal short-axis view by two-dimensional (**A**) and color Doppler imaging (**B**). *Bottom,* Parasternal long-axis view of the same outlet VSD *(yellow arrow),* showing the defect by two-dimensional (**C**) and the left-to-right shunt (L2RS) by color Doppler imaging (**D**). *Ao,* Aorta; *AoV,* aortic valve; *LA,* left atrium; *LV,* left ventricle; *RA,* right atrium; *RV,* right ventricle; *RVOT,* right ventricular outflow tract. (See accompanying Video 141.10, *A-D*)

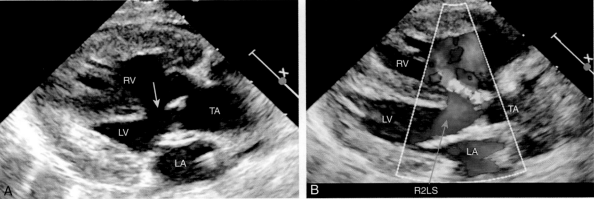

Figure 141.11. Outlet ventricular septal defect (VSD; *yellow arrow*) in a patient with truncus arteriosus visualized by transthoracic echocardiography in the parasternal long-axis view by two-dimensional (**A**) and color Doppler imaging (**B**). Color Doppler shows the right-to-left shunt (R2LS) across the VSD and a regurgitant jet from the dysplastic truncal valve. *LA,* left atrium; *LV,* left ventricle; *RV,* right ventricle; *TA,* truncus arteriosus. (See accompanying Video 141.11, *B*)

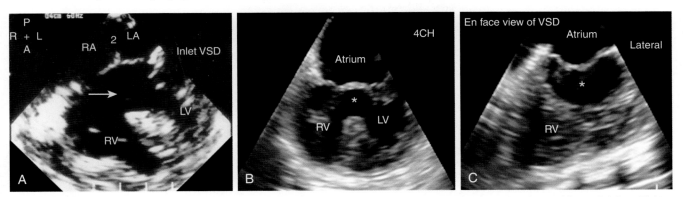

Figure 141.12. A, Inlet ventricular septal defect (VSD; *arrow*) shown in the four-chamber view along with a secundum atrial septal defect. *Right,* Inlet VSD *(asterisk)* is present in atrioventricular septal defect (AVSD), as seen in this complete AVSD from the four-chamber view (**B**) and in an en face view (C**).** *LA,* left atrium; *LV,* left ventricle; *RA,* right atrium; *RV,* right ventricle.

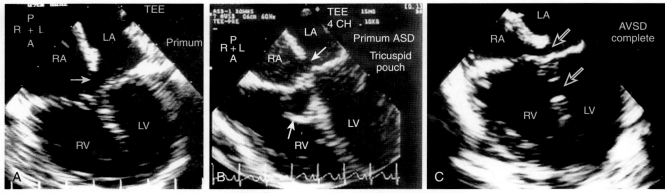

Figure 141.13. Three types of atrioventricular septal defects (AVSDs) seen from the four-chamber (4 CH) view. **A,** Primum atrial septal defect *(arrow).* **B,** Intermediate AVSD with primum atrial septal defect *(top arrow),* inlet ventricular septal defect, and atrioventricular valve pouch tissue *(bottom arrow).* **C,** Complete AVSD with primum ASD *(top arrow)* and inlet ventricular septal defect *(bottom arrow)* without valve pouch tissue. *A,* Anterior; *ASD,* atrial septal defect; *L,* left; *LA,* left atrium; *LV,* left ventricle; *P,* posterior; *R,* right; *RA,* right atrium; *RV,* right ventricle; *TEE,* transesophageal echocardiography.

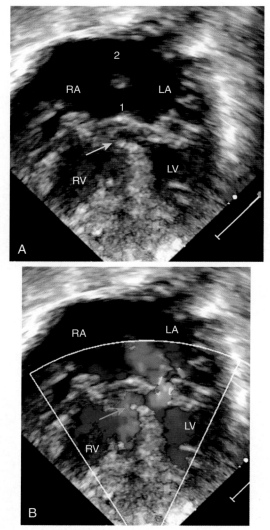

Figure 141.14. Intermediate atrioventricular (AV) septal defect visualized from the apical four-chamber view. **A,** Two-dimensional imaging showing primum atrial septal defect *(1)* and inlet ventricular septal defect with atrioventricular valve pouch tissue *(yellow arrow)*, as well as an additional secundum atrial septal defect *(2)*. **B,** Color Doppler imaging showing left-to-right shunt *(blue arrow)* across the inlet ventricular septal defect. *LA,* Left atrium; *LV,* left ventricle; *RA,* right atrium; *RV,* right ventricle. (See accompanying Video 141.14)

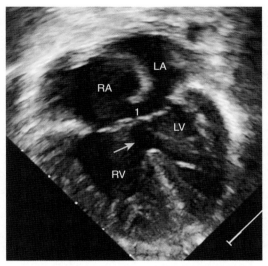

Figure 141.15. Complete atrioventricular septal defect visualized from the apical four-chamber view. Two-dimensional imaging shows primum atrial septal defect *(1)* and inlet ventricular septal defect *(arrow)*. *LA,* Left atrium; *LV,* left ventricle; *RA,* right atrium; *RV,* right ventricle. (See accompanying Video 141.15)

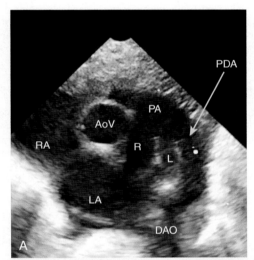

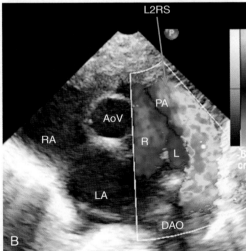

Figure 141.16. Large patent ductus arteriosus (PDA) visualized from a parasternal short-axis "three finger" view. **A,** Two-dimensional imaging shows the PDA extending from the descending aorta (DAO) to the pulmonary artery (PA). **B,** Color Doppler imaging demonstrates the large left-to-right shunt (L2RS) across the PDA. *AoV,* Aortic valve; *L,* left pulmonary artery; *LA,* left atrium; *R,* right pulmonary artery; *RA,* right atrium. (See accompanying Video 141.16)

REFERENCES

1. Hoffman JI, Kaplan S. The incidence of congenital heart disease. *J Am Coll Cardiol.* 2002;39:1890–1900.
2. Helgason H, Jonsdottir G. Spontaneous closure of atrial septal defects. *Pediatr Cardiol.* 1999;20:195–199.
3. Van Hare GF, Soffer LJ, Sivakoff MC, et al. Twenty-five-year experience with ventricular septal defect in infants and children. *Am Heart J.* 1987;114:606–614.
4. McMahon CJ, Feltes TF, Fraley JK, et al. Natural history of growth of secundum atrial septal defects and implications for transcatheter closure. *Heart.* 2002;87:256–259.
5. Arora R. Transcatheter closure of patent ductus arteriosus. *Rev Cardiovasc Ther.* 2005;3:865–874.
6. Holzer R, Balzer D, Cao QL, et al. Amplatzer muscular ventricular septal defect I: device closure of muscular ventricular septal defects using the Amplatzer muscular ventricular septal defect occluder. *J Am Coll Cardiol.* 2004;43:1257–1263.
7. Holzer R, de Giovanni J, Walsh KP, et al. Transcatheter closure of perimembranous ventricular septal defects using the Amplatzer membranous VSD occluder: immediate and midterm results of an international registry. *Catheter Cardiovasc Interv.* 2006;68:620–628.
8. Shah D, Azhar M, Oakley CM, et al. Natural history of secundum atrial septal defect in adults after medical or surgical treatment: a historical prospective study. *Br Heart J.* 1994;71:224–227. discussion 228.
9. Phillips SJ, Okies JE, Henken D, et al. Complex of secundum atrial septal defect and congestive heart failure in infants. *J Thorac Cardiovasc Surg.* 1975;70:696–700.
10. Campbell M. Natural history of atrial septal defect. *Br Heart J.* 1970;32:820–826.
11. Kazmouz S, Kenny D, Cao QL, et al. Transcatheter closure of secundum atrial septal defects. *J Invasive Cardiol.* 2013;25:257–264.
12. Silverman NH, Zuberbuhler JR, Anderson RH. Atrioventricular septal defects: Cross-sectional echocardiographic and morphologic comparisons. *Int J Cardiol.* 1986;13:309–331.
13. Van Praagh S, Carrera ME, Sanders SP, et al. Sinus venosus defects: unroofing of the right pulmonary veins—anatomic and echocardiographic findings and surgical treatment. *Am Heart J.* 1994;128:365–379.
14. Raghib G, Ruttenberg HD, Anderson RC, et al. Termination of left superior vena cava in left atrium, atrial septal defect, and absence of coronary sinus: a developmental complex. *Circulation.* 1965;31:906–918.
15. Jarmakani MM, Graham Jr TP, Canent Jr RV, et al. Effect of site of shunt on left heart-volume characteristics in children with ventricular septal defect and patent ductus arteriosus. *Circulation.* 1969;40:411–418.
16. Lucas Jr RV, Adams Jr P, Anderson RC, et al. The natural history of isolated ventricular septal defect: a serial physiologic study. *Circulation.* 1961;24:1372–1387.
17. Jacobs JP, Burke RP, Quintessenza JA, et al. Congenital heart surgery nomenclature and database project: ventricular septal defect. *Ann Thorac Surg.* 2000;69:S25–S35.
18. Soto B, Becker AE, Moulaert AJ, et al. Classification of ventricular septal defects. *Br Heart J.* 1980;43:332–343.
19. Ramaciotti C, Vetter JM, Bornemeier RA, et al. Prevalence, relation to spontaneous closure, and association of muscular ventricular septal defects with other cardiac defects. *Am J Cardiol.* 1995;75:61–65.
20. Roberson DA, Muhiudeen IA, Cahalan MK, et al. Intraoperative transesophageal echocardiography of ventricular septal defect. *Echocardiography.* 1991;8:687–697.

21. Wu MH, Wang JK, Chang CI, et al. Implication of anterior septal malalignment in isolated ventricular septal defect. *Br Heart J*. 1995;74:180–185.
22. Rhodes LA, Keane JF, Keane JP, et al. Long follow-up (to 43 years) of ventricular septal defect with audible aortic regurgitation. *Am J Cardiol*. 1990;66:340–345.
23. Colon M, Anderson RH, Weinberg P, et al. Anatomy, morphogenesis, diagnosis, management, and outcomes for neonates with common arterial trunk. *Cardiol Young*. 2008;18(suppl 3):52–62.

24. Jacobs JP, Burke RP, Quintessenza JA, et al. Congenital heart surgery nomenclature and database project: atrioventricular canal defect. *Ann Thorac Surg*. 2000;69:S36–S43.
25. Malviya MN, Ohlsson A, Shah SS. Surgical versus medical treatment with cyclooxygenase inhibitors for symptomatic patent ductus arteriosus in preterm infants. *Cochrane Database Syst Rev*. 2013;3. CD003951.

142 Obstructive Lesions

Leo Lopez, Wyman W. Lai

Obstructive lesions along the outflow tracts of the right ventricle (RV) and left ventricle (LV) can be found at the level of the semilunar valve, below the valve within the subarterial outflow chamber, or above the valve along the great arteries. Based on a meta-analysis of nearly 40 published studies evaluating the incidence of congenital heart disease (CHD) over many decades, pulmonary stenosis (PS) represents the fourth most common CHD (occurring in 73 per 100,000 live births), coarctation of the aorta (CoA) the sixth most common (occurring in 41 per 100,000 live births), and aortic stenosis (AS) the seventh most common (occurring in 40 per 100,000 live births).[1] Among almost 600,000 patients evaluated at the Cardiovascular Program of Boston Children's Hospital from 1988 to 2002, a pulmonary valve (PV) abnormality is the fourth most common diagnosis with a frequency of 5.7%, and an aortic valve (AoV) abnormality is the fifth most common with a frequency of 5.5%.[2] In patients with left ventricular outflow obstruction, valvar AS is the most common subgroup, followed by CoA, subvalvar AS, and supravalvar AS. CoA may present as an isolated anomaly or in association with other cardiac lesions, particularly a bicuspid AoV, other left-sided obstructive lesions, or a ventricular septal defect (VSD). RV outflow obstructive lesions include valvar PS, double-chambered RV (DCRV), supravalvar PS, and peripheral pulmonic stenosis (PPS). Aortic obstruction is more commonly seen than obstruction along the main or branch pulmonary arteries.

ANATOMY OF THE OUTFLOW TRACTS AND THORACIC AORTA

The normal outflow tract can be divided into three anatomic segments: the subarterial region, the semilunar valve, and the proximal great artery. The conus or infundibulum represents the subarterial muscular chamber separating the atrioventricular (AV) valve from the corresponding semilunar valve. In the normal heart, the subpulmonary conus is separated from the trabecular segment of the RV chamber at the infundibular os defined by the moderator, septal, and parietal bands.

The normal semilunar valve consists of three leaflets with three-dimensional attachments in a semilunar or crownlike fashion within the arterial root extending from the ventriculoarterial junction to the sinotubular junction. Hence, the term *annulus* used for the semilunar valve in echocardiography is in fact a diagnostician construct without a true anatomic correlate because this area represents only the most proximal attachments of the semilunar valve at the ventriculoarterial junction. The leaflets are separated by three commissures extending during diastole from the center of the valve at the level of the ventriculoarterial junction to the arterial wall at the level of the sinotubular junction.

The thoracic aorta may be divided into five segments: (1) ascending aorta, including the aortic root; (2) proximal transverse arch, between the right innominate (brachiocephalic) and left common carotid arteries; (3) distal transverse arch, between the left common carotid and left subclavian arteries; (4) isthmus, between the left subclavian artery and the ligamentum or ductus arteriosus; and (5) descending aorta. The aortic arch is left sided (traveling to the left of the trachea) in more than 99% of patients. Several generally benign variants in branching pattern are found, including (1) common origin of the right innominate and left common carotid arteries (incorrectly referred to as a "bovine arch"), (2) aortic origin of the left vertebral artery, and (3) aberrant right subclavian artery with separate origin of the right subclavian artery distal to the left subclavian artery origin.

Clinical Presentation

Obstructive lesions are associated with a pressure-overloaded ventricle, often accompanied by progressive hypertrophy and fibrosis. Patients with these problems generally present with a systolic murmur whose location is determined by the affected outflow tract and whose frequency and intensity are determined by the degree of obstruction. Occasionally, a systolic click is heard. Symptoms in children are rare, though severe obstruction can be associated with chest pain, syncope, or exercise intolerance, particularly for left ventricular outflow obstruction. Rarely, older children and adults present with signs of right ventricular or left ventricular failure because severe hypertrophy can result in progressive diastolic and systolic dysfunction.

The presentation of CoA later in life is usually an incidental finding, although life-threatening complications such as intracranial bleed, aortic dissection, or infective endarteritis do occur. The more benign presentation usually involves a systolic murmur; absent or weak femoral pulses with brachiofemoral delay; upper extremity hypertension; hypertensive retinopathy; exercise intolerance; or leg fatigue or claudication.[3] Electrocardiography may show left ventricular hypertrophy (LVH), and the classic chest radiographic findings are the "3" sign and rib notching.

Valvar Aortic Stenosis

Congenital valvar AS is most frequently associated with a bicuspid AoV, which likely represents the most common CHD with an incidence of 0.4% to 2% in the general population.[4–6] A truly bicuspid AoV with only two leaflets is uncommon, appearing in only 11% of patients in one international multicenter registry.[7] Instead, a bicuspid AoV usually results from fusion of two of the three leaflets or underdevelopment of one of the three commissures (known as a raphe), leading to the use of the terms *functionally bicuspid* or *bicommissural AoV* for these lesions. Fusion occurs most frequently at the intercoronary commissure between the right and left coronary leaflets (70%) (Fig. 142.1A) followed by the commissure between the right and noncoronary leaflets (28%) (Fig. 142.1B)

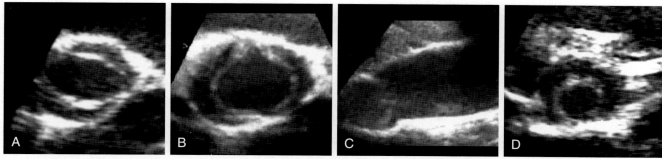

Figure 142.1. A, Parasternal short-axis image of a bicommissural aortic valve (AoV) with fusion of the right and left coronary leaflets (intercoronary commissure). Notice the horizontal orientation of the aortic opening. (See accompanying Video 142.1.) **B,** Parasternal short-axis image of a bicommissural AoV with fusion of the commissure between the right and noncoronary leaflets. Notice the vertical orientation of the aortic opening. **C,** High parasternal long-axis image of ascending aortic dilatation in association with a bicommissural AoV. **D,** Parasternal short-axis image in a neonate with valvar aortic stenosis and a unicommissural AoV in which the only patent commissure is between the left and noncoronary leaflets.

and the commissure between the left and noncoronary leaflets (rare).[8] In adults, valvar AS appears to progress more rapidly in the setting of fusion of the intercoronary commissure,[9] though studies in children have shown faster progression of AS and regurgitation as well as an earlier need for intervention when the right and non-coronary leaflets are fused.[10] Common associations include CoA,[4] subvalvar AS, VSD, coronary anomaly, Turner syndrome,[11] and aortic dilatation and aneurysm formation[12,13] (Fig. 142.1C). Other AoV morphologic abnormalities associated with valvar AS include a dysplastic tricuspid AoV and a hypoplastic aortic "annulus."

Echocardiographic evaluation of valvar AS must involve assessment of leaflet and commissural morphology, best seen in parasternal views. A bicuspid AoV with a horizontally oriented systolic opening in short-axis views is generally associated with fusion of the intercoronary commissure (see Fig. 142.1A and Video 142.1), whereas a more vertically oriented systolic opening is associated with fusion of the commissure between the right and noncoronary leaflets (see Fig. 142.1B). Incomplete commissural separation can restrict lateral mobility of the leaflets, resulting in a systolic doming appearance in long-axis views. The degree of obstruction is assessed by measuring peak and mean gradients using continuous-wave Doppler interrogation in the apical, right sternal border, and suprasternal views, though one must be cognizant of the known discrepancies between the maximum instantaneous gradient measured by echocardiography and the peak-to-peak gradient measured by catheterization as well as the effects of pressure recovery.[14] Although criteria for valvar AS severity have not been established for children, guidelines published for adults with valvar AS, including calculation of AoV area by the continuity equation, have been applied to the pediatric population.[15] Three-dimensional echocardiography has also proven to be helpful in children as well as adults[16] (Video 142.2). Other important components of the echocardiographic evaluation include assessment of the degree of LVH, the presence of endocardial fibroelastosis, and the size of the ascending aorta (see Fig. 142.1C).

Aortic Coarctation

CoA is typically juxtaductal in location, involving the aortic isthmus. The length of the narrowed segment may be discrete or long segment. Narrowing or hypoplasia of the transverse arch is more commonly found in patients presenting as fetuses or early in childhood, whereas discrete narrowing with the presence of collaterals is more often seen in patients presenting later. The vast majority of patients with CoA are now diagnosed as infants. The diagnosis of CoA is 1.7 times more common in males, but CoA occurs in 12% to 17% of patients with Turner syndrome. In several large series of patients with CoA, 14% to 27% had significant AS or

aortic regurgitation (AR).[17] Complications are common in patients after CoA repair, and age at repair appears to be a risk factor. Late cardiovascular complications include systemic hypertension, reco-arctation, dissection, aneurysm, rupture, and early coronary artery disease.[18]

The hallmark of CoA is luminal narrowing of the aorta due to a posterior "shelf" or a circumferential membrane. A helpful anatomic definition of narrowing is a diameter of the proximal transverse arch of 60% or less of the ascending aorta, distal transverse arch of 50% or less of the ascending aorta, or isthmus narrowing helpful anatomic definition of narrowing is a diameter of the proximal transverse arch of 40%.[19] Echocardiography is a useful diagnostic tool for CoA, but imaging of the aortic isthmus and proximal descending aorta is difficult in older children and adults (Video 142.3). In these cases, other imaging modalities such as magnetic resonance imaging (MRI) (Fig. 142.2 and Video 142.4) or computed tomography (CT) are indicated.

Goals of the echocardiographic examination include evaluation of aortic arch sidedness and branching pattern, severity and length of CoA, size of other aortic segments (including aneurysms), other left-sided structures (including AoV morphology), collaterals, LV size (including LV mass) and function, and associated lesions. The arch is best visualized from the suprasternal and high left sternal border windows, but it may be seen in neonates even from the subcostal window. Aortic branching is evaluated in suprasternal short-axis imaging, with a normal pattern visualized as a bifurcating first brachiocephalic artery to the right (opposite to the sidedness of the arch). Absence of normal bifurcation may raise the suspicion of an aberrant right subclavian artery. The region of the CoA and proximal descending aorta is sometimes better seen in a sagittal plane at the high left sternal border window using the main pulmonary artery as a "window" for imaging. A juxtaductal CoA can involve the origin of the left subclavian artery. If present, an aberrant subclavian artery may be above or below the site of CoA.

Doppler interrogation for the CoA gradient is best performed in the suprasternal view, occasionally with the transducer positioned toward the neck or right subclavicular region to align the ultrasound beam with the long axis of the descending aorta or aortic isthmus. The Doppler tracing of significant CoA shows a high-velocity systolic peak followed by gradual deceleration throughout diastole (Fig. 142.3A). Peak and mean gradients are measured, and in the setting of multiple levels of obstruction, the gradient proximal to the CoA site (measured by pulsed wave Doppler) should be subtracted from the total gradient. An important aspect of echocardiographic screening for CoA is the Doppler pattern of the descending aorta at the level of the diaphragm, where a low-velocity signal with continuous antegrade diastolic flow may be seen (Fig. 142.3B).

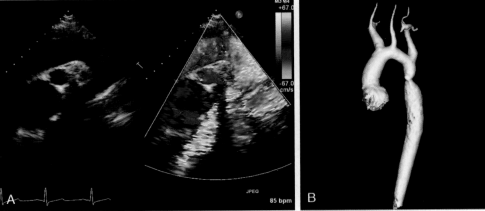

Figure 142.2. A, Suprasternal notch long-axis Color Compare image of an adolescent with mild coarctation of the aorta and a bicuspid aortic valve without stenosis or regurgitation. Aliasing of the color Doppler flow jet is seen across the region of stenosis, which is not well visualized on two-dimensional imaging. (See accompanying Video 142.3.) **B,** Three-dimensional volume rendering of a gadolinium-enhanced magnetic resonance angiogram of the same patient demonstrating discrete narrowing of the aortic isthmus with mild poststenotic dilatation of the proximal descending aorta without aneurysm. (See accompanying Video 142.4.)

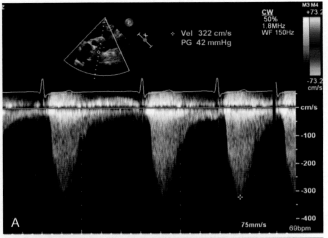

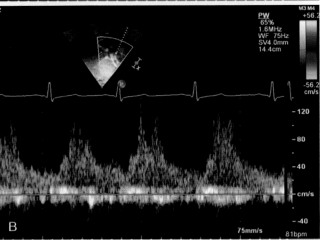

Figure 142.3. A, Suprasternal notch continuous-wave Doppler of the same adolescent patient showing a peak instantaneous gradient of 42 mm Hg across the region of coarctation with gradual deceleration of flow throughout diastole. The systolic blood pressure gradient was 20 to 25 mm Hg by upper- and lower-extremity blood pressure measurements. **B,** Doppler tracing of the descending aorta of the same patient at the level of the diaphragm showing low-velocity flow with continuous antegrade diastolic flow.

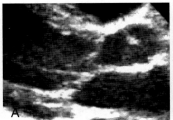 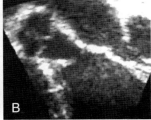

Figure 142.4. A, Parasternal long-axis image of subvalvar aortic stenosis secondary to a subaortic fibromuscular ridge. **B,** Apical image of subvalvar aortic stenosis secondary to a subaortic fibromuscular ridge extending to the anterior mitral leaflet. (See accompanying Video 142.5.)

Subvalvar Aortic Stenosis

Many people have classified subvalvar AS as an acquired heart disease rather than a congenital one because it is rarely diagnosed in the newborn period.[20] Nevertheless, it is a progressive disease that is associated with abnormalities in left ventricular outflow tract (LVOT) morphology such as a steep aortoseptal angle, an elongated mitral-aortic intervalvular fibrosa, exaggerated aortic override, prominent LVOT muscle bundles, and abnormal MV attachments to the ventricular septum.[21,22] Subvalvar AS in isolation most frequently presents as a discrete fibrous or fibromuscular shelf from the ventricular septum below the AoV (Fig. 142.4A), occasionally extending to the anterior mitral leaflet in a diaphragmatic fashion (Fig. 142.4B and Video 142.5). Occasionally, the muscular component is so prominent that it results in a tunnel-like outflow tract with significant obstruction. When a VSD is present, the subaortic obstruction frequently results from posterior deviation of the conal septum, often associated with aortic coarctation or interrupted aortic arch.[23] Other mechanisms for subvalvar AS with a VSD include an endocardial fold or fibromuscular ridge at the crest of the muscular septum[24] or abnormal MV attachments to the ventricular septum (particularly in unrepaired or repaired AV canal defects). Other associations with subvalvar AS include a bicuspid AoV, a DCRV,[25] and AR, which is usually not progressive in adults[26] but can be rapidly progressive in children and require early surgical intervention.[27] Echocardiographic evaluation of patients with subvalvar AS must involve assessment of the mechanism and location of the obstruction in apical and parasternal views as well as the degree

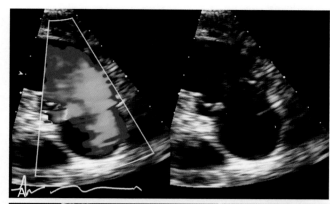

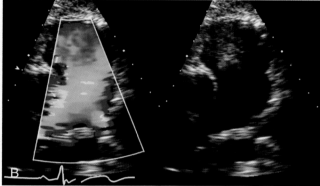

Figure 142.5. A, Angled parasternal long-axis Color Compare demonstrating doming pulmonary valve and mild valvar pulmonary stenosis. **B,** Parasternal short-axis color compare of the same patient with a dilated main pulmonary artery and severe left pulmonary artery hypoplasia.

of the obstruction in apical, right sternal border, and suprasternal views. In addition, AR and other associated abnormalities must be excluded.

Supravalvar Aortic Stenosis

Although it occasionally presents as a familial autosomal-dominant lesion or as a sporadic idiopathic disorder, supravalvar AS is usually associated with Williams syndrome, a constellation of clinical problems including abnormal calcium metabolism, developmental delay, failure to thrive, and abnormal facial features.[28] Three anatomic subtypes have been described: the most common hourglass type frequently involving dilatation of the aortic root and ascending aorta on either side of the narrowing, the membranous or diaphragmatic type, and the rare tubular type with diffuse hypoplasia of the ascending aorta.[29] The obstruction is usually progressive over time, and the degree of obstruction must be assessed by measuring the maximum gradient in apical, right sternal border, and suprasternal views. Patients with Williams syndrome can also have branch pulmonary artery stenosis, aortic coarctation, and renal artery stenosis. Other associations include abnormalities of the AoV, coronary arteries (including dilatation, ostial stenosis, or ostial entrapment by a tethered leaflet), aortic arch branches, and branch pulmonary arteries, and echocardiography must involve careful evaluation of these structures.

Valvar Pulmonary Stenosis

Valvar PS most commonly presents either as thin but doming leaflets with bicuspid morphology and poststenotic dilatation of the main pulmonary artery. Fusion or underdevelopment of a

commissure can result in a thickened raphe with tethering to the arterial wall at the sinotubular junction, often making it difficult to distinguish this lesion from supravalvar PS. In fact, underdevelopment of the distal commissures can result in a more circular attachment of the valve at the pulmonary root rather than the usual semilunar attachments.[30] Occasionally, valvar PS presents as dysplastic leaflets with thickened leaflet edges, annular hypoplasia, and a small main pulmonary artery. In these cases, the leaflets are attached to the root in a semilunar fashion. Hence, echocardiographic evaluation must include characterization of the PV leaflets as well as the pulmonary root and pulmonary arteries (Fig. 142.5). Because most patients with significant valvar PS can be treated with transcatheter pulmonary balloon valvotomy, it is important to distinguish valvar PS from supravalvar PS, a frequently challenging task when the presentation occurs during the neonatal period. The degree of obstruction is measured by continuous-wave Doppler interrogation of the pulmonary outflow tract in subcostal views, modified apical views with anterior angulation, and parasternal views. An atrial septal defect or patent foramen ovale is commonly found in these patients, and the atrial septum must be evaluated during the echocardiogram.

Double-Chambered Right Ventricle

A DCRV is an obstructive lesion involving anomalously prominent muscle bundles, usually located at the infundibular os and dividing the RV into two chambers: a proximal high-pressure inflow chamber and a distal low-pressure outflow chamber.[31] Unlike tetralogy of Fallot with anterior deviation of the conal septum resulting in subvalvar PS and an underdeveloped subpulmonary conus, the subpulmonary conus in a DCRV is expanded and well developed. Like subvalvar AS, the obstruction in a DCRV may not be present early in life, though a congenital anatomic substrate can be identified echocardiographically with superior displacement and hypertrophy of the moderator band contributing to progressive hypertrophy at the infundibular os.[32] Others, however, have suggested that the anomalous muscle bundles in a DCRV are in fact distinct from the normal moderator band.[33] The most common association is a membranous VSD, occurring in up to 67% of these patients[34] (Video 142.6). More important, DCRV occurs in up to 10% of patients undergoing VSD surgery,[35] necessitating careful assessment of the RV chamber in all patients with a VSD. As discussed previously, another common association is subvalvar AS, occurring in 25% of patients with a DCRV and VSD.[25] In fact, up to 88% of these patients will have a fixed subaortic ridge at the crest of the ventricular septum with or without obstruction. The obstruction in a DCRV is usually progressive and almost always requires surgical intervention. The usual presentation is during childhood or adolescence, though cases of adult presentation have been reported.[36]

Aside from characterization of the prominent muscle bundles and subpulmonary conus in multiple views, echocardiography must evaluate the degree of obstruction, usually in subcostal views or modified apical views with anterior angulation. Parasternal views may not be as helpful because of the anterior location of the prominent muscle bundles and perpendicular orientation of the flow along the obstruction in these views. Transesophageal echocardiography may help separate the flow acceleration from the VSD versus the subpulmonary obstruction (Fig. 142.6). A careful evaluation of the ventricular septum is crucial to identify an associated VSD. In most instances, the VSD is related to the proximal high-pressure chamber, and the gradient across the VSD will be low if there is significant obstruction associated with the DCRV. In the rare instance when the VSD is related to the low-pressure chamber, there will be turbulent flow across the VSD and will not reflect the degree of obstruction at the abnormal muscle bundles. In addition, careful assessment of the LVOT, particularly at the crest of the ventricular septum in the setting of a VSD, is needed to exclude subvalvar AS.

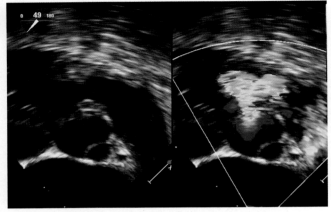

Figure 142.6. Transesophageal right ventricular outflow tract view of double-chambered right ventricle with Color Compare demonstrating left-to-right flow across a membranous ventricular septal defect and muscular narrowing at the infundibular os.

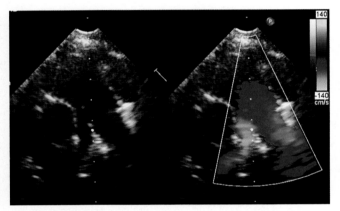

Figure 142.7. Parasternal short-axis Color Compare demonstrating diffuse right pulmonary artery hypoplasia in a patient with dextrocardia and right lung hypoplasia.

Supravalvar and Peripheral Pulmonic Stenosis

Congenital supravalvar PS is commonly seen in Noonan syndrome, and PPS (also known as branch pulmonary artery stenosis) is most commonly seen in congenital syndromes such as Williams, Rubella, or Alagille syndromes.[37] The pathogenesis of these lesions is incompletely understood. In addition, branch pulmonary artery hypoplasia may be seen in the setting of lung hypoplasia (Fig. 142.7). Echocardiography should include evaluation of arterial size at the site of narrowing, the sizes of other pulmonary artery segments, Doppler gradients, and signs of right ventricular hypertension (including tricuspid regurgitation gradient) or failure. As noted earlier, supravalvar PS must be distinguished from valvar PS, which may involve tethering of the valve at the sinotubular junction. Mild PPS is a physiologic finding in early infancy during the period of remodeling of the branch pulmonary arteries (Fig. 142.8). Branch pulmonary artery stenosis may be unilateral or bilateral.

The main and branch pulmonary arteries are generally imaged from parasternal and suprasternal views, although subcostal imaging may be useful in neonates and young children. For Doppler interrogation, care must be taken to align the ultrasound beam with the long axis of the pulmonary artery, and a different window from the one used to measure arterial diameter is required. With unilateral PPS, flow to the stenotic pulmonary artery is reduced, and the gradient tends to underestimate the severity of the

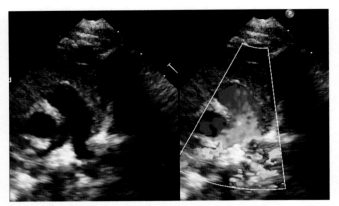

Figure 142.8. Parasternal short-axis Color Compare demonstrating mild bilateral pulmonary artery hypoplasia in a young infant, often "physiologic" peripheral pulmonic stenosis.

obstruction. Additional imaging modalities, such as MRI and CT, may be needed to visualize the pulmonary arteries in older children and adults.

Please access ExpertConsult to view the corresponding videos for this chapter.

REFERENCES

1. Hoffman JI, Kaplan S. The incidence of congenital heart disease. *J Am Coll Cardiol.* 2002;39:1890–1900.
2. Triedman JK. Methodological issues for database development: trends. In: Keane JF, Lock JE, Fyler DC, eds. *Nadas' Pediatric Cardiology.* 2nd ed. Philadelphia: Saunders Elsevier; 2006:323–336.
3. Rosenthal E. Coarctation of the aorta from fetus to adult: curable condition or life long disease process? *Heart.* 2005;91:1495–1502.
4. Campbell M. Calcific aortic stenosis and congenital bicuspid aortic valves. *Br Heart J.* 1968;30:606–616.
5. Roberts WC. The congenitally bicuspid aortic valve: a study of 85 autopsy cases. *Am J Cardiol.* 1970;26:72–83.
6. Ward C. Clinical significance of the bicuspid aortic valve. *Br Heart J.* 2000;83:81–85.
7. Kong WK, Delgado V, Poh KK, et al. Prognostic implications of raphe in bicuspid aortic valve anatomy. *JAMA Cardiol.* 2017;2:285. 2-92.
8. Fernandes SM, Sanders SP, Khairy P, et al. Morphology of bicuspid aortic valve in children and adolescents. *J Am Coll Cardiol.* 2004;44:1648–1651.
9. Beppu S, Suzuki S, Matsuda H, et al. Rapidity of progression of aortic stenosis in patients with congenital bicuspid aortic valves. *Am J Cardiol.* 1993;71:322–327.
10. Fernandes SM, Khairy P, Sanders SP, Colan SD. Bicuspid aortic valve morphology and interventions in the young. *J Am Coll Cardiol.* 2007;49:2211–2214.
11. Miller MJ, Geffner ME, Lippe BM, et al. Echocardiography reveals a high incidence of bicuspid aortic valve in Turner syndrome. *J Ped.* 1983;102:47–50.
12. Nistri S, Sorbo MD, Basso C, Thiene G. Bicuspid aortic valve: abnormal aortic elastic properties. *J Heart Valve Dis.* 2002;11:369–373.
13. Fedak PW, de Sa MP, Verma S, et al. Vascular matrix remodeling in patients with bicuspid aortic valve malformations: implications for aortic dilatation. *J Thor Cardiovasc Surg.* 2003;126:797–806.
14. Heinrich RS, Fontaine AA, Grimes RY, et al. Experimental analysis of fluid mechanical energy losses in aortic valve stenosis: importance of pressure recovery. *Ann Biomed Eng.* 1996;24:685–694.
15. Bonow RO, Carabello BA, Chatterjee K, et al. ACC/AHA 2006 guidelines for the management of patients with valvular heart disease. *J Am Coll Cardiol.* 2006;48(3):e1–e148.
16. Bharucha T, Fernandes F, Slorach C, et al. Measurement of effective aortic valve area using three-dimensional echocardiography in children undergoing aortic balloon valvuloplasty for aortic stenosis. *Echocardiography.* 2012;29:484–491.
17. Stewart AB, Ahmed R, Travill CM, Newman CG. Coarctation of the aorta life and health 20-44 years after surgical repair. *Br Heart J.* 1993;69:65–70.
18. Oliver JM, Gallego P, Gonzalez A, et al. Risk factors for aortic complications in adults with coarctation of the aorta. *J Am Coll Cardiol.* 2004;44:1641–1647.
19. Machii M, Becker AE. Hypoplastic aortic arch morphology pertinent to growth after surgical correction of aortic coarctation. *Ann Thor Surg.* 1997;64:516–520.
20. Leichter DA, Sullivan I, Gersony WM. "Acquired" discrete subvalvular aortic stenosis: Natural history and hemodynamics. *J Am Coll Cardiol.* 1989;14:1539–1544.
21. Kleinert S, Geva T. Echocardiographic morphometry and geometry of the left ventricular outflow tract in fixed subaortic stenosis. *J Am Coll Cardiol.* 1993;22:1501–1508.

22. Sigfusson G, Tacy TA, Vanauker MD, Cape EG. Abnormalities of the left ventricular outflow tract associated with discrete subaortic stenosis in children: an echocardiographic study. *J Am Coll Cardiol.* 1997;30:255–259.

23. Salem MM, Starnes VA, Wells WJ, et al. Predictors of left ventricular outflow obstruction following single-stage repair of interrupted aortic arch and ventricular septal defect. *Am J Cardiol.* 2000;86:1044–1047.

24. Silverman NH, Gerlis LM, Ho SY, Anderson RH. Fibrous obstruction within the left ventricular outflow tract associated with ventricular septal defect: a pathologic study. *J Am Coll Cardiol.* 1995;25:475–481.

25. Vogel M, Smallhorn JF, Freedom RM, et al. An echocardiographic study of the association of ventricular septal defect and right ventricular muscle bundles with a fixed subaortic abnormality. *Am J Cardiol.* 1988;61:857–860.

26. Stassano P, Di Tommaso L, Contaldo A, et al. Discrete subaortic stenosis: long-term prognosis on the progression of the obstruction and of the aortic insufficiency. *Thorac Cardiovasc Surg.* 2005;53:23–27.

27. Coleman DM, Smallhorn JF, McCrindle BW, et al. Postoperative follow-up of fibromuscular subaortic stenosis. *J Am Coll Cardiol.* 1994;24:1558–1564.

28. Williams JC, Barratt-Boyes BG, Lowe JB. Supravalvular aortic stenosis. *Circulation.* 1961;24:1311–1318.

29. Stamm C, Li J, Ho SY, et al. The aortic root in supravalvular aortic stenosis: the potential surgical relevance of morphologic findings. *J Thor Cardiovasc Surg.* 1997;114:16–24.

30. Stamm C, Anderson RH, Ho SY. Clinical anatomy of the normal pulmonary root compared with that in isolated pulmonary valvular stenosis. *J Am Coll Cardiol.* 1998;31:1420–1425.

31. Restivo A, Cameron AH, Anderson RH, Allwork SP. Divided right ventricle: a review of its anatomical varieties. *Ped Cardiol.* 1984;5:197–204.

32. Wong PC, Sanders SP, Jonas RA, et al. Pulmonary valve-moderator band distance and association with development of double-chambered right ventricle. *Am J Cardiol.* 1991;68:1681–1686.

33. Lucas Jr RV, Varco RL, Lillehei CW, et al. Anomalous muscle bundle of the right ventricle. Hemodynamic consequences and surgical considerations. *Circulation.* 1962;25:443–455.

34. Hachiro Y, Takagi N, Koyanagi T, et al. Repair of double-chambered right ventricle: surgical results and long-term follow-up. *Ann Thor Surg.* 2001;72:1520–1522.

35. Simpson Jr WF, Sade RM, Crawford FA, et al. Double-chambered right ventricle. *Ann Thor Surg.* 1987;44:7–10.

36. McElhinney DB, Chatterjee KM, Reddy VM. Double-chambered right ventricle presenting in adulthood. *Ann Thor Surg.* 2000;70:124–127.

37. Bacha EA, Kreutzer J. Comprehensive management of branch pulmonary artery stenosis. *J Intervent Cardiol.* 2001;14:367–375.

143 The Adult With Unrepaired Complex Congenital Heart Defects

Rachel Wald, Samuel Siu, Erwin Oechslin

Most complex congenital heart disease (CHD) present with cyanosis in early childhood and necessitate intervention before adulthood. In contrast, adults with acyanotic complex CHD can escape detection for many decades because they often do not have major associated lesions. The echocardiographic approach should be tailored to the indication: a sequential and segmental approach should be used for an initial diagnostic study. If the study is to be used for preprocedural planning, prior discussion with the interventional cardiologist or surgeon is beneficial to ensure that necessary data are obtained. In a follow-up study when the diagnosis has been well established, a typical adult imaging sequence can be followed. Access to the patient's clinical record at the time of echocardiography provides the sonographer and interpreting cardiologist with important details regarding the underlying anatomy and the nature of previous interventions. In adults with limited acoustic windows, supplemental data from transesophageal echocardiography (TEE), cardiovascular magnetic resonance imaging (CMRI), and/or cardiac computed tomography (CT) may be required. Adults with neurodevelopmental and neurocognitive deficits and disorders, those who may be anxious, or those with multiple chest incisions may not tolerate prolonged imaging.

In this chapter, we focus on two areas: (1) summary of sequential, segmental analysis for assessment of complex CHD and (2) diagnostic features of cyanotic and acyanotic forms of complex adult CHD. The consensus recommendations of the International Society for Adult Congenital Heart Disease provide a comprehensive and structured approach in echocardiography evaluation of adults with CHD.[1] Recommendations about TEE and three-dimensional (3D) echocardiography in patients with CHD have also been published.[2,3]

SUMMARY OF THE SEQUENTIAL, SEGMENTAL APPROACH TO COMPLEX CONGENITAL HEART DISEASE

In the sequential, segmental approach, chambers and vessels are recognized according to their intrinsic morphologic "rightness" and

morphologic "leftness" and not determined by their right- or left-sided position in the chest, relative position to other chambers, or by the connection to the systemic or pulmonary circulation.[4,5] The heart is considered in three segments (atria, the ventricles, and the great arteries; characteristics are summarized in Table 143.1). The atrioventricular (AV) valves always connect with the corresponding ventricles: the tricuspid valve is more apically positioned than the mitral (Video 143.1; *arrows*) with the exception of AV septal defect (AVSD) or double-inlet LV.

Abdominal or cardiac situs: Determination of the abdominal situs and atrial arrangement (cardiac situs) from the subcostal view is the first step (Fig. 143.1). Because the features that distinguish between the left atrium (LA) and right atrium (RA) are usually not visualized on transthoracic echocardiography (TTE) (see Table 143.1), cardiac situs can be inferred by the following features: (1) the cardiac and abdominal situs are usually concordant, and (2) the RA almost always receives the inferior vena cava (IVC; with the exception of an interrupted IVC). Based on the relationship of the abdominal aorta and IVC, there are three types of cardiac situs: solitus (normal); (Fig. 143.2A), situs inversus (Fig. 143.2B and Video 143.2), and isomerism (heterotaxy syndrome, when the caval vein and aorta are on the same side of the spine; Fig. 143.3).

Cardiac position: Cardiac position is best assessed in the subcostal view and includes two terms that are not interchangeable: location of the heart within the chest (levoposition, dextroposition, mesoposition) and cardiac orientation. Abnormal location of the heart within the mediastinum may also be a result of other factors, including thoracic abnormalities, mediastinal and thoracic structures, and surgical procedures. Cardiac orientation describes the base-apex long axis of the heart (levocardia, dextrocardia, or mesocardia).

Definition of the connection: The AV and ventriculoarterial (VA) connections are defined after successful identification of the three segments (atria, ventricles, and great arteries; see Table 143.1). The AV connection can be concordant, discordant,

TABLE 143.1 The Three Segments and Their Morphologic Features

ATRIAL	Right Atrium	Left Atrium
Appendage	Broad based, triangular	Narrow, fingerlike, tubular
Terminal crest	Present	Absent
Pectinate muscles	Many; extends toward the atrioventricular valve or Eustachian valve	Few; confined to the left atrial appendage
Fossa Ovalis	Rim around the fossa ovalis	
VENTRICULAR	**Right Ventricle**	**Left Ventricle**
Atrioventricular valve	Apical attachment of the tricuspid valve to the septum	
Ventricular Crest	Present	Absent
Semilunar to atrioventricular valve fibrous continuity	Absent	Present
Trabeculations	Coarse apical trabeculations; moderator band, septomarginal trabeculation	Fine apical trabeculations
Chordal attachment to the septum	Present	Absent
ARTERIAL SEGMENT	**Aorta**	**Pulmonary**
	Supplies neck vessels or arch	Bifurcates to branch pulmonary arteries

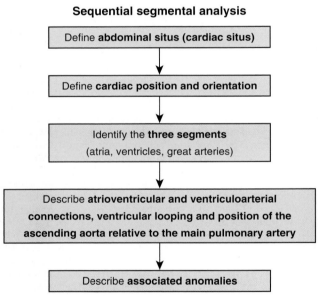

Sequential segmental analysis

Define **abdominal situs (cardiac situs)**

↓

Define **cardiac position and orientation**

↓

Identify the **three segments**
(atria, ventricles, great arteries)

↓

Describe **atrioventricular and ventriculoarterial connections, ventricular looping and position of the ascending aorta relative to the main pulmonary artery**

↓

Describe **associated anomalies**

Figure 143.1. Sequential segmental analysis.

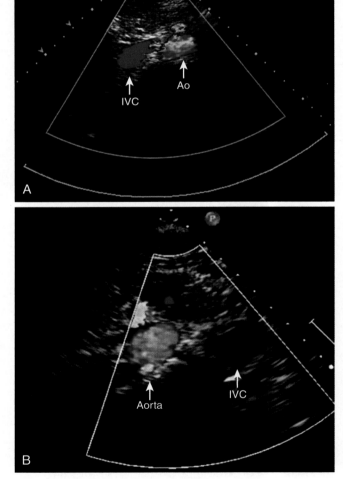

Figure 143.2. Subcostal views to identify abdominal situs. **A,** Situs solitus: the inferior vena cava (IVC) is on the right, and the aorta (Ao) is on the left of the spine. **B,** Abdominal situs inversus: the IVC is on the left, and the aorta is on the right of the spine.

ambiguous, or univentricular. Concordant AV and VA connections are the normal state. Discordant AV and VA connections are features of physiologically or congenitally corrected transposition of the great arteries (cc-TGA), which is a circulation in series (acyanotic) (see Fig. 143.4A). Concordant AV and discordant VA connections are features of complete transposition of the great arteries (c-TGA) which is a circulation in parallel (cyanotic) (see Fig. 143.4B). The AV connection is ambiguous, neither concordant nor discordant, when the cardiac situs is isomeric or indeterminate. Univentricular connections can exist with any type of cardiac situs and can be absent right (Fig. 143.5A and Video 143.3) or absent left AV valve or double-inlet ventricle (Fig. 143.5B and Video 143.4). When there is overriding of the AV valve (malalignment of the annulus of one of the AV valve or atrial septum relative to the ventricular septum), the 50% rule will determine whether the connection is biventricular (overriding <50%, concordant connection with overriding of the AV valve) or a univentricular connection (overriding of one AV valve >50%; see Fig. 143.5B

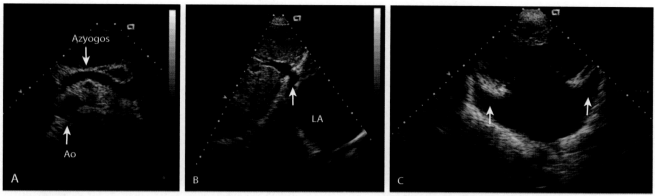

Figure 143.3. Left atrial isomerism. **A,** Subcostal view with the aorta on the right of the spine and absent suprarenal inferior vena cava with azygos continuation. **B,** Direct connection of the hepatic veins to the right-sided left atrium. **C,** Apical four-chamber view with bilateral left atrial appendages *(arrows)*. *Ao,* Aorta; *LA,* left atrium.

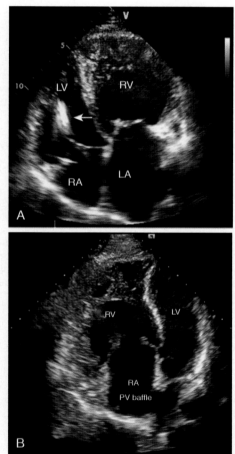

Figure 143.4. Apical four-chamber-views to image atrioventricular (AV) connections and ventricular looping. **A,** Cardiac situs solitus and discordant AV connection in physiologically "corrected" transposition of the great arteries. The right ventricle (RV) is on the left of the left ventricle (LV), which indicates a ventricular L-loop. **B,** Cardiac situs solitus and ventricular D-loop in a patient who has an undergone atrial switch (Mustard) procedure. The atria are connected with the corresponding ventricles (concordant AV connections). The *arrow* indicates the pacemaker lead in the subpulmonic LV. *LA,* LEFT atrium; *PV,* pulmonary venous; *RA,* right atrium.

and Video 143.4). The receiving ventricle can be a morphologic RV, LV (see Fig. 143.5B and Video 143.4), or indeterminate ventricle. The VA connection (concordant, discordant, double outlet, or common arterial trunk) is best determined by a short-axis sweep that defines the plane of the ventricular septum in relation to the great arteries. The pulmonary artery (PA) is identified by its bifurcation, and the aorta is identified by the origin of neck vessels. The relationship between the ascending aorta and the main PA is described in the parasternal short-axis (PSAX) view. Normally, the RV outflow tract is anterior and loops around the aorta on the PSAX views (Fig. 143.6B). When the ascending aorta and pulmonary artery arise in parallel as seen on parasternal long-axis (PLAX) or apical views or seen en face on PSAX views with the aorta anteriorly positioned, transposition of the great arteries (TGA) should be suspected. The position of the ascending aorta should then be described relative to the PA (e.g., anterior to the right, anterior to the left, anteroposterior, or side-by-side arrangement).

Ventricular looping: Ventricular looping determines the distribution of the coronary artery pattern and conduction system. The apical four-chamber view differentiates D-(dextro) loop (normal; morphologic RV right of morphologic LV) (see Fig. 143.4B and Video 143.2) versus L-(levo) loop (morphologic RV left of mor- phologic LV) (see Fig. 143.4A and Video 143.1). Importantly, the transducer has to be positioned according to the standard orientation and should not be reversed in an attempt to familiarize image display.

Associated malformations: Description of associated cardiac malformation is the last step and includes but is not restricted to cardiac shunts (at any level), valvular function, LV or RV outflow tract obstruction, anomalous systemic or pulmonary venous connection(s), aortic coarctation, aortopulmonary vessels, and iatrogenic (palliative) shunts. Coronary anomalies are very difficult to ascertain by TTE in adults, although variations in coronary artery patterns are commonly seen in cyanotic CHD and should be sought before intervention using complementary imaging modalities as necessary.

Cyanotic Complex Congenital Heart Disease

Central cyanosis in an adult with unrepaired CHD is a result of one of three major mechanisms, which need not be mutually exclusive: central mixing of pulmonary and systemic blood flow, reduction of pulmonary blood flow, or Eisenmenger physiology resulting in reversal of an intracardiac shunt. We will review some of the more common cyanotic lesions, the most complex forms of CHD (single-ventricle physiology), and palliative shunts.

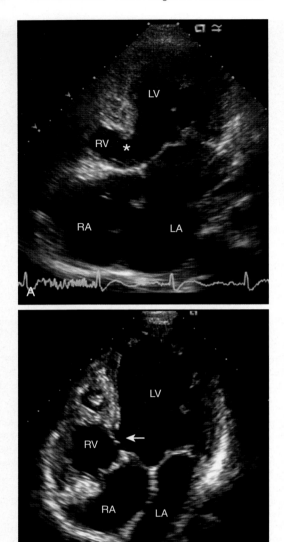

Figure 143.5. Univentricular connections: **A,** Apical four-chamber view of tricuspid atresia, secundum atrial septa defect, and ventricular septal defect (VSD) *(asterisk)*. Note absence of the right atrioventricular (AV) valve (tricuspid valve). **B,** Apical four-chamber view of double-inlet left ventricle (LV): both AV valves predominantly connect to the LV because of malalignment of the interatrial and ventricular septum with overriding of the right-sided AV valve (>50% overriding). Note the VSD and straddling of the right-sided AV valve with chords attached to both sides of the interventricular septum *(arrow)*. The right- and left-sided AV valves are on the same plane. *LA,* Left atrium; *RA,* right atrium; *RV,* hypoplastic right ventricle.

Tetralogy of Fallot

Tetralogy of Fallot (ToF) is the most common form of cyanotic CHD with survival to adulthood and is defined by the presence of pulmonary outflow tract stenosis (at multiple levels), malalignment ventricular septal defect (VSD), dextroposition of the aorta with override of the ventricular septum, and RV hypertrophy (see Fig. 143.6 and Video 143.5). Anterosuperior deviation of the infundibular (outlet) septum is the intrinsic anatomic defect that results in a malalignment-type VSD, partial commitment of the aorta to the RV, and subpulmonary outflow obstruction (Fig. 143.6B). Hypertrophy of the septoparietal trabeculation may be an additional diagnostic feature.[6] The PLAX view typically

demonstrates the malalignment outlet VSD and the override of the aorta (see Fig. 143.6A and Video 143.5). If override of the aorta is greater than 50%, it would be described as "double-outlet RV" rather than ToF.[7]

The deviation of the infundibular septum anteriorly and superiorly is best seen in the PSAX view, and subvalvar pulmonary stenosis often begins at this level with usual extension to include valvar and supravalvular levels (Fig. 143.6C). The parasternal and subcostal short-axis views are useful to delineate the level of RV outflow tract obstruction and provides suitable alignment for Doppler interrogation of the level of obstruction (Fig. 143.6C and D). Valvular and supravalvular pulmonary obstruction can be well-depicted on the PSAX view. Delineation of branch pulmonary artery stenosis usually require CMRI or CT. Importantly, the severity of pulmonary obstructive gradient may be underestimated in the presence of right-to-left shunting at the VSD level. Associated defects that should be assessed include atrial septal defect (ASDs; pentalogy of Fallot), additional VSDs, AVSD, right-sided aortic arch (with mirror-image branching or aberrant left subclavian artery contributing to a vascular ring), and anomalous origins of the coronary arteries. Enlargement of the aortic root and ascending aorta are common and generally benign associated findings.[8,9] Surgical repair should be considered, even with a late diagnosis, to improve long-term outcome and typically includes relief of subvalvar and supravalvar pulmonary stenoses, pulmonary valvotomy, and VSD patch closure. Although echocardiography can typically establish the diagnosis of ToF in adults, multimodality imaging should be used for characterization of the vascular anatomy (PAs, aortic arch ± aortopulmonary collaterals) and the coronary artery pattern and patency.[10,11]

Complete Transposition of the Great Arteries

Complete or "classic" TGA, the second most common cyanotic congenital heart defect after ToF, denotes concordant AV connection and discordant VA connection with a subaortic RV and subpulmonic LV. If left untreated, c-TGA is almost uniformly fatal in the first year of life; however, if adequate mixing exists later, death typically occurs as a result of pulmonary vascular disease.[12,13] Although the typical adult with complete TGA will have undergone atrial or arterial switch surgeries, the unrepaired state of this lesion illustrates important features of segmental diagnosis. Cardiac situs solitus is the most common presentation, with the aorta positioned anterior and to the right of the PA. The parallel course of the great arteries is the characteristic feature in the PLAX view. The aorta originating from the RV gives rise to the neck arteries, whereas a short artery bifurcating first confirms the PA, which originates from the LV. Associated lesions include shunts (patent foramen ovale (PFO)/secundum ASD, VSD, or PDA), outflow tract obstruction (RVOT or LVOT), arch anomalies, valve abnormalities (dysplastic or common AV valves), juxtaposition of the atrial appendages, or anomalous pulmonary venous connections.[14] The coronary arteries are never in the normal position, and anatomic variants are commonly encountered.

Univentricular Heart

The "univentricular heart" represents a heterogeneous spectrum of defects unified by the absence of two well-developed ventricles with commitment of majority of atrial flow to one functionally single ventricle. Typically, there are a dominant ventricle and a second rudimentary or accessory chamber (see Fig. 143.5 and Video 143.4); a truly solitary ventricle is relatively rare. Echocardiography can characterize the dominant ventricle as LV (characterized by smooth walls, fine trabeculations, lack of septal attachments of the chordae of the AV valve), RV (characterized by course trabeculations and chordal attachments of the valve to the septal surface), or indeterminate. The position of the accessory

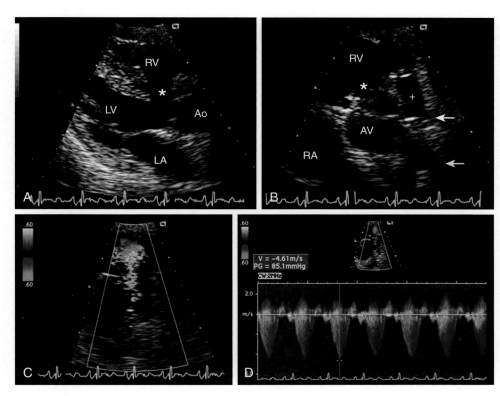

Figure 143.6. Unrepaired tetralogy of Fallot. **A,** Parasternal long-axis view showing malalignment of the aortic valve annulus relative to the ventricular septum with malalignment ventricular septal defect (VSD) and overriding of the aorta *(asterisk).* Parasternal short-axis view shows anterior and superior deviation of the infundibular septum resulting in malalignment VSD *(asterisk)* and subpulmonary outflow tract obstruction *(+).* The *white arrow* indicates the muscle bundles in the right ventricular outflow tract. The *yellow arrow* shows bifurcation of the main pulmonary artery (PA) to the right and left PA. **C,** Color Doppler flow mapping demonstrates flow acceleration at the level of the subpulmonary outflow tract. **D,** Continuous-wave Doppler demonstrates severe right ventricular outflow tract obstruction. *Ao,* Aortic root; *AV,* aortic valve; *LA,* left atrium; *LV,* left ventricle; *RV,* right ventricle.

chamber is anterior (undeveloped RV) in the LV type and posterior in the RV type (undeveloped LV). The AV connection may be a single, a double, or a common inlet. In the case of a single inlet (absent right or left AV valve), AV valve morphology follows the ventricular type. In the case of double-inlet ventricle, right- and left-sided AV valves is the common designation because tricuspid or mitral valve configurations does not apply (see Fig. 143.5B and Video 143.4). Additional features to define include the location and number of intracardiac septal defects as well as the location and function of the semilunar valves and great arteries. Survival to adult life without surgical intervention is uncommon but can occur with balanced physiology, and mortality rates are higher for those with univentricular hearts of RV than those with LV morphology.[15] A cyanotic adult with a univentricular heart typically has had a palliative shunt earlier in life and is almost invariably deemed to be at prohibitively high risk of needing a Fontan procedure.

Palliative Shunts

Systemic pulmonary palliative shunts serve to augment pulmonary blood flow. Common types include the Blalock-Taussig-Thomas shunt connection from the subclavian artery to the PA (typically on the side opposite to the side of the arch) (Fig. 143.7A and B), the Waterston shunt from the ascending aorta to the right PA, and the Potts shunt from the descending aorta to the left PA (Fig. 143.7C and D). All of the aforementioned shunts are best imaged in the suprasternal window with addition of the high parasternal or "ductal" cut for the Blalock-Taussig-Thomas shunt visualization and the PSAX view for imaging the Waterston shunt. Diastolic flow reversal in the thoracic and abdominal aorta can be an important sign of shunt patency. Complications of these shunts include pulmonary arterial hypertension and branch PA stenosis. Glenn shunts may be "classic" with a connection from the right superior vena cava to a disconnected right PA, "bidirectional" if the main PA is not ligated leaving continuity between the right and left PA, or "bilateral" in the event of right and left superior vena cavae (without a bridging innominate vein).

Doppler interrogation of a patent Glenn shunt demonstrates low velocity respirophasic flow. Pulmonary arteriovenous malformations can develop in the lung ipsilateral to a classic Glenn shunt (because of the absence of hepatic factor) and can be inferred by a late positive bubble appearance after injection of agitated saline into the right arm.

ACYANOTIC COMPLEX CONGENITAL HEART DEFECTS

Ebstein Anomaly

Ebstein anomaly features a syndrome including a dysplastic tricuspid valve, disease of the right and left myocardium, and abnormal conduction system. It represents a very broad spectrum, varying from the severe neonatal form, which has a dismal prognosis, to the milder form, which may only become manifest in adult life, if at all.[16,17] Rotational displacement of the dysplastic septal and posterior tricuspid valve leaflets is the anatomic landmark caused by failure of delamination of the tricuspid valve tissue from the underlying myocardium, which results in apical attachments of the mural (posterior) and septal leaflets. This apical displacement of the AV junction gives rise to an inlet portion of the RV, which is attenuated, resulting in two components: an "atrialized" RV and a "functional" RV (Fig. 143.8 and Video 143.6). The degree of adherence of the mural and septal leaflets determines the spectrum of disease severity, ranging from mild forms with minimal displacement of the septal leaflet to an imperforate membrane. The anterior leaflet is rarely displaced but is often redundant, or "sail-like" (see Fig. 143.8A and Video 143.6).[18] The anatomically normal tricuspid valve demonstrates some apical displacement relative to the hinge point of the mitral valve; however, this offset does not typically exceed the threshold of 8 mm/m[2].[19]

The diagnosis of Ebstein anomaly is often apparent from the apical four-chamber view, but additional views are necessary to fully appreciate valve morphology and size of the functional RV. The malformed tricuspid valve leaflets often result in stenosis or

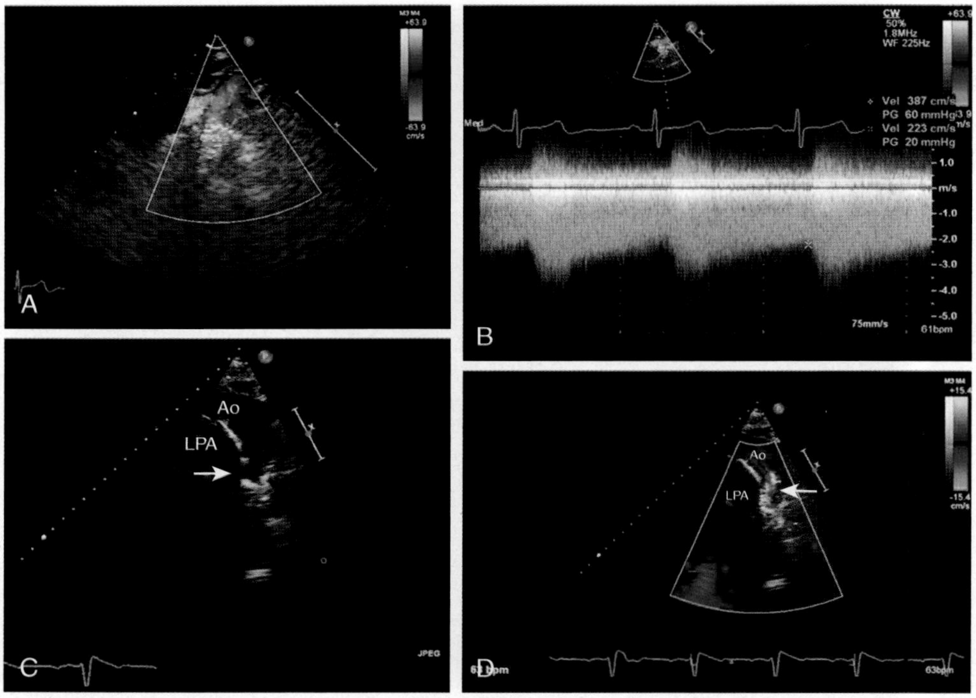

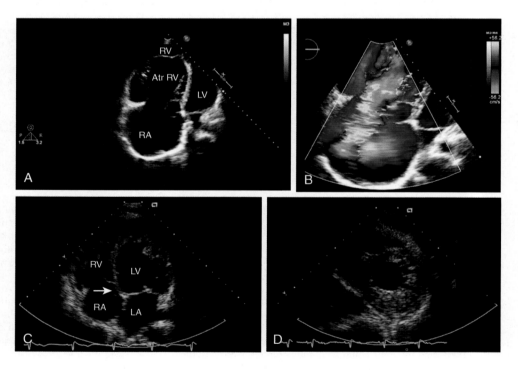

Figure 143.7. Palliative shunts **A** and **B,** Left Blalock-Taussig-Thomas shunt with continuous flow demonstrated by continuous-wave Doppler. **C** and **D,** Potts anastomosis *(arrow).* Note the diastolic backward flow from the left pulmonary artery (LPA) to the proximal thoracic descending aorta (Ao) caused by the suprasystemic pressure in the LPA during diastole.

Figure 143.8. Ebstein anomaly. **A,** Severe form of Ebstein anomaly with severe apical displacement of the septal leaflet resulting a small functional right ventricle (RV), a large atrialized RV (Atr RV). The anterior tricuspid valve leaflet is redundant and "sail-like." The left ventricle is small. **B,** corresponding color Doppler image demonstrates free tricuspid regurgitation. **C,** Mild form of Ebstein anomaly with left ventricular noncompaction. Apical four-chamber view demonstrates only mild displacement (9 mm/m^2) of the septal leaflet of the tricuspid valve *(arrow).* Note the thickening of the midventricular lateral and apical myocardium. **D,** Parasternal short-axis view at early systole demonstrates severe thickening of the midventricular and apical inferolateral segments with features of noncompaction. *LA,* Left atrium; *LV,* left ventricle; *RA,* right atrium.

regurgitation. However, the latter is far more common (see Fig. 143.8B). Fenestrations, particularly of the anterior leaflet, are commonly present. In addition, tethering of the anterior leaflet is often seen and is caused by chordal attachments to the ventricular free wall or displaced papillary muscles. The anterior leaflet is generally elongated and, if redundant, may obstruct the right ventricular outflow tract. Associated lesions may include atrial-level shunts (PFO or ASD), VSDs, or noncompaction of the LV (see Fig. 143.8C and D and Video 143.7).[19] Echocardiography assessment of the tricuspid valve and CMRI assessment of the ventricular volumes and systolic

function are complementary imaging modalities and guide surgical decision making regarding the timing of surgery and suitability for valve repair versus valve replacement.[2,20,21] Tricuspid valve repair (cone repair) is the preferred surgical approach in experienced centers.[22] Echocardiographers should familiarize themselves with type of tricuspid valve repair performed at their respective institution and the echocardiography data required. Surgery may also include closure of intracardiac shunts, plication of the atrialized portion of the RV, reduction right atrioplasty, and/or a bidirectional Glenn connection to offload a diminutive functional RV.

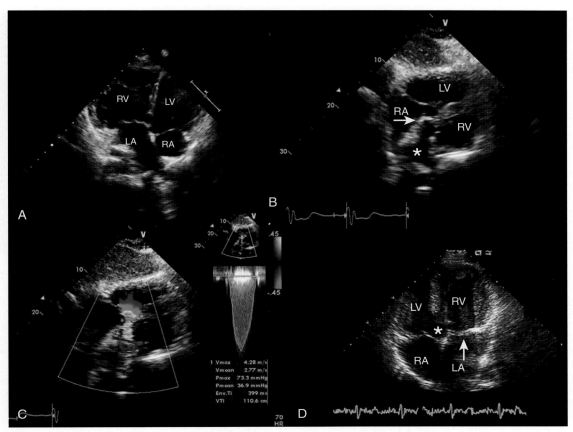

Figure 143.9. Physiologically "corrected" transposition of the great arteries (TGA) with associated cardiac anomalies. **A,** Apical four-chamber view, obtained from the right lateral position, of a patient with situs inversus and dextrocardia. The more apically positioned atrioventricular valve on the right is the anatomic landmark for the tricuspid valve, which communicates with the corresponding right ventricle (RV). The right-sided RV indicates ventricular D-loop and d-TGA. **B,** Subcostal view in situs solitus and levocardia. An anterior sweep of the transducer allows imaging the left ventricular outflow tract with parallel alignment of the blood flow and ultrasound beam. Note the subvalvular membrane *(arrow)* causing obstruction of the pulmonary (left ventricular) outflow tract. The *asterisk* indicates bifurcation of the pulmonary artery. **C,** Color Doppler mapping demonstrates flow acceleration at the level of the subvalvular membrane in the left ventricular outflow tract. Continuous-wave Doppler documents a mean systolic gradient of 37 mm Hg. **D,** Apical four-chamber view in cardiac situs solitus and levocardia. Physiologically "corrected" TGA and a membranous ventricular septal defect ventricular septal defect extending to the inlet septum *(asterisk)*. The *arrow* indicates the tricuspid valve, which is more apically positioned than the mitral valve. *LA,* Left atrium; *LV,* left ventricle; *RA,* right atrium.

Physiologically "Corrected" Transposition of the Great Arteries

Physiologically or congenitally "corrected" TGA is characterized by discordant AV and VA connections. Because the two discordant connections "cancel each other out" with respect to the circulation, the patients are acyanotic with circulations in series and can remain undiagnosed until adulthood in the absence of a murmur or any associated defect. The discordant AV and VA connections cannot be considered an *anatomic* correction because the subaortic ventricle is a RV supporting the systemic circulation, and the subpulmonic ventricle is the LV connected to the pulmonary artery.[23] Physiologically "corrected" TGA is more appropriate and indicates physiologic, but not anatomic, correction. Most patients have cardiac situs solitus and a ventricular L-loop (see Fig. 143.4A and Video 143.1), but 5% of the patients have cardiac situs inversus and dextrocardia or mesocardia with ventricular D-loop (Fig. 143.9A; see Video 143.2). Similar to the case with univentricular hearts, only one ventricle is seen on the PLAX view, reflecting the side by side orientation of LV and RV in patients with cc-TGA. The parallel course of the great arteries is typical, and the aorta is usually anterior and to the left in patients with cardiac situs solitus (Fig. 143.10A). More than 90% of patient with cc-TGA have associated congenital heart defects,[24,25] the classical triad being

VSD (denoted by the *asterisk* in Video 143.1), LV (subpulmonary) outflow tract obstruction (Fig. 143.9B–D), and anomalies of the tricuspid valve. Dysplastic tricuspid valves are very common and occur with or without apical displacement of the septal and posterior leaflets. This Ebstein-like malformation of the tricuspid valve is different from patients with classic Ebstein anomaly and is less amenable to repair. Long-term outcome is determined by the complexity and severity of associated CHDs and severity of tricuspid regurgitation. Complete heart block or failure of the subaortic RV can be the first presentation. Moderate to severe regurgitation of the subaortic tricuspid valve is associated with surgical morbidity and mortality and poor outcomes.[26,27] An association between end-diastolic diameters of the subaortic RV and subpulmonic LV and major adverse outcomes has been recently reported.[28]

LIMITATIONS IN ECHOCARDIOGRAPHIC ASSESSMENT OF COMPLEX CONGENITAL HEART DISEASE AND THE ROLE OF NEW TECHNOLOGY

Extracardiac vascular structures, such as the pulmonary vessels, aortopulmonary collaterals, and aortic arch or descending aorta are suboptimally assessed on TTE and require supplemental cross-sectional imaging by CMRI or CT. CMRI can provide additional

Figure 143.10. Parallel position of the great arteries. **A,** Parasternal short-axis view in a patient with situs solitus and physiologically "corrected" transposition of the great arteries (TGA). The aorta (asterisk) is anterior and to the left of the pulmonary trunk (+). **B,** Anterior sweep of a modified apical four-chamber view showing situs inversus and physiologically "corrected" TGA. Note the transducer is reversed with mirror-imaged arrangement of the great arteries! The right ventricle (RV) and the aorta are on the right and not on the left as one could assume from the images (i.e., there is a ventricular D-loop). Ao, Aortic root; LV, left ventricle; PA, pulmonary artery with bifurcation.

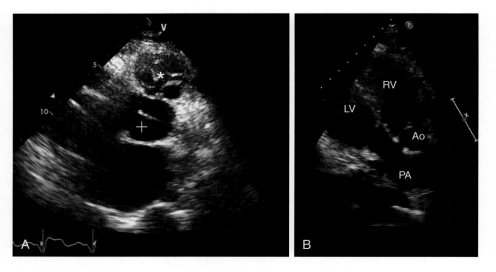

information about flow characteristics, can quantify shunt and regurgitant fraction, and is considered to be the reference standard for evaluation of ventricular volumes, systolic function, and mass in adults with CHD.[29,30] CT is the supplemental modality of choice for patients with pacemakers or metallic stents or coils and for evaluation of coronary artery anatomy.[29] In adults with congenital lesions, 3D echocardiography may provide incremental utility in understanding structural relationships, assessing chamber sizes, and determining systolic function. However, this incremental utility is critically dependent on good visualization of cardiac structure, which is more likely in pediatric than adult patients. Therefore, 3D echocardiography should be considered as complementary to two-dimensional echocardiographic imaging in evaluating adults with complex congenital disease.[3]

Please access ExpertConsult to view the corresponding videos for this chapter.

REFERENCES

1. Li W, West C, McGhie J, et al. Consensus recommendations for echocardiography in adults with congenital heart defects from the International Society of Adult Congenital Heart Disease (ISACHD). *Int J Cardiol.* 2018;272:77–83.
2. Puchalski MD, Lui GK, Miller-Hance WC, et al. Guidelines for performing a comprehensive transesophageal echocardiographic: examination in children and all patients with congenital heart disease. *J Am Soc Echocardiogr.* 2019;32:173–215.
3. Simpson J, Lopez L, Acar P, et al. Three-dimensional echocardiography in congenital heart disease. *J Am Soc Echocardiogr.* 2017;30:1–27.
4. Anderson RH, Becker AE, Freedom RM, et al. Sequential segmental analysis of congenital heart disease. *Pediatr Cardiol.* 1984;5:281–287.
5. Van Praagh R. The segmental approach clarified. *Cardiovasc Intervent Radiol.* 1984;7:320–325.
6. Bashore TM. Adult congenital heart disease: right ventricular outflow tract lesions. *Circulation.* 2007;115:1933–1947.
7. Mahle WT, Martinez R, Silverman N, et al. Anatomy, echocardiography and surgical approach to double outlet right ventricle. *Cardiol Young.* 2008;18(suppl 3):39–51.
8. Niwa K, Siu SC, Webb GD, Gatzoulis MA. Progressive aortic root dilatation in adults late after repair of tetralogy of Fallot. *Circulation.* 2002;106:1374–1378.
9. Mongeon FP, Gurvitz MZ, Broberg CS, et al. Aortic root dilatation in adults with surgically repaired tetralogy of Fallot: a multicenter cross-sectional study. *Circulation.* 2013;127:172–179.
10. Antonetti I, Lorch D, Coe B, et al. Unrepaired tetralogy of Fallot with major aortopulmonary collateral arteries in an adult patient. *Congenit Heart Dis.* 2013;8:E24–E30.
11. Valente AM, Cook S, Festa P, et al. Multimodality imaging guidelines for patients with repaired tetralogy of Fallot. *J Am Soc Echocardiogr.* 2014;27:111–141.
12. Chan E, Alejos J. Pulmonary hypertension in patients after repair of transposition of the great arteries. *Congenit Heart Dis.* 2010;5:161–164.
13. Liebman J, Cullum L, Belloc NB. Natural history of transposition of the great arteries. Anatomy and birth and death characteristics. *Circulation.* 1969;40:237–262.
14. Cohen MS, Eidem BW, Cetta F, et al. Multimodality imaging guidelines of patients with transposition of the great arteries. *J Am Soc Echocardiogr.* 2016;29:571–621.
15. Moodie DS, Ritter DG, Tajik AJ, O'Fallon WM. Long-term follow-up in the unoperated univentricular heart. *Am J Cardiol.* 1984;53:1124–1128.
16. Anderson RH. Understanding Ebstein's malformation. *Cardiol Young.* 2015;25:137–138.
17. Tretter JT, Anderson RH. Ebstein's or Prescher's anomaly. *Eur Heart J.* 2018;39:972–973.
18. Zuberbuhler JR, Allwork SP, Anderson RH. The spectrum of Ebstein's anomaly of the tricuspid valve. *J Thorac Cardiovasc Surg.* 1979;77:202–211.
19. Attenhofer Jost CH, Connolly HM, Dearani JA, et al. Ebstein's anomaly. *Circulation.* 2007;115:277–285.
20. Qureshi MY, O'Leary PW, Connolly HM. Cardiac imaging in Ebstein anomaly. *Trends Cardiovasc Med.* 2018;28:403–409.
21. Yalonetsky S, Tobler D, Greutmann M, et al. Cardiac magnetic resonance imaging and the assessment of Ebstein anomaly in adults. *Am J Cardiol.* 2011;107:767–773.
22. Holst KA, Dearani JA, Said S, et al. Improving results of surgery for Ebstein anomaly: where are we after 235 cone repairs. *Ann Thorac Surg.* 2018;105:160–168.
23. Warnes CA. Congenitally corrected transposition: the uncorrected misnomer. *J Am Coll Cardiol.* 1996;27:1244–1245.
24. Anderson KR, Danielson GK, McGoon DC, Lie JT. Ebstein's anomaly of the left-sided tricuspid valve: pathological anatomy of the valvular malformation. *Circulation.* 1978;58:I87–I91.
25. Graham Jr TP, Bernard YD, Mellen BG, et al. Long-term outcome in congenitally corrected transposition of the great arteries: a multi-institutional study. *J Am Coll Cardiol.* 2000;36:255–261.
26. Mongeon FP, Connolly HM, Dearani JA, et al. Congenitally corrected transposition of the great arteries ventricular function at the time of systemic atrioventricular valve replacement predicts long-term ventricular function. *J Am Coll Cardiol.* 2011;57:2008–2017.
27. Beauchesne LM, Warnes CA, Connolly HM, et al. Outcome of the unoperated adult who presents with congenitally corrected transposition of the great arteries. *J Am Coll Cardiol.* 2002;40:285–290.
28. Geenen LW, van Grootel RWJ, Akman K, et al. Exploring the prognostic value of novel markers in adults with a systemic right ventricle. *J Am Heart Assoc.* 2019;8. e013745.
29. Crean A. Cardiovascular MR and CT in congenital heart disease. *Heart.* 2007;93:1637–1647.
30. Kilner PJ, Geva T, Kaemmerer H, et al. Recommendations for cardiovascular magnetic resonance in adults with congenital heart disease from the respective working groups of the European Society of Cardiology. *Eur Heart J.* 2010;31:794–805.

144 Adult Congenital Heart Disease With Prior Surgical Repair

Yamuna Sanil, Pooja Gupta, Richard Humes

An extensive variety of operations are used to correct or palliate congenital heart disease (CHD), often cloaked in the language of acronyms and eponyms. This chapter provides simple guidance for clinicians and sonographers in deciphering this occasionally confusing area. The approach to an adult postoperative patient should include some knowledge and history of what has been previously done for the patient. Attempting an echocardiogram without this knowledge can a time-consuming, frustrating experience and can lead to errors. Familiarity and experience with the echocardiographic appearance of postoperative CHD is an essential element to performing a good-quality study.[1,2]

HISTORICAL PERSPECTIVE AND TIMELINE

Repair of congenital heart disease has evolved tremendously over the past 60 to 70 years, resulting in improved survival for many defects that would be ultimately lethal if left untreated. The recent advances in the care of patients with CHD have been driven by technology and innovative thinking.[3,4] Diagnostic techniques such as echocardiography, cardiac magnetic resonance imaging (CMRI), computed tomography (CT), and cardiac catheterization have also undergone significant advancements that have aided in this effort. The general trend in recent years has been to repair the CHD early and not perform the so-called palliative operations that were done in the past. As techniques have improved for managing small infants on cardiopulmonary bypass (CPB), this has now become possible. A listing of some of these operations and the timeline in which they were developed is shown in Table 144.1. The early attempts to repair CHD were done without the use of CPB; a "closed heart" operation done on the beating heart.[5-7] These operations were frequently palliative. Most of the early palliative operations were considered definitive at the time because no repair was yet available. The advent of CPB allowed the heart to be open and still for a more complex but complete repair. Beginning in the mid-1950s, this ushered in a rapidly expanding area of innovation in surgical technique. Experience in this technique continued and in the late 1970s expanded again with advances in bypass technology that allowed smaller infants to be placed on the bypass machine.[8] With this advancement, the age at operation began to drop rapidly, and more operations could be performed in the first few months of life. Additionally, infants for whom there was previously no initial lifesaving palliation now could undergo successful repair as infants. Other more subtle technological advances, such as the use of cold-blood cardioplegic solutions to quiet the myocardium during bypass that was introduced in 1979, have helped to preserve myocardial function and improve outcome after surgery. As a result, patients repaired after 1980 are more likely to have better overall myocardial function, depending on the length and complexity of the operation.

BASIC CONCEPTS OF SURGICAL REPAIR

The concepts used by some of these creative operations are very simply stated: (1) holes, abnormal communications—close them (patch, suture); (2) obstruction to normal flow—open up the narrowed area (resection, valvotomy, conduit); (3) too little pulmonary blood flow—add some (from the systemic circulation); (4) too much pulmonary blood flow—restrict it (close the hole, band the pulmonary arteries); and (5) only one pumping chamber—use it for the systemic circulation (Box 144.1). Overall, the surgical repairs may be divided into three categories: palliative, anatomic, and nonanatomic.

Palliative Operations

Currently, these operations are typically performed as the initial, or sometimes only, step in patients with complex CHD. Palliative operations usually involve some control of pulmonary blood flow. It may be performed without bypass and can be accomplished in a short operative time and is therefore lower risk. Examples of these palliative operations are shown in Fig. 144.1.

Control of pulmonary blood flow is an important consideration in the repair of CHD, particularly complex defects. Excessive pulmonary blood flow results in an infant who is well oxygenated ("pink") but may be in heart failure from pulmonary edema. The

TABLE 144.1 Significant Milestones in the Management of Congenital Heart Disease[a]

Year	Physician(s)	Procedure
1938	Gross	Ligation of PDA
1944	Blalock, Taussig	Systemic pulmonary shunt
1945	Gross, Crafoord, Nylin	Repair of coarctation
1952	Muller	Pulmonary artery band
1953	Gibbon	Repair of ASD
1954	Lillehei	Repair of VSD
1954	Glenn	SVC-to-PA shunt
1955	Lillihei, Kirklin	Repair of ToF
1959	Senning	Atrial correction of TGA
1960	Waterston	Aortopulmonary shunt
1963	Mustard	Atrial correction of TGA
1964	Rastelli	Conduit replacement of PA
1966	Rashkind	Balloon atrial septostomy
1971	Fontan, Kreutzer	Repair of tricuspid atresia
1973	Heymann, Rudolf	PGE1 to open PDA
1976	Jatene	Arterial switch of TGA
1983	Norwood	Palliation of HLHS
1988	deLeval	Total cavopulmonary anastomosis
1990	Marcelletti	Extracardiac Fontan
1999	Sano	RV-to-PA shunt

[a]It is very helpful to know the timeline for various surgical repairs, particularly in patients in whom a detailed surgical history is not available. For example, a 40-year-old patient with d-transposition of great arteries is more likely to have had an atrial switch procedure (Mustard procedure) as opposed to an arterial switch operation (Jatene surgery). This table lists the timeline for various surgical procedures. Other landmark events in this field are use of prostaglandin (PGE1) (described in 1973, but clinical trials begun in 1978) and the use of two-dimensional echocardiography in the late 1970s.

ASD, Atrial septal defect; HLHS, hypoplastic left heart syndrome; PA, pulmonary artery; PDA, patent ductus arteriosus; RV, right ventricular; SVC, superior vena cava; TGA, transposition of the great arteries; ToF, tetralogy of Fallot; VSD, ventricular septal defect.

surgical solution to this is to restrict the pulmonary blood flow by closing the offending shunt or by placing a palliative band around the main pulmonary artery (PA band), restricting blood flow to the lung. The band serves to protect the lung beds from excessive blood flow and increased pressure. Previously, pulmonary banding was routinely performed in young infants with shunt lesions because it did not require bypass. The child was allowed to grow to an age and size at which bypass could be safely performed. Because of the increasing ability to use bypass in infants, PA banding is no longer used in great numbers and is reserved mostly for complicated cases in which a complete repair cannot be safely performed. Smaller, premature babies are one group in whom PA banding is still used.

Insufficient pulmonary blood flow and an intracardiac right-to-left shunt will result in cyanosis ("blue baby"). If a complete repair is not immediately possible, surgical palliation may be performed to create an additional source of blood for the pulmonary arteries. This can be done with an aortopulmonary shunt. Types of aortopulmonary shunts include Blalock-Taussig shunt, Waterston shunt, and Pott shunt. The modified Blalock-Taussig shunt is the most commonly performed shunt currently. The Waterston and Pott shunts were abandoned because of complications, including excessive pulmonary blood flow and PA distortion. The classic Glenn shunt involved anastomosis of the superior vena cava (SVC) to the right pulmonary artery (RPA) and disconnection of the RPA from the main pulmonary artery (MPA). Although the classic Glenn shunt is now abandoned as a technique, this operation demonstrated that blood could flow into the lungs passively without a ventricular pump and was an important precursor to the concept of single ventricle repair, described later in this chapter. The classic Glenn shunt was later modified as a bidirectional Glenn shunt in which the

SVC is anastomosed to the RPA but the RPA remains connected to MPA as the second stage for Fontan operation.

Anatomic Operations

The goal of an anatomic correction is to repair the CHD such that the patient has a four-chamber heart and two pumping ventricles. The repair might be simple, such as septal defect closure, or complex, when a combination of defects is present. It may be approached in one stage or in more than one stage. These operations are usually final. Most are now accomplished in the first year of life. Usually, CPB is needed.

If there are simple shunt defects ("holes"), they are most frequently repaired either by direct suture closure or by a patch. The patch material could be autologous pericardium or prosthetic material such as Dacron. Primary repair is preferable, but some factors (i.e., unusual location of defect, prematurity) preclude early primary repair and require initial palliation. Shunts may be thought of as "high pressure" (e.g., when a high-pressure chamber or vessel [left ventricle or aorta] is connected to a chamber or vessel that is normally under low pressure [right ventricle or PA]). Examples of high-pressure shunts are ventricular septal defects (VSDs) and patent ductus arteriosus (PDA). When pressure and flow are transmitted through the shunt from a high-pressure to a low-pressure area, the need for early surgery or palliation is greater, and operation should take place early to protect the pulmonary vasculature. By contrast, a "low-pressure" shunt (e.g., when a low-pressure area is connected to another low-pressure area, such as an atrial septal defect) rarely requires early surgery, and repair can usually wait until the patient is older and bigger.

If the cardiac defect is an obstruction and involves a cardiac valve, repair might involve either opening up the valve leaflets (valvotomy) or resecting the valve or obstructive muscle. The timing of these operations or interventional catheterization procedures often depends on the degree of obstruction. Therefore, the echocardiographic valvular gradient becomes an important factor in determining the need and timing of repair. The narrow or obstructed area might also be repaired with a patch or by interposition of a conduit or prosthetic valve. Conduits and artificial valves have an obvious disadvantage because of their inability to grow with the patient. Therefore, valves and conduits placed early in life will ultimately require replacement. There may be then the need for multiple operations because of the rapid growth seen in the pediatric age group.

Nonanatomic Operations

Nonanatomic repair most often includes a staged approach to a single usable ventricle, referred to as a "Fontan" operation. In

---

BOX 144.1 Fontan or Single-Ventricle Concept

Holes	Close them	Patch or suture
Obstruction to flow	Open it	Resection, valvotomy, or conduit
Too little pulmonary flow	Add flow from systemic circulation	Central shunt, Blalock-Taussig shunt, Waterston shunt, Potts shunt
Too much pulmonary flow	Restrict it	Close the shunt or band the pulmonary arteries
Only one pumping chamber	Use it for systemic circulation	Fontan operation

---

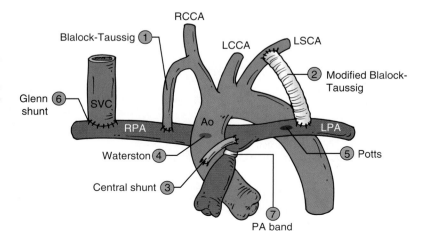

Figure 144.1. Palliative operations. *1,* The classic Blalock-Taussig shunt is an anastomosis of the subclavian artery to the ipsilateral pulmonary artery (PA). *2,* The modified Blalock-Taussig shunt uses a prosthetic tube interpositioned between the subclavian artery and PA. *3,* A central shunt is a prosthetic tube that connects the ascending aorta (Ao) to the main (central) PA. *4,* The Waterston shunt is a side-to-side anastomosis between the ascending Ao and right pulmonary artery (RPA). *5,* The Potts shunt is a side-to-side anastomosis between the ascending Ao and left pulmonary artery (LPA). *6,* A classic Glenn shunt is an anastomosis between the superior vena cava (SVC) and RPA. *7,* Used to restrict pulmonary blood flow, a PA band is a constricting band placed around the MPA. *LCCA,* Left common cardiac artery; *LSCA,* left subclavian artery; *RCCA,* right common cardiac artery.

these instances, the one available ventricular pump is used for the systemic circulation. The pulmonary ventricle is bypassed, and the entire venous return from the SVC and inferior vena cava (IVC) goes directly into the pulmonary arteries, separating the systemic and pulmonary circulation. The net result is a patient with relatively normal oxygen saturations but no pulmonary pump. A completed Fontan operation is currently accomplished in three stages. If a patient has had three operations within the first few years of life, it is highly likely that he or she had some variation of single-ventricle repair. Older adults who had an operation before 1985 may have had this done in two stages, with the later stage at an older age.

The first stage of the Fontan operation is done to gain control of the pulmonary circulation. The kind of operation varies depending on the cardiac anatomy and status of the pulmonary blood flow. This could involve placement of a band around the MPA to restrict pulmonary blood flow or placement of an aortopulmonary shunt to increase pulmonary blood flow. If the systemic outflow tract is inadequate, pulmonary outflow is used to reconstruct the systemic outflow tract (Norwood procedure). Hence, a source of pulmonary blood flow in the form of a shunt is needed. It may be a Blalock-Taussig shunt or a right ventricle to PA shunt (Sano modification), which is favored by some centers. In either case, mixed arterial and venous blood is delivered to the aorta and the body. In patients with CHD in whom the pulmonary blood flow and pressure are in an acceptable range and there is no systemic outflow tract obstruction, the first-stage operation can sometimes be skipped.

The second stage of the Fontan operation involves connection of the SVC to the PA. This is referred to as "hemi-Fontan" or "bidirectional Glenn shunt" and is typically performed around 6 months of age. The lower body venous return via IVC still enters the systemic circulation, resulting in continued desaturation after this stage. The third and final stage of the Fontan operation is often referred to as "completion of Fontan," in which the venous return from the IVC is now directed into the pulmonary arteries, completing the separation of the systemic and pulmonary circulations. This final stage is performed between 18 months to 3 years of age, depending on the modification of the Fontan connection performed and the systemic venous anatomy. There is some variation between different institutions in terms of the timing for this final operation. The Fontan circuit may be fenestrated in certain cases to allow a small right-to-left shunt at the atrial level.

IMPORTANT ECHOCARDIOGRAPHIC CONSIDERATIONS IN THE POSTOPERATIVE PATIENT

Some of the unique concepts pertaining to surgical repair of CHD that may influence the performance and interpretation of the echocardiographic study follow:

- The pulmonary valve is expendable, and pulmonary insufficiency is very well tolerated for many years before some form of intervention is required.
- The primary goal of surgical repair in many cases of CHD is to control the pulmonary blood flow. Therefore, a detailed examination of pulmonary arteries, pulmonary blood flow, and pulmonary pressures is important. Determination of pulmonary pressure can be done using tricuspid regurgitant flow velocities or using the VSD shunt gradient if present.
- Patches placed in the heart become endothelialized over time and become part of the heart. A relatively large patch placed in an infant heart will be a very small part of the adult heart and may be invisible on the echocardiogram. During the echocardiographic study, thorough evaluation for any residual shunts should be performed. This finding has clinical implications for endocarditis prophylaxis.[9]
- Detailed examination of all available chambers and valves during an echocardiographic study is crucial in the management of a patient with CHD.

- Patients with CHD may often have "missing parts." Do not assume that the inability to image a chamber or valve is caused by inadequate technique or echocardiographic window. The chamber or valve might not be present as a part of the CHD. For example, the pulmonary valve may be "missing" in postoperative patients with tetralogy of Fallot (ToF) that was repaired with a transannular patch.
- The route taken by the blood flow in and out of the heart may vary in patients with CHD. It is important to trace the blood flow from the point of entry into the heart to the exit point out of the heart by following the segmental analysis, as described in Chapter 140.
- Many postoperative adult patients with CHD have poor acoustic windows, and transthoracic echocardiography may be suboptimal. Transesophageal echocardiogram may play an important role[10] (refer to Chapter 140), and CMRI is rapidly gaining utility for this cohort of patients.[11,12] CT is a good option when CMRI is contraindicated in certain cases.

REPRESENTATIVE CASE EXAMPLES

A few case scenarios are discussed here to help develop an understanding of commonly encountered postoperative patients with CHD. Exhaustive examples of every congenital heart operation are beyond the scope of this chapter.

Case 1

A 33-year-old male patient is seen at an outpatient cardiology clinic. He states that he is currently doing well and has had two previous operations for a heart defect that he was born with. He describes the defect as a "hole in the heart." He thinks that the first operation was done at around 2 months of age and the second one at 4 years of age. On examination, he has a grade 2 of 6 to-and-fro murmur at the upper left sternal border. The electrocardiogram (ECG) reveals sinus rhythm with right bundle branch block. He has a midline scar (median sternotomy) and a scar on his right side between the ribs (right lateral thoracotomy) (Figs. 144.2 and 144.3; Videos 144.1 to 144.5).

Repair of Conotruncal Defects

A variety of defects, including ToF, truncus arteriosus, double-outlet right ventricle, and so, on may be bundled together under the category of "conotruncal" defects because they share some common anatomic features. These defects are also frequently repaired

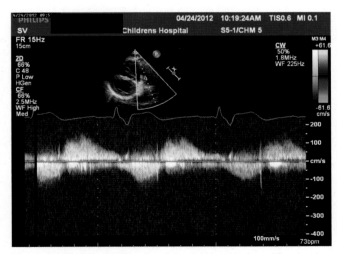

Figure 144.2. Spectral Doppler of the right ventricular outflow tract demonstrates the "to-and-fro" nature of the flow in this area.

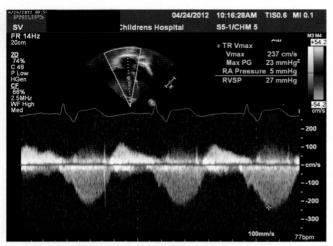

Figure 144.3. Spectral Doppler of the tricuspid regurgitation signal allows a prediction of the right ventricular systolic pressure, which is normal in this case. This is a typical finding, despite the volume overload from the pulmonary regurgitation.

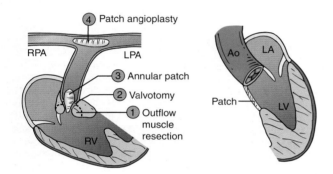

Figure 144.4. Repair of tetralogy of Fallot. The repair involves several steps including right ventricular outflow muscle resection *(1)*, pulmonary valvotomy *(2)*, a possible patch across the pulmonary annulus *(3)*, and possible enlargement of the proximal pulmonary arteries with a patch *(4)*. In addition, the ventricular septal defect must be closed to direct left ventricular blood to the aorta (Patch). *Ao*, Aorta; *LA*, left atrium; *LPA*, left pulmonary artery; *LV*, left ventricle; *RPA*, right pulmonary artery, *RV*, right ventricle.

in a similar fashion and usually as a four-chamber heart. Common features include the presence of a large VSD and a variable degree of pulmonary outflow obstruction. As a result, the surgical repair involves closure of the VSD so that left ventricular blood is pumped to the aorta and right ventricular blood is pumped to the pulmonary arteries. The technical variations found in the operative approaches to the repair usually revolve around the repair of the pulmonary outflow obstruction. This may be accomplished by either resection of the subpulmonary obstruction (with or without pulmonary valvotomy) (Fig. 144.4) or placement of a right ventricle to PA conduit as shown in Fig. 144.5. Typically, ToF repair involves an incision across the stenotic pulmonary valve and placement of an overlay patch to make the narrow outflow tract widely patent, referred to as *transannular patch*. This patch successfully relieves the obstruction but results in loss of valve action and free pulmonary insufficiency. In the current era, primary repair is performed during infancy.[13] When a transannular patch is used for primary repair, there is often a need for pulmonary valve replacement at a later time. Standards for the timing of this are still open to discussion. Patients frequently require pulmonary valve replacement in their late teens or early adulthood. Right ventricular volumes measured

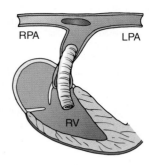

Figure 144.5. Conotruncal defects: relief of obstruction with a right ventricle to pulmonary artery conduit. *LPA*, Left pulmonary artery; *RPA*, right pulmonary artery; *RV*, right ventricle.

on CMRI are currently used to determine a surgical threshold.[14] A conduit is used in special circumstances, such as when the native pulmonary outflow tract cannot be used for various anatomical reasons. These reasons might be pulmonary valve atresia, certain cases of double-outlet right ventricle, transposition of the great arteries with VSD and pulmonary stenosis, or for rare coronary artery anomalies in ToF, when incision in the outflow tract may endanger the coronary artery integrity and myocardial perfusion.

Postoperative Complications

With improved surgical techniques, the overall prognosis for these patients is good.[15,16] The VSD is amenable to surgical repair and is virtually never a problem. The aortic root is frequently larger than normal in patients with repaired conotruncal defects.[17] Most significant issues in a postoperative patient involve the pulmonary outflow tract and the branch pulmonary arteries. Patients may develop ventricular dysfunction, aortic insufficiency, residual pulmonary stenosis, or, more frequently, pulmonary regurgitation, frequently of a severe degree.[18–20] Significant pulmonary regurgitation leads to enlargement of the right ventricle over time.[21,22] In the absence of pulmonary outflow obstruction, elevated right ventricular systolic pressures may be seen in patients with peripheral pulmonary stenosis, which may be difficult to image during the echocardiographic study. These patients are at increased risk of life-threatening arrhythmias and heart block.[23–25]

Postoperative Echocardiography Checklist (Conotruncal Defects)

1. Right ventricular dilatation or dysfunction
2. Pulmonary outflow obstruction
3. Pulmonary regurgitation
4. Peripheral pulmonary stenosis
5. Aortic root size and regurgitation
6. Right ventricular systolic pressure
7. Residual VSD shunt

Case 2

A 38-year-old male patient complains of frequent palpitations and generalized fatigue. He reports having an operation at age 3 years to "fix his arteries that were backward." He has a midline scar (median sternotomy). His ECG shows a low atrial rhythm with a rate of 45 beats/min and right ventricular hypertrophy (Fig. 144.6 and Videos 144.6 to 144.9).

Repair of D-Transposition of the Great Arteries

In older adult patients, d-transposition of the great arteries (d-TGA) was likely repaired with an atrial switch operation (Mustard or

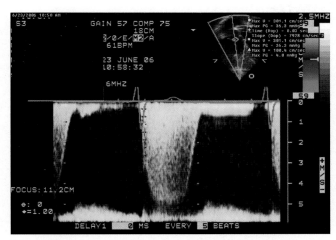

Figure 144.6. Continuous-wave Doppler of the tricuspid regurgitant signal shows a high velocity. In this instance, this *does not* infer that there is pulmonary hypertension because this is the systemic, not the pulmonary atrioventricular valve, in this arrangement.

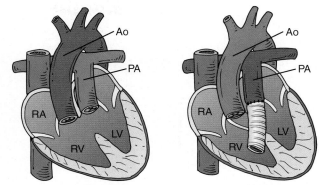

Figure 144.8. D-transposition of the great arteries with ventricular septal defect: Rasteli operation . Repair is performed by closing the ventricular septal defect directing left ventricular flow to the aorta and placing a conduit from the right ventricle to the pulmonary artery. *Ao,* Aorta; *LV,* left ventricle; *PA,* pulmonary artery; *RA,* right atrium; *RV,* right ventricle.

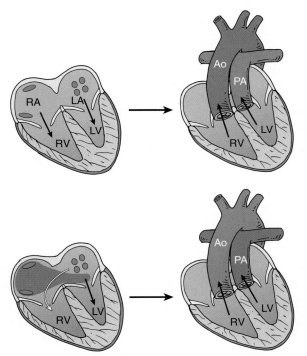

Figure 144.7. D-transposition of the great arteries: atrial switch operation. The Mustard or Senning operation is accomplished by constructing an atrial baffle, which incorporates the inferior and superior caval flow and redirects it to the mitral valve, where it then can exit the heart through the pulmonary artery. Pulmonary venous blood will flow anterior to this baffle, toward the tricuspid valve, completing the atrial switch. Whereas the Senning operation uses mostly infoldings of the atria to create the baffle, the Mustard operation uses a trouser-shaped baffle of autologous material. Echocardiographically, the two operations are difficult to distinguish from one another. *Ao,* Aorta; *LV,* left ventricle; *PA,* pulmonary artery; *RA,* right atrium; *RV,* right ventricle.

Senning) that rerouted blood at the atrial level with a complex intraatrial baffle[26,27] (Fig. 144.7). The transposed great arteries were unchanged during surgical repair. Blood was routed from the right atrium to the left ventricle and out the PA using two separate channels that came together at the level of the mitral valve. These two channels directed the SVC and IVC blood and are referred to as SVC baffle and IVC baffle, respectively. Blood from the left atrium was routed to the right ventricle and out the aorta. It is important to note here that the right ventricle became the systemic pump. Patients with d-TGA and a VSD might have been repaired by closing the VSD to the aorta and placing a conduit from the right ventricle to the PA (Fig. 144.8), referred to as "Rastelli operation." The original concept of a pulmonary conduit was first devised for this anatomy and has been since then used in repair of other conotruncal abnormalities.[28] In the late 1970s and early 1980s, the "arterial switch" (Jatene operation) compared with previously performed "atrial switch" operation (Mustard or Senning) became prevalent and at present is the operation of choice for almost all forms of d-TGA.[29] This is conceptually a simpler repair in which the abnormal arterial position is corrected by switching it back to a normal location over their respective ventricles (Fig. 144.9).

Postoperative Complications

The Mustard or Senning (atrial switch) operation was very successful in the early years of its use. The survival rate was high, and patients tended to be clinically well in their pediatric years.[30] In later years, the atrial baffle proved to be a source of problems and potential obstruction.[31,32] Obstruction could occur anywhere along the SVC baffle (rarely in the IVC baffle). SVC obstruction frequently results in blood being shunted through the azygos vein down to the IVC and may not produce any symptoms. More serious consequences arose from obstruction of pulmonary venous blood flow to the tricuspid valve. The hemodynamics in this situation would be analogous to mitral stenosis in the normal heart. After a Mustard operation, the right ventricle is the systemic ventricle and is predisposed to ventricular failure. Rhythm problems are frequent because of the presence of multiple suture lines and complex intraatrial baffle after Mustard repair.[33–35] Arrhythmia in these patients predicts a poor prognosis, including sudden cardiac death.[36]

The Rastelli operation predisposes the patient to conduit failure and need for replacement. When done in a young person, the patient will outgrow the conduit and relative stenosis may develop. Right ventricular function may also decline over time. The Jatene operation creates a near-normal heart. Problems are few in most cases.[37] However, manipulating the pulmonary arteries to accomplish the arterial switch may lead to suprapulmonary or peripheral PA stenosis.[38] Less commonly, narrowing along the anastomotic area (both suprapulmonary and supraaortic) may be seen.[39] In some cases, progressive aortic root dilatation with

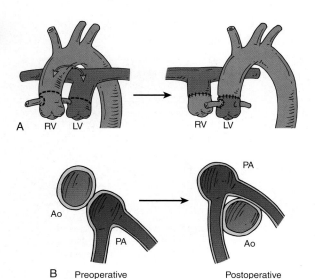

Figure 144.9. d-Transposition of the great arteries: arterial switch operation. **A,** The great arteries are transected above the semilunar valve. The coronary arteries are removed with a button of tissue from the aorta (Ao). After mobilization of the pulmonary arteries (PAs), the Ao is moved posteriorly and reattached to the pulmonary stump with reanastomosis of the coronary arteries to this neoaorta. The mobilized PAs are brought forward over the Ao and reattached to the neopulmonary artery, completing the arterial switch. **B,** Diagrams generally depict an arterial switch as a side-to-side rearrangement. However, the arteries are actually in an anteroposterior orientation and need to be moved thusly. The resultant rearrangement results in a straddling of the Ao by the PAs. *LV,* left ventricle; *RV,* right ventricle.

aortic insufficiency has been seen.[40] The coronary arteries are also explanted from the transposed aorta and reimplanted into the neoaortic sinuses. Rarely, patients may develop problems at the coronary ostia, resulting in stenosis and ischemia.[41]

Postoperative Echocardiography Checklist (d-Transposition of the Great Arteries)

1. Systemic ventricular function
2. Supraaortic and pulmonary valve area, PA branches, and pulmonary blood flow
3. Aortic root and pulmonary root sizes
4. Right ventricular systolic pressure
5. In postoperative atrial switch (Mustard-Senning): atrial baffle: systemic venous baffle (including the SVC and IVC), pulmonary venous baffle, degree of tricuspid regurgitation and systemic (right ventricular) ventricular function.

Case 3

A 22-year-old female patient with a history of repaired CHD is seen in the office and wants to discuss pregnancy. She used to see a pediatric cardiologist but has not followed up for more than 5 years. She says that she has had three previous heart operations and describes her heart as "only half a heart." She feels generally well but is mildly obese and not very active (Videos 144.10 to 144.14).

The Fontan-Type Operation for Single Ventricle

In the setting of CHD, when one of the pumping chamber or a particular valve or valves are missing or critically small, four-chamber repair cannot be performed. Hearts that cannot be fixed anatomically with four chambers and two pumping ventricles require

---

BOX 144.2 Fontan Operation

GOALS OF THE FONTAN OPERATION
1. Separate systemic and pulmonary circulations.
2. Remove volume load from the (single) pumping chamber.

FONTAN OPERATIVE CONCEPT
1. Direct the systemic venous blood to the lungs.
2. No pumping chamber in the pulmonary circuit.

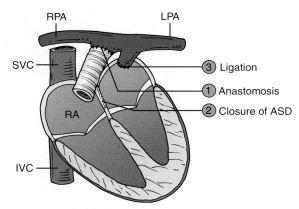

Figure 144.10. Modified Fontan-Kreutzer operation. The original early Fontan operation incorporated several bovine valves to direct flow. It was successful, but problems ultimately developed with the valves. Throughout the 1980s and early 1990s, the operation was done as shown, usually anastomosing the right atrial appendage to the inferior portion of the pulmonary artery and possibly augmenting this anastomosis with additional material (1). The result was a very broad connection from the atrium to the pulmonary artery. Any atrial communication was closed (2), as well as isolating any patent right-sided atrioventricular valve (3). If the pulmonary flow was still present, this was ligated. *ASD,* Atrial septal defect; *IVC,* inferior vena cava; *LPA,* left pulmonary artery; *RA,* right atrium; *RPA,* right pulmonary artery; *SVC,* superior vena cava.

Fontan-type repair, in which they have only one pumping chamber used for systemic circulation (Box 144.2). Knowledge of this operation is important because, although not frequently encountered, it is a unifying concept that, when taken as a whole, encompasses many different patients and a variety of CHD. Because of the improved survival of these patients, it is now more likely that they will be encountered as adults. A wide variety of complex lesions result in single-ventricle physiology such as (1) hypoplastic left heart syndrome, (2) hypoplastic right heart syndrome, (3) tricuspid valve atresia or mitral valve atresia, (4) double-inlet single ventricle, (5) common-inlet single ventricle, and (6) complex atrioventricular (AV) valve straddling that results in one hypoplastic ventricle.

The concept of partial circulatory bypass of the right heart was first introduced in 1958 by Glenn.[42] The concept was later modified and popularized by Fontan and Kreutzer.[43] The original procedures involved connecting the right atrium to the right ventricular outflow tract with an interposed valved conduit. Later the operation was modified to a direct anastomosis of the right atrium to the pulmonary arteries without a valve (Fig. 144.10).[44] This was a reasonable palliation, but over time, it resulted in poor flow hemodynamics and rhythm problems as the right atrium dilated. Further modifications were introduced to troubleshoot the right atrial enlargement. Newer modifications led to direct connection of the SVC and IVC to the pulmonary arteries using a tunnel through the right atrium, referred to as "lateral tunnel" (*total cavopulmonary anastomosis*)[45,46] (Fig. 144.11). The Fontan operation is usually performed in three stages,

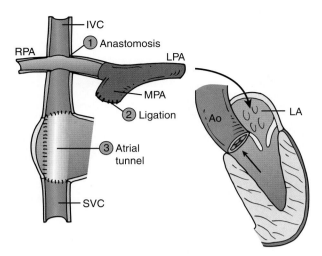

Figure 144.11. In a newer technique advocated by de Leval in 1988, the superior vena cava (*SVC*) was directly connected to the pulmonary artery (1) as the second stage of single-ventricle repair. Somewhat different techniques have evolved that are fundamentally the same but slightly different in construction and are called the bidirectional Glenn or the hemi-Fontan. Other sources of pulmonary flow are generally ligated (2) at this time. In the third stage, often called completion of Fontan, the inferior vena cava (*IVC*) blood is incorporated into the pulmonary circuit. Frequently, this is done with a tunnel running through the right atrium (3). However, with complex anatomy or simply by the surgeon's preference, the IVC anastomosis may also be accomplished using an extracardiac tunnel to complete the Fontan. This is the extracardiac Fontan. *Ao,* Aorta; *LA,* left atrium; *LPA,* left pulmonary artery; *MPA,* main pulmonary artery; *RPA,* right pulmonary artery.

with completion between 18 months to 3 years of age. One other newer modification of Fontan repair used in patients with complex systemic venous anomalies is called the *extracardiac Fontan*, in which a conduit outside the heart is used to direct the IVC blood into the pulmonary arteries.[47] This modification is increasingly used in patients with systemic venous anomalies and in older patients undergoing revision of their old-style Fontan connection. When pulmonary pressures are high or ventricular function is questionable, the tunnel may be fenestrated to allow a pop-off of flow into the systemic atrium from the atriopulmonary connection.

Despite these technical differences and modifications, the basic result is the same: the systemic venous blood (blue blood) flows passively into the pulmonary arteries, the pulmonary venous blood (red blood) passes through the only ventricle and is pumped to the body, and there is complete separation of systemic and pulmonary circulation, resulting in near normal saturations.

Postoperative Complications

Fontan surgery is a palliative surgery[48,49] and not an anatomic repair with improved early outcomes.[50,51] Postoperative problems include consequences associated with higher-than-normal venous pressures such as varicose veins, protein-losing enteropathy, and ascites and liver damage. Numerous rhythm problems are also encountered.[52,53] Ventricular dysfunction[54] and AV valve regurgitation can be particularly problematic and may contribute to increased morbidity and mortality in this group during young adulthood.[55] Pregnancy in patients with Fontan palliation is considered moderate to high risk, with adverse outcomes for both the patient and the fetus.[56]

Postoperative Echocardiography Checklist (Fontan: Single-Ventricle Repair)

Complex single ventricles may be relatively easier to image, contrary to what most people think. It certainly requires experience and knowledge, which can only be gained by performing studies in many patients. Echocardiographic evaluation of a patient after Fontan repair should be reserved for specialists trained in this area.[57] However, for an experienced echocardiographer, there are fewer things to image, and it is a quicker study.

1. Evaluate the site of repair or cavopulmonary anastomosis
2. Systemic ventricular function
3. Valvular integrity and function (AV or semilunar valves)
4. Presence or absence of a fenestration
5. Pericardial effusion

Please access ExpertConsult to view the corresponding videos for this chapter.

REFERENCES

1. Lai WW, Geva T, Shirali GS, et al. Guidelines and standards for performance of a pediatric echocardiogram. *J Am Soc Echocardiogr.* 2006;19:1413–1430.
2. Lopez L, Colan SD, Frommelt PC, et al. Recommendations for quantification methods during the performance of a pediatric echocardiogram. *J Am Soc Echocardiogr.* 2010;23:465–495. quiz 576–577.
3. Freedom RM, Lock J, Bricker JT. Pediatric cardiology and cardiovascular surgery: 1950–2000. *Circulation.* 2000;102:IV58–IV68.
4. Boneva RS, Botto LD, Moore CA, et al. Mortality associated with congenital heart defects in the United States: trends and racial disparities. 1979–1997. *Circulation.* 2001;103:2376–2381.
5. Gross RE. Surgical management of the patent ductus arteriosus: with summary of four surgically treated cases. *Ann Surg.* 1939;110:321–356.
6. Blalock A, Taussig HB. The surgical treatment of malformations of the heart in which there is pulmonary stenosis or pulmonary atresia. *J Am Med Assoc.* 1984;251:2123–2138.
7. Rashkind WJ, Miller WW. Creation of an atrial septal defect without thoracotomy. A palliative approach to complete transposition of the great arteries. *J Am Med Assoc.* 1966;196:991–992.
8. Castaneda A. Congenital heart disease: a surgical-historical perspective. *Ann Thorac Surg.* 2005;79:S2217–S2220.
9. Wilson W, Taubert KA, Gewitz M, et al. Prevention of infective endocarditis: guidelines from the American heart association. *Circulation.* 2007;116:1736–1754.
10. Ayres NA, Miller-Hance W, Fyfe DA, et al. Indications and guidelines for performance of transesophageal echocardiography in the patient with pediatric acquired or congenital heart disease. *J Am Soc Echocardiogr.* 2005;18:91–98.
11. Partington SL, Valente AM. Cardiac magnetic resonance in adults with congenital heart disease. *Methodist Debakey Cardiovasc J.* 2013;9:156–162.
12. Orwat S, Diller GP, Baumgartner H. Imaging of congenital heart disease in adults: choice of modalities. *Eur Heart J Cardiovasc Imag.* 2014;15:6–17.
13. Hirsch JC, Mosca RS, Bove EL. Complete repair of tetralogy of Fallot in the neonate: results in the modern era. *Ann Surg.* 2000;232:508–514.
14. Geva T. Indications and timing of pulmonary valve replacement after tetralogy of Fallot repair. *Semin Thorac Cardiovasc Surg Pediatr Card Surg Annu.* 2006:11–22.
15. Murphy JG, Gersh BJ, Mair DD, et al. Long-term outcome in patients undergoing surgical repair of tetralogy of Fallot. *N Engl J Med.* 1993;329:593–599.
16. Waien SA, Liu PP, Ross BL, et al. Serial follow-up of adults with repaired tetralogy of Fallot. *J Am Coll Cardiol.* 1992;20:295–300.
17. Warnes CA, Child JS. Aortic root dilatation after repair of tetralogy of Fallot: pathology from the past? *Circulation.* 2002;106:1310–1311.
18. Vogel M, Sponring J, Cullen S, et al. Regional wall motion and abnormalities of electrical depolarization and repolarization in patients after surgical repair of tetralogy of Fallot. *Circulation.* 2001;103:1669–1673.
19. Ghai A, Silversides C, Harris L, et al. Left ventricular dysfunction is a risk factor for sudden cardiac death in adults late after repair of tetralogy of Fallot. *J Am Coll Cardiol.* 2002;40:1675–1680.
20. Geva T, Sandweiss BM, Gauvreau K, et al. Factors associated with impaired clinical status in long-term survivors of tetralogy of Fallot repair evaluated by magnetic resonance imaging. *J Am Coll Cardiol.* 2004;43:1068–1074.
21. Frigiola A, Redington AN, Cullen S, et al. Pulmonary regurgitation is an important determinant of right ventricular contractile dysfunction in patients with surgically repaired tetralogy of Fallot. *Circulation.* 2004;110:II153–II157.
22. Therrien J, Siu SC, McLaughlin PR, et al. Pulmonary valve replacement in adults late after repair of tetralogy of Fallot: are we operating too late? *J Am Coll Cardiol.* 2000;36:1670–1675.
23. Gatzoulis MA, Balaji S, Webber SA, et al. Risk factors for arrhythmia and sudden cardiac death late after repair of tetralogy of Fallot. *Lancet.* 2000;356:975–981.

24. Khairy P, Landzberg MJ, Gatzoulis MA, et al. Value of programmed ventricular stimulation after tetralogy of Fallot repair. *Circulation.* 2004;109:1994–2000.

25. Gatzoulis K, Frogoudaki A, Brili S, et al. Implantable defibrillators: from the adult cardiac to the grown up congenital heart disease patient. *Int J Cardiol.* 2004;97(suppl 1):117–122.

26. Senning A. Surgical correction of transposition of the great vessels. *Surgery.* 1959;45:966–980.

27. Mustard WT. Successful two-stage correction of transposition of the great vessels. *Surgery.* 1964;55:469–472.

28. Rastelli GC, Wallace RB, Ongley PA. Complete repair of transposition of the great arteries with pulmonary stenosis. *Circulation.* 1969;39:83–95.

29. Jatene AD, Fontes VF, Paulista PP, et al. Successful anatomic correction of transposition of the great vessels. A preliminary report. *Arq Bras Cardiol.* 1975;28:461–464.

30. Wilson NJ, Clarkson PM, Barratt-Boyes BG, et al. Long-term outcome after the mustard repair for simple transposition of the great arteries. *J Am Coll Cardiol.* 1998;32:758–765.

31. Daehnert I, Hennig B, Wiener M, et al. Interventions in leaks and obstructions of the interatrial baffle late after Mustard and Senning correction for transposition of the great arteries. *Catheter Cardiovasc Interv.* 2005;66:400–407.

32. Ward CJ, Mullins CE, Nihill MR, et al. Use of intravascular stents in systemic venous and systemic venous baffle obstructions. *Circulation.* 1995;91:2948–2954.

33. Dos L, Teruel L, Ferreira IJ, et al. Late outcome of Senning and Mustard procedures for correction of transposition of the great arteries. *Heart.* 2005;91:652–656.

34. Khairy P, Landzberg MJ, Lambert J, et al. Long-term outcomes after the atrial switch for surgical correction of transposition. *Cardiol Young.* 2004;14:284–292.

35. Gelatt M, Hamilton RM, McCrindle BW, et al. Arrhythmia and mortality after the Mustard procedure: a 30-year single- center experience. *J Am Coll Cardiol.* 1997;29:194–201.

36. Kammeraad JA, van Deurzen CH, Sreeram N, et al. Predictors of sudden cardiac death after Mustard or Senning repair for transposition of the great arteries. *J Am Coll Cardiol.* 2004;44:1095–1102.

37. von Bernuth G. 25 years after the first arterial switch procedure: mid-term results. *Thorac Cardiovasc Surg.* 2000;48:228–232.

38. Williams WG, Quaegebeur JM, Kirklin JW, et al: outflow obstruction after the arterial switch operation, *J Thorac Cardiovasc Surg.* 114:975–987, discussion 87–90, 1997.

39. Prifti E, Crucean A, Bonacchi M, et al. Early and long-term outcome of the arterial switch operation for transposition of the great arteries: predictors and functional evaluation. *Eur J Cardio Thorac Surg.* 2002;22:864–873.

40. McMahon CJ, Ravekes WJ, Smith EO, et al. Risk factors for neo-aortic root enlargement and aortic regurgitation following arterial switch operation. *Pediatr Cardiol.* 2004;25:329–335.

41. Raisky O, Bergoend E, Agnoletti G, et al. Late coronary artery lesions after neonatal arterial switch operation. *Eur J Cardio Thorac Surg.* 2007;31:894–898.

42. Glenn WW. Circulatory bypass of the right side of the heart. IV. Shunt between superior vena cava and distal right pulmonary artery. *N Engl J Med.* 1958;259:117–120.

43. Fontan F, Baudet E. Surgical repair of tricuspid atresia. *Thorax.* 1971;26:240–248.

44. Norwood WI, Kirklin JK, Sanders SP. Hypoplastic left heart syndrome: experience with palliative surgery. *Am J Cardiol.* 1980;45:87–91.

45. de Leval MR, Kilner P, Gewillig M, et al. Total cavopulmonary connection: a logical alternative to atriopulmonary connection for complex Fontan operations. *J Thorac Cardiovasc Surg.* 1988;96:682–695.

46. Bove EL, de Leval MR, Migliavacca F, et al. Computational fluid dynamics in the evaluation of hemodynamic performance of cavopulmonary connections after the Norwood procedure for hypoplastic left heart syndrome. *J Thorac Cardiovasc Surg.* 2003;126:1040–1047.

47. Nakano T, Kado H, Ishikawa S, et al. Midterm surgical results of total cavopulmonary connection. *J Thorac Cardiovasc Surg.* 2004;127:730–737.

48. Fontan F, Kirklin JW, Fernandez G, et al. Outcome after a "perfect" Fontan operation. *Circulation.* 1990;81:1520–1536.

49. de Leval MR. The Fontan circulation: what have we learned? What to expect? *Pediatr Cardiol.* 1998;19:316–320.

50. Gentles TL, Mayer Jr JE, Gauvreau K, et al. Fontan operation in five hundred consecutive patients. *J Thorac Cardiovasc Surg.* 1997;114:376–391.

51. Gentles TL, Gauvreau K, Mayer Jr JE, et al. Functional outcome after the Fontan operation: factors influencing late morbidity. *J Thorac Cardiovasc Surg.* 1997;114:392–403.

52. van den Bosch AE, Roos-Hesselink JW, Van Domburg R, et al. Long-term outcome and quality of life in adult patients after the Fontan operation. *Am J Cardiol.* 2004;93:1141–1145.

53. Collins 2nd RT, Fram RY, Tang X, et al. Hospital utilization in adults with single ventricle congenital heart disease and cardiac arrhythmias. *J Cardiovasc Electrophysiol.* 2014;25:170–186.

54. Cedars A, Joseph S, Ludbrook P. Heart failure in adults who had the Fontan procedure: Natural history, evaluation, and management. *Curr Treat Options Cardiovasc Med.* 2013;15:587–601.

55. Petko M, Myung RJ, Wernovsky G, et al. Surgical reinterventions following the Fontan procedure. *Eur J Cardio Thorac Surg.* 2003;24:255–259.

56. Canobbio MM, Mair DD, van der Velde M, et al. Pregnancy outcomes after the Fontan repair. *J Am Coll Cardiol.* 1996;28:763–767.

57. Stout KK, Daniels CJ, Aboulhosn JA, et al. AHA/ACC Guideline for the management of adults with congenital heart disease. *J Am Coll Cardiol.* 2018;73(12). 2019.

145 Hypertension

Brian D. Hoit

Systemic arterial hypertension is a major cause of cardiovascular morbidity and mortality and is the number one attributable risk factor for death throughout the world.[1] The adverse effects of hypertension result from structural and functional changes in the heart and arteries and from acceleration of atherosclerosis. Pressure overload–induced concentric left ventricular (LV) hypertrophy, although initially adaptive (by normalizing increased wall stress), is associated with alterations in gene expression and myocardial architecture, systolic and diastolic dysfunction, and eventually heart failure. Aortic thickening and atherosclerosis, dilatation, and increased stiffness may give rise to abnormal ventricular–vascular coupling, increased LV afterload, aortic insufficiency, and dissection. Echocardiography plays a critical role in the management of patients with hypertension because of its ability to quantify LV volumes, function and mass, cardiac mechanics, and arterial dynamics (Fig. 145.1).

LEFT VENTRICULAR SIZE, CHAMBER FUNCTION, AND MASS

M-Mode Echocardiography

Historically, M-mode echocardiography was the first modality used for measurements of end-diastolic and end-systolic LV minor diameters and end-diastolic posterior and septal wall thicknesses. This in turn allowed for direct calculation of LV fractional shortening and relative wall thickness (RWT) and by assuming spherical ventricular geometry, LV volumes, ejection fraction, and mass (Table 145.1).[2]

Concentric hypertrophy is defined as increased LV mass (>95 g/m^2 for women, >115 g/m^2 for men) and a RWT greater than 0.42, and concentric remodeling is defined as an increased RWT with a normal LV mass index. Increased LV mass with a normal RWT characterizes eccentric hypertrophy, which may be seen later in the course of hypertensive heart disease (Table 145.2).

Although temporal and spatial resolutions are excellent, M-mode echocardiography is limited in that a one-dimensional "ice-pick" view of the heart is produced, which is suitable only for ventricles with uniform geometry and wall motion. Moreover, unrealistic spherical geometry is assumed when either the Teichholz or cubed formula is used, and coupled with the potential for tangential imaging, overestimations of volume and mass result.

Two- and Three-Dimensional Echocardiography

Two-dimensional (2D) echocardiography overcomes many of these limitations but increases measurement complexity, requires epicardial definition, and is not free of the need for geometric assumptions or errors owing to foreshortened apical views (see Table 145.1).[2] Thus, although accuracy is increased, volumes and mass are underestimated, and reproducibility remains problematic. In contrast, real-time three-dimensional (3D) echocardiography (RT3DE) accurately and reproducibly measures LV volumes, ejection fraction, and mass compared with the reference standard, cardiac magnetic resonance imaging. However, the relatively low temporal and spatial resolution and limited sector size remain barriers to the implementation of RT3DE in daily clinical practice.[3,4]

Ultrasound tissue characterization using videodensitometry or integrated backscatter detects ultrastructural changes in the hypertrophied left ventricle and is a marker of increased fibrosis, altered collagen architecture, and early myocardial dysfunction. LV hypertrophy in patients with hypertension is associated with reduced cyclic variation of integrated backscatter, and regression of LV mass with blockade of the renin-angiotensin system may normalize the abnormal ultrasonic backscatter parameters.[5,6]

LV hypertrophy is also accompanied by abnormal coronary flow reserve. Reduced coronary flow reserve in patients with hypertension may be detected using either transthoracic Doppler assessment of the left anterior descending (LAD) coronary or intramyocardial velocity before and after hyperemic stimulation with adenosine or dipyridamole.[7] Although LAD flow can be reliably obtained, high-frequency transducers (4–8 MHz) with dynamic pulse repetition frequency and adequate time-spatial resolution are needed to adequately visualize the intramyocardial arterioles.[8] However, the procedure is time consuming and requires expertise, and measurements are restricted to the LAD territory. Coronary flow reserve has also been measured with quantitative myocardial contrast echocardiography by analysis of microbubble refilling curves in an intramyocardial region of interest, but this technique has not found application in clinical practice.[9]

CARDIAC MECHANICS

LV systolic function as assessed by LV fractional shortening or ejection fraction is often normal or increased in patients with hypertension. However, these indices measure endocardial motion and therefore assess chamber mechanics, not myocardial mechanics. In contrast, LV midwall shortening,[10] which more accurately reflects sarcomeric shortening, is reduced in hypertensive hypertrophy and concentric remodeling (Table 145.3). Similarly, systolic annular tissue Doppler velocity (Sm) and deformational indices (i.e., strain, strain rate) are often reduced in patients with hypertension with normal or increased LV ejection fraction.[11,12]

Abnormalities of LV longitudinal systolic deformation are seen both in prehypertension and early in the course of hypertension, whereas circumferential and radial strains are similar to hearts of both athletes with physiological hypertrophy and control participants.[12–14] Reduced global area, longitudinal, and radial (but not circumferential) strains measured with RT3DE are reported in patients with hypertension and are independently correlated with

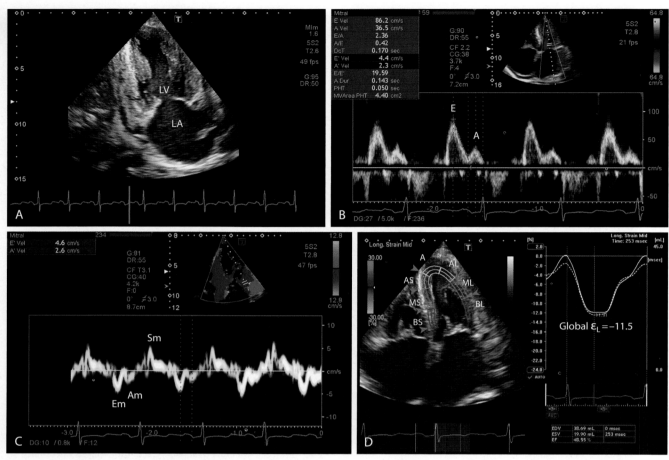

Figure 145.1. Echocardiography images of a patient with preserved systolic chamber function, left ventricular hypertrophy and pseudonormal filling, and reduced global longitudinal strain. **A,** Two-chamber view of the left atrium (LA) and left ventricle (LV). **B,** Transmitral Doppler early (E) and late diastolic (A) velocities. **C,** Lateral annular tissue velocities during early (Em) and late diastole (Am) and systole (Sm). **D,** Longitudinal strain (*solid line*, ε_L) derived from the four-chamber view. The *dashed line* represents the left ventricular volume–time curve. *A*, apical cap; *AL*, apical lateral; *AS*, apical septum; *BL*, basal anterolateral; *BS*, basal inferoseptum; *ML*, mid anterolateral; *MS*, mid inferoseptum.

TABLE 145.1 Echocardiographic Measures of Left Ventricular Size, Chamber Function, and Mass[a]

Modality	Index	Equation
M-mode	LV volume (prolate ellipse)	$\pi/3 \ (EDD)^3$
	LV volume (Teichholz)	$[7/(2.4 + EDD)]/(EDD)^3$
	LV fractional shortening	$(EDD - ESD)/EDD$
	LV midwall shortening	$(EDD + IVSd/2 + PWd/2) - (ESD + \text{inner shell})$, in which inner shell = $[(EDD + IVSd/2 + PWd/d)^3 - EDD^3 + ESD^3]^{1/3} - ESD$
	RWT	$(2 \times PWd)/EDD$
	LV mass	$0.8 \times \{[(EDD + IVSd + PWd)^3 - (EDD)^3]\} + 0.6$
2D	LV and LA volume	Biplane method of discs recommended; single-plane method of discs and area-length methods are alternatives
	LV stroke volume	$EDV - ESV$
	LV ejection fraction	$(EDV - ESV)/EDV$
	LV mass (area-length)	$1.05\{[5/6 \ A_1(a + t)] - [5/6 \ A_2(a)]\}$

[a]In which $b = \sqrt{A_2/\varpi}$, $t = \sqrt{A_1/\varpi} - b$, and A_1 and A_2 are the short axis end-diastolic and end-systolic areas, respectively.
EDD, Left ventricular end-diastolic dimension; *ESD*, left ventricular end-systolic dimension; *IVSd*, septal wall thickness in diastole; LV, left ventricular; *PWd*, posterior left ventricular wall thickness in diastole; *RWT*, relative wall thickness.

blood pressure and LV mass index.[15] However, rotational indices (twist, rotation, torsion) during systole remain normal or are increased in patients with hypertension with normal to increased LV ejection fraction and may represent a compensatory mechanism for the reduced longitudinal myocardial shortening associated with hypertension.[16] Although patients with hypertension with concentric hypertrophy and concentric remodeling have increased torsional dynamics, torsion is reduced in the more advanced stage characterized by eccentric hypertrophy.[17]

LV diastolic dysfunction, one of the earliest abnormalities of hypertensive heart disease, may occur in the absence of LV hypertrophy and may help risk stratify patients with hypertension. Doppler waveforms of transmitral and pulmonary venous flows coupled with mitral annular tissue Doppler during early diastole (E'; also referred to as Em), left atrial volume measurements, and tricuspid regurgitant velocity are commonly used to describe patterns of impaired relaxation, pseudonormal, and restrictive filling (grades I through III, respectively), reflecting abnormalities in the rate of LV relaxation, LV diastolic passive stiffness, and left atrial pressure.[18] However, these indices are load dependent, and because they measure phenomena after isovolumic LV relaxation (i.e., after mitral valve opening), they are influenced by left atrial pressure. In addition, tissue Doppler of mitral annular velocities assumes that a measurement at a single (or multiple) site accurately represents global LV relaxation. Importantly, the E/E' ratio predicted independently cardiovascular events in a hypertensive population without known cardiac disease.[19] Global strain rate during isovolumic relaxation (SR_{IVR}) correlates with hemodynamic indices of LV relaxation, and the ratio of transmitral E velocity to SR_{IVR} predicts LV filling pressures more accurately than the E/E' ratio.[20]

Deformational and torsional indices during diastole have also been described in patients with hypertension. The ratio of early to late diastolic longitudinal segmental strains and strain rates are reduced in symptomatic patients with hypertension (and indeed may predict symptomatic status) with diastolic dysfunction and are correlated with relative wall thickness and LV mass index.[21] A promising measure involves torsional dynamics during early diastole. Untwisting (or recoil) represents the release of restoring forces that develop during systole and provides an accurate estimate of LV isovolumic relaxation. The time to peak negative twist velocity is prolonged, and early diastolic untwisting and untwisting rate are reduced pari passu with increasing LV mass index.[17,22]

ARTERIAL DYNAMICS

Hypertension accelerates age-related arterial stiffness, an important predictor of cardiovascular morbidity and mortality. Arterial stiffening requires the LV to generate greater forces and, by ventricular–vascular coupling (i.e., the matching of LV ejection with the systemic vasculature), increases LV end-systolic stiffness and reduces contractile efficiency. Arterial stiffening results in an increase in the speed and magnitude of reflected waves, which amplifies late systolic aortic pressure (i.e., LV afterload); the pulse pressure widens and pulsatile shear increases, contributing to structural changes in the arteries, LV hypertrophy, diastolic dysfunction, subendocardial ischemia, and reduced cardiac reserve.

TABLE 145.2 Forms of Left Ventricular Hypertrophy

		Left Ventricular Mass	
		Normal: men ≤115 g/m² Women ≤95 g/m²	Increased: men >115 g/m² Women >95 g/m²
Relative wall thickness	Increased (≥0.42)	Concentric remodeling	Concentric hypertrophy
	Normal (<0.42)	Normal	Eccentric hypertrophy

TABLE 145.3 Echocardiographic Indices of Ventricular Mechanics in Patients With Hypertension

Modality	Indices	Directional change
SYSTOLIC FUNCTION		
M-mode, 2DE, RT3DE	LV dimension/volume; shortening/ejection fraction, LA volume	N or ↑
	Midwall fractional shortening	↓
Tissue Doppler imaging	Systolic annular velocity, Sm	↓
Strain imaging: deformation	ε_L	↓
	ε_C, ε_R	N or ↓
Strain imaging: torsional indices	Rotation, twist, torsion	N or ↑
DIASTOLIC FUNCTION		
Spectral Doppler	Diastolic transmitral flow, PV flow	Grade I: E/A <0.8, DT >200 ms, Ar-A <0
		Grade II: E/A 0.8–1.5, DT 160–200 ms, Ar-A ≥30 ms
		Grade III: E/A ≥2, DT <160 ms, Ar-A ≥30 ms
Tissue Doppler imaging	Early diastolic annular velocity, Em (also referred to as E')	↓
Strain imaging: deformation	Early/late diastolic strain	↓
	SR_E, SR_{IVR}	↓
Strain imaging: torsional indices	Untwist, untwist rate	↓
	Time to PNTV	↑
VENTRICULAR REMODELING		
M-mode, 2D, RT3DE	LV mass index, RWT, LA volume index	↑
Tissue characterization	IBS	↓
Coronary flow reserve	Color-flow Doppler	↓
	Quantitative MCE	↓

$\varepsilon\Lambda$, Longitudinal strain; εX, circumferential strain; εP, radial strain; *Ar-A*, pulmonary vein atrial systolic reverse wave duration-transmitral atrial systolic wave duration; *E/A*, early to late diastolic transmitral flow ratio; *IBS*, integrated backscatter; *MCE*, myocardial contrast echo; *PNTV*, peak negative twist velocity; *RWT*, regional wall thickness; *RT3DE*, real-time three-dimensional echocardiography; SR_E, strain rate during early diastole; SR_{IVR}, strain rate during isovolumic relaxation; *2D*, two-dimensional.

TABLE 145.4 Echocardiographic Indices of Arterial Dynamics in Patients With Hypertension

Modality	Indices	Directional Change
M-mode	Aortic strain (%)= 100 [(ASD – ADD)/ADD]	↓
	Aortic distensibility (cm²/g) = (2 × aortic strain)/PP	↓
2D, RT3DE	E_{ES} (mm Hg/mL) = ESP/ESV	↑
	E_A (mm Hg/mL) = ESP/SV	↑
	V-V coupling = E_A/E_{ES}	N or ↓
Tissue Doppler imaging	Ejection work density = Area of the pressure-strain loop	↓
	Peak aortic εP	↓
	Systolic expansion velocity	↓
	Early diastolic retraction velocity	↓

ADD, Aortic diastolic diameter; *ASD*, aortic systolic diameter; E_A, arterial elastance; E_{ES}, end-systolic elastance; *ESP*, end-systolic pressure (= systolic blood pressure × 0.9); *ESV*, end-systolic volume; *PP*, pulse pressure; *SV*, stroke volume; *V-V*, ventricular-vascular. Other abbreviations as in Table 145.2.

Echocardiographic assessment of arterial dynamics has been validated against and complements the techniques of pulsed wave velocity and analysis of augmented central pulse pressure using tonometry, arguably the gold standard methods used to measure arterial mechanics.

M-mode measurement of aortic diameters and tissue Doppler strain imaging (tissue velocity and radial strain) of the thoracic aorta have been used to analyze aortic stiffness (reduced velocity and strain denote increased stiffness), and 2D and 3D echocardiography have been used to analyze arterial elastance (a measure of the arterial input impedance) and ventricular–vascular coupling (Table 145.4).[23–27] Using these techniques, increased arterial stiffness and reduced aortic wall strain in patients with hypertension have been shown to be associated with LV hypertrophy, diastolic dysfunction, and increased pulse pressure. Progressive vascular stiffening in patients with hypertension measured with brachial-ankle pulse wave velocity is associated with impairment of speckle-tracking echocardiography–determined systolic (reduced global LV longitudinal strain) and diastolic (reduced early LV diastolic strain rate) myocardial function and attenuation of compensatory (i.e., increased) torsion.[28] M-mode echocardiography–determined arterial stiffness (aortic strain and distensibility) was shown to correlate well with pulsed-wave velocity and to be associated with resistant but not controlled hypertension.[29] 2D echocardiography coupled with radial artery applanation tonometry has been used to demonstrate changes in arterial elastance (Ea, end-systolic pressure/stroke volume), ventricular end-systolic elastance (Ees, end-systolic pressure/end-systolic volume), and ventricular–vascular coupling (Ea/Ees) after chronic antihypertensive therapy from a coupling ratio that maximized cardiac output to one that optimized mechanical work efficiency.[26] Finally, measurement of Ea, Ees, ventricular–vascular coupling, and systemic arterial compliance (stroke volume/pulse pressure) were shown to be feasible with RT3D echocardiography,[25] and these measurements (i.e., carotid tonometry and RT3DE) have recently been shown to be reproducible and sensitive to changes in LV elastance in patients with hypertension.[30]

REFERENCES

1. Chobanian AV, Bakris GL, Black HR, et al. The seventh report of the Joint National Committee on the Prevention, Detection, Evaluation, and Treatment of High Blood Pressure. *J Am Med Assoc*. 2003;289:2560–2572.
2. Lang RM, Badano LP, Mor-Avi V, et al. Recommendations for cardiac chamber quantification by echocardiography in adults. *J Am Soc Echocardiogr*. 2015;28:1–39.
3. Sugeng L, Mor-Avi V, Weinert L, et al. Quantitative assessment of left ventricular size and function: side-by-side comparison of real-time three-dimensional echocardiography and computed tomography with magnetic resonance reference. *Circulation*. 2006;114:654–661.
4. Mor-Avi V, Sugeng L, Weinert L, et al. Fast measurement of left ventricular mass with real-time three-dimensional echocardiography: comparison with magnetic resonance imaging. *Circulation*. 2004;110:1814.
5. Di Bello V, Giorgi D, Talini E, et al. Incremental value of ultrasonic tissue characterization (backscatter) in evaluation of left ventricular myocardial structure and mechanics in essential arterial hypertension. *Circulation*. 2003;107:74–80.
6. Ciulla MM, Paliotti R, Esposito A, et al. Different effects of antihypertensive therapies based on losartan and atenolol on ultrasound and biochemical markers of myocardial fibrosis. *Circulation*. 2004;110:552–557.
7. Galderisi M, de Simone G, Cicala S, et al. Coronary flow reserve in hypertensive patients with appropriate and inappropriate left ventricular mass. *J Hypertens*. 2003;21:1–6.
8. Youn HJ, Lee JM, Park CS, et al. The impaired flow reserve capacity of penetrating intramyocardial coronary arteries in apical hypertrophic cardiomyopathy. *J Am Soc Echocardiogr*. 2005;18:128–132.
9. Wei K, Jayaweera AR, Firoozan S, et al. Quantification of myocardial blood flow with ultrasound-induced destruction of microbubbles administered as a constant venous infusion. *Circulation*. 1998;97:473–483.
10. Shimizu G, Hirota Y, Kita Y, et al. Left ventricular midwall mechanics in systemic arterial hypertension. *Circulation*. 1991;83:1676–1684.
11. Narayanan A, Aurigemma GP, Chinali M, et al. Cardiac mechanics in mild hypertensive heart disease: a speckle-strain imaging study. *Circ Cardiovasc Imag*. 2009;2:382–390.
12. Di Bello V, Talini E, Dell'Omo G, et al. Early left ventricular mechanics abnormalities in prehypertension: a two-dimensional strain echocardiography study. *Am J Hypertens*. 2010;23:405–412.
13. Galderisi M, Lomoriello VS, Santoro A, et al. Differences of myocardial systolic deformation and correlates of diastolic function in competitive rowers and young hypertensives. *J Am Soc Echocardiogr*. 2010;23:1190–1198.
14. Kouzu H, Yuda S, Muranaka A, et al. Left ventricular hypertrophy causes different changes in longitudinal, radial, and circumferential mechanics in patients with hypertension. *J Am Soc Echocardiogr*. 2011;24:192–199.
15. Galderisi M, Esposito R, Schiano-Lomoriello V, et al. Correlates of global area strain in native hypertensive patients: a three-dimensional speckle-tracking echocardiography study. *Eur Heart J Cardiovasc Imag*. 2012;13:730–738.
16. Ahmed MI, Desai RV, Gaddam KK, et al. Relation of torsion and myocardial strains to LV ejection fraction in hypertension. *JACC Cardiovasc Imag*. 2012;5:273–2781.
17. Camelli M, Lisi M, Righini FM, et al. Left ventricular remodeling and torsion dynamics in hypertensive patients. *Int J Cardiovasc Imag*. 2013;29:79–86.
18. Nagueh SF, Smiseth OA, Appleton CP, et al. Recommendations for the evaluation of left ventricular diastolic function by echocardiography. *J Am Soc Echocardiogr*. 2016;29:277–314.
19. Sharp AS, Tapp RJ, Thom SA, et al. Tissue Doppler E/E' ratio is a powerful predictor of primary cardiac events in a hypertensive population. *Eur Heart J*. 2010;31:747–752.
20. Wang J, Khoury KS, Thohan V, et al. Global diastolic strain rate for the assessment of left ventricular relaxation and filling pressures. *Circulation*. 2007;115:1376–1383.
21. Pavlopoulos H, Nihoyannopoulos P. Abnormal segmental relaxation patterns in hypertensive disease and symptomatic diastolic dysfunction detected by strain echocardiography. *J Am Soc Echocardiogr*. 2008;21:899–906.
22. Takeuchi M, Borden WB, Nakai H, et al. Reduced and delayed untwisting of the left ventricle in patients with hypertension and left ventricular hypertrophy. *Eur Heart J*. 2007;28:2756–2762.
23. Eren M, Gorgulu S, Uslu N, et al. Relation between aortic stiffness and left ventricular diastolic function in patients with hypertension, diabetes, or both. *Heart*. 2004;90:37–43.
24. Vitarelli A, Giordano M, Germano G, et al. Assessment of ascending aorta wall stiffness in hypertensive patients by tissue Doppler imaging and strain Doppler echocardiography. *Heart*. 2010;96:1469–1474.
25. Scali MC, Basso M, Gandolfo A, et al. Real time 3D echocardiography for assessment of ventricular and vascular function in hypertensive and heart failure patients. *Cardiovasc Ultrasound*. 2012;10(27).
26. Osranek M, Eisenbach JH, Khandheria BK, et al. Arterioventricular coupling and ventricular efficiency after antihypertensive therapy. *Hypertension*. 2008;51:275–281.
27. Kuznetsova T, D'Hooge J, Kloch-Badelek M, et al. Impact of hypertension on ventricular-arterial coupling and regional myocardial work at rest and during isometric exercise. *J Am Soc Echocardiogr*. 2012;25:882–890.
28. Hwang J-W, Kang S-J, Lim H-S. Impact of arterial stiffness on regional myocardial function assessed by speckle tracking echocardiography in patients with hypertension. *J Cardiovasc Ultrasound*. 2012;20:90–96.
29. Pabuccu T, Baris N, Ozpelit E, et al. The relationship between resistant hypertension and arterial stiffness. *Clin Exp Hypertens*. 2012;34:57–62.
30. Bonnet B, Jourdan F, duCailar G, et al. Noninvasive evaluation of left ventricular elastance according to pressure-volume curves modeling in arterial hypertension. *Am J Physiol Heart Circ Physiol*. 2017;313:H237–H243.

146 Diabetes Mellitus

Peter A. Kahn, Julius M. Gardin

PATHOPHYSIOLOGY

Death and disability caused by cardiac dysfunction are among the most common complications of diabetes mellitus (DM).[1] DM can cause pathophysiologic changes in the heart both directly, through its effects on the myocardium (e.g., through deposition of advanced glycosylation products, reactive oxygen species, impaired calcium handling by cells), and secondarily through its effects on the coronary circulation and on the cardiac autonomic nerves, which can be affected along with other nerves as part of diabetic neuropathy.[2–4] In addition, DM can indirectly exacerbate these myocardial and coronary processes through its well-known association with lipid disorders and hypertension, often as part of the *metabolic syndrome,* the precise mechanisms of which are becoming increasingly known.[4] More directly, DM can produce and also exacerbates cardiac changes that accompany the aging process such as loss of cardiac myocytes with resultant swelling or hypertrophy in remaining myocytes, resulting in left ventricular (LV) remodeling, characterized by hypertrophy and increased wall thickness (concentric LV remodeling or hypertrophy).[5] Additionally, collagen deposition, an attempted repair mechanism, can cause further derangement of the myocardium, thereby further contributing to reduced LV function.

Metabolic disturbances that are characteristic of DM directly and indirectly result in myocyte loss, myocyte hypertrophy, collagen deposition, and fibrosis.[2,6] A DM-associated microangiopathy

also contributes to this decline in cardiac muscle function, or diabetic cardiomyopathy.[7] This microangiopathy is associated with endothelial changes and oxidative stress, accompanied by a depletion of endothelial progenitor cells. Despite these clear causative mechanisms, no precise definition in the echocardiographic literature is available for diabetic cardiomyopathy beyond cardiac dysfunction in the setting of diabetes.[3] Fig. 146.1 represents an attempt to put the pathophysiologic cardiovascular derangements related to DM in perspective. DM can predispose patients to a constellation of findings related to these pathophysiologic mechanisms, including ischemic heart disease, heart failure, and atrial fibrillation, all of which are detectible by echocardiography.[8]

TIME COURSE OF DIABETES MELLITUS: ANATOMIC AND ECHOCARDIOGRAPHIC OVERVIEW

Table 146.1 summarizes the progressive abnormalities of LV anatomy and systolic and diastolic function that occur during the early, intermediate, and late stages of diabetic cardiomyopathy.[2] In the early stages of DM, the cardiac tissue appears to be relatively normal without fibrosis or hypertrophy of the myocytes.[9] In the intermediate stage of DM, advanced glycosylation products, fibrosis, and hypertrophy of the myocytes all cause a decrease in LV relaxation, and possibly compliance, as well as

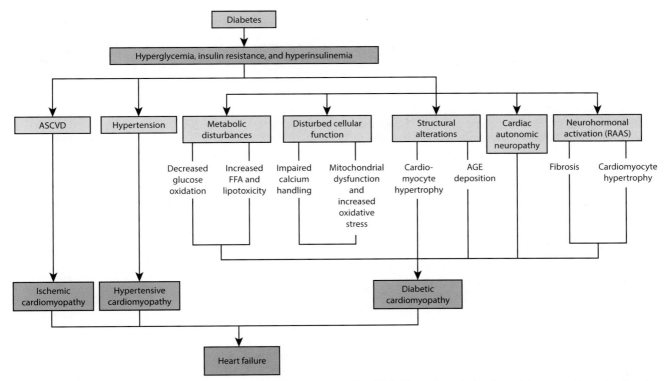

Figure 146.1. Pathophysiologic mechanisms of heart failure in diabetes mellitus (DM). Hyperglycemia, insulin resistance, and hyperinsulinemia, the main physiologic disturbances in DM, contribute to atherosclerotic cardiovascular disease (ASCVD), hypertension, and multiple derangements of cellular metabolism, function, and structure, as well as activation of the renin–angiotensin–aldosterone system (RAAS). The different cardiomyopathies that result from these processes clinically present as heart failure in DM. *AGE,* Advanced glycation end-product; *FFA,* free fatty acids. (Reproduced with permission from Low Wang CC, et al: Cardiovascular disease in diabetes mellitus: Atherosclerotic cardiovascular disease and heart failure in type 2 diabetes mellitus—Mechanisms, management, and clinical considerations, *Circulation* 133:2459–2502, 2016.)

TABLE 146.1 Diabetic Myocardial Disease: Echocardiography Doppler Findings

	Anatomic	Systolic Function	Diastolic Function
Early stage	Echocardiography • Normal LV dimensions, volumes, wall thickness, and mass	Echocardiography • Normal resting LVEF Strain • Decreased peak LV GLS (<−18%) and SR (≤0.90 sec⁻¹) TDI • Blunted rise in mitral annular S′ with supine bicycle exercise; possible decreased resting annular S′	Pulsed Doppler • Normal transmitral E, E/A, and IVRT Strain • Decreased peak global early diastolic SR (<1.0 sec⁻¹) and LA strain. TDI • Decreased mitral annular E′ and E′/A′ (<1.0) • Blunted rise in mitral annular E′ with supine bicycle exercise

Intermediate stage	Echocardiography
	• Possible increases in LV wall thickness (concentric), LV mass index, and LA volume index (>28 mL/m² BSA)
		Echocardiography
		• Normal resting LVEF
		• Blunted rise in LVEF with supine bicycle exercise
		• Increased global MPI (Tei index)
		Strain
		• As for early stage
		• TDI
		• As for early stage
			Pulsed or color M-mode Doppler
			• Grade 1 diastolic dysfunction
			  • Decreased E (<0.6 m/s), E/A (<1.0), Vₚ (<45 cm/s)
			  • Increased IVRT (>90 ms) and DT (>250 ms)
			• Possible grade 2 diastolic dysfunction
			  • Increased E/E′ (>15)
			  • Normal E, E/A, IVRT, Vₚ
			Strain
			• As for early stage
			TDI
			• As for early stage

Late stage	Echocardiography
	• LV concentric remodeling or LVH (concentric or eccentric)
	• Increased LV dimensions, volume index, and LV mass index
	• Increased LA volume index (>28 mL/m² BSA)
		Echocardiography
		• Possibly decreased LVEF
		Strain
		• As for early stage
		TDI
		• As for early stage
			Pulsed or color M-mode Doppler
			• Grade 2 diastolic dysfunction (as for intermediate stage)
			• Possible grade 3 diastolic dysfunction (if LVEF is decreased)
			  • Increased E and E/A (>1.0)
			  • Decreased IVRT (<60 m/s), DT (<150 ms), and Vₚ (<45 cm/s)
			Strain
			• As for early stage
			TDI
			• As for early stage

DT, Deceleration time; *E*, peak transmitral early diastolic filling velocity; *E/A*, E to peak transmitral late diastolic filling velocity; *E′′*, peak early diastolic annular tissue Doppler velocity; *E′/A′*, E′ to peak late diastolic annular tissue Doppler velocity; *GLS*, global longitudinal strain; *IVRT*, isovolumic relaxation time; *LV*, left ventricular; *LA*, left atrial; *LVEF*, left ventricular ejection fraction; *MPI*, myocardial performance index; *S′*, peak left ventricular systolic annular tissue Doppler velocity; *SR*, strain rate; *TDI*, tissue Doppler imaging; *Vₚ*, left ventricular inflow propagation rate.
Adapted with permission from Stoddard MF: Echocardiography in the evaluation of cardiac disease resulting from endocrinopathies, renal disease, obesity, and nutritional deficiencies. In Otto CM, editor. *The Practice of Clinical Echocardiography*. 4th ed. Philadelphia: Elsevier Saunders, 2012.

resting LV diastolic dysfunction.[9] In the later stage of DM, cardiac remodeling has occurred, leading to increased cardiac mass, concentric LV hypertrophy, increased volume, and decreased LV compliance.[2]

Echocardiographically, in the early stages of DM, although the heart may appear anatomically normal, changes reflecting mild systolic and diastolic dysfunction are apparent when examined via exercise tissue Doppler imaging (TDI) peak annular early diastolic (E′) and peak systolic (S′) mitral annular velocities and resting speckle-tracking echocardiography (STE) assessment of strain and strain rate (SR).[10–14] In the intermediate stage, early LV and left atrial anatomic changes, including a decrease in systolic function with exercise and abnormalities in resting diastolic function (grade 1 and possibly grade 2), become evident. In the late stages of DM, cardiac anatomic remodeling is evident and is accompanied by more advanced LV diastolic function and possible decreased resting LV ejection fraction (EF).[15] Studies with myocardial contrast echocardiography similarly demonstrate impairment of transmural myocardial blood flow reserve; however, these measurements reportedly did not correlate with function.[16]

Left Ventricular Systolic Function

The earliest manifestations of LV systolic dysfunction in DM (see Table 146.1) are generally decreases in peak global longitudinal strain (GLS) and strain rate (SR) as well as in peak LV S′ (with exercise and possibly at rest). Each of these measures may be reduced in DM before any traditional echocardiography measurements, including measures of LV diastolic dysfunction.[10,12,13,17,18] The advent of STE has afforded clinicians the ability to determine whether latent cardiac dysfunction is present using either exercise or dobutamine stress. This preclinical dysfunction can, through the use of STE, be assessed before more advanced diabetic cardiac dysfunction becomes apparent (Figs. 146.2 and 146.3).[10,12,18] It has been suggested that abnormal GLS and strain rate may precede abnormalities in circumferential strain and strain rate.[12] The decrease in longitudinal strain has also been reported to correlate with the duration of the DM.[17] As DM progresses to its later stages, there is a progression to reduced exercise-induced and, finally, resting LV EF.

Left Ventricular Diastolic Function

The earliest changes in diastolic function detected in DM (see Table 146.1) are decreases in exercise-induced mitral annular E′, E′/A′ ratio, and peak global early diastolic strain rate.[11] Grade 1 diastolic dysfunction is characterized by delayed relaxation of the myocardium, that is, an increased isovolumic relaxation time (IVRT), accompanied by decreased peak transmitral E wave velocity and a reduced E/A ratio.[2] Left atrial strain has also been shown to be decreased in patients with DM compared with control patients and

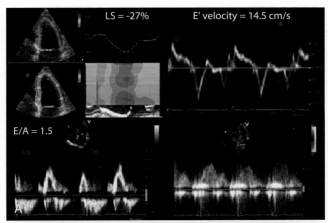

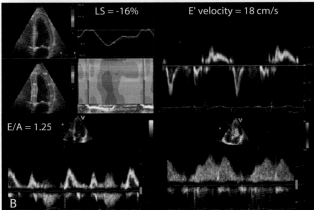

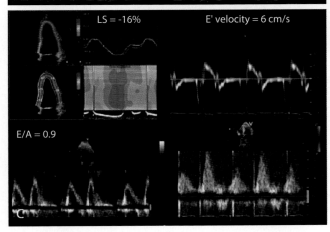

Figure 146.2. Examples of longitudinal systolic strain and diastolic functional assessment in three male patients with diabetes mellitus with normal longitudinal systolic and diastolic function (**A**), longitudinal systolic dysfunction and normal diastolic function (**B**), and longitudinal systolic dysfunction and grade II diastolic dysfunction (**C**). In each panel, the *upper left corner* shows strain imaging, *upper right corner* shows mitral annular tissue Doppler, *lower left corner* shows mitral blood inflow spectral Doppler, and *lower right corner* shows pulmonary venous spectral Doppler. *LS,* Longitudinal strain. (Reproduced with permission from Ernande L, et al: Diastolic dysfunction in patients with type 2 diabetes mellitus: Is it really the first marker of diabetic cardiomyopathy? *J Am Soc Echocardiogr* 24:1268–1275, 2011.)

represents another marker in the diagnosis of subclinical DM as well as the determination of disease progression (Fig. 146.3).[18]

TWIST AND TORSION AS MEASURES OF CARDIAC FUNCTION IN DIABETES

Work in the field of STE has suggested potential utility in evaluating twist and torsion as measures of disease progression in DM.[19–21] Reduced twist and untwisting have been previously identified as a consequence of LV hypertrophy, which is seen in the intermediate to later stages of DM.[22] Peak LV torsion measured by echocardiography has been reported to be significantly greater in patients with mild LV diastolic dysfunction ($n = 45$; 29.7 degrees $\pm$ 9.0 degrees) compared with control participants ($n = 32$; 15.6 degrees $\pm$ 4.0 degrees), with normalization in moderate ($n = 49$; 19.3 degrees $\pm$ 4.8 degrees) and severe diastolic dysfunction (n = 22; 17.3 degrees $\pm$ 9.3 degrees).[23]

RIGHT VENTRICULAR FUNCTION

DM is associated with subclinical right ventricular (RV) systolic and diastolic dysfunction—including reduced peak systolic strain rate and peak early diastolic strain rate—in the basal and apical segments of the RV free wall.[24] Three-dimensional echocardiography has also demonstrated that RV and right atrial myocardial deformation and function are all reduced in patients with DM.[25] Furthermore, patients with DM present with impaired diastolic function, and particularly impaired relaxation, in both ventricles before the development of systolic dysfunction.[14] These changes in RV function have been attributed to the effects of DM on myocardial function in addition to ventricular interdependence.

Aortic Valve and Aortic Elasticity

In addition to the anatomic changes noted, DM is a risk factor for aortic stenosis (AS). In patients with moderate calcific AS over a 2.5-year follow-up period, a greater mean decrease in aortic valve area in patients with DM (0.25 cm^2/year) compared with individuals without DM (0.14 cm^2/year, P = .0016) has been reported.[26] In patients with AS, DM exacerbates hypertrophic remodeling produced by pressure overload, resulting in increased LV mass and larger cavity dimensions along with reduced systolic strain.[27] Furthermore, the elasticity of the aorta may be diminished and stiffness increased in DM, serving to diminish perfusion.[28]

PREDICTORS OF TREATMENT SUCCESS AND MORTALITY

Although DM therapy and outcomes are best judged using traditional endocrinology benchmarks such as hemoglobin A1c values, echocardiography can be an important tool in the assessment of disease progression and the cardiovascular effects of therapy in DM. Various DM treatment strategies have been evaluated using echocardiography. For example, metformin, rosiglitazone, canagliflozin, and empagliflozin all have been demonstrated to have positive effects on cardiac remodeling through various mechanisms, such as improved microcirculation, improved LV relaxation, and reductions in epicardial fat.[29–32] Additionally, stress echocardiography has been demonstrated to be predictive of mortality in patients with DM and represents an important evaluative and potentially prognostic tool.[33]

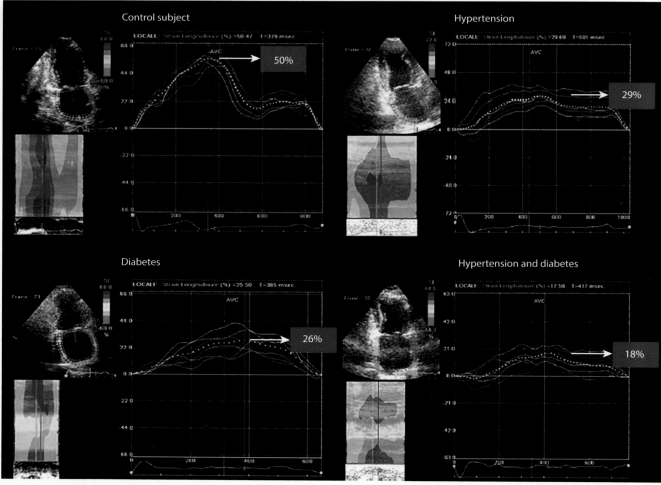

Figure 146.3. Left atrial strain curves obtained from the apical four-chamber view in four patients representative of the study groups (Reproduced with permission Mondillo S, et al: Early detection of left atrial strain abnormalities by speckle-tracking in hypertensive and diabetic patients with normal left atrial size, *J Am Soc Echocardiogr* 24:898–908, 2011.)

REFERENCES

1. Kengne AP, Turnbull F, MacMahon S. The Framingham Study, diabetes mellitus and cardiovascular disease: turning back the clock. *Progress Cardiovasc Diseases.* 2010;53:45–51.
2. Fang ZY, Prins JB, Marwick TH. Diabetic cardiomyopathy: evidence, mechanisms, and therapeutic implications. *Endocr Rev.* 2004;25:543–567.
3. Lee MMY, McMurray JJV, Lorenzo-Almoros A, et al. Diabetic cardiomyopathy. *Heart.* 2019;105:337–345.
4. Low Wang CC, Hess CN, Hiatt WR, Goldfine AB. Cardiovascular disease in diabetes mellitus: atherosclerotic cardiovascular disease and heart failure in type 2 diabetes mellitus—mechanisms, management, and clinical considerations. *Circulation.* 2016;133:2459–2502.
5. Regan TJ, Lyons MM, Ahmed SS, et al. Evidence for cardiomyopathy in familial diabetes mellitus. *J Clin Invest.* 1977;60:884–899.
6. Diamant M, Lamb HJ, Groeneveld Y, et al. Diastolic dysfunction is associated with altered myocardial metabolism in asymptomatic normotensive patients with well-controlled type 2 diabetes mellitus. *J Am Coll Cardiol.* 2003;42:328–335.
7. Zhao C, Wang M, Siu C, et al. Myocardial dysfunction in patients with type 2 diabetes mellitus: role of endothelial progenitor cells and oxidative stress. *Cardiovasc Diabetol.* 2012;11:147.
8. Wang Y, Marwick TH. Update on echocardiographic assessment in diabetes mellitus. *Curr Cardiol Rep.* 2016;18:85.
9. van Heerebeek L, Hamdani N, Handoko ML, et al. Diastolic stiffness of the failing diabetic heart: importance of fibrosis, advanced glycation end products, and myocyte resting tension. *Circulation.* 2008;117:43–51.
10. Ernande L, Rietzschel ER, Bergerot C, et al. Impaired myocardial radial function in asymptomatic patients with type 2 diabetes mellitus: a speckle-tracking imaging study. *J Am Soc Echocardiogr.* 2010;23:1266–1272.
11. Ha JW, Lee HC, Kang ES, et al. Abnormal left ventricular longitudinal functional reserve in patients with diabetes mellitus: implication for detecting subclinical myocardial dysfunction using exercise tissue Doppler echocardiography. *Heart.* 2007;93:1571–1576.
12. Ng AC, Delgado V, Bertini M, et al. Findings from left ventricular strain and strain rate imaging in asymptomatic patients with type 2 diabetes mellitus. *Am J Cardiol.* 2009;104:1398–1401.
13. Ernande L, Bergerot C, Rietzschel ER, et al. Diastolic dysfunction in patients with type 2 diabetes mellitus: is it really the first marker of diabetic cardiomyopathy? *J Am Soc Echocardiogr.* 2011;24:1268–1275.
14. Karamitsos TD, Karvounis HI, Dalamanga EG, et al. Early diastolic impairment of diabetic heart: the significance of right ventricle. *Int J Cardiol.* 2007;114:218–223.
15. Marwick TH. Diabetic heart disease. *Heart.* 2006;92:296–300.
16. Moir S, Hanekom L, Fang ZY, et al. Relationship between myocardial perfusion and dysfunction in diabetic cardiomyopathy: a study of quantitative contrast echocardiography and strain rate imaging. *Heart.* 2006;92:1414–1419.
17. Nakai H, Takeuchi M, Nishikage T, et al. Subclinical left ventricular dysfunction in asymptomatic diabetic patients assessed by two-dimensional speckle tracking echocardiography: Correlation with diabetic duration. *Eur J Echocardiogr.* 2009;10:926–932.
18. Mondillo S, Cameli M, Caputo ML, et al. Early detection of left atrial strain abnormalities by speckle-tracking in hypertensive and diabetic patients with normal left atrial size. *J Am Soc Echocardiogr.* 2011;24:898–908.
19. Tan YT, Wenzelburger F, Lee E, et al. The pathophysiology of heart failure with normal ejection fraction: exercise echocardiography reveals complex abnormalities of both systolic and diastolic ventricular function involving torsion, untwist, and longitudinal motion. *J Am Coll Cardiol.* 2009;54:36–46.
20. Geyer H, Caracciolo G, Abe H, et al. Assessment of myocardial mechanics using speckle tracking echocardiography: fundamentals and clinical applications. *J Am Soc Echocardiogr.* 2010;23:351–369; quiz 453–355.
21. Enomoto M, Ishizu T, Seo Y, et al. Myocardial dysfunction identified by three-dimensional speckle tracking echocardiography in type 2 diabetes patients relates to complications of microangiopathy. *J Cardiol.* 2016;68:282–287.
22. Takeuchi M, Borden WB, Nakai H, et al. Reduced and delayed untwisting of the left ventricle in patients with hypertension and left ventricular hypertrophy: a study using two-dimensional speckle tracking imaging. *Eur Heart J.* 2007;28:2756–2762.

23. Park SJ, Miyazaki C, Bruce CJ, et al. Left ventricular torsion by two-dimensional speckle tracking echocardiography in patients with diastolic dysfunction and normal ejection fraction. *J Am Soc Echocardiogr.* 2008;21:1129–1137.

24. Kosmala W, Przewlocka-Kosmala M, Mazurek W. Subclinical right ventricular dysfunction in diabetes mellitus—an ultrasonic strain/strain rate study. *Diabet Med.* 2007;24:656–663.

25. Tadic M, Celic V, Cuspidi C, et al. Right heart mechanics in untreated normotensive patients with prediabetes and type 2 diabetes mellitus: a two- and three-dimensional echocardiographic study. *J Am Soc Echocardiogr.* 2015;28:317–327.

26. Kamalesh M, Ng C, El Masry H, et al. Does diabetes accelerate progression of calcific aortic stenosis? *Eur J Echocardiogr.* 2009;10:723–725.

27. Lindman BR, Arnold SV, Madrazo JA, et al. The adverse impact of diabetes mellitus on left ventricular remodeling and function in patients with severe aortic stenosis. *Circ Heart Fail.* 2011;4:286–292.

28. Seyfeli E, Duru M, Saglam H, et al. Association of left ventricular diastolic function abnormalities with aortic elastic properties in asymptomatic patients with

type 2 diabetes mellitus: a tissue Doppler echocardiographic study. *Int J Clin Pract.* 2008;62:1358–1365.

29. Fitchett D, Zinman B, Wanner C, et al. Heart failure outcomes with empagliflozin in patients with type 2 diabetes at high cardiovascular risk: results of the EMPA-REG OUTCOME(R) trial. *Eur Heart J.* 2016;37:1526–1534.

30. Andersson C, Sogaard P, Hoffmann S, et al. Metformin is associated with improved left ventricular diastolic function measured by tissue Doppler imaging in patients with diabetes. *Eur J Endocrinol.* 2010;163:593–599.

31. Pala S, Esen O, Akcakoyun M, et al. Rosiglitazone, but not pioglitazone, improves myocardial systolic function in type 2 diabetic patients: a tissue Doppler study. *Echocardiography.* 2010;27:512–518.

32. Matsutani D, Sakamoto M, Kayama Y, et al. Effect of canagliflozin on left ventricular diastolic function in patients with type 2 diabetes. *Cardiovasc Diabetol.* 2018;17:73.

33. Cortigiani L, Borelli L, Raciti M, et al. Prediction of mortality by stress echocardiography in 2835 diabetic and 11 305 nondiabetic patients. *Circulation Cardiovasc Imag.* 2015;8(5).

147 End-Stage Renal Disease

Mark Goldberger

EPIDEMIOLOGY

Chronic renal disease is a major public health problem. The end-stage renal disease (ESRD) population is increasing in size. More than 26 million people (13%) in the United States have chronic kidney disease (CKD), and most are undiagnosed. Another 20 million are at increased risk of the disease. Cardiovascular disease is the leading cause of death in patients with ESRD. Cardiovascular mortality is 5 to 30 times higher in dialysis patients than in individuals from the general population who are the same age, sex, and race. The total annual cost of treating ESRD in the United States was $26.8 billion in 2008. Patients with chronic renal failure (CRF) have significant cardiovascular morbidities, including hypertension, left ventricular hypertension (LVH), congestive heart failure (CHF), calcification, and pericarditis. These conditions can be readily assessed and evaluated by echocardiography[1] (Tables 147.1 and 147.2).

Hypertension and Left Ventricular Hypertension

Hypertension is prevalent in patients with CRF, reaching up to 90% in some published series. LVH is also a common finding among patients with CRF. LVH has a prevalence of approximately 32% in patients with chronic renal insufficiency and rises to approximately 75% at the time of initiation of dialysis therapy.[2]

Major risk factors for the development of LVH include hypertension, increasing age, anemia, and chronic volume overload. Left atrial dilatation is increasingly recognized as an adverse prognostic factor in CKD patients. The cause of left atrial dilatation in patients with CRF is multifactorial; these patients have diastolic dysfunction (which occurs in approximately 75% of those with stages 3–5 CKD), volume overload, and inflammation as causes.[3]

Kidney transplantation has been shown to cause regression of LVH. In one study, 24 patients followed for 1 year after transplantation with serial echocardiograms had a reduction from 75% to 52.1% in the incidence of LVH[4] (Fig. 147.1).

Congestive Heart Failure

The incidence of CHF increases with declining renal function. The diagnosis of CHF in CKD patients is challenging because volume-overloaded patients with CKD can have clinical signs, such as effort intolerance, fatigue, and edema. These signs are also present in non-CKD patients with CHF. Thus, echocardiography plays a key role in the evaluation of these patients because LVH, diastolic and systolic dysfunction, and valvular and pericardial disease can be readily assessed using echocardiography. LV diastolic function is a frequent finding in patients with CKD. Diastolic dysfunction is associated with the development of CHF and increased mortality. Myocardial fibrosis is one of the causes of the development of diastolic dysfunction. Patients with CKD are exposed to several factors that help facilitate the development of CHF. Volume overload is related to excess fluid accumulation because of reduced renal function. Pressure overload develops because of hypertension and vascular stiffness. The heart is subjected to increased LV wall stress from these factors. The myocardium is exposed to various factors that lead to dysfunction and subsequent cardiac abnormalities. Hemodialysis can result in progressive LV systolic dysfunction.[5]

Patients with CKD develop CHF and other cardiovascular disorders because of the cardiorenal syndrome. Cardiorenal syndromes are disorders of the heart and kidneys, in which acute or chronic dysfunction in one organ may induce acute or chronic dysfunction in the other[6] (Fig. 147.2 and Box 147.1).

Valvular Heart Disease

Valvular heart disease is very common in patients with common renal disease. Based on epidemiologic data, it is estimated that mitral annular calcification is present in 10% to 50% of patients undergoing dialysis, and 25% to 60% of dialysis patients have aortic calcification. Aortic valve calcification in dialysis patients occurs 10 to 20 years earlier in patients with ESRD compared with the general population.[7]

Aortic stenosis (AS) is the most common valvular stenosis in these patients. AS progresses faster, with an estimated incidence of 3.3% per year. The current Kidney Disease Improving Global Outcomes guidelines recommend yearly echocardiograms for renal patients with AS. Regurgitant lesions are also quite common. In one study, 40% of dialysis patients had moderate or severe mitral regurgitation, and 18% had moderate to severe tricuspid regurgitation. Aortic regurgitation occurred less frequently; only 4% of the study patients had moderate aortic regurgitation.[8]

The degree of valvular regurgitation is influenced by many factors, including the volume status of the patient. A study of 21 patients on

TABLE 147.1 Types of Cardiac Disease in Chronic Kidney Disease

CVD Type	Pathologic or Structural Manifestation	Risk Factors	Indicators or Diagnostic Tests	Clinical Sequelae
Arterial disease	Atherosclerosis: Luminal narrowing of arteries because of plaques	Dyslipidemia Diabetes mellitus Hypertension Other traditional and nontraditional risk factors	Inducible ischemia on nuclear imaging Cardiac catheterization	Myocardial infarction Angina Sudden cardiac death Heart failure
	Arteriosclerosis: Diffuse dilatation and wall hypertrophy of larger arteries with loss of arterial elasticity	Hypertension Volume overload Hyperparathyroidism Hyperphosphatemia Other factors predisposing to medial calcification	Vascular calcification Increased pulse pressure Aortic pulse-wave velocity Cardiac computed tomography Other arterial imaging	Myocardial infarction Angina Sudden cardiac death Heart failure LVH
Cardiomyopathy	LVH: adaptive hypertrophy to compensate for increased cardiac demand	Pressure overload Increased afterload because of hypertension, valvular disease, and arteriosclerosis Volume overload Volume retention because of progressive kidney disease ± anemia	Echocardiography CMRI	Myocardial infarction Angina Sudden cardiac death Heart failure
	Decreased LV contractility	Ischemic heart disease Hypertension LVH Other traditional and nontraditional risk factors	Echocardiography	Cardiorenal syndrome Sudden cardiac death Heart failure Myocardial infarction Angina
	Impaired LV relaxation	Hypertension Anemia and volume overload Abnormal mineral metabolism Other arteriosclerosis risk factors Other traditional and nontraditional risk factors	Echocardiography	Heart failure Myocardial infarction Angina Sudden cardiac death
Structural disease	Pericardial effusion	Delayed or insufficient dialysis	Echocardiography	Heart failure Hypotension
	Aortic and mitral valve disease	CKD stages 3–5 Abnormal calcium, phosphate, and PTH metabolism Aging Dialysis vintage	Echocardiography	Aortic stenosis Endocarditis Heart failure
	Mitral annular calcification	CKD stages 3–5 Abnormal calcium, phosphate, and PTH metabolism	Echocardiography Uniform echodense rigid band located near the base of the posterior mitral leaflet	Arrhythmia Embolism Endocarditis Heart failure
	Endocarditis	Valvular disease Chronic venous catheters	Echocardiography	Arrhythmia Heart failure Embolism
Arrhythmia	Atrial fibrillation	Ischemic heart disease Cardiomyopathy	Electrocardiography	Hypotension Embolism
	Ventricular arrhythmia	Ischemic heart disease Cardiomyopathy Electrolyte abnormalities	Electrocardiography Electrophysiology study	Sudden cardiac death

CKD, Chronic kidney disease; *CMRI,* cardiovascular magnetic resonance imaging; *CVD,* cardiovascular disease; *LV,* left ventricular; *LVH,* left ventricular hypertension; *PTH,* parathyroid hormone.
From Gilbert S, Weiner DE: Cardiac function and cardiovascular disease in chronic kidney disease. In *National Kidney Foundation Primer on Kidney Disease.* 6th ed. St Louis: Saunders; 2013:491.

dialysis assessed the effects of aggressive ultrafiltration on the severity of valvular regurgitations. In that cohort, 13 patients had no mitral regurgitation, and 14 patients had no detectible tricuspid regurgitation. The degree of regurgitation decreased in the remaining patients.[9]

Infectious endocarditis is also a known complication in dialysis patients.

Pericarditis

Renal failure is associated with pericardial effusions, pericarditis, and (rarely) chronic constrictive pericarditis. Up to 20% of patients with renal failure can develop pericardial disease. Echocardiography is the test of choice to diagnose pericardial effusions. There are two major types of CRF-related pericardial disease.

Uremic pericarditis occurs in 6% to 10% of patients with renal failure before dialysis begins or afterward. The cause is inflammation of the pericardium, which is correlated with the degree of azotemia. Dialysis-associated pericarditis has been reported in up to 13% of patients who are on maintenance dialysis. The causes of dialysis-associated pericarditis include inadequate dialysis and fluid overload. Treatment includes intensive hemodialysis. Serial echocardiograms are recommended to follow-up on the size of the effusion[10] (Fig. 147.3).

Pulmonary Hypertension

Pulmonary hypertension is being recognized and diagnosed with increasingly frequency in patients with CKD. Causes include

TABLE 147.2 Echocardiographic Findings in Chronic Kidney Disease

Valvular Disease	Structural Abnormalities	Diastolic Dysfunction	Systolic Dysfunction
Conventional M-mode, 2D, and Doppler echocardiography	Conventional M-mode, 2D, and Doppler echocardiography	Strain or tissue Doppler imaging	Strain imaging
Aortic valve calcification (in 28%–60% with ESRD)	Concentric LV hypertrophy	↓Global and mid (< 1.2 sec) LV peak early diastolic SR	↓Global (<−15%) and regional LV longitudinal strain
Mitral annular calcification (in 10%–36% on hemodialysis)	Eccentric LV hypertrophy	↑Regional Tei index	
	Asymmetric LV hypertrophy		↓Peak global (<0.7 s) and regional LV SR
Aortic regurgitation (in 13% with CKD)	LV hypertrophy (in 70% with ESRD; in 34%–78% with CKD)		
Mitral regurgitation (in 38% with CKD)	LV hypertrophy—2.5×–4× more common in women than men		
Aortic and mitral stenosis	LA enlargement		
Tricuspid and pulmonic insufficiency (secondary to pulmonary hypertension as opposed to calcification)	LV enlargement		
	Dilated cardiomyopathy (associated with secondary hyperparathyroidism)		
	Ultrasonic integrated backscatter	Conventional Doppler echocardiography	Conventional 2D echocardiography
	↑Myocardial acoustic reflectivity	Grade 1 diastolic dysfunction:	↓LVEF (in 33% of new dialysis patients)
		↓E (<0.6 m/s)	Global or regional myocardial stunning with hemodialysis
		↓E/A ratio (< 1.0)	
		↑IVRT (>90 ms)	
		Grade 2 (pseudonormal) and grade 3 (restrictive) diastolic dysfunction occur	

2D, Two-dimensional; *CKD*, chronic kidney disease; *ESRD*, end-stage renal disease; *IVRT*, isovolumic resting time; *LA*, left atrial; *LV*, left ventricular; *LVEF*, left ventricular ejection fraction; *SR*, strain rate.
From Stoddard MF: Echocardiography in the evaluation of cardiac disease resulting from endocrinopathies, renal disease, obesity, and nutritional deficiencies. In Otto CM, editor. *The Practice of Clinical Echocardiography*. 4th ed., Philadelphia: Saunders; 2012:746.

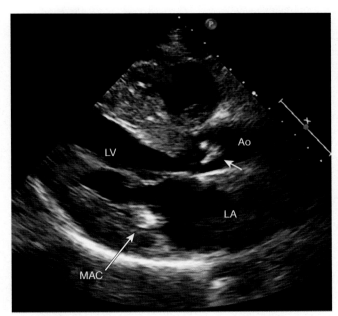

Figure 147.1. Hypertensive heart disease. *Ao,* Aorta; *LA,* left atrium; *LV,* left ventricle; *MAC,* mitral annular calcification (From Otto C: Cardiomyopathies, hypertensive and pulmonary heart disease. In Otto CM, editor. *Textbook of Clinical Echocardiography*. 5th ed, St. Louis: Saunders; 2013:245.)

hypertension, chronic fluid overload, myocardial stiffness, and placement and utilization of arteriovenous fistulas. The prevalence of pulmonary hypertension ranges from 9% to 39% in individuals with stage 5 CKD, 18% to 69% in hemodialysis patients, and 0% to 42% in patients on peritoneal dialysis (PD) therapy.[11] The diagnosis of pulmonary hypertension using echocardiography is discussed in other chapters of this book.

Mobile Calcific Calcinosis of the Heart

Calcinosis is a known complication of ESRD. The heart is subjected to abnormal calcification in ESRD, including extensive calcification of the valves and the mitral valve annulus. Arterial calcification is another cardiac manifestation of ESRD. Mobile cardiac calcinosis has been identified by echocardiography as another cardiac syndrome associated with ESRD. Calcinosis has been associated with strokes and peripheral emboli[12] (Fig. 147.4).

GUIDELINES
Kidney Disease Outcomes Quality Initiative Clinical Practice Guidelines for Cardiovascular Disease in Dialysis Patients

The Kidney Disease Outcomes Quality Initiative[13] provides the following guidelines:

1. Echocardiograms should be performed in all patients at the initiation of dialysis, when patients have achieved dry weight, ideally within 1–3 months of dialysis initiation (A), and at 3-yearly intervals thereafter (B).
2. Special considerations for echocardiographic evaluation in dialysis patients:
   a. Dry weight optimization should be achieved before testing to enhance the interpretation of results (B).
   b. The interpretation of repeat echocardiographic evaluations should be done with consideration of the relationship between the echocardiographic examination and either the hemodialysis treatment or the presence or absence of PD fluid in the peritoneal cavity (B).
3. Asymptomatic dialysis patients on the transplantation waitlist with moderate or more severe AS (aortic valve area ≤1 cm²) should have annual Doppler echocardiograms (because AS progresses faster in dialysis patients than that in the general population) (C).

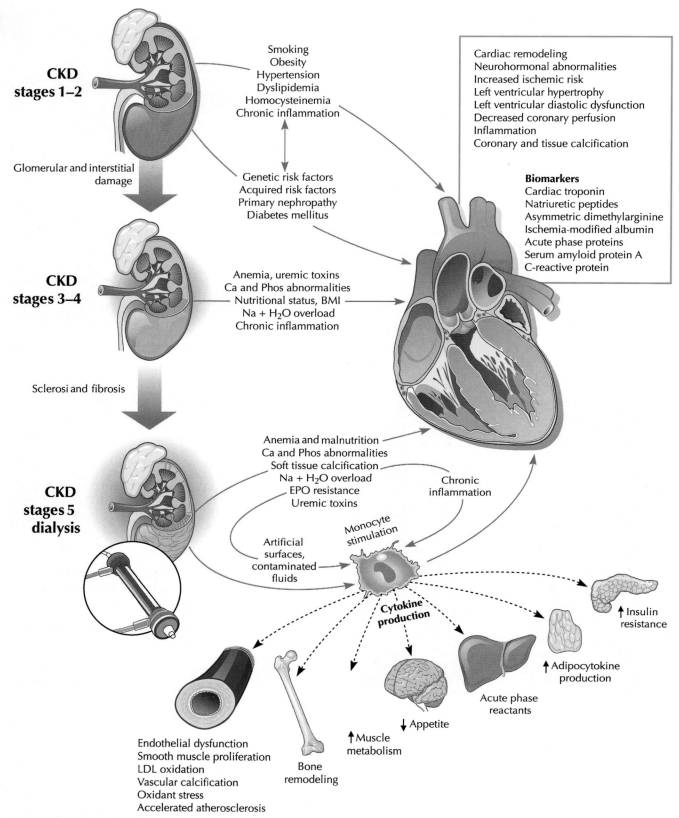

Figure 147.2. The cardiorenal syndrome. *BMI,* Body mass index; *Ca,* calcium; *CKD,* chronic kidney disease; *EPO,* erythropoietin; *H₂O,* water; *LDL,* low-density lipoprotein; *Na,* sodium; *Phos,* phosphorus (From Ronco C, et al: Cardiorenal syndrome, *J Am Coll Cardiol* 19:1527–1539, 2008.)

4. Newly or increasingly symptomatic (e.g., displaying dyspnea, angina, fatigue, and unstable intradialytic hemodynamics) patients with valvular heart disease should be reevaluated by echocardiography.
5. Dialysis patients should be evaluated for the presence of cardio-myopathy in the same manner as the general population, using echocardiographic testing (C).

BOX 147.1 Definition and Classification of the Cardiorenal Syndromes

CHRONIC CARDIORENAL SYNDROME (TYPE 2)

Chronic abnormalities in cardiac function leading to renal dysfunction

ACUTE RENOCARDIAC SYNDROME (TYPE 3)

Acute worsening of renal function causing cardiac dysfunction

CHRONIC RENOCARDIAC SYNDROME (TYPE 4)

Chronic abnormalities in renal function leading to cardiac disease

SECONDARY CARDIORENAL SYNDROMES (TYPE 5)

Systemic conditions causing simultaneous dysfunction of the heart and kidney

From Ronco C, et al: Cardiorenal syndrome, *J Am Coll Cardiol* 19:1527–1539, 2008.)

2012 Kidney Disease: Improving Global Outcomes Clinical Practice Guideline for the Evaluation and Management of Chronic Kidney Disease

These guidelines include the following[14]:

1. We recommend that all patients with CKD be considered at increased risk for cardiovascular disease (1A).
2. We suggest that clinicians be familiar with the limitations of noninvasive cardiac tests in adults and interpret the results accordingly.

Cardiac Disease and Evaluation and Management among Kidney and Liver Transplantation Candidates

These guidelines include the following[15]:

1. Noninvasive stress testing may be considered in kidney trans-plantation candidates with no active cardiac conditions based on the presence of multiple coronary artery disease risk factors, regardless of functional status. Relevant risk factors among transplantation candidates include diabetes mellitus, previous cardiovascular disease, more than 1 year on dialysis, left ven-tricular hypertrophy, age older than 60 years, smoking, hyper-tension, and dyslipidemia. The specific number of risk factors that should be used to prompt testing remains to be determined, but the committee considers three or more as reasonable (class IIb; level of evidence: C).

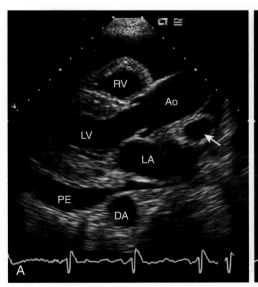
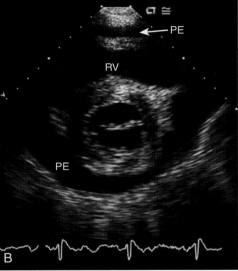

Figure 147.3. Pericardial effusion on echocardiography. *A,* parasternal long-axis view; *B,* short-axis view. *Ao,* Aorta; *DA,* descending aorta; *LA,* left atrium; *LV,* left ventricle; *PE,* pulmonary embolism; *RV,* right ventricle (From Otto C: Pericardial disease. In Otto CM, ed. *Textbook of Clinical Echocardiography.* 5th ed. St Louis: Saunders; 2013:256.)

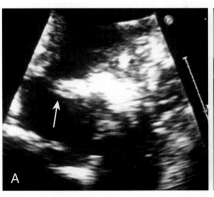
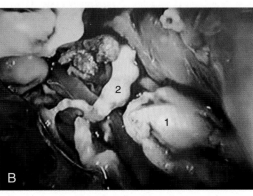

Figure 147.4. A and **B,** Mobile cardiac calcific calcinosis *(arrow)* (Modified from Kubota H, et al: Cardiac swinging calcified amorphous tumors (1 and 2) in end-stage renal disease patients, *Ann Thorac Surg* 90:1692–1694, 2010.)

2. It is reasonable to perform preoperative assessment of left ventricular function followed by echocardiography in potential kidney transplantation candidates (class IIa, level of evidence: B). There is no evidence for or against surveillance by repeated left ventricular function tests after listing for cardiac transplantation.

REFERENCES

1. Go AS, Mozaffarian D, Roger VL, et al. Heart disease and stroke statistics—2014 update: a report from the American Heart Association. *Circulation.* 2014;129:e28–e292.
2. Park M, Hsu CY, Li Y, et al. Associations between kidney function and subclinical cardiac abnormalities in CKD. *J Am Soc Nephrol.* 2012;23:1725–1734.
3. Paoletti E, Zoccali C. A look at the upper heart chamber: the left atrium in chronic kidney disease. *Nephrol Dial Transplant.* 2013.
4. Ferreira SR, Moises VA, Tavares A, et al. Cardiovascular effects of successful renal transplantation: a 1-year sequential study of left ventricular morphology and function, and 24-hour blood pressure profile. *Transplantation.* 2002;74:1580–1587.
5. Herzog CA, Asinger RW, Berger AK, et al. Cardiovascular disease in chronic kidney disease. A clinical update disease in chronic kidney disease. (KDIGO). *Kidney Int.* 2011;80(6):572–586.
6. Ronco C, Haapio M, House AA, et al. Cardiorenal syndrome. *J Am Coll Cardiol.* 2008;19:1527–1539.
7. London GM, Pannier B, Marchais SJ, et al. Calcification of the aortic valve in the dialyzed patient. *J Am Soc Nephrol.* 2000;11:778–783.
8. Stinebaugh J, Lavie CJ, Milani RV, et al. Doppler echocardiographic assessment of valvular heart disease in patients requiring hemodialysis for end-stage renal disease. *South Med J.* 1995;88:65–71.
9. Cirit M, Ozkahya M, Cinar CS, et al. Disappearance of mitral and tricuspid regurgitation in hemodialysis patients after ultrafiltration. *Nephrol Dial Transplant.* 1998;12:389–392.
10. Maisch B, Sererovic PM, Ristic AD, et al. Guidelines on the diagnosis and management of pericardial diseases executive summary. *Eur Heart J.* 2004;25:587–610.
11. Bolignano MD, Rastelli MD, Agarwal R, et al. Pulmonary hypertension in CKD. *Am J Kidney Dis.* 2013;61:612–622.
12. Kubota H, Fujioka Y, Yoshino H, et al. Cardiac swinging calcified amorphous tumors in end-stage renal disease patients. *Ann Thorac Surg.* 2010;90:1692–1694.
13. K/DOQI Workgroup: K/DOQI clinical practice guidelines for cardiovascular disease in dialysis patients. *Am J Kidney Dis.* 2005;45(4 suppl 3):S1–S153.
14. Levin A, Stevens PE. Summary of KDIGO CKD Guideline: behind the scenes, need for guidance, and a framework for moving forward. *Kidney Int.* 2014;85:49–61.
15. Lentine KL, Costa SP, Weir MR, et al. Cardiac disease and evaluation and management among kidney and liver transplantation candidates. *J Am Coll Cardiol.* 2012;60:434–480.

148 Obesity

Francine Erenberg, Sudhir Ken Mehta

Approximately 93.3 million, or 39.8% of adults in the United States, are obese.[1] It is estimated by the World Health Organization that more than 650 million adults worldwide are obese and that this number has tripled since 1975. Because of a number of physiologic and metabolic changes associated with obesity, these individuals are at increased risk for cardiovascular (CV) disease. These changes include insulin resistance and hyperinsulinemia, type 2 diabetes mellitus, lipid abnormalities, hypertension, obstructive sleep apnea, systemic inflammation, sympathetic nervous system activation, and endothelial dysfunction. Additionally, obesity is an independent risk factor for development of heart failure even after accounting for comorbid conditions such as diabetes mellitus and hypertension.[2]

Most definitions of obesity are based on cut points of body mass index (BMI), which is weight in kilograms divided by height in meters squared, with obesity set at a BMI greater than or equal to 30 kg/m² in adults and greater than the 95th percentile of age and sex specific charts for children and youth. It should be recognized that BMI does not measure body fat directly, and the relationship between BMI and body fat varies by sex, age, and race. In addition to BMI, abdominal obesity or central obesity (CO) also plays a major role in CV morbidity and mortality. Otherwise normal individuals with a normal BMI but increased body fat and CO (so-called "normal weight obesity") have diminished insulin sensitivity, higher serum C-reactive protein, and impaired left ventricular (LV) systolic and diastolic function.[3] CO with normal BMI in patients with coronary artery disease has been associated with elevated mortality rates. Conversely, an increase in lean body mass that is associated with obesity appears to offer some protection from CV mortality in certain populations (the so-called obesity paradox).

PATHOPHYSIOLOGY

Far from being a passive energy storage site, adipose tissue synthesizes and releases proinflammatory markers into the bloodstream, instigating a low-level, chronic inflammatory state, which in turn may induce insulin resistance and endothelial dysfunction (Fig. 148.1). Extensive capillary networks surrounding adipose tissue require extra blood flow that can ultimately add to the total circulatory volume. An increase in skeletal muscle mass also accompanies obesity to support the resulting increase in body weight. Except during fasting state, skeletal muscle, with its higher metabolic activity, has significantly higher resting blood flow than the adipose tissue. This extra blood flow, or preload, adds further to the total circulatory blood volume, resulting in higher LV volume and higher cardiac output primarily through increase in stroke volume. Ensuing increase in LV mass (LVM), eccentric and concentric, is also an independent predictor of CV risk with a 1.3-fold risk for death or CV events for each mild, moderate, and severe category of LVM.[4] Increasing adipose tissue in the epicardium and myocardium leads to myocyte degeneration, pressure-induced atrophy, and conduction defects and contributes to a higher LVM. The frequent association of hypertension with obesity adds to LV dilatation and hypertrophy.

Lean body mass, primarily composed of organs and skeletal muscle, is the foremost determinant of energy requirements and correlates strongly with LVM. Conversely, increased adipose tissue is primarily responsible for adverse metabolic and energy-related changes that may alter the myocardial function. Epicardial accumulation of the adipose tissue in and around the heart may add to diastolic and systolic ventricular dysfunction. Although congestive heart failure in obese individuals may occur as a result of either diastolic or systolic dysfunction, systolic dysfunction, when measured only by LVEFs, is rare with obesity alone (obesity cardiomyopathy).[5] Diastolic dysfunction linked to obesity is seen independent of LVM. The active myocardial relaxation is a result of calcium homeostasis and myocardial energetics. A lower cardiac energetics, as measured by the ratio of phosphocreatine to adenosine triphosphate, at rest and during dobutamine stress, may help explain the lower LV peak filling rates associated with obesity.[6]

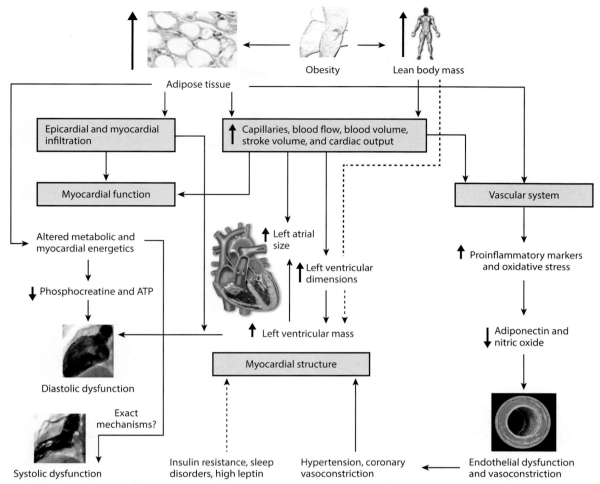

Figure 148.1. Summary of potential pathways by which obesity can influence cardiac and vascular structure and function. The *broken lines* indicate a significant association. *ATP,* Adenosine triphosphate.

CARDIAC ASSESSMENT BY ECHOCARDIOGRAPHY

Echocardiographic assessment in obesity begins with gathering information on the patient's age, gender, weight, height, and blood pressures because these factors may affect measured parameters associated with obesity. Clinical information, including history and physical examination, helps ascertain the etiology of abnormalities seen on imaging and differentiate individuals with associated comorbidities, including aortic stenosis, mitral stenosis, and hypertrophic cardiomyopathy.

On echocardiography, increasing BMI is associated with several LV structural changes, including increased LV end systolic and diastolic volumes and LVM. These changes are progressive with increasing BMI. Thus, over time, many obese individuals have mild left atrial (LA) and LV enlargement as well as mild LV hypertrophy. Although obese individuals have higher blood volume, enlargement of the left atrium invariably signifies higher LV filling pressures. Both eccentric hypertrophy and concentric hypertrophy are reported.

Chamber Quantification

When indexing the chamber sizes, it should be implicit that LA and LV growth may not be linear to the body surface area (BSA). Therefore, LA and LV sizes and LVM, when not indexed, may be higher as compared with nonobese control participants, but with indexing these same measurements to BSA, the chamber sizes may

appear normal or even be underestimated in severely obese individuals. Furthermore, if indexed measurements are made after significant weight loss, the chamber sizes are often overestimated when corrected for the (new) BSA, giving a false impression of increasing chamber size particularly after bariatric surgery or liposuction. Similarly, exercise intervention that may have the consequence of improving LV filling properties may accompany an increase in skeletal muscle with little or no change in weight or BMI, resulting in confounding results if indexed measurements are used.

Indexing of LVM to body size by weight, height, or BSA has limited success because of the nonlinear relationship between body size and LVM. Allometric approaches such as LVM/height[2,7] were found to be more sensitive indicators for future CV events, although there was an inverse relationship with height during the first 10 years of life. LVM/height[2,7] tends to overcorrect for height by artificially increasing LVM index in short patients and by lowering LVM index in tall patients. Indexing with height[1,7] may be superior in predicting CV outcomes[7] and may also be a reliable indicator of obesity-associated LV hypertrophy in children.[8]

Left Ventricular Systolic and Diastolic Function

In general, the left ventricular ejection fraction (LVEF) remains normal. Despite reported normal LVEFs, LV systolic function, when measured by more sensitive methods such as tissue Doppler imaging, strain and strain rate, and calibrated integrated backscatter parameters,

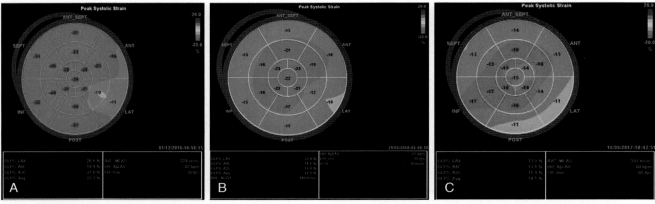

Figure 148.2. Change in average left ventricular systolic strain in an overweight/obese patient with weight gain. **A,** Body mass (BMI) of 30.5 kg/m². **B,** BMI of 33.1 kg/m². **C,** BMI of 35.6 kg/m².

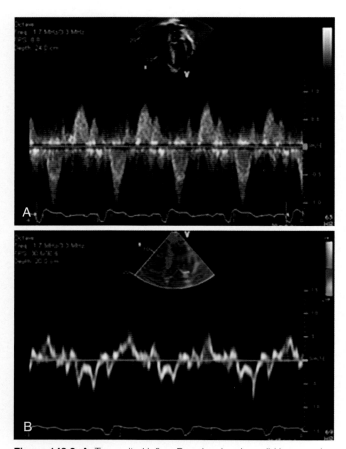

Figure 148.3. A, Transmitral inflow Doppler showing mild increase in "A" wave velocity but normal E/A ratio preserved. **B,** Mitral annulus tissue Doppler from the same obese patient showing lower mitral annulus early diastolic velocity (e′) and a higher mitral annulus late diastolic velocity (a′).

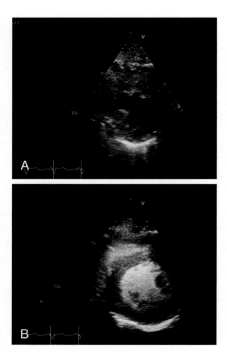

Figure 148.4. Parasternal short-axis image of the left ventricle (LV) in an obese patient. **A,** Standard two-dimensional imaging. **B,** Contrast-enhanced image in the same patient shows improved LV endocardial border detection.

show subclinical systolic dysfunction even in overweight (BMI, 25–29.9) or mildly obese (BMI, 30–35) individuals even though these individuals have a higher preload (Fig. 148.2). BMI correlates significantly with global longitudinal LV strain, e′ waves, and systolic myocardial velocities. Overweight and mildly obese individuals show reduced myocardial systolic and e′ velocity, reduced LV basal septal strain, and increased reflectivity by calibrated integrated backscatter suggesting the presence of underlying myocardial fibrosis. In severely

obese (BMI >35), additional reduction in the myocardial velocities are noted in the LV basal inferior and average LV strain.[9]

Many obese individuals have comorbidities such as diabetes mellitus and hypertension, themselves associated with impaired LV systolic function, abnormal global longitudinal strain, and abnormal tissue Doppler indices. Obesity has been seen to be independently associated with an additive detrimental effect on LV myocardial dysfunction.[10] These indices may prove to be more useful in assessing cardiac changes with weight loss. As myocardial velocities change with increasing age, an awareness of patient's age is warranted during the proper interpretation of lower e′ and higher a′ waves.

A lower LVEF with obesity, or "obesity cardiomyopathy," is extremely rare and invariably signifies a long-standing morbid obesity with associated comorbidities. Left ventricular diastolic dysfunction (LVDD) is a common finding in individuals who are obese, as well as in those with related comorbidities, including hypertension and diabetes mellitus.[11–13] Consensus recommendations of the American Society of Echocardiography and the European Association of Cardiovascular Imaging from 2016 provide recommendations for assessment of LVDD, including mitral E- and A-wave Doppler, pulmonary vein Doppler, and tissue Doppler imaging.[14]

Increased preload that tends to increase the early diastolic filling at the mitral valve (E) may not manifest itself because of altered LV filling pressure in the setting of the higher LVM often seen in obesity. This tends to lower the E wave velocity while significantly increasing the late diastolic transmitral blood flow (A) during atrial contraction, resulting in an overall lower E/A ratio. Thus, diastolic function measurements based on the transmitral flow alone may be equivocal in certain obese patients. In such instances, tissue Doppler diastolic velocity are more diagnostic. In the early stages of increasing weight gain and increasing stroke volume, alterations are seen in the myocardial velocities—a lower mitral annulus early diastolic velocity (e′) and a higher mitral annulus late diastolic velocity (a′). A lower e′ results in higher E/e′, reflecting higher LV filling pressures (Fig. 148.3). Isovolumic relaxation time is frequently prolonged in obese individuals.

Childhood obesity has been correlated with increased structural abnormalities in adulthood regardless of adult BMI, including increased LV mass index and LA volume index. In children who were obese and followed into adulthood, indices of LV function, including global longitudinal strain and mitral e′, were associated more with adult overweight or obesity, independent of childhood obesity.[15]

TECHNICAL ISSUES ASSOCIATED WITH IMAGING

Obese patients often present with technical challenges for echocardiographic imaging, including poor acoustic windows, which limit ability to obtain diagnostic images. It is estimated that 10% to 20% of echocardiographic images are technically suboptimal, particularly for measurement of LV wall motion and systolic function, and a large portion of this group is made up of those who are obese. This has led to the development of a group of ultrasound-enhancing (contrast) agents designed to improve LV opacification and LV endocardial border definition in patients with technically suboptimal echocardiographic images. These agents consist of microbubbles with a thin and relatively permeable shell typically filled with some type of high-molecular-weight gas that slows diffusion and dissolution within the bloodstream. The design of these agents is intended to preserve gas within the bubble after administration to increase the duration of opacification. Use of these has increased visualization of LV structure and function, LVEF, and segmental wall motion analysis.[16] (Fig. 148.4).

REFERENCES

1. Hales CM, Carroll MD, Fryar CD, et al. *Prevalence of Obesity Among Adults and Youth: United States, 2015–2016. NCHS Data Brief, No 288.* Hyattsville, MD: National Center for Health Statistics; 2017.
2. Kenchaiah S, Evans JC, Levy D, et al. Obesity and the risk of heart failure. *N Engl J Med.* 2002;347:305–313.
3. Kosmala W, Jedrzejuk D, Derzhko R, et al. Left ventricular function impairment in patients with normal-weight obesity: contribution of abdominal fat deposition, profibrotic state, reduced insulin sensitivity, and proinflammatory activation. *Circ Cardiovasc Imag.* 2012;5:349–356.
4. Barbieri A, Bursi F, Mantovani F, et al. Prognostic impact of left ventricular mass severity according to the classification proposed by the ASE/EAE. *J Am Soc Echocardiogr.* 2011;24:1383–1391.
5. Owan T, Litwin SE. Is there a cardiomyopathy of obesity. *Curr Heart Fail Rep.* 2007;4:221–228.
6. Rider OJ, Francis JM, Ali MK, et al. Effects of catecholamine stress on diastolic function and myocardial energetics in obesity. *Circulation.* 2012;125:1511–1519.
7. Chirinos JA, Segers P, De Buyzere ML, et al. Left ventricular mass: allometric scaling, normative values, effect of obesity, and prognostic performance. *Hypertension.* 2010;56:91–98.
8. Mehta SK. Left ventricular mass by echocardiographic measures in children and adolescents. *Cardiol Young.* 2013;23:727–773.
9. Wong CY, O'Moore-Sullivan T, Leano R, et al. Alterations of left ventricular myocardial characteristics associated with obesity. *Circulation.* 2004;110:3081–3087.
10. Ng ACT, Prevedello F, Dolci G, et al. Impact of diabetes and increasing body mass index category on left ventricular systolic and diastolic function. *J Am Soc Echocardiogr.* 2018;31:916–925.
11. Powell BD, Redfield MM, Bybee KA, et al. Association of obesity with left ventricular remodeling and diastolic dysfunction in patients without coronary artery disease. *Am J Cardiol.* 2006;98:116–120.
12. Russo C, Jin Z, Homma S, et al. Effect of obesity and overweight on left ventricular diastolic function: a community-based study in an elderly cohort. *J Am Coll Cardiol.* 2011;57:1368–1374.
13. Cil H, Bulur S, Türker Y, et al. Impact of body mass index on left ventricular diastolic dysfunction. *Echocardiography.* 2012;29:647–651.
14. Nagueh SF, Smiseth OA, Appleton CP, et al. Recommendations for the evaluation of left ventricular diastolic function by echocardiography. *Eur Heart J Cardiovasc Imag.* 2016;17:1321–1360.
15. Yan H, Huynh QL, Venn AJ, et al. Associations of childhood and adult obesity with left ventricular structure and function. *Int J Obesity.* 2017;41:560–568.
16. Mulvagh SL, Rakowski H, Vannan MA, et al. American Society of Echocardiography consensus statement on the clinical applications of ultrasonic contrast agents in echocardiography. *J Am Soc Echocardiogr.* 2008;21:1179–1201.

149 Rheumatic Fever and Rheumatic Heart Disease

Ferande Peters, Bijoy K. Khandheria

Acute rheumatic fever (ARF) is an inflammatory disorder that occurs after a throat infection with group A β-hemolytic streptococcus infection (GAS).[1] Rheumatic heart disease (RHD) is a chronic disorder in which the heart valves are damaged after an episode of ARF, or as is frequently the case, no identifiable history of ARF. The latter scenario has been defined as latent or subclinical RHD.[2]

EPIDEMIOLOGY

Currently, ARF and RHD are not commonly encountered in the United States and all developed countries. When cases are encountered, they are usually found among immigrants. In contrast, the incidence of ARF in children ages 5 to 14 years worldwide is estimated to range from 300,000 to 350,000 per year.[3] The majority of these cases are found in sub-Saharan Africa, but because of the paucity of epidemiologic studies, accurate estimates of ARF are lacking. The highest documented rates of ARF and RHD in the world are in indigenous Australians.[3]

Pathogenesis

ARF occurs after a GAS infection. In the absence of previous ARF or RHD, a small minority of individuals (0.3%–3%) with GAS throat infections develop ARF, RHD, or both.[4] The pathogenesis of ARF is complex and may be multifactorial. The general consensus is that the development of ARF requires four key factors—a susceptible host, GAS infection with specific strains that are thought to be rheumatogenic (M subtypes 1, 3, 5, 6, or 18), an abnormal immune response, and environmental factors (e.g., poverty and overcrowding)—that contribute to this interaction (Fig. 149.1).[5,6]

DIAGNOSIS
Acute Rheumatic Fever

The revised Jones criteria of 2015 offer an integrated clinical approach to improve the diagnosis of ARF.[7] Similar to prior iterations of the Jones criteria, evidence of a preceding streptococcal infection (throat culture serology) with either two major criteria or one major and two minor criteria are required for the diagnosis of ARF.[8] However, before the application of any criteria, the clinician should determine the patient's risk for ARF. If an individual comes from a community that has a low prevalence of RHD (<1

case in 1000) or ARF (<2 cases in 100,000), she or he is classified as low risk. Individuals who are not from low-risk communities are grouped together as moderate to high risk. The criteria proposed in the 2015 iteration differs for low-risk populations versus those deemed moderate to high risk (Table 149.1) with regard to joint manifestations, the temperature level, and the erythrocyte sedimentation rate (ESR) level.[7,8] The rationale for these changes is based on the desire to improve the detection of ARF in moderate- and high-risk populations by using more sensitive criteria.

The second major change in the revised Jones criteria of 2015 is that echocardiography is germane to the diagnosis of carditis and that the absence of echocardiographic evidence suggestive of ARF excludes the diagnosis of ARF.[8] The identification of valvular regurgitation that is not detectable with clinical examination—termed *subclinical carditis*—now constitutes a major criteria in all populations.[9–12] An additional advantage of echocardiography is the detection of concomitant subclinical pericardial effusions and left ventricular (LV) dysfunction and the differentiation of physiological murmurs from pathology, especially in febrile or hyperdynamic states.[10,11] The latter scenario can often lead to an incorrect conclusion that ARF may be present, as was the case in a study by Abernethy and coworkers.[10] The most important advantage of echocardiography is that it can identify an alternative diagnosis, such as mitral valve prolapse or congenital heart disease.[10,11]

There are two major limitations to echocardiography being used as diagnostic criteria. First, it is a relatively expensive examination that is not widely available in poorer communities where the prevalence of ARF is high. Second, unless end users of echocardiography have adequate training, misdiagnosis may easily occur, especially because adequately trained cardiologists or sonographers are unlikely to be working in rural or semirural areas.

The aim of echocardiography in assessing valvulitis in ARF is first to integrate the morphologic abnormality of the mitral or aortic valve with the presence of pathological regurgitation and second to differentiate morphologic features of ARF from chronic RHD. This is most pertinent to the mitral valve as the morphologic echocardiographic features of the aortic valve are similar in ARF and RHD (Table 149.2). Morphologic mitral valve thickening may be focal and may represent valvulitis. Vasan and coworkers reported nodules detected on the body or the tips of the leaflets in almost 25% of patients with ARF.[13] They postulated that these nodules represent the echocardiographic equivalents of the verrucae seen either at surgery or in autopsy specimens.[14] It is essential that the echocardiographer integrate the morphologic abnormalities with Doppler evaluation of regurgitation (Figs. 149.2 and 149.3; Video 149.1).

Within the correct clinical context, the presence of any chronic rheumatic morphologic changes on the mitral valve implies that recurrent carditis may require exclusion. An important caveat when interpreting Doppler data is that a minimum of one view is required to satisfy the required jet length and characterize the timing of regurgitation. However, the color jet needs to be evaluated in multiple views at standard technical settings, with the

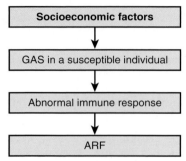

Figure 149.1. Pathogenesis of acute rheumatic fever (ARF). *GAS,* Group A β-hemolytic streptococcus infection.

TABLE 149.1 Revised Jones Criteria of 2015

Low-Risk Population	Moderate- to High-Risk Population
Major	Major
Carditis	Carditis
Polyarthritis	Polyarthralgia, monoarthritis, polyarthritis
Chorea	Chorea
Erythema marginatum	Erythema marginatum
Subcutaneous nodules	Subcutaneous nodules
Minor	Minor
Prolonged PR interval	Prolonged PR interval
Polyarthralgia	Monoarthralgia
Fever >38.5°C	Fever >38°C
ESR >60	ESR >30
CRP >3 mg/dL	CRP >3 mg/dL

CRP, C-reactive protein; *ESR,* erythrocyte sedimentation rate.

TABLE 149.2 Key Morphologic and Functional Criteria in Acute Rheumatic and Rheumatic Heart Disease

	ARF Morphology	Chronic RHD Morphology	Pathological Regurgitation
Mitral	• Annular dilatation • Leaflet tip prolapse • Leaflet beading or nodularity • Chordal elongation or rupture	• Leaflet thickening • Restricted leaflet motion • Leaflet calcification • Chordal shortening, thickening or fusion	• Detection in two or more views • Jet length >–2 cm • Pan systolic jet • Jet velocity >3 m/s
Aortic	• Leaflet thickening or irregularity • Restricted leaflet motion • Leaflet prolapse • Coaptation defect	• Leaflet thickening or irregularity • Restricted leaflet motion • Leaflet prolapse • Coaptation defect	• Detection in two or more views • Jet length >–1 cm • Pan diastolic jet • Jet velocity >3 m/s

ARF, Acute rheumatic fever; *RHD,* rheumatic heart disease.

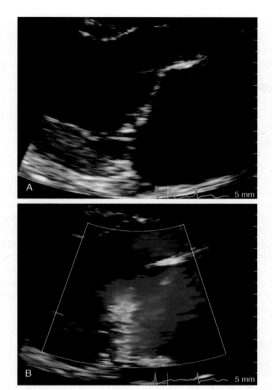

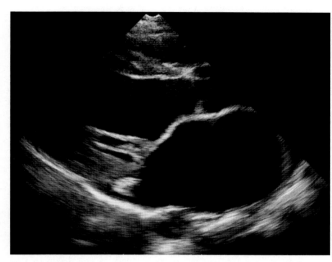

Figure 149.3. Left parasternal view demonstrating the prolapse of the anterior leaflet with prominent thickened chordae attached to both leaflets.

Figure 149.2. A, Left parasternal view demonstrating prolapse of the anterior leaflet of the mitral valve, with failure of coaptation of the anterior and posterior leaflet tips. **B,** Left parasternal view demonstrating an eccentric jet of mitral regurgitation caused by prolapse of the anterior leaflet.

imager using color M-mode and continuous-wave Doppler of the regurgitant jet to aid in timing the duration of the regurgitant jet. Other echocardiographic features of carditis include the presence of LV dysfunction out of keeping with the degree of valvular regurgitation, which is suggestive of myocarditis and the presence of a pericardial effusion.

It is essential that the echocardiographer avoid several pitfalls in the diagnosis of ARF (Box 149.1). ARF most commonly affects the mitral and aortic valves; involvement of the tricuspid and pulmonary valves is uncommon. Mitral regurgitation (MR) is the most common lesion encountered in ARF; its mechanisms are multifactorial and should be carefully evaluated using echocardiography to identify the mechanisms at play, particularly in patients who may require surgery (Fig. 149.4).[15] Currently, the assessment and quantification of valvular regurgitation should be based on the American Society of Echocardiography (ASE) guidelines on valvular regurgitation despite the lack of modern studies on ARF that determine long-term outcomes based on using this approach.

Identifying the severity of MR is of paramount importance, as is identifying the degree of LV remodeling and ejection fraction. The impact of valvular regurgitation is usually commensurate with the degree of ventricular remodeling and dysfunction. Although myocarditis may occur, the major dysfunction is most often valvular related and can be reversed with surgery.[16,17] Although the ejection fraction is a less reliable marker of contractile dysfunction in MR, identification of an abnormality using echocardiography may warrant surgery in some patients with worsening New York Heart Association functional class despite the absence of clinical heart failure. A second clinical scenario in which an integrated approach using echocardiography is effective is to determine if the degree of symptoms is commensurate with the degree of valvular and

---

BOX 149.1 Avoiding Pitfalls in the Diagnosis and Assessment of Acute Rheumatic Fever

DETECTING REGURGITATION
- Differentiate physiological from pathological regurgitation.
- Ensure all technical settings are correct.
- Evaluation must be performed using multiple views.
- Interpret findings judiciously when high-output states such as anemia and fever are present.
- Caution should be exercised when only Doppler regurgitation is found in the absence of other clinical features of acute rheumatic fever.
- Avoid diagnosing isolated tricuspid or pulmonary regurgitation as evidence of carditis in the absence of left-sided involvement.

MORPHOLOGIC ASSESSMENT AND MEASUREMENTS
- Ensure correct gain settings and avoid harmonic imaging.
- Use high-frequency imaging, such as zoom mode to evaluate nodules.
- Differentiate true prolapse from leaflet malcoaptation, ideally avoiding sole assessment using an apical four-chamber view.
- The presence of restricted leaflet motion may point to previous rheumatic involvement and is not a feature of de novo acute carditis.
- Diagnosing myocarditis as the cause of left ventricular dysfunction in the presence of hemodynamically significant valvular regurgitation.
- Detecting myocardial abnormality or pericardial effusion in the absence of valvular abnormality should be viewed with caution as evidence of rheumatic carditis.

---

ventricular dysfunction. This is particularly important when concomitant fever and anemia may be present in young children or adults and may alter the hemodynamics. Assessment of the tricuspid valve and the degree of regurgitation is very important in patients undergoing left-sided valvular surgery because this may mandate a concomitant tricuspid annuloplasty.

Recurrent Acute Rheumatic Fever

The incidence of recurrent ARF after a strep throat infection is 50% in patients with a history of ARF compared with 0.3% to 3% in

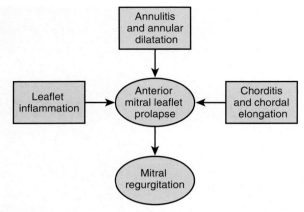

Figure 149.4. Mechanisms of mitral regurgitation in acute rheumatic fever.

those who have never had ARF. The recurrence rate is highest in the first 5 years after the first episode of ARF and can be decreased by secondary prevention with penicillin. The revised Jones criteria of 2015 suggests recurrent ARF may be diagnosed in individuals with documented prior ARF or echocardiographic evidence of RHD who have evidence of streptococcal infection and two major, one major and two minor, or three minor criteria.[7] These patients may have features of chronic rheumatic disease, such as diastolic doming of the anterior leaflet and shortened posterior leaflets with diminished leaflet motion, which are not found in ARF (Videos 149.2 and 149.3).

Subclinical Carditis in Acute Rheumatic Fever

As previously mentioned, patients with suspected carditis but no murmurs can have valvular regurgitation on echocardiographic Doppler imaging for a variety of reasons. This clinical scenario is called subclinical carditis, which has been reported within the context of other clinical manifestations of ARF and must not be confused with subclinical RHD.[18] The reported prevalence of subclinical carditis varies. It has been reported in up to 53% of cases, although a more accurate assessment by a meta-analysis of more than 1700 cases found it to be 18.1%.[19] Patients with chorea have been shown to have a high incidence of subclinical carditis, and using echocardiography is advantageous.

Rheumatic Heart Disease

Chronic RHD most commonly affects the mitral valve followed by the aortic and, less commonly, the tricuspid valve. Pulmonary involvement is infrequent. Contemporary data from the Remedy multicenter international study has revealed that multivalvular left-sided disease with mixed lesions is the most common lesion encountered.[19] The most common isolated lesion before age 20 years is MR; thereafter it is mitral stenosis. Isolated aortic stenosis was found to be very uncommon.[20–23] In most instances of chronic RHD, a preceding history of ARF is uncommon, and patients are detected either because of an incidental murmur, or they manifest with symptomatic valvular disease and its complications: heart failure, atrial fibrillation, and pulmonary hypertension.[24,25] Clues to a rheumatic pathology are based on the profile of the patient. This includes whether they originate from geographical areas where RHD is prevalent and their age. Younger individuals are more likely to have RHD.[24,25] In older individuals, especially in multivalvular disease and even isolated lesions such as mitral stenosis, differentiation from degenerative valvular disease, radiation, and certain drug-related valvulopathies is required. Thus, it behooves the imager to carefully analyze the entire morphology of the respective valve, bearing in mind some

of the chronic morphologic changes of RHD (see Table 149.2). The presence of doming of leaflets and a predilection of pathology for the leaflet tips and its proximal surroundings with relative sparing of the bases of leaflets are additional clues more suggestive of a rheumatic process. The hemodynamic assessment of stenosis or regurgitation in RHD should be performed in accordance with current ASE guidelines.

The detection of clinically overt disease is often not difficult; however, the identification of subclinical RHD and its milder forms in children and young adults in endemic areas can be challenging. The past two decades have witnessed numerous echocardiographic studies on screening for RHD in various parts of the world.[20–23] These studies have attempted to document the prevalence of RHD, but they have also been problematic because of the lack of standardized criteria for diagnosing RHD. Different definitions of RHD can result in dramatically different burdens of diseases in the same cohort.[24,25] Recently, the World Heart Federation proposed guidelines for the diagnosis of RHD that were based on expert consensus to standardize disease definitions.[26] The details of these criteria should be consulted because they represent the minimum criteria to diagnose RHD. Currently, routine screening is not advocated because of several socioeconomic factors coupled with several diagnostic and therapeutic uncertainties relating to the screening process.

THERAPY

Treatment of Acute Rheumatic Fever

Pharmacologic therapy with penicillin is essential to eradicate the GAS infection. In allergic patients, macrolides are an alternative therapy. Aspirin and corticosteroids are used as adjunctive therapy for arthritis and pericarditis. Surgery is needed in ARF when patients develop heart failure secondary to significant valvular regurgitation. Earlier work by Essop and associates showed that LV dysfunction improved with correction of MR by mitral valve surgery in young individuals.[16] Surgical repair has included both mitral valve repair and mitral valve replacement. The ideal option is mitral valve repair, which avoids the risks of a prosthetic valve and warfarin usage in young patients who often live in rural settings or female patients who are yet to enter or are in their childbearing years. Importantly, mitral valve repair in the presence of acute carditis carries an increased risk of failure.[27] Secondary prevention with intramuscular penicillin or oral daily penicillin is the mainstay of prevention and has been shown to decrease recurrent ARF episodes, decrease RHD progression, and even reverse mild disease. However, its true benefit in subclinical disease is unknown.

CONCLUSIONS

An understanding of the various spectrums of ARF and chronic RHD is essential to allow for correct diagnosis and intervention in these clinical scenarios. Echocardiography is an additive tool that, if used in a responsible and judicious manner, is additive to the clinical assessment of both ARF and RHD.

Please access ExpertConsult to view the corresponding videos for this chapter.

REFERENCES

1. Carapetis JR, Steer AC, Mulholland EK, et al. The global burden of group A streptococcal diseases. *Lancet Infect Dis.* 2005;5:685–694.
2. Tibazarwa KB, Volmink JA, Mayosi BM. Incidence of acute rheumatic fever in the world: a systematic review of population-based studies. *Heart.* 2008;94:1534–1540.
3. World Health Organization. *The Current Evidence for the burden of Group A Streptococcal Diseases.* Geneva: World Health Organization; 2005:1–52.
4. Rheumatic fever and rheumatic heart disease. *World Health Organization Tech Rep Ser.* 2004;923:1–122.
5. Carapetis JR, McDonald M, Wilson NJ. Acute rheumatic fever. *Lancet.* 2005;366:155–168.

6. Kaplan MH, Bolande R, Rakita L, Blair J. Presence of bound immunoglobulins and complement in the myocardium in acute rheumatic fever: Association with cardiac failure. *N Engl J Med.* 1964;271:637–645.

7. Jones TD. The diagnosis of acute rheumatic fever. *J Am Med Assoc.* 1944;126:481–484.

8. Gewitz MH, Baltimore RS, Tani LY, et al. Revision of the Jones Criteria for the diagnosis of acute rheumatic fever in the era of Doppler echocardiography. *Circulation.* 1992;131:1806–1818.

9. Folger Jr GM, Hajar R, Robida A, et al. Occurrence of valvar heart disease in acute rheumatic fever without evident carditis: colour-flow Doppler identification. *Br Heart J.* 1992;67:434–438.

10. Abernethy M, Bass N, Sharpe N, et al. Doppler echocardiography and the early diagnosis of carditis in acute rheumatic fever. *Aust N Z J Med.* 1994;24:530–535.

11. Wilson NJ, Neutze JM. Echocardiographic diagnosis of subclinical carditis in acute rheumatic fever. *Int J Cardiol.* 1995;50:1–6.

12. Taranta A, Kleinberg E, Feinstein AR, et al. Rheumatic fever in children and adolescents: a long-term epidemiologic study of subsequent prophylaxis, streptococcal infections, and clinical sequelae: V. Relation of the rheumatic fever recurrence rate per streptococcal infection to pre-existing clinical features of the patients. *Ann Intern Med.* 1964;60:58–67.

13. Vasan RS, Shrivastava S, Vijayakumar M, et al. Echocardiographic evaluation of patients with acute rheumatic fever and rheumatic carditis. *Circulation.* 1996;94:73–82.

14. Kinsley RH, Girdwood RW, Milner S. Surgical treatment during the acute phase of rheumatic carditis. *Surg Ann.* 1981;13:299–323.

15. Marcus RH, Sareli P, Pocock WA, et al. Functional anatomy of severe mitral regurgitation in active rheumatic carditis. *Am J Cardiol.* 1989;63:577–584.

16. Essop MR, Wisenbaugh T, Sareli P. Evidence against a myocardial factor as the cause of left ventricular dilation in active rheumatic carditis. *J Am Coll Cardiol.* 1993;22:826–829.

17. Gentles TL, Colan SD, Wilson NJ, et al. Left ventricular mechanics during and after acute rheumatic fever: contractile dysfunction is closely related to valve regurgitation. *J Am Coll Cardiol.* 2001;37:201–207.

18. Tubridy-Clark M, Carapetis JR. Subclinical carditis in rheumatic fever: a systematic review. *Int J Cardiol.* 2007;119:54–58.

19. Zühlke L, Karthikeyan G, Engel ME, et al. Clinical outcomes in 3343 children and adults with rheumatic heart disease from 14 low- and middle-income countries: two-year follow-up of the global rheumatic heart disease registry (the REMEDY Study). *Circulation.* 2016;134:1456–1466.

20. Marijon E, Ou P, Celermajer DS, et al. Prevalence of rheumatic heart disease detected by echocardiographic screening. *N Engl J Med.* 2007;357:470–476.

21. Carapetis JR, Hardy M, Fakakovikaetau T, et al. Evaluation of a screening protocol using auscultation and portable echocardiography to detect asymptomatic rheumatic heart disease in Tongan schoolchildren. *Nat Clin Pract Cardiovasc Med.* 2008;5:411–417.

22. Steer AC, Kado J, Wilson N, et al. High prevalence of rheumatic heart disease by clinical and echocardiographic screening among children in Fiji. *J Heart Valve Dis.* 2009;18:327–335.

23. Reeves BM, Kado J, Brook M. High prevalence of rheumatic heart disease in Fiji detected by echocardiography screening. *J Paediatr Child Health.* 2011;47:473–478.

24. Mirabel M, Celermajer DS, Ferreira B, et al. Screening for rheumatic heart disease: evaluation of a simplified echocardiography-based approach. *Eur Heart J Cardiovasc Imag.* 2012;13:1024–1029.

25. Marijon E, Celermajer DS, Tafflet M, et al. Rheumatic heart disease screening by echocardiography: the inadequacy of World Health Organization criteria for optimizing the diagnosis of subclinical disease. *Circulation.* 2009;120:663–668.

26. Reményi B, Wilson N, Steer A, et al. World Heart Federation criteria for echocardiographic diagnosis of rheumatic heart disease—an evidence-based guideline. *Nat Rev Cardiol.* 2012;9:297–309.

27. Skoularigis J, Sinovich V, Joubert G, et al. Evaluation of the long-term results of mitral valve repair in 254 young patients with rheumatic mitral regurgitation. *Circulation.* 1994;90(II):167–174.

150 Systemic Lupus Erythematosus

Rajeev V. Rao, Kwan-Leung Chan

In 1924, Emanuel Libman and Benjamin Sacks demonstrated noninfectious, nonrheumatic verrucous endocarditis in an autopsy series of four young patients with multiple symptoms. The seminal description highlighted the constellation of polyarthritis, pericarditis, fever, and cutaneous eruptions common in these patients and that the endocardial lesions extended into the mural endocardium.[1] Since the original description by Libman and Sacks of their eponymous endocarditis, systemic lupus erythematosus (SLE) is now recognized to be a complex, heterogeneous, multisystem autoimmune disorder with a wide range of potential cardiac manifestations (Fig. 150.1). A comprehensive systematic approach is essential in the assessment of patients with SLE because the findings can be subtle and nonspecific. Indeed, none of the cardiac findings are pathognomonic for the disease.

CAUSE AND PATHOPHYSIOLOGY

The cause of SLE is unknown and is likely related to genetic, immunologic, environmental, and hormonal factors. Genetic factors play a role with the most common predisposition occurring at the major histocompatibility complex whereby genes that encode for antigen-presenting cells are affected.[2] The derangement in adaptive immunity that forms the pathologic hallmark of SLE involves polyclonal B-cell activation, hypergammaglobulinemia, and autoantibody production, resulting in immune-complex formation with self-antigens. The production of these autoantibodies likely plays an important role in the pathogenesis, and their presence can be used in the detection of the disease as well as in monitoring disease activity.[3]

Valves

The classic Libman-Sacks valvular and mural lesions can either be active or healed. Active lesions more commonly seen in patients with recent disease onset may demonstrate focal necrosis, fibrinous clumps, and inflammatory mononuclear infiltrates, whereas healed lesions are often associated with calcification of the valves involved.[3–5] Multiple mechanisms of valvular dysfunction may be operative in SLE (Table 150.1),[4,6] and the prevalence of cardiac involvement does not appear to correlate with the severity of disease activity.[5] The presence of antiphospholipid antibodies is associated with cardiac involvement according to a recent meta-analysis of echocardiographic studies in patients with SLE.[7] The importance of immune-complex deposition is highlighted by the deposition of C3 and immunoglobulin on direct immunofluorescence.[4,6] The role of antiphospholipid syndrome in the pathogenesis of valvular lesions in SLE is discussed separately (see Chapter 151).

Myocardium

Myocardial involvement is nonspecific, and mononuclear invasion into the perivascular and interstitial space in addition to myocyte injury and associated fibrosis has been described.[5] The myocardial dysfunction may be a consequence of the disease process but can also be caused by hydroxychloroquine therapy, which can be part of the treatment,[8] and cardiac myocyte cytoplasmic vacuolization, interstitial fibrous connective tissue on light microscopy, and lamellar lysosomal structures on electron microscopy are the typical pathological findings.[9] Coronary artery disease (CAD)

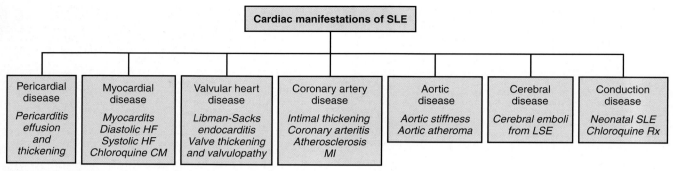

Figure 150.1. Cardiovascular manifestations of systemic lupus erythematosus (SLE). *CM,* Cardiomyopathy; *HF,* heart failure; *LSE,* Libman-Sacks endocarditis; *MI,* myocardial infarction; *Rx,* treatment.

TABLE 150.1 Mechanisms of Valvular Dysfunction in Systemic Lupus Erythematosus and Consequences

Mechanism	Clinical Consequence
Healing of verrucous valvular lesions leading to leaflet retraction	Valvular regurgitation and rarely stenosis
Large valvular verrucous lesion	Obstruction of valvular orifice leading to stenosis or malcoaptation of leaflets leading to regurgitation
Infective endocarditis	Caused by underlying abnormal valve or immunosuppression
Chordal rupture in presence of verrucae	Valvular regurgitation
Papillary muscle dysfunction caused by acute myocardial infarction	Valvular regurgitation
Mitral valve prolapse	Valvular regurgitation

Modified with permission from Roberts WC, High ST: The heart in systemic lupus erythematosus, *Curr Probl Cardiol* 24:1–56, 1999.

TABLE 150.2 Prevalence of Cardiac Abnormalities in Systemic Lupus Erythematosus

Site of Involvement	Prevalence (%)
Pericarditis or effusion	11–54
Myocarditis	7–10
Valvular heart disease	15–75
Coronary artery disease	6–10

Modified with permission from Doria A, et al: Cardiac involvement in systemic lupus erythematosus, *Lupus* 14:683–686, 2005.

can result from intimal narrowing due to coronary arteritis or atherosclerosis.[4–6]

Pericardium

Pericardial involvement is predominantly fibrinous in the acute phase and may become fibrous in the chronic phase.

PREVALENCE AND OUTCOME

The estimated incidence of SLE using data from Olmstead county, Minnesota, during the period 1980 to 1992, adjusting for age and sex to the 1970 US white population, was 5.56 per 100,000 (95% confidence interval, 3.93–7.19), which was more than triple the incidence in the 1950 to 1979 cohort.[8] The overall prevalence of SLE using California and Pennsylvania hospital administrative databases is 107 to 150 per 100,000 and approximately 1.8 to 2.5 per 1,000 women.[10] In terms of cardiovascular morbidity and mortality, a large Toronto cohort from 1997 to 2005 with a 9-year follow-up reported a standardized mortality ratio of 3.46 for patients with SLE.[11] Cardiovascular morbidity in SLE consists of a 2- to 10-fold increase in risk of nonfatal myocardial infarction associated with prolonged hospitalization and increased in-hospital mortality rate. Patients with SLE have accelerated atherosclerosis demonstrating no specific pattern of coronary involvement.[1,12] Young women with SLE have a 2.5-fold increased risk of congestive heart failure (CHF) hospitalization and a 3.5-fold increase in CHF-associated mortality

compared with patients with CHF without SLE.[1,12] It is prudent to aggressively manage the traditional risk factors of atherosclerosis in these patients.

DIAGNOSTIC APPROACH

Patients with SLE often have multiple constitutional symptoms, including musculoskeletal and cutaneous manifestations, many of which are criteria for the diagnosis of SLE.[13,14] Because much of the cardiac involvement in SLE is clinically silent, there should be a low threshold to initiate cardiac investigations in patients with suspected or proven SLE irrespective of cardiac symptomatology. Echocardiography should be performed in patients with SLE because of its ability to provide a comprehensive cardiac assessment. A recent study showed that only 25% of young patients with new-onset SLE had echocardiograms, and 18% of them were diagnosed to have cardiac disease. There was a positive correlation of echocardiogram use with the prevalence of cardiac disease, suggesting that echocardiography may be underused in these patients.[15]

Initial investigations include routine hematology and biochemistry to assess for cytopenias and renal function. Urinalysis and urine protein quantification should be performed when renal involvement is documented. Serology includes the use of the sensitive antinuclear antibody assay in addition to specific markers such as the Smith antigen (anti-Sm) and double-stranded DNA (anti-dsDNA). Inflammatory markers such as the erythrocyte sedimentation rate or C-reactive protein may also be used to monitor disease activity.

CARDIAC MANIFESTATIONS

The prevalence of cardiac abnormalities varies widely depending on the type of involvement (Table 150.2).

Pericardium

The pericardium is most frequently affected and pericarditis is usually present at the onset or during relapse of the disease.[4]

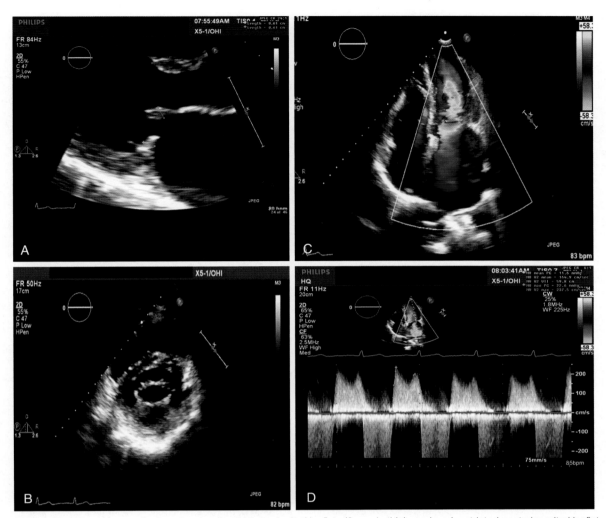

Figure 150.2. A, Parasternal long-axis view showing the thickened mitral leaflets (6 mm in thickness) and restricted posterior mitral leaflet motion in a patient with lupus-associated valve disease. **B,** Short-axis view of the mitral valve (MV) showing restricted posterior MV leaflet with no commissural fusion. **C,** Apical four-chamber view demonstrating mixed MV disease with moderate mitral stenosis and regurgitation. **D,** Continuous-wave Doppler of mitral inflow demonstrating increased transvalvular mitral gradients. (See accompanying Video 150.2.)

Pericardial effusion may be seen as a consequence of the serositis and is rarely symptomatic. On the other hand, symptomatic effusion is associated with reduced survival. A recent study of 85 Chinese patients with SLE showed pericardial effusion in 22 (25.9%) patients and pericardial thickening in 5 (5.9%) patients.[16] Therapy consists of nonsteroidal antiinflammatory drugs for mild disease; symptomatic effusion may require higher steroid doses in addition to pericardiocentesis.[4]

Myocardium

There is a spectrum of SLE-associated myocardial involvement ranging from increased left ventricular (LV) mass and excess hypertrophy to myocarditis.[14,17] Myocarditis, reported in 3% to 9% of patients, usually occurs early in the course of the disease and is associated with higher disease activity.[18] Longer disease duration and higher disease activity are associated with diastolic abnormalities[19] and LV systolic dysfunction.[20] Myocarditis can lead to heart failure, arrhythmia, myocardial dysfunction, dilated cardiomyopathy, and even LV pseudoaneurysm.[18,21] Myocardial involvement can be clinically overt or silent but important to recognize because immediate therapy is indicated. Overall, 40% of patients with myocarditis may die or have residual myocardial dysfunction despite aggressive treatment.[18] Independent of the

disease activity, myocardial dysfunction can occur as a result of the treatment with hydroxychloroquine and is potentially reversible on cessation of the drug.[8] Hydroxychloroquine-associated cardiomyopathy is rare but typically manifests as a restrictive cardiomyopathy with biatrial enlargement, a restrictive filling pattern, and thickened atrioventricular valves. Cardiac magnetic resonance imaging (CMRI) frequently shows stress perfusion deficits and thickened LV walls with patchy late gadolinium enhancement; these findings may not correlate with symptoms, indicating that CMRI may be used to detect subclinical cardiac involvement.[10,22]

Valves

Valvular heart disease from SLE can range from mild valvular thickening with normal function to overt valvulopathy with vegetations and severe regurgitation or stenosis (Fig. 150.2). Galve and coworkers[23] prospectively followed 74 patients with SLE for almost 5 years with echocardiography and demonstrated a prevalence of 18% of valvular abnormalities consisting of two types of involvement with vegetation in seven patients and valvular thickening with associated stenosis or regurgitation in six patients. The patients with vegetations were younger with a shorter duration of disease activity.

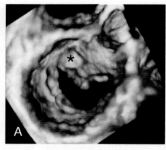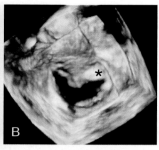

Figure 150.3. Transesophageal three-dimensional echocardiographic images of the mitral valve from the left atrial perspective (**A**) and the left ventricular perspective (**B**) in an 18-year-old woman with long-standing lupus showing mild diffuse thickening of both leaflets and nodular calcification (*asterisks*) at the medial aspect of the anterior mitral leaflet. (See accompanying Video 150.3.)

Transthoracic echocardiography (TTE) is able to detect SLE-associated vegetations (Libman-Sacks endocarditis) with a sensitivity of 63% and a specificity of 58%.[24] Transesophageal echocardiography (TEE) is superior to TTE in assessing SLE-associated valve disease.[25] In a prospective study of 69 patients, TEE detected valve thickening, in 51% of patients at baseline, and 52% of patients during follow-up,[25] defined as greater than 3 mm for the mitral or tricuspid valves and greater than 2 mm for the aortic valve with involvement of at least two cusps or with associated regurgitation or vegetation. The diffuse thickening of leaflets and the lack of commissural fusion distinguish SLE valve disease from rheumatic valvular disease.[23] The potential incremental diagnostic value of real time three-dimensional TEE in this disease remains to be defined because there are only case reports of its use in this entity[26] (Fig. 150.3). Early detection of SLE-related vegetations may prompt the early and aggressive use of corticosteroids and immunosuppressive therapy because a recent study has shown a strong association of this finding with cerebral microemboli and neuropsychiatric events.[27] Surgical intervention including valve repair or mechanical valve replacement may be considered in patients with severe valvulopathy.[4]

Patients with SLE have premature and accelerated atherosclerosis, which correlates with disease duration and activity,[28] and CAD may arise through a number of mechanisms, including atherosclerosis and vasculitis, which have important therapeutic implications but difficult to determine clinically.[4] In addition, the pattern of cardiac involvement may be influenced by the effect of corticosteroid therapy. Increased aortic stiffness predates atherosclerosis in patients with SLE and appears to be ameliorated with cyclophosphamide therapy, suggesting a role for aggressive immunosuppression.[29]

Pulmonary Hypertension

The prevalence of SLE-associated pulmonary hypertension is low, and thus screening echocardiography is not currently recommended for asymptomatic patients.[30] The presence of high SLE disease activity, Raynaud phenomenon, anticardiolipin antibodies, serositis and anti-RNP antibodies are predictors of pulmonary hypertension in patients with SLE, and these features can be used to identify high-risk patients who should be screened for pulmonary hypertension.[30]

In summary, SLE affects all aspects of the cardiovascular system. Echocardiography plays an integral role in the diagnosis, monitoring, and management of SLE-associated cardiac disease.

Please access ExpertConsult to view the corresponding videos for this chapter.

REFERENCES

1. Libman E, Sacks B. A hitherto undescribed form of valvular and mural endocarditis. *Arch Intern Med.* 1924;33:701–737.
2. Barcellos LF, May SL, Ramsay PP, et al. High-density SNP screening of the major histocompatibility complex in systemic lupus erythematosus demonstrates strong evidence for independent susceptibility regions. *PLoS Genet.* 2009;5. e1000696.
3. Frieri M. Mechanisms of disease for the clinician: systemic lupus erythematosus. *Ann Allergy Asthma Immunol.* 2013;110:228–232.
4. Doria A, Iaccarino L, Sarzi-Puttini P, et al. Cardiac involvement in systemic lupus erythematosus. *Lupus.* 2005;14:683–686.
5. Jain D, Halushka MK. Cardiac pathology of systemic lupus erythematosus. *J Clin Pathol.* 2009;62:584–592.
6. Roberts WC, High ST. The heart in systemic lupus erythematosus. *Curr Probl Cardiol.* 1999;24:1–56.
7. Zuily S, Regnault V, Selton-Suty C, et al. Increased risk for heart valve disease associated with antiphospholipid antibodies in patients with systemic lupus erythematosus: meta-analysis of echocardiographic studies. *Circulation.* 2011;124:215–224.
8. Uramoto KM, Michet CJ, Thumboo J, et al. Trends in the incidence and mortality of systemic lupus erythematosus. *Arthritis Rheum.* 1999;42:46–50.
9. Abbasi S, Tarter L, Farzaneh-Far R, Farzaneh-Far A, Hydroxychloroquine. A treatable cause of cardiomyopathy. *J Am Coll Cardiol.* 2012;60:786.
10. Chakravarty EF, Bush TM, Manzi S, et al. Prevalence of adult systemic lupus erythematosus in California and Pennsylvania in 2000: estimates obtained using hospitalization data. *Arthritis Rheum.* 2007;56:2092–2094.
11. Urowitz MB, Gladman DD, Tom BDM, et al. Changing patterns in mortality and disease outcomes for patients with systemic lupus erythematosus. *J Rheumatol.* 2008;35:2152–2158.
12. Symmons DPM, Gabriel SE. Epidemiology of CVD in rheumatic disease, with a focus on RA and SLE. *Nat Rev Rheumatol.* 2011;7:399–408.
13. Hochberg MC. Updating the American College of Rheumatology revised criteria for the classification of systemic lupus erythematosus. *Arthritis Rheum.* 1997;40:1725.
14. Pieretti J, Roman MJ, Devereux RB, et al. Systemic lupus erythematosus predicts increased left ventricular mass. *Circulation.* 2007;116:419–426.
15. Chang JC, Knight AM, Xiao R, et al. Use of echocardiography at diagnosis and detection of acute cardiac disease in youth with systemic lupus erythematosus. *Lupus.* 2018;27:1348–1357.
16. Yu X-H, Li Y-N. Echocardiographic abnormalities in a cohort of Chinese patients with systemic lupus erythematosus: a retrospective analysis of eighty-five cases. *J Clin Ultrasound.* 2011;39:519–526.
17. Zawadowski GM, Klarich KW, et al. A contemporary case series of lupus myocarditis. *Lupus.* 2012;21:1378–1384.
18. Tanwani J, Tselios K, Gladman DD, et al. Lupus myocarditis: a single center experience and a comparative analysis of observational cohort studies. *Lupus.* 2018;27:1296–1302.
19. Shang Q, Yip GW-K, Tam L-S, et al. SLICC/ACR damage index independently associated with left ventricular diastolic dysfunction in patients with systemic lupus erythematosus. *Lupus.* 2012;21:1057–1062.
20. Yip GW-K, Shang Q, Tam L-S, et al. Disease chronicity and activity predict subclinical left ventricular systolic dysfunction in patients with systemic lupus erythematosus. *Heart.* 2009;95:980–987.
21. Hoff LS, Pimentel CQ, Faillace BLR, et al. Left ventricular pseudoaneurysm associated with systemic lupus erythematosus. *Lupus.* 2019;28(5):681–684.
22. Burkard T, Trendelenburg M, Daikeler T, et al. The heart in systemic lupus erythematosus—a comprehensive approach by cardiovascular magnetic resonance tomography. *PLoS One.* 2018;13. e0202105.
23. Galve E, Candell-Riera J, Pigrau C, et al. Prevalence, morphologic types, and evolution of cardiac valvular disease in systemic lupus erythematosus. *N Engl J Med.* 1988;319:817–823.
24. Roldan CA, Qualls CR, Sopko KS, Sibbitt WL. Transthoracic versus transesophageal echocardiography for detection of Libman-Sacks endocarditis: a randomized controlled study. *J Rheumatol.* 2008;35:224–229.
25. Roldan CA, Shively BK, Crawford MH. An echocardiographic study of valvular heart disease associated with systemic lupus erythematosus. *New Engl J Med.* 1996;335:1424–1430.
26. Vatankulu MA, Erdogan E, Tasal A, et al. The role of real time 3D transesophageal echocardiography in assessing Libman-Sacks endocarditis. *Echocardiography.* 2012;29. E216–217.
27. Roldan CA, Sibbitt WL, Qualls CR, et al. Libman-Sacks endocarditis and embolic cerebrovascular disease. *JACC Cardiovasc Imag.* 2013;6:973–983.
28. Roman MJ, Shanker B-A, Davis A, et al. Prevalence and correlates of accelerated atherosclerosis in systemic lupus erythematosus. *New Engl J Med.* 2003;349:2399–2406.
29. Roldan CA, Joson J, Sharrar J, et al. Premature aortic atherosclerosis in systemic lupus erythematosus: a controlled transesophageal echocardiographic study. *J Rheumatol.* 2010;37:71–78.
30. Ruiz-Irastorza G, Garmendia M, Villar I, et al. Pulmonary hypertension in systemic lupus erythematosus: prevalence, predictors and diagnostic strategy. *Autoimmun Rev.* 2013;12:410–415.

151 Antiphospholipid Syndrome

Rajeev V. Rao, Kwan-Leung Chan

The pathogenic role of antiphospholipid antibodies (APLAs) in thrombotic events was recognized 30 years ago in a study of 65 patients with systemic lupus erythematous (SLE).[1] The antiphospholipid syndrome (APS) is a clinical entity composed of venous or arterial thrombotic events or pregnancy-associated complications in the presence of APLAs. The frequent subgroups of APLA are lupus anticoagulant, anticardiolipin antibodies, and anti–β-2-glycoprotein I antibodies (Box 151.1).

The original definition and classification of APS were developed in 1999 and updated in 2006 to reflect greater knowledge of the role of specific antibodies in thrombosis as well as defining specific organ involvement for future studies[2,3] (Table 151.1). The diagnosis of APS is based on the presence of at least one clinical and one laboratory criterion. Early literature proposed the concept of the primary APS and secondary APS, with the latter referring to APS in the presence of another underlying disease, most commonly SLE.[4] The 2006 consensus statement recommended against the use of the term "secondary APS" because APS and SLE may be manifestations of one disease and not necessarily two coexisting diseases. Furthermore, similar clinical features are present in patients with primary and secondary APS.[5–7] Although APLA has been shown to be an important pathogenic contributor to valvular heart disease in patients with SLE, the consensus statement did not include valvular disease or any other cardiac abnormalities in the diagnostic criteria because the cardiac findings are nonspecific, affected by confounding factors such as age and hypertension, and not consistently associated with APLA.[3]

DEMOGRAPHICS AND PRESENTING SYMPTOMS

As mentioned previously, it may not be appropriate to categorize APS into primary and secondary forms, and the association of APS with SLE is well recognized.[1,3,5] Among patients presenting with thrombotic events, 5% to 20% of them have APLA,[7] but the prevalence of APLA is 1% to 10% in the general population and higher in patients with autoimmune diseases such as rheumatoid arthritis and SLE (at 16% and 30% to 40%, respectively).[7] The risk of thrombosis in patients with APLA is variable and may be related to the type and magnitude of circulating autoantibodies. Asymptomatic patients with APLA have a low annual rate of thrombotic events (0%–4%), and many of these patients can remain free of symptoms for years.[8] Carriers of all three subgroups of APLA have been shown to have more frequent pregnancy-related complications, and they may deserve more aggressive treatment.[9] Patients with lupus with APLAs are at the high end of the range of thrombotic events. Valvular heart disease occurs in about one-third of the patients with APS but appears to be more frequent when associated with SLE.[10–13]

The spectrum of clinical presentation can also be quite variable, ranging from asymptomatic APLA carrier to catastrophic APS with multiple small-vessel thrombosis involving different organs and a mortality rate of 50% (Fig. 151.1). Recurrent arterial and venous thromboembolism is the hallmark with deep vein thrombosis (DVT) and stroke or transient ischemic attack representing the most common venous and arterial sites of involvement.[8] Additional non-APS manifestations include cutaneous findings such as livedo reticularis, nephropathy, and cardiac abnormalities.

PATHOPHYSIOLOGY

APS is an autoimmune systemic disease characterized by the presence of APLA, which are a family of heterogeneous autoantibodies directed against phospholipid-binding plasma proteins (see Box 151.1). Binding of APLAs to endothelial cells leading to thrombosis through expression of tissue factor by monocytes and endothelial cells and activation of the complement system has been demonstrated and the inflammatory response may be a key component of APS.[7,8] Platelets also play a role in the pathogenesis of APS through expression of glycoprotein IIb/IIIa and synthesis of thromboxane A2, which is a procoagulant.[8] Because there are many carriers of APLA without clinical thrombotic events, a "two-hit hypothesis" has been proposed. An incident such as minor injury, pregnancy, malignancy, or infection is believed to be the required trigger to initiate the thrombotic process in susceptible carriers of APLA.[14]

DIAGNOSTIC APPROACH

The initial workup begins with a strong clinical suspicion surrounding a thrombotic event or pregnancy-related complication. Clinical history involves a review of prior thrombotic events and surrounding circumstances in addition to a detailed pregnancy-related history. Physical examination should assess for cutaneous manifestations (livedo reticularis), valvular dysfunction, and evidence of pulmonary thromboembolic disease. A complete hematologic panel, including complete blood count, international normalized ratio (INR), and activated partial thromboplastin time (aPTT) with a mixing study, is performed if the aPTT is abnormal. The presence of APLA can prolong the aPTT, thus creating the effect of a coagulopathy. The failure of a 1:1 mix of patient's plasma and normal plasma to normalize this coagulopathy suggests the presence of an extrinsic anticoagulant, and this is often the first clue to the presence of APLA in an asymptomatic patient. There are multiple antibodies that can act as "lupus anticoagulants," and the actual binding is not to the phospholipids themselves but epitopes on the proteins to which the phospholipids are attached.[7] Serology should include immunoglobulin (Ig) M and IgG subtypes of anticardiolipin, lupus anticoagulant activity, and IgG and IgM subtypes of β2-glycoprotein I (see Table 151.1). Chest imaging should be obtained when a suspicion of pulmonary embolism exists.

CARDIAC MANIFESTATIONS

Cardiac involvement in APS is diverse and includes ventricular dysfunction, ventricular hypertrophy, coronary thrombosis, premature atherosclerosis, intracardiac thrombi, valvular abnormalities, and pulmonary hypertension.[14] Although none of the cardiac manifestations are specific enough to be included in the classification criteria (see Table 151.1), valvular disease can be the most striking feature in patients with APS with involvement usually of the left-sided valves, particularly the mitral valve[15–17] (Fig. 151.2). Large, mobile valvular masses or vegetations can be seen in 10% to 40% of patients and may be difficult to differentiate from infective vegetations.[17] In addition to valvular vegetations, focal or diffuse thickening of valve leaflets has been observed.[15] In contrast with rheumatic valvular disease, significant valvular stenosis is uncommon despite diffuse thickening of the valve leaflets, and valvular regurgitation is far more common because of improper coaptation resulting from leaflet thickening or interference by the vegetations.[16] Destruction of the valve leaflets or annulus is absent, and this is a clear distinction from infective endocarditis.[17] The morphologic features of valvular disease in APS are summarized in Box 151.2.

Acute coronary syndrome (ACS) can occur but is far less common than cerebrovascular disease.[8] Patients with APS have an increased risk of myocardial infarction, and APS should be considered in young patients with ACS with normal coronary arteries and no conventional atherosclerotic risk factors.[18] Other important features of cardiac APS are intracardiac thrombi and biopsy evidence of myocardial microthrombosis without vasculitis, and thrombus can occur in normally contracting left ventricle.[19–21] Dense spontaneous contrast, a precursor of thrombosis, in the left atrium has been demonstrated by transesophageal echocardiography (TEE) in 10% of patients with APS with no apparent reason for

stasis.[22] Finally, pulmonary hypertension can occur as a result of recurrent pulmonary embolism from DVT or less commonly from in situ right ventricular thrombosis. Left untreated, right ventricular dysfunction and tricuspid regurgitation may develop.

MANAGEMENT

Management of patients with APS depends on the clinical scenario, bearing in mind the wide spectrum of presentation.[23] Asymptomatic carriers of APLA without a prior obstetric mishap or thrombotic event require no therapy or probably aspirin only. Whereas patients with a first venous thrombotic event with definite APS warrant anticoagulation with a target INR of 2.0 to 3.0, patients with arterial events may require a higher target INR of 3.0 to 4.0, although there are no data showing superiority of the higher anticoagulation target.[7,8] Recurrent thrombotic events despite therapeutic anticoagulation are a treatment dilemma. A higher anticoagulation target (INR, 3.0–4.0), concomitant use of antiplatelet agent, low-molecular weight heparin, or direct oral anticoagulant (DOAC) agents can be tried, but there are no trial data to support any of these strategies.[7,8] The role of the new DOACs is unclear, and they need to be used with caution.[24] The management of APS-associated valve disease is also uncertain. Espínola-Zavaleta and colleagues reported a 1-year follow-up TEE study on 29 patients with APS showing that antithrombotic therapy failed to modify the valvular lesions in 22 patients.[25] New lesions occurred in 7 patients despite the treatment. In a 5-year follow-up study by Turiel and associates, the

---

BOX 151.1 Frequent Subgroups of Antiphospholipid Antibody

- Lupus anticoagulant
- Anticardiolipin antibodies
- Anti–β2-glycoprotein I antibodies

TABLE 151.1 Diagnostic Criteria for the Antiphospholipid Syndrome

Clinical criteria	Vascular thrombosis	• One or more clinical episodes of arterial, venous, or small-vessel thrombosis *and* • Thrombosis must be confirmed by unequivocal findings of appropriate imaging studies or histopathology *and* • For histopathologic confirmation, thrombosis should be present without significant vessel wall inflammation
	Pregnancy criteria	• One or more unexplained deaths at or beyond the 10th week of gestation of a morphologically normal fetus, documented by ultrasonography or by direct examination of the fetus *or* • One or more premature births of a morphologically normal neonate before the 34th week of gestation because of eclampsia, severe preeclampsia, or recognized features of placental insufficiency *or* • Three or more unexplained consecutive spontaneous abortions before the 10th week of gestation, with exclusion of maternal anatomic or hormonal abnormalities and paternal and maternal chromosomal causes
Laboratory criteria	Anticardiolipin Antibody	IgG and/or IgM isotype in serum or plasma present in medium or high titer (i.e., >40 GPL or MPL or >99th percentile) on two or more occasions at least 12 weeks apart, measured by a standardized ELISA
	Anti–β2-glycoprotein I antibody	IgG and/or IgM isotype in serum or plasma (in titer >99th percentile) present on two or more occasions at least 12 weeks apart, measured by a standardized ELISA
	Lupus anticoagulant (LA)	LA present in plasma on two or more occasions at least 12 weeks apart, detected according to established guidelines
Diagnosis of definite APS		APS is present if at least one clinical and one laboratory criterion is present and <5 years elapsed between the positive laboratory criteria and clinical event

APS, Antiphospholipid syndrome; *ELISA,* enzyme-linked immunosorbent assay; *GPL,* anti-B2-glycoprotein/anticardiolipin IgG level; *Ig,* immunoglobulin; *MPL,* anti-B2-glycoprotein/anticardiolipin IgM level;.
Adapted with permission from Miyakis S, et al: International consensus statement on an update of the classification criteria for definite antiphospholipid syndrome (APS), *J Thromb Haemost* 4:295–306, 2006.

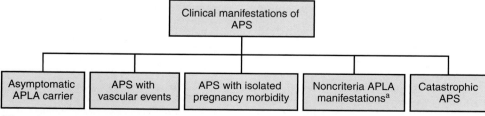

aThrombocytopenia, hemolytic anemia, livedo reticularis, APLA nephropathy, cardiac valve disease.

Figure 151.1. Clinical manifestations of antiphospholipid syndrome (APS). *APLA,* Antiphospholipid antibody (Modified from George D, Erkan D: Antiphospholipid syndrome, *Prog Cardiovasc Dis* 52(2):115–125, 2009.)

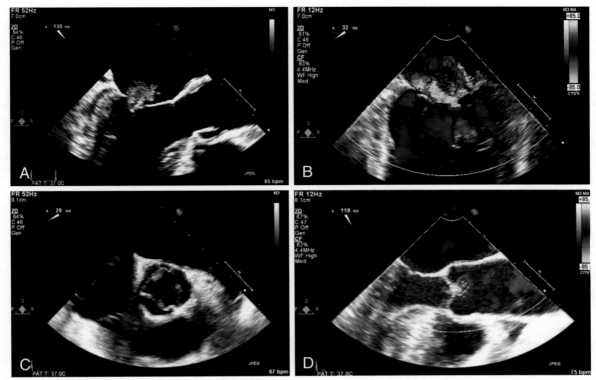

Figure 151.2. Transesophageal echocardiography in a patient with antiphospholipid antibody syndrome with both mitral and aortic vegetations. **A,** Midesophageal long-axis view demonstrates a large 1.5-cm × 1.4-cm heterogeneous echogenic mass attached to the posterior mitral valve leaflet. **B,** Color Doppler midesophageal bicommissural view of the mitral valve demonstrates mild mitral regurgitation associated with the valvular mass. **C,** Midesophageal short-axis view of the aortic valve demonstrates masses on the noncoronary (0.9 × 0.5 cm) and right coronary (0.4 × 0.3 cm) cusps. **D,** Color Doppler midesophageal long-axis view of the aortic valve demonstrates mild aortic regurgitation associated with the vegetations. (See accompanying Video 151.2.)

BOX 151.2 Morphologic Features of Cardiac Valve Disease in Antiphospholipid Syndrome

- Valve thickness >3 mm
- Localized thickening of proximal and middle portion of the valve leaflets
- Nodules on the atrial surface of the mitral valve and/or the aortic surface of the aortic valve
- Rheumatic valvular disease and infective endocarditis should be excluded

Modified with permission from: Miyakis S, et al: International consensus statement on an update of the classification criteria for definite antiphospholipid syndrome (APS), *J Thromb Haemost* 4:295–306, 2006.

---

lack of efficacy of antiplatelet and antithrombotic agents on the APS-associated valvular disease was again demonstrated, although higher intensity anticoagulation appeared to reduce the incidence of new valve lesions.[26] The role of antiinflammatory or immunosuppressive therapy with corticosteroids or cyclophosphamide in the treatment of valvular thickening or vegetations has not been properly evaluated. Valve replacement or valve repair with excision of valvular vegetations is associated with high perioperative mortality and morbidity rates, as well as a high rate of recurrence. A conservative approach with medical treatment is generally preferred, and lifelong anticoagulation is recommended in patients after valve surgery.[7,8]

Please access ExpertConsult to view the corresponding video for this chapter.

REFERENCES

1. Harris EN, Gharavi AE, Boey ML, et al. Anticardiolipin antibodies: detection by radioimmunoassay and association with thrombosis in systemic lupus erythematosus. *Lancet.* 1983;2:1211–1214.
2. Wilson WA, Gharavi AE, Koike T, et al. International consensus statement on preliminary classification criteria for definite antiphospholipid syndrome: report of an international workshop. *Arthritis Rheum.* 1999;42:1309–1311.
3. Miyakis S, Lockshin MD, Atsumi T, et al. International consensus statement on an update of the classification criteria for definite antiphospholipid syndrome (APS). *J Thromb Haemost.* 2006;4:295–306.
4. Gleason CB, Stoddard MF, Wagner SG, et al. A comparison of cardiac valvular involvement in the primary antiphospholipid syndrome versus anticardiolipin-negative systemic lupus erythematosus. *Am Heart J.* 1993;125:1123–1129.
5. Zuily S, Regnault V, Selton-Suty C, et al. Increased risk for heart valve disease associated with antiphospholipid antibodies in patients with systemic lupus erythematosus: meta-analysis of echocardiographic studies. *Circulation.* 2011;124:215–224.
6. Vianna JL, Khamashta MA, Ordi-Ros J, et al. Comparison of the primary and secondary antiphospholipid syndrome: a European multicenter study of 114 patients. *Am J Med.* 1994;96:3–9.
7. George D, Erkan D. Antiphospholipid syndrome. *Prog Cardiovasc Dis.* 2009;52(2):115–125.
8. Ruiz-Irastorza G, Crowther M, Branch W, Khamashta MA. Antiphospholipid syndrome. *Lancet.* 2010;376:1498–1509.
9. Lazzaroni MG, Fredi M, Andreoli L, et al. Triple antiphospholipid (aPL) antibodies positivity is associated with pregnancy complications in aPL carriers: a multicenter study on 62 pregnancies. *Front Immunol.* 1948;10:2019.
10. Brenner B, Blumenfeld Z, Markiewicz W, Reisner SA. Cardiac involvement in patients with primary antiphospholipid syndrome. *J Am Coll Cardiol.* 1991;18:931–936.
11. Cervera R, Khamashta MA, Font J, et al. High prevalence of significant heart valve lesions in patients with the "primary" antiphospholipid syndrome. *Lupus.* 1991;1:43–47.
12. Galve E, Ordi J, Barquinero J, et al. Valvular heart disease in the primary antiphospholipid syndrome. *Ann Intern Med.* 1992;11:293–298.
13. Hojnik M, George J, Ziporen L, Shoenfeld Y. Heart valve involvement (Libman-Sacks endocarditis) in the antiphospholipid syndrome. *Circulation.* 1996;93:1579–1587.

14. Tenedios F, Erkan D, Lockshin MD. Cardiac involvement in the antiphospholipid syndrome. *Lupus.* 2005;14:691–696.

15. Reisner SA, Brenner B, Haim N, et al. Echocardiography in nonbacterial thrombotic endocarditis: from autopsy to clinical entity. *J Am Soc Echocardiogr.* 2000;13:876–881.

16. Qaddoura F, Connolly H, Grogan M, et al. Valve morphology in antiphospholipid antibody syndrome: echocardiographic features. *Echocardiography.* 2005;22:255–259.

17. Silbiger JJ. The cardiac manifestations of antiphospholipid syndrome and their echocardiographic recognition. *J Am Soc Echocardiogr.* 2009;22:1100–1108.

18. Murphy JC, Bhindi R, Ward M. An unusual cause of embolic myocardial infarction. *Eur Heart J.* 2012;33:960.

19. Sacré K, Brihaye B, Hyafil F, et al. Asymptomatic myocardial ischemic disease in antiphospholipid syndrome: a controlled cardiac magnetic resonance imaging study. *Arthritis Rheum.* 2010;62:2093–2100.

20. Abanador-Kamper N, Wolfertz J, et al. Disseminated intracardiac thrombosis: a rare manifestation of antiphospholipid syndrome. *Eur Heart J Cardiovasc Imag.* 2012;13:537.

21. Ames PRJ, Margarita A, Alves JD. Antiphospholipid antibodies and atherosclerosis: insights from systemic lupus erythematosus and primary antiphospholipid syndrome. *Clin Rev Allergy Immunol.* 2009;37:29–35.

22. Turiel M, Muzzupappa S, Gottardi B, et al. Evaluation of cardiac abnormalities and embolic sources in primary antiphospholipid syndrome by transesophageal echocardiography. *Lupus.* 2000;9:406–412.

23. Uthman I, Noureldine MHA, Ruiz-Irastorza G, Khamashta M. Management of antiphospholipid syndrome. *Ann Rheum Dis.* 2019;78:155–161.

24. Andrade D, Cervera R, Cohen H, et al. 15th International Congress on Antiphospholipid Antibodies task force on antiphospholipid syndrome treatment trends report. *Antiphospholipid Syndrome.* 2017:317–338.

25. Espínola-Zavaleta N, Vargas-Barrón J, Colmenares-Galvis T, et al. Echocardiographic evaluation of patients with primary antiphospholipid syndrome. *Am Heart J.* 1999;137:973–978.

26. Turiel M, Sarzi-Puttini P, Peretti R, et al. Five-year follow-up by transesophageal echocardiographic studies in primary antiphospholipid syndrome. *Am J Cardiol.* 2005;96:574–579.

152 Carcinoid Heart Disease

Fei Fei Gong, Vera H. Rigolin

Carcinoid tumors are rare neuroendocrine tumors that secrete vasoactive compounds, including serotonin.[1] The estimated incidence of carcinoid tumors is reported between 1.0 and 8.4 per 100,000.[1] Carcinoid tumors are classified based on their embryologic site of origin: foregut (bronchus, stomach, proximal duodenum), midgut (distal duodenum, jejunum, ileum, appendix, ascending colon), and hindgut (transverse and descending colon, rectum). Midgut tumors arising from the ileum and appendix are the most common.[2–4] Carcinoid syndrome occurs in 30% to 40% of patients and results from the release of vasoactive compounds into the systemic circulation, leading to intermittent episodes of flushing, diarrhea, bronchospasm, and hypotension.[5] Up to two-thirds of patients with carcinoid syndrome develop carcinoid heart disease, and carcinoid heart disease may also be the presenting problem in up to 20% of patients with carcinoid tumors.[1,6]

CARCINOID HEART DISEASE

The pathogenesis of carcinoid heart disease remains poorly understood, but vasoactive substances secreted by neuroendocrine cells, including serotonin, prostaglandins, histamine, and bradykinin, are believed to play an important role.[5] In particular, plasma serotonin levels and urine levels of the primary serotonin metabolite 5-hydroxyindoleacetic acid (5-HIAA) are higher in patients with carcinoid heart disease.[7,8] Urine 5-HIAA level of 300 μmol/24 hours or greater is an independent predictor of the development or progression of carcinoid heart disease.[9] Most patients with carcinoid heart disease have liver metastases whose vasoactive compounds reach the heart and systemic circulation via the hepatic vein. However, patients with primary ovarian carcinoid can also develop cardiac involvement in the absence of liver metastases because these compounds can drain directly into the inferior vena cava.[6,10]

Typical cardiac lesions are described as fibrous, plaquelike areas of endocardial thickening that deposit most commonly on the surface of valve leaflets but may also affect the subvalvular apparatus and cardiac chambers.[5,6] Right-sided valvular lesions predominate because vasoactive substances are normally inactivated in the lungs. However, left-sided lesions can be seen in up to 15% of patients and are thought to occur in the setting of right-to-left intracardiac shunts, bronchial carcinoids,

or high levels of circulating vasoactive substances.[5,6] Patients with carcinoid heart disease often present with a murmur or symptoms of right heart failure. The onset of carcinoid heart disease is a marker for increased mortality rates in patients with carcinoid tumors, who have a median survival time of 14 months.[6,8]

ECHOCARDIOGRAPHIC FEATURES OF CARCINOID HEART DISEASE

Echocardiographic features of carcinoid heart disease are well described.[8,10–12] Characteristic findings include thickening of the valves from the leaflet tip to the base, resulting in straightened and stiffened leaflets. The chordae and papillary muscles can also become thickened, shortened, or fused. These changes result in retraction and impaired coaptation, leading to a combination of both valvular regurgitation and stenosis.

The tricuspid valve is most often affected with tricuspid regurgitation the most common abnormality. In severe cases, leaflets appear "frozen" with limited motion in both systole and diastole (Fig. 152.1A and Video 152.1A). This leads to severe tricuspid regurgitation (Fig. 152.1B and Video 152.1B) with the typical "dagger-shaped" appearance of the spectral Doppler profile (Fig. 152.2) secondary to rapid pressure equilibration between the right atrium and right ventricle. Mild or moderate tricuspid stenosis may also be present, and dilatation of the right atrium and right ventricle are commonly seen. Isolated leaflet involvement has also been described, resulting in an eccentric jet of tricuspid regurgitation.

The pulmonary valve is the next most commonly affected valve (Fig. 152.3 and Video 152.3). Both pulmonary regurgitation and pulmonary stenosis may be present. Plaque deposition at the pulmonary root may restrict orifice size and be associated with poststenotic dilatation of the pulmonary artery. The use of Doppler imaging enhances detection of pulmonic valve involvement, especially if the valve is poorly visualized[8] (Fig. 152.4). The severity of pulmonary stenosis may be underestimated in the setting of severe tricuspid regurgitation owing to low cardiac output.[6] Tricuspid and pulmonary stenosis and regurgitation are graded the same as for all other causes.

Left-sided valvular lesions are far less frequent but are often associated with a patent foramen ovale. Myocardial metastases

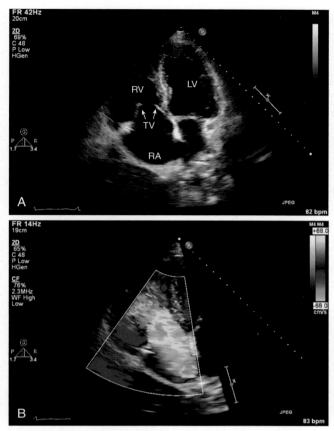

Figure 152.1. Tricuspid valve leaflets are thickened and retracted, causing failure of coaptation (**A**) and resulting in severe tricuspid regurgitation with laminar flow (**B**). *LV*, Left ventricle; *RA*, right atrium; *RV*, right ventricle; *TV*, tricuspid valve. (See accompanying Video 152.1 and video 152-1B.)

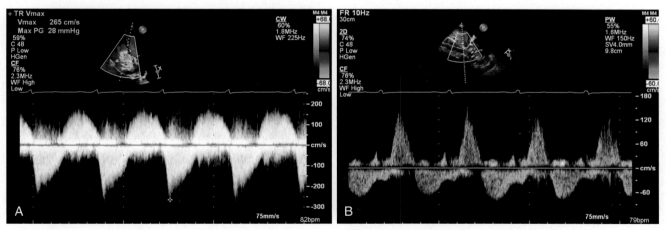

Figure 152.2. The "dagger"-shaped spectral Doppler signal (**A**) and systolic flow reversal in the hepatic vein (**B**) indicating severe tricuspid regurgitation.

occur in approximately 4% with carcinoid heart disease and can be seen both with and without valvular involvement. Recent recommendations encourage initial assessment with transthoracic echocardiography (TEE) for all patients with carcinoid syndrome with clinical features of cardiac involvement, increased B-type natriuretic peptides, or increased 5-HIAA levels, with regular echocardiographic monitoring thereafter.[5]

VALVULAR INTERVENTIONS FOR CARCINOID HEART DISEASE

Valve replacement is recommended when severe valvular dysfunction is associated with symptoms or progressive right ventricular dilatation or dysfunction,[5] and survival has improved over the past decades for patients with carcinoid heart disease who undergo earlier valve replacement.[13] The choice of surgical prosthesis requires individualization. Early concern surrounding carcinoid involvement of bioprosthetic valves led to greater use of mechanical prostheses. However, in one large series, reoperation rates and survival over approximately 4.5 years of follow-up was similar for bioprosthetic and mechanical valves.[14] This finding may be due in large part to improvements in the medical management of carcinoid heart disease. TEE should be performed early postoperatively to establish baseline valvular function and then every 3 to 12 months depending on the clinical scenario[5] (Fig. 152.5 and Video 152-5A-5B).

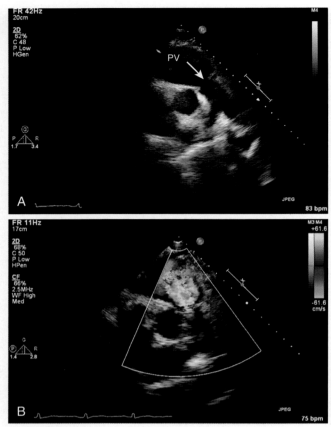

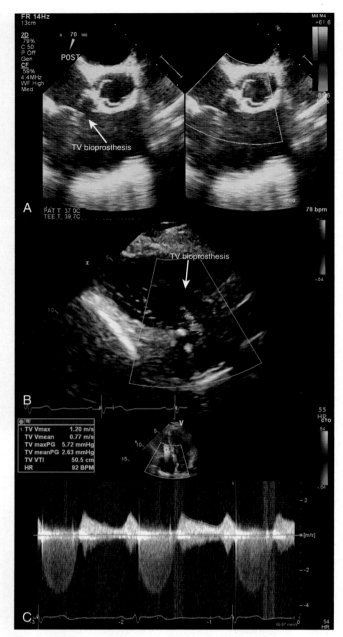

Figure 152.3. Carcinoid heart disease affecting the pulmonary valve leading to poor leaflet coaptation (**A**) and severe pulmonary regurgitation (**B**). *PV*, Pulmonary valve. (See accompanying videos 152-3A and 3B.)

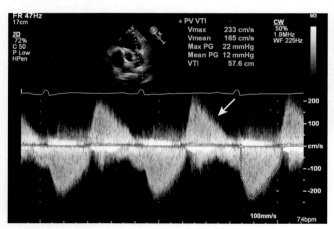

Figure 152.4. Spectral Doppler signal of the patient in Fig. 152.3 with pulmonary valve involvement. There are mild pulmonary stenosis with a mean transpulmonary gradient of 12 mm Hg and a short pulmonary regurgitation deceleration time *(arrow)*, indicating significant pulmonary regurgitation.

Figure 152.5. Intraoperative transesophageal echocardiogram after a bioprosthetic tricuspid valve (TV) replacement (**A**) showing trivial tricuspid regurgitation. A transthoracic echocardiogram of the same patient 3 years later showing a well-seated bioprosthesis with mild tricuspid regurgitation (**B**) and a mean gradient of 2.6 mm Hg (**C**). (See accompanying videos 152-5A and 5B.)

Transcatheter techniques have also been used to treat patients deemed at high surgical risk, including transcatheter pulmonary valve replacement[15–17] and pulmonary and tricuspid valve-in-valve replacement for bioprosthetic valve degeneration.[18] Balloon valvuloplasty may also be an option for patients with symptoms of pulmonic stenosis and elevated right-sided heart pressures to palliate symptoms and decrease the severity of tricuspid regurgitation and right-sided pressures. Balloon valvuloplasty has been reported to be successful in a handful of cases.[19,20]

SUMMARY

Carcinoid heart disease is characterized by fibrous, plaquelike areas of endocardial thickening that affect valve leaflets as well as the subvalvular apparatus and mural endocardium. Tricuspid and pulmonary valve involvement are most common, with leaflet thickening and retraction contributing to malcoaptation and the development of both valvular regurgitation and stenosis. Valvular replacement is recommended upon development of heart failure symptoms or progressive right heart enlargement or dysfunction. Echocardiography is integral in the diagnosis of cardiac involvement in patients with carcinoid syndrome and the serial monitoring of patients both before and after valvular replacement.

Please access ExpertConsult to view the corresponding videos for this chapter.

REFERENCES

1. Kulke MH, Mayer RJ. Carcinoid tumors. *N Engl J Med*. 1999;340:858–868.
2. Anderson AS, Krauss D, Lang R. Cardiovascular complications of malignant carcinoid disease. *Am Heart J*. 1997;134:693–702.
3. Yao JC, Hassan M, Phan A, et al. One hundred years after "carcinoid": epidemiology of and prognostic factors for neuroendocrine tumors in 35,825 cases in the United States. *J Clin Oncol*. 2008;26:3063–3072.
4. Luis SA, Pellikka PA. Carcinoid heart disease: diagnosis and management. *Best Pract Res Clin Endocrinol Metab*. 2016;30:149–158.
5. Davar J, Connolly HM, Caplin ME, et al. Diagnosing and managing carcinoid heart disease in patients with neuroendocrine tumors: an expert statement. *J Am Coll Cardiol*. 2017;69:1288–1304.
6. Bhattacharyya S, Davar J, Dreyfus G, et al. Carcinoid heart disease. *Circulation*. 2007;116:2860–2865.
7. Robiolio PA, Rigolin VH, Wilson JS, et al. Carcinoid heart disease: correlation of high serotonin levels with valvular abnormalities detected by cardiac catheterization and echocardiography. *Circulation*. 1995;92:790–795.
8. Pellikka PA, Tajik AJ, Khandheria BK, et al. Carcinoid heart disease: clinical and echocardiographic spectrum in 74 patients. *Circulation*. 1993;87:1188–1196.
9. Bhattacharyya S, Toumpanakis C, Chilkunda D, et al. Risk factors for the development and progression of carcinoid heart disease. *Am J Cardiol*. 2011;107:1221–1226.
10. Howard RJ, Drobac M, Rider WD, et al. Carcinoid heart disease: diagnosis by two-dimensional echocardiography. *Circulation*. 1982;66:1059–1065.
11. Bhattacharyya S, Toumpanakis C, Burke M, et al. Features of carcinoid heart disease identified by 2- and 3-dimensional echocardiography and cardiac MRI. *Circ Cardiovasc Imag*. 2010;3:103–111.
12. Roberts WC. A unique heart disease associated with a unique cancer: carcinoid heart disease. *Am J Cardiol*. 1997;80:251–256.
13. Moller JE, Pellikka PA, Bernheim AM, et al. Prognosis of carcinoid heart disease: analysis of 200 cases over two decades. *Circulation*. 2005;112:3320–3327.
14. Connolly HM, Schaff HV, Abel MD, et al. Early and late outcomes of surgical treatment in carcinoid heart disease. *J Am Coll Cardiol*. 2015;66:2189–2196.
15. Heidecker B, Moore P, Bergsland EK, et al. Transcatheter pulmonic valve replacement in carcinoid heart disease. *Eur Heart J Cardiovasc Imag*. 2015;16:1046.
16. Loyalka P, Schechter M, Nascimbene A, et al. Transcatheter pulmonary valve replacement in a carcinoid heart. *Tex Heart Inst J*. 2016;43:341–344.
17. Kesarwani M, Ports TA, Rao RK, et al. First-in-human transcatheter pulmonic valve implantation through a tricuspid valve bioprosthesis to treat native pulmonary valve regurgitation caused by carcinoid syndrome. *JACC Cardiovasc Interv*. 2015;8:e161–e163.
18. Khan JN, Doshi SN, Rooney SJ, et al. Transcatheter pulmonary and tricuspid valve-in-valve replacement for bioprosthesis degeneration in carcinoid heart disease. *Eur Heart J Cardiovasc Imag*. 2016;17:114.
19. Obel O, Coltart DJ, Signy M. Balloon pulmonary valvuloplasty in carcinoid syndrome. *Heart*. 2000;84:E13.
20. Carrilho-Ferreira P, Silva D, Almeida AG, et al. Carcinoid heart disease: outcome after balloon pulmonary valvuloplasty. *Can J Cardiol*. 2013;29:751. e7–9.

153 Amyloid

Revathi Balakrishnan, Muhamed Saric

The term *amyloidosis* (from Greek ἄμυλον: *amylon*, starch) was popularized in the 19th century by the German pathologist Rudolf Virchow because of amyloid's affinity for staining dyes with starch.[1] It is clearly a misnomer because amyloid deposits are made of protein and not starch. In general, amyloidosis entails typically extracellular infiltration by one of a variety of misfolded proteins, which all share the same β-pleated sheet configuration.[2] This misfolded protein configuration is visualized as apple-green birefringence under polarized light when tissue specimens are stained with Congo red.[3] Several dozen proteins have been shown to be amyloidogenic. Amyloidosis is a multiorgan disorder; the degree of myocardial involvement varies because amyloidogenic proteins are not equally cardiotropic.

Amyloid light-chain (AL) amyloidosis is the most common form of amyloidosis. It results from accumulation of clonal immunoglobulin light-chain deposits in multiple myeloma and similar disorders.[4] Only 10% to 15% of patients with multiple myeloma develop AL amyloidosis.[5] Cardiac involvement occurs in up to half of patients with AL amyloidosis, and half of these patients will develop restrictive, nondilated cardiomyopathy.[6] Only 5% of patients with AL amyloidosis present with isolated cardiac disease without other signs of systemic involvement.[7]

Amyloid A (AA) amyloidosis is the result of deposition of serum AA protein in patients with chronic inflammatory disorders, such as rheumatoid arthritis or inflammatory bowel disease. It primarily affects the kidneys, and rarely, the heart.[8]

Amyloidosis-related to transthyretin (TTR) deposits takes two forms: hereditary familial systemic amyloidosis and senile systemic amyloidosis.

Hereditary familial systemic TTR amyloidosis is caused by autosomal dominant mutations in the TTR gene.[9] Peripheral neuropathy and autonomic dysfunction are primary manifestations;

cardiac involvement is less aggressive than that in AL disease. Isolated cardiac involvement of familial amyloidosis is associated with a mutation in the isoleucine 122 location.[10]

Senile systemic TTR amyloidosis is an age-related, slowly progressive form caused by deposition of amyloid derived from wild-type TTR. It primarily manifests as cardiac amyloidosis but can also occur in multiple organ systems, including the brain, lung, liver, and kidney. It is less aggressive than AL amyloid.[11]

OTHER AMYLOIDOGENIC PROTEINS

Other forms of cardiac amyloidosis include isolated atrial amyloidosis (caused by endocardial deposition of atrial natriuretic peptide)[4] and hemodialysis-related amyloidosis (caused by the accumulation of β2-microglobulin in the setting of chronic uremia).[12]

CLINICAL PRESENTATION

Cardiac amyloidosis is often first suspected as a discordant combination of a markedly increased left ventricular (LV) wall thickness on cardiac imaging (e.g., echocardiography) and the absence of electrocardiographic voltage criteria for LV hypertrophy (Fig. 153.1 and Video 153.1A). In advanced amyloidosis, the electrocardiogram may even demonstrate low QRS voltage (≤0.5 mV in limb leads and ≤1.0 mV in precordial leads). Cardiac magnetic resonance imaging demonstrates characteristic diffuse, predominantly subendocardial enhancement on delayed images. This late enhancement may reflect fibrosis rather than amyloid deposition per se.[13] The diagnosis of amyloidosis is confirmed by tissue biopsy, which is typically fat pad or endomyocardial biopsy (Fig. 153.2).

Figure 153.1. Echocardiographic and electrocardiographic appearance of amyloidosis. Note the apparent discordance between marked thickening of the left ventricular walls on transthoracic echocardiogram in the parasternal long-axis view (**A**) and the low QRS voltage on the electrocardiogram (**B**). (See accompanying Video 153.1A.) *LA,* Left atrium; *LV,* left ventricle; *RV,* right ventricle.

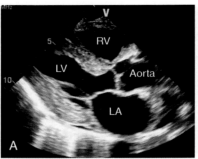
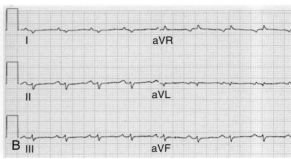

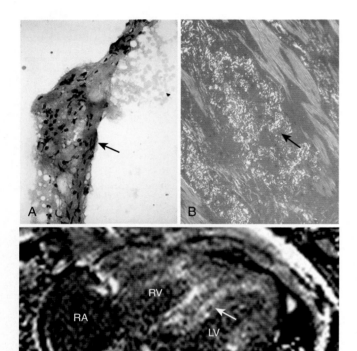

Figure 153.2. Histopathology and magnetic resonance imaging (MRI) of amyloidosis. Congo red–stained tissue samples demonstrating amyloid deposits *(arrows)* in a fat pad biopsy specimen (**A**) and the myocardium (**B**). Note in **B** the extracellular location of amyloid deposits between myofibrils. **C,** Cardiac MRI–delayed images demonstrate diffuse late gadolinium enhancement throughout the left and right ventricles (RVs) consistent with amyloidosis. The deposits are predominantly subendocardial *(arrow)*. *LA,* Left atrium; *LV,* left ventricle; *RA,* right atrium. (Courtesy of Dr. Robert Donnino, New York University Division of Cardiology and Veterans Administration New York Harbor Healthcare System.)

ECHOCARDIOGRAPHIC FEATURES
Structural Changes

Concentric wall thickening of a nondilated left ventricle in the absence of hypertension, aortic stenosis, or other known causes of apparent LV hypertrophy is the hallmark of cardiac amyloidosis.[14,15] In the early era of two-dimensional (2D) echocardiography, when only fundamental (nonharmonic) imaging was available, granular sparkling of the myocardium was reported to be suggestive of cardiac amyloidosis.[16] Modern harmonic 2D imaging often gives a speckled appearance to the myocardium, even in the absence of amyloidosis. Switching from harmonic to fundamental imaging can help avoid overdiagnosis of amyloidosis. An increase in the thickness of the right ventricular wall, interatrial septum, and the atria; biatrial enlargement; thickened valves; and pericardial and pleural effusions are also common findings.

Functional Changes

Cardiac amyloidosis typically presents as heart failure with a preserved left ventricular ejection fraction (LVEF). LV diastolic dysfunction is the predominant feature and eventually progresses to restrictive cardiomyopathy (Fig. 153.3). Although LVEF is preserved until terminal stages of the disease, subtle systolic dysfunction is detectable early on by strain imaging (Fig. 153.4 and Video 153.4).

Mitral Tissue Doppler

Pulsed-wave tissue Doppler velocity measured at the septal annulus and lateral mitral annulus in the apical views reflects the longitudinal excursion of the mitral annulus in systole and diastole and can provide evidence of systolic and diastolic impairment in the presence of a preserved ejection fraction.[13] Normal values of tissue Doppler velocity at the septal and lateral mitral annulus typically decrease with age. For instance, at 60 years of age or older, normal early diastolic (e′) wave values are 10.4 ± 2.1 cm/s at the septal annulus and 12.9 ± 3.5 cm/s at the lateral annulus.[13] In cardiac amyloidosis, very low e′ velocities are frequently seen; these velocities are typically less than 8 cm/s (see Fig. 153.3A). Furthermore, the ratio of early diastolic (e′) to late diastolic (a′) mitral annular tissue Doppler velocity (e′/a′ ratio) progressively diminishes as cardiac amyloidosis advances.

Mitral Inflow Pattern

With disease progression, the mitral inflow filling pattern progresses from impaired relaxation early on to the pseudonormal and restrictive filling pattern seen in advanced disease. Initially, isovolumic relaxation is impaired with an increased dependence on atrial contraction, which results in an impaired relaxation pattern with a decreased early diastolic flow across the mitral valve (E wave) relative to the atrial (A) wave (E/A ratio <1 and e′/a′ <1). As myocardial infiltration progresses, LV wall compliance decreases, and left atrial pressures increases; this initially leads to a pseudonormal inflow pattern (1 <E/A <2 with e′/a′ <1) and then to a restrictive inflow pattern with E/A greater than 2, E-wave deceleration time less than 150 ms, and a very low e′ (see Fig. 153.3B).[17]

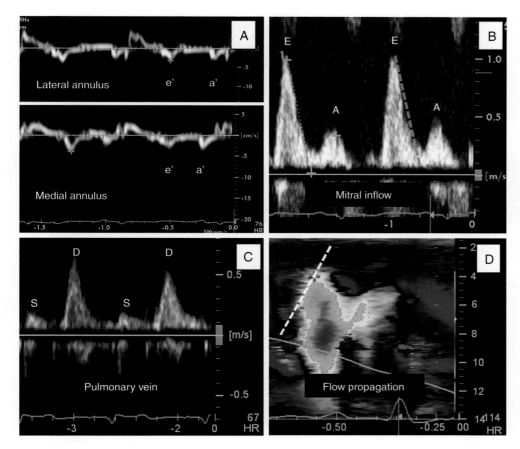

Figure 153.3. Diastolic dysfunction in amyloidosis. **A,** Tissue Doppler imaging at both the lateral and medial (septal) annulus demonstrates very low e′ velocities (<5 cm/s). **B,** Mitral inflow demonstrates a restrictive filling pattern: E/A greater than 2 and rapid E-wave deceleration (<150 ms; *dashed line*). **C,** Pulmonary vein flow velocity pattern demonstrates an S/D less than one pattern, which is indicative of elevated left atrial pressure. **D,** In this patient, mitral flow propagation velocity recording demonstrates paradoxically normal slope of the first aliasing velocity (*dashed line*) of 55 cm/s. A normal slope of the first aliasing velocity does not exclude the diagnosis of amyloidosis.

Elevated mid-diastolic flow (>20 cm/s) can also be indicative of elevated left atrial pressure and advanced diastolic dysfunction.[18] In contrast to constrictive pericarditis, there are no marked respiratory variations in peak mitral E-wave velocities in patients with cardiac amyloidosis.

Pulmonary Vein Pattern

In a patient with sinus rhythm, pulmonary venous flow demonstrates two anterograde (systolic [S] and diastolic [D]) and one retrograde (atrial reversal [AR]) waves. In general, the peak velocity of the S wave is influenced by changes in left atrial pressure, contraction, and relaxation, whereas the D wave is influenced by changes in LV compliance; D wave changes occur in parallel with the mitral E wave.[16] As filling pressures rise with progression of cardiac amyloidosis, the S velocity decreases, and the D velocity increases, which results in a S/D ratio less than 1 (see Fig. 153.3C). As LV diastolic pressure increases, peak velocity and duration of the AR wave tend to increase. LV diastolic pressure is likely elevated whenever the AR wave outlasts the mitral A wave by at least 30 ms.[19] In atrial fibrillation, which frequently accompanies cardiac amyloidosis, there is a loss of the AR wave, and the peak velocity of the S wave diminishes even if the left atrial pressure is normal.

Mitral Flow Propagation

Early diastolic flow propagation velocity from the mitral valve to the cardiac apex reflects the relaxing properties of the left ventricle, especially when the left ventricle is dilated. Color M-mode images are acquired in the apical four-chamber view, with the M-mode scan through the center of the left ventricle and the color Nyquist limit set to approximately 40 cm/s. The slope of the first aliasing velocity (Vp) in early diastole is then measured.[16] The normal Vp is more than 50 cm/s. Because of the presence of abnormal relaxation in cardiac amyloidosis, it is expected that the Vp would be diminished. Nonetheless, patients with amyloidosis often have a normal Vp, likely because the LV cavity size is normal (see Fig. 153.3D).

Left Ventricular Strain Imaging

On strain imaging, amyloidosis is characterized by diminished longitudinal strain in the basal and mid-LV segments with characteristic apical sparing ("cherry-on-top phenomenon"; Fig. 153.4 and Video 153.4). The loss of global longitudinal function occurs because amyloid fibrils deposit predominantly in the subendocardial region, which is primarily responsible for longitudinal deformation. The normal range of global longitudinal peak systolic strain[20] is below −18 ± 2%; patients with amyloidosis typically have peak longitudinal strain values above −12%. The loss of longitudinal function occurs early in the course of amyloidosis and reflects systolic dysfunction despite preserved LVEF and fractional shortening.[2] The exact mechanism for apical sparing is yet to be fully elucidated. Nonetheless, apical sparing has been shown to be both sensitive (93%) and specific (82%) for the diagnosis of amyloidosis compared with other disorders with increased LV wall thickness, such as hypertrophic cardiomyopathy and aortic stenosis.[21]

Please access ExpertConsult to view the corresponding videos for this chapter.

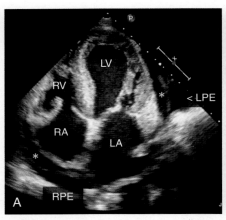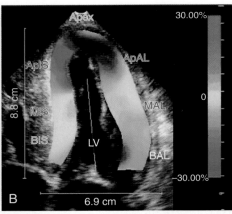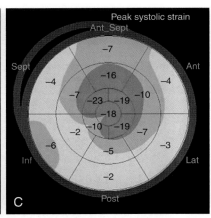

Figure 153.4. Two-dimensional echocardiography and strain imaging of amyloidosis. **A,** Transthoracic echocardiogram in the apical four-chamber view demonstrates typical features of amyloidosis: increased left ventricular and right ventricular wall thickness, biatrial enlargement, thickened valves *(arrow)*, pericardial effusion *(asterisk)*, and pleural effusions. **B** and **C,** Speckle-based longitudinal strain imaging demonstrates the phenomenon of apical sparing (relative preservation of apical longitudinal strain in the setting of otherwise decreased left ventricular longitudinal strain). Global longitudinal strain in this patient was diminished to −10%. *Ant,* Anterior; *ApAL,* pical anterolateral segment; *ApIS,* apical inferior septal segment; *BAL,* basal anterolateral segment; *BIS,* basal inferoseptal segment; *Inf,* inferior; *LA,* left atrium; *Lat,* lateral; *LPE,* left pleural effusion; *LV,* left ventricle; *MIS,* mid inferoseptal segment; *Post,* posterior; *RA,* right atrium; *RA,* right ventricle; *RPE,* right pleural effusion; *Sept,* septal. (See accompanying Video 153.4.)

REFERENCES

1. Virchow R. Zur Cellulose-Frage. *Virchows Arch Pathol Anat.* 1854;6:416–426.
2. Desai HV, Aronow WS, Peterson SJ, et al. Cardiac amyloidosis: approaches to diagnosis and management. *Cardiol Rev.* 2010;18:1–11.
3. Kyle RA. Amyloidosis: a convoluted story. *Br J Haematol.* 2001;114:529–538.
4. Sedaghat D, Zakir RM, Cohen J, et al. Multiple myeloma and the heart: a long-distance relationship. *J Clin Ultrasound.* 2009;37:179–184.
5. Kyle RA, Gertz MA. Primary systemic amyloidosis: clinical and laboratory features in 474 cases. *Semin Hematol.* 1995;32:45–59.
6. Falk RH. Diagnosis and management of the cardiac amyloidosis. *Circulation.* 2005;112:2047–2060.
7. Dubrey SW, Cha K, Anderson J, et al. The clinical features of immunoglobulin light-chain (AL) amyloidosis with heart involvement. *Q J Med.* 1998;91:141–157.
8. Gillmore JD, Lovat LB, Persey MR, et al. Amyloid load and clinical outcome in AA amyloidosis in relation to circulating concentration of serum amyloid A protein. *Lancet.* 2001;358:24–29.
9. Lachmann HJ, Booth DR, Booth SE, et al. Misdiagnosis of hereditary amyloidosis as AL (primary) amyloidosis. *N Engl J Med.* 2002;346:1786–1791.
10. Jacobson DR, Pastore R, Pool S, et al. Revised transthyretin Ile 122 allele frequency in African-Americans. *Hum Genet.* 1996;98:236–238.
11. Ng B, Connors LH, Davidoff R, et al. Senile systemic amyloidosis presenting with heart failure: a comparison with light chain-associated amyloidosis. *Arch Intern Med.* 2005;165:1425–1429.
12. Gal R, Korzets A, Schwartz A, et al. Systemic distribution of beta 2-microglobulin-derived amyloidosis in patients who undergo long-term hemodialysis. Report of seven cases and review of the literature. *Arch Pathol Lab Med.* 1994;118:718–721.
13. Hosch W1, Kristen AV, Libicher M, et al. Late enhancement in cardiac amyloidosis: correlation of MRI enhancement pattern with histopathological findings. *Amyloid.* 2008;15:196–204.
14. Rahman JE, Helou EF, Gelzer-Bell R, et al. Noninvasive diagnosis of biopsy-proven cardiac amyloidosis. *J Am Coll Cardiol.* 2004;43:410–415.
15. Sokol I, Vincelj J, Saric M. Echocardiographic assessment of diagnosis and prognosis of biopsy-proven amyloid cardiomyopathy. *Med Arh.* 2005;59:388–390.
16. Siqueira-Filho AG, Cunha CL, Tajik AJ, et al. M-mode and two-dimensional echocardiographic features in cardiac amyloidosis. *Circulation.* 1981;63:188–196.
17. Nagueh SF, Appleton CP, Gillebert TC, et al. Recommendations for the evaluation of left ventricular diastolic function by echocardiography. *J Am Soc Echocardiogr.* 2009;22:107–133.
18. Ha JW, Oh JK, Redfield MM, et al. Triphasic mitral inflow velocity with mid-diastolic filling: clinical implications and associated echocardiographic findings. *J Am Soc Echocardiogr.* 2004;17:428–431.
19. Abdalla I, Murray RD, Lee JC, et al. Duration of pulmonary venous atrial reversal flow velocity and mitral inflow a wave: a new measure of severity of cardiac amyloidosis. *J Am Soc Echocardiogr.* 1998;11:1125–1133.
20. Mor-Avi V, Lang RM, Badano LP, et al. Current and evolving echocardiographic techniques for the quantitative evaluation of cardiac mechanics. *J Am Soc Echocardiogr.* 2011;24:277–313.
21. Phelan D, Collier P, Thavendiranathan P, et al. Relative apical sparing of longitudinal strain using two-dimensional speckle-tracking echocardiography is both sensitive and specific for the diagnosis of cardiac amyloidosis. *Heart.* 2012;98:1442–1448.

154 Sarcoidosis

Hena N. Patel, Amit R. Patel

Sarcoidosis is a systemic inflammatory disorder characterized by the formation of noncaseating granulomas in multiple organs.[1] Although its cause remains uncertain, accumulating evidence suggests that it is caused by an immunologic response to an unidentified antigenic trigger in genetically susceptible individuals.[2] The annual incidence of sarcoidosis has been estimated at 5 to 40 cases per 100,000 in the United States and Europe with a threefold higher risk in blacks than in whites, particularly in women.[1,3] Although the disease can occur at any age, it is most common in individuals between 25 to 60 years of age.[3] The lungs, skin, and eyes are most commonly affected; however, the disease can also involve the liver, spleen, parotid gland, and heart.

Cardiac sarcoidosis (CS) affects at least one-quarter of patients, portends a worse prognosis, and accounts for significant mortality and morbidity from this disease.[4,5] Granulomatous infiltration into the basal interventricular septum can result in conduction abnormalities such as advanced atrioventricular block and bundle branch block. Similarly, regions of prior infiltration are thought to evolve into scar formation that serves as a substrate for reentrant ventricular tachycardia[6] and atrial arrhythmias.[7] Cardiac involvement in sarcoidosis is associated with an increased risk of life-threatening arrhythmias and death, even if the involvement is not clinically manifested.[8,9] Absence of extracardiac sarcoidosis does not exclude isolated CS.[5]

The clinical presentation of CS can be diverse, ranging from asymptomatic to palpitations or syncope from conduction abnormalities and atrial or ventricular arrhythmias, symptomatic heart failure, and sudden cardiac death.[10,11] Identifying patients with CS is of importance, as treatment with glucocorticoids may slow the progression of heart failure and implantable cardioverter-defibrillators may improve survival.[12]

However, cardiac involvement can be difficult to detect because CS is a patchy disease that often involves only small amounts of the myocardium without causing obvious abnormalities in left ventricular (LV) function.[6] Electrocardiography has an estimated sensitivity of 33% to 58% and a specificity of 22% to 71%.[13,14] Ambulatory Holter monitoring carries a sensitivity of 50% to 67% and a specificity of 80% to 97%.[5] Cardiac biopsies are highly specific but have a sensitivity of only 20% to 30% for detecting CS because of myocardial sampling errors related to the patchy nature of granuloma infiltration into the myocardium.[15]

The diagnosis of CS often uses clinical criteria, such as the Japanese Ministry of Health and Welfare criteria, which were originally published in 1993 and later modified in 2007. More recently, the Heart Rhythm Society published an expert consensus statement in which cardiac magnetic resonance imaging (CMRI) and positron emission tomography (PET) play an integral role in the diagnosis and management of patients with suspected CS.[16] Current approaches utilize both clinical criteria and imaging to estimate the likelihood of CS rather than providing a definitive diagnosis. In addition, imaging can be used to identify patients who may require additional treatments, such as immunosuppressive therapies, and to follow response to therapy.

ECHOCARDIOGRAPHIC FINDINGS OF CARDIAC SARCOIDOSIS

Transthoracic echocardiography (TTE) is a valuable, widely available modality that often provides the first suspicion for CS in a diagnostic workup.[5,17] Expected findings in an affected heart are reduced LV ejection fraction, LV dilatation, focal basal septal wall thinning, wall motion abnormalities, diastolic dysfunction, right ventricular (RV) involvement, pericardial effusion, and valvular disease. Although there is no one pathognomonic echocardiographic finding, several echocardiographic changes may raise suspicion for CS.

Regions of the heart with the greatest predilection for granulomatous deposition include the interventricular septum, particularly the basal portion, as well as the basal LV posterior wall, the LV free wall, and the papillary muscles.[9,18] Atrial involvement has also been reported to be present in 20% of cases. The cardiac manifestations are variable and can include overall normal LV systolic function, globally hypokinetic systolic dysfunction, dilated or restrictive cardiomyopathy, or regional wall motion abnormalities in a noncoronary pattern. The most characteristic findings on echocardiography are thinning or scarring of the basal portion of the interventricular septum, with associated focal akinesia of that area (Fig. 154.1). Bright echogenicity of the LV may reflect granulomatous inflammation and scarring, especially in the intraventricular septum and free wall. Regional wall thickening secondary to edema or granulomatous infiltration may be present and can mimic LV hypertrophy.[19] Wall motion abnormalities in a noncoronary distribution are also characteristic of CS.[8] Scar and edema in the conduction system may occur and can lead to severe arrhythmias. Of note, the visual extent of myocardial involvement has not been shown to consistently correlate with prognosis.[12]

LV diastolic dysfunction is frequently seen with CS. Increased LV stiffening from chronic myocardial inflammation leads to diastolic dysfunction, starting with impaired relaxation and progressing to restrictive LV filling over time. However, diastolic dysfunction is not sensitive or specific enough to reliably detect cardiac involvement with sarcoidosis. In fact, diastolic dysfunction has been reported to be present in 14% to 33% of individuals with sarcoidosis in the absence of cardiac involvement.[8,20] Others have suggested that diastolic dysfunction is present in the majority of patients with extracardiac sarcoidosis and may be related to aging rather than the presence of CS.[21]

Aneurysms, particularly at the inferolateral LV wall, are also common. Ventricular aneurysms are reported to occur in 10% of patients with CS[22] and more commonly are found in the septal and anterior wall segments. Ventricular aneurysms are of significance for a couple of reasons. They have the ability to be arrhythmogenic because they are associated with frequent arrhythmias, which may resolve after resection of the aneurysm. In addition, an intraventricular thrombus can develop in up to 17% of patients with severely reduced ventricular function and ventricular aneurysm, most commonly arising along the inferior wall.[23] Contrast-echocardiography can enhance the visibility of aneurysmal deformities.

Isolated RV involvement is rare and can be difficult to identify by TTE. Granulomatous inflammation can lead to global RV

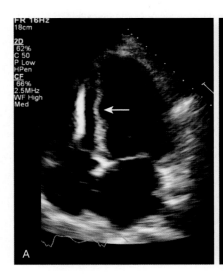 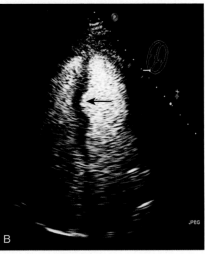

Figure 154.1. A, Apical four-chamber view with an aneurysmal *(arrow)* segment in the midinterventricular septum. **B,** The same view after opacification with microbubble contrast. The *arrow* indicates the aneurysmal segment.

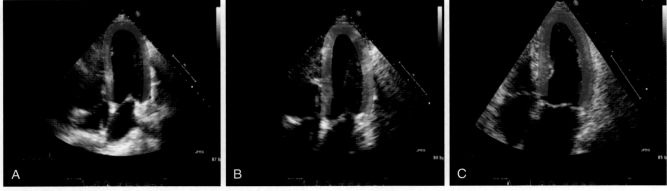

Figure 154.2. Apical four-chamber views color coded for longitudinal strain are shown for three individuals. Segments with normal longitudinal strain are *blue*, and segments with reduced longitudinal strain are encoded in *red* or *white*. **A** and **B,** Images acquired from individuals with cardiac sarcoidosis. **C,** An image from an individual with extracardiac sarcoidosis without cardiac involvement.

systolic dysfunction or wall motion abnormalities of any portion of the RV.[24] Echocardiographic features of right-sided CS can also mimic arrhythmogenic RV cardiomyopathy.[25] More commonly, RV involvement occurs secondary to LV dysfunction or comorbid lung disease resulting in elevated right-sided pressures, including pulmonary hypertension (PH) and RV enlargement.[25]

PH is a complication of sarcoidosis and is associated with increased mortality rate with or without cardiac involvement. The prevalence of PH in patients with CS has ranged from 6% in outpatients to 74% in patients referred for lung transplant and may be secondary to LV dysfunction or pulmonary involvement.[22] However, PH can be difficult to estimate by echocardiography, particularly when the tricuspid regurgitation signal is poor, and invasive assessment with right heart catherization may be needed to estimate right-sided pressures in dyspneic patients.

Valvular disease in CS patients can also be detected by echocardiography. Direct valvular involvement by CS is rare; however, sarcoid infiltration of the papillary muscles can lead to papillary dysfunction with secondary valvular abnormality such as mitral regurgitation or prolapse.[22] Mitral regurgitation can also develop secondary to LV dilatation.[23]

Pericardial involvement of CS is rare and present in less than 10% of patients. It usually presents as an asymptomatic pericardial effusion. Small pericardial effusions are seen in about 20% of patients with CS[22]; however, significant pericardial effusion has been reported in 2% to 8% of patients at autopsy. These effusions are usually not hemodynamically significant, but cases of cardiac tamponade have been observed as the initial manifestation of CS.[23] Constrictive pericarditis is also rare, but there are several reports of granulomatous infiltration of the pericardium requiring pericardiectomy.[26] Symptomatic patients require careful assessment of the echocardiographic features of these processes.

NOVEL ECHOCARDIOGRAPHIC TECHNIQUES FOR THE DETECTION OF CARDIAC SARCOIDOSIS

Myocardial strain imaging is an established advanced echocardiography technique that has the potential to identify subtle myocardial changes from granulomatous infiltration without the influence of tethering and translation and improve the detection of CS[27] (Fig. 154.2). An increased detection rate of subclinical CS has been reported with the use of global longitudinal strain (GLS) analysis even in asymptomatic patients.[27] Several retrospective echocardiography studies of asymptomatic sarcoidosis patients without CS and preserved LV ejection fraction found reduced GLS as a strong and independent predictor of adverse cardiovascular events.[28–30] Reduced GLS in CS has been shown to correlate with

late gadolinium enhancement on CMRI.[29] Three-dimensional (3D) speckle-tracking radial strain may also be useful in distinguishing CS from dilated cardiomyopathy, although further validation is needed.[24,31] Strain imaging may also provide a method to assess response to therapy and follow patients with CS in the future. Longitudinal strain measured using either echocardiography or CMRI has been shown to improve after treatment with corticosteroid therapy despite the absence of improvement in more conventional imaging parameters.[32–34]

The role of RV strain has not yet been established but appears promising.[35] Manifest RV dysfunction is known to negatively affect outcomes in sarcoidosis patients, and subtle RV changes are likely the initial presenting features of sarcoidosis.[36] RV function assessment by longitudinal strain improves detection of RV involvement and has a predictive value for adverse outcomes in patients with sarcoid even without known cardiac involvement or PH.[36] GLS may be useful to detect sarcoidosis-related LV and RV dysfunction at an earlier and potentially modifiable stage and has notable potential in CS.[35,36] The currently available data are mostly limited to case reports and retrospective observational studies, so further prospective studies are needed to establish the role strain imaging in CS.

Other investigated echocardiography applications include exercise echocardiography to detect abnormalities in exercise-induced LV dysfunction as a marker of occult CS and integrated backscatter, which measures cardiac acoustic properties.[37,38] Abnormal backscatter may represent early granuloma presence and inflammation. In one study, patients with CS were noted to have a decrease in cycle dependent variation of integrated back scatter in the basal septum despite the absence of other abnormalities on two-dimensional (2D) echocardiography.[37]

MULTIMODALITY IMAGING FOR CARDIAC SARCOIDOSIS

Based on expert consensus, echocardiography has an important role in screening for suspected CS despite its poor sensitivity, especially in the early disease stages.[9] Notably, echocardiographic abnormalities were present in only 25% of patients with CMRI and cardiac F(18)-fluorodeoxyglucose positron emission tomography (FDG PET) evidence of CS.[5] Thus, CMRI and FDG PET have emerged as valuable advanced imaging modalities for the screening and risk stratification of CS. In addition to detecting areas of wall thinning or aneurysm and regional wall motion abnormalities, CMRI can also accurately identify even small areas of myocardial damage on the basis of late gadolinium enhancement (LGE).[39] The absence of LGE is associated with a high negative predictive value for excluding CS along with an excellent prognosis.[16] FDG PET with resting myocardial perfusion imaging can also be used for the diagnosis of cardiac (and extracardiac) disease, with a reported sensitivity of 85% to 100% and specificity of 38.5% to 90.9% for CS.[40] The serial assessment of inflammation via FDG PET may be used to follow response to therapy, thereby guiding the choice and duration of therapy. Further, CMRI and FDG PET have a better predictive rate for adverse clinical outcomes among patients with preserved ejection fraction and are also useful in identifying patients who have higher risk of adverse events such as ventricular tachycardia or death, in whom preventive therapies such as defibrillators may need stronger consideration.[16,27] Recently, CMRI has been combined with FDG PET either separately through co-registration of distinctly acquired scans or in combination via a PET-CMRI hybrid scanner.[41] This combined modality allows an accurate assessment of function by CMRI, identification of fibrosis or scar by CMRI using LGE, and assessment of inflammation by FDG PET.[16] Although clinical applicability is currently limited, the potential to combine these imaging techniques may be important for future applications.

CONCLUSION

CS is a potentially life-threatening disorder that can be difficult to diagnose. Despite its limited sensitivity, echocardiography has a central role in the evaluation and management of CS patients. Echocardiography provides valuable information related to patient prognosis and treatment response. If there is suspicion for CS, a comprehensive echocardiographic evaluation of the LV and RV walls should be performed, with attention to asymmetry, thinning, or reduced function. Full assessment of valvular function and cardiac pressures, including direct and indirect signs of PH, should also be obtained. Although a major limitation of echocardiography in the evaluation of CS is its inability to reliably identify individuals with early CS, advances in 2D and 3D myocardial strain imaging are promising. Further studies are needed to establish the role that these advanced techniques may have in the care of patients with CS. Last, the integration of echocardiography with advanced imaging modalities such as CMRI and PET should also be explored further to improve patient management.

Acknowledgments

The authors thank Drs. Amit V. Patel and Gillian Murtagh for their contributions to the previous edition of this chapter.

REFERENCES

1. Iannuzzi MC. Sarcoidosis. *J Am Med Assoc.* 2011;305:391.
2. McGrath DS, Goh N, Foley PJ, du Bois RM. Sarcoidosis: genes and microbes—Soil or seed? *Sarcoidosis Vasc Diffus Lung Dis.* 2001;18:149–164.
3. Morimoto T, Azuma A, Abe S, et al. Epidemiology of sarcoidosis in Japan. *Eur Respir J.* 2008;31:372–379.
4. Iwai K, Tachibana T, Takemura T, et al. Pathological studies on sarcoidosis autopsy. I. Epidemiological features of 320 cases in Japan. *Acta Pathol Jpn.* 1993;43:372–376.
5. Mehta D, Lubitz SA, Frankel Z, et al. Cardiac involvement in patients with sarcoidosis. *Chest.* 2008;133:1426–1435.
6. Banba K, Kusano KF, Nakamura K, et al. Relationship between arrhythmogenesis and disease activity in cardiac sarcoidosis. *Hear Rhythm.* 2007;4:1292–1299.
7. Viles-Gonzalez JF, Kar S, Douglas P, et al. The clinical impact of incomplete left atrial appendage closure with the Watchman device in patients with atrial fibrillation. *J Am Coll Cardiol.* 2012;59:923–929.
8. Fahy GJ, Marwick T, McCreery CJ, et al. Doppler echocardiographic detection of left ventricular diastolic dysfunction in patients with pulmonary sarcoidosis. *Chest.* 1996;109:62–66.
9. Burstow DJ, Tajik AJ, Bailey KR, et al. Two-dimensional echocardiographic findings in systemic sarcoidosis. *Am J Cardiol.* 1989;63:478–482.
10. Silverman KJ, Hutchins GM, Bulkley BH. Cardiac sarcoid: a clinicopathologic study of 84 unselected patients with systemic sarcoidosis. *Circulation.* 1978;58:1204–1211.
11. Blankstein R, Waller AH. Evaluation of known or suspected cardiac sarcoidosis. *Circ Cardiovasc Imag.* 2016;9:e000867.
12. Birnie DH, Sauer WH, Bogun F, et al. HRS expert consensus statement on the diagnosis and management of arrhythmias associated with cardiac sarcoidosis. *Heart Rhythm.* 2014;11:1304–1323.
13. Chapelon-Abric C, de Zuttere D, Duhaut P, et al. Cardiac sarcoidosis: a retrospective study of 41 cases. *Medicine.* 2004;83:315–334.
14. Okayama K, Kurata C, Tawarahara K, et al. Diagnostic and prognostic value of myocardial scintigraphy with thallium-201 and gallium-67 in cardiac sarcoidosis. *Chest.* 1995;107:330–334.
15. Uemura A, Morimoto S, Hiramitsu S. Histologic diagnostic rate of cardiac sarcoidosis: evaluation of endomyocardial biopsies. *Am Heart J.* 1999;138:299–302.
16. Hulten E, Aslam S, Osborne M, et al. Cardiac sarcoidosis—State of the art review. *Cardiovasc Diagn Ther.* 2016;6:50–63.
17. Youssef G, Beanlands RSB, Birnie DH, Nery PB. Cardiac sarcoidosis: applications of imaging in diagnosis and directing treatment. *Heart.* 2011;97:2078–2087.
18. Bargout R, Kelly RF. Sarcoid heart disease: clinical course and treatment. *Int J Cardiol.* 2004;97:173–182.
19. Yazaki Y, Isobe M, Hiramitsu S, et al. Comparison of clinical features and prognosis of cardiac sarcoidosis and idiopathic dilated cardiomyopathy. *Am J Cardiol.* 1998;82:537–540.
20. Patel AR, Klein MR, Chandra S, et al. Myocardial damage in patients with sarcoidosis and preserved left ventricular systolic function: an observational study. *Eur J Heart Fail.* 2011;13:1231–1237.
21. Focardi M, Picchi A, Nikiforakis N, et al. Assessment of cardiac involvement in sarcoidosis by echocardiography. *Rheumatol Int.* 2009;29:1051–1055.
22. Sekhri V, Sanal S, DeLorenzo LJ, et al. Cardiac sarcoidosis: a comprehensive review. *Arch Med Sci.* 2011;4:546–554.
23. Yamano T, Nakatani S. Cardiac sarcoidosis: what can we know from echocardiography? *J Echocardiogr.* 2007;5:1–10.
24. Smedema J-P, van Geuns R-J, Ainslie G, et al. Right ventricular involvement in cardiac sarcoidosis demonstrated with cardiac magnetic resonance. *ESC Heart Fail.* 2017;4:535–544.
25. Patel MB, Mor-Avi V, Murtagh G, et al. Right heart involvement in patients with sarcoidosis. *Echocardiography.* 2016;33:734–741.
26. Darda S, Zughaib ME, Alexander PB, et al. Cardiac sarcoidosis presenting as constrictive pericarditis. *Texas Heart Inst J.* 2014;41:319–323.
27. Murtagh G, Laffin LJ, Patel KV, et al. Improved detection of myocardial damage in sarcoidosis using longitudinal strain in patients with preserved left ventricular ejection fraction. *Echocardiography.* 2016;33:1344–1352.
28. Joyce E, Ninaber MK, Katsanos S, et al. Subclinical left ventricular dysfunction by echocardiographic speckle-tracking strain analysis relates to outcome in sarcoidosis. *Eur J Heart Fail.* 2015;17:51–62.
29. Joyce E, Delgado V, Ninaber MK, Marsan NA. The invisible made visible: multimodality imaging in the evaluation of cardiac sarcoidosis. *Eur Heart J.* 2013;34. 1278–1278.
30. Felekos I, Aggeli C, Gialafos E, et al. Global longitudinal strain and long-term outcomes in asymptomatic extracardiac sarcoid patients with no apparent cardiovascular disease. *Echocardiography.* 2018;35:804–808.
31. Tsuji T, Tanaka H, Matsumoto K, et al. Capability of three-dimensional speckle tracking radial strain for identification of patients with cardiac sarcoidosis. *Int J Cardiovasc Imag.* 2013;29:317–324.
32. Nakano S, Kimura F, Osman N, et al. Improved myocardial strain measured by strain-encoded magnetic resonance imaging in a patient with cardiac sarcoidosis. *Can J Cardiol.* 2013;29:1531.
33. Shah BN, De Villa M, Khattar RS, Senior R. Imaging cardiac sarcoidosis: the incremental benefit of speckle tracking echocardiography. *Echocardiography.* 2013;30. E213–214.
34. Lo A, Foder K, Martin P, Younger JF. Response to steroid therapy in cardiac sarcoidosis: insights from myocardial strain. *Eur Hear J Cardiovasc Imag.* 2012;13. E3–E3.
35. Kurmann R, Mankad SV, Mankad R. Echocardiography in sarcoidosis. *Curr Cardiol Rep.* 2018;20:118.
36. Joyce E, Kamperidis V, Ninaber MK, et al. Prevalence and correlates of early right ventricular dysfunction in sarcoidosis and its association with outcome. *J Am Soc Echocardiogr.* 2016;29:871–878.
37. Hyodo E. Early detection of cardiac involvement in patients with sarcoidosis by a non-invasive method with ultrasonic tissue characterisation. *Heart.* 2004;90:1275–1280.
38. Yasutake H, Seino Y, Kashiwagi M, et al. Detection of cardiac sarcoidosis using cardiac markers and myocardial integrated backscatter. *Int J Cardiol.* 2005;102:259–268.
39. Kouranos V, Tzelepis GE, Rapti A, et al. Complementary role of CMR to conventional screening in the diagnosis and prognosis of cardiac sarcoidosis. *JACC Cardiovasc Imag.* 2017;10:1437–1447.
40. Chareonthaitawee P, Beanlands RS, Chen W, et al. Joint SNMMI-ASNC expert consensus document on the role of 18F-FDG PET/CT in cardiac sarcoid detection and therapy monitoring. *J Nucl Med.* 2017;58:1341–1353.
41. Nekolla SG, Martinez-Moeller A, Saraste A. PET and MRI in cardiac imaging: from validation studies to integrated applications. *Eur J Nucl Med Mol Imag.* 2009;36(suppl 1):S121–S130.

155 Cardiac Involvement in Hypereosinophilic Syndrome

Scipione Carerj, Luca Longobardo, Ludovica Carerj, Maurizio Cusmà-Piccione, Concetta Zito

In 1936, the Swiss physician Wilhelm Loeffler described a patient with progressive cardiac failure, eosinophilia, and inflammatory endocardial thickening.[1] Subsequently, in 1968, Hardy and Anderson[2] coined the term *hypereosinophilic syndromes* (HESs) encompassing different entities with marked blood eosinophilia in the absence of helminthiasis or allergic disorders.

IDIOPATHIC HYPEREOSINOPHILIC SYNDROME

In 1975, Chusid and colleagues[3] established diagnostic criteria for idiopathic HES (IHES) (Box 155.1), substantially based on the finding of persistent hypereosinophilia (>1500/mm^3 for >6 months) with signs and symptoms of multisystemic organ dysfunction in the absence of other known causes of eosinophilia. Recent advances in the understanding of molecular pathogenesis of hypereosinophilia made it possible to distinguish two forms of IHES, according to the different mechanisms responsible for eosinophilia: myeloproliferative (M-HES) and lymphocytic (L-HES) variants of HES.[4] The former has been related to genetic abnormalities leading to clonal expansion of the myeloid lineage, including eosinophils, subsequent to the activation of a tyrosine kinase. The latter has been associated to an overproduction of cytokines (interleukin-5 [IL]5]), stimulating growth of eosinophils, by abnormal circulating T cells.

In IHES, a variety of organs other than the heart are usually involved, including the lungs, bone marrow, and brain. Cardiac manifestations of IHES are frequent, involving 50% to 60% of the patients and represent the leading cause of morbidity and mortality.[5–7] Particularly, heart failure, sudden death, and thromboembolism are the main cardiovascular manifestations, implying a worse prognosis and increased mortality rate.[8] Cardiac damage is the result of myocardial infiltration with eosinophils or eosinophil-derived mediators, as confirmed by biopsy specimens revealing the presence of degranulated eosinophils and eosinophil cationic protein in the endocardium, as well as activated eosinophils at the myocardial interstitium. These mediators lead to endothelial damage and stimulate thrombus formation.[9]

SECONDARY HYPEREOSINOPHILIC SYNDROME

The pathologic findings occur less commonly in patients with secondary hypereosinophilia related to parasitic disease, hypersensitivity, and tumor, although a smaller proportion of patients with such secondary hypereosinophilia manifest cardiac disease by two-dimensional echocardiography.[10] As widely reported, typical cardiac findings include endocardial fibrosis and mural thrombosis, which is most frequent in the apices of both ventricles.

BOX 155.1 Diagnostic Criteria for Hypereosinophilic Syndromes

- Eosinophil counts >1500/mm^3 for ≥6 months or younger than 6 months with evidence of organ damage
- Lack of evidence for parasitic, allergic, or other recognized causes of eosinophilia
- Symptoms and signs of organ system involvement

Clinical presentation depends on the stages of eosinophilic endomyocardial disease, which are as follows:

1. Necrotic stage, characterized by hypereosinophilia with systemic illness (20%–30%) and acute carditis (20%–50%)
2. Thrombotic stage with thromboemboli (10%–20%)
3. Fibrotic stage (late stage) with restrictive myopathy (10%) and valve regurgitations

To date, HES is included in the current classification of cardiomyopathies into the secondary forms.[11]

DEMOGRAPHICS AND PRESENTING SYMPTOMS

According to the most recent World Health Organization report about eosinophilic disorders, incidence rate of HES is approximately 0.036 per 100,000.[7] The majority of patients (~75%) described in reports from Europe and North America were white, with a variable age of onset occurring from early childhood to extreme old age, although the majority (70%) of patients have onset between the ages of 20 and 50 years.[12] Before IHES was distinguished into M-HES and L-HES, a greater prevalence of IHES was found in men, with a male-to-female ratio ranging from 4:1 to 9:1.[12] Recently, this male-to-female ratio has been confirmed in M-HES, whereas a sex ratio close to 1:1 has been reported in L-HES.[13]

The principal clinical features include fatigue, weight loss, fever, cough, and rash. Mucosal ulcerations are suggestive of M-HES, whereas transient angioedema has been more frequently reported in L-HES. Vascular manifestations, resulting from vasculitis or thrombosis of both small and large vessels, have been also described in IHES. Musculoskeletal manifestations, including arthralgias and myalgia, are other common findings.

Although early cardiac involvement may be asymptomatic, overt cardiac dysfunction occurs in more than half of patients and may be right or left sided or both.[14] In this respect, symptoms and signs of congestive heart failure, including dyspnea, ascites, and peripheral edema, have been commonly observed in patients with IHES. In addition, systemic embolism, potentially leading to neurologic or renal dysfunction, has been reported. It has been reported that the median survival time in patients with IHES was about 22.2 months.[7] Death mostly results from heart failure (65% of deaths at autopsy), often with associated renal, hepatic, or respiratory involvement.

PATHOPHYSIOLOGY

In IHES, a variety of organs are usually involved besides the heart, including the lungs, bone marrow, and brain. Cardiac pathology consists of an acute eosinophilic myocarditis, fibrinoid vasculitis of the intramural coronary arteries, mural thrombosis along damaged endocardium, fibrotic endocardial thickening, and ultimately, endomyocardial fibrosis with ventricular obliteration. Cardiac involvement is often biventricular, with mural endocardial thickening of the inflow portions and apex of the ventricles, resulting in increased ventricular stiffness and reduced size of ventricular cavities, both associated with elevated ventricular filling pressure. Atrioventricular valvular regurgitation may occur because of involvement of the supporting apparatus of the mitral or tricuspid

> **BOX 155.2** Echocardiographic Features of Hypereosinophilic Syndrome
>
> - Wall thickening with layering of the endocardial echoes. This is most evident at the apex of one or both ventricles in the region of papillary muscles at posterior mitral and anterior tricuspid valve leaflets.
> - Mitral and/or tricuspid valve regurgitation
> - Obliteration of the apex by thrombus
> - Enlargement of the atria, with ventricular chambers generally normal or small
> - Systolic function often preserved or impaired with diastolic dysfunction
> - Pericardial effusion of variable degree

valves by endocardial scarring or thrombus. Mitral and tricuspid stenosis may also occur and likely results from entrapment of the subvalvular apparatus in the fibrous material.[15]

DIAGNOSIS

The electrocardiogram (ECG) most commonly shows nonspecific ST-segment and T-wave abnormalities. Published case reports highlight presentations with unusual ECG changes mimicking acute myocardial infarction.[16] Arrhythmias, especially atrial fibrillation, and conduction defects, particularly right bundle branch block, may also be present. The chest radiograph may reveal cardiomegaly and pulmonary congestion or, less commonly, pulmonary infiltrates.

The echocardiogram commonly demonstrates (1) wall thickening with layering of endocardial echoes (Box 155.2), most evident at the apex of one or both ventricles (Fig. 155.1), in the region of papillary muscles at the posterior mitral and anterior tricuspid valve leaflets, causing regurgitation of those valves; (2) obliteration of the apex by a thrombus that may extend up to the inflow tract of the atrioventricular valves, impeding normal leaflet function, with an appearance of a "clenched fist" or "ace of spades"; (3) hypercontractility of basal myocardial segments in contrast to the abnormal apex (Merlon sign)[17]; (4) enlargement of the atria with inversion of the normal ventricular-to-atrial size ratio (markedly dilated atria in contrast to obliterated ventricles)[18]; (5) on M-mode echocardiography, the initial rapid motion of septum and posterior wall followed by a flat endocardial reflection (square root sign); (6) systolic function, preserved or impaired, and diastolic dysfunction with restrictive pattern; and (7) pericardial effusion of variable degree.[14,19]

Contrast echocardiography, which can accurately delineate ventricular shape and endocardial border, may be used for better evaluation of apical obliteration provoked by thrombus or fibrosis. Furthermore, it has been reported that two-dimensional speckle-tracking LV global longitudinal strain was reduced in a cohort of 32 patients with HES, all with normal conventional echocardiographic findings compared with healthy control participants, and the cut-off value of 17.0% or less was the best predictor of LV endocardial dysfunction; on the contrary, authors did not find any significant difference about radial and circumferential strain.[20]

Despite the good diagnostic accuracy of echocardiogram, when compared with endomyocardial biopsies, the gold standard technique for the diagnosis, it has been reported that echocardiograms and endomyocardial biopsies agree for presence or absence of cardiac involvement only 60% of the time, and biopsy detected cardiac involvement in a significant percentage of patients in whom the echocardiogram was negative for findings of HES.[21]

Endomyocardial biopsy allows the evaluation of histologic findings that include variable degrees of an acute inflammatory eosinophilic myocarditis involving the myocardium and endocardium; thrombosis, fibrinoid change, and inflammatory reaction involving small intramural coronary vessels; mural

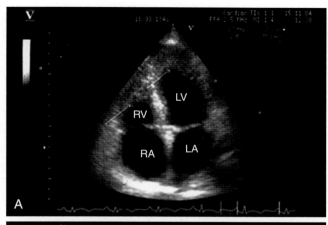

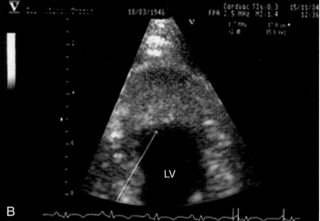

Figure 155.1. A, Apical four-chamber view, obliteration of apices of both ventricles. **B,** Left atrial thrombus. *LA,* Left atrium; *LV,* left ventricle; *RA,* right atrium; *RV,* right ventricle.

thrombi, often containing eosinophils; and fibrotic thickening of up to several millimeters. On electron microscopy, a characteristic cardiac myocytolytic change showing disruption at the intercellular junction has been observed.[22]

However, endomyocardial biopsy is an invasive procedure, and sometimes it may fail to obtain adequate samples in the last stage of the disease and may be difficult to perform. In this respect, cardiac magnetic resonance imaging (MRI), allowing accurate tissue characterization by means of gadolinium-delayed enhancement and better thrombus detection, may decrease the need for endomyocardial biopsies for the diagnosis of IHES.[23,24] Indeed, it has been reported that MRI was able to detect HES in a significant percentage of patients with normal ECGs and echocardiograms,[23] and some authors suggested that it may be considered as a surrogate to myocardial biopsies (Fig. 155.2 and Video 155.2).[25] Box 155.3 summarizes all investigations needed for the diagnosis and classification of HES.

TREATMENT

The three primary goals for the management of IHES are (1) reduction of peripheral and tissue levels of eosinophils, (2) prevention of end-organ damage, and (3) prevention of thromboembolic events in patients at risk. Corticosteroids appear to have a beneficial effect on acute myocarditis, and together with cytotoxic drugs (hydroxyurea in particular), may improve survival.[26] Patients not responding to standard therapy have been successfully treated with interferon, acting through induction of apoptosis of eosinophils. Moreover,

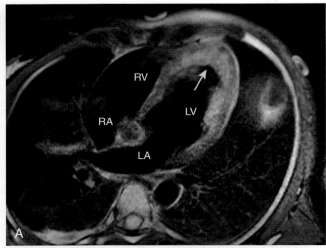

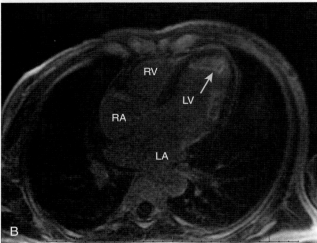

Figure 155.2. Cardiac magnetic resonance images (CMRI) in a patient with hypereosinophilic syndrome. **A** and **B,** CMRI demonstrates increased left ventricular size with decreased systolic function (left ventricular ejection fraction, 36%) and a combination of left ventricular apical edema, diffuse apical thrombus (arrows), and subendocardial enhancement consistent with eosinophilic myocarditis. *LA,* Left atrium; *LV,* left ventricle; *RA,* right atrium; *RV,* right ventricle. (See accompanying Video 155.2.)

thrombosis or fibrosis. In these regards, valve replacement with bioprosthesis is preferred because of increased risk of thrombosis with mechanical prosthesis. However, variable operative mortality rates (15%–29%) are reported.

Please access ExpertConsult to view the corresponding video for this chapter.

after recent advances concerning the pathogenesis of IHES, a targeted therapy according to the IHES variants has been proposed. In this respect, the use of a tyrosine kinase inhibitor, such as imatinib mesylate, has been introduced for M-HES variant based on the identification in this subgroup of a deregulated tyrosine kinase activity.[27] At the same time, a monoclonal anti–IL5 antibody, such as mepolizumab, has been used for L-HES variant to counterbalance the overproduction of IL-5 by T-cells.

As adjunctive therapy, diuretics, vasodilators, and, occasionally, inotropic agents are indicated in the management of congestive heart failure. In earlier stages, moreover, angiotensin-converting enzyme inhibitors and β-blockers may be used to prevent the development of overt ventricular dysfunction. In addition, particularly in patients with ventricular thrombosis, anticoagulation therapy is indicated to prevent pulmonary and systemic embolism and to limit apical thrombotic obliteration.

When the fibrotic stage has been reached, surgical therapy appears to offer significant palliation of symptoms. Valve replacement, thrombectomy, and endomyocardectomy may provide benefit to patients with valvular compromise and endomyocardial

REFERENCES

1. Loeffler W. Endocarditis parietalis fibroplastica mit Bluteosinophilie. *Schweiz Med Wochenschr.* 1936;65:817–820.
2. Hardy WR, Anderson RE. The hypereosinophilic syndromes. *Ann Intern Med.* 1968;68:1220–1229.
3. Chusid MJ, Dale DC, West BC, et al. The hypereosinophilic syndrome: analysis of fourteen cases with review of the literature. *Medicine.* 1975;54:1–27.
4. Kahn JE, Blétry O, Guillevin L. Hypereosinophilic syndromes. *Best Pract Res Clin Rheumatol.* 2008;22:863–882.
5. Corssmit EP, Trip MD, Durrer JD. Löffler's endomyocarditis in the idiopathic hypereosinophilic syndrome. *Cardiology.* 1999;91:272–276.
6. Child JS, Perloff JK. The restrictive cardiomyopathies. *Cardiol Clin.* 1988;6:289–316.
7. Shomali W, Gotlib J. World Health Organization-defined eosinophilic disorders: 2019 update on diagnosis, risk stratification, and management. *Am J Hematol.* 2019;94:1149–1167.
8. Gupta PN, Valiathan MS, Balakrishnan KG, et al. Clinical course of endomyocardial fibrosis. *Br Heart J.* 1989;62:450–454.
9. Weller PF, Bubley GJ. The idiopathic hypereosinophilic syndrome. *Blood.* 1994;83:2759–2779.
10. Ommen SR, Seward JB, Tajik AJ. Clinical and echocardiographic features of hypereosinophilic syndromes. *Am J Cardiol.* 2000;86:110–113.
11. Maron BJ, Towbin JA, Thiene G, et al. Contemporary definitions and classification of the cardiomyopathies. *Circulation.* 2006;113:1807–1816.
12. Wilkins HJ, Crane MM, Copeland K, et al. Hypereosinophilic syndrome: an update. *Am J Hematol.* 2005;80:148–157.
13. Rothenberg ME, Klion AD, Roufosse FE, et al. Treatment of patients with the hypereosinophilic syndrome with mepolizumab. *N Engl J Med.* 2008;358:1215–1228.
14. Karnak D, Kayacan O, Beder S, et al. Hypereosinophilic syndrome with pulmonary and cardiac involvement in a patient with asthma. *CMAJ (Can Med Assoc J).* 2003;168:172–175.
15. Weyman AE, Rankin R, King H. Loeffler's endocarditis presenting as mitral and tricuspid stenosis. *Am J Cardiol.* 1977;40:438–444.
16. Jin X, Ma C, Liu S, et al. Cardiac involvements in hypereosinophilia-associated syndrome: case reports and a little review of the literature. *Echocardiography.* 2017;34:1242–1246.
17. Berenszte in CS, Piñeiro D, Marcotegui M, et al. Usefulness of echocardiography and Doppler echocardiography in endomyocardial fibrosis. *J Am Soc Echocardiogr.* 2000;13:385–392.
18. Nemes A, Marton I, Domsik P, et al. Characterization of left atrial dysfunction in hypereosinophilic syndrome—Insights from the motion analysis of the heart and great vessels by 3D speckle tracking echocardiography in pathological cases. *Rev Port Cardiol.* 2016;35:277–283.

19. Kocaturk H, Yilmaz M. Idiopathic hypereosinophilic syndrome associated with multiple intracardiac thrombi. *Echocardiography*. 2005;22:675–676.
20. Yamamoto T, Tanaka H, Kurimoto C, et al. Very early stage left ventricular endocardial dysfunction of patients with hypereosinophilic syndrome. *Int J Cardiovasc Imag*. 2016;32:1357–1361.
21. Butterfield JH, Kane GC, Weiler CR. Hypereosinophilic syndrome: endomyocardial biopsy versus echocardiography to diagnose cardiac involvement. *Postgrad Med*. 2017;129:517–523.
22. Hayashi S, Isobe M, Okubo Y, et al. Improvement of eosinophilic heart disease after steroid therapy: successful demonstration by endomyocardial biopsied specimens. *Heart Ves*. 1999;14:104–108.
23. Miszalski-Jamka T, Szczeklik W, Karwat K, et al. MRI-based evidence for myocardial involvement in women with hypereosinophilic syndrome. *Magn Reson Med Sci*. 2015;14:107–114.

24. Salemi VM, Rochitte CE, Shiozaki AA, et al. Late gadolinium enhancement magnetic resonance imaging in the diagnosis and prognosis of endomyocardial fibrosis patients. *Circ Cardiovasc Imag*. 2011;4:304–311.
25. Perazzolo Marra M, Thiene G, Rizzo S, et al. Cardiac magnetic resonance features of biopsy-proven endomyocardial diseases. *JACC Cardiovasc Imag*. 2014;7:309–312.
26. Roufosse F, Cogan E, Goldman M. The hypereosinophilic syndrome revisited. *Ann Rev Med*. 2003;54:169–184.
27. Druker BJ, Talpaz M, Resta DJ, et al. Efficacy and safety of a specific inhibitor of the BCR-ABL tyrosine kinase in chronic myeloid leukemia. *N Engl J Med*. 2001;344:1031–1037.

156 Endocrine Disease

Talal S. Alnabelsi, Steve W. Leung, Vincent L. Sorrell

Endocrine diseases can result in cardiovascular alterations in response to changes in homeostasis. Diabetes mellitus is the most common endocrine disease and is discussed in detail in another chapter. In this chapter, we cover the other major endocrine diseases along with their effects on the heart. There are no pathognomonic echocardiographic findings related to endocrine diseases such as hypothyroidism, hyperthyroidism, acromegaly, hypercortisolism, and hyperaldosteronism. However, some echocardiographic features are commonly seen and have been described (Table 156.1). These features are likely caused by a combination of the intrinsic effects of the circulating hormones on the myocardium and the effects of changes in cardiac preload or afterload. Correction of these hormonal abnormalities usually resolves these abnormal echocardiographic changes.

HYPOTHYROIDISM

Hypothyroidism is a common endocrine disorder resulting from a decrease in circulating thyroid hormone levels, which causes a reduction in the body's basal metabolic rate. Decreases in thyroid hormone levels can be caused by a decrease in their production by the thyroid gland (primary), a decrease in thyroid-stimulating hormone (TSH) by the pituitary gland (secondary), or a decrease in thyrotropin-releasing hormone (TRH) from the hypothalamus (tertiary). The severity of hypothyroidism can vary from subclinical hypothyroidism to myxedema. The systemic effects of hypothyroidism are extensive and can involve virtually every organ system. Common manifestations include weight gain, hair loss, depression, constipation, cold intolerance, and nonpitting edema. Delayed tendon relaxation during reflex testing can be seen on physical examination and is most easily demonstrated using the Achilles tendon reflex test (Video 156.1).

The cardiovascular effects of hypothyroidism include a decrease in the resting heart rate, impaired ventricular filling, and reduced myocardial contractility. There is also an increase in peripheral vascular resistance. Electrocardiography can demonstrate sinus bradycardia and low voltage. Chest radiography can demonstrate an enlarged cardiac silhouette because of the presence of a pericardial effusion (Fig. 156.1).

Echocardiographic abnormalities can be detected in the subclinical stages of hypothyroidism, and they comprise evidence of diastolic dysfunction and particularly impaired relaxation.[1] Parameters of diastolic dysfunction that have been reported by Doppler echocardiography include prolongation of the isovolumic relaxation time (IVRT), decrease in the peak early diastolic filling velocity (E) with an associated increase in E-wave deceleration time, increased peak late diastolic filling velocity (A) resulting in a decrease in the E/A ratio, and a low early diastolic mitral annular velocity (e°).[2] These Doppler findings have been described in the right ventricle (RV) as well as the left ventricle (LV).[3] More recently, let atrial (LA) emptying function and passive ejection fraction has been shown to be impaired in patients with subclinical hypothyroidism.[4] Systolic dysfunction can be seen in overt hypothyroidism but is not apparent in milder forms of the disease.[5] Unexplained bradycardia combined with marked left ventricular systolic dysfunction on two-dimensional echocardiography (with or without a pericardial effusion) should raise the suspicion of hypothyroidism.

Patients with myxedema can have severe systolic and diastolic dysfunction, as well as the presence of a pericardial

TABLE 156.1 Common Echocardiographic Findings in Endocrine Disease

Disease	Left Ventricular Mass	Systolic Function	Diastolic Function	Other
Hypothyroidism	→	↓[a]	Impaired	Pericardial effusion[a]
Hyperthyroidism	→	↑	Normal or increased	Left ventricular hypertrophy (rare) Reduced LVEF[a]
Acromegaly	↑	↓[a]	Impaired	—
Hypercortisolism	↑	→	Impaired	—
Hyperaldosteronism	↑	→	Impaired	—

[a]Severe disease only.
LVEF, Left ventricular ejection fraction.

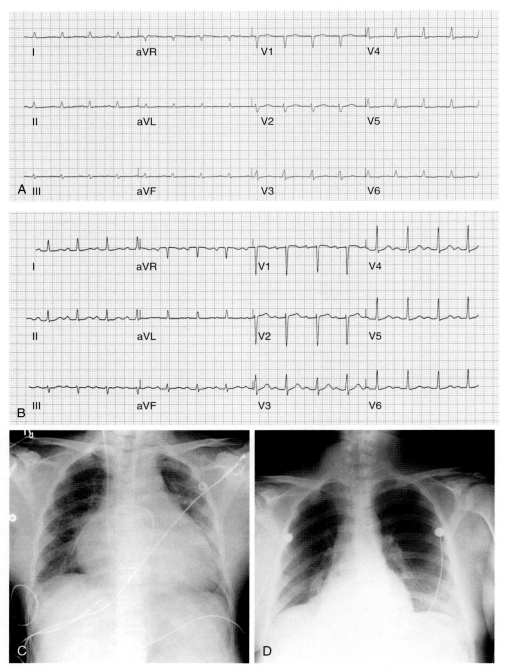

Figure 156.1. Hypothyroidism. **A,** Twelve-lead electrocardiogram (ECG) of a patient with profound hypothyroidism in heart failure. Note the low-voltage, widened QRS, and flattened T waves. **B,** Twelve-lead ECG from the same patient 5 months later after thyroid hormone replacement. The ECG is now normal except for first-degree atrioventricular block. **C,** Chest radiograph on admission in heart failure with a pericardial effusion. **D,** Chest radiograph before discharge 3 weeks later with normal cardiac silhouette. (See accompanying Video 156.1(See accompanying Videos 156.1, 156.2, and 156.3).) (Reproduced with permission from Crawford MH, et al, editors: *Cardiology*. 2nd ed. St. Louis: Mosby; 2004.)

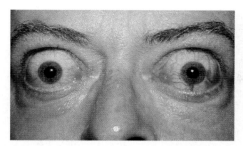

Figure 156.2. Exophthalmos of both eyes with lid retraction caused by hyperthyroidism. (Reproduced from Spalton D, et al: *Atlas of Clinical Ophthalmology*. 3rd ed. St Louis: Mosby; 2004.)

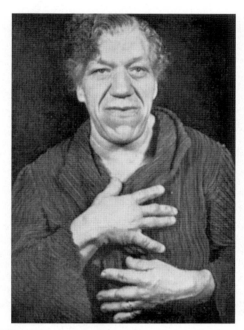

Figure 156.3. Typical appearances of acromegaly. The face shows enlarged supraorbital ridges, nose, lips, and jaw. Note the patient's spadelike hands. (Reproduced with permission from Ignatavicius DD, Workman ML: *Medical-Surgical Nursing: Critical Thinking for Collaborative Care*. 4th ed. Philadelphia: Saunders; 2002.) (See accompanying Video 156.4.)

effusion (Videos 156.2 and 156.3). Although large pericardial effusions can be seen in severe hypothyroidism, these are rarely associated with cardiac tamponade physiology.[6] With thyroid hormone replacement therapy, most of these cardiac findings (diastolic, systolic dysfunction, and pericardial effusion) are reversed.[1,7]

HYPERTHYROIDISM

Thyrotoxicosis is an excess in circulating thyroid hormones, resulting in increased tissue metabolic rate and demand for oxygen. Thyrotoxicosis resulting from thyroid gland overactivity is referred to as hyperthyroidism. Thyrotoxicosis can occur in the absence of hyperthyroidism caused by the release of stored thyroid hormones from a damaged thyroid gland (postpartum thyroiditis, amiodarone-induced thyroiditis). Secondary hyperthyroidism is less common and occurs because of increased levels of TSH or TRH, which increases production of thyroid hormones. Common signs and symptoms include unintentional weight loss, heat intolerance, sweating, anxiety, tremors, hair

loss, palpitations, diarrhea, and exophthalmos (mainly in Graves disease; Fig. 156.2). In contrast to hypothyroidism, hyperthyroidism results in increased resting heart rate, enhanced left ventricular contractility, increased blood volume, and decreased peripheral vascular resistance, translating into a high-output cardiac state.[8] These patients are at an increased risk of developing atrial fibrillation as well, especially in patients with a dilated left atrium.[9]

Three decades earlier, M-mode echocardiography demonstrated an increase in the maximum left ventricular shortening and lengthening velocities, which corresponds to enhanced systolic and diastolic function, respectively.[10] The IVRT has been noted to be shortened but returns to normal after patients return to an euthyroid state with therapy.[11] More recent data mostly support these findings, although evidence of impaired relaxation with increased left ventricular mass was reported in 34% of patients (n = 50).[12] Additionally, longitudinal and circumferential strain by speckle tracking was demonstrated to be reduced in patients with subclinical hyperthyroidism despite an often enhanced left ventricular ejection fraction (LVEF) in overt hyperthyroidism.[13] However, patients demonstrate markedly limited exercise capacity caused by an inability to augment output during exercise.[14]

Pulmonary hypertension is also commonly noted in hyperthyroidism and can be due in part to the increased cardiac output in the absence of a concomitant reduction in pulmonary vascular resistence.[15,16] Prolonged increases in heart rate or cardiac output can cause patients to develop a dilated cardiomyopathy because of a tachycardia-mediated process or a high-output failure mechanism, respectively. This can be corrected by normalization of thyroid hormone levels.

ACROMEGALY

Acromegaly is a rare endocrine disorder caused by the overproduction of growth hormone, typically arising from pituitary adenomas. The increased level of growth hormone promotes insulinlike growth factor-1 production in the liver, which induces growth of musculoskeletal tissues and internal organs. Patients with acromegaly have characteristic clinical features (e.g., macrognathia, macroglossia), including musculoskeletal changes (Fig. 156.3).

Cardiovascular manifestations of acromegaly are termed *acromegalic cardiomyopathy,* and their extent depends on the stage at which the disease is diagnosed. Research from the 1990s and the early 2000s showed evidence of increased myocardial wall thickness, left ventricular mass, and chamber size. Global systolic function as measured by fractional shortening and LVEF are preserved.[17] Diastolic dysfunction (increased IVRT, decreased E, decreased e'/a', abnormal Tei index) is also commonly associated with acromegaly.[18] As noted in other endocrinologic diseases, the increase in myocardial wall thickness and impaired diastolic function has been found to be a biventricular process involving both the RV and the LV.[19] More recently, however, echocardiographic and cardiac magnetic resonance imaging (MRI) data have failed to show a difference in left ventricular wall thickness and left ventricular mass between patients with and without acromegaly.[20,21] This raises the question of whether the previously reported differences are attributed to underlying comorbidities such as obesity and hypertension. LA volume, however, appears to be significantly enlarged in patients with acromegaly independent of the diastolic function. Finally, patients with acromegaly can develop heart failure with a modest decline in ejection fraction along with an enlarged chamber size thought to be caused by the prolonged high-output state (Video 156.4).[22] Patients who are treated either surgically or medically can demonstrate reversal of myocardial hypertrophy as well as normalization of diastolic function.[23]

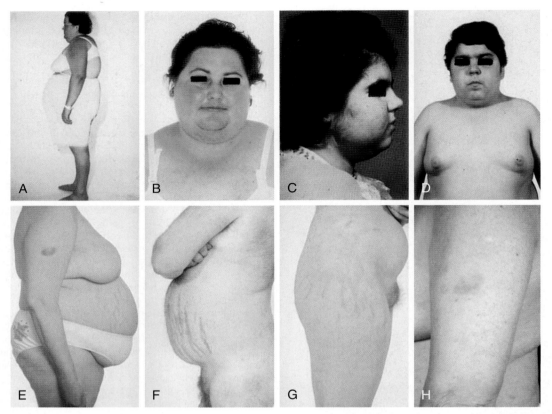

Figure 156.4. Hypercortisolism: clinical features of Cushing syndrome. **A,** Centripetal and some generalized obesity and dorsal kyphosis in a 30-year-old woman with Cushing disease. **B,** The same patient as in *A*, showing moon facies, plethora, hirsutism, and enlarged supraclavicular fat pads. **C,** Facial rounding, hirsutism, and acne in a 14-year-old young woman with Cushing disease. **D,** Central and generalized obesity and moon facies in a 14-year-old young man with Cushing disease. **E** and **F,** Typical centripetal obesity with livid abdominal striae seen in a 41-year-old woman (**E**) and a 40-year-old man (**F**) with Cushing syndrome. **G,** Striae in a 24-year-old patient with congenital adrenal hyperplasia treated with excessive doses of dexamethasone as replacement therapy. **H,** Typical bruising and thin skin of a patient with Cushing syndrome. In this case, the bruising occurred without obvious injury. (Reproduced with permission from Stewart PM, Krone NP: In Melmed S, et al, editor: *Williams Textbook of Endocrinology*. Philadelphia: Saunders; 2011:479–544.)

HYPERCORTISOLISM

Hypercortisolism is caused by the overproduction of cortisol, a glucocorticoid hormone. The increase in production can be caused by an adrenal adenoma (primary) or adrenal hyperplasia (secondary) induced by an increase in circulating corticotropin hormone either from the pituitary gland (Cushing disease) or from an ectopic tumor. Characteristic clinical manifestations include moon facies, buffalo hump, central obesity, striae formation, hirsutism, and amenorrhea in women (Fig. 156.4). Patients on chronic steroid therapies can also develop similar physical findings.

On echocardiography, these patients have significant left ventricular hypertrophy (LVH) with an increase in relative wall thickness and a slight decrease in chamber size but no significant difference in LVEF.[24] This contrasts with MRI data, which reported a subclinical biventricular and LA systolic dysfunction.[25] There is also an association with diastolic dysfunction as described by increased IVRT, decreased E/A, prolonged E-wave deceleration time, decreased e′, decreased e′/a′, and increased Tei index.[26] The hypertrophy and diastolic dysfunction do not appear to correlate with blood pressure or urinary cortisol levels but do correlate with the duration of the disease and typically reverse after normalization of cortisol levels.[27]

HYPERALDOSTERONISM

Hyperaldosteronism is caused by the excess production of aldosterone, a mineralocorticoid hormone. This can either be caused by adrenal adenoma (primary or Conn syndrome) or be induced by an overactive renin–angiotensin system (secondary). Aldosterone increases the reabsorption of sodium and water in the distal tubules and the secretion of potassium in the collecting tubules of the kidneys (Fig. 156.5) Resistant hypertension and hypokalemia are common manifestations.

Commonly found on echocardiography is significant concentric LVH with increased interventricular septal and posterior wall thickness, increased relative wall thickness, and increased left ventricular mass index.[28] These patients often have evidence of impaired diastolic function with a decreased E velocity and E/A ratio. In contrast to patients with essential hypertension, the degree of LVH and diastolic function dysfunction is more pronounced despite similar elevations in systemic blood pressure. This suggests that LVH relies not only on cardiac load or output but also on the activation of the renin–angiotensin system.[29] After adrenalectomy to treat hyperaldosteronism, LVH typically regresses.[30]

CONCLUSION

Endocrine disorders often result in a multitude of cardiovascular consequences partly caused by direct hormonal effects on cardiac myocytes. Echocardiography can be vital in detecting certain cardiovascular abnormalities ranging from subtle changes in relaxation parameters to overt systolic and diastolic dysfunction. With the development of new echocardiographic techniques such as comprehensive myocardial deformation imaging and three-dimensional echocardiography, continued investigation of these patient

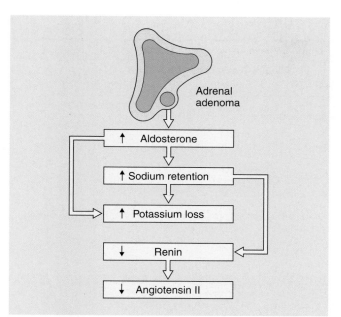

Figure 156.5. Mechanism of pathophysiologic changes in primary hyperaldosteronism. The autonomous production and release of aldosterone from the tumor lead to excessive sodium retention and potassium wasting; these occur largely as a result of the effects of aldosterone on the distal tube of the kidney. Renin release from the kidney is therefore inhibited, which leads to a fall in circulating levels of angiotensin II. (Reproduced with permission from Besser CM, Thorner MO: *Comprehensive Clinical Endocrinology*. 3rd ed. St Louis: Mosby; 2002.)

populations is warranted and may reveal further insight into their cardiovascular effects.

Please access ExpertConsult to view the corresponding videos for this chapter.

REFERENCES

1. Malhotra Y, Kaushik RM, Kaushik R. Echocardiographic evaluation of left ventricular diastolic dysfunction in subclinical hypothyroidism: a case–control study. *Endocr Res.* 2017;42:198–208.
2. Tiryakioglu SK, Tiryakioglu O, Ari H, et al. Left ventricular longitudinal myocardial function in overt hypothyroidism: a tissue Doppler echocardiographic study. *Echocardiography.* 2010;27:505–511.
3. Kosar F, Sahin I, Aksoy Y, et al. Usefulness of pulsed-wave tissue Doppler echocardiography for the assessment of the left and right ventricular function in patients with clinical hypothyroidism. *Echocardiography.* 2006;23:471–477.
4. Dereli S, Bayramoğlu A, Özer N, et al. Evaluation of left atrial volume and functions by real time 3D echocardiography in patients with subclinical hypothyroidism before and after levothyroxine therapy. *Echocardiography.* 2019;6:916–923.
5. Chen X, Zhang N, Zhang WL, et al. Meta-analysis on the association between subclinical hypothyroidism and the left ventricular functions under Doppler echocardiography. *Zhonghua Liuxingbingxue Zazhi.* 2011;32:1269–1274.
6. Kabadi UM, Kumar SP. Pericardial effusion in primary hypothyroidism. *Am Heart J.* 1990;120:1393–1395.
7. Virtanen VK, Saha HH, Groundstroem KW, et al. Thyroid hormone substitution therapy rapidly enhances left-ventricular diastolic function in hypothyroid patients. *Cardiol.* 2001;96:59–64.
8. Graettinger JS, Muenster JJ, Selverstone LA, et al. A correlation of clinical and hemodynamic studies in patients with hyperthyroidism with and without congestive heart failure. *J Clin Invest.* 1959;38:1316–1327.
9. Iwasaki T, Naka M, Hiramatsu K, et al. Echocardiographic studies on the relationship between atrial fibrillation and atrial enlargement in patients with hyperthyroidism of Graves' disease. *Cardiol.* 1989;76:10–17.
10. Friedman MJ, Okada RD, Ewy GA, et al. Left ventricular systolic and diastolic function in hyperthyroidism. *Am Heart J.* 1982;104:1303–1308.
11. Mintz G, Pizzarello R, Klein I. Enhanced left ventricular diastolic function in hyperthyroidism: noninvasive assessment and response to treatment. *J Clin Endocrinol Metab.* 1991;73:146–150.
12. Anakwue RC, Onwubere BJ, Ike V, et al. Echocardiographic assessment of left ventricular function in thyrotoxicosis and implications for the therapeutics of thyrotoxic cardiac disease. *Ther Clin Risk Manag.* 2015;11:189–200.
13. Tadic M, Ilic T, Cuspidi C, et al. Subclinical hyperthyroidism impacts left ventricular deformation: 2D and 3D echocardiographic study. *Scand Cardiovasc J.* 2015;49(2):74–81.
14. Forfar JC, Muir AL, Sawers SA, et al. Abnormal left ventricular function in hyperthyroidism: evidence for a possible reversible cardiomyopathy. *N Engl J Med.* 1982;307:1165–1170.
15. Siu CW, Zhang XH, Yung C, et al. Hemodynamic changes in hyperthyroidism-related pulmonary hypertension. *J Clin Endocrinol Metab.* 2007;92:1736–1742.
16. Tudoran C, Tudoran M, Vlad M, et al. Echocardiographic evolution of pulmonary hypertension in female patients with hyperthyroidism. *Anatol J Cardiol.* 2018;20:174–181.
17. Hradec J, Marek J, Kral J, et al. Long-term echocardiographic follow-up of acromegalic heart disease. *Am J Cardiol.* 1993;72:205–210.
18. Baykan M, Erem C, Gedikli O, et al. Assessment of the Tei index by tissue Doppler imaging in patients with acromegaly. *Echocardiography.* 2008;25:374–380.
19. Fazio S, Cittadini A, Sabatini D, et al. Evidence for biventricular involvement in acromegaly: a Doppler echocardiographic study. *Eur Heart J.* 1993;14:26–33.
20. dos Santos Silva CM, Gottlieb I, Volschan I, et al. Low frequency of cardiomyopathy using cardiac magnetic resonance imaging in an acromegaly contemporary cohort. *J Clin Endocrinol Metab.* 2015;100(12):4447–4455.
21. Popielarz-Grygalewicz A, Gasior JS, Konwicka A, et al. Heart in acromegaly: the echocardiographic characteristics of patients diagnosed with acromegaly in various stages of the disease. *Int J Endocrinol.* 2018;6935054.
22. Damjanovic SS, Neskovic AN, Petakov MS, et al. High output heart failure in patients with newly diagnosed acromegaly. *Am J Med.* 2002;112:610–616.
23. Merola B, Cittadini A, Colao A, et al. Chronic treatment with the somatostatin analog octreotide improves cardiac abnormalities in acromegaly. *J Clin Endocrinol Metab.* 1993;77:790–793.
24. Muiesan ML, Lupia M, Salvetti M, et al. Left ventricular structural and functional characteristics in Cushing's syndrome. *J Am Coll Cardiol.* 2003;41:2275–2279.
25. Kamenický P, Redheuil A, Roux C, et al. Cardiac structure and function in Cushing's syndrome: a cardiac magnetic resonance imaging study. *J Clin Endocrinol Metab.* 2014;99:E2144–E2153.
26. Baykan M, Erem C, Gedikli O, et al. Assessment of left ventricular diastolic function and Tei index by tissue Doppler imaging in patients with Cushing's Syndrome. *Echocardiography.* 2008;25:182–190.
27. Pereira AM, Delgado V, Romijn JA, et al. Cardiac dysfunction is reversed upon successful treatment of Cushing's syndrome. *Eur J Endocrinol.* 2010;162:331–340.
28. Rossi GP, Sacchetto A, Pavan E, et al. Remodeling of the left ventricle in primary aldosteronism due to Conn's adenoma. *Circulation.* 1997;95:1471–1478.
29. Cesari M, Letizia C, Angeli P, et al. Cardiac remodeling in patients with primary and secondary aldosteronism: a tissue Doppler study. *Circ Cardiovasc Imag.* 2016;9. e004815.
30. Rossi GP, Cesari M, Cuspidi C, et al. Long-term control of arterial hypertension and regression of left ventricular hypertrophy with treatment of primary aldosteronism. *Hypertension.* 2013;62:62–69.

157 Chagas Cardiomyopathy

Rachel Marcus, Federico M. Asch

EPIDEMIOLOGY OF CHAGAS DISEASE

First described by the Brazilian physician Carlos Chagas in 1909, Chagas cardiomyopathy is the result of a chronic myocarditis caused by infection with the parasite *Trypanosoma cruzi*. The chief mode of transmission is via the bite of a *Triatomine* species insect (kissing bug), although other modes of transmission such as congenital, transfusion-related, and oral have become more common. The disease is typically referred to as an illness of non-island nations of Latin America. There are an estimated 6 million individuals with Chagas disease.[1] Both domestic rural to urban migration and international migration from Latin America have led to a broader distribution of infected individuals. There are an estimated

TABLE 157.1 Stages of Chagas Heart Disease

Acute Phase	Chronic Phase				
	Indeterminate Form		Chagas Cardiomyopathy		
	A	B1	B2	C	D
• Infected with *Trypanosoma cruzi* • Findings of acute Chagas disease	• Positive serology • Normal ECG • No heart disease • No heart failure	• Structural abnormalities • Abnormal laboratory results (abnormal ECG or echocardiograph) • Normal LV function • No heart failure	• LV dysfunction • No heart failure	• LV dysfunction • Current or prior heart failure	• Refractory heart failure despite optimal medical management

LV, Left ventricular.
Reproduced with permission from Acquatella, H, et al: Recommendations for multimodality cardiac imaging in patients with Chagas disease, *J Am Soc Echocardiogr* 31:3–25, 2018; Filho P, et al: Left ventricular global performance and diastolic function in indeterminate and cardiac forms of Chagas' disease, *J Am Soc Echocardiogr* 20:1338–1343, 2007.

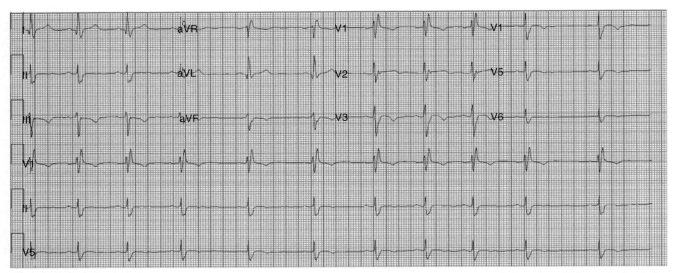

Figure 157.1. Typical electrocardiogram (ECG) of a patient with Chagas cardiomyopathy showing right bundle branch and left anterior fascicular blocks. This 27-year-old El Salvadorian man presented with palpitations and was found to have frequent premature ventricular contractions (which were not captured in this ECG) and bifascicular block with normal left ventricular function. Serologic analysis was confirmed positive for Chagas disease.

300,000 seropositive individuals in the United States, 80,000 in Europe, and smaller numbers in Japan, Australia, and Canada.[2]

Chagas Disease Stages

Chagas disease is divided into three stages: acute, indeterminate, and chronic.

Initial phase. Most commonly, after an insect bite and hematogenous spread of parasite, an acute febrile illness follows, which is accompanied by nonspecific symptoms and is therefore frequently undiagnosed. In a small number of patients (<5%), a more serious illness occurs, including myopericarditis with pericardial effusion and meningoencephalitis.[3]

Intermediate phase. Virtually all patients then pass into the "indeterminate phase" of the illness, characterized by two distinct positive serologic assays and the absence of end-organ manifestation of the disease.

Chronic phase. After 15 to 30 years, 20% to 30% of individuals develop cardiac manifestations of the illness,[4] which can lead to complications such as stroke, arrhythmias, and heart failure.

Chagas Cardiomyopathy Stages

Chagas cardiomyopathy is stratified into stages A through D (Table 157.1): stage A (abnormal serology with normal electrocardiogram [ECG]), stage B1 (abnormal serology, cardiac disease such as abnormal ECG but with normal ejection fraction), stage B2 (abnormal EF, no symptoms), stage C (abnormal echocardiography with clinical heart failure), and stage D (refractory heart failure). Individuals with normal ECGs are thought to progress to Chagas cardiomyopathy at a rate of 1.8% to 5% per year.[5–7]

PATHOPHYSIOLOGY OF CHAGAS DISEASE

The pathophysiology of Chagas disease is inflammatory, and the cardiac manifestations are the result of myocardial fibrosis, neuronal damage, autonomic dysfunction, and microvascular disease. The cumulative damage explains the frequent occurrence of ventricular dysfunction, tachyarrhythmias, bradyarrhythmias, stroke, and sudden cardiac death associated with Chagas cardiomyopathy.

The diagnosis of Chagas disease is contingent upon positive serologic testing results performed on two different assays. These may be two assays of the same type using different antigens or

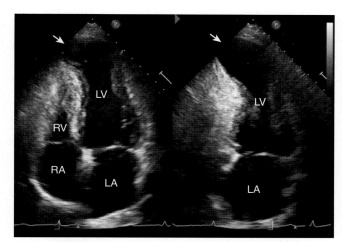

Figure 157.2. Left ventricular apical aneurysm. Four-chamber apical view of a patient with Chagas heart disease with a large left ventricular apical aneurysm *(arrows)*. *LA,* Left atrium; *LV,* left ventricle; *RA,* right atrium; *RV,* right ventricle. (Reproduced with permission from Acquatella H, et al: Recommendations for multimodality cardiac imaging in patients with Chagas disease. *J Am Soc Echocardiogr* 31:3–25, 2018.)

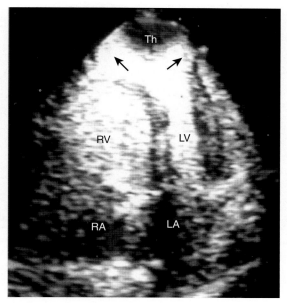

Figure 157.3. Left ventricular apical aneurysm with thrombus. Contrast echocardiogram for left ventricular opacification in a patient with Chagas heart disease and biventricular damage shows a large apical aneurysm *(arrows)* with a thrombus (Th). Contrast infusion allows to define the extension of the aneurysm and size of the thrombus. The right ventricle is more dilated than the left ventricle. (Reproduced with permission from Acquatella H, et al: Recommendations for multimodality cardiac imaging in patients with Chagas disease, *J Am Soc Echocardiogr* 31:3–25, 2018.) (See accompanying Videos 157.2 and 157.3)

two distinct techniques. After identified with Chagas disease, the hallmark of the diagnosis of Chagas cardiomyopathy is an abnormal ECG. Findings that are suggestive of Chagas disease include right bundle branch block with or without left anterior fascicular block (Fig. 157.1), frequent premature ventricular contractions, atrial fibrillation, first-degree atrioventricular block, or higher-degree heart block.[8] As will be discussed further later in this chapter, there can be echocardiographic manifestations of the disease even with a normal ECG.

ECHOCARDIOGRAPHIC FINDINGS IN ACUTE CHAGAS DISEASE

The prevalence of echocardiographic abnormalities in acute Chagas disease is difficult to know, as most patients do not present for medical care in the setting of this nonspecific febrile illness. In the few series reported of acute Chagas disease with echocardiographic examination, pericardial effusion was the most common finding on echo (42%–88%), including some cases of tamponade requiring pericardial drainage. Most patients have normal left ventricular (LV) systolic function. Signs of congestion caused by heart failure or cardiac tamponade were observed in 24%, diminished LV ejection fraction (LVEF) in 35%, and regional wall motion abnormalities in 28% of patients, although ECG abnormalities were the most frequent finding.[9]

ECHOCARDIOGRAPHIC FINDINGS IN INDETERMINATE CHAGAS DISEASE (STAGE A)

A patient with a normal ECG has a prognosis similar to a noninfected patient. Therefore, particularly in resource-poor environments, no additional testing beyond ECG has been recommended if the ECG is normal. Nevertheless, significant numbers of patients with a normal ECG can show abnormal regional LV function.[10,11] Although the prognostic implications of an abnormal imaging test in the setting of a normal ECG are not known, echocardiography is a reasonable option as part of the initial evaluation of a Chagas patient to complement the ECG.[12] Aside from two-dimensional (2D) imaging, several additional modalities have been used to assess for subclinical myocardial disease, including evaluation of diastolic function[13] (which is abnormal in up to 10% of stage A patients) and speckle tracking/strain analysis of both the LV and

right ventricle (RV). Myocardial strain is a sensitive method to detect asymptomatic disease, but its implications for risk of progression to stage B have not yet been determined.[14]

ECHOCARDIOGRAPHIC FINDINGS IN CHRONIC CHAGAS CARDIOMYOPATHY (STAGES B-D)
Left Ventricle

Chagas cardiomyopathy is an inflammatory scarring cardiomyopathy in which the extent of LV impairment and scar relates directly to symptom status, risk for arrhythmia, and death. The landmark lesions are LV aneurysms; they are mostly apical, although they could be present in any wall or even the RV (Fig. 157.2). However, focal and global hypokinesis are most frequent as the disease progresses[11] (Video 157.1). Aneurysms are often small and therefore difficult to image without careful off-axis imaging of the apex or intravenous (IV) injection of ultrasound enhancing agents (Video 157.2). The addition of three-dimensional imaging, echocardiography contrast, or both to the 2D study is particularly helpful for LV function or if the apex is not well visualized.

The classic apical aneurysm, known as a "punch-hole" lesion (a very focal outpouching at the apex surrounded by normal contractile tissue), is associated with thromboembolic events. Careful assessment of the apex for associated thrombus is critical (echocardiography contrast may be needed) because thrombus can be found in up to 23% of patients with aneurysms[15] (Fig. 157.3 and Video 157.3). Importantly, in patients with cardiomyopathy, this imaging finding is very characteristic and, when present, is highly suggestive of Chagas disease as the etiologic diagnosis. LV apical aneurysms are found in 8.5% of asymptomatic patients, but this increases to 55% (ranging from 47%–64%) in patients with moderate or severe LV systolic dysfunction.[16] Of note, the

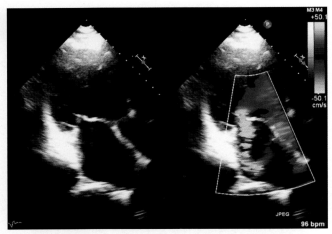

Figure 157.4. Secondary (functional) mitral regurgitation in Chagas cardiomyopathy. Apical two-chamber view shows inferolateral aneurysm and a large posteriorly directed jet of mitral regurgitation as a result of posterior leaflet tethering. (See accompanying Video 157.4).

presence of an apical aneurysm increases the risk for cardioembolic stroke, particularly in older patients with reduced LVEF. Basal inferior or inferolateral scars are associated with ventricular tachyarrhythmias.[17] Secondary (functional) mitral regurgitation that appears "ischemic" is common, particularly because of basal inferolateral aneurysm or LV dilatation and associated leaflet tethering (Fig. 157.4 and Video 157.4).

LVEF has been the most widely used prognostic variable derived from 2D echocardiography, either alone or as part of risk-scoring systems.[18] New data from the BENznidazole Evaluation For Interrupting Trypanosomiasis (BENEFIT) trial echocardiography substudy identified other predictors of death. A wall motion score index of 2 or higher is associated with a ninefold increase in risk of death compared with a normal score of 1, and an abnormal left atrial volume was also an independent indicator of risk of death.[19]

Right Ventricle

Although abnormalities in the LV are most common, evaluation of the RV is also of high importance: RV Tei index (>0.56) provides incremental prognostic information to that of more traditional risk factors, such as New York Heart Association functional class and LV function.[20] The value of RV strain is still unclear in Chagas disease, though it has been found to be abnormal in some patients in the indeterminate phase with no other echocardiographic abnormalities.[14,21] Occasionally, RV apical aneurysm is the only detectable abnormality.[22]

Additional echocardiography imaging modalities such as assessment of diastolic function and strain are an important part of the echocardiography examination of patients with established Chagas cardiomyopathy. Diastolic dysfunction with elevated LA pressures based on E/e' ratio greater than 15 is a strong predictor of death.[23] Abnormalities found by global longitudinal strain imaging correlate highly with degree of fibrosis assessed by magnetic resonance imaging and with risk of ventricular arrhythmia.[24]

Please access ExpertConsult to view the corresponding videos for this chapter.

REFERENCES

1. Chagas disease in Latin America. An epidemiological update based on 2010 estimates. *Wkly Epidemiol Rec.* 2015;90:33–43.
2. Gascon J, Bern C, Pinazo MJ. Chagas disease in Spain, the United States, and other nonendemic countries. *Acta Trop.* 2010;115:22–27.
3. Tanowitz H, Kirchoff L, Simon D, et al. Chagas' disease. *Clin Microbiol Rev.* 1992:400–419.
4. Pinto Dia JC. The indeterminate form of human chronic Chagas' disease: a clinical epidemiological review. *Revista Soc Brasil Med Tropical.* 1989;22:147–156.
5. Espinosa R, Carrasco HA, Belandria F, et al. Life expectancy analysis in patients with Chagas' disease: prognosis after one decade (1973–1983). *Int J Cardiol.* 1985;8:45–56.
6. Goldsmith R, Zarate RJ, Zarate LG. Clinical and epidemiologic studies of Chagas' disease in Rural Communities of Oaxaca, Mexico, and an eight-year follow up: II. *Bull Pan Am Health Organ.* 1992;26.
7. Maguire J, Hoff R, Sherlock I, et al. Cardiac morbidity and mortality due to Chagas' disease: prospective electrocardiographic study of a Brazilian community. *Circulation.* 1987;75:1140–1145.
8. Rojas L, Glisic M, Pletsch-Borba L, et al: Electrocardiographic abnormalities in Chagas disease in the general population: a systematic review and meta-analysis, PLoS Negl Trop Dis 12:e0006567
9. Alarcón de Noya B, Díaz-Bello Z, Colmenares C, et al. Large urban outbreak of orally acquired acute Chagas disease at a school in Caracas, Venezuela. *J Infect Dis.* 2010;201:1308–1315.
10. Carrasco HA, Barboza JS, Inglessi G, et al. Left ventricular cineangiography in Chagas' disease: detection of early myocardial damage. *Am Heart J.* 1982;104:595–602.
11. Viotti R, Vigliano C, Laucella S, et al. Value of echocardiography for diagnosis and prognosis of chronic Chagas disease cardiomyopathy without heart failure. *Heart.* 2004;90:655–660.
12. Acquatella H, Asch F, Barbosa M, et al. Recommendations for multimodality cardiac imaging in patients with Chagas disease. *J Am Soc Echocardiogr.* 2018;31:3–25.
13. Filho P, Romano MM, Gomes Furtado R, et al. Left ventricular global performance and diastolic function in indeterminate and cardiac forms of Chagas' disease. *J Am Soc Echocardiogr.* 2007;20:1338–1343.
14. Barbosa M, Costa Rocha M, Vidigal D, et al. Early detection of left ventricular contractility abnormalities by two-dimensional speckle tracing strain in Chagas disease. *Echocardiography.* 2014;31:623–630.
15. Nunes M, Barbosa M, Rocha M. Peculiar aspects of cardiogenic embolism in patients with Chagas' cardiomyopathy: a transthoracic and transesophageal echocardiographic study. *J Am Soc Echocardiogr.* 2005;18:761–767.
16. Acquatella H. Echocardiography in Chagas heart disease. *Circulation.* 2007;115:1124–1131.
17. Sarabanda A, Sosa E, Simõe M, et al. Ventricular tachycardia in Chagas' disease: a comparison of clinical, angiographic, electrophysiologic and myocardial perfusion disturbances between patients presenting with either sustained or nonsustained forms. *Int J Cardiol.* 2005;22:9–19. 102.
18. Rassi A, Little W, Xavier S, et al. Development and validation of a risk score for predicting death in Chagas' heart disease. *N Engl J Med.* 2006;355:799–808.
19. Schmidt A, Romano M, Marin-Neto J, et al. Effects of trypanocidal treatment on echocardiographic parameters in chagas cardiomyopathy and prognostic value of wall motion score: a BENEFIT Trial substudy. *J Am Soc Echocardiogr.* 2018;2:286–295.
20. Nunes MC, Rocha MO, Ribeiro AL, et al. Right ventricular dysfunction is an independent predictor of survival in patients with dilated chronic Chagas' cardiomyopathy. *Int J Cardiol.* 2008;127:372–379.
21. Barros M, Machado F, Ribeiro A, et al. Detection of early right ventricular dysfunction in Chagas' disease using Doppler tissue imaging. *J Am Soc Echocardiogr.* 2002;15:1197–1201.
22. Oliveira JS, Mello De Oliveira JA, Frederigue U, et al. Apical aneurysm of Chagas' heart disease. *Br Heart J.* 1981;46:432–437.
23. Nunes M, Colosimo E, Padilha Reis R, et al. Different prognostic impact of the tissue Doppler-derived E/e' ratio on mortality in Chagas cardiomyopathy patients with heart failure. *J Heart Lung Transplant.* 2012;31:634–641.
24. Barros M, Leren I, Edvardsen T, et al. Mechanical dispersion assessed by strain echocardiography is associated with malignant arrhythmias in Chagas cardiomyopathy. *J Am Soc Echocardiogr.* 2016;29:368–374.

158 Sickle Cell Disease

Nina Rashedi, Ankit A. Desai, Amit R. Patel

Sickle cell disease (SCD) is an autosomal recessive disease that affects millions of people worldwide and approximately 1 in 500 African Americans and 1 in 1200 Hispanic Americans.[1] It is caused by a β-globin gene mutation, resulting in systemic complications caused by vaso-occlusive episodes and hemolysis.[2] Cardiopulmonary complications have surfaced as leading causes of morbidity and premature mortality, with a median life span of 45 years of age. Common cardiopulmonary abnormalities in individuals with SCD include evidence of pulmonary hypertension (PH), right ventricular (RV) and left ventricular (LV) dilatation, and increased LV mass.[3] Recently, significant attention has been placed on the use of noninvasive cardiovascular imaging to further elucidate these observations, including important prognostic and diagnostic characteristics. Characteristics such as an elevated peak tricuspid regurgitation velocity and the presence of diastolic dysfunction are examples of the utility of echocardiography to risk stratify this patient population. Importantly, clinical practice guidelines from several national organizations have been published in the past decade that addresses the use of echocardiography in SCD. Although the National Institutes of Health guidelines in 2014 were unable to make a recommendation for or against the use of echocardiography alone as a screening PH test because of insufficient evidence, American Thoracic Society guidelines the same year recommended a screening echocardiogram in all children with SCD for the purposes of diagnosis and intensification of therapies.[4] This chapter thus focuses on published cardiovascular features of SCD, in particular highlighting the knowledge derived from and the utility of echocardiography.

LEFT VENTRICULAR STRUCTURE AND SYSTOLIC FUNCTION

Myocardial abnormalities occur frequently in adults with SCD, and several reports have used echocardiography to describe early pathophysiological characteristics in children. A Brazilian study that performed echocardiography in 45 patients with SCD younger than 20 years of age and another 109 patients without SCD revealed higher z-scores for LV (13.1-fold higher) and RV (5.2-fold) chamber dimensions, LV mass and wall thickness, and left atrial diameter (4.9-fold) in children with SCD over the control group.[5] This observed chamber dilatation and increase in wall mass have also been observed in adults with SCD along with increased stroke volume, all of which have been associated with chronic anemia.[1] Another study evaluating echocardiographic findings in a young population with SCD as part of an outpatient screening protocol showed a 25% to 30% prevalence of both mild tricuspid regurgitation jet velocity elevation and varying degrees of LV dilatation, which were associated with markers of SCD morbidity.[6] This LV remodeling has been associated with impaired LV filling[7,8] with increasing age, a concept that needs further investigation and validation in SCD.

Although cardiopulmonary causes are the primary determinant of increased mortality rates in patients with SCD, the presence and effects of heart failure in SCD have largely been underrecognized. Furthermore, published reports demonstrate, in part, conflicting observations. Both heart failure with reduced left ventricular ejection fraction (LVEF) and heart failure with preserved LVEF have been reported in patients with SCD. Most SCD studies to date have confirmed that the majority of patients likely have a preserved

ejection fraction based on screening echocardiography. In fact, studies using three-dimensional (3D) echocardiography with speckle tracking (Fig. 158.1) have confirmed the presence of normal longitudinal, radial and circumferential components of 3D strain with normal angle and torsion.[9] Interestingly, two-dimensional echocardiography strain has revealed reduction in longitudinal shortening during acute crisis but unaltered LV myocardial performance because of relatively preserved circumferential shortening and increased radial thickening.[10] Although there is a general consensus that LV systolic function determined by ejection fraction is typically preserved, measures of LV contractility using load-independent techniques have shown both normal and abnormal findings. End-systolic stress volume index, for example, was shown to be abnormal in patients with SCD, but the relationship of end-systolic wall stress to velocity of circumferential shortening has revealed mixed results. Although systolic LV function appears to be largely preserved, Doppler and tissue Doppler imaging reveal evidence of significant diastolic dysfunction in children and in adults.[5,11–13]

Changes in absolute right and left ventricular global longitudinal strain (RVGLS, LVGLS) have been demonstrated as more sensitive markers of systolic function than ejection fraction. Indeed, it has been shown that absolute RVGLS was increased in children with SCD compared with control participants despite normal tricuspid annular plane systolic excursion. The increased RVGLS points to an early compensatory mechanism of the right ventricle during childhood in response to upstream myocardial insults as well as elevated cardiac output.[14] Another study showed that RV systolic annular velocity was higher in the patients with SCD than in control participants.[15] The increased RV preload caused by anemia may also play a role in augmentation of the RV function as detected by increased RVGLS. After early compensatory augmented RV systolic function in childhood as manifested by the increased RVGLS, RVGLS may normalize in young adulthood and later decline, a concept that has not been well studied. It is possible that the right ventricle, which is not designed to pump against high resistance, cannot sustain augmented function, resulting in eventual decline in function in later adulthood.

LEFT VENTRICULAR DIASTOLIC DYSFUNCTION

The presence of LV diastolic dysfunction is an independent risk factor for death with a risk ratio of 4.8 (95% confidence interval, 1.9–12.1; $P < .001$).[12] Importantly, the combination of diastolic dysfunction and echocardiography-derived estimates of elevated pulmonary artery pressures (Fig. 158.2) increases this mortality risk ratio to more than 13.[1] As expected, LV diastolic abnormalities are associated with older age, increases in blood pressure, increased LV mass, and higher creatinine levels.[1] A comprehensive noninvasive cardiac imaging study using same-day echocardiography, cardiovascular magnetic resonance imaging (CMRI), and arterial tonometry revealed the association of increased LV mass and diastolic dysfunction linked significantly to afterload including relative systemic hypertension and central aortic stiffness in SCD. Importantly, the study did not find any significant association between diastolic dysfunction and direct myocardial damage from microvascular disease, iron deposition, fibrosis, and changes related to chronic anemia, all of which have been previously postulated as etiologies for the cardiac relaxation abnormalities.[16]

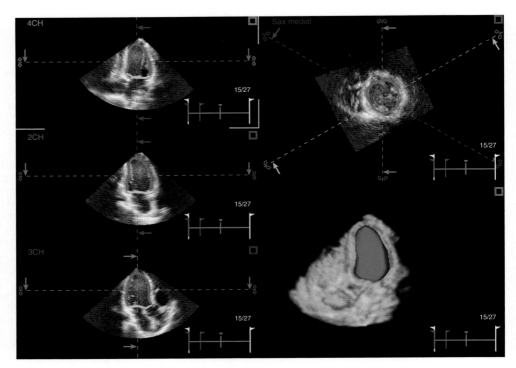

Figure 158.1. Three-dimensional echocardiography in sickle cell disease. (Adapted with permission from Ahmad H, et al: Evaluation of myocardial deformation in patients with sickle cell disease and preserved ejection fraction using three-dimensional speckle tracking echocardiography, *Echocardiography* 29:962–969, 2012.)

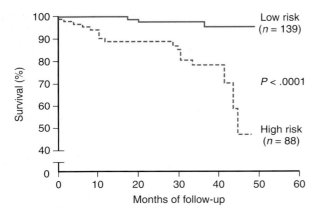

Figure 158.2. Survival in individuals with sickle cell disease is reduced with the presence of left ventricular diastolic dysfunction with pulmonary hypertension. (Adapted with permission from Sachdev V, et al: Diastolic dysfunction is an independent risk factor for death in patients with sickle cell disease, *J Am Coll Cardiol* 49:472–479, 2007.)

Prospective validation studies of echocardiography-derived measures of LV diastolic dysfunction in patients with SCD are lacking. Using current definitions of echocardiography-defined diastolic function and dysfunction, which includes criteria for left atrial volumes, may not be accurately applied to SCD in which a majority of the patients develop large left atrial volumes associated with chronic anemia and a high-output state. 3D speckle-tracking echocardiography–derived LV filling parameters have been demonstrated to be significantly different from normal control participants, reflecting an increase in both early and atrial filling volumes and slowing in active relaxation, depicted by a decrease in filling volume fractions at fixed times and an increase in rapid filling duration.[9] Based on studies of PH in SCD using right heart catheterization (RHC), LV diastolic dysfunction is present in nearly half of the patients undergoing the invasive procedure.[1,17–19] Using noninvasive tissue Doppler thresholds, the prevalence of LV diastolic dysfunction varies significantly between 15% and 33% in children and adults with SCD.[7,17,20–22] Although significant variation in measurements of echocardiography-derived filling pressures have been reported in the past, a tissue Doppler-derived E/e′ ratio greater than 15 has been associated with elevated LV filling pressure in the setting of LV systolic dysfunction. However, the majority of patients with SCD have preserved ejection fraction. In heart failure with normal ejection fraction, an increased E/e′ ratio above 8 was found to be a useful noninvasive predictor of diastolic dysfunction.[1] A retrospective review of patients undergoing echocardiography and RHC within 72 hours reported a positive association between elevated E/e′ ratios and a pulmonary capillary wedge pressure greater than 15 mm Hg.[1] Receiver operating characteristic analysis showed that a cutoff value of 8.2 had a sensitivity of 78% and specificity of 71% (positive predictive value, 65%; negative predictive value, 82%; area under the curve, 0.72) for predicting an elevated wedge pressure.

Another echocardiographic study showed a strong trend toward low lateral and septal e′ values consistent with diastolic dysfunction in patients with SCD. Notably, lower lateral and septal e′ values were most prevalent in older patients with SCD. The decreasing lateral and septal e′ values with increasing age further suggest that diastolic function worsens with age. A restrictive diastolic filling pattern was also observed despite the young age of these patients. Multiple studies have suggested that the left atrium is dilated in patients with SCD. Together the pattern of diastolic dysfunction, left atrial dilatation, and normal systolic function observed in young patients with SCD suggest that some patients with SCD may have restrictive physiology.[23]

PULMONARY HYPERTENSION

PH represents a major cause of early death in adult patients with SCD.[1,17–19] PH affects approximately 10% of adult patients with SCD, particularly those with the SS genotype. Despite various contributors to PH, postmortem SCD studies demonstrate pulmonary vascular obliteration and smooth muscle hypertrophy, histopathology typically seen in patients with group 1 pulmonary arterial hypertension.[24] Up until the past few years, most SCD studies have evaluated

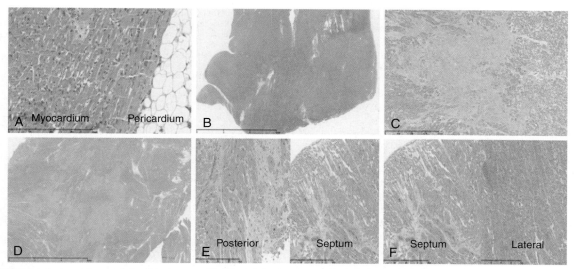

Figure 158.3. Histologic evidence of significant myocardial fibrosis in six patients (**A–F**) with sickle cell disease. (Adapted with permission Desai AA, et al: Mechanistic insights and characterization of sickle cell disease-associated cardiomyopathy, *Circ Cardiovasc Imag* 7:430–437, 2014.)

PH noninvasively, primarily screening for an elevated peak tricuspid regurgitant jet velocity (TRV, ≥2.5 m/s) on transthoracic echocardiography. In recent years, studies have used RHC for confirmation (defined using the older threshold of mean pulmonary artery pressure, mPAP ≥25 mm Hg, which is 2/3 dPAP + 1/3 sPAP, where dPAP is diastolic pulmonary artery pressure, and sPAP is systolic pulmonary artery pressure). The cause of PH, however, remains unclear in most patients. Catheterization-based studies have shed some insight into the prevalence of the disease in SCD, but PH is often identified after patients have progressed to advanced disease.

Although RHC is required for confirmation, echocardiography remains a useful noninvasive screening tool for PH in patients with SCD. Using the Bernoulli equation, the TRV provides a calculated estimate of RV and pulmonary artery systolic pressures. However, use of a TRV threshold of 2.5 m/s or greater is associated with a low positive predictive value in SCD as demonstrated by several studies. Part of this observation is explained by the high-output state of patients with SCD caused by anemia and low viscosity caused by anemia, which can affect estimates of pulmonary vascular resistance and the fact that TRV is not always measurable on echocardiography.[1,19] Several suggested echocardiographic parameters or maneuvers for the detection of PH in SCD include a higher TRV threshold, mean tricuspid regurgitant jet gradient, end-diastolic pulmonary regurgitation gradient, measures of RV systolic function and time intervals, tissue Doppler imaging, strain-rate echocardiography, saline contrast to enhance the tricuspid regurgitant jet or pulmonary regurgitation signals, and incorporation of pulmonary-artery stroke distance (the velocity–time integral measured from the pulmonic value as an estimate of stroke volume) as an indicator of cardiac output.

Several screening studies have been performed evaluating the prevalence of an elevated peak TRV alone with the presence of RHC-defined PH in patients with SCD at steady-state (i.e., not during or near the time of a sickle crisis). For each study, catheterization was indicated if patients' echocardiography demonstrated a TRV of 2.5 m/s or above. Most studies have revealed that approximately 25% to 30% of patients have screening echocardiography that demonstrates a TRV of 2.5 m/s or greater and approximately10% of patients with a value of 3.0 m/s or greater. However, subsequent RHC has confirmed PH in only about 6% to 11% patients with SCD.[1,18,19,25]

Although a TRV of 2.5 m/s or greater in adults with SCD is a relatively poor predictor of RHC-defined PH in patients with SCD, the threshold remains strongly associated with poor outcomes and

functional status in patients with SCD. A TRV of 2.5 m/s or greater is associated with an approximate 9- to 16-fold risk ratio for early death in adults with SCD, high NT-proBNP (N-terminal pro-B-type natriuretic peptide) levels, and decreased functional capacity. A TRV of 3 m/s or greater is more specific for RHC-defined PH but is only present in about 10% of adults with SCD and remains associated with a significant risk ratio for death of about 10.[1,18] Elevations of TRV between 2.5 and 3 m/s continue to represent poor prognostic markers of SCD, but their diagnostic values remain indeterminate.

Of adult patients screened with borderline TRV values of 2.5 to 3 m/s, American Thoracic Society (ATS) guidelines recommend additional risk stratification with NT-proBNP and 6-minute walk testing. Additional testing can increase the positive predictive value of the TRV. A prospective multicenter French study found that positive predictive value of TRV in asymptomatic individuals to be only 25% when using a cutoff of 2.5 m/s. However, the combination of a TRV of at least 2.5 m/s and either an NT proBNP level greater than 164 pg/mL or a 6-minute walk distance less than 333 m improved the positive predictive values to 62%.[19]

OTHER CARDIAC FINDINGS

Although predisposed to lifelong sickle cell crises involving hypoxia and reperfusion abnormalities, the presence of myocardial infarctions from atherosclerotic coronary artery disease has been rare. Hence, regional wall motion abnormalities on echocardiography are also not common is SCD. Instead, these patients seem to have evidence of myocardial fibrosis (Fig. 158.3) and abnormal myocardial perfusion reserve, suggesting abnormalities in the microvasculature.[16] In addition to microvascular dysfunction, individuals with SCD have evidence of aortic stiffness despite the presence of a normal systemic blood pressure.[16] Although patients with SCD can require a high burden of blood transfusions, the presence of myocardial siderosis is infrequent, in contrast to patients with β-thalassemia.

SCREENING CONSIDERATION

Given the significant cardiovascular abnormalities present in SCD, many experts agree on obtaining a screening echocardiogram for all patients with SCD. Using only chest pain, dyspnea, or other cardiorespiratory symptoms without echocardiography to identify patients at risk for cardiovascular complications is confounded by symptoms of chronic anemia, vaso-occlusive pain crises, and systemic involvement of the disease. The timing of the initial screening echocardiogram and the utility of repeat echocardiograms for screening purposes have not been studied nor defined. The importance of a screening echocardiogram during childhood is highlighted by the significant prognostic implications and studies that have reported findings in children. Additionally, because many of the echocardiography-based abnormalities such as diastolic dysfunction and elevated TRV are associated with increasing age, repeat echocardiogram in adults can be considered despite the lack of rigorous data in this rare disease. For translation into practice, the ATS guidelines state for risk stratification to perform a baseline study and interval of every 1 to 3 years.[4] We also support consideration of RHC in SCD, in particular in patients with TRV of 3 m/s or greater. If any other abnormal findings are suspected or observed, we also suggest a low threshold for pursuing further cardiovascular testing such as CMRI to help define the underlying cause of even subtle LV dysfunction and RHC to confirm the presence and severity of PH.

LIMITATIONS

Garnering meaningful cardiovascular observations has been marred by significant challenges in investigating patients with SCD. First, many patients have an increased lifetime burden of vaso-occlusive crises, which are associated with severe pain, hospitalization, and significant swings in heart rate, blood pressure, oxygen saturation, and respiratory status. These crises can significantly impact the load on the heart and limit the interpretations from conventional observations on echocardiography. Additionally, for more advanced studies such as with contrast or invasive catheterizations, obtaining appropriate intravenous access has been challenging across many clinical studies. Furthermore, a large proportion of urban patient populations with SCD are complicated by significant socioeconomic challenges, which further limit successful participation in clinical trials. Despite more than 60 years of research, progress has been limited, and SCD remains a dramatic example of health disparities in the United States.

REFERENCES

1. Gladwin MT, Sachdev V. Cardiovascular abnormalities in sickle cell disease. *J Am Coll Cardiol.* 2012;59:1123–1133.
2. Gladwin MT. Cardiovascular complications and risk of death in sickle-cell disease. *Lancet.* 2016;387:2565–2574.
3. Haywood LJ. Cardiovascular function and dysfunction in sickle cell anemia. *J Natl Med Assoc.* 2009;101:24–30.
4. Klings ES, Machado RF, Barst RJ, et al. An official American Thoracic Society clinical practice guideline: diagnosis, risk stratification, and management of pulmonary hypertension of sickle cell disease. *Am J Respir Crit Care Med.* 2014;189:727–740.
5. Ribera MC, Ribera RB, Koifman RJ, Koifman S. Echocardiography in sickle cell anaemia patients under 20 years of age: a descriptive study in the Brazilian Western Amazon. *Cardiol Young.* 2015;25:63–69.
6. Allen KY, Jones S, Jackson T, et al. Echocardiographic screening of cardiovascular status in pediatric sickle cell disease. *Pediatr Cardiol.* 2019;40:1670–1678.
7. Balfour IC, Covitz W, Arensman FW, et al. Left ventricular filling in sickle cell anemia. *Am J Cardiol.* 1988;61:395–399.
8. Gerry JL, Baird MG, Fortuin NJ. Evaluation of left ventricular function in patients with sickle cell anemia. *Am J Med.* 1976;60:968–972.
9. Ahmad H, Gayat E, Yodwut C, et al. Evaluation of myocardial deformation in patients with sickle cell disease and preserved ejection fraction using three-dimensional speckle tracking echocardiography. *Echocardiography.* 2012;29:962–969.
10. Sengupta SP, Jaju R, Nugurwar A, et al. Left ventricular myocardial performance assessed by 2-dimensional speckle tracking echocardiography in patients with sickle cell crisis. *Indian Heart J.* 2012;64:553–558.
11. Zilberman MV, Du W, Das S, Sarnaik SA. Evaluation of left ventricular diastolic function in pediatric sickle cell disease patients. *Am J Hematol.* 2007;82:433–438.
12. Sachdev V, Machado RF, Shizukuda Y, et al. Diastolic dysfunction is an independent risk factor for death in patients with sickle cell disease. *J Am Coll Cardiol.* 2007;49:472–479.
13. Ntim WO, Upadhya B, Cruz J. Diastolic dysfunction is an independent risk factor for death in patients with sickle cell disease. *J Am Coll Cardiol.* 2007;50:378. author reply 378–379.
14. Whipple NS, Naik RJ, Kang G, et al. Ventricular global longitudinal strain is altered in children with sickle cell disease. *Br J Haematol.* 2018;183:796–806.
15. Barbosa MM, Vasconcelos MC, Ferrari TC, et al. Assessment of ventricular function in adults with sickle cell disease: role of two-dimensional speckle-tracking strain. *J Am Soc Echocardiogr.* 2014;27:1216–1222.
16. Desai AA, Patel AR, Ahmad H, et al. Mechanistic insights and characterization of sickle cell disease-associated cardiomyopathy. *Circ Cardiovasc Imag.* 2014;7:430–437.
17. Fonseca GH, Souza R, Salemi VM, et al. Pulmonary hypertension diagnosed by right heart catheterisation in sickle cell disease. *Eur Respir J.* 2012;39:112–118.
18. Machado RF, Gladwin MT. Pulmonary hypertension in hemolytic disorders: pulmonary vascular disease: the global perspective. *Chest.* 2010;137:30S–38S.
19. Parent F, Bachir D, Inamo J, et al. A hemodynamic study of pulmonary hypertension in sickle cell disease. *N Engl J Med.* 2011;365:44–53.
20. Anthi A, Machado RF, Jison ML, et al. Hemodynamic and functional assessment of patients with sickle cell disease and pulmonary hypertension. *Am J Respir Crit Care Med.* 2007;175:1272–1279.
21. Caldas MC, Meira ZA, Barbosa MM. Evaluation of 107 patients with sickle cell anemia through tissue Doppler and myocardial performance index. *J Am Soc Echocardiogr.* 2008;21:1163–1167.
22. Eddine AC, Alvarez O, Lipshultz SE, et al. Ventricular structure and function in children with sickle cell disease using conventional and tissue Doppler echocardiography. *Am J Cardiol.* 2012;109:1358–1364.
23. Niss O, Quinn CT, Lane A, et al. Cardiomyopathy with restrictive physiology in sickle cell disease. *JACC Cardiovasc Imag.* 2016;9:243–252.
24. Manci EA, Culberson DE, Yang YM, et al. Causes of death in sickle cell disease: an autopsy study. *Br J Haematol.* 2016;123:359–365.
25. Mehari A, Gladwin MT, Tian X, et al. Mortality in adults with sickle cell disease and pulmonary hypertension. *J Am Med Assoc.* 2012;307:1254–1256.

159 Human Immunodeficiency Virus

Daniel Bamira, Muhamed Saric

Cardiovascular manifestations of human immunodeficiency virus (HIV) and acquired immunodeficiency syndrome (AIDS) have been reported since the early years of the pandemic.[1] Before the introduction of highly active antiretroviral therapy (HAART), many of the cardiovascular findings resulted from immunosuppression and direct myocardial infection. Common examples of these findings include myocardial and pericardial disease, cardiac tumors, and dilated cardiomyopathy (DCM; Box 159.1). With the advent of HAART and prolonged survival, these findings have become less prevalent, but lipid and metabolic abnormalities, acceleration of coronary disease, and other atherosclerotic disorders have become more common.[2–5] Echocardiographically, there are no pathognomonic findings specific for HIV-associated heart disease. Instead, findings of myocardial, pericardial, or valvular disease secondary to HIV infection are noted.

MYOCARDIAL DISEASE

Myocarditis and DCM in patients with advanced HIV infections occur because of opportunistic infections, autoimmune response, drug-related toxicity, or directly from the HIV virus itself and are frequently associated with a poor prognosis.[6,7] An autopsy study performed before the era of HAART demonstrated an incidence of myocarditis in approximately one-third of patients with AIDS, with a specific cause found in fewer than 20% of these patients.[8]

Myocardial biopsy has been helpful in detecting and treating specific co-infections such as fungal, mycobacterial, or viral pathogens when identified in a case of active myocarditis. Most cases of myocarditis in HIV are clinically silent, and some authors hypothesize that this condition may contribute to HIV-associated DCM.[5,9,10]

In the pre-HAART era, the prevalence of HIV-associated cardiomyopathy was as high as 30% by echocardiographic and autopsy studies and tended to be diagnosed later in the course of the disease, especially in patients with a history of opportunistic infections. Mean survival times of those with HIV-associated cardiomyopathy was 101 days (95% confidence interval [CI] 42–146) compared with 472 days (95% CI, 383–560) for those without it.[11] Since then, there have been vast improvements in both longevity and quality of life[4,7,12]; however, HIV-associated cardiomyopathy seems to remain a distinct condition with worse prognosis than many other forms of cardiomyopathy.[13]

Transthoracic Echocardiography

Myocarditis and DCM are common findings. Some studies have described the effects on the myocardium of both the HIV infection and its treatment in asymptomatic individuals, including diastolic dysfunction and increased left ventricular (LV) mass. After adjusting for race and hypertension, HIV-infected individuals in one study had a statistically significant increase in LV mass of 8 g/m^2 compared with control participants, who had similar left ventricular ejection fraction (LVEF). This finding was associated with lower nadir CD4 T-cell count. In this same report, 50% of patients with HIV showed mild diastolic dysfunction compared with only 29% of control participants.[14] In another study, patients taking HIV protease inhibitors (PIs) demonstrated an increased incidence of cardiac morphologic changes. Significantly higher wall thickness and parameters of diastolic dysfunction were seen in HIV patients receiving protease inhibitors as part of antiretroviral therapy (ART) compared with the non-PI group.[15]

Stress Echocardiography

A study from 2011 investigated the role of dobutamine stress echocardiography in patients with HIV-associated cardiomyopathy. Patients with a LVEF less than 45% (mean LVEF 28% ± 11%) were evaluated for the presence of inotropic contractile reserve (ICR). Whereas the presence of ICR in this population was associated with subsequent improvement in LVEF, its absence was a predictor of cardiac death in addition to advanced New York Heart Associated class IV heart failure.[16]

Strain Imaging

Children and young adults with long-standing HIV (mean duration of HAART, 14.6 years) were shown to have impaired strain and strain rate despite having normal LV systolic function, not associated with a specific difference in LV mass.[17] This suggests that subclinical cardiac abnormalities may be common even in the era of effective ART.

PERICARDIAL DISEASE

Pericardial effusion is the most common cardiac manifestation of HIV and is seen in approximately 20% of cases in the pre-ART era.[3,18] Echocardiography is crucial in diagnosing these effusions, in providing support of pericardial drainage, and in the follow-up of these patients. Pericardial effusions and pericarditis can be from infectious causes (viral, fungal, bacterial, mycobacterial); malignant; or as is most often the case, can be nonspecific in nature. Nutritionally related causes such as hypoalbuminemia may also contribute to these effusions in this population.

Although most of these nonspecific effusions resolve spontaneously, even a transient effusion is a prognosticator of poor outcomes. One study reported a 36% survival at 6 months after the onset of effusions compared with 93% survival in those who never had one. The presence of a pericardial effusion appears to be an indicator of more advanced HIV disease.[3,19] More recently, in a large echocardiographic study performed between 2004 to 2006 with 85% of patients on ART, only two asymptomatic patients were diagnosed with pericardial effusions, and both were deemed small.[20,21] In contrast, a study published in 2016 using cardiac magnetic resonance imaging demonstrated mostly small pericardial effusions in 57% of HIV-infected patients versus 21% of control participants. In ART-naïve patients, there was a 77% incidence of pericardial effusions, although this was not statistically significant.[20,22]

ENDOCARDIAL AND VALVULAR DISEASE

Infective endocarditis (IE) in patients with HIV is primarily seen in injection drug users. Patients with HIV with severe immunosuppression and left-sided lesions carry greater risk for death.

Echocardiographic findings: Clinical factors and presentation are often similar in patients with IE regardless of HIV status.[10,23–25]

CARDIAC TUMORS

In the general population, metastatic tumors are more common than primary cardiac tumors. Certain malignancies, including Kaposi sarcoma and lymphoma, are common in HIV-infected patients, which increase the probability for cardiac involvement. Kaposi sarcoma is rarely confined to the heart; it is usually associated with mucocutaneous disease. Cardiac manifestation includes the pericardium, epicardium, or myocardium.[10,26] Primary cardiac lymphoma in this population is typically B-cell lymphoma (Fig. 159.1 and Video 159.1) and can be aggressive.[27]

Echocardiographic findings: Echocardiography plays a significant role with regard to cardiac tumors because they may present with pericardial effusions and tamponade, wall motion abnormalities, wall thickening, distinct masses, obstructive lesions, and heart failure symptoms.[10,28]

PULMONARY HYPERTENSION

HIV-associated pulmonary hypertension was first described in 1987, affecting these patients at 1000 times great rate than the general population (1 in 200 people with HIV vs 1 in 200,000 without HIV).[4,29,30] This disease has significant morbidity, including right heart failure and poor quality of life, and early studies showed a 50% 1-year mortality rate, with a median survival period from diagnosis to death of 6 months.[29,31] The underlying pathophysiology of HIV-associated pulmonary hypertension shares characteristics with various pulmonary arterial hypertension causes and is likely multifactorial.[4,32] The most specific form of HIV-associated pulmonary hypertension is classified as the World Health Organization class IA. HAART improves symptoms in some studies; however, overall improvement in the post-ART era have been mixed without great decrease in the prevalence of this disease.[5,33]

Figure 159.1. Left ventricular lymphoma in a patient with human immunodeficiency virus and Epstein-Barr infection. **A,** Noncontrast transthoracic echocardiography (TTE) image in parasternal long-axis view demonstrates intracavitary left ventricular lymphoma *(asterisk).* **B,** Microbubble contrast TTE imaging in the apical four-chamber view demonstrates contrast uptake by the lymphoma *(asterisk). LA,* Left atrium; *LV,* left ventricle; *RV,* right ventricle. (See accompanying Video 159.1.)

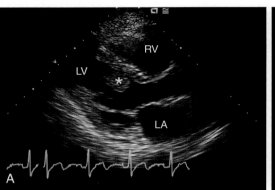
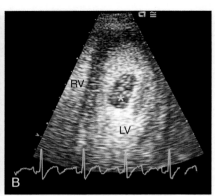

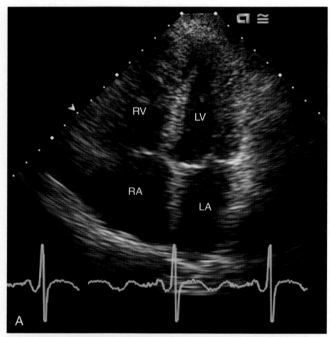

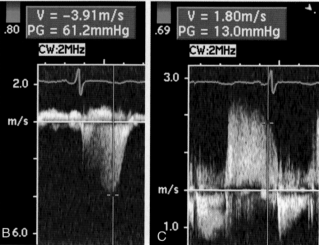

Figure 159.2. Human immunodeficiency virus–associated pulmonary arterial hypertension (World Health Organization class IA). **A,** Dilated and hypertrophied right ventricle (RV) and right atrium (RA) in a patient with severely elevated pulmonary artery (PA) systolic pressure **(B)** and elevated PA diastolic pressure **(C).** *LA,* Left atrium; *LV,* left ventricle. (Video 159.2A corresponds to panel A.)

Echocardiographic findings: General morphologic and functional findings of pulmonary hypertension are observed (Fig. 159.2 and Video 159.2A). Echocardiography plays a critical role in screening for and monitoring progression of this disease.

ATHEROSCLEROSIS

Because of the widespread use of HAART, many of the aforementioned cardiovascular manifestations of HIV have become rare. The combination of prolonged survival and medication side effects have instead led to increasing metabolic abnormalities and accelerated atherosclerosis.

Echocardiographic findings: Stress echocardiography can be used in diagnosis and prognostication of accelerated disease in this population while providing valuable data with regards to exercise capacity. Because the accelerated atherosclerosis in this population leads to coronary disease at a younger age, echocardiography is especially helpful in that it can be performed without exposing these patients to radiation. As HIV transitions into more of a chronic disease, these patients will benefit from the increasingly available percutaneous cardiac interventions that rely heavily on echocardiography for guidance.

Please access ExpertConsult to view the corresponding videos for this chapter.

REFERENCES

1. Autran B, Gorin I, Leibowitch M, et al. AIDS in a Haitian woman with cardiac Kaposi's sarcoma and Whipple's disease. *Lancet.* 1983;1:767–768.
2. Carr A, Cooper DA. Adverse effects of antiretroviral therapy. *Lancet.* 2000;356:1423–1430.
3. Harmon WG, Dadlani GH, Fisher SD, Lipshultz SE. Myocardial and pericardial disease in HIV. *Curr Treat Options Cardiovasc Med.* 2002;4:497–509.
4. Boccara F. Cardiovascular complications and atherosclerotic manifestations in the HIV-infected population: type, incidence and associated risk factors. *AIDS.* 2008;22(suppl 3):S19–S26.
5. Ho JE, Hsue PY. Cardiovascular manifestations of HIV infection. *Heart.* 2009;95:1193–1202.
6. Liu QN, Reddy S, Sayre JW, et al. Essential role of HIV type 1-infected and cyclooxygenase 2-activated macrophages and T cells in HIV type 1 myocarditis. *AIDS Res Hum Retroviruses.* 2001;17:1423–1433.
7. Sagar S, Liu PP, Cooper Jr LT. Myocarditis, *Lancet.* 2012;379:738–747.
8. Anderson DW, Virmani R, Reilly JM, et al. Prevalent myocarditis at necropsy in the acquired immunodeficiency syndrome. *J Am Coll Cardiol.* 1988;11:792–799.
9. Hofman P, Drici MD, Gibelin P, et al. Prevalence of toxoplasma myocarditis in patients with the acquired immunodeficiency syndrome. *Br Heart J.* 1993;70:376–381.
10. Sudano I, Spieker LE, Noll G, et al. Cardiovascular disease in HIV infection. *Am Heart J.* 2006;151:1147–1155.
11. Currie PF, Jacob AJ, Foreman AR, et al. Heart muscle disease related to HIV infection: prognostic implications. *BMJ.* 1994;309:1605–1607.
12. Pugliese A, Isnardi D, Saini A, et al. Impact of highly active antiretroviral therapy in HIV-positive patients with cardiac involvement. *J Infect.* 2000;40:282–284.
13. Felker GM, Thompson RE, Hare JM, et al. Underlying causes and long-term survival in patients with initially unexplained cardiomyopathy. *N Engl J Med.* 2000;342:1077–1084.

14. Hsue PY, Hunt PW, Ho JE, et al. Impact of HIV infection on diastolic function and left ventricular mass. *Circ Heart Fail*. 2010;3:132–139.
15. Meng Q, Lima JA, Lai H, et al. Use of HIV protease inhibitors is associated with left ventricular morphologic changes and diastolic dysfunction. *J Acquir Immune Defic Syndr*. 2002;30:306–310.
16. Wever-Pinzon O, Bangalore S, Romero J, et al. Inotropic contractile reserve can risk-stratify patients with HIV cardiomyopathy: a dobutamine stress echocardiography study. *JACC Cardiovasc Imag*. 2011;4:1231–1238.
17. Sims A, Frank L, Cross R, et al. Abnormal cardiac strain in children and young adults with HIV acquired in early life. *J Am Soc Echocardiogr*. 2012;25:741–748.
18. Estok L, Wallach F. Cardiac tamponade in a patient with AIDS: a review of pericardial disease in patients with HIV infection. *Mt Sinai J Med*. 1998;65:33–39.
19. Heidenreich PA, Eisenberg MJ, Kee LL, et al. Pericardial effusion in AIDS. Incidence and survival. *Circulation*. 1995;92:3229–3234.
20. Glesby MJ. Pericardial disease. In: Myerson MGM, ed. *Cardiovascular Care in Patients with HIV*. Cham: Springer International Publishing; 2019:153–157.
21. Lind A, Reinsch N, Neuhaus K, et al. Pericardial effusion of HIV-infected patients? Results of a prospective multicenter cohort study in the era of antiretroviral therapy. *Eur J Med Res*. 2011;16:480–483.
22. Ntusi N, O'Dwyer E, Dorrell L, et al. HIV-1-related cardiovascular disease is associated with chronic inflammation, frequent pericardial effusions, and probable myocardial edema. *Circ Cardiovasc Imag*. 2016;9. e004430.
23. Nel SH, Naidoo DP. An echocardiographic study of infective endocarditis, with special reference to patients with HIV. *Cardiovasc J Afr*. 2014;25:50–57.
24. Gebo KA, Burkey MD, Lucas GM, et al. Incidence of, risk factors for, clinical presentation, and 1-year outcomes of infective endocarditis in an urban HIV cohort. *J Acquir Immune Defic Syndr*. 2006;43:426–432.
25. Cicalini S, Forcina G, De Rosa FG. Infective endocarditis in patients with human immunodeficiency virus infection. *J Infect*. 2001;42:267–271.
26. Stotka JL, Good CB, Downer WR, Kapoor WN. Pericardial effusion and tamponade due to Kaposi's sarcoma in acquired immunodeficiency syndrome. *Chest*. 1989;95:1359–1361.
27. Mendiolaza J, Baltasar JF, Anis A, et al. Left ventricular non-Hodgkin lymphoma visualized on contrast echocardiography. *J Clin Ultrasound*. 2007;35:462–464.
28. Goldfarb A, King CL, Rosenzweig BP, et al. Cardiac lymphoma in the acquired immunodeficiency syndrome. *Am Heart J*. 1989;118:1340–1344.
29. Mesa RA, Edell ES, Dunn WF, Edwards WD. Human immunodeficiency virus infection and pulmonary hypertension: two new cases and a review of 86 reported cases. *Mayo Clin Proc*. 1998;73:37–45.
30. Kim KK, Factor SM. Membranoproliferative glomerulonephritis and plexogenic pulmonary arteriopathy in a homosexual man with acquired immunodeficiency syndrome. *Hum Pathol*. 1987;18:1293–1296.
31. Mehta NJ, Khan IA, Mehta RN, Sepkowitz DA. HIV-related pulmonary hypertension: Analytic review of 131 cases. *Chest*. 2000;118:1133–1141.
32. Limsukon A, Saeed AI, Ramasamy V, et al. HIV-related pulmonary hypertension. *Mt Sinai J Med*. 2006;73:1037–1044.
33. Zuber JP, Calmy A, Evison JM, et al. Pulmonary arterial hypertension related to HIV infection: improved hemodynamics and survival associated with antiretroviral therapy. *Clin Infect Dis*. 2004;38:1178–1185.

160 Cardiotoxic Effects of Cancer Therapy

Tyler B. Moran, Juan Carlos Plana

Cardiac toxicity by chemotherapeutic drugs was first described more than 50 years ago after the introduction of daunomycin, an anthracycline, as an antimitotic agent.[1] The early recognition of heart failure as a side effect of anthracyclines led oncologists to limit the cumulative dose of chemotherapy and prompted them to find a method to serially monitor the occurrence of left ventricular dysfunction (LVD).[2] Initially, endomyocardial biopsy and left ventricular ejection fraction (LVEF) were the methods most commonly used for the identification of anthracycline-induced cardiomyopathy.[3,4] The role of endomyocardial biopsy has vanished over time because of risks inherent in its invasive nature and costs involved. As a result, noninvasive estimation of LVEF has become the most widely used method for monitoring cardiac function during and after cancer therapy.[5] The success in the treatment and the resultant increase in survival seen in the past decade in patients diagnosed with some forms of cancer have created a new cohort of patients with sufficient survival to develop cardiovascular complications of cancer therapy. If we use the example of breast cancer, the most common malignancy in women in the United States, one in eight women will develop breast cancer over the course of their lifetime. The age-adjusted death rate is 22.6 per 100,000.[6] With increased survival within recent years, the American Cancer Society estimates there are now more than 3.8 million breast cancer survivors in the United States.[7] Because of this extended survival, cardiac toxicity in the form of heart failure becomes the main determinant of quality of life and early death in these patients.[8] Moreover, a patient diagnosed with breast cancer and treated at an early stage has a higher probability of dying from cardiac disease than from recurrence of cancer.[9] To adequately address the burden imposed by heart failure, a combined approach of early identification and treatment of LVD is required, with the hope of preventing the morbidity and mortality associated with progression to the congestive heart failure syndrome in these patients.[10]

CANCER THERAPEUTICS–RELATED CARDIAC DYSFUNCTION

Historically, the term *cardiotoxicity* was used to describe the development of LVD in the setting of the administration of cardiotoxic chemotherapeutic regimens. However, the term is nonspecific, as chemotherapeutic agents may affect the heart in ways different from LVD, including pericardial disease, hypertension, pulmonary hypertension, and QT prolongation.[11] The American Society of Echocardiography (ASE) and the European Association of Cardiovascular Imaging (EACVI) defined in their expert consensus the term *cancer therapeutics–related cardiac dysfunction* (CTRCD) as a decrease in the LVEF of greater than 10 absolute points to a value less than 53%. In 2016, the American Society of Clinical Oncology published its clinical practice guidelines on prevention and monitoring of cardiac dysfunction in survivors of adult cancers. The guidelines state that the existing American College of Cardiology/American Heart Association guidelines for management of stage B disease recommend initiation of pharmacotherapy for individuals with reduced LVEF regardless of cause. They make the point that the exact absolute reduction of ejection fraction (EF) points is irrelevant as long as there is adjudication of stage B heart failure demonstrating the presence of a reduced LVEF.

ANTHRACYCLINE–MEDIATED CARDIAC DYSFUNCTION

Although a comprehensive discussion of all cancer therapeutics associated with CTRCD is beyond the scope of this review, we will focus on two of the most commonly encountered and historically important agents: anthracyclines and trastuzumab. CTRCD secondary to anthracyclines has long been attributed to the production of reactive oxygen species (ROS). However, in the past decade, considerable evidence supports the role of the enzyme topoisomerase 2.[12] There are two topoisomerase 2 isoenzymes in mammalian species: TOP2α and TOP2β. It has been demonstrated that the antitumoral effect of doxorubicin is mediated by the formation of a ternary complex consisting of TOP2α, doxorubicin, and DNA.[13] TOP2α is expressed only in cells with a high mitotic rate, such as neoplastic cells, which explains the high efficacy of anthracyclines. In contrast, TOP2β is expressed in normal tissue, including cardiac cells. The role of TOP2β in anthracycline cardiotoxicity was demonstrated in a *Top2β* knockout animal.[14] Formation of the ternary complexes leads to DNA fragmentation. The resultant overproduction of ROS and defective mitochondrial biogenesis ultimately leads to apoptosis of myocardial cells. The incidence of heart failure, which is the major complication of anthracycline-mediated cardiotoxicity, fluctuates between 2.2% and 5.1% depending on the series.[15] The curves of cardiotoxicity with doxorubicin showed an incidence of heart failure that was appreciably low until the cumulative dose reaches 450 mg/m^2.[16] This finding promoted the common belief that CTRCD was unlikely with doxorubicin doses lower than 450 mg/m^2. Nevertheless, there was evidence of a rate of 26% of mild left ventricular (LV) dysfunction at 6 months (EF <50% by cardiac magnetic resonance imaging [CMRI]) in patients who were treated with doses previously thought to be benign (50–375 mg/m^2).[17]

The pathophysiology of CTRCD secondary to anthracyclines involves early and cumulative dose-dependent myocyte damage, which is mediated largely by cellular apoptosis. Overall, anthracycline cardiomyopathy, which includes doxorubicin, epirubicin, and idarubicin, has been linked to a poor prognosis, with 2-year mortality rates up to 60%.[18] These agents are now considered to have increased potential for long-term cardiac dysfunction and increased morbidity and mortality and, as a result, warrant a higher level of long-term scrutiny.[6,19]

TRASTUZUMAB–ASSOCIATED CARDIAC DYSFUNCTION

In contrast to anthracyclines, a number of agents, such as trastuzumab, do not directly cause myocyte apoptosis at the time of administration in a cumulative dose-dependent fashion. The typical anthracycline-induced cell damage seen in cardiac biopsies is not seen in patients treated with these agents. In many instances, these agents have been continued for decades without the progressive cardiac dysfunction that would be expected with anthracyclines. Functional recovery of myocardial function is frequently seen after their interruption. Nevertheless, recent data recognize a cohort of patients that would have higher risk of trastuzumab-related CTRCD (older adult patients, patients with more than two traditional cardiovascular risk factors, patients with borderline baseline LVEF and combination chemotherapy and/or radiotherapy).[20]

The amplification of the *HER2/neu (ErbB2)* gene represents an essential process in this subgroup of breast cancer and is associated with a more malignant behavior and prognosis. Trastuzumab (Herceptin) is a humanized monoclonal antibody that targets the HER2 protein acting as an inhibitor of the tyrosine kinase receptor encoded by the *ErbB2* gene.[21] The development of this monoclonal antibody, approved in 1998, was one of the most significant breakthroughs in the history of translational research. Multiple large-scale studies have proven that trastuzumab significantly reduces the risks of recurrence and early death in patients with *HER2*-positive breast cancers. An incidence of heart failure has been reported in up to 12% of treated patients.[22]

COMBINED CHEMOTHERAPY

The addition of trastuzumab to anthracyclines therapy increases the toxicity risk. Slamon and colleagues[23] compared three chemotherapy protocols in patients with metastatic *HER2*-positive breast cancer, reporting a rate of 27% of LVD in the group of combined

trastuzumab–anthracycline compared with 13% in the trastuzumab paclitaxel protocol and 8% in the trastuzumab-free group. The incidence of severe cardiac dysfunction with New York Heart Association class III or IV was the highest at 16%, among the patients who received trastuzumab and anthracycline, compared with 3% in patients who received anthracyclines without trastuzumab and 2% among those who received trastuzumab and paclitaxel.[23] Animal studies done with a model of cardiac stress mediated by anthracyclines and hemodynamic overload showed that *ErbB2* knockout mice were significantly more susceptible to cardiac toxicity and heart failure. These findings support the crucial role of the *ErbB2* gene in the activation of cardioprotective pathways to permit myocyte survival during acute stress signaling activation.[24] A reduction in these cardioprotective pathways after trastuzumab treatment probably facilitates myocyte loss after exposure to anthracyclines. This premise is consistent with clinical findings evidencing increased cardiotoxicity after exposure to trastuzumab in patients with underlying myocardial disease in whom the cardiac stress signals are presumably already activated.[25] In the American Society of Clinical Oncology Clinical Practice Guideline, patients treated even with low-dose anthracycline (<250 mg/m^2, epirubicin <600 mg/m^2) followed by trastuzumab are considered at increased risk of developing cardiac dysfunction, and routine surveillance with echocardiography as the modality of choice can be considered even in asymptomatic patients.[20]

Immune Checkpoint Inhibitor–Associated Cardiac Toxicity

The advent of cancer immunotherapy including immune checkpoint inhibitors (ICIs) led to improved outcomes for advanced-stage cancers, including metastatic melanoma, renal cell cancer, and non–small cell lung cancer, as well as Hodgkin and non-Hodgkin lymphomas. These antibodies result in stimulation of previously inactive cytotoxic T cells to target tumor cells. Although these treatments are generally well tolerated, unfortunately, a small proportion of these patients develop significant cardiac complications, including atrial fibrillation, ventricular tachycardia, heart block, heart failure, and myocarditis.[26] The incidence of myocarditis based on Bristol-Myers Squibb safety database was initially found to be fairly low at approximately 0.09% with single ICI therapy; however, more recent data suggest it may be a bit higher and at least 1%.[27] Those who have ICI-associated myocarditis experience significant complications, and in one study, 46% a had major adverse cardiac event (MACE), defined as a composite of cardiovascular death, cardiac arrest, cardiogenic shock, and hemodynamically significant complete heart block.[27] Importantly, the study found nearly all patients with myocarditis had elevated troponin (94%), and treatment with higher-dose steroids was associated with lower rates of MACE.[27] A high index of suspicion is necessary when evaluating these patients because presenting symptoms can be nonspecific and may overlap with typical cancer therapy–associated symptoms, including malaise, fever, nausea, and vomiting. Clearly, further research is necessary to help guide detection and management in this rare but potentially fatal ICI-associated cardiac toxicity.

ECHOCARDIOGRAPHIC EVALUATION OF PATIENTS RECEIVING CANCER THERAPY

Echocardiography has been established as the cornerstone in the imaging evaluation of patients in preparation for, during, or after cancer therapy. This is because of its wide availability, versatility, lack of radiation exposure, and low cost compared with other modalities. In addition to the evaluation of left and right ventricular dimensions and systolic and diastolic function at rest and during stress, it also allows a comprehensive evaluation of cardiac valves, the aorta, and the pericardium, making it the imaging modality of choice in the evaluation of the cancer patient.[1]

Two-Dimensional Echocardiography

LVEF is the most common method used to evaluate cardiac function at baseline and during treatment.[5] LVEF is most commonly evaluated with echocardiography.[28] However, the technique is affected by the quality of the acoustic window, the use of geometric assumptions to calculate LV volumes, load dependency, and operator expertise.[29] Thavendiranathan et al.[30] evaluated the temporal variability of two-dimensional (2D) EF for sequential assessment of LVEF. They found a 95% confidence interval (CI) for 2D EF of approximately 10 points of EF. This is particularly problematic because this is the same magnitude of change that is used to adjudicate the presence of CTRCD.[31] In addition, the reported intra- and interobserver variabilities are significantly high, with ranges that fluctuate between 6% to 11% and 8% to 16%, respectively, depending on the series.[30]

Contrast-Enhanced Echocardiography

The use of contrast agents is crucial for the assessment of LV volumes and function when the endocardium is not well visualized.[32] The presence of endocardial dropout is especially frequent in patients with breast cancer because of the common occurrence of mastectomy and chest radiation. The ASE and the EACVI recommend the use of ultrasonic contrast agents when two or more contiguous LV segments are not seen on noncontrast images.[33,34] Nahar and associates[35] compared LVEF quantification by radionuclide angiography with four different 2D echocardiography techniques (fundamental, fundamental with contrast, harmonic, and harmonic with contrast), reporting an incremental correlation with each method. However, harmonic imaging with contrast provided the closest correlation.[36] Also, compared with standard 2D imaging, contrast enhancement increased the feasibility of biplane volume analysis from 79% to 95% and narrowed the limits of LVEF agreement between echo and CMRI from −18.1% to 8.3% to −7.7% to 4.1%.[36] Intra- and interobserver reproducibility also benefited from contrast use, achieving correlation indices (r) greater than 0.9.[32] It is important to realize that there are no established values for normal LV volumes with enhanced echocardiography. A study examining baseline prechemotherapy echocardiograms on female patients with breast cancer classified 51% of contrast-enhanced end-diastolic volume as abnormal even though LV dimensions were within the normal range by unenhanced 2D volume measurements.

Three-Dimensional Echocardiography

The main pitfalls of 2D echocardiography for ventricular volumes and LVEF quantification are geometric assumptions and foreshortening of the LV. Real-time three-dimensional (3D) echocardiography has emerged as a good alternative because of its ability to capture full ventricular volumes, which allows easy identification of the true apex and the use of automatic endocardial detection algorithms.

Real-time 3D echocardiography has also proven to be a reproducible tool, making it an ideal method for the successive evaluations required in chemotherapy patients, which are acquired at different time points and analyzed by different observers. In the study by Thavendiranathan and associates[30] discussed previously, noncontrast 3D volumes and LVEF had the best intra- and interobserver as well as lower test–retest variability. 3D LVEF provided an upper CI limit of 4.9%, which is just below the 5% threshold in asymptomatic patients (Fig. 160.1 and Video 160.1).

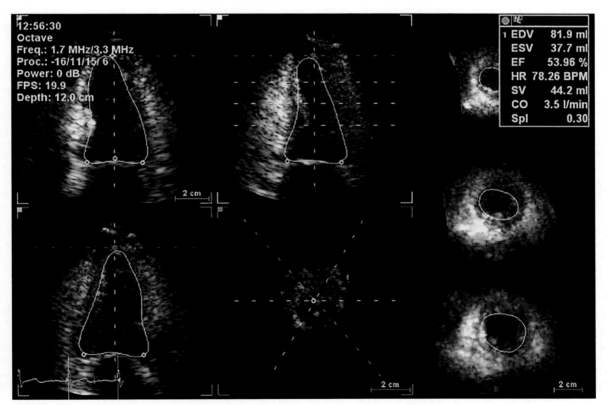

Figure 160.1. Three-dimensional echocardiography for the estimation of left ventricular volumes and ejection fraction (EF) in a 61-year-old woman before the initiation of trastuzumab-based regimen. Her EF is 53% (low normal). *CO,* Cardiac output; *EDV,* end-diastolic volume; *ESV,* end-systolic volume; *EF,* ejection fraction; *FPS,* frames per second; *HR,* heart rate; *Spl,* sphericity index; *SV,* stroke volume. (Also see accompanying Video 160.1.)

Walker and coworkers[37] evaluated the role of 3D in patients with breast cancer. They found that whereas 2D TTE demonstrated a weak correlation with CMRI for LVEF assessment ($r = 0.31$ at baseline; $r = 0.42$ at 12 months), 3D TTE showed a strong correlation compared with CMRI ($r = 0.91$ at baseline; $r = 0.90$ at 12 months).

Stress Echocardiography for Evaluation of Cardiotoxicity

Although both exercise and dobutamine stress echocardiograms have been applied for identification of anthracycline cardiotoxicity, the results of these studies have been inconclusive and contradictory. In 31 patients with cancer studied before, during, and after 6 months of chemotherapy, low-dose dobutamine provided no additional value for the early detection of cardiotoxicity.[38,39] In contrast, a prospective study of LV contractile reserve by repeated low-dose dobutamine stress echocardiography in 49 women with breast cancer showed that a reduction in LVEF with dobutamine greater than 5% appeared to be a threshold that discriminated the risk of a future drop in LVEF.[40] It is reasonable to assess the presence of ischemia in patients with risk factors or known history of coronary artery disease with planned regimens associated with ischemia (e.g., anti–vascular endothelial growth factor therapy inhibitors).

Strain Imaging

As previously described, LVEF is the most common method of monitoring cardiac function during cancer treatment. However, LVEF fails to identify small changes in LV function. The evaluation of LV mechanics using strain has emerged as a reproducible and accurate method for comprehensive evaluation of systolic function.[41-43] Strain has also proved to be a useful technique in the detection of subclinical myocardial dysfunction in multiple clinical entities.

Global longitudinal strain (GLS) has proven to be an early independent predictor of later reduction in LVEF after exposure to chemotherapeutic drugs. In one study of 81 women with breast cancer treated with anthracyclines followed by taxanes and trastuzumab and evaluated every 3 months for a period of 15 months, a decrease in longitudinal strain below −19% during the initial anthracycline treatment predicted the occurrence of subsequent cardiotoxicity.[44] Negishi and colleagues[45] evaluated the optimal myocardial deformation index to predict cardiotoxicity (defined as a 10% drop in LVEF) at 12 months in 81 consecutive patients exposed to trastuzumab. In their study, an 11% drop in GLS (95% CI, 8.3%–14.6%) was the strongest predictor of later cardiotoxicity with an area under the curve of 0.87, a sensitivity of 65%, and a specificity of 94%.[45] It was concluded that a relative reduction less than 8% was of no clinical significance, and a relative reduction greater than 15% was of definite clinical significance[45] (Figs. 160.2 to 160.5). A recent meta-analysis by Oikonomou and associates of 21 studies with 1783 patients concluded that measurement of GLS after initiation of potentially cardiotoxic chemotherapy with anthracyclines with or without trastuzumab had good prognostic performance for subsequent CTRCD.[46] However, risk of bias in the original studies, publication bias, and limited data on the incremental value of GLS and its optimal cutoff value highlights the need for larger prospective multicenter studies.

There has been also interest in the role of GLS in patients with myocarditis from ICIs. The International ICI Myocarditis cohort study reported that GLS is abnormal in patients with preserved and reduced EF. A lower GLS is associated with MACE among all myocarditis cases.[47]

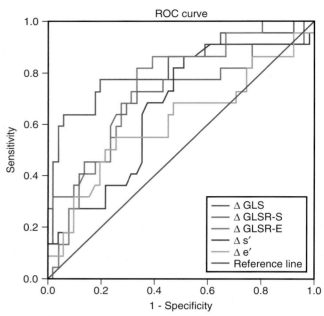

Figure 160.2. Receiver operating characteristic curves (ROC) to predict subsequent decrease in ejection fraction (EF). Discriminative abilities of the deformation parameters were evaluated to predict the subsequent decrease in EF. *GLS,* Global longitudinal strain; *GLSR-E,* global longitudinal early diastolic strain rate; *GLSR-S,* global longitudinal peak systolic strain rate. (Modified with permission from Negishi K, et al: Independent and incremental value of deformation indices for prediction of trastuzumab-induced cardiotoxicity, *J Am Soc Echocardiogr* 26:493–498, 2013.)

Diastolic Function and Cardiotoxicity

Several small prospective studies have demonstrated that changes in LV diastolic parameters precede LVEF drop during and after anthracycline treatment,[48-50] and changes in tissue Doppler parameters may be more sensitive than standard Doppler measurements to detect diastolic dysfunction in this population.[51] It is important to recognize that fluctuations in early diastolic velocity of the mitral annulus by pulsed-tissue Doppler (E′ wave) can be a result of changes in preload as a consequence of chemotherapy (nausea, vomiting, and diarrhea) and not necessarily related to cardiotoxicity affecting the diastolic properties of the heart. Current evidence does not support the role of these indices for the prediction of later cardiotoxicity.[49,52]

CONCLUSIONS

Every patient scheduled to receive a cardiotoxic regimen should obtain a baseline echocardiogram. 3D echocardiography has the lowest temporal variability and as a result is the modality of choice for the longitudinal assessment of EF where available. GLS is a promising technique for the early recognition of cardiotoxicity. We recommend following the algorithms proposed in the expert consensus on the multimodality imaging of adult patients during and after cancer therapy[53] as well as the American Society of Clinical Oncology guidelines[20] for the initiation, surveillance, and follow-up of cancer treatment.

Please access ExpertConsult to view the corresponding video for this chapter.

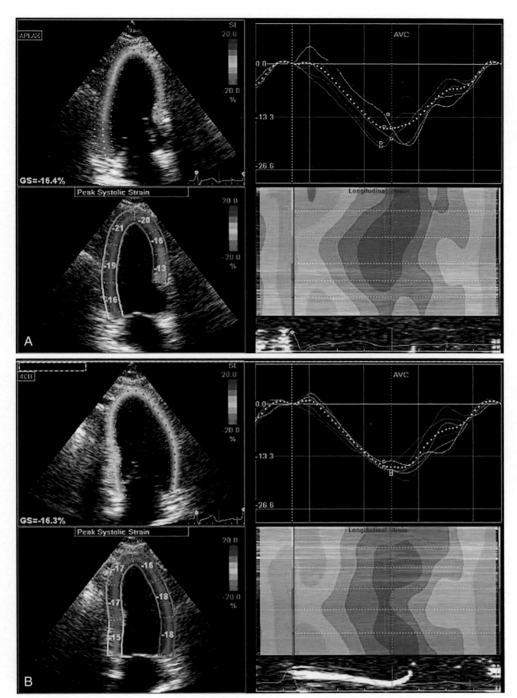

Figure 160.3. Global longitudinal strain (GLS) obtained at baseline in the patient described in Fig. 160.1 in the apical three-(AP3) (**A**), four-(AP4) (**B**), and two-(AP2)

Continued

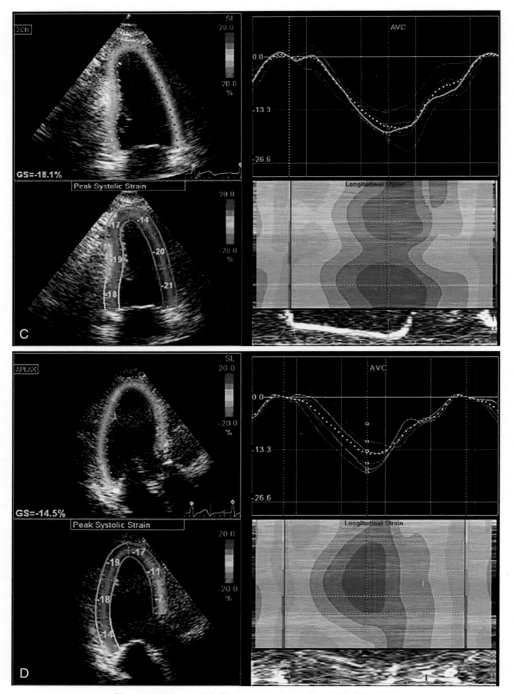

Figure 160.3, cont'd (**C**) chamber views. The AP3- (**D**), AP4-

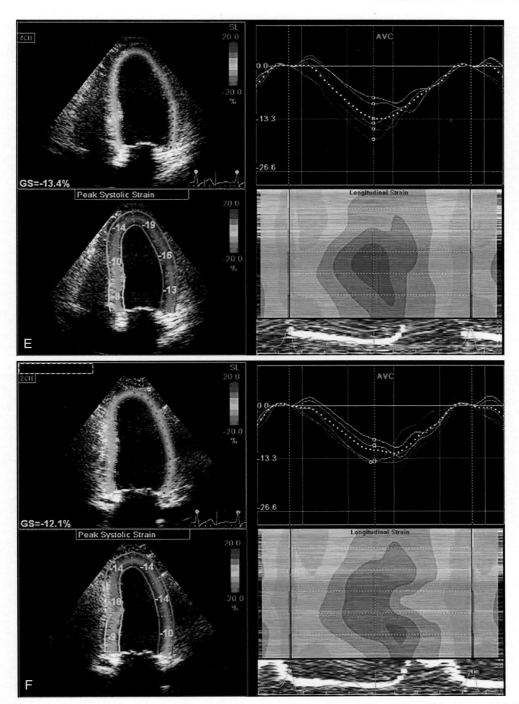

Figure 160.3, cont'd (**E**), and AP2- (**F**) derived GLS 3 months into treatment with trastuzumab. The GLS has fallen from −16.9% to −13.3% (21% relative decrease). *AVC,* aortic valve closure; *GS,* global strain.

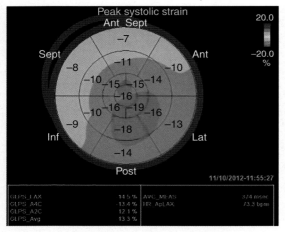

Figure 160.4. Bull's-eye display of the global longitudinal strain 3 months after the initiation of treatment. *Ant,* Anterior; *Inf,* inferior; *Lat,* lateral; *Post,* posterior; *Sept,* septal.

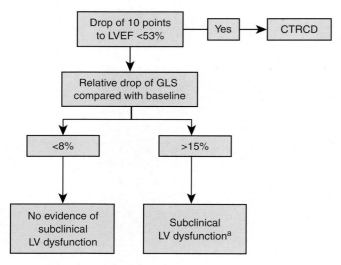

[a] The data supporting the initiation of cardioprotection for the treatment of subclinical LV dysfunction are limited.

Figure 160.5. Early detection of cardiotoxicity using strain imaging. *CTRCD,* Cancer therapeutics–related cardiac dysfunction; *EF,* ejection fraction; *GLS,* global longitudinal strain; *LV,* left ventricular; *LVEF,* left ventricular ejection fraction (Reproduced with permission from Plana JC, et al: Expert consensus for multimodality imaging evaluation of adult patients during and after cancer therapy, *J Am Soc Echocardiogr* 27:911–939, 2014.)

REFERENCES

1. Tan C, Tasaka H, Yu KP, et al. Daunomycin, an antitumor antibiotic, in the treatment of neoplastic disease: clinical evaluation with special reference to childhood leukemia. *Cancer.* 1967;20:333–353.
2. Lefrak EA, Pitha J, Rosenheim S, Gottlieb JA. A clinicopathologic analysis of Adriamycin cardiotoxicity. *Cancer.* 1973;32:302–314.
3. Ramos A, Meyer RA, Korfhagen J, et al. Echocardiographic evaluation of Adriamycin cardiotoxicity in children. *Cancer Treat Rep.* 1976;60:1281–1284.
4. Billingham ME, Bristow MR, Glatstein E, et al. Adriamycin cardiotoxicity: endomyocardial biopsy evidence of enhancement by irradiation. *Am J Surg Pathol.* 1977;1:17–23.
5. Lenzhofer R, Dudczak R, Gumhold G, et al. Noninvasive methods for the early detection of doxorubicin-induced cardiomyopathy. *J Cancer Res Clin Oncol.* 1983;106:136–142.
6. Toriola AT, Colditz GA. Trends in breast cancer incidence and mortality in the United States: implications for prevention. *Breast Cancer Res Treat.* 2013;138:665–673.
7. Street W. Cancer facts & figures 2019. *Am Cancer Soc.* 2019;76.
8. Mann DL, Krone RJ. Cardiac disease in cancer patients: an overview. *Prog Cardiovasc Dis.* 2010;53:80–87.
9. Hanrahan EO, Gonzalez-Angulo AM, Giordano SH, et al. Overall survival and cause-specific mortality of patients with stage T1abN0M0 breast carcinoma. *J Clin Oncol.* 2007;25:4952–4960.
10. Atherton JJ. Stage B heart failure: rationale for screening. *Heart Fail Clin.* 2012;8:273–283.
11. Chang H-M, Moudgil R, Scarabelli T, et al. Cardiovascular complications of cancer therapy: best practices in diagnosis, prevention, and management—Part 1. *J Am Coll Cardiol.* 2017;70:2536–2551.
12. De Graff WG, Myers LS, Mitchell JB, Hahn SM. Protection against Adriamycin cytotoxicity and inhibition of DNA topoisomerase II activity by 3,4-dihydroxybenzoic acid. *Int J Oncol.* 2003;23(7):159–163.
13. Tewey KM, Rowe TC, Yang L, et al. Adriamycin-induced DNA damage mediated by mammalian DNA topoisomerase II. *Science.* 1984;226:466–468.
14. Lyu YL, Kerrigan JE, Lin C-P, et al. Topoisomerase II mediated DNA double-strand breaks: implications in doxorubicin cardiotoxicity and prevention by dexrazoxane. *Cancer Res.* 2007;67:8839–8846.
15. Von Hoff DD, Layard MW, Basa P, et al. Risk factors for doxorubicin-induced congestive heart failure. *Ann Intern Med.* 1979;91:710–717.
16. Ewer MS, Von Hoff DD, Benjamin RS. A historical perspective of anthracycline cardiotoxicity. *Heart Fail Clin.* 2011;7:363–372.
17. Drafts BC, Twomley KM, D'Agostino R, et al. Low to moderate dose anthracycline-based chemotherapy is associated with early noninvasive imaging evidence of subclinical cardiovascular disease. *JACC Cardiovasc Imag.* 2013;6:877–885.
18. Felker GM, Thompson RE, Hare JM, et al. Underlying causes and long-term survival in patients with initially unexplained cardiomyopathy. *N Engl J Med.* 2000;342:1077–1084.
19. Knobf MT. The influence of endocrine effects of adjuvant therapy on quality of life outcomes in younger breast cancer survivors. *Oncol.* 2006;11:96–110.
20. Armenian SH, Lacchetti C, Barac A, et al. Prevention and monitoring of cardiac dysfunction in survivors of adult cancers. *J Clin Oncol.* 2017;35:893–911.
21. Baselga J, Norton L, Albanell J, et al. Recombinant humanized anti-HER2 antibody (Herceptin) enhances the antitumor activity of paclitaxel and doxorubicin against HER2/neu overexpressing human breast cancer xenografts. *Cancer Res.* 1998;58:2825–2831.
22. Bowles EJA, Wellman R, Feigelson HS, et al. Risk of heart failure in breast cancer patients after anthracycline and trastuzumab treatment: a retrospective cohort study. *JNCI J Natl Cancer Inst.* 2012;104:1293–1305.
23. Slamon DJ, Leyland-Jones B, Shak S, et al. Use of chemotherapy plus a monoclonal antibody against her2 for metastatic breast cancer that overexpresses HER2. *N Engl J Med.* 2001;344:783–792.
24. Crone SA, Zhao Y-Y, Fan L, et al. ErbB2 is essential in the prevention of dilated cardiomyopathy. *Nat Med.* 2002;8:459–465.
25. Chien KR. Herceptin and the heart: a molecular modifier of cardiac failure. *N Engl J Med.* 2006;354(8):789–790.
26. Escudier M, Cautela J, Malissen N, et al. Clinical features, management, and outcomes of immune checkpoint inhibitor–related cardiotoxicity. *Circulation.* 2017;136:2085–2087.
27. Mahmood SS, Fradley MG, Cohen JV, et al. Myocarditis in patients treated with immune checkpoint inhibitors. *J Am Coll Cardiol.* 2018;71:1755–1764.
28. Oreto L, Todaro MC, Umland MM, et al. Use of echocardiography to evaluate the cardiac effects of therapies used in cancer treatment: what do we know? *J Am Soc Echocardiogr.* 2012;25:1141–1152.
29. Jannazzo A, Hoffman J, Lutz M. Monitoring of anthracycline-induced cardiotoxicity. *Ann Pharmacother.* 2008;42:99–104.
30. Thavendiranathan P, Grant AD, Negishi T, et al. Reproducibility of echocardiographic techniques for sequential assessment of left ventricular ejection fraction and volumes. *J Am Coll Cardiol.* 2013;61:77–84.
31. Stanton T, Leano R, Marwick TH. Prediction of all-cause mortality from global longitudinal speckle strain: comparison with ejection fraction and wall motion scoring. *Circ Cardiovasc Imag.* 2009;2:356–364.
32. McGowan JH, Cleland JGF. Reliability of reporting left ventricular systolic function by echocardiography: a systematic review of 3 methods. *Am Heart J.* 2003;146:388–397.
33. Yu EH, Sloggett CE, Iwanochko RM, et al. Feasibility and accuracy of left ventricular volumes and ejection fraction determination by fundamental, tissue harmonic, and intravenous contrast imaging in difficult-to-image patients. *J Am Soc Echocardiogr.* 2000;13:216–224.
34. Mulvagh SL, Rakowski H, Vannan MA, et al. American Society of echocardiography consensus Statement on the clinical Applications of ultrasonic contrast agents in echocardiography. *J Am Soc Echocardiogr.* 2008;21:1179–1201.
35. Nahar T, Croft L, Shapiro R, et al. Comparison of four echocardiographic techniques for measuring left ventricular ejection fraction. *Am J Cardiol.* 2000;86:1358–1362.
36. Senior R, Becher H, Monaghan M, et al. Contrast echocardiography: evidence-based recommendations by European association of echocardiography. *Eur J Echocardiogr.* 2008;10:194–212.
37. Walker J, Bhullar N, Fallah-Rad N, et al. Role of three-dimensional echocardiography in breast cancer: comparison with two-dimensional echocardiography, multiple-gated acquisition scans, and cardiac magnetic resonance imaging. *J Clin Oncol.* 2010;28:3429–3436.
38. Bountioukos M. Repetitive dobutamine stress echocardiography for the prediction of anthracycline cardiotoxicity. *Eur J Echocardiogr.* 2003;4:300–305.

39. Cottin Y. Dobutamine stress echocardiography identifies anthracycline cardiotoxicity. *Eur J Echocardiogr.* 2000;1:180–183.
40. Civelli M, Cardinale D, Martinoni A, et al. Early reduction in left ventricular contractile reserve detected by dobutamine stress echo predicts high-dose chemotherapy-induced cardiac toxicity. *Int J Cardiol.* 2006;111:120–126.
41. Korinek J, Wang J, Sengupta PP, et al. Two-dimensional strain—a Doppler-independent ultrasound method for quantitation of regional deformation: validation in vitro and in vivo. *J Am Soc Echocardiogr.* 2005;18:1247–1253.
42. Yeon SB, Reichek N, Tallant BA, et al. Validation of in vivo myocardial strain measurement by magnetic resonance tagging with sonomicrometry. *J Am Coll Cardiol.* 2001;38:555–561.
43. Urheim S, Edvardsen T, Torp H, et al. Myocardial strain by Doppler echocardiography: validation of a new method to quantify regional myocardial function. *Circulation.* 2000;102:1158–1164.
44. Sawaya H, Sebag IA, Plana JC, et al. Assessment of echocardiography and biomarkers for the extended prediction of cardiotoxicity in patients treated with anthracyclines, taxanes, and trastuzumab. *Circ Cardiovasc Imag.* 2012;5:596–603.
45. Negishi K, Negishi T, Hare JL, et al. Independent and incremental value of deformation indices for prediction of trastuzumab-induced cardiotoxicity. *J Am Soc Echocardiogr.* 2013;26:493–498.
46. Oikonomou EK, Kokkinidis DG, Kampaktsis PN, et al. Assessment of prognostic value of left ventricular global longitudinal strain for early prediction of chemotherapy-induced cardiotoxicity: a systematic review and meta-analysis. *JAMA Cardiol.* 2019;4:1007.
47. Awadalla M, Mahmood S, Groarke J, et al. Decreased global longitudinal strain with myocarditis from immune checkpoint inhibitors and occurrence of major adverse cardiac events. *J Am Coll Cardiol.* 2019;73(9 suppl 1):1532.
48. Stoddard MF, Seeger J, Liddell NE, et al. Prolongation of isovolumetric relaxation time as assessed by Doppler echocardiography predicts doxorubicin-induced systolic dysfunction in humans. *J Am Coll Cardiol.* 1992;20:62–69.
49. Dorup I. Prospective longitudinal assessment of late anthracycline cardiotoxicity after childhood cancer: the role of diastolic function. *Heart.* 2004;90:1214–1216.
50. Marchandise B, Schroeder E, Bosly A, et al. Early detection of doxorubicin cardiotoxicity: interest of Doppler echocardiographic analysis of left ventricular filling dynamics. *Am Heart J.* 1989;118:92–98.
51. Tassanmangina S, Codorean D, Metivier M, et al. Tissue Doppler imaging and conventional echocardiography after anthracycline treatment in adults: early and late alterations of left ventricular function during a prospective study. *Eur J Echocardiogr.* 2006;7:141–146.
52. Rohde LE, Baldi A, Weber C, et al. Tei index in adult patients submitted to Adriamycin chemotherapy: failure to predict early systolic dysfunction: diagnosis of Adriamycin cardiotoxicity. *Int J Cardiovasc Imag.* 2007;23:185–191.
53. Plana JC, Galderisi M, Barac A, et al. Expert consensus for multimodality imaging evaluation of adult patients during and after cancer therapy. *J Am Soc Echocardiogr.* 2014;27:911–939.

161 Pregnancy and the Heart

Tasneem Z. Naqvi, Afsoon Fazlinezhad, Uri Elkayam

During normal pregnancy, the maternal cardiovascular system undergoes significant hemodynamic changes to ensure an uncomplicated pregnancy and a healthy fetus. Evaluation of these changes needs precise and safe diagnostic modalities.[1] Echocardiography is the modality of choice to evaluate cardiac structure and function in pregnant women. Transthoracic echocardiography (TTE) is noninvasive and safe; does not involve radiation; is easily available, affordable, and portable; and can provide accurate assessment of cardiac morphology and function. Transesophageal echocardiography is seldom performed during pregnancy; however, when necessary, it can be performed safely, although careful monitoring of maternal oxygen saturation is necessary if midazolam is used for sedation. However, the risk of vomiting and aspiration as well as sudden increases in intraabdominal pressure should be considered and fetal monitoring performed.[2] Physiological exercise testing is an integral part of follow-up of patients with adult congenital heart disease and valve disease and may be combined with stress echocardiography for additional information.[2]

PHYSICAL EXAMINATION FINDINGS IN NORMAL PREGNANCY

Many healthy pregnant women experience shortness of breath, syncope, dizziness, and fatigue, and at later stages of pregnancy bilateral pedal edema, that mimic the presence of significant heart disease. On cardiac examination, the heart rate increases, particularly in the second trimester of pregnancy. Slight elevation of jugular venous pressure may be detected in the middle of the second trimester. Prominent first and second heart sounds may be detected that may suggest an atrial septal defect or an increase pulmonary artery pressure. Up to 3/6 ejection systolic flow murmur from increased flow through the left and right ventricular (RV) outflow tracts can be heard along with a bounding arterial pulse, a prominent apical impulse that may be shifted laterally because of the gravid uterus, and an RV impulse caused by volume overload; a third heart sound may also be present.[3] Continuous murmurs, either a cervical venous hum best heard over the right supraclavicular area, or a mammary murmur (continuous or systolic) caused by increased flow in the mammary arteries, may also be heard over the breast late in pregnancy or during lactation period. When disproportionate or unexplained dyspnea or new cardiovascular signs or symptoms occur during pregnancy or when a new pathological murmur or diastolic murmur is heard, echocardiography is indicated.[2]

PHYSIOLOGIC CHANGES WITH PREGNANCY

Pregnancy has prominent effects on the cardiovascular system.[4] These include increase in blood volume, red cell mass, heart rate, and cardiac output related to changes in afterload, preload, and peripheral vascular resistance, and these effects are sustained into the postpartum period.[1] Pregnancy in women with cardiovascular disease is associated with impaired physiological adaptation and hence results in adverse material and fetal outcomes.[5] Blood volume increases by 10% to 15% by 7 weeks of gestation and rises until around 32 weeks to a 30% to 50% increase in total plasma volume.[6] About 75% of this increase has occurred by the end of the first trimester. The red cell mass also increases until the end of pregnancy to about 20%, resulting in anemia of pregnancy. Overall, cardiac output increases 30% to 50% during normal pregnancy, beginning during the first trimester and peaking at around 25 to 35 weeks of gestation.[7–12]

The increase in stroke volume accounts for much of the increase in cardiac output in the first two trimesters. An elevation in heart rate becomes a more important factor in the third trimester of pregnancy. Blood pressure (BP) decreases at 7 weeks' gestation and continues to fall until it reaches nadir by midpregnancy, reaching about 5 to 10 mm Hg (~10%) below baseline. The decrease in the BP is related to the decrease in systemic vascular resistance (SVR), which is noted as early as 5 weeks of gestation, falling to around 35% to 40% at 20 weeks, when it plateaus. Afterward, BP gradually increases and returns to its prepregnancy level at term.[7,9] Increased level of estrogen, progesterone, and relaxin with some vasodilatory properties and increased production of vascular nitric oxide are probable contributors to reduced SVR during pregnancy. Uteroplacental shunting and

TABLE 161.1 Echocardiographic Changes During Pregnancy

Echocardiographic Variable	Change During Pregnancy
LVD and volume	Increases
LV wall thickness and LV mass	Increases
LVEF	Unchanged
LV fractional shortening	Unchanged
LV radial and longitudinal strain rate	Increases
Aortic root diameter	Mildly increases
RV dimension and volume	Increases
RVEF	Unchanged
Left atrial size and volume	Increases
Stroke volume as measured using LVOT VTI	Increases
Mitral E-wave velocity	Increases and then decreases
Mitral A-wave velocity	Increases
Peak pulmonary artery systolic pressure estimated using TR jet	Unchanged

LV, Left ventricular; *LVD,* left ventricular dimension; *LVEF,* left ventricular ejection fraction; *LVOT,* left ventricular outflow tract. *RV,* right ventricular; *RVEF,* right ventricular ejection fraction; *TR,* tricuspid regurgitation; *VTI,* velocity time integral.

decrease in vascular responsiveness to the pressor effect of angiotensin II and norepinephrine are other contributors.[7,8]

The physiological adaptations to pregnancy influence the evaluation and interpretation of cardiac function and clinical status. Maternal cardiac dysfunction is related to impaired uteroplacental flow and suboptimal fetal outcome.[5,9] Increase in blood volume is offset by a reduction in SVR, causing no change in pulmonary artery pressures.[10] These cardiovascular changes resolve after delivery, with hemodynamics largely returning to baseline level by 24 weeks postpartum.[7,11]

ECHOCARDIOGRAPHIC FINDINGS DURING NORMAL PREGNANCY

In response to the hemodynamic changes in pregnancy, the heart undergoes major Morphologic and functional adaptations that can be detected by TTE (Table 161.1).

Left Ventricular Relative Wall Thickness

The increase in circulating volume during pregnancy is thought to lead to an increase in left ventricular (LV) mass and a proportional increase in LV wall thickness. The ratio between ventricular end-diastolic radius and wall thickness, represented by the relative wall thickness (RWT), remains stable during normal pregnancy and is referred to as eccentric remodeling.[12] This is in contrast to concentric remodeling, which occurs in hypertensive pregnancy when RWT increases more than LV end-diastolic radius.[1,13]

Cardiac Chamber Dimensions

Left Ventricle

To accommodate the increased preload, there is a 5% to 10% increase in LV end-diastolic dimension[9,10] (Fig 161.1). Along with an increase in LV dimensions, there is a corresponding increase in LV wall thickness and LV mass, reaching a maximum increase of 23.6% in the third trimester followed by a sharp drop in LV mass late in the third trimester.[14–17] Increase in LV mass is significantly higher in preeclamptic and pregnancies complicated by pregnancy-induced hypertension compared with normotensive pregnancies (*P* < .0001).[14]

This physiologic hypertrophy is thought to normalize the elevated level of systolic wall stress. During normotensive pregnancies, interventricular septal thickness does not change up to the early third trimester compared with reference, but thickness

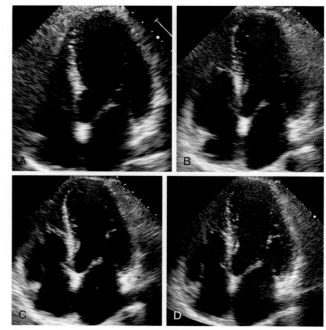

Figure 161.1. Cardiac dimension changes during normal pregnancy (first to third trimesters). Changes in cardiac dimensions during pregnancy are shown in the apical four-chamber view. Images obtained during the first trimester (**A**), second trimester (**B**), third trimester (**C**), and postpartum (**D**) are shown. Note the increases in left atrial, right atrial, right ventricular, and left ventricular size, which are most noticeable in the third trimester (**C**) in this case example.

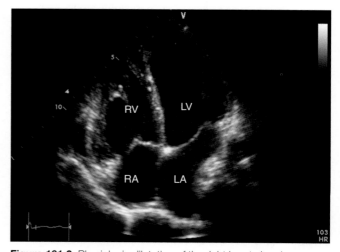

Figure 161.2. Physiologic dilatation of the right heart chambers during pregnancy. Apical four-chamber view shows physiologic right atrial (RA) and right ventricular (RV) dilatation with normal systolic function in the third trimester of pregnancy. *LA,* Left atrium; *LV,* left ventricle. (See accompanying Video 161.2.)

statistically significantly increases between 29 and 35 weeks of gestation by 0.09 cm.[1]

Right Ventricle

Similar to the left ventricle, the right ventricle increases in size over the course of pregnancy because of the increased preload[15] (Fig 161.1). This increase in size can be detected in the apical four-chamber view at the basal or mid-RV level (Fig. 161.2 and Video 161.2).

Left Atrium

The left atrium starts to increase in size gradually between 22 and 28 weeks of gestation, with the maximal atrial size seen at term. Studies have shown an increase in the left atrial (LA) anteroposterior diameter in the parasternal long-axis view, LA area in the four-chamber view, LA volume in the apical four- and two-chamber views, or by three-dimensional (3D) echocardiography.[16,23]

Left Ventricular Outflow Tract

Serial studies in pregnant women show a slight increase in LV outflow tract diameter as pregnancy progresses. These changes are on the order of 2 to 3 mm[16] but are detectable by two-dimensional (2D) TTE.

Aorta

There is a parallel increase in aortic root diameter and the aorta.[16] Expression of estrogen receptors in the aorta results in fragmentation of reticulin fibers, reduced amount of acid mucopolysaccharides, and loss of the normal arrangement of elastin fibers, predisposing women to aortic dissection, particularly if they have an aortopathy.[16] Risk factors for aortic dilatation are hypertension and advanced maternal age. Pregnancy is a high-risk period for all patients with aortic pathology.

Left Ventricular Contractility and Ejection Fraction

The change in LV contractility in pregnancy is a controversial subject. Most studies have found no significant change in ejection fraction (EF).[9,17] Some have found a decrease in the ratio of wall stress to velocity of circumferential fiber contraction (VCFC), implying enhanced intrinsic myocardial contractility,[7] but others have concluded that EF or contractility as measured by fractional shortening (FS) and VCFC decline slightly, especially in the late third trimester.[32,33] The gravid uterus pushes the diaphragm upward, making it difficult to obtain true apical views, especially during the third trimester. On the other hand, later in pregnancy, the left ventricle becomes more globular in shape, and the biplane EF calculation for an elliptical-shaped left ventricle becomes more unreliable.[17]

Three-Dimensional Echocardiography and Left Ventricular Mechanics

We found an increase in LV and RV volumes in the second and third trimester using 3D TTE along with a slight but insignificant decrease in LVEF in the third trimester using 3D echocardiography.[18] Others have shown a decrease in longitudinal LV shortening, as measured by longitudinal tissue Doppler strain, toward the end of pregnancy and an increase in LV globularity.[26] However, our own observations using speckle-tracking strain rate indicate an increase in cardiac contractility as demonstrated by an increase in LV radial and longitudinal rate of deformation, particularly during first and second trimesters. Other studies using strain (longitudinal, radial, and circumferential and area strain) by 3D echocardiography showed strain to reduce by the third trimester before returning to normal postpregnancy. Savu and colleagues also observed increased LV and RV longitudinal strain rate in the first trimester.[26] Earlier studies[31,32] found that FS and VCFC decreased during normal pregnancy and that the load-adjusted index of contractility, the ESS–VCFC relationship, did not change during normotensive pregnancy[1,34] or that the LV contractility (VCFC adjusted for end-systolic wall stress) was lower during pregnancy than at 6 months postpartum.[32]

Cong and associates[34] evaluated global LV strain in normal pregnancies. Global longitudinal strain (GLS), global circumferential strain (GCS), global radial strain (RS), and global area strain (GAS) showed a significant decrease in the second and third trimesters and increased again postpartum (Fig. 161.3). This behavior was found in almost all ventricular walls. The biggest differences were found in the anterior and some segments of the inferoseptal and anteroseptal walls. Among the strain components, GAS showed the strongest associations with 3D EF, sphericity index, and LV mass index. GAS showed strong correlations with GLS (r = 0.81; $P < .01$) and GCS (r = 0.82; $P < .01$). It is noteworthy that these results were derived from the 3D approach based on direct volumetric quantification, which does not depend on any geometry assumption of the LV and is relatively operator independent because of its semiautomatic methods. GAS is a novel 3D speckle-tracking echocardiography index that corresponds to the percentage of deformation in LV endocardial surface area. Since it has integrated longitudinal and circumferential deformation, Seo and coworkers inferred that GAS might decrease the tracking error and emphasize synergistically the magnitude of deformation.[19]

These partially discrepant findings appear related to the load dependency in normal hearts along with tethering effect of neighboring segments that may produce different results when evaluated by tissue Doppler imaging.[20] In contrast, speckle tracking is a 2D technique independent of the angle dependency of Doppler and of motion of surrounding segments. Speckle-tracking strain rate is the most sensitive and load-independent parameter of LV contractility. These data support that myocardial contractility is maintained in normotensive pregnant women.

Right Ventricular Systolic Function

Few echocardiographic studies have evaluated RV function during pregnancy. Savu and associates, using tissue Doppler strain rate imaging of the RV free wall[26] and the speckle-tracking strain rate of the entire right ventricle, found an increase in RV longitudinal strain rate in the first and second trimesters and a decrease in the third trimester, indicating an increase in RV contractility during pregnancy. We also found no change in RVEF using 3D echocardiography but an increase in RV systolic and diastolic volumes in the second and third trimesters of pregnancy along with an increase in stroke volume.

Cardiac Output

The increase in cardiac output results in elevated antegrade flow velocities across the LV outflow tract and the RV outflow tract. Increased flow velocities are seen in normal pregnancy that can reach as high as 2 m/s, resulting in a corresponding increase in time velocity integral of aortic and pulmonary flow. This, along with increased LV outflow tract diameter, results in increased stroke volume. Measurements of cardiac output using Doppler echocardiography correlate well with measurements obtained by invasive heart catheterization using the thermodilution method.[21] Cardiac output changes significantly with different maternal positions. Uterine enlargement beyond about 20 weeks can compress the inferior vena cava (IVC). Echocardiography should be performed in the left lateral decubitus position so that the uterus is displaced off the IVC. This can be accomplished by placing a wedge or a pillow under the woman's right side. Immediately after delivery, cardiac output may transiently increase to as much as 80% above prelabor values because of relief of IVC compression and autotransfusion from the placenta. The hemodynamic changes that develop during pregnancy return toward baseline values postdelivery. Most of the changes resolve early after delivery, although complete resolution of all measurable pregnancy-associated effects may take as long as 6 months.[22]

Diastolic Function

Because of the effect of preload on LV diastolic function, studies have shown variable effects of pregnancy on diastolic function.

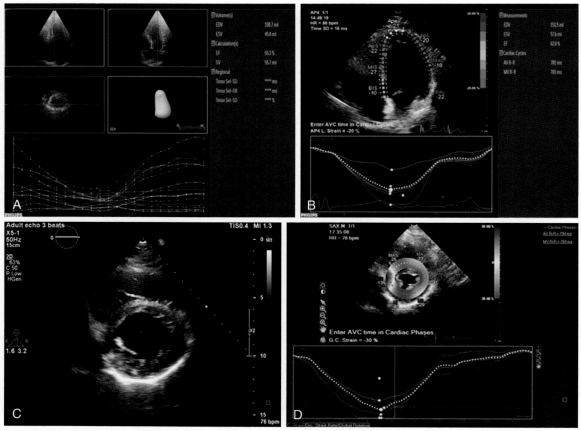

Figure 161.3. Three-dimensional (3D) left ventricular (LV) volumes and two-dimensional speckle-tracking strain during normal pregnancy. **A,** 3D LV analysis and strain imaging during third trimester of pregnancy show normal LV systolic function, preserved LV synchrony, and mildly increased LV volumes. **B,** Normal apical four-chamber longitudinal LV strain. Parasternal short-axis view at the distal LV level shows robust radial LV function (**C**) with preserved circumferential strain (**D**). (See accompanying Video 161.3, which corresponds to panel C.)

LV remodeling during pregnancy is also associated with changes in diastolic function during normal pregnancy.[22–24] The isovolumic relaxation time (IVRT) shortens markedly during pregnancy, and it seems to be independent of the heart rate because IVRT remains short postpartum, when the heart rate returns to normal and may be related to an increase in early diastolic LV relaxation, possibly from hormonal influences and increased availability of nitric oxide.[15]

Mitral Inflow and Pulmonary Venous Flow

The mitral inflow E and A waves are a result of the suction force, LV preload, and the pressure gradients between the left atrium and LV during ventricular diastole.[23] During the first trimester of pregnancy, the increase in preload leads to increased volume in the left atrium, whereas the decrease in peripheral vascular resistance leads to a decrease in afterload, both resulting in an increase in mitral inflow E wave velocity and mitral A wave inflow velocity (Fig. 161.4) as well as mitral E-wave duration. As pregnancy progresses, there is a gradual reduction of E-wave velocity, perhaps from an increase in LV wall thickness, causing reduced LV compliance. To maintain cardiac output, LA contraction becomes more important, and peak A-wave velocity continues to rise. The change in hemodynamics results in a pattern where mitral inflow E-wave velocity increases slightly during the first trimester and then decreases gradually from around week 15, reaches its nadir around week 36, and remains decreased 6 months postpartum.[24] In contrast, mitral inflow A wave velocity increases throughout pregnancy and reaches its peak in the third trimester (see Fig. 161.4). It has been shown that in the presence of a heightened atrial preload, such as occurs with fluid loading, atrial contractility increases, and both

mitral forward flow and the pulmonary vein atrial velocity increase at atrial contraction on mitral inflow or mitral annulus.[42] In addition, both reductions of septal and lateral E′ velocities are observed near term[43] (Fig. 161.5). The pulmonary vein inflow profile is notable for an increase in peak systolic forward flow velocity, again reflecting the increase in preload.[41] The peak pulmonary venous A-wave velocity also increases as a result of the increase in LA function (Fig. 161.6). Studies have found no change in the duration of pulmonary A wave, although technical difficulty with measuring pulmonary vein duration could account for no measurable change being observed.[41]

Pulmonary Artery Systolic Pressure

Pulmonary artery systolic pressure is estimated using the tricuspid regurgitant jet. The estimated pulmonary artery systolic pressure remains in the normal range in all stages of pregnancy because the increase in pulmonary blood flow is offset by a decrease in pulmonary vascular resistance (Fig. 161.7).

Valve Function

The mitral annulus and tricuspid annulus diameters increase with pregnancy. This along with an increase in LV preload corresponds to an increase in valve regurgitation. Valve regurgitation is often seen during the third trimester.[25] As pregnancy progresses and blood volume increases, any baseline physiologic valve regurgitation without necessarily any changes in the valve function is accentuated, especially in tricuspid valve (Fig. 161.8 and Video 161.8). In contrast, physiologic mitral regurgitation, despite the

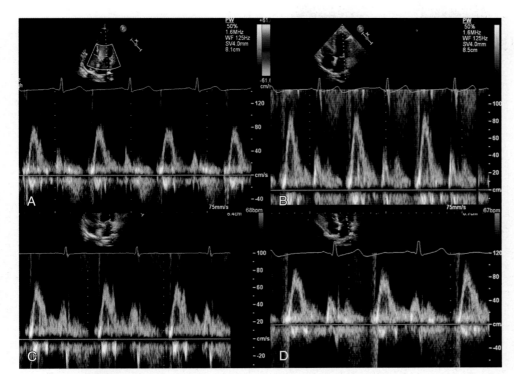

Figure 161.4. Mitral inflow Doppler parameters during normal pregnancy. Changes in mitral inflow pulsed-wave Doppler during pregnancy. Images obtained during the first trimester (**A**), second trimester (**B**), third trimester (**C**), and postpartum (**D**) are shown. There is an increase E-wave velocity in early to midpregnancy (**A** and **B**) followed by a decrease in the third trimester (**C**). There is a progressive increase in atrial velocity. This results in a reduction in E/A ratio during pregnancy.

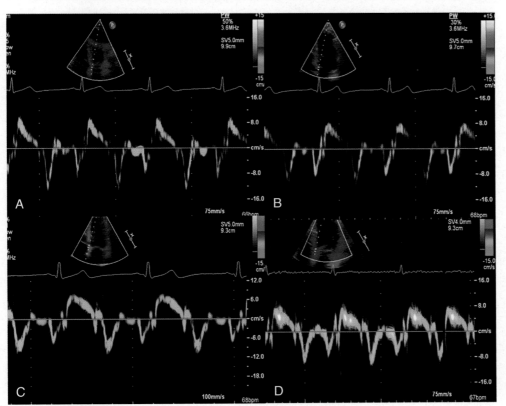

Figure 161.5. Mitral annular tissue Doppler during normal pregnancy. Changes in medial mitral annular tissue Doppler velocities during pregnancy. Images obtained during the first trimester (**A**), second trimester (**B**), third trimester (**C**), and postpartum (**D**) are shown. There is an increase E' wave velocity in early to midpregnancy (**A** and **B**) followed by a decrease in the third trimester (**C**).

extra volume load, often appears less during pregnancy because of the decrease in SVR, but all preexisting pathologic mitral regurgitations revealed increase severity by chamber dilatation anemia and high cardiac output of pregnancy.[26–28] Tricuspid regurgitation and pulmonic regurgitation are seen in almost all pregnant women, whereas mitral regurgitation is detected in one-quarter of pregnant women. The degree of regurgitation is usually trace or mild. Aortic regurgitation is almost never seen.

Pericardial Effusion

A small pericardial effusion is seen on echocardiography in up to 25% of normal pregnancies in the first and second trimesters and in approximately 40% of pregnant women during the third trimester.[29] This does not appear to have any hemodynamic significance (Fig. 161.9 and Videos 161.9 and 161.9E). Although diseases of the pericardium may occur sporadically during pregnancy, there is no

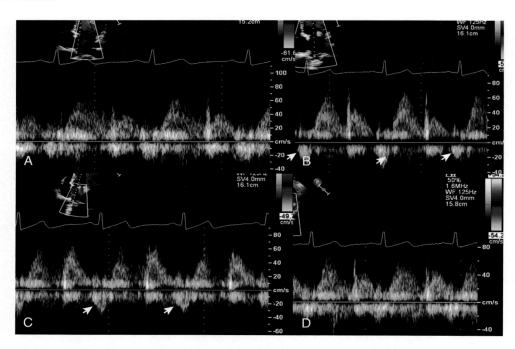

Figure 161.6. Pulmonic vein Doppler during normal pregnancy. Changes in pulmonary vein inflow pulsed-wave Doppler during pregnancy. Images obtained during the first trimester (**A**), second trimester (**B**), third trimester (**C**), and postpartum (**D**) are shown. There is an increase in S-wave velocity in early to midpregnancy (**A** and **B**). There is a progressive increase in atrial reversal velocity during pregnancy secondary to increased atrial contraction (**B** and **C**, *white arrows*).

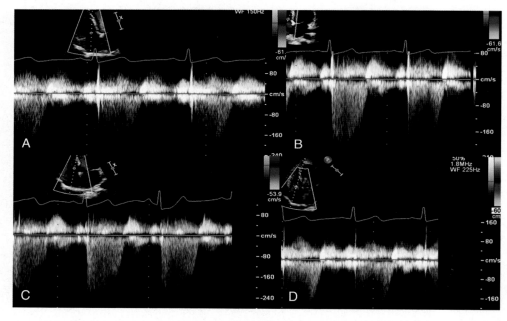

Figure 161.7. Tricuspid regurgitation (TR) during normal pregnancy. Changes in TR and peak pulmonary artery systolic pressure measured by tricuspid inflow continuous-wave Doppler during pregnancy. Images obtained during the first trimester (**A**), second trimester (**B**), third trimester (**C**), and postpartum (**D**) are shown. There is an increase in the severity of TR within physiologic range as shown by the density of the TR signal in the second and third trimesters (**B** and **C**). The peak pulmonary artery remains in the physiologic range throughout pregnancy.

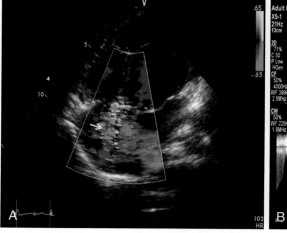
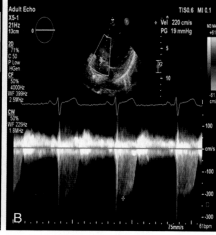

Figure 161.8. Pulmonary artery pressure and tricuspid regurgitation during normal pregnancy. Apical four-chamber color Doppler view in the third trimester shows moderate physiologic TR (**A**, *yellow arrow*) and normal right ventricular–right atrial systolic velocity of 2.2 m/s corresponding to a peak systolic pressure gradient of 19 mm Hg (**B**). (See accompanying Video 161.8.)

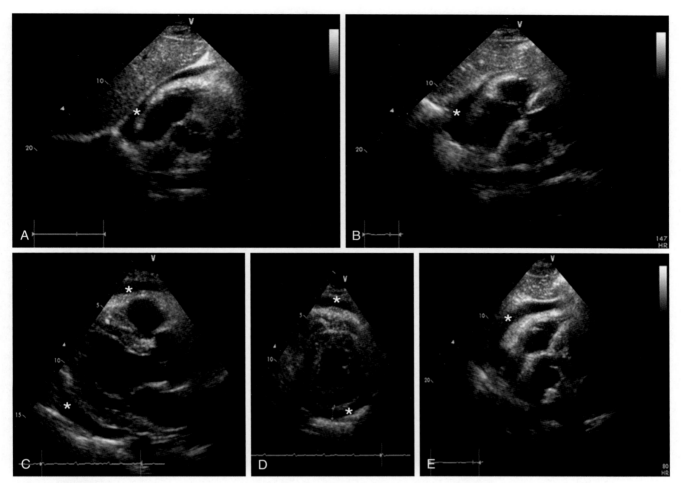

Figure 161.9. Pericardial effusion during normal pregnancy. Images obtained during the first trimester (**A**), second trimester (**B**), and third trimester (**C–E**) during a normal pregnancy. Trace pericardial effusion is seen inferior to the right atrium in the in subcostal view in the first trimester (**A**, *white asterisk*), becoming small in the second trimester (**B**, *asterisk*) and small to moderate in the third trimester in the parasternal long-axis (**C**, *asterisk*), midparasternal short-axis (**D**, *asterisk*), and subcostal (**E**, *asterisk*) views. The effusion resolved postpartum. (See accompanying Videos 161.9B and 161.9E.)

evidence that pregnancy increases the susceptibility to pericardial diseases.

In general, these effusions are asymptomatic, benign, and transient, and they resolve spontaneously without therapy. In the absence of signs or symptoms of acute pericarditis or cardiac tamponade, neither diagnostic testing (generally with echocardiography) nor specific treatment is required.

The following observations have been made regarding pericardial effusions in pregnancy:

- The effusion is usually small to moderate in size, with separation of the pericardial layers of less than 10 mm. When sampled, these effusions are usually found to be a transudate (hydropericardium).
- Slightly elevated BP or nonspecific ST-T changes have been reported in association with pericardial effusion.
- The clinical examination and electrocardiogram are generally normal.
- The pericardial effusion is usually transient and disappears within 2 months after delivery.
- In the absence of signs or symptoms of acute pericarditis or cardiac tamponade, treatment is not required.[30]

The signs and symptoms of cardiac tamponade may be masked during pregnancy because of the physiologic increase in circulating blood volume. This may lead to a larger pericardial effusion being present before signs or symptoms are detected.

Use of Echocardiography Image-Enhancing Agent (IEA) in Pregnancy

Echocardiographic IEAs are not used during pregnancy because no safety data are available. Studies have suggested that the theoretically small potential risk associated with nonthermal bioeffects from acoustic cavitation may be considered to prohibit the use in the first trimester pregnant women.

Fetal Effects of Cardiac Ultrasound

There have been no reports of documented adverse fetal effects for diagnostic ultrasonography procedures themselves, including duplex Doppler imaging. The US Food and Drug Administration has limited the spatial-peak temporal average intensity of ultrasound transducers to 720 mW/cm^2. At this intensity, the theoretical increase in temperature elevation for the fetus may be as high as 2°C (35.6°F). However, it is highly unlikely that any sustained temperature elevation will occur at any single fetal anatomic site. The risk of temperature elevation is lowest with B-mode imaging and is higher with color Doppler and spectral Doppler applications.[31–34]

FINAL INTERPRETATION OF ECHOCARDIOGRAPHIC FINDINGS IN UNCOMPLICATED PREGNANCY

At the time of echocardiography report, the age of pregnancy should be reported to help the referring physician place the findings in context. For example, the magnitude of valvular regurgitation may be artificially reduced with the reduced SVR during midpregnancy and then apparently increases during late pregnancy as SVR approaches prepregnancy levels. Similarly, mild mitral valve prolapse may be masked by the chamber dilatation of pregnancy. In women with lesions known to be masked by the physiologic changes of pregnancy, the echocardiogram should be repeated after the sixth postpartum month when the hemodynamic changes have returned to baseline.[39]

Please access ExpertConsult to view the corresponding videos for this chapter.

REFERENCES

1. De Haas S, Ghossein-Doha C, Geerts L, van Kuijk SMJ, van Drongelen J, Spaanderman MEA. Cardiac remodeling in normotensive pregnancy and in pregnancy complicated by hypertension: systematic review and meta-analysis. *Ultrasound Obstet Gynecol.* 2017;50:683–696.
2. ESC Guidelines for the management of cardiovascular diseases during pregnancy. *Eur Heart J.* 2018;39:3165–3241.
3. Mishra M, Chambers JB, Jackson G. Murmurs in pregnancy. An audit of echocardiography. *BMJ.* 1992;304:1413–1414.
4. Naqvi TZ, Elkayam U. Serial echocardiographic assessment of the human heart in normal pregnancy. *Circulation: Cardiovascular Imaging.* 2012;5:283–285.
5. Wald RM, Silversides CK, Kingdom J, et al. Maternal cardiac output and fetal Doppler predict adverse neonatal outcomes in pregnant women with heart disease. *J Am Heart Assoc.* 2015;4. e002414.
6. Ouzounian JG, Elkayam U. Physiologic changes during normal pregnancy and delivery. *Cardiol Clin.* 2012;30:317–329.
7. Gilson GJ, Samaan S, Crawford MH, Qualls CR, Curet LB. Changes in hemodynamics, ventricular remodeling, and ventricular contractility during normal pregnancy: a longitudinal study. *Obstet Gynecol.* 1997;89:957–962.
8. Hunter S, Robson SC. Adaptation of the maternal heart in pregnancy. *Br Heart J.* 1992;68:540–543.
9. Katz DR, Karliner JS, Resnik R. Effects of a natural volume overload state (pregnancy) on left ventricular performance in normal human subjects. *Circulation.* 1978;58:434–441.
10. Robson SC, Hunter S, Boys RJ, Dunlop W. Serial study of factors influencing changes in cardiac output during human pregnancy. *Am J Physiol.* 1989;256:1060–1065.
11. Mabie WC, DiSessa TG, Crocker LG, Sibai BM, Arheart KL. A longitudinal study of cardiac output in normal human pregnancy. *Am J Obstet Gynecol.* 1994;170:849–856.
12. Meah VL, Cockcroft JR, Backx K, Shave R, Stohr EJ. Cardiac output and related haemodynamics during pregnancy: a series of meta-analyses. *Heart.* 2016;102:518–526.
13. Grindheim G, Estensen ME, Langesaeter E, Rosseland LA, Toska K. Changes in blood pressure during healthy pregnancy: a longitudinal cohort study. *J Hypertens.* 2012;30:342–350.
14. Adam K. Pregnancy in women with cardiovascular diseases. *Methodist Debakey Cardiovasc J.* 2017;13:209–215.
15. Sladek SM, Magness RR, Conrad KP. Nitric oxide and pregnancy. *Am J Physiol.* 1997;272:441–463.
16. Ashrafi R, Curtis SL. Heart Disease and Pregnancy. *Cardiol Ther.* 2017;6:157–173.
17. Robson SC, Hunter S, Boys RJ, Dunlop W. Serial changes in pulmonary haemodynamics during human pregnancy: a non-invasive study using Doppler echocardiography. *Clin Sci.* 1991;80:113–117.
18. Robson SC, Dunlop W, Hunter S. Haemodynamic changes during the early puerperium. *Br Med J.* 1987;294:1065.
19. Melchiorre K, Sharma R, Thilaganathan B. Cardiac structure and function in normal pregnancy. *Current Opin Obstet Gynecol.* 2012;24:413–421.
20. Melchiorre K, Sharma R, Khalil A, Thilaganathan B. Maternal cardiovascular function in normal pregnancy: evidence of maladaptation to chronic volume overload. *Hypertension.* 2016;67:754–762.
21. Pandey AK, Banerjee AK, Das A, et al. Evaluation of maternal myocardial performance during normal pregnancy and postpartum. *Indian Heart J.* 2010;62:64–67.
22. Schannwell CM, Zimmermann T, Schneppenheim M, Plehn G, Marx R, Strauer BE. Left ventricular hypertrophy and diastolic dysfunction in healthy pregnant women. *Cardiology.* 2002;97:73–78.
23. Valensise H, Novelli GP, Vasapollo B, et al. Maternal cardiac systolic and diastolic function: relationship with uteroplacental resistances. A Doppler and echocardiographic longitudinal study. *Ultrasound Obstet Gynecol.* 2000;15:487–497.
24. Grossman W. Cardiac hypertrophy: useful adaptation or pathologic process? *Am J Med.* 1980;69:576–584.
25. Soma-Pillay P, Louw MC, Adeyemo AO, Makin J, Pattinson RC. Cardiac diastolic function after recovery from pre-eclampsia. *Cardiovascular J Afr.* 2018;29:27–31.
26. Savu O, Jurcuţ R, Giuşcă S, et al. Morphological and functional adaptation of the maternal heart during pregnancy. *Circ Cardiovasc Imaging.* 2012;5:289–297.
27. Yosefy C, Shenhav S, Feldman V, Sagi Y, Katz A, Anteby E. Left atrial function during pregnancy: a three-dimensional echocardiographic study. *Echocardiography.* 2012;29:1096–1101.
28. Poppas A, Shroff SG, Korcarz CE, et al. Serial assessment of the cardiovascular system in normal pregnancy. Role of arterial compliance and pulsatile arterial load. *Circulation.* 1997;95:2407–2415.
29. Easterling TR, Benedetti TJ, Schmucker BC, Carlson K, Millard SP. Maternal hemodynamics and aortic diameter in normal and hypertensive pregnancies. *Obstet Gynecol.* 1991;78:1073–1077.
30. Nolte JE, Rutherford RB, Nawaz S, Rosenberger A, Speers WC, Krupski WC. Arterial dissections associated with pregnancy. *J Vasc Surg.* 1995;21:515–520.
31. Geva T, Mauer B, Striker L, Kirshon B, Pivarnik JM. Effects of physiologic load of pregnancy on left ventricular contractility and remodeling. *Am Heart J.* 1997;133:53–59.
32. Estensen ME, Beitnes JO, Grindheim G, et al. Altered maternal left ventricular contractility and function during normal pregnancy. *Ultrasound Obstet Gynecol.* 2013;41:659–666.
33. Mone SM, Sanders SP, Colan SD. Control mechanisms for physiological hypertrophy of pregnancy. *Circulation* 1996;94:667–672
34. Cong J, Fan T, Yang X, et al. Structural and functional changes in maternal left ventricle during pregnancy, a three-dimensional speckle-tracking echocardiography study. *Cardiovasc Ultrasound.* 2015;13(6):1–10.
35. Naqvi TZ, Lee MS, Aldridge M, Rafie R, Bamba A, Narayanan M. Normal cardiac adaptation during pregnancy—assessment by velocity vector imaging and three dimensional echocardiography in healthy pregnant women. *Circulation.* 2013;128:A16377.
36. Seo Y, Ishizu T, Enomoto Y, Sugimori H, Aonuma K. Endocardial surface area tracking for assessment of regional LV wall deformation with 3D speckle tracking imaging. *JACC Cardiovasc Imaging.* 2011;4:358–365.
37. Jacques D, Pinsky MR, Severyn D, Gorscan III J. Influence of acute alterations in loading on mitral annular velocity by tissue Doppler echocardiography and its associated ability to predict filling pressures. *Chest.* 2004;126:1910–1918.
38. Easterling TR, Carlson KL, Schmucker BC, Brateng DA, Benedetti TJ. Measurement of cardiac output in pregnancy by Doppler technique. *Am J Perinatol.* 1990;7:220–222.
39. Liu S, Elkayam U, Naqvi TZ. Echocardiography in pregnancy: part I. *Curr Cardiol Rep.* 2016;18(92):1–10.
40. Naqvi TZ. Diastolic function assessment incorporating new techniques in Doppler echocardiography. *Rev Cardiovasc Med.* 2003;4:81–99.
41. Mesa A, Jessurun C, Hernandez A, et al. Left ventricular diastolic function in normal human pregnancy. *Circulation.* 1999;99:511–517.
42. Fok WY, Chan LY, Wong JT, Yu CM, Lau TK. Left ventricular diastolic function during normal pregnancy: assessment by spectral tissue Doppler imaging. *Ultrasound Obstet Gynecol.* 2006;28:789–793.
43. Kametas NA, McAuligge F, Hancock J, Chambers J, Nicolaides KH. Maternal left ventricular mass and diastolic function during pregnancy. *Ultrasound Obstet Gynecology.* 2001;18:460–466.
44. Campos O, Andrade JL, Bocanegra J, et al. Physiologic multivalvular regurgitation during pregnancy: a longitudinal Doppler echocardiographic study. *Int J Cardiol.* 1993;40:265–272.
45. So GJ, Lee JM, Shaban NM, et al. Normal echocardiographic measurements in uncomplicated pregnancy, a single center experience. *J Cardiovasc Dis Res.* 2014;5:3–8.
46. Gatzoulis M, Webb G, Daubeney P. *Diagnosis and Management of Adult Congenital Heart Disease.* 3rd. Elsevier; 2011.
47. Liu S, Elkayam U, Naqvi TZ. Echocardiography in pregnancy: Part 1. *Curr Cardiol Rep.* 2016;18:92.
48. Abduljabbar HS, Marzouki KM, Zawawi TH, Khan AS. Pericardial effusion in normal pregnant women. *Acta Obstet Gynecol Scand.* 1991;70:291–294.
49. Ristić AD, Seferovic PM, Ljubić A, et al. Pericardial disease in pregnancy. *Herz.* 2003;28:209–215.
50. Committee Opinion. Diagnostic imaging during pregnancy and lactation. *Obstet Gynecol.* 2017;130:e210–216.
51. Barnett SB, Duck F, Ziskin M. World Federation of ultrasound in Medicine and Biology. Symposium on Safety of ultrasound in Medicine: ultrasound contrast agents. Safety of ultrasound contrast agents. *Ultrasound Med Biol.* 2007;33:171–234.
52. Miller DL, Averkiou MA, Brayman AA, et al. Bioeffects considerations for diagnostic ultrasound contrast agents. *J Ultrasound Med.* 2008;27:611–632.
53. Miller DL. The Safe Use of Contrast-Enhanced Diagnostic Ultrasound. In: ter Haar G, ed. *The Safe Use of Ultrasound in Medical Diagnosis.* London, England: British Institute of Radiology; 2012:105–124.

162 Cocaine

Sudhir Ken Mehta, Swaminatha V. Gurudevan

Cocaine use is a leading cause of cardiovascular disease in young adults in the United States. The National Survey on Drug Use and Health in 2008 estimated that there were 1.9 million cocaine users in the United States. Cocaine use accounts for 24% of all drug abuse–related visits to emergency departments.[1]

PATHOPHYSIOLOGY

Cocaine is a sympathomimetic drug that inhibits catecholamine reuptake at sympathetic nerve terminals, leading to increased levels of neuronal catecholamines. In addition, it augments the release of catecholamines from central and peripheral stores. This results in a dose-dependent increase in heart rate and blood pressure. Furthermore, cocaine increases myocardial oxygen demand by acting as an inotropic agent. Concurrently, through adrenergic stimulation and by releasing endothelin-1 and inhibiting nitric oxide production from endothelial cells, it acts as a powerful vasoconstrictor. The ensuing vasoconstriction of the coronary microcirculation[2] limits myocardial oxygen supply. The resulting imbalance in myocardial oxygen demand and supply may lead to ischemia or infarction (Fig. 162.1).

Cocaine may also lead to acceleration of atherosclerosis. Among individuals presenting with acute chest pain in the emergency department, cocaine users had more pronounced atherosclerosis than the general population.[3] Coronary vasoconstriction is more pronounced in atherosclerotic segments, although most individuals presenting with cocaine-induced myocardial ischemia do not have significant coronary artery disease.

Recent data from myocardial contrast echocardiography have shed new light on the specific mechanism by which cocaine causes coronary vasoconstriction. Gurudevan and colleagues studied 10 normal individuals using myocardial contrast echocardiography to evaluate myocardial perfusion at baseline and after a low-dose intranasal cocaine challenge.[2] The administration of cocaine caused a measurable rise in blood pressure and heart rate with a corresponding decrease in myocardial perfusion. Fig. 162.2 demonstrates the perfusion of the interventricular septum at baseline, after administration of low-dose dobutamine, and after administration of low-dose intranasal cocaine. In this study, the decrease in perfusion in the interventricular septum was demonstrated to be secondary to vasoconstriction of terminal feed arteries in the coronary circulation and a decrease in microvascular conductance.

Cocaine users have a higher incidence of myocardial ischemia and infarction, aortic dissection, arrhythmias, and sudden death. Thrombogenic effects of cocaine originate from platelet activation,

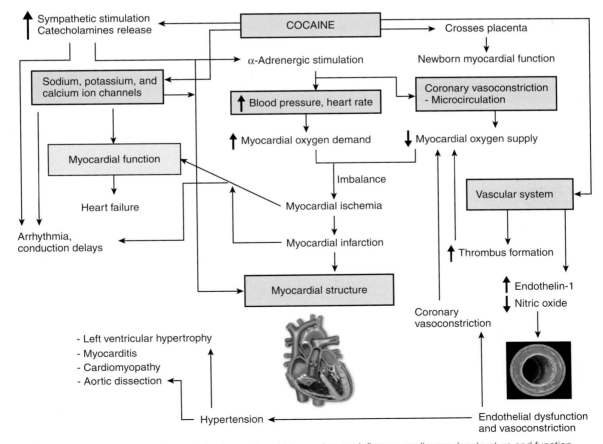

Figure 162.1. Summary of potential pathways by which cocaine can influence cardiovascular structure and function.

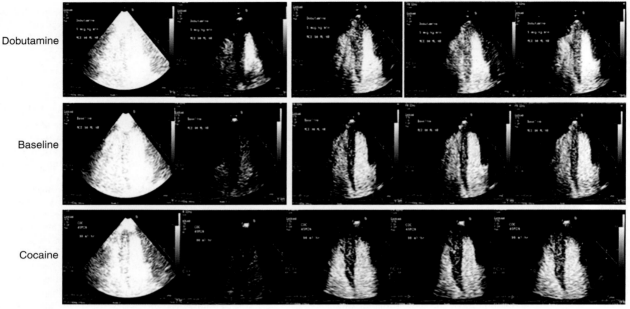

Figure 162.2. Myocardial contrast echocardiography in a human at baseline *(center)* and after the administration of low-dose dobutamine *(top)* and low-dose intranasal cocaine *(bottom)*. Five frames are shown. The first frame is a flashed pulse of ultrasound at end-systole that destroys all intramyocardial bubbles. The baseline and sequential end-systolic pulsing intervals are shown in the four subsequent images. There is a measurable decrease in both peak video intensity and the rate of rise of video intensity during cocaine administration compared with baseline. In contrast, dobutamine *(top)* causes an increase in both peak video intensity and rate of rise of video intensity in the same person.

aggregation, and α-granule release. Cocaine also increases plasminogen activator inhibitor activity and fibrinogen levels. Myocardial ischemia results from vasoconstriction of coronary arteries, from accelerated atherosclerosis, or through the initiation of in situ coronary thrombus formation. Cocaine-induced arrhythmias may result from myocardial ischemia, excessive catecholamines, or as a direct result of ion channel alterations. Excess catecholamines can cause malignant tachycardias, including torsades de pointes, ventricular tachycardia, and fibrillation. Chronic cocaine use is associated with ventricular hypertrophy, myocarditis, and dilated cardiomyopathy, including Takotsubo cardiomyopathy.

CLINICAL ASSESSMENT

Before performing an echocardiographic examination, it is crucial for the clinician to obtain a detailed clinical history and physical examination of the patient with suspected cocaine-induced cardiac toxicity. Myocardial ischemia or infarction secondary to epicardial coronary artery disease and aortic dissection must be ruled out in all patients presenting with a history of chest pain, particularly young male smokers. Aortic dissection in the setting of cocaine use is often the result of both untreated or inadequately controlled hypertension and underlying connective tissue disease in addition to the drug effect.

Acute cocaine toxicity may present with signs of seizures, hemorrhagic and ischemic strokes, rhabdomyolysis, mesenteric ischemia, myocardial infarction (MI), congestive heart failure, arrhythmias, aortic dissection, and renal failure. Pregnant women, patients infected with human immunodeficiency virus, individuals with alcoholism, and smokers are at a higher risk for manifesting cardiovascular toxicity.

ECHOCARDIOGRAPHY

Echocardiography is a useful tool for the clinician who suspects cocaine-induced myocardial dysfunction. Echocardiography may demonstrate alterations in global and regional left ventricular (LV) function. Myocardial contrast echocardiography may illustrate regional wall motion abnormalities better than standard echocardiography through the improvement of endocardial border definition. Regional wall motion abnormalities secondary to edema and fibrosis can also be seen in asymptomatic cocaine abusers.

MI of the anterior wall is the most common serious cardiac complication of cocaine abuse. It is unrelated to the dose, route of administration, or frequency of cocaine use, and it most often occurs during the first 3 to 4 hours of cocaine use. The recognition of regional wall motion abnormalities can be a challenge in the presence of LV hypertrophy, which is not uncommon among cocaine users.

Cardiac troponin I is a useful biomarker of myocardial necrosis especially in young patients with chest pain who may not have electrocardiographic abnormalities. Cocaine users are known to have higher troponin I levels and have higher in-hospital mortality rates when presenting with acute coronary syndromes. Independent of coronary blood flow, cocaine use can have a direct negative inotropic effect on the myocardium secondary to alteration of ion channels, apoptosis, and fibrosis in the myocardium.

Long-term cocaine use can lead to prolonged transmitral deceleration time and concentric LV hypertrophy with high LV mass and thickened posterior wall but normal diastolic dimensions. Ultimately, cocaine abusers may develop a dilated cardiomyopathy with or without frank signs of heart failure. A high LV end-systolic volume and lower ejection fraction may be an indicator of cardiomyopathy or myocarditis.

The precise cause of myocarditis and cardiomyopathy remains unclear, although subclinical myocardial changes, including myocardial edema and fibrosis, have been identified in asymptomatic cocaine addicts evaluated by cardiovascular magnetic resonance. Based on limited evidence, chronic cocaine use may be associated with regional LV diastolic dysfunction, suggested by a decrease in early (E) and an increase in late diastolic filling (A) at the mitral valve in addition to a lower average diastolic strain, both of which are seen in chronic cocaine abusers.

COCAINE USE IN PREGNANCY

Short- and long-term adverse cardiac effects of cocaine abuse during pregnancy are similar in pregnant women, except that cocaine crosses the placenta and can affect the developing fetus. Based on limited short-term studies, infants during the first 2 days of life exhibited LV filling abnormalities that were more pronounced in those with heavy in utero cocaine exposure. Unless exposed to high levels of intrauterine cocaine, the diastolic alterations resolve in most infants during the first 2 to 6 months of life.[4] These infants have not been shown to exhibit any systolic dysfunction. A higher rate of arrhythmias has also been reported in these infants, although use of multiple drugs by these mothers makes it a challenge to isolate the specific effect of cocaine.

TREATMENT

Treatment of a patient with suspected cocaine-induced cardiac toxicity is similar to the general treatment of patients with acute coronary syndromes. The mainstay of initial therapy is antiplatelet therapy with aspirin and/or thienopyridines and anticoagulation with heparin or low-molecular-weight heparin. Nitroglycerin may be useful to relieve symptoms of angina and reverse the effects of cocaine-induced vasoconstriction. The use of β-blockers in cocaine-induced MI is controversial. Earlier data suggested that β-blockers used in the setting of cocaine intoxication may cause unopposed α-adrenergic stimulation that could potentiate cocaine-induced coronary artery vasoconstriction and systemic arterial hypertension, particularly in acute situations.[5] More recent data suggest that β-blockers are safe when used in patients with cocaine-induced chest pain.[6] Future studies using myocardial contrast echocardiography will examine the specific effect of β-blockers on myocardial perfusion in the setting of cocaine use.

Acknowledgment

The authors wish to acknowledge the late Ronald G. Victor, MD, PhD, for his creative insight, mentorship, and focus without which a seminal work of research that greatly contributed to this publication would not be possible.

REFERENCES

1. U.S. Department of Health and Human Services, National Institutes of Health. *Cocaine: Abuse and Addiction, National Institute of Drug Abuse Research Report Series.* NIH, Pub; 2010:1–7. No. 10-4166.
2. Gurudevan SV, Nelson MD, Rader F, et al. Cocaine induced vasoconstriction in the human coronary microcirculation. *Circulation.* 2013;128:598–604.
3. Ebersberger U, Sudarski S, Schoepf UJ, et al. Atherosclerotic plaque burden in cocaine users with acute chest pain. *Atherosclerosis.* 2013;229:443–448.
4. Mehta SK, Super DM, Connuck D, et al. Diastolic alterations in infants exposed to intrauterine cocaine: a follow-up study by color kinesis. *J Am Soc Echocardiogr.* 2002;15:1361–1366.
5. Fareed FN, Chan G, Hoffman RS. Death temporally related to the use of a beta adrenergic receptor antagonist in cocaine associated myocardial infarction. *J Med Toxicol.* 2007;3:169–172.
6. Ibrahim M, Maselli DJ, Hasan R, Hamilton A. Safety of β-blockers in the acute management of cocaine-associated chest pain. *Am J Emerg Med.* 2013;31:613–616.

163 Incidental Noncardiovascular Findings on Echocardiography

Bernard Kadosh, Astha Tejpal, Kudrat Gill, Ahmadreza Alizadeh, Roberto M. Lang

HEART AND PERICARDIUM

There are many well-described typical cardiac tumors (both primary and metastatic to the heart) that are discussed elsewhere in this text. However, intra- and extracardiac masses can present in various ways, requiring close attention on the part of the echocardiographer. Fig. 163.1A demonstrates a large pericardial tumor seen in the subcostal view that is compressing right-sided structures. Fig. 163.1B shows a two-chamber view with deformation of the right atrium by an apparent mass causing extrinsic compression. Transesophageal echocardiography (TEE) allows for a detailed assessment of the superior vena cava in the bicaval view, which is shown with a mass traversing into the right atrium (Fig. 163.1C). Although the causes of these masses may be unknown without histopathologic assessment, recognition of their presence may warrant further investigation.

LUNGS AND PLEURAL SPACE

The lungs have a typical sliding appearance as they expand across the chest wall and can be recognized by the presence of A lines and B lines, as well as characteristic M-mode patterns.[1] In the presence of a pneumothorax, however, the low acoustic impedance of air causes ultrasound waves to be mostly reflected back. Thus, the absence of typical lung findings and failure to visualize deeper structures may suggest this diagnosis.[2] The property of low impedance causes a distinct sonographic appearance termed "dirty shadowing," which is highly suggestive of the presence of air (Fig. 163.1D).[3] This is in contrast to pleural effusions that are commonly seen as an anechoic collection posterior to the aorta and bordered by the diaphragm or chest wall (Fig. 163.1E). Atelectatic lung (Fig. 163.1F) can be seen flapping in the effusion, sometimes with partially aerated lung tissue expanding with respiration, which is known as the "curtain sign."[4,5]

STOMACH AND COLON

Normally, the colon is fixated by suspensory ligaments that prevent its interposition between the liver and diaphragm. Rarely, a loop of bowel can be seen in this location, a finding that has been termed the Chilaiditi sign, after the Greek radiologist Dimítrios Chilaiditi. Fig. 163.2A demonstrates this finding while attempting to visualize the inferior vena cava (IVC). Although this is usually a benign condition, Chilaiditi syndrome is the association of this phenomenon with chronic abdominal pain, nausea, and constipation.[6]

The stomach is often seen on parasternal and subcostal views. Hiatal hernias can be mistaken for masses with extrinsic compression on the heart.[7,8] Having the patient consume a carbonated beverage during the study will fill the stomach with

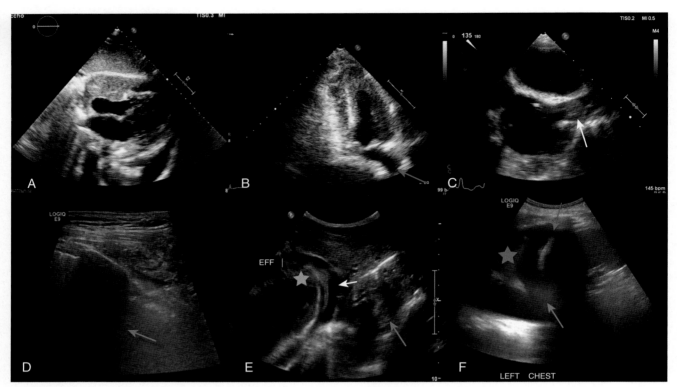

Figure 163.1. A, Transthoracic echocardiogram shows a pericardial tumor compressing the right heart. **B,** Extracardiac mass impinging the left atrium *(red arrow)*. **C,** Transesophageal echocardiogram shows an superior vena cava mass in the bicaval view *(white arrow)*. **D,** Right-sided pneumothorax creating "dirty shadowing" *(blue arrow)*. **E,** Right pleural effusion *(small white arrow)* between the right lung *(blue star)* and liver *(blue arrow)*. **F,** Hepatization of lung tissue *(blue star)* seen with atelectasis. The collapsed lung *(red arrow)* has an ultrasound density similar to tissue and floats within the hypoechoic pleural effusion *(blue arrow)*. *EFF,* effusion.

Figure 163.2. A, Subcostal view of the heart with probe positioned toward the liver shows a round mass with an echogenic center and hypoechoic space surrounding it *(red circle)*. Cine loop imaging demonstrated peristalsis. These findings are consistent with bowel loop. **B,** Hiatal hernia seen on transthoracic echocardiogram posterior to the left atrium after consumption of a carbonated drink *(blue oval)*.

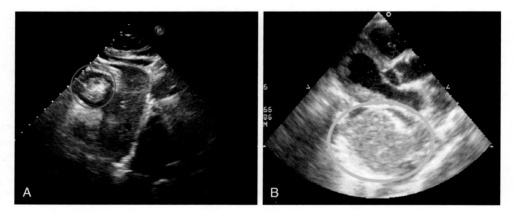

bubble contrast and allow for visualization of a hiatal hernia just posterior to the left atrium (Fig. 163.2B).

Liver, Gallbladder, and Pancreas

The subcostal view affords the visualization of these structures that may be associated with numerous pathologies. Hepatic steatosis results from abnormal accumulation of triglycerides in the hepatocytes. A normal liver has nearly the same echogenicity as the adjacent kidney. Because of ultrasound beam scattering by lipid droplets, a fatty liver looks much brighter relative to the renal cortex (Fig. 163.3A) with poor visualization of the internal hepatic vasculature.[9] The progression of fatty liver disease may lead to the development of a cirrhotic liver. This is typically characterized by nodularity of the liver surface with a coarse echotexture as smooth hepatocytes are replaced by fibrotic tissue (Fig. 163.3B).[10,11]

Ascites is often seen in this clinical context as demonstrated in Fig. 163.3C showing the falciform ligament, which is enhanced in the presence of anechoic fluid. The differential diagnosis of echo-free space around the heart anterior to the right ventricle includes ascites, pericardial effusion, pleural effusion, and pericardial cyst. The falciform ligament is a thin anteroposterior peritoneal fold connecting the liver to the abdominal wall just to the right of the midline, primarily seen in the subxiphoid view.[12] Undulations of the ligament can be seen, which are thought to be caused by transmission of cardiac motion to the ascitic fluid via the diaphragm. Cardello and coworkers found that visualization of this structure on echocardiography was associated with a confirmatory diagnosis of ascites, allowing differentiation from other fluid collections.[13]

Cysts and solid lesions are commonly seen in the liver with a wide differential, including hemangioma and abscess as well as benign and malignant tumors. Ultrasound findings of these

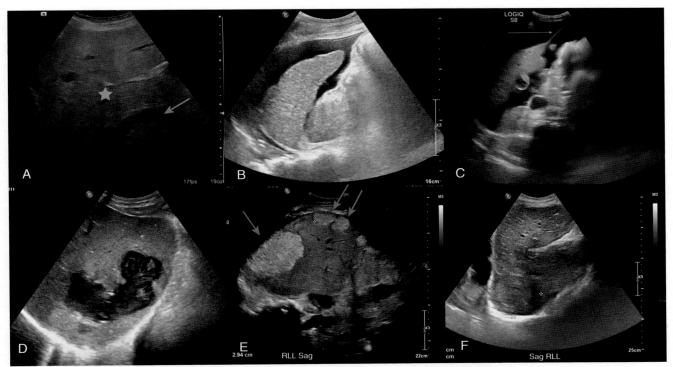

Figure 163.3. A, Hepatic steatosis. The liver *(blue star)* is hyperechoic compared with the renal cortex *(blue arrow).* **B,** Liver with nodular contour surrounded by ascitic fluid consistent with cirrhosis. **C,** Falciform ligament is seen connecting the liver with the anterior abdominal wall. Anechoic ascitic fluid outlines the falciform ligament. **D,** Hepatic abscess seen as complex fluid collection in the liver. **E,** Multiple echogenic masses seen in the liver, confirmed to be hepatocellular carcinoma (HCC) *(red arrows)* with magnetic resonance imaging. **F,** Isoechoic mass in posterior segment of the right hepatic lobe, also HCC *(red arrow).*

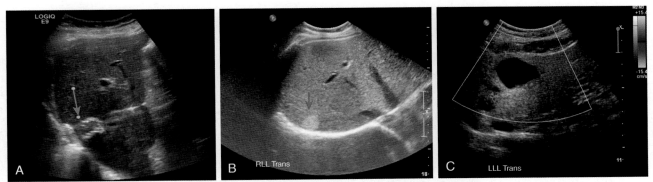

Figure 163.4. A, Typical appearance of a calcified hepatic echinococcal cyst *(blue arrow)* representing the inactive late stage form. **B,** Hemangioma. Hyperechoic mass in the posterior segment of the right liver lobe *(red arrow).* **C,** Anechoic, well-circumscribed, avascular structure in the liver, consistent with a hepatic cyst. *LLL Trans,* left liver lobe; *RLL Trans,* right liver lobe.

types are usually suggestive of the diagnosis but are rarely pathognomonic. Fig. 163.3D shows a complex fluid collection with internal echogenic strands, later found to be a hepatic abscess. Hepatocellular carcinoma has variable sonographic appearance depending on the degree of necrosis and presence of fibrosis, fat, or calcification.[14] It appears as irregular masses of varying echogenicity in our examples (Figs. 163.3E and F).

Echococcal cysts have a more typical appearance depending on what stage they present, usually appearing with a calcified rim in later stages (Fig. 163.4A).[15] Hemangiomas may have a well-defined homogenous hyperechoic appearance (Fig. 163.4B) in contrast to hepatic cysts (Fig. 163.4C), which are hypoechoic lesions without a wall.

The gallbladder can be differentiated from a cyst by the presence of a wall. It may be filled with sludge that appears as a layering of echogenic debris (Fig. 163.5A) or gallstones that appear as bright foci within the gallbladder lumen, casting a shadow posteriorly (Fig. 163.5B). Nonmobile filling defects within the gallbladder are usually caused by polyps, but an irregular mass with vascularity on Doppler interrogation should raise suspicion for gallbladder carcinoma (Figs. 163.5C and D).

The pancreas is a notoriously difficult structure to image without contrast enhancement techniques.[16] Because of its anatomic proximity to the duodenum and stomach, as well as the aorta and its mesenteric branches, tumors can remain undetected until they grow to a substantial extent. Figs. 163.6A and B show a heterogenous mass on the pancreatic head without apparent vascularity on color Doppler.

Spleen and Kidney

Retroperitoneal structures may be visualized while obtaining apical views of the heart. Splenic cysts are seen as completely anechoic

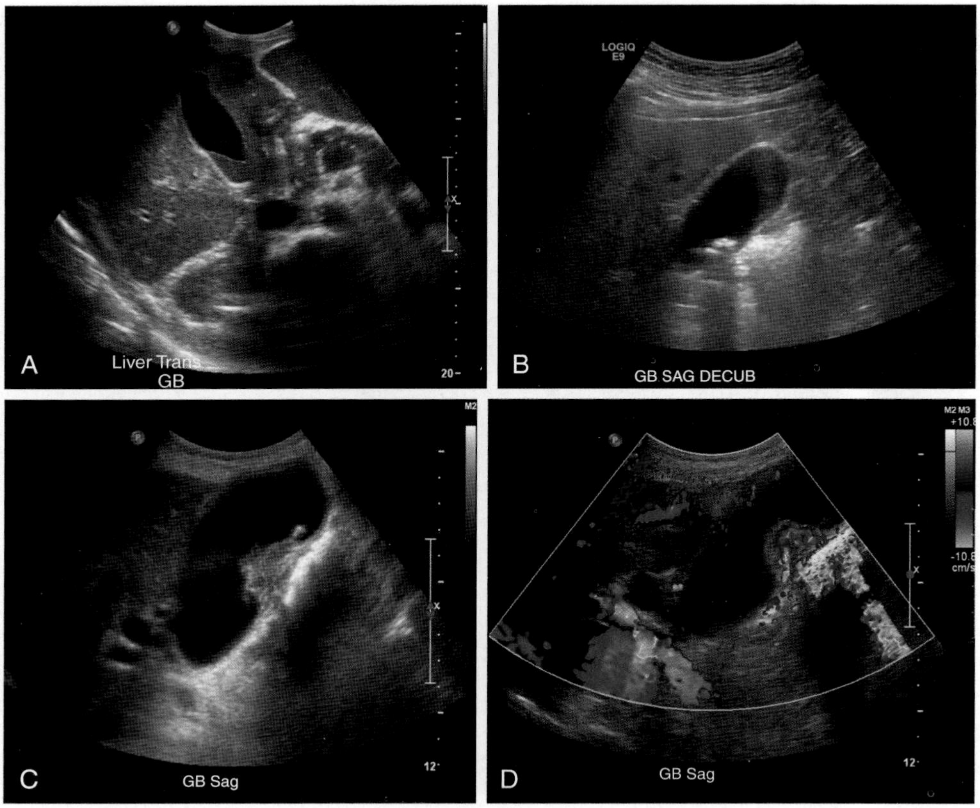

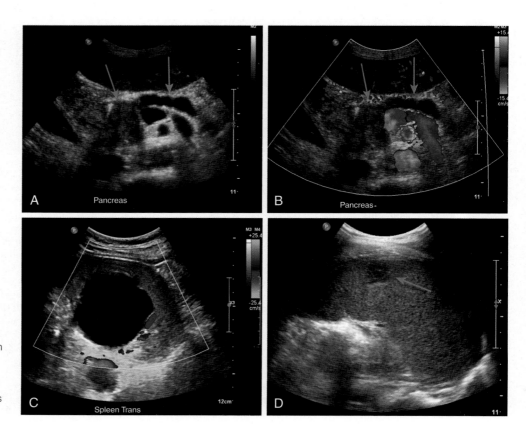

Figure 163.5. A, Layering of echogenic debris can be seen within the gallbladder consistent with sludge. **B,** Gallstones are visualized in the gallbladder as echogenic foci within the gallbladder lumen with posterior acoustic shadowing. **C,** Focal irregular mass in the gallbladder is concerning for malignancy. **D,** Color Doppler shows the vascular nature of the mass, which is also supportive of a tumor. *Decub,* Decubitus; *GB,* gallbladder; *Sag,* sagittal.

Figure 163.6. A and **B,** Hypoechoic mass *(red arrow)* in the pancreatic head with a dilated pancreatic duct *(blue arrow),* consistent with pancreatic carcinoma. **C,** Splenic cystic lesion with color Doppler over the cyst showing its avascular nature. **D,** Splenic infarcts are often seen as wedge-shaped hypoechoic lesions within the spleen *(blue arrow).*

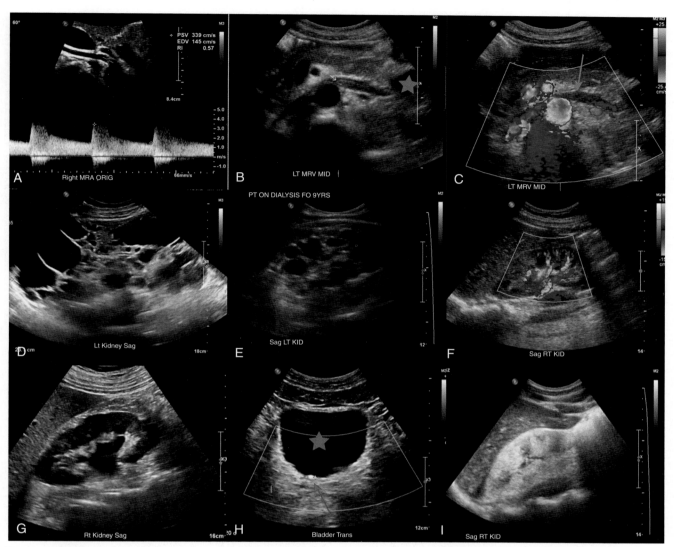

Figure 163.7. A, Elevated renal artery velocity of 339 cm/s secondary to renal artery stenosis. **B,** Left kidney *(blue star)*. Hypoechoic clot seen distending the left renal vein *(white arrow)* with lack of color flow within the clot (**C,** *blue arrow*). **D,** Markedly enlarged kidney replaced by innumerable cysts caused by polycystic kidney disease. **E,** Multiple cysts seen within the renal parenchyma consistent with acquired renal cystic disease. **F,** Focal hyperechoic change and deceased flow in the right kidney caused by pyelonephritis. **G,** Hydronephrosis secondary to a 7-mm uretero-vesicular junction stone (**H,** *red arrow*) causing obstructive uropathy. Bladder *(blue star).* **I,** HIV nephropathy.

avascular structures.[11] Fig. 163.6C shows a splenic cyst with a lack of color-flow Doppler within the cyst, supporting the lack of vascularity. Splenic infarcts classically appear as wedge-shaped hypoechoic lesions within the spleen (Fig. 163.6D).

Vascular Doppler ultrasound can be used to assess for renal artery stenosis. Elevated velocities within the renal artery are seen when the vessel is stenotic (Fig. 163.7A). Renal vein thrombosis is identified on ultrasonography as a hypoechoic filling defect that demonstrates no flow on color Doppler imaging (Figs. 163.7B and C).

Numerous renal cysts are seen in adult polycystic kidney disease (Fig. 163.7D) and acquired cystic disease of hemodialysis, but they are distinguished by kidney size. The kidneys are enlarged in adult polycystic kidney disease and are of normal size or atrophic in dialysis-related cystic disease. Fig. 163.7E shows a renal ultrasound performed on a patient with end-stage renal disease who had been on hemodialysis for 9 years and developed cystic degeneration.

Pyelonephritis is difficult to diagnose on ultrasonography. Focal changes in parenchymal echogenicity and diminished vascular flow are the most common sonographic findings (Fig. 163.7F).[17] Kidney

stones appear as echogenic structures with posterior acoustic shadowing. Obstructive uropathy is characterized by fluid-filled dilated pelvicalyceal system, and secondary hydronephrosis can be seen as well (Fig. 163.7G). Ureteral calculi are usually obscured by bowel gas, but stones at the ureterovesical junction are well seen through the anechoic bladder window (Fig. 163.7H).

Medical renal disease is a broad term that encompasses a wide differential but is suggested by increased echogenicity of the renal parenchyma. Clinical correlation and further studies are required to determine the specific cause. Fig. 163.7I shows an example of an enlarged kidney with a hyperechoic renal cortex, likely representing HIV nephropathy by history.

Renal cell carcinoma is known to metastasize to the heart via direct extension from the renal vein.[18–21] Fig. 163.8A shows a transesophageal echocardiogram in the bicaval view that revealed a mass invading the right atrium from the IVC, resulting in bulging of the interatrial septum. Color-flow doppler revealed turbulence in the IVC caused by obstruction by the tumor (Fig. 163.8B), which was surgically resected. The gross specimen

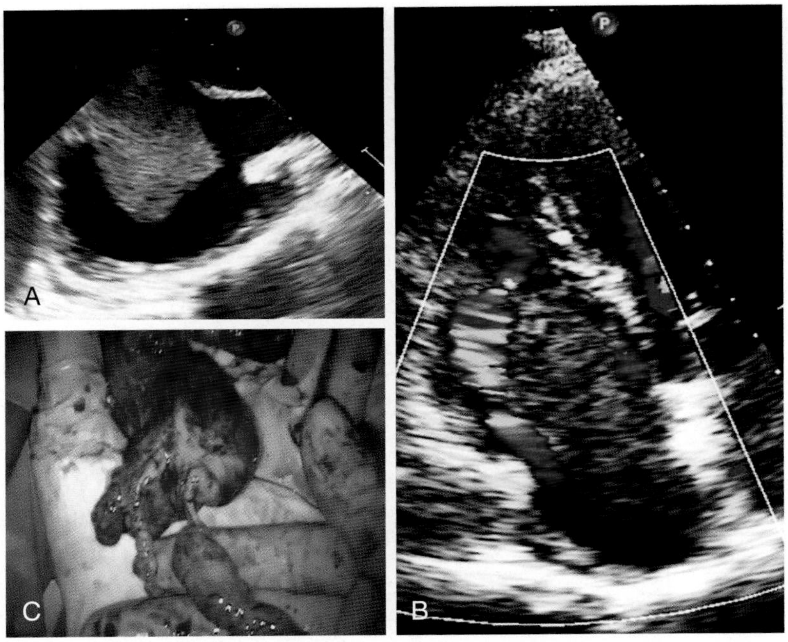

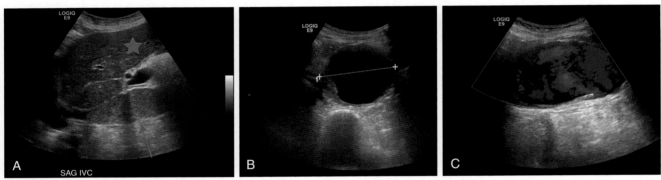

Figure 163.8. Renal cell carcinoma (RCC). **A,** Transesophageal echocardiogram, bicaval view of a mass invading the inferior vena cava (IVC) and the right atrium resulting in bulging of the interatrial septum toward the left atrium. This large echogenic mass was seen in this isolated view of the IVC as well. Color-flow Doppler shows turbulent flow in the IVC caused by obstruction by the tumor (**B**). A gross specimen removed during surgery, which was confirmed to be RCC by histologic analysis (**C**).

Figure 163.9. A, Distended inferior vena cava with a large hypoechoic mass consistent with thrombus *(blue arrow).* The *blue star* indicates the liver. **B,** Transverse view of the abdominal aorta demonstrates aneurysmal dilatation and is measured to be 7.43 cm. **C,** The aneurysmal abdominal aorta is seen again in sagittal view with color Doppler.

(Fig. 163.8C) was later confirmed to be renal cell carcinoma by histologic analysis.

Vena Cava and Aorta

TEE allows for dynamic assessment of posterior structures that are not normally well visualized by ultrasonography. Assessment of the IVC from the transgastric view revealed complete occlusion of the vessel caused by a large thrombus in a patient with lower extremity edema (Fig. 163.9A). The aorta is routinely assessed for atheromas, dissection, and aneurysm. Care should be taken to visualize as much of the descending aorta as possible while completing TEE. Figs. 163.9B and C show an abdominal aortic aneurysm of 7.43 cm incidentally found in an asymptomatic patient.

CONCLUSIONS

The fidelity and precision of echocardiography has greatly improved in recent years, allowing for better visualization of structures and pathologic entities than was previously possible. Here we tried to show either common or typical-appearing abnormalities that can be incidentally discovered during cardiac imaging. This work is not meant to be an exhaustive list, and we encourage interested physicians to study the source material referenced here. We hope that this summary provides an introduction to extracardiac findings, facilitates diagnosis, and inspires clinicians with a keen eye to broaden the scope of echocardiography practice.

Acknowledgments

The authors would like to thank Drs. Itzhak Kronzon, Robert J. Siegel, Hezzy Shmueli, and Neil L. Coplan for their contributions to the previous editions this chapter.

REFERENCES

1. Broaddus VC, Mason RJ, Nadel JA, eds. *Murray and Nadel's Textbook of Respiratory Medicine.* 6th ed. Vol. 2. Philadelphia: Elsevier Saunders; 2016.
2. Buttar S, Cooper D, Olivieri P, et al. Air and its sonographic appearance: understanding the artifacts. *J Emerg Med.* 2017;53:241–247.
3. Rubin JM, Adler RS, Bude RO, et al. Clean and dirty shadowing at US: a reappraisal. *Radiology.* 1991;181:231–236.
4. Lee FCY. The curtain sign in lung ultrasound. *J Med Ultrasound.* 2017;25:101–104.
5. Mann DL, Thompson K, Kaiser J. Cross-sectional echocardiographic characterization of atelectatic lung segments: differentiation from extracardiac tumors. *Chest.* 1990;97:404–406.
6. Moaven O, Hodin RA. Chilaiditi syndrome: a rare entity with important differential diagnoses. *Gastroenterol Hepatol.* 2012;8:276–278.

7. D'Cruz IA, Hancock HL. Echocardiographic characteristics of diaphragmatic hiatus hernia. *Am J Cardiol*. 1995;75:308–310.

8. Koskinas KC, Oikonomou K, Karapatsoudi E, Makridis P. Echocardiographic manifestation of hiatus hernia simulating a left atrial mass: case report. *Cardiovasc Ultrasound*. 2008;6:46.

9. Zhang YN, Fowler KJ, Hamilton G, et al. Liver fat imaging: a clinical overview of ultrasound, CT, and MR imaging. *Br J Radiol*. 2018;91:20170959.

10. Heller MT, Tublin ME. The role of ultrasonography in the evaluation of diffuse liver disease. *Radiol Clin North Am*. 2014;52:1163–1175.

11. Rumack CM, Wilson SR, Charboneau JW, Levine D. *Diagnostic Ultrasound: General Adult*. 4th ed. St. Louis: Elsevier Saunders; 2014.

12. Kerut EK, Dearstine M, Hanawalt C. Utility of identification of the falciform ligament in the echocardiography laboratory. *Echocardiography*. 2007;24:887–888.

13. Cardello FP, Yoon D-HA, Halligan RE, Richter H. The falciform ligament in the echocardiographic diagnosis of ascites. *J Am Soc Echocardiogr*. 2006;19:1074.e3–4.

14. Kee K-M, Lu S-N. Diagnostic efficacy of ultrasound in hepatocellular carcinoma diagnosis. *Expert Rev Gastroenterol Hepatol*. 2017;11:277–279.

15. Brunetti E, Tamarozzi F, Macpherson C, et al. Ultrasound and cystic echinococcosis. *Ultrasound Int Open*. 2018;4:E70–E78.

16. Sofuni A, Tsuchiya T, Itoi T. Ultrasound diagnosis of pancreatic solid tumors. *J Med Ultrason*. 2020;47(3):359–376.

17. Edell SL, Bonavita JA. The sonographic appearance of acute pyelonephritis. *Radiology*. 1979;132:683–685.

18. Abraham KP, Reddy V, Gattuso P. Neoplasms metastatic to the heart: review of 3314 consecutive autopsies. *Am J Cardiovasc Pathol*. 1990;3:195–198.

19. Chiles C, Woodard PK, Gutierrez FR, Link KM. Metastatic involvement of the heart and pericardium: CT and MR imaging. *Radiographics*. 2001;21:439–449.

20. Makhija Z, Deshpande R, Desai J. Unusual tumours of the heart: diagnostic and prognostic implications. *J Cardiothorac Surg*. 2009;4(4).

21. Ananthasubramaniam K, Karthikeyan V. Images in cardiology: metastatic renal cell cancer detected by transoesophageal echocardiography. *Heart*. 2000;83:710.

164 Evaluation of Patients Undergoing Transcatheter Aortic Valve Replacement

Federico M. Asch

Transcatheter aortic valve replacement (TAVR) has emerged as a new option for the treatment of patients with severe symptomatic aortic stenosis (AS). Although initially approved for patients considered inoperable or at greatly increased risk for surgical aortic valve replacement (SAVR), recent clinical trials have proved that TAVR is noninferior or even superior to SAVR in patients at intermediate and low surgical risk. Echocardiography plays an essential role in TAVR patient selection, intraprocedural monitoring, and postprocedural follow-up, with three-dimensional (3D) echocardiography playing an increasingly important role.

Two types of transcatheter heart valves (THVs) are currently available: mechanically expandable and self-expanding. Each THV comes in various sizes, to be implanted according to the patient's aortic annulus and root size. A description of valve structure, delivery techniques, and clinical experience with these valves is beyond the scope of this chapter, so readers are referred to each THV's labeling material or the European Association of Echocardiography/American Society of Echocardiography (ASE) recommendations for the use of echocardiography in new transcatheter interventions for valvular heart disease for additional detail.[1]

PATIENT SELECTION

The presence of severe AS must first be established using the current guidelines.[2] Pivotal trials have been limited to patients with high transvalvular velocities and mean gradients ($\geq$ 4 m/s and $\geq$40 mm Hg, respectively). Although severity grading is usually a straightforward process, it can be challenging in patients with low-flow, low-gradient (LFLG) AS. On one hand, the aortic valve opening may be limited by the low-flow condition, therefore exaggerating the severity of disease (pseudo-severe AS); on the other hand, the low-flow state may present with low gradients despite a severely stenotic valve. In this scenario, dobutamine stress echocardiography is a useful tool to differentiate between "real severe" and moderate, "pseudo-severe" AS. The inotropic effect of dobutamine (provided there is contractile reserve, defined as improvement in stroke volume >20%) restores a "normal flow state" and allows proper estimation of gradients, peak velocities, and valve area.[3]

A detailed stepwise approach for evaluation of AS, as recommended by European Association of Cardiovascular Imaging/ASE guidelines (Fig. 164.1).[2] LFLG AS is usually defined as a mean transvalvular gradient less than 35 mm Hg, an effective orifice area less than 1.0 cm[2], and left ventricular ejection fraction (LVEF) 40% or greater. The True or Pseudo-Severe Aortic Stenosis - transcatheter aortic valve implant (TOPAS-TAVI) study has shown the benefit of TAVR in such patients.[4] Although in this study, dobutamine echocardiography was critical for patient selection for TAVR (distinction of severe vs pseudo-severe AS), patients had improved outcomes after TAVR regardless of the presence or absence of contractile reserve.[5] More recently, LFLG AS has also been described in patients with preserved LVEF.[6]

PREPROCEDURAL IMAGING

Accurate preprocedural aortic annular sizing is essential to optimize TAVR results by maximizing the postprocedural orifice area and decrease the risk of patient–prosthesis mismatch while minimizing paravalvular leak (PVL).[7,8] For annular sizing before TAVR, the virtual ring formed by the basal cusp attachment (corresponding to the hinge point of the aortic cusps) is measured, providing the primary determinant of valve size. Given the frequently oval shape of the aortic annulus, two-dimensional (2D) echocardiography significantly underestimates its maximum diameter and cross-sectional area.[9] The annulus measured by TTE using the conventional long-axis orientation is in average 1 mm smaller than that measured by 2D TEE, which is, in turn, 1.5 mm smaller than the corresponding multislice computed tomography (MSCT) measurement; 3D TEE annular measurements, however, more closely approximate those obtained with MSCT.[8] Therefore, THV sizing should be determined by a 3D imaging technique such as MSCT (preferred) or 3D TEE. Multiplanar reconstruction of 3D volume sets permits the measurement of orthogonal diameters as well as the annular perimeter and area (Fig. 164.2).

In the screening process, 3D imaging by either technique is also needed to measure the coronary ostium height and the distance from the annulus to the sinotubular junction because these measurements help determine which THV is best suited for the patient. A coronary height of 10 to 11 mm (or larger than the length of the calcified leaflet) is desirable to prevent ostium obstruction at the time of THV deployment. Preprocedural assessment should also include evaluation of the degree of upper septal hypertrophy (septal bulge), which can predispose to valve malposition or displacement, assessing the mitral valve because it may be damaged during TAVR, and documenting baseline left ventricular (LV) function. In summary, preprocedural echocardiography is typically limited to TTE, with TEE restricted to patients in whom MSCT is suboptimal or contraindicated.

PROCEDURAL IMAGING

Early in the history of TAVR, the procedure used to be highly dependent on TEE guidance for valve sizing and positioning. However, the more recent use of MSCT as a mandatory part of the preprocedural evaluation has simplified the procedure to an extent that TEE is only required in a minority of complicated cases. Nowadays, most cases are performed under moderate sedation with TTE used after implantation to determine the presence and severity of residual aortic regurgitation (AR) or PVL and to evaluate changes in LV wall motion or presence of new pericardial effusion. Escalation to TEE may be needed if any procedural complications are suspected. These include, but are not limited to, moderate or severe PVL, coronary ostium occlusion, aortic annular rupture, THV migration, and acute mitral regurgitation.

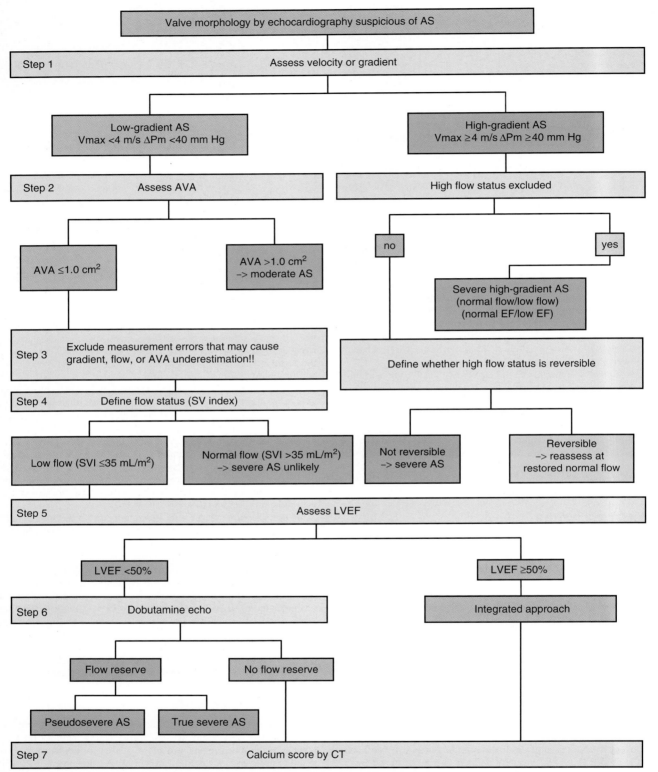

Figure 164.1. Stepwise evaluation of aortic stenosis (AS) according to flow, gradients, and ejection fraction (EF). *AVA,* Aortic valve area; *CT,* computed tomography; *LVEF,* left ventricular ejection fraction; *SVI,* stroke volume index. (Reproduced with permission from Baumgartner H, et al: Recommendations on the echocardiographic assessment of aortic valve stenosis, *J Am Soc Echocardiogr* 30:372–392, 2017.)

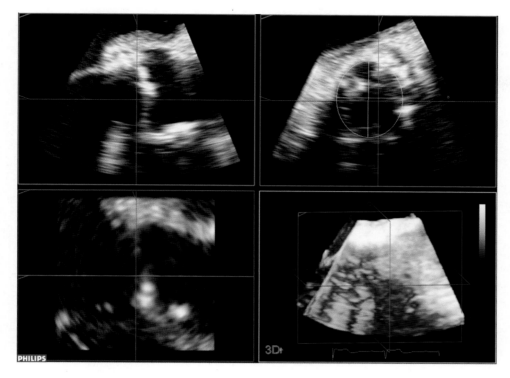

Figure 164.2. Annular sizing with three-dimensional (3D) transesophageal echocardiography. 3D reconstruction allows for proper plane selection at the annulus levels in at least two planes (*green lines* in *upper right* and *lower left panels*), such that the optimal short axis is displayed *(upper left panel)*. In this oval-shaped annulus, the annulus area and perimeter can be easily measured *(red oval)*, as well as the maximum *(full line)* and minimum diameters *(dashed line)*. These measurements are used for proper valve sizing of transcatheter heart valve devices.

TABLE 164.1 Strengths and Weaknesses of each Imaging Modality to Evaluate Transcatheter Heart Valve Function

	TTE	TEE 2D+ 3D	4D CT
Leak severity	++	++	-
Leak location	+	++	-
Valve hemodynamics	++	+	-
Malpositioning	-	+	++
Eccentric annulus	-	++	++
Aortic root geometry	-	+	++
Frame integrity	-	+/-	++
Leaflet thrombosis	-	++	++
Leaflet degeneration	+/-	++	-
Leaflet coaptation	-	++	-

2D, Two-dimensional; *3D,* three-dimensional; *4D,* four-dimensional; *CT,* computed tomography; *TTE,* transthoracic echocardiography.

POSTPROCEDURAL FOLLOW-UP

Follow-up of patients with THV is similar to that for surgical prostheses and is performed with TTE for valve hemodynamics and regurgitation. TEE, MSCT, or both will be needed if valve dysfunction or thrombosis are suspected as each of them has a higher value to evaluate specific features of the THV (Table 164.1).

Hemodynamic Evaluation

Key hemodynamic parameters to be followed are peak and mean gradient, effective orifice area (EOA, calculated with the continuity equation), and the Doppler velocity index (DVI, defined as the ratio of velocities proximal to and distal to the valve).[10] As is true for all aortic valves, multiple windows including apical, right parasternal, and suprasternal as well as imaging and nonimaging (PEDOF) probes should be used.[2] The calculation of EOA and DVI requires special attention to detail because they depend on formulas that involve multiple measurements. They both include left ventricular outflow tract (LVOT) and aortic valve velocities (TVIs are preferred but alternatively peak velocities can be used), so increases in

flow for any physiological conditions would not affect the calculations (changes in velocities proximal and distal to the THV would be directly proportional). DVI is preferred in daily practice because it avoids using the LVOT diameter (DVI = LVOT/AoV velocities), a measurement that is particularly challenging because of the artifacts created by the THV stent. Therefore, longitudinal follow-up of an individual patient should be performed by direct, side-to-side comparison of gradients or velocities and DVI.

When used, the LVOT diameter is best measured just proximal to or at the proximal end of the stent, with the leading edge–to–leading edge technique, although different approaches have been used. It is important that the LVOT sample volume be carefully placed at the same plane where the LVOT diameter is being measured. To date, favorable hemodynamics, which appear to be stable over 5 years, have been demonstrated for both the SAPIEN and CoreValve THVs, as well as to other valves with shorter follow-up data such as LOTUS, PORTICO, or ACURATE. Normal mean gradients are specific to each THV and for each size and are typically between 8 and 15 mm Hg. Normal THV hemodynamic function has been defined by the second Valve Academic Research Consortium (VARC 2) criteria based on mean gradient (normal <20 mm Hg), EOA (normal >0.9–1.1 cm^2), and DVI (>0.35) following a specific algorithm (Fig. 164.3).[10] Most important, direct comparison of any follow-up with early post-TAVR gradients and DVI is critical to detect changes that could reflect valve degeneration or thrombosis.

Aortic Regurgitation and Paravalvular Leak

Identification and grading of severity of PVL is important, given the poor prognosis of those with moderate or severe PVL after THV implantation. PVL is common, but with recent advances in THV design and implantation techniques, the incidence of moderate or severe regurgitation has decreased enormously (<5% for most currently available devices). Accurate assessment of post-TAVR AR may be difficult because of the coexistence of valvular and paravalvular jets and, more importantly because PVL may consist of multiple jets with highly eccentric trajectories. These eccentric jets tend to appear much larger by color Doppler in the LVOT than they actually are, so the severity of AR should never be graded purely

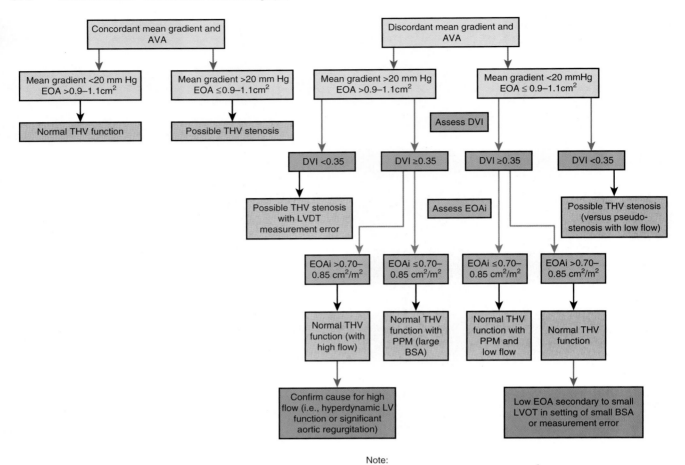

Note:
Use lower values of EOA for BSA <1.6 m^2
Use lower values of EOAi for BMI ≥30 kg/m^2

Figure 164.3. Transcatheter heart valve hemodynamic evaluation as recommended by the second Valve Academic Research Consortium (VARC 2). *BMI,* Body mass index; *BSA,* body surface area; *DVI,* Doppler velocity index; *EOA,* effective orifice area; *EOAi,* indexed effective orifice area; *LV,* left ventricular; *LVOT,* left ventricular outflow tract; *PPM,* prosthesis–patient mismatch; *THV,* transcatheter heart valve. (Reproduced with permission from Kappetein AP, et al: Updated standardized endpoint definitions for transcatheter aortic valve implantation, *Eur Heart J* 33:2403–2418, 2012.)

on the basis of the jet width, jet extension, or jet-to-LVOT ratio but rather on a comprehensive manner that includes qualitative and quantitative parameters obtained by color and spectral Doppler, hemodynamics, and so on.[11]

It is essential that multiple imaging windows (parasternal long and short axes, apical five and three chamber, with nonstandard variations of these views) be used. Short-axis views with color Doppler should be recorded at multiple levels to identify the exact plane of the PVL jet's origin. It is critical that the circumferential extent of regurgitant jets get recorded at the plane of the aortic annulus (vena contracta of the PVL). These PVL jets "spread out" as soon as they reach the LVOT; therefore, a short-axis plane that is even 1 mm into the LVOT will exaggerate the severity of PVL (Fig. 164.4).

The severity of PVL from the circumferential extent is estimated as mild (<10% of the stent circumference is leaking), moderate (10%–29%), or severe (≥30%). However, severity grading should not rely on a single parameter but rather on an integrated approach as recommended by the recent ASE recommendations (Fig. 164.5)[10] that includes pressure half-time, assessment of the abdominal and descending thoracic aorta for retrograde flow, and calculations of regurgitant volume and fraction using integrated Doppler (continuity equation) as well as jet characteristics by color Doppler. Applying the proximal isovelocity surface area

approach to THVs is difficult, so its mere presence usually reflects significant regurgitation. More recently, it has been suggested that direct planimetry of the vena contracta of the regurgitant jet(s) with 3D echocardiography may be helpful.[12] Although this approach is promising, it may be limited because of the spatial and temporal resolution of 3D color Doppler.

Leaflet Thrombosis

Subclinical leaflet thrombosis after TAVR was recently described in a randomized trial and subsequently demonstrated in a series of registries involving all transcatheter and surgical bioprostheses.[13] Although in some series, it has been linked with a higher incidence of stroke or transient ischemic attack, its real clinical significance is still unclear. Although it has been mostly described in the initial 45 days after implant, it is still unknown whether early valve thrombosis is linked with longer-term valve degeneration. The computed tomography hallmarks were noted to be hypoattenuated leaflet thickening associated with reduced leaflet motion.[14] Leaflet thickening typically starts from and is wider in the periphery (THV stent), decreasing toward the leaflet edge. Similar findings can be seen with TEE, in cases in which CT is of suboptimal quality or contraindicated (Fig. 164.6). These lesions typically disappear after treatment with anticoagulation.

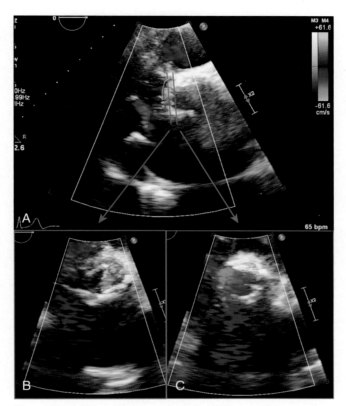

Figure 164.4. Effect of aortic regurgitation (AR) eccentricity on color Doppler jet recording in assessing the severity of pulmonary vascular resistance with para-valvular leak (PVL) after transcatheter aortic valve replacement. Scanning of the whole stented valve in short axis is needed to identify the vena contracta of the jet(s). Proper plane selection of the short axis is critical. In the case of an eccentric jet in the left ventricular outflow tract (LVOT) (**A**, *curved arrow*), the plane below the valve ring (**B**, *red*) shows a large color jet as it spreads in the LVOT, overestimating the severity of AR. By selecting the proper short axis at the aortic annulus, the regurgitant orifice is best depicted (**C,** *green arrow*), more consistent with mild PVL. Similarly, a high short-axis view at the aortic root level (not shown) could be misinterpreted because of normal diastolic flow in the sinuses of Valsalva or coronary arteries; flows in these locations, however, are of lower velocity and are not aliased. (Adapted from Zoghbi WA, et al: Guidelines for the evaluation of valvular regurgitation after percutaneous valve repair or replacement, *J Am Soc Echocardiogr* 32:431–475, 2019.)

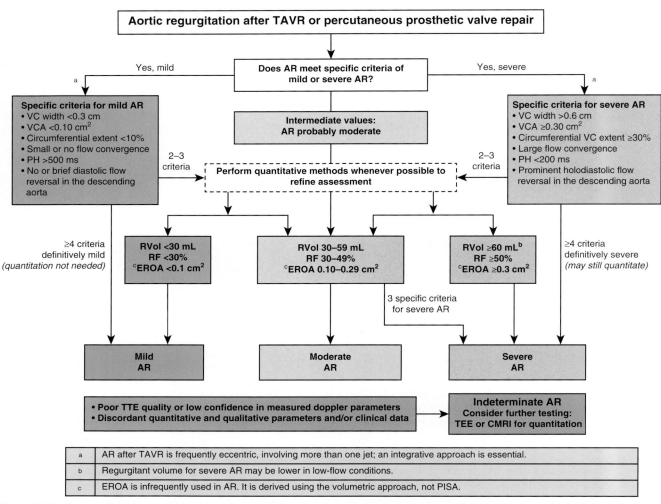

Figure 164.5. Suggested algorithm to guide implementation of integration of multiple parameters of the severity of aortic regurgitation (AR) after transcatheter aortic valve replacement (TAVR) or prosthetic aortic valve repair. Good-quality echocardiographic imaging and complete data acquisition are assumed. If imaging is technically difficult, consider transesophageal echocardiography (TEE) or cardiac magnetic resonance imaging (CMRI). The severity of AR may be indeterminate because of poor image quality, technical issues with data, internal inconsistency among echocardiography findings, or discordance with clinical findings. *EROA,* Effective regurgitant orifice area; *PH,* pulmonary hypertension; *PISA,* proximal isovelocity surface area; *RF,* regurgitant fraction; *RVol,* regurgitant volume; *TTE,* transthoracic echocardiography; *VC,* vena contracta; *VCA,* vena contracta area. (Reproduced from Zoghbi WA, et al: Guidelines for the evaluation of valvular regurgitation after percutaneous valve repair or replacement, *J Am Soc Echocardiogr* 32:431–475, 2019.)

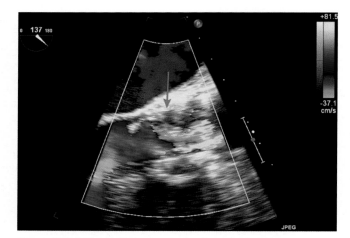

Figure 164.6. Transcatheter heart valve thrombosis. This transesophageal echocardiography still frame in midsystole of a two-dimensional echocardiography with color Doppler is an example of a leaflet that remains closed in systole (restricted leaflet motion, reduced leaflet motion). The *red arrow* shows a large thrombus attached to the aortic surface of the leaflet (leaflet thickening, hypoattenuated leaflet thickening). Color Doppler shows forward flow through the normal leaflet (from the left ventricle on the *left* to the aorta on the *right*) but no flow through the thrombosed, immobile leaflet.

Acknowledgments

We thank Drs. Linda D. Gillam, Konstantinos Koulogiannis, and Leo Marcoff for their contributions to the previous edition of this chapter.

REFERENCES

1. Zamorano JL, Badano LP, Bruce C, et al. EAE/ASE recommendations for the use of echocardiography in new transcatheter interventions for valvular heart disease. *J Am Soc Echocardiogr.* 2011;24:937–965.
2. Baumgartner H, Hung J, Bermejo J, et al. Recommendations on the echocardiographic assessment of aortic valve stenosis. *J Am Soc Echocardiogr.* 2017;30:372–392.
3. Asch FM, Weissman NJ. Aortic stenosis and the failing heart. *Expert Rev Cardiovasc Ther.* 2006;4:25–31.
4. Ribeiro HB, Lerakis S, Gilard M, et al. Transcatheter aortic valve replacement in patients with low-flow, low-gradient aortic stenosis: the TOPAS-TAVI Registry. *J Am Coll Cardiol.* 2018;71:1297–1308.
5. Maes F, Lerakis S, Barbosa Ribeiro H, et al. Outcomes from transcatheter aortic valve replacement in patients with low-flow, low-gradient aortic stenosis and left ventricular ejection fraction less than 30%: a substudy from the TOPAS-TAVI Registry. *JAMA Cardiol.* 2019;4:64–70.
6. Clavel MA, Magne J, Pibarot P. Low-gradient aortic stenosis. *Eur Heart J.* 2016;37:2645–2657.
7. Athappan G, Patvardhan E, Tuzcu EM, et al. Incidence, predictors, and outcomes of aortic regurgitation after transcatheter aortic valve replacement: meta-analysis and systematic review of literature. *J Am Coll Cardiol.* 2013;61:1585–1595.
8. Kasel AM, Cassese S, Bleiziffer S, et al. Standardized imaging for aortic annular sizing: implications for transcatheter valve selection. *JACC Cardiovasc Imag.* 2013;6:249–262.
9. Piazza N, de Jaegere P, Schultz C, et al. Anatomy of the aortic valvar complex and its implications for transcatheter implantation of the aortic valve. *Circ Cardiovasc Interv.* 2008;1:74–81.
10. Kappetein AP, Head SJ, Généreux P, et al. Updated standardized endpoint definitions for transcatheter aortic valve implantation. *Eur Heart J.* 2012;33:2403–2418.
11. Zoghbi WA, Asch FM, Bruce C, et al. Guidelines for the evaluation of valvular regurgitation after percutaneous valve repair or replacement. *J Am Soc Echocardiogr.* 2019;32:431–475.
12. Gonçalves A, Almeria C, Marcos-Alberca P, et al. Three-dimensional echocardiography in paravalvular aortic regurgitation assessment after transcatheter aortic valve implantation. *J Am Soc Echocardiogr.* 2012;25:47–55.
13. Makkar RR, Fontana G, Jilaihawi H, et al. Possible subclinical leaflet thrombosis in bioprosthetic aortic valves. *N Engl J Med.* 2015;373:2015–2024.
14. Jilaihawi H, Asch FM, Manasse E, et al. Systematic CT methodology for the evaluation of subclinical leaflet thrombosis. *JACC Cardiovasc Imaging.* 2017;10:461–470.

165 Mitral Valve Balloon Valvuloplasty

Ernesto E. Salcedo, Edward A. Gill, Robert A. Quaife, John D. Carroll

Mitral stenosis (MS) is the most common form of rheumatic valve disease and produces significant disability, particularly in young and middle-aged adults.[1,2] Patients with severe MS usually develop fatigue, heart failure, atrial fibrillation, and thromboembolism. Of the many causes of MS, rheumatic mitral stenosis (RMS) remains the most common, usually presenting in patients between the ages 20 and 40 years, several years after an attack of rheumatic fever. In developed countries RMS is primarily seen in the immigrant population.[3] Degenerative mitral valve stenosis (DMS), the other common form of MS, is more often seen in older adults, and its prevalence is increasing.[4] Unlike RMS, DMS is typically not amenable to percutaneous mitral valve balloon valvuloplasty (MVBV).

Echocardiography is the diagnostic tool of choice to determine the presence, type, and severity of MS; to determine the best therapeutic options; and to follow patients with MS.[5] The hemodynamics of MS has been reviewed with several associated problems such as pregnancy, in obese patients, and with resultant pulmonary hypertension.[6]

MVBV and surgery are complementary interventions used at different times in the management of patients with MS. There are clear indications for surgical mitral valve repair or replacement in MS; however, surgery has been replaced by MVB) as the procedure of choice for managing severe, symptomatic rheumatic MS. The 2014 American Heart Association (AHA)/American College of Cardiology (ACC)[7] and the 2017 European Society of Cardiology/European Association for Cardio-Thoracic Surgery[8] (Table 165.1) guidelines for the management of valvular heart disease delineate the central role of MVBV in the management of severe MS. The recent

TABLE 165.1 Guidelines for Interventions in Mitral Stenosis

(Class I Indications)	Level of Evidence
2014 ACC/AHA GUIDELINES FOR INTERVENTIONS IN MITRAL STENOSIS [7]	
1. Percutaneous mitral balloon commissurotomy is recommended for symptomatic patients with severe MS (MVA ≤1.5 cm^2, stage D) and favorable valve morphology in the absence of left atrial thrombus or moderate to severe MR.	A
2. Mitral valve surgery (repair, commissurotomy, or valve replacement) is indicated in severely symptomatic patients (NYHA class III to IV) with severe MS (MVA ≤1.5 cm^2, stage D) who are not high risk for surgery and who are not candidates for or who have failed previous percutaneous mitral balloon commissurotomy.	B
2017 ESC/EACTS GUIDELINES FOR INTERVENTIONS IN MITRAL STENOSIS [8]	
1. Percutaneous mitral balloon commissurotomy is indicated in symptomatic patients without unfavorable characteristics for PMC.	B
2. Percutaneous mitral balloon commissurotomy is indicated in all symptomatic patients with a contraindication or a high risk for surgery.	C
3. Mitral valve surgery is indicated in symptomatic patients who are not suitable for percutaneous mitral balloon commissurotomy.	C

ACC, American College of Cardiology; *AHA,* American Heart Association; *EACTS,* European Association for Cardio-Thoracic Surgery; *ESC,* European Society of Cardiology; *MR,* mitral regurgitation; *MS,* mitral stenosis; *MVA,* mitral valve area; *NYHA,* New York Heart Association; *PMC,* percutaneous mitral commissurotomy.

TABLE 165.2 Rheumatic Versus Degenerative Mitral Stenosis

	Rheumatic	Degenerative
Age group	Younger	Older
History of rheumatic fever	Yes (not always)	No
Commissural fusion	Yes	No
Mitral annulus calcification	No (usually)	Yes
Extension of calcification to surrounding tissues	Uncommon	Common
Main leaflet thickening	Tips	Base
Valve geometry	Funnel shape	Tunnel shape

2019 American Association for Thoracic Surgery/ACC/American Society of Echocardiography (ASE)/Society for Cardiovascular Angiography and Interventions/Society of Thoracic Surgeons Expert Consensus System of Care Document includes percutaneous mitral balloon commissurotomy as one of seven interventional procedures requiring care under a Comprehensive Valve Center.[9]

MVBV is most effective in patients with rheumatic MS, and echocardiography plays an essential role in determining MVBV suitability according to well-stablished scoring parameters. In patients with degenerative MS, other transcatheter procedures are being used, including the deployment of valves designed for transcatheter aortic valve replacement (TAVR) as valve in mitral

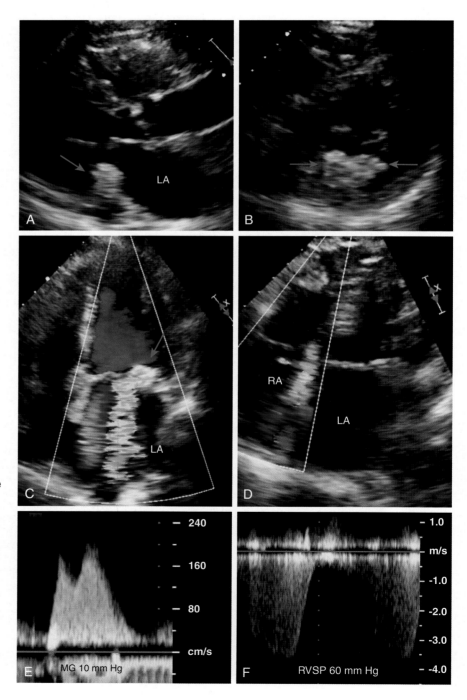

Figure 165.1. Degenerative or calcific mitral stenosis. **A,** Parasternal long-axis view of the left ventricle (LV) with severe calcification of the mitral annulus *(red arrow)*. Note the enlarged left atrium. **B,** Parasternal short-axis of the LV. Note the dense and extensive calcification of the posterior mitral annulus *(red arrows)*. **C,** Apical four-chamber view illustrates the dense calcification of the mitral anulus *(red arrow)* and the presence of associated moderate mitral regurgitation. **D,** Another apical four-chamber view illustrates the presence of associated tricuspid regurgitation. **E,** The presence of a mean transmitral gradient of 10 mm Hg is noted, and the associated pulmonary hypertension is documented **F**. *RA*, Right atrium; *RVSP*, right ventricular systolic pressure.

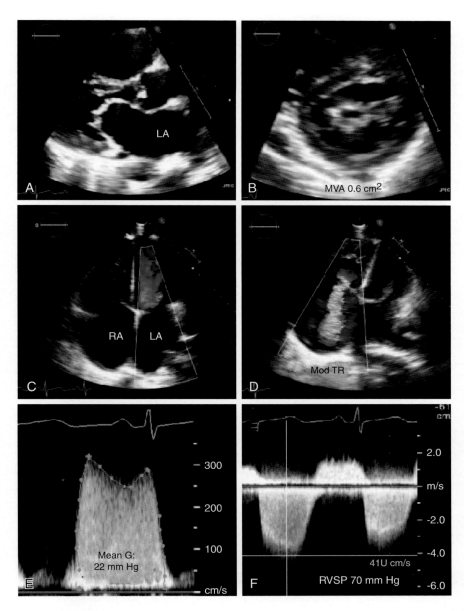

Figure 165.2. Rheumatic mitral stenosis (MS) severity. A 22-year-old woman with rheumatic heart disease, including tricuspid regurgitation, mitral stenosis, and mixed aortic valve disease with resultant pulmonary hypertension, who presented with decompensated heart failure and atrial fibrillation. **A,** Left parasternal view of the mitral valve shows the typical doming and funnel-shaped mitral valve with an associated large left atrium (LA). The Wilkins score was measured at 8. **B,** Parasternal short-axis view of the mitral valve demonstrates bicommissural fusion and a very small mitral orifice size with a mitral valve area (MVA) of 0.6 cm² by planimetry. **C,** Color Doppler apical four-chamber view demonstrates absence of mitral regurgitation. **D,** Moderate (Mod) tricuspid regurgitation (TR). **E,** Apical Doppler transmitral mean gradient of 22 mm Hg consistent with severe MS. **F,** Severe pulmonary hypertension as demonstrated by the TR-derived right ventricular systolic pressure (RVSP) of 70 mm Hg. *G,* Gradient; *RA,* right atrium.

anulus calcification (MAC) or valve-in-ring interventions.[10,11] A similar approach is being used in patients with mitral bioprosthesis stenosis.[12,13]

This chapter describes the role of echocardiography in the management of MS with MVBV. Patient selection, intraprocedural guidance, detection and prevention of procedural complications, and evaluation of results and follow-up are discussed.

PATIENT SELECTION FOR MITRAL VALVE BALLOON VALVULOPLASTY

Proper medical, interventional, and surgical management of patients with MS requires characterization of the cause, stage, valve anatomy, valve hemodynamics, hemodynamic consequences, and determination of the presence and severity of symptoms. Candidates for MVBV have symptoms of heart failure, rheumatic valve changes with commissural fusion and diastolic doming of the mitral valve leaflets, and severe MS with a mitral valve area (MVA) of 1.5 cm² or less. Absence of more than mild mitral regurgitation (MR) and absence of left atrial (LA) thrombus[14] are also prerequisites.

DETERMINING THE CAUSE OF MITRAL STENOSIS

Native valve MS can be rheumatic, or nonrheumatic. Nonrheumatic causes include DMS with MAC,[4,15–18] radiation–induced MS,[19] and congenital MS.[20–23] Rare causes of MS include LA myxoma,[24] LA mases,[25] amyloidosis,[26] carcinoid syndrome,[27] systemic lupus erythematosus,[28,29] endomyocardial fibroelastosis,[30] and endocarditis.[31] MS can also occur in the setting of prosthetic mitral valve dysfunction,[32] which typically is not treatable by MVBV.

The first step in determining suitability for MVBV is to exclude nonrheumatic MS. Most of the nonrheumatic causes of MS have characteristic echocardiographic findings and are relatively easy to differentiate from rheumatic MS; these are not discussed here. However, differentiating rheumatic from degenerative MS is not always straightforward, and this distinction has important implications regarding eligibility for MVBV. Preprocedural cardiac computed tomography (CCT) is being increasingly used for the planning of valve in MAC with very promising results.[33] Table 165.2 and Figs. 165.1 and 165.2 illustrate and summarize the main differences between rheumatic and degenerative MS.

TABLE 165.3 Wilkins Score to Determine Mitral Valve Balloon Valvuloplasty Suitability[a]

Grade	Mobility	Thickening	Calcification	Subvalvular Thickening
1	Highly mobile valve with only leaflet tips restricted	Leaflets near normal in thickness (4–5 mm)	A single area of increased echo brightness	Minimal thickening just below the mitral leaflets
2	Leaflet mid and base	Midleaflets normal, considerable thickening of margins (5–8 mm)	Scattered areas of brightness confined to leaflet margins	Thickening of chordal structures extending to one-third of the chordal length
3	Valve continues to move forward in diastole, mainly from the base	Thickening extending through the entire leaflet (5–8 mm)	Brightness extending into the midportions of the leaflets	Thickening extended to distal third of the chords
4	No or minimal forward movement of the leaflets in diastole	Considerable thickening of all leaflet tissue (>8–10 mm)	Extensive brightness throughout much of the leaflet tissue	Extensive thickening and shortening of all chordal structures extending down to the papillary muscles

[a]The total echocardiographic score is derived from an analysis of mitral leaflet mobility, valvar and subvalvar thickening, and calcification, which are graded from 0 to 4 according to these criteria. This gives a total score of 0 to 16. See also Fig. 165.5.
Reproduced with permission from Wilkins GT, et al: Percutaneous balloon dilatation of the mitral valve: an analysis of echocardiographic variables related to outcome and the mechanism of dilatation, *Br Heart J* 60:299–308, 1988.

Leaflet mobility	2	3	3
Subvalvular thickening	2	3	4
Leaflet thickening	2	3	3
Leaflet calcium	2	2	3
Wilkins score	8 (favorable)	11 (equivocal)	13 (unfavorable)

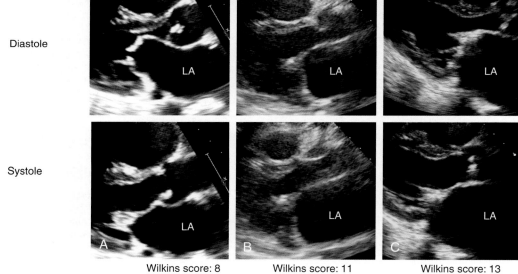

Diastole

Systole

Wilkins score: 8   Wilkins score: 11   Wilkins score: 13

Figure 165.3. Wilkins score: three different patients with variable Wilkins scores. In each patient, a diastolic and systolic frame is included to emphasize leaflet motion. Patient A has a Wilkins score of 8, favorable for mitral valve balloon valvuloplasty (MVBV); patient B has uncertain eligibility for MVBV with a score of 10; and patient C with a Wilkins score of 13 is unlikely to benefit from MVBV. *LA,* Left atrium.

DETERMINING MS SEVERITY

Candidates for MVBV have evidence of severe MS as described by the ASE guidelines for the assessment of valve stenosis.[5] The following echocardiographic or Doppler indices of MS severity are required (see Fig. 165.2):

1. *Mean mitral gradient* from continuous-wave Doppler diastolic mitral flow. Mitral gradient, although reliably assessed by

Doppler, is not the best marker of the severity of MS because it is dependent on the MVA as well as several other factors that influence transmitral flow rate, such as heart rate, cardiac output, and associated MR. Because of this, the 2014 AHA/ACC guidelines on valvular heart disease explicitly state that the gradient is an ancillary method of determining the severity of MS. Severe MS typically has a mean diastolic transmitral gradient of more than 5 to 10 mm Hg.

2. *MVA planimetry* using two-dimensional (2D) echocardiography of the mitral orifice has the advantage of being a direct measurement of MVA, and unlike other methods, it is not affected by flow conditions, cardiac chamber compliance, or associated valvular lesions. Severe MS is MVA of 1.5 cm^2 or less.

3. *Pressure halftime (PHT)* is defined as the time interval in milliseconds between the maximum mitral gradient in early diastole and the time point at which the gradient is half the maximum initial value. Severe MS is a diastolic PHT of 150 ms or greater.

4. *Other markers of MS severity* include increased LA volume and pulmonary hypertension (pulmonary artery systolic pressure ≥50 mm Hg).

The determination of severity may require exercise when the resting gradient does not meet the severity level or the patient appears to be symptomatic with activities. Exercise not only increases cardiac output but also decreases the diastolic filling time. Furthermore, some patients with MS may restrict their activities to avoid breathlessness, and exercise provides an objective assessment of hemodynamics as well as symptoms. Therefore, baseline measurement of mean mitral gradient and estimated pulmonary systolic pressure is compared with immediate postexercise measurements.[34] The results are integrated with the presence of symptoms with exercise to determine the physiologic impact of the patient's MS.

Determining Mitral Valve Balloon Valvuloplasty Eligibility

Wilkins Score

The Wilkins score[35] (Table 165.3 and Fig. 165.3), the most common method to assess MVBV suitability, describes the mitral valve anatomic predictors (leaflet mobility, subvalvular thickening, leaflet thickening, and leaflet calcification) to determine successful MVBV in patients with rheumatic MS. In the original Wilkins series (*n* = 22 patients), all patients with echocardiographic scores greater than 11 had suboptimal results, and all those with scores less than 9 had optimal results. The score failed to predict outcome in those with scores of 9 to 11. Of note, the Wilkins score does not include two important variables for determining suitability for MVBV: the presence of more than mild MR and the presence and degree of commissural fusion.

Iung and Cornier Score

A simpler echocardiographic or fluoroscopic score for MS was introduced by the Iung and Cormier score.[36] This score was derived from 1514 patients divided in three groups:

Group 1: pliable noncalcified anterior mitral leaflet and mild subvalvular disease (i.e., thin chordae ≥10 mm long)

Group 2: pliable noncalcified anterior mitral leaflet and severe subvalvular disease (i.e., thickened chordae <10 mm long)

Group 3: calcification of mitral valve of any extent, as assessed by fluoroscopy, whatever the state of the subvalvular apparatus

This single-center series comprising patients with varied characteristics demonstrates the efficacy of MVBV with 90% good immediate results. The multivariate model showed that the prediction of immediate results for MVBV is multifactorial, based on anatomic, clinical, and procedural variables.

Nunes Score

Nunes and coworkers[37] (*n* = 325 patients) described a score including the ratio between the commissural areas and the maximal excursion of the leaflets from the annulus in diastole. Independent predictors of outcome were assigned a point value proportional to their regression coefficients: MVA of 1 cm^2 or less, maximum

leaflet displacement of 12 mm or less, commissural area ratio of 1.25 or greater, and subvalvular involvement. Three risk groups were defined: low (score of 0–3), intermediate (score of 5), and high (score of 6–11), with observed suboptimal MVBV results of 16.9%, 56.3%, and 73.8%, respectively.[38] The authors conclude that this scoring system incorporating new quantitative echocardiographic parameters more accurately predicts outcome after MVBV than existing models. Long-term post-MVBV event-free survival was predicted by age, degree of MR, and postprocedural hemodynamic data.

Intraprocedural Guidance

Transesophageal echocardiography (TEE) guidance has become standard for most structural heart disease interventions.[39-41] Real-time three-dimensional (3D) TEE guidance assists during the septal puncture, the guidance of wire catheters, and balloon navigation in the left atrium and into the left ventricle, with optimal positioning of the balloon in the left ventricle before inflation, during balloon inflation, and for immediate postballoon assessment of results and potential complications.[42] Intracardiac echocardiography (ICE) has also been successfully used in the past[43] and may see a resurgence with the development of 3D ICE.

TEE guidance is frequently done with general anesthesia, and this often results in a lower transmitral pressure gradient. The use of the gradient to decide whether or not successful MVBV has been achieved may therefore be compromised. Additionally, MVA by the PHT method should not be used to assess the procedural success immediately after MVBV because the left heart chamber compliance has not yet changed to accommodate increased transmitral blood flow after successful MVBV.

Careful intraprocedural assessment of the degree of reduction in the severity of MS is especially important when using the Inoue balloon, which allows a stepwise approach with 1-mm increments in the volume of fluid used to inflate the balloon to an increasingly larger diameter. Therefore, the guidance of the procedure and the assessment of the impact of serial balloon inflations involves assessment of the degree of splitting of fused commissures along with an assessment of the degree of MR. The mechanism of hemodynamic and clinical improvement of MVBV is the achievement of a commissurotomy. This also is the reason MVBV is not routinely used in nonrheumatic MS and in bioprosthetic MS.

The echocardiographer providing image guidance support during a MVBV needs to have clear understanding of the sequence of steps required during a MVBV as well as the fluoroscopic and echocardiographic appearance of devices and catheters used during the intervention. This knowledge allows the echocardiographer to anticipate the imaging needs of the interventionalist during each phase of the intervention.

The approaches that are most commonly used for MVBV are the antegrade transvenous approach (the Inoue balloon technique,[44] the double-balloon technique,[45] the Cribier technique[46]) and the retrograde transarterial approach (Stefanadis technique[47]). The Inoue technique, first described in 1984, is the most widely used method for MVBV, and in this chapter, it serves as the standard technique to describe the use of echocardiography for guidance of this intervention.

Table 165.4 and Figs. 165.4 to 165.9 summarize the interventional tasks and the echocardiographic guidance goals to perform a MVBV. Pre-, intra-, and postprocedural MVBV tasks are described and illustrated. Fig. 165.10 illustrates the sustained drop in transmitral valve gradients after MVBV.

Complications of Mitral Valve Balloon Valvuloplasty

The most serious risks of MVBV include cardiac perforation with associated cardiac tamponade and embolic stroke. The

TABLE 165.4 Mitral Valve Balloon Valvuloplasty Procedural Guidance

Interventional Task	Echocardiography, Doppler, or TEE Goals
PREPROCEDURAL CATHETERIZATION LABORATORY ASSIGNMENTS (SEE FIGS. 165.4 AND 165.5)	
1. Before procuring femoral vein access should wait for TEE confirmation of lack of contraindications and appropriateness to proceed with MVBV	Confirm and determine the severity of MS: mean gradient and MV area by planimetry
	Confirm commissure fusion
	Confirm absence of more than mild MR
	Confirm valve suitability for MVBV
	Confirm absence of left atrial and LAA thrombus
	Measure RVSP from TR jet
	Determine the absence or presence and size of pericardial effusion
INTRAPROCEDURAL ASSIGNMENTS (SEE FIGS. 165.6 TO 165.10)	
1. Transseptal puncture	Use biplane TEE to illustrate septal tenting in desired septal puncture site
2. Guidewire introduced to the LA	Demonstrate distal portion of wire "parked" in LUPV
3. Atrial septum is dilated	Demonstrate further tenting and "release" after the dilator enters LA; confirm that the tip of the dilator is 1–2 cm into the LA
4. Balloon is introduced to the LA	Preferably with 3D TEE; follow the balloon as it enters the LA and encircles the base of the LA near the mitral annulus circumference
5. Balloon is advanced into the LV	The catheter is partially withdrawn until its tip is near the MV orifice, through which it is advanced into the LV
6. Balloon is positioned in the center of the subvalvular mitral apparatus	The catheter is positioned in the center of the LV, away from the septum or lateral wall
7. Balloon is inflated sequentially	The sequential inflation and pullback of the balloon are followed on 2D or 3D
8. Balloon is deflated and pulled back to the LA	The balloon is followed as it is being pulled back into the LA, making sure its tip does not interfere with MV function; the presence and severity of MR, mean gradient, and planimetric MV area are assessed
9. Repeat MVBV if required	Repeat MVBV is considered if there is incomplete commissural splitting, the valve area is <1 cm^2, and the MR is not more than mild
Postprocedural Assignments (see Fig. 165.11)	
	Confirm the size, location, and direction of ASD flow
	Final assessment of MS severity: MVA, mean gradient, TR and RVSP
	Final assessment of MR severity
	Final assessment of pericardial effusion or other complications if present

2D, Two-dimensional; *3D,* three-dimensional; *ASD,* atrial septal defect; *LA,* left atrium; *LAA,* left atrial appendage; *LUPV,* left upper pulmonary vein; *LV,* left ventricle; *MR,* mitral regurgitation; *MS,* mitral stenosis; *MV,* mitral valve; *MVBV,* mitral valve balloon valvuloplasty; *RVSP,* right ventricular systolic pressure; *TEE,* transesophageal echocardiography; *TR,* tricuspid regurgitation.

creation of acute severe MR is also a potential complication of the procedure, frequently requiring emergent mitral valve replacement. The procedure-related mortality ranges rate from 0% to 2.7% with lower mortality rates reported recently. The most frequent cause of procedure-related death has been left ventricular (LV) perforation, almost exclusively a complication associated with the double-balloon technique, which requires LV guidewires. Cardiac perforation caused by inadvertent atrial perforation during transseptal catheterization may occur with the Inoue technique as well, but this tends to be less severe and has not resulted in death.

Embolic stroke occurs in 1.1% to 5.4% of cases. The incidence of embolic events has decreased with the routine preprocedure TEE by excluding patients with LA thrombi. Significant MR occurs in 3.3% to 10.5% of patients undergoing balloon mitral commissurotomy (Fig. 165.11). Fortunately, MR infrequently requires emergency surgery (0.3%–3.3% of cases). Iatrogenic atrial septal defects are usually small without clinical consequences. Their frequency has been reduced with the use of the Inoue balloon catheter system and rarely require transcatheter or surgical repair.[48–50]

Acute severe MR is the most frequent indication for emergency surgery after MVBV. It results in acute hemodynamic compromise that may immediately progress to cardiogenic shock or acute pulmonary edema. Most patients can be stabilized with nitroprusside and intraaortic balloon counterpulsation. Some patients may require respiratory care support followed by urgent mitral valve replacement (MVR). In a recent series by Pillai and coworkers,[51] 1224 MVBV procedures done over the 18-year period were analyzed, and 85 patients (6.9%) with acute severe MR and cardiogenic shock were found. Of the 85 patients, 84 underwent MVR. Anterior mitral leaflet tear was observed in 65 (75%) cases, paracommissural with annular tear in 8 (9.4%), chordal injury in 7 (8%), and torn posterior leaflet in 5 (5.8%). Of note, none of the present valve scoring systems could predict the occurrence of severe MR.

CONCLUSIONS

Mitral balloon valvuloplasty has replaced surgical mitral repair and replacement as the procedure of choice for the treatment of severe symptomatic rheumatic MS in carefully selected patients whose obstructions are principally caused by commissural fusion without extensive leaflet or subvalvular deformities. Echocardiography plays a central role in guiding the MVBV procedure with a significant impact on the pre-, intra-, and postprocedural echocardiographic assignments. In addition, echocardiography plays a fundamental role in determining the presence, severity, and type of procedural complications. Finally, echocardiography is ideally qualified to provide detailed information for the continuous success of the MVBV procedure.

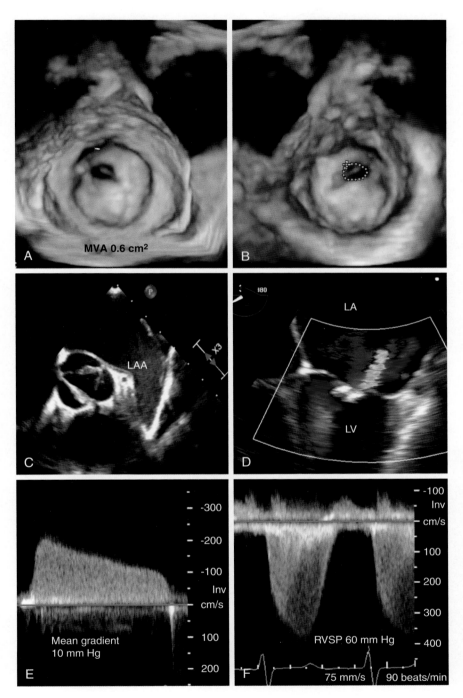

Figure 165.4. Preprocedural check: transesophageal echocardiography obtained in the catheterization laboratory preceding mitral valve balloon valvuloplasty. **A** and **B,** Left atrial and left ventricular three-dimensional views of the mitral orifice confirm the presence of severe mitral stenosis (mitral valve area [MVA, 0.6 cm²) and the presence of bicommissural fusion. **C,** Dense spontaneous contrast but no left atrial appendage (LAA) thrombus. **D,** Absence of significant mitral regurgitation. **E,** Under general anesthesia, the mean mitral valve gradient (10 mm Hg) and right ventricular systolic pressure (**F**; 60 mm Hg) were lower than those seen in the echocardiography laboratory without sedation or anesthesia (see Fig. 165.2). *RVSP,* Right ventricular systolic pressure.

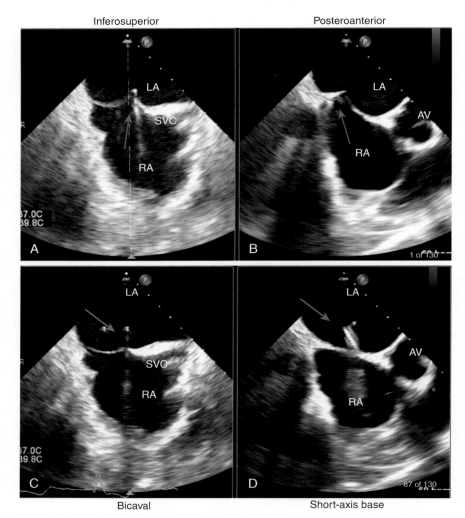

Figure 165.5. Interatrial septum tenting and puncture. Orthogonal biplane transesophageal echocardiography images with **A** and **B** illustrating tenting *(red arrows)* of the membrane of the fossa ovalis. Note that the bicaval images demonstrate the tenting occurring along the inferosuperior axis and in this particular case is in the middle of the fossa. The short-axis base images demonstrate tenting in the posterior aspect of the fossa. **C** and **D,** The moment when the septal puncture has occurred, the tenting is no longer apparent, and the tip of the catheter now sits in the left atrial cavity *(green arrows)*. *AV,* Aortic valve; *LA,* left atrium; *RA,* right atrium; *SVC,* superior vena cava.

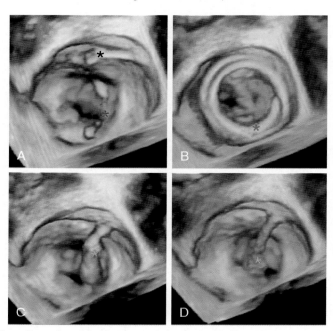

Figure 165.6. Balloon positioning. These three-dimensional transesophageal echocardiography images of the mitral valve from the left atrium perspective illustrate the sequential steps to advance the balloon through the mitral valve. **A,** The catheter *(black asterisk)* is delivered about 2 cm into the left atrial cavity. A guidewire *(red asterisk)* sits in the floor of the left atrium (LA). **B,** The balloon catheter is fully advanced into the LA, encircling the mitral annulus. **C,** After the catheter has been partially retracted, the balloon *(orange asterisk)* is pointing to the mitral valve orifice. **D,** The balloon *(orange asterisk)* is advanced through the narrow mitral orifice.

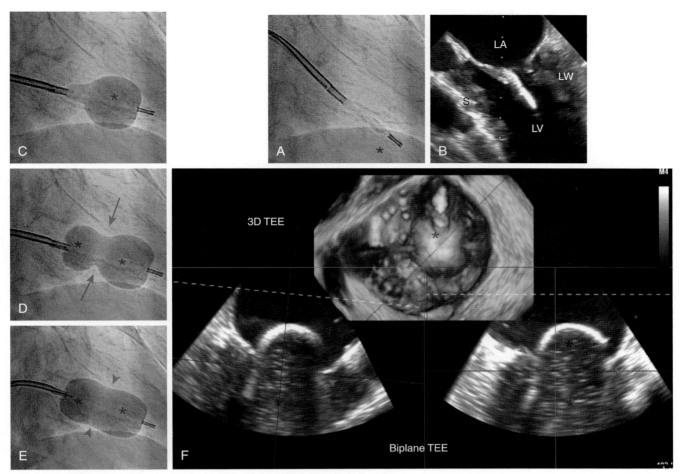

Figure 165.7. Fluoroscopy and transesophageal echocardiography (TEE) mitral valve balloon valvuloplasty (MVBV) balloon inflation. Fluoroscopic and two- and three-dimensional (3D) TEE imaging of a patient undergoing MVBV. **A** and **B,** The balloon catheter going through the left atrium (LA) into the left ventricle (LV), the *red asterisk* marking its tip. Note that the fluoroscopic image shows no soft tissue, whereas the TEE image shows the catheter to be in the center of the LV cavity. **C,** Fluoroscopic image of the first sequential phase of balloon inflation of the distal segment *(blue asterisk)*. **D,** Second phase of balloon inflation in which the proximal balloon *(green asterisk)* is inflated, but there is still a "waist" *(red arrows)* before the commissure split. **E** and **F,** Fluoroscopic and echocardiographic images of the third phase of the balloon inflation when the commissures are split. The *red arrowheads* depict only a small residual "waist." *LA,* Left atrium; *LW,* lateral wall; *S,* septum.

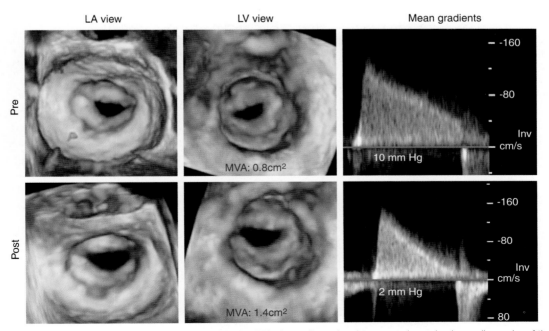

Figure 165.8. Before and after mitral valve balloon valvuloplasty (MVBV), three-dimensional transesophageal echocardiography of the mitral valve area (MVA) as seen from the left atrium (LA) and left ventricle (LV) demonstrates commissure splitting with an increased MVA from 0.8 to 1.4 cm². The transmitral mean gradient decreased from 10 to 4 mm Hg.

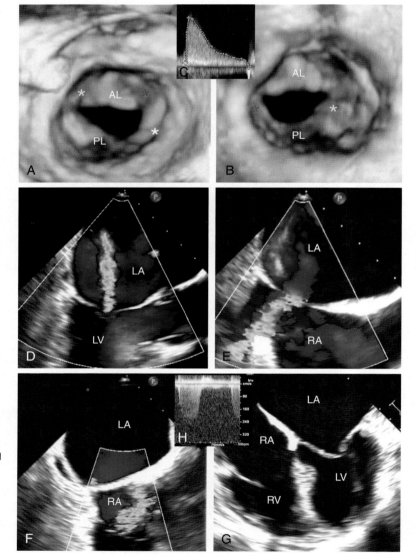

Figure 165.9. Postprocedural final check. A final comprehensive check is made after completing the mitral valve balloon valvuloplasty (MVBV) procedure. **A** and **B,** Mitral valve orifice size as seen from the left atrium (LA and left ventricle (LV). The open anterior leaflet (AL) and posterior (PL) leaflet and the split medial *(yellow asterisk)* and lateral *(red asterisk)* commissures are noted. **C**, The transmitral valve gradient, which decreased from 8 to 3 mm Hg after MVBV. **D,** Mild residual mitral regurgitation. **E**, Moderate-sized atrial septal defect in the area of septal puncture. It was noted to be unidirectional, so a closure device was not necessary. **F**, Mild tricuspid regurgitation with a right ventricular systolic pressure (RVSP) of 30 mm Hg, which was unchanged from the pre-MVBV RVSP. **G,** Midesophageal four-chamber view highlights the absence of pericardial effusion. *RA,* Right atrium; *RV,* right ventricle.

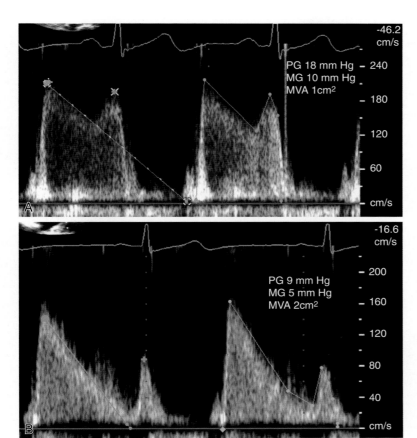

Figure 165.10. Pre and post gradients. This figure illustrates the post–mitral valve balloon valvuloplasty (MVBV) sustained (2-year) improvement in mitral valve area (MVA) and mean and peak transmitral gradients (MG and PG). MVA immediately after MVBV. (Reproduced from Thomas JD, Weyman, AE: Mitral pressure half-time: a clinical tool in search of theoretical justification, *J Am Coll Cardiol* 10:923–929, 1987.)

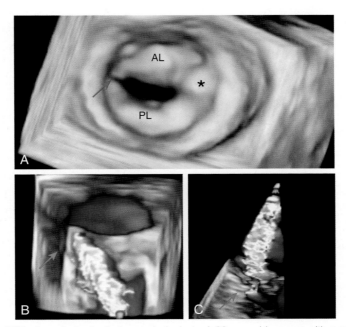

Figure 165.11. Mitral regurgitation (MR) after mitral valve balloon valvuloplasty. A 66-year-old woman with symptomatic mitral stenosis Elevated left-sided filling pressures (left atrium [LA], 14/23; mean, 16). Successful balloon valvuloplasty to 28 mm with Inoue balloon, yet emergence of moderate MR noted and inability to split the medial commissure. **A,** En face view of the mitral valve from the LA. The *red arrow* points to the split lateral commissure. The *black asterisk* points to the calcified and unsplit medial commissure. **B** and **C,** The MR jet originating from the lateral commissure. Repeating another valvuloplasty would have been unwise because of the risk of producing extension of the splitting of the lateral commissure into the mitral annulus with the potential for acute severe MR. The medial commissure, because of dense calcification, was unlikely to split. *AL,* Anterior leaflet; *PL,* posterior leaflet.

REFERENCES

1. Hollenberg SM. Valvular heart disease in adults: etiologies, classification, and diagnosis. *FP Essent.* 2017;457:11–16.
2. Domenech B, Pomar JL, Prat-Gonzalez S, et al. Valvular heart disease epidemics. *J Heart Valve Dis.* 2016;25:1–7.
3. Carroll JD, Feldman T. Percutaneous mitral balloon valvotomy and the new demographics of mitral stenosis. *J Am Med Assoc.* 1993;270:1731–1736.
4. Al-Taweel A, Almahmoud MF, Khairandish Y, Ahmad M. Degenerative mitral valve stenosis: diagnosis and management. *Echocardiography.* 2019;36:1901–1909.
5. Baumgartner H, Hung J, Bermejo J, et al. Echocardiographic assessment of valve stenosis: EAE/ASE recommendations for clinical practice. *J Am Soc Echocardiogr.* 2009;22:1–23.
6. Abbo KM, Carroll JD. Hemodynamics of mitral stenosis: a review. *Cathet Cardiovasc Diagn.* 1994;(suppl 2):16–25.
7. Nishimura RA, Otto CM, Bonow RO, et al. 2014 AHA/ACC guideline for the management of patients with valvular heart disease: executive summary: a report of the American College of Cardiology/American Heart Association Task Force on practice guidelines. *Circulation.* 2014;129:2440–2492.
8. Falk V, Baumgartner H, Bax JJ, et al. ESC/EACTS Guidelines for the management of valvular heart disease. *Eur J Cardio Thorac Surg.* 2017;52:616–664. 2017.
9. Nishimura RA, O'Gara PT, Bavaria JE, et al. AATS/ACC/ASE/SCAI/STS expert consensus systems of care document: a proposal to optimize care for patients with valvular heart disease. *J Am Coll Cardiol.* 2019;73:2609–2635. 2019.
10. Guerrero M, Eleid M, Foley T, et al. Transseptal transcatheter mitral valve replacement in severe mitral annular calcification (transseptal valve-in-MAC). *Ann Cardiothorac Surg.* 2018;7:830–833.
11. Maisano F, Taramasso M. Mitral valve-in-valve, valve-in-ring, and valve-in-MAC: the good, the bad, and the ugly. *Eur Heart J.* 2019;40:452–455.
12. Kasel AM, Frangieh AH. Transcatheter aortic valve-in-valve procedures using current-generation balloon-expandable valves: what's the optimal valve positioning strategy for a better outcome. *JACC Cardiovasc Interv.* 2019;12:1618–1620.
13. Shivaraju A, Michel J, Frangieh AH, et al. Transcatheter aortic and mitral valve-in-valve implantation using the Edwards Sapien 3 heart valve. *J Am Heart Assoc.* 2018;7.
14. Manjunath CN, Srinivasa KH, Panneerselvam A, et al. Incidence and predictors of left atrial thrombus in patients with rheumatic mitral stenosis and sinus rhythm: a transesophageal echocardiographic study. *Echocardiography.* 2011;28:457–460.
15. Banovic M, DaCosta M. Degenerative mitral stenosis: from pathophysiology to challenging interventional treatment. *Curr Probl Cardiol.* 2019;44:10–35.
16. Reddy YNV, Murgo JP, Nishimura RA. Complexity of defining severe "stenosis" from mitral annular calcification. *Circulation.* 2019;140:523–525.
17. Tsutsui RS, Banerjee K, Kapadia S, et al. Natural history of mitral stenosis in patients with mitral annular calcification. *JACC Cardiovasc Imag.* 2019;12:1105–1107.
18. Tsutsui RS, Simsolo E, Saijo Y, et al. Severe mitral stenosis in patients with severe mitral annular calcification: an area of unmet need. *JACC Cardiovasc Interv.* 2019;12:2566–2568.
19. Anselmino M, Lupia E, Goffi A, et al. Isolated radiation-induced mitral stenosis: a yet undescribed valvulopathy. *J Cardiovasc Surg.* 2009;50:251–252.
20. Baird CW, Marx GR, Borisuk M, et al. Review of congenital mitral valve stenosis: analysis, repair techniques and outcomes. *Cardiovasc Eng Technol.* 2015;6:167–173.
21. Burzo ML, De Matteis G, Nicolazzi MA, et al. The strange case of congenital mitral stenosis in an adult man with cor triatriatum. *Echocardiography.* 2019;36:2122–2125.
22. Collins-Nakai RL, Rosenthal A, Castaneda AR, et al. Congenital mitral stenosis. A review of 20 years' experience. *Circulation.* 1977;56:1039–1047.
23. Naeim HA, Taha EA, Taha RA, et al. Isolated adult congenital uni-leaflet severe mitral valve stenosis, a case report, and review of literature. *J Cardiol Cases.* 2019;19:177–181.
24. Jagtap SV, Salunkhe P, Mane A, et al. Cardiac myxoma with cartilaginous differentiation—an uncommon variant presented as mitral stenosis. *Indian J Pathol Microbiol.* 2019;62:599–601.
25. Capuano F, Sechi S, De Luca A, Sinatra R. Severe mitral valve stenosis due to a giant left atrial mass. *Eur J Cardio Thorac Surg.* 2019;6:1207.
26. Frumkin D, Taube ET, Stangl K, Knebel F. Rapid progression of aortic and mitral stenosis in a patient with AA amyloidosis: a case report. *Eur Heart J Case Rep.* 2019;3:ytz051.
27. Hegglin R, Zollinger H. [Clinical, pathological and anatomical demonstrations: mitral stenosis, Libman-Sacks syndrome and metastasizing small intestine carcinoid]. *Cardiologia.* 1956;28:151–167.
28. Gouya H, Cabanes L, Mouthon L, et al. Severe mitral stenosis as the first manifestation of systemic lupus erythematosus in a 20-year-old woman: the value of magnetic resonance imaging in the diagnosis of Libman-Sacks endocarditis. *Int J Cardiovasc Imag.* 2014;30:959–960.
29. Hussain R, Neligan MC. Systemic lupus erythematosus a rare cause of mitral stenosis. *Thorac Cardiovasc Surg.* 1993;41:125–126.
30. Bartkevich S, Kopel L, Lemos S, et al. [Fibroelastosis of the left atrium simulating mitral stenosis]. *Arq Bras Cardiol.* 1972;25:135–139.
31. Roberts CS, Milligan GP, Stoler RC, et al. Mitral stenosis produced by infective endocarditis involving a previously anatomically normal valve. *Proc Bayl Univ Med Ctr.* 2019;32:387–389.
32. Fernandez J, Laub GW, Adkins MS, et al. Early and late-phase events after valve replacement with the St. Jude Medical prosthesis in 1200 patients. *J Thorac Cardiovasc Surg.* 1994;107:394–406.
33. Attizzani GF, Fares A, Tam CC, et al. Transapical mitral valve implantation for the treatment of severe native mitral valve stenosis in a prohibitive surgical risk patient: importance of comprehensive cardiac computed tomography procedural planning. *JACC Cardiovasc Interv.* 2015;8:1522–1525.
34. Kern MJ, Kim M, Yu J, Seto AH. Evaluation of the severity of mitral stenosis in patient with pulmonary hypertension: role of exercise hemodynamics. *Catheter Cardiovasc Interv.* 2019;94:301–307.
35. Wilkins GT, Weyman AE, Abascal VM, et al. Percutaneous balloon dilatation of the mitral valve: an analysis of echocardiographic variables related to outcome and the mechanism of dilatation. *Br Heart J.* 1988;60:299–308.
36. Iung B, Cormier B, Ducimetiere P, et al. Immediate results of percutaneous mitral commissurotomy. A predictive model on a series of 1514 patients. *Circulation.* 1996;94:2124–2130.
37. Nunes MC, Tan TC, Elmariah S, et al. The echo score revisited: impact of incorporating commissural morphology and leaflet displacement to the prediction of outcome for patients undergoing percutaneous mitral valvuloplasty. *Circulation.* 2014;129:886–895.
38. Palacios IF. Percutaneous mitral balloon valvuloplasty: worldwide trends. *J Am Heart Assoc.* 2019;8. e012898.
39. Silvestry FE, Kerber RE, Brook MM, et al: Echocardiography-guided interventions, *J Am Soc Echocardiogr* 2009;22:213–231; quiz 316–317.
40. Zamorano JL, Badano LP, Bruce C, et al. EAE/ASE recommendations for the use of echocardiography in new transcatheter interventions for valvular heart disease. *Eur J Echocardiogr.* 2011;12:557–584.
41. Salcedo EE, Carroll JD. *Echocardiography in Patient Assessment and Procedural Guidance in Structural Heart Disease Interventions.* Philadelphia: Lippincott Williams and Wilkins; 2012.
42. Eng MH, Salcedo EE, Kim M, et al. Implementation of real-time three-dimensional transesophageal echocardiography for mitral balloon valvuloplasty. *Catheter Cardiovasc Interv.* 2013;82:994–998.
43. Green NE, Hansgen AR, Carroll JD. Initial clinical experience with intracardiac echocardiography in guiding balloon mitral valvuloplasty: technique, safety, utility, and limitations. *Catheter Cardiovasc Interv.* 2004;63:385–394.
44. Inoue K, Owaki T, Nakamura T, et al. Clinical application of transvenous mitral commissurotomy by a new balloon catheter. *J Thorac Cardiovasc Surg.* 1984;87:394–402.
45. Al Zaibag M, Ribeiro PA, Al Kasab S, Al Fagih MR. Percutaneous double-balloon mitral valvotomy for rheumatic mitral-valve stenosis. *Lancet.* 1986;1:757–761.
46. Cribier A, Eltchaninoff H, Koning R, et al. Percutaneous mechanical mitral commissurotomy with a newly designed metallic valvulotome: immediate results of the initial experience in 153 patients. *Circulation.* 1999;99:793–799.
47. Stefanadis CI, Stratos CG, Lambrou SG, et al. Retrograde nontransseptal balloon mitral valvuloplasty: immediate results and intermediate long-term outcome in 441 cases—a multicenter experience. *J Am Coll Cardiol.* 1998;32:1009–1016.
48. Harrison JK, Wilson JS, Hearne SE, Bashore TM. Complications related to percutaneous transvenous mitral commissurotomy. *Cathet Cardiovasc Diagn.* 1994;(suppl 2):52–60.
49. Ben Farhat M, Betbout F, Gamra H, et al. [Complications of percutaneous mitral commissurotomy. Personal experience and review of the literature]. *Arch Mal Coeur Vaiss.* 1996;89:417–423.
50. Complications and mortality of percutaneous balloon mitral commissurotomy. A report from the National Heart, Lung, and Blood Institute Balloon Valvuloplasty Registry. *Circulation.* 1992;85:2014–2024.
51. Pillai AA, Balasubramanian VR, Munuswamy H, Seenuvaslu S. Acute severe mitral regurgitation with cardiogenic shock following balloon mitral valvuloplasty: echocardiographic findings and outcomes following surgery. *Cardiovasc Interv Ther.* 2019;34:260–268.

166 Percutaneous Mitral Edge-to-Edge Repair

Renuka Jain, Bijoy K. Khandheria

The percutaneous mitral edge-to-edge repair[1] is based on the principle of surgical edge-to-edge repair, also known as the Alfieri technique, introduced in 1991 by the Italian surgeon Ottavio Alfieri, who successfully treated a patient with anterior leaflet prolapse.[2,3] Using a stitch, he approximated the edges of the middle portions of the anterior and posterior leaflets to create a double-orifice mitral valve (MV). The surgical group subsequently reported[4] a series of 260 patients, of whom 80% underwent the Alfieri technique and had additional mitral annuloplasty, which was associated with reduced rate of reoperation within a follow-up period of 5 years.[5]

The initial percutaneous edge-to-edge repair system is referred to as the MitraClip (Abbott). Since then at least one additional system has been developed, namely the PASCAL system (Edwards LifeScience). The mitral leaflet–grasping device in both systems may be generically referred to as a "mitral clip." In this chapter, percutaneous edge-to-edge repair is described for the MitraClip, but similar principles apply to the PASCAL system.

The percutaneously implanted MitraClip has been the most studied device for the transcatheter treatment of mitral regurgitation (MR). The Endovascular Valve Edge-to-Edge Repair Study I (EVEREST I) demonstrated efficacy, safety, and clear hemodynamic improvement in patients with moderate to severe and severe MR.[6] In the EVEREST II trial,[1,7,8] the percutaneous approach was safer than surgery (30-day rate of major adverse cardiac events, 15% vs 48%; $P < .001$). Although patients treated with the MitraClip more commonly required surgery to treat residual MR by the first year of follow-up, a limited number of surgeries were needed, and there was no difference in the prevalence of moderate to severe and severe MR or mortality at 4 years.[8] Other studies[9–12] confirmed the efficacy of the MitraClip in primary (degenerative) MR. More recently, the MitraClip device has been demonstrated to show benefit in patients with secondary (functional) MR.[13,14]

INDICATIONS

Patient selection criteria for the percutaneous mitral edge-to-edge repair procedure is based entirely on echocardiography. Transthoracic echocardiography (TTE) is an initial appropriate screening tool for presence and severity of MR. Determination of suitability for edge-to-edge repair is determined based on morphologic features of MV visualized on transesophageal echocardiography (TEE). As the procedural experience has increased, the

suitability criteria have expanded (Table 166.1) into optimal, challenging, and unsuitable morphologies[15] for both primary and secondary MR (Fig. 166.1).

TRANSESOPHAGEAL ECHOCARDIOGRAPHY

Multiplane TEE is the gold-standard modality for preoperative assessment as well as intraprocedural guidance for percutaneous mitral edge-to-edge repair insertion.[15–18] To perform a comprehensive examination of the MV, it is essential to understand how transesophageal probe maneuvers change the imaging plane with respect to the MV.

Two-dimensional (2D) TEE has long been used to visualize the scallops of the MV. In the standard midesophageal four-chamber view (typically at a transducer angle of 0 degrees), A1, A2, P1, and P2 scallops are best visualized. From this position, flexion and withdrawal of the transducer tip allow visualization of the aortic root and anterolateral portions of the mitral leaflets at 120 degrees (A2 and P2). Similarly, retroflexion and advancement of the transducer tip allow visualization of the posteromedial portions of the leaflets (A3 and P3). The midesophageal plane at an angle between 45 and 90 degrees (intercommissural, also referred to as bicommissural, view) provides the opportunity for mitral leaflets to be examined with a plane parallel to the mitral orifice and to confirm MV pathology. Through the major axis of the valve orifice, P3, A2, and P1 may be evaluated on the TEE image from left to right. Subsequently, by manual rotation of the probe in a clockwise direction, the entire anterior leaflet can be visualized (A1, A2, and A3). Counterclockwise probe rotation provides visualization of the entire posterior leaflet (P1, P2, and P3). Other imaging planes and transducer positions, such as the transgastric short-axis view, may be used for additional imaging and to assist with the assessment of the MV.[16]

Three-dimensional (3D) TEE is superior to 2D TEE in visualizing the entire anatomy of the MV in real time, the "surgeon's view" with the aortic root at the 12 o'clock position, establishing the anterior landmark (Fig. 166.2). From this view, the different scallops can be seen in their entirety along with surrounding structures and anatomic landmarks. Adding color to the 3D TEE view can help localize and quantify severity of MR, particularly multiple jets. Although 2D TEE is adequate for vena contracta, direct measurement of vena contracta area using 3D TEE

TABLE 166.1 Suitability Criteria for the MitraClip Procedure That Encompasses Both Primary and Secondary Mitral Regurgitation

Optimal Morphology	Challenging Morphology	Unsuitable Morphology
Central A2 or P2 pathology	Peripheral A1/P1 or A3/P3 pathology	Cleft or perforation
No calcification of leaflets	Calcification present but not in grasping zone	Calcification in grasping zone
MVA >4 cm^2	MVA 3–4 cm^2	MVA <3 cm^2 or MG >5 mm Hg
Posterior leaflet >10 mm	Posterior leaflet 7–10 mm	Posterior leaflet <7 mm
Tenting height <11 mm; coaptation reserve >2 mm	Tenting height ≥11 mm	
Normal leaflets and mobility	Carpentier IIIB (restricted motion in diastole)	Carpentier IIIA (restricted motion in systole and diastole)
Flail gap <10 mm; flail width <15 mm	Flail width >15 mm (with sufficient valve area to tolerate multiple clips)	Multiple segments, Barlow's valve

MVA, Mitral valve area; *MG,* mean gradient.
Adapted from Nyman CB, et al: Transcatheter mitral valve repair using the edge-to-edge clip, *J Am Soc Echocardiogr* 31:434–453, 2018.

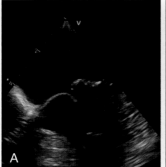 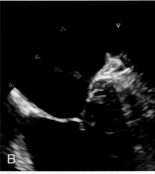 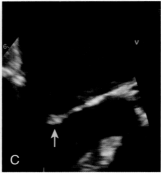 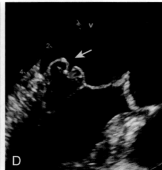

Figure 166.1. Morphologic criteria for the MitraClip device using two-dimensional transesophageal echocardiography. **A,** Optimal: isolated P2 flail with a flail gap smaller than 10 mm. **B,** Optimal: reduced coaptation with adequate coaptation length and depth. **C,** Unsuitable: anterior leaflet calcification at the grasping zone *(arrow)*. **D,** Unsuitable: multiple segments with severe billowing *(arrow)*. (See accompanying Video 166.1.)

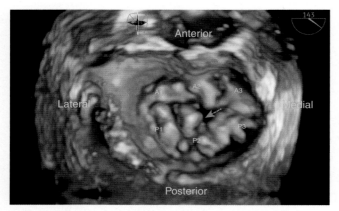

Figure 166.2. Three-dimensional transesophageal echocardiography mitral valve en face ("surgeon's view") from the left atrium, with appropriate anatomic landmarks. This patient has severe prolapse and flail of the P2 scallop *(arrow)*. (See accompanying Video 166.2.)

demonstrates that jets are not spherical (Fig. 166.3), and geometric assumptions may be challenging with multiple jets.[19–21] The assessment of the severity of MR follows the current guidelines for MV evaluation[17] and encompasses and both 2D and 3D quantitative methods.

PROCEDURE

The percutaneous mitral edge-to-edge repair procedure is divided into seven important steps.

Transseptal Puncture

Transseptal puncture represents one of the most important aspects of the percutaneous mitral edge-to-edge repair procedure. The optimal puncture site is located superiorly and posteriorly in the interatrial septum. The most important TEE planes to identify the correct site are the short-axis view at the base for anteroposterior orientation (~30–60 degrees), bicaval view for superoinferior orientation (~90–120 degrees), and four-chamber view (~0 degrees) to direct the height above the MV. Because it combines the short-axis view with the long-axis view, 3D simultaneous biplane ("x-plane") can also be used for determination of the correct puncture site. The position of the transseptal needle is visualized as tenting of the interatrial septum toward the left atrium (LA). In fibroelastic disease, the puncture site needs to be 4 to 5 cm above the mitral annulus to secure adequate space for a catheter and mitral clip maneuvering (Fig. 166.4). On the other hand, in functional MR, the puncture site may need to be more inferior and closer to the annular plane

because of extensive tethering and because the line of coaptation is below the plane of the mitral annulus.

A patent foramen ovale should be avoided because this entry is too far anterior. An atrial septal defect also is not suitable for the percutaneous mitral edge-to-edge repair procedure; any defect that is larger than the sheath size will prohibit effective support of steerable guide catheter and maneuvering.

Steerable Guide Catheter Introduction Into the Left Atrium

A steerable guide catheter with a dilator is advanced into the LA over a wire and placed in the left upper pulmonary vein under fluoroscopic and TEE guidance. The dilator has a cone-shaped tip and therefore may be easily identified because it has an echogenic appearance with TEE. A radiopaque echo-bright double ring characterizes the tip of the guide catheter. The advancement of the catheter should be followed constantly with TEE as well and fluoroscopic monitoring to avoid left atrial free wall damage. After the catheter is placed in the LA, the dilator is retrieved first followed by the wire. The guide catheter placement should be monitored throughout the procedure; maintain at least 2 cm in the LA to adequately support and maneuver the clip delivery system (Fig. 166.5A).

Advancement of the Clip Delivery System Into the Left Atrium

The clip delivery system is advanced via the catheter under fluoroscopic guidance through the steerable guide catheter (Fig. 166.5B). 2D and 3D TEE are necessary to ensure that the tip of the catheter remains across the interatrial septum and that the clip delivery system will not cause damage to the left atrial free wall. It is important always to monitor the distance of the clip delivery system from the atrial wall with 2D and 3D TEE.

Steering and Positioning of the Mitral Clip Above the Mitral Valve

After the clip delivery system has been inserted into the LA, the system needs to be maneuvered to position clip over the MV. The posterior withdrawal of the catheter and retraction of the whole system will help the correct positioning of the clip delivery system above the MV, rotating the system medially. The midesophageal intercommissural view and the rotation of the system in the anterior and posterior direction are important for the adjustment of the MitraClip.

To ensure correct MitraClip alignment, both arms of the device should be visualized in full length in the long-axis view; no device arms should be seen in the intercommissural view. The MitraClip

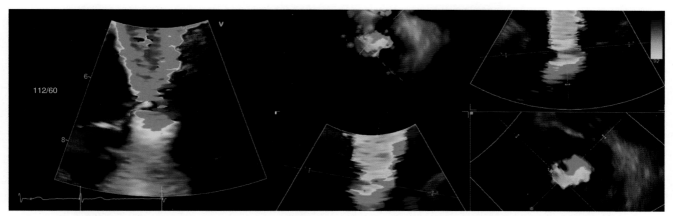

Figure 166.3. Two- and three-dimensional transesophageal views of mitral regurgitation (MR) used for quantitation of MR severity. Note in the three-dimensional reconstruction that the MR effective orifice area is not a circle, but rather ovaloid, along the coaptation line of the valve.

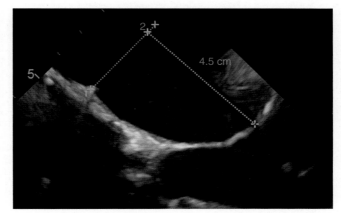

Figure 166.4. Two-dimensional transesophageal echocardiography (0-degree view) demonstrates a 4.5-cm height between transseptal puncture and the mitral annulus.

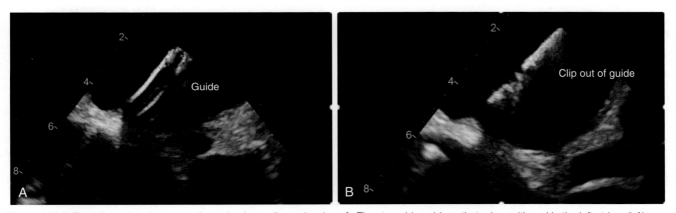

Figure 166.5. Two-dimensional transesophageal echocardiography view. **A,** The steerable guide catheter is positioned in the left atrium (LA). **B,** The MitraClip delivery system is then advanced from the guide catheter into the LA.

should split the regurgitation jet in both orthogonal views, and the tip of the device should be directed toward the largest proximal isovelocity surface area. If 3D imaging is difficult, the transgastric view may be important to determine orientation of the device. A single 3D en face view allows visualization of correct alignment and proper orientation perpendicular to the line of MV coaptation (Fig. 166.6); the combination of 2D and 3D TEE views ensures proper alignment of the clip arms before advancement of the clip into the ventricle.

Advancement of the MitraClip Into the Left Ventricle

Advancement of the MitraClip into the left ventricle (LV) may be monitored with 2D imaging using the intercommissural and midesophageal long-axis views simultaneously. The arms are often closed slightly for advancement into the ventricle and then reopened after this step is completed. Under fluoroscopic and TEE guidance, crossing of the MV is monitored. The orientation

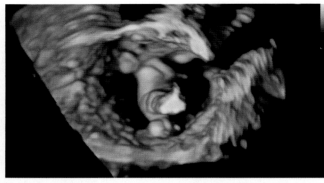

Figure 166.6. Three-dimensional transesophageal echocardiography mitral valve en face ("surgeon's view") from the left atrium demonstrates the mitral clip arms perpendicular to the leaflets. (See accompanying Video 166.6.)

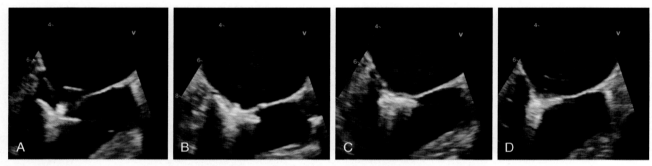

Figure 166.7. Two-dimensional transesophageal echocardiography (120 degrees) demonstrates grasping of the mitral leaflets by the clip. **A,** The clip arms are aligned perpendicular to the leaflets. **B,** The system is retracted back to the mitral valve until the leaflets are resting on the clip arms. **C,** Minor rotation reveals that the anterior leaflet is resting on the clip arm with more than 9 mm of leaflet tissue. **D,** Grippers are released, and the clip is slowly closed.

of the device and delivery system must be monitored from the LV because the device may rotate during its transition from the LA to the ventricle. The most important views are the inter-commissural and long-axis views because they provide proper mediolateral and anteroposterior orientation of the clip, respectively. To visualize the MitraClip in relation to the MV and the line of coaptation, 3D TEE from either the LA or LV presents direct views. It is easiest to maintain a left atrial 3D mitral view, which may be used if the device orientation cannot be judged adequately; decreasing gains can allow arms to be visualized even in ventricle from this view. The intercommissural and long-axis views are useful to verify that the device is splitting the mitral regurgitant jet and both mitral leaflets are freely moving above the device arms.

Grasping of the Leaflets and Assessment of Proper Leaflet Insertion

After correct positioning of the clip arms, grasping of the leaflets between the device arms is monitored using a midesophageal long-axis view (Fig. 166.7). It is always important to acquire a longer loop during the grasping of the leaflets. Furthermore, it is recommended to initially close the MitraClip only up to 60 to 90 degrees in angulation and subsequently fully close the device after determination of proper leaflet insertion and demonstration of regurgitation reduction. Insertion of the posterior leaflet is commonly best seen in the long-axis view and the insertion of the anterior leaflet in the four-chamber view. The intercommissural view has an additive role. After the leaflets are well positioned

between the device arms and there is clear reduction of MR, the MitraClip can be closed.

Assessment of Result and MitraClip Release

After positioning and closing the clip arms, it is important to evaluate four key aspects of the MV. First, one must determine the structural difference of the MV (i.e., capture of the flail leaflet tip in degenerative disease), improving coaptation in secondary disease. Second, the clip must be interrogated for adequate insertion (9-mm leaflet tissue for the MitraClip XT system, 4-mm leaflet tissue for the MitraClip NT system); this should be assessed in multiple 2D views and by reviewing the images from the clip grasp. Third, evaluation of the grade of residual MR may lead to further adjustment after a MitraClip implantation or the addition of a second clip. It is important to understand that the area of color jets is larger with multiple jets, which commonly occurs because of the addition of multiple jet areas after a MitraClip is implanted, than if there is a single jet. This may potentially lead to overestimating residual regurgitation in patients with multiple jets.[21] Finally, adequate clip placement should not lead to mitral stenosis; an assessment of MV area should be performed before release of the clip (>2 cm^2 is considered adequate MV area before release; a mean gradient <5 mm Hg is also considered procedural success).[22] This can be performed using 3D reconstructions in esophageal views (Fig. 166.8) or in transgastric views. Initial evaluation of the MitraClip result is usually performed under general anesthesia; therefore, it is important to realize that hemodynamic conditions may be different than in preoperative assessment. In addition, the artifact caused by the

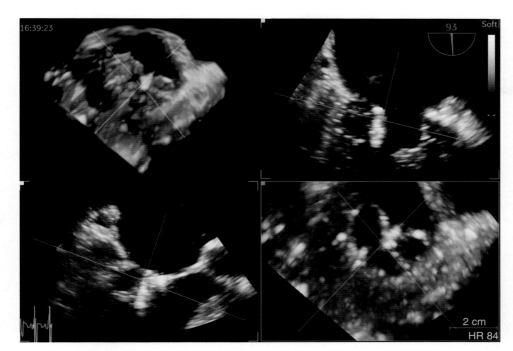

Figure 166.8. After the clip is closed, three-dimensional transesophageal echocardiography is used to reconstruct an on-plane view of the mitral valve (MV) to ensure an adequate MV area. (See accompanying Video 166.8.)

MitraClip using 2D echocardiography also may influence imaging. New studies will discover the gold standard imaging index for best assessment after MitraClip insertion.

Additional MitraClip Implantation

When a second MitraClip is required, the orientation of the second device should be optimized by 2D or, when available, 3D TEE while clip is in the LA. Fluoroscopy has greater value in the guidance of inserting the additional device, which should always be aligned as parallel as possible to the first device. Folding of leaflet tissue between two clips should be avoided because it may cause significant residual MR.

CONCLUSIONS

The MitraClip procedure remains the most studied and established edge-to-edge transcatheter repair for MR, and long-term follow-up is excellent when the procedure is successful (Fig. 166.9). A similar device is in early feasibility trials (Edwards PASCAL system), which is also based on the Alfieri method.[23] Echocardiography

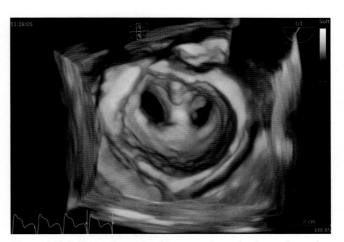

Figure 166.9. Three-dimensional transesophageal echocardiography mitral valve en face ("surgeon's view") from the left atrium after clip release demonstrates a double-orifice mitral valve. (See accompanying Video 166.9.)

TABLE 166.2 Complications of the MitraClip Procedure

Complication	Cause	Prevention	Treatment
Pericardial effusion or tamponade	Cardiac perforation during transseptal puncture or advancement of guidewire, dilator, or CDS	Appropriate location for transseptal puncture; continuous TEE monitoring during guidewire, dilator, or CDS advancement	Pericardial drainage
Thrombus formation	Presence of foreign material	Prompt anticoagulation after transseptal puncture and maintenance of appropriate ACT (250–300 s)	Administration of additional anticoagulation
Partial clip detachment (complete detachment is rare)	Insufficient leaflet grasping, clip malposition, or device malfunction	Appropriate clip positioning; TEE assessment of adequate leaflet insertion and grasping	Additional clip placement in close approximation of the partially detached clip to address the MR and stabilize the clip (for complete detachment, percutaneous or open surgical retrieval)
Entrapment of the MitraClip in the chordae tendineae or chordal injury	Inappropriate movement of the clip within the LV, most common when the clip is moved outside the central aspect of the valve	Appropriate positioning and clip arm orientation under TEE guidance within the LA; when in the LV, if significant repositioning or movement is required, clip eversion and withdrawal back into LA	Clip arm eversion and withdrawal into the LA; in case of chordal entrapment, advancement of the CDS farther into the LV, below the level of the papillary muscle before closure and subsequent withdrawal may be attempted
IASD	Transseptal puncture and dilatation by the SGC	Avoid need for repeat transseptal puncture by optimizing position for first septal puncture	Most resolve spontaneously and require no intervention; in the presence of hypoxia caused by right-to-left shunting, closure should be considered
Major bleeding and vascular injury	Large-bore catheter	Placement of a vascular closure device.; appropriate management after sheath removal	Supportive; vascular injury may require intervention
GI injury	Prolonged TEE examination	Appropriate application of lubricant; minimize extensive or excessive probe manipulation	Upper endoscopy; may require surgical intervention

ACT, Activated clotting time; *CDS,* clip delivery system; *GI,* gastrointestinal; *IASD,* iatrogenic atrial septal defect; *LV,* left ventricle; *LA,* left atrium; *MR,* mitral regurgitation; *SGC,* steerable guide catheter; *TEE,* transesophageal echocardiography.
Adapted with permission from Nyman CB, et al: Transcatheter mitral valve repair using the edge-to-edge clip, *J Am Soc Echocardiogr* 31:434–453, 2018.

remains critical to determining appropriateness of transcatheter edge-to-edge repair, guiding all critical steps, and managing all complications of the procedure (Table 166.2).

Please access ExpertConsult to view the corresponding videos for this chapter.

Acknowledgments

The authors gratefully acknowledge Julia Grapsa, MD, PhD; Ilias D. Koutsogeorgis, MD; Petros Nihoyannopoulos, MD; and Ferande Peters, MD, who were the authors of this chapter in the previous edition.

REFERENCES

1. Feldman T, Foster E, Glower DD, et al. Percutaneous repair or surgery for mitral regurgitation. *N Engl J Med.* 2011;364:1395–1406.
2. Maisano F, Redaelli A, Pennati G, et al. The hemodynamic effects of double-orifice valve repair for mitral regurgitation: a 3D computational model. *Eur J Cardio Thorac Surg.* 1999;15:419–425.
3. Alfieri O, Denti P. Alfieri stitch and its impact on mitral clip. *Eur J Cardio Thorac Surg.* 2011;39:807–808.
4. Maisano F, La Canna G, Colombo A, et al. The evolution from surgery to percutaneous mitral valve interventions: the role of the edge-to-edge technique. *J Am Coll Cardiol.* 2011;58:2174–2182.
5. Alfieri O, Maisano F, De Bonis M, et al. The double-orifice technique in mitral valve repair: a simple solution for complex problems. *J Thorac Cardiovasc Surg.* 2001;122:674–681.
6. Feldman T, Kar S, Rinaldi M, et al. Percutaneous mitral repair with the MitraClip system: safety and midterm durability in the initial EVEREST (Endovascular Valve Edge-to-Edge REpair Study) cohort. *J Am Coll Cardiol.* 2009;54:686–694.
7. Foster E, Kwan D, Feldman T, et al. Percutaneous mitral valve repair in the initial EVEREST cohort: Evidence of reverse left ventricular remodeling. *Circ Cardiovasc Imag.* 2013;6:522–530.
8. George JC, Varghese V, Dangas G, et al. Percutaneous mitral valve repair: Lessons from the EVEREST II (Endovascular valve edge-to-edge REpair study) and beyond. *JACC Cardiovasc Interv.* 2011;4:825–827.
9. Reichenspurner H, Schillinger W, Baldus S, et al. Clinical outcomes through 12 months in patients with degenerative mitral regurgitation treated with the MitraClip device in the ACCESS-EUrope Phase I trial. *Eur J Cardio Thorac Surg.* 2013;44:e280–e288.
10. Maisano F, Franzen O, Baldus S, et al. Percutaneous mitral valve interventions in the real world: early and 1-year results from the ACCESS-EU, a prospective, multicenter, nonrandomized post-approval study of the MitraClip therapy in Europe. *J Am Coll Cardiol.* 2013;62:1052–1061.
11. Baldus S, Schillinger W, Franzen O, et al. MitraClip therapy in daily clinical practice: initial results from the German transcatheter mitral valve interventions (TRAMI) registry. *Eur J Heart Fail.* 2012;14:1050–1055.
12. Franzen O, Baldus S, Rudolph V, et al. Acute outcomes of MitraClip therapy for mitral regurgitation in high-surgical-risk patients: emphasis on adverse valve morphology and severe left ventricular dysfunction. *Eur Heart J.* 2010;31:1373–1381.
13. Obadia JF, Messika-Zeitoun G, Leurent G, et al. Percutaneous repair or medical treatment for secondary mitral regurgitation. *N Engl J Med.* 2018;379:2297–2306.
14. Stone GW, Lindenfeld J, Abraham WT, et al. Transcatheter mitral-valve repair in patients with heart failure. *N Engl J Med.* 2018;379:2307–2318.
15. Nyman CB, Mackensen GB, Jelacic S, et al. Transcatheter mitral valve repair using the edge-to-edge clip. *J Am Soc Echocardiogr.* 2018;31:434–453.
16. Zoghbi WA, Adams D, Bonow RO, et al. Recommendations for noninvasive evaluation of native valvular regurgitation. *J Am Soc Echocardiogr.* 2017;30:303–370.
17. Hahn RT, Abraham T, Adams MS, et al. Guidelines for performing a comprehensive transesophageal echocardiographic examination. *J Am Soc Echocardiogr.* 2013;26:921–964.
18. Faletra F, Grimaldi A, Pasotti E, et al. Real-time 3-dimensional transesophageal echocardiography during double percutaneous mitral edge-to-edge procedure. *JACC Cardiovasc Imag.* 2009;2:1031–1033.
19. Hyodo E, Iwata S, Tugcu A, et al. Direct measurement of multiple vena contracta areas for assessing the severity of mitral regurgitation using 3D TEE. *JACC Cardiovasc Imag.* 2012;5:669–676.
20. Altiok E, Hamada S, Brehmer K, et al. Analysis of procedural effects of percutaneous edge-to-edge mitral valve repair by 2D and 3D echocardiography. *Circ Cardiovasc Imag.* 2012;5:748–755.
21. Lin BA, Forouhar AS, Pahlevan NM, et al. Color Doppler jet area overestimates regurgitant volume when multiple jets are present. *J Am Soc Echocardiogr.* 2010;23:993–1000.
22. Zoghbi WA, Asch FM, Bruce C, et al. Guidelines for the evaluation of valvular regurgitation after percutaneous valve repair or replacement. *J Am Soc Echocardiogr.* 2019;32:431–475.
23. Praz F, Spargias K, Chrissoheris M, et al. Compassionate use of the PASCAL transcatheter mitral valve repair system for patients with severe mitral regurgitation: a multicentre, prospective, observational, first-in-man study. *Lancet.* 2017;390:773–780.

167 Transcatheter Mitral Valve Replacement

Muhamed Saric

Mitral valve (MV) disease is the most prevalent form of valvular disease worldwide. Moderate to severe and severe native mitral regurgitation (MR) are the most prevalent forms of significant valvular disease in the developed countries. In 2006, it was estimated that moderate to severe and severe MR are approximately 20 times more prevalent than severe aortic stenosis (AS) in the United States (Fig. 167.1), yet the number of patients with severe AS exceeds the number of patients with MR treated with surgical or transcatheter procedures.[1]

Transcatheter mitral valve replacement (TMVR) is an emerging technology using transapical or transeptal approaches to replace either failed surgical MV repairs and bioprosthesis or diseased native MVs. They are currently approved for high-risk and inoperable patients. Procedural risks include an incomplete seal, resulting in paravalvular regurgitation, left ventricular (LV) outflow tract obstruction, and rarely ejection of the transcatheter valve into the adjacent cardiac chamber.

TRANSCATHETER REPLACEMENT OF FAILED SURGICAL MITRAL VALVE REPAIRS AND BIOPROSTHESES

Transcatheter replacement of failed surgical mitral repairs and replacements uses existing transcatheter aortic valve replacement (TAVR) technology with some modifications.[2] Historically, when a surgical bioprosthesis failed, resulting in either prosthetic stenosis or regurgitation, the only therapeutic option was to perform a redo surgery. Such a surgery caries an operative risk of morbidity and mortality that is higher than of the original procedure. Over the past decade, transcatheter replacements of failed surgical repairs, and bioprostheses have emerged as an alternative to redo surgery.[3] They were first developed for failed aortic bioprostheses[4] but were soon applied in the mitral position as well.[5] In the mitral space, these percutaneous approaches are referred to as valve-in-valve (ViV; Fig. 167.2) and valve-in-ring (ViR; Fig. 167.3) procedures.[6]

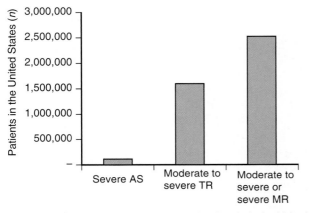

Figure 167.1. Prevalence of significant valvular disease in the United States. *AS,* Aortic stenosis; *TR,* tricuspid regurgitation. (Adapted from Stuge O, Liddicoat J: Emerging opportunities for cardiac surgeons within structural heart disease, *J Thorac Cardiovasc Surg* 132:1258–1261, 2006.)

ViV and ViR have same procedural steps: (1) a TAVR valve (e.g., a balloon-expandable Edwards Sapien [Edwards Lifesciences] bioprosthesis) is loaded backward in the delivery system; (2) the TAVR valve is then advanced into the failed surgical mitral repair or replacement using either a transapical or transvenous–transeptal approach; and (3) the TAVR valve is then deployed in the mitral position. The existing surgical annuloplasty ring or surgical bioprosthetic sewing ring serves the same role as aortic root calcification in anchoring the transcatheter valve.

Transthoracic echocardiography and transesophageal echocardiography (TEE) play an essential role in preprocedural diagnosis by demonstrating the mechanism and severity of surgical MV repair or replacement failure. TEE is indispensable for intraprocedural ViV and ViR guidance and for assessment of procedural success.

TRANSCATHETER REPLACEMENT OF NATIVE MITRAL VALVE

Transcatheter replacement of native MV refers to either placement of a TAVR valve in a mitral annual calcification (valve-in-MAC) or placement of a transcatheter valve specifically designed for native MV, typically unaffected by significant annular calcification (TMVR sensu stricto).

Valve in Mitral Annual Calcification

The valve-in-MAC (Fig. 167.4) procedure is used to treat either mitral stenosis or MR due to degenerative mitral annular and leaflet calcifications. Surgical repairs or replacement therapies for such disorders often carry a prohibitive operative risk. Valve-in-MAC has emerged as an alternative to surgery; however, it is also a high-risk procedure.[7] Valve-in-MAC uses the same technology and procedural steps described for ViV and ViR earlier.

TRANSCATHETER MITRAL VALVE REPLACEMENT FOR NONCALCIFIC NATIVE MITRAL VALVE DISEASE

This technology is less developed than TAVR technology because design requirements for transcatheter mitral prostheses are more challenging. Whereas for AS, TAVR technology relies on native valvular calcifications for prosthesis anchoring, TMVR design must rely on different anchoring approaches because the most common forms of native MR are not calcific in nature.[8] Some are deployed transapically (Fig. 167.5), and others use a transvenous–transeptal (Fig. 167.6) delivery approach. None of the currently designed transcatheter MVs are approved for routine clinical use; however, many are undergoing clinical trials.

The Intrepid system (Medtronic) is an example of transapical TMVR. It requires mini thoracotomy for surgical exposure of the LV apex. The surgeon ascertains proper transapical access site by poking the LV apex, which is visualized by TEE (see Fig. 67.5A). Next, the TMVR delivery capsule is advanced through the apical access site into the left heart (see Fig. 167.5B) and then partly opened in the left atrium to assure proper orientation of the prosthesis (see Fig. 167.5C). Finally, the Intrepid TMVR bioprosthesis is deployed inside the native MV apparatus (see Fig. 167.5D).

The Caisson system (LivaNova) is an example of a transvenous–transeptal TVMR. The system consists of an anchor that is placed first and a bioprosthetic valve that is then placed inside the anchor.

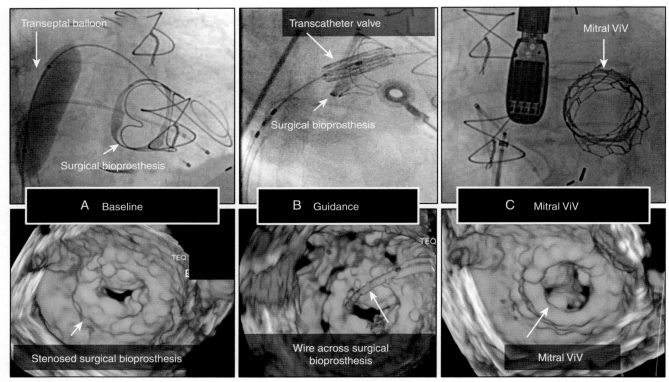

Figure 167.2. Transcatheter mitral valve-in-valve (ViV) procedure. Fluoroscopic *(top row)* and three-dimensional (3D) transesophageal echocardiography (TEE) *(bottom row)* guidance of the transcatheter mitral ViV procedure. The left atrial side of the mitral valve is visualized on 3D TEE from the so-called surgical view. **A,** Baseline. **B,** Guidance. **C,** Mitral ViV. (See accompanying Video 167.2.)

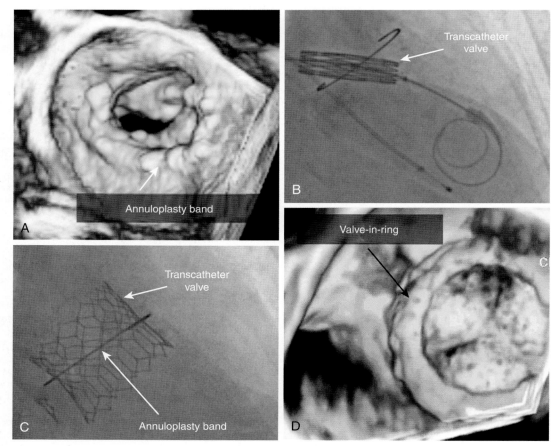

Figure 167.3. Transcatheter mitral valve-in-ring (ViR) procedure. Fluoroscopic and three-dimensional (3D) transesophageal echocardiography (TEE) guidance of the transcatheter mitral ViR procedure. The left atrial side of the mitral valve is visualized on 3D TEE from the so-called surgical view. **A,** Failed surgically implanted annuloplasty band (incomplete ring). **B** and **C,** Fluoroscopic guidance of the ViR procedure; the transcatheter valve is being positioned in **B** and is fully deployed in **C**. **D,** 3D TEE image of a ViR procedure from the surgical view. (See accompanying Video 167.3.)

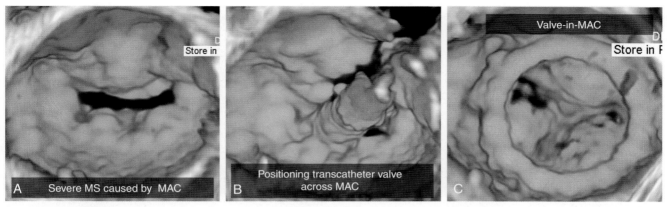

Figure 167.4. Transcatheter valve-in-mitral annual calcification (MAC) procedure. Three-dimensional transesophageal echocardiography imaging of the mitral valve-in-MAC procedure from the surgical view. **A,** Diastolic frame of a severely stenosed native mitral valve caused by MAC. **B,** Positioning of the transcatheter valve across the native mitral valve. **C,** Successfully deployed valve-in-MAC. *MS,* Mitral stenosis. (See accompanying Video 167.4.)

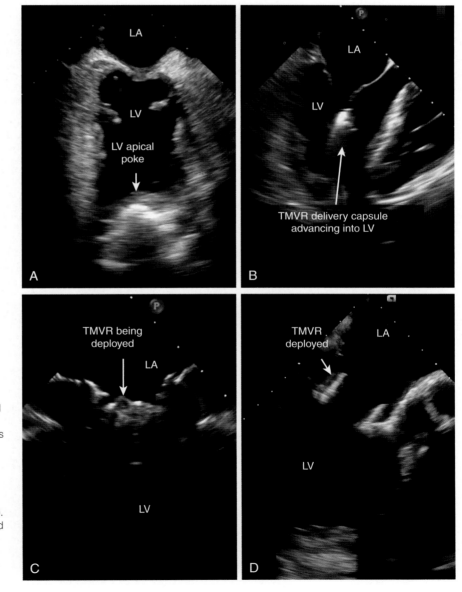

Figure 167.5. Transapical transcatheter mitral valve replacement (TMVR). Transesophageal echocardiography imaging of procedural steps in midesophageal views. **A,** First, the surgeon performs an apical poke to ascertain the location of transapical access. **B,** In the next step, the TMVR delivery capsule is advanced into the left ventricle (LV) and then across the native mitral valve (MV) into the left atrium (LA). **C,** Thereafter, the TMVR valve is partly opened in the LA and then pulled back toward the mitral annulus. **D,** Finally, the TMVR valve is fully deployed and anchored in the native MV apparatus. (See accompanying Video 167.5.)

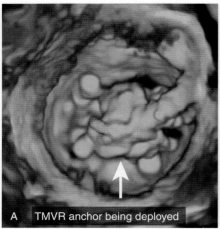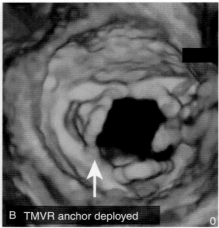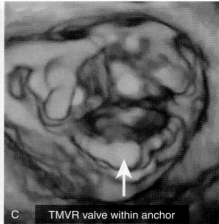

Figure 167.6. Transvenous–transeptal transcatheter mitral valve replacement (TMVR). Three-dimensional (3D) transesophageal echocardiography (TEE) imaging in the surgical view of the procedural step in implantation of transvenous–transeptal TMVR. **A,** After obtaining femoral transvenous access and performing transeptal puncture, the TMVR anchor is brough into the left atrium (LA) and oriented under 3D TEE guidance. **B,** In the next step, the TMVR anchor is fully deployed withing the native mitral annuls. **C,** Finally, a TMVR bioprosthesis is deployed inside the anchor. (See accompanying Video 167.6.)

Femoral transvenous access is obtained, and then transeptal puncture is performed to gain access into the left atrium. A folded anchor is then advanced inside the left atrium, oriented under two- and three-dimensional TEE guidance (see Fig. 167.6A) and then deployed inside the native mitral annulus (see Fig. 167.6B). Finally, using a separate delivery sheath, a bioprosthesis is the deployed inside the anchor (see Fig. 167.6C).

Please access ExpertConsult to view the corresponding videos for this chapter.

REFERENCES

1. Stuge O, Liddicoat J. Emerging opportunities for cardiac surgeons within structural heart disease. *J Thorac Cardiovasc Surg.* 2006;132:1258–1261.
2. Edelman JJ, Khan JM, Rogers T, et al. Valve-in-valve TAVR: state-of-the-art review. *Innovations.* 2019;14:299–310.
3. Alter EL, Jilaihawi H, Williams MR, et al: Imaging in mitral valve interventions: MitraClip and beyond. https://www.acc.org/latest-in-cardiology/articles/2018/08/06/13/25/imaging-in-mv-interventions.
4. Dvir D, Webb J, Brecker S, et al. Transcatheter aortic valve replacement for degenerative bioprosthetic surgical valves: results from the global valve-in-valve registry. *Circulation.* 2012 Nov 6;126:2335–2344.
5. Shivaraju A, Michel J, Frangieh AH, et al. Transcatheter aortic and mitral valve-in-valve implantation using the Edwards Sapien 3 heart valve. *J Am Heart Assoc.* 2018;7:14.
6. Long A, Mahoney P. Transcatheter mitral valve-in-valve and valve-in-ring replacement in high-risk surgical patients: feasibility, safety, and longitudinal outcomes in a single-center experience. *J Invasive Cardiol.* 2018;30:324–328.
7. Guerrero M, Dvir D, Himbert D, et al. Transcatheter mitral valve replacement in native mitral valve disease with severe mitral annular calcification: results from the first multicenter global registry. *JACC Cardiovasc Interv.* 2016;9:1361–1371.
8. Del Val D, Ferreira-Neto AN, Wintzer-Wehekind J, et al. Early experience with transcatheter mitral valve replacement: a systematic review. *J Am Heart Assoc.* 2019;8. e013332.

168 Transcatheter Valve-in-Valve Implantation

Itzhak Kronzon, Carlos E. Ruiz, Gila Perk

Surgical valve replacement is frequently required in patients with severe native valve disorders not amenable to valve repair. Until recently, valve replacement invariably required open-heart surgery with cardiopulmonary bypass. This major surgery was associated with morbidity, mortality, long hospital stays, and disability. The surgical prosthetic valves commonly used are less than perfect, and the long-term results are still suboptimal. Most prosthetic valves that are surgically implanted are either mechanical or biological (tissue valves). Although the mechanical valves are durable and can potentially last for a lifetime, they require full, lifelong anticoagulation therapy, which may result in bleeding tendency and limitation of strenuous sports and physical activity. Bioprosthetic valves were introduced with the hope that anticoagulation would not be required. Unfortunately, biological valves degenerate and fail within years after their surgical implantation and become stenotic, insufficient, or both. Valve failure is more rapid in young patients. Therefore, bioprosthetic valves are more frequently recommended in older adult patients (who have higher prevalence of coronary disease and other comorbidities). However, with improved patient care and better survival of cardiac patients, many individuals will require one or more major open-heart surgeries to replace a failed valve. The repeat procedure carries relatively high morbidity and mortality, with long hospitalizations and frequently incomplete recovery.

VALVE-IN-VALVE PROCEDURE

During the past decade, an alternative procedure has been developed: transcutaneous, transcatheter delivery of an expandable prosthetic valve to be deployed within a failed prosthetic valve. This procedure, also known as "valve in valve" (ViV),[1] should be distinguished from transcutaneous implantation of a prosthetic valve within a native malfunctioning valve, such as transcatheter aortic valve replacement (TAVR) or transcatheter pulmonic valve replacement, which are discussed elsewhere in this book.

The (ViV) procedure gained growing acceptance into medical practice; in 2017, the Food and Drug Administration approved expanded indication for the Edwards Sapien 3 transcatheter bioprosthetic valve for aortic and mitral ViV procedures in patients at high surgical risk or greater. Failed aortic bioprosthetic valves can be treated with either balloon expandable or self-expandable valves.

IMAGING

Multimodality imaging before and during the procedure is frequently essential. This includes fluoroscopy, two- and three-dimensional (2D and 3D) transesophageal echocardiography (TEE) and computed tomography (CT). Fusion imaging techniques are quite useful. This includes the Cardiac Navigator system for fluoroscopy and CT image fusion as well as the EchoNav system for 2D and 3D TEE and fluoroscopy fusion (both by Philips). The fusion technology superimposes the TEE or CT images on the fluoroscopic screen and thus enables the operator to navigate the catheters, wires, and devices into the target sites defined by these images.

Accurate demonstration of the internal dimension, perimeter, and shape of the failed prosthetic ring are essential for prosthetic valve selection. These can be evaluated from the 3D echocardiographic or CT images. Color and spectral Doppler are essential for the evaluation of the failed valve hemodynamics. The exact degree of stenosis and regurgitation can be quantified. The site of regurgitation is important. Paravalvular leaks may require device closure, not valve replacement.

PROCEDURAL GUIDANCE

In right-sided ViV procedures,[1] access to the right heart is obtained by a central venous approach. The procedure can be performed, if indicated, in patients who underwent tricuspid valve replacement with a bioprosthesis or even tricuspid valve repair using a prosthetic ring. Pulmonic ViV procedures are frequently done with the Melody valve.[2]

For left-sided valves, the approach to the damaged, malfunctioning aortic bioprosthesis can be retrograde via a peripheral large artery. This is very similar to the TAVR procedure.[3] The approach to the mitral valve can be antegrade via a central venous approach and transseptal puncture or transapical puncture of the left ventricle with a retrograde approach to the failed prosthetic valve.[1] In cases

of prosthetic valve stenosis, balloon dilatation of the prosthesis may be required.

Balloon-Expandable Transcatheter Valves

Under fluoroscopic and echocardiographic real-time surveillance, the failed prosthetic valve is crossed by a wire. A catheter with the collapsed new valve over a deflated balloon is advanced over the wire and placed with the collapsed valve at the failed prosthesis orifice. The balloon is then inflated to expand the new valve in the desired position, supported in place by the failed prosthesis, which holds it securely. It should be emphasized that after the new valve is inflated, it cannot be recollapsed or repositioned, underscoring the importance of exact positioning before balloon inflation. For ViV procedures in the mitral and tricuspid positions, a balloon-expandable valve is typically the only transcatheter option.

Self-Expanding Transcatheter Valves

For ViV procedures in the aortic position, either balloon-expandable or self-expanding transcatheter valves can be used. The advantage of self-expanding valves (e.g., Medtronic CoreValve) is that they can be repositioned before final deployment to assure proper position.

After the ViV is deployed, Doppler echocardiography is used to demonstrate residual valvular regurgitation and to assess the new transvalvular gradient and valve area.

COMPLICATIONS

The complication rate depends on anatomic factors, patient comorbidities, and operator skill and experience. Any structural intervention may have complication related to access and manipulation of intracardiac catheters. Cardiac rupture and tamponade may result from intracardiac manipulation of large-bore catheters or from failed transseptal puncture. During the manipulation of the collapsed valve across the atrial septum, a large atrial septal defect can be created that may require closure using a device. The apical puncture may be responsible for bleeding into the pericardial sac or into the left pleural cavity. Device closure of the apical puncture site is frequently performed. Arrhythmia and conduction abnormalities are common. Residual regurgitation, especially paravalvular, is occasionally noted; fortunately, in most cases, it is not severe. Detachment and even complete dislodgement of the

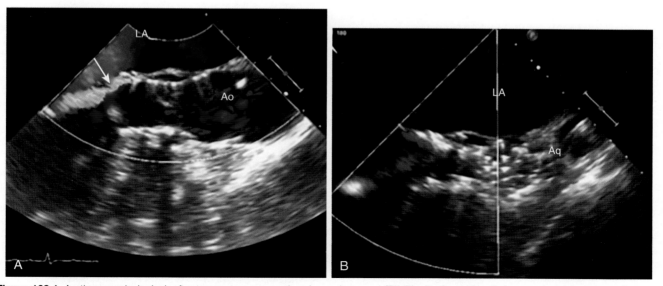

Figure 168.1. Aortic paravalvular leak after transcutaneous aortic valve replacement (TAVR) with CoreValve. **A,** Long-axis, midesophageal transesophageal echocardiographic image, diastolic frame. Note the significant paravalvular aortic regurgitation *(arrow)*. **B,** After the implantation of an additional CoreValve, there is no aortic regurgitation. *Ao,* Aorta; *LA,* left atrium.

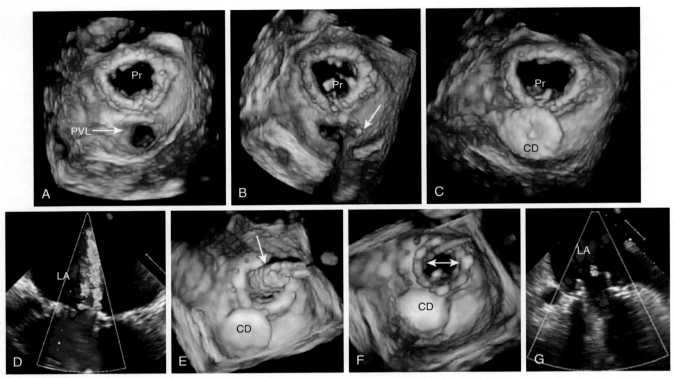

Figure 168.2. Mitral paravalvular leak closure and valve-in-valve implant, transesophageal echocardiography, two-dimensional, and real-time three-dimensional images. **A,** Mitral valve en face view, left atrial (LA) perspective. A tissue prosthesis is noted (Pr). There is a large paravalvular leak (PVL). **B,** After percutaneous left ventricular apical puncture, a catheter *(arrow)* is advanced from the left ventricle to the left atrium across the PVL. **C,** The PVL closure device (CD) is deployed. **D,** Color Doppler demonstrates significant valvular (and no residual paravalvular) mitral regurgitation (MR). **E,** A balloon catheter with a collapsed percutaneous valve *(arrow)* is advanced across the mitral bioprosthesis orifice. **F,** With balloon inflation, the new valve *(double-headed arrow)* is deployed in the bioprosthesis orifice. **G,** At the end of the procedure, only minimal MR is seen. (See accompanying Videos 168.2C–G.)

newly installed valve occur very rarely. An important consideration with ViV implantation is the degree of residual stenosis and possible patient–prosthesis mismatch. A serious complication that can be seen with mitral ViV procedure is left ventricular outflow tract (LVOT) obstruction.[4] It has been described in multiple series of mitral ViV and can cause severe hemodynamic collapse, even necessitating emergency surgical intervention, which carries an extremely high risk. Preprocedure CT imaging with computer modeling of the expected "neo-LVOT" has been used to assess the risk of postprocedure LVOT obstruction.

Fig. 168.1 demonstrates a patient with previous TAVR performed with a CoreValve. After the procedure, the patient complained of shortness of breath. The arterial blood pressure was 157/45 mm Hg. TEE demonstrated significant aortic regurgitation. Another CoreValve was advanced into a slightly more superior position and was deployed. At the end of the procedure, the blood pressure was 135/70 mm Hg, and the aortic insufficiency jet was no longer seen. The mean systolic gradient across the newly placed valve was 9 mm Hg.

Fig. 168.2 shows a ViV procedure in a patient with severe mitral bioprosthetic insufficiency. After a needle puncture of the left ventricular apex, a wire was advanced from the left ventricle across the mitral valve into the left atrium. This wire was snared in the left atrium to another wire, which was advanced from the femoral vein across the atrial septum (after transseptal puncture). A catheter that carried a collapsed valve over a deflated balloon was advanced into the mitral bioprosthetic orifice. With the collapsed valve in good position, the balloon was inflated, and the valve was expanded for deployment. When all the catheters were removed, there was no significant residual mitral regurgitation or stenosis. At the end of the procedure, the transseptal puncture site was closed with an Amplatzer closure device, and the apex puncture site was

closed with another closure device. A few days later, the patient left the hospital in good condition.

CONCLUSION

ViV replacement of a failed bioprosthesis is feasible in the aortic, mitral, tricuspid, or pulmonic position. Multimodality imaging includes fluoroscopy, transthoracic and transesophageal 2D and real-time 3D echocardiography, CT, and fusion technologies. Although ViV implantation frequently offers immediate relief and restoration of valvular hemodynamics, the long-term follow-up results and prognosis are still being investigated. With rapidly accumulated experience, the performance of the valve in valve in comparison with surgically implanted valves will define its routine use in patients with failed bioprostheses.

Please access ExpertConsult to view the corresponding videos for this chapter.

REFERENCES

1. Murdoch DJ, Webb JG. Transcatheter valve-in-valve implantation for degenerated surgical bioprosthesis. *J Thorac Dis.* 2018;10(suppl 30):S3573–S3577.
2. Gillespie MJ, Rome JJ, Daniel S, et al. Melody valve implant within failed bioprosthetic valves in the pulmonary position: a multicenter experience. *Circ Cardiovasc Interv.* 2012;5:862–870.
3. Ruiz CE, Laborade LC, Condonato JF, et al. First percutaneous transcatheter aortic valve-in-valve implant with three-year follow-up. *Catheter Cardiovasc Interv.* 2008;72:143–148.
4. Wang DD, Eng MH, Greenbaum AB, et al. Validating a prediction modeling tool for left ventricular outflow tract (LVOT) obstruction after transcatheter mitral valve replacement. *Catheter Cardiovasc Interv.* 2018;92:379–387.

169 Atrial and Ventricular Septal Defect Closure

Todd Mendelson, Carlos L. Alviar, Muhamed Saric

ATRIAL SEPTAL DEFECT CLOSURE

Aside from the bicuspid aortic valve, an atrial septal defect (ASD) is the most common congenital cardiac anomaly in adults with an approximate prevalence of 1 per 1000 individuals.[1] This chapter focuses on echocardiographic imaging during ASD closure. Embryology, classification, diagnosis, and hemodynamic significance of ASDs are discussed in detail in the congenital heart disease section of this book. Briefly, there are four main types of ASDs (listed in decreasing order of frequency): secundum ASD, primum ASD, sinus venosus ASD, and unroofed coronary sinus. When indicated, ASDs can be closed either surgically or via a percutaneous approach. According to most recent guidelines,[2] the primary indication for ASD closure is the presence of right atrial or right ventricular enlargement, especially in the presence of symptoms (classes I and II). Secundum ASDs are the only ASDs for which percutaneous closure with current devices is indicated. All other ASDs are closed surgically in eligible patients. Indications for percutaneous or surgical ASD closure in adults with isolated secundum ASD are summarized in Table 169.1. The primary contraindication of ASD closure is the presence of irreversible, severe pulmonary arterial hypertension and no evidence of left-to-right shunt (class III). During ASD closure attempts, an occlusion test may be performed. ASD is transiently closed using sizing balloon while the patient's hemodynamic parameters are monitored. Closure is aborted if hemodynamic instability or signs of acute pulmonary edema develop.[3]

Surgical Atrial Septal Defect Closure

The earliest surgical closure of an ASD was reported in the early 1950s.[4] Surgical ASD closure was the first successful open-heart operation (performed under general hypothermia and inflow occlusion) even before the advent of cardiopulmonary bypass (CPB).[5] Subsequently, ASD closure became the very first type of cardiac surgery to use CPB.[6] Surgical closure can be accomplished by either direct suture or using a patch. It is recommended that the surgical ASD closure be performed by surgeons with expertise and special training in congenital heart disease.[2] Surgery remains the only recommended means of closing primum, sinus venosus, and coronary sinus types of ASDs. Surgery is an alternative to percutaneous closure of secundum ASDs.

Percutaneous Atrial Septal Defect Closure

Percutaneous closure of an ASD was first described in the mid-1970s.[7] Currently, percutaneous closure has become the most common means of repairing secundum ASDs. All currently available ASD closure devices in the United States are only approved for secundum-type ASDs. These devices have a similar basic structure; they all contain two disks connected by a waist. Some are approved for simple secundum ASDs with a solitary hole, whereas others are specifically designed for secundum ASDs with multiple holes, referred to as fenestrated or cribriform (sieve-like) ASDs. The three most commonly used devices (Fig. 169.1) are:

- The Amplatzer atrial septal occluder (St. Jude Medical) is used to close nonfenestrated secundum ASDs. It contains a larger left atrial disk connected to a smaller right atrial disk. The waist connecting the two disks ranges from 4 to 38 mm in diameter. When selecting an appropriate device size, the waist diameter of the device should correspond to the ASD diameter.
- The Gore Cardioform atrial septal occluder (WL Gore & Associates) contains two equal-sized disks connected by a spiral shaft; disk diameter ranges from 15 to 35 mm. An appropriately selected Gore device should have a disk diameter that at is at least twice the ASD diameter.
- The Amplatzer multifenestrated atrial septal occluder (St. Jude Medical) contains two equal-sized disks connected by a thin shaft for use with cribriform ASDs. Disk diameters range from 18 to 35 mm. An appropriately selected device should have a disk size of a sufficient diameter to cover the entire ASD.

Role of Echocardiography in Percutaneous Atrial Septal Defect Closure

Echocardiography is an essential part of the percutaneous ASD closure process because it is needed before, during, and after percutaneous ASD closure.

Before Atrial Septal Defect Closure

Both transthoracic echocardiography (TTE) and transesophageal echocardiography (TEE) can establish the presence of an ASD, define its type, size the defect, and determine shunt direction and its hemodynamic significance. Three-dimensional (3D) echocardiography overcomes many limitations of two-dimensional (2D) echocardiography by providing accurate visualization of the size and shape of the defect and its rims on unique en face views. Proper ASD sizing is essential in selecting the device size to avoid complications from using an undersized or oversized closure device (e.g., incomplete defect closure, device embolization, or disk erosion into surrounding cardiac structures).

TABLE 169.1 Indications for Percutaneous or Surgical Closure of Isolated Secundum Atrial Septal Defect in Adults

	Class I	Class IIA	Class IIB	Class III
Symptoms	Symptomatic	Asymptomatic		
Right heart enlargement	Present			
Qp:Qs ratio	>1.5:1 (net left > right shunt)			<1.0 (net right > left shunt)
PA pressure	<50% systemic		>50% systemic	>2/3 systemic
PVR	<1/3 systemic		>1/3 systemic	>2/3 systemic
Cyanosis at rest or with exercise	Absent			

PA, Pulmonary artery; *PVR*, pulmonary vascular resistance; *Qp*, pulmonic flow; *Qs*, systemic flow.

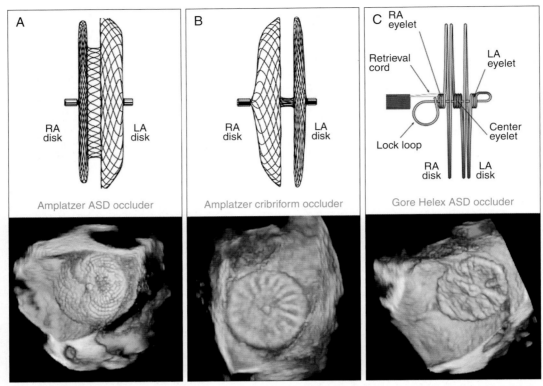

Figure 169.1. Secundum atrial septal defect (ASD) occluders. The three devices most commonly used for percutaneous ASD closure are depicted. The *bottom images* in each panel represent en face three-dimensional transesophageal echocardiographic zoom views of the left atrial disk. **A,** Amplatzer atrial septal occluder. **B,** Amplatzer cribriform occluder. **C,** Gore Helex atrial septal occluder. (Recently, Gore replaced the Helex device with a Cardioform device, which is similar in appearance to the Helex device depicted in Panel C.) *LA,* Left atrium; *RA,* right atrium.

In general, when deciding on the size of an ASD closure device, the maximum diameter of a secundum ASD cannot exceed the device-specific cutoff value, which is 38 mm when using an Amplatzer atrial septal occluder and 17 mm when using a Gore Cardioform device. Furthermore, there should be sufficient ASD rims to anchor the device. Anatomically, there are six distinct ASD rims listed in a clockwise direction: superior vena cava (SVC) rim, aortic (anterior) rim, atrioventricular rim, inferior vena cava (IVC) rim, posteroinferior rim, and posterosuperior rim.[8,9]

Historically, the device size was selected based on an invasive measurement of a so-called stop-flow ASD diameter by gradually inflating a sizing balloon placed across an ASD until no color Doppler flow across the ASD is seen on TEE. More recently, device selection is based on direct ASD diameter measurements by 2D and 3D TEE.

On 2D TEE, ASD should be visualized in multiple views; in each view, the maximum ASD diameter during atrial diastole as well as the size of the two visible ASD rims should be measured. At approximately 0 degrees (four-chamber view), the atrioventricular and posterosuperior ASD rims are seen. At approximately 60 degrees (short-axis view at the level of the aortic valve), the aortic and posteroinferior rims are seen. At 90 to 120 degrees (bicaval view), the SVC and IVC rims are visualized (Fig. 169.2 and Video 169.2).

The term "sufficient rim" denotes a minimum rim width capable of securely anchoring the closure device. For the Amplatzer atrial septal occluder, the rims should be at least 5 mm; for the Amplatzer multifenestrated atrial septal occluder, the SVC and the aortic rim should be at least 9 mm. Absence of the IVC rim is considered a contraindication for device closure of a secundum ASD. Absence of the aortic rim is a major risk factor for device erosion into surrounding structure, especially when using the Amplatzer atrial septal occluder.[10]

3D TEE is especially well suited for accurate characterization of ASD size, shape, and rim (Fig. 169.3). On 3D zoom en face views, the full extent of ASD and its relations to surrounding cardiac structures are demonstrated from both the right atrial and left atrial perspectives. The so-called tilt up then left (TUPLE) maneuver can be used to place ASD images in anatomically correct orientation, which then facilitates characterization of ASD anatomy.[11] On 3D TEE imaging, one can easily determine the size of a secundum ASD (circular, ovoid, or irregular), its location within the floor of the fossa ovalis, and the presence or absence of associated anomalies such as an atrial septal aneurysm involving the remainder of the fossa ovalis.[12]

During Atrial Septal Defect Closure

During the procedure, venous access is gained via the femoral vein. Subsequently, the interventionalist may opt to advance a sizing balloon across the ASD to confirm the ASD size using the stop-flow technique described earlier (Fig. 169.4A and B). Thereafter, a delivery catheter is advanced into the right atrium and then through the ASD into the left atrium under fluoroscopic and echocardiographic guidance. A collapsed ASD closure device attached to its delivery cable is advanced through the delivery catheter, and the left atrial disk is opened first and positioned against the left atrial side of ASD. In the next step, the right atrial disk is opened to anchor the device within the ASD (see Fig. 169.4C and D).

2D and 3D TEE imaging, or alternatively, intracardiac echocardiography (ICE), is used to ascertain proper positioning of the closure device. On 3D TEE, the near-field left atrial disk is easier to visualize than the far-field right atrial disk. After the proper positioning of the ASD closure device is determined, the device is unscrewed from its delivery cable and released.

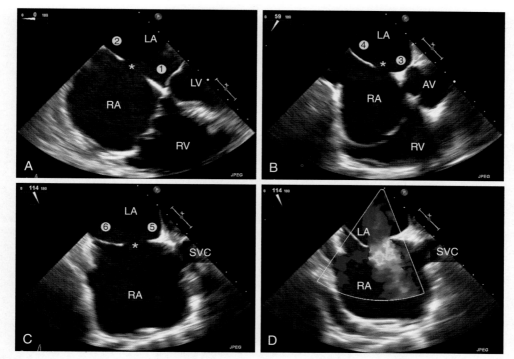

Figure 169.2. Secundum atrial septal defect (ASD) and its rims on two-dimensional transesophageal echocardiography. **A,** Secundum ASD *(asterisk)* seen at 0 degrees in the midesophageal four-chamber view. Atrioventricular *(1)* and posterosuperior *(2)* ASD rims are seen. **B,** Secundum ASD *(asterisk)* seen at 59 degrees in the midesophageal short-axis view at the level of the aortic valve (AV). Aortic *(3)* and posteroinferior *(4)* ASD rims are seen. **C,** Secundum ASD *(asterisk)* seen at 114 degrees in the midesophageal bicaval view. Superior vena cava (SVC) *(5)* and inferior vena cava (IVC) *(6)* ASD rims are seen. **D,** Color Doppler imagining at 114 degrees in the midesophageal bicaval view demonstrates a left-to-right shunt across the secundum ASD (from the left atrium [LA] to the right atrium [RA]). *LV,* Left ventricle; *RV,* right ventricle. (See accompanying Video 169.2).

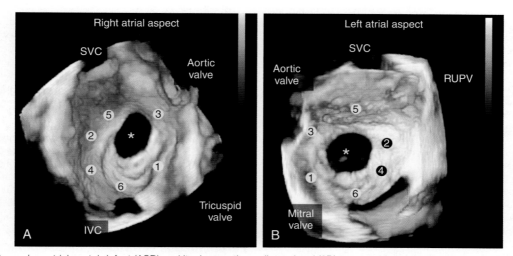

Figure 169.3. Secundum atrial septal defect (ASD) and its rims on three-dimensional (3D) transesophageal echocardiography (TEE). 3D TEE zoom images of a secundum ASD *(asterisk)* from the right atrial (**A**) and left atrial (**B**) perspectives. The ASD is located in the anterosuperior portion of the fossa ovalis. The remainder of fossa ovalis is aneurysmal. ASD rims are clearly seen: atrioventricular rim *(1)*, posterosuperior rim *(2)*, aortic rim *(4)*, posteroinferior rim *(4)*, SVC rim *(5)*, and inferior vena cava (IVC) rim *(5)*. On these 3D TEE images, the ASD was placed in proper anatomic orientation using the so-called tilt up then left (TUPLE) maneuver, which is demonstrated in accompanying Video 169.3. *RUPV,* Right upper pulmonary vein; *SVC,* superior vena cava.

After Atrial Septal Defect Closure

Immediately after device release, 2D and 3D TEE are used to check for device position, residual shunt, and presence of any complications such as a pericardial effusion. When ASD closure is successful, color Doppler imaging demonstrates complete absence of any flow around the device (no peridevice leak between the edges of the closure device and ASD rims; Fig. 169.4E). In contrast, small amounts of color Doppler flow through the device are normal; they typically resolve over time as the device endothelializes (Fig. 169.4F). On completion of percutaneous ASD closure, the patient is placed on antiplatelet therapy for several weeks. Regular follow-up

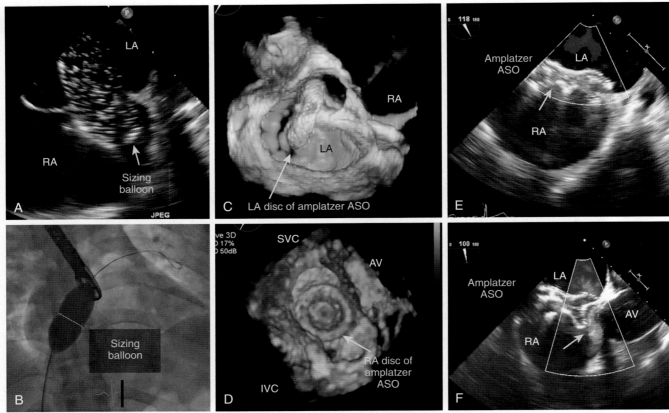

Figure 169.4. Percutaneous atrial septal defect (ASD) closure. Balloon sizing of a secundum ASD seen on two-dimensional transesophageal echocardiography (**A**) and fluoroscopy (**B**). Video 169.4A demonstrates that the balloon is inflated enough to prevent any shunt across the ASD. The diameter of the balloon at that moment is referred to as the stop-flow diameter. Deployment of an Amplatzer atrial septal occluder: first the left atrial disk is opened (**C**), followed by deployment of the right atrial disk (**D**). After device deployment, color Doppler is used to assess proper closure. **E,** Successful ASD closure with only small amount of flow *(arrow)* through the device. Video 169.4E corresponds to this panel. **F,** Incomplete ASD closure with abnormal flow *(arrow)* around the device (paradevice leak). Video 169.4F corresponds to this panel. *ASO,* Atrial septal occluder; *AV,* aortic valve; *IVC,* inferior vena cava; *LA,* left atrium; *RA,* right atrium; *SVC,* superior vena cava.

after closure, typically with TTE, is recommended to ensure the absence of device migration, erosion, or other complications.

VENTRICULAR SEPTAL DEFECT CLOSURE

Ventricular septal defects (VSDs) can be divided according to their cause as either congenital or acquired.[13] Acquired VSDs are less common than the congenital ones and are typically caused by myocardial infarction or trauma.[14,15] VSDs can also be classified according to their anatomic location in perimembranous (also known as infracristal or subaortic), muscular (which can be subdivided into inlet, trabecular and infundibular, or supracristal), and atrioventricular or Gerbode defect, which entails a communication between the left ventricle and the right atrium.[16]

Perimembranous VSDs represent the majority of cases in postneonates; they usually have a windsock appearance due to evagination of the membranous septum.[17] Muscular VSDs may be either acquired or congenital,[18] and they can be either solitary or multiple (when they may be referred to as "Swiss cheese VSDs"). When indicated, VSDs are typically closed surgically, although percutaneous closure options are being developed. According to current guidelines,[19] primary indications (classes I and II) and contraindications (class III) to close a VSD are summarized in Table 169.2. VSD closure is contraindicated in patients with severe irreversible pulmonary arterial hypertension (class III).

Surgical Ventricular Septal Defect Closure

Surgery has been the classic approach to close VSDs. Steady improvements in surgical techniques have led to remarkable improvements in the prognosis and survival of patients with VSDs in the past 50 years.[20] However, a surgical VSD closure remains a major procedure requiring CPB and carries significant risk to the patient. Such risks are particularly high in patients with post–myocardial infarction VSDs who are frequently hemodynamically unstable and whose VSD borders are friable and difficult to suture.[21]

Percutaneous Ventricular Septal Defect Closure

The use of percutaneous catheter-based devices has emerged as a nonsurgical option to treat VSDs in selected patients.[22] The first case of percutaneous VSD closure was reported in 1988 using a double-umbrella device.[23] Devices are currently approved in the United States for percutaneous closures of congenital VSDs that are not located in the proximity of heart valves in patients with high risk for surgical VSD closure.

Thus, congenital muscular VSDs are the principal VSD type amenable to percutaneous closure (Fig. 169.5). Postinfarction muscular VSDs have been closed percutaneously in an off-label manner.[24] In addition, percutaneous closure devices have been used to close residual ventricular defects after prior attempts at surgical closure as well as for traumatic or iatrogenic defects occurring

TABLE 169.2 Indications for Ventricular Septal Defect Closure in Adults

	Class I	Class IIA	Class IIB	Class III
LV volume overload	Present			
Qp:Qs ratio	>1.5:1 (net left > right shunt)		>1.5:1 (net left > right shunt)	<1.0 (net right > left shunt)
PA pressure	<50% systemic		>50% systemic	>2/3 systemic
PVR	<1/3 systemic		>1/3 systemic	>2/3 systemic
SPECIAL CIRCUMSTANCES				
VSD-related AR		Surgical closure of perimembranous or supracristal VSD is reasonable in adults when there is worsening AR caused by VSD		
VSD-related IE			Surgical closure of a VSD may be reasonable in adults with a history of IE caused by VSD if not otherwise contraindicated	

AR, Aortic regurgitation; *IE,* infective endocarditis; *PA,* pulmonary artery; *PVR,* pulmonary vascular resistance; *Qp,* pulmonic flow; *Qs,* systemic flow.

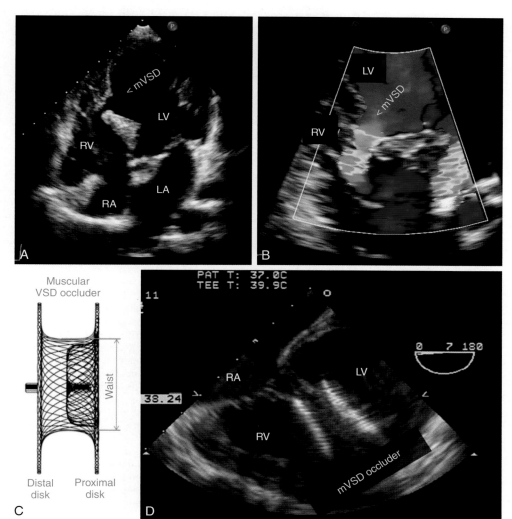

Figure 169.5. Congenital muscular ventricular septal defect (mVSD). **A,** Transthoracic echocardiogram (TTE) in the apical four-chamber view demonstrates a congenital mVSD. Note that the contractility of the surrounding interventricular septum is normal in congenital mVSD. This is in contrast to postinfarction mVSD, which is located within an area of interventricular septal hypokinesis or akinesis. **B,** TTE with color Doppler in the apical four-chamber view demonstrates a left-to-right shunt across a congenital mVSD. **C,** The Amplatzer mVSD occluder device approved in the United States for closure of congenital mVSDs. Note the two symmetrical disks separated by a waist. **D,** Transesophageal echocardiogram in the four-chamber midesophageal view demonstrates an Amplatzer mVSD occluder. *LA,* Left atrium; *LV,* left ventricle; *RA,* right atrium; *RV,* right ventricle. (See accompanying Video 169.5.)

after surgical aortic valve replacement.[25,26] Notably, because of their anatomic proximity to the aortic valve, perimembranous VSDs and VSD associated with aortic valve prolapse are generally not amenable to transcatheter device closure unless surgical intervention is contraindicated.[27]

Different types of percutaneous devices have been tried for VSD closure, with some of them yielding disappointing results, including the Rashkind double umbrella, the Bard Clamshell, the Button device, and the Gianturco coils.[28] Currently, the Amplatzer Muscular VSD Occluder (St. Jude Medical) is the only device

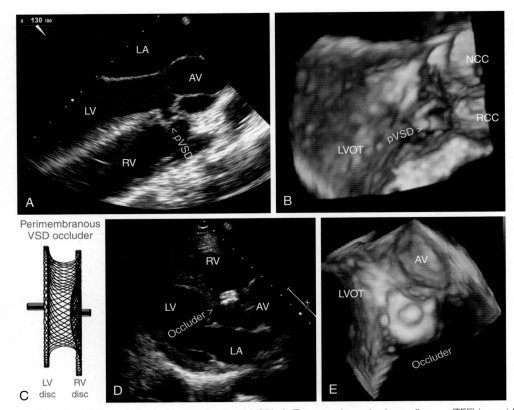

Figure 169.6. Congenital perimembranous ventricular septal defect (pVSD). **A,** Transesophageal echocardiogram (TEE) in a midesophageal view at 130 degrees demonstrates a windsock appearance of a congenital pVSD. **B.** 3D TEE zoom view demonstrates an en face view of a congenital pVSD just below the right coronary cusp (RCC) of the aortic valve. **C,** The Amplatzer pVSD occluder device approved outside the United States for closure of congenital pVSDs. Note the two asymmetrical disks separated by a waist. **D,** Transthoracic echocardiogram in the parasternal long-axis view demonstrates an Amplatzer pVSD occluder. Note in the video clip that there is no color flow around or across the device. **E,** 3D TEE zoom view demonstrates an en face view of an Amplatzer pVSD occluder. The device was implanted outside the United States. *AV,* Aortic valve; *LA,* left atrium; *LV,* left ventricle; *LVOT,* left ventricular outflow tract; *NCC,* noncoronary cusp of aortic valve; *RV,* right ventricle. (See accompanying Video 169.6.)

specifically approved for VSD closure in the United States. It features two disks of equal diameter separated by a waist that is positioned across the VSD. It comes in different sizes with a width diameter ranging from 14 to 18 mm. An Amplatzer device with eccentric disk configuration specifically designed for closure of perimembranous VSDs (Fig. 169.6) has been used outside the United States.[29]

Role of Echocardiography in Percutaneous Ventricular Septal Defect Closure

Echocardiography plays an important role before, during, and after percutaneous VSD closure. Before closure, both TTE and TEE can establish the presence of a VSD, define its type, size the defect, and determine its hemodynamic significance. 3D echocardiography may overcome limitations of 2D echocardiography[30] by providing accurate visualization of the size and shape of the defect on unique en face views of a VSD.[31,32] Proper VSD sizing is essential in selecting the device size to avoid complications from using an undersized or oversized closure device (e.g., incomplete defect closure or complete heart block).

Intraprocedural TEE, along with fluoroscopy, is essential for percutaneous VSD closure. 2D and 3D TEE, or alternatively, ICE, is crucial for procedural guidance. In general, percutaneous VSD closure is a complex procedure requiring both arterial and venous access. After arterial puncture, a catheter is delivered to the left ventricle in a retrograde fashion passing through the aortic valve,

and its tip is placed across the VSD. Subsequently, using techniques of guidewire snaring and exteriorizing to form an arteriovenous loop, an antegrade device delivery sheath is brought to the heart via the IVC after a venous puncture. The closure device is then advanced and carefully positioned across the VSD from the right ventricular side. The distal disk of the closure device is opened first and located on the left ventricular aspect of the VSD; this is followed by the deployment of the proximal disk on the right ventricular side.[33]

After percutaneous VSD closure, color Doppler imaging in conjunction with 2D and 3D imaging is essential for evaluating procedural success and possible complications. Successful VSD closure is characterized by a complete absence of any peridevice leak (a flow around the device between the VSD rims and the edge of the device). In contrast, small amounts of color Doppler flow through the device are normal and will resolve as the device endothelializes over time.

Please access ExpertConsult to view the corresponding videos for this chapter.

REFERENCES

1. Saric M, Benenstein R. Three-dimensional echocardiographic guidance of percutaneous procedures. In: Nanda N, ed. *Comprehensive Textbook of Echocardiography*. 1st ed. New Delhi: Jaypee Brothers Medical Publishers; 2013.
2. Stout KK, Daniels CJ, Aboulhosn JA, et al: 2018 AHA/ACC guideline for the management of adults with congenital heart disease, Circulation 139:e698–e800, 2019.

3. Javed U1, Levisman J, Rogers JH. A tale of two balloons: assessment of hemodynamics with atrial septal defect temporary balloon occlusion. *J Invasive Cardiol.* 2012;24:248–249.
4. Cohn LH. Fifty years of open-heart surgery. *Circulation.* 2003;107:2168–2170.
5. Lewis FJ, Taufic M. Closure of atrial septal defects with the aid of hypothermia: experimental accomplishments and the report of one successful case. *Surgery.* 1953;33:52–59.
6. Gibbon Jr JH. Application of a mechanical heart and lung apparatus to cardiac surgery. *Minn Med.* 1954;37:171–185.
7. King TD, Mills NL. Nonoperative closure of atrial septal defects. *Surgery.* 1974;75:383–388.
8. Amin Z. Transcatheter closure of secundum atrial septal defects. *Catheter Cardiovasc Interv.* 2006;68:778–787.
9. Mathewson JW, Bichell D, Rothman A, et al. Absent posteroinferior and anterosuperior atrial septal defect rims: factors affecting nonsurgical closure of large secundum defects using the Amplatzer occluder. *J Am Soc Echocardiogr.* 2004;17:62–69.
10. Amin Z. Echocardiographic predictors of cardiac erosion after Amplatzer septal occluder placement. *Catheter Cardiovasc Interv.* 2014;83:84–92.
11. Saric M, Perk G, Purgess JR, et al. Imaging atrial septal defects by real-time three-dimensional transesophageal echocardiography: step-by-step approach. *J Am Soc Echocardiogr.* 2010;23:1128–1135.
12. Razzouk L, Saric M, Slater JN. Placement of a large Gore-Helex atrial septal occluder device in a patient with deficient aortic rim and large atrial septal aneurysm. *Closing Remarks Newsletter.* 2013;XXII.
13. Anderson RH, Becker AE, Tynan M. Description of ventricular septal defects—or how long is a piece of string? *Int J Cardiol.* 1986;13:267–278.
14. Fraisse A, Piechaud JF, Avierinos JF, et al. Transcatheter closure of traumatic ventricular septal defect: an alternative to surgical repair? *Ann Thorac Surg.* 2002;74:582–584.
15. Birnbaum Y, Fishbein MC, Blanche C, Siegel RJ. Ventricular septal rupture after acute myocardial infarction. *N Engl J Med.* 2002;347:1426–1432.
16. Minette MS, Sahn DJ. Ventricular septal defects. *Circulation.* 2006;114:2190–2197.
17. Razzouk L, Applebaum RM, Okamura C, Saric M. The windsock syndrome: subpulmonic obstruction by membranous ventricular septal aneurysm in congenitally corrected transposition of great arteries. *Echocardiography.* 2013;30:E243–E248.
18. Saric MKI. Ventricular septal defect and Eisenmenger syndrome. In: Lang RGS, Kronzon I, Khanderia BK, eds. *Dynamic Echocardiography: A Case-Based Approach.* 1st ed. New York: Springer; 2010:446–450.
19. Stout KK, Daniels CJ, Aboulhosn JA, et al: 2018 AHA/ACC Guideline for the management of adults with congenital heart disease, Circulation 139:e698–e800, 2019.
20. Gilboa SM, Salemi JL, Nembhard WN, et al. Mortality resulting from congenital heart disease among children and adults in the United States, 1999 to 2006. *Circulation.* 2010; 122:2254–2263.
21. Halpern DG, Perk G, Ruiz C, et al. Percutaneous closure of a post-myocardial infarction ventricular septal defect guided by real-time three-dimensional echocardiography. *Eur J Echocardiogr.* 2009;10:569–571.
22. Lock JE, Block PC, McKay RG, et al. Transcatheter closure of ventricular septal defects. *Circulation.* 1988;78:361–368.
23. Holzer R, Balzer D, Amin Z, et al. Transcatheter closure of postinfarction ventricular septal defects using the new Amplatzer muscular VSD occluder: results of a U.S. Registry. *Catheter Cardiovasc Interv.* 2004;61:196–201.
24. Pesonen E, Thilen U, Sandstrom S, et al. Transcatheter closure of post-infarction ventricular septal defect with the Amplatzer Septal Occluder device. *Scand Cardiovasc J.* 2000;34:446–448.
25. Thanopoulos BD, Tsaousis GS, Konstadopoulou GN, Zarayelyan AG. Transcatheter closure of muscular ventricular septal defects with the Amplatzer ventricular septal defect occluder: initial clinical applications in children. *J Am Coll Cardiol.* 1999;33:1395–1399.
26. Rigby ML, Redington AN. Primary transcatheter umbrella closure of perimembranous ventricular septal defect. *Br Heart J.* 1994;72:368–371.
27. Diab KA, Cao QL, Hijazi ZM. Device closure of congenital ventricular septal defects. *Congenit Heart Dis.* 2007;2:92–103.
28. Masura J, Gao W, Gavora P, et al. Percutaneous closure of perimembranous ventricular septal defects using the eccentric Amplatzer device: multicenter follow-up study. *Pediatr Cardiol.* 2005;26:216–219.
29. Hagler DJ, Edwards WD, Seward JB, Tajik AJ. Standardized nomenclature of the ventricular septum and ventricular septal defects, with applications for two-dimensional echocardiography. *Mayo Clin Proc.* 1985;60:741–752.
30. Dall'Agata A, Cromme-Dijkhuis AH, Meijboom FJ, et al. Three-dimensional echocardiography enhances the assessment of ventricular septal defect. *Am J Cardiol.* 1999;83:1576–1579. A8.
31. van den Bosch AE, Ten Harkel DJ, McGhie JS, et al. Feasibility and accuracy of real-time 3-dimensional echocardiographic assessment of ventricular septal defects. *J Am Soc Echocardiogr.* 2006;19:7–13.
32. Holzer R, de Giovanni J, Walsh KP, et al. Transcatheter closure of perimembranous ventricular septal defects using the Amplatzer membranous VSD occluder: Immediate and midterm results of an international registry. *Catheter Cardiovasc Interv.* 2006;68:620–628.
33. Hijazi ZM, Hakim F, Haweleh AA, et al. Catheter closure of perimembranous ventricular septal defects using the new Amplatzer membranous VSD occluder: initial clinical experience. *Catheter Cardiovasc Interv.* 2002;56:508–515.

170 Transcatheter Closure of Cardiac Pseudoaneurysms

Itzhak Kronzon, Carlos E. Ruiz, Gila Perk

Left ventricular (LV) pseudoaneurysm is a rare but serious complication of myocardial infarction (MI), cardiac surgery, trauma, and infection. Medical treatment alone is frequently not effective and is associated with as much as 50% mortality. Until recently, the recommended treatment was surgical closure. These surgeries carried high risk because of abnormal hemodynamics, necrotic substrates, and the comorbidities of these patients. Recently, transcatheter closure has been shown to be an acceptable alternative to open surgical intervention. Multimodality imaging, including three-dimensional (3D) echocardiography, identifies the location, size, and shape of the defect and can assess, guide, and follow up the closure procedure. This chapter discusses the use of transcatheter procedures in the treatment of an important complication of acute MI, namely LV pseudoaneurysm. Medical treatment of these patients carries very poor outcomes with high mortality rates. Surgery can close the defect but still involves high mortality rates. Transcatheter closure of these conditions is feasible and may be an effective alternative therapy in those patients with hemodynamic instability

and other comorbidities. Real-time 3D echocardiography is an important imaging modality in the diagnosis and the assessment of this structural heart disease and has a significant role in guiding and monitoring the interventional procedure.

PATHOPHYSIOLOGY OF LEFT VENTRICULAR PSEUDOANEURYSM

LV free wall rupture is the most common acute tear of the left ventricle in patients with acute MI. Unfortunately, acute free wall tear leads to severe intrapericardial bleeding in most patients, which rapidly results in cardiac tamponade and death. Accordingly, free wall tear accounts for 14% to 20% of all MI-related deaths. In contrast, it is seen in only 7% of all in-hospital MI-related deaths.[1] In other words, most cases of death from acute free wall rupture occur before arrival in the hospital.

On rare occasions, the rupture is contained by pericardial and fibrous tissue, creating a LV pseudoaneurysm. Characteristically, the orifice of the pseudoaneurysm is narrow, with a characteristic to-and-fro blood flow: from the left ventricle into the pseudoaneurysm during systole and from the pseudoaneurysm into the left ventricle during diastole. The pseudoaneurysm wall is made of adherent pericardial or fibrous tissue, without any myocardial or endocardial layers. Thus, the wall is thin and may easily rupture and cause bleeding into the chest cavity and death.

A meta-analysis reviewed the charts and reports of 290 patients with LV pseudoaneurysms.[2] It demonstrated that approximately two-thirds of all LV pseudoaneurysms occur after MI. Pseudoaneurysms are more common in men (75%) and in whites (75%), and the average age of these patients is 60 years. The presenting symptoms in infarct-related pseudoaneurysm included congestive heart failure in 36%, chest pain in 30%, shortness of breath in 25%, and sudden death in 3%. Twelve percent were asymptomatic at the time of presentation.

In this meta-analysis, the maximal diameter of the pseudoaneurysm varied from 1.5 to 20 cm. The pseudoaneurysm involved the posterior and lateral walls more commonly than the anterior wall. It appears that the risk of rupture is higher in the first 3 months after infarction. Later, pseudoaneurysms become chronic and stable and may remain intact for years.[3]

Besides rupture, which may result in bleeding, exsanguination, and cardiac tamponade, other complications include heart failure, arrhythmia, clot formation and embolization, and compression of coronary arteries, which may result in ischemia and compression of extracardiac structures.[4] Pseudoaneurysms can also occur after mitral valve replacement, with a rupture near the posterior aspect of the mitral ring. Other conditions that may lead to LV pseudoaneurysm formation include aortic valve replacement, endocarditis with abscess formation, and penetrating cardiac trauma. Several recent case reports have described apical LV pseudoaneurysm after transcatheter aortic valve implantation.[4–6]

ECHOCARDIOGRAPHIC IMAGING

Echocardiography suggests or establishes the diagnosis in most cases. It shows a loculated echo-free space, which communicates with the left ventricle via a narrow neck or tract. The ratio between the neck diameter and the maximal pseudoaneurysm diameter is less than 0.5 in typical cases.[7] This ratio is used to differentiate a pseudoaneurysm from a true aneurysm. In the latter, the ratio between the communication diameter and the maximal cavity diameter is more than 0.5. It should be noted, however, that exceptions to this numerical rule do exist: The neck of a true aneurysm may be less than 50% of its maximal diameter, whereas the neck of a pseudoaneurysm may be more than 50% of its maximal cavity diameter. Thus, when in doubt, the only accurate way to resolve the differential diagnosis is the demonstration of all cardiac layers in a true aneurysm wall, as oppose to pericardial and fibrous tissue in the wall of a pseudoaneurysm. This information can be obtained only during surgery or at autopsy.[4]

Spectral and color Doppler echocardiography can demonstrate the characteristic to-and-fro flow in the communicating tract (from the left ventricle to the pseudoaneurysm during systole and from the pseudoaneurysm to the ventricle during diastole). Occasionally, when there is an echo-free space near the left ventricle but the communication is not clearly seen, color Doppler and contrast echocardiography can be used to demonstrate the abnormal communication.[8] Therefore, when making the diagnosis of "loculated pericardial effusion," the possibility of pseudoaneurysm should always be considered and explored. Transesophageal echocardiography (TEE), especially real-time 3D TEE, can better demonstrate the anatomy of the pseudoaneurysm and define the size and shape of the communication.

OTHER IMAGING MODALITIES

Other diagnostic imaging modalities include chest radiography, which demonstrates abnormal cardiac silhouette in 65%; cardiac computed tomography (CT); magnetic resonance imaging (MRI); radionuclide studies; and contrast left ventriculography.[4,7–9] The selection of each of these modalities depends on personal experience and preference, availability, and the patient's condition and comorbidities (e.g., MRI is contraindicated in patients with a pacemaker or automatic implanted defibrillator; CT requires contrast injection and ionizing radiation). It is common to use more than one modality for accurate diagnosis and treatment planning.

CLINICAL COURSE AND TREATMENT OPTIONS

Infarction-related pseudoaneurysm is an ominous complication. Until recently, surgery was considered the treatment of choice; however, it is frequently unsuccessful. Suturing into the necrotic myocardium may be unsteady and fail. The quoted surgical mortality rate is 15% to 23%. Medical therapy has higher mortality rate of 30% to 45%.[2]

Transcatheter repair of pseudoaneurysm is now another treatment option. It is best done under fluoroscopic as well as two-dimensional (2D) and real-time 3D TEE and transthoracic echocardiographic surveillance and guidance.[4,7–9,10] The 3D image can be helpful in the selection of the closure device. Other imaging modalities such as CT scan are frequently used as well in preparation for a surgical or transcatheter procedure.

Fig. 170.1 shows a case of an anterior wall infarct with a large pseudoaneurysm. After establishing the diagnosis, a decision was made to close the pseudoaneurysm via an apical approach. CT imaging shows the pseudoaneurysm, which is connected to the left ventricle by a narrow neck (arrow). Using 3D real-time TEE, a direct percutaneous needle puncture of the pseudoaneurysm was performed. Thereafter, a wire followed by a catheter was advanced from the puncture site through the communicating tract into the LV cavity. A closure device (Amplatzer, Abbott) was then deployed to close the communication. On withdrawal of all catheters, another Amplatzer closure device was deployed at the pseudoaneurysm puncture site. The patient recovered without complications.

The aneurysmal cavity can be approached from the LV cavity or by chest wall puncture, as in the case described. The selection of the approach and the nature of the closure method depend on the site, size, and shape of the pseudoaneurysm and on operator preference and experience. Smaller pseudoaneurysms can be closed by a coil or even by the combination of coil (to clot the pseudoaneurysm cavity) and a closure device to close the communication.

Fig. 170.2 shows a case of LV outflow pseudoaneurysm as a result of endocarditis in a patient with a prosthetic aortic valve. The endocarditis was successfully treated medically, and there were no residual signs or markers of infection. 2D and 3D echocardiography clearly demonstrated the 2.5- × 1.7-cm pseudoaneurysm cavity, which communicated with the LV outflow tract through a small perforation in the intervalvular fibrosa. A characteristic to-and-fro flow was documented by color and spectral Doppler. After LV apical puncture, a wire followed by a catheter were advanced into the pseudoaneurysm cavity via the communication. Coils were used to completely eliminate the pseudoaneurysm cavity (Fig. 170.3). Pseudoaneurysm can also be observed in the right ventricle, in the atria, and in arteries and veins.

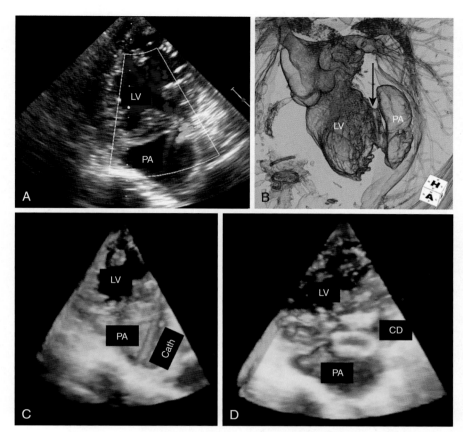

Figure 170.1. Postinfarction left ventricular pseudoaneurysm (PA). Color Doppler interrogation of the left ventricular PA. **A,** Systolic frame, with blood flow from the left ventricle (LV) into the PA. **B,** Three-dimensional computed tomography demonstrates the characteristic PA with a narrow neck and wider aneurysm cavity. *Arrow* indicates the communication tract between the PA and the LV. **C,** A catheter (Cath) seen entering from the chest wall into the PA cavity and across the communication tract into the left ventricle. **D,** The closure device (CD) in place, sealing the PA communication. *Ao,* Aorta.

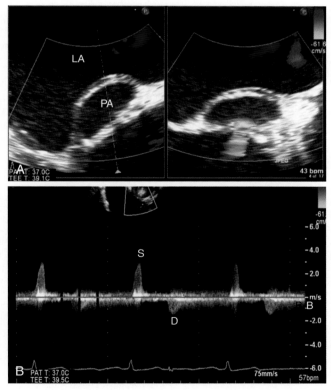

Figure 170.2. Left ventricular outflow tract pseudoaneurysm (PA). **A,** Diastolic frame, transesophageal echocardiographic midesophageal long-axis view. Color Doppler shows to-and-fro flow from the PA to the left ventricular outflow tract. (See accompanying Video 170.2A.) **B,** Continuous-wave Doppler demonstrates the characteristic to-and-fro flow. *D,* Diastolic blood flow; *LA,* left atrium; *S,* systolic blood flow.

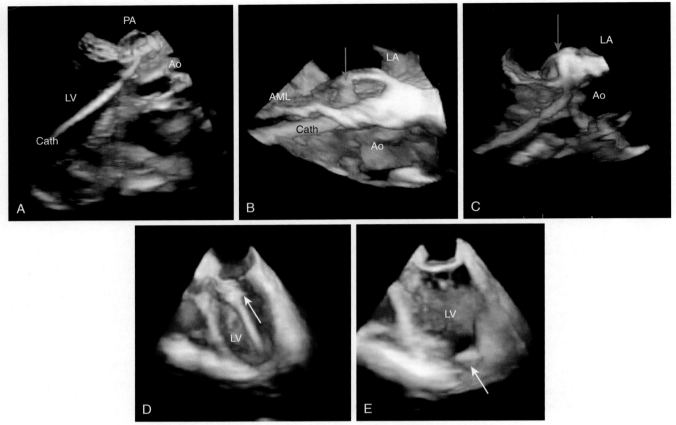

Figure 170.3. Closure of left ventricular outflow tract aneurysm. **A,** Real-time, three-dimensional transesophageal echocardiography shows a catheter (Cath) advanced from the left ventricular apex to the pseudoaneurysm (PA) track. **B,** Magnified image. The tip of the catheter can be seen in the pseudoaneurysm cavity *(arrow)*. **C,** The pseudoaneurysm cavity is filled with coils and obliterated. **D,** The catheter with a closure device *(arrow)* is withdrawn toward the apex. **E,** The device occludes the apical perforation *(arrow)*. *AML,* Anterior mitral leaflet; *Ao,* aorta; *LA,* left atrium; *LV,* left ventricle. (See accompanying Video 170.3.)

CONCLUSION

Recent advances in cardiac imaging allow for better evaluation of cardiac anatomy and pathology. Real-time 3D echocardiography and other imaging modalities can provide accurate online information that may lead to better diagnosis and treatment of LV pseudoaneurysm. At present, there are no written guidelines for pseudoaneurysm closure. The outcomes of transcutaneous versus surgical closure results have not yet been studied. It is hoped that the less invasive approach will lead to better results and improved survival of patients with these complications.

Please access ExpertConsult to view the corresponding videos for this chapter.

REFERENCES

1. Reddy SG, Roberts WC. Frequency of rupture of the left ventricular free wall or ventricular septum among necropsy cases of fatal acute myocardial infarction since the introduction of coronary care units. *Am J Cardiol.* 1989;63:906–911.
2. Frances C, Romero A, Grady D. Left ventricular pseudoaneurysm. *J Am Coll Cardiol.* 1998;32:557–561.
3. Yoo TC, Malouf JP, Oh JK, et al. Clinical profile and outcome in 52 patients with cardiac pseudoaneurysms. *Ann Intern Med.* 1998;128:299–305.
4. Hulten EA, Blankstein R. Pseudoaneurysm of the heart. *Circulation.* 2012;125(5):1920–1925.
5. Feldman T, Pearson P, Smart SS. Percutaneous closure of post TAVR LV apical pseudoaneurysm. *Catheter Cardiovasc Interv.* 2016;88(3):479–485.
6. Okuyama K, Chakravarty T, Makkar RR. Percutaneous transapical pseudoaneurysm closure following transcatheter aortic valve replacement. *Catheter Cardiovasc Interv.* 2018;91:159–164.
7. Gatewood RP, Nanda NC. Differentiation of left ventricular pseudoaneurysm from true aneurysm with two dimensional echocardiography. *Am J Cardiol.* 1980;46:869–878.
8. Tunick PA, Slater W, Kronzon I. The hemodynamics of left ventricular pseudoaneurysm: color Doppler echocardiographic study. *Am Heart J.* 1989;117:116–117.
9. Narayan RL, Vaishnava P, Goldman ME, et al. Percutaneous closure of left ventricular pseudoaneurysm. *Ann Thorac Surg.* 2012;94:e123–e125.
10. Dudiy Y, Jelnin V, Einhorn BN, et al. Percutaneous closure of left ventricular pseudoaneurysm. *Circ Cardiovasc Interv.* 2011;4:322–326.

171 Echocardiographic Imaging of Left Atrial Appendage Occlusion

Alan F. Vainrib, Muhamed Saric

Atrial fibrillation (AF) is the most common cardiac arrhythmia in the world, affecting more than 3 million people in the United States alone. AF is defined as a supraventricular tachyarrhythmia characterized by uncoordinated atrial activation and consequent deterioration of mechanical atrial function.[1] The incidence of AF in the United States is projected to increase to 7.56 million by 2050 as the population ages.[2] AF may be considered valvular or nonvalvular in cause. Stroke and other manifestations of systemic thromboembolism can occur in both valvular and nonvalvular AF. As per the 2014 intersociety guidelines, nonvalvular AF is defined as "AF in the absence of rheumatic mitral stenosis, a mechanical or bioprosthetic heart valve, or mitral valve repair."[3] The need for a distinction between "valvular" and "nonvalvular" AF stems from the possibility of two distinct pathogenic mechanisms of thrombogenesis. The left atrial appendage (LAA) is the site of thrombus formation in approximately 91% of patients with nonvalvular AF and 57% of patients with valvular AF.[4] Even though most AF-related thrombi form locally in the LAA, systemic anticoagulation has been the preferred method of thromboembolism prevention. However, systemic anticoagulants may be associated with significant bleeding risk (≤1.4% to >3% per year) and are contraindicated in certain patients.[5] Both surgical and percutaneous approaches to LAA closure devised as alternatives to systemic anticoagulation are discussed in this chapter.

LEFT ATRIAL APPENDAGE ANATOMY SPECIFIC TO LEFT ATRIAL APPENDAGE OCCLUSION

The LAA is a remnant of the primitive embryonic let atrium (LA). The remainder of the adult LA derives from the primitive pulmonary veins. The LAA is a complex structure and arises from the anterolateral portion of the LA. The interface between the LAA and the LA is the anatomic orifice, which is typically ovoid, separated from the left-sided pulmonary veins by the ligament of Marshall (also referred to as the left lateral or "Coumadin" ridge). The orifice then progresses to the neck region, then to the body, and ultimately ends in the apex. The LAA may additionally contain one or more lobes, defined as protrusions from its main body. The so-called "landing zone" region within the LAA is a virtual region specific for placement of endocardially delivered LAA occlusion devices.

There are multiple anatomic variants of the LAA that may impact LAA closure. These include the windsock, cactus, cauliflower (or broccoli), and chicken wing morphologies.[6] The chicken wing LAA typically has a broad orifice or landing zone region and a shallow depth, which poses a unique challenge to percutaneous endocardially delivered intra-LAA closure devices. This is in contrast to epicardially delivered or extra-LAA closure devices, which are less affected by LAA anatomic variations.

SURGICAL LEFT ATRIAL APPENDAGE CLOSURE

The first surgical amputation of the LAA was likely performed in New York by the renowned cardiothoracic surgeon John L. Madden at King's County hospital in February 1948.[7] However, soon after this, surgical LAA amputation was no longer favored because of poor postoperative outcomes, and the newly discovered vitamin K antagonists demonstrated efficacy in providing systemic anticoagulation.[8]

After more than 40 years of dormancy, enthusiasm for surgical LAA closure was reborn in the 1990s by Cox with the Maze procedure, which included LAA removal and became routine during mitral valve surgery.[9,10] Multiple techniques and devices have been developed for surgical LAA exclusion. These have included stapled excision, LAA removal with neck ligation, stump oversew, purse-string techniques, radiofrequency tissue fusion, and the AtriClip (Atricure) a novel LAA exclusion clip.[11–13] Because surgical LAA closure is typically performed as an adjunct to other cardiac surgeries, the number of eligible patients for this type of therapy may be limited.

COMMON STEPS FOR ALL PERCUTANEOUS LEFT ATRIAL APPENDAGE OCCLUSION PROCEDURES

All percutaneous LAA occluder implantation procedures require peripheral venous access, typically via a femoral vein; however, a superior vena cava (SVC) approach has been described.[14] Subsequently, transseptal puncture is performed to access the LA from the right atrium (RA). After transseptal puncture, specific steps for deployments of individual occluder devices are taken. From the transfemoral approach, a delivery catheter and dilator are passed through the inferior vena cava into the RA and then temporarily placed in the SVC. Under fluoroscopic and transesophageal echocardiography (TEE) guidance, a needle–catheter assembly is then withdrawn from the SVC into the RA and positioned against the interatrial septum. Echocardiographic guidance is crucial for proper transseptal puncture. Typically, the ideal location for transseptal puncture in LAA closure procedures is the inferoposterior portion of the interatrial septum, which provides the most direct route to the anterolaterally located LAA. When the echocardiographer provides real-time TEE imaging to an interventionalist, it is useful to label superior, inferior, anterior, and posterior location in the echocardiographic image (Fig. 171.1). After proper position is confirmed, the needle is advanced, creating a transseptal puncture. Subsequently, the dilator and sheath are then advanced into the LA together to avoid wall injury. A wire is then inserted into the LAA that is typically positioned in the left superior pulmonary vein, and finally the dilator and sheath are removed.

Atrial septal aneurysm (ASA) and marked lipomatous atrial septal hypertrophy (LASH) may present anatomic challenges to successful transseptal puncture. ASA is associated with a highly mobile interatrial septum and may increase the risk for LA wall perforation. In the presence of LASH, the thin central portion of the fossa ovalis should be punctured if possible, as opposed to the hypertrophied limbs.[15] Three-dimensional (3D) TEE imaging using 3D zoom of the interatrial septum may be helpful in guiding TS puncture to the inferior and posterior location. A step-by-step approach for the production of high-quality views of the interatrial septum by 3D TEE has been previously described using the TUPLE (tilt up then left) maneuver.[16]

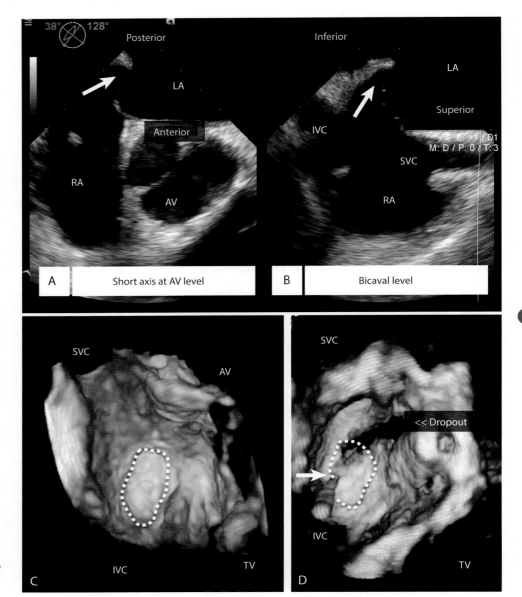

Figure 171.1. Two-dimensional transesophageal echocardiography (TEE) images with biplane imaging demonstrate the interatrial septum in the midesophageal short-axis and bicaval views during the transseptal puncture portion of a left atrial appendage (LAA) occlusion procedure (**A** and **B**). Note the tenting in the inferior and posterior portion of the fossa ovalis, which is the ideal location for puncture. (Videos 171.1A and 171.B correspond to **A** and **B**.) Three-dimensional TEE of the interatrial septum from the right atrial perspective at baseline before transseptal puncture (**C**) and after transseptal puncture (**D**). This view demonstrates the anatomic location of the fossa ovalis (*white dotted circles*) at baseline (**C**) and catheter-related dropout (**D**). AV, Aortic valve; *LA,* left atrium; *IVC,* inferior vena cava; *PA,* pulmonary artery; *RA,* right atrium; *SVC,* superior vena cava; *TV,* tricuspid valve. (Reprinted with permission from Vainrib AF, et al: Left atrial appendage occlusion/exclusion: Procedural image guidance with transesophageal echocardiography, *J Am Soc Echocardiogr* 31:454–474, 2018.)

Percutaneous Left Atrial Appendage Occlusion Devices

Percutaneous LAA occlusion devices may be purely endocardially delivered such as the Watchman Classic and Watchman FLX (Boston Scientific), WaveCrest (Biosense Webster), and Amulet (St. Jude Medical), or both endocardially and pericardially delivered such as the Lariat (Sentre-HEART).

Watchman Procedure (Classic and FLX)

The Watchman and Watchman FLX devices are constructed using self-expanding nickel titanium (also referred to as Nitinol) with covered by a permeable polyester fabric. The Watchman shape is crownlike, with its the outer portion surrounded by multiple protrusions that are referred to as fixation barbs (Watchman) or anchors (Watchman FLX). The Watchman family of devices are delivered purely endocardially using fluoroscopic and echocardiographic guidance. Both Watchman classic and Watchman FLX devices are each available in five sizes (classic; 21, 24, 27, 30, and 33; FLX; 20, 24, 27, 31, and 34 mm). The Watchman FLX has a longer covering of polyethylene terephthalate (PET) fabric, more anchors, an atraumatic closed end, and a shorter device length.

TEE is essential for preprocedural LAA sizing. LAA orifice size and LAA depth are measured on two-dimensional (2D) TEE imaging at 0, 45, 90, and 135 degrees (Fig. 171.2) to determine the maximal LAA orifice diameter and appendage depth. For the Watchman, the LAA orifice is measured from the top of the mitral valve annulus or circumflex coronary artery to a point 2 cm below the tip of the left upper pulmonary vein limbus. Depth is measured from the plane of the LAA orifice to the LAA apex.

The Watchman procedure begins with venous access and transseptal puncture as described earlier. Subsequently, the Watchman 12-Fr delivery system with a pigtail catheter is advanced into the LA over the wire and then placed into the LAA. Next, iodinated contrast is injected into the LAA to define its anatomy on fluoroscopy. The Watchman device is then positioned and delivered in the LAA ostium. The Watchman FLX is initially positioned while partially deployed, a configuration referred to as the "ball." The Watchman classic is fully deployed using the position of the distal end of the delivery sheath.

Before device release, four PASS (position, anchor, size, and seal) criteria must be met (Fig. 171.3). When assessing for paradevice leak (PDL), a low Nyquist limit (~30 cm/s) is recommended to detect low-velocity flow.[17] 3D TEE with color Doppler imaging may also

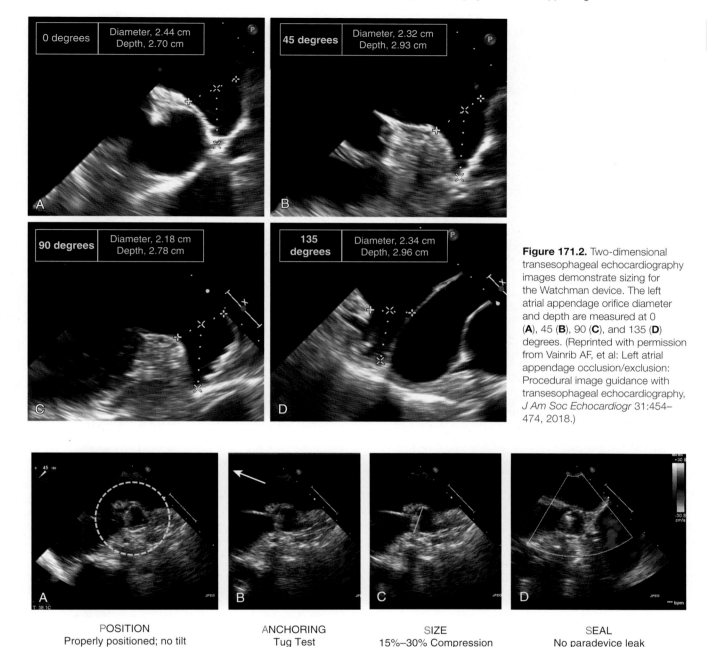

Figure 171.2. Two-dimensional transesophageal echocardiography images demonstrate sizing for the Watchman device. The left atrial appendage orifice diameter and depth are measured at 0 (**A**), 45 (**B**), 90 (**C**), and 135 (**D**) degrees. (Reprinted with permission from Vainrib AF, et al: Left atrial appendage occlusion/exclusion: Procedural image guidance with transesophageal echocardiography, *J Am Soc Echocardiogr* 31:454–474, 2018.)

POSITION
Properly positioned; no tilt

ANCHORING
Tug Test

SIZE
15%–30% Compression

SEAL
No paradevice leak

Figure 171.3. Before release of the Watchman left atrial appendage (LAA) occluder device, four so-called PASS (position, anchor, size, and seal) criteria must be met. **A,** First, the Watchman device must be properly positioned within the LAA orifice (i.e., not tilted). **B,** Second, the device cannot demonstrate excessive motion on the "tug test" (i.e., the device is pulled backward while still attached to the threaded insert and visualized using fluoroscopy and echocardiography). **C,** Third, compression measurements are performed at 0, 45, 90, and 135 degrees. A line is drawn from shoulder to shoulder with the threaded insert in view (this is located in the center of the device) to ensure that the device is measured at the location of its maximal width. **D,** Finally, a paradevice leak smaller than 5 mm is considered an adequate seal between the device and the LAA. If any of the PASS criteria are not met, the Watchman device can be recaptured and then repositioned, or a new device size may be selected. (Reprinted with permission from Vainrib AF, et al: Left atrial appendage occlusion/exclusion: Procedural image guidance with transesophageal echocardiography, *J Am Soc Echocardiogr* 31:454–474, 2018.)

be performed, which provides additional information regarding the circumferential extent of PDL (Fig. 171.4). Suboptimal implantation and device-related complications may include device shoulder (Fig. 171.5) and device-associated thrombus (Fig. 171.6).

After Watchman device deployment, the delivery catheter is withdrawn from the LAA and LA. At this point, color Doppler may be applied to the interatrial septum to assess the size of transseptal related atrial septal defect (ASD). ASDs less than 10 mm in size are common. Transseptal-related ASDs larger than 10 mm are unusual and may require percutaneous closure with an ASD occluder device.

Amulet Procedure

The Amulet device is constructed from self-expanding nitinol covered in handsewn polyester mesh. The device consists of a lobe and disk that are connected by a central articulating waist. The lobe

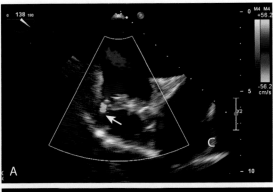

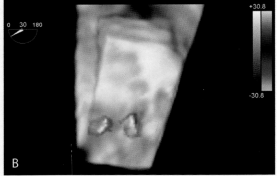

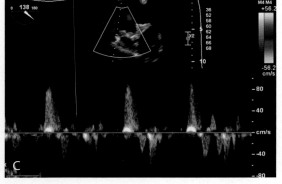

Figure 171.4. Color and spectral Doppler demonstrate a paradevice leak on the inferior edge of a Watchman left atrial appendage (LAA) occluder. **A,** Leak on 2D TEE (arrow; also Video 171.4A). **B,** Leak on 3D TEE consists of two small jets. **C,** Spectral pulsed-wave Doppler confirms a communication is present between the left atrium and LAA, adjacent to a Watchman LAA occluder. (Reprinted with permission from Vainrib AF, et al: Left atrial appendage occlusion/exclusion: Procedural image guidance with transesophageal echocardiography, *J Am Soc Echocardiogr* 31:454–474, 2018.)

portion of the Amulet serves as the key anchoring mechanism and is implanted approximately 10 to 12 mm distal to the anatomic LAA. The Amulet is supported within the LAA by stabilizing wires located circumferentially on the lobe. The disk portion of the device is deployed in the LA and abuts the LAA orifice, which provides an additional seal. The Amulet comes in eight sizes, which correspond to the lobe diameter (16, 18, 20, 22, 25, 28, 31, and 34 mm). The wider range of Amulet sizes may accommodate both larger and small LAA sizes than the Watchman. The "proximal end screw,"

located in the center of the device, is similar to the "threaded insert" of the Watchman. This portion is recessed, which serves to reduce the risk of device-associated thrombus. TEE is essential for preprocedural LAA sizing (Fig. 171.7). The Amulet "ball" is positioned in the "Amulet landing zone" of the LAA (10–12 mm from the LAA ostium). The device lobe and disk are then sequentially deployed (Fig. 171.8).

WaveCrest

The WaveCrest 1.3 device consists of a self-expanding nitinol frame with 20 anchoring points, covered by an expanded polytetrafluoroethylene (ePTFE, also known as Gore-Tex) fabric. It comes in three sizes (22, 27, and 32 mm). The steps for guidance of the WaveCrest device are similar to those for the Watchman and Amulet devices. However, during TEE imaging, the WaveCrest device creates acoustic shadowing because of the presence of air between layers of WaveCrest ePTFE fabric may partly hinder echocardiographic assessment of device seal. Acoustic shadowing diminishes and echocardiographic imaging improves after device endothelialization (Fig. 171.9).[18]

Lariat Procedure

Percutaneous LAA closure with the Lariat device consists of both endocardially and epicardially delivered magnetic tipped wires that unite at the distal LAA wall. This creates a rail for delivery of a pretied suture that ultimately ligates the LAA. Because this device does not leave any device in contact with the bloodstream,[19] it does not typically require postprocedural warfarin therapy.[20,21]

TEE is important for preprocedural LAA sizing (Fig. 171.10). The Lariat procedure typically begins with pericardial access, which is typically performed using fluoroscopic guidance only. However, TEE imaging of the right ventricle (RV) during pericardial access can be helpful to demonstrate that the right RV has not been punctured. Subsequently, transseptal puncture is performed using 2D and 3D TEE guidance as described earlier. A wire is then inserted into the LA and positioned in the left superior pulmonary vein, and the dilator and sheath are removed. Through a Lariat delivery catheter, a 15-mm balloon-tipped catheter (EndoCATH) backloaded with a magnet-tipped 0.025-inch guidewire is advanced into the LAA. The magnet wire tip is then advanced toward the LAA apex and the deflated balloon placed at the ostium of the LAA. The balloon is subsequently inflated, acting as a target for snare placement, and provides support to prevent slippage of the suture during tightening.[22] Next, an end-to-end magnet union is created between the radiopaque markers on the distal tips of the pericardial and endocardial wires. The Lariat snare is then advanced epicardially over the LAA to the ostium and tightened.

On echocardiography, Color Doppler is applied to the area of the ligated LAA, to assess for residual communication between the LA and LAA. Color Doppler flows of greater than 5 mm using a low (<40 cm/s) Nyquist limit may require device alteration. After adequate ligation of the LAA is confirmed on echocardiography (Figs. 171.11 and 171.12), the endocardial balloon catheter and endocardial wire are removed from the LAA. Finally, the epicardial suture is released from the snare and tightened, which excludes the LAA. On 3D TEE, the ligated LAA demonstrates what we refer to as a "bowtie" appearance. At the end of the procedure, an assessment of ASD at the site of transseptal puncture is performed, similar to the other percutaneous LAA closure devices.

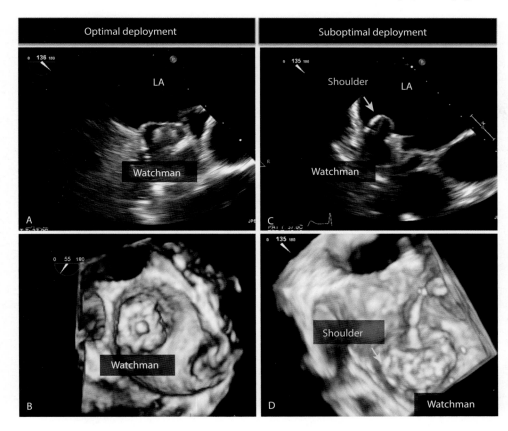

Figure 171.5. Two-dimensional transesophageal echocardiography (TEE) images at 135-degree view and three-dimensional TEE demonstrate optimal and suboptimal Watchman device deployment. The device should be optimally be deployed parallel to the left atrial appendage orifice (**A** and **B**). (Videos 171.5 and 171.5B correspond to **A** and **B**.) If the device is excessively tilted, a device "shoulder" will be visualized (**C** and **D**). To ensure an adequate seal, the extent of the shoulder cannot be greater than 40% to 50% of the device height. (Videos 171.5C and 171.5D correspond to **C** and **D**.) *LA,* Left atrium. (Reprinted with permission from Vainrib AF, et al: Left atrial appendage occlusion/exclusion: Procedural image guidance with transesophageal echocardiography, *J Am Soc Echocardiogr* 31:454–474, 2018.)

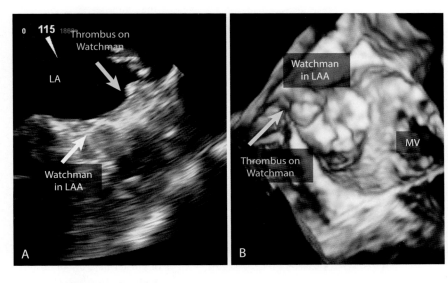

Figure 171.6. Two- (**A**) and three-dimensional (**B**) transesophageal echocardiography images demonstrate a Watchman associated thrombus. The thrombus originates at the "threaded-insert" portion of the Watchman device and propagates outward. (Videos 171.6A and 171.6B correspond to this figure.) *LA,* Left atrium; *LAA,* left atrial appendage; *MV,* mitral valve. (Reprinted with permission from Vainrib AF, et al: Left atrial appendage occlusion/exclusion: Procedural image guidance with transesophageal echocardiography, *J Am Soc Echocardiogr* 31:454–474, 2018.)

POSTPROCEDURAL FOLLOW-UP TRANSESOPHAGEAL ECHOCARDIOGRAPHY

After an endocardial LAA closure device (Watchman, Amulet, or WaveCrest) is implanted, it takes approximately 45 days for device endothelialization to occur. With this in mind, a 45-day follow-up TEE examination is typically performed in clinical practice, mirroring the major clinical trials evaluating the Watchman.[23,24]

CONCLUSIONS

Although the history of mechanical LAA closure for thromboprophylaxis in AF has been complex, advances in structural heart intervention have led to a recent interest in minimally invasive LAA exclusion. Recent noninferiority studies have supported the concept that local therapy on the LAA appears to be a feasible and effective alternative to systemic anticoagulation. Percutaneous LAA occlusion creates a new option for stroke risk reduction in patients who are either high risk or ineligible for systemic anticoagulation in nonvalvular AF. In conjunction with fluoroscopy, high-quality 2D and 3D TEE imaging is critical for successful implantation of all of the percutaneous LAA occluder devices. The echocardiographer is essential in these procedures. Echocardiographers identify exclusion criteria, delineate LAA anatomy, provide LAA landing zone measurements for device sizing, guide the location of transseptal puncture and position of catheters, and assess procedural success and complications.

Please access ExpertConsult to view the corresponding videos for this chapter.

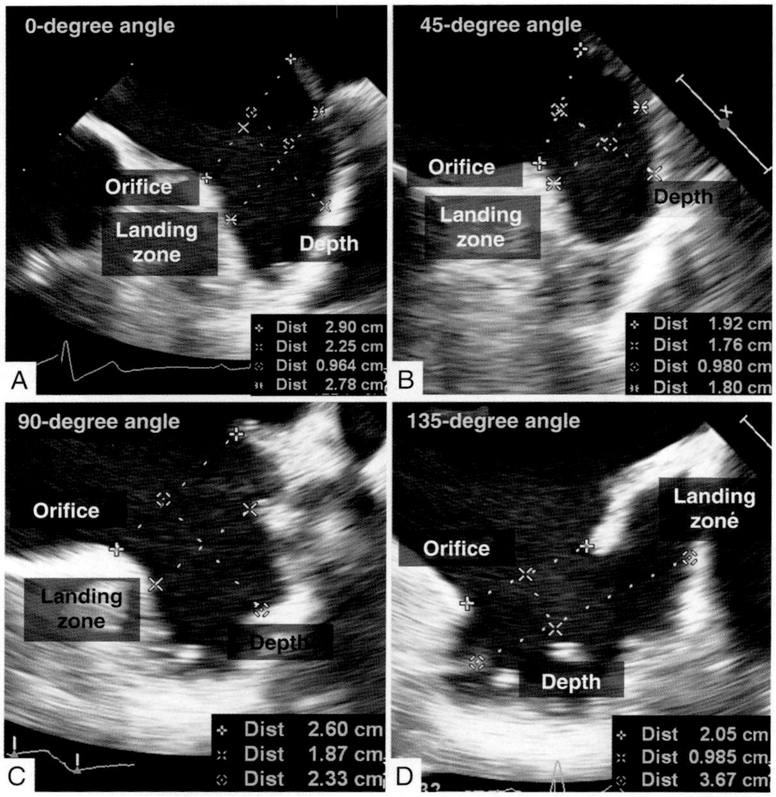

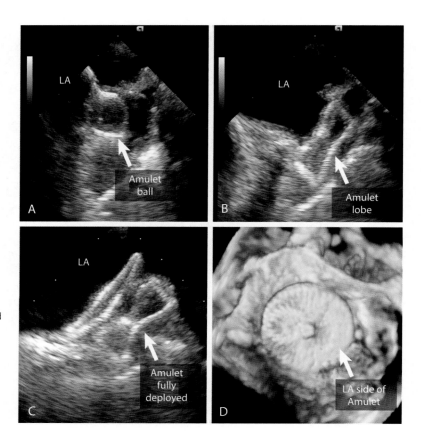

Figure 171.7. Two-dimensional transesophageal echocardiography demonstrates sizing for the Amulet device. The left atrial appendage (LAA) ostium diameter, landing zone diameter, and depth are measured at 0 (**A**), 45 (**B**), 90 (**C**), and 135 (**D**) degrees. Note that the landing zone diameter is measured 10 to 12 mm from the ostium and that the depth is measured from the ostium to the LAA wall in a plane perpendicular to the ostium. (Reprinted with permission from Vainrib AF, et al: Left atrial appendage occlusion/exclusion: Procedural image guidance with transesophageal echocardiography, *J Am Soc Echocardiogr* 31:454–474, 2018.)

Figure 171.8. Two- and three-dimensional transesophageal echocardiography demonstrates the stages of Amulet deployment. First, the partially deployed Amulet lobe also known as the "ball" is deployed (**A**). Subsequently, the lobe is fully deployed (**B**). Finally, the disk is deployed, and the Amulet is released (**C** and **D**). (Video 171.8 corresponds to this figure.) *LA,* Left atrium. (Reprinted with permission from Vainrib AF, et al: Left atrial appendage occlusion/exclusion: Procedural image guidance with transesophageal echocardiography, *J Am Soc Echocardiogr* 31:454–474, 2018.)

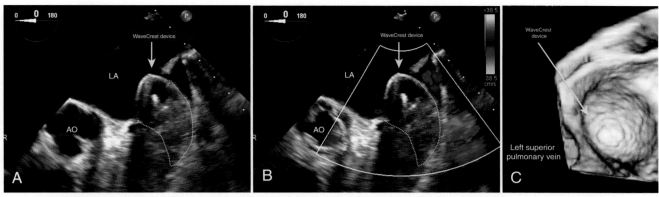

Figure 171.9. Forty-five-day follow-up two-dimensional transesophageal echocardiography (TEE) imaging in the midesophageal left atrial appendage view at 0 degrees (**A**) demonstrates a better visualized WaveCrest device compared with intraprocedural TEE as air between fabric layers has receded. Color Doppler shows no significant paradevice leak (**B**, Videos 171.9A and 171.9B). Three-dimensional TEE imaging also improves on 45-day follow up compared with intraprocedural study (**C**; Video 171.9C). *AO,* Aorta; *LA,* left atrium. (Reprinted with permission from Vainrib AF, et al: Echocardiographic guidance of the novel WaveCrest left atrial appendage occlusion device, *CASE* 2:297–300, 2018.)

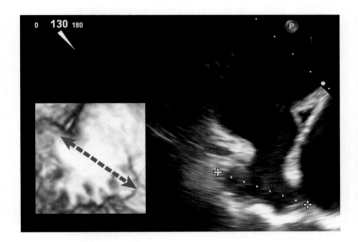

Figure 171.10. Three-dimensional computed tomographic volume-rendered image superimposed on a two-dimensional transesophageal echocardiography image demonstrates the left atrial appendage maximum width *(blue double arrow)*, which should be 45 mm or less. (Reprinted with permission from Vainrib AF, et al: Left atrial appendage occlusion/exclusion: Procedural image guidance with transesophageal echocardiography, *J Am Soc Echocardiogr* 31:454–474, 2018.)

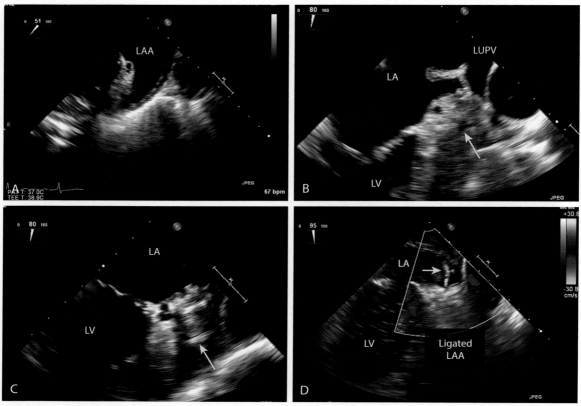

Figure 171.11. Transesophageal echocardiography (TEE) assessment of LARIAT closure of the left atrial appendage (LAA). **A,** Two-dimensional TEE appearance of the LAA before LARIAT closure. **B,** Typical appearance of the LAA after LARIAT ligation. **C,** Appearance of a ligated LAA in another patient. In this patient, the presence of a pericardial effusion outlines the ligated appendage *(arrow)*. **D,** After the LARIAT snare is deployed but before removal of the endocardial catheter from the LAA, a small degree of central leak *(arrow)* may be seen on color Doppler imaging. (See accompanying Videos 171.11B–D.) *LA,* Left atrium; *LV,* left ventricle; *LUPV,* left upper pulmonary vein. (Reprinted with permission from Vainrib AF, et al: Left atrial appendage occlusion/exclusion: Procedural image guidance with transesophageal echocardiography, *J Am Soc Echocardiogr* 31:454–474, 2018.)

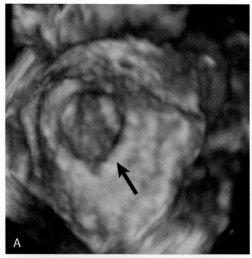

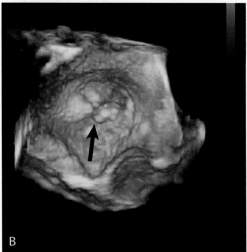

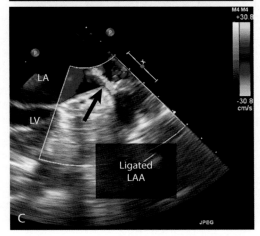

Figure 171.12. A, Three-dimensional transesophageal echocardiography (TEE) appearance of left atrial appendage (LAA) at baseline and after ligation. Three-dimensional TEE zoom imaging demonstrates the en face view of the LAA orifice seen from the left atrial perspective. At baseline, there is a widely patent orifice of the LAA *(arrow)*. **B,** After completion of the LARIAT suture ligation, the LAA orifice is completely closed. The *arrow* points to the location of the suture. Note the "bowtie" appearance of the ligated LAA orifice. **C,** After completion of the LARIAT procedure, there are typically no residual leaks between the left atrium and LAA. If there is residual leak, it is typically solitary and central, as shown in this panel *(arrow)*. (Video 171.12C corresponds to **C**.) *LA,* Left atrium; LV, left ventricle. (Reprinted with permission from Vainrib AF, et al: Left atrial appendage occlusion/exclusion: Procedural image guidance with transesophageal echocardiography, *J Am Soc Echocardiogr* 31:454–474, 2018.)

REFERENCES

1. Fuster V, Ryden LE, Cannom DS, et al. ACCF/AHA/HRS focused updates incorporated into the ACC/AHA/ESC 2006 guidelines for the management of patients with atrial fibrillation. *J Am Coll Cardiol.* 2011;57:e101–198. 2011.
2. Naccarelli GV, Varker H, Lin J, Schulman KL. Increasing prevalence of atrial fibrillation and flutter in the United States. *Am J Cardiol.* 2009;104:1534–1539.
3. January CT, Wann LS, Alpert JS, et al. AHA/ACC/HRS guideline for the management of patients with atrial fibrillation. *J Am Coll Cardiol.* 2014;64:e1–76. 2014.
4. Blackshear JL, Odell JA. Appendage obliteration to reduce stroke in cardiac surgical patients with atrial fibrillation. *Ann Thorac Surg.* 1996;61:755–779.
5. Hughes M, Lip GY, et al. Risk factors for anticoagulation-related bleeding complications in patients with atrial fibrillation: a systematic review. *QJM.* 2007;100:599–607.
6. Beigel R, Wunderlich NC, Ho SY, et al. The left atrial appendage: anatomy, function, and noninvasive evaluation. *JACC Cardiovasc Imag.* 2014;7:1251–1265.
7. Madden JL. Resection of the left auricular appendix: a prophylaxis for recurrent arterial emboli. *J Am Med Assoc.* 1949;140:769–772.

8. Leonard FC, Cogan MA. Failure of ligation of the left auricular appendage in the prevention of recurrent embolism. *N Engl J Med.* 1952;246:733–735.
9. Cox JL. The surgical treatment of atrial fibrillation. IV. Surgical technique. *J Thorac Cardiovasc Surg.* 1991;101:584–592.
10. Sakellaridis T, Argiriou M, Charitos C, et al. Left atrial appendage exclusion—where do we stand? *J Thorac Dis.* 2014;6(suppl 1):S70–S77.
11. Johnson WD, Ganjoo AK, Stone CD, et al. The left atrial appendage: our most lethal human attachment! Surgical implications. *Eur J Cardio Thorac Surg.* 2000;17:718–722.
12. Healey JS, Crystal E, Lamy A, et al. Left Atrial Appendage Occlusion Study (LAAOS): results of a randomized controlled pilot study of left atrial appendage occlusion during coronary bypass surgery in patients at risk for stroke. *Am Heart J.* 2005;150:288–293.
13. Emmert MY, Puippe G, Baumuller S, et al. Safe, effective and durable epicardial left atrial appendage clip occlusion in patients with atrial fibrillation undergoing cardiac surgery: first long-term results from a prospective device trial. *Eur J Cardio Thorac Surg.* 2014;45:126–131.
14. Aizer A, Young W, Saric M, et al. Three-dimensional transesophageal echocardiography to facilitate transseptal puncture and left atrial appendage occlusion via upper extremity venous access. *Circ Arrhythm Electrophysiol.* 2015;8:988–990.
15. Laura DM, Donnino R, Kim EE, et al. Lipomatous atrial septal hypertrophy: a review of its anatomy, pathophysiology, multimodality imaging, and relevance to percutaneous interventions. *J Am Soc Echocardiogr.* 2016;29:717–723.
16. Saric M, Perk G, Purgess JR, Kronzon I. Imaging atrial septal defects by real-time three-dimensional transesophageal echocardiography: step-by-step approach. *J Am Soc Echocardiogr.* 2010;23:1128–1135.
17. Tzikas A, Holmes Jr DR, Gafoor S, et al. Percutaneous left atrial appendage occlusion: the Munich consensus document on definitions, endpoints, and data collection requirements for clinical studies. *Europace.* 2017;19:4–15.
18. Vainrib AF, Bamira D, Benenstein RJ, et al. Echocardiographic guidance of the novel WaveCrest left atrial appendage occlusion device. *CASE.* 2018;2:297–300.
19. Bartus K, Han FT, Bednarek J, et al. Percutaneous left atrial appendage suture ligation using the LARIAT device in patients with atrial fibrillation: initial clinical experience. *J Am Coll Cardiol.* 2013;62:108–118.
20. Massumi A, Chelu MG, Nazeri A, et al. Initial experience with a novel percutaneous left atrial appendage exclusion device in patients with atrial fibrillation, increased stroke risk, and contraindications to anticoagulation. *Am J Cardiol.* 2013;111:869–873.
21. Patel TK, Yancy CW, Knight BP. Left atrial appendage exclusion for stroke prevention in atrial fibrillation. *Cardiol Res Pract.* 2012:610827. 2012.
22. Singh SM, Dukkipati SR, d'Avila A, et al. Percutaneous left atrial appendage closure with an epicardial suture ligation approach: a prospective randomized pre-clinical feasibility study. *Heart Rhythm.* 2010;7:370–376.
23. Holmes DR, Reddy VY, Turi ZG, et al. Percutaneous closure of the left atrial appendage versus warfarin therapy for prevention of stroke in patients with atrial fibrillation: a randomised non-inferiority trial. *Lancet.* 2009;374:534–542.
24. Holmes Jr DR, Kar S, Price MJ, et al. Prospective randomized evaluation of the Watchman Left Atrial Appendage Closure device in patients with atrial fibrillation versus long-term warfarin therapy: the PREVAIL trial. *J Am Coll Cardiol.* 2014;64:1–12.

172 Periprosthetic Leaks

Nadeen N. Faza, Stephen H. Little

Paravalvular regurgitation (PVR) is a serious and underdiagnosed problem of prosthetic valves. It occurs in 7% to 17% of surgical mitral prosthetic valves and 2% to 10% of aortic prosthetic valves. Approximately 74% of PVR occur in the first year after implantation.[1–4] Anatomic risk factors for development of PVR include history of endocarditis, significant mitral annular calcification, corticosteroid use, and presence of mechanical prosthetic valves.[5–8] Although the vast majority of cases of PVR are asymptomatic, up to 5% of the cases are complicated by heart failure, hemolytic anemia, or infective endocarditis.[4,5,9] Per the American College of Cardiology/American Heart Association guidelines, percutaneous PVR closure is indicated in patients with symptomatic heart failure (New York Heart Association functional class III to IV) or persistent hemolytic anemia who have anatomic features that are suitable for percutaneous repair at a center of expertise.[10] Studies have demonstrated successful use of transcatheter-based repair techniques in high-risk surgical patients, with 90% success in defect closure and improved patients' outcome.[11,12] Periprocedural imaging is invaluable in determining suitability for percutaneous closure in addition to planning and guiding the intervention. Echocardiography plays a pivotal role in diagnosing PVR, assessing candidacy and guiding transcatheter closure, and identifying immediate postprocedural complications in addition to postprocedural follow-up.

CLOSURE DEVICES

The PVR closure procedure is a technically challenging procedure. The ideal closure device is one that conforms to the tortuous course of the defect, achieves complete occlusion of the defect, is easily deliverable, and has a low risk of embolization. Periprocedural imaging aids in device selection by determining the size, extent, and course of the defect. Commonly used closure devices include the Amplatzer vascular plug II, Amplatzer Atrial Septal Defect Occluder, Amplatzer Ventricular Septal Defect Occluder, and Patent Ductus Arteriosus Occluder.

PREPROCEDURAL PLANNING
Echocardiography

Echocardiography is the primary imaging modality for diagnosis and quantitation of PVR. A detailed discussion of the echocardiographic evaluation of prosthetic valve function and PVR is provided elsewhere in this book.

Electrocardiographically Gated Multidetector Computed Tomography

Electrocardiographically gated multidetector computed tomography (MDCT) is a key imaging modality for the anatomic characterization of the paravalvular defect for procedural planning.[13] It enables localization and sizing of the defect. This is important because undersizing of the defect and hence the occluder devices used can lead to complications such as device embolization or migration and PVR.

Three-Dimensional Printing

With increasing complexity of transcatheter structural interventions, use of three-dimensional (3D) printing to simulate patient-specific valve geometry may provide useful data in the preprocedural planning phase.[14] This rapidly evolving technology entails the integration volumetric transesophageal echocardiography (TEE) images or MDCT data to a create patient-specific 3D printed model of prosthetic valve, which in turn enables accurate device selection and prediction of potential complications resulting from the interaction between the valve and the implanted device (Fig. 172.1).[15]

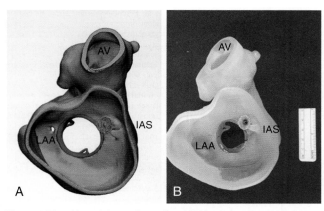

Figure 172.1. Use of three-dimensional (3D) printing for predicting size of paravalvular regurgitation (PVR) closure device and its interaction with the prosthetic valve after deployment. **A,** A patient-specific digital model designed using multidetector computed tomography images. **B,** A 3D-printed model showing a closure device deployed in an anteromedial PVR. Aortic valve; *IAS,* interatrial septum; *LAA,* left atrial appendage.

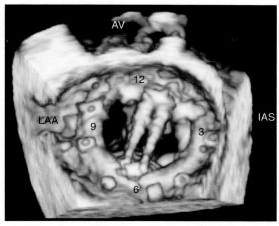

Figure 172.2. Three-dimensional en face surgical view of the mitral valve. The aortic valve (AV) marks the anterior border at 12 o'clock, the left atrial appendage (LAA) marks the lateral border at 9 o'clock, the interatrial septum (IAS) marks the medial border at 3 o'clock, and the posterior atrial wall marks the posterior border of the mitral prosthetic valve at 6 o'clock. The landmarks facilitate communication with the interventional cardiologists.

INTERVENTIONAL ECHOCARDIOGRAPHY

A comprehensive TEE examination at the start of the procedure is essential to confirm the findings of the preprocedural imaging studies and rule out the presence of infective endocarditis, significant valve instability (dehiscence involving more than one-fourth to one-third of the valve ring), or intracardiac thrombi, all of which represent contraindications to the procedure.

Mitral Valve

Localization

Because of its higher spatial resolution, TEE (with two-dimensional [2D] and 3D imaging) is superior in anatomic assessment and localization of PVR compared with TTE.[16] PVR can be single or multiple and can assume different shapes; they can be crescentic, oblong, and fenestrated and can form serpiginous tracts. Therefore, detailed imaging of the valve in multiple planes in addition to the use of 3D imaging is key in unmasking the full extent of the defect.

A standard clock-face view provided by an en face TEE view of the mitral valve is used when describing the location of PVR. In this view, the aortic valve is located anteriorly, the interatrial septum is located medially, and the left atrial appendage is located laterally (Fig. 172.2). The PVR is described in relation to these anatomic landmarks.

Quantification

Determining the degree of PVR is more challenging compared with native valve regurgitation. The area of proximal flow coverage is often shadowed by the prosthesis and difficult to measure. The use of the proximal isovelocity surface area radius (PISA) method, therefore, has not been validated in prosthetic valves. If a large area of flow converge is visualized, however, severe regurgitation should be suspected. Most PVR jets are eccentric, and this leads to underestimation of their severity based on measurement of the jet area due to the Coanda effect. Other parameters, including jet width (vena contracta), jet area, and density, can be used.[17,18] An additional specific sign for the presence of severe mitral regurgitation is the presence of systolic flow reversal in the pulmonary venous flow.[17]

The American Society of Echocardiography (ASE) guidelines on evaluation of prosthetic valves recommend estimating the proportion of the regurgitant area to the circumference of the prosthetic ring, in which PVR is defined as mild if it occupies less than 10% of the prosthesis and severe if it occupies more than 20%.[17] In case of multiple defects, there is no well-established method to quantify severity of PVR. In such cases, the guidelines recommend determining the proportion of the regurgitation area to the prosthesis circumference.[17] Continuous-wave Doppler interrogation across the mitral valve is used to assess transmitral gradients. If the pressure gradient is elevated in the absence of imaging features of prosthetic valve obstruction, then significant PVR contributing to a high-flow diastolic state should be a consideration.

Aortic Valve

Localization

It can be challenging to localize the origin of an aortic PVR because of the significant acoustic shadowing caused by the prosthesis (especially on parasternal TTE views and long-axis TEE views). It is therefore important to sweep the valve with color Doppler imaging and thoroughly examine the valve in apical TTE views and deep transgastric TEE views. Acoustic shadowing is often minimal in these views. Determining the origin of an eccentric jet is important because this represents the target for percutaneous closure.

Quantification

Short-axis imaging below the valve may overestimate the severity of aortic regurgitation in eccentric jets. Deep transgastric views during TEE are essential for assessment of regurgitant jets; however, jet area and length are recommended parameters to assess the severity of regurgitation. The application of these methods is described in detail in the ASE guideline on residual regurgitation quantitation[19] (Fig. 172.3).

INTRAPROCEDURAL GUIDANCE

TEE with real-time 3D imaging with its superior spatial resolution is the principal imaging modality used for procedural guidance and detection of immediate complications and is fundamental in

Doppler parameters			
Qualitative	**Mild**	**Moderate**	**Severe**
Proximal flow convergence (CD)	Absent	May be present	Often present
AR velocity waveform density (CWD)	Soft	Dense	Dense
Diastoic flow reversal (PWD) in			
- Proximal descending aorta	- Brief, early diastolic	- May be holodiastolic	- Holodiastolic (end-diasrolic velocity
- Abdominal aorta	- Absent	- Absent	≥20 cm(s)
			- Present
Semi-quantitative			
Vena contracta width (cm) (CD)	<0.3	0.3-0.6	>0.6
Vena contracta area (cm²) (2D/3D CD)	<0.10	0.10-0.29	≥0.30
Circumferential extent of PVR (%) (CD)	<10	10-29	≥30
Jet deceleration rate (PHT, ms) (CWD)	Variable	Variable	Steep
	Usually >500	200-500	Usually <200
Quantitative			
Regurgitant volume (mL)	<30	30-59	>60 (May be lower in low flow states)
Regurgitant fraction (%)	<30	30-49	>50
EROA (cm²)	<0.10	0.10-0.29	>0.30

A

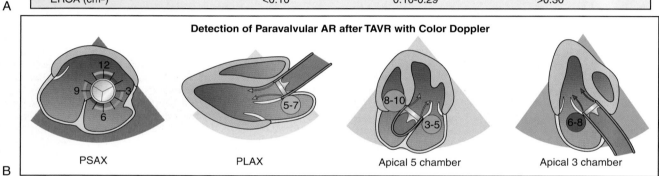

B

Figure 172.3. Quantification (**A**) and localization (**B**) of aortic paravalvular regurgitation as specified in the guidelines. *CD,* Color Doppler; *CWD,* continous wave Doppler; *EROA,* effective regurgitant orifice area; *PLAX,* parasternal long axis; *PSAX,* parasternal short axis; *PVR,* paravalvular regurgitation; *PWD,* pulsed wave Doppler. (Adapted with permission from Zoghbi WA, et al: Guidelines for the evaluation of valvular regurgitation after percutaneous valve repair or replacement, *J Am Soc Echocardiogr* 32:431–475, 2019.)

improving the accuracy of the procedure, thereby improving safety and outcomes.

Mitral Paravalvular Regurgitation Closure

Transseptal Approach

The transseptal approach is the most common approach used in mitral PVR closure devices. Both the short-axis midesophageal and the bicaval views allow visualization of the interatrial septum during transseptal puncture. Use of biplane imaging, which allows the simultaneous visualization of two orthogonal views, is helpful in guiding the transseptal puncture (Fig. 172.4). 3D imaging is also used to determine optimal location of transseptal puncture. The ideal transseptal site is based on the location of the PVR. For example, a more superior transseptal site may improve the catheter angulation to cross a lateral PVR site, whereas a relatively inferior transseptal site may facilitate catheter positioning within an anterior or medial PVR site.

Catheter Positioning and Crossing the Defect

Optimizing 2D TEE images to obtain a 3D surgical view of the mitral prosthesis enables accurate assessment of the exact anatomic location of the paravalvular defect. Improving frame rate

can be achieved by multibeat acquisition, in addition to optimizing the focus and depth of view. Stitching artifact can be avoided by a breath-hold (ventilator-hold) technique, which can be performed in the catheterization laboratory when the patient is under general anesthesia. Application of 3D color Doppler allows visualization and localization of the paravalvular jets and differentiating it from echocardiographic dropout.

Visualization of the intracardiac catheters is best achieved by real-time 3D imaging.[20] The catheters can be visualized by 3D TEE as they cross the interatrial septum. Use of real-time 3D imaging enables complete visualization of the delivery system, including the entire length of the catheter, in the left atrium with inclusion of key anatomic landmarks. This facilitates communication with the interventionist as the catheters and wires are being positioned in relation to the PVR.[20]

A 3D zoomed view is then used to focus on the valve and the paravalvular defect(s). The catheter itself can lead to shadowing with areas of dropout identified beyond the catheter. In such cases, it is important to adjust the imaging angle to ensure adequate visualization of the prosthetic valve in its entirely as the defect is being crossed by the wire. In the presence of large defects or when multiple closure devices are anticipated, two wires are positioned in the defect before device deployment in anticipation of the need for additional devices. This facilitates additional device deployment, especially because deploying the first device can result

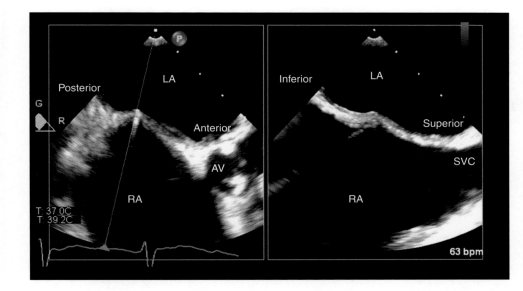

Figure 172.4. Use of biplane imaging facilitates transseptal puncture by providing two orthogonal views to allow exact localization of the optimal puncture site for crossing paravalvular regurgitation. *AV,* Aortic valve; *LA,* left atrium; *RA,* right atrium; *SVC,* superior vena cava.

in unpredictable alteration to the geometry of the paravalvular defect. When multiple paravalvular defects are present, real-time 3D confirms that the targeted defect is being crossed.

Device Deployment

TEE further guides the deployment process. Biplane views are particularly helpful in centering the occluder device because it provides two simultaneous orthogonal views of the prosthetic valve and the closure device. The 3D surgical view of the mitral valve guides optimal positioning of the device. The midesophageal commissural view (45–65 degrees) helps in evaluating the position of the device in the medial-lateral direction, and the midesophageal long-axis view (120–140 degrees) helps in positioning the device in the anteroposterior direction. The long-axis view also aids is assessing for left ventricular outflow tract (LVOT) obstruction when a device is placed anteriorly.

Prosthetic leaflet impingement, a feared complication reported in up to 4% of cases, can be immediately detected by TEE.[21] This occurs more commonly with the setting of mechanical and stentless prostheses and with the use of larger occluder devices. TEE affirms valve function and leaflet motion after positioning an occluder device and before its release from the delivery system. The interaction between the ventricular disk of the occluder and the prosthetic valve is evaluated by assessing prosthetic valve motion by TEE and fluoroscopy. If the prosthetic valve leaflet or disk is entrapped in diastole by the presence of an occluder, it leads to prosthetic valve obstruction with increased gradients (Fig. 172.5). Conversely, if the occluder device creates prosthetic valve leaflet or disk entrapment in systole, it leads to significant transvalvular regurgitation. Positioning the device under direct 3D real-time guidance helps to avoid interference with prosthetic valve function.

In the event that the prosthetic valve motion is hindered by the presence of an occluder, the device needs to be readjusted in a way to allow for deployment closer to the atrioventricular plane. Alternatively, a smaller device can be used to circumvent this important complication.

A tug test is usually performed to assess the stability of the PVR closure device to prevent device embolization. This is performed before releasing the device by pushing on the device with the catheter while simultaneously pulling the delivery system. TEE and fluoroscopy can confirm device stability during the tug test. If the device is unstable, repositioning the device or substituting it for a device is warranted to avoid device embolization. Visualization of the PVR closure device on 2D and 3D TEE provides additional insight into the stability of the device. Interference with prosthetic leaflet function can occur after a device is released from the delivery cases. In such instances, it is not possible to retrieve the device.

After a closure device is positioned and before its release from the delivery system, the transmitral valve gradients are measured and compared with the baseline values (Fig. 172.6). The gradients should be similar or lower because of the decrease in transmitral flow. If the gradients are increased, this should raise suspicion for prosthetic valve obstruction.[22] It is important to re-image the device and valve and assess the valve function and degree of regurgitation because of potential occluder device shifts after release. The process of catheter positioning and device deployment and release is demonstrated in Fig. 172.7.

Assessment of Residual Regurgitation

After a device is deployed, imaging of the prosthetic valve and the PVR closure device allows assessment of any residual PVR jets. Precise quantification of residual MR can be challenging because it is further complicated by added ultrasound shielding created by the prosthetic valve and the closure device.[23] Use of real-time 3D TEE with color imaging can be useful (Fig. 172.8). If the residual regurgitation is significant, the device should be repositioned and the degree of regurgitation reassessed. If the degree of regurgitation remains significant, the device should be replaced with a larger one or additional devices.[24]

It is important to differentiate PVR from normal retrograde jets, including mechanical washing jets and closing volume jets. Closing volume jets are trivial regurgitant jets located at the edges of the occluder and are caused by its motion. Washing jets are located inside the valve ring, focused around the hinge points, and are internally directed. This is in contrast to PVR jets, which are located outside the prosthetic valve ring and are externally directed. The washing jets serve to reduce the risk of valve thrombosis and are not considered to be pathological. This concept applies both to mitral and aortic prosthetic valves.

Hemodynamic Assessment After Deployment

After device release, the transvalvular gradients are assessed to confirm the absence of valve obstruction. The following parameters aid in confirming significant reduction in PVR:

- An increase in LVOT stroke volume (measured in deep transgastric TEE view)
- The appearance of a new antegrade S wave in pulmonary venous flow (Fig. 172.9)

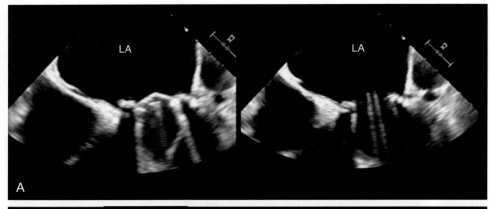

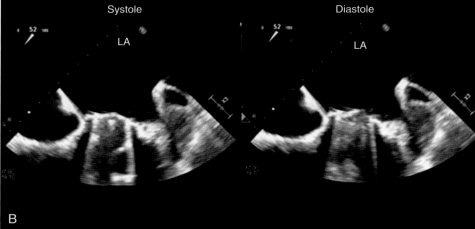

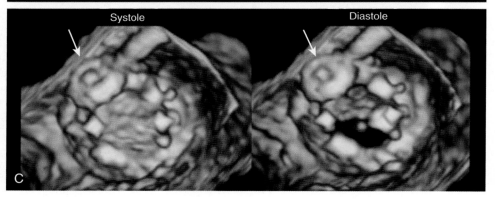

Figure 172.5. A, Normal mechanical prosthetic disk motion in systole and diastole. **B,** Closure device *(arrow)* causing interference with disk motion in diastole, leading to valve obstruction. **C,** Three-dimensional images of mechanical leaflet impingement in diastole. The disk is "stuck" in a closed position in diastole, leading to valve obstruction. *LA,* Left atrium.

- The presence of new spontaneous echo contrast within the LA
- A small decrease in the left ventricular (LV) ejection fraction. This is related to a decrease in regurgitant volume, decreased LV preload, and decreased end-diastolic volume with preserved LV systolic function, leading to a decrease in LV ejection fraction function.

Aortic Paravalvular Regurgitation Closure

The retrograde approach is used in transcatheter aortic PVR closure. It is important for evaluate the aorta for the presence of significant atherosclerosis or aortic dissection at baseline.

Catheter Positioning and Crossing the Defect

The catheter and wire are visualized in ascending aorta using the long-axis midesophageal view (120 degree). Biplane imaging, showing two orthogonal views, is very helpful in confirming wire position in the paravalvular space. Changing the imaging angle

may be necessary if the catheter causes echocardiographic dropout, precluding optimal visualization of the defect and wire. Similar to mitral PVR procedure, if the use of more than one occlusion device is anticipated, then passing two guidewires across the defect may be helpful. The catheter itself can create shadowing with areas of dropout identified beyond the catheter. The wire is followed as it crosses to the LV cavity. PVR closure in transcatheter aortic valve replacement cases can be more challenging because of the length of the valve frame and the tortuous course of the paravalvular defect, making it more technically difficult to deploy an occluder device.

Device Deployment

In aortic cases, it is important to ensure that there is no interaction between the closure device and the mitral valve. This is performed by assessment for worsening mitral regurgitation or stenosis before the device is released. Additionally, it is important to ensure that the closure device does not interact with the aortic or mitral prosthetic

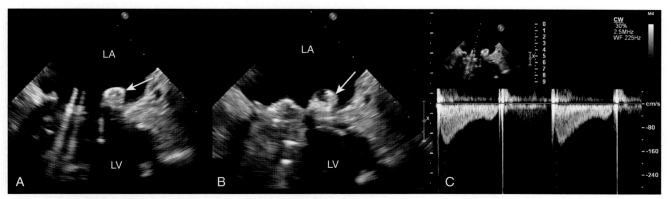

Figure 172.6. Assessment of prosthetic valve function after release of the closure device (*arrows* in **A** and **B**). Normal prosthetic valve disk motion is noted in diastole (**A**) and systole (**B**) with acceptable transmitral gradients of 4 mm Hg (**C**). *LA,* Left atrium; *LV,* left ventricle

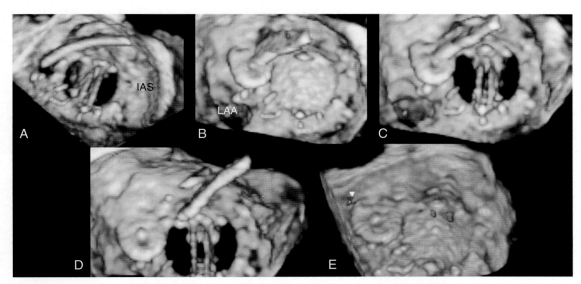

Figure 172.7. Mitral paravalvular regurgitation (PVR) closure. The catheter is positioned in close proximity to the defect and a wire is used to cross the defect (**A**). After device deployment, the prosthetic valve function is assessed in systole (**B**) and diastole (**C**) to ensure no interference with the prosthetic valve function. The occluder device is then released (**D**). Three-dimensional color Doppler further allows assessment of residual PVR (*arrowhead*) (**E**). *IAS,* interatrial septum; *LAA,* left atrial appendage.

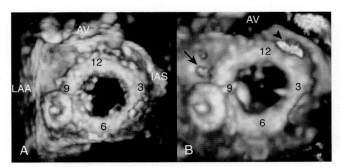

Figure 172.8. Three-dimensional (3D) transesophageal echocardiography color Doppler assessment enables evaluation of residual paravalvular regurgitation (PVR) after closure device deployment. After occluder device deployment in a posterolateral defect at 8 o'clock (**A**), 3D color assessment (**B**) reveals trace residual PVR anterior to the device at the 10 o'clock position *(arrow)* with an additional mild anteromedial defect at the 1 o'clock position *(arrowhead)*. *AV,* Aortic valve; *IAS,* interatrial septum; *LAA,* left atrial appendage.

disks, causing either impingement or transvalvular regurgitation. Deep transgastric views of the LVOT and aortic valve enables calculation of aortic valve gradients. Before release, the stability of the device is assessed with a tug test by the interventional cardiologist. The process of catheter positioning and device deployment and release is demonstrated in Figs. 172.10 and 172.11.

Assessment of Residual Regurgitation

Evaluating any residual PVR is important because the presence of significant residual PVR necessitates the use of a larger device or additional devices. Long- and short-axis views of the aortic valve are helpful in assessment. Similar to preprocedural assessment, the same principles can be applied in the assessment of residual aortic regurgitation after closure device deployment.

Hemodynamic Assessment After Deployment

In addition, it is important to assess prosthetic valve function by measuring transvalvular gradients to ensure lack of interference with prosthetic valve function. These can be obtained from deep transgastric views.

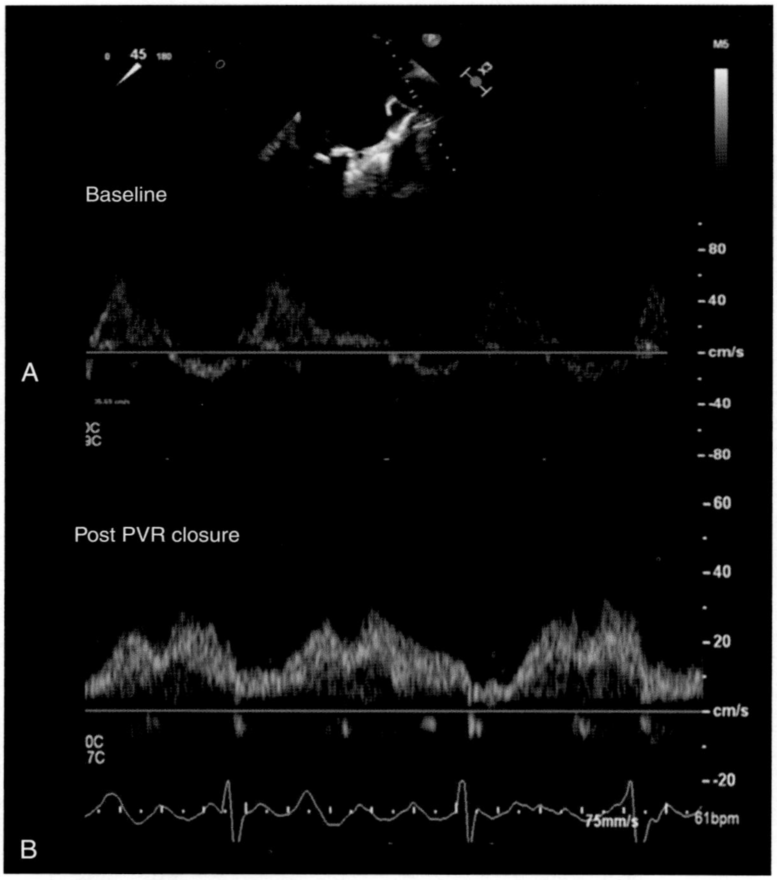

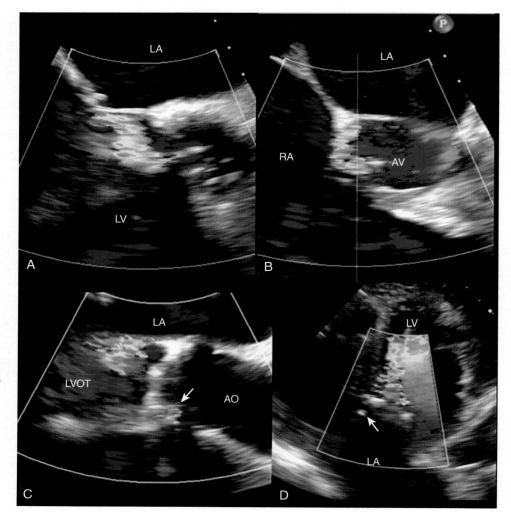

Figure 172.9. Pulsed-wave Doppler interrogation of the left upper pulmonary vein at baseline reveals systolic flow reversal, consistent with severe mitral regurgitation (MR) (**A**). After paravalvular regurgitation (PVR) closure, an upright systolic wave is noted, indicative of a reduction in MR and left atrial pressure (**B**).

Figure 172.10. Localization of an aortic paravalvular regurgitation (PVR) can be challenging and often requires sweeping through different planes. An eccentric regurgitant jet is noted (**A**). Short-axis views do not show the origin of the jet (**B**). Further sweeping reveals the anterior origin of the PVR *(arrow)* (**C**). Deep transgastric views aid in localization of the PVR *(arrow)* (**D**). *AO,* Ascending aorta; *AV,* aortic valve; *LA,* left atrium; *LV,* left ventricle; *LVOT,* left ventricular outflow tract; *RA,* right atrium.

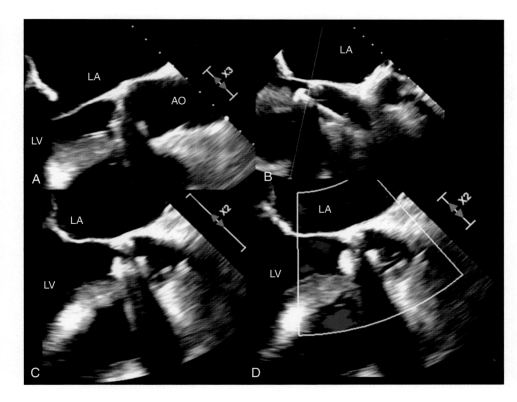

Figure 172.11. Aortic paravalvular regurgitation (PVR) closure. The catheter is advanced into the PVR by a retrograde aortic approach (**A**). The ventricular disk of the occluder device is deployed (**B**), followed by the aortic disk of the device (**C**). Color Doppler assessment reveals trace residual PVR. *AO,* Aorta; *LA,* left atrium; *LV,* left ventricle.

POSTDEPLOYMENT DETECTION OF COMPLICATIONS

TEE is central in the evaluation of immediate complications after deployment of a PVR closure device. Timely detection of such complications is important because some of these can potentially be life threatening or require emergent intervention. 2D and 3D TEE confirm device location and stability by ensuring that the device is well seated with no excessive motion. Device embolization and migration occurs in fewer than 1% of cases.[21] This can result from device undersizing or inexact deployment and can be readily detected on TEE.

Pericardial effusion can result from cardiac perforation caused by wire-related injuries sustained during manipulation in the left atrium and left ventricle. Therefore, it is important to continuously monitor the pericardium throughout the procedure, especially in the setting of hemodynamic compromise.

TEE can also detect less frequent complications. In mitral PVR closure procedures, these complications include the presence of an interatrial septal defect with right-to-left shunting, left coronary artery trauma, coronary sinus trauma, and mitral annular rupture. In aortic PVR closure procedures, these include aortic dissections and coronary obstruction.

FOLLOW-UP

Transthoracic echocardiography (TTE) plays an essential role in the follow-up of patients after PVR closure. It is recommended that yearly TTE is obtained to determine efficacy of the procedure and presence of complications. Similar to baseline TTE, residual PVR can be challenging to diagnose and is limited by acoustic shadowing from the valve and device, which can mask regurgitant jets. Additional imaging is recommended if there a suspicion for significant PVR.

CONCLUSION

Transcatheter PVR closure has emerged as a viable option for patients who are deemed poor surgical candidates. Echocardiography is the key imaging modality for diagnosing PVR, determining suitability for a catheter-based intervention, facilitating procedural guidance, and enabling timely detection of procedural complications.

REFERENCES

1. Kumar R, Jelnin V, Kliger C, Ruiz CE. Percutaneous paravalvular leak closure. *Cardiol Clin.* 2013;31:431–440.
2. Ionescu A, Fraser AG, Butchart EG. Prevalence and clinical significance of incidental paraprosthetic valvar regurgitation: a prospective study using transoesophageal echocardiography. *Heart.* 2003;89:1316–1321.
3. Hammermeister K, Sethi GK, Henderson WG, et al. Outcomes 15 years after valve replacement with a mechanical versus a bioprosthetic valve: final report of the Veterans Affairs randomized trial. *J Am Coll Cardiol.* 2000;36:1152–1158.
4. Dávila-Román VG, Waggoner AD, Kennard ED, et al. Prevalence and severity of paravalvular regurgitation in the artificial valve endocarditis reduction trial (AVERT) echocardiography study. *J Am Coll Cardiol.* 2004;44:1467–1472.
5. Rallidis LS, Moyssakis IE, Ikonomidis I, Nihoyannopoulos P. Natural history of early aortic paraprosthetic regurgitation: a five-year follow-up. *Am Heart J.* 1999;138:351–357.
6. O'Rourke DJ, Palac RT, Malenka DJ, et al. Outcome of mild periprosthetic regurgitation detected by intraoperative transesophageal echocardiography. *J Am Coll Cardiol.* 2001;38:163–166.
7. Vongpatanasin W, Hillis LD, Lange RA. Prosthetic heart valves. *N Engl J Med.* 1996;335:407–416.
8. Jindani A, Neville EM, Venn G, Williams BT. Paraprosthetic leak: a complication of cardiac valve replacement. *J Cardiovasc Surg.* 1991;32:503–508.
9. Cruz-Gonzalez I, Rama-Merchan JC, Arribas-Jimenez A, et al. Paravalvular leak closure with the Amplatzer Vascular Plug III device: immediate and short-term results. *Revista Española Cardiología.* 2014;67:608–614.
10. Nishimura RA, Otto CM, Bonow RO, et al. 2017. AHA/ACC focused update of the 2014 AHA/ACC guideline for the management of patients with valvular heart disease. *J Am Coll Cardiol.* 2017;70:252–289.
11. Sorajja P, Cabalka AK, Hagler DJ, Rihal CS. Percutaneous repair of paravalvular prosthetic regurgitation: acute and 30-day outcomes in 115 patients. *Circ Cardiovasc Interv.* 2011;4:314–321.
12. Ruiz CE, Jelnin V, Kronzon I, et al. Clinical outcomes in patients undergoing percutaneous closure of periprosthetic paravalvular leaks. *J Am Coll Cardiol.* 2011;58:2210–2217.
13. O'Neill AC, Martos R, Murtagh G, et al. Practical tips and tricks for assessing prosthetic valves and detecting paravalvular regurgitation using cardiac CT. *J Cardiovasc Comput Tomogr.* 2014;8:323–327.
14. Little SH, Vukicevic M, Avenatti E, et al. 3D printed modeling for patient-specific mitral valve intervention: repair with a clip and a plug. *JACC Cardiovasc Interv.* 2016;9:973–975.

15. Vukicevic M, Mosadegh B, Min JK, Little SH. Cardiac 3D printing and its future directions. *JACC Cardiovasc Imag.* 2017;10:171–184.
16. Cortés M, García E, García-Fernandez MA, et al. Usefulness of transesophageal echocardiography in percutaneous transcatheter repairs of paravalvular mitral regurgitation. *Am J Cardiol.* 2008;101:382–386.
17. Zoghbi WA, Chambers JB, Dumesnil JG, et al. Recommendations for evaluation of prosthetic valves with echocardiography and Doppler ultrasound. *J Am Soc Echocardiogr.* 2009;22:975–1014. quiz 1082-4.
18. Yildiz M, Duran NE, Gökdeniz T, et al. The value of real-time three-dimensional transesophageal echocardiography in the assessment of paravalvular leak origin following prosthetic mitral valve replacement. *Türk Kardiyol Dern Arş.* 2009;37:371–377.
19. Zoghbi WA, Asch FM, Bruce C, et al. Guidelines for the evaluation of valvular regurgitation after percutaneous valve repair or replacement. *J Am Soc Echocardiogr.* 2019;32:431–475.
20. Perk G, Lang RM, Garcia-Fernandez MA, et al. Use of real time three-dimensional transesophageal echocardiography in intracardiac catheter based interventions. *J Am Soc Echocardiogr.* 2009;22:865–882.
21. Eleid MF, Cabalka AK, Malouf JF, et al. Techniques and outcomes for the treatment of paravalvular leak. *Circ Cardiovasc Interv.* 2015;8. e001945.
22. Quader N, Davidson CJ, Rigolin VH. Percutaneous closure of perivalvular mitral regurgitation: how should the interventionalists and the echocardiographers communicate? *J Am Soc Echocardiogr.* 2015;28:497–508.
23. Cavalcante JL, Rodriguez LL, Kapadia S, et al. Role of echocardiography in percutaneous mitral valve interventions. *JACC Cardiovasc Imag.* 2012;5:733–746.
24. Lazaro C, Hinojar R, Zamorano JL. Cardiac imaging in prosthetic paravalvular leaks. *Cardiovasc Diagn Ther.* 2014;4:307–313.

173 Echocardiography-Guided Biopsy of Intracardiac Masses

Steven A. Goldstein, Muhamed Saric

Endomyocardial biopsy (EMB) is a commonly performed procedure for the evaluation of cardiac tissue for transplant monitoring (Video 173.1), myocarditis, drug toxicity, cardiomyopathy, and secondary cardiac involvement by systemic diseases and for diagnosis of cardiac masses.[1,2] This chapter discusses only the role of EMB of cardiac masses. Although lesion morphology and location often suggest a diagnosis, histologic evaluation is required before the initiation of potentially toxic chemotherapy or to guide possible surgical approach for resection. There are numerous case reports of EMB being performed for tissue diagnosis of cardiac tumors.[3–19] The majority of these are malignant or metastatic (Table 173.1).

A scientific statement from the American Heart Association (AHA), the American College of Cardiology (ACC), and the European Society of Cardiology (ESC) recommends that "EMB is reasonable in the setting of suspected tumors, with the exception of typical myxomas" (class of recommendation: IIa; level of evidence: C).[20] The AHA/ACC/ESC suggests that EMB for suspected cardiac tumor is appropriate if the following conditions are met: (1) the diagnosis cannot be established by noninvasive modalities (e.g., cardiac magnetic resonance imaging) or less invasive (noncardiac) biopsy; (2) the tissue diagnosis can be expected to influence the course of therapy; (3) the chances of successful biopsy are believed to be reasonably high; and (4) the procedure is performed by an experienced operator. Guidance with transesophageal echocardiography (TEE) is advised when possible.

TECHNIQUE OF ECHOCARDIOGRAPHY GUIDANCE

Lesions have been biopsied in all four cardiac chambers, though the vast majority are performed in right-sided tumors. Although

left-sided EMB is possible,[21–23] it is usually avoided because of the potential for systemic embolism. Biopsy samples can be obtained from the right atrium or right ventricle via the venous route through jugular, subclavian, or femoral veins. From the left atrium or left ventricle, samples can be obtained via transseptal puncture or by direct access through a peripheral artery, usually the femoral or brachial artery.[14,24]

EMB is performed using a bioptome, a biopsy forceps threaded into the heart through a catheter. EMB is typically guided by both fluoroscopy and echocardiography in cardiac catheterization suites. The advantages of fluoroscopy include high temporal resolution and the ability to visualize the tip of the bioptome. However, fluoroscopy guidance also has its limitations. The inability to directly visualize the anatomic or spatial location of the bioptome with respect to the target mass is a major limitation. As a result of this limitation of fluoroscopic guidance, echocardiography has been used as a complementary method of imaging to guide biopsy of intracardiac masses (Figs. 173.1 and 173.2; see Video 173.1).

Numerous original articles and case reports have demonstrated the value of 2D transthoracic echocardiography (TTE) to guide EMB.[3–19] However, TTE may be difficult to perform in patients

TABLE 173.1 Malignant Primary or Metastatic Cardiac Tumors Reported in the Literature as Diagnosed by Endomyocardial Biopsy

Malignant Primary Tumors	Metastatic Tumors
Angiosarcoma	Adenocarcinoma
Fibrosarcoma	Cervical carcinoma
Granulocytic sarcoma (chloroma)	Endometrial carcinoma
Leiomyosarcoma	Lymphoma
Lymphoma	Melanoma
Malignant fibrous histiocytoma	Squamous cell carcinoma
Rhabdomyosarcoma	
Sarcoma not otherwise specified	
Synovial sarcoma	

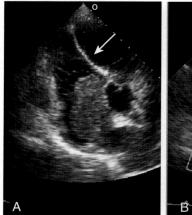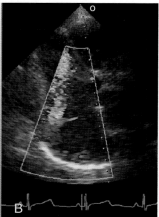

Figure 173.1. A, Transthoracic echocardiogram (TTE) modified short-axis view illustrating a biopsy catheter *(arrow)* contacting a right atrial tumor. **B,** TTE with color Doppler illustrates turbulent flow diverted around the large tumor mass.

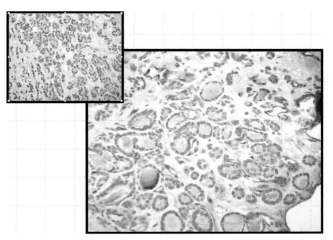

Figure 173.2. Histology of the biopsy specimen derived from the patient shown in Fig. 173.1, documenting the mass to be thyroid carcinoma. The *inset* in the *upper left corner* is a hematoxylin and eosin stain of the tumor, and the *larger panel* is a special stain for vessels (the tumor cells in this patient were negative for vascular marker).

in the catheterization laboratory who are supine. Further difficulty may be imposed in patients with chest tubes, bandages, obesity, chronic lung disease, mastectomy, and so on. In addition, TTE imaging with the operator's hands and the ultrasound probe on the chest prevent simultaneous fluoroscopic imaging. Therefore, over the past decade, such biopsies have usually been performed preferentially with the aid of TEE.[1,22,25–33]

Transesophageal Echocardiography and Transthoracic Echocardiography Guidance

Although the shaft of the biopsy catheter is usually seen in multiple views, the tip (jaws of the bioptome) is only seen in selected views. Orienting the bioptome is facilitated by using simultaneous orthogonal views provided by biplane imaging. Scanning is a dynamic process, and following the relatively rapid motion of the bioptome tip through a three-dimensional structure such as the right atrium or right ventricle requires experience. Sometimes the shaft but not the bioptome tip is imaged. The key to guiding biopsies of intracardiac masses is the ability to assess the bioptome tip in relation to the target mass. This may also require repositioning of the sheath to permit the bioptome tip to approach the target mass at an appropriate angle (Fig. 173.3). Determining the precise spatial

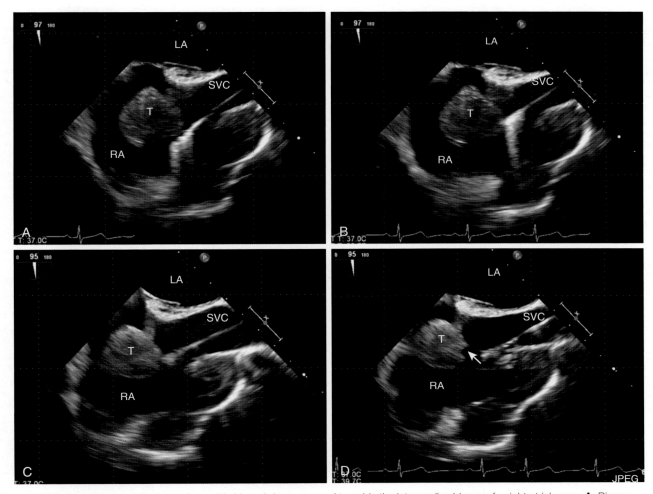

Figure 173.3. Transesophageal echocardiographic bicaval view was used to guide the intracardiac biopsy of a right atrial mass. **A,** Biopsy catheter passing beyond the mass, not contacting it. **B,** The biopsy catheter has been redirected and is approaching the mass nearly perpendicularly. **C,** The catheter immediately after being withdrawn containing the biopsy specimen. **D,** The "bite" *(arrow)* resulting from the biopsy. *LA,* Left atrium; *RA,* right atrium; *SVC,* superior vena cava; *T,* tumor.

BOX 173.1 Complications of Endomyocardial Biopsy

- Cardiac chamber perforation (with possible cardiac tamponade)
- Hematoma
- Tricuspid valve damage
- Arteriovenous fistula
- Vasovagal reaction
- Pneumothorax
- Arrhythmia
- Heart block
- Pulmonary embolism

---

relationship between the mass and the bioptome typically requires multiple views, and biplane imaging is helpful. The opening and closing of the bioptome jaws at the surface of the mass is critical and better appreciated with TEE than with fluoroscopy. It should be recognized, however, that although this is usually possible, the bioptome tip cannot always be visualized with certainty, even with TEE guidance.

The risks of EMB depend on the clinical status of the patient and experience of the operator. The potential complications of EMB are listed in Box 173.1.[34] The use of echocardiographic guidance may reduce the likelihood of several of these complications. Moreover, echocardiography has the advantage of rapidly detecting complications such as wall perforation, effusion, and tricuspid valve damage if they occur.

Intracardiac Echocardiography

Intracardiac echocardiography is also becoming increasingly used to guide EMB.[35,36]

Please access ExpertConsult to view the corresponding video for this chapter.

REFERENCES

1. Silvestry FE, Kerber RE, Brook MM, et al. Echocardiography-guided interventions. *J Am Soc Echocardiogr*. 2009;22:213–231.
2. Leone O, Veinot JP, Angelini A, et al. 2011. Consensus statement on endomyocardial biopsy from the Association for European Cardiovascular Pathology and the Society for Cardiovascular Pathology. *Cardiovasc Pathol*. 2012;21:245–274.
3. Flipse TR, Tazelaar HD, Holmes DJ. Diagnosis of malignant cardiac disease by endomyocardial biopsy. *Mayo Clin Proc*. 1990;65:1415–1422.
4. Gelb AB, Van Meter SH, Billingham ME, et al. Infantile histiocytoid cardiomyopathy—myocardial or conduction system hamartoma: what is the cell type involved? *Hum Pathol*. 1993;24:1226–1231.
5. Salka S, Siegel R, Sagar KB. Transvenous biopsy of intracardiac tumor under transesophageal echocardiographic guidance. *Am Heart J*. 1993;125:1782–1784.
6. Poletti A, Cocco P, Valente M, et al. In vivo diagnosis of cardiac angiosarcoma by endomyocardial biopsy. *Cardiovasc Pathol*. 1993;2:89–91.
7. Takach TJ, Reul GJ, Ott DA, et al. Primary cardiac tumors in infants and children: immediate and long-term operative results. *Ann Thorac Surg*. 1996;62:559–564.
8. Amory J, Chou TM, Redberg RF, et al. Diagnosis of primary cardiac leiomyosarcoma by endomyocardial biopsy. *Cardiovasc Pathol*. 1996;5:113–117.
9. Nardi P, Gaspardone A, Chiariello L, et al. Percutaneous transvenous biopsy for the diagnosis of a right atrial myxoma. *G Ital Cardiol*. 1999;29:308–311.
10. Bittira B, Tsang J, Huynh T, et al. Primary right atrial synovial sarcoma manifesting as transient ischemic attacks. *Ann Thorac Surg*. 2000;69:1949–1951.
11. Owa M, Higashikata T, Shimada H, et al. Primary cardiac malignant fibrous histiocytoma in the right ventricular infundibulum treated with a cavo-pulmonary shunt and coronary embolization. *Jpn Circ J*. 2000;64:982–984.
12. Chan KL, Veinot J, Leach A, et al. Diagnosis of left atrial sarcoma by transvenous endocardial biopsy. *Can J Cardiol*. 2001;17:206–208.
13. Alter P, Grimm W, Tontsch D, et al. Diagnosis of primary cardiac lymphoma by endomyocardial biopsy. *Am J Med*. 2001;110:593–594.
14. Veinot JP. Diagnostic endomyocardial biopsy pathology—general biopsy considerations and its use for myocarditis and cardiomyopathy. *Can J Cardiol*. 2002;18:55–65.
15. Fuzellier JF, Saade YA, Torossian PF, et al. Primary cardiac lymphoma: diagnosis and treatment. Report of 6 cases and review of the literature. *Arch Mal Coeur Vaiss*. 2005;98:875–880.
16. Vujin B, Benc D, Srdic S, et al. Rhabdomyosarcoma of the heart. *Herz*. 2006;31:798–800.
17. Abramowitz Y, Hiller N, Perlman G, et al. The diagnosis of primary cardiac lymphoma by right heart catheterization and biopsy using fluoroscopic and transthoracic echocardiographic guidance. *Int J Cardiol*. 2007;118. e39–e40.
18. Fealey ME, Edwards WD, Miller DV, et al. Hamartomas of mature cardiac myocytes: report of 7 new cases and review of literature. *Hum Pathol*. 2008;39:1064–1071.
19. Miller ES, Hoekstra AV, Hurteau JA, et al. Cardiac metastasis from poorly differentiated carcinoma of the cervix: a case report. *J Reprod Med*. 2010;55:78–80.
20. Cooper LT, Baughman KL, Feldman AM, et al. The role of endomyocardial biopsy in the management of cardiovascular disease. *J Am Coll Cardiol*. 2007;50:1914–1931.
21. Wong CW, Ruygrok P, Sutton T, et al. Transseptal fine needle aspiration of a large left atrial tumour. *Heart Lung Circ*. 2010;19:438–439.
22. Satya K, Kalife G, Navarijo J, et al. Transseptal biopsy of a left atrial mass with 3-dimensional transesophageal echocardiographic guidance. *Texas Heart Inst J*. 2012;39:707–710.
23. Schneider CM, Buiatti A, Schwamborn K, Dirschinger RJ. Diagnosis of a rare cardiac human herpesvirus-8 positive B-cell lymphoma manifestation: a case report of transoesophageal echocardiography-guided trans-septal catheter biopsy. *Eur Heart J Case Reports*. 2018;2:1–5.
24. Yilmaz A, Kindermann I, Kindermann M, et al. Comparative differences of left and right ventricular endomyocardial biopsy: differences in complication rate and diagnostic performance. *Circulation*. 2010;122:900–909.
25. Scott PJ, Ettles DF, Rees MR, et al. The use of combined transesophageal echocardiography and fluoroscopy in the biopsy of a right atrial mass. *Br J Radiol*. 1990;63:222–224.
26. Starr SK, Pugh DM, O'Brien-Ladner A, et al. Right atrial mass biopsy guided by transesophageal echocardiography. *Chest*. 1993;104:969–970.
27. Azuma T, Ohira A, Akagi H, et al. Transvenous biopsy of a right atrial tumor under transesophageal echocardiographic guidance. *Am Heart J*. 1996;131:402–404.
28. Malouf JF, Thompson RC, Maples WJ, et al. Diagnosis of right atrial metastatic melanoma by transesophageal echocardiographic-guided transvenous biopsy. *Mayo Clin Proc*. 1996;71:1167–1170.
29. Hammoudeh AJ, Chaaban F, Watson RM, et al. Transesophageal echocardiography-guided transvenous endomyocardial biopsy used to diagnose primary cardiac angiosarcoma. *Cathet Cardiovasc Diagn*. 1996;37:347–349.
30. Savoia MT, Liguori C, Nahar T, et al. Transesophageal echocardiography-guided transvenous biopsy of a cardiac sarcoma. *J Am Soc Echocardiogr*. 1997;10:752–755.
31. Burling F, Devlin G, Heald S. Primary cardiac lymphoma diagnosed with transesophageal echocardiography-guided endomyocardial biopsy. *Circulation*. 2000;101:E179–E181.
32. Scholte AJ, Frissen PH, van der Wouw PA. Transesophageal echocardiography-guided transvenous biopsy of an intracardiac tumor. *Echocardiography*. 2004;21:721–723.
33. Hosokawa Y, Kodani E, Kusama Y, et al. Cardiac angiosarcoma diagnosed by transvenous endomyocardial biopsy with the aid of transesophageal echocardiography and intra-procedural consultation. *Int Heart J*. 2010;51:367–369.
34. Han J, Park Y, Lee H, et al. Complications of 2-D echocardiography guided transfemoral right ventricular endomyocardial biopsy. *J Korean Med Sci*. 2006;21:989–994.
35. Park K-I, Kim MJ, Oh JK, et al. Intracardiac echocardiography to guide biopsy for two cases of intracardiac masses. *Korean Circ J*. 2015;45:165–168.
36. Zanobi M, Dello Russo A, Saccocci M, et al. Endomyocardial biopsy guided by intracardiac echocardiography as a key step in intracardiac mass diagnosis. *BMC Cardiovasc Disorders*. 2018;18(1–5).

174 Vacuum Extraction of Intracardiac Masses

Joseph M. Venturini, Atman P. Shah

The management of intracardiac masses is clinically challenging. Much of the difficulty arises from the fact that it is often difficult to describe the precise character and location of cardiac masses by current imaging techniques. Possible causes of intracardiac masses typically include tumor, thrombus, vegetation, or foreign body. Therefore, traditional management of cardiac masses often has included a trial of anticoagulation and eventual surgical embolectomy. However, many patients with cardiac masses are too ill for surgical embolectomy, or their comorbidities make a surgical approach exceedingly high risk. Furthermore, given that thrombus may be difficult to distinguish from tumor, clinicians are often challenged with a choice of sending a patient for cardiac surgery who may only need anticoagulation. Therefore, physicians are increasingly turning to percutaneous vacuum-assisted approaches for removal of unwanted intracardiac material.[1-12] When percutaneous approaches are attempted, the use of real-time, three-dimensional (3D) transesophageal echocardiography (TEE) is vital for procedure efficacy and safety.[10]

ANGIOVAC

The AngioVac system (AngioDynamics) is a negative-pressure device designed to assist in the removal of intravascular material (Fig. 174.1). The suction for the system is created with the assistance of a centrifugal pump system that is typically used for extracorporeal bypass. This pump can create up to 80 mm Hg of suction at high flow. The suction, or outflow, cannula is 22 Fr and has a balloon-actuated funnel at its distal tip (Fig. 174.2). This cannula is delivered to the heart through a 26-Fr sheath inserted in either the right internal jugular vein or either of the common femoral veins. To avoid massive blood loss, the system is designed to reinfuse blood via a second venous cannula,

typically a 17-Fr sheath that inserted in the contralateral femoral vein. All blood is passed through a thrombus filter before reinfusion.

Procedure

The removal of intracardiac material with the AngioVac is typically performed with the assistance of general anesthesia and TEE guidance. After endotracheal intubation and initial TEE, vascular access is obtained. The suction cannula can be advanced to the right atrium of the heart from either the right internal jugular vein or either of the common femoral veins (Fig. 174.3). Although an angled AngioVac Cannula is available (see Fig. 174.2), the cannula is difficult to steer after it is in the heart. Therefore, the choice of access site is selected to enable the AngioVac system to access the mass as directly as possible. For example, if the unwanted material or mass is adherent to the interatrial septum, it is often simpler to approach from the inferior vena cava (IVC) (Fig. 174.4). However, if the mass is low in the atrium or adherent to the tricuspid valve annulus, it may be easier to approach from the superior vena cava. After vascular access is obtained in the desired vein, the venotomy is dilated to allow for placement of a 26-Fr sheath.

Site selection for the reinfusion cannula is at the discretion of the operator. If a femoral approach is planned, most operators place the reinfusion cannula in the contralateral common femoral vein. If a jugular approach is planned, most operators use one of the femoral veins for reinfusion. However, in cases with very large masses or material that are unlikely to be completely removed via the cannula, it is sometimes necessary to suck the mass or material into the cone of the cannula and then drag it out of the body while maintaining suction. If this approach is used from a femoral (IVC) approach, it may be beneficial to have the reinfusion cannula in the

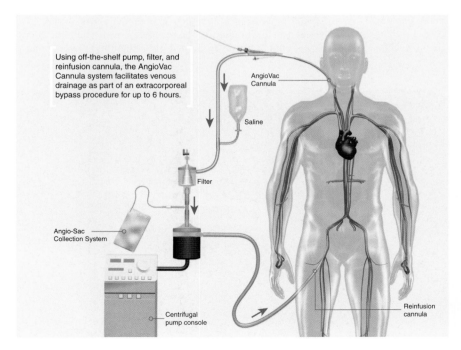

Using off-the-shelf pump, filter, and reinfusion cannula, the AngioVac Cannula system facilitates venous drainage as part of an extracorporeal bypass procedure for up to 6 hours.

AngioVac Cannula

Saline

Filter

Angio-Sac Collection System

Centrifugal pump console

Reinfusion cannula

Figure 174.1. The AngioVac circuit. The circuit consists of a suction AngioVac cannula, an extracorporeal circuit including a centrifugal pump and filter, and a reinfusion cannula.

internal jugular vein to avoid pulling the material against the flow created by the reinfusion cannula in the IVC.

When the 26-Fr sheath and reinfusion cannula are in place, therapeutic anticoagulation is achieved with a goal activated clotting time of at least 250 seconds. The reinfusion cannula and AngioVac cannula are connected to a primed circuit and centrifugal pump (see Fig. 174.1). The AngioVac cannula is then inserted via the 26-Fr sheath. The cannula can be advanced either over a guidewire or without. The cannula is delivered to the heart under fluoroscopy. The balloon on the tip of the cannula is then inflated to low pressure to open the inflow funnel (see Fig. 174.2). With the assistance of a perfusionist, the centrifugal pump is turned on to create flow in the AngioVac circuit and suction at the tip of the AngioVac cannula. The cannula is advanced into the right atrium with a combination of fluoroscopy and TEE guidance (see Fig. 174.3). The tip of the cannula is then directed toward the unwanted material.

Ideally, the unwanted material in the heart is removed quickly after enabling suction from the tip of the AngioVac cannula. If the size of the material allows, it will be pulled through the cannula and will be lodged in the thrombus filter. However, in many instances, the material is too large to pass through the cannula en bloc and

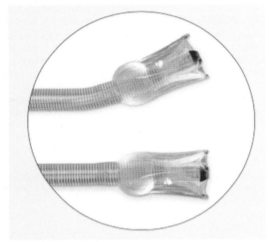

Figure 174.2. Tip of the AngioVac inflow Cannula. The tip of the AngioVac Cannula has a balloon-actuated tip that results in flowing of the inflow tip. The cannula also comes in an angled (20-degree) tip.

instead obstructs flow either at the tip of the cannula or within the circuit itself (Fig. 174.5). When this happens, flow in the circuit will stop. In some cases, continued suction from the centrifugal pump will eventually pull the material in to the filter, and flow will recover. However, often the cannula must be removed and flushed. The centrifugal pump must be stopped when the cannula is removed to avoid pulling air into the circuit and reinfusing air into the central venous system.

If initial approaches with the AngioVac cannula fail to remove the material, alternative approaches may be required. If the material or mass is adherent to the wall of the atrium, the suction of AngioVac cannula may not be sufficient to pull it off the wall. In these cases, a guidewire or snare may be used to dislodge the material while simultaneously positioning the AngioVac cannula near the material (Fig. 174.6). If the cannula is not easily directed to the mass or material, the tip of the cannula may be directed by snaring the tip of the cannula from another access site in an effort to direct the tip of the cannula. The use of these techniques allows for removal of different sizes and locations of intracardiac material (Fig. 174.7).

After the intracardiac material has been removed from the heart, flow in the circuit is stopped. The AngioVac cannula is removed from the patient and inserted into a container of heparinized saline. The circuit is then restarted briefly to reinfuse the blood contained in the circuit while pulling saline into the circuit. After reinfusion, the flow is again stopped. The material that has been collected into the filter may be sent for analysis. The 26-Fr sheath and reinfusion cannula are removed. Hemostasis is typically achieved with figure-of-8 sutures or manual pressure.

Complications

Complications resulting from vacuum-assisted removal of intracardiac material can be divided into three general categories: vascular access issues, embolic phenomena, and iatrogenic cardiac injury. Of these complications, vascular complications are the most common. The procedure requires two large-bore venous access sites and therapeutic anticoagulation, so minor bleeding does occur occasionally. However, given the size of the sheaths and the degree of anticoagulation, major vascular complications may occur. Careful vascular access technique is necessary to ensure that venous access in achieved cleanly without compromise of nearby arterial structures.

Distal embolization of either part or the entire intracardiac material can occur during attempted removal. Embolic debris most commonly travels from the right atrium into the pulmonary

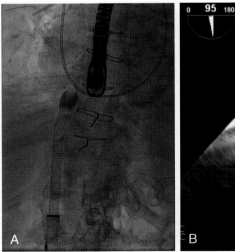

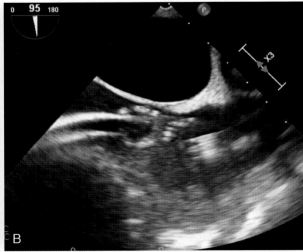

Figure 174.3. The AngioVac cannula inserted in the right atrium from a femoral venous approach. **A,** Fluoroscopy image. **B,** Transesophageal echocardiography image.

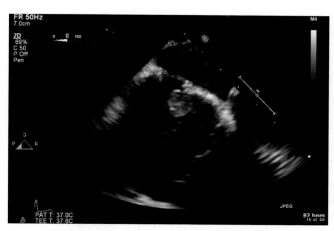

Figure 174.4. Transesophageal echocardiography image of an intracardiac mass adherent to the interatrial septum. These masses are more easily approached from a femoral approach when using the AngioVac system.

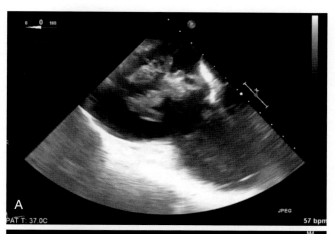

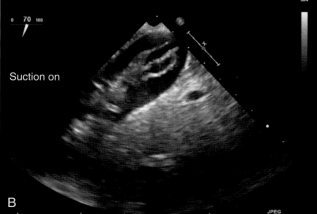

Figure 174.5. Suction removal of a large, mobile right atrial thrombus in transit. The serpiginous thrombotic material was identified in the right atrium (**A**). When the inflow cannula engaged the material, it occluded flow and became stuck on the end of the cannula. The cannula was pulled back into the inferior vena cava (**B**) and eventually out of the body. Large, serpiginous thrombus in transit in the right atrium. Large thrombus being pulled down the inferior vena cava after lodging into the inflow cannula. Removal of the large thrombus stuck in the inflow cannula by removing the cannula from the body with suction ongoing. (See accompanying Video 174.5.)

circulation and results in pulmonary embolism (PE).[13] The size and extent of PE determine the clinical implications of this complication. In some cases, pulmonary thrombectomy may be required to correct hypoxia or hemodynamic compromise. However, the clinical risks associated with embolism are substantially higher in the presence of a patent foramen ovale (PFO) or other transient right-to-left intracardiac shunt. In these cases, embolic material may pass into the systemic circulation and result in stroke, myocardial infarction, or injury to another distal capillary bed. For this reason, it is recommended that the presence of PFO be excluded before any attempted percutaneous removal of intracardiac material.

Direct cardiac injury is a rare, but feared, complication. The mechanism of injury typically involves collision trauma from the AngioVac cannula funnel or suction trauma resulting from transient tissue entrapment within the cannula tip. The most vulnerable structures to injury are the thin tissue of the right atrial free wall, the interatrial septum, and the tricuspid valve leaflets. If the free wall of the right atrium is injured, hemopericardium and cardiac tamponade may develop rapidly. Careful monitoring for pericardial effusion throughout the case and in the postprocedure period is vital. Rapid identification and subsequent pericardial drain placement are the mainstays of treatment. In many cases, surgical repair can be avoided. Many of these defects are small and can be managed with reversal of anticoagulation and close monitoring with a pericardial drain in place. In some cases, percutaneous closure of the free-wall defect can be performed with the off-label use of cardiac occluder devices.

Iatrogenic interatrial septal injury is typically identified during the procedure with the assistance of real-time TEE guidance. The management of this complication is dictated by the size, severity, and direction of the resulting interatrial shunt. If the iatrogenic defect is believed to result in a physiologically significant shunt, percutaneous repair during the index procedure may be considered. 3D TEE assessment of these defects is vital; the specific shape and size of the defect determine the likelihood of successful percutaneous repair with cardiac occluder devices.

Tricuspid valve and subvalvular apparatus injury likely occur as a result of suction trauma when the valve is pulled into the tip

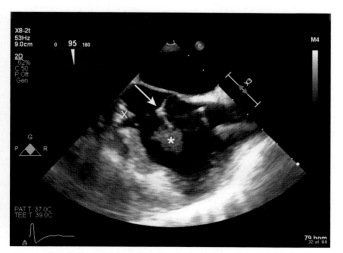

Figure 174.6. Supplemental use of a snare device *(arrow)* delivered through the inflow cannula (X) to disrupt and remove adherent intracardiac material *(asterisk)*. Three-dimensional transesophageal echocardiography images of an intravascular snare being used to disrupt an adherent right atrial mass for vacuum removal with the AngioVac system. Disruption of adherent right atrial material with an intravascular snare delivered through the inflow cannula. (See accompanying Video 174.6.)

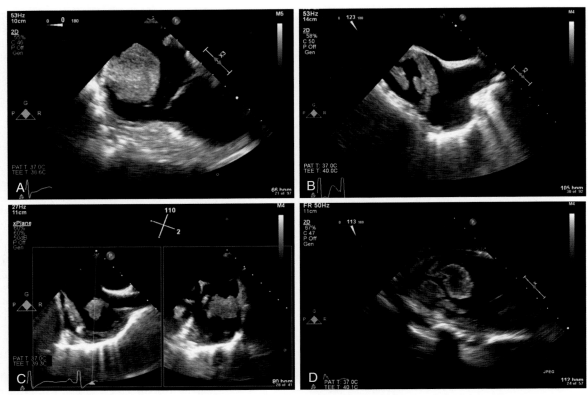

Figure 174.7. A range of intracardiac masses amenable to removal with the AngioVac system. **A,** A large right atrial mass that was adherent to the right atrial free wall. **B,** A large, serpiginous thrombus in transit. **C,** A thrombus attached to a pacemaker lead in the right atrium. **D,** A complex right ventricular (RV) apical thrombus in the setting of severe RV dysfunction.

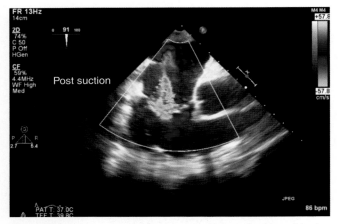

Figure 174.8. Severe tricuspid valve regurgitation after tricuspid valve injury at the time of vacuum-assisted removal of a right atrial mass. (See accompanying Video 174.8.)

of the AngioVac cannula. The resulting valve dysfunction can be identified at the time of the procedure with TEE.[14] The first sign of injury is typically the presence of new or worsened tricuspid regurgitation (Fig. 174.8). Management is usually supportive, although the presence of new tricuspid valve dysfunction should result in an adjustment of approach or abortion of the procedure.

OTHER DEVICES

The INARI FlowTriever (Inari Medical) and Penumbra thrombectomy system (Penumbra) are designed for removal of thrombotic material from the Iliocaval system and pulmonary arteries. These devices may be used for removal of intracardiac material in some cases, although the specific indications and best practice use for this indication is still being defined.

CONCLUSIONS

Percutaneous vacuum-assisted removal of intracardiac material can be accomplished with careful procedure planning and meticulous technique. The use of real-time 3D TEE guidance is pivotal for procedure safety and success.

Please access ExpertConsult to view the corresponding videos for this chapter.

REFERENCES

1. Ram H, Gerlach RM, Conte AH, et al. The AngioVac device and its anesthetic implications. *J Cardiothorac Vasc Anesth.* 2017;31:1091–1102.
2. Todoran T, Sobieszcyzyk P, Levy M, et al. Percutaneous extraction of right atrial mass using the AngioVac aspiration system. *J Vasc Interv Radiol.* 2011;22:1345–1347.
3. Divekar A, Scholz T, Fernandez J. Novel percutaneous transcatheter intervention for refractory active endocarditis as a bridge to surgery—angiovac aspiration system. *Catheter Cardiovasc Interv.* 2013;81:1008–1012.
4. Moriarty J, Al-Hakim R, Bansal A, Park J. Removal of caval and right atrial thrombi and masses using the AngioVac device: initial operative experience. *J Vasc Interv Radiol.* 2016;27:1584–1591.
5. Wallenhorst P, Rutland J, Gurley J, Guglin M. Use of AngioVac for removal of tricuspid valve vegetation. *J Hear Valve Dis.* 2018;27:120–123.
6. Hameed I, Lau C, Khan F, et al. AngioVac for extraction of venous thromboses and endocardial vegetations: a meta-analysis. *J Card Surg.* 2019;34:170–180.
7. Badri AA, Kliger C, Weiss D, et al. Right atrial vaccum-assisted thrombectomy: Single-center experience. *J Invasive Cardiol.* 2016;26:196–201.
8. Patnaik S, Rammohan H, Shah M, et al. Percutaneous embolectomy of serpentine thrombus from the right atrium. *Tex Hear Inst J.* 2016;43:524–527.

9. Schultz J, Andersen A, Grove EL, et al. Case report large solid right atrial thrombus treated by angiovac catheter-based suction thrombectomy. *Case Reports Cardiol*. 2018;3–5.

10. Enezate TH, Kumar A, Aggarwal K, et al. Non-surgical extraction of right atrial mass by AngioVac aspiration device under fluoroscopic and transesophageal echocardiographic guidance. *Cardiovasc Diagn Ther*. 2017;7:331–335.

11. Kiani S, Saboyon D, Lloyd M, et al. Outcomes of percutaneous vacuum-assisted debulking of large vegetations as an adjunct to lead extraction. *Pacing Clin Electophysiol*. 2019;42:1032–1037.

12. Grimm JC, Parsee AM, Brinker JA, et al. Utilization of AngioVac and snare for eradication of a mobile right atrial thrombus. *Ann Thorac Surg*. 2015;99:698–700.

13. Del Rosario T, Basta M, Agarwal S. Angiovac suction thrombectomy complicated by thrombus fragmentation and distal embolization leading to hemodynamic collapse: a case report. *AA Case Rep*. 2017;8:206–209.

14. Boisen ML, Iyer MH. Transesophageal echocardiography diagnosis of tricuspid valve injury during AngioVac percutaneous pulmonary embolectomy. *Cardiovasc Imaging Case Reports*. 2018;2:181–185.

175 Systematic Echocardiographic Approach to Left Ventricular Assist Device Therapy

Karima Addetia, Roberto M. Lang

As the population ages, the prevalence of heart failure continues to escalate.[1] Heart failure with reduced ejection fraction (HFrEF) comprises approximately 50% of the admission diagnoses for heart failure. The American College of Cardiology/American Heart Association categorizes heart failure into four stages labeled A to D. Patients with stage D heart failure have the worst outcomes. Clinically, they have persistent symptoms despite optimal doses of guideline-directed medical therapy and cardiac resynchronization devices when appropriate.[2] These patients, classified as "advanced" or "end stage," may be eligible for advanced therapies such as mechanical assist devices and cardiac transplantation. Unfortunately, the number of patients with stage D HFrEF far surpasses donor heart availability, such that cardiac transplantation is not an option for many patients, and alternative options must be considered. The ventricular assist device (VAD) is one such alternative.

The left ventricular (LV) assist device or LVAD is a battery-operated pump that conducts blood from the left ventricle via an inflow cannula implanted at the LV apex to the aorta by way of an outflow graft with direct anastomosis to the ascending aorta. In so doing, it augments cardiac output in the failing heart by reducing the afterload on the left ventricle and decreasing filling pressures, pulmonary artery pressures, and mitral regurgitation (MR; Fig. 175.1). Patients eligible for LVADs generally have stage D HFrEF (explained earlier) with New York Heart Association class III to IV symptoms and LV ejection fraction (EF) less than 25%, with or without cardiac resynchronization therapy with most often a dilated left ventricle.

According to the INTERMACS registry,[3] more than 20,000 LVADs have been implanted in the United States with more than 2500 new implants occurring every year. VADs can be commissioned for short- (hours to days) or long- (months to years) term support. VADs are differentiated based on a number of factors: (1) location of implant (intracorporeal versus extracorporeal), (2) implantation approach (percutaneous versus surgical), (3) flow characteristics (pulsatile versus continuous), (4) pump mechanism (volume displacement, axial, centrifugal), and (5) ventricle supported (left, right, both).[2]

Transthoracic echocardiography (TTE) is the noninvasive imaging modality of choice for the assessment of patients with continuous-flow (CF) LVADs. The purpose of this chapter is to focus on the echocardiographic imaging recommendations for CF LVADs. Most of the data supporting the use of echocardiography in these patients come from the experience with axial-flow pumps (HeartMate II), which are described in more detail later.

THE LEFT VENTRICULAR ASSIST DEVICE

Three types of CF LVADs are currently approved for implantation in the United States: the Heartmate II (Abbott Laboratories), which houses an axial-based pump, and the HeartWare (Medtronic) and HeartMate III, both of which house a centrifugal-based pump. CF LVADs have been shown to have improved device performance and patient survival profiles compared with the earlier pulsatile-flow devices. The axial pump generates flow parallel to the axis of rotor or impeller rotation using a propeller in pipe mechanism while the centrifugal pump generates flow perpendicular to the axis of rotation with a spinning bladed disk.[4] Studies based on two-dimensional (2D) and three-dimensional (3D) echocardiographic measurements have shown that the HeartWare Ventricular Assist System (HVAD) results in less of a reduction in LV chamber diameter and 3D volumes with increasing pump speed compared with the Heart Mate II pump.[5–7] Both pumps, however, have been shown to provide similar overall flows in the normal working range of speed[8] so that the differential shape changes seen in

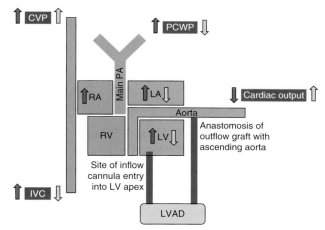

Figure 175.1. End-stage heart failure with reduced ejection fraction is associated with a low-output state with high pulmonary venous pressures, left ventricular end-diastolic pressures, central venous pressures, right atrial pressures *(green arrows),* and a deviated interventricular septum (IVS) to the right. With left ventricular assist device (LVAD) implantation, the IVS should move leftward as blood is drawn from the left ventricle to the ascending aorta. Cardiac output increases, and left atrial and ventricular pressures decrease *(yellow arrows).* At the same time, the venous return to the right ventricle (RV) increases, and right atrial pressure also increases *(yellow arrows).* The extent to which these pressures (the central venous and right atrial pressures) remain high varies depending on a variety of factors, including the extent of right ventricular dysfunction before LVAD insertion. *CVP,* Central venous pressure; *IVC,* inferior vena cava; *LA,* left atrium; *LV,* left ventricle; *PA,* pulmonary artery; *PCWP,* pulmonary capillary wedge pressure; *RA,* right atrium.

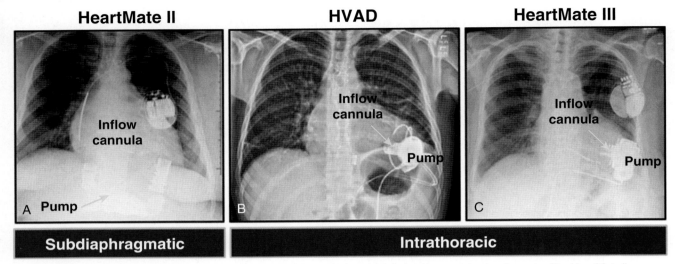

Figure 175.2. Appearance and location of the most common left ventricular assist device types on chest radiography. The HeartMate II pump is located subdiaphragmatically (**A**), and the HeartWare Ventricular Assist System (HVAD) (**B**) and HeartMate III (**C**) pumps are inserted intrathoracically at the left ventricular apex.

these studies during unloading may be attributable to the location of the pumps in the thorax. The HeartMate II pump is located subdiaphragmatically, likely resulting in inferior displacement of the LV apex because of the pull of the inflow cannula. In contrast, the HVAD and HeartMate III pumps are inserted intrathoracically at the LV apex, resulting in less distortion of the LV apex[6] (Fig. 175.2). LVADs can be used as (1) a bridge to cardiac transplantation, (2) a bridge to cardiac transplant candidacy, 3) a bridge to recovery, and (4) destination therapy.

LEFT VENTRICULAR ASSIST DEVICE IMAGING PROTOCOL
Preoperative Assessment

Echocardiographic examination of LVAD candidates should include a comprehensive 2D, Doppler, and color Doppler assessment. Findings that may impact patient outcomes and device function include the presence of LV thrombus, any ascending aortic pathology, dilatation or dysfunction of the right ventricle, presence of significant tricuspid regurgitation (TR), presence of significant pulmonary hypertension, significant aortic or mitral stenosis, or regurgitation and presence of an interatrial communication. If significant MR is present, the mechanism needs to be elucidated. Primary MR may not improve with LV unloading, and the mitral valve may need to be repaired or replaced at the time of LVAD implantation. Similarly, significant TR may need to be intervened upon before LVAD placement.[9] Significant aortic regurgitation (AR) is a very important comorbidity (see later) and usually requires either oversewing of the valve or valve replacement before LVAD placement. Interatrial septal defects should be ruled out with an agitated saline study before LVAD placement, and if clinical suspicion remains, the interatrial septum should be evaluated on transesophageal echocardiography (TEE) preoperatively. Unloading of the left ventricle after LVAD results in a decrease in both LV and left atrial (LA) pressures. Right atrial (RA) pressures, on the other hand, as described in Fig. 175.1, may remain the same or increase in the presence of increased venous return after LVAD-assisted improvement in cardiac output. The pressure differential created across a defective interatrial septum forms the perfect milieu for paradoxical embolization or hypoxia (with right-to-left shunting), and both of these complications can occur immediately after implantation or months later. If found on preoperative imaging, these interatrial septal defects can be closed at the time of LVAD implantation.

Postoperative Assessment

Imaging patients after LVAD insertion can be challenging, especially during the immediate postoperative period. Generally, a standard echocardiographic protocol (2D and Doppler) is adopted with certain additions or modifications and off-axis views to adequately assess LVAD function. These modifications or additions are discussed sequentially later. The first screen of the stored echocardiogram on a patient with an LVAD should document the type of LVAD (e.g., HeartMate II, HeartWare, HeartMate III), the LVAD speed in revolutions per minute (rpm), and the power and pulsatility index of the device. Any changes made during the study should also be recorded (Table 175.1).

LEFT HEART CHAMBER SIZE AND FUNCTION AND INTERVENTRICULAR SEPTUM POSITION

Both the LV end-diastolic (LVEDD) and end-systolic (LVESD) diameters in the parasternal long-axis view are good measures of LV decompression. Optimal unloading by the LVAD is suggested by reduction in LV diameters by 20% to 30% and LV volumes by 40% to 50%.[10,11] Slight leftward interventricular and interatrial septal positions also indicate adequate LV and LA decompression. If the LV cavity is too small (generally LVEDD ≤37 mm per the current guidelines), then the cavity may be underfilled, or the speed of the LVAD too high, and this needs to be communicated to the heart failure specialist so that appropriate action can be taken. Causes of a small LV cavity include an LVAD speed that is too high and dehydration (such as in the setting of poor intake, diarrheal illness, or vomiting). Alternatively, if the LV cavity is inadequately decompressed, the septum may be directed rightward and the LV cavity dilated (Fig. 175.3).

THE RIGHT VENTRICLE

Right ventricular (RV) failure before LVAD implantation is a harbinger for pump failure and a poor prognosis in the postoperative period.[12] After LVAD implantation, RV failure can occur

TABLE 175.1 Left Ventricular Assist Device Imaging Protocol (in Addition to the Standard Imaging Protocol)

Annotate LVAD Type and Speed Setting

Parasternal long-axis view
- LV diameters in diastole and systole
- Aortic and ascending aorta
- Aortic regurgitation (specify diastolic vs continuous)
- Aortic valve opening (2D and M-mode)
- Mitral regurgitation
- Tricuspid regurgitation
- Inflow cannula position can sometimes be noted here; CW Doppler flow through the inflow cannula may be possible on off-axis views
- Pericardial effusion or substernal fluid collection

Right upper sternal view
- Outflow cannula location: try to visualize anastomosis site with ascending aorta here using both 2D and color Doppler
- Obtain PW and CW Doppler flows through the outflow cannulaParasternal short-axis view
- Aortic valve opening
- Aortic regurgitation
- Short-axis for LV function and wall motion
- Inflow cannula may be seen in this view; off-axis imaging may be required
- Pericardial effusion

Apical four-chamber view
- View of all four chambers to assess IVS position and RV-to-LV ratio
- LV function views
- Mitral regurgitation (often difficult to assess because of interference from the LVAD cannula)
- RV size and function from the RV-focused view
- Degree of tricuspid regurgitation
- LV thrombus
- Inflow cannula position: may require off-axis imaging; consider CW Doppler through the cannula if alignment is adequate
- Tricuspid regurgitation gradient
- Pericardial effusionSubcostal view
- Pericardial effusion
- IVC diameter and collapse
- Pleural effusions
- Ascites

2D, Two-dimensional; *CW,* continuous-wave; *IVC,* inferior vena cava; *IVS,* interventricular septum; *LV,* left ventricular; *LVAD,* left ventricular assist device; *PW,* pulsed-wave; *RV,* right ventricular;

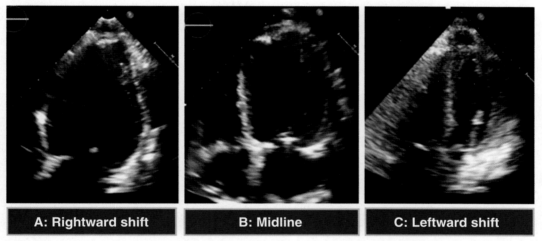

| A: Rightward shift | B: Midline | C: Leftward shift |

Figure 175.3. If the left ventricle in a patient with a left ventricular assist device (LVAD) is inadequately decompressed, the septum may be directed rightward and the left ventricular (LV) cavity dilated (**A**). A midline or slightly leftward shift in the interventricular and interatrial septal positions is suggestive of adequate LV unloading (**B**). However, if the LV cavity is too small and the septum is shifted to the left, then the cavity is underfilled, or the speed of the LVAD is too high (**C**).

early or late (Fig. 175.4). When the LVAD is first placed, there is an almost immediate decompression of the LV with varying degrees of reduction in LV filling parameters and increase in cardiac output. The extracardiac output returns to the right ventricle as increased venous return and can have a variable of effects on subsequent RV size function depending on baseline RV performance and degree of venous return increase.[13] Echocardiographic assessment of the right ventricle in the LVAD recipient is not different than in patients without an LVAD. Parameters include dimensions, fractional area change, myocardial performance index tricuspid annular systolic excursion (TAPSE), and systolic annular motion of the tricuspid valve (S′) all performed from the RV-focused view. There is evidence that the right-to-left ventricular end-diastolic diameter ratio may provide added value in identifying patients with increased risk of RV failure before and after LVAD implantation.[14–16] Select studies have shown an added benefit in the use of free-wall strain to stratify patients who are more likely to develop RV failure.[17,18] Typically, in patients with significant RV failure, the

RV and the tricuspid annulus appear dilated often with TR and a leftward shift of the interventricular septum (IVS).

THE AORTIC VALVE

Aortic valve opening (AVO) in CF LVADs depends on the systolic function of the native LV, the LVAD pump speed, and the preload and afterload on the heart.[19] By directing blood flow from the LV apex into the ascending aorta via the outflow graft, the LVAD bypasses the left ventricle and eliminates the normal pressure differential across the aortic valve that is responsible for AVO, altering the behavior of the aortic valve during the cardiac cycle. The frequency and degree of AVO in these patients depend on LVAD speed, native LV function, patient volume status, and peripheral vascular resistance and can range from no AVO to intermittent AVO to normal AVO occurring with every beat depending on the clinical situation. AVO can also occur with normal or reduced excursion. The frequency of AVO can be assessed visually in the parasternal long- or short-axis view or with M-mode though the aortic valve from the same views (Fig. 175.5).

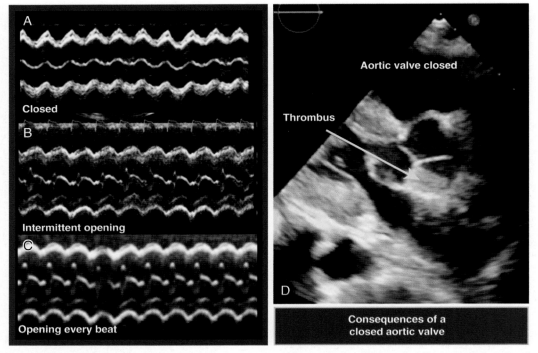

Figure 175.4. M-mode tracings of the aortic valve taken from the parasternal long-axis view *(left panel)*. **A** illustrates a closed aortic valve, **B** suggests that there is intermittent opening of the aortic valve, and **C** shows an M-mode tracing in a patient with aortic valve opening with every beat. **D,** A still image taken from the parasternal long-axis view showing one of the complications of a closed aortic valve. The *arrow* is pointing to thrombosis of the noncoronary cusp.

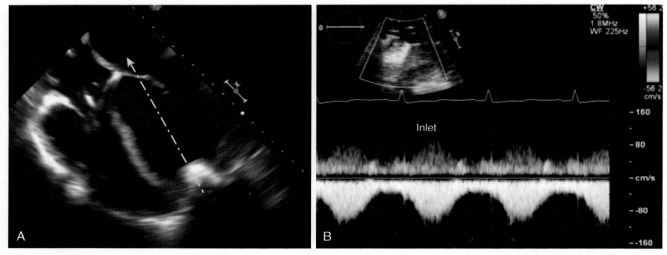

Figure 175.5. A, The correct orientation of the left ventricular assist device inflow cannula (toward the mitral valve as illustrated by the *yellow dashed arrow*). **B,** A continuous-wave Doppler pulse is directed into the inflow cannula, depicting the velocities through the cannula that are normal.

Stored clips should include 10 cardiac cycles to allow an approximation of the number of times the aortic valve opens. If the aortic valve opens three times in 10 beats, then AVO can be reported as approximately 30%. Increasing frequency of AVO can be associated with LV functional recovery. In patients with a closed aortic valve, evaluation for thrombus in the aortic root or sinus of Valsalva is important because stasis of blood flow can occur in this region (see Fig. 175.5).

The LVAD outflow cannula continuously deposits blood into the ascending aorta, resulting in a high retrograde aorta-to-LV gradient and exposing the aortic valve to high pressures over time, eventually leading to AR.[20] Higher LVAD speeds lead to higher transvalvular pressures and more AR. AR, in turn, leads to LVAD inefficiency

because a portion of the blood that is supposed to be distributed to the systemic circulation regurgitates back into the LV cavity. Prolonged exposure to high LVAD speeds has also been shown to result in aortic valve leaflet deterioration, calcification, and commissural fusion, contributing to worsening AR even in patients who did not have AR before LVAD implantation. This is especially true when the aortic valve remains closed.[20,21] Because of the absence of normal "cardiac cycles" in patients with LVADs, AR is often continuous (systolic and diastolic) so that the conventional methods for AR assessment such as vena contracta width, jet height, and proximal isovelocity surface area often underestimate the hemodynamic significance of AR, although these parameters are still used to quantitate AR in these patients.

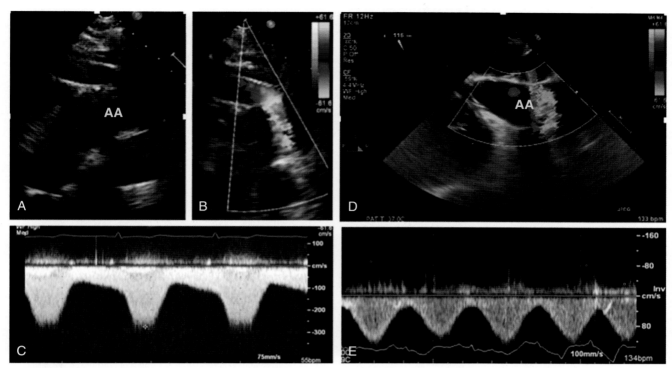

Figure 175.6. The appearance of the outflow cannula with the transthoracic transducer located in the right parasternal window without (**A**) and with Color Doppler imaging (**B**). **C,** The velocity across the outflow cannula. **D,** The appearance of the outflow cannula from the transesophageal perspective with color Doppler imaging. **E,** The continuous-wave Doppler velocity is captured in the image. *AA,* Ascending aorta.

This is further complicated by the fact that these patients have low systemic pressures and high diastolic pressures, making it difficult to obtain a true measurement of AR. When possible, the regurgitation volume and fraction should also be calculated. "De novo" AR occurs in approximately 25% to 33% of patients 12 months after CF LVAD implantation and is associated with adverse outcomes.[22,23] Furthermore, it tends to occur more commonly in patients with aortic valves that do not open (66% of such cases in one study) than in those that do (8% occurrence in the same study).[24] With the increasing use of LVADs for destination therapy, deterioration of the aortic valve is a serious long-term complication with no durable long-term solutions at this time. Recent recommendations suggest that the LVAD speed should be low enough so that AVO is intermittent (i.e., every second to third beat).[23] This has been shown to decrease the severity of AR in the long term. Importantly, however, in patients with severely reduced LV function, the aortic valve may not open at any speed. In patients with pre-LVAD AR, surgical intervention to correct AR may be considered before LVAD implantation.

MITRAL AND TRICUSPID REGURGITATION

Unloading of the left ventricle with resultant decrease in LV size should result in reduction of functional MR with decreased papillary muscle displacement and improved leaflet coaptation. Lack of improvement in MR may suggest inadequate LV unloading or interference of the inflow cannula with the submitral apparatus. TR is often a function of the RV size and tricuspid annular dimension. With high LVAD speeds, TR has the potential to worsen because of shifting of the IVS to the left or dilatation of the right heart chambers. In a normally functioning LVAD, optimization of pump speed with the RAMP study (discussed later) can help to avoid or rectify this.

INFLOW CANNULA

The inflow cannula is implanted at the LV apex and should be directed toward the mitral valve so that an invisible line drawn from

the cannula opening to the mitral valve bisects the mitral valve leaflets (Fig. 175.6). Interrogation of the LVAD cannula should be performed in both modified and standard four- and two-chamber views on TTE and on the midesophageal view on TEE to assess cannula orientation and proximity to the IVS (four-chamber view) and its anteroposterior location (two-chamber view). Sometimes the modified or standard parasternal long-axis view can also be used to assess cannula position and alignment. 3D echocardiography can complement 2D imaging, especially in the modified parasternal long-axis view, to assess cannula alignment. Color, pulsed-wave (PW), and continuous-wave (CW) Doppler can be used to assess inflow cannula flows. Normal color Doppler assessment of the inflow cannula should reveal nonturbulent, laminar flow through the cannula. PW and CW Doppler interrogation of the inflow cannula should show lower diastolic velocities and a higher systolic velocity. The presence of a diastolic velocity component is necessary for good functioning in CF LVAD.[19,23] Cannula velocities are slightly pulsatile because of the residual inherent LV contraction even in the presence of a closed aortic valve. Peak inflow cannula velocities should be less than about 2 m/s. Higher inflow velocities can be suggestive of inflow cannula obstruction. Clinically, LVAD cannula obstruction is also accompanied by low-flow alarms and increased power surges. These alarms act as a warning to the patient. The most common causes of obstruction include thrombosis of the inflow cannula, inlet occlusion by myocardial trabeculations, and cannula malposition caused by LV underfilling or kinking. Importantly, normal values of inflow cannula flow velocities are defined based on the device (see Fig. 175.6).

OUTFLOW CANNULA

The outflow cannula is typically imaged in the right parasternal location or from the high left parasternal location at the level of the ascending aorta (Fig. 175.7). In this view, the outflow graft and sometimes its end-to-side anastomosis with the ascending aorta can be seen. Color Doppler enhancement sometimes helps with the

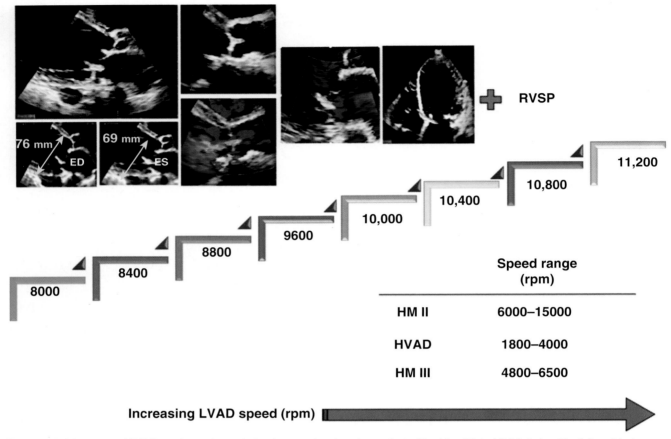

Figure 175.7. Incremental RAMP study used to optimize the speed settings in a patient with a HeartMate (HM) II device. The left ventricular assist device (LVAD) speed is increased in increments (illustrated as steps in a staircase), and at each speed level, a number of echocardiographic views are obtained. These tend to be center specific (as is the RAMP study adoption and specific protocol). Views obtained at each speed setting include the parasternal long-axis view for left ventricular dimensions, aortic valve opening, aortic regurgitation, and mitral regurgitation. Apical views may be added to assess septal position and right ventricular size and tricuspid regurgitation degree and to estimate right ventricular systolic pressure. Expected speed ranges for the different devices are illustrated in the figure (right). *ED,* end-diastole; *ES,* end-systole; *HVAD,* HeartWare Ventricular Assist System; *RVSP,* right ventricular systolic pressure.

localization of the outflow cannula in difficult cases. The outflow cannula should be interrogated using color Doppler, PW Doppler, and CW Doppler. Normal outflow graft velocities are device dependent with abnormal velocities generally falling in the greater than 2 m/s range

LVAD surveillance TTE examinations are recommended approximately 2 weeks after device implantation or before hospitalization discharge, followed by surveillance TTE at 1, 3, 6, and 12 months after implantation and every 6 to 12 months thereafter.[23]

RECOVERY OF THE MYOCARDIUM

Myocardial recovery has been reported in fewer than 5% to 11% of patients on LVAD support.[25,26] Echocardiographic parameters associated with myocardial recovery include improvement in LV EF (some say >45%) and LVEDD (≤55 mm).[11,19,27] Documentation of myocardial recovery is a complex process. Improvement in echocardiographic parameters is only one of many factors considered in the assessment for myocardial recovery. Other parameters include cardiopulmonary exercise testing, pharmacologic exercise testing on partial versus full LVAD support, and invasive hemodynamic testing. At this time there is no uniformly acceptable LVAD weaning protocol. Of note, AVO has been studied as a surrogate for LV performance. High speeds in patients with CF LVADs can unload the LV to the point at which the LV pressure consistently

less than the mean aortic pressure, resulting in aortic valve closure throughout the cardiac cycle. The speed setting at which this occurs is partly related to LV contractility. The ability to maintain AVO at higher speeds is an indicator of myocardial recovery.[25]

ECHOCARDIOGRAPHIC ASSESSMENT OF LEFT VENTRICULAR ASSIST DEVICE COMPLICATIONS

Data from the Randomized Evaluation of Mechanical Assistance for the Treatment of Congestive Heart Failure (REMATCH) trial suggests that 35% of patients have LVAD failure 2 years after device implantation, making it the second most common cause of death.[28,29] Careful scanning and interpretation of echocardiographic images in these patients can sometimes provide timely clues toward possible LVAD malfunction. LVAD complications can be divided into those that occur in the immediate postoperative period and those that occur later during the follow-up period. Immediate complications are often heralded by hypotension and include (1) pericardial effusion or tamponade; (2) thrombosis; (3) inadequate LV filling or unloading or suction events; (4) RV failure; (5) pump failure or malfunction, including inflow–outflow obstruction; (6) AR; and (7) LVAD-mediated MR. Many of these can still occur in the follow-up period. Of course, pericardial effusion or tamponade in the follow-up period can occur for the same reasons that they do in native hearts. RV failure that occurs more than 48 hours after LVAD implantation is referred to as late RV failure.

TABLE 175.2 Echocardiographic Approach to Left Ventricular Assist Device Alarms

Left Ventricular Assist Device Alarm	Echocardiographic Parameters	Diagnosis
Low flow	• Decreased LV size • IVS midline or leftward	Hypovolemia Suction events
Low flow	• Decrease LV size • IVS leftward • RV dilatation	Right heart failure
Low flow	• Large or loculated effusion with compression	Tamponade
Low flow Increased power	• Increased LV size • IVS rightward • Increased AVO • Mitral regurgitation	Inflow cannula or outflow cannula obstruction
High flow Low cardiac output	• Increased LV size • IVS midline or rightward • Aortic regurgitation	Significant aortic regurgitation
High flow	• Increased LV size • IVS rightward • Increased AVO • Mitral regurgitation	Thrombus

AVO, Aortic valve opening; *IVS,* interventricular septum; *LV,* left ventricular; *RV,* right ventricular.

TTE should be performed in any patient with an acute illness, LVAD alarms, abnormal device parameters, or symptoms of heart failure. Low pump flow with low power could suggest cannula obstruction or low LV preload, as may occur with hypovolemia, tamponade, severe TR, or RV dysfunction. Low pump flows with high power and high cannula velocities could suggest cannula obstruction. High pump flow with or without more frequent AVO, rightward septal deviation, and worsened MR may suggest cannula obstruction, device malfunction, or pump thrombosis. High pump flows with a low systemic cardiac output state raises concern for de novo severe aortic insufficiency (Table 175.2).

Pericardial tamponade is a medical emergency and a clinical diagnosis in which echocardiography is complementary. It is often, but not always, heralded by hypotension. It may be elusive in post-LVAD patients because effusions are often loculated. The echocardiographer must search for fluid collections, which may be compressing one or more of the cardiac chambers. A substernal fluid collection, for instance, may impair filling of the RV outflow tract, and a posterior fluid collection may restrict filling of the left atrium. TEE may be helpful in these patients because these fluid collections can accumulate posteriorly and be difficult to find on TTE. The typical Doppler parameters suggestive of interventricular dependence such as respirophasic variations in mitral and tricuspid inflow patterns are often not reliable in patients with LVADs because of the hemodynamic alterations associated with the presence of these devices. The diagnosis is therefore dependent on a high clinical suspicion.

The risk of thrombus formation is 9% to 16% in patients with an implanted LVAD,[30] likely because of the chronic low flow state in these patients. Thrombosis can occur in the LV apex; in and around the inflow cannula; and in the aortic root, especially in patients with no AVO or with suture closure of the aortic valve. Sometimes contrast microbubbles can help reveal thrombi in these areas. Thrombus formation in the inflow cannula is difficult to assess on TTE. Increased inflow cannula velocities may hint at this possibility but generally the activation of low-flow alarms, presence of hemolysis on bloodwork, or alternative imaging with cardiac computed tomography (CT) or a RAMP study (see later) is needed in order to diagnose inflow cannula thrombosis.

When the patient's condition deteriorates (e.g., when he or she contracts fever, vomiting, diarrhea, decreased oral intake, or illness), the intravascular volume may change, altering the hemodynamics of the LVAD. The IVS is a good marker of LV unloading. Under normal conditions, the IVS should be midline. A midline or slightly leftward IVS is consistent with adequate LV and LA unloading. A rightward shift of the septum is suggestive

of inadequate LV unloading, which in the immediate postoperative setting could suggest speed that is too low, device malfunction, or cannula obstruction or thrombosis. A leftward shift in the IVS is suggestive of excessive LV unloading, which may be caused by high LVAD speed, intravascular volume depletion (hypovolemia), or RV dysfunction (see Fig. 175.3). When the LV cavity is small, the chances of "suction events" increases. This is a situation in which the LV myocardium obstructs flow through the inflow cannula. In these patients, the inflow cannula is often directed toward the IVS instead of the mitral valve. This complication can usually be quickly reversed by decreasing the LVAD pump speed or, depending on the clinical situation, increasing LV preload.

RV failure has been reported in up to 44% of LVAD recipients postimplant[31] and can be acute (<48 hours), early (48 hours–14 days), or late (>14 days).[32] Echocardiographic indices of RV failure include RV dilatation and dysfunction; worsening TR; and IVS deviation toward the LV, including signs of an elevated central venous pressure such as elevated RA pressures, dilated IVC, and ascites. Reported pre-LVAD echocardiographic predictors of early and late RV failure are listed in Table 175.3. In the preoperative assessment, it is important to document RV size and function because poor RV indices can be associated with increased postoperative risk of RV failure and trigger early consideration for RV mechanical support. RV-to-LV end-diastolic diameter ratio greater than 0.75 on pre-LVAD assessment has been associated with RV failure after surgery. Similarly, TAPSE values of 7.5 or less have also been associated with increased risk of RV failure after LVAD insertion. Limited data suggest that RV free-wall strain values greater than −14% may be predictive of poorer outcomes in these patients.[17] In assessment of the RV, it is generally accepted that no one parameter is sufficient to characterize its function.[23] Multiparameter assessment is considered the optimal approach.

Inflow cannula assessment can be difficult on TTE. Flow into the apical cannula during LVAD filling should be unidirectional. Inflow cannula regurgitation on color Doppler assessment or elevated CW Doppler velocities should raise the suspicion for inflow cannula obstruction, LVAD pump malfunction, or outflow graft twisting or obstruction. The latter can lead to an increase in afterload to the LVAD and inflow valve regurgitation. Inflow cannula obstruction is often associated with LV dilatation, increased AVO and interventricular septal deviation to the right. Color Doppler assessment of the inflow cannula can be used to visualize the regurgitation and turbulence at the inlet during LV systole. Outflow cannula obstruction can be caused by graft malposition, twisting, occlusion, external compression, and thrombosis. Findings of outflow cannula obstruction as they relate to the LV and aortic

TABLE 175.3 Echocardiographic Predictors of Right Ventricular Failure as Reported in the Literature and the Limitations to Their Use in Clinical Practice

Parameter	Limitations
Fractional area change	• Poor reproducibility • Tedious
RV-to-LV end-diastolic diameter ratio	• Poor reproducibility • View dependent
TAPSE	• Sensitive to loading conditions • Values do not correlate well with RV function in the postcardiac surgery period • Reduced reliability in the presence of significant TR
RV strain	• Intervendor variability • Requires good views of the RV free wall • Limited data

LV, left ventricular; *RV,* right ventricular; *TR,* tricuspid regurgitation; *TAPSE,* tricuspid annular systolic excursion.

valve are similar to those for inflow cannula obstruction. In these patients, abnormal (elevated or diminished) CW velocities may be recorded at the outflow graft anastomosis to the ascending aorta.

Significant AR is often accompanied by high-flow alarms and low cardiac output. If significant AR is suspected, TEE may prove useful for confirmation in these patients if TTE images are difficult.

RAMP STUDIES

The RAMP study is one example of an LVAD speed optimization protocol that generally involves the use of TTE at stepwise incremental device speed settings to determine the best speed setting for the particular device. Details of the protocol vary from center to center. Views obtained at each speed setting include parasternal long-axis views for LV dimensions, AVO, AR, and MR. Apical views may be added to assess septal position and RV size or TR degree. In some cases, concomitant right heart catheterization may also be used. In a normally functioning LVAD, increasing LVAD speed results in augmented LV unloading, decreased LV diameters, and shifting of the IVS to the left with a decrease in MR degree. At the same time AVO decreases, AR worsens, and RV size increases.[33] Current targets for device speed settings include mean arterial pressure greater than 65 mm Hg, intermittent AVO, minimal AR, midline IVS position, and no more than mild MR to ensure optimal LV unloading.[34] Fig. 175.7 illustrates a RAMP study used to optimize the speed settings in a patient with a HeartMate II device. Expected speed ranges for the different devices are also illustrated in the figure.[35]

RAMP studies can also be used to diagnose device malfunction.[24] For example, instances of device thrombosis have been diagnosed using a RAMP study. In these patients, the LVAD does not unload the LV normally, and LV size does not decrease with increased speed settings. Of course, echocardiography is not used in isolation to make these diagnoses. Patients with device thrombosis also often demonstrate intravascular hemolysis with high levels of lactate dehydrogenase and low haptoglobin. Ultimately, other modalities such as cardiac CT and fluoroscopy or in extreme situations surgical exploration may be required to make or confirm the diagnosis.

SUMMARY

TTE is an important, noninvasive first step in the evaluation of patients with CF LVADs. It is used to assess the heart before LVAD implantation, in the immediate postoperative period to evaluate any hemodynamic deterioration, and in follow-up to ensure optimal device function. TEE is often used in the intraoperative

setting and may also be used pre- and postoperatively to confirm or verify findings unclear on TTE. When the clinical status of the patient deteriorates or LVAD flow or power alarms are activated, the device should be re-imaged. All echocardiograms performed on LVAD patients should assess the degree of LV unloading, RV size and function, IVS position, AVO, AR degree, mitral and tricuspid valvular dysfunction, inflow and outflow cannula function, and any thrombosis or pericardial effusion. With increasing heart failure diagnoses and the projected increased used of LVADs for destination therapy, echocardiographers may encounter more of these devices in the future.

REFERENCES

1. Benjamin EJ, Muntner P, Alonso A, et al. Heart disease and stroke statistics—2019 update. *Circulation.* 2019;139. e56–e528.
2. Yancy CW, Jessup M, Bozkurt B, et al. ACCF/AHA guideline for the management of heart failure. *J Am Coll Cardiol.* 2013;62. e147–239, 2013.
3. Kirklin JK, Pagani FD, Kormos RL, et al. Eighth annual INTERMACS report: special focus on framing the impact of adverse events. *J Heart Lung Transplant.* 2017;36:1080–1086.
4. Han JJ, Acker MA, Atluri P. Left ventricular assist devices. *Circulation.* 2018;138:2841–2851.
5. Addetia K, Uriel N, Maffessanti F, et al. 3D morphological changes in LV and RV during LVAD RAMP studies. *JACC Cardiovasc Imag.* 2018;11(2 pt 1):159–169.
6. Lalonde SD, Alba AC, Rigobon A, et al. Clinical differences between continuous flow ventricular assist devices: a comparison between HeartMate II and HeartWare HVAD. *J Card Surg.* 2013;28:604–610.
7. Sauer AJ, Meehan K, Gordon R, et al. Echocardiographic markers of left ventricular unloading using a centrifugal-flow rotary pump. *J Heart Lung Transplant.* 2014;33:449–450.
8. Uriel N, Sayer G, Addetia K, et al. Hemodynamic RAMP tests in patients with left ventricular assist devices. *JACC Heart Fail.* 2016;4:208–217.
9. Piacentino 3rd V, Williams ML, Depp T, et al. Impact of tricuspid valve regurgitation in patients treated with implantable left ventricular assist devices. *Ann Thorac Surg.* 2011;91:1342–1346.
10. Levin HR, Oz MC, Chen JM, et al. Reversal of chronic ventricular dilation in patients with end-stage cardiomyopathy by prolonged mechanical unloading. *Circulation.* 1995;91:2717–2720.
11. Rasalingam R, Johnson SN, Bilhorn KR, et al. Transthoracic echocardiographic assessment of continuous-flow left ventricular assist devices. *J Am Soc Echocardiogr.* 2011;24:135–148.
12. Topilsky Y, Oh JK, Shah DK, et al. Echocardiographic predictors of adverse outcomes after continuous left ventricular assist device implantation. *JACC Cardiovasc Imaging.* 2011;4:211–222.
13. Meineri M, Van Rensburg AE, Vegas A. Right ventricular failure after LVAD implantation: prevention and treatment. *Best Pract Res Clin Anaesthesiol.* 2012;26:217–229.
14. Kukucka M, Stepanenko A, Potapov E, et al. Right-to-left ventricular end-diastolic diameter ratio and prediction of right ventricular failure with continuous-flow left ventricular assist devices. *J Heart Lung Transplant.* 2011;30:64–69.
15. Neyer J, Arsanjani R, Moriguchi J, et al. Echocardiographic parameters associated with right ventricular failure after left ventricular assist device. *J Heart Lung Transplant.* 2016;35:283–293.
16. Vivo RP, Cordero-Reyes AM, Qamar U, et al. Increased right-to-left ventricle diameter ratio is a strong predictor of right ventricular failure after left ventricular assist device. *J Heart Lung Transplant.* 2013;32:792–799.
17. Grant AD, Smedira NG, Starling RC, Marwick TH. Independent and incremental role of quantitative right ventricular evaluation for the prediction of right ventricular failure after left ventricular assist device implantation. *J Am Coll Cardiol.* 2012;60:521–528.
18. Kato TS, Jiang J, Schulze PC, et al. Serial echocardiography using tissue Doppler and speckle tracking imaging to monitor right ventricular failure before and after left ventricular assist device surgery. *JACC Heart Fail.* 2013;1:216–222.
19. Estep JD, Stainback RF, Little SH, et al. The role of echocardiography and other imaging modalities in patients with left ventricular assist devices. *JACC Cardiovasc Imag.* 2010;3:1049–1064.
20. Aggarwal A, Raghuvir R, Eryazici P, et al. The development of aortic insufficiency in continuous-flow left ventricular assist device-supported patients. *Ann Thorac Surg.* 2013;95:493–498.
21. Jorde UP, Uriel N, Nahumi N, et al. Prevalence, significance, and management of aortic insufficiency in continuous flow left ventricular assist device recipients. *Circ Heart Fail.* 2014;7:310–319.
22. Cowger J, Pagani FD, Haft JW, et al. The development of aortic insufficiency in left ventricular assist device-supported patients. *Circ Heart Fail.* 2010;3:668–674.
23. Stainback RF, Estep JD, Agler DA, et al. Echocardiography in the management of patients with left ventricular assist devices. *J Am Soc Echocardiogr.* 2015;28:853–909.
24. Uriel N, Morrison KA, Garan AR, et al. Development of a novel echocardiography ramp test for speed optimization and diagnosis of device thrombosis in continuous-flow left ventricular assist devices: the Columbia ramp study. *J Am Coll Cardiol.* 2012;60:1764–1775.

25. Estep JD, Chang SM, Bhimaraj A, et al. Imaging for ventricular function and myocardial recovery on nonpulsatile ventricular assist devices. *Circulation.* 2012;125:2265–2277.

26. Maybaum S, Mancini D, Xydas S, et al. Cardiac improvement during mechanical circulatory support: a prospective multicenter study of the LVAD Working Group. *Circulation.* 2007;115:2497–2505.

27. Dandel M, Weng Y, Siniawski H, et al. Long-term results in patients with idiopathic dilated cardiomyopathy after weaning from left ventricular assist devices. *Circulation.* 2005;112(9 Suppl):I37–I45.

28. Horton SC, Khodaverdian R, Chatelain P, et al. Left ventricular assist device malfunction: an approach to diagnosis by echocardiography. *J Am Coll Cardiol.* 2005;45:1435–1440.

29. Rose EA, Gelijns AC, Moskowitz AJ, et al. Long-term use of a left ventricular assist device for end-stage heart failure. *N Engl J Med.* 2001;345:1435–1443.

30. Ammar KA, Umland MM, Kramer C, et al. The ABCs of left ventricular assist device echocardiography: a systematic approach. *Eur Heart J Cardiovasc Imag.* 2012;13:885–899.

31. Drakos SG, Janicki L, Horne BD, et al. Risk factors predictive of right ventricular failure after left ventricular assist device implantation. *Am J Cardiol.* 2010;105:1030–1035.

32. Raina A, Patarroyo-Aponte M. Prevention and treatment of right ventricular failure during left ventricular assist device therapy. *Crit Care Clin.* 2018;34:439–452.

33. Topilsky Y, Oh JK, Atchison FW, et al. Echocardiographic findings in stable outpatients with properly functioning HeartMate II left ventricular assist devices. *J Am Soc Echocardiogr.* 2011;24:157–169.

34. Park SJ, Milano CA, Tatooles AJ, et al. Outcomes in advanced heart failure patients with left ventricular assist devices for destination therapy. *Circ Heart Fail.* 2012;5:241–248.

35. Tchoukina I, Smallfield MC, Shah KB. Device management and flow optimization on left ventricular assist device support. *Crit Care Clin.* 2018;34:453–463.

176

Extracorporeal Membrane Oxygenation, Impella, and Other Circulatory Mechanical Support

Benjamin B. Kenigsberg, Alexander I. Papolos, Raymond F. Stainback, Preetham Kumar

MECHANICAL CIRCULATORY SUPPORT

Mechanical circulatory support (MCS) refers to nonpharmacologic cardiac assist systems that provide hemodynamic support in the treatment of patients with cardiogenic shock. Temporary MCS is used as a bridge to myocardial recovery, durable MCS, and heart transplantation or to provide time for clinical decision making. Despite having been in use for more than 40 years, the most common form of MCS remains the intraaortic balloon pump (IABP) (Getinge).[1] More contemporary MCS includes intracardiac systems that can be implanted percutaneously (Impella, ABIOMED; the TandemHeart, CardiacAssist), peripheral or central extracorporeal membrane oxygenation (ECMO), and centrally inserted (via sternotomy) temporary ventricular assist systems.

At this time, no specific form of MCS has demonstrated clear superiority in the management of cardiogenic shock.[2] Each MCS method has unique hemodynamic and mechanical characteristics that affect its clinical use and peri-implantation echocardiographic evaluation.[3] As a result, cardiologist and echocardiographer exposure to MCS devices is heterogenous and based on patient- and center-specific parameters. This chapter reviews the most prevalent types of MCS, with a focus on echocardiographic assessment (Table 176.1). Of note, in all patients being considered for MCS, baseline echocardiographic assessment should include assessing biventricular function, presence of severe valvular disease, intracardiac thrombus, and identification of alternative pathophysiologic mechanism for hemodynamic shock.

EXTRACORPOREAL MEMBRANE OXYGENATION

In ECMO, a cardiopulmonary bypass circuit is used to provide extended cardiac and/or respiratory support for days to weeks.[4] ECMO cannulas can be positioned in a venoarterial (VA) or venovenous (VV) configuration and are connected to an externalized adjustable continuous-flow centrifugal pump and oxygenator. VA-ECMO is the only single MCS technique that provides biventricular (combined right ventricular [RV] and left ventricular [LV]) hemodynamic assistance, albeit indirectly by diverting blood flow away from both ventricles. VA-ECMO can

TABLE 176.1 Peri-implant Echocardiographic Assessment and Monitoring of Mechanical Circulatory Support Devices[a]

MCS System	Preimplant Contraindications	Insertion Guidance	Postimplant Complications
ECMO	None	Often TTE/TEE; TEE for dual-lumen VV-ECMO	VV-ECMO: recirculation from adjacent cannulas VA-ECMO: LV pressure loading and reduced LV ejection
Impella	Severe AR, mechanical aortic valve, aortic dissection, LV thrombus	Fluoroscopy TTE to confirm postimplant position	Malpositioning (incorrect depth or interference with MV function) Suction event from LV decompression or malpositioning
IABP	Severe AR, aortic dissection	Fluoroscopy	Malpositioning
TandemHeart RV Support	Left atrial thrombus, severe pulmonic regurgitation or stenosis, severe tricuspid stenosis	Fluoroscopy, TEE, or both Fluoroscopy and often TEE	Suction events from LA decompression Pulmonic regurgitation Malpositioning

[a]Preimplantation assessment for all types of percutaneous mechanical circulatory support (MCS) should include left ventricular (LV) and right ventricular (RV) function, LV and RV size, severe valvular stenosis and regurgitation, ventricular septal defect, and peripheral vascular disease.

AR, Aortic regurgitation; *ECMO,* extracorporeal membrane oxygenation; *IABP,* intraaortic balloon pump; *MV,* mitral valve; *TEE,* transesophageal echocardiography; *TTE,* transthoracic echocardiography; *VA,* venoarterial; *VV,* venovenous.

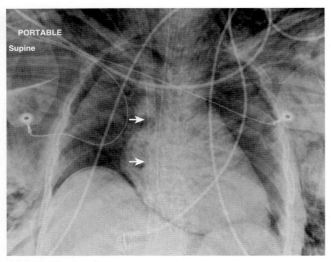

Figure 176.1. Chest radiograph showing a single dual-lumen venovenous extracorporeal membrane oxygenation cannula *(arrows)* inserted via the right internal jugular vein in a patient with acute respiratory distress syndrome.

be done peripherally, via an inflow cannula extending into the venae cavae and an outflow cannula in a femoral or iliac artery, or centrally, with the inflow cannula in the right atrium and the outflow cannula in the aorta. VV-ECMO can also be peripheral, with both the inflow and outflow cannulas in the venous system; notably, VV-ECMO provides only pulmonary support without cardiac bypass.

Echocardiography is frequently used to guide cannula insertion, assess the adequacy of support, evaluate for complications, and determine the timing of ECMO weaning.[5,6] During implantation, either transthoracic echocardiography (TTE) or transesophageal echocardiography (TEE) can be used to verify that the venous inflow catheter is positioned correctly, typically at the vena cava–right atrial junction. Notably, adequate VV-ECMO cannula positioning requires the inflow and outflow ports to be spatially distanced from each other, typically with one in the superior vena cava and one in the inferior vena cava to prevent recirculation of blood. Alternatively, a single dual-lumen VV-ECMO cannula can be placed from the right internal jugular vein. The inflow ports of the dual-lumen cannula are located in the distal and proximal portions of the cannula, drawing from the inferior and superior vena cava, and the outflow port resides in the midportion of the cannula, which is positioned in the right atrium oriented toward the tricuspid valve.[7] Crucially,

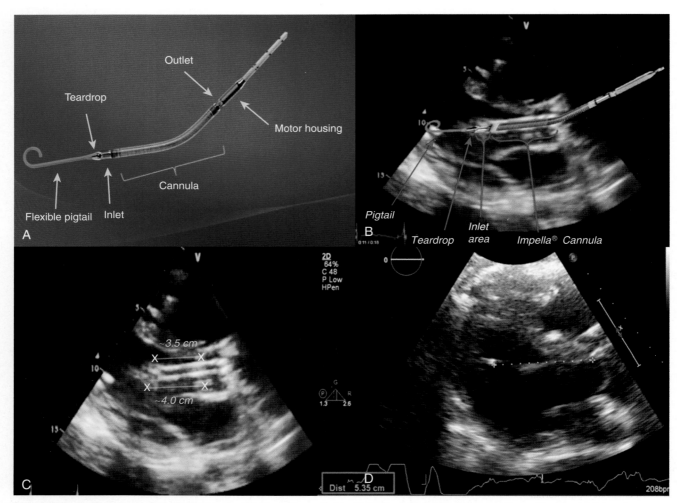

Figure 176.2. A, Anatomy of the Left-side Impella 5.0 Heart Pump. **B,** Identifying the Impella Heart Pump regions with echocardiography: transthoracic echocardiography parasternal long-axis view of an Impella with an overlying graphic of the Impella. **C,** How to measure the depth of the Impella Heart Pump in the left ventricle (LV). Recommended positioning depth should be 3.5 cm with measurement from the aortic annulus to the mid-inlet, or 4 cm with measurement from the aortic annulus to the teardrop. **D,** Impella Heart Pump too deep in the LV. The Impella extends 5.35 cm from the aortic annulus to the teardrop, indicating that it has been inserted too far into the LV. (Courtesy of ABIOMED Inc., 2019.)

echocardiographic guidance of catheter placement should ensure that the distal end of the cannula is not positioned in the RV, in the coronary sinus, or through a patent foramen ovale into the left atrium.[8] Technically, a subxiphoid TTE view of the inferior vena cava or a midesophageal TEE view of both venae cavae can allow visualization of the guide wires before cannula insertion and after insertion to optimize the orientation of the outflow port (Fig. 176.1).

After ECMO initiation, the Extracorporeal Life Support Organization (ELSO) guidelines suggest frequent echocardiographic assessment both during support and during weaning trials.[9] Echocardiographic findings may refine prognostication and guide clinical decision making regarding weaning of ECMO support. Doppler assessment during ECMO weaning trials suggests that the combination of LV outflow tract velocity time integral 10 cm or greater, LV ejection fraction (LVEF) greater than 25%, and lateral mitral annulus peak systolic velocity 6 cm/s or greater is predictive of successful ECMO weaning.[10] Notably, Doppler-derived assessment of LV filling pressure, such as mitral inflow E and tissue Doppler e′, do not clearly predict outcomes.[10] Similarly, an assessment of RV parameters during ECMO support identified three-dimensional echocardiography of RV ejection fraction (RVEF) as the most predictive parameter; specifically, an RVEF greater than 25% was associated with successful weaning and lower risk of all-cause mortality.[11] Protocolized TEE-guided ECMO weaning has also been attempted, in which weaning trials were discontinued if ventricular dilatation developed.[12] Finally, baseline RV dilatation before VV-ECMO insertion for refractory acute respiratory distress syndrome is an independent predictor of intensive care unit death.[13] Notably, hemodynamic support by VA-ECMO does not preclude the use of other forms of MCS. Instead, MCS devices are often used concurrently with VA-ECMO to unload the left ventricle.[14]

IMPELLA

The Impella is a percutaneously inserted continuous-flow intravascular microaxial device for short-term ventricular support. A motor housed within the catheter spins an Archimedes screw that draws blood from an inlet cage positioned in the let ventricle that subsequently ejects the blood into the ascending aorta. The Impella catheter must be precisely positioned for it to provide mechanical support, minimize hemolysis, and avoid disrupting the mitral apparatus. The catheter itself is not tethered to any internal structure and is prone to migration. Therefore, catheter position should be assessed and optimized under echocardiographic guidance after insertion, device manipulation, change in patient clinical status, and specific device alarms. Important echocardiographic contraindications are severe aortic regurgitation, mechanical aortic valve, aortic dissection, and LV thrombus, given the device's anatomic location extending from the LV cavity to the aorta. Although the Impella device traverses the aortic valve, severe aortic stenosis does not contraindicate insertion.[15] Typically, the smaller diameter Impella 2.5 and CP are inserted under fluoroscopic guidance in the cardiac catheterization laboratory; however, limited data suggest that TEE can also be used to guide placement.[16] The larger diameter Impella 5.0 is typically inserted via direct surgical cutdown to the subclavian artery.

Postimplantation Impella positioning is almost exclusively guided by cardiac ultrasonography. Only limited evidence from patients with aortic valve prostheses suggests that cardiac device positioning can be verified by supine chest radiography.[17] The transthoracic parasternal long-axis and transesophageal midesophageal long-axis views are the most reliable for determining Impella depth (Fig. 176.2). A multibeat acquisition of the catheter while panning through the LV cavity can help to minimize foreshortening. The depth of the catheter is measured from the proximal edge of the inlet cage to the aortic annulus (see Fig. 176.2). The inlet cage itself cannot be well visualized directly by ultrasonography. However, the proximal edge of the inlet cage connects to the cannula portion of the catheter, which appears as a pair of echogenic parallel lines referred to by the manufacturer as the "railroad tracks." Depth is thus measured from the aortic annulus to the end of the cannula (i.e., end of the railroad tracks). The optimal depth is 3.5 cm, and readjustment should be considered for a margin of error greater than 0.5 cm.

An additional method to ensure proper depth is to interrogate the aortic root with color Doppler from the long-axis view. A mosaic pattern of flow will be seen coming from the Impella outlet cage in the aortic root. In the absence of aortic regurgitation, this flow pattern should be limited to the aortic side of the valve. If it is observed below the valve, the device is too deep and should be pulled back (Fig. 176.3).

After the Impella depth has been optimized, the spatial relationship between the catheter and intracardiac structures should be assessed. The cannula portion of the catheter is built with a 30-degree bend. The purpose of the bend is to angle the catheter toward the anteroseptal apex of the left ventricle and away from the papillary muscles and mitral valve. If the catheter is angled incorrectly, it is possible for the pigtail at its distal tip to get caught in the mitral apparatus or for a segment of the catheter to restrict mitral valve opening. It is therefore important to evaluate mitral valve function by two-dimensional (2D) and color Doppler imaging (Fig. 176.4). Furthermore, crowding of the inlet or outlet cages increases shear stress on the blood pumped through the catheter, accelerating the rate of hemolysis caused by the device. Attention to the size and function of the left and right ventricles, as well as interventricular septal position, should be included in the echocardiographic assessment of the Impella catheter because low-flow and suction alarms can occur in patients with RV failure or dilatation.

Repositioning of the Impella catheter should be done under real-time echocardiographic guidance. During manipulation of the catheter, it is important to remember that the distance advanced or withdrawn is not necessarily transmitted in a one-to-one fashion because slack may be present in or introduced into the catheter. A suprasternal notch view of the aortic arch may reveal slack that is causing the catheter to be mobile within the aortic lumen instead of taut against the lesser curvature of the aortic arch (Fig. 176.5).

INTRAAORTIC BALLOON PUMP

The IABP uses diastolic counterpulsation to both augment coronary perfusion and reduce systemic vascular resistance, thereby indirectly augmenting cardiac output by approximately 0.5 LPM.[18] An IABP is inserted (typically peripherally via the femoral artery or less often the axillary or subclavian artery) into the descending aorta and is attached to an externalized gas pump that drives balloon inflation and deflation. Important echocardiographic contraindications for IABP include aortic dissection, given the balloon's anatomic position in the descending aorta, and significant aortic regurgitation because the counterpulsation mechanism propels blood back toward the aortic valve and may exacerbate aortic insufficiency.

IABP positioning is typically assessed by fluoroscopy or radiography because the device has a radiopaque marker on its distal tip. However, IABPs have also been placed by TEE guidance when radiography is not readily available (Fig. 176.6).[19] Echocardiography can identify the mobile echogenic structure in the descending thoracic aorta, particularly during early diastolic inflation, because of the sonographic impedance of the air-filled balloon (Fig. 176.7). The device should be positioned in the descending thoracic aorta to avoid proximal occlusion of the left subclavian artery and distal occlusion of the renal arteries.

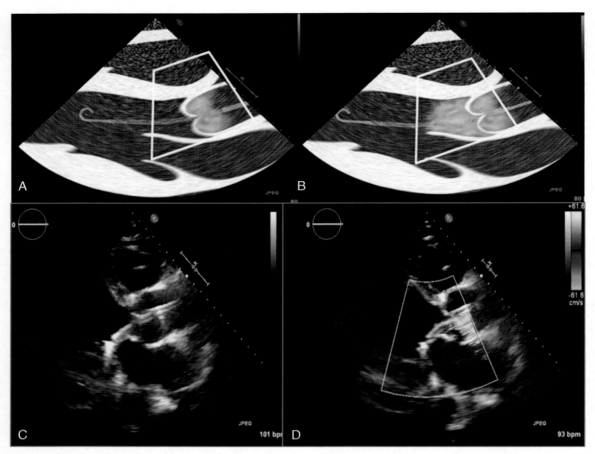

Figure 176.3. Graphical representation of color Doppler interrogation of Impella heart pump with the device appropriately positioned (**A**) and the device inserted too far into the left ventricle (**B**), with the outlet below the aortic valve. **C,** Transthoracic echocardiography parasternal long-axis image of Impella oriented inferiorly with device inlet adjacent to the mitral valve, and (D) color Doppler image consistent with device outlet above the aortic annulus. (Parts A and B courtesy of ABIOMED Inc., 2019).

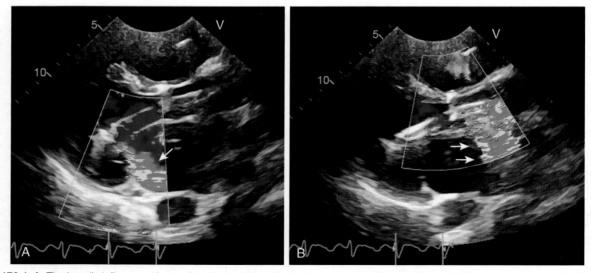

Figure 176.4. A, The Impella inflow zone is angulated toward the mitral valve apparatus with associated significant mitral regurgitation *(arrow)*, which may be caused by device interference, ischemia, or both. **B,** Color Doppler of the device in the same patient shows the characteristic "waterfall" color Doppler artifact within the left atrium *(double arrows)* from the impeller mechanism; this should not be confused with mitral regurgitation.

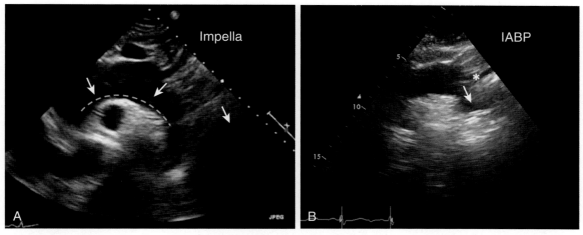

Figure 176.5. The transthoracic echocardiography suprasternal notch view can be used to identify the Impella device (**A**) along the lesser curve of the aortic arch *(arrows)* or the intraaortic balloon pump tip position *(single arrow)*, ideally just distal to the left subclavian artery *(asterisk)* (**B**).

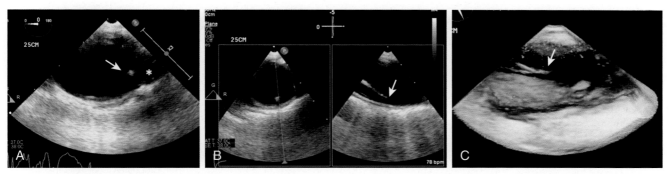

Figure 176.6. Transesophageal echocardiography (TEE) imaging can be useful for confirming intraaortic balloon pump (IABP) position. **A,** Intraoperative TEE demonstrated the IABP tip *(arrow)* too close to the left subclavian artery *(asterisk)*. After slight pullback, the IABP is better positioned (**B** and **C**). Note: The characteristic IABP tip position varies during the cardiac cycle, and its precise location can be difficult with planar imaging alone but is improved using simultaneous orthogonal plane (**B**) or using three-dimensional imaging (**C**).

TANDEMHEART

TandemHeart (Cardiac Assist) is a percutaneously inserted ventricular support device with an externalized continuous-flow centrifugal pump. The inflow cannula is typically positioned in the left atrium via a transseptal puncture from the femoral vein, with the outflow cannula delivering up to 5 LPM of flow into the femoral artery (Fig. 176.8). Echocardiographic contraindications to placement include left atrial thrombus. Notably, because of the intracardiac positioning of the device, neither severe aortic or mitral valvular disease nor LV thrombus precludes device implantation.

During TandemHeart placement, transseptal puncture and left atrial cannula positioning are guided by fluoroscopy, TEE, or both. A midesophageal bicaval view confirms the presence of the wire in the right atrium, and a midesophageal aortic valve short-axis view (40–50 degrees) can be used to guide the transseptal puncture to avoid aortic injury.[20] Transseptal puncture can also be guided by intracardiac ultrasonography.[21] After implantation, echocardiographic assessment should focus on left atrial size and cannula position to prevent suction events that can interfere with hemodynamic support.

RV SUPPORT

Two percutaneous RV support devices are currently used in clinical practice. The Impella RP is an intravascular microaxial ventricular

support device, similar to left-sided Impella systems, that is placed via a femoral vein. Blood is drawn through an inflow port in the inferior vena cava and is then ejected into the pulmonary artery. The ProtekDuo is a dual-lumen cannula that is inserted via the right internal jugular vein and terminates in the main pulmonary artery.[22] With this system, blood is drawn through an inflow port in the right atrium via an extracorporeal pump, to which an oxygenator can be attached, and is then ejected through the outflow port in the main pulmonary artery. Both devices are placed via wire exchange over a pulmonary arterial catheter.

Before the insertion of either device, a preimplantation echocardiogram should be performed to evaluate valvular integrity, RV size and function, and mural or vena caval thrombi. Severe pulmonic regurgitation or severe stenosis of either the pulmonic or tricuspid valve are contraindications to device implantation. TEE is frequently used to help guide placement of both devices, which is best achieved with the midesophageal short-axis view (30–60 degrees). Each device's outflow port should optimally sit in the distal main pulmonary artery so as to remain clear of the pulmonic valve but not beyond the pulmonary arterial bifurcation, which could result in preferential perfusion of one of the lungs. After implantation, serial imaging is commonly indicated to assess response to therapy, ability to wean from support, and device positioning. Short-axis views should be obtained by 2D and color-flow Doppler imaging to evaluate for pulmonic regurgitation and

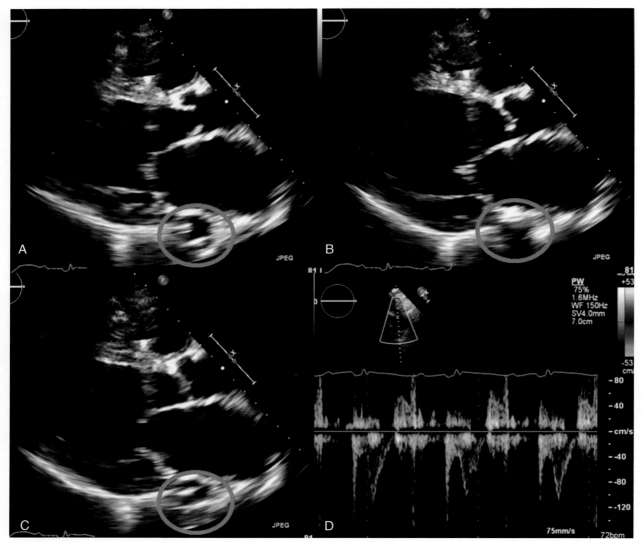

Figure 176.7. Intraaortic balloon pump (IABP) findings during echocardiography. Transthoracic echocardiography images in the parasternal long-axis view, with the *red circle* outlining the descending thoracic aorta, show the IABP deflated during systole (**A**), inflated during early diastole (**B**); note the shadowing posterior to the descending aorta caused by air filling the intraaortic balloon), and deflated during late diastole (**C**). **D,** Pulsed-wave Doppler tracing in the proximal descending aorta shows antegrade systolic flow and retrograde flow in early diastole.

confirm device position, in addition to standard assessment of RV size and function.

Clinicians should keep in mind that these devices partially bypass the right ventricle in terms of volume load, but they do so at the expense of increasing flow through the pulmonary circulation. Therefore, when these devices are used in patients with RV dysfunction caused by pulmonary hypertension, they can progressively worsen RV pressure loading, dilatation, and failure.

Acknowledgment

Stephen N. Palmer, PhD, ELS, contributed to the editing of the manuscript.

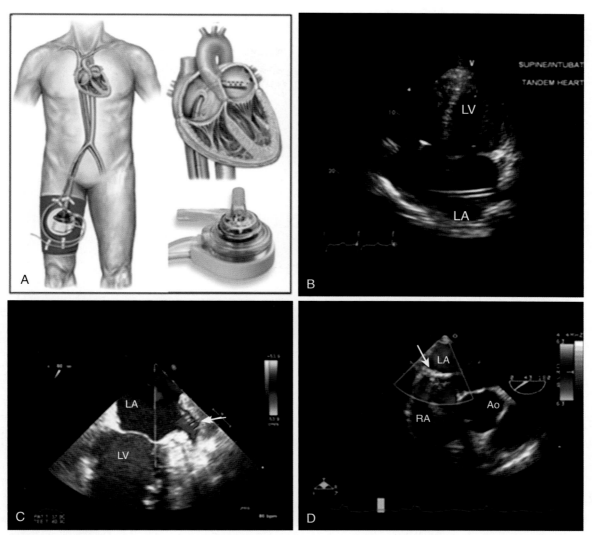

Figure 176.8. A, Illustration of the TandemHeart system, including the extracorporeal continuous-flow pump. **B,** Transthoracic echocardiography apical four-chamber view shows the device's inflow cannula within the left atrium. **C,** Transesophageal echocardiography (TEE) shows the distal cannula's multiple-port inflow zone within the left atrial appendage *(arrow)*. **D,** TEE shows the transatrial septal portion of the inflow conduit *(arrow)*. (Part A courtesy of CardiacAssist, Inc. Part D reproduced with permission from Stainback RF, et al: Echocardiography in the management of patients with left ventricular assist devices: recommendations from the American Society of Echocardiography, *J Am Soc Echocardiogr* 28:853–909, 2015.)

REFERENCES

1. Shah M, Patnaik S, Patel B, et al. Trends in mechanical circulatory support use and hospital mortality among patients with acute myocardial infarction and non-infarction related cardiogenic shock in the United States. *Clin Res Cardiol.* 2018;107:287–303.
2. Thiele H, Jobs A, Ouweneel DM, et al. Percutaneous short-term active mechanical support devices in cardiogenic shock: a systematic review and collaborative meta-analysis of randomized trials. *Eur Heart J.* 2017;38:3523–3531.
3. Stainback RF, Estep JD, Agler DA, et al. Echocardiography in the management of patients with left ventricular assist devices: recommendations from the American Society of Echocardiography. *J Am Soc Echocardiogr.* 2015;28:853–909.
4. Guglin M, Zucker MJ, Bazan VM, et al. Venoarterial ECMO for adults: JACC scientific expert panel. *J Am Coll Cardiol.* 2019;73:698–716.
5. Donker DW, Meuwese CL, Braithwaite SA, et al. Echocardiography in extracorporeal life support: a key player in procedural guidance, tailoring and monitoring. *Perfusion.* 2018;33(1 Suppl):31–41.
6. Platts DG, Sedgwick JF, Burstow DJ, et al. The role of echocardiography in the management of patients supported by extracorporeal membrane oxygenation. *J Am Soc Echocardiogr.* 2012;25:131–141.
7. Javidfar J, Brodie D, Wang D, et al. Use of bicaval dual-lumen catheter for adult venovenous extracorporeal membrane oxygenation. *Ann Thorac Surg.* 2011;91:1763–1768.

8. Giraud R, Banfi C, Bendjelid K. Echocardiography should be mandatory in ECMO venous cannula placement. *Eur Heart J Cardiovasc Imag.* 2018;19:1429–1430.
9. Extracorporeal Life Support Organization (ELSO): Guidelines for adult cardiac failure. https://www.elso.org/Portals/0/IGD/Archive/FileManager/e76ef78eabcu sersshyerdocumentselsoguidelinesforadultcardiacfailure1.3.pdf.
10. Aissaoui N, Luyt CE, Leprince P, et al. Predictors of successful extracorporeal membrane oxygenation (ECMO) weaning after assistance for refractory cardiogenic shock. *Intensive Care Med.* 2011;37:1738–1745.
11. Huang KC, Lin LY, Chen YS, et al. Three-dimensional echocardiography-derived right ventricular ejection fraction correlates with success of decannulation and prognosis in patients stabilized by venoarterial extracorporeal life support. *J Am Soc Echocardiogr.* 2018;31:169–179.
12. Cavarocchi NC, Pitcher HT, Yang Q, et al. Weaning of extracorporeal membrane oxygenation using continuous hemodynamic transesophageal echocardiography. *J Thorac Cardiovasc Surg.* 2013;146:1474–1479.
13. Lazzeri C, Cianchi G, Bonizzoli M, et al. Right ventricle dilation as a prognostic factor in refractory acute respiratory distress syndrome requiring veno-venous extracorporeal membrane oxygenation. *Minerva Anestesiol.* 2016;82:1043–1049.
14. Meani P, Gelsomino S, Natour E, et al. Modalities and effects of left ventricle unloading on extracorporeal life support: a review of the current literature. *Eur J Heart Fail.* 2017;19(Suppl 2):84–91.

15. Singh V, Yadav PK, Eng MH, et al. Outcomes of hemodynamic support with Impella in very high-risk patients undergoing balloon aortic valvuloplasty. *Int J Cardiol.* 2017;240:120–125.

16. Crowley J, Cronin B, Essandoh M, et al. Transesophageal echocardiography for Impella placement and management. *J Cardiothorac Vasc Anesth.* 2019;33:2663–2668.

17. Ouweneel DM, Sjauw KD, Wiegerinck EM, et al. Assessment of cardiac device position on supine chest radiograph in the ICU: introduction and applicability of the aortic valve location ratio. *Crit Care Med.* 2016;44:e957–963.

18. Scheidt S, Wilner G, Mueller H, et al. Intra-aortic balloon counterpulsation in cardiogenic shock. Report of a co-operative clinical trial. *N Engl J Med.* 1973;288:979–984.

19. Kaplan LJ, Weiman DS, Langan N, et al. Safe intraaortic balloon pump placement through the ascending aorta using transesophageal ultrasound. *Ann Thorac Surg.* 1992;54:374–375.

20. Pretorius M, Hughes AK, Stahlman MB, et al. Placement of the TandemHeart percutaneous left ventricular assist device. *Anesth Analg.* 2006;103:1412–1413.

21. Alkhouli M, Rihal CS, Holmes Jr DR. Transseptal techniques for emerging structural heart interventions. *JACC Cardiovasc Interv.* 2016;9:2465–2480.

22. Kapur NK, Esposito ML, Bader Y, et al. Mechanical circulatory support devices for acute right ventricular failure. *Circulation.* 2017;136:314–326.

177 Post Heart Transplant Echocardiographic Evaluation

S. Carolina Masri, James N. Kirkpatrick

Cardiac transplantation remains the gold standard therapy for patients with end-stage heart failure that is refractory to optimal medical therapy (American College of Cardiology/American Heart Association stage D heart failure).[1] Since the first cardiac transplantation in 1967, considerable advances in immunosuppressive therapy have led to improved long-term survival, with recent reports of 1-year survival rates after heart transplantation of almost 90% and a conditional half-life of 13 years.[2] Today approximately 5074 heart transplantations are performed annually in the world.[3] Echocardiography is an important tool that serves a significant role in identifying and managing patients who undergo cardiac transplantation. In this chapter, the use of echocardiography in all stages of transplantation evaluation is discussed, including screening, perioperative monitoring, and posttransplantation surveillance.

SCREENING

The role of echocardiography in pretransplantation screening involves evaluation of both the recipient and the donor.

Recipient Evaluation

Echocardiography with Doppler interrogation is instrumental in identifying the cause of heart failure, establishing candidacy for transplantation, and monitoring for the progression of disease. Patients with elevated and irreversible pulmonary vascular resistance (>2.5 Wood units) are at significantly higher risk for fatal right heart failure after heart transplantation compared with patients who have a pulmonary vascular resistance of less than 2.5 Wood units (40.6% vs 3.8%, respectively).[4] Pulmonary hypertension and pulmonary vascular resistance are typically evaluated by right heart catheterization in all pretransplantation evaluations. However, there is evidence to suggest echocardiography may be used as a noninvasive method to assess hemodynamics, including pulmonary hypertension and vascular resistance.[5]

Donor Evaluation

Evaluation of the potential donor heart is critical for the outcomes after transplantation. Since its first reported use in 1988 for pretransplantation donor evaluation, echocardiography (transthoracic and transesophageal) has served an instrumental role in this evaluation because of its portability and accurate assessment of ventricular function, as well as its evaluation of valvular and structural (including congenital) abnormalities.[6,7]

Left ventricular (LV) systolic dysfunction, as identified on echocardiography, accounts for approximately 26% of all unused donor hearts presented for transplantation.[8] It should be noted that LV systolic dysfunction in the absence of coronary artery disease is a common finding in patients with brain death caused by intracranial pathologies (e.g., intracranial hemorrhage); studies have reported a frequency of up to 42%.[9,10] This phenomenon is thought to occur as a consequence of the neuronal and humoral catecholamine surge induced by brain death. Apical sparing has been noted in these clinical circumstances because of the decreased sympathetic nerve terminals and reduced myocardial norepinephrine content in the LV apex.[11] Ventricular dysfunction in the absence of coronary artery disease has also been identified in patients with metabolic derangements, including acidosis, anemia, hypothyroidism, and hypoxia. In these patients, LV systolic dysfunction may be a transient phenomenon, and serial imaging has been used to identify improvements in contractile function, particularly after hemodynamic and metabolic correction.[12] The use of low-dose dobutamine stress echocardiography has been studied to identify myocardial reserve in donor hearts with LV dysfunction. Those donor hearts with improvement in systolic function had excellent posttransplant outcomes, suggesting that this may be an approach to identify donors with reversible cardiac dysfunction.[13]

The effect of left ventricular hypertrophy (LVH) on posttransplant survival has provided conflicting results. Although a single study showed LV wall thickness greater than 1.4 cm was associated with reduced survival,[14] others found a favorable survival in most recipients of allografts with LVH, including moderate to severe LVH (>1.4 cm).[15] However, the presence of LVH in combination with older age (older than 55 years) or prolonged ischemic time (>4 hours) was found to increase the posttransplant mortality rate.[15]

Limitations of donor heart evaluation with echocardiography include difficulties in image acquisition in organ donors who are receiving mechanical ventilation and in those with chest trauma.

PERIOPERATIVE MONITORING

Surgical approaches for heart transplantation include the biatrial and bicaval anastomoses. The original surgical technique, biatrial anastomosis, involves retention of biatrial tissue of the recipient ("atrial cuffs") for direct anastomosis with the donor heart atria. Although this is advantageous in maintaining the recipient vena cavae and pulmonary veins the biatrial technique results in atrial distortion that is readily seen on echocardiography (Fig. 177.1) and has been associated with atrial thrombus formation, atrial arrhythmias, tricuspid valve incompetence, and possible loss of donor heart sinoatrial and atrioventricular nodal tissue. The biatrial anastomosis appears as an echo-dense ridge at the site along the suture line. Residual suture material may sometimes also be seen at the anastomotic site. The bicaval approach, introduced in the 1990s, involves complete removal of the recipient atria, except for a cuff of tissue around the pulmonary vein orifices. The donor heart is then anastomosed at the level of the superior and/or inferior vena cavae and pulmonary veins. In routine echocardiographic evaluation, hearts transplanted with the bicaval technique may be difficult to distinguish from nontransplanted hearts. The bicaval technique results in improved atrioventricular geometry, decreased incidence of atrial arrhythmias, and decreased sinus node dysfunction or heart block requiring permanent pacing.[16]

POSTTRANSPLANTATION SURVEILLANCE

The European Association of Cardiovascular Imaging recommends a comprehensive echocardiography examination at 6 months after heart transplantation as a baseline study, which can be compared with subsequent follow-up examinations.[17] The posttransplantation course is governed by complications related to immunosuppression, including infection, acute cellular and antibody-mediated rejection, and cardiac allograft vasculopathy (CAV). These complications can generally be classified into early and late occurrences.

Structure and Function of the Normal Cardiac Allograft

Normal reference values for healthy transplants were recently published. The data demonstrated that echocardiographic parameters

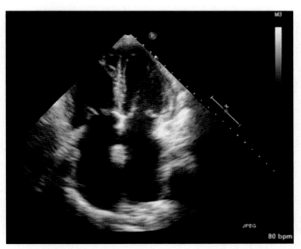

Figure 177.1. Biatrial anastomoses in heart transplantation.

for transplant recipients differ from values found in healthy normals.[18] (Table 177.1).

Left Ventricle

Early after heart transplantation, LV mass increases from edema and usually resolves after 3 months.[19] After this period, an increase of LV mass has several potential causes, including chronic tachycardia, hypertension secondary to immunosuppression treatment, and repeated episodes of rejection.[20] Heart transplant patients exhibit diastolic LV volumes in the lower normal range. The presence of postoperative dyskinetic septal motion is a common finding.

In the absence of complications, the allograft ventricular systolic ejection fraction remains preserved in the majority of the patients over a 10- to 15-year period. Decreased LV systolic function during the first year is a predictor of allograft rejection or CAV. A reduction late after heart transplantation correlates with CAV progression.[21]

In cardiac allografts with normal global systolic function, deformation indices measured by longitudinal strain and strain rate are reduced compared with normal healthy controls (mean, −16.5% +/- 3.3% (Figs. 177.2 and 177.3). The strain values remain stable over a longer period in transplant patients with normal LV function and absence of CAV. On the other hand, the LV global circumferential strain remains within the normal range.[18,22]

The interpretation of diastolic function is more challenging because of many factors, and studies evaluating conventional diastolic function have failed to find any single parameter that correctly diagnoses diastolic dysfunction.[23] The presence of high heart rate in the denervated heart results in frequent fusion of E and A waves. Pulmonary flows may be affected by contraction of the remnant recipient atrial tissue, leading to decreased pulmonary flow in systole (lower S velocity), and Ar (atrial reversal) velocity can be increased if recipient contraction occurs at end-diastole.[24]

Immediately after heart transplantation, diastolic function is abnormal, characterized by decrease in E′ and a′ velocities by tissue Doppler imaging (TDI), shorter isovolumic relaxation time and E-wave deceleration time, and increase of the E/A ratio. The presence of restrictive physiology immediately after heart transplantation is common and may be related to ischemic myocardial injury, donor recipient mismatch, and recipient pulmonary hypertension. These indices recover gradually after transplantation but remain lower than the normal population even after 1 year.[25] The persistence of abnormal diastolic function is likely caused by immune-mediated injury, fibrosis, and allograft vasculopathy.

Right Ventricle

The right ventricular (RV) size is increased immediately after heart transplant because of afterload mismatch with relatively higher

TABLE 177.1 References Values of Ventricular Function in Heart Transplant Patients Compared with Reference Values

Ventricular Function Parameter	Heart Transplant Patients	Normal Reference	P Value
LEFT VENTRICLE			
LVEF (%)	62.1 +/- 7.0	63.9 +/- 4.9	< .01
LVGCS (%)	−22.9 +/- 6.3	−23.3 +/- 1.3	NS
LVGLS (%)	−16.5 +/- 3.3	−19.7 +/- 1.8	< .0001
RIGHT VENTRICLE			
RVFAC (%)	40 +/- 8	49.7 +/- 8	< .0001
TAPSE (mm)	15 +/- 4	24 +/- 4	< .0001
S′ right ventricle	9.7 +/- 6.0	14.1 +/- 2.3	< .0001
RIMP	0.29 +/- 0.18	0.26 +/- 0.01	NS
RV LS free wall (%)	−16.9 +/- 4.2	−29.0 +/- 4.5	< .001

LVEF, Left ventricular ejection fraction; *LVGCS,* left ventricular global circumferential strain; *LVGLS,* left ventricular lobal longitudinal strain; *NS,* not significant; *RIMP,* right index of myocardial performance; *RVFAC,* right ventricular fractional area change; *RVLS,* right ventricular longitudinal strain; *TAPSE,* tricuspid annular plane systolic excursion.

pulmonary pressures in the recipients and is related to ischemic time and cause of donor death. The RV systolic function measured by tricuspid annular plane systolic excursion (TAPSE), Doppler tissue imaging, and fractional area change are all lower than in healthy control participants.[26] These values remains similar up to

15 years after heart transplantation. RV systolic function measured by longitudinal strain of the RV free wall is also decreased compared with normal control participants (−16.9 ± 4.2% vs −20%, respectively).[18] However, it is known that after cardiac surgery, RV longitudinal parameters are abnormal, and they are not sensitive markers to evaluate RV global systolic function.[27,28] Despite abnormal right-sided function, in the absence of severe tricuspid regurgitation, clinical signs and symptoms of heart failure are usually not present.

Atria

The atrial geometry and function are related to the surgical technique as already described. In the original surgical technique, biatrial anastomosis, LA enlargement is more evident, and the biatrial anastomosis appears as an echo-dense ridge at the site along the suture line. In the bicaval approach, the geometry and atrial function are comparable to those in normal control participants. The LA contraction appears to contribute more to LV stroke volume than in nontransplant patients. In the bicaval group, atrial volumes correlate with allograft age. This may reflect the fact that, with increased allograft age, diastolic dysfunction develops with increased filling pressures. Atrial volume should be measured using the biplane algorithm or three-dimensional echocardiography.

Few studies have evaluated the atrial function using strain in patients with bicaval anastomoses. The atrial reservoir function is markedly reduced compared with normal control participants.

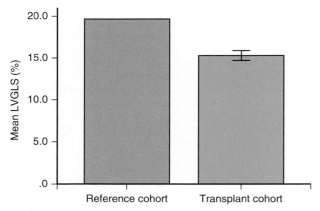

Figure 177.2. Left ventricular global longitudinal strain (LVGLS) parameters in heart transplant patients compared with normal reference values. Bars represent mean of the reference population and heart transplant patients, respectively. Error bars represent 95% confidence interval of the mean in heart transplant patients. Strain values should be interpreted as negative values.[18]

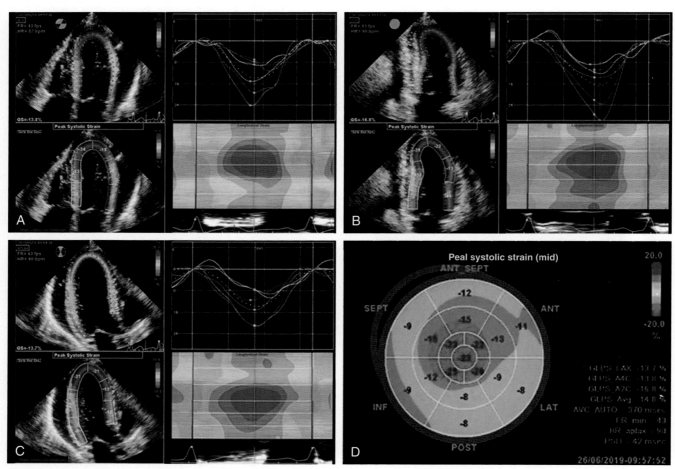

Figure 177.3. Computation of peak left ventricular global longitudinal strain (LVGLS) using the speckle-tracking technique in a transplanted heart without history of rejection or transplant vasculopathy on three conventional apical views: four-chamber (**A**), two-chamber (**B**), and apical long-axis (**C**). Left ventricular segmental values of longitudinal strain are displayed both as numbers and as parametric colorization on a bull's eye display (**D**). *ANT,* Anterior; *INF,* inferior; *LAT,* lateral; *POST,* posterior; *SEPT,* septal.

The most pronounced reduction in atrial reservoir function assessed by speckle-tracking echocardiography (STE) was seen in heart transplant recipients with elevated filling pressures. Further studies are needed to evaluate atrial strain regarding its ability to identify increased ventricular filling pressure in this population.[29]

Valve Function

The echocardiographic appearance of the mitral, tricuspid, aortic, and pulmonary valves is typically normal after transplantation. Valvular regurgitation is common, particularly tricuspid regurgitation, which may result from several mechanisms. Immediately after transplantation, tricuspid regurgitation is secondary to pulmonary hypertension, and its severity decreases with improvement of pulmonary vascular resistance. Other frequent causes of tricuspid regurgitation are persistence of elevated pulmonary pressures, tricuspid annulus enlargement caused by RV dilatation, and damage to the valve apparatus during endomyocardial biopsies or from endocarditis. Tricuspid regurgitation seems to be more prevalent with biatrial anastomosis because of the alteration of right atrial morphology and annulus dilatation.

Aorta and Pulmonary Artery

The anastomoses of the donor heart to the aorta and pulmonary artery can be visualized (Fig. 177.4 and Video 177.4). In a normal heart transplant, Doppler flow velocities at the aortic and pulmonic level are usually normal. Occasionally, there is mismatch between the diameter of the donor and recipient pulmonary artery, and the suture line in the proximal artery may be seen as a narrowing. However, there is usually no significant gradient. The anastomosis at the level of aorta may be a site of potential surgical complications. An echocardiographic evaluation of the aorta assessing diameter and potential wall thinning or leaking (with paraaortic fluid collections) is recommended.

Superior and Inferior Vena Cava and Pulmonary Veins

In patients with bicaval anastomosis, special attention should be paid to the superior vena cava to evaluate for possible obstruction at the surgical anastomosis that has been described in 2.4% of the cases. Obstruction of inferior vena caval and pulmonary vein anastomoses can also be detected by echocardiography (Fig. 177.5).

Pericardium

Small to moderate pericardial effusions are seen after transplantation in approximately two-thirds at 3 months and in 25% of the patients at 6 months (Fig. 177.6 and Video 177.6). Large and clinically significant effusions are less common and are associated with undersized hearts or absence of previous cardiac surgery.[30] The natural history of these effusions varies and required serial evaluation regarding the extent, location, and hemodynamic impact. In cases of newly detected pericardial effusions, graft rejection, infection, or neoplasm should be considered as possible causes. Cardiac perforation should also be considered if the patient has recently undergone biopsy (Fig. 177.7 and Video 177.7).

EARLY ALLOGRAFT FAILURE

Early graft dysfunction occurs within 24 hours after heart transplant surgery and is the leading cause of 30-day mortality after transplant.[31] Graft dysfunction is classified as primary (PGD) in the absence of obvious cause or as secondary when attributed to a cause such as hyperacute rejection, pulmonary hypertension, or known surgical complications.

PGD is currently defined as LV, RV, or biventricular dysfunction. A severity scale is used for PGD of the -LV. For

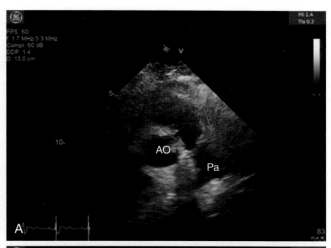

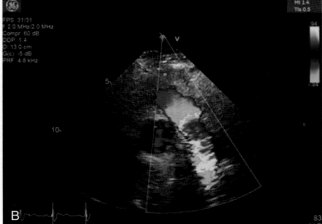

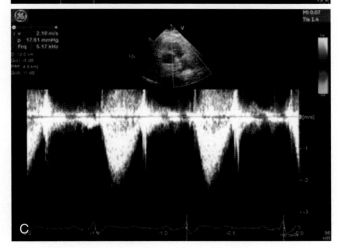

Figure 177.4. A, Two-dimensional echocardiography acquisitions focused on the pulmonary artery (Pa) in a heart transplant recipient. The suture lines can be easily identified *(arrows)*. **B,** Color Doppler of the main pulmonary artery demonstrates turbulent flow. **C,** Continuous-wave Doppler demonstrates high velocity (peak velocity 2.1 m/s) across the vessel which is consistent with mild pulmonary artery stenosis. *Ao,* Aorta. (See accompanying Video 177.4.)

mild and moderate categories, it relies on the requirement of inotropic support and ventricular dysfunction identified by echocardiography or right heart catheterization to demonstrate hemodynamic compromise. The echocardiographic criteria used includes presence of a left ventricular ejection fraction

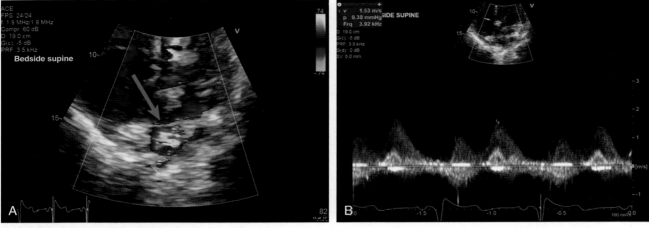

Figure 177.5. Two-dimensional echocardiographic imaging (apical four-chamber view) of a patient with a recent heart transplant. **A,** Color Doppler of the right upper pulmonary vein demonstrates turbulent flow *(arrow)*. **B,** Continuous-wave Doppler demonstrates high velocity (peak velocity, 1.5 m/s; peak gradient, 9 mm Hg) across the vessel, which is consistent with a mild pulmonary vein stenosis. (See accompanying Video 177.5.)

(LVEF) of less than 40%. The diagnosis of severe PGD includes the need of mechanical support, including extracorporeal membrane oxygenation or ventricular assist devices in any form (percutaneous or surgical).[32]

Secondary graft failure can occur because of reperfusion injury during surgery; prolonged cold ischemia time; or, less commonly, the presence of hyperacute rejection. Echocardiographic evaluation demonstrates reduced global systolic function (LVEF <40%) or increased RV volume with systolic dysfunction (TAPSE <15 mm or a RV ejection fraction <45%).[32]

Isolated RV failure can be detected by echocardiography and is defined by the presence of RV dysfunction with normal or near normal LV systolic function.

ACUTE GRAFT REJECTION

Acute cardiac allograft rejection (ACAR) is a common problem after heart transplantation, mainly early after surgery. The contribution of rejection to posttransplant mortality has decreased over time, but it still occurs in up to 30% of patients during the first year and continues to reduce long-term survival in transplant recipients.[3] Acute rejection results from recognition of non–self-histocompatibility antigens and elaboration of an immune response against heart muscle or endothelium and leads to compromised cardiac function and graft loss.

ACAR involves (1) cellular rejection (most common) characterized by lymphocytic infiltration with or without myocyte necrosis and (2) antibody-mediated rejection, a less understood process, which involves deposition of immunoglobulins and complement in the microvasculature.

Endomyocardial biopsy (EMB) is the current standard of care for diagnosis of rejection based on International Society for Heart and Lung Transplantation (ISHLT) guidelines.[33] Although this intervention is relatively safe in experience hands, approximately 0.5% to 1% of patients can have complications, including myocardial perforation, pericardial tamponade, tricuspid valve injury, and access-site complications. In addition, EMB is associated with sampling error and histologic "false-negative" ACAR, occurring in up to 20% of the patients.

Although echocardiography is not currently considered a first-line tool for surveillance of acute rejection, it does serve an adjunctive role in monitoring for rejection.[17] Initial studies focused on morphologic features such as change in LV wall thickness, increased LV mass, myocardial echogenicity, and development

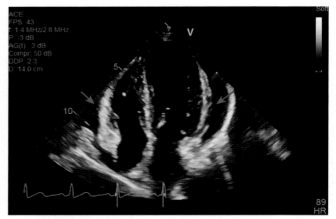

Figure 177.6. Pericardial effusion, apical four-chamber view. A 45-year-old woman underwent heart transplantation. A circumferential pericardial effusion *(arrows)* was found in a routine echocardiogram 10 days later. (See accompanying Video 177.6.)

of pericardial effusion that in the setting of rejection may be the result of increased interstitial edema.[34] However, it was recognized that these findings occur late in the natural history of rejection. In the era of antirejection calcineurin inhibitors, acute rejection may present in a subtle fashion without frank symptoms. Decline of LV systolic function is not an early indicator of graft dysfunction, and there is no correlation between the magnitude of LVEF decline and acute cellular rejection grade on biopsy.[35]

Abnormalities of diastolic function are the earliest changes that occur in acute rejection.[36] The Doppler changes include decreased pressure halftime, decreased isovolumetric relaxation time, and increased E velocity. However, these parameters have low specificity for rejection because of their dependence on loading conditions and heart rate. Small studies using TDI of the mitral annulus have shown that a reduction in early and late diastolic velocities (E′ and A′) and lower systolic velocities (S′) correlate with acute episodes of rejection. Although TDI measurements are sensitive markers of rejection, their specificity is low, reflecting the baseline abnormal diastolic function inherent in transplant physiology. No single diastolic parameter appears reliable enough to predict graft rejection[37] (Table 177.2).

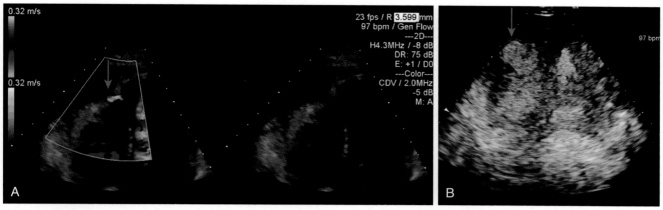

Figure 177.7. A, Two-dimensional echocardiographic imaging (apical four-chamber view) shows small right ventricular (RV) free wall rupture after endomyocardial biopsy. Color Doppler imaging shows the RV free wall rupture into the pericardial space with effusion *(arrow)*. **B,** Contrast-enhanced transthoracic echocardiogram (apical four-chamber sweep) shows extrusion of the contrast into the pseudoaneurysm of the RV free wall *(arrow)*. (See accompanying Video 177.7.)

Because transplantation rejection is generally a focal process, strain echocardiographic imaging detecting myocardial deformation may more reliably identify small changes in ACAR (see Table 177.2). Recent studies found that global longitudinal peak systolic strain and strain rate are reduced in patients with proven acute rejection. Marciniak and coworkers found that lateral wall peak systolic longitudinal strain was −21% ± 6% in patients with ACR grade 1B or less compared with −13% ± 5% in patients with greater than grade 1B ACR (*P* < .05). Peak systolic radial strain rate was also reduced in ACR grade 1B or greater.[38] In another study, a mean systolic strain cutoff value of −27.4% predicted grade 1B or greater ACR with a sensitivity of 82.2% and specificity of 82.3%.[39]

One of the limitations of using TDI strain and strain rate parameters is the dependence on transducer angle; therefore, imaging can be challenging to acquire with poor reproducibility. Two-dimensional (2D) STE overcomes this limitation, and this technique has been evaluated for ACAR. Sato and coworkers used 2D STE to measure LV torsion for the detection of ACR. This study demonstrated that a reduction of torsion of greater than 25 percentage points from baseline was able to predict ACR grade 2R or greater with a high specificity and negative predictive value (NPV) of 95.1% and 92.9%, respectively.[40] A prospective study of 34 consecutives patients, pairing 235 biopsies and echocardiograms, found an independent relationship between ACR degree 2R or greater and two combined parameters: RV free-wall longitudinal strain and LV global longitudinal strain (threshold values of <17% and <15.5%, respectively, with NPV 98.8% for both indices).[41] On the contrary, a retrospective study using speckle-tracking strain and strain rate measurements obtained from 30 patients with asymptomatic biopsy-proven rejection and 14 control transplants was not able to show significant differences in circumferential and longitudinal strain or strain rate between baseline, rejection, and resolution studies.[42] These studies had different methodologies and different referent EMB cutoff values (moderate vs mild and moderate ACR) and the limitations of small sample size, single-center experience, and limited number of moderate or greater ACR episodes. Future studies aimed to standardize surveillance strategy and deformation assessment are needed before specific recommendations can be done.

CHRONIC GRAFT REJECTION

Although infection and acute allograft rejection can present at any time, late complications of cardiac transplantation largely encompass CAV and malignancy. CAV is a diffuse disease affecting not only the epicardial vessels but also the microvasculature. When CAV progresses, it is extremely difficult to treat, and retransplantation is the only option. CAV is multifactorial in origin and is associated with immune-mediated phenomena, in addition to nonimmunologic phenomena including older donor age, cytomegalovirus infection, hyperlipidemia, and impaired glycemic control. Because of cardiac denervation, it may advance silently before it manifests clinically as ischemia, infarction, ventricular dysfunction, heart failure, or ventricular arrhythmia and sudden cardiac death.

The incidence of CAV is 29% at 5 years and 47% at 10 years and can develop as early as 1 year after transplantation.[43] Therefore, routine screening is paramount.

Current guidelines recommend annual or biannual coronary angiography with longer intervals if multiple angiograms are normal.[33] Despite being the current gold standard for detecting CAV, angiography is limited for the detection of early disease and microvasculature lesions. Intravascular ultrasound (IVUS) has demonstrated an association in multiple studies between changes in maximal thickness (>0.5 cm) in 1 year and increased cardiac events and mortality.[44] Current guidelines recommend using IVUS, in conjunction with coronary angiography, at 4 to 6 weeks and again at 1-year posttransplantation as an option to detect rapidly progressing CAV or exclude significant disease when the angiogram is uncertain.

The use of stress echocardiography is recommended also in the guidelines for detection of CAV.

Exercise stress echocardiography has a low sensitivity for detecting CAV because of the inability of the denervated heart to reach target heart rates with exercise with a limited sensitivity of 15% to 33%.[45] Dobutamine stress echocardiography (DSE) has been the most common test used for noninvasive screening of CAV. Earliest studies with DSE reported a sensitivity of 70% to 80% for detecting significant CAV compared with coronary angiography. A negative stress test result indicates a low likelihood of prognostically relevant CAV and low rate of occurrence of major adverse cardiac events at 1 year.[46,47]

However, two recent studies including more than 500 patients questioned the adequacy of DSE to detect angiographic CAV, particularly for mild lesions. The sensitivity of DSE was only 6.5% for ISHLT CAV1, 27% for CAV2, and 24% for ISHLT CAV3.[48,49] Ischemia on DSE did not predict cardiovascular outcomes. Small studies suggest improved performance when DSE is used in combination with STE or contrast perfusion for determination of coronary flow reserve.[50,51] The adoption of these techniques is limited by lack of widespread expertise in these imaging modalities.

TABLE 177.2 Selected Studies Evaluating Efficacy of Echocardiographic Imaging for Detecting Acute Rejection in Heart Transplantation

Author (Year)	Number of Biopsies (prevalence of ACR)	Method (parameter cut-off value)	EMB Grade to Define ACR	Sensitivity (%)	Specificity (%)	NPV
Sun et al[53] (2005)		2D and standard Doppler (>2 of PE, IVRT <90 ms, E/A >1.7)	>1B			
	223 (37%)	<6 months posttransplantation		57	54	68
	183 (27%)	>6 months posttransplantation		60	93	86
	264 (29%)	PW-TDI (Mitral annulus Aa velocity <9.0 cm/s)		67	49	78
Palka et al[54] (2005)	44 (27%)	PW and color M-mode TDI	>3A			
		(e′ septal MV annulus <12 cm/s)		69	46	80
		IVRT increased with rejection		88	58	93
Marciniak et al[38] (2007)	31 (32%)	Color TDI	≥1B			
		(LVPW radial peak systolic strain ≤30%)		85	90	93
		LVPW radial peak systolic SR, 3.0 ⁻¹)		80	86	90
Kato et al[39] (2010)	35 (11.3%)	TDI-derived strain rate (Systolic strain, −27.4%)	≥1B	82.2	82.3	82.3
		(Peak early diastolic strain rate, −2.8 s-1)		75.6	74.9	75
Sato et al[40] (2011)	32 (8.9%)	Speckle strain (>25% reduction in LV torsion)	>2	73.7	95.1	92.9
Mingo-Santos et al[41] (2015)	62 (26.4%)	2D-STE				
		(LV longitudinal strain <15.5%)	>2R	85.7	81.4	25
		(Free-wall RV longitudinal strain <17%)		85.7	91.1	98.8
Ruiz Ortiz et al[55] (2015)	20 (59%)	2D-STE	2R			
		(Average radial strain <25%)		100	48	100

2D, Two-dimensional; *Aa,* peak late diastolic velocity; *ACR,* acute cellular rejection; *E/A,* ratio of peak early diastolic velocity to peak late diastolic velocity; *EMB,* endomyocardial biopsy; *IVRT,* isovolumetric relaxation time; *LV,* left ventricular; *LVPW,* left ventricular posterior wall; *MV,* mitral valve; *NPV,* negative predictive value; *PE,* pericardial effusion; *PW-TD,* pulsed-wave tissue Doppler imaging; *RV,* right ventricular; *SR,* strain rate; *STE,* speckle-tracking echocardiography; *TDI,* tissue Doppler imaging.

Please access ExpertConsult to view the corresponding videos for this chapter.

REFERENCES

1. Yancy CW, Jessup M, Bozkurt B, et al. 2013 ACCF/AHA guideline for the management of heart failure. *J Am Coll Cardiol.* 2013;62:e147–239.
2. Lund LH, Edwards LB, Dipchand AI, et al. The Registry of the International Society for heart and Lung transplantation: thirty-third adult heart transplantation report—2016. *J Heart Lung Transplant.* 2016;35:1158–1169.
3. Lund LH, Khush KK, Cherikh WS, et al. The Registry of the International Society for heart and Lung transplantation: thirty-fourth adult heart transplantation report—2017. *J Heart Lung Transplant.* 2017;36:1037–1046.
4. Costard-Jackle A, Fowler MB. Influence of preoperative pulmonary artery pressure on mortality after heart transplantation: testing of potential reversibility of pulmonary hypertension with nitroprusside is useful in defining a high risk group. *J Am Coll Cardiol.* 1992;19:48–54.
5. Kuppahally SS, Michaels AD, Tandar A, et al. Can echocardiographic evaluation of cardiopulmonary hemodynamics decrease right heart catheterizations in end-stage heart failure patients awaiting transplantation? *Am J Cardiol.* 2010;106:1657–1662.
6. Zaroff J. Echocardiographic evaluation of the potential cardiac donor. *J Heart Lung Transplant.* 2004;23(9 Suppl):S250–S252.
7. Venkateswaran RV, Bonser RS, Steeds RP. The echocardiographic assessment of donor heart function prior to cardiac transplantation. *Eur J Echocardiogr.* 2005;6:260–263.
8. Zaroff JG, Rordorf GA, Ogilvy CS, Picard MH. Regional patterns of left ventricular systolic dysfunction after subarachnoid hemorrhage: evidence for neurally mediated cardiac injury. *J Am Soc Echocardiogr.* 2000;13:774–779.
9. Khush KK, Menza R, Nguyen J, et al. Donor predictors of allograft use and recipient outcomes after heart transplantation. *Circ Heart Fail.* 2013;6:300–309.
10. Mohamedali B, Bhat G, Zelinger A. Frequency and pattern of left ventricular dysfunction in potential heart donors: implications regarding use of dysfunctional hearts for successful transplantation. *J Am Coll Cardiol.* 2012;60:235–236.
11. Dujardin KS, McCully RB, Wijdicks EF, et al. Myocardial dysfunction associated with brain death: clinical, echocardiographic, and pathologic features. *J Heart Lung Transplant.* 2001;20:350–357.
12. Venkateswaran RV, Townend JN, Wilson IC, et al. Echocardiography in the potential heart donor. *Transplantation.* 2010;89:894–901.
13. Bombardini T, Arpesella G, Maccherini M, et al. Medium-term outcome of recipients of marginal donor hearts selected with new stress-echocardiographic techniques over standard criteria. *Cardiovasc Ultrasound.* 2014;12:20.
14. Kuppahally SS, Valantine HA, Weisshaar D, et al. Outcome in cardiac recipients of donor hearts with increased left ventricular wall thickness. *Am J Transplant.* 2007;7:2388–2395.
15. Wever Pinzon O, Stoddard G, Drakos SG, et al. Impact of donor left ventricular hypertrophy on survival after heart transplant. *Am J Transplant.* 2011;11:2755–2761.
16. Zeltsman D, Acker MA. Surgical management of heart failure: an overview. *Ann Rev Med.* 2002;53:383–391.
17. Badano LP, Miglioranza MH, Edvardsen T, et al. European Association of Cardiovascular Imaging/Cardiovascular Imaging Department of the Brazilian Society of Cardiology recommendations for the use of cardiac imaging to assess and follow patients after heart transplantation. *Eur Heart J Cardiovasc Imag.* 2015;16:919–948.
18. Ingvarsson A, Werther Evaldsson A, Waktare J, et al. Normal reference ranges for transthoracic echocardiography following heart transplantation. *J Am Soc Echocardiogr.* 2018;31:349–360.
19. Kou S, Caballero L, Dulgheru R, et al. Echocardiographic reference ranges for normal cardiac chamber size: results from the NORRE study. *Eur Heart J Cardiovasc Imag.* 2014;15:680–690.
20. Goodroe R, Bonnema DD, Lunsford S, et al. Severe left ventricular hypertrophy 1 year after transplant predicts mortality in cardiac transplant recipients. *J Heart Lung Transplant.* 2007;26:145–151.
21. Wilhelmi M, Pethig K, Wilhelmi M, et al. Heart transplantation: echocardiographic assessment of morphology and function after more than 10 years of follow-up. *Ann Thorac Surg.* 2002;74:1075–1079.

22. Saleh HK, Villarraga HR, Kane GC, et al. Normal left ventricular mechanical function and synchrony values by speckle-tracking echocardiography in the transplanted heart with normal ejection fraction. *J Heart Lung Transplant.* 2011;30:652–658.

23. Okada DR, Molina MR, Kohari M, et al. Clinical echocardiographic indices of left ventricular diastolic function correlate poorly with pulmonary capillary wedge pressure at 1 year following heart transplantation. *Int J Cardiovasc Imaging.* 2015;31:783–794.

24. Nagueh SF, Smiseth OA, Appleton CP, et al. Recommendations for the evaluation of left ventricular diastolic function by echocardiography. *J Am Soc Echocardiogr.* 2016;29:277–314.

25. Dandel M, Hummel M, Muller J, et al. Reliability of tissue Doppler wall motion monitoring after heart transplantation for replacement of invasive routine screenings by optimally timed cardiac biopsies and catheterizations. *Circulation.* 2001;104(12 suppl 1):I1184–I191.

26. Clemmensen TS, Eiskjaer H, Logstrup BB, et al. Echocardiographic assessment of right heart function in heart transplant recipients and the relation to exercise hemodynamics. *Transpl Int.* 2016;29:909–920.

27. Haddad F, Doyle R, Murphy DJ, Hunt SA. Right ventricular function in cardiovascular disease, part II: Pathophysiology, clinical importance, and management of right ventricular failure. *Circulation.* 2008;117:1717–1731.

28. Haddad F, Hunt SA, Rosenthal DN, Murphy DJ. Right ventricular function in cardiovascular disease, part I: Anatomy, physiology, aging, and functional assessment of the right ventricle. *Circulation.* 2008;117:1436–1448.

29. Bech-Hanssen O, Pergola V, Al-Admawi M, et al. Atrial function in heart transplant recipients operated with the bicaval technique. *Scand Cardiovasc J.* 2016;50:42–51.

30. Hauptman PJ, Couper GS, Aranki SF, et al. Pericardial effusions after cardiac transplantation. *J Am Coll Cardiol.* 1994;23:1625–1629.

31. Stehlik J, Edwards LB, Kucheryavaya AY, et al. The Registry of the International Society for Heart and Lung transplantation: 27th official adult heart transplant report—2010. *J Heart Lung Transplant.* 2010;29:1089–1103.

32. Kobashigawa J, Zuckermann A, Macdonald P, et al. Report from a consensus conference on primary graft dysfunction after cardiac transplantation. *J Heart Lung Transplant.* 2014;33:327–340.

33. Costanzo MR, Dipchand A, Starling R, et al. The International Society of heart and Lung transplantation guidelines for the care of heart transplant recipients. *J Heart Lung Transplant.* 2010;29:914–956.

34. Sagar KB, Hastillo A, Wolfgang TC, et al. Left ventricular mass by M-mode echocardiography in cardiac transplant patients with acute rejection. *Circulation.* 1981;64:II217–II220.

35. Streeter RP, Nichols K, Bergmann SR. Stability of right and left ventricular ejection fractions and volumes after heart transplantation. *J Heart Lung Transplant.* 2005;24:815–818.

36. Yun KL, Niczyporuk MA, Daughters GT, et al. Alterations in left ventricular diastolic twist mechanics during acute human cardiac allograft rejection. *Circulation.* 1991;83:962–973.

37. Mena C, Wencker D, Krumholz HM, McNamara RL. Detection of heart transplant rejection in adults by echocardiographic indices: a systematic review of the literature. *J Am Soc Echocardiogr.* 2006;19:1295–1300.

38. Marciniak A, Eroglu E, Marciniak M, et al. The potential clinical role of ultrasonic strain and strain rate imaging in diagnosing acute rejection after heart transplantation. *Eur J Echocardiogr.* 2007;8:213–221.

39. Kato TS, Oda N, Hashimura K, et al. Strain rate imaging would predict subclinical acute rejection in heart transplant recipients. *Eur J Cardiothorac Surg.* 2010;37:1104–1110.

40. Sato T, Kato TS, Komamura K, et al. Utility of left ventricular systolic torsion derived from 2-dimensional speckle-tracking echocardiography in monitoring acute cellular rejection in heart transplant recipients. *J Heart Lung Transplant.* 2011;30:536–543.

41. Mingo-Santos S, Monivas-Palomero V, Garcia-Lunar I, et al. Usefulness of two-dimensional strain parameters to diagnose acute rejection after heart transplantation. *J Am Soc Echocardiogr.* 2015;28:1149–1156.

42. Ambardekar AV, Alluri N, Patel AC, et al. Myocardial strain and strain rate from speckle-tracking echocardiography are unable to differentiate asymptomatic biopsy-proven cellular rejection in the first year after cardiac transplantation. *J Am Soc Echocardiogr.* 2015;28:478–485.

43. Nikolova AP, Kobashigawa JA. Cardiac allograft vasculopathy: the enduring enemy of cardiac transplantation. *Transplantation.* 2019;103:1338–1348.

44. Tuzcu EM, Kapadia SR, Sachar R, et al. Intravascular ultrasound evidence of angiographically silent progression in coronary atherosclerosis predicts long-term morbidity and mortality after cardiac transplantation. *J Am Coll Cardiol.* 2005;45:1538–1542.

45. Collings CA, Pinto FJ, Valantine HA, et al. Exercise echocardiography in heart transplant recipients: a comparison with angiography and intracoronary ultrasonography. *J Heart Lung Transplant.* 1994;13:604–613.

46. Mehra MR, Crespo-Leiro MG, Dipchand A, et al. International Society for Heart and Lung Transplantation working formulation of a standardized nomenclature for cardiac allograft vasculopathy-2010. *J Heart Lung Transplant.* 2010;29:717–727.

47. Bacal F, Moreira L, Souza G, et al. Dobutamine stress echocardiography predicts cardiac events or death in asymptomatic patients long-term after heart transplantation: 4-year prospective evaluation. *J Heart Lung Transplant.* 2004;23:1238–1244.

48. Chirakarnjanakorn S, Starling RC, Popovic ZB, et al. Dobutamine stress echocardiography during follow-up surveillance in heart transplant patients: diagnostic accuracy and predictors of outcomes. *J Heart Lung Transplant.* 2015;34:710–717.

49. Clerkin KJ, Farr MA, Restaino SW, et al. Dobutamine stress echocardiography is inadequate to detect early cardiac allograft vasculopathy. *J Heart Lung Transplant.* 2016;35:1040–1041.

50. Eroglu E, D'Hooge J, Sutherland GR, et al. Quantitative dobutamine stress echocardiography for the early detection of cardiac allograft vasculopathy in heart transplant recipients. *Heart.* 2008;94(e3).

51. Tona F, Caforio AL, Montisci R, et al. Coronary flow reserve by contrast-enhanced echocardiography: a new noninvasive diagnostic tool for cardiac allograft vasculopathy. *Am J Transplant.* 2006;6:998–1003.

52. Lang RM, Badano LP, Mor-Avi V, et al. Recommendations for cardiac chamber quantification by echocardiography in adults. *J Am Soc Echocardiogr.* 2015;28:1–39. e14.

53. Sun JP, Abdalla IA, Asher CR, et al. Non-invasive evaluation of orthotopic heart transplant rejection by echocardiography. *J Heart Lung Transplant.* 2005;24:160–165.

54. Palka P, Lange A, Galbraith A, et al. The role of left and right ventricular early diastolic Doppler tissue echocardiographic indices in the evaluation of acute rejection in orthotopic heart transplant. *J Am Soc Echocardiogr.* 2005;18:107–115.

55. Ruiz Ortiz M, Pena ML, Mesa D, et al. Impact of asymptomatic acute cellular rejection on left ventricle myocardial function evaluated by means of 2D speckle tracking echocardiography in heart transplant recipients. *Echocardiography.* 2015;32:229–237.

178   Pulmonary Hypertension

Gregory M. Scalia

CLINICAL MANIFESTATIONS

Pulmonary hypertension, defined hemodynamically, refers to a broad range of conditions with a final common feature of raised arterial pulmonary pressures. Symptoms are nonspecific and include lethargy, reduced exercise capacity, and breathlessness. Clinical signs, when present, are compelling—edema and ascites, precordial heave, altered heart sounds, and arrhythmia. Unfortunately, clinical symptoms and signs are detected months or indeed years after the onset of the process (Fig. 178.1).[1] With the advent of specific pulmonary vasodilator drugs for some causes of pulmonary hypertension, early diagnosis is now critical.[2] The pivotal role of echocardiography in the identification, stratification, triage, and response to therapy and prognostication is now well accepted.[3]

DEFINITIONS OF PULMONARY HYPERTENSION: INVASIVE AND NONINVASIVE

Historically, the formal diagnosis of pulmonary hypertension, usually investigated for the assessment of breathlessness and right heart failure, required invasive intravascular assessment of pressures by right heart catheterization. So entrenched are the dictums of invasive pulmonary hypertension diagnosis that virtually all trials of

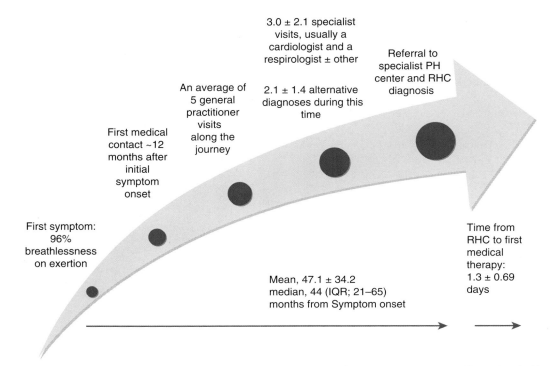

Figure 178.1. Delays in presentation and investigation of pulmonary hypertension (PH). *RHC, right heart catheterization.* (Reproduced with permission from Strange G, et al: Time from symptoms to definitive diagnosis of idiopathic pulmonary arterial hypertension: the delay study, *Pulm Circ* 3:89–94, 2013.)

BOX 178.1 Abbreviations

CTEPH, chronic thromboembolic pulmonary hypertension
ePLAGS, echocardiographic pulmonary to left atrial global strain ratio
ePLAR, echocardiographic pulmonary to left atrial ratio
LAP, left atrial pressure
LVEDP, left ventricular end-diastolic pressure
PAP, pulmonary artery pressure
PAD_P, diastolic pulmonary artery pressure
PAP_M, mean pulmonary artery pressure
PAP_S, systolic pulmonary artery pressure
PCWP, pulmonary capillary wedge pressure
PVR, pulmonary vascular resistance
RVOT, right ventricular outflow tract
RVOTVTI, right ventricular outflow tract pulsed-wave Doppler velocity time integral
RVSP, right ventricular systolic pressure
TPG, transpulmonary gradient
TRV_{max}, tricuspid regurgitation maximum continuous-wave Doppler velocity

---

TABLE 178.1 Hemodynamic Definitions and Updated Clinical Classification of Pulmonary Hypertension From the World Symposium on Pulmonary Hypertension

Definitions	Characteristics
Precapillary PH	PAP_M >20 mm Hg PAWP ≤15 mm Hg PVR ≥3 WU
Isolated postcapillary PH	PAP_M >20 mm Hg PAWP >15 mm Hg PVR <3 WU
Combined pre- and postcapillary PH	PAP_M >20 mm Hg PAWP >15 mm Hg PVR ≥3 WU

PAP_M, Mean pulmonary artery pressure; *PAWP,* pulmonary artery wedge pressure; *PH,* pulmonary hypertension; *PVR,* pulmonary vascular resistance.
Reproduced with permission from Simonneau G, et al: Haemodynamic definitions and updated clinical classification of pulmonary hypertension, *Eur Respir J* 53(1):1801913, 2019.

---

modern sophisticated pulmonary hypertension pharmaceutical therapies have mandated these invasive parameters for enrolment. Consequently, guidelines for prescribing and coverage of these drugs continue to require right heart catheterization. Paradoxically, for more than 30 years, echocardiography has been the workhorse for identification, quantification, and triage of patients with these symptoms, who will subsequently be diagnosed with pulmonary hypertension.

The absolute values of these invasive parameters that define pulmonary hypertension and its subcategories and physiologies have recently evolved. When first defined in 1973, pulmonary hypertension was defined by an arbitrary mean pulmonary artery pressure (PAP_M) cut-off of 25 mm Hg or greater.[4] Unlike the systemic circulation, where systolic and diastolic pressure measurements define systemic hypertension, PAP_M (PAP_M = PAP_D + 1/3 [PAP_S − PAP_D]) has remained the benchmark in the catheterization laboratory. This invasive value of PAP_M 25 mm Hg or greater has for 40 years been the basis for recruitment in drug trials and subsequent prescribing guidelines (Box 178.1).

In recent years, large cohort studies, metanalyses, and massive database machine learning analyses[5] have focused attention on the prognostic effects of slightly less elevated levels of PAP_M (20–25 mm Hg). Very large datasets of invasive measurements from normal pulmonary circulations have shown values of PAP_M 14.0 ± 3.3 mm Hg.[6] Two standard deviations above the mean value represents about 20 mm Hg. Indeed, participants with PAP_M from 20 to 25 mm Hg have shown a linear increase in adverse prognostic outcomes in several cohort studies.[7,8] Based on these data, the 6th World Symposium on Pulmonary Hypertension in Nice in 2018[9] redefined pulmonary hypertension as having invasively measured PAP_M greater than 20 mm Hg (Table 178.1).

Peak tricuspid regurgitation velocity (m/s)	Presence of other echo "PH signs"	Echocardiographic probability of pulmonary hypertension
≤2.8 or not measurable	No	Low
≤2.8 or not measurable	Yes	Intermediate
2.9–3.4	No	Intermediate
2.9–3.4	Yes	High
>3.4	Not required	High

Figure 178.2. Echocardiographic probability of pulmonary hypertension in symptomatic patients with a suspicion of pulmonary hypertension. *PH,* Pulmonary hypertension. (Reproduced with permission from Galie N, et al: 2015 ESC/ERS guidelines for the diagnosis and treatment of pulmonary hypertension, *Eur Heart J* 37:67–119, 2016.)

The ventricles	Pulmonary artery[a]	Inferior vena cava and right atrium[a]
Right ventricle/ left ventricle basal diameter ratio >1.0	Right ventricular outflow Doppler acceleration time <105 ms and/or midsystolic notching	Inferior cava diameter >21 mm with decreased inspiratory collapse (<50% with a sniff or <20% with quiet inspiration)
Flattening of the interventricular septum (left ventricular eccentricity index >1.1 in systole and/or diastole)	Early diastolic pulmonary regurgitation velocity >2.2 m/s	Right atrial area (end-systole) >18 cm²
	PA diameter >25 mm	

Figure 178.3. Echocardiographic signs suggesting pulmonary hypertension used to assess the probability of pulmonary hypertension in addition to the tricuspid regurgitation velocity measurement. *PA,* Pulmonary artery; (Reproduced with permission from Galie N, et al: 2015 ESC/ERS guidelines for the diagnosis and treatment of pulmonary hypertension, *Eur Heart J* 37:67–119, 2016.)

After being diagnosed, pulmonary hypertension immediately must be categorized by physiology and hemodynamic state. *Precapillary* pulmonary hypertension represents obstruction to transpulmonary flow through the lung microvasculature. By invasive definition, the calculated pulmonary vascular resistance (PVR = transpulmonary gradient $(PAP_M – PCWP)$/cardiac output) is defined as 3 Woods units or greater with normal left atrial pressure (LAP) (<15 mm Hg). *Postcapillary* pulmonary hypertension (or pulmonary hypertension secondary to left heart disease) is defined invasively as PAP_M greater than 20 mm Hg with PCWP 15mm Hg or greater. If isolated, *postcapillary* pulmonary hypertension has normal transpulmonary flow, with PVR less than 3 Woods units. After long periods, patients with *postcapillary* pulmonary hypertension can develop secondary vascular changes in the lung microcirculation, causing *mixed* pulmonary hypertension, with PAP_M greater than 20mm Hg with PCWP 15 mm Hg or greater and PVR 3 Woods units or greater. High cardiac output states can raise PAP_M greater than 20 mm Hg with normal PVR values. Such conditions would not satisfy the current criteria for pulmonary hypertension.

ECHOCARDIOGRAPHY ASSESSMENT OF PRESSURES

Echocardiography is ubiquitous in our community, and noninvasive assessment of right ventricular systolic pressure (RVSP) is available on most standard transthoracic studies. Continuous-wave (CW) Doppler interrogation of the tricuspid regurgitation (TR) jet, with the appropriate Bernoulli equation, is considered by many to be the entry level for most patients. In the European Society of Cardiology guidelines,[10] echocardiography is regarded as a screening tool to predict whether pulmonary hypertension is present or not. Participants with a tricuspid regurgitation maximum continuous-wave Doppler velocity (TRV_{max}) 2.8 m/s or less are considered unlikely to have pulmonary hypertension, but those with TRV_{max} 3.4 m/s or greater are highly likely to have pulmonary hypertension when invasively assessed (Fig. 178.2). The very large "grey zone" from TRV_{max} 2.8 to 3.4 m/s requires ancillary echocardiography features to increase or decrease the posttest probability of pulmonary hypertension being present (Fig. 178.3).

Interrogation of the TR jet velocity requires optimization of the co-linearity of the CW Doppler cursor.[11] Parasternal short-axis or right ventricular (RV)–focused four-chamber views are usually best. Care must be taken to measure the modal velocity rather the fluffy higher velocities. Indeed, measuring the "chin," not the "beard" (Fig. 178.4) can greatly improve the accuracy of assessment.[12] It should be noted that absence of TR is no guarantee that pulmonary hypertension is not present. Indeed, up to 50% of patients with pulmonary hypertension have inadequate TR to generate a CW Doppler peak velocity.[13] Alternative clues can be obtained from other Doppler and anatomic parameters.

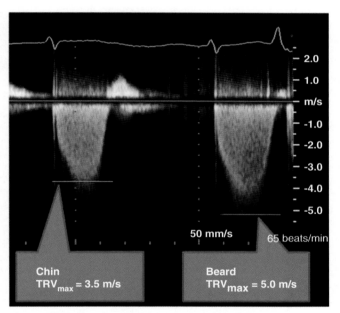

Figure 178.4. Measurement of the dense "beard" yields much more accurate estimations of true right ventricular systolic pressure than the fluffy "beard." *TRV_max,* Tricuspid regurgitation maximum continuous-wave Doppler velocity. (Kyranis SJ, et al: Improving the echocardiographic assessment of pulmonary pressure using the tricuspid regurgitant signal—the "chin" vs the "beard," *Echocardiography* 35:1085–1096, 2018.)

Pulmonary artery acceleration time, measured by pulsed-wave Doppler in the RVOT, can generate PAP_M via the formula of Dabestani (PAP_M = 90 – [0.62 × acceleration time]).[14] This technique performs reasonably well[15,16] but not as effectively as TRV_{max} calculations.[17]

DEFINITION OF PHYSIOLOGIES

Differentiating *precapillary* from *postcapillary* physiology is of the utmost clinical significance. *Precapillary* pulmonary

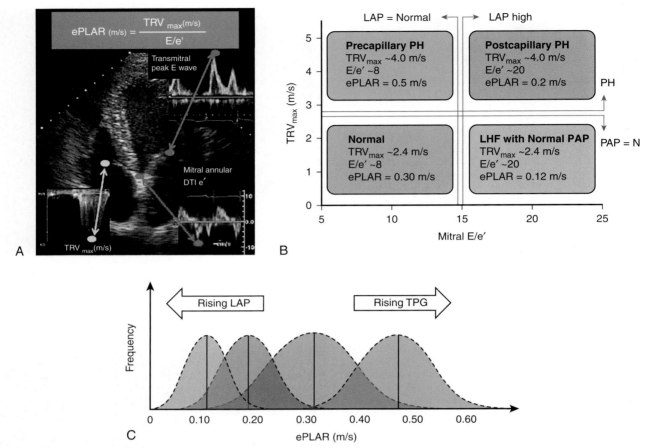

Figure 178.5. Echocardiographic pulmonary to left atrial ratio (ePLAR) explanation and example data. **A,** The ePLAR comprises three simple measurements: peak tricuspid regurgitation continuous wave velocity (m/s) divided by the transmitral peak pulsed-wave Doppler E wave (cm/s): peak Doppler tissue imaging mitral septal annular e′-wave (cm/s). **B,** The four nominal patient subsets clinically encountered are demonstrated, with predicted bell curves displayed. **C,** Normal individuals *(red)* have normal PAP_{mean} (<25 mm Hg), normal tricuspid regurgitation, maximum continuous-wave Doppler velocity (TRV_{max}) (e.g., 2.4 m/s), normal left atrial pressure (LAP) (<15 mm Hg), normal E/e′ (e.g., 8), and predicted calculated ePLAR values of approximately 0.30 m/s. Patients with left heart failure (LHF) with normal pulmonary arterial pressures (PAP_{mean} <25 mm Hg) have normal TRV_{max} (e.g., 2.4 m/s) with a high E/e′ (e.g., 20) yielding ePLAR values of approximately 0.12 m/s *(orange)*. Patients with postcapillary pulmonary hypertension (PH) secondary to raised LAP have high TRV_{max} (e.g., 4.0 m/s) and high E/e′ (e.g., 20), yielding ePLAR values of approximately 0.20 m/s *(blue)*. Patients with precapillary PH have high TRV_{max} (e.g., 4.0 m/s) with a normal E/e′ (e.g., 8), yielding the highest of ePLAR values, approximately 0.50 m/s in this example *(green)*. **C,** ePLAR is higher than normal in patients with precapillary physiology (rising transpulmonary gradient [TPG]) and lower than normal in patients with postcapillary physiology (rising LAP). (Reproduced with permission from Scalia GM, et al: ePLAR—the echocardiographic pulmonary to left atrial ratio—a novel non-invasive parameter to differentiate pre-capillary and post-capillary pulmonary hypertension, *Int J Cardiol* 212:379–386, 2016.)

hypertension is caused by obstructive disease of the pulmonary capillary tree, great vessels, or both. Pulmonary arterial hypertension (previously known as primary pulmonary hypertension) is the archetype and most feared of these conditions. Spontaneous sclerosing changes to the capillary walls lead to progressively increasing PVR and relentlessly advancing right heart failure. Until the advent of modern pulmonary vasodilator drugs, the prognosis was short and grave.[18] Related conditions include the pulmonary vascular changes of scleroderma and other connective tissue diseases. Obstruction of the pulmonary large- and medium-sized vessels by recurrent pulmonary emboli also leads to *precapillary* pulmonary hypertension with pulmonary hypertension will have *postcapillary* physiology.[19] With the aging population, systolic (heart failure with reduced ejection fraction) and diastolic (heart failure with preserved ejection fraction) left ventricular dysfunction is ubiquitous. Raised filling pressures (left ventricular end-diastolic pressure and LAPas measured by pulmonary capillary wedge pressure) raise pulmonary venous pressure and, by a backpressure effect, pulmonary arterial pressure, in the setting of normal PVR. These

patients benefit from standard heart failure therapies and diuretics. Modern pulmonary vasodilator drugs actually are deleterious to this patient group.[20]

ECHOCARDIOGRAPHIC ASSESSMENT OF PHYSIOLOGIES

Assessment of PVR by echocardiography is an optimal goal in noninvasive categorization of pulmonary hypertension patients as a surrogate for catheter-based testing. Transpulmonary gradient divided by cardiac output by catheter is mimicked by TRV_{max} divided by RVOTVTI to generate this flow-dependent parameter.[21] This parameter works best in less severe cases (PVR <8 Woods units).[22] A value for TRV_{max}/RVOTVTI greater than 0.275 is highly likely to represent a PVR greater than 6WU.[23] Slight modifications of this formula (TRV_{max}^2/RVOTVTI) have yielded slightly better prediction in some cases.[23] In the younger population, the simple TRV_{max}/RVOTVTI formula correlates with PVR measured by cardiac catheterization in children and young adults with cardiomyopathy.[24]

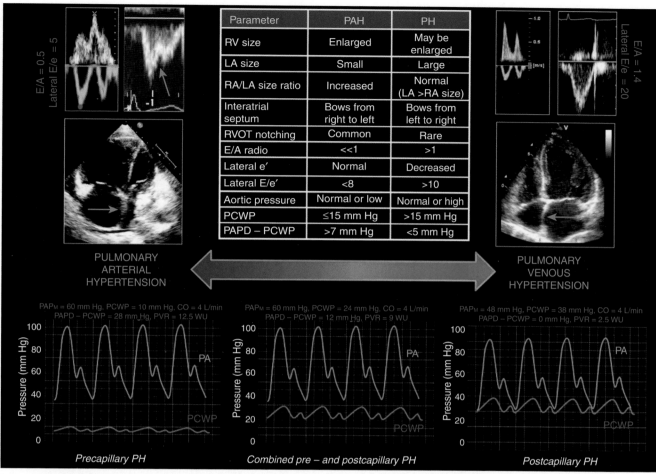

Parameter	PAH	PH
RV size	Enlarged	May be enlarged
LA size	Small	Large
RA/LA size ratio	Increased	Normal (LA >RA size)
Interatrial septum	Bows from right to left	Bows from left to right
RVOT notching	Common	Rare
E/A radio	<<1	>1
Lateral e′	Normal	Decreased
Lateral E/e′	<8	>10
Aortic pressure	Normal or low	Normal or high
PCWP	≤15 mm Hg	>15 mm Hg
PAPD – PCWP	>7 mm Hg	<5 mm Hg

PULMONARY ARTERIAL HYPERTENSION

PULMONARY VENOUS HYPERTENSION

PAP$_M$ = 60 mm Hg, PCWP = 10 mm Hg, CO = 4 L/min
PAPD – PCWP = 28 mm Hg, PVR = 12.5 WU

PAP$_M$ = 60 mm Hg, PCWP = 24 mm Hg, CO = 4 L/min
PAPD – PCWP = 12 mm Hg, PVR = 9 WU

PAP$_M$ = 48 mm Hg, PCWP = 38 mm Hg, CO = 4 L/min
PAPD – PCWP = 0 mm Hg, PVR = 2.5 WU

Precapillary PH   *Combined pre – and postcapillary PH*   *Postcapillary PH*

Figure 178.6. *Left,* Prototypical echocardiographic and invasive hemodynamic findings from a patient with precapillary pulmonary hypertension (PH). The right atrium (RA) and right ventricle (RV) are severely enlarged, and the left ventricle (LV) and left atrium (LA) are small and underfilled. The interatrial septum bows from right to left. On mitral inflow, the E/A ratio is less than 1 because of underfilling of the LA and decreased compliance of the LV caused by extrinsic compression from the enlarged RV. There is notching in the right ventricular outflow tract (RVOT) profile on pulsed-wave Doppler imaging caused by increased pulmonary artery (PA) stiffness. Pulmonary capillary wedge pressure (PCWP) is normal, and the PAD$_P$ (diastolic pulmonary artery pressure)-PCWP gradient is severely increased. *Right,* Prototypical echocardiographic and invasive hemodynamic findings from a patient with postcapillary PH. The LA is enlarged, and the interatrial septum bows from left to right. On mitral inflow, the E/A ratio is greater than 1, and the E/e′ ratio is increased, suggestive of grade 2 diastolic dysfunction with impaired LV relaxation and elevated LV filling pressures. There is no notching in the RV outflow tract profile. PCWP is elevated, and there is no gradient between the PAD$_P$ and PCWP. *CO,* Cardiac output; *PAH,* pulmonary arterial hypertension; *PAP$_M$,* mean pulmonary artery pressure; *PVR,* pulmonary vascular resistance. (Adapted with permission McLaughlin VV, et al: Management of pulmonary arterial hypertension, *J Am Coll Cardiol* 65:1976–1997, 2015.)

Echocardiographic parameters that approximate transpulmonary gradient *without* a flow-related element (i.e., without cardiac output or RVOTVTI) have been recently proposed. These include echocardiographic surrogates for both elements of transpulmonary gradient—pulmonary artery pressure and LAP. The new parameter ePLAR (echocardiographic pulmonary to left atrial ratio) defined as ePLAR (m/s) = TRV$_{max}$ (m/s)/mitral septal annular E/e′, is proposed as an echocardiographic surrogate for TPG (transpulmonary gradient) and its interaction with LAP[25] (Fig. 178.5). This "analogue" of the PAP$_M$/LAP gradient (TPG) with its units "meters/second" is conceptually appropriate because Doppler flow velocities are directly related to pressure gradients by the Bernoulli equation.

In *precapillary* pulmonary hypertension, the PAP (and TRV$_{max}$) increases without significant elevations of LAP (and therefore E/e′). The ePLAR quotient thus is expected to be higher than normal. In *postcapillary* pulmonary hypertension, both the PAP (and TRV$_{max}$) and the LAP (and E/e′) increase. Numerically, the magnitude of the E/e′ changes are an order-of-magnitude greater than any increase in TRV$_{max}$. This drives ePLAR lower than in normal participants

in *postcapillary* cases. Validated in multiple populations, higher ePLAR levels (>0.3 m/s) are associated with *precapillary* physiologies and lower levels (<0.3 m/s) with *postcapillary* physiologies.[26] Recently, ePLAGS (echocardiographic pulmonary to left atrial global strain ratio) has similarly demonstrated excellent differentiation of *precapillary* from *postcapillary* pulmonary hypertension, particularly in mixed physiology cases.[27]

Anatomic characteristic seen on echocardiograms can also steer the diagnosis toward *precapillary* or *postcapillary* physiology (Fig. 178.6). The atrial volume ratio (LA$_{volume}$)/(RA$_{volume}$) has been shown to be higher in *precapillary* cases than *postcapillary* cases (1.0360.69 vs 0.5060.19; *P* < .001).[28] It is important to rule out shunts in such an algorithm because elevation of the relative atrial index (RA$_{area}$/LA$_{area}$) similarly has been shown to be highly related to interatrial shunting.[29] Finally, the atrial workload distribution (mitral E/ e′ × [(LA$_{volume}$)/(RA$_{volume}$)]) has been shown to differentiate *precapillary* from *postcapillary* physiology in a small cohort.[30] Combined approaches, considering PVR, ePLAR, and anatomic considerations, probably are most desirable and have been proposed by several authors.[2,31] Considering anatomic features (relative right and left heart sizes) and Doppler parameters increases or decreases the likelihood of *precapillary* physiology.

ACUTE RISES IN PULMONARY VASCULAR RESISTANCE

In acute pulmonary embolism, particularly with massive or submassive thrombus burden, the naïve right ventricle is not prepared for abrupt changes in PVR. Impaired RV function in the setting of modest rises in TRV_{max}, particularly with the classical McConnell sign, may provide important echocardiographic clues.[32] Indeed, significant pulmonary hypertension in the setting of acute pulmonary embolism is suggestive of chronicity and the diagnosis of preexisting chronic thromboembolic pulmonary hypertension. RV dysfunction has pivotal implications for treatment (the use of lysis) and prognosis.[33] Infrequently, thrombus or tumor may be seen in the right heart, inferior vena cava, or proximal pulmonary arteries. Marked elevations of ePLAR and other echocardiographic parameters consistent with *precapillary* physiology have been reported in massive pulmonary embolism.[34]

ECHOCARDIOGRAPHY PREDICTION OF PROGNOSIS

Clinical and echocardiographic features of decompensation of RV function portend a poor prognosis. Initially, RV hypertrophy develops to preserve function. RV wall thickness should be measured in diastole in the subcostal view, with a wall thickness greater than 5 mm considered abnormal.[35] Strain (percentage change in free-wall length) of the right ventricle is assessed on most modern scanners with speckle tracking strain has prognostic relevance in the setting of pulmonary hypertension. An RV global strain 15% or less has been significantly associated with reduced survival (hazard ratio [HR], 1.66; 95% confidence interval [CI], 1.03–2.67; $P = .044$).[36] Recently, the simplified biventricular index (the ratio of $RV_{end-diastolic area}/LV_{end-diastolic area}$ on four-chamber view) has been shown to be predictive of outcome in patients with pulmonary hypertension. Values 0.93 or greater have been shown to have significantly higher all-cause mortality (hazard ratio, 1.84; 95% CI, 1.14–2.96; $P = .019$).[36]

The presence of a pericardial effusion in pulmonary hypertension is an ominous sign of right heart decompensation. The pericardial lymphatics drain via the coronary sinus to the right atrium.[37] The association of *precapillary* pulmonary hypertension with connective tissue disorders such as scleroderma raises the possibility also that pericardial effusions may be incidental to the pulmonary hypertension and are actually a serositis.

ECHOCARDIOGRAPHY ASSESSMENT OF THERAPY

Regular echocardiographic monitoring in patients with pulmonary hypertension emphasizes the need for test–retest accuracy. Small inaccuracies in the acquisition of TRV_{max} are amplified by the Bernoulli equation.[12] Great care should be taken to minimize potential confounding factors because critical therapeutic decisions are made based on these data.

CONCLUSION

Pulmonary hypertension is a hemodynamic status, defined by invasive measures but most commonly identified by echocardiography. Indeed, the detection and characterization of pulmonary hypertension by echocardiography are among principal responsibilities of echocardiographers. Care must be taken to generate accurate data, with due cognizance of the potential for error and exaggeration inherent in the Bernoulli equation. Differentiating *precapillary* from *postcapillary* physiology with echocardiography is now feasible, with many tools and techniques available. These data will then guide and monitor treatments that, in the modern era, give hope and comfort to patients with previously ominous disease states.

REFERENCES

1. Strange G, Gabbay E, Kermeen F, et al. Time from symptoms to definitive diagnosis of idiopathic pulmonary arterial hypertension: the delay study. *Pulm Circ.* 2013;3(1):89–94.
2. McLaughlin VV, Shah SJ, Souza R, Humbert M. Management of pulmonary arterial hypertension. *J Am Coll Cardiol.* 2015;65(18):1976–1997.
3. Parasuraman S, Walker S, Loudon BL, et al. Assessment of pulmonary artery pressure by echocardiography—a comprehensive review. *Int J Cardiol Heart Vasc.* 2016;12:45–51.
4. Hoeper MM, Bogaard HJ, Condliffe R, et al. Definitions and diagnosis of pulmonary hypertension. *J Am Coll Cardiol.* 2013;62(25 Suppl):D42–D50.
5. Strange G, Stewart S, Celermajer DS, et al. Threshold of pulmonary hypertension associated with increased mortality. *J Am Coll Cardiol.* 2019;73(21):2660–2672.
6. Kovacs G, Berghold A, Scheidl S, Olschewski H. Pulmonary arterial pressure during rest and exercise in healthy subjects: a systematic review. *Eur Respir J.* 2009;34(4):888–894.
7. Valerio CJ, Schreiber BE, Handler CE, et al. Borderline mean pulmonary artery pressure in patients with systemic sclerosis: transpulmonary gradient predicts risk of developing pulmonary hypertension. *Arthritis Rheum.* 2013;65(4):1074–1084.
8. Douschan P, Kovacs G, Avian A, et al. Mild elevation of pulmonary arterial pressure as a predictor of mortality. *Am J Respir Crit Care Med.* 2018;197(4):509–516.
9. Simonneau G, Montani D, Celermajer DS, et al. Haemodynamic definitions and updated clinical classification of pulmonary hypertension. *Eur Respir J.* 2019;53(1):1801913.
10. Galie N, Humbert M, Vachiery JL, et al. 2015 ESC/ERS guidelines for the diagnosis and treatment of pulmonary hypertension: the Joint Task Force for the diagnosis and treatment of pulmonary hypertension of the European Society of Cardiology (ESC) and the European Respiratory Society (ERS): endorsed by: association for European Paediatric and Congenital Cardiology (AEPC), International Society for heart and lung Transplantation (ISHLT). *Eur Heart J.* 2016;37(1):67–119.
11. Amsallem M, Sternbach JM, Adigopula S, et al. Addressing the controversy of estimating pulmonary arterial pressure by echocardiography. *J Am Soc Echocardiogr.* 2016;29(2):93–102.
12. Kyranis SJ, Latona J, Platts D, et al. Improving the echocardiographic assessment of pulmonary pressure using the tricuspid regurgitant signal—the "chin" vs the "beard. *Echocardiography.* 2018;35(8):1085–1096.
13. O'Leary JM, Assad TR, Xu M, et al. Lack of a tricuspid regurgitation Doppler signal and pulmonary hypertension by invasive measurement. *J Am Heart Assoc.* 2018;7(13).
14. Dabestani A, Mahan G, Gardin JM, et al. Evaluation of pulmonary artery pressure and resistance by pulsed Doppler echocardiography. *Am J Cardiol.* 1987;59(6):662–668.
15. Wang YC, Huang CH, Tu YK. Pulmonary hypertension and pulmonary artery acceleration time: a systematic review and meta-analysis. *J Am Soc Echocardiogr.* 2018;31(2):201–210 e3.
16. Yared K, Noseworthy P, Weyman AE, et al. Pulmonary artery acceleration time provides an accurate estimate of systolic pulmonary arterial pressure during transthoracic echocardiography. *J Am Soc Echocardiogr.* 2011;24(6):687–692.
17. Hellenkamp K, Unsöld B, Mushemi-Blake S, et al. Echocardiographic estimation of mean pulmonary artery pressure: a comparison of different approaches to assign the likelihood of pulmonary hypertension. *J Am Soc Echocardiogr.* 2018;31(1):89–98.
18. McLaughlin VV, Hoeper MM, Channick RN, et al. Pulmonary arterial hypertension-related morbidity is prognostic for mortality. *J Am Coll Cardiol.* 2018;71(7):752–763.
19. Chung K, Strange G, Codde J, et al. Left heart disease and pulmonary hypertension: are we seeing the full picture? *Heart Lung Circ.* 2018;27(3):301–309.
20. Gerges C, Gerges M, Skoro-Sajer N, et al. Hemodynamic thresholds for precapillary pulmonary hypertension. *Chest.* 2016;149(4):1061–1073.
21. Abbas AE, Fortuin FD, Schiller NB, et al. A simple method for noninvasive estimation of pulmonary vascular resistance. *J Am Coll Cardiol.* 2003;41(6):1021–1027.
22. Rajagopalan N, Simon MA, Suffoletto MS, et al. Noninvasive estimation of pulmonary vascular resistance in pulmonary hypertension. *Echocardiography.* 2009;26(5):489–494.
23. Abbas AE, Franey LM, Marwick T, et al. Noninvasive assessment of pulmonary vascular resistance by Doppler echocardiography. *J Am Soc Echocardiogr.* 2013;26(10):1170–1177.
24. Markush D, Ross RD, Thomas R, Aggarwal S. Noninvasive echocardiographic measures of pulmonary vascular resistance in children and young adults with cardiomyopathy. *J Am Soc Echocardiogr.* 2018;31(7):807–815.
25. Scalia GM, Scalia IG, Kierle R, et al. ePLAR—the echocardiographic pulmonary to left atrial ratio—a novel non-invasive parameter to differentiate pre-capillary and post-capillary pulmonary hypertension. *Int J Cardiol.* 2016;212:379–386.
26. Waldie AM, DG Platts GM. Scalia, Incremental value of ePLAR—echocardiographic pulmonary to left atrial ratio—in the diagnosis of chronic thromboembolic pulmonary hypertension. *Int J Cardiol.* 2016;221:141–143.
27. Venkateshvaran A, Manouras A, Kjellström B, Lund LH. The additive value of echocardiographic pulmonary to left atrial global strain ratio in the diagnosis of pulmonary hypertension. *Int J Cardiol.* 2019;292:205–210.

28. Saito N, Kato S, Saito N, et al. Distinction between precapillary and postcapillary pulmonary hypertension by the atrial volume ratio on transthoracic echocardiography. *J Ultrasound Med.* 2018;37(4):891–896.
29. Kelly NF, Walters DL, Hourigan LA, et al. The relative atrial index (RAI)—a novel, simple, reliable, and robust transthoracic echocardiographic indicator of atrial defects. *J Am Soc Echocardiogr.* 2010;23(3):275–281.
30. Vijiiac AE, Deaconu AI, Iancovici S, et al. The atrial workload distribution—a novel echocardiographic parameter for the differentiation of pre-capillary from postcapillary pulmonary hypertension. *J Hypertens Res.* 2018;4(1):22–33.
31. Opotowsky AR, Ojeda J, Rogers F, et al. A simple echocardiographic prediction rule for hemodynamics in pulmonary hypertension. *Circ Cardiovasc Imaging.* 2012;5(6):765–775.
32. McConnell MV, Solomon SD, Rayan ME, et al. Regional right ventricular dysfunction detected by echocardiography in acute pulmonary embolism. *Am J Cardiol.* 1996;78(4):469–473.
33. Agnelli G, Becattini C. Acute pulmonary embolism. *N Engl J Med.* 2010;363(3):266–274.
34. Scalia IG, Riha AZ, Kwon A, et al. Dramatic normalization of the echocardiographic pulmonary-to-left atrial ratio with thrombolysis in a case of life-threatening submassive pulmonary emboli. *CASE (Phila).* 2017;1(4):124–127.
35. Rudski LG, Lai WW, Afilalo J, et al. Guidelines for the echocardiographic assessment of the right heart in adults: a report from the American Society of Echocardiography endorsed by the European Association of Echocardiography, a registered branch of the European Society of Cardiology, and the Canadian Society of Echocardiography. *J Am Soc Echocardiogr.* 2010;23(7):685–713. quiz 786–788.
36. Goda A, Ryo K, Delgado-Montero A, et al. The prognostic utility of a simplified biventricular echocardiographic index of cardiac remodeling in patients with pulmonary hypertension. *J Am Soc Echocardiogr.* 2016;29(6):554–560.
37. Raymond RJ, Hinderliter AL, Willis PW, et al. Echocardiographic predictors of adverse outcomes in primary pulmonary hypertension. *J Am Coll Cardiol.* 2002;39(7):1214–1219.

179 Echocardiography in Patients With Heart Failure With Preserved Ejection Fraction

Jonathan Buggey, Brian D. Hoit

The American College of Cardiology Foundation (ACCF) and American Heart Association (AHA) define heart failure with preserved ejection fraction (HFpEF) as the clinical syndrome of heart failure (HF) with evidence of a left ventricular ejection fraction (LVEF) 50% or greater.[1] An estimated 6.5 million adult Americans have HF, and over the past 30 years, there has been a rise in the prevalence of HFpEF from 41% to 56%, surpassing the prevalence of HF with reduced ejection fraction (EF).[2,3] The diagnosis of HFpEF remains challenging because it involves the exclusion of other dyspnea-causing disease processes and the demonstration of increased left ventricular (LV) filling pressures.[1] Because echocardiography provides important information regarding LV and left atrial (LA) structure, function, and hemodynamics, the ACCF/AHA make a class I recommendation to perform two-dimensional (2D) echocardiography with Doppler during the initial evaluation of all patients with HF (Fig. 179.1).[1]

PATHOPHYSIOLOGY

Echocardiography detects and quantifies the hallmarks of HFpEF, namely preserved LVEF, diastolic dysfunction, and elevated LV filling pressures at rest or with exertion. Importantly, although more than 80% of patients with HFpEF have diastolic dysfunction, the majority of patients with critical diastolic dysfunction do not have symptomatic HFpEF[3]; indeed, one prospective study reported a HF incidence of only 12% over the course of 6 years for patients with moderate or severe diastolic dysfunction.[4]

Conceptually, normal diastolic function implies an active (i.e., energy-requiring) LV relaxation in early diastole that, in addition to restoring forces (Fig. 179.2), contributes importantly to the gradient for flow from the left atrium to the left ventricle at normal levels of LA pressure (i.e., filling vis-a-tergo) and that becomes quantitatively more critical during exercise.[5] In addition, a normally compliant passive diastolic pressure–volume relation maintains normal ventricular diastolic pressures over a wide range of ventricular filling. In contrast, in diastolic dysfunction, the rate of LV relaxation is slowed, restoring forces are decreased, and the gradient for filling at rest and especially with exercise (when the increased heart rate preferentially shortens diastole) is at the expense of an increase in LA pressure (i.e., filling vis-a-fronte). Thus, in patients with HFpEF,

when delayed LV relaxation is coupled with an increase in passive ventricular stiffness, an abnormal increase in LA pressure is required to achieve the same degree of LV filling. The development of LA hypertension not only contributes to the symptoms of dyspnea but also predisposes the patient to the development of LA remodeling, pulmonary hypertension, right ventricular (RV) dysfunction, and atrial fibrillation.[5]

With these consequences in mind, in the initial evaluation of patients with normal LVEF, the American Society of Echocardiography (ASE) recommends assessment of diastolic function using an algorithm comprised of four indices: average E/e′ ratio greater than 14, mitral septal e′ velocity less than 7 cm/s or lateral e′ velocity less than 10 cm/s, tricuspid regurgitation (TR) velocity greater than 2.8 m/s, and LA volume index greater than 34 mL/m². If a patient meets zero or one criterion, diastolic function is normal, and if a patient meets three or more criteria, diastolic function is abnormal. Meeting two criteria would yield an indeterminate assessment and often requires incorporation of other variables such as E/A ratio, pulmonary vein Doppler systolic/diastolic ratio, and atrial systolic reversal duration, the ratio of the isovolumic relaxation time (IVRT) divided by the time (t) from the early diastolic transmitral flow velocity (E) to the early diastolic annular tissue velocity (e′), LV mass index, and LV or LA strain.[6] Developed by expert consensus, the algorithm yielded a sensitivity and specificity of 69% and 81%, respectively, for the estimation of LV filling pressures when validated against invasive left heart catheterization.[7] Limitations of this approach in the HFpEF population (which often includes older hypertensive women with atrial fibrillation and obesity) include an overlap between delayed LV relaxation and normal aging, the effect of atrial fibrillation on transmitral velocities, and an underestimation of LA volume when indexed for increased total body size.[8] However, indices such as E/e′ and estimated pulmonary artery systolic pressure (PASP) are relatively age independent and play an important diagnostic role.[6] Nevertheless, the accurate diagnosis of HFpEF remains challenging.

PHENOTYPING

It has become widely accepted that the HFpEF syndrome consists of a very heterogenous group of patients; as such, pharmacologic treatment strategies have yielded mixed results.[9] Identifying specific

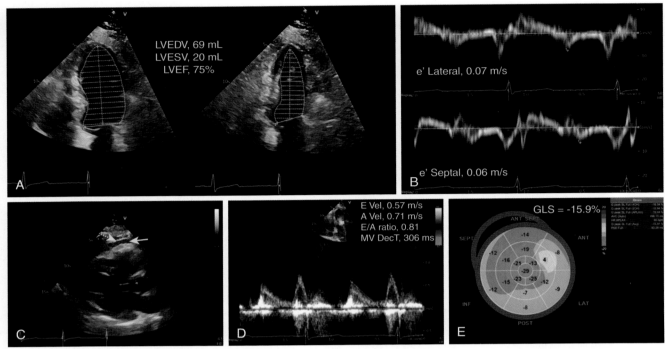

Figure 179.1. Echocardiographic findings in heart failure with preserved ejection fraction (HFpEF). The patient is a 62-year-old female patient with HFpEF, body mass index of 38 kg/m^2, and prior coronary artery disease with coronary artery bypass surgery. Invasive hemodynamics revealed a normal pulmonary capillary wedge pressure at rest (11 mm Hg) with significant elevation with exercise (25 mm Hg). **A,** The ventricular ejection fraction (LVEF) is 50% or greater as quantified using Simpson's biplane method. **B,** The lateral and septal mitral valve annular tissue velocities are reduced. **C,** There is evidence of increased epicardial fat *(large arrow)* visualized at end-diastole of the parasternal long-axis view and located beneath the pericardium *(dashed arrow)*. **D,** The transmitral valve inflow velocities are consistent with grade 1 diastolic dysfunction (E/A ratio, 0.8; E-wave deceleration time, 306 ms; maximum E-wave velocity [E Vol], 0.57 m/s). **E,** Left ventricular global longitudinal strain (GLS) is mildly abnormal at −15.9%, with several impaired myocardial segments. *A Vel,* A wave velocity; *LVEDV,* left ventricular end-diastolic volume; *LVESV,* left ventricular end-systolic volume; *MV DecT,* mitral valve deceleration time.

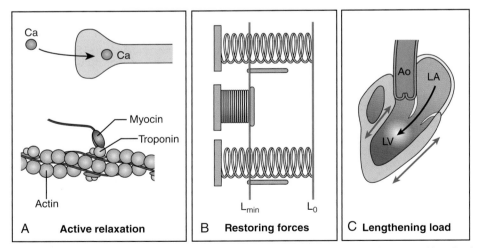

Figure 179.2. The three independent determinants of e′, which are left ventricular relaxation, restoring forces, and lengthening load. **A,** Rate of relaxation reflects decay of active fiber force. **B,** Restoring forces, which account for diastolic suction, are illustrated by an elastic spring, which is compressed to a dimension (L$_{min}$) less than its resting length (L$_0$) and recoils back to resting length when the compression is released. **C,** Lengthening load is the pressure in the left atrium at mitral valve opening, which "pushes" blood into the left ventricle (LV) and thereby lengthens the ventricle. *AO,* Aorta; *LA,* left atrium. (Based on Nagueh SF, et al: Recommendations for the evaluation of left ventricular diastolic function by echocardiography, *J Am Soc Echocardiogr* 29:277–314, 2016.)

phenotypes of the HFpEF syndrome is important for prognostication and may help to guide future therapies. Of note, at present, published phenotypes are not universally accepted. Furthermore, infiltrative cardiomyopathies (e.g., amyloidosis), restrictive pericarditis, and valvular disease (e.g., aortic stenosis) are considered by some as specific types of "HFpEF"; however, these entities have disease-specific prognoses and treatment strategies and for our purposes are not included as HFpEF phenotypes. This definition is aligned with the prospective comparison of angiotensin receptor neprilysin inhibitors with angiotensin receptor blockers Global

Outcomes in HF With Preserved Ejection Fraction (PARAGON-HF) trial definition of HFpEF, which excludes patients with isolated right-sided HF, pericardial constriction, genetic hypertrophic cardiomyopathy, infiltrative cardiomyopathy, and hemodynamically significant valvular heart disease.[10] Furthermore, the phenotypes presented here are in line with contemporary published views.[8]

The Obesity Phenotype

In a single-center retrospective analysis, obese (body mass index [BMI] ≥35 kg/m^2) patients with HFpEF had similar LV end-diastolic volumes when indexed for body surface area (BSA) compared with nonobese HFpEF patients (BMI <30 kg/m^2) but larger RV size and greater LV concentric remodeling, nonindexed volumes, and mass. Furthermore, obese patients with HFpEF were younger and had a greater degree of ventricular interaction, evidenced by interventricular flattening at end-diastole and a significantly higher LV eccentricity index compared with nonobese patients with HFpEF.[11] Secondary analysis of the Phosphodiesterase-5 Inhibition to Improve Clinical Status and Exercise Capacity in Heart Failure with Preserved Ejection Fraction (RELAX) randomized clinical trial also found obese HFpEF patients to be younger and have larger LV volumes, dimensions, and mass, as well as worse New York Heart Association (NYHA) functional class and 6-minute walk test distance results compared with nonobese patients with HFpEF.[12] The mechanism by which obesity plays a role in the development of HFpEF is complex, but there is a body of literature that suggests epicardial fat, which may be measured using echocardiography in the parasternal long- and short-axis views, may play a significant role as a mediator of direct inflammation on the myocardium.[13]

The Ischemia/Microvascular Dysfunction Phenotype

A retrospective analysis found that HFpEF patients with concomitant epicardial coronary artery stenosis 50% or greater were significantly more likely to be male, with lower LVEF and higher mortality during follow up than those without coronary artery disease (CAD).[14] Although regional wall motion abnormalities provided clues to the presence of CAD, the ability of stress echocardiography to identify epicardial CAD in patients with HFpEF was poor, with an overall accuracy of 66%.[14] In another study, analysis of 559 patients with HFpEF over 5 years found that LVEF declined more in patients with CAD, and 39% of patients with HFpEF had an LVEF less than 50% at some point after their initial diagnosis.[15] One potential mechanism for these findings may be underlying microvascular dysfunction, which was recently evaluated in HFpEF (without epicardial CAD) using coronary flow reserve (CFR) during adenosine stress Doppler echocardiography in the PRevalance Of MIcrovascular dysfunction in Heart Failure with Preserved Ejection Fraction (PROMIS-HFpEF) study.[16] The investigators found that 75% of patients had microvascular dysfunction (CFR <2.5), which was associated with higher N-terminal pro-brain natriuretic peptide (NT-proBNP) levels (1050 vs 597 pg/mL), and worse RV function as assessed by lower tricuspid annular plane systolic excursion (TAPSE) and tricuspid annular systolic velocity (RV S′) measurements.[16] The identification of CAD in patients with HFpEF is important because revascularization (when feasible) has been shown to improve the LVEF trajectory and mortality.[15]

The Pulmonary Hypertension and Right Ventricular Dysfunction Phenotype(s)

Although some investigators distinguish between the pulmonary hypertension (PH) and RV dysfunction phenotypes,[8] the development of RV dysfunction is closely correlated to PH, and the two entities share significant overlap.[17] In general, there is a high prevalence of PH in patients with HFpEF, with studies citing a range of

TABLE 179.1 Differential Diagnoses of Heart Failure With Preserved Ejection Fraction and Their Echocardiographic Clues

Differential Diagnosis	Echocardiographic Clues
Hypertrophic cardiomyopathy	Asymmetric hypertrophy, ↑↑LV wall thickness, LVOT obstruction, SAM
Restrictive cardiomyopathy	Small LV cavity, ↑LV wall thickness, sparkling myocardium, apical sparing, severely reduced tissue Doppler, PE
Pulmonary arterial hypertension	↑RVSP with no sign of increased LV filling pressure, isolated right heart dilatation, PA dilatation, RVOT Doppler midsystolic notch
Constrictive pericarditis	Pericardial thickening, septal bounce, annulus paradoxus and annulus reversus, ↑respiratory variation in mitral/tricuspid flow, absence of IVC collapse
Valvular heart disease	Morphologic valvular abnormalities, color Doppler
Coronary artery disease	Regional wall motion abnormality and thinning
Chronic thromboembolic pulmonary hypertension	↑RVSP with no sign of increased LV filling pressure, isolated right heart dilatation, PA dilatation, RVOT Doppler midsystolic notch
High-output HF	↑Doppler-derived cardiac output

HF, Heart failure; *IVC,* inferior vena cava; *LVOT,* left ventricular outflow obstruction; *PA,* pulmonary artery; *PE,* pericardial effusion; *RVOT,* right ventricular outflow; *RVSP,* right ventricular systolic pressure; *SAM,* systolic anterior motion of the mitral valve.

Reproduced with permission from Obokata M, et al: The role of echocardiography in heart failure with preserved ejection fraction: What do we want from imaging? *Heart Fail Clin* 15:241–256, 2019.

18% to 83% of patients with HFpEF being affected.[18,19] Patients with HFpEF with PH tend to have worse exercise capacity and increased mortality rate than without.[18,19] Furthermore, RV dysfunction among patients with HFpEF ranges from 18% to 28% depending of the echocardiographic criteria used (e.g., TAPSE <16 mm, fractional area change <35%, or RV S′ <9.5 cm/s). Multiple studies have found that RV dysfunction is associated with increased mortality rates and higher rates of HF hospitalizations.[19,20] An emerging parameter to associate these two entities is the ratio of TAPSE to PASP, which reflects right ventricular–vascular coupling, with values below 0.36 mm/mm Hg representing abnormal coupling.[21] Values below this threshold in patients with HFpEF are able to predict a component of precapillary PH (sensitivity, 86%; specificity, 79%) and have been associated with increased mortality.[22]

DIAGNOSTIC VALUE

In a symptomatic patient, echocardiography is useful first in excluding other possible causes of dyspnea (Table 179.1) and quantifying the LVEF. It should be noted that 2D echocardiography has limited reliability for LVEF assessment. In one study with experienced echocardiographers, the interobserver correlation coefficient for visually estimated LVEF was only 0.78,[23] and others have found that LVEF is quantified using the recommended biplane Simpson method in only 46% of patients with HF.[24] LV volumes and EF are more accurately and reproducibly measured using 3D rather than 2D echocardiography.[25]

Although the identification of diastolic dysfunction is an important step, the ultimate goal in the diagnosis of HFpEF is to identify patients with elevated LV and LA filling pressures. One of the most widely studied echocardiographic measure is the E/e′ ratio, which compared with other echocardiographic parameters, performs the best at detecting diastolic dysfunction and elevated

LV filling pressures.[26] However, although this index has high specificity for the identification of elevated LV filling pressures (77%–100%), its sensitivity is highly variable (0%–73%).[8]

Another echocardiographic parameter that has been evaluated in the diagnosis of HFpEF is LA strain. In one study, abnormal LA strain during ventricular systole (the reservoir phase) was 89% sensitive but only 55% specific for the diagnosis of HFpEF.[27] Kurt and coworkers[28] used the ratio of E/e′ to LA reservoir strain as an estimation of "LA stiffness" and in a small cohort of patients found that a ratio above 0.99 was 85% sensitive and 78% specific (area under the curve [AUC], 0.85) in identifying patients with HFpEF versus diastolic dysfunction without HF. However, this index requires further validation.

The need for a simpler and accurate tool to aid in the diagnosis of HFpEF remains. Recently, parameters were identified in 414 patients with unexplained dyspnea that were subsequently incorporated into a simple scoring system to aid in the diagnosis of HFpEF (Table 179.2).[29] The combination of the E/e′ ratio greater than 9 and estimated PASP greater than 35 mm Hg with four clinical parameters (BMI >30 kg/m², use of two or more antihypertensive medications, atrial fibrillation, or age older than

60 years old), provided excellent discrimination of patients with HFpEF from control participants (AUC, 0.84); the odds of having HFpEF increased twofold for every 1-point increase in the score.[29]

Further complicating the diagnosis, patients with HFpEF may display normal LV filling pressures at rest and only develop abnormalities and symptoms with exercise. The ASE recommends diastolic stress testing in patients with grade 1 diastolic dysfunction (i.e., delayed LV relaxation with normal LA pressure) when resting echocardiography does not explain the symptoms of dyspnea. According to the ASE, diastolic dysfunction is identified when three indices are met during exercise: average E/e′ greater than 14 or septal E/e′ ratio > 15, peak TR velocity greater than 2.8 m/s, and septal e′ velocity less than 7 cm/s (Fig. 179.3).[6] The test result is considered normal if average (or septal) E/e′ remains below 10 and peak TR velocity is less than 2.8 m/s with peak exercise. In a small prospective trial of patients with unexplained dyspnea, the use of just the exercise E/e′ ratio greater than 14 significantly improved the sensitivity for the diagnosis of HFpEF to 90%.[30] Collectively, 2D and Doppler echocardiography serve vital roles in the diagnosis of HFpEF through the exclusion of other dyspnea-causing causes and the identification of diastolic dysfunction and elevated LV filling pressures either at rest or with exertion.

PROGNOSTIC VALUE

In addition to aiding in diagnosis, echocardiography may be helpful in identifying high-risk patients with HFpEF and predicting clinical outcomes. In the Treatment of Preserved Cardiac Function Heart Failure with an Aldosterone Antagonist (TOPCAT) trial, several echocardiographic parameters were found to be associated with the primary endpoint of HF hospitalization, cardiovascular death, or aborted cardiac arrest in patients with HFpEF. These included increased LV mass index, concentric LV hypertrophy, E/A ratio greater than >1.6, E/e′ ratio 10 or greater, and TR velocity greater than 2.9 m/s).[31] The most robust associations were seen with an E/e′ ratio of 10 or greater and E/A greater than 1.6, which remained significantly associated with the primary outcome after multivariable adjustments. Other investigators have also shown correlations between E/e′ ratio and all-cause mortality and cardiovascular hospitalization among patients with HFpEF.[32]

An increasingly used technique to identify subclinical myocardial dysfunction in patients with preserved LVEF is LV global longitudinal strain (GLS). Compared with hypertensive patients with normal LVEF, absolute LV GLS measured using

TABLE 179.2 Description of H₂FPEF Score for the Diagnosis of Failure With Preserved Ejection Fraction

	Variable	Cut-Off Value	Points
H₂	Heavy	BMI >30 kg/m²	2
	Hypertensive	Two or more antihypertensive medications	1
F	Atrial fibrillation	Paroxysmal or persistent	3
P	Pulmonary hypertension	Estimated PASP >35 mm Hg	1
E	Older adult	Age older than 60 years	1
F	Filling pressures	E/e′ >9	1
Total Score[a]			**(0–9)**

[a]A low score is 0 to 1, an intermediate score is 2 to 5, and a high score is 6 to 9.

BMI, Body mass index; *PASP,* pulmonary artery systolic pressure.

Adapted from Reddy YNV, et al: A simple, evidence-based approach to help guide diagnosis of heart failure with preserved ejection fraction, *Circulation* 138:861–870, 2018.

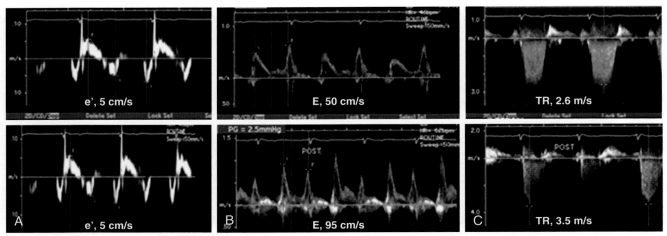

Figure 179.3. Exercise diastolic stress test. Mitral septal annulus (**A**), mitral inflow (**B**), and tricuspid regurgitation (TR) velocity (**C**) at rest *(top)* and immediately after treadmill exercise test *(bottom)*. At rest, E/e′ is 10, and pulmonary artery systolic pressure (PASP) is normal. With exercise, e″ remains the same, and the E velocity increased such that the E/e′ ratio increased to 19 along with an increase of PASP to 49 mm Hg or greater (TR velocity, 3.5m/s). (Reproduced with permission from Nagueh SF, et al: Recommendations for the evaluation of left ventricular diastolic function by echocardiography: an update from the American Society of Echocardiography and the European Association of Cardiovascular Imaging, *J Am Soc Echocardiogr* 29:277–314, 2016.)

speckle-tracking echocardiography (STE) was lower in patients with HFpEF.[33] Furthermore, impaired LV strain has been associated with worse peak oxygen consumption and increased natriuretic peptide levels, HF hospitalizations, and cardiovascular death.[33,34] Although the ASE does not currently recommend LV GLS measurement as a *formal* marker of diastolic or systolic dysfunction, it does recognize that many patients with HFpEF have abnormal LV GLS and that this marker significantly correlates with LV relaxation.[6] STE can also be used to quantify the degree and rate of LV twist and untwist, which is a direct reflection of the LV torque provided by the left-handed helix subepicardial fibers, and has been shown to be normal in patients with HFpEF versus HFrEF.[35] It has been postulated that despite reduced LV GLS, the preservation of circumferential strain and twist is the reason patients with HFpEF maintain normal LVEF.[36]

As mentioned previously, a more novel echocardiographic technique being applied to patients with HFpEF is the measurement of LA strain. The LA plays a crucial role in maintaining appropriate LV filling through its actions as a reservoir, conduit, and "booster pump"; as such, abnormal LA mechanics have been implicated in the pathophysiology of HFpEF.[37] Among the patients with HFpEF in the TOPCAT trial, LA strain was also found to be associated with more HF hospitalizations and the composite endpoint of cardiovascular death, HF hospitalization, or aborted sudden cardiac death.[38]

CONCLUSIONS

The use of echocardiography is important in the diagnosis of HFpEF through a comprehensive assessment of LV and LA structure and function. Specifically, echocardiography is key in the identification of diastolic dysfunction and elevated LV filling pressures and excluding other dyspnea-causing etiologies to help establish a diagnosis of HFpEF. Within the HFpEF population, various echocardiographic indices have been shown to accurately predict LV filling pressures, exercise tolerance, and important clinical events such as HF hospitalizations and death.

REFERENCES

1. Yancy CW, Jessup M, Bozkurt B, et al. 2013 ACCF/AHA guideline for the management of heart failure: Executive summary: a report of the American College of Cardiology Foundation/American Heart Association Task Force on practice guidelines. *Circulation.* 2013;128(16):1810–1852.
2. Vasan RS, Xanthakis V, Lyass A, et al. Epidemiology of left ventricular systolic dysfunction and heart failure in the Framingham study: an echocardiographic study over 3 decades. *JACC Cardiovasc Imaging.* 2018;11(1):1–11.
3. Benjamin EJ, Blaha MJ, Chiuve SE, et al. Heart disease and stroke statistics—2017 update: a report from the American Heart Association. *Circulation.* 2017;135(10):e146–e603.
4. Kane GC, Karon BL, Mahoney DW, et al. Progression of left ventricular diastolic dysfunction and risk of heart failure. *JAMA.* 2011;306(8):856–863.
5. Borlaug BA. The pathophysiology of heart failure with preserved ejection fraction. *Nat Rev Cardiol.* 2014;11(9):507–515.
6. Nagueh SF, Smiseth OA, Appleton CP, et al. Recommendations for the evaluation of left ventricular diastolic function by echocardiography: an update from the American Society of Echocardiography and the European Association of Cardiovascular Imaging. *J Am Soc Echocardiogr.* 2016;29(4):277–314.
7. Balaney B, Medvedofsky D, Mediratta A, et al. Invasive validation of the echocardiographic assessment of left ventricular filling pressures using the 2016 diastolic guidelines: head-to-Head comparison with the 2009 guidelines. *J Am Soc Echocardiogr.* 2018;31(1):79–88.
8. Obokata M, Reddy YNV, Borlaug BA. The role of echocardiography in heart failure with preserved ejection fraction: what do we want from imaging? *Heart Fail Clin.* 2019;15(2):241–256.
9. Shah SJ, Kitzman DW, Borlaug BA, et al. Phenotype-specific treatment of heart failure with preserved ejection fraction: a multiorgan roadmap. *Circulation.* 2016;134(1):73–90.
10. Solomon SD, Rizkala AR, Gong J, et al. Angiotensin receptor neprilysin inhibition in heart failure with preserved ejection fraction: rationale and design of the PARAGON-HF trial. *JACC Heart Fail.* 2017;5(7):471–482.
11. Obokata M, Reddy YNV, Pislaru SV, et al. Evidence supporting the existence of a distinct obese phenotype of heart failure with preserved ejection fraction. *Circulation.* 2017;136(1):6–19.
12. Reddy YNV, Lewis GD, Shah SJ, et al. Characterization of the obese phenotype of heart failure with preserved ejection fraction: a RELAX trial ancillary study. *Mayo Clin Proc.* 2019;94(7):1199–1209.
13. Packer M. Epicardial adipose tissue may mediate deleterious effects of obesity and inflammation on the myocardium. *J Am Coll Cardiol.* 2018;71(20):2360–2372.
14. Hwang SJ, Melenovsky V, Borlaug BA. Implications of coronary artery disease in heart failure with preserved ejection fraction. *J Am Coll Cardiol.* 2014;63(25 Pt A):2817–2827.
15. Dunlay SM, Roger VL, Weston SA, et al. Longitudinal changes in ejection fraction in heart failure patients with preserved and reduced ejection fraction. *Circ Heart Fail.* 2012;5(6):720–726.
16. Shah SJ, Lam CSP, Svedlund S, et al. Prevalence and correlates of coronary microvascular dysfunction in heart failure with preserved ejection fraction: PROMIS-HFpEF. *Eur Heart J.* 2018;39(37):3439–3450.
17. Hoeper MM, Lam CSP, Vachiery JL, et al. Pulmonary hypertension in heart failure with preserved ejection fraction: a plea for proper phenotyping and further research. *Eur Heart J.* 2017;38(38):2869–2873.
18. Lam CS, Roger VL, Rodeheffer RJ, et al. Pulmonary hypertension in heart failure with preserved ejection fraction: a community-based study. *J Am Coll Cardiol.* 2009;53(13):1119–1126.
19. Gorter TM, Hoendermis ES, van Veldhuisen DJ, et al. Right ventricular dysfunction in heart failure with preserved ejection fraction: a systematic review and meta-analysis. *Eur J Heart Fail.* 2016;18(12):1472–1487.
20. Mohammed SF, Hussain I, AbouEzzeddine OF, et al. Right ventricular function in heart failure with preserved ejection fraction: a community-based study. *Circulation.* 2014;130(25):2310–2320.
21. Guazzi M, Bandera F, Pelissero G, et al. Tricuspid annular plane systolic excursion and pulmonary arterial systolic pressure relationship in heart failure: an index of right ventricular contractile function and prognosis. *Am J Physiol Heart Circ Physiol.* 2013;305(9):H1373–H1381.
22. Gorter TM, van Veldhuisen DJ, Voors AA, et al. Right ventricular-vascular coupling in heart failure with preserved ejection fraction and pre- vs. post-capillary pulmonary hypertension. *Eur Heart J Cardiovasc Imaging.* 2018;19(4):425–432.
23. Blondheim DS, Beeri R, Feinberg MS, et al. Reliability of visual assessment of global and segmental left ventricular function: a multicenter study by the Israeli Echocardiography Research Group. *J Am Soc Echocardiogr.* 2010;23(3):258–264.
24. Pellikka PA, She L, Holly TA, et al. Variability in ejection fraction measured by echocardiography, gated single-photon emission computed tomography, and cardiac magnetic resonance in patients with coronary artery disease and left ventricular dysfunction. *JAMA Netw Open.* 2018;1(4). e181456.
25. Lang RM, Badano LP, Mor-Avi V, et al. Recommendations for cardiac chamber quantification by echocardiography in adults: an update from the American Society of Echocardiography and the European Association of Cardiovascular Imaging. *Eur Heart J Cardiovasc Imaging.* 2015;16(3):233–270.
26. Kasner M, Westermann D, Steendijk P, et al. Utility of Doppler echocardiography and tissue Doppler imaging in the estimation of diastolic function in heart failure with normal ejection fraction: a comparative Doppler-conductance catheterization study. *Circulation.* 2007;116(6):637–647.
27. Aung SM, Guler A, Guler Y, et al. Left atrial strain in heart failure with preserved ejection fraction. *Herz.* 2017;42(2):194–199.
28. Kurt M, Wang J, Torre-Amione G, Nagueh SF. Left atrial function in diastolic heart failure. *Circ Cardiovasc Imaging.* 2009;2(1):10–15.
29. Reddy YNV, Carter RE, Obokata M, et al. A simple, evidence-based approach to help guide diagnosis of heart failure with preserved ejection fraction. *Circulation.* 2018;138(9):861–870.
30. Obokata M, Kane GC, Reddy YN, et al. Role of diastolic stress testing in the evaluation for heart failure with preserved ejection fraction: a simultaneous invasive-echocardiographic study. *Circulation.* 2017;135(4):825–838.
31. Shah AM, Claggett B, Sweitzer NK, et al. Cardiac structure and function and prognosis in heart failure with preserved ejection fraction: findings from the echocardiographic study of the treatment of preserved cardiac function heart failure with an Aldosterone Antagonist (TOPCAT) trial. *Circ Heart Fail.* 2014;7(5):740–751.
32. Nauta JF, Hummel YM, van der Meer P, et al. Correlation with invasive left ventricular filling pressures and prognostic relevance of the echocardiographic diastolic parameters used in the 2016 ESC heart failure guidelines and in the 2016 ASE/EACVI recommendations: a systematic review in patients with heart failure with preserved ejection fraction. *Eur J Heart Fail.* 2018;20(9):1303–1311.
33. Kraigher-Krainer E, Shah AM, Gupta DK, et al. Impaired systolic function by strain imaging in heart failure with preserved ejection fraction. *J Am Coll Cardiol.* 2014;63(5):447–456.
34. Hasselberg NE, Haugaa KH, Sarvari SI, et al. Left ventricular global longitudinal strain is associated with exercise capacity in failing hearts with preserved and reduced ejection fraction. *Eur Heart J Cardiovasc Imaging.* 2015;16(2):217–224.
35. Wang J, Khoury DS, Yue Y, et al. Preserved left ventricular twist and circumferential deformation, but depressed longitudinal and radial deformation in patients with diastolic heart failure. *Eur Heart J.* 2008;29(10):1283–1289.
36. Nagueh SF, Chang SM, Nabi F, et al. Cardiac imaging in patients with heart failure and preserved ejection fraction. *Circ Cardiovasc Imaging.* 2017;10(9).
37. Singh A, Addetia K, Maffessanti F, et al. LA strain for categorization of LV diastolic dysfunction. *JACC Cardiovasc Imaging.* 2017;10(7):735–743.
38. Santos AB, Roca GQ, Claggett B, et al. Prognostic relevance of left atrial dysfunction in heart failure with preserved ejection fraction. *Circ Heart Fail.* 2016;9(4). e002763.

Index

Page numbers followed by "*b*" indicate boxes, "*f*" indicate figures, "*t*" indicate tables.